BONE MARROW TRANSPLANTATION

BONE MARROW TRANSPLANTATION

EDITED BY

STEPHEN J. FORMAN, MD, FACP

Director, Department of Hematology and Bone Marrow Transplantation
City of Hope National Medical Center
Duarte, California

KARL G. BLUME, MD, FACP

Director, Bone Marrow Transplantation Program
Stanford University School of Medicine
Stanford, California

E. DONNALL THOMAS, MD, FACP

Fred Hutchinson Cancer Research Center
Seattle, Washington

BOSTON • BLACKWELL SCIENTIFIC PUBLICATIONS
Oxford London Edinburgh Melbourne Paris Berlin Vienna

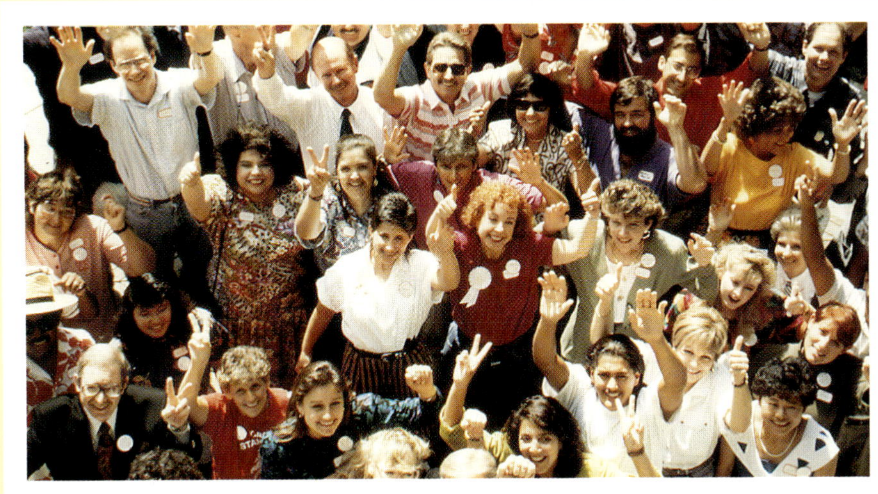

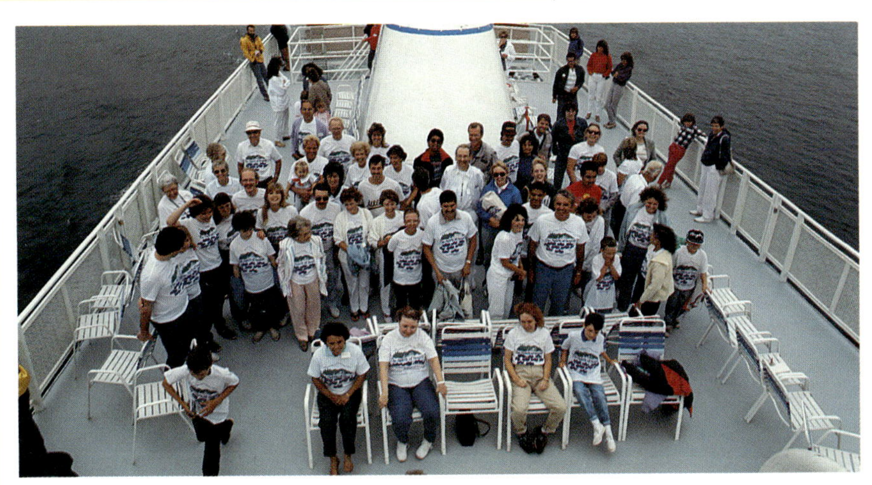

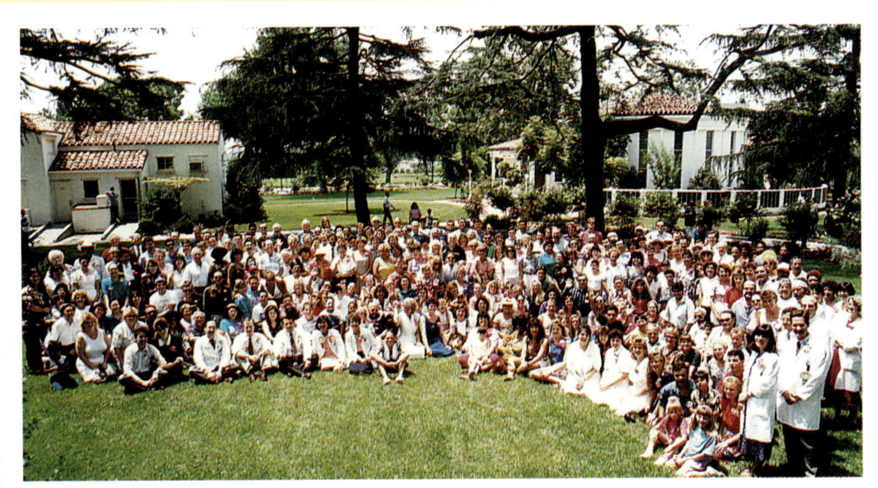

BLACKWELL SCIENTIFIC PUBLICATIONS

EDITORIAL OFFICES:
238 Main Street, Cambridge, Massachusetts 02142, USA
Osney Mead, Oxford OX2 OEL, England
25 John Street, London WC1N 2BL, England
23 Ainslie Place, Edinburgh EH3 6AJ, Scotland
54 University Street, Carlton, Victoria 3053, Australia
Arnette SA, 1 rue de Lille, 75007 Paris, France
Blackwell-Wissenschaft, Düsseldorfer str. 38, D-10707 Berlin, Germany
Blackwell MZV, Feldgasse 13, A-1238 Vienna, Austria

DISTRIBUTORS:

USA
Blackwell Scientific Publications
238 Main Street
Cambridge, Massachusetts 02142
(Telephone orders: 800-759-6102 or 617-876-7000)

Canada
Times Mirror Professional Publishing
130 Flaska Drive
Markham, Ontario L6G 1B8
(Telephone orders: 800-268-4178 or 416-470-6739)

Australia
Blackwell Scientific Publications (Australia) Pty Ltd
54 University Street
Carlton, Victoria 3053
(Telephone orders: 03-347-5552)

Outside North America and Australia
Blackwell Scientific Publications, Ltd.
c/o Marston Book Services, Ltd.
P.O. Box 87
Oxford OX2 ODT
England
(Telephone orders: 44-865-791155)

TYPESET BY HURON VALLEY GRAPHICS
PRINTED AND BOUND BY BRAUN-BRUMFIELD, INC.

PRINTED IN THE UNITED STATES OF AMERICA

93 94 95 96 97 5 4 3 2 1

LIBRARY OF CONGRESS CATALOGING-IN-PUBLICATION DATA

Bone marrow transplantation / edited by Stephen J. Forman, Karl G.
Blume, E. Donnall Thomas.
p. cm.
Includes bibliographical references and index.
ISBN 0-86542-253-2
1. Bone marrow—Transplantation. I. Forman, Stephen J.
II. Blume, Karl G. III. Thomas, E. Donnall.
[DNLM: 1. Bone Marrow Transplantation. WH 380 B71192122 1994]
RD123.5.B652 1994
617.4'4—dc20
DNLM/DLC
for Library of Congress 93-26102

Dedication

This book is dedicated to our patients and their families, whose courage and trust enabled them to choose a difficult, dangerous, and sometime unproven therapy that offered the only chance in their fight against a fatal disease. Many thousands of patients are currently alive after undergoing successful BMT that would have been impossible without the fortitude of our patients, who took the risks and thereby paved the way for the current and future increasing application of this therapy.

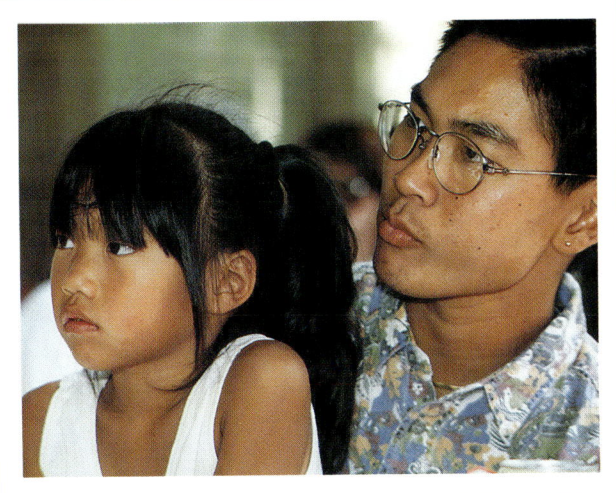

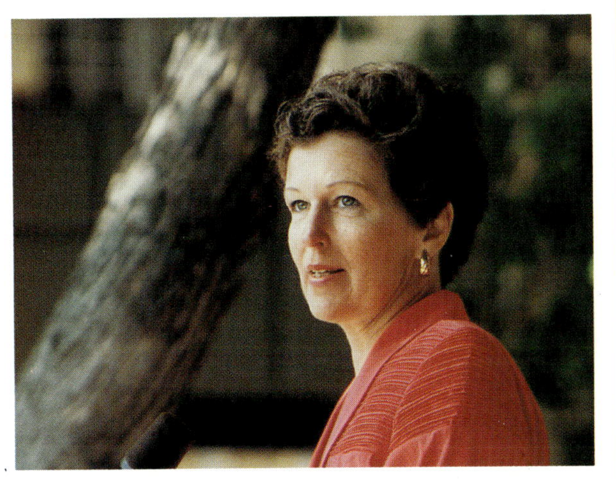

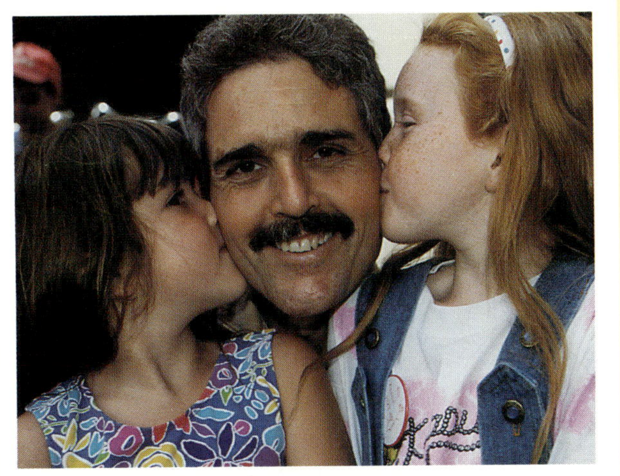

Contents

Contributors

CLAUDIO ANASETTI, MD

Associate Member and Director, Unrelated Donor Marrow Transplant Program, Fred Hutchinson Cancer Research Center, Seattle, Washington

KAREN H. ANTMAN, MD

Chief, Division of Medical Oncology, Professor of Medicine, College of Physicians and Surgeons of Columbia University, New York, New York

FREDERICK R. APPELBAUM, MD

Professor of Medicine, University of Washington School of Medicine, Seattle, Washington, Director, Clinical Research Division, Fred Hutchinson Cancer Research Center, Seattle, Washington

JAMES O. ARMITAGE, MD

Professor and Chairman, Department of Internal Medicine, University of Nebraska Medical Center, Omaha, Nebraska

ANN M. ARVIN, MD

Professor of Pediatrics, Infectious Diseases Division, Department of Pediatrics, Stanford University School of Medicine, Stanford, California

BART BARLOGIE, MD

Professor of Medicine, Department of Medicine, Division of Hematology/Oncology, University of Arkansas for Medical Sciences, Little Rock, Arkansas

MICHAEL J. BARNETT, B.M.

Clinical Associate Professor, Division of Hematology, British Columbia Cancer Agency, Vancouver General Hospital, and University of British Columbia, Vancouver, British Columbia, Canada

CHARLES M. BAUM, MD, PhD

Assistant Professor and Director of Stem Cell Biology and Gene Therapy, Emory University School of Medicine, Department of Internal Medicine, Atlanta, Georgia

S.I. BEARMAN, MD

Associate Professor of Medicine, Clinical Director, Bone Marrow Transplant Program, University of Colorado, Denver, Colorado

ERNEST BEUTLER, MD

Chairman, Department of Molecular and Experimental Medicine, The Scripps Research Institute, La Jolla, California

PHILIP J. BIERMAN, MD

Assistant Professor of Medicine, Department of Internal Medicine, Section of Hematology/Oncology, University of Nebraska Medical Center, Omaha, Nebraska

KARL G. BLUME, MD

Professor of Medicine, Director, Bone Marrow Transplantation Program, Stanford University Hospital, Stanford, California

B.A. BOLONESI, PA, C

Bone Marrow Transplant Program, University of Utah, Salt Lake City, Utah

RALEIGH A. BOWDEN, MD

Associate Professor of Pediatrics, University of Washington School of Medicine, Associate Member, Fred Hutchinson Cancer Research Center, Seattle, Washington

E. RANDOLPH BROUN, MD

Assistant Professor of Medicine, Division of Hematology/Oncology, Indiana University, Indianapolis, Indiana

C. DEAN BUCKNER, MD

Professor of Medicine, University of Washington School of Medicine, Member and Head Autologous Marrow Transplant and Supportive Care Program, Fred Hutchinson Cancer Research Center, Seattle, Washington

WILLIAM H. BURNS, MD

Associate Professor of Oncology and Medicine, The Johns Hopkins University School of Medicine, Baltimore, Maryland

RICHARD CHAMPLIN, MD

Professor of Medicine, University of Texas—MD Anderson Hospital, Houston, Texas

NELSON CHAO, MD

Assistant Professor of Medicine, Stanford University Medical Center, Stanford, California

MICHAEL L. CLEARY, MD

Associate Professor of Pathology, Stanford University Medical Center, Stanford, California

REGINALD A. CLIFT, FIMLS

Staff Scientist, Fred Hutchinson Cancer Research Center, Seattle, Washington

MARTIN J. CLINE, MD

Bowyer Professor of Medical Oncology, University of California at Los Angeles, Los Angeles, California

PETER F. COCCIA, MD

Ittner Professor of Pediatrics, Chief, Section of Pediatric Hematology/Oncology, Director, Pediatric Bone Marrow Transplantation Program, University of Nebraska Medical Center, Omaha, Nebraska

STEPHEN W. CRAWFORD, MD

Associate Professor, Pulmonary and Critical Care Medicine, University of Washington School of Medicine, Associate Member, Fred Hutchinson Cancer Research Center, Seattle, Washington

H. JOACHIM DEEG, MD

Associate Member, Program in Transplantation Biology, Clinical Research Division, Fred Hutchinson Cancer Research Center, Seattle, Washington

BO DUPONT, MD, DSc

Professor of Immunology, Cornell University Graduate School of Medical Sciences, Member, Memorial Sloan-Kettering Cancer Center, Director, Clinical Histocompatibility Testing Laboratory, Memorial Hospital, New York, New York

CONNIE J. EAVES, PhD

Deputy Director, Terry Fox Laboratory, British Columbia Cancer Agency, Professor of Medical Genetics, University of British Columbia, Vancouver, British Columbia, Canada

ALLEN C. EAVES, MD, PhD, FRCP(C), FACP

Professor, Departments of Medicine and Pathology, Head, Division of Clinical Hematology, University of British Columbia, Vancouver General Hospital, and British Columbia Cancer Agency, Director, Terry Fox Laboratory, Vancouver, British Columbia, Canada

ANTHONY ELIAS, MD

Assistant Professor of Medicine, Department of Medicine, Harvard Medical School, Dana-Farber Cancer Institute, Boston, Massachusetts

ALEXANDER FEFER, MD

Professor of Medicine, University of Washington School of Medicine, Member, Fred Hutchinson Cancer Research Center, Seattle, Washington

HOWARD A. FINE, MD

Chief of the Brain Tumor Center, Department of Medicine, Harvard Medical School, Dana-Farber Cancer Institute, Boston, Massachusetts

LLOYD D. FISHER, PhD

Member and Director, Clinical Statistics, Fred Hutchinson Cancer Research Center, Professor, Department of Biostatistics, University of Washington, Director, Biostatistics/Epidemiology Core, Center for AIDS Research, University of Washington, Seattle, Washington

STEPHEN J. FORMAN, MD

Director, Department of Hematology and Bone Marrow Transplantation, Staff Physician, Department of Medical Oncology and Therapeutics Research, City of Hope National Medical Center, Duarte, California

WILHELM FRIEDRICH, MD

Privat Dozent, Department of Pediatrics, University of Ulm, Ulm, Germany

GOSTA GAHRTON, MD

Professor of Medicine, Karolinska Institutet, Department of Medicine, Huddinge University Hospital, Huddinge, Sweden

ELIANE GLUCKMAN, MD

Professor of Hematology, Head, Bone Marrow Transplant Unit, Hospital St. Louis, Paris, France

JAN W. GRATAMA, MD

Department of Clinical and Tumor Immunology, Dr. Daniel den Hoed Cancer Center, Rotterdam, The Netherlands

JOHN G. GRIBBEN, MD, PhD, MRCP(UK), MRCPath

Division of Tumor Immunology, Dana-Farber Cancer Institute, Boston, Massachusetts, Assistant Professor, Department of Medicine, Harvard Medical School, Cambridge, Massachusetts

ROBERT C. HACKMAN, MD

Associate Professor of Pathology, University of Washington School of Medicine, Assistant Member and Acting Clinical Laboratory Director, Fred Hutchinson Cancer Research Center, Seattle, Washington

JOHN A. HANSEN, MD

Professor of Medicine, University of Washington School of Medicine, Member, Clinical Research Division, Fred Hutchinson Cancer Research Center, Seattle, Washington

H. KENT HOLLAND, MD

Assistant Professor of Medicine, Director, Cell Separator Laboratory, Bone Marrow Transplantation Program, Emory University School of Medicine, Atlanta, Georgia

JILL HOWS, FRCP, FRCPath

Consultant Haematologist, South Mead Hospital, Westbury-n-Trym, Bristol, England

SUNDAR JAGANNATH, MD

Professor of Medicine, Department of Medicine, Division of Hematology/Oncology, University of Arkansas for Medical Sciences, Little Rock, Arkansas

RICHARD J. JONES, MD

Associate Professor of Oncology, The Johns Hopkins University School of Medicine, Baltimore, Maryland

ROY B. JONES, PhD, MD

Associate Professor of Medicine, Director, Bone Marrow Transplantation Program, University of Colorado Health Sciences Center, Denver, Colorado

NANCY A. KERNAN, MD

Associate Attending, Memorial Sloan-Kettering Cancer Research Center, New York, New York

JOHN KERSEY, MD

Professor and Director, Bone Marrow Transplant Program, University of Minnesota, Minneapolis, Minnesota

ROBERT KORNGOLD, PhD

Associate Professor, Department of Microbiology and Immunology, Jefferson Medical College, Philadelphia, Pennsylvania

WILLIAM KRIVIT, MD, PhD

Professor of Pediatrics, University of Minnesota, Member, Institute of Human Genetics, University of Minnesota Hospital and Clinic, Minneapolis, Minnesota

GWYNN LONG, MD

Assistant Professor of Medicine, Bone Marrow Transplantation Program, Stanford University Hospital, Stanford, California

GUIDO LUCARELLI, MD

Director, Department of Hematology and Bone Marrow Transplantation, Hospital of Pesaro, Pesaro, Italy

PAUL MARTIN, MD

Professor of Medicine, University of Washington School of Medicine, Member, Fred Hutchinson Cancer Research Center, Seattle, Washington

ERNEST A. MCCULLOCH, MD, FRSC

Professor Emeritus of Medicine, Professor Emeritus of Medical Biophysics, University Professor Emeritus, University of Toronto, Toronto, Canada

GEORGE B. MCDONALD, MD

Professor of Medicine, University of Washington School of Medicine, Member and Head, Gastroenterology/Hepatology Section, Fred Hutchinson Cancer Research Center, Seattle, Washington

PHILIP B. MCGLAVE, MD

Professor of Medicine, Director, Adult Bone Marrow Transplantation Program, Department of Medicine, University of Minnesota Medical School, Minneapolis, Minnesota

HANS A. MESSNER, MD, PhD FRCP(C)

Professor of Medicine, University of Toronto, Director of the Bone Marrow Transplant Program, Princess Margaret Hospital, Toronto, Canada

A. DUSTY MILLER, PhD

Affiliate Associate Professor, Department of Pathology, University of Washington, Member, Program in Molecular Medicine, Fred Hutchinson Cancer Research Center, Seattle, Washington

SONIA NADER, MD

Department of Pediatrics, Infectious Disease Division, Stanford University School of Medicine, Stanford, California

LEE M. NADLER, MD

Division of Tumor Immunology, Dana-Farber Cancer Institute, Boston, Massachusetts, Professor, Department of Medicine, Harvard Medical School, Cambridge, Massachusetts

ROBERT S. NEGRIN, MD

Assistant Professor of Medicine, Stanford University Medical Center, Stanford, California

JOHN NEMUNAITIS, MD

Director, Cytokine Research, Baylor Medical Center/Sammons Cancer Center, Director, Clinical Research, Texas Oncology, Dallas, Texas

CRAIG R. NICHOLS, MD

Associate Professor, Department of Medicine, Division of Hematology/Oncology, Indiana University, Indianapolis, Indiana

JOYCE C. NILAND, PhD

Director of Biostatistics, City of Hope National Medical Center, Duarte, California, Clinical Associate Professor, Department of Preventive Medicine, University of Southern California School of Medicine, Los Angeles, California

RICHARD J. O'REILLY, MD

Chairman, Department of Pediatrics, Chief, Bone Marrow Transplantation Service, Memorial Sloan-Kettering Cancer Center, New York, New York

HARRY OPENSHAW, MD

Director, Department of Neurology, City of Hope National Medical Center, Duarte, California

ROBERTSON PARKMAN, MD

Head, Division of Research Immunology/Bone Marrow Transplantation, Children's Hospital, Los Angeles, and Professor of Pediatrics and Microbiology, University of Southern California School of Medicine, Los Angeles, California

BRUNO PEAULT, PhD

Institut d'Embryologie Cellulaire et Moleculaire du CNRS et du College de France, Nogent cur Marne Cedex, France

WILLIAM P. PETERS, MD, PhD

Director, Bone Marrow Transplantation Program, Division of Hematology/Oncology, Associate Professor of Medicine, Duke University Medical Center, Durham, North Carolina

FINN BO PETERSEN, MD

Professor of Medicine, Bone Marrow Transplant Program, University of Utah, Salt Lake City, Utah

LAWRENCE D. PETZ, MD

Professor of Pathology and Laboratory Medicine, University of California, Los Angeles, School of Medicine, Director of Transfusion Medicine, UCLA Medical Center, Los Angeles, California

GORDON LEIGH PHILLIPS, MD

Director, Leukemia/Bone Marrow Transplant Program of British Columbia, Professor of Medicine, University of British Columbia, Vancouver, British Columbia, Canada

NORMA K.C. RAMSAY, MD

Professor and Director, Pediatric Bone Marrow Transplant Program, University of Minnesota, Minneapolis, Minnesota

C. PATRICK REYNOLDS, MD, PhD

Associate Professor, Division of Hematology/Oncology, Department of Pediatrics, Childrens Hospital of Los Angeles, University of Southern California School of Medicine, Los Angeles, California

JEROME RITZ, MD

Associate Professor of Medicine, Harvard Medical School, Division of Tumor Immunology, Dana-Farber Cancer Institute, Boston, Massachusetts

SCOTT ROWLEY, MD, FACP
Associate Member and Director, Clinical Cryobiology Laboratory, Fred Hutchinson Cancer Research Center, Seattle, Washington

DAVID H. SACHS, MD
Director, Transplantation Biology Research Center, Professor, Department of Surgery, Massachusetts General Hospital/ Harvard Medical School, Boston, Massachusetts

JEAN E. SANDERS, MD
Professor of Pediatrics, University of Washington School of Medicine, Member, Fred Hutchinson Cancer Research Center, Seattle, Washington

GEORGE E. SALE, MD
Professor of Pathology, University of Washington School of Medicine, Member, Fred Hutchinson Cancer Research Center, Seattle, Washington

REIN SARAL, MD
Professor of Medicine, Director, Bone Marrow Transplantation Program, Emory University School of Medicine, Atlanta, Georgia

GERHARD M. SCHMIDT, MD
Department of Hematology and Bone Marrow Transplantation, City of Hope National Medical Center, Duarte, California

SARAH JANE SCHWARZENBERG, MD
Associate Professor of Pediatrics, University of Minnesota, Minneapolis, Minnesota

ROBERT C. SEEGER, MD
Professor, Division of Hematology/Oncology, Department of Pediatrics, Childrens Hospital of Los Angeles, University of Southern California School of Medicine, Los Angeles, California

BRENDA SHANK, MD
Chairman and Professor, Radiation Oncology Department, Mount Sinai School of Medicine, Director, Radiation Oncology Department, Mount Sinai Hospital, New York, New York

ELSA G. SHAPIRO, PhD
Assistant Professor of Pediatric Neurology, University of Minnesota Hospital and Clinic, Minneapolis, Minnesota

ELIZABETH J. SHPALL, MD
Associate Professor of Medicine, University of Colorado School of Medicine, Denver, Colorado

MARGARET C. SHUHART, MD
Senior Fellow in Medicine, Fred Hutchinson Cancer Research Center, Seattle, Washington

HOWARD M. SHULMAN, MD
Professor of Pathology, University of Washington School of Medicine, Member, Fred Hutchinson Cancer Research Center, Seattle, Washington

JACK W. SINGER, MD
Clinical Professor of Medicine, University of Washington School of Medicine, Executive Vice President and Scientific Director, Cell Therapeutics, Seattle, Washington

NEAL E. SLATKIN, MD
Staff Physician, Department of Neurology, City of Hope National Medical Center, Duarte, California

SHERRILL SLICHTER, MD
Scientific Director, Puget Sound Blood Center, Professor of Medicine, University of Washington Medical School, Seattle, Washington

TRUDY N. SMALL, MD
Assistant Member, Department of Pediatrics, Bone Marrow Transplantation Service, Memorial Sloan-Kettering Cancer Center, New York, New York

IRENA SNIECINSKI, MD
Associate Professor of Pathology, Director, Department of Transfusion Medicine, City of Hope National Medical Center, Duarte, California

DAVID S. SNYDER, MD
Associate Director, Department of Hematology and Bone Marrow Transplantation, City of Hope National Medical Center, Duarte, California

JONATHAN SPRENT, MD, PhD
Member, Department of Immunology, The Scripps Research Institute, La Jolla, California

PATRICK J. STIFF, MD
Associate Professor of Medicine, Director, Bone Marrow Transplantation Program, Loyola University Medical Center, Maywood, Illinois

RAINER STORB, MD
Professor of Medicine, University of Washington School of Medicine, Member and Program Head, Transplantation Biology, Fred Hutchinson Cancer Research Center, Seattle, Washington

SAMUEL STROBER, MD
Professor, Department of Medicine, Division of Immunology and Rheumatology, Department of Medicine, Stanford University School of Medicine, Stanford, California

KEITH M. SULLIVAN, MD
Professor of Medicine, University of Washington School of Medicine, Member, and Medical Director, Outpatient Department and Long-term Follow-up Program, Fred Hutchinson Cancer Research Center, Seattle, Washington

MEGAN SYKES, MD
Assistant Professor, Department of Surgery and Medicine, Massachusetts General Hospital/Harvard Medical School, Boston, Massachusetts

E. DONNALL THOMAS, MD
Professor of Medicine, Emeritus, University of Washington School of Medicine, Member, Fred Hutchinson Cancer Research Center, Seattle, Washington

NOBUKO UCHIDA, PhD
Howard Hughes Medical Institute, Stanford University School of Medicine, Stanford, California

GEORGIA B. VOGELSANG, MD
Associate Professor of Oncology, The Johns Hopkins University, Baltimore, Maryland

KENNETH WEINBERG, MD
Department of Pediatrics, Division of Research Immunology and Bone Marrow Transplantation, Childrens Hospital of Los Angeles, and University of Southern California School of Medicine, Los Angeles, California

SALLY WEISDORF, MD
Associate Professor of Pediatrics, Graduate Faculty In Nutrition, School of Food Science and Nutrition, University of Minnesota, Minneapolis, Minnesota

IRVING L. WEISSMAN, MD
Professor, Department of Pathology and Developmental Biology, Stanford University School of Medicine, Stanford, California

DAVID WELLISCH, MD
Department of Medical Psychology, Department of Psychiatry, University of California at Los Angeles School of Medicine, Los Angeles, California

JOHN REID WINGARD, MD
Professor of Medicine, Clinical Director of Bone Marrow Transplantation Program, Emory University School of Medicine, Atlanta, Georgia

DEANE L. WOLCOTT, MD
Associate Clinical Professor, Department of Psychiatry and Behavioral Sciences, University of California at Los Angeles School of Medicine, Los Angeles, California, Director, Psychosocial Services, The Cedars–Sinai Comprehensive Cancer Center, Los Angeles, California

SOO YOUNG YANG, PhD
Associate Professor of Immunology, Cornell University Graduate School of Medical Sciences, Associate Member, Memorial Sloan-Kettering Cancer Center, and Associate Director, Clinical Histocompatibility Testing Laboratory, Memorial Hospital, New York, New York

ANDREW M. YEAGER, MD
Professor of Pediatrics, Director, Division of Pediatric Hematology/Oncology and Bone Marrow Transplantation, Emory School of Medicine, Atlanta, Georgia

JOHN A. ZAIA, MD
Director, Virology and Infectious Diseases, Division of Pediatrics, City of Hope National Medical Center, Duarte, California

Foreword

The observations of the Danish investigator, Fabricious-Moeller, in guinea pigs in 1922 (Experimental studies of the hemorrhagic diathesis from x-ray sickness. Copenhagen: Levin and Munksgaard, 1922) and those of Jacobson and colleagues in mice 27 years later (Effects of spleen protection on mortality following x-irradiation. J Clin Med 1949;34:1538) that the shielding of hematopoietic tissue could alleviate the myelosuppressive effects induced by total body irradiation planted the seeds of what has subsequently produced an ever-widening spectrum of research in the fundamentals of hematopoiesis, transplantation immunology and immunogenetics. These investigations continue to provide increasing insights into the cellular and molecular mechanisms of normal and neoplastic lympho hematopoiesis.

The past 35 years have, in parallel, also seen the clinical application of hematopoietic stem cell transplantation evolve from its beginning as a highly experimental procedure to a well-established and potentially curative therapeutic modality for the treatment of malignancy, diseases of marrow failure, and selected genetic diseases. The editors, with the aid of a number of prominent and established investigators, have assembled an excellent comprehensive volume on bone marrow transplantation. The opening chapters on the scientific foundation of marrow transplantation, based on animal and human studies, and an overview of transplantation immunology are written by pioneers in bone marrow transplantation and provide an excellent background for the subsequent chapters. These in-depth discussions range from mechanisms of human hematopoiesis, biostatistical methods in marrow transplantation, to discussion of various aspects of supportive care and prevention and treatment of the immunological, infectious and psychological complications of marrow transplantation in the various hematopoietic malignancies and disorders, selected genetic diseases, and selected solid tumors. The volume concludes with a chapter on the future of bone marrow transplantation in the 21st Century.

In summary, this comprehensive treatise on clinical bone marrow transplantation provides a solid background on its rationale and beginnings as well as discussions on current problems and their solutions. This volume will have a wide interest and be a valuable reference for all the clinicians and scientists who are interested in cancer therapy, hematology, and genetic diseases. This book undoubtedly will help those involved in bone marrow transplantation appreciate the past efforts, review the current state-of-the-art, and look to future investigations in this most promising and fulfilling discipline.

George W. Santos, MD
Professor of Oncology and Medicine
Johns Hopkins University Oncology Center
Baltimore, Maryland

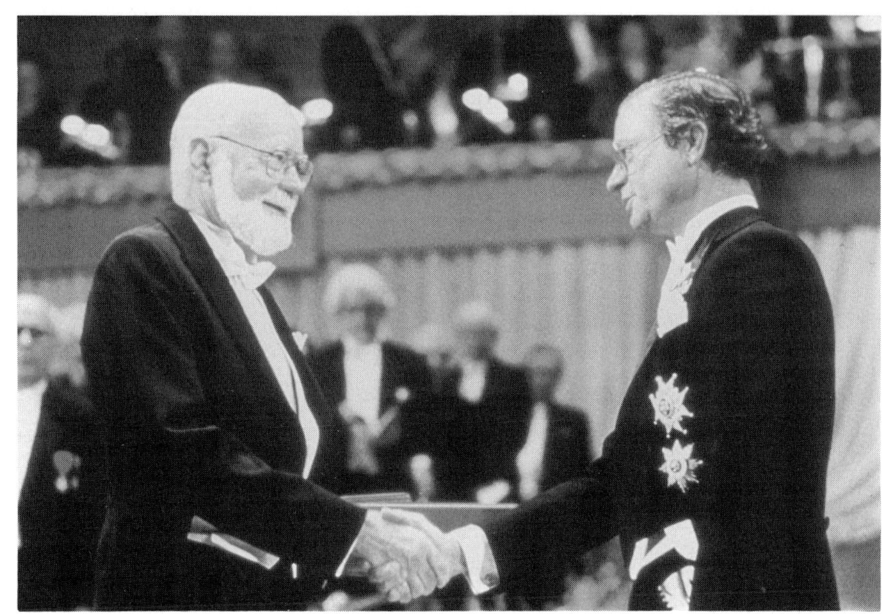

Dr. E. Donall Thomas and King Carl Gustaf of Sweden. Dr. Thomas and Dr. Joseph Murray (not shown in the picture) shared the Nobel Prize for Physiology or Medicine, 1990, recognizing the field of organ transplantation. Dr. Thomas was honored for endeavors in experimental and clinical bone marrow transplantation. Their prizes emphasize the importance of patient related research.

PREFACE

The widespread application of bone marrow transplantation (BMT) to treatment of a steadily increasing number of life-threatening hematological, oncological, hereditary, and immunological disorders is the culmination of more than four decades of research by many investigators. Early attempts in the 1950s to transplant living cells from one individual to another were carried out in the face of considerable skepticism. It was generally accepted as axiomatic that the immunological barrier to "foreign tissue" could never be overcome.

The horrors of Nagasaki and Hiroshima spurred interest in studies of the lethal effects of irradiation. It was discovered that mice given total body irradiation in doses lethal to the marrow could be protected from death by shielding the spleen or by an infusion of marrow, and that the marrow of such animals contained living cells of donor origin. These observations suggested that patients with leukemia might be given a lethal exposure of total body irradiation, which would destroy the malignant cells along with the remaining normal marrow. The exposure would also destroy the immune system, making it possible to protect against lethality by a transplant of normal marrow cells.

The theory was correct, but results were disappointing. Because the procedure was both unproved and dangerous, only those patients who had no other options were considered. Except for a few patients with an identical twin donor, there were no survivors beyond a few months. Understanding of the human leukocyte antigen (HLA) system was not yet available, and little was known about the complication we now call graft-versus-host disease (GVHD). Thus, after a brief period of enthusiasm, most investigators abandoned this seemingly hopeless pursuit.

Fortunately, work in animal models continued. Studies in inbred rodents defined the genetics of the major histocompatibility system and the fundamental rules of transplantation biology. Immunosuppressive drugs were developed to limit the severity of the immune reactions between donor and host. Demonstration of successful marrow transplants in the canine model using littermates matched for the major histocompatibility complex set the stage for successful transplantation of marrow between human siblings. Thus, it is clear that a long series of experimental studies in animals ultimately made human marrow transplantation possible.

By the late 1960s, much was known about the HLA system, more effective antibiotics were available, and platelet transfusions were becoming routine. Thus began the modern era of human BMT. The past 25 years have witnessed an almost exponential growth in the number of transplants being performed and the number of diseases being considered for BMT. Initially, most grafts employed marrow from an HLA-identical sibling. Autologous marrow, long known to be effective in animal systems, is now being used with increasing frequency following intensive cancer chemotherapy. Hematopoietic progenitor cells from the peripheral blood are now being used for BMT, either alone or to supplement marrow. As a result of increasing national and international cooperation, large panels of volunteer marrow donors of known HLA type are becoming available to patients whose own marrow cannot be used or who do not have a family donor.

Currently, thousands of transplants are being performed each year worldwide. With the demonstration that marrow could be transplanted and that the cure rate would be substantial, the logical step was taken to treat patients early during the course of their respective disease (i.e., in leukemia when the burden of malignant cells was relatively low and when the patient was in excellent clinical condition). With improved patient selection, development of improved tissue typing methods, availability of potent antimicrobial agents, advances in supportive care, and improved prevention of GVHD, the results of BMT have continued to improve.

Marrow transplantation is now being applied to a long list of diseases with a wide range of results depending on the disease, the type of transplant, and the stage of the disease. For some of the diseases, BMT has already proven to be the most effective therapy (e.g., some leukemias and severe aplastic anemia), whereas for others it is the only available curative treatment (e.g., thalassemia). In very rare genetic disorders, one successful BMT may establish the success of the treatment. For other more common disorders, controlled trials are necessary to define the proper role of allogeneic or autologous BMT, or therapy not involving BMT.

Only through rigorous study and long-term follow-up can novel approaches be confirmed as effective (or ineffective). For those working in the field of marrow transplantation, a source of intellectual satisfaction has been the interdisciplinary nature of the studies. A view of the wide-ranging disciplines involved can be gleaned by reading the chapter titles for this book. A successful BMT program is always a team effort. There must be cooperation between blood banks, referring physicians, radiation oncologists, immunologists, and physicians from many subspecialties. A dedicated support staff of technicians, data managers, and, above all, nurses, is crucial. The nursing team in particular is responsible for the day-to-day care of patients. Nurses not only provide bedside management of complex protocol studies, but also bear the burden of emotional support through the difficult hospital period. They are the most readily available source of information for patients and families day and night. Without a strong nursing team, the entire BMT program is jeopardized.

Most important are the patients who come to the transplant center with the courage to accept days, weeks, and sometimes months of discomfort in the hope of surviving a fatal disease. We must ensure that we acknowledge and respect the dignity and individuality of each patient, that we provide adequate information for informed decision making and then include patients and families in the decision process. The greatest reward for clinical investigators is to see patients reintegrated into their personal, social, and professional lives, free of their disease and its complications.

Stephen J. Forman
Karl G. Blume
E. Donnall Thomas

GLOSSARY

ABC	ATP-Binding Cassette
ABMT	Autologous Bone Marrow Transplantation
α-TIF	α-Transinducing Factor
ACV	Acyclovir
ADA	Adenosine Deaminase
ADCC	Antibody Dependent Cell-mediated Cytotoxicity
AIDS	Acquired Immune Deficiency Syndrome
ALC	Absolute Lymphocyte Count
ALD	Adrenoleukodystrophy
ALL	Acute Lymphoblastic Leukemia
AML	Acute Myeloblastic Leukemia—also Acute Myeloid Leukemia
AMM	Agnogenic Myeloid Metaplasia
ANC	Absolute Neutrophil Count
APC	Antigen-presenting Cell
APL	Acute Promyelocytic Leukemia
ara-C	Cytosine Arabinoside
ARDS	Adult Respiratory Distress Syndrome
ATG	Anti-thymocyte Globulin
B2M	Beta$_2$-microglobulin
BACT	BCNU, Cytosine-Arabinoside, Cyclophosphamide, Thioguanine
BAL	Bronchoalveolar Lavage
BAVC	BCNU, Amsacrine, VP16, Cytosine-Arabinoside
BCAA	Branched Chain Amino Acid
BCNU	1,3-Bis(2-Chloroethyl)-1-nitrosourea (Carmustine)
BCR	Breakpoint Cluster Region
BEAM	BCNU, Etoposide, Cytosine Arabinoside, Melphalan
BED	Biologically Effective Dose
BEE	Basic Energy Expenditure
BEP	Bleomycin, Etoposide, Cisplatin
BFU-E	Burst Forming Units—Erythroid
BLS	Bare Lymphocyte Syndrome
BM	Bone Marrow
BMT	Bone Marrow Transplantation
BU	Busulfan
BUN	Blood Urea Nitrogen
CALGB	Cancer and Acute Leukemia Group
CBV	Cyclophosphamide, BCNU, Etoposide (VP16)
CCI	Corrected Count Increment
CCSG	Childrens Cancer Study Group
CDC	Complement-dependent Cytotoxicity
CFU-B	B lymphocyte Colony Forming Units
CFU-BLAST	Blast Forming Colony Units
CFU-GM	Colony Forming Unit–Granulocyte Macrophage
CFU-GEMM	Colony Forming Unit–Granulocyte/Erythroid/Macrophage/Megakaryocytic
CFU-MEG	Colony Forming Unit–Megakaryocytic
CFU-Mix	Colony Forming Unit–Mixed
CFU-S	Colony Forming Unit–Spleen
CFU-T	T lymphocyte Colony Forming Units
CFU-T	Colony Forming Unit–Thymus
CHOP	Cyclophosphamide, Hydroxydaunomycin, Vincristin, Prednisone
CID	Combined Immunodeficiency Syndrome
CIPRO	Ciprofloxacin
CML	Chronic Myelogenous Leukemia
CMMoL	Chronic Myelomonocytic Leukemia
CMV	Cytomegalovirus
CMV-IG	CMV-Antibody Enriched Intravenous Immunoglobulin
CMV-IP	Cytomegalovirus-Associated-Interstitial Pneumonia
Con A	Concanavilin A
CP	Chronic Phase
CNS	Central Nervous System
CPR	Cardiopulmonary Resuscitation
CR	Complete Remission
CREG	Cross-Reactive Group
CSP	Cyclosporine A
CT	Computerized Tomography
CTL	Cytotoxic T-Lymphocytes
CVB	Cyclophosphamide, VP16, BCNU
CY	Cyclophosphamide
DFS	Disease-free Survival
DFCC	Dana Farber Cancer Center
DIC	Disseminated Intravascular Coagulation
DLA	Dog Leukocyte Antigen
DLCL	Diffuse Large Cell Lymphoma
DLCO	Diffusion Capacity
DNA	Deoxyribonucleic Acid

DPT	Diptheria Pertussis Tetanus
DTH	Delayed-type Hypersensitivity
EACA	Epsilon Amino Caproic Acid
EBMT	European BMT Group
EBNA	Epstein-Barr (Virus) Nuclear Antigen
EBV	Epstein-Barr Virus
ECG	Electrocardiogram
ECOG	Eastern Cancer Oncology Group
ED	Early Death also Extensive Disease
EDAP	Etoposide, Dexamethasone, Cytosine Arabinoside, Cisplatin
EFS	Event-free Survival
ELISA	Enzyme-linked Immunosorbent Assay
EORTC	European Organization for Research on the Treatment of Cancer
EPO	Erythropoietin
ET	Essential Thrombocythemia
5-FU	5-Fluorouracil
FA	Fanconi Anemia
FAB	French-American British Classification
FACS	Fluorescence-activated Cell Sorter
FEV_1	Forced Expiratory Ventilation in one Second
FHCRC	Fred Hutchinson Cancer Research Center
FISH	Fluorescence in-situ Hybridization
FMF	Flow Microfluorometry
FSCL	Follicular Small Cleaved Cell Lymphoma
FSH	Follicle Stimulating Hormone
FVC	Forced Volume Capacity
G-6-PD	Glucose-6-Phosphate Dehydrogenase
G-CSF	Granulocyte Colony Stimulating Factor
GH	Growth Hormone
GCV	Ganciclovir
GLD	Globoid Cell Leukodystrophy
GM-CSF	Granulocyte-Macrophage Colony Stimulating Factor
GVHD	Graft-versus-Host Disease
GVL (E)	Graft-versus-Leukemia (Effect)
4-HC	4-Hydroperoxycyclophosphamide
HBV	Hepatitis B Virus
HCV	Hepatitis C Virus
HD-AC	High-dose ara-C
HD-CY	High-dose Cyclophosphamide
HHV6	Human Herpes Virus 6
HIV	Human Immunodeficiency Virus
HLA	Human Leukocyte Antigen
HPP	High Proliferative Potential
HSC	Hematopoietic Stem Cell
HSV	Herpes Simplex Virus
HTC	Homozygous Typing Cells
HVG	Host-versus-Graft
IBMTR	International Bone Marrow Transplant Registry
IDUA	α-L-Iduronide Iduronolydrolase
IE	Immediate Early (Antigen Expression)
IEF	Isoelectric Focusing
Ig	Immunoglobulin
IGF-1	Insulin-like Growth Factor 1
IIP	Idiopathic Interstitial Pneumonia
IL-1	Interleukin-1
IP	Interstitial Pneumonia
IVIg	Intravenous Immunoglobulin
JCML	Juvenile Chronic Myelogenous Leukemia
KLH	Keyhole Limpet Hemocyanin
KPS	Karnofsky Performance Score
LAK	Lymphokine Activated Killer (Cells)
LAT	Latency-associated Factor
LIN	Lineage
LH	Luteinizing Hormone
LMP	Low Molecular Weight Problems
L-PAM	L-Phenylalanine Mustard
LPC	Leukemic Progenitor Cell
LTC-IC	Long Term Culture Initiating Cells
M-CSF	Macrophage Colony Stimulating Factor
MDR	Multidrug Resistance
MDS	Myelodysplastic Syndrome
MHC	Major Histocompatibility Complex
MEG-CSA	Megakaryocyte Colony Stimulating Activity
MEG-GPA	Megakaryocyte Growth Promoting Activity
MEL	Melphalan
MGF	Mast-cell Growth Factor
MLC	Mixed Leukocyte Culture
MLD	Metachromatic Leukodystrophy
MLS	Maroteaux-Lamy Syndrome
MM	Multiple Myeloma
MMR	Measles, Mumps, Rubella
MoAB	Monoclonal Antibody
MOPP	Mustargen, Vincristine, Prednisone, Procarbazine
MP	Melphalan/Prednisone
MP	Methylprednisone
MRD	Minimal Residual Disease
m-RNA	Messenger Ribonucleic Acid
MSKCC	Memorial Sloan-Kettering Cancer Center

MTD	Maximum Tolerated Dose
MTX	Methotrexate
NHL	Non-Hodgkin's Lymphoma
NK	Natural Killer (Cells)
NMDP	National Marrow Donor Program
NPC	Non-protein Calories
NRM	Non-relapse Mortality
NS	Natural Suppressor (Cells)
PAIS	Psychological Adjustment to Illness Scale
PBMC	Peripheral Blood Mononuclear Cells
PBPC	Peripheral Blood Progenitor Cells
PCR	Polymerase Chain Reaction
PD	Protective Dose
PEC	Cisplatin, Etoposide, Cyclophosphamide
Ph	Philadelphia (Chromosome)
PHA	Phytohemagglutanin A
PLT	Platelet
PNET	Primitive Neuroectodermal Tumor
POG	Pediatric Oncology Group
PR	Partial Remission
PRP	Polyribosylphosphate
PSE	Prednisone
PTX	Pentoxifylline
PV	Polycythemia Vera
QOL	Quality of Life
RA	Refractory Anemia
RAEB	Refractory Anemia with Excess Blasts
RAEB-T	Refractory Anemia with Excess Blasts in Transformation
RARS	Refractory Anemia with Ringed Sideroblasts
RBC	Red Blood Cell
RDA	Recommended Daily Allowance
REE	Resting Energy Expenditure
RIA	Radioimmune Assay
RFLP	Restriction Fragment Length Polymorphism
RFS	Relapse-free Survival
RNA	Ribonucleic Acid
RQ	Respiratory Quotient
RR	Relative Risk, Relative Relapse, or Resistant Relapse
RRT	Regimen-related Toxicity
RSV	Respiratory Syncytial Virus
RT_3U	Resin T_3 Uptake
SAA	Severe Aplastic Anemia
SAC	*Staphylococcus Aureus* Cowan Strain A
SAS-SR	Social Adjustment Scale–Self Report
SBA	Soy Bean Agglutinin
SCF	Stem Cell Factor
SCID	Severe Combined Immunodeficiency Syndrome
SCID-hu	Severe Combined Immunodeficiency Syndrome/ Human (Mouse)
SCLC	Small-cell Lung Cancer
SEAS	Sleep, Energy, Appetite Scale
SECSG	Southeastern Cancer Study Group
SER	Symptom Experience Report
SIP	Sickness Impact Profile
SLF	Steel Factor
SSOP	Sequence–Specific Oligonucleotide Probe
SWOG	Southwest Oncology Group
STL	Steel Factor
TAI	Thoracoabdominal Irridiation
TBI	Total Body Irradiation
TCA	Tricarbonic Acid (Cycle)
TCD	T-cell Depletion
TCR	T-cell Receptor
TdT	Terminal Deoxynucleotidyl Transferase
T-GVHD	Transfusion-Induced Graft-versus-Host Disease
TIL	Tumor-infiltrating Lymphocytes
TLI	Total Lymphoid Irradiation
TMP-SMX	Trimethoprim-Sulfamethoxazole
TNF-α	Tumor Necrosis Factor-alpha
TPN	Total Parenteral Nutrition
TSH	Thyroid-stimulating Hormone
URU	Upper Respiratory Infection
UV	Ultraviolet (Light)
VAD	Vincristine, Adriamycin, Decadron
VIP	Etoposide, Ifosfamide, Cisplatin
VLCFA	Very Long Chain Fatty Acids
VNTR	Variable Number of Tandem Repeat
VOD	Veno-occlusive Disease
VP16	Etoposide
VZV	Varicella Zoster Virus
WAS	Wiscott-Aldrich Syndrome
WBC	White Blood Cell

Credits

Frontmatter photos, reprinted with the permission of the patients, are from City of Hope National Medical Center, Stanford University School of Medicine (© Joel Simon, photographer, P.O. Box 1042, Menlo Park, CA 94026-1042, *telephone* (415) 321-8458), and the Fred Hutchinson Cancer Research Center (courtesy of R.J. McDougall).

Notice

The indications and dosages of all drugs in this book have been recommended in the medical literature and conform to the practices of the general medical community. The medications described do not necessarily have specific approval by the Food and Drug Administration for use in the diseases and dosages for which they are recommended. The package insert for each drug should be consulted for use and dosage as approved by the FDA. Because standards of usage change, it is advisable to keep abreast of revised recommendations, particularly those concerning new drugs.

Part I
Scientific Basis

Chapter 1

The Scientific Foundation of Marrow Transplantation Based on Animal Studies

Rainer Storb and E. Donnall Thomas

It should be noted that marrow grafting could not have reached clinical application without animal research, first in inbred rodents and then in outbred species, particularly the dog.
E. Donnall Thomas, The Nobel Prizes, 1990; Les Prix Nobel, Norstedts Tryckeri AB, Stockholm, 1991, p. 227

With modern demonstration of conservation of so many genes across species, it is apparent that human beings have much in common with all animals and other living things. It should be no surprise, therefore, that so many of the biological principles underlying transplantation immunology are transferable from one species to another. The successful application in humans of not only bone marrow transplantation (BMT), but also transplantation of other organs has been achieved as a result of extensive animal studies.

The experiments of Alexis Carrel at the beginning of this century established a paradigm of biology—that cells or organs transferred from one individual to another would always be recognized as foreign and therefore be rejected. That this paradigm might not always be true was suggested by Owen, who noted that freemartin cattle contained cells of different genetic origin. The paradigm was further undermined by the hypothesis of Burnett and by the animal experiments of Medawar and colleagues. They provided the scientific basis for an understanding of tolerance induced in utero or in newborns. However, their studies indicated that tolerance between genetically divergent animals could not be achieved once the immune system had developed sufficiently to distinguish self from non-self. The numerous studies of transplantation biology performed before 1960 are presented in the monograph by Woodruff (1). Studies of BMT and immunosuppressive drugs would eventually provide at least a partial solution to the immunological barrier against transplantation.

Marrow Transplant Studies in the Murine Model

The possibility of BMT came first from studies in the mouse. At the end of World War II following the atomic bomb explosions, there was a great deal of interest in how radiation damages living organisms. It became recognized that the marrow is the organ most sensitive to radiation and that death following low-lethal exposures was due to marrow failure. Jacobson and associates (2) made the observation that mice could withstand an otherwise lethal exposure to whole-body irradiation if the spleen were protected by a lead foil. Shortly thereafter, Lorenz and colleagues (3) found that similar radiation protection could be conferred by infusion of bone marrow. At first it was thought that the radioprotective effect was due to a humoral factor derived from the spleen or marrow, which stimulated marrow recovery.

In the mid-1950s, several reports offered a different explanation for the "radiation protection" effect. In 1955, Main and Prehn (4) showed that a mouse given lethal irradiation and a marrow infusion from a different strain would accept a subsequent skin graft from the donor, and in 1956, Trentin (5) showed that the skin graft acceptance was specific for the donor strain. Also in 1956, Ford and associates (6) showed that the cytogenetic characteristics of the marrow in such mice were those of the donor and not the recipient, and Nowell and colleagues (7) demonstrated the presence of rat granulocytes in mice protected with rat marrow. These experiments made it clear that protection against radiation was due to the transfer of living cells and that a form of tolerance had been induced.

In 1958, Schwartz and Dameshek (8) found that 6-mercaptopurine could induce a form of specific immune tolerance in rabbits when given at the time of antigen exposure. This observation was followed by the development of azathioprine by Elion and associates (9). Murray (10) showed that these agents could prolong the life of kidney grafts in dogs. These studies of immunosuppression by drugs led the way to solid organ grafts and to control of the graft-versus-host (GVH) reaction following a marrow graft.

The availability of inbred mice made possible a wide range of studies of immunology, immunogenetics, and radiation biology, too numerous to review completely herein. The book by van Bekkum and de Vries (11) summarizes many of the early observations. Some of the more important studies demonstrated that:

1. Marrow given intravenously was just as effective in repopulating the marrow spaces as marrow given by any other route (12).
2. Marrow, an immunologically competent organ, could mount an immune attack against the host, resulting in graft-versus-host disease (GVHD) (11).
3. The severity of the immune reaction of donor cells against the host was controlled by genetic factors (13).
4. Methotrexate (MTX) could prevent or ameliorate the GVH reaction (14,15).
5. Cyclophosphamide (CY) alone could provide immunosuppression sufficient for allogeneic engraftment (16).

Finally, in mice, the importance of the thymus, T cells, B cells, and other lymphoid subsets in immunogenetics and transplantation biology began to be understood (17–19).

Marrow Transplant Studies in Other Animal Models

Other animal species have had important roles in transplantation biology. The inbred rat has made possible the extension of observations in the mouse, particularly the study of immunosuppressive drugs (20). Busulfan was first introduced into marrow transplant preparative regimens in the rat (21). The rabbit has been widely used in studies of skin grafting and in studies of humoral immunity (1,8). The pig has been particularly informative in liver transplantation (22) and in studies of chimerism after marrow grafting (23). The monkey has provided important information on the pathology of GVHD (24). In preclinical studies applicable to human patients, the dog has been the most widely used and informative species.

Marrow Transplant Studies in the Canine Model

For more than three decades the dog has served as a random-bred animal model for studies of principles and techniques of BMT applicable to humans. Early studies of radiation and marrow grafting in dogs, carried out before the modern knowledge of the histocompatibility complex, identified the problems of graft rejection and GVHD and resulted in some long-term canine chimeras that survived in good health for a number of years (Figure 1-1) (25,26).

The dog offers several advantages over other animal species for transplantation research. Dogs are generally available and relatively inexpensive. They can be kept disease-free in a suitable colony and are easy to work with. They are large enough to obtain serial blood and marrow samples and organ biopsies and to allow external gamma-camera scanning of the infusion of radiolabeled antibodies. Large canine families are regularly available for genetic studies of istocompatibility antigens, and they provide matched littermate pairs, stimulating HLA-identical human sibling pairs. The major canine histocompatibility complex, DLA, is now well defined. An added attraction of the dog is the availability of animals with spontaneous malignant and nonmalig-

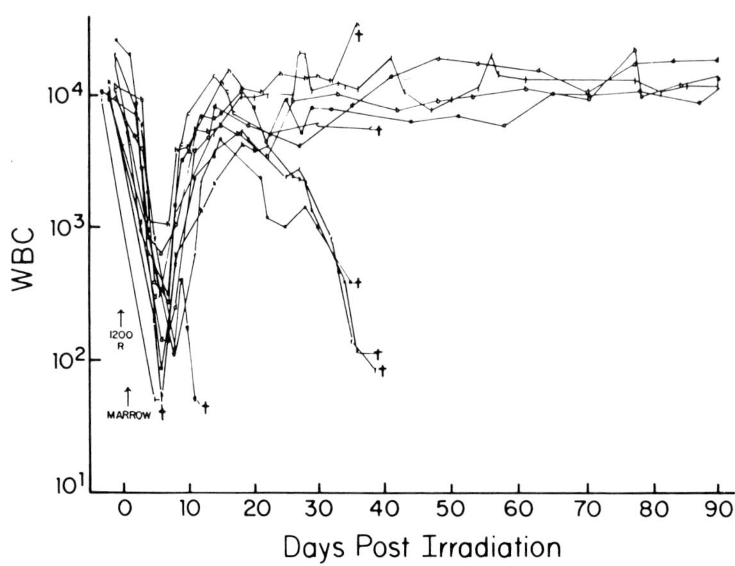

Figure 1-1. Results of marrow transplants in dogs before tissue typing became available. Eleven dogs were given TBI, 12 R (measured in air), and post-grafting MTX. This figure shows the white blood cell count in these animals demonstrate failure of engraftment, graft rejection, or GVHD (with normal counts) all followed by death (+). Some animals became long-term survivors. (Reproduced by permission from Crouch BG, van Putten LM, van Bekkum DW, de Vries MJ. Treatment of total-body x-irradiated monkeys with autologous and homologous bone marrow. J Natl Cancer Inst 1961;27: 53–65.)

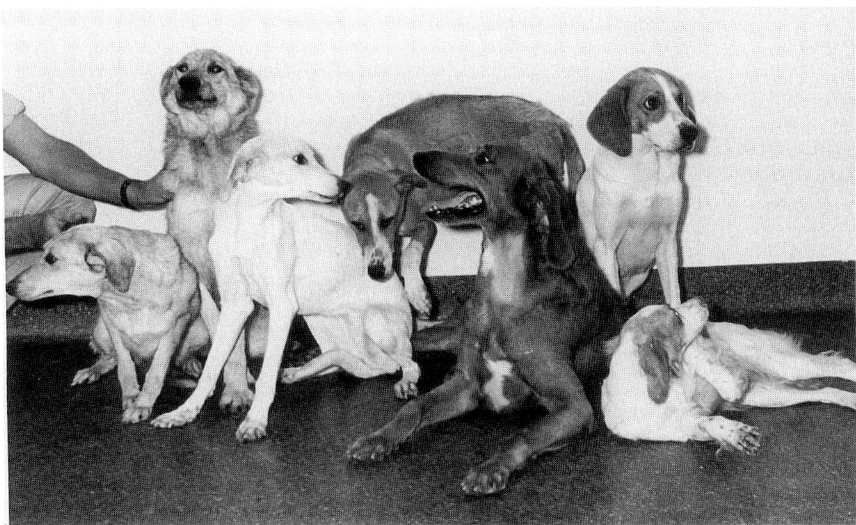

Figure 1-2. Recipients of allogeneic marrow grafts 2 to 12 years after transplant. Dogs with graying hair color were conditioned by 9.2 Gy TBI, whereas the large hound was conditioned by cyclophosphamide.

nant hematological diseases resembling those encountered in humans.

Conditioning Regimens

Conditioning programs serve to suppress the recipient's immune system for acceptance of the marrow graft and to eradicate the recipient's underlying disease that made treatment by BMT necessary. Total body irradiation (TBI) has been the most commonly used conditioning program for BMT. Dogs not given a marrow infusion usually die from complications of marrow failure when exposed to a TBI dose of 4 Gy, although dogs given intensive care may occasionally survive that exposure (27). Consistent survival following otherwise lethal doses of TBI can be obtained when dogs are given an infusion of autologous marrow, fresh or cryopreserved (28,29). Successful allogeneic marrow grafts from DLA-identical littermates are consistently obtained only after a TBI dose of more than 9 Gy, delivered at a dose rate of 7 cGy/min (30). Grafts from DLA-nonidentical unrelated or littermate donors require TBI doses in excess of 15 Gy (31). Dogs with successful grafts have, as a rule, been complete chimeras (i.e., cells from marrow, peripheral blood, lymph nodes, and bronchoalveolar fluid have all been of donor origin).

The fact that many leukemic recurrences were seen after human marrow grafting stimulated research into increasing the dose of TBI by the use of dose fractionation. Hematopoietic cells are less capable of undergoing DNA repair after a dose of fractionated TBI than other tissue cells. Thus, administering multiple fractions of, for example, 200 cGy of TBI with at least 3-hour interfraction intervals would lead to severe marrow toxicity, whereas other organs would be much less affected. Bodenberger and colleagues (32) administered doses of TBI ranging from 18 to 23 Gy, given in fractions of 4.5 to 9 Gy, at rates of 4 cGy/min over periods of 3 to 7 days. Most dogs survived these very high doses of TBI with the help of a subsequent infusion of autologous marrow. Deeg and associates (33) explored fractions of 1.5 to 2 Gy, given at intervals of 3 to 6 hours, for total doses of 12 to 21 Gy, with dose rates ranging from 2 to 20 cGy/min. The acute radiation toxicity of single- and fractionated-dose TBI regimens was comparable at equal total doses. Lower dose rates permitted higher total doses and vice versa. Long-term complications were significantly less in dogs given fractionated TBI compared with those given a single exposure. Late radiation deaths were related to liver failure, malnutrition, and pancreatic atrophy. Although the effects of fractionated and single-dose TBI on the myeloid elements of the marrow are comparable, the immunosuppressive effects of fractionated TBI are inferior to those of single-dose TBI. Studies in dogs have shown a much higher rate of graft failure when fractionated TBI was used in preparation for the transplant (34).

Consistent with findings in mice, rats, and monkeys, the alkylating agent CY can be substituted for TBI to prepare dogs for allogeneic marrow transplants (35). CY-conditioned dogs often show persisting mixtures of host and donor hematopoietic cells. This finding may be undesirable in efforts to condition patients with hematopoietic malignancies for marrow transplants, but can be disregarded in patients with nonmalignant disorders of the marrow.

Following studies with busulfan (BU) in the rat, the BU derivative, dimethylbusulfan, was studied extensively in dogs (36,37). The major advantage of dimethylbusulfan over BU is that it can be injected intravenously. The LD_{99} was 7.5 mg/kg in the absence of autologous marrow infusion. When autologous marrow was infused, dogs were able to survive a dose of 10 mg/kg. Marrow grafts were not successful when donors were DLA-nonidentical. However, when DLA-identical littermate marrow was used, approximately half the animals showed long-term sustained engraftment. The other half rejected their grafts, presumably as a result of disparity for minor histocompatibility antigens outside of DLA. Graft failure could be prevented by the addition of immunosuppression with antithymocyte serum to the dimethylbusulfan preparative regimen.

Resistance to DLA-nonidentical Marrow Grafts

Graft resistance reflects the action of host cells that are insensitive to the usual doses of TBI and do not require prior sensitization to donor histocompatibility antigens to destroy an allogeneic marrow graft. Although the phenomenon of hybrid resistance—rejection of marrow grafts from homozygous parents by the F1 hybrid recipients—had been well described in mice, studies in the dog model drew attention to allogeneic resistance (reviewed in 38). After 9.2 Gy of TBI, grafts of 4×10^8 marrow cells/kg were successful when donors were genotypically DLA-identical littermates, but usually did not succeed in DLA-nonidentical recipients (31). The genetic determinants involved in resistance appear to be separate from but linked to the recognized antigens of the DLA complex. The recipient cells mediating resistance appear to be large granular lymphocytes that do not express classic T-cell markers. They are not susceptible to treatment of recipients with antithymocyte serum or cyclosporine (CSP). Also, injections of recipients with silica particles, L-asparaginase, *Corynebacterium parvum*, or CY to overcome resistance were either unsuccessful in enhancing engraftment or gave inconsistent results (31,38). Success was achieved by treating the recipients with a monoclonal antibody directed against a leukocyte adhesion molecule, CD44 (39). The mechanism of this enhancement is currently under investigation.

Hematopoietic engraftment could be achieved by increasing the radiation dose or by adding viable peripheral blood mononuclear cells to the marrow inoculum (31). Similar success was seen when donor thoracic duct cells were added, indicating that the graft-enhancing effect is mediated by donor lymphocytes, either through immunological destruction of the host cells involved in resistance or by providing an accessory function promoting both differentiation and self-renewal of hematopoietic stem cells (31). In vitro irradiated mononuclear cells were ineffective.

Hematopoietic Precursor Cells From Sources Other Than the Marrow

Dogs, as well as mice, guinea pigs, rats, and baboons, have circulating pluripotent hematopoietic stem cells in their blood (40,41). These cells can be collected effectively with leukapheresis techniques and are capable of repopulating marrow in otherwise lethally irradiated animals. Long-term repopulation of canine marrow by cells of donor type has been shown (41,42).

The Role of Histocompatibility Matching

Histocompatibility is an important factor governing graft acceptance, development of lethal GVHD, or eventual survival of the recipient after BMT. DLA is similar to the major histocompatibility complex in other species. Two serologically determined loci, DLA-A and DLA-B, and a third locus, DLA-D, defined by mixed leukocyte culture, have been recognized (43,44). The molecular structure of the canine histocompatibility complex also resembles that of other species (45,46). There is considerable polymorphorism of antigens at each of the loci.

The dog was the first random-bred species in which the prospective value of in vitro histocompatibility typing for the outcome of marrow transplants was shown (47). Littermates genotypically identical for DLA survived significantly longer after BMT than their DLA-nonidentical counterparts. Despite DLA genotypic identity, GVHD was severe in some animals, indicating the need for immunosuppression after grafting (48). Presumably, GVHD in this setting is directed at "minor" transplantation antigens other than DLA. These studies emphasized the need for immunosuppression after transplantation, even in histocompatible situations. Encouraged by findings in dogs, human BMT began in the late 1960s to use siblings who were genotypically identical with their recipients for HLA. Subsequent studies in unrelated dogs of different breeds suggested that long-term survival can be achieved in some recipients of phenotypically DLA-identical unrelated marrow, although with a higher incidence of GVHD (49).

The Influence of Transfusions on Subsequent Marrow Grafts

Transfusions given before a marrow graft can influence the outcome (reviewed in 31). Marrow rejection was seen in all dogs given three preceding whole blood transfusions from their littermate marrow donors before TBI. Even with only one preceding transfusion from the DLA-identical marrow donor, 75% of dogs rejected a subsequent marrow graft. These results can be explained by sensitization of recipients to polymorphic minor histocompatibility antigens outside of DLA, which are undetected by the usual in vitro histocompatibility typing techniques. Sensitizing cells seem to be dendritic cells contained in the transfused blood. The 100% incidence of rejection after three transfusions of whole blood from the marrow donor is consistent with at least two polymorphic histocompatibility systems outside of DLA being involved in sensitization. The notion that several minor polymorphic loci have a role in sensitization made it likely that graft rejection would be a problem after blood transfusions from unrelated donors. Under those circumstances, graft rejection would be seen if one or more of the blood transfusion donors had minor antigens in common with the marrow donor and if these antigens were not present on the cells of the recipient. Indeed, our studies showed that 9 preceding blood transfusions from randomly selected, unrelated donors resulted in rejection of marrow from DLA-identical littermates in 40% of cases.

Subsequent studies in dogs pointed the way to avoiding or overcoming transfusion-induced sensitization. The use of buffy coat–poor blood products reduced the incidence of rejection, presumably because of the removal of antigen-presenting mononuclear cells from the transfusion. The combination of an alkylating agent and antithymocyte serum successfully overcame transfusion-induced sensitization. Most recent studies have shown that the sensitizing ability of blood transfusions can be abrogated by treatment of blood products with either ultraviolet light irradiation (50) or gamma irradiation (51). In the future, therefore, problems resulting from transfusion-induced sensitization should be significantly diminished in magnitude.

Graft-versus-host Disease

Theoretically, GVHD can be expected in all allogeneic marrow graft recipients because of the multiple differences of polymorphic histocompatibility antigens. T cells in the marrow inoculum recognize host histocompatibility antigens as foreign, become sensitized, proliferate, and attack the tissue cells of the recipient, thereby producing the clinical picture of GVHD in skin, gut, and liver.

Studies in dogs showed that GVHD can occur even among DLA-identical littermates (reviewed in 52). When transplants are carried out between DLA-nonidentical recipient pairs, GVHD occurs more rapidly and is fatal in all animals when no postgrafting immunosuppression is given (Figure 1-3). The incidence of GVHD after grafts between unrelated dogs phenotypically DLA-identical was much higher than that seen among DLA-identical littermates. This finding is likely to be related to the greater degree of disparity for minor histocompatibility antigens in the unrelated pairs.

On the basis of studies in mice (14,15), MTX was used in dogs and was shown to be effective in preventing GVHD in some recipients (25). The drug was more effective when given for 3 months after grafting than when given for shorter periods (Figure 1-4). Eventually, it could be discontinued. Azathioprine and 6-mercaptopurine were somewhat effective, but were inferior to MTX. Procarbazine, CY, cytosine arabinoside, 15-deoxyspergualine, and prednisone were all ineffective in preventing GVHD. Antithymocyte serum had only a marginal effect on GVHD when given prophylactically, but was of value in treating established GVHD. On the basis of the early canine studies, MTX was administered prophylactically in most human marrow transplant recipients during the 1970s, and antithymocyte globulin was used to treat acute GVHD, once established.

In the late 1970s, the immunosuppressive drug CSP became available and was found to be as effective as MTX in preventing GVHD in dogs. The equivalency of the two drugs was subsequently confirmed in randomized prospective human studies. A very effective prophylactic regimen in the dog was a combination of a short course of MTX and long-term CSP after BMT (Figure 1-5) (53,54). This combination was then used in human patients in 1981. Randomized prospective trials showed the combination to be more effective than either drug alone. This is now a frequently used regimen for GVHD prophylaxis.

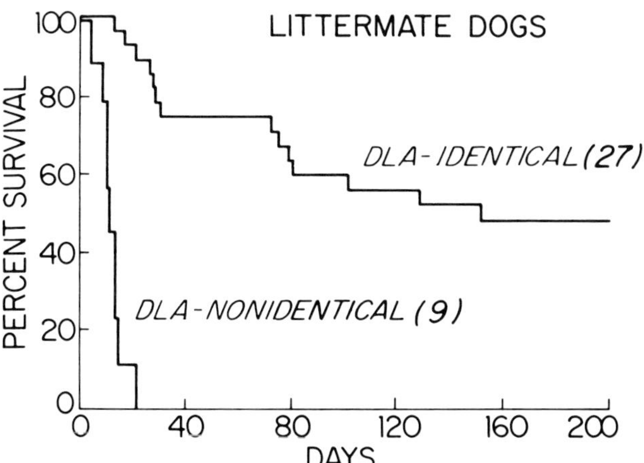

Figure 1-3. Survival of dogs given 9.2 Gy TBI and hematopoietic grafts from either DLA-identical or DLA-haploidentical littermates. No immunosuppression was given after transplant.

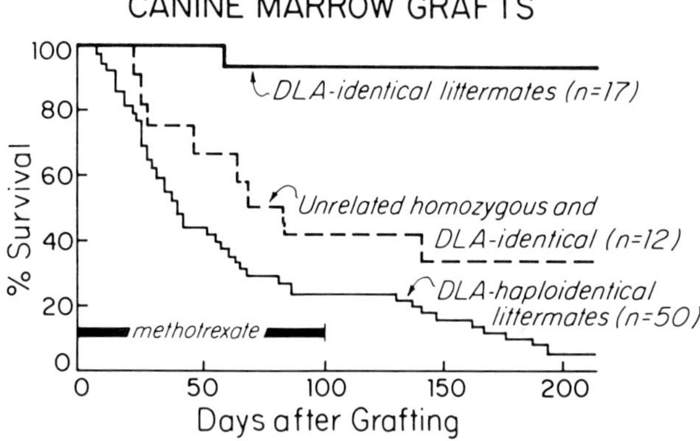

Figure 1-4. Survival of dogs given 9.2 Gy TBI and hematopoietic grafts from genotypically DLA-identical littermates, phenotypically DLA-identical unrelated donors, or DLA-haploidentical littermates. All dogs were given immunosuppression with intermittent methotrexate for 100 days after grafting.

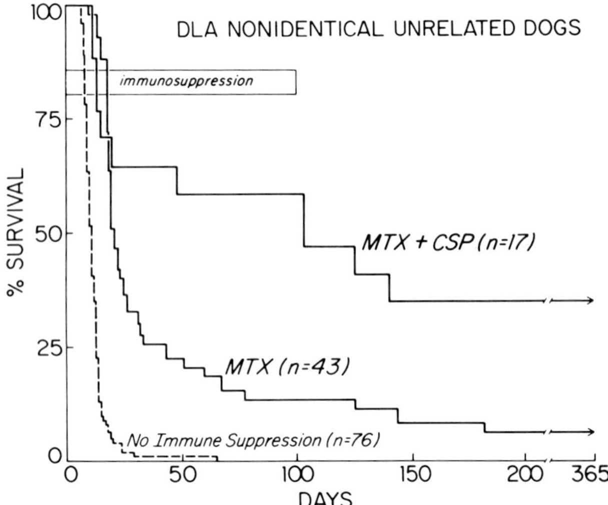

Figure 1-5. Survival of dogs given 9.2 Gy TBI and hematopoietic grafts from DLA-identical unrelated donors. Dogs were given no immunosuppression, methotrexate for 100 days after grafting, or a short course of methotrexate (0.4 mg/kg IV) on days 1, 3, 6, and 11, along with cyclosporine from day 0 to day 100.

Graft-host Tolerance

Lifelong graft-host tolerance has been documented repeatedly in canine recipients of marrow allografts, even though immunosuppressive therapy was discontinued after a few weeks or months. These dogs have served in studies on the nature of the operational tolerance involved in maintaining the stable chimeric state (55–58). In vitro tests showed that donor lymphocytes circulating in recipient dogs were specifically nonresponsive to lymphocytes of host origin while responding to those from unrelated animals. In turn, lymphocytes from dogs with GVHD showed strong reactivity to host lymphocytes in mixed leukocyte culture. Serum blocking factors were ruled out as a mechanism of maintaining unresponsiveness in stable chimeras, and results of further studies suggested that clonal abortion was operative whereby newly generated lymphocytes potentially reactive with host tissue are removed. Transplantation studies with a combination of marrow and peripheral blood cells showed that tolerance to host tissue could be transferred, a finding which is in agreement with the concept of suppressor cells. Consistent with findings in mice, grafts of solid organs from marrow donors could be transplanted into recipients without the need of immunosuppression.

Reconstitution of Immunological Function

Extensive studies were carried out on the recovery of humoral and cellular immune responses after canine BMT (59). Regardless of the type of graft, dogs were found to be profoundly immunodeficient for the first 200 to 300 days after transplantation. Thereafter, immunological reconstitution appeared to be nearly complete except for dogs with chronic GVHD. As a clinical correlate to these observations on immune function, long-term chimeras regained their health and were able to live in an unprotected environment without an increased incidence of infection.

Secondary Malignant Tumors and Other Long-range Irradiation Effects

Many canine chimeras have been observed for more than 10 years after BMT. Careful studies on gonadal function in canine chimeras have not been carried out. However, as a rule, chimeras prepared with TBI appeared to be sterile, but some dogs have become impregnated and others have sired normal litters. Chimeras prepared with CY had normal fertility. Radiation-induced cataracts developed in most dogs.

The increased risk of development of cancer after irradiation has been known since the days of the early radiologists, a knowledge that has been extended by the observations in the victims of the atomic bomb explosions in Hiroshima and Nagasaki. There has therefore been concern about the possibility of the development of malignant tumors after TBI in preparation for marrow grafting. A comparison of the cumulative cancer incidence among 153 long-term canine irradiation chimeras and 242 untreated dogs observed for 6 to 188 months (median, 81) showed a 5 times higher incidence of cancer in irradiation chimeras (60) (Figure 1-6). No tumor was seen in a smaller number of chemotherapy-conditioned animals followed for a comparable period. The canine findings suggested that TBI should be avoided whenever possible in conditioning of human marrow transplant recipients for nonmalignant disease.

Marrow Grafting for Spontaneous Canine Diseases

Diseases such as hemolytic anemia associated with hereditary pyruvate kinase deficiency; cyclic neutro-

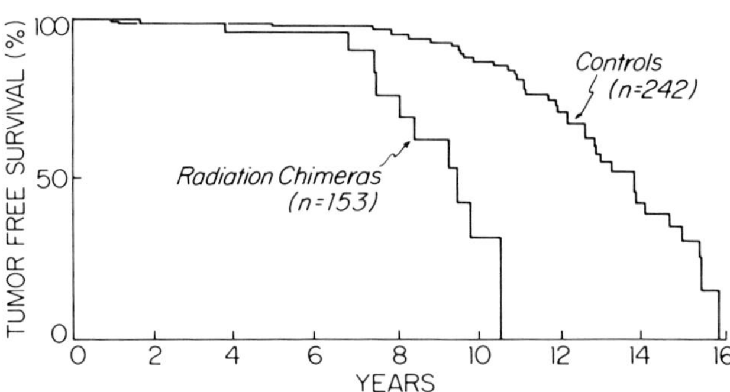

Figure 1-6. Kaplan-Meier product limit estimates of tumor-free survival of otherwise normal dogs (controls) and dogs given 9.2 Gy TBI followed by either autologous or allogeneic hematopoietic grafts (radiation chimeras).

penia; hemophilia, spontaneous malignancies, including lymphoma, leukemia, and nonhematopoietic solid tumors; as well as inborn errors of metabolism are valuable models for studying the use of therapeutic marrow transplantation.

It was possible to show that cyclic neutropenia is not the result of a defect of marrow regulation, but rather of a stem-cell defect that is correctable by BMT (61,62). Orthotopic transplantation of a normal liver into a hemophilic dog completely corrected the factor VIII deficiency (63). Marrow grafting studies ruled out the hematopoietic and lymphoid systems as sources of factor VIII production (64). Severe life-threatening hemolytic anemia due to pyruvate kinase deficiency has been corrected by marrow grafting (65,66); increased iron stores in the liver associated with the hemolytic process decreased with time after transplantation. Studies in canine lymphosarcomas have shown that one fourth of dogs at an otherwise incurable stage of disease could be cured by autologous marrow grafts following TBI (67). BMTs in dogs with ceroid lipofuscinosis and GM_1 gangliosidosis, although technically successful, showed that these genetic defects are not reversible using this approach (reviewed in 68). Fucosidosis and mucopolysaccharidosis have been shown to be correctable.

Gene Transfer

The ability of pluripotent stem cells not only to self-renew but also to differentiate into the various committed hematopoietic precursors has made them potential targets for attempts at somatic gene therapy. It is now reasonable to contemplate the replacement of missing or defective genes in hematopoietic tissues to cure potentially lethal hereditary or acquired disorders. Currently, retroviral vectors represent the preferred method for gene transduction because they provide high efficiency of transduction and stable integration of the provirus into the host genome. Gene transduction into long-term repopulating marrow cells has been shown in the mouse. In 1991, Schuening and colleagues (69) reported successful long-term gene transfer into canine hematopoietic cells. Amphotropic helper-free retrovirus vectors containing the bacterial neomycin phosphotransferase gene (neo) and the human adenosine deaminase (ADA) gene were used to transduce canine marrow cells, which were kept in a long-term culture system. The marrow was then transplanted into the dog of origin after an otherwise lethal dose of TBI consisting of 9.2 Gy. The longest surviving dogs are now approaching 3 years after BMT. Their marrows show intermittently between 1 to 11% neomycin-resistant CFU-GM colonies. Concurrent polymerase chain reaction analysis demonstrates the presence of both the neo and human ADA genes in marrow cells, granulocytes, and blood and lymph node lymphocytes. These findings provide evidence for gene transduction into pluripotent hematopoietic stem cells. Peripheral blood samples of all dogs were free of helper virus, and no long-term side effects of the gene transduction were observed. Similar findings have now been reported by Carter and associates (70).

Radiolabeled Monoclonal Antibodies

Monoclonal antibodies directed against antigens on tumor cells offer an opportunity for directed anticancer therapy. Monoclonal antibodies injected in vivo can concentrate on tumor cells, but they generate only a limited antitumor effect because some tumor cells lack target antigens, whereas others, although coated by antibody, are not killed. Studies are ongoing with antibodies linked to toxins, such as the ricin-A chain, for more effective cancer cell kill. Another possible way to use monoclonal antibodies is to attach them to short-lived radioactive isotopes. Not only cells expressing the target antigens, but also neighboring cells, which may be antigen-negative, would be killed.

Studies in dogs have shown appropriate antibody isotope conjugates to localize preferentially in marrow and spleen, and to some extent also in lymph nodes; the amount of isotope in the marrow compared with other organs achieved a ratio of 28:1 or more (71,72). Such radiolabeled antibodies can produce fatal marrow aplasia, which can then be reversed by infusion of cryopreserved autologous marrow several days later when very little radioactivity is left. These studies are continuing, and various combinations of chemotherapy, TBI, and radiolabeled antibody are being explored for their efficacy in preparing dogs for grafts of T-cell–depleted marrow. It is hoped that refinements of this approach, particularly the use of high-energy beta-emitting isotopes with short linear energy transfer, will ultimately result in less toxic and more efficient conditioning programs, which would not only provide better eradication of malignant disease, but also lessen the problem of graft failure.

References

1. Woodruff, MFA. The transplantation of tissues and organs. Springfield, Illinois: Charles C. Thomas, 1960.
2. Jacobson LO, Marks EK, Robson MJ, Gaston EO, Zirkle RE. Effect of spleen protection on mortality following x-irradiation. J Lab Clin Med 1949;34:1538–1543.
3. Lorenz E, Uphoff D, Reid TR, Shelton E. Modification of irradiation injury in mice and guinea pigs by bone marrow injections. J Natl Cancer Inst 1951;12:197–201.
4. Main JM, Prehn RT. Successful skin homografts after the administration of high dosage X radiation and homologous bone marrow. J Natl Cancer Inst 1955;15: 1023–1029.
5. Trentin JJ. Mortality and skin transplantability in x-irradiated mice receiving isologous or heterologous bone marrow. Proc Soc Exp Biol Med 1956;92:688–693.
6. Ford CE, Hamerton JL, Barnes DWH, Loutit JF. Cytological identification of radiation-chimaeras. Nature 1956;177:452–454.
7. Nowell PC, Cole LJ, Habermeyer JG, Roan PL. Growth and continued function of rat marrow cells in x-radiated mice. Cancer Res 1956;16:258–261.

8. Schwartz R, Dameshek W. Drug-induced immunological tolerance. Nature 1959;183:1682–1683.
9. Elion GB, Callahan S, Bieber S, Hitchings GH, Rundles RW. A summary of investigations with 6-(1-methyl-4-nitro-5-imidazolyl) thiopurine (BW57-322). Cancer Chemother Rep 1961;14:93–98.
10. Murray JE. The first successful organ transplants in man. In: Frängsmyr T, Lundeberg B, eds. The Nobel Prizes. Stockholm: Norstedts Tryckeri AB, 1992: 204–214.
11. van Bekkum DW, de Vries MJ. Radiation chimaeras. Radiobiological Institute of the Organisation for Health Research TNO, Rijswijk Z.H. Netherlands. New York: Academic Press, 1967.
12. van Bekkum DW, Vos O, Weyzen WWH. Homo- et hétérogreffe tissues hématopoiétiques chez la souris. Rev d'Hémat 1956;11:477–485.
13. Uphoff DE. Genetic factors influencing irradiation protection by bone marrow. I. The F1 hybrid effect. J Natl Cancer Inst 1957;19:123–125.
14. Uphoff DE. Alteration of homograft reaction by A-methopterin in lethally irradiated mice treated with homologous marrow. Proc Soc Exp Biol Med 1958;99: 651–653.
15. Lochte HL Jr, Levy AS, Guenther DM, Thomas ED, Ferrebee JW. Prevention of delayed foreign marrow reaction in lethally irradiated mice by early administration of methotrexate. Nature 1962;196:1110–1111.
16. Santos GW, Owens AH Jr. Allogeneic marrow transplants in cyclophosphamide treated mice. Transplant Proc 1969;1:44–46.
17. Good RA, Dalmasso AP, Martinez C, Archer OK, Pierce JC, Papermaster BW. The role of thymus in development of immunologic capacity in rabbits and mice. J Exp Med 1962;116:773–796.
18. Miller JFAP. Immunological significance of the thymus of the adult mouse. Nature 1962;195:1318–1319.
19. Cooper MD, Perey DY, Peterson RDA, Gabrielsen AE, Good RA. The two component concept of the lymphoid system. In: Bergsma D, Good RA, eds. Immunologic deficiency disease in man. Philadelphia: Lea and Febiger, 1968:175–197.
20. Santos GW, Owens AH Jr. A comparison of the effects of selected cytotoxic agents on allogeneic skin graft survival in rats. Bull Johns Hopkins Hosp 1965;116:327–340.
21. Santos GW, Tutschka PJ. Marrow transplantation in the busulfan treated rat—preclinical model of aplastic anemia. J Natl Cancer Inst 1974;54:1781–1785.
22. Calne RY, Sells RA, Pena JR, et al. Induction of immunological tolerance by porcine liver grafts. Nature 1969;223:472–476.
23. Popitz-Bergez FA, Sakamoto K, Pennington LR, et al. Bone marrow transplantation in miniature swine. II. Effect of selective genetic differences on marrow engraftment and recipient survival. Transplantation 1988;45:27–31.
24. Crouch BG, van Putten LM, van Bekkum DW, de Vries MJ. Treatment of total-body x-irradiated monkeys with autologous and homologous bone marrow. J Natl Cancer Inst 1961;27:53–65.
25. Thomas ED, Collins JA, Herman EC Jr, Ferrebee JW. Marrow transplants in lethally irradiated dogs given methotrexate. Blood 1962;19:217–228.
26. Epstein RB, Bryant J, Thomas ED. Cytogenetic demonstration of permanent tolerance in adult outbred dogs. Transplantation 1967;5:267–272.
27. Thomas ED, LeBlond R, Graham T, Storb R. Marrow infusions in dogs given midlethal or lethal irradiation. Radiat Res 1970;41:113–124.
28. Mannick JA, Lochte HL Jr, Ashley CA, Thomas ED, Ferrebee JW. Autografts of bone marrow in dogs after lethal total-body radiation. Blood 1960;15:255–266.
29. Cavins JA, Kasakura S, Thomas ED, Ferrebee JW. Recovery of lethally irradiated dogs following infusion of autologous marrow stored at low temperatures in dimethyl-sulphoxide. Blood 1962;20:730–734.
30. Storb R, Raff RF, Appelbaum FR, et al. What radiation dose for DLA-identical canine marrow grafts? Blood 1988;72:1300–1304.
31. Storb R, Deeg HJ. Failure of allogeneic canine marrow grafts after total body irradiation: allogeneic "resistance" vs transfusion induced sensitization. Transplantation 1986;42:571–580.
32. Bodenberger U, Kolb HJ, Reider I, et al. Fractionated total body irradiation and autologous bone marrow transplantation in dogs: hemopoietic recovery after various marrow cell doses. Exp Hematol 1980;8:384–394.
33. Deeg HJ, Storb R, Longton G, et al. Single dose or fractionated total body irradiation and autologous marrow transplantation in dogs: effects of exposure rate, fraction size and fractionation interval on acute and delayed toxicity. Int J Radiat Oncol Biol Phys 1988;15:647–653.
34. Storb R, Raff RF, Appelbaum FR, et al. Comparison of fractionated to single-dose total body irradiation in conditioning canine littermates for DLA-identical marrow grafts. Blood 1989;74:1139–1143.
35. Storb R, Epstein RB, Rudolph RH, Thomas ED. Allogeneic canine bone marrow transplantation following cyclophosphamide. Transplantation 1969;7:378–386.
36. Kolb HJ, Storb R, Weiden PL, et al. Immunologic, toxicologic and marrow transplantation studies in dogs given dimethyl myleran. Biomedicine 1974;20:341–351.
37. Storb R, Weiden PL, Graham TC, Lerner KG, Nelson N, Thomas ED. Hemopoietic grafts between DLA-identical canine littermates following dimethyl myleran. Evidence for resistance to grafts not associated with DLA and abrogated by antithymocyte serum. Transplantation 1977;24:349–357.
38. Schuening F, Storb R, Goehle S, et al. Facilitation of engraftment of DLA-nonidentical marrow by treatment of recipients with monoclonal antibody directed against marrow cells surviving radiation. Transplantation 1987; 44:607–613.
39. Sandmaier BM, Storb R, Appelbaum FR, Gallatin WM. An antibody that facilitates hematopoietic engraftment recognizes CD44. Blood 1990;76:630–635.
40. Cavins JA, Scheer SC, Thomas ED, Ferrebee JW. The recovery of legally irradiated dogs given infusions of autologous leukocytes preserved at −80°C. Blood 1964; 23:38.
41. Storb R, Epstein RB, Ragde H, Thomas ED. Marrow engraftment by allogeneic leukocytes in lethally irradiated dogs. Blood 1967;30:805–811.
42. Gerhartz HH, Nothdurft W, Carbonell F, Fliedner TM. Allogeneic transplantation of blood stem cells concentrated by density gradients. Exp Hematol 1985;13: 136–142.
43. Bull RW, Vriesendorp HM, Cech R, et al. Joint Report of the Third International Workshop on Canine Immunogenetics. II. Analysis of the serological typing of cells. Transplantation 1987;43:154–161.

44. Deeg HJ, Raff RF, Grosse-Wilde H, et al. Joint Report of the Third International Workshop on Canine Immunogenetics: I. Analysis of homozygous typing cells (HTCs). Transplantation 1986;41:111–117.
45. Sarmiento UM, Storb RF. Restriction fragment length polymorphism of the major histocompatibility complex of the dog. Immunogenetics 1988;28:117–124.
46. Sarmiento UM, Sarmiento JI, Storb R. Allelic variation in the DR subregion of the canine major histocompatibility complex. Immunogenetics 1990;32:13–19.
47. Epstein RB, Storb R, Ragde H, Thomas ED. Cytotoxic typing antisera for marrow grafting in littermate dogs. Transplantation 1968;6:45–58.
48. Storb R, Rudolph RH, Thomas ED. Marrow grafts between canine siblings matched by serotyping and mixed leukocyte culture. J Clin Invest 1971;50:1272–1275.
49. Storb R, Weiden PL, Graham TC, Lerner KG, Thomas ED. Marrow grafts between DLA-identical and homozygous unrelated dogs. Evidence for an additional locus involved in graft-versus-host disease. Transplantation 1977;24:165–174.
50. Deeg HJ, Aprile J, Graham TC, Appelbaum FR, Storb R. Ultraviolet irradiation of blood prevents transfusion-induced sensitization and marrow graft rejection in dogs. Concise report. Blood 1986;67:537–539.
51. Bean MA, Storb R, Graham T, et al. Prevention of transfusion-induced sensitization to minor histocompatibility antigens on DLA-identical canine marrow grafts by gamma irradiation of marrow donor blood. Transplantation 1991;52:956–960.
52. Storb R, Thomas ED. Graft-versus-host disease in dog and man: the Seattle experience. In: Möller G, ed. Immunological reviews, no. 88. Copenhagen: Munksgaard, 1985:215–238.
53. Deeg HJ, Storb R, Weiden PL, et al. Cyclosporin A and methotrexate in canine marrow transplantation: engraftment, graft-versus-host disease, and induction of tolerance. Transplantation 1982;34:30–35.
54. Deeg HJ, Storb R, Appelbaum FR, Kennedy MS, Graham TC, Thomas ED. Combined immunosuppression with cyclosporine and methotrexate in dogs given bone marrow grafts from DLA-haploidentical littermates. Transplantation 1984;37:62–65.
55. Tsoi M-S, Storb R, Weiden PL, Graham TC, Schroeder M-L, Thomas ED. Canine marrow transplantation: are serum blocking factors necessary to maintain the stable chimeric state? J Immunol 1975;114:531–539.
56. Atkinson K, Storb R, Weiden PL, Deeg HJ, Gerhard-Miller L, Thomas ED. In vitro tests correlating with presence or absence of graft-vs-host disease in DLA nonidentical canine radiation chimeras: evidence that clonal abortion maintains stable graft-host tolerance. J Immunol 1980;124:1808–1814.
57. Deeg HJ, Atkinson K, Weiden PL, Storb R. Mechanisms of tolerance in canine radiation chimeras. Transplant Proc 1987;19(suppl 7):75–81.
58. Weiden PL, Storb R, Tsoi M-S, Graham TC, Lerner KG, Thomas ED. Infusion of donor lymphocytes into stable canine radiation chimeras: implications for mechanism of transplantation tolerance. J Immunol 1976;116:1212–1219.
59. Ochs HD, Storb R, Thomas ED, et al. Immunologic reactivity in canine marrow graft recipients. J Immunol 1974;113:1039–1057.
60. Deeg HJ, Prentice R, Fritz TE, et al. Increased incidence of malignant tumors in dogs after total body irradiation and marrow transplantation. Int J Radiat Oncol Biol Phys 1983;9:1505–1511.
61. Weiden P, Robinett B, Graham TC, Adamson JW, Storb R. Canine cyclic neutropenia. A stem cell defect. J Clin Invest 1974;53:950–953.
62. Dale DC, Graw RG Jr. Transplantation of allogeneic bone marrow in canine cyclic neutropenia. Science 1974;183:83–84.
63. Marchioro TL, Hougie C, Ragde H, Epstein RB, Thomas ED. Hemophilia: role of organ homografts. Science 1969;163:188–190.
64. Storb R, Marchioro TL, Graham TC, Willemin M, Hougie C, Thomas ED. Canine hemophilia and hemopoietic grafting. Blood 1972;40:234–238.
65. Weiden PL, Storb R, Graham TC, Schroeder ML. Severe hereditary haemolytic anaemia in dogs treated by marrow transplantation. Br J Haematol 1976;33:357–362.
66. Weiden PL, Hackman RC, Deeg HJ, Graham TC, Thomas ED, Storb R. Long-term survival and reversal of iron overload after marrow transplantation in dogs with congenital hemolytic anemia. Blood 1981;57:66–70.
67. Weiden PL, Storb R, Deeg HJ, Graham TC, Thomas ED. Prolonged disease-free survival in dogs with lymphoma after total-body irradiation and autologous marrow transplantation consolidation of combination-chemotherapy-induced remissions. Blood 1979;54:1039–1049.
68. Deeg HJ, Storb R. Bone marrow transplantation in dogs. In: Makowka L, Cramer DV, Podesta LG, eds. Handbook of animal models in transplantation research. Boca Raton, Florida: CRC Press, 1993 (in press).
69. Schuening FG, Kawahara K, Miller DA, et al. Retrovirus-mediated gene transduction into long-term repopulating marrow cells of dogs. Blood 1991;78:2568–2576.
70. Carter RF, Abrams-Ogg ACG, Dick JE, et al. Autologous transplantation of canine long-term marrow culture cells genetically marked by retroviral vectors. Blood 1992;79:356–364.
71. Appelbaum FR, Brown P, Sandmaier B, et al. Antibody-radionuclide conjugates as part of a myeloblative preparative regimen for marrow transplantation. Blood 1989;73:2202–2208.
72. Bianco JA, Sandmaier B, Brown P, et al. Specific marrow localization of an ^{131}I-labeled anti-myeloid antibody in normal dogs: effects of a "cold" antibody pretreatment dose on marrow localization. Exp Hematol 1989;17:929–934.

Chapter 2

The Evolution of the Scientific Foundation of Marrow Transplantation Based on Human Studies

E. Donnall Thomas

Science does not stop at the laboratory door. In fact, the body of knowledge that constitutes science is increased by insights and information gathered at all stages of development and application of technology. The scientific foundation of marrow transplantation biology was established in pioneering studies conducted with rodents, was enlarged by developmental studies in dogs, and has been enormously expanded by experience derived from the treatment of sick people. This chapter describes some of the discoveries that came about as a result of marrow transplantation in human patients. These insights provided feedback to investigators working with mice and dogs. Chapter 1 describes the evolution of knowledge based on animal studies, but it should be kept in mind that the developments in human and nonhuman animals parallel each other, and that experiments in one species often dictated the next studies in others.

Following the demonstration in mice that marrow grafting could be accomplished after lethal irradiation, it seemed logical to apply this technique to the treatment of human hematological malignancy using intensive chemotherapy or irradiation followed by marrow infusion to protect the recipient from otherwise lethal marrow aplasia. The first attempts, reported in 1957, were largely unsuccessful; only one transient graft was successful (1). Nevertheless, those studies contributed one important discovery—that relatively large amounts of marrow could be infused intravenously into human patients without ill effect provided that the marrow was properly anticoagulated and screened to break up particles.

The next important observation was made in 1959. Two patients with advanced acute lymphoblastic leukemia were given supralethal total-body irradiation (TBI) and a marrow infusion from an identical twin (syngeneic graft) (2). Hematological recovery occurred in two weeks, showing clearly that a compatible marrow graft could protect against the lethal marrow aplasia produced by irradiation. In those first two patients, leukemia recurred in a few months, indicating that irradiation alone might not be sufficient to eradicate leukemia and that additional chemotherapy might be necessary. The authors also discussed the potential role of an immunological reaction of the graft against the leukemia if allogeneic rather than syngeneic marrow was used. Barnes and colleagues (3), in the initial effort to treat leukemia in mice by irradiation and a syngeneic marrow graft, had encountered the same problem and had postulated that to cure leukemia, a reaction of the graft against the leukemia might be necessary.

Important early observations were made by Mathe and by Thomas and their colleagues (reviewed in 4,5). Their initial attempts to achieve marrow grafts in leukemic patients after presumably lethal TBI of 400 to 600 cGy failed to result in engraftment. Their studies demonstrated that more irradiation would be necessary to achieve engraftment in human patients and that successful engraftment depends on destroying not only the marrow to make "room" for the graft, but also on the immune system of the recipient. These observations were confirmed and expanded in the canine model. Using a highcr irradiation exposure, Mathe and associates (4) achieved the first enduring human marrow graft, only to have the patient die of multiple complications and infections that we now know as chronic graft-versus-host disease (GVHD). The human histocompatibility system had not been characterized at that time. Such early attempts to perform marrow grafting in patients made it clear that some form of matching of donor and recipient would be necessary.

Early marrow grafting studies in animals involved sacrifice of the donor. In early human studies there was concern about whether effective quantities of marrow could be obtained from living donors. As it turned out, procurement of marrow for grafting from human donors is relativly simple and much easier than procurement of solid organs. Quantities of marrow sufficient for engraftment can be obtained by needle aspiration from the iliac crests (6). With anticoagulation, screening to break up particles, and proper attention to volume, marrow can be administered intravenously to the recipient without consequence. Anesthesia for the donor is of concern. Donors have given marrow on more than one occasion. Marrow can be cryopreserved for long periods (7). More recently, cells for engraftment can be obtained from the white cell fraction of peripheral blood, especially after administration of growth factors, such as granulocyte or granulocyte macrophage colony stimulating factors, which increase the number of circulating progenitor cells (8,9) (see Chapter 21).

Total body irradiation was used in the first human marrow graft recipients because studies in mice had shown it to be effective in destroying normal marrow and permitting engraftment. It is easy to achieve homogenous TBI with 250-kv x-ray machines in mice because of their small size. It quickly became apparent that the achievement of reasonably uniform TBI in animals the size of humans would be difficult because of the absorption of radiation energy by tissue. Initially this problem was solved by the use of cobalt-60 irradiators, especially dual-opposing sources (10). Later, as linear accelerators became available, TBI could be performed satisfactorily with high-energy irradiators. Because of the necessity for large fields for TBI, dose rates were usually low (i.e., 5–25 cGy min).

Santos and Owens (11) carried out studies in the mouse showing that cyclophosphamide (CY) alone was an effective immunosuppressant capable of allowing allogeneic engraftment. CY was effective in permitting engraftment and long-term survival in patients with severe aplastic anemia (12,13). CY alone was also effective in securing engraftment in human patients with acute leukemia, but the antileukemic effect was inadequate and the disease recurred (14,15). To achieve the greatest immunosuppression and the greatest antileukemic effect, investigators decided to combine CY with TBI (16).

Three other critical developments contributed to the success of human marrow transplantation. One was the development of the knowledge and technology needed to provide supportive care to patients without marrow function. A major obstacle in the development of organ transplantation had always been the demands of supporting patients through the early post-transplant period. For patients receiving kidney transplants, this problem was resolved by dialysis; however, such organ substitution was difficult to achieve for marrow recipients. Marrow transplantation is usually employed in clinical settings in which the patient's marrow has failed or is so diseased that its function is severely compromised. In addition, the cytotoxic and immunosuppressive regimens used in preparation for marrow grafting effectively destroy any remaining marrow function. Transplanted marrow requires 2 to 4 weeks to become functionally useful; during this time, the patient has a dwindling supply of cellular elements necessary for hemostasis and infection prevention and control. The necessary support came about through the development of new antibiotics to treat infections, particularly those caused by gram-negative organisms; the development of platelet collection and transfusion technology to prevent bleeding; and more effective isolation techniques to prevent infections (reviewed in 5).

The second critical development was elucidation of the human histocompatibility system. Dausset (17) was the first to recognize human leukocyte antigens (HLA) and their importance in histocompatibility. In the 1960s, several brilliant investigators made great progress in the definition and recognition of the antigens controlled by loci of chromosome 6, the complex "super gene" that represents the major histocompatibility system in humans. The rapid development of human kidney transplantation stimulated interest in tissue typing; however, we now know that tissue typing is only of moderate importance for the success of kidney transplants, but is absolutely critical to the success of human marrow grafts.

The third critical development was the demonstration in an outbred species that matching at the major histocompatibility complex would predict a successful outcome of a marrow graft. In the late 1950s and early 1960s, we found that marrow grafts between littermate dogs occasionally resulted in long-term engraftment, but that most such transplants resulted in graft failure or GVHD. By 1968, we had developed canine antisera for tissue typing (18). These antisera permitted identification of canine littermates whose cells reacted in the same pattern with the battery of antisera. Littermates matched by these sera made successful donor-recipient pairs, whereas recipients of marrow from mismatched donors never became long-term survivors (19). These studies indicated the feasibility of marrow grafting between compatible human sibling pairs, a diseased recipient, and a normal donor.

Thus, at the end of the 1960s, the stage was set for the beginning of the "modern" era of marrow transplantation. In November 1968, the Minneapolis team carried out a marrow graft based on knowledge of human histocompatibility typing in an infant with severe immunological deficiency who, because of the nature of this disease, did not require intensive treatment before transplantation to prevent graft rejection (20). The Seattle team carried out a sibling transplant for a leukemic patient given lethal TBI in March 1969 (5). Within a few years, many similar transplants were carried out. These and other early transplants demonstrated that patients with severe aplastic anemia could be successfully engrafted and cured after preparation with CY alone and that patients with advanced acute leukemia could be transplanted and cured after preparation with CY and TBI.

Many problems remained, however. Transplantation studies in animals had predicted many of these problems, but their specific characteristics and solutions had to be worked out in human patients. One theoretically simple problem was of great practical importance. Patients receiving a marrow graft require frequent blood sampling and transfusions of blood products, intravenous antibiotics, nutrition support by hyperalimentation, and fluid and electrolyte administration. Long-term vascular access was difficult if not impossible in animals; human patients, however, have cleaner skin and access to good nursing care. Quinton and colleagues (21) devised the arteriovenous silastic shunt for repeated vascular access for dialysis. Hickman and associates (22) then developed a Teflon shunt with a Dacron cuff, which made long-term venous access possible. This rather simple technical development not only made intravenous support of these patients possible, but also enhanced patient comfort because it made repeated venipunctures unnecessary.

Animal studies did not fully predict the extreme sensitivity of transplanted human marrow to the influence of histocompatibility differences. The engrafted marrow is an immunologically competent organ and can mount an attack against the "foreign" host, resulting in the clinical manifestations that we recognize as GVHD. Studies in inbred mice showed that GVHD could range in severity from very mild to lethal depending on the strains chosen as donor and recipient. In the dog, acute GVHD occurred, but with matching for the major histocompatibility system and with postgrafting immunosuppression with methotrexate (MTX) to suppress the graft-versus-host reaction, most animals survived with permanent engraftment. In humans, GVHD proved to be severe even when donor and recipient were genotypically matched for HLA, the major histocompatibility system comparable to H-2 in the mouse and DLA in the dog. With human matched-sibling grafts, there is a high probability of severe acute GVHD unless some form of immunosuppression is given after the graft (5). Because animal studies indicated that MTX given immediately after the graft was useful in attenuating GVHD, this was the first agent used for this purpose in human patients. Even with postgrafting MTX, severe acute GVHD developed in one third to one half of graft recipients. Other agents used include corticosteroids, CY, and, more recently, cyclosporine. The most effective regimen currently is the combination of a short course of MTX combined with 6 months of cyclosporine, which has reduced the incidence of severe GVHD to 15 to 20% of patients (23). After human solid organ grafts it is necessary to continue immunosuppression indefinitely, but after a marrow graft, it is usually possible to discontinue immunosuppression after a few months, except for those patients in whom chronic GVHD develops.

Chronic GVHD is a problem in human marrow graft recipients that was not anticipated fully from animal studies, in part because of the difficulty in maintaining sick animals for adequate periods of time. Clinically it may involve the skin, the gut, and the liver and is associated with a sicca syndrome and impairment of immunological capability. Fortunately, many cases are mild and respond to continued corticosteroid therapy, but others are progressive and are associated with opportunistic infections (24). Lack of a comparable animal model has hampered the development of new methods of treating severe chronic GVHD.

Opportunistic infections are another problem of great clinical significance to human marrow graft recipients. Animal marrow graft recipients demonstrated susceptibility to infections, but the severity and extent of immunoincompetence and infections in human marrow graft recipients proved to be greater than anticipated. Human marrow graft recipients, even those receiving a syngeneic or an autologous graft, are severely immunoincompetent for days or weeks, and the duration is extended for allogeneic recipients. Immunosuppressive regimens after grafting, especially those used for the treatment of GVHD, compound the problem. Human marrow graft recipients are plagued by a long list of infections that are rare in healthy individuals. Responsible organisms include bacteria such as coagulase-negative staphylococcus; a variety of viral agents, especially cytomegalovirus; fungi such as *Candida* and *Aspergillus;* and protozoa such as *Pneumocystis carinii* (25).

These infections, which are common in marrow graft recipients, became of greater general importance when the acquired immune deficiency syndrome (AIDS), which is also characterized by immunoincompetence, became epidemic. There has been significant progress in control of these infections, as demonstrated by the use of acyclovir for Herpes simplex (26), ganciclovir for cytomegalovirus (27,28), and trimethoprim-sulfamethoxazole for *Pneumocystis carinii* (29). Nevertheless, all marrow graft recipients are at risk of infection for a period of weeks to months until immune competence returns.

One interesting consequence of the severe, prolonged immunoincompetence that sometimes occurs in marrow transplant recipients is the occasional development of B-cell malignancies associated with Epstein-Barr virus. Several such cases have occurred, usually in patients who received intensive immunosuppressive therapy in an attempt to control severe GVHD (30). The disease is rapidly progressive and almost always fatal. This problem was not observed in animal models.

Finally, the diseases treated by human marrow transplantation are unique to humans. An exact laboratory model of the human therapeutic situation would require the existence of animal populations analogous to human families, with frequently occurring spontaneous tumors similar to those encountered in humans. Clearly, such a model cannot be achieved. For example, the life span of most laboratory animals would not permit tumor models with evolutionary development as is seen in chronic myeloid leukemia. There is no good animal model comparable to severe idiopathic aplastic anemia, and the discovery that this disease can be cured by a compatible marrow graft after immunosuppression with CY alone could only be made in human patients. Models of genetic diseases of the marrow are available in animal species and have been informative, but human patients with a disease such as Thalassemia major, who have been treated with long-term transfusion therapy and who may have hepatitis, present unique problems (31). Canine lymphosarcomas and viral leukemias in mice are useful models, but there is no good animal model for human acute lymphoblastic leukemia, acute myeloid leukemia, or chronic myeloid leukemia. Most studies of marrow transplantation in animal models are carried out in young, healthy subjects. Human patients tend to be heavily treated before being referred for marrow transplantation. Older human patients present unique problems, especially in terms of treatment-related toxicity and in the severity of GVHD. The long life span of human patients after marrow grafting allows observation of growth, development, and physiological changes not possible in animal models (32). Although most long-term human graft recipients are healthy, a few complications, including liver or lung disease and secondary malignancies, have been observed after long periods (33).

This chapter summarizes some of the experiences that have been more or less unique to marrow grafting in human subjects. Other chapters will provide much greater details about all aspects of human marrow transplantation.

References

1. Thomas ED, Lochte HL Jr, Lu WC, Ferrebee JW. Intravenous infusion of bone marrow in patients receiving radiation and chemotherapy. N Engl J Med 1957;257:491–496.
2. Thomas ED, Lochte HL Jr, Cannon JH, Sahler OD, Ferrebee JW. Supralethal whole body irradiation and isologous marrow transplantation in man. J Clin Invest 1959;38:1709–1716.
3. Barnes DWH, Corp MJ, Loutit JF, Neal FE. Treatment of murine leukaemia with x-rays and homologous bone marrow. Preliminary communication. Br Med J 1956; 2:626–627.
4. Mathe G, Amiel JL, Schwarzenberg L, Catton A, Schneider M. Adoptive immunotherapy of acute leukemia: experimental and clinical results. Cancer Res 1965;25:1525–1531.
5. Thomas ED, Storb R, Clift RA, et al. Bone-marrow transplantation. N Engl J Med 1975;292:832–843; 895–902.
6. Thomas ED, Storb R. Technique for human marrow grafting. Blood 1970;36:507–515.
7. Buckner CD, Appelbaum FR, Thomas ED. Bone marrow and fetal liver. In: Karow AM Jr, Pegg DE, eds. Organ preservation for transplantation. New York: Marcel Dekker, 1981:355–375.
8. Kessinger A, Armitage JO, Landmark JD, Smith DM, Weisenburger DD. Autologous peripheral hematopoietic stem cell transplantation restores hematopoietic function following marrow ablative therapy. Blood 1988;71:723–727.
9. Juttner CA, To LB, Haylock DN, et al. Autologous blood stem cell transplantation. Transplant Proc 1989;21: 2929–2931.
10. Ferrebee JW, Thomas ED. Factors affecting the survival of transplanted tissues. Am J Med Sci 1958;235:369–386.
11. Santos GW, Owens AH Jr. Allogeneic marrow transplants in cyclophosphamide treated mice. Transplant Proc 1969;1:44–46.
12. Thomas ED, Buckner CD, Storb R, et al. Aplastic anaemia treated by marrow transplantation. Lancet 1972;1:284–289.
13. Storb R, Anasetti C, Appelbaum F, et al. Marrow transplantation for severe aplastic anemia and thalassemia major. Semin Hematol 1991;28:235–239.
14. Santos GW, Sensenbrenner LL, Burke PJ, et al. Marrow transplantation in man following cyclophosphamide. Transplant Proc 1971;3:400–404.
15. Graw RG Jr, Yankee RA, Rogentine GN, et al. Bone marrow transplantation from HL-A-matched donors to patients with acute leukemia. Toxicity and antileukemic effect. Transplantation 1972;14:79–90.
16. Buckner CD, Clift RA, Fefer A, et al. Marrow transplantation for the treatment of acute leukemia using HL-A-identical siblings. Transplant Proc 1974;6:365–366.
17. Dausset J. Iso-leuco-anticorps. Acta Haematol 1958;20: 156–166.
18. Epstein RB, Storb R, Ragde H, Thomas ED. Cytotoxic typing antisera for marrow grafting in littermate dogs. Transplantation 1968;6:45–58.
19. Storb R, Rudolph RH, Thomas ED. Marrow grafts between canine siblings matched by serotyping and mixed leukocyte culture. J Clin Invest 1971;50:1272–1275.
20. Gatti RA, Meuwissen HJ, Allen HD, Hong R, Good RA. Immunological reconstitution of sex-linked lymphopenic immunological deficiency. Lancet 1968;2:1366–1369.
21. Quinton W, Dillard D, Scribner BH. Cannulation of blood vessels for prolonged hemodialysis. Trans Am Soc Artif Intern Organs 1960;6:104–113.
22. Hickman RO, Buckner CD, Clift RA, Sanders JE, Stewart P, Thomas ED. A modified right atrial catheter for access to the venous system in marrow transplant recipients. Surg Gynecol Obstet 1979;148:871–875.
23. Storb R, Deeg HJ, Pepe M, et al. Methotrexate and cyclosporine versus cyclosporine alone for prophylaxis of graft-versus-host disease in patients given HLA-identical marrow grafts for leukemia: long-term follow-up of a controlled trial. Blood 1989;73:1729–1734.
24. Sullivan KM, Witherspoon RP, Storb R, et al. Alternating-day cyclosporine and prednisone for treatment of high-risk chronic graft-v-host disease. Blood 1988;72: 555–561.
25. Meyers JD, Thomas ED. Infection complicating bone marrow transplantation. In: Rubin RH, Young LS, eds. Clinical approach to infection in the immunocompromised host. New York: Plenum Press, 1988:525–556.
26. Meyers JD, Wade JC, Shepp DH, Newton B. Acyclovir treatment of varicella-zoster virus infection in the compromised host. Transplantation 1984;37:571–574.
27. Schmidt GM, Horak DA, Niland JC, Duncan SR, Forman SJ, Zaia JA. A randomized, controlled trial of prophylactic ganciclovir for cytomegalovirus pulmonary infection in recipients of allogeneic bone marrow transplants. N Engl J Med 1991;324:1005–1011.
28. Goodrich JM, Bowden RA, Fisher L, Keller C, Schoch G, Meyers JD. Ganciclovir prophylaxis to prevent after allogeneic marrow transplant. Ann Intern Med 1993; 118:173–178.
29. Hughes WT, Kuhn S, Chaudhary S, et al. Successful chemoprophylaxis for pneumocystis carinii pneumonitis. N Engl J Med 1977;297:1419–1426.
30. Zutter MM, Durnam DM, Hackman RC, et al. Secondary T-cell lymphoproliferation after marrow transplantation. Am J Clin Pathol 1990;94:714–721.
31. Lucarelli G, Galimberti M, Polchi P, et al. Bone marrow transplantation in patients with thalassemia. N Engl J Med 1990;322:417–421.
32. Sanders JE, the Seattle Marrow Transplant Team. The impact of marrow transplant preparative regimens on subsequent growth and development. Semin Hematol 1991;28:244–249.
33. Sullivan KM, Witherspoon RP, Storb R. Buckner CD, Sanders J, Thomas ED. Long-term results of allogeneic bone marrow transplantation. Transplant Proc 1989; 21:2926–2928.

Chapter 3
Overview of Marrow Transplantation Immunology

Paul Martin

Immunology has a central role in allogeneic bone marrow transplantation (BMT). Any appreciation of the immunological mechanisms involved in engraftment, graft-versus-host disease (GVHD), the development of tolerance, immune reconstitution, and control of malignancy requires some understanding of the immunogenetic basis for immune reactions provoked by grafting tissue from one individual to another. Insight into the cellular basis of alloreactivity requires an understanding of immune recognition, the development of the immune system, and the nature of immune responses. This chapter will introduce readers to the immunology of marrow transplantation. Citations are made to other chapters that provide detailed information, as well as references to the extensive literature on this subject.

Fundamental Differences Between Marrow Transplantation and Solid Organ Transplantation

Marrow transplantation differs fundamentally from grafting of most other organs. In solid organ transplantation, the graft generally contains only limited numbers of cells with immunological function, and the primary clinical concern rests with preventing rejection. The immune system in solid organ transplant recipients remains of host origin. Thus, lifelong administration of immunosuppressive medication is required to prevent rejection not only by cellular and humoral mechanisms in the host at the time of transplantation, but also by elements generated from immunological progenitors after transplantation. The preparative regimen administered before BMT eliminates most, although not all, progenitors and mature elements of the host immune system. The transplanted marrow contains large numbers of progenitors and mature cellular elements, which replace those of the host. Thus, the immune system in a BMT recipient is generated by the graft and originates from the donor. The primary clinical concerns rest not only with preventing rejection by host cells that survive the conditioning regimen, but also with preventing donor cells from causing immune-mediated injury in the recipient (i.e., GVHD), while allowing immunological reconstitution for recognition and control of pathogens. Immunosuppressive medications are administered after BMT primarily to prevent GVHD (see Chapter 10). Eventually it becomes possible to discontinue such treatment. Subsequent persistence of durably engrafted donor lymphoid and hematopoietic cells without GVHD while maintaining an ability to respond to other antigens indicates that a state of immunological "tolerance" has been achieved between the donor and the recipient.

Immunogenetic Basis of Alloreactivity

Immune reactions provoked by grafting tissue from one individual to another are caused by transplantation or histocompatibility antigens (see Chapter 4). Genes encoding transplantation antigens are located both within and outside the major histocompatibility complex (MHC). The human MHC is located on the short arm of chromosome 6 and contains a series of genes encoding two distinct types of highly polymorphic cell surface glycoproteins, termed *human leukocyte antigens* (HLAs). HLA class I antigens are encoded by three loci (HLA-A, HLA-B, and HLA-C) and contain a single polymorphic α-chain noncovalently associated with β2-microglobulin. More than 41 HLA-A, 61 HLA-B, and 18 HLA-C alleles have been described. HLA class II antigens are encoded by three loci (HLA-DR, HLA-DQ, and HLA-DP) and contain a single polymorphic β chain noncovalently associated with a polymorphic (DQ and DP) or a nonpolymorphic (DR) α-chain. The α-chains of HLA-DR, HLA-DQ, and HLA-DP antigens are encoded by the respective DRA, DQA, and DPA genes, whereas the β-chains are encoded by the respective DRB1, DQB, and DPB genes. More than 60 HLA-DRB1, 14 DQA, 19 DQB, 8 DPA, and 38 DPB alleles have been described.

The genes encoding HLA class I and class II antigens are tightly linked; as a result, they are inherited in families as "haplotypes" with low recombination frequencies. For a given patient, there is a 0.25 probability that any one sibling inherited the same paternal haplotype and the same maternal haplotype, thereby being "HLA-genotypically identical." Because of the highly polymorphic nature of HLA antigens, the probability that two unrelated individuals will have the same HLA-A, -B, -C, -DR, -DQ, and -DP alleles is extremely low.

MHC class I and II antigens have similar structures. The general structure consists of a floor formed by β-pleated sheets overlaid by two α-helices in parallel orientation, leaving a groove or pocket between for binding of small peptides. The polymorphic residues of these glycoproteins are located both in the floor and on the α-helices. "Minor histocompatibility antigens" or transplantation antigens encoded by genes outside the MHC represent the small, endogenous, polymorphic peptides that bind to MHC molecules. In general, the peptides that bind MHC class I antigens originate from intracellular proteins, whereas those that bind MHC class II antigens originate from extracellular sources. Unlike MHC antigens, minor histocompatibility antigens recognized by T cells cannot be detected with antibodies and have not been defined biochemically. Genetic studies in mice have identified more than 40 loci that encode minor histocompatibility antigens, most of which have only two or three known alleles. Because these loci are not genetically linked, there is a high probability of at least some disparity for minor histocompatibility antigens between siblings. Because of the greater diversity of alleles in the population than within families, the probability of disparity between two unrelated individuals is even higher.

Cellular Basis of Alloreactivity

The principal effectors of immune responses are T and B lymphocytes. In T cells, immune recognition is mediated by the T-cell receptor, whereas in B cells, immune recognition is mediated by immunoglobulin molecules. Each T cell and B cell expresses only one type of receptor for recognizing antigen. Both types of cells utilize similar mechanisms for generating an enormous diversity of clonally distributed receptors. This diversity is generated initially by somatic rearrangements that link V (variable), D (diversity), and J (joining) segments in various combinations to encode distinct receptors.

Immune progenitors destined to become T cells originate from stem cells in the marrow and migrate to the thymus. Within the thymus, developing T cells that express receptors which recognize "self" antigens are deleted by a process termed *negative selection*. Those cells that express receptors capable of recognizing foreign peptide antigens in association with self-MHC molecules are preferentially selected for export to the peripheral blood, lymph nodes, spleen, and other organs. This process of "positive selection" is mediated by thymic epithelial cells. Negative selection is mediated by marrow-derived macrophages and dendritic cells and also to some extent by thymic epithelial cells. The interaction with thymic epithelial cells causes T-cell precursors to become nonresponsive or "anergic" to self-MHC molecules. By preventing the emergence of autoimmune T cells, negative selection and induction of anergy in the thymus represent the principal mechanisms for maintaining self-tolerance.

MHC class I and II antigens are recognized by two distinct types of T cells. T cells that express CD4 recognize MHC class II molecules and minor histocompatibility antigens bound to MHC class II molecules, whereas T cells that express CD8 recognize MHC class I molecules and minor histocompatibility antigens bound to MHC class I molecules. These recognition patterns reflect the fact that CD4 molecules on T cells bind directly to MHC class II molecules on antigen-presenting cells, whereas CD8 molecules bind to MHC class I molecules. Thus, CD4 and CD8 have been described as "associative recognition structures" for T-cell activation.

Both T cells and B cells exhibit two general types of immune responses. "Primary" responses occur when the immune system first encounters a specific antigen. The immune response after an initial encounter with antigen develops during a period of several weeks and results in the expansion of specific clones with receptors capable of recognizing the antigen. These "memory" cells remain poised to respond quickly should the same antigen be encountered again. The "secondary" responses that occur after a repeated encounter with antigen develop during a period of several days and show greater intensity than the original primary response.

Donor Selection for Allogeneic Marrow Transplantation

The immunogenetic relationship between the donor and the recipient profoundly influences the outcome of BMT (see Chapter 51). With the constraints of current practice, however, these differences are most apparent when analyzing immunological outcome, such as graft rejection and the incidence and severity of GVHD, and are less apparent when analyzing disease-free survival. Best results are seen after BMT from HLA-genotypically matching sibling donors, but only 30% of patients have such a donor. Some patients without an HLA-identical sibling have an HLA-haploidentical family member with limited disparity between the nonshared haplotypes. Previous studies have shown that patients receiving HLA-haploidentical transplants incompatible for one HLA-A, HLA-B, or HLA-DR antigen have disease-free survival similar to that of patients transplanted with marrow from HLA-genotypically identical siblings. Patients receiving transplants incompatible at two or three of these loci had a significantly lower probability of survival. BMT from HLA-phenotypically identical unrelated donors is an alternative for patients who lack a donor in the family.

Unrelated BMT has been made feasible by the development of large registries of HLA-typed individuals willing to serve as marrow donors. Selection of unrelated donors has been based on matching for HLA-A, HLA-B, and HLA-DR, whereas the necessity of matching for HLA-C, HLA-DQ, and HLA-DP remains to be evaluated. With currently available registries in the United States and in other countries, it is now possible to identify an HLA-A, HLA-B, HLA-DR–phenotypically identical unrelated donor for approximately 20% of patients. If a single HLA-A, HLA-B, or HLA-DR disparity is allowed, then it might be possible to identify a donor for more than 90% of patients. Studies have suggested that disease-free survival for patients transplanted with marrow from an HLA-A, HLA-B, HLA-DR–identical unrelated donor may be comparable to that for similar patients transplanted from an HLA-genotypically identical sibling. In addition, limited data have suggested that the presence of a single HLA-A, HLA-B, or HLA-DR disparity may not adversely affect survival after unrelated BMT if the disparate HLA-A or HLA-B antigens are serologically cross-reactive or if the disparate HLA-DR antigens have the same private specificity by serological testing.

Outcomes Influenced by Genetic Disparity Between Donor and Recipient

Engraftment

Graft rejection after BMT may be manifested as either the lack of initial engraftment or the development of pancytopenia and marrow aplasia after initial engraftment. Graft rejection is usually fatal because spontaneous reconstitution with host hematopoietic cells seldom occurs, and patients generally cannot tolerate the preparative regimen for another BMT. The diagnosis of graft rejection can be difficult because lack of initial engraftment and pancytopenia can also be caused by drug toxicity and certain viral infections. Detection of host T cells in association with graft failure is usually interpreted to indicate rejection. The risk of graft failure depends on the degree of genetic disparity between the donor and the recipient. With HLA-genotypically identical BMT, the risk of graft failure is approximately 2%, and the risk of graft rejection is probably less than 1%. With HLA-haploidentical donors, the risk of graft failure is higher (3–15%) and varies according to whether the donor and recipient have equivalent or nonequivalent disparity with each other. With HLA-heterozygous donors for HLA-homozygous recipients, the disparity for rejection is greater than the disparity for GVHD, and the risk of rejection is 15%. With HLA-homozygous donors for HLA-heterozygous recipients, the disparity for rejection is less than the disparity for GVHD, and the risk of rejection is 5%.

The risk of graft rejection is greatly influenced by transfusion-induced alloimmunization of the recipient against the donor before BMT. This alloimmunization presumably occurs when transfusion donors have transplantation antigens in common with the marrow donor. Alloimmunization of the patient can be detected by the presence of cytotoxic antibodies that recognize donor T cells or B cells. In this situation, rejection may be caused either by memory T cells that survive the conditioning regimen or by antibody-mediated destruction of donor cells.

Three additional factors influence the risk of rejection: (1) the pretransplant immunosuppressive regimen, (2) the post-transplant immunosuppressive regimen, and (3) the presence of T cells in the donor marrow. Patients with aplastic anemia who are prepared for BMT with a regimen of cyclophosphamide (CY) alone have a higher risk of rejection than patients with malignancy who are prepared with multiple agents, often including total body irradiation (TBI). The increased incidence of rejection with less intensive preparative regimens results from survival of larger numbers of host T lymphocytes. Post-transplant administration of immunosuppressive agents such as methotrexate (MTX) and cyclosporine (CSP) decreases the risk of rejection by interfering with the function of host cells that survive the conditioning regimen. The presence of T cells in the donor marrow also helps eliminate or inactivate these residual host cells, which would otherwise remain capable of causing rejection. Graft failure occurs in approximately 10% of patients when T cells are removed from the donor marrow to prevent GVHD in HLA-identical recipients, although marked variation has been seen among different studies.

Graft-versus-Host Disease

The development of acute GVHD represents a major determinant of outcome after allogeneic BMT (see Chapter 26). Patients with GVHD limited to grade I or II severity have a 20% 6-month risk of transplant-related mortality, which is comparable to the risk of transplant-related mortality in patients with no GVHD. Patients with grade III GVHD, however, have a 60% risk of transplant-related mortality at 6 months, whereas grade IV GVHD is almost uniformly fatal. The risk of grades III to IV GVHD depends primarily on the degree of genetic disparity between the recipient and the donor. The type of post-transplant immunosuppression and compliance with the prophylactic regimen represent additional important determinants of risk. Alloimmunization of the donor by prior pregnancy or possibly by transfusion has also been associated with an increased risk of GVHD, probably caused by "memory" T cells with specificity for antigens shared by the fetus or the transfusion donor and the BMT recipient.

With a regimen of MTX and CSP, patients transplanted from an HLA-genotypically identical sibling have an approximately 15% risk for development of grades III to IV acute GVHD. Patients transplanted from an HLA-haploidentical family member with no detectable HLA-A, HLA-B, or HLA-DR disparity have an approximately 25% risk for development of grades III to IV GVHD, whereas those with disparity at one or two of these loci have estimated risks of 35 and 50%, respectively. Patients transplanted from an HLA-phenotypically identical unrelated donor have an estimated 35% risk for development of grades III to IV acute GVHD, whereas those with disparity at a single HLA-A, HLA-B, or HLA-DR locus have an approximately 50% risk.

During the afferent phase of GVHD, donor CD8 cells are activated when there is recipient disparity for MHC class I antigens or for minor antigens presented by MHC class I molecules in the host. Donor CD4 cells are activated when there is recipient disparity for MHC class II antigens or for minor antigens presented by MHC class II molecules in the host. The initial alloactivation of donor cells induced by MHC disparity can occur as early as 24 to 48 hours after BMT and is followed by rapid, interleukin-2 (IL2)–dependent clonal proliferation. Cells from both the CD4 and the CD8 subsets are able to produce lymphokines and to generate cytolytic activity. The respective contributions of cytolytic T cells, natural killer (NK) cells, macrophages, and cytokines in mediating tissue damage during the efferent phase of GVHD remain controversial.

Acute GVHD can be prevented by removing mature T cells from the donor marrow (see Chapter 11). In HLA-identical recipients given no post-transplant immunosuppression, the incidence of grades II to IV acute GVHD decreases from approximately 80% with unmodified marrow to 20% or less when 95 to 99% of T cells are removed. In HLA-mismatched recipients, the incidence of grades II to IV GVHD can be reduced to 20% or less if at least 99.9% of T cells are removed. There is relatively little published information concerning the effects of T-cell depletion on chronic GVHD, although the incidence in some studies appears to be much lower than usually seen in patients transplanted with unmodified marrow. Because of the increased risk of graft failure and other complications, removal of T cells from the donor marrow to prevent GVHD has not been shown to improve disease-free survival after BMT. Research studies are attempting to determine whether the donor cells that cause GVHD can be distinguished from those needed to facilitate engraftment. In the past, most clinical trials have employed methods aimed at global T-cell depletion even though GVHD is initiated by the relatively small subset of donor cells that are specifically alloreactive against host histocompatibility antigens. In the future, it may be possible to employ specific depletion of alloreactive cells as a means of preventing GVHD.

Development of Tolerance

T cells that develop in the host thymus after BMT do not cause acute GVHD because of induction of anergy and negative selection mediated by host thymic epithelial cells. Host marrow–derived macrophages and dendritic cells may survive for several months after transplantation and may also contribute to negative selection among developing T cells. Negative selection by donor marrow–derived macrophages and dendritic cells prevents development of T cells that could recognize and destroy the graft. Failure of negative selection mechanisms in the thymus may allow development of donor cells capable of recognizing MHC class II antigens, thereby causing chronic GVHD. In the absence of chronic GVHD, prophylactic immunosuppressive treatment can be discontinued without complications, indicating either that the originally infused donor T cells, which recognize host alloantigens, have a finite life span, or that regulatory mechanisms develop to prevent them from causing immune-mediated injury (see Chapter 17).

Immune Reconstitution

The preparative regimen for BMT causes extensive ablation of host immunity and profound but transient immunodeficiency develops in all patients until reconstitution with donor cells (see Chapter 36). This reconstitution can occur initially by adoptive transfer of memory cells in the graft, but long-term reconstitution of immunity against certain pathogens probably represents the acquisition of new memory cells generated by exposure to antigens after BMT. The time for restoration varies for different components and functions of the immune system. In healthy patients, immunological function returns to normal by one year after BMT, and immunization with diphtheria, pertussis, tetanus, and pneumonococcal vaccines will generate normal responses. As a precaution, however, immunization with live viral vaccines such as measles, mumps, rubella, and oral polio is avoided, even in healthy patients. Full immunocompetence does not develop in patients with chronic GVHD until chronic GVHD resolves. For this reason, infections represent the major cause of morbidity and mortality among patients with chronic GVHD.

Optimal reconstitution of immunological function after BMT requires at least some degree of MHC compatibility between the donor and the recipient. This requirement stems from the fact that epithelial cells in the thymus favor the development of T cells that can recognize peptide antigens presented by MHC antigens of the host. In the periphery, however, marrow-derived dendritic cells represent the population most effective for activating T cells. If there were no MHC compatibility between the donor and the recipient, the T cells activated by antigen presented on marrow-derived cells would not be able to recognize antigen presented on nonmarrow-derived tissues. For this reason, current clinical practice generally considers related BMT to be feasible only when the donor and the recipient share at least one MHC haplotype. Likewise, unrelated BMT is not undertaken if there is disparity for more than one HLA-A, HLA-B, or HLA-DR antigen.

Currently, BMT is limited to patients with malignancy or certain nonmalignant disorders involving marrow-derived tissues. Thus, the preparative regimen is designed to eliminate malignant cells or abnormal marrow-derived cells of the host and to permit engraftment of the donor marrow. In the future, BMT may be developed as a method for facilitating transplantation of other tissues from the same donor. The rationale for this approach follows from the fact that T cells developing after BMT are tolerant of histocompatibility antigens of both the donor and the recipient because of negative selection by epithelial cells and marrow-derived cells in the thymus. For this purpose, the continued presence of some donor marrow–derived cells in the host thymus would suffice to prevent the development of T cells that could recognize a solid organ graft from the same donor, and complete elimination of host marrow–derived cells would not be necessary. Moreover, complete elimination of host-derived marrow cells would then require some degree of MHC compatibility between the donor and the recipient to allow optimal immune function after BMT. Preservation of some host-derived marrow cells together with the donor marrow would allow complete MHC incompatibility between the donor and the recipient, thereby broadening considerably the availability of donors without jeopardizing immune function after BMT. These considerations have led to intensive research exploring methods that would allow mixed reconstitution with both donor and host marrow cells.

Graft-versus-leukemia Effects

Myelosuppression represents the dose-limiting toxicity of many agents used for the treatment of malignancy. By circumventing this limitation, BMT allows the administration of chemotherapy and irradiation at doses two to three-fold higher than would otherwise be possible. It has been recognized, however, that the therapeutic advantage of allogeneic BMT results not only from the ability to deliver more intensive treatment but also from antineoplastic effects mediated by the graft (see Chapter 19). Clinical evidence for a "graft-versus-leukemia" (GVL) effect came initially from retrospective observations that leukemic relapse occurred less frequently in patients in whom GVHD developed, compared with those in whom it did not. The association between acute or chronic GVHD and reduced risk of relapse was most readily detectable in patients with lymphoid malignancies in relapse at the time of BMT.

Two other clinical observations have supported the concept that certain cells in an allogeneic marrow graft can help eliminate malignant cells that survive the conditioning regimen. Patients with acute myeloid leukemia (AML) in remission who were transplanted with HLA-genotypically identical marrow and given both MTX and CSP had a lower incidence of GVHD but a higher relapse rate than those given CSP alone. Removal of T cells in the donor marrow has also been associated with an increased risk of relapse. The risk of relapse after T-cell–depleted BMT for acute leukemia is comparable to the risk in patients in whom GVHD does not develop after BMT with unmodified marrow. Thus, the increased risk of relapse associated with T-cell depletion in patients with acute leukemia could simply reflect a decreased incidence of GVHD. Taken together, the data in patients with AML given MTX and CSP and the data in patients with acute leukemia transplanted with T-cell–depleted marrow confirm earlier suggestions that the occurrence of GVHD *per se* has an antileukemic effect.

The most striking association between T-cell depletion and increased risk of post-transplant relapse has occurred in patients transplanted for treatment of chronic myeloid leukemia (CML). Multivariate analyses have shown that the increased relapse risk cannot be explained entirely by a decreased incidence of GVHD. In patients with CML, donor T cells may therefore exert an antileukemic effect that is independent of overt GVHD.

The diversity of clinical observations emphasizes the likelihood that multiple mechanisms account for the antileukemic effects of an allogeneic BMT. Thus, alloantigens expressed by malignant cells can serve as direct targets for GVHD effector cells, or GVHD may activate other effectors such as NK cells and lymphokine-activated killer cells that have cytotoxic activity against leukemic cells. Certain leukemic cells have been demonstrated to express unique antigens that can serve as targets for immunocompetent donor cells. Finally, certain cytokines elaborated during GVHD may have effects on the proliferation and differentiation of malignant cells. From a clinical standpoint, the central question is whether GVL effects can be separated from GVHD. Initial attempts to decrease the risk of relapse by manipulations designed to increase the incidence and severity of GVHD did not succeed. With new insights gained from ongoing laboratory research, future clinical trials may demonstrate the feasibility of manipulating the immune system to prevent leukemic relapse without increasing the morbidity and mortality caused by GVHD.

Summary and Conclusions

Although this overview of the immunology of BMT focused on the individual outcomes of engraftment, GVHD, tolerance induction, immune reconstitution, and control of malignancy, these topics remain highly interconnected as different aspects of a single overall process. Nowhere has this lesson been better emphasized than in the discovery that the beneficial effects of T-cell depletion in decreasing the risk of GVHD were offset by the detrimental effects of increased graft failure and leukemic relapse and possibly impaired immune reconstitution. Thus, evaluation of interventions designed to influence one particular immunological outcome of BMT will require equivalent scrutiny of other immunological outcomes.

Historically, clinical BMT has evolved from the knowledge and understanding gained from animal studies. Murine models have the advantages of well-defined immunogenetics and a wealth of reagents for dissecting the cellular and humoral mechanisms involved in BMT immunology, whereas canine and non-human primate models more closely mimic the problems of BMT in a large outbred species. The wide range of experimental manipulations afforded by animal models has enabled rapid progress in the understanding of BMT immunology in all of its interconnected complexity. These insights provide a rational foundation for the ongoing development of BMT as a therapeutic method in humans.

Chapter 4
Histocompatibility

Bo Dupont and Soo Young Yang

It has been known for more than a century that autografts taken from and returned to the same animal become vascularized and accepted, whereas allografts exchanged between genetically different individuals of the same species are rejected. Rejection is a consequence of interactions between the immune system of the transplanted individual (recipient) and the histocompatibility antigens of the transplant (donor). Studies utilizing pure inbred strains of mice established that more than 20 different genetic systems are involved in rejection of a transplant.

A major breakthrough in transplantation immunology occurred during the late 1930s, when the British pathologist, Peter Gorer, identified antibodies that detected the H_2 antigens of the mouse (1). The genetic system identified by these alloantigens included the most important antigens involved in tissue rejection; they were therefore named the major histocompatibility antigens. The genes encoding these antigens constitute the major histocompatibility complex (MHC). The MHC has been identified in all vertebrates and consists of a number of closely linked genetic loci that constitute a genetic system which is inherited as a genetic unit. These genes are mapped within the H_2 region of chromosome 17 in mice, and, in humans, in a region analogous to H_2, called HLA (abbreviation for human leukocyte antigen system A) and located on the short arm of chromosome 6. The MHC contains a very large number of genes, many of which are not involved in immune function or transplant rejection.

The major histocompatibility antigens can be divided into two groups: (1) the MHC class I antigens, composed of an MHC-encoded α-chain (45 kd) associated with β_2-microglobulin (β2M), and (2) the MHC class II antigens composed of two MHC-encoded molecules, the α-chain and the β-chain (2). The MHC antigens serve the biological function of presenting peptide antigens to T lymphocytes. The MHC antigens are therefore centrally placed in evoking an immune response. Nearly all the genes encoding the MHC antigens are highly polymorphic, with many different allelic forms. T lymphocytes from one individual will recognize allelic differences in nonself MHC antigens, resulting in an immune response, which is called alloreactivity. This chapter will describe the genetics, the structure-function relationship, and the characterization (i.e., typing) of the human MHC antigens, HLA.

MHC Antigens and Immune Response

The immune system of an animal recognizes the presence of foreign or abnormal structures and generates an immune response. The immune response is mediated primarily by three types of cells: T lymphocytes, B lymphocytes, and macrophages. B-lymphocyte recognition of antigen is mediated by the idiotype of the antibody that will recognize unprocessed antigen. In contrast, T lymphocytes will recognize processed peptide fragments that are presented to the antigen (peptide)-specific, clonally distributed T-cell receptor (TCR). Most peripheral blood T cells express a TCR composed of an α/β-chain heterodimer, and both chains are encoded by a family of genes that somatically rearrange during T-cell development. This rearrangement results in an enormous diversification of TCRs very similar to that occurring in immunoglobulin genes. However, although antibodies will bind antigens directly, TCRs are limited to the recognition of peptide antigens that are presented by self-MHC molecules (i.e., MHC restriction of antigen presentation) (3).

Both MHC class I and II molecules present peptide antigens to the TCR (4,5). Class I molecules bind peptides of approximately 9 amino acids in length, whereas class II molecules bind peptides that are slightly larger (e.g., 13–17 amino acids), but only one or two amino acid residues are critical for binding (6–11). Each MHC molecule can bind and present a large array of peptides, and most proteins can be predicted to contain at least one peptide that can bind to any particular MHC molecule. Allelic variants of MHC molecules, however, will bind different combinations of peptides. The exquisite specificity of TCR for a particular combination of peptide/MHC antigen constitutes the molecular basis for an individual's T-lymphocyte–dependent immune responses.

T lymphocytes develop and mature in the thymus, where they first encounter self-MHC molecules and undergo positive and negative selection. As a consequence of T-cell selection in the thymus, a unique spectrum of α/β TCRs will develop in each individual of a species. This process is determined by somatic rearrangement in TCR genes, the combination of MHC alleles inherited by the individual, and the array of peptides that can bind to and be presented by the MHC molecules.

T lymphocytes with α/β TCR can be divided into two major subsets: $CD4^+$, $CD8^-$ and $CD8^+$, $CD4^-$. These T-cell subsets are functionally distinct due to their differences in MHC restriction. $CD4^+$ T cells recognize peptide antigens presented by class II, whereas $CD8^+$ T cells are class I–restricted. During T-cell development in the thymus, T cells with TCR specificity for peptide/class I are selected due to specific binding and interactions between CD8/class I, whereas T cells with specificity for peptide/class II have selective CD4/class II interactions.

The molecular basis for peptide antigen presentation to TCR was revealed by resolution of the crystal structure of the human class I antigen, HLA-A2 (12). This finding demonstrated that the class I molecule on its surface has a peptide-binding groove, which is available for binding to the TCR. A similar structure has been predicted for the MHC class II molecule (13). TCR recognition of peptide/MHC can therefore be predicted to utilize similar mechanisms independently of the CD4 or CD8 phenotype or peptide antigen presentation by class I or II molecules.

There are, however, major differences in the function of $CD4^+$ and $CD8^+$ T lymphocytes. A major function of $CD8^+$ T cells is to kill target cells that express a particular peptide. The antigen-specific cytotoxic T cells serve the function of eliminating infected or transformed cells, consistent with the presence of class I molecules on virtually all somatic cells. The $CD4^+$ class II–restricted T cells include helper T cells, which produce lymphokines and cytokines necessary for the function of many other cells of the immune system. The class II molecules are constitutively expressed on "professional" antigen-presenting cells such as monocytes, macrophages, mature B lymphocytes, and dendritic cells. The class II antigens can also be induced by cytokines (e.g., interferon-γ, tumor necrosis factor) on other cells, such as fibroblasts, endothelial, and epithelial cells. $CD4^+$ T cells will therefore be recruited to an inflammatory focus, where exogenous peptides will be processed and presented as peptide/class II complexes.

Development and selection of TCRs with specificity for peptide/MHC class I or peptide/MHC class II occur in the thymus (i.e., positive and negative selection). The CD8 and CD4 molecules are intimately involved in these processes. Mature, peripheral antigen-specific T cells with an α/β TCR utilize either CD4 or CD8 as a coreceptor, which will bind to MHC class II or I, respectively, during peptide/MHC interactions. MHC restriction to MHC class I or II therefore depends on which coreceptor is present on the T cell. However, there are also differences in the source of peptides that bind to class I or II molecules. In general, class I molecules bind peptides derived from proteins synthesized by the cell (i.e., endogenous peptides), whereas class II molecules bind peptides derived from exogenous, internalized proteins (i.e., exogenous peptides).

Antigen Processing and Presentation

The many different cellular events that lead to peptide binding to MHC molecules are called antigen processing (14,15). Differences in antigen processing for class I and II molecules, particularly differences in the cytoplasmic compartments where class I and II molecules assemble and bind peptides, are responsible for the peptides that will be presented on the cell surface by class I or II molecules. The primary source of peptides presented by class I molecules is cytosolic and nuclear proteins. Peptides derived from these proteins are transported from the cytosol to the endoplasmic reticulum (ER). Correct folding and transport of the class I molecule to the cell surface require association of the class I heavy chain molecule (45 kd) with β2M in the presence of peptide, and this process occurs in the endoplasmic reticulum. In the absence of peptide, class I molecules assemble inefficiently and are unstable if they reach the cell surface.

The mechanisms by which cytosolic peptides are generated from antigenic proteins and transported into the ER are not yet understood completely. This process does not require an acidic compartment or lysosomal proteases, and lysosomal peptides are normally not presented by class I molecules. There is, however, increasing evidence that cytosolic proteasomes may constitute the proteolytic machinery that generates antigenic peptides for presentation by class I molecules (16). The so called low molecular weight proteins (LMPs) are subunits of the proteasomes, and some LMPs are encoded by genes within the MHC class II region (17,18). Currently, direct evidence for a role of LMPs or proteasomes in generating class I restricted peptides has not yet been obtained.

Recently, several genes encoding putative peptide transporters have been identified (19–21). These genes are also encoded in the MHC, adjacent to the proteasome subunits, and mutation in these "peptide supply factors" markedly impairs antigen presentation by class I molecules. The putative peptide transports are homologous to known adenosine triphosphate (ATP)–dependent membrane transport systems, which contain the ATP-binding cassette (ABC) motif (22). These molecules transport peptides from the cytosol into the ER, where the peptides become available for binding to MHC class I molecules.

In complete contrast to class I molecules, the class II molecules are very effective in presenting peptides generated in the endosomal and lysosomal compartments. Extracellular antigens are taken up by endocytosis, and the proteins are then degraded by acidic proteases (e.g., cathepsins) (23). The MHC class II molecules consist of an α/β-heterodimer expressed on the cell surface. The α- and β-chains assemble immediately in the ER by a process that is independent of peptides. The α/β-heterodimer immediately combines with the nonpolymorphic glycoprotein called the invariant chain (Ii) (CD74). The α/βIi complexes are transported from the ER via the Golgi and transgolgi network (TGN) to the endocytic compartments, where the Ii is removed by proteolysis (24). Therefore, one of the functions of Ii is to prevent peptide binding to class II in the ER. The Ii also has additional functions involved in transport of class II molecules to the precise endocytic compartments where they become available for peptide binding. A diagrammatic representation of antigen processing and MHC class I and II assembly and transport to the cell surface is shown in Figure 4-1.

Antigenic Peptides, Class I and II Molecules

The class I and II molecules described are distinct with regard to their biosynthesis, assembly, peptide binding, and transport to the cell surface. The class I molecules require peptides for their correct assembly in the ER. In contrast, the class II molecules assemble together with Ii in the ER in absence of peptide, and this complex is transported to postgolgi compartments where the α/β-heterodimer binds peptide and the Ii is released. Antigenic proteins can be expected to generate at least one peptide that will bind to any particular class I or II molecule. The source of peptides presented by either class I or II molecules depends on the intracellular compartment where the peptide is available for binding to MHC molecules. Peptides generated from proteins synthesized in the cytosol, such as viral antigens or mutated self-antigens, can be assembled with the class I molecules following transport into the ER. As a result of these requirements, most exogenous antigenic proteins will not be presented by class I molecules, because endocytosed proteins are not normally delivered to the cytosol. There are, however, some exceptions to this rule, but the general principle that class I molecules present endogenous peptides is valid.

The class II molecules, in contrast to class I, are very efficient at presenting endocytosed (exogenous) peptide antigens to T cells. The class II molecules are even more versatile, because they can also present peptides derived from endogenously synthesized proteins. Therefore, during virus infection, endogenous, virus-derived peptides will be presented by class I MHC molecules to peptide-antigen specific cytolytic, $CD8^+$ T cells. In addition, MHC class II–positive, "professional" antigen-presenting cells (e.g., macrophages) will process exogenous, virus-derived proteins that can be presented by class II molecules to $CD4^+$ T cells. However, a virus-infected, class II–positive cell will also be able to present virus-derived peptides by class II molecules and thereby generate $CD4^+$ T-cell helper functions to a broad spectrum of virus-specific peptides.

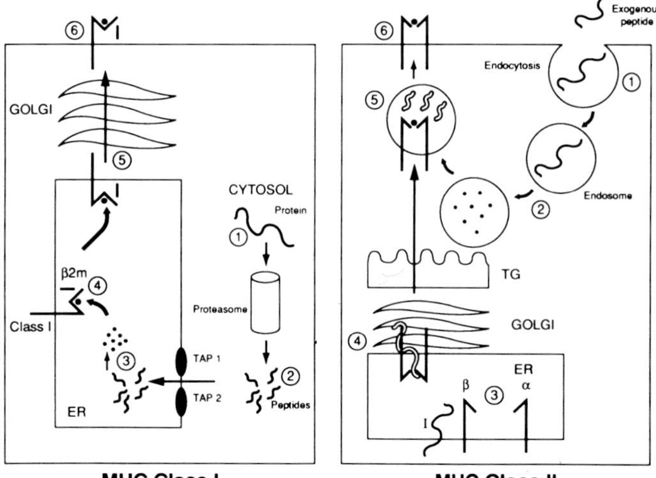

Figure 4-1

Alloreactivity

Rejection of an allograft is an immunological process that in most instances is mediated by T lymphocytes (25–30). Although the initial immune response may be limited to $CD4^+$ or $CD8^+$ T cells, both major T-cell subsets normally participate in the complex set of phenomena involved in tissue or organ rejection. The molecular basis for T-cell–mediated alloreactivity is currently not well understood. Alloantigen activation of T lymphocytes occurs when the TCR recognize non-self MHC molecules (i.e., alloreactivity to major transplantation antigens), but alloreactivity can also occur when the donor and the recipient are identical for MHC but different for non-MHC alloantigens (i.e., alloreactivity to minor transplantation antigens). The current model for peptide antigen-specific TCR-mediated T-cell activation can readily explain alloreactivity to minor histocompatibility antigens. The TCRs will recognize differences in self-peptides between the donor and the recipient, and these peptides will be presented in an MHC-restricted fashion by self-MHC class I and II molecules because the donor and the recipient are identical for MHC. The self-peptides can, for example, be normally occurring cellular proteins that have genetically determined allelic forms for which the donor and the recipient are different. Other peptides could be mutated self-proteins resulting from malignant cell transformation or viral proteins produced as a consequence of virus infection.

Differences in MHC antigens between donor and recipient are, however, the most potent genetic factors involved in development of alloreactivity and graft rejection. The molecular basis for alloreactivity to major transplantation antigens (i.e., MHC antigens) is currently not well understood. It is attractive to develop a model for TCR-mediated alloreactivity to non-self MHC molecules, which mimics the normal TCR-mediated T-cell activation to peptide/self-MHC. Such a model would be consistent with the observations that some allospecific T cells can crossreactively recognize foreign antigen presented by self-MHC molecules (31,32), and antigen-specific T cells can also, in some instances, recognize specific alloantigens (33,34). The major issue of contention for accepting this model concerns the nature of MHC restriction that occurs during an alloresponse to MHC antigens. The molecular interactions that occur within the trimolecular complex consisting of MHC-peptide-TCR are currently incompletely understood. Most peptides presented by, for example, class I molecules are nonopeptides (i.e., 9 amino acid residues in length), and the residue in position 2 from the N-terminal of the peptide and the residue in position 9 are the major anchoring residues for peptide-MHC binding. Two or three of the intervening residues are important for TCR contact. The MHC restricting elements are formed by combinations of amino acid residues on the MHC molecule, which can accommodate contact with the TCR. It has been shown that the putative TCR contact residues on MHC molecules are limited. It has been demonstrated, for example, that some point mutations in MHC molecules do not cause alloreactivity, whereas others do (32–38).

Amino acid residues particularly important in eliciting an alloantigen response are mapped to the α-helices of the MHC molecules surrounding the peptide binding groove, whereas others are located in the floor of the peptide binding groove. Substitutions in amino acid residues on the α-helixes will presumably be involved in TCR/MHC contact, whereas substitutions in residues in the peptide binding groove will affect peptide binding. The most likely explanation for alloreactivity to non-self MHC molecules is therefore that the alloantigenic determinants are formed by a new spectrum of peptides presented to the TCRs in context of foreign MHC molecules. The MHC restricting elements would be formed by a combination of TCR contact residues on the MHC molecules, which by chance can accommodate the TCRs with a given peptide specificity. The spectrum of TCRs that combines the capacity to interact with peptide and MHC will elicit the alloreactive T-cell response. Some of the MHC restricting elements would be formed by a particular combination of residues on the α-helixes, which by chance have affinity for the peptide-specific TCR. Other peptide-specific TCRs may, as the MHC restricting element, utilize contact residues, which are shared between self-MHC and one particular allo-MHC molecule. It is well established that HLA alleles of a single gene may differ only for a single amino acid residue (e.g., HLA-B*4401 vs B*4403) and the most divergent alleles still have at least 80% amino acid identity. TCR cross-reactivity between peptide/self-MHC and allo-MHC could therefore readily be explained. One particular antigen-specific TCR may, for example, have the same self-MHC restricting element as the allo-MHC, which binds a new peptide with affinity for the same TCR.

This model for TCR recognition of allo-MHC antigens combines the hypothesis of mimicry between peptide/self-MHC and peptide/allo-MHC with the observation that the frequency of alloreactive T cells is significantly higher than the frequency of peptide-specific T cells generated in response to a single protein antigen.

Genetics of the HLA Complex

The human MHC, HLA, is located on the short arm (p) of chromosome 6 in the 6p21.31 to 6p21.33 region. The physical map of the HLA region has been determined by a combination of cosmic walking and genomic mapping using pulsed field gel electrophoresis and spans approximately 4,000 kilobases (kb) of DNA. The HLA region can be divided into three regions: (1) the class I region, (2) the class III region, and (3) the class II region. The class I region is the most telomeric, and the class II region is centromeric (39). A diagrammatic representation of the physical map of the HLA region is shown in Figure 4-2. A complete listing of all known HLA class I and II genes is shown in Table 4-1.

Class I Region

This region spans approximately 2,000 kb and encodes the genes for the 45-kd α-chain of the class I molecules. The HLA region does not contain the gene encoding the class I light chain, β-2-microglobin (β_2M), which is located on chromosome 15. The class I molecules known to be peptide-presenting cell surface molecules are named HLA-A, HLA-B, and HLA-C. The class I region also contains a number of additional, structurally related class I genes, of which HLA-E, HLA-F, and HLA-G are intact and potentially functional. In con-

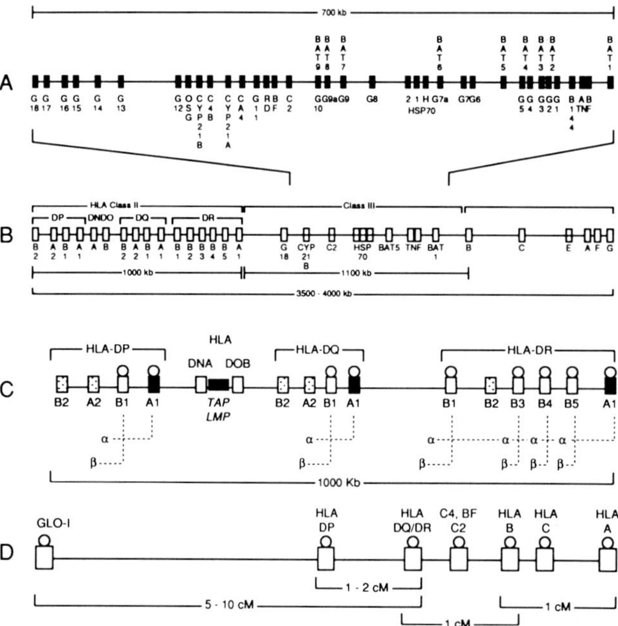

Figure 4-2

Table 4-1.
Names for Genes in the HLA Region

Name	*Previous Name*	*Molecular Characteristics*
HLA-A	. . .	Class I α-chain
HLA-B	. . .	Class I α-chain
HLA-C	. . .	Class I α-chain
HLA-E	E,'6.2'	Associated with class I 6.2-kB *Hin*dIII fragment
HLA-F	F,'5.4'	Associated with class I 5.4-kB *Hin*dIII fragment
HLA-G	G,'6.0'	Associated with class I 6.0-kB *Hin*dIII fragment
HLA-H	H,AR,'12.4'	Class I pseudogene associated with 5.4-kB *Hin*dIII fragment
HLA-J	cda12	Class I pseudogene associated with 5.9-kB *Hin*dIII fragment
HLA-DRA	DRα	DR α-chain
HLA-DRB1	DRβI,DR1B	DR β1-chain determining specificities DR1, DR2, DR3, DR4, DR5, etc.
HLA-DRB2	DRβII	Pseudogene with DR β-like sequences
HLA-DRB3	DRβIII,DR3B	DR β3-chain determining DR52 and Dw24, Dw25, Dw26 specificities
HLA-DRB4	DRβIV,DR4B	DR β4-chain determining DR53
HLA-DRB5	DRβIII	DR β5-chain determining DR51
HLA-DRB6	DDRBX,DRBσ	DRB pseudogene found on DR1, DR2, and DR10 haplotypes
HLA-DRB7	DRBψ1	DRB pseudogene found on DR4, DR7, and DR9 haplotypes
HLA-DRB8	DRBψ2	DRB pseudogene found on DR4, DR7, and DR9 haplotypes
HLA-DRB9	M4.2β exon	DRB pseudogene, isolated fragment
HLA-DQA1	DQα1,DQ1A	DQ α-chain as expressed
HLA-DQB1	DQβ1,DQ1B	DQ β-chain as expressed
HLA-DQA2	DXα,DQ2A	DQ α-chain–related sequence, not known to be expressed
HLA-DQB2	DXβ,DQ2B	DQ β-chain–related sequence, not known to be expressed
HLA-DQB3	DVβ,DQB3	DQ β-chain–related sequence, not known to be expressed
HLA-DOB	DOβ	DO β-chain
HLA-DMA	RING6	DM α-chain
HLA-DMB	RING7	DM β-chain
HLA-DNA	DZα,DOα	DN α-chain
HLA-DPA1	DPα1,DP1A	DP α-chain as expressed
HLA-DPB1	DPβ1,DP1B	DP β-chain as expressed
HLA-DPA2	DPα2,DP2A	DP α-chain–related pseudogene
HLA-DPB2	DPβb2,DP2B	DP β-chain–related pseudogene
TAP1	RING4,Y3,PSF1	ABC (ATP binding cassette) transporter
TAP2	RING11,Y1,PSF2	ABC (ATP binding cassette) transporter
LMP2	RING12	Proteasome-related sequence
LMP7	RING10	Proteasome-related sequence

trast, the genes encoding the class I genes HLA-H and HLA-J are pseudogenes. Whereas HLA-A, HLA-B, and HLA-C genes are highly polymorphic, occurring in multiple allelic forms, HLA-E, HLA-F, and HLA-G exhibit low polymorphism, and their functions are poorly understood. The HLA-A, HLA-B, and HLA-C antigens are expressed on most nucleated somatic cells and to varying degrees on platelets. HLA-E, HLA-F, and HLA-G are expressed with tissue specificity, and their α-chains associate with β2M. Only HLA-G is transported to the cell surface, but its expression is limited to the cytotrophoblast. HLA-E transcripts have been detected in lymphoid and nonlymphoid cells, whereas HLA-F transcripts are found in resting T cells and transformed B-cell lines, but not in liver or fibroblasts.

Class II Region

The most centromeric segment of HLA is the class II region, which spans approximately 1,000 kb. It contains all the genes encoding the known HLA class II molecules, HLA-DR, HLA-DQ, and HLA-DP. This region also includes genes involved in antigen processing, such as the proteasome-related genes encoding LMPs, and genes involved in peptide transport, the ABC (ATP binding cassette) transporters. Currently, two LMP genes, LMP2 and LMP7, are known to be located in the class II region, as well as two transporter genes, TAP1 and TAP2. A number of additional nonclass II genes that have no obvious association with the immune system have been identified in the class II region. Some of these genes have known functions such as the collagen gene type 11A2, located centromeric to HLA-DP, and the RING 3 gene homologous to the *Drosophila* gene, female sterile homeotic, which is located close to the class II α gene. Several additional genes of unknown function have recently been identified in the class II region.

The HLA class II molecules are heterodimers consisting of the two HLA-encoded polypeptide chains α (designated A-genes) and β (designated B genes). There are a variable number of expressed HLA-DR molecules, all of which have the same DR α-chain encoded by the DRA locus. The genomic organization of the HLA-DR region is shown in Figure 4-3. This figure demonstrates that the number of expressed DR genes depends on the genetic origin of the allele expressed by the DRB1 locus. For example, the HLA-DR region that encodes the DRB1 alleles DRB1*0101, *0102, *0103, *1001, and some of the HLA-DR haplo-

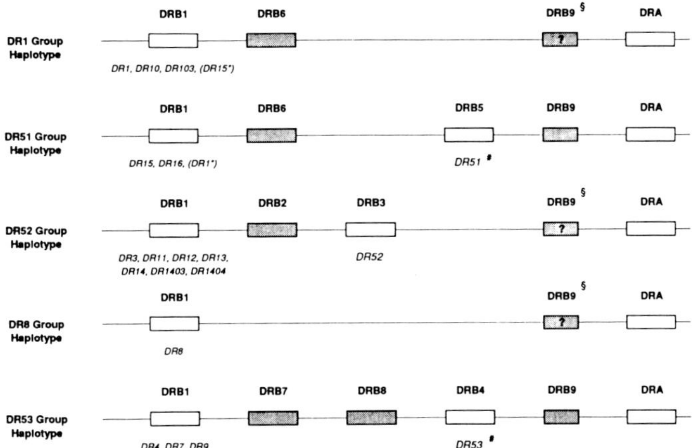

Figure 4-3 Genomic Organization of the HLA-DR region and encoded products (specificities).

types with DRB1*15 only express the DR α/β-heterodimer encoded by the DRA and DRB1 loci. In contrast, HLA-DR regions encoding the DRB1 alleles corresponding to the serological specificities DR4, DR7, and DR9 have two species of DR α/β-heterodimers encoded by DRA with DRB1 and DRA with DRB4, respectively. The DRA, DRB4–encoded molecules give rise to HLA-DR molecules expressing the serological specificity DR53. It is also demonstrated in Figure 4-3 that the different HLA-DR regions contain variable numbers of pseudogenes. For example, HLA-DR regions encoding the DRB1 alleles corresponding to the serological specificity DR8 contain only one DRB pseudogene, DRB9. In contrast, HLA-DR regions that express DR53-associated alleles contain three DRB pseudogenes: DRB7, DRB8, and DRB9.

The HLA-DQ region of class II contains five genes; two DQA genes, DQA1 and DQA2; and three DQB genes, DQB1, DQB2, and DQB3. Only the DQA1 and DQB1 gene products are known to be expressed as the HLA-DQ α/β-heterodimeric class II molecules.

The HLA-DP region is the most centromeric component of the class II region and contains the two DPA genes, DPA1 and DPA2, and the two DPB genes, DPB1 and DPB2. Only the DPA1 and DPB1 genes encode the HLA-DP class II α/β-heterodimeric molecule.

The class II region contains additional class II genes, such as the α-chain–like genes DMA and DNA and the β-chain–like genes DMB and DOB. The function of these genes is currently unknown.

Class III Region

At least 36 genes have now been located to the class III region, which is located between the class I and II regions. It spans approximately 700 kb. This genetic region contains genes encoding proteins with known immune functions such as the structural genes for some of the serum complement components C2, C4, Bf, the two genes encoding tumor necrosis factor, TNF-α and TNF-β (lymphotoxin), and at least two heat shock proteins, Hsp 70 2 and 1H. C4 is encoded by two genes, C4A and C4B. Centromeric to each of the C4 genes are the genes encoding the steroid hormone biosynthesis enzyme, 21-hydroxylase, CYP21. CYP21B located next to C4B is functional and gives rise to the enzyme, whereas CYP21A located next to C4A is a pseudogene. The C4/CYP21 region is characterized by frequent gene duplications and deletions. The region of the genes encoding C2 and Bf, which are closely related genes, also contains a gene, RD, which encodes a 42-kd intracellular protein characterized by a dipeptide repeat with the basic residues R or K next to an acidic one (D or E). The telomeric segment of the class III region contains two genes BAT2 (G2) and BAT3 (G3), encoding large proline-rich proteins with molecular masses of 228 and 110 kd, respectively. Their function is currently unknown, as is the function of the many additional BAT (or G) genes located in this region.

Genetic Recombination

The HLA region is normally inherited as a genetic unit. The genes, however, can be separated by genetic recombination (i.e., crossover of genetic material between homologous chromosomes during meiotic division). This recombination occurs quite rarely, as established from testing a large number of families for segregation of HLA class I and II antigens. It has been determined that the frequency of genetic recombination between HLA-A and HLA-B is approximately 1%. In most instances of HLA-A/HLA-B recombination, the recombinational event occurs between the HLA-A and the HLA-C locus; the HLA-A allele is separated from the original HLA-C, HLA-B segment of the class I region. Genetic recombination between HLA-C and HLA-B is very rare; only a few families have been reported during the past 20 years. Genetic recombination between the HLA class I and II region also occurs with a frequency of approximately 1%, resulting in formation of a recombinant HLA-B/HLA-DR haplotype. The HLA-B/HLA-DR recombinations probably occur very rarely within the class III region but seem to occur between HLA-B and class III or between class III and HLA-DR. Genetic recombination within the class II region also occurs. Separation of the HLA-DR, HLA-DQ segment from the HLA-DP region is the most common form of recombination. HLA-DR, HLA-DQ/DP recombination has a frequency of approximately 1 to 2%. In summary, the HLA complex can be considered as a single genetic unit that is inherited as a bloc of genes from a parent to a child.

HLA Haplotypes, Genotypes, and Phenotypes

The genetic unit of HLA class I, III, and II regions on one chromosome is called an HLA haplotype. The two HLA haplotypes present in one individual are called the HLA genotype. The genes encoding the HLA class I antigens, HLA-A, HLA-B, HLA-C, and the class II antigens, HLA-DR, HLA-DQ, HLA-DP, are codominantly expressed as cell-surface molecules. Therefore, the HLA antigens are transmitted as dominantly inherited, Mendelian traits, and each child will express one set of paternal and one set of maternal HLA antigens corresponding to the HLA genes inherited by one paternal and one maternal HLA haplotype. A diagrammatic representation of HLA haplotype segregation in a family is depicted in Figure 4-4. The father's two HLA haplotypes are labeled "a" and "b" and the mother's are labeled "c" and "d." Accordingly, the father's HLA genotype is "ab" and the mother's is "cd." There are then four possible genotypes for their children: ac, ad, bc, and bd. The probability of an offspring inheriting any one of these four possible HLA genotypes is 0.25. Accordingly, the chance of any one sibling within a family being HLA-genotypically identical with any other sibling is 25%. The chances of sharing one HLA haplotype between siblings is 50%, and the chance of two siblings being completely different with regard to HLA haplotypes is 25%. Consequently, a child will always differ genetically from each of the parents for one HLA haplotype, and children will always share one HLA haplotype with each of their parents. The only exception to this rule involves children who have inherited an HLA recombinant haplotype.

Because the HLA gene products are codominantly expressed, each individual will express two different sets of HLA-A molecules, one encoded by the HLA-A gene inherited from the father and one set of HLA-A molecules encoded by the maternally inherited HLA-A gene. Similarly, each individual will express

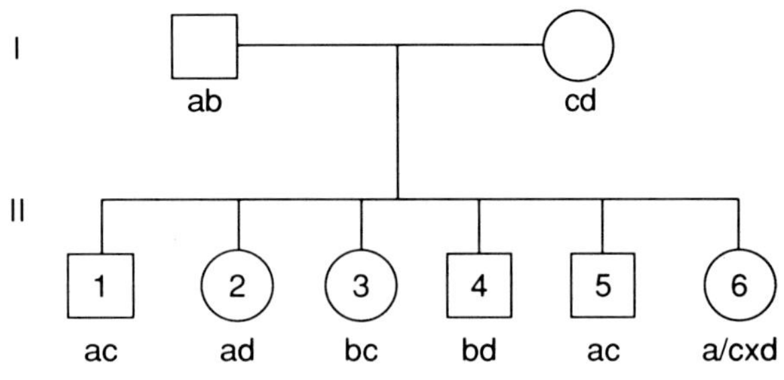

a: A1, B8, Cw8, DR3, DR52, DQ2
b: A3, B7, Cw7, DR2, DQ6
c: A2, B44, Cw3, DR4, DR53, DQ7
d: A3, B35, Cw4, DR1, DQ5

R cxd: A2, B35, Cw4, DR1, DQ5

a, b, c, d: parental HLA haplotypes

ab, ac, cd, ad, bc, bd: HLA genotypes

Figure 4-4

two sets of HLA-B molecules, two HLA-C molecules, and two sets of HLA class II antigens. This combination of HLA antigens constitutes the person's HLA phenotype. Most people are HLA-heterozygous for each HLA locus (e.g., they express two different HLA-A alleles). Sometimes, however, a father and a mother express the same HLA allele on one of their HLA haplotypes (e.g., both parents express HLA-A2). A child who inherits the two HLA haplotypes that express HLA-A2 will then be homozygous for the HLA-A2 antigen.

Some HLA haplotypes are relatively common. For example, the HLA-A1, HLA-B8, HLA-DR3 haplotype is quite frequent in the Caucasian population from Northern Europe. Therefore, an individual by chance may have inherited the same HLA haplotype from each of the parents, resulting in the person being homozygous for the HLA-A1, HLA-B8, HLA-DR3 haplotype. Such individuals are commonly referred to as HLA-homozygous. An individual can be homozygous for one allele at a single HLA locus (e.g., homozygous for HLA-A2) or HLA-homozygous for an entire HLA haplotype (e.g., HLA-A1, HLA-B8, HLA-DR3). The genetic region containing HLA spans nearly 4,000 kb of DNA, and it is highly unlikely that two unrelated individuals would be identical for all the genes contained within this stretch of DNA. There are, however, instances in which an individual could be truly genetically homozygous for the whole HLA region (e.g., HLA homozygosity as a result of inbreeding, as seen in some offspring from brother-sister or first cousin matings). The term *homozygosity* for an HLA antigen is frequently used when the individual expresses the same HLA antigen detected by conventional, serological HLA typing. The expression "homozygosity for HLA-A2" may therefore not necessarily imply that the person expresses exactly the same HLA-A2 allele inherited from the paternal and maternal HLA haplotype. For example, currently, 12 different HLA-A2 alleles have been identified (designated A*0201–A*0212) (Table 4-2). An individual is only truly HLA-A2-homozygous if the same HLA-A2 allele was inherited from both parents (e.g., A*0201/A*0201).

The HLA Linkage Group

The HLA region is genetically linked to several other genes, such as gene-encoding superoxide dismutase 2 (SOD2), phosphoglucomutase 3 (PDM3), malic enzyme 1 (ME1), neuraminidase (NEU), and glyoxalase 1 (GLOI). Of particular interest is the gene for the enzyme GLOI, which is located centromeric to HLA. The two isoforms of GLOI (GLOI.1 and GLOI.2) have been used as genetic markers in HLA genotyping.

HLA Polymorphism

Genetic polymorphism is defined as the occurrence in a population of two or more genetically determined forms of a gene in frequencies such that the rare event could not be maintained by mutation alone. The different forms of the gene are called alleles.

Table 4-2.
Designations of HLA-A, HLA-B and HLA-C Alleles

HLA Alleles	*HLA Specificity*	*Previous Equivalents*
A*0101	A1	...
A*0201	A2	A2.1
A*0202	A2	A2.2F
A*0203	A203	A2.3
A*0204	A2	...
A*0205	A2	A2.2Y
A*0206	A2	A2.4a
A*0207	A2	A2.4b
A*0208	A2	A2.4c
A*0209	A2	A2-0ZB
A*0210	A210	A2-LEE
A*0211	A2	A2.5
A*0212	A2	...
A*0301	A3	A3.1
A*0302	A3	A3.2
A*1101	A11	A11E
A*1102	A11	A11K
A*2301	A23(9)	...
A*2401	A24(9)	...
A*2402	A24(9)	...
A*2403	A2403	A9.3
A*2501	A25(10)	...
A*2601	A26(10)	...
A*2901	A29(19)	...
A*2902	A29(19)	A29.2
A*3001	A30(19)	A30.3
A*3002	A30(19)	A30.2
A*31011	A31(19)	...
A*31012	A31(19)	...
A*3201	A32(19)	...
A*3301	A33(19)	Aw33.1
A*3401	A34(10)	...
A*3402	A34(10)	...
A*3601	A36	...
A*4301	A43	...
A*6601	A66(10)	...
A*6602	A66(10)	...
A*6801	A68(28)	Aw68.1
A*6802	A68(28)	Aw68.2
A*6901	A69(28)	...
A*7401	A74(19)	...
B*0701	B7	B7.1
B*0702	B7	B7.2
B*0703	B703	BPOT
B*0801	B8	...
B*1301	B13	B13.1
B*1302	B13	B13.2
B*1401	B14	...
B*1402	B65(14)	...
B*1501	B62(15)	...
B*1502	B75(15)	...
B*1503	B72(15)	...
B*1504	B62(15)	Bw62-G
B*1801	B18	...
B*2701	B27	27f
B*2702	B27	27e,27K,B27.2
B*2703	B27	27d,27J
B*2704	B27	27b,27C,B27.3
B*2705	B27	27a,27W,B27.1
B*2706	B27	27D,B27.4
B*2707	B27	B27-HS
B*3501	B35	...
B*3502	B35	...
B*3503	B35	...
B*3504	B35	...
B*3505	B35	B35-G
B*3506	B35	B35-K
B*3701	B37	...
B*3801	B38(16)	B16.1
B*3901	B3901	B16.2
B*3902	B3902	B39.2
B*4001	B60(40)	...
B*4002	B40	B40*
B*4003	B40	B40-G1
B*4004	B40	B40-G2
B*4005	B4005	BN21
B*4101	B41	...
B*4201	B42	...
B*4401	B44(12)	B44.1
B*4402	B44(12)	B44.2
B*4403	B44(12)	B44.1:New
B*4501	B45(12)	...
B*4601	B46	...
B*4701	B47	...
B*4801	B48	...
B*4901	B49(21)	...
B*5001	B50(21)	...
B*5101	B51(5)	...
B*5102	B5102	B5.35
B*5103	B5103	BTA
B*5201	B52(5)	...
B*5301	B53	...
B*5401	B54(22)	...
B*5501	B55(22)	...
B*5502	B55(22)	...
B*5601	B56(22)	...
B*5602	B56(22)	...
B*5701	B57(17)	...
B*5702	B57(17)	Bw57.2
B*5801	B58(17)	...
B*7801	B7801	B'SNA'.Bx1
B*7901	...	B"X"-HS
Cw*0101	Cw1	Cw1.1
Cw*0102	Cw1	Cw1.2
Cw*0201	Cw2	Cw2.1
Cw*02021	Cw2	Cw2.2
Cw*02022	Cw2	Cw2.2
Cw*0301	Cw3	...
Cw*0302	Cw3	...
Cw*0401	Cw4	...
Cw*0501	Cw5	...
Cw*0601	Cw6	...
Cw*0701	Cw7	...
Cw*0702	Cw7	JY328
Cw*0801	Cw8	...
Cw*0802	Cw8	...
Cw*1201	...	Cx52
Cw*1202	...	Cb-2
Cw*1301	...	CwBL18
Cw*1401	...	Cb-1
E*0101	...	JTW15
E*0102	...	HLA-6.2
E*0103	...	M32507
E*0104	...	M32508

The genes encoding the HLA class I and II molecules are highly polymorphic. Nearly all of the genes have many alleles, and the HLA region represents the most polymorphic genetic system in humans. The mechanisms by which the extensive genetic polymorphism of the HLA antigens have developed and are maintained are currently not known. It is believed that HLA polymorphism has had a role in protecting the species during the course of evolution. The assumption has been made that certain HLA alleles provide protection against deleterious infections during infancy and childhood, which would then result in the transmission of the protective HLA alleles from generation to generation. Different ethnic groups and ethnic subgroups would have been exposed to different infectious agents and other environmental factors, which may have contributed to the differences in HLA alleles in different geographic regions.

The molecular basis for HLA polymorphism is due to differences in nucleotide sequences within the coding regions of the individual HLA genes. Representative DNA clones for most of the currently known HLA genes were isolated during the years 1980 to 1984. Molecular cloning of the HLA class I and II genes has made it possible to obtain precise definitions of the HLA alleles for each of the HLA genes. The HLA alleles are currently defined by a unique sequence of nucleotides present in the coding region of the individual HLA gene. The nucleotide sequences correspond to specific amino acid residues in the expressed cell-surface molecules. Therefore, the HLA phenotype of an individual can now be defined by direct determination of the nucleotide sequences for each of the HLA class I and II genes.

HLA Terminology

The HLA terminology is designated by the World Health Organization (WHO) Nomenclature Committee for Factors of the HLA system, which updates the HLA nomenclature at regular intervals (40). The most recent listing of recognized HLA class I alleles is shown in Table 4-2. This Table also indicates the serological HLA antigens that correspond to the different alleles. For example, only one HLA-A1 allele, A*0101, has been identified, and this allele corresponds to the serological specificity HLA-A1. In contrast, there are currently 7 different HLA-B27 alleles, designated B*2701 to B*2707, which all encode HLA-B27 molecules that are serologically detectable by anti-B27 antisera or monoclonal antibodies. The currently identified HLA class II alleles are listed for HLA-DR, HLA-DQ and HLA-DP in Tables 4-3, 4-4 and 4-5, respectively.

Gene Frequencies and Genetic Linkage Disequilibrium

It is well established that the antigen frequency for a given HLA allele varies considerably among ethnic

Table 4-3.
Designations of HLA-DR Alleles

HLA Alleles	*HLA-DR Serological Specificities*	*HLA-D–associated (T-cell–defined) Specificities*	*Previous Equivalents*
DRA*0101	...	...	DRα,PDR-α-2
DRA*0102	...	...	DR-H
DRB1*0101	DR1	Dw1	...
DRB1*0102	DR1	Dw20	DR1-NASC
DRB1*0103	DR103	Dw'BON'	DR1-CETUS,DRB1*BON
DRB1*1501	DR15(2)	Dw2	DR2B Dw2
DRB1*1502	DR15(2)	Dw12	DR2B Dw12
DRB1*1503	DR15(2)	...	...
DRB1*1601	DR16(2)	Dw21	DR2B Dw21
DRW1*1602	DR16(2)	Dw22	DR2B Dw22
DRB1*0301	DR17(3)	Dw3	...
DRB1*0302	DR18(3)	Dw'RSH'	...
DRB1*0303	DR18(3)	...	...
DRB1*0401	DR4	Dw4	...
DRB1*0402	DR4	Dw10	...
DRB1*0403	DR4	Dw13	DR4 Dw13A, 13.1
DRB1*0404	DR4	Dw14	DR4 Dw14A, 14.1
DRB1*0405	DR4	Dw15	...
DRB1*0406	DR4	Dw'KT2'	...
DRB1*0407	DR4	Dw13	DR4 Dw13B, 13.2
DRB1*0408	DR4	Dw14	DR4-CETUS, Dw14B, 14.2
DRB1*0409	DR4	...	...
DRB1*0410	DR4	...	DR4.CB
DRB1*0411	DR4	...	DR4.EC
DRB1*0412	DR4	...	AB2
DRB1*11011	DR11(5)	Dw5	DRw11.1

Table 4-3 (continued)

HLA Alleles[a]	*HLA-DR Serological Specificities*	*HLA-D–associated (T-cell–defined) Specificities*	*Previous Equivalents*
DRB1*11012	DR11(5)	Dw5	. . .
DRB1*1102	DR11(5)	Dw'JVM'	DRw11.2
DRB1*1103	DR11(5)	. . .	DRw11.3
DRB1*11041	DR11(5)	Dw'FS'	. . .
DRB1*11042	DR11(5)	. . .	. . .
DRB1*1105	DR11(5)	. . .	. . .
DRB1*1201	DR12(5)	Dw'DB6'	. . .
DRB1*1202	DR12(5)	. . .	DRw12b
DRB1*1301	DR13(6)	Dw18	DRw6aI
DRB1*1302	DR13(6)	Dw19	DRw6cI
DRB1*1303	DR13(6)	Dw'HAG'	. . .
DRB1*1304	DR13(6)	. . .	RB1125-14
DRB1*1305	DR13(6)	. . .	DRw6'PEV'
DRB1*1306	DR13(6)	. . .	DRB1*13.MW
DRB1*1401	DR14(6)	Dw9	DRw6bI
DRB1*1402	DR14(6)	Dw16	. . .
DRB1*1403	DR1403	. . .	JX6
DRB1*1404	DR1404	. . .	DRB1*LY10, DRw6b.2
DRB1*1405	DR14(6)	. . .	DRB1*14c
DRB1*1406	DR14(6)	. . .	DRB1*14.GB,14.6
DRB1*1407	DR14(6)	. . .	14.7
DRB1*1408	DR14(6)	. . .	AO1,14.8
DRB1*1409	DR14(6)	. . .	AB4
DRB1*1410	. . .	. . .	AB3
DRB1*0701	DR7	Dw17	. . .
DRB1*0702	DR7	Dw'DB1'	. . .
DRB1*0801	DR8	Dw8.1	. . .
DRB1*08021	DR8	Dw8.2	DRw8-SPL
DRB1*08022	DR8	Dw8.2	DRw8b
DRB1*08031	DR8	Dw8.3	DRw8-TAB
DRB1*08032	DR8	Dw8.3	. . .
DRB1*0804	DR8	. . .	RB1066–1, DR8-V86
DRB1*0805	DR8	. . .	DR8-A74
DRB1*09011	DR9	Dw23	. . .
DRB1*09012	DR9	Dw23	. . .
DRB1*1001	DR10	. . .	. . .
DRB3*0101	DR52	Dw24	DR2 III, DRw6a III
DRB3*0201	DR52	Dw25	DRw6b III
DRB3*0202	DR52	Dw25	pDR5b.3
DRB3*0301	DR52	Dw26	. . .
DRB4*0101	DR53	Dw4, Dw10, Dw13, Dw14, Dw15, Dw17, Dw23	. . .
DRB5*0101	DR51	Dw2	DR2A Dw2
DRB5*0102	DR51	Dw12	DR2A Dw12
DRB5*0201	DR51	Dw21	DR2A Dw21
DRB5*0202	DR51	Dw22	DR2A Dw22
DRB6*0101	. . .	. . .	DRBσ*0101, DRBX11
DRB6*0201	. . .	. . .	DRBX21, DRBVI
DRB6*0202	. . .	. . .	DRBσ*0201, DRBX22, DRB6III

groups. Most HLA alleles occur in all ethnic groups, and only very few if any HLA alleles are limited to a single ethnic group. The frequency of an HLA allele also varies within an ethnic group, dependent on the geographic location of the population.

The antigen phenotype frequency for a given HLA-allele in a population can be converted to an estimation of the gene frequency in the population according to the formula:

$$g = 1 - \sqrt{1-f}$$

where g is the gene frequency and f is the antigen phenotype frequency in the population (41). The expected frequency (h) for a given HLA-A, HLA-B haplotype would then be $h = p \times q$, where p is the gene frequency for the HLA-A allele and q is the gene frequency for the HLA-B allele. When such calculations are performed for different combinations of

Table 4-4.
Designations of HLA-DQ Alleles

HLA Alleles	*HLA-DQ Serological Specificities*	*HLA-D–associated (T cell–defined) Specificities*	*Previous Equivalents*
DQA1*0101	...	Dw1,w9	DQA 1.1,1.9
DQA1*0102	...	Dw2,w21,w19	DQA 1.2,1.19,1.AZH
DQA1*0103	...	Dw18,w12,w8,Dw'FS'	DQA 1.3, 1.18, DRw8-DQw1
DQA1*0104	...	...	...
DQA1*0201	...	Dw7,w11	DQA 2,3.7
DQA1*03011	...	Dw4,w10,w13,w14,w15	DQA 3,3.1,3.2
DQA1*03012	...	Dw23	DQA 3,3.1,3.2,DR9-DQw3
DQA1*0302	...	Dw23	DQA 3,3.1, 3.2, DR9-DQw3
DQA1*0401	...	Dw8,Dw"RSH"	DQA 4.2,3.8
DQA1*0501[e]	...	Dw3,w5,w22	DQA 4.1,2
DQA1*05011	...	Dw3	DQA 4.1,2
DQA1*05012	...	Dw5	DQA 4.1,2
DQA1*05013	...	Dw22	DQA 4.1,2
DQA1*0601	...	Dw8	DQA 4.3
DQB1*0501	DQ5(1)	Dw1	DQB 1.1, DRw10-DQw1.1
DQB1*0502	DQ5(1)	Dw21	DQB 1.2, 1.21
DQB1*05031	DQ5(1)	Dw9	DQB 1.3, 1.9, 1.3.1
DQB1*05032	DQ5(1)	Dw9	DQB 1.3, 1.9, 1.3.2
DQB1*0504	...	...	DQB 1.9
DQB1*0601	DQ6(1)	D12,w8	DQB 1.4, 1.12
DQB1*0602	DQ6(1)	Dw2	DQB 1.5, 1.25
DQB1*0603	DQ6(1)	Dw18, Dw"FS'	DQB 1.6, 1.18
DQB1*0604	DQ6(1)	Dw19	DQB 1.7, 1.19
DQB1*0605	DR6(1)	Dw19	DQB 1.8, DQBSLE, 1.19b, 2013–24
DQB1*0606	...	...	DQB1*WA1
DQB1*0201	DQ2	Dw3, w7	DQB 2
DQB1*0301	DQ7(3)	Dw4, w5, w8, w13	DQB3.1
DQB1*0302	DQ8(3)	Dw4, w10, w13, w14	DQB 3.2
DQB1*03031	DQ9(3)	Dw23	DQB 3.3
DQB1*03032	DQ9(3)	Dw23, w11	DQB 3.3
DQB1*0304	DQ7(3)	...	DQB1*03HP,*03new
DQB1*0401	DO4	Dw15	DQB 4.1, Wa
DQB1*0402	DQ4	Dw8, Dw'RSH'	DOB 4.2, Wa

HLA-A and HLA-B alleles, it is found that the expected HLA-A, HLA-B haplotype frequencies in most instances differ from the observed frequencies in the population. The difference between the expected and the observed haplotype frequencies (i.e., $h - pq \neq 0$) is called the DELTA value and is a numerical representation of the phenomenon of genetic linkage disequilibrium. Genetic linkage disequilibrium is also called nonrandom gametic association. If a DELTA value is greater than 0, the genetic linkage disequilibrium is termed *positive;* if it is less than 0 it is termed *negative.* If the DELTA value for a particular HLA-A, HLA-B haplotype is positive, the HLA haplotype occurs in the population with a frequency that is higher than expected from the gene frequencies of the alleles in the population. Similarly, if the DELTA value is negative, the HLA-A, HLA-B haplotype occurs less frequently than expected from the gene frequencies of the HLA-A and the HLA-B alleles in the population.

As a result of differences in HLA antigen frequencies among populations and differences in genetic linkage disequilibrium between the different alleles in the populations, there are major ethnic differences in HLA antigen frequencies as well as differences in HLA haplotype frequencies in different geographic regions, even within the same ethnic group. The phenomenon of genetic linkage disequilibrium occurs throughout the HLA complex: There is genetic linkage disequilibrium between HLA-A, HLA-C, HLA-B, HLA-DR, and HLA-DQ. In some instances, genetic linkage disequilibrium has been observed to extend to the alleles at the HLA-DP locus. A complete description of HLA antigen frequencies and HLA haplotypes observed within ethnic groups is beyond the scope of this chapter. A few typical examples are described to illustrate the extensive degree of HLA polymorphism and how this impacts on the degree of histocompatibility testing needed for HLA matching of two unrelated individuals.

The most common HLA-A antigen is A2, with 12 different alleles (A*0201–A*0212). A2 is the most common HLA antigen in Caucasoids, where the A*0201 allele accounts for 96% of the A2 antigens. A2 is also the most common HLA-A antigen in Negroids, where it has a frequency similar to A30. A24 is the most common

Table 4-5.
Designations of HLA-DP Alleles

HLA Alleles	*Associated HLA-DP Specificities*	*Previous Equivalents*
DPA1*0101	...	LB14/LB24,DPA1
DPA1*0102	...	pSCα-318
DPA1*0103	...	DPw4α1
DPA1*0201	...	DPA2,pDAα13B
DPA1*02021	...	2.21
DPA1*02022	...	2.22
DPA1*0301	...	3.1
DPA1*0401	...	4.1
DPB1*0101	DPw1	DPB1,DPw1a
DPB1*0201	DPw2	DPB2.1
DPB1*02011	DPw2	DPB2.1
DPB1*02012	DPw2	DPB2.1
DPB1*0202	DPw2	DPB2.2
DPB1*0301	DPw3	DPB3
DPB1*0401	DPw4	DPB4.1,DPw4a
DPB1*0402	DPw4	DPB4.2,DPw4b
DPB1*0501	DPw5	DPB5
DPB1*0601	DPw6	DPB6
DPB1*0801	...	DPB8
DPB1*0901	...	DPB9,DP'Cp63'
DPB1*1001	...	DPB10
DPB1*1101	...	DPB11
DPB1*1301	...	DPB13
DPB1*1401	...	DPB14
DPB1*1501	...	DPB15
DPB1*1601	...	DPB16
DPB1*1701	...	DPB17
DPB1*1801	...	DPB18
DPB1*1901	...	DPB19
DPB1*2001	...	Oos, DPB-JA
DPB1*2101	...	DPB-GM, DPB30, NewD
DPB1*2201	...	DPB1*AB1,NewH
DPB1*2301	...	DPB32,NewB
DPB1*2401	...	DPB33,NewC
DPB1*2501	...	DPB34,NewE
DPB1*2601	...	DPB31, WA2
DPB1*2701	...	DPB23, WA3
DPB1*2801	...	DPB21
DPB1*2901	...	DPB27, NewG
DPB1*3001	...	DPB28
DPB1*3101	...	DPB22,NewF
DPB1*3201	...	DPB24,NewI
DPB1*3301	...	DPB25
DPB1*3401	...	DPB26
DPB1*3501	...	DPB29
DPB1*3601	...	New A,SSK2

HLA-A antigen in Mongoloids, where A2 is the second most common HLA-A antigen. A*0201 is also the most frequent A2 allele in Negroid and Mongoloid populations. A*0202 has so far been observed only in Blacks, and A*0203 and A*0207 only in Chinese, but population data on A2 alleles are currently limited (42). The HLA-B antigens, B8, B7, and B44, are very common among Caucasians of Northern European and British extraction. The HLA haplotypes A1;B8;DR3, A3;B7;-DR2, A29;B44;DR7, and A2;B44;DR4 are particularly common in this ethnic subpopulation. In contrast, the HLA haplotypes A30 or A31;B18;DR3, A1;B57;DR7, A30 or A31;B13,DR7, and A2;B18;DR13 are common in Southern European populations. The HLA haplotypes A24;B14;DR1, A33;B14;DR1, and A26;B38;DR4 are frequently found in Ashkenazi Jews. Some HLA haplotypes are observed nearly exclusively among Caucasians; for example, A3;B47;DR7 (which carries a deletion of the CYP21B gene) and A25;B18;DR2 (which carries a null allele at the complement C2 gene in the HLA class III region) (Table 4-6).

It has become possible to identify precisely the HLA alleles by determining the nucleotide sequences encoding the molecules. The previously described analysis of HLA-A2 alleles illustrates this process. Similarly, at least two B*44 alleles, *4401 and *4403, exist. B*4401 is common in all ethnic groups, whereas B*4403 is observed only very rarely in non-Caucasian individuals. HLA-B13 has two alleles: *1301 and *1302; *1301 is the Mongoloid and *1302 is the Caucasian allele (43). This distinction is very important with regard to matching by HLA typing for organ or tissue transplantation. For example, a potential Caucasian donor for an Oriental patient, both having the HLA haplotype A2;B13;DR7, will most likely be different for the two HLA-B13 alleles. The potential Caucasian donor could furthermore also be different from the Oriental recipient for the A2 allele A*0201, which is the most likely Caucasian allele, and the patient could carry the A*0203 allele, which is commonly observed in Chinese. Another example of common HLA antigen incompatibilities undetected by conventional HLA typing by serological methods is illustrated by the example of two unrelated Caucasian individuals with the HLA genotype, A2;B44;DR7/A29;B44;DR7. Due to genetic linkage disequilibrium within HLA, the most likely combination of HLA alleles would be A*0201;-B*4403;DRB1*0701/A*2902;B*4401;DRB1*0701, because A*0201;B*4403 and A*2902;B*4401 are very common Caucasian HLA haplotypes with strong

Table 4-6.
HLA-A, HLA-B, and HLA-DR Haplotypes: Caucasoids

HLA-A	*HLA-B*	*HLA-DR*
1	8	3
3	7	2
2 or 24	7	2
29	44	7
23	44	7
2	44	4
2	44	2 or 11
30 or 31	18	3
2	18	11
3 or 11	35	1
...	35	2, 4, 11, 13, 14
2	62	4 or 11
1 or 24	61	2 or 8
2 or 30	13	7
2	51	2 or 11
1	57	7
1	41	8

positive genetic linkage disequilibrium. However, the allele combination A*0201;B*4401 also occurs with reasonable frequency. The identification of homozygosity for B*4401 or heterozygosity for B*4401/B*4403 in both the potential donor and the recipient should be determined (44).

Population analysis for HLA antigens in different Oriental and other Mongoloid groups has increased during the last 10 years, and the information currently available is of the same depth as for Caucasian populations. The most common HLA antigen in Orientals is A24. The HLA haplotype A24;B54;DR4 is very common in Japanese, as is A24;B52;DR2. A characteristic Mongoloid HLA-B antigen is B46, which so far has been identified in only very few Caucasian individuals. The HLA haplotype A2;B46;DR8 is characteristic for Japanese, whereas A2;B46;DR9 is the characteristic Chinese B46-positive haplotype. Other characteristic Oriental haplotypes are A33;B58;DR3, A2;B59;DR4, and B7;DR1. Other common HLA haplotypes occurring in Mongoloid populations have the HLA-B antigens B35, B39, B60, B61 and B51 (Table 4-7). The HLA-B antigens B75, B76, and B77, which genetically are closely related to B62, are characteristic for individuals from Southeast Asia (e.g., Thailand). Two different B56 alleles have been identified, of which B*5601 is preferentially observed in Japanese, whereas B*5602 is typical in Caucasians. B48 is most common in the Mongoloid, Eskimo population, whereas B*4005 (BN) is typical for Native American Indians and Mexicans.

Population studies of Negroid populations are limited. Most data are available for African-American Black populations and South African Blacks. Some typical HLA haplotypes observed in these populations are listed in Table 4-8. The A36 antigen, which is closely related to A1, is most commonly observed on the A36;B53;DR11 haplotype. Another characteristic haplotype is A30;B42;DR3. This haplotype nearly always carries the DRB1*0302 or DRB1*0303 alleles, which are the two DRB1*03 alleles encoding the serological specificity DR18. The characteristic Caucasian DRB1*03 allele is DRB1*0301, which encodes the serological specificity DR17. The HLA-A antigens A34, A43, and A66 are serologically related to A10 and are identified in South African Blacks. A74 is serologically related to the A19 antigens (A29, A30, A31, A32, A33) and typically occurs on the HLA haplotype A74;B72;DR3.

Table 4-7.
HLA-A, HLA-B, HLA-DR Haplotypes: Mongoloids

HLA-A	*HLA-B*	*HLA-DR*
24	52	2
24	52	4
24	54	4
2 or 11	54	4
. . .	54	2 or 14
24	7	1
2	7	1
2 or 30	13	7 or 12
2, 11, or 24	35	4
. . .	35	2, 9, or 12
2	46	8
2	46	9
33	58	3
2	59	4
2 or 24	60	12 or 14
2, 24, or 26	61	9 or 11
2	62	2 or 9
11	62	4

Table 4-8.
HLA-A, HLA-B, HLA-DR Haplotypes: Negroids[a]

HLA-A	*HLA-B*	*HLA-DR*
36	58	11
2, 3, or 28	58	11 or 14
11 or 24	35	1 or 14
1	8	3
30	42	3
74	72	3
. . .	72	7 or 11
28	14	7
3	7	2
. . .	7	1 or 13
. . .	49	11

[a]HLA antigens predominantly observed in negroid populations: A34, 43, 66 (A10-like antigens); A74 (A19-like antigen); A36 (A1-like antigen).

Polymorphism and Genetic Linkage Disequilibrium in the HLA Class II Region

All currently known class II molecules (HLA-DR, HLA-DQ, and HLA-DP) are highly polymorphic, and the class II alleles are listed in Tables 4-3, 4-4, and 4-5 (45–49). The polymorphism in the HLA-DR molecules is due to allelic variations in the DRB genes, whereas HLA-DQ and HLA-DP polymorphism is caused by allelic variation in both the α-chain genes and the β-chain genes. There is extensive genetic linkage disequilibrium within the HLA-DR/HLA-DQ region. The DRB alleles, which nonrandomly associate with particular DQA and DQB alleles, vary among ethnic groups, and significant geographic variations exist within one ethnic group. Examples of typical DR-DQ haplotypes are shown in Tables 4-9, 4-10, 4-11, and 4-12. These tables also indicate the major ethnic groups in which the haplotypes are commonly observed. There are, however, numerous other DR-DQ haplotypes, and the association to ethnic groups is far from absolute. The examples of DR-DQ haplotypes listed in these four tables are grouped according to their supertypic serological HLA-DR specificity (i.e., generic HLA-DR specificity). Table 4-9 provides an example of 8 different DR-DQ haplotypes, which all encode the serological, supertypic HLA-DR specificity, DR2. Four of these haplotypes encode the supertypic serological specificity DR15, and 4 encode the DR16 specificity. The 8 DR2 haplotypes, however, are only the most com-

Table 4-9.
DRB1, DRB5, DQA1, and DQB1 Haplotypes Associated with HLA-DR1, HLA-DR2, and HLA-DR10

DR Specificity	HLA-DRB Allele		HLA-DQ Allele		Ethnic Association		
	*DRB1**	*DRB5**	*DQA1**	*DQB1**	*C*	*N*	*M*
DR1	0101	. . .	0101	0501	+	+	+
	0102	. . .	0101	0501	+	+	+
	0103	. . .	0101	0501	+		
DR10	1001	. . .	0101	0501	+	+	+
DR15	1501	0101	0102	0602	+	+	+
	1502	0102	0103	0601	+		+
	1502	0101	0102	0601			+
	1503	0101	0102	0602		+	
DR16	1601	0201	0102	0502	+		
	1602	0202	0102	0502			+
	1602	0101	0102	0502		+	+
	1602	0202	0501	0301			+

monly observed, and the ethnic association of a given DR-DQ haplotype is indicated only as a general guide. For example, the haplotype DRB1*1503-DRB5*0101-DQA1*0102-DQB1*0602 is commonly found among African-American Blacks but can also be observed in Caucasians.

The genetic linkage disequilibrium within the DR-DQ subregion of the HLA class II region sometimes extends to the HLA-DP region. Genetic linkage disequilibrium spanning from HLA-DR to HLA-DP is currently established for very few haplotypes. For example, in Caucasians, the HLA-haplotypes B*0801-DRB1*0301-DQA1*0501-DQB1*0201-DPB1*0101 and B*4401-DRB1*07-DQA1*0201-DQB1*0201-DPB1*1101

Table 4-10.
DRB1, DRB3, DQA1, and DQB1 Haplotypes Associated with HLA-DR3 and HLA-DR6

DR Specificity		HLA-DRB Allele		HLA-DQ Allele		Ethnic Association		
		*DRB1**	*DRB3**	*DQA1**	*DQB1**	*C*	*N*	*M*
DR3								
	DR17	0301	0101	0501	0201	+	+	
	DR17	0301	0202	0501	0201	+	+	+
	DR18	0302	0101	0401	0402		+	
DR6								
	DR13	1301	0101	0103	0603	+	+	+
		1302	0301	0102	0604	+	+	
		1302	0301	0102	0501	+	+	
		1303	0101	0501	0301	+	+	
		1303	0101	0201	0201		+	
		1305	0101	0201	0201		+	
	DR14							
		1401	0202	0101	0503	+	+	+
		1401	0202	0101	0602		+	
		1402	0101	0501	0301			+
		1403	0101	0501	0301	+		+

Table 4-11.
DRB1, DRB3, DQA1, and DQB1 Haplotypes Associated with HLA-DR5 and HLA-DR8

DR Specificity		HLA-DRB Allele		HLA-DQB Allele		Ethnic Association		
		*DRB1**	*DRB3**	*DQA1**	*DQB1**	*C*	*N*	*M*
DR5								
	DR11	1101	0202	0501	0301	+	+	+
		1101	0202	0102	0602	+	+	
		1102	0202	0501	0301	+	+	
		1102	0301	0501	0301		+	
		1103	0202	0501	0301	+		
		1104	0202	0501	0301	+	+	
	DR12	1201	0202	0501	0301	+	+	+
		1201	0202	0101	0501	+	+	
		1201	0101	0101	0501		+	
		1202	0301	0601	0301			+
DR8		0801	. . .	0401	0402	+	+	
		0802	. . .	0401	0402	+		+
		0803	. . .	0103	0601			+
		0804	. . .	0401	0402	+	+	

illustrate extended HLA haplotypes where genetic linkage disequilibrium exists for the HLA alleles from the HLA-B locus to the HLA-DPB locus. Similarly, in Japan, the HLA haplotype A24-B52-DRB1*1502-DQA1*0103-DQB1*0601-DPB1*0901 is characteristic for this ethnic subgroup.

Clinical Histocompatibility Testing

Clinical histocompatibility testing, which is commonly referred to as "tissue typing," is the determination of an individual's HLA class I and II specificities (50). Such testings are routinely performed for the purpose of HLA matching of donors and recipients for organ and tissue transplantation.

Table 4-12.
DRB1, DQA1, and DQB1 Haplotypes Associated with HLA-DR4, HLA-DR7, and HLA-DR9

DR Specificity	HLA-DRB Allele	HLA-DQ Allele		Ethnic Association		
	*HLA DRB1**	*DQA1**	*DQB1**	*C*	*N*	*M*
DR4	0401	0301	0301	+		+
	0401	0301	0302	+		+
	0402	0301	0302	+	+	+
	0403	0301	0301	+		
	0404	0301	0302	+		
	0405	0301	0302		+	+
	0406	0301	0302			+
	0407	0301	0302	+		
DR7	0701	0201	0201	+	+	+
	0701	0201	0303	+	+	+
	0701	0301	0201		+	
DR9	0901	0301	0201	+	+	
	0901	0301	0303	+		+

Table 4-13.
Complete Listing of Recognized HLA Specificities

A	*B*	*C*	*D*	*DR*	*DQ*	*DP*
A1	B5	Cw1	Dw1	DR1	DQ1	DPw1
A2	B7	Cw2	Dw2	DR103	DQ2	DPw2
A203	B703	Cw3	Dw3	DR2	DQ3	DPw3
A210	B8	Cw4	Dw4	DR3	DQ4	DPw4
A3	B12	Cw5	Dw5	DR4	DQ5(1)	DPw5
A9	B13	Cw6	Dw6	DR5	DQ6(1)	DPw6
A10	B14	Cw7	Dw7	DR6	DQ7(3)	
A11	B15	Cw8	Dw8	DR7	DQ8(3)	
A19	B16	Cw9(w3)	Dw9	DR8	DQ9(3)	
A23(9)	B17	Cw10(w3)	Dw10	DR9		
A24(9)	B18		Dw11(w7)	DR10		
A2403	B21		Dw12	DR11(5)		
A25(10)	B22		Dw13	DR12(5)		
A26(10)	B27		Dw14	DR13(6)		
A28	B35		Dw15	DR14(6)		
A29(19)	B37		Dw16	DR1403		
A30(19)	B38(16)		Dw17(w7)	DR1404		
A31(19)	B39(16)		Dw18(w6)	DR15(2)		
A32(19)	B3901		Dw19(w6)	DR16(2)		
A33(19)	B3902		Dw20	DR17(3)		
A34(10)	B40		Dw21	DR18(3)		
A36	B4005		Dw22			
A43	B41		Dw23	DR51		
A66(10)	B42					
A68(28)	B44(12)		Dw24	DR52		
A69(28)	B45(12)		Dw25			
A74(19)	B46		Dw26	DR53		
	B47					
	B48					
	B49(21)					
	B50(21)					
	B51(5)					
	B5102					
	B5103					
	B52(5)					
	B53					
	B54(22)					
	B55(22)					
	B56(22)					
	B57(17)					
	B58(17)					
	B59					
	B60(40)					
	B61(40)					
	B62(15)					
	B63(15)					
	B64(14)					
	B65(14)					
	B67					
	B70					
	B71(70)					
	B72(70)					
	B73					
	B75(15)					
	B76(15)					
	B77(15)					
	B7801					
	Bw4					
	B46					

The HLA class I molecules are expressed on most somatic cells. The amount of class I antigen expressed on different tissues varies greatly. Some cells (e.g., endocrine cells) express a very small amount and some cells (e.g., corneal endothelium and villous trophoblasts) express no class I antigens. Erythrocytes have minimal if any class I antigens, whereas lymphocytes, granulocytes, monocytes, and even platelets express class I antigens. The HLA class II antigens are expressed only on some cells, mostly "professional" antigen-presenting cells such as B lymphocytes, monocytes, macrophages, dendritic cells, and Langerhans cells of the skin. HLA-A, HLA-B, and HLA-C typing can be performed readily on peripheral blood T and B lymphocytes, whereas serological typing for HLA-DR and HLA-DQ antigens is performed on B lymphocytes. HLA typing by serology is routinely performed using highly selected, HLA antigen-specific alloantisera or monoclonal antibodies. Most commonly, complement fixing, cytotoxic antibodies are used in the complement-dependent lymphocytotoxicity assay. HLA-DP antigens cannot be identified by this procedure due to lack of high-quality HLA-DP-specific antibodies. A complete listing of currently recognized HLA specificities detected by serological methods is given in Table 4-13. Some HLA specificities are broad, supertypic antigens. For example, the HLA-A9 specificity can be detected by some antisera, however, the A9 group of antigens can be further divided into A23(9) and A24(9) (the broad specificity is indicated in parentheses). Similarly, HLA-A10 can be further divided into the HLA-A specificities A25(10), A26(10), A34(10), and A66(10). A listing of broad HLA antigen specificities and their subdivisions and associated antigens is given in Table 4-14.

The alloantibodies that detect the Bw4 and Bw6 HLA epitopes illustrate a different phenomenon. Bw4 and Bw6 are serologically detectable, mutually exclusive epitopes present on nearly all HLA-B molecules and on a few HLA-A molecules. The distribution of the Bw4 and Bw6 epitopes among the HLA class I antigens is shown in Table 4-15. The Bw4 and Bw6 epitopes are due to nucleotide substitutions within codons 77 to 83 of the α_1-helix of the class I heavy chain molecule. The Bw4 motif (amino acid sequence) in this region is NLRIALR, and the Bw6 motif is SLRNLRG.

Cellular In Vitro Assays Detecting Alloreactivity

Identification of HLA class II region products (i.e., the HLA-D region) was originally made by their capacity to induce T-lymphocyte activation in vitro in the mixed lymphocyte culture (MLC) reaction (reviewed in 51). The MLC test is routinely performed using mixtures of peripheral blood mononuclear cells (PBMC) from two different individuals, during which the PBMC from the alloantigen-presenting donor (i.e., stimulator cells) are prevented from cell proliferation by inactivation with irradiation. Cell proliferation in the responder cells is measured by incorporation of ^{3}H- or ^{14}C-labeled thymidine. It is well established that MLC tests between HLA-genotypically identical siblings do not result in cell proliferation. This assay system is commonly used for confirmation of HLA identity in family studies. Modifications in the MLC test using cells from HLA-D region homozygous cell donors as stimulator cells (i.e., HLA-D homozygous typing cells [HTC]) have been used as a typing

Table 4-14.
Broad HLA Specificities, "Splits," and Associated Antigens

Original Broad Specificities[a]	*Splits and Associated Antigens*[b]
A2	A203#, A210#
A9	A23,A24,A2403#
A10	A25,A26,A34,A66
A19	A29,A30,A31,A32,A33,A74
A28	A68,A69
B5	B51,B52
B7	B703#
B12	B44,B45
B14	B64,B65
B15	B62,B63,B75,B76,B77
B16	B38,B39,B3901#,B3902#
B17	B57,B58
B21	B49,B50,B4005#
B22	B54,B55,B56
B40	B60,B61
B70	B71,B72
Cw3	Cw9,Cw10
DR1	DR103#
DR2	DR15,DR16
DR3	DR17,DR18
DR5	DR11,DR12
DR6	DR13,DR14,DR1403#,DR1404#
DQ1	DQ5,DQ6
DQ3	DQ7,DQ8,DQ9
Dw6	Dw18,Dw19
Dw7	Dw11,Dw17

[a]The listing of broad specificities in parentheses after a narrow specificity (e.g., HLA-A23(9)) is optional.
[b]The following is a list of those specificities that arose as clear-cut splits of other specificities and of associated antigens (#), which are variants of the orginial broad specificity and not splits as previously defined.

Table 4-15.
Bw4 and Bw6 Epitopes and Associated Specificities

Epitope	*Associated Specificities*
Bw4	B5,B5102,B5103
	B13, B17, B27, B37, B38(16), B44(12), B47, B49(21), B51(15), B52(5), B53, B57(17), B58(17), B59, B63(15), B77(15)
	A9, A23(9), A24(9), A2403, A25(10), A32(19)
Bw6	B7, B703, B8, B14, B18, B22, B35, B39(16), B3901, B3902, B40, B4005, B41, B42, B45(12), B46, B48, B50(21), B54(22), B55(22), B56(22), B60(40), B61(40), B62(15), B64(14), B67, B70, B71(70), B72(70), B73, B75(15), B76(15), B7801

procedure for HLA-D, and the HLA-Dw specificities listed in Table 4-13 were defined by this methodology.

Another functional in vitro assay for alloactivation of T cells was used for the identification of the HLA-DPw specificities (see Table 4-13). It is now well established that the HLA class II region is composed of many expressed class II genes, and all HLA class II molecules can induce alloactivation of T cells (52). The cellular in vitro assays for alloreactivity, such as MLC testing, HTC typing for HLA-Dw, and primed lymphocyte typing (PLT) for detection of HLA-DPw specificities, therefore do not provide the exact and unambiguous assignment of HLA class II region alleles as the DNA typing procedures. It is, for example, well recognized that the HLA-DR antigens are responsible for most of the T-cell activation which occurs in the MLC test, but a contribution of HLA-DQ antigens and probably also HLA-DP antigens may occur under certain conditions. The MLC test is therefore a very valuable supplemental test for confirmation of HLA-D region identity among HLA-genotypically identical siblings and is also a useful assay for establishing HLA-D region compatibility between HLA-phenotypically identical relatives. The application of MLC testing for confirmation of HLA-D region compatibility among unrelated individuals is, however, not an efficient assay because of difficulties in data interpretation, particularly with regard to evaluation of nonresponsiveness in the MLC test. A large proportion of patients who are potential candidates for unrelated marrow transplantation suffer from leukemia or aplastic anemia, conditions in which peripheral blood mononuclear cells contain abnormal cells or abnormal distribution of T-lymphocyte subsets. This abnormality has an impact on the culture conditions in the in vitro assay and also affects the T-cell subsets responding in MLC. An enhanced contribution of minor histocompatibility antigen differences (e.g., differences in normal or abnormal self-peptides) to T-cell activation in the MLC test probably also occurs when performing the assay on PBMC between unrelated individuals. A significant proportion of MLC tests performed between unrelated, HLA-phenotypically identical pairs tested prior to BMT therefore result in false-positive and false-negative test results.

HLA-DNA Typing

The nucleotide sequences have been determined for the coding regions of all currently defined HLA class I and II alleles, and their allele designations are listed in Tables 4-2, 4-3, 4-4, and 4-5. During the years 1984 to 1988, DNA typing techniques for detection of HLA specificities were developed based on restriction fragment length polymorphism (RFLP). Most of the sites in genomic DNA where the restriction endonucleases act (i.e., the restriction sites) are located in the introns of the HLA genes, and the RFLP obtained primarily reflect genetic linkage disequilibrium between the location of the restriction sites and the allelic variation in the coding regions (i.e., exons) of the HLA genes (53). Therefore, HLA typing by RFLP is at best an indirect measurement of presence or absence of a given HLA allele. The technical breakthrough resulting in the development of the DNA polymerase chain reaction (PCR) (54,55) has made it possible to amplify a particular gene or a gene segment by the use of synthetic oligonucleotide primers and DNA-polymerase. It is therefore possible to construct DNA primers by selecting nucleotide sequences within the individual HLA class I and II genes that will amplify the DNA corresponding to a single HLA gene (56,57). The specific HLA allele present in this gene can then be identified by nucleotide sequence analysis of the coding region. Although an HLA typing procedure based on complete sequencing of the extracellular domains of the individual HLA allele is the ultimate goal for clinical histocompatibility testing, such a technique has not yet been developed for practical, large-scale application.

Currently, HLA-DNA typing for HLA class II alleles is routinely performed with techniques utilizing a combination of PCR amplification of HLA genes and allele-specific or sequence-specific oligonucleotides for identification of absence or presence of a particular nucleotide sequence within one allele. The most commonly used technique applied for DNA typing of HLA-DR, HLA-DQ, and HLA-DP alleles is called PCR-SSOP typing (45–49). In this test, the HLA class II gene segment corresponding to the most variable domain of the coding region is PCR-amplified (e.g., exon 2 for the DR genes). Sequence-specific oligonucleotide probes (SSOPs) corresponding to the different HLA-DR alleles or combinations of alleles are then tested for hybridization to the amplified DNA. If hybridization occurs with one SSOP, it signifies that the nucleotide sequence corresponding to the SSOP is present in the HLA-DR allele. The hybridization pattern obtained with a set of SSOPs defines the presence or absence of one particular HLA allele. There are several variations of this technique; one variation utilizes allele-specific DNA amplification, where the SSOP is used as a primer in the DNA amplification.

The PCR-SSOP HLA class II typing technique can be designed according to particular clinical needs. It may, for example, only be necessary to obtain HLA class II information for HLA-DR at a level of resolution corresponding to the HLA-DR specificities listed in Table 4-13. PCR-SSOP typing corresponding to this level of DR typing is commonly referred to as "generic DR typing." An initial screening at this level of potential unrelated donor-recipient pairs is commonly performed to reduce the number of potential donors on whom detailed HLA-DR allele specific typing is performed.

A similar PCR-SSOP technique for HLA class I typing is currently being developed and may be introduced in clinical histocompatibility testing during the coming years.

Conclusions

Histocompatibility and alloreactivity are very large topics covering most areas of modern immunology, including immunogenetics. It is not possible to comprehensively discuss all the different subjects in depth, and interested readers may wish to gain more specific details. The accompanying list of references has been selected with this in mind. Some of the references refer to historically important original publications; others refer to recent comprehensive reviews for a particular area. Finally, some references have been selected because they contain recent information on HLA alleles and nucleotide sequencing or particularly useful reference lists. The most comprehensive publications on HLA immunogenetics and analysis of HLA polymorphism are contained in a series of publications entitled "Histocompatibility Testing," which has been published following each of the 11 International Histocompatibility Workshops (1964–1991). This chapter was written specially to inform clinical investigators, practicing hematologists, and others who wish to obtain background information on histocompatibility testing in relation to BMT. It is well established that HLA-genotypically identical siblings are the preferred allogeneic marrow donors for patients. It is also known that HLA-phenotypically identical combinations can be used and the outcome of such transplants is very similar to the HLA-identical sibling group. The dramatic increase in the number of HLA-matched unrelated BMTs performed since 1987 demonstrates that this approach for donor selection is feasible. The level of HLA matching needed for successful unrelated BMT with a clinical outcome similar to HLA-identical related combinations is currently unknown. The establishment of such requirements is one of the most important goals for the immediate future.

References

1. Gorer PA. The detection of antigenic differences in mouse enythrocytes by employment of immune sera. Br Med Bull 1936;17:50–53.
2. Klein J. The natural history of the major histocompatibility complex. New York: Wiley and Sons, 1986.
3. Zinkernagel RM, Doherty PC. MHC-restricted cytotoxic T-cells: studies on the biological role of polymorphic major transplantation antigens determining T-cell restriction specificity, function, and responsiveness. Adv Immunol 1979;27:51–177.
4. Unanue ER. Antigen-presenting function of the macrophage. Annu Rev Immunol 1984;2:395–428.
5. Townsend A, Bodmer H. Antigen recognition by class I-restricted T lymphocytes. Annu Rev Immunol 1989;7: 601–624.
6. Maryanski JL, Verdini AS, Weber PC, Salemme FR, Corradin G. Competitor analogs for defined T cell antigens: peptides incorporating a putative binding motif and polyproline or polyglycine spacers. Cell 1990;60:63–72.
7. Van Bleek GM, Nathenson SG. Isolation of an endogenously processed immunodominant viral peptide from the class I H-2K^b molecule. Nature 1990;348:213–216.
8. Falk K, Rotzschke O, Stevanovic S, Jung G, Rammensee H-G. Allele-specific motifs revealed by sequencing of self-peptides eluted from MHC molecules. Nature 1991;351:290–296.
9. Jardetzky TS, Lane WS, Robinson RA, Madden DR, Wiley DC. Identification of self peptides bound to purified HLA-B27. Nature 1991;353:326–329.
10. Jardetzky TS, Gorga JC, Busch R, Rothbard J, Strominger JL, Wiley DC. Peptide binding to HLA-DR1: a peptide with most residues substituted to alanine retains MHC binding. EMBO J 1990;9:1797–1803.
11. Rudensky AY, Preston-Hurlburt P, Hong S-C, Barlow A, Janeway CA Jr. Sequence analysis of peptides bound to MHC class II molecules. Nature 1991;353:622–627.
12. Bjorkman, PJ, Saper MA, Samraoui B, Bennett WS, Strominger JL, Wiley DC. Structure of human class I histocompatibility antigen, HLA-A2. Nature 1987;329: 506–512.
13. Brown JH, Jardetzky T, Saper MA, Samraoui B, Bjorkman PJ, Wiley DC. A hypothetical model of the foreign antigen binding site of class II histocompatibility molecules. Nature 1988;332:845–850.
14. Long EO. Antigen processing for presentation to CD4$^+$ T cells. New Biologist 1992;4:274–282.
15. Brodsky FM, Guagliardi LE. The cell biology of antigen processing and presentation. Annu Rev Immunol 1991;9:707–744.
16. Goldberg AL, Rock KL. Proteolysis, proteasomes and antigen presentation. Nature 1992;357:375–379.
17. Monaco JJ, McDevitt HO. Identification of a fourth class of proteins linked to the murine major histocompatibility complex. Proc Natl Acad Sci USA 1982;79: 3001–3005.
18. Brown MG, Driscoll J, Monaco JJ. Structural and serological similarity of MHC-linked LMP and proteasome (multicatalytic proteinase) complexes. Nature 1991;353:355–357.
19. Spies T, Bresnhan M, Bahram S, et al. A gene in the human major histocompatibility complex class II region controlling the class I antigen presentation pathway. Nature 1990;348:744–747.
20. Powis SJ, Townsend ARM, Deverson EV, et al. Restoration of antigen presentation to the mutant cell line RMA-S by an MHC-linked transporter. Nature 1991; 354:529–531.
21. Monaco JJ, Cho S, Attaya M. Transport protein genes in the murine MHC: possible implications for antigen processing. Science 1990;250:1723–1726.
22. Higgins CF, Hiles ID, Salmond GPC, et al. A family of related ATP-binding subunits coupled to many distinct biological processes in bacteria. Nature 1986;323:448–450.
23. Allen PM, Babbitt BP, Unanue ER. T-cell recognition of lysozyme: the biochemical basis of presentation. Immunol Rev 1987;98:171–187.
24. Teyton L, Peterson PA. Invariant chain: a regulator of antigen presentation. Trends Cell Biol 1992;2:52–56.
25. Medawar PB. The behaviour and fate of skin autografts and skin homografts in rabbits. J Anat 1944;78:176–199.
26. Billingham RE, Brent L, Medawar PB. Actively acquired tolerance of foreign cells. Nature 1953;172:603–606.
27. Hasek M. Parabiosis of birds during embryonic development. Cesk Biol 1953;265–270.
28. Michison NA. Passive transfer of transplantation immunity. Proc R Soc Lond 1954;142:72–87.

29. Miller JFAP. Effect of neonatal thymectomy on the immunological responsiveness of the mouse. Proc R Soc Lond [Biol] 1962;156:415–428.
30. Good RA, Dalmasso AP, Martinez C, Archer OK, Pierce JC, Papermaster BW. The role of the thymus in development of immunologic capacity in rabbits and mice. J Exp Med 1962;116:773–795.
31. Lombardi G, Sidhu S, Batchelor JR, Lechler RI. Allorecognition of DR1 by T cells from a DR4/Drw13 responder mimics self-restricted recognition of endogenous peptides. Proc Natl Acad Sci USA 1989;86:4190–4194.
32. Singer A, Kruisbeck AM, Andrysiak PM. T cell accessory cell interactions that initiate allospecific cytoxic T lymphocyte responses: existence of both Ia-restriction and Ia-unrestricted cellular interaction pathways. J Immunol 1984;132:2199–2209.
33. Eckels DD, Gorski J, Rothbard J, Lamb JR. Peptide-mediated modulation of T cell allorecognition. Proc Natl Acad Sci USA 1988;85:8191–8195.
34. Matis LA, Sorger SB, McElligott DL, Fink PJ, Hedrick SM. The molecular basis of alloreactivity in antigen-specific histocompatibility complex–restricted T cell clones. Cell 1987;51:59–69.
35. McMichael AJ, Gotch FM, Santos-Aguado J, Strominger JL. Effect of mutations and variations of HLA-A2 on recognition of a virus peptide epitope by cytoxic T lymphocytes. Proc Natl Acad Sci USA 1988;85:9194–9198.
36. Jelachich ML, Cowen EP, Turner RV, Coligan JE, Biddison WE. Analysis of the molecular basis of HLA-A3 recognition by cytotoxic T cells using defined mutants of the HLA-A3 molecule. J Immunol 1989;141:1108–1113.
37. Hogan KT, Clayberger C, Bernhard EJ, et al. A panel of unique HLA-A2 mutant molecules define epitopes recognized by HLA-A2 specific antibodies and cytotoxic T lymphocytes. J Immunol 1989;142:2097–2104.
38. Santos-Aguado J, Crimmins MAV, Menzter SJ, Burakoff SJ, Strominger JL. Alloreactivity studied with mutants of HLA-A2. Proc Natl Acad Sci USA 1989;86:8936–8940.
39. Trowsdale J, Ragoussis J, Campbell RD. Map the human MHC. Immunology Today 1991;12:443–446.
40. Bodmer JG, Marsh SGE, Albert ED, et al. Nomenclature for factors of the HLA system. Tissue Antigens 1992; 39:161–173.
41. Mattiuz PL, Ihde D, Piazza A, Ceppellini R, Bodmer WF. New approaches for the population genetics and segregation analysis of the HL-A system. In: Terasaki PI, ed. Histocompatibility testing 1970. Copenhagen: Munksgaard, 1970:193–205.
42. Fernandez-Vina MA, Falco M, Sun Y, Stastny P. DNA typing for HLA class I alleles: I. Subsets of HLA-A2 and of -A28. Hum Immunol 1992;33:163–173.
43. Kato K, Dupont B, Young SY. Localization of nucleotide sequence which determines mongoloid subtype of HLA-B13. Immunogenetics 1989;29:117–120.
44. Fleischhauer K, Kernan NA, O'Reilly RJ, Dupont B, Yang SY. Bone marrow allograft rejection by allocytotoxic T lymphocytes recognizing a single amino acid in HLA-B44. New Engl J Med 1990;323:1818–1822.
45. Lee KW, Johnson AH, Hurley CK. Two divergent routes of evolution gave rise to the DRw13 haplotypes. J Immunol 1990;145:3119–3125.
46. Fernandez-Vina MA, Gao X, Moraes ME, et al. Alleles at four HLA class II loci determined by oligonucleotide hybridization and their associations in five ethnic groups. Immunogenetics 1991;34:299–312.
47. Gao X, Serjeantson SW. Heterogenity in HLA-DR2-related DR, DQ haplotypes in eight populations of Asia-Oceania. Immunogenetics 1991;34:401–408.
48. Schreuder GMTH, Van Berg-Loonen PM, Verdnyn W, et al. Increasing complexity of HLA-DR2 as detected by serology and oligonucleotide typing. Hum Immunol 1991;32:141–149.
49. Begovich AB, McClure GR, Suraj VC, et al. Polymorphism, recombination, and linkage disequilibrium within the HLA class II region. J Immunol 1992;148:249–258.
50. Zachary AA, Teresi GA, eds. Laboratory manual, ed 2. Lenexa: American Society for Histocompatibility and Immunogenetics, 1990.
51. Dupont B, Hansen JA, Yunis EJ. Human mixed lymphocyte culture reaction: genetics, specificity and biological implications. Adv Immunol 1976;23:107–202.
52. Flomenberg N. Functional polymorphisms of HLA class II gene products detected by T-lymphocyte clones: summary of the Tenth International Histocompatibility Workshop Cellular Studies. In: Dupont B, ed. Immunobiology of HLA, vol 1. Histocompatibility testing 1987. New York: Springer-Verlag, 1989:532–550.
53. Simons MJ, Wheeler R, Cohen D, LaLonel JM, Dupont B. Restriction fragment length polymorphism of HLA genes: summary of the Tenth International Workshop Southern Blot Analysis. In: Dupont B, ed. Immunobiology of HLA, vol 1. Histocompatibility testing 1987. New York: Springer-Verlag, 1989:959–1023.
54. Mullis KB, Faloona FA. Specific synthesis of DNA in vitro via a polymerase-catalysed chain reaction. Methods Enzymol 1987;155:335–350.
55. Saiki RK, Scharf S, Faloona FA, et al. Enzymatic amplification of β-globin genomic sequences and restriction site analysis for diagnosis of sickle cell anemia. Science 1985;230:1350–1354.
56. Zemmour J, Parham P. HLA class I nucleotide sequences, 1992. Tissue Antigens 1992;40(5):221–228.
57. Marsh SGE, Bodmer JG. HLA class II nucleotide sequences, 1992. Tissue Antigens 1992;40(5)229–243.

Chapter 5
Mechanisms of Human Hematopoiesis

Hans A. Messner and Ernest A. McCulloch

Allogeneic and autologous bone marrow transplantations (BMTs) have become the treatment of choice for a number of malignant and nonmalignant blood disorders, and more recently for some solid tumors. Transplants are performed to reconstitute marrow function in patients with hematological and immunological deficiencies, to treat hematopoietic malignancies, to correct genetic defects manifested in hematopoietic cells, and to permit wide-field radiation and dose escalation of chemotherapy in the treatment of selected solid tumors. The outcome of BMT has shown a slow but significant improvement over the past two decades (1). Increased survival is mainly attributable to advances in the management of transplant-related complications with more effective immunosuppressive therapy, drugs with antiviral activity, and more stringently tested blood products.

BMT is not only of direct benefit to a suitable recipient, but also important in the investigation of human hematopoietic stem cells and their interactions with various cell populations that form the complex regulatory network of hematopoiesis. The existence and separability of a subpopulation of human marrow cells with reconstituting ability was demonstrated for autologous transplants (2). Grafts were established successfully by infusion of a positively selected population of CD34-positive cells. The short hematopoietic recovery period leaves little doubt that the early increase in blood counts resulted from the infused cell population rather than from the residual hematopoietic cells. However, it remains unclear whether engraftment is sustained by these transfused cells or whether long-term reconstitution is a function of hematopoietic stem cells that resided in the patient during the myeloablative regimen and survived.

The interaction of repopulating cells with cells of the regulatory network was suggested by observations in allogeneic BMTs. For instance, grafts that are depleted of T lymphocytes have a significantly higher rate of failure compared with unmanipulated marrow (3–8). Cells of the graft-derived regulatory network may also influence the proliferative potential of malignant hematopoietic cells that may have escaped the myeloablative effect of the preparative regimen. In some hematopoietic malignancies, such as chronic myeloid leukemia (CML), a significantly higher relapse rate resulted from the infusion of T-cell–depleted grafts (9,10). A more recent study exploited this observation therapeutically. A small number of patients with CML who relapsed after allogeneic BMT were treated with repeated infusions of lymphocytes derived from the original marrow donor (11). Hematopoietic and cytogenetic remissions were achieved. Observations of this nature may ultimately lead to the development of novel therapeutic strategies to control malignant cell populations.

The Hematopoietic System

Adequate and timely production of blood cells under steady-state conditions and during periods of increasing demand is controlled through the interaction of hematopoietic progenitors with a network of cells that provide growth support and function in a regulatory capacity (Figure 5-1). Current understanding of this complex system is based on studies that have used a variety of assays in animal models and humans. Early transplantation studies documented the ability of bone marrow cells to repopulate lethally irradiated animals (12). The spleen colony assay provided the first method to quantitate pluripotent progenitors (13). It became feasible to dissect the system further by developing culture systems for hematopoietic cells (14–27). Semisolid and liquid suspension cultures permitted identification and characterization of multipotent and single lineage progenitors and facilitated examination of their interaction with growth-promoting cells that include T lymphocytes, monocytes, and stromal cells. The ability to segregate proliferating from growth-promoting cells led to the recognition of growth-promoting activities for various progenitor populations. Some, such as erythropoietin (EPO), granulocyte-macrophage colony stimulating factor (GM-CSF), granulocyte colony stimulating factor (G-CSF), and interleukin-3 (IL-3), have now entered the realm of clinical practice. Unfortunately, conventional clonogenic culture assays do not seem to evaluate cells with repopulating ability. By definition, these cells can be identified only by marrow transplant studies. The recently reported successful growth of human hematopoietic progenitors in mice with severe combined immunode-

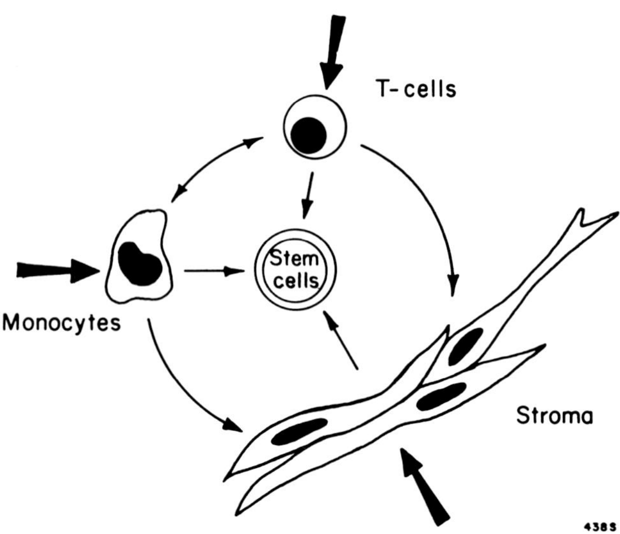

Figure 5-1. Regulatory cell-cell interactions—a model depicting the interactive network of hematopoiesis.

ficiency syndrome (SCID) may be an approach to solve this question (28,29).

Repopulation Studies

Classic marrow transplantation studies (12,13) demonstrated the presence of cells in murine hematopoietic tissues that were able to repopulate lethally irradiated animals. Subsequent studies (30,31) have shown that approximately 10^5 nucleated marrow cells are necessary to reestablish hematopoiesis in murine-irradiated hosts. This number of cells can be considered a repopulation unit. More recently, it was feasible to characterize the immunological phenotype of murine cells with repopulating capabilities. These cells are $Thy1^+$, and $SCA1^+$ and do not express any lineage-related markers (LIN^-) (32). As few as 30 of these highly selected cells are able to reestablish and sustain hematopoiesis in a lethally irradiated recipient; however, these cells appear to require T lymphocytes to establish fully functioning grafts.

Complete engraftment can be sustained by a limited number of hematopoietic clones. Introduction of genetic markers into individual hematopoietic stem cells provided a method of tracing their progeny (33). A period of instability in the clonal composition of the graft was observed early after BMT (34). Some clones that participated transiently in the production of blood cells disappeared, whereas others emerged. The clonal composition of the graft stabilized after some weeks and remained constant for the life span of the animals. In addition, the marrow of engrafted animals appears to contain repopulating cells at a number that is sufficient to reestablish hematopoiesis in a second generation of recipients. These observations suggest that murine hematopoietic clones can be expanded to function for at least two successive generations of BMT recipients.

This view is supported by the limited human data available. Three cases are known in which a BMT recipient served as donor for the original donor (Powles R, Huebsch L, Thomas D. Personal communications). Successful secondary grafts were established in all three cases. These data are consistent with a model of hematopoiesis in which the production of blood cells is sustained by a limited number of clones that persist for the life span of the individual. The alternative model of clonal succession is less likely. In this model, hematopoietic clones would have a limited life span and need to be replaced by newly recruited, previously not active hematopoietic stem cells and their progeny.

Spleen Colony Assay

The spleen colony assay described by Till and McCulloch (13) permitted quantitation of multipotent cells with self-renewal and differentiation capability. The assay detects a heterogenous group of pluripotent progenitors. Some appear to be more primitive (35,36) and reflect more likely hematopoietic precursors with repopulating capacity, whereas others display only limited self-renewal. The assay was applied to study hematopoietic defects of two mutant strains of genetically anemic mice, denoted w/w^v and sl/sl^d. Both mutations result in changes of the coat color and in sterility. The experiments indicated that proliferation of hematopoietic progenitors is regulated by genes intrinsic to spleen colony forming cells and influenced by genes that determine the functional program of stromal cells required for growth support. The proliferative ability of spleen colony forming cells was found to be linked to the w-locus (37), the necessary microenvironmental support to the sl-locus (38). The described mutation in either locus prevented the formation of spleen colonies.

Recent studies have provided the molecular details for this interaction. The w-locus was found to be associated with the proto-oncogene c-kit (39,40), which encodes a receptor on the surface of hematopoietic progenitors that binds to its ligand (kit-ligand) found on the surface of stromal cells. The kit-ligand is encoded by the sl-locus (41–46). C-kit and kit-ligand may have a similar role in human hematopoiesis. The receptor can be identified on normal hematopoietic progenitors and leukemic blood cell populations (47,48). The soluble human kit-ligand has growth-promoting activities for clonogenic hematopoietic progenitors (49–52). It is also known to synergize with other hematopoietic growth factors (53,54).

Mutations in the equivalent human genes may be responsible for certain hematopoietic defects. Although there is as yet no defect identified that resembles the sl/sl^d mutation, the description of the "piebald" syndrome suggests a lesion that is consistent with a w/w^v-like mutation, at least with respect to hair color (55).

Cell Culture Studies

The development of cell culture assays for early hematopoietic progenitors opened new avenues in the investigation of early hematopoietic events. Although pioneered in murine models, the assays were adapted rapidly to use for human cells. They led to the currently acknowledged model of hematopoiesis that describes a hierarchical order of clonogenic progenitor cells. Primitive multipotent cells with high proliferative potential give rise to clonogenic precursors that are restricted to a single hematopoietic lineage. Their proliferation, differentiation, and maturation is influenced by hormone-like substances that are derived from multiple sources, such as T lymphocytes, monocytes, and stromal cells.

Semisolid Culture Systems for Clonogenic Hematopoietic Progenitors

Semisolid culture systems are currently available for clonogenic progenitors at various levels of differentiation. The most primitive progenitor population that can be identified by this technology is denoted as CFU-BLAST, which gives rise to colonies composed of cells with blast-like morphology (25,27). Some cells within these blast colonies remain CD34-positive, indicating their early developmental status (56). Long-term observation of blast colonies under unchanged conditions shows that they acquire properties of megakaryocytes, erythroblasts, and granulocytes within 6 to 8 weeks (56). Lymphoid cells were not observed within these colonies. When recloned under identical conditions, blast cell colonies give rise to secondary multilineage or single lineage colonies (27,56). Unfortunately, it is not yet feasible to expand these populations of primitive cells any further and to preserve their pluripotency and self-renewal capacity indefinitely.

Multipotent progenitors with little or no self-renewal (CFU-GEMM) form colonies within 14 days of culture that may contain granulocytes, erythroblasts, megakaryocytes, and macrophages (57). Detailed studies on the cellular composition of multilineage colonies showed that rare multilineage colonies may contain T lymphocytes in addition to myeloid cells. T lymphocytes were seen only if T-cell growth factor was present in the cultures (58,59). A common origin for myeloid and lymphoid cells within individual colonies was strongly suggested by studies performed on peripheral blood samples of G-6-PD–heterozygous individuals (59). Identical isoenzymes were observed for the myeloid and lymphoid components, suggesting that a small number of common progenitors for myelopoiesis and lymphopoiesis exists in normal hematopoietic tissues.

Clonogenic progenitors with restriction to a single lineage can be identified for all known components of myelopoiesis and lymphopoiesis. These progenitors are denoted as granulocyte-macrophage colony forming units (CFU-GM), erythroid burst-forming units (BFU-E), megakaryocyte colony forming units (CFU-MEG), T-lymphocyte colony-forming units (CFU-T), and B-lymphocyte colony forming units (CFU-B).

Colony formation by the various progenitor populations is dependent on defined culture conditions. Apart from nutrients, growth is influenced by a number of growth-promoting activities that are produced naturally by cells that are part of the hematopoietic network. The first description that products of peripheral blood cells may promote growth of human marrow (60,61) led to a relentless pursuit of molecules with this function. Nearly 20 of these factors have been described and characterized. The group of molecules described first (GM-CSF, G-CSF, and M-CSF) were named operationally colony stimulating factors. More recent additions to this growing list of molecules influencing hematopoietic cells are called interleukins (IL), acknowledging that they mediate the communication between groups of leukocytes. They function by interacting with their respective target cells through specific receptors. Some of the interleukins demonstrate a wide spectrum of activities and stimulate multipotent progenitors as well as lineage-restricted clonogenic precursors. For example, IL-3 and GM-CSF both influence colony formation by CFU-GEMM, CFU-GM, BFU-E, and CFU-MEG (62). Other interleukins have a narrowly defined activity profile directing growth, development, and function of a single hematopoietic lineage. EPO is a representative of this group.

The complicated processes of differentiation and maturation involved in the transition from a primitive progenitor population to cells with lineage-restricted function are viewed as being under the influence of a cascade of interleukins. Resting primitive progenitors are activated by exposure to IL-1. The process of activation is associated with a series of secondary events, including expression and up-regulation of receptors for other interleukins, such as IL-3 and GM-CSF. Timely exposure of receptor-bearing cells to these factors will lead to their proliferation and further development. The ultimate lineage-specific maturation may require interaction with molecules such as EPO, G-CSF, or M-CSF. The terminal lineage development may also be influenced by the concentration in which a factor is made available to respective target cells. This influence was convincingly demonstrated for CFU-GM–derived daughter cells (63). At the doublet stage, cells were mechanically separated and exposed to either high or low concentrations of GM-CSF. Cells cultured with high concentrations developed predominantly into neutrophilic granulocytes. Cells grown in low concentrations more frequently gave rise to macrophages.

Independent of their specific composition of nutrients and stimulators, semisolid culture systems provide an environment for differentiation and terminal maturation. Self-renewal, even by CFU-BLASTS, is limited to one or two generations. It is therefore unlikely that the described systems are suitable for unlimited expansion of hematopoietic stem cells. One of the reasons may relate to the absence of a stromal support system. Such a layer can be established in liquid suspension cultures.

Long-term Bone Marrow Cultures

Liquid suspension cultures of marrow are able to sustain the production of clonogenic hematopoietic progenitors for weeks (64–67). The conditions promote the formation of a layer of stromal cells that appears to be essential for the continued proliferation of clonogenic cells. Formation of the stromal layer fosters an intimate cell-to-cell contact between progenitors and the stromal support. This direct contact is likely important for some of the signals necessary to induce and maintain proliferation. The required frequent media changes may provide a separate source of signals. It has been well documented that immediately following the exchange, cells appear to enter into cycle, whereas they have a higher tendency to be dormant prior to the next exchange (68). Hematopoietic progenitor cells and cells that form the stromal support system appear not to be derived from a common progenitor cell population. As shown in transplant studies, the majority of cells within the stromal layer formed by marrow samples of BMT recipients appear to be of host origin (69–72), whereas proliferating hematopoietic cells are donor-derived. The system is therefore ideal to evaluate the function of progenitor and support cells separately. For this purpose, one can establish preformed stromal layers, irradiate these layers to prevent further proliferation, and use them to identify cells that are able to repopulate the culture. Cells that are CD34-positive, HLA-DR–negative, and free of lineage-related determinants (LIN^-) are able to maintain production of hematopoietic progenitors under these conditions (73). Cells of this phenotype likely represent the currently known most primitive hematopoietic progenitor population.

The long-term culture system was successfully used to investigate early progenitors in hematopoietic malignancies. Seminal contributions were made, particularly for CML. At diagnosis of this disease, hematopoiesis is usually sustained solely by members of a single Philadelphia chromosome (Ph)–positive malignant clone. The fate of the normal hematopoietic clones was unclear; they were considered either to be ablated or at least completely suppressed. Long-term culture studies on marrow samples from patients with CML revealed two phenomena: (1) Ph-positive cells declined rapidly and (2) polyclonal Ph-negative clonogenic progenitors emerged (74). The culture system therefore provided the opportunity to be used as a novel purging technique for the purpose of autografting for patients with CML.

The hypothesis was tested clinically (75). Ph-negative grafts were established in 20 patients treated. Although some patients have relapsed in the interim, the approach bears promise (see Chapter 56). The survival of normal progenitors in CML was also documented by immunological separation techniques. $CD34^+$, $HLA\text{-}DR^-$, and lineage-negative cells were found to reestablish hematopoiesis on preformed irradiated stromal layers. Resulting myeloid clonogenic progenitors gave rise to colonies composed of cells that did not show the bcr/abl rearrangement typically observed in CML cells (McGlave P. Personal communication). A direct analysis of $CD34^+$, $Thy1^+$, and LIN^- cells revealed that this population may be bcr/abl–negative when evaluated using the highly sensitive polymerase chain reaction (PCR) (Negrin RS. Personal communication). On the basis of this information, it might be possible to perform autologous marrow transplants with positively selected progenitor populations rather than following purging procedures to eliminate contaminating malignant cells.

Bone Marrow Grafts

Marrow grafts are traditionally established by infusing unmanipulated suspensions of aspirable, donor-derived marrow cells into the respective recipient. The marrow suspension consists of a complex mixture of cells that includes the essential population of repopulating cells as well as cells that are part of the regulatory network of hematopoiesis, such as T lymphocytes.

The question was asked early on whether infusion of complete marrow was essential or whether hematopoiesis could be reestablished by transplantation of a selected population of marrow cells. It has been demonstrated in a murine BMT model that T-cell–depleted marrow cell suspensions were effective in repopulating host marrow without causing graft-versus-host disease (GVHD) (76). The same separation technique based on differences in sedimentation velocity of T cells and hematopoietic progenitors was used clinically. This initial approach resulted in poor engraftment (77). The subsequent use of more effective separation techniques, such as antibody-mediated T-cell removal, demonstrated the feasibility of engrafting patients with T-cell–depleted marrow while substantially reducing the frequency and severity of GVHD. However, these studies also showed that the use of unmanipulated marrow may be advantageous to recipients. BMT of complete marrow resulted in a lower rate of graft failure and, more importantly, a significantly lower relapse rate. The latter was of particular importance for patients with CML. These observations strongly supported the view that T cells have an important role in the engraftment process and participate in the control of malignant cells.

Manipulations of autografts were introduced to ablate residual malignant cells in the graft. Most commonly, grafts are exposed to drugs such as 4-hydroperoxycyclophosphamide. This procedure appears to eliminate the more mature progenitors CFU-GEMM, BFU-E, CFU-GM, and CFU-MEG without compromising cells with repopulating ability (78).

Alternative methods of purging include exposure to monoclonal antibodies with appropriate lineage specificity (79,80). A cocktail of multiple antibodies directed against various B-cell determinants, for instance, was found to be effective in removing disease-propagating cells from the graft prior to infusion into patients with non-Hodgkin's lymphoma (81). Unfortunately, this approach requires the testing of appropriate reagents and methods for each disease.

A more recently developed technique may be more universally applicable. It is based on the positive selection of a residual normal progenitor population with marrow-repopulating ability. Murine hematopoiesis can be reestablished by injection of a small number of Thy1$^+$, SCA1$^+$, LIN$^-$ progenitors (32). Studies in baboons yielded similar results with positively selected CD34$^+$ cells (82). This technique has now been adopted successfully for human autografts (2) and represents the first step for selective preparation of repopulating cells. Preclinical studies suggest that cells that are CD34-positive, HLA-DR–negative, and depleted of cells that carry lineage-associated markers have a high probability of being free of contaminating malignant cells.

Enrichment of repopulating cells has other advantages. The volume of frozen cells can be reduced to approximately 5 mL at significant cost saving with respect to storage. In addition, the negligibly small amount of dimethyl sulfoxide causes less discomfort to patients at the time of administration.

Peripheral Blood as a Source of Repopulating Cells

The effectiveness of peripheral blood cells to repopulate lethally irradiated animals was originally demonstrated in the dog model (83). Long-term reconstitution of myelopoiesis and lymphopoiesis was observed (83–85). Introduction of the concept of peripheral blood cell infusions as a source of repopulating cells was initially described for patients with aplastic anemia (86). The frequency of graft failures following preparation with chemotherapy alone was significantly reduced by this maneuver. More recently, the technique was applied for autologous reconstitution (87). The rationale to use peripheral blood as a source of repopulating cells was based on the assumption that peripheral blood may be less likely to contain malignant cells compared with marrow (88). The procedure of collecting cells is simple and can be performed on an out-patient basis. The yield can be improved if each collection is performed in the recovery phase after chemotherapy (89–91) or following the use of growth factors (92,93). Hematopoietic recovery appears to be at least as rapid as that following infusion of marrow (94). The combined administration of marrow- and blood-derived repopulating cells may be the most effective method of reconstitution (95).

The Role of Hematopoietic Growth Factors in BMT

The availability of various hematopoietic growth factors for clinical trials has provided the opportunity to determine whether engraftment can be improved by their timely administration to BMT recipients. On the basis of the reproducible observation that plasma from patients with severe aplastic anemia contains activities that promote colony formation of hematopoietic progenitors in culture (96), a study was conducted to determine the presence of endogenous stimulating activities in the plasma of BMT recipients (97). Plasma samples collected longitudinally from 34 recipients of allografts contained activities that promoted growth of CFU-MEG, CFU-GM, and occasionally also BFU-E (Figure 5-2). The activity profiles peaked between day 7 and 21 after BMT. Patients who showed sustained activities as late as day 30 usually demonstrated a delayed return of their peripheral blood counts.

The observation of endogenously produced G-CSF was confirmed in a recent report on 12 patients (98). In a double-blind, randomized study (Messner HA. Unpublished data), we investigated whether these activity profiles could be altered by administration of GM-CSF. Recipients of allografts with lymphoid malignancies received either GM-CSF or placebo for 14 days following infusion of marrow. Plasma samples collected from patients in both groups contained biologically active quantities of G-CSF, EPO, and megakaryocyte colony stimulating activity. The concentrations were independent of the observed GM-CSF levels. A preliminary evaluation of engraftment parameters did not reveal any differences in the time to recovery for both groups. This finding differs from observations in autologous BMTs, in which administration of GM-CSF (99–101) and G-CSF (102,103) resulted in a considerable shortening of the neutropenic phase. The reason for this difference is not clear. It may relate to the administration of methotrexate (MTX) for GVHD prophylaxis to recipients of allografts. Alternatively, autograft recipients may not produce growth factors in concentrations observed after allografts. This possibility is currently under study at our institution. The previously cited report (98) did not reveal any differences between recipients of allografts and autografts with respect to their endogenous G-CSF production.

Engraftment

Infusion of allogeneic marrow results in profound changes within the recipient. Apart from replacing the hematopoietic and immune system, transplants have facilitated the identification of cells that are derived from marrow components but are not hematopoietically active. These cells include pulmonary alveolar macrophages (104), von Kupffer cells in the liver, osteoclasts, Langerhans cells of the skin, and microglia cells of the brain. Some of these cell populations convert slowly into donor cells, suggesting a slow endogenous turnover. Hematopoietic and immunological recovery of BMT recipients occur at variable speeds and are influenced by a number of conditions, including the nature and status of the primary disease, previously administered chemotherapy and

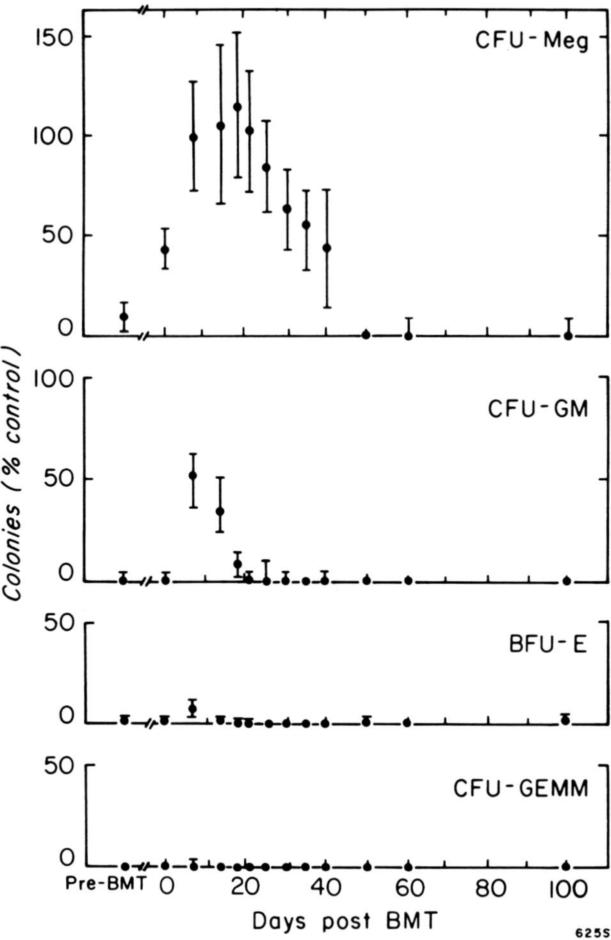

Figure 5-2. Colony formation by normal nonadherent bone marrow cells plated with plasma obtained from BMT recipients before and serially after BMT. The cultures did not contain any other exogenous source of growth factors. Data are expressed as percent of normal control values. Control specimens for CFU-Meg and CFU-GM were plated with 30% normal human plasma and 10% PHA-LCM. Controls for BFU-E and CFU-GEMM also contained 1 U EPO. The following control values (mean ± SEM) per 2×10^5 mononuclear cells were observed: CFU-Meg, 63 ± 12; CFU-GM, 189 ± 24; BFU-E, 217 ± 22; CFU-GEMM, 25 ± 3. (Reproduced by permission from Yamasaki K, Solberg LA Jr, Jamal N, et al. Hemopoietic colony growth-promoting activities in the plasma of bone marrow transplant recipients. J Clin Invest 1988;82:255–261.)

radiation, the choice of the preparative regimen, the type of GVHD prophylaxis, viral complications (particularly related to cytomegalovirus infections after BMT), and the use of antiviral agents.

Recovery of Myelopoiesis

Small clusters of hematopoietic cells can be observed in biopsy specimens within 10 to 14 days following BMT (105). The marrow cellularity increases rapidly over the following 2 to 4 weeks and shows morphological evidence of all myeloid components. However, it may require 6 to 12 months before cellularity reaches normal density. The increase of mature blood cells in the peripheral circulation varies considerably from patient to patient. A study at the Princess Margaret Hospital (Figure 5-3) (106) revealed a median time of 23 days to reach 1.0×10^9/L neutrophilic granulocytes. The times for individual patients varied from 12 to 45 days. Reticulocytes of 100×10^9/L were observed after 12 to 72 days, with a median of 24 days. The pattern of platelet recovery showed an even wider range. The median time to reach 100×10^9 platelets/L was 39 days; however, 25% of patients required 3 to 6 months to produce this number. Patients with chronic GVHD appear to be particularly slow in their platelet recovery. Despite individual variations, during the early post-BMT period, the majority of recipients will eventually give rise to normal peripheral blood counts. Hematopoietic cells after BMT are usually of donor origin. Coexistence of donor- and host-derived cells can be observed in some patients (107).

Failure to establish or sustain a functioning marrow graft is relatively uncommon in patients transplanted with unmanipulated marrow for hematopoietic malignancies. In contrast, engraftment problems are more common in patients with severe aplasia or recipients of T-lymphocyte–depleted allografts. Poor engraft-

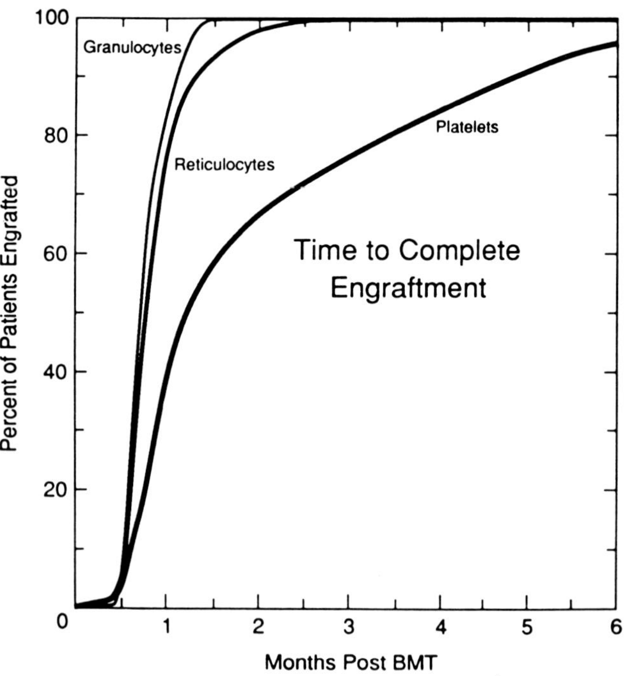

Figure 5-3. Kaplan-Meier product-limit estimates of time to engraftment of granulocytes, reticulocytes, and platelets for 121 patients achieving complete engraftment. (Reproduced by permission from Fyles GM, Messner HA, Lockwood G, et al. Long-term results of bone marrow transplantation for patients with AML, ALL, and CML prepared with single dose total body irradiation of 500 cGy delivered with a high dose rate. Bone Marrow Transplantation 1991;8:453–463.)

ment or early rejection in patients with aplastic anemia appears to be related to the activity of residual host-derived T lymphocytes, cells that may have been responsible for development of the original marrow aplasia. This problem is less common in patients who receive GVHD prophylaxis with cyclosporin (CSP)-containing schedules. The reasons for graft failure in recipients of T-lymphocyte–depleted marrow are less well understood. Perhaps T lymphocytes foster engraftment by producing growth factors that are required for the engraftment process. This view is supported by the observation of various growth factors in the circulation of recipients of unmanipulated allografts (97,98).

In contrast to normal peripheral blood counts and marrow cellularity, the frequency of clonogenic progenitors remains significantly reduced compared with normal control subjects (108–111). Even long-term follow-up of individual patients for 10 to 12 years shows that the frequency of clonogenic progenitors does not increase over time. When evaluated for their cycle state, nearly all clonogenic cells proliferate actively (109), which is in contrast to the cycle status of progenitors in normal donors, in whom a resting population can be identified. This observation suggests that the marrow of BMT recipients operates with little or no reserve. It agrees with the assessment by Turhan and colleagues (112) that a smaller than normal number of clones participates in hematopoiesis after BMT. Long-term follow-up of these patients will determine whether this sustained stress-like status may result in late complications, such as secondary hematopoietic malignancies. Development of acute myeloid leukemia (AML) in donor cells of one patient transplanted for aplastic anemia (113) and one patient transplanted for CML (Messner HA. Unpublished data) serves as a caution.

Recovery of Immune Function

Development of normal immune function after BMT occurs with some delay (114–117). During this period, patients remain at risk for life-threatening infectious complications. Evidence for the recovery of some normal immunity can be observed within 3 to 4 months following BMT. Serum complement and serum immunoglobulin G (IgG) and IgM levels return to normal during this time. The recovery of normal IgA levels is often delayed, and a chronic IgA deficiency is observed for many patients with chronic GVHD. Recovery of cellular immune function is even slower and may take up to 2 years (118).

Clonogenic Progenitors and Engraftment

The question of whether engraftment can be predicted by donor- or host-related clonogenic progenitors has not yet been answered satisfactorily. Until recently, it was not possible in allografts to link time to engraftment or quality of engraftment to well-recognized clonogenic progenitors (110,119,120). As shown in a number of reports, the total number of cells within a graft was more important than a subpopulation of clonogenic cells (86,110,121,122). This observation is consistent with the view that multipotent clonogenic progenitors (e.g., CFU-GEMM) and single lineage precursors (e.g., CFU-GM, BFU-E, CFU-MEG) are not responsible for the permanent repopulation of marrow after BMT. This hypothesis was confirmed in autografts in which these progenitors were dramatically reduced by purging procedures without influencing the engraftment process (87). However, at least in autotransplants, an association can be demonstrated between clonogenic cells and recovery (123). New studies are required to evaluate the predictive value of long-term culture repopulating cells that are characterized by the described $CD34^+$, $HLA\text{-}DR^-$, and LIN^- immunological phenotype.

Alternatively, the difficulty of detecting specific donor-derived populations as predictors of engraftment may be a testimony to the complexity of the system. As mentioned, spleen colony formation in the mouse model requires not only intact colony forming cells, but also an intact permissive stroma. Evaluation of stroma-related parameters in human hematopoiesis remains cumbersome and indirect. Although it is possible to grow layers of growth-supporting stromal cells in long-term culture, this technique has not been used routinely to evaluate its influence on engraftment. In one study from Toronto, clonogenic progenitors of recipients were studied prior to administration of the respective ablative regimen. The frequency of multilineage and single lineage colonies (Figure 5-4) in the majority of patients was lower than those observed for their respective donors (110,124). This observation is expected for patients with aplastic anemia. The low frequency in patients with leukemia may relate to previous chemotherapy or to the disease process. Among clonogenic cells, the frequency of CFU-MEG was the only parameter that predicted time to engraftment. Patients with a low number of CFU-MEG engrafted significantly more slowly. The reason for this observation is not understood. Perhaps the frequency of CFU-MEG reflects the function of the stromal support system. When injured by pretransplant therapy, the stroma may not provide the environment that permits expansion of megakaryocytes, representing the most sensitive hematopoietic lineage. This microenvironmental component may impose limits that cannot be overcome by the presence of long-range factors that stimulate megakaryocytopoiesis. As indicated, the plasma of patients with a slow platelet recovery usually contains high levels of megakaryocyte-stimulating activities.

Interactions of Graft-derived Cells with Residual Malignant Host Cells

BMTs facilitate administration of chemotherapy at high doses and wide-field irradiation to patients with hematopoietic malignancies. Observations during the past two decades have demonstrated that myeloablative treatments represent only one of the mecha-

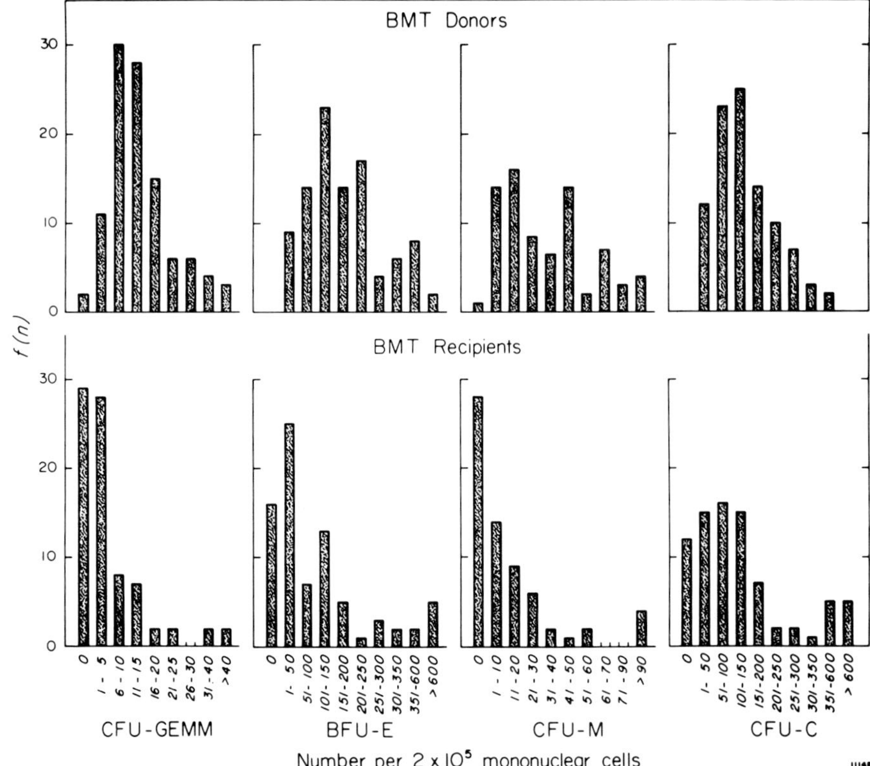

Figure 5-4. Frequency of clonogenic progenitors in BMT recipients prior to BMT and of their respective donors. (Reproduced by permission from Messner HA, Yamasaki K. Conditions affecting the growth of hemopoietic progenitors after bone marrow transplantation. In: Testa NG, Gale RP, eds. Hematopoiesis: long-term effects of chemotherapy and radiation, vol 8. New York: Marcel Dekker, 1988:377–388.)

nisms that are essential for control of malignant cell populations. It became apparent that graft-derived cells have a major role in the interaction with residual malignant cells. The higher relapse rate in syngeneic transplants, in recipients with little or no GVHD, and in patients transplanted with T-cell–depleted marrow emphasize the control function of graft-derived T lymphocytes (see Chapter 11).

Similarly, patients treated with prolonged immunosuppression may show persistence or recurrence of the primary malignancy. This finding was documented for patients who received a BMT for CML (125). Discontinuation of intensive immunosuppression may result in the spontaneous disappearance of the Ph chromosome–positive malignant clone. As mentioned, involvement of cells that are part of the immune surveillance system has been further documented by Kolb and associates (11). Patients with CML who relapsed after BMT were treated with interferon and multiple infusions of lymphocytes obtained from the original marrow donor. Some of these patients experienced development of GVHD, transient marrow hypoplasia, and reduction of peripheral blood counts. Upon recovery, cells were found to be of donor origin. The index case is now 3.5 years after the procedure and remains bcr/abl–negative by PCR (Kolb H. Personal communication). If confirmed in a larger series, this observation may represent the most important advance in our understanding of disease control following BMT. It raises the question of whether the same effect can be achieved with T-cell infusion without requiring a previous allograft.

The observation that patients transfused with donor lymphocytes respond with a hypoplastic phase of the marrow may lead to intriguing speculations about the biological phenomenon associated with aplastic anemia in patients who respond to immunosuppressive therapy. It is conceivable that the aplastic phase in those patients represents the strongest possible defense mechanism against development of a hematopoietic malignancy. Under these conditions, the activated T-cell population may suppress not only the malignant population, but also normal hematopoietic progenitors. This suppression can be terminated by administration of antithymocyte globulin (ATG) or CSP. Reports that describe development of myelodysplastic syndromes, paroxysmal nocturnal hemoglobinuria, or AML in patients with aplastic anemia treated with ATG may suggest that the malignant clone had not been eliminated (126,127).

Summary and Future Directions

BMT has become an important clinical modality in the treatment of patients with hematopoietic malignancies, selected solid tumors, and other disorders of the blood-forming system. Hematopoiesis may not return to normal when assessed by current identifiable clonogenic progenitors. Production of blood cells is maintained by a lower number of hematopoietic clones compared with normal individuals. Observations over 15 to 20 years have shown, however, that blood cell production was sustained. Three BMT recipients are known to have served as donors for their original marrow donors; in all cases it was possible to repopulate marrow in the secondary recipient. This finding supports the view that hematopoietic clones show extensive expandability. Cells that are responsible for sustained engraftment are present in low frequency and appear to belong to a population of $CD34^+$, $HLA\text{-}DR^-$, LIN^- cells. Identification of this population is of importance because it may facilitate positive selection and separation from contaminating malignant cells for the purpose of autologous BMT. In allogeneic BMT, combination of marrow repopulating cells and cells of the donor-derived immune surveillance system may lead to a tailor-made composition of grafts that have optimal repopulating ability and maximal potential to control residual malignant cells within the host.

References

1. Horowitz MM, Bortin MM. Allogeneic bone marrow transplantation (BMT) for leukemia: has outcome improved in the last 10 years? Exp Haemato 17:545.
2. Berenson DJ, Bensinger WI, Hill RS, et al. Engraftment after infusion of $CD34^+$ marrow cells in patients with breast cancer or neuroblastoma Blood 1991;77:1717–1722.
3. Martin PJ, Hansen JA, Buckner CD, et al. Effects of in vitro depletion of T cells in HLA-identical allogeneic marrow grafts. Blood 1985;66:664–672.
4. Patterson J, Prentice HG, Brenner MK, et al. Graft rejection following HLA matched T-lymphocyte depleted bone marrow transplantation. Br J Haematol 1986;63:221–230.
5. Guyotat D, Duton L, Ersham A, et al. Graft rejection after T cell depleted marrow transplantation: role of fractionated irradiation. Br J Haematol 1987;65:499–507.
6. Martin PJ, Hansen JA, Torok-Storb B, et al. Graft failure in patients receiving T cell depleted HLA-identical allogeneic marrow transplants. Bone Marrow Transplantation, 1988;3:445–456.
7. Butturini A, Gale RP. T-cell depletion in bone marrow transplantation for leukemia: current results and future directions. Bone Marrow Transplantation 1988;3:185–192.
8. Martin PJ. The role of donor lymphoid cells in allogeneic marrow engraftment. Bone Marrow Transplantation 1990;6:283–289.
9. Apperley JF, Mauro F, Goldman JM, et al. Bone marrow transplantation for chronic myeloid leukemia in chronic phase: importance of a graft-versus-leukemia effect. Br J Haematol 1988;69:239–245.
10. Hughes TP, Goldman JM. Biological importance of residual leukemia cells after BMT for CML: does the polymerase chain reaction help? Bone Marrow Transplantation 1990;5:3–6.
11. Kolb HJ, Mittermuller J, Clemm Ch, et al. Donor leukocyte transfusions for treatment of recurrent chronic myelogenous leukemia in marrow transplant patients. Blood 1990;76:2462–2465.
12. Lorenz E, Uphoff DE, Reid TR, et al. Modification of irradiation injury in mice and guinea pigs by bone marrow infusions. JNCI 1951;12:197–201.
13. Till JE, McCulloch EA. A direct measurement of the radiation sensitivity of normal mouse bone marrow cells. Radiat Res 1961;14:213–222.
14. Pluznik DN, Sachs L. The cloning of normal "mast" cells in tissue culture. J Cell Comp Physiol 1965; 66:319–324.
15. Bradley TR, Metcalf D. The growth of mouse bone marrow cells in vitro. Aust J Exp Biol Med Sci 1966;44:287–300.
16. Senn JS, McCulloch EA, Till JE. Comparison of the colony forming ability of normal and leukemic human marrow in cell culture. Lancet 1967;2:597.
17. Stephenson JR, Axelrad AA, McLeod DL, et al. Induction of colonies of hemoglobin synthesizing cells by erythropoietin in vitro. Proc Natl Acad Sci USA 1971;68:1542–1546.
18. Tepperman AD, Curtis JE, McCulloch EA. Erythropoietic colonies in cultures of human marrow. Blood 1974;44:659–669.
19. Iscove NN, Sieber F, Winterhalter K. Erythroid colony formation in culture of mouse and human bone marrow: analysis of the requirement for erythropoietin by gel filtration and affinity chromatography on agarose concanavalin A. J Cell Physiol 1974;83:309–320.
20. Metcalf D, MacDonald HR, Odartchenko N, et al. Growth of mouse megakaryocyte colonies in vitro. Proc Natl Acad Sci USA 1975;72:1744–1748.
21. Vainchenker W, Bouget J, Guichard J, et al. Megakaryocyte colony formation from human bone marrow precursors. Blood 1979;54:940–945.
22. Messner HA, Jamal N, Izaguirre C. The growth of large megakaryocyte colonies from human bone marrow. J Cell Physiol 1982;1(suppl):45–51.
23. Fauser AA, Messner HA. Granuloerythropoietic colonies in human bone marrow, peripheral blood and cord blood. Blood 1978;52:1243–1248.
24. Metcalf D, Johnson GR, Mandel TE. Colony formation in agar by multipotential hemopoietic cells. J Cell Physiol 1979;98:401–420.
25. Nakahata T, Ogawa M. Identification in culture of a class of hemopoietic colony-forming units with extensive capability to self renew and generate multipotential hemopoietic colonies. Proc Natl Acad Sci USA 1982;79:3843–3847.
26. Keller GM, Phillips RA. Detection in vitro of a unique multi-potent hemopoietic progenitor. J Cell Physiol 1982;1(suppl):31–36.
27. Nakahata T, Ogawa M. Hemopoietic colony-forming cells in umbilical cord blood with extensive capability to generate mono and multipotential hemopoietic progenitors. J Clin Invest 1982;70:1324–1328.
28. McCune JM, Namikawa R, Kaneshima H, et al. The SCID- hu mouse: murine model for the analysis of human hematolymphoid differentiation and function. Science 1988;241:1632–1639.
29. Kamel-Reid S, Dick J. Engraftment of immune-deficient mice with human hematopoietic stem cells. Science 1988;242:1706–1709.

30. Boggs DR, Boggs SS, Saxe DF, et al. Hematopoietic stem cells with high proliferative potential—assay of their concentration in marrow by the frequency and duration of cure of W/W^v mice. J Clin Invest 1982;70:242–253.
31. Harrison DE, Clinton MA. Loss of stem cell repopulating ability upon transplantation—effects of donor age, cell number, and transplantation procedure. J Exp Med 1982;156:1767–1779.
32. Spangrude GJ, Heimfeld S, Weissman IL. Purification and characterization of murine hemopoietic stem cells. Science 1988;241:58–62.
33. Lemischka IR, Raulet DH, Mulligan RC. Developmental potential and dynamic behaviour of hematopoietic stem cells. Cell 1986;45:917–927.
34. Jordan CT, Lemischka IR. Clonal and systematic analysis of long-term hemopoiesis in the mouse. Genes Dev 1990;4:220–232.
35. Worton RG. Physical separation of hemopoietic stem cells. Doctoral Thesis, Department of Medical Biophysics, University of Toronto, 1969.
36. Magli MC, Iscove NN, Odartchenko N. Transient nature of early haemopoietic spleen colonies. Nature 1982;295:527–529.
37. McCulloch EA, Siminovitch L, Till JE. Spleen colony formation in anemic mice of genotype W/W^v. Science 1964;144:844–846.
38. McCulloch EA, Russell ES, Siminovitch L, et al. The cellular basis of the genetically determined hemopoietic defect in anemic mice of genotype Sl/Sl^d. Blood 1965;26:399–410.
39. Chabot B, Stephenson DA, Chapman VM, et al. The proto-oncogene c-kit encoding a transmembrane tyrosine kinase receptor maps to the mouse W Locus. Nature 1988;88–89.
40. Geissler EN, Ryan MA, Housman DE. The dominant white-spotting (W) locus of the mouse encodes the c-kit proto-oncogene. Cell 1988;55:185–192.
41. Williams DE, Eisenman J, Baird A, et al. Identification of a ligand for the c-kit proto-oncogene. Cell 1990;63: 167–174.
42. Copeland MG, Gilbert DJ, Cho BC, et al. Mast cell growth factory maps near the steel locus on mouse chromosome 10 and is deleted in a number of steel alleles. Cell 1990;63:175–183.
43. Flanagan JG, Leder P. The kit ligand: a cell surface molecule altered in steel mutant fibroblasts. Cell 1990;63:185–194.
44. Zsebo KM, Williams DA, Geissler EN, et al. Stem cell factor is encoded by the SI locus of the mouse and is the ligand of the c-kit tyrosine kinase receptor. Cell 1990;63:213–224.
45. Huang E, Nocka K, Beier DR, et al. The hematopoietic growth factor KL is encoded by the SI locus and is the ligand of the c-kit receptor, the gene product of the W locus. Cell 1990;63:525–533.
46. Anderson DM, Lyman SD, Baird A, et al. Molecular cloning of mast cell growth factor, a hematopoietin that is active in both membrane bound and soluble forms. Cell 1990;63:235–243.
47. Wong C, Curtis JE, Geissler NE, et al. The expression of the proto-oncogene c-kit in the blast cells of acute myeloblastic leukemia. Leukemia 1989;3:699–702.
48. Andre C, d'Auriol L, Lacombe C, et al. C-kit mRNA expression in human and murine hematopoietic cell lines. Oncogene 1989;4:1047–1049.
49. Broxmeyer HE, Hangoc G, Cooper S, et al. Influence of murine mast cell growth factor (c-kit ligand) on colony formation by mouse marrow hematopoietic progenitor cells. Exp Hematol 1991;19:143–146.
50. Migliaccio G, Migliaccio AR, Valinsky J, et al. Stem cell factor (SCF) induces proliferation and differentiation of highly enriched murine hematopoietic cells. Proc Natl Acad Sci USA 1991;88:7420–7424.
51 Broxmeyer HE, Cooper S, Lu L, et al. Effects of murine mast cell growth factor (c-kit proto-oncogene ligand) on colony formation by human marrow hematopoietic progenitor cells. Blood 1991;77:2142–2149.
52. Migliaccio G, Migliaccio AR, Druzin ML, et al. Effects of recombinant human stem cell factor (SCF) on the growth of human progenitor cells in vitro. J Cell Physiol 1991;148:503–509.
53. Bernstein ID, Andrews RG, Zsebo KM. Recombinant human stem cell factor enhances the formation of colonies by CD34$^+$LIN$^-$ cells, and the generation of colony-forming cell progeny from CD34$^+$LIN$^-$ cells cultured with interleukin 3, granulocyte colony-stimulating factor, or granulocyte-macrophage colony stimulating factor. Blood 1991;77:2316–2321.
54. McNiece IK, Langley KE, Zsebo KM. Recombinant human stem cell factor synergises with GM-CSF, G-CSF, IL-3 and Epo to stimulate human progenitor cells of the myeloid and erythroid lineages. Exp Hematol 1991;19:226–231.
55. Giebel LB, Spritz RA. Mutation of the kit (mast/stem cell growth factor receptor) proto-oncogene in human Piebaldism. Proc Natl Acad Sci USA 1991;88:8696–8699.
56. Hirota Y, Jamal N, Messner HA. Differentiation profiles of normal blast cell colonies derived from mononucleated cells, T-cell depleted nonadherent cells and CD33-negative, CD34-positive normal human bone marrow cells. Int J Cell Cloning 1993 (in press).
57 Fauser AA, Messner HA. Identification of megakaryocytes, macrophages, and eosinophils in colonies of human bone marrow containing neutrophilic granulocytes and erythroblasts. Blood 1979;53:1023–1027.
58. Messner HA, Izaguirre C, Jamal N. Identification of T-lymphocytes in human mixed hemopoietic colonies. Blood 1981;58:402–405.
59. Lim B, Jamal N, Tritchler D, Messner HA. G-6-PD isoenzyme analysis of myeloid and lymphoid cells in human multilineage colonies. Blood 1984;63:1481–1487.
60. Chervenick PA, Boggs DE. Bone marrow colonies: stimulation in vitro by supernatant from incubated human blood cells. Science 1970;169:691–692.
61. Iscove NN, Senn JS, Till JE, et al. Colony formation by normal and leukemic human marrow cells in culture: effect of conditioned medium from human leukocytes. Blood 1971;37:1–5.
62. Messner HA, Yamasaki K, Jamal N, et al. Growth of human hemopoietic colonies in response to recombinant gibbon interleukin 3: comparison with human recombinant granulocyte and granulocyte-macrophage colony stimulating factor. Proc Natl Acad Sci USA 1987;84:6765–6769.
63. Metcalf D. Control of hemopoietic cell proliferation and differentiation. In: Cummingham D, Goldwasser E, Watson J, Fox C, eds. Progress in clinical and biological research, vol 66. New York: Alan R. Liss, 1981;66:473–483.
64. Dexter TM, Lajtha LG. Proliferation of haemopoietic stem cells in vitro. Br J Haematol 1974;28:525–530.
65. Dexter TM, Allen TD, Lajtha LG. Conditions controlling

the proliferation of haemopoietic stem cells in vitro. J Cell Physiol 1977;91:335–344.
66. Reimann J, Burger H. In vitro proliferation of haemopoietic cells in the presence of adherent cell layers II. Differential effect of adherent cell layers derived from different organs. Exp Hematol 1979;7:52–58.
67. Gartner S, Kaplan HS. Long term culture of human bone marrow cells. Proc Natl Acad Sci USA 1980;77: 4756–4759.
68. Eaves CJ, Cashman JD, Kay RJ, et al. Evidence that human marrow stromal cells produce TGF-β and thereby arrest the cycling of primitive populations of normal hemopoietic progenitors. Blood 1988;72(suppl 1):84a.
69. Simmons PJ, Przepiorka D, Thomas ED, et al. Host origin of marrow stromal cells following allogeneic bone marrow transplantation. Nature 1987;328:429–432.
70. Lim B, Izaguirre CA, Aye MT, et al. Characterization of reticulo-fibroblastoid colonies (CFU-RF) derived from bone marrow and long term culture adherent layers. J Cell Physiol 1986;127:45–54.
71 Castro-Malaspina M, Gay RE, Resnick G, et al. Characterization of human bone marrow fibroblast colony-forming cells (CFU-F) and their progency. Blood 1980;56:289–301.
72. Singer JW, Keating A, Cuttner J, et al. Evidence for a stem cell common to hematopoiesis and its in vitro microenvironment: studies of patients with clonal hematopoietic neoplasia. Leuk Res 1984;4:535–545.
73. Sutherland HJ, Eaves HJ, Eaves CJ, et al. Characterization and partial purification of human marrow cells capable of initiating long-term hematopoiesis in vitro. Blood 1989;74:1563–1570.
74. Coulombel L, Kalousek, Eaves CJ. Long term marrow culture reveals chromosomally normal hematopoietic progenitor cells in patients with Philadelphia chromosome-positive chronic myelogenous leukemia. N Engl J Med 1983;308:1493–1498.
75. Barnett MJ, Eaves CJ, Philips GL, et al. Successful autografting in chronic myeloid leukemia after maintenance of marrow in culture. Bone Marrow Transplantation 1989;4:345–351.
76. Phillips RA, Miller RG. Physical separation of hemopoietic stem cells from cells causing graft-versus-host disease. I. Sedimentation properties of cells causing graft-versus-host disease. J Immunol 1970;105:1168–1174.
77. Abu-Zahra H, Amato D, Aye MT, et al. Bone marrow transplantation in patients with acute leukemia. Ser Haematol 1972;5:189–204.
78. Kaizer H, Stuart RK, Brookmeyer R, et al. Autologous bone marrow transplantation in acute leukemia: a phase I study of in vitro treatment of bone marrow with 4-hydroperoxycyclophosphamide to purge tumor cells. Blood 1985;65:1504–1510.
79. DeFabritiis F, Bregni M, Lipton J, et al. Elimination of clonogenic Burkitt's lymphoma cells from human bone marrow using 4-HC in combination with monoclonal antibodies and complement. Blood 1985;65:1064–1077.
80. Ramsay N, LeBien T, Nesbit M, et al. Autologous bone marrow transplantation for patients with acute lymphoblastic leukemia in second or subsequent remission: results of bone marrow treated with monoclonal antibodies BA-1, BA-2, and BA-3 plus complement. Blood 1985;66:508–513.
81. Takvorian T, Canellos GP, Ritz J, et al. Prolonged disease free survival after autologous bone marrow transplantation in patients with a poor prognosis. N Engl J Med 1987;316:1499–1505.
82. Berenson RJ, Andrews RG, Bensinger WI, et al. Antigen CD34+ marrow cells engraft lethally irradiated baboons. J Clin Invest 1988;81:951–955.
83. Cavins ED, Scheer SC, Thomas ED, et al. The recovery of lethally irradiated dogs given infusions of autologous leukocytes preserved at −80°C. Blood 1964;23:38–43.
84. Nelson B, Calvo W, Fliedner TM, et al. The repopulation of lymph nodes of dogs after 1200 R whole body X-irradiation and intravenous administration of mononuclear blood leukocytes. Am J Pathol 1976;84:259–282.
85. Nothdurft W, Bruch C, Fliedner TM, et al. Studies on the regeneration of the CFUc population in blood and bone marrow of lethally irradiated dogs after autologous transfusion of cryopreserved mononuclear blood cells. Scand J Haematol 1977;19:470.
86. Storb R, Prentice Rl, Thomas ED. Marrow transplantation for treatment of aplastic anemia—an analysis of factors associated with graft rejection. N Engl J Med 1977;296:61–66.
87. Körbling M, Dörken B, Ho AD, et al. Autologous transplantation of blood-derived hemopoietic stem cells after myeloablative therapy in a patient with Burkitt's lymphoma. Blood 1986;67:529–532.
88. Sharp JG, Armitage J, Crouse D, et al. Are occult tumor cells present in peripheral stem cell harvests of candidates for autologous transplantation? In: Dicke KA, Spitzer G, Jagannath S, Evinger-Hodges MJ, eds. Autologous bone marrow transplantation: proceedings of the Fourth International Symposium. 1989:693.
89. Juttner CA, To LB, Haylock DN, et al. Approaches to blood stem cell mobilisation. Initial Australian clinical results. Bone Marrow Transplantation 1990;5(suppl 1):21–23.
90. Craig JIQ, Parker AC, Anthony RS. The effects of various chemotherapy regimens on the levels of peripheral blood stem cells in patients with lymphoma. Bone Marrow Transplantation 1990;5(suppl 1):30–31.
91. Espigado I, Rodriquez JM, Carmona M, et al. Peripheral blood stem cell collection: comparison of two protocols. Bone Marrow Transplantation 1990;5(suppl 1):21.
92. Siena S, Bregni M, Brando B, et al. Circulation of CD34+ hematopoietic stem cells in the peripheral blood of high-dose cyclophosphamide-treated patients: enhancement by intravenous recombinant human granulocyte-macrophage colony-stimulating factor. Blood 1989;74: 1905–1914.
93. Körbling M, Haas R, Knauf W, et al. Therapeutic efficacy of autologous blood stem cell transplantation (ABSCT): the role of cytotoxic cytokine stem cell mobilization. Bone Marrow Transplantation 1990;5(suppl 1):39–40.
94. Lopez M, Mortel O, Pouillart P, et al. Infusion of autologous peripheral blood nucleated cells hastens hematological recovery after high dose chemotherapy and autologous transplantation of bone marrow. Bone Marrow Transplantation 1990;5(suppl 1):44–45.
95. Lopez M, Pouillart P, Du Puy Montbrun MC, et al. Fast hematological reconstitution after combined infusion of autologous marrow purged with mafosfamide and autologous peripheral blood stem cells in a patient with Ewing sarcoma. Bone Marrow Transplantation 1988;3:172–174.
96. Solberg L, Jamal N, Messner HA. Characterization of human megakaryocytic colony formation in human plasma. J Cell Physiol 1985;124:67–74.

97. Yamasaki K, Solberg LA Jr, Jamal N, et al. Hemopoietic colony growth-promoting activities in the plasma of bone marrow transplant recipients. J Clin Invest 1988;82:255–261.
98. Cairo MS, Suen Y, Sener L, et al. Circulating granulocyte colony-stimulating factor (G-CSF) levels after allogeneic and autologous bone marrow transplantation: endogenous G-CSF production correlates with myeloid engraftment. Blood 1992;79:1869–1873.
99. Nemunaitis J, Singer JW, Buckner CD, et al. Use of recombinant human granulocyte-macrophage colony-stimulating factor in autologous marrow transplantation for lymphoid malignancies. Blood, 1988;72:834–836.
100. Devereux S, Linch DC, Gribben JG, McMillan A, Patterson K, Goldstone AH. GM-CSF accelerates neutrophil recovery after autologous bone marrow transplantation for Hodgkin's disease. Bone Marrow Transplantation 1989;4:49–54.
101. Brandt SJ, William PP, Atwater SK, et al. Effect of recombinant human granulocyte-macrophage colony-stimulating factor on hematopoietic reconstitution after high-dose chemotherapy and autologous bone marrow transplantation. N Engl J Med 1988;318:869–876.
102. Sheridan WP, Wolf M, Lusk J, et al. Granulocyte colony-stimulating factor and neutrophil recovery after high-dose chemotherapy and autologous bone marrow transplantation. Lancet 1989;2:891–895.
103. Taylor K, Jagannath S, Spizer G, et al. Recombinant human granulocyte colony-stimulating factor hastens granulocyte recovery after high-dose chemotherapy and autologous bone marrow transplantation in Hodgkin's disease. J Clin Oncol 1993 (in press).
104. Thomas ED, Ramberg RE, Sale GE, et al. Direct evidence for a bone marrow origin of the alveolar macrophage in man. Science 1976;192:1016–1018.
105. van der Berg H, Kluin PM, Vossen JM. Early recognition of haematopoiesis after allogeneic bone marrow transplantation: A prospective histopathological study of bone marrow biopsy specimens. J Clin Pathol 1990;43:365–369.
106. Fyles GM, Messner HA, Lockwood G, et al. Long-term results of bone marrow transplantation for patients with AML, ALL and CML prepared with single dose total body irradiation of 500 cGy delivered with a high dose rate. Bone Marrow Transplantation 1991;8:453–463.
107. Petz LD, Yam P, Wallace RB, et al. Mixed hematopoietic chimerism following bone marrow transplantation for hematologic malignancies. Blood 1987;70:1331–1337.
108. Li S, Champlin R, Fitchen JH, Gale RP. Abnormalities of myeloid progenitor cells after "successful" bone marrow transplantation. J Clin Invest 1985;75:234–241.
109. Arnold R, Schmeisser T, Heit W, et al. Hemopoietic reconstitution after bone marrow transplantation. Exp Hematol 1986;14:271–277.
110. Messner HA, Curtis JE, Minden MD, et al. Clonogenic hemopoietic precursors in bone marrow transplantation. Blood 1987;70:1425–1432.
111. Vellenga E, Sizoo W, Hagenbeek A, Lowenberg B. Different repopulation kinetics of erythroid (BFU-E), myeloid (CFU-GM) and T lymphocyte (TL-CFU) progenitor cells after autologous and allogeneic bone marrow transplantation. Br J Haematol 1987;65:137–142.
112. Turhan AG, Humphries RK, Philips GL, et al. Clonal hematopoiesis demonstrated by X-linked DNA polymorphisms after allogeneic bone marrow transplantation. N Engl J Med 1989;320:1655–1661.
113. Browne PV, Lawler M, Humphries P, et al. Donor cell leukemia after bone marrow transplantation for severe aplastic anemia. N Engl J Med 1991;325:710–713.
114. Elfenbein GJ, Anderson PN, Humphrey RL, et al. Immune system reconstitution following allogeneic bone-marrow transplantation in man: a multiparameter analysis. Transplant Proc 1976;8:641–646.
115. Noel DR, Witherspoon RP, Storb R, et al. Does graft-versus-host disease influence the tempo of immunologic recovery after allogeneic human marrow transplantation? An observation on 56 long-term survivors. Blood 1978;51:1087–1105.
116. Witherspoon RP, Lum LG, Storb R. Immunologic reconstitution after human marrow grafting. Semin Hematol 1984;21:2–10.
117. Small TN, Keever CA, Weiner-Fedus S, et al. B-cell differentiation following autologous, conventional, or T-cell depleted bone marrow transplantation: a recapitulation of normal B-cell ontogeny. Blood 1990;76: 1647–1656.
118. Witherspoon RP, Matthews D, Storb R, et al. Recovery of in vivo cellular immunity after human marrow grafting. Transplantation 1984;37:145–150.
119. Torres A, Alonso MC, Gomez-Villagran JL, et al. No influence of numbers of donor CFU-GM on granulocyte recovery in bone marrow transplantation of acute leukemia. Blut 1985;50:89–94.
120. Atkinson K, Norrie S, Chan P, et al. Lack of correlation between nucleated bone marrow cell dose, marrow CFU-GM dose or marrow CFU-E dose and the rate of HLA identical sibling marrow engraftment. Br J Haematol 1985;60:245–251.
121. Ringden O, Nilsson B. Death by graft-versus-host disease associated with HLA mismatch, high recipient age, low marrow cell dose, and splenectomy. Transplantation 1985;40:39–44.
122. Niederwieser D, Gratwohl A, Oberholzer M, et al. Bone marrow cell dose and kinetics of recovery following allogeneic marrow transplantation in man. Blut 1983;47:355–360.
123. Spitzer G, Verma DS, Fisher R, et al. The myeloid progenitor cell—its value in predicting hematopoietic recovery after autologous bone marrow transplantation. Blood 1980;55:317–323.
124. Messner HA, Yamasaki K. Conditions affecting the growth of hemopoietic progenitors after bone marrow transplantation. In: Testa NG, Gale RP, eds. Hematopoiesis: long-term effects of chemotherapy and radiation, vol 8. New York: Marcel Dekker, 1988:377–388.
125. Messner HA, Meharchand JM, Minden MD, et al. Cyclosporin and relapse rate in patients transplanted for chronic myeloid leukemia (CML). J Cell Biochem (suppl 14A):
126. Tichelli A, Gratwohi A, Wursch A, Nissen C, Speck B. Late hematological complications in severe aplastic anemia. Br J Haematol 1988;69:413–418.
127. De Planque MM, Kalvin PM, Brand A, et al. Evolution of acquired severe aplastic anemia to myelodysplasia and subsequent leukemia in adults. Br J Haematol 1988;70:55–62.

Chapter 6
Isolation and Characterization of Hematopoietic Progenitor and Stem Cells

Charles M. Baum, Nobuko Uchida, Bruno Peault, and Irving L. Weissman

Although it had been known since the 1950s that irradiation-induced hematopoietic failure could be ameliorated by injection of genetically marked donor bone marrow cells, resulting in radioprotection and blood cell reconstitution, it was not until the landmark studies of Till and McCulloch, beginning in 1961, that the concepts concerning and the definitions of hematopoietic stem cells (HSC) became clarified (1). By analyzing the number and nature of cells giving rise to myeloerythroid and megakaryocytic spleen colonies in the irradiated mouse, Till and McCulloch found that each spleen colony was derived from a single clonogenic precursor; that each colony could contain granulocytic, monocytic, erythroid, and megakaryocytic elements; and that the spleens of these animals also contained cells capable of secondary spleen colony formation (2–4). From these experiments, they proposed that a cell type involved in spleen colony formation (CFU-S) was the HSC, that a single HSC was capable of multilineage differentiation, and that self-renewal of HSCs was one of the outcomes of cell division by these clonogenic precursors (2–4). Later work by Abramson and colleagues (5) demonstrated that lymphocytes in the thymus and in the periphery can be members of the same clone as the splenic myeloerythroid and megakaryocytic CFU-S progeny. On the basis of the known radioprotective activities of marrow, HSCs would be defined as (1) having the capacity for radioprotection, with fewer cells required for protection and with increased purification of the marrow suspension; (2) being capable of developing myeloid, erythroid, and lymphoid elements; and (3) having the capacity for self-renewal (6–9). There have been studies suggesting that although the CFU-S described by Till and McCulloch could include HSCs, radioprotection and long-term reconstitution could be mediated by different cell types—radioprotection by nonrenewing lineage-committed progenitors, and self-renewal by long-lived pre-CFU-S or pre-HSC cells (10,11).

From the foregoing, it is clear that the choice of assay for populations of cells believed to contain or consist of HSCs is critical to the assay result, because it is likely that different assays disclose activities of different populations. For example, the methylcellulose assay believed to detect HSCs involves the formation of colonies in vitro by clonogenic precursors that include multiple myeloerythroid and megakaryocytic lineages in each colony, or blast cell colonies (12,13). The CFU-S assay is more indicative of HSC function, especially if one looks for the cell type that is responsible for the appearance of colonies late (i.e., 12 days after injection of test cells), but not early (i.e., 8 days after injection) after lethal irradiation, under the hypothesis that more primitive cells, including HSCs, will take longer to give rise to day-12 CFU-S (14,15). Pre-CFU-S are defined as precursor cells capable of giving rise to CFU-S in secondary transplantation (from marrow or spleen) into lethally irradiated mice (16–18). It has been shown that some but not all late CFU-S contain pre-CFU-S activities (3,19). Radioprotection is yet another assay of HSC function (7,20,21). Therefore, data from several different assays, both in vitro and in vivo, must be evaluated for any particular cell population suspected of including HSCs.

Hematopoietic cells have been subfractionated based on size, density, and their expression of particular cell surface molecules (22). Cells expressing the stem cell antigen (Sca-1), low levels of Thy-1.1, and lacking markers of mature lineage commitment, although heterogeneous as to self-renewal capacity and some other properties, are capable of multilineage reconstitution. Both radioprotection and HSC renewal are properties expressed by this cell population (21–24).

Identification of the Marrow Clonogenic Precursors That Initiate Marrow Stromal Cultures

Marrow precursors for the pre-B and B-cell lineages are identified in mice by their ability to form B-lineage colonies on Whitlock-Witte stromal feeder layers (25,26). Utilizing a cloned marrow stromal line capable of supporting Whitlock-Witte cultures (27), it was shown that the cells capable of initiating these long-term, stromal-dependent, B-lineage cultures express no surface markers of the B-cell lineage, or of any other blood cell lineages (Lin^-). It was noted that the Thy-1 gene product, normally expressed at high levels on mouse thymic and peripheral T cells, as well as some fibroblasts and neurons, was expressed at very low levels on approximately 1% of marrow cells. The $Thy\text{-}1^{lo}$ Lin^- population, representing 0.15 to 0.20% of marrow cells, contained all of the activity in initiating Whitlock-Witte pre-B cultures (25). At limit dilution, approximately 1 in 11 of these cells was clonogenic and could initiate stromal cultures, compared with 1 in 1,100 unfractionated marrow cells (25). Approximately 1 in 30 of these same $Thy\text{-}1^{lo}$ Lin^- cells was capable of giving rise to a day-10 splenic colony (25). Thus, the $Thy\text{-}1^{lo}$ Lin^- population was simultaneously enriched in clonogenic B-cell precursors and clonogenic myeloerythroid precursors measured by the Till and McCulloch spleen colony assay.

Because neither of these results indicated that every $Thy\text{-}1^{lo}$ Lin^- cell gave rise to a colony (28–30), it was clear that additional purification would be required. To test the thymic progenitor activity of this population, an assay was developed for clonogenic thymic precursors (31–33). Thymic colonies derived from clonogenic marrow precursors injected into irradiated mice at limit dilution were detected using monoclonal antibodies directed against donor allele–specific markers (32). Approximately 1 in 36,000 unfractionated marrow cells was capable of initiating a single thymic focus when injected intravenously, or approximately 1 in 5,100 when injected intrathymically. Only two marrow subpopulations injected intravenously contained thymic progenitors—$Thy\text{-}1^{lo}$ Lin^- (1/600) and $Thy\text{-}1^{lo}$ Lin^+ (1/21,000) (32). Thus, the $Thy\text{-}1^{lo}$ Lin^- population was highly enriched for clonogenic T-cell, B-cell, and myeloerythroid progenitors.

THY-1.1^{lo} LIN$^-$ SCA-1$^+$ Mouse Marrow Cells Include Mouse HSCs

Further marrow fractionation was accomplished using the Sca-1 antibody (34), which marked a subset of marrow cells (2 to 8%) and 25 to 35% of $Thy\text{-}1.1^{lo}$ Lin^- marrow cells (22). Clonogenic precursors for thymus (CFU-T), spleen colonies (CFU-S), and marrow long-term stromal cultures were contained within the $Thy\text{-}1.1^{lo}$ Lin^- $Sca\text{-}1^+$ subset (21).

HSCs are generally thought to provide protection from myeloablative procedures that normally would result in "hematopoietic death," as well as long-term repopulation of T cells, B cells, and myeloerythroid cells. Therefore, purified populations of cells that include stem cells should share these properties. For example, as shown in Figure 6-1, approximately 200,000 unselected marrow cells are required to save 95 to 100% of lethally irradiated congenic mice (PD_{95}), and 40,000 cells are required to save approximately half the mice (PD_{50}). $Thy\text{-}1.1^{lo}$ Lin^- $Sca\text{-}1^+$ cells, representing 0.05% of marrow cells (1/2,000), were highly enriched for this activity; the PD_{95} was approximately 100 cells, whereas the PD_{50} was 20 to 30 cells (21). In all cases, radioprotected mice survived at least 6 months, and in all cases for which radioprotection occurred and was analyzed, donor-derived T cells, monocytes, granulocytes, and B cells were identified (21,35). Thus, the $Thy\text{-}1.1^{lo}$ Lin^- $Sca\text{-}1^+$ population, representing approximately 1 in 2,000 cells, was roughly 2,000-fold enriched for radioprotective and long-term multilineage reconstitutive activity.

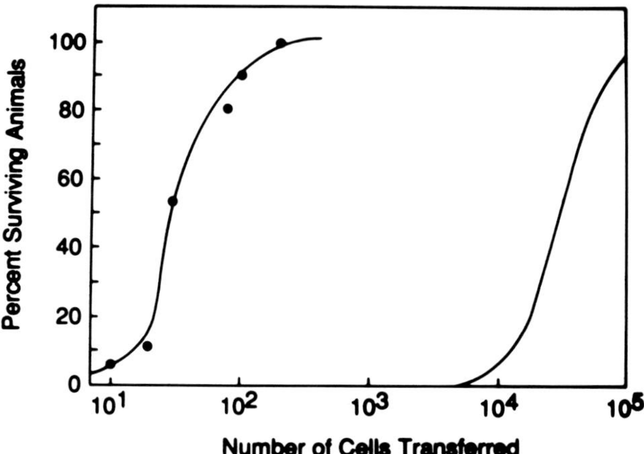

Figure 6-1. Radioprotection from lethal irradiation by purified $Thy\text{-}1.1^{lo}$ Lin^- $Sca\text{-}1^+$ stem cells. Groups of 10 to 20 mice were lethally irradiated (900 cGy) and reconstituted with graded number of $Thy\text{-}1.1^{lo}$ Lin^- $Sca\text{-}1^+$ hematopoietic stem cells intravenously. The figure shows the percent of animals surviving lethal irradiation (see text for details). (Reproduced by permission from Spangrude GJ, Heimfeld S, Weissman IL. Purification and characterization of mouse hematopoietic stem cells. Science 1988;241:58–62.)

To test whether any other cell population contained either HSC or pre-HSC activity, Ly-5.1 marrow cells were divided into the $Thy\text{-}1.1^+$ versus the Thy 1.1^-, the Lin^+ versus the Lin^-, or the $Sca\text{-}1^+$ versus the $Sca\text{-}1^-$ subsets, and injected into lethally irradiated Ly-5.2 hosts either alone or with 100,000 Ly-5.2 marrow cells. When isolated cell populations were injected alone, $Thy\text{-}1.1^+$ (but not $Thy\text{-}1.1^-$), Lin^- (but not Lin^+), and $Sca\text{-}1^+$ (but not $Sca\text{-}1^-$) cells gave rise to radioprotection (36). Furthermore, $Thy\text{-}1.1^-$, Lin^+, or $Sca\text{-}1^-$ populations did not give rise to donor-derived cells in lethally irradiated Ly-5.2 hosts radioprotected with syngeneic marrow cells. Finally, at all doses tested, the animals that were radioprotected with $Thy\text{-}1^{lo}$ Lin^- $Sca\text{-}1^+$ cells gave rise to T cells, B cells, granulocytes, and macrophages for at least 3 months following injection.

To test whether all clonogenic cells in the $Thy\text{-}1^{lo}$ Lin^- $Sca\text{-}1^+$ fraction are multipotent, 1, 5, 10, or 20 $Thy\text{-}1^{lo}$ Lin^- $Sca\text{-}1^+$ cells from Ly-5.2 donors were injected into lethally irradiated congenic hosts (Ly-5.1), with either 100 host-type $Thy\text{-}1.1^{lo}$ Lin^- $Sca\text{-}1^+$ cells or 200,000 host-type marrow cells (23,24). Using the Poisson distribution, the limit dilution number for a single clonogenic hit giving rise to greater than 1% of cells of donor type in the bloodstream at any time after irradiation and reconstitution is approximately 15 to 25 cells, centering on 22 cells (24). A wide heterogeneity of results was seen. Although all reconstitutions included myeloid and lymphoid cells, some animals did not reconstitute the T-cell lineage (23,24). The lack of T-cell reconstitution could be either due to a failure of seeding of the thymus by donor-marked HSCs or their progeny, or there might be heterogeneity of HSCs (33). The degree of reconstitution varied from 1% to greater than 60%. In those cases where myelopoiesis was sustained, donor-type marrow or isolated Thy-1.1^{lo} Lin$^-$ Sca-1$^+$ cells could retransfer to secondary lethally irradiated hosts full reconstitution in all lineages, as well as radioprotection (23,24). In approximately two thirds of the animals, myelopoiesis was not sustained (<28 wk); in these animals, reconstitution in the lymphoid lineages also often waned. Furthermore, these mice did not contain retransferable donor-derived HSC activity (24). Despite the heterogeneity in outcomes, all Thy-1.1^{lo} Lin$^-$ Sca-1$^+$ cells tested were multilineage progenitors that gave rise to lymphoid and myeloid cells.

How Many HSC Clones are Active at One Time?

The answer to this question in normal mice is unknown. However, by retroviral marking marrow cells isolated from donors treated with 5-fluorouracil (5-FU) in culture in the presence of packaged, defective murine leukemia virus genomes, unique retroviral integrants could be found in hosts transplanted following irradiation (37–40). Although such retroviruses cannot provide analysis at the level of a single cell, each hematopoietic clone was identified using restriction endonuclease cleavage followed by genomic Southern blot hybridization using probes from the transfecting sequence. It is relatively straightforward to quantitate these Southern blots, so that the level of unique integrants per cell can be calculated and the outcome of the clone can be recorded (39). In most studies, a common retroviral integrant could be found in B cells, thymic T cells, and myeloerythroid cells, often at a frequency of one copy/cell (39). Thus, the progeny of a single stem-cell clone can dominate hemolymphopoiesis. Furthermore, either in the same animal at a later time, or on retransplantation of marrow to a secondary animal, new clones can succeed, showing that the marrow contained more than a single integrant (40). The limit-dilution analysis of nontreated marrow implies that approximately 1 of 20 Thy-1.1^{lo} Lin$^-$ Sca-1$^+$ cells can form a clonogenic event in vivo, and one fourth to one third of these cells give rise to self-renewing clones (24). Thus, one would expect that only 1 in 60 to 1 in 90 Thy-1.1^{lo} Lin$^-$ Sca-1$^+$ cells normally contributes to long-lived, multilineage reconstitutions, the range observed when single-cell injections were carried out (23). Whether this process is a product of heterogeneity of seeding as well as heterogeneity of self-renewal potential or burst size is not yet known.

Heterogeneity of THY-1.1^{lo} LIN$^-$ SCA-1$^+$ Cells

Approximately one fourth to one third of Thy-1.1^{lo} Lin$^-$ Sca-1$^+$ adult marrow cells give rise to long-lived multilineage and self-renewing hematopoiesis, suggesting heterogeneity of separable HSCs. A mitochondrial dye, rhodamine 123 (Rh123), has been useful in separating marrow progenitor populations (7,18,41). Spangrude and Johnson (19) showed that Thy-1.1^{lo} Lin$^-$ Sca-1$^+$ marrow cells separated on the basis of the intensity of staining and retention of Rh123 correlate with their biological potentials. Their initial assay was (1) the ability of clones to give rise to both myeloid and T-lymphoid cells when injected directly into a lethally irradiated host's thymus, and (2) the ability to give large secondary spleen colonies in a retransfer from either marrow or spleen after injection of such marked cells. In both cases, large burst size and sustained hematopoiesis was a property of Rh123^{lo} Thy-1.1^{lo} Lin$^-$ Sca-1$^+$ cells, whereas Rh123^{hi} Thy-1.1^{lo} Lin$^-$ Sca-1$^+$ cells responded poorly in experiments that required large burst size or sustained hematopoiesis in secondary transfers (19). Li and associates (42) recently confirmed and extended this finding, demonstrating that in primary hosts Rh123^{lo} Lin$^-$ Sca-1$^+$ cells provide long-term multilineage outcomes of large burst size, whereas Rh123^{hi} Lin$^-$ Sca-1$^+$ marrow cells gave rise to limited multilineage differentiation.

Hematopoietic cells have been fractionated based on size and density using techniques such as velocity sedimentation, elutriation, and forward light scatter (21). Velocity sedimentation of marrow has shown that subsets of CFU-S can be isolated that differ in their proliferative capacities in vitro (22,43). Elutriation of marrow cells, which separates cells by size and density, has been used in an attempt to divide cells responsible for radioprotection versus cells responsible for long-term reconstitution (10). Male elutriated marrow cells were injected into lethally irradiated female mice, using Y chromosome sequences as a marker of chimerism. These investigators (10) reported that the smallest cells, contained within the 25 mL/minute elutriator fraction (FR 25), had undetectable CFU-S activity but were capable of long-term multilineage reconstitution if they were combined with a marrow fraction that was radioprotective. That is, FR 25 cells were neither radioprotective nor contained detectable CFU-S activity, but when injected with the blast cell fraction (called "Rotor-off") from the same donor marrow, these cells contributed to long-term reconstitutions in lymphoid and myeloid tissues (10). The day-12 CFU-S activity peaked in fraction 29 (FR 29), decreased somewhat in fraction 33 (FR 33), but stayed roughly level in the "Rotor-off," blast-cell fraction.

An independent analysis of HSC activities of FR 25, FR 29, FR 33, and "Rotor-off" shows that the distribution of Thy-1.1^{lo} Lin^- Sca-1^+ cells maps very well with the distribution of day-12 CFU-S activity in the 4 eluted fractions. When unselected marrow was injected, both long-term reconstitution and radioprotection correlate with the number of Thy-1.1^{lo} Lin^- Sca-1^+ cells contained within each elutriator fraction. In addition, the Thy-1.1^+, but not Thy-1.1^- cells, from FR 25 contain radioprotective and long-term reconstitutive activity in lethally irradiated hosts (24). In this study, it was not possible to divide the cells responsible for radioprotection from those responsible for long-term reconstitution.

Within the Thy-1.1^{lo} Lin^- Sca-1^+ population of mouse HSCs, there exists heterogeneity in terms of size, cell cycle status, Rh123 staining, and relative radioprotective effect, as well as long-term reconstitution ability. This heterogeneity appears to be intrinsic to the cell population isolated, because cells isolated by physical or DNA content parameters differ in their outcomes following injection into lethally irradiated animals. It is not clear that the heterogeneity exists in vivo; for example, cells in cycle might express different classes of homing receptors than resting cells, and in the artifactual circumstance of preparing and injecting cell suspensions, these cells might home differentially to marrow, resulting in differences in long-term reconstitution.

Regardless of whether the different physical and reconstituting properties are intrinsic, any intrinsic status for the cells could depend on its microenvironment, as well as its life history. A model that explains the data gathered to date is presented in Figure 6-2. This is only one of many models that explains the data, but it should suggest experiments to test its validity. There are several elements to this model. First, there would be a specific microenvironment for HSCs, and the number of HSC microenvironments is limited in normal mice. In this view, the HSCs residing in the self-renewing (S) stroma occupy a physically limited niche. As shown in Figure 6-2A, when an HSC undergoes cell divisions, not all of its progeny HSCs may occupy the S niche, but are pushed into the next niche, bordered by expansion (E) stroma. Although HSCs in both S and E niches could express the same profile of receptors, S and E stroma could provide different stimuli to HSCs. For example, S stroma would promote self-renewal of HSC, whereas E stroma provides microenvironments for extensive proliferation of HSCs with diminished self-renewal. As expansion in the E niche occurs, daughter cells would enter the regions where maturation occurs, presumably governed by maturation stroma (M). The number of available S niches would presumably regulate the number of injected HSCs that can engraft and expand in the context of bone marrow transplantation (BMT). Second, in the transition between the self-renewing microenvironment and the lineage-committing microenvironment, cells would be multipotent, but a significant fraction would have lost the capacity to self-renew when placed back in vivo, either because of a failure to home to these preset niches or due to a developmental change that is intrinsic, perhaps via the expression or function of cytokine receptors. Third, it is reasonable to propose that the vast majority of HSCs in the self-renewing microenvironment are sessile and that a limited fraction are called on to enter the proliferative and differentiative pool. This fraction could be increased by local or distant events that activate these microenvironmental niches. Cells that have undergone a renewing division, perhaps by virtue of their movement out of the microenvironment, may be changed such that a certain number of cell divisions can be accomplished by HSCs without losing the capacity for large-scale self-renewal or differentiation. This proposal is consistent with several hypotheses of HSC aging and with experiments in which serial retransplantation of marrow has a limit (44).

Heterogeneity of HSCs During Ontogeny

The outcomes of hematolymphopoiesis during embryonic and fetal development can differ from that found in postfetal and adult life (45–47). Perhaps the best known example is the switch of globins from embryonic to fetal to adult types in humans, and at least fetal to adult in mouse (48–51). Fetal versus adult B-cell and T-cell outcomes are also known (52–55). Perhaps the best example of successive outcomes in T lymphopoiesis has been defined in the mouse (47). During mouse fetal life, successive waves of immunocompetent T cells appear and disappear from the thymus and then seed the periphery, based on the particular T-cell receptor $V\gamma$ elements they rearrange and express, as well as the tissues to which they home and in which they reside (Figure 6-3A) (54,56). In mice, the order of successive rearrangements and expressions that is best known includes the $V\gamma3$ T cells first, which seed the skin; the $V\gamma4$ T cells next, which seed the female reproductive epithelium and both male and female tongue epithelium; the $V\gamma2/3$, which at least seeds the spleen; the $V\gamma5$ next, which seeds the intestinal epithelia; and then the switch to the highly diverse $\alpha\beta$ T-cell receptor (TCR) expressing cells, which seed the lymphoid organs and provide the most enduring and quantitatively largest subset of T cells in the body. As shown in Figure 6-3B, the order of appearance of these $V\gamma$ genes maps closely to their order on the $V\gamma$ chromosome; $V\gamma3$ is placed most closely to the $J\gamma1$ to which it will rearrange, followed by $V\gamma4$, $V\gamma2$, then $V\gamma5$.

At both the population and the clonogenic level, fetal HSCs placed in the fetal thymic microenvironment give rise to fetal ($V\gamma3$, $V\gamma4$) as well as the more mature ($V\gamma2$, $V\gamma5$, TCR$\alpha\beta$) outcomes. HSCs from late fetal and adult life placed in the fetal thymic microenvironment give rise to the more mature outcomes (55). Neither fetal nor adult HSCs could give

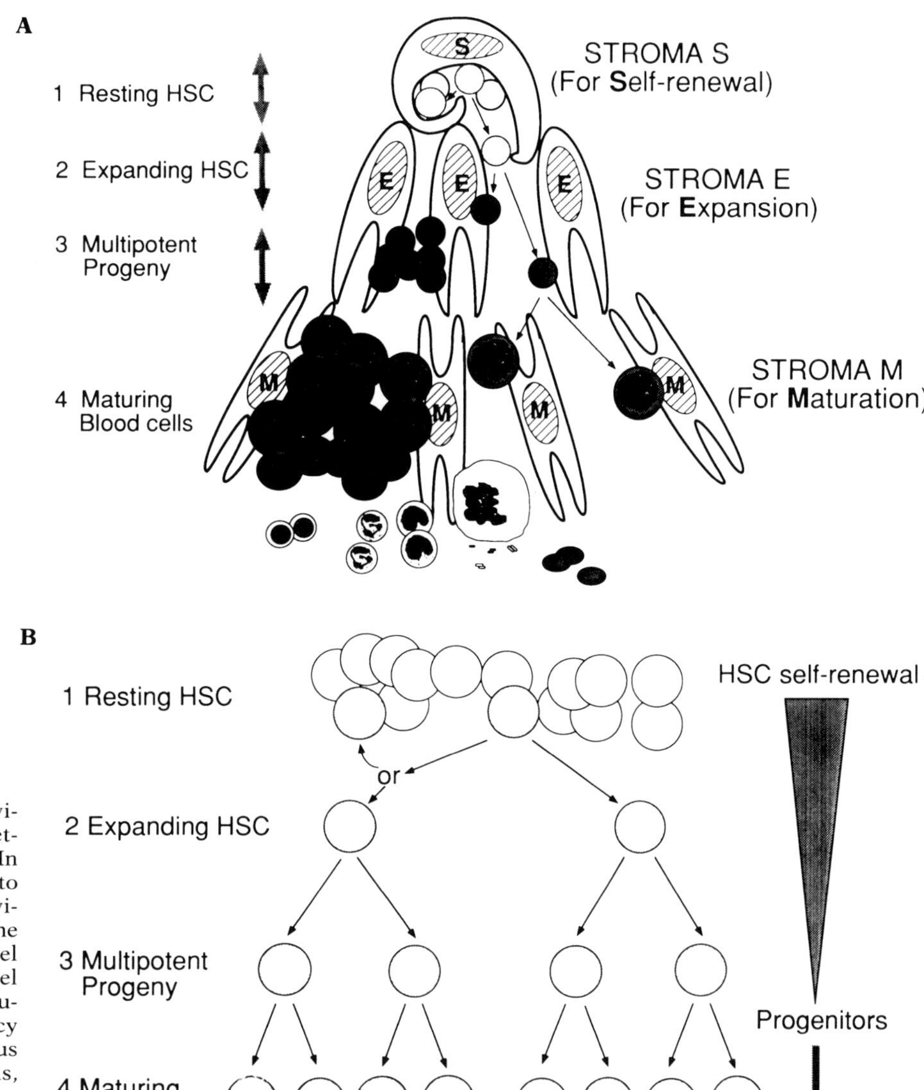

Figure 6-2. A model of microenvironmental determination of HSC heterogeneity (see text for details). (A) In this model, HSCs are subdivided into functional subsets by the microenvironments in which they reside. (B) The dynamics represented by this model could be derived from the model shown in (A), wherein stromal influences largely govern the frequency and distribution of renewing versus expanding HSCs, or other models, wherein these changes could be intrinsic to HSCs.

rise to the fetal outcome in the adult thymus, although both could give rise to the full variety of adult thymocytes and the full variety of adult peripheral T cells (55). Because each clone developing in the fetal thymus from fetal HSCs gives rise to both fetal and mature outcomes, the commitment to the fetal outcome does not mean that the cell is limited to that outcome. Furthermore, when the Vγ4 element rearranges to Jγ1 to make the fetal TCR, an enzymatic system that includes the enzyme terminal deoxynucleotidyl transferase (TdT) (57,58) adds extra nucleotides at the Vγ4-Jγ1 junction, which add to the diversity of specificities of that TCR (see Figure 6-3B) (59). However, the Vγ4 TCRs derived from day 13 or 14 fetal HSCs very rarely have N-nucleotides added. With increasing donor age, the isolated HSCs gave rise to Vγ4 T cells containing more N-nucleotide insertions (60). Thus, early fetal seeding of the reproductive and lingular epithelium is of T cells, all bearing exactly the same receptor specificity (61–63), whereas later T cells entering the same sites appear to be capable of antigen recognition diversity.

Response of HSCs and Related Cells to Hematopoietic Cytokines

HSC subsets have been defined by Rh123 staining, elutriation profile, and DNA synthesis (cell cycle) status. In addition, at least three other progenitors have been isolated—the Thy-1^{lo} Lin$^-$ Sca-1$^-$ primitive myeloid and erythroid progenitors (64), the Thy-1^{lo} B220$^+$ B-lineage progenitors (64,65), and the Thy-1^{lo} B220$^-$ Mac-1$^+$ myelomonocytic progenitors (64). The

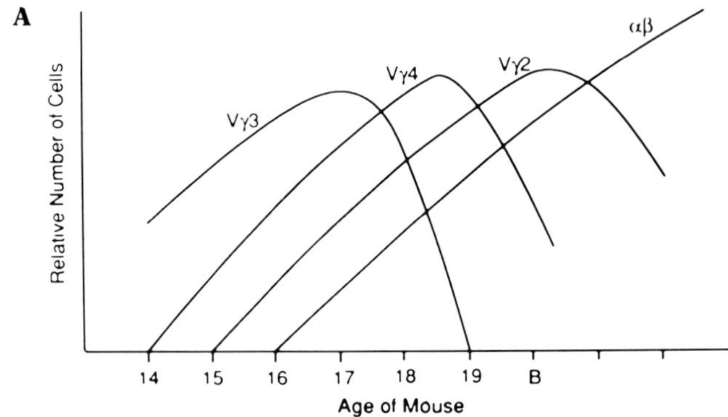

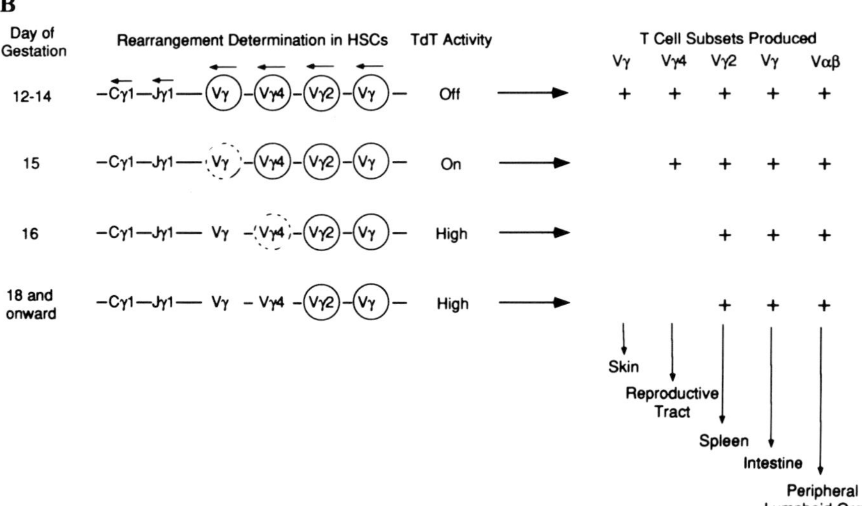

Figure 6-3. Differentiation of $\gamma\delta$ T cells during development. (A) Sequential waves of thymocytes during mouse development. (B) A model of chromosomal determinative events at the level of HSCs that concern T-cell development. Determination of T-cell receptor gene rearrangement and N nucleotide insertion at the level of HSC is shown. *Circles* indicate chromosomal closure to the recombination machinery. Vγ genes without circles represent closed loci, which are not accessible for the recombination machinery. The outcome of T-cell development and distribution is shown on the right. (Reproduced by permission from Ikuta K, Uchida N, Friedman J, Weissman IL. Lymphocyte development from stem cells. Annu Rev Immunol 1992;**10**:759–783.)

response of Thy-1.1^{lo} Lin$^-$ Sca-1$^+$ cells and Thy-1.1^{lo} Lin$^-$ Sca-1$^-$ cells to a number of hematopoietic cytokines has been tested (66). Although Thy-1.1^{lo} Lin$^-$ Sca-1$^+$ cells do not respond to any cytokine given singly (including steel factor [SLF]), interleukin-1 (IL-1), IL-3, IL-6, G-CSF, GM-CSF, M-CSF (66), IL-7 (24), IL-5 (67), and the Thy-1^{lo} Lin$^-$ Sca-1$^-$ myeloerythroid progenitors can respond in vitro by forming populations that contain myeloerythroid and megakaryocytic elements when incubated with IL-3, or any combination of factors that include IL-3 (66). The addition of IL-1, IL-3, or IL-6 in pairs also does not cause Thy-1.1^{lo} Lin$^-$ Sca-1$^+$ cells to respond, although the presence of all three factors causes a limited response; the addition of G-CSF, GM-CSF, and M-CSF can result in 50% of HSCs going into a proliferative cycle, the outcome of which is predominantly myeloid (66). In contrast, the addition of IL-1, IL-3, or IL-6 to SLF causes a significant fraction of HSCs to proliferate along the myeloid or erythroid lineages, with very massive burst sizes. SLF alone appears to provide long-term survival to nondividing HSCs, compared with no factor treatment. Isolated HSCs from adult mice have been useful for the study of cytokines that act on them alone or act as comitogens with other factors for their expansion and commitment to, at least, the myeloid/erythroid lineages. Because multilineage in vitro methylcellulose colonies can derive from non-HSC myeloid/erythroid progenitors, it is not a reliable measure of HSCs. In contrast, in vitro initiation of long-term cultures on Dexter or Whitlock-Witte stromal cells with retransfer activity is correlated strongly with HSC activity (68,69).

The Special Case of Steel Factor

It has long been believed that two mutations that cause profound anemias in mice are complementary to each other. The mutant forms of two genes, *Sl* and *W* (for Steel and dominant White spotting, respectively), when expressed in homozygotes, can result in lethal or pathogenic outcomes. In the lethal forms, mice die in late fetal or early postnatal life, with defects in the hematopoietic system, in brain and neural crest development, and in the formation of gonads (70,71). The mutant *W* locus codes for an intrinsic anemia, which can be transferred with marrow hematopoietic cells, whereas the steel gene codes for a marrow stromal microenvironmental defect. Thus, normal marrow cells cannot mature efficiently in *Sl/Sl* hosts, but *Sl/Sl* marrow cells can mature in normal hosts (72–75). The *W* locus gene, also known as c-*kit* (76–79), encodes a receptor with a cytoplasmic tyrosine kinase. Its ligand is the hematopoietic factor encoded by the *steel* locus, variably called Steel factor (SLF), stem-cell factor (SCF), mast cell growth factor (MCGF), or kit ligand (80–85). The factor can be expressed in membrane-bound or soluble forms. The full lethal form, *Sl/Sl*, reflects a deletion of the gene; the pathogenic but not full-lethal Sl^d defect is due to a deletion of the transmembrane form, leading to an anemia in which only the soluble form is expressed (86). This finding indicates that the membrane-bound form may be more effective or more efficient than the soluble form in promoting hematopoiesis (Figure 6-4).

The developing fetal liver of *Sl/Sl* mice contains 10-fold fewer hematopoietic cells compared with age-matched heterozygote and normal homozygote littermates (87). The Thy-1.1^{lo} Lin^- Sca-1^+ subset was present in these mice at levels reduced to approximately one third the level of the non-*Sl/Sl* littermates. The number of these cells doubled in the fetal liver between days 13 to 15 gestation at roughly the same rate as they did in the normal or heterozygote littermates (87). Despite the fact that most, if not all, HSCs express c-kit, generation of HSCs occurs in the fetal liver of mice that lack SLF or its receptor (87,88). Thus, it would appear that other growth factors, in addition to SLF, are critical to HSC generation.

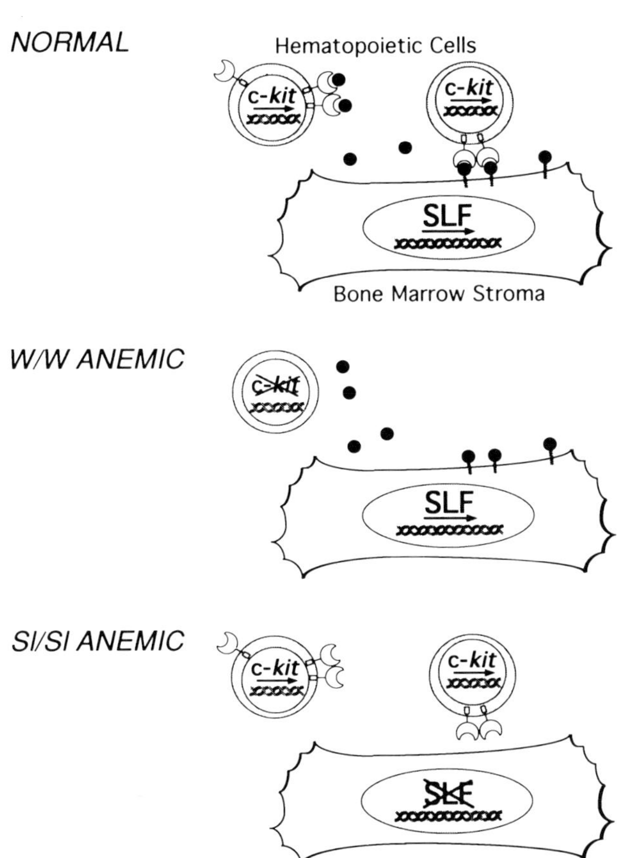

Figure 6-4. Steel *c-kit* model.

Steel factor with or without other local cytokines has an important role in the survival of HSCs once generated, and as a comitogen in their movement out of the HSC pool into progeny pools. Normal mice treated with recombinant soluble SLF conjugated to polyethyleneglycol for one week continuously in vivo exhibit a progressive loss of Thy-$1.1^{lo}$$Lin^-$Sca-$1^+$ cells by phenotype and function from the marrow and a progressive gain in their appearance in the blood and spleen, the latter presumably by passage through the blood. After one week of SLF therapy, spleen cellularity doubled and the number of Thy-1.1^{lo} Lin^- Sca-1^+ cells increased four-fold, whereas a 20-fold increase in Thy-1.1^{lo} Lin^- Sca-1^+ cells was observed in the peripheral blood (89). Nevertheless, the total body content of Thy-1.1^{lo} Lin^- Sca-1^+ HSCs increased by only approximately 25 to 30%. Because the most effective form of SLF is the membrane-bound form, it is conceivable that high concentrations of exogenously provided SLF will not only stimulate cells bearing c-*kit* receptors, but also release them from microenvironments wherein adhesion may in part be mediated by membrane-bound SLF on stromal cells and membrane-bound c-*kit* on HSCs.

Treatment of baboons with STL factor showed that the WBC count and $CD34^+$ cells increased, as did the content of methylcellulose colony forming cells in peripheral blood (90). A more modest elevation in marrow cellularity and methylcellulose colony formation was observed. The mast cell content of skin, marrow, and other tissues was elevated. The lack of massive self-renewal of HSCs in mice treated with high levels of SLF over a long period may imply that factors in addition to SLF are required for self-renewing HSC divisions. On the basis of the possibility that other factors may have a role in HSC dynamics, Mathews and colleagues (91) cloned molecules encoding other cytoplasmic domain protein tyrosine kinases and are searching for their ligands from a mouse fetal HSCs–enriched complementary DNA library in the hope of finding stem cell–restricted growth factors.

The Role of HSCs in Mouse BMT

It is part of the conventional wisdom that marrow transplants include mature cells for immediate use, lineage-restricted or oligolineage-restricted progenitors for short-term differentiation of mature cells, and HSCs for long-term establishment and maintenance of the hematopoietic system. Purified Thy-1.1^{lo} Lin^- Sca-1^+ HSCs provide radioprotection to hosts roughly to the extent that they are represented in marrow, suggesting that for radioprotection the most important cell type transferred was HSCs (21). Lethally irradiated Ly-5.1 mice injected with Thy-1.1^{lo} Lin^-

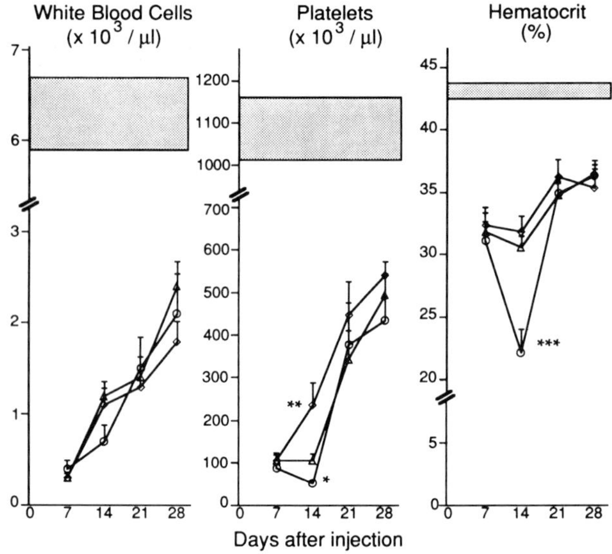

Figure 6-5. Hematopoietic recovery in lethally irradiated mice transplanted with purified Thy-1.1^{lo} Lin$^-$ Sca-1$^+$ cells. The irradiated mice were injected with either 100 (*circles*), 500 (*triangles*), or 1,000 (*diamonds*) Thy-1.1^{lo} Lin$^-$ Sca-1$^+$ cells. The normal values of WBC, platelet counts, and percent of hematocrit of unirradiated mice are represented by the *shaded boxes*. Data represent mean ± SE obtained from 7 to 11 mice with 100 or 500 Thy-1.1^{lo} Lin$^-$ Sca-1$^+$ cells injected, and from 4 to 5 mice with 1,000 Thy-1.1^{lo} Lin$^-$ Sca-1$^+$ cells injected in each data point. * = 100 vs 500 Thy-1.1^{lo} Lin$^-$ Sca-1$^+$ cells injected, $p < 0.006$; ** = 500 vs 1,000 Thy-1.1^{lo} Lin$^-$ Sca-1$^+$ cells injected, $p < 0.02$; and *** = 100 vs 500 Thy-1.1^{lo} Lin$^-$ Sca-1$^+$ cells injected, $p < 0.01$. (Uchida N, Fleming WH. Unpublished data).

Sca-1$^+$ cells from C57BL/Thy-1.1 donors showed that the time to appearance of white blood cells (granulocytes and monocytes), platelets, and red blood cells sufficient to maintain hematocrit in mice injected with 100, 500, or 1,000 Thy-1.1^{lo} Lin$^-$ Sca-1$^+$ cells varied only slightly; by days 21 to 28, no significant differences could be found (Figure 6-5) (Uchida N, Fleming WH. Unpublished data). Using allelic Ly-5 markers, the white cells found on day 14 and the white cells, B cells, and T cells found as late as week 29 were largely, if not completely, donor-derived. Perhaps most interestingly, 500 Thy-1.1^{lo} Lin$^-$ Sca-1$^+$ cells injected into lethally irradiated congenic mice gave rise to donor-derived white cells, platelets, and red blood cells at levels very close to that found when 1×10^6 marrow cells (the number of marrow cells containing 500 Thy-1.1^{lo} Lin$^-$ Sca-1$^+$ cells) were injected (see Figure 6-5).

These experiments suggest that both during early and late phases of hematopoiesis, the cells of central importance in donor-derived reconstitution as well as radioprotection were the Thy-1.1^{lo} Lin$^-$ Sca-1$^+$ HSCs, and that the direct effects of adding other progenitors and mature cells were not major. Marrow populations depleted of cells with stem-cell phenotype show minimal effect on life span following lethal irradiation, with approximately 6-day prolongation in life, but no significant long-term radioprotective effects (36). Specific studies delineating the biological activities of lineage-committed and oligolineage-committed non-HSC progenitors transplanted along with the minimal radioprotective dose of HSCs in the presence or absence of cytokines designed to expand some of these populations could reveal important adjunctive roles for non-HSC progenitors. Furthermore, the Rh123^{hi} and Rh123^{lo} subsets of Thy-1^{lo} Lin$^-$ Sca-1$^+$ HSCs may have differential capacities for blood cell/element production and HSC/progenitor renewal at different phases after BMT.

Allogeneic BMT In Mice

BMT across allogeneic or semiallogeneic MHC barriers has been carried out and has several important clinical and biological consequences in both mouse and humans (see Chapters 18, 19, and 26). In the mouse, studies of BMTs across allogeneic barriers have shown that lethal irradiation is not sufficient to suppress all elements that interfere with the transplantation of hematopoietic cells (92). The most potent MHC barrier was found to be active in situations where other tissue transplants normally succeed—the transplantation of inbred parent strain marrow or tissues to crosses between that inbred strain (e.g., strain A) and another inbred strain (e.g., strain B) to form (A × B) F1 hybrids (92–94). Cudkowicz and colleagues (92) proposed that a set of transplantation antigens is present on hematopoietic progenitors and that radio-resistant effector cells in F1 hosts recognize these recessive antigens as foreign and block the ability of transplanted hematopoietic progenitors to survive or expand (93). These results led to an intensive search to elucidate the hybrid-histocompatibility (Hh) determinants, the cells that recognize the Hh determinants, and the receptor cells used to recognize these determinants (95). Several different investigators have shown that natural killer (NK) cells are involved in recognizing Hh determinants (96–98).

In clinical BMT, allogeneic marrow depleted of T cells fails to engraft more often than allogeneic marrow containing T cells (see Chapters 3 and 11). Addition of T cells to marrow in the mouse induces graft-versus-host disease (GVHD), which can overcome the previously described Hh-related barriers (95). It seems likely that either the marrow T cells or the added peripheral T cells enable engraftment by inactivating or depleting the population of cells bearing NK antigens, although the details of which cells are engraftment-facilitating and whether they also suppress or possess GVHD activity is still to be determined. It is clear that the donor population need not include T cells to provide a GVHD activation of T cells that provide secreted hematopoietic cytokines, because autologous or Ly-5 congenic transplants with Thy-1.1^{lo} Lin$^-$ Sca-1$^+$ cells only is sufficient for radioprotection, multilineage reconstitution, and long-term self-renewal of HSCs (21,23).

When Thy-1.1^{lo} Lin^{-} Sca-1^{+} cells are transplanted in a parent → F1 or an allogeneic combination along with treatment of the host with antibodies that eliminate the Hh-type resistance, engraftment occurs in the absence of GVHD (Jerabek L, Weissman L. Unpublished data). Because GVHD across either major or minor histocompatibility barriers is a major limitation to the successful and widespread use of allogeneic BMT in the treatment of human diseases, the fact that pure HSC transplants can engraft without GVHD is most promising for the future of BMT in humans.

Isolation and Characterization of Human Hematopoietic Progenitor and Stem Cells

Isolation and characterization of human hematopoietic progenitor and stem cells have been hindered by the paucity of hematopoietic assay systems available, particularly in vivo model systems. As described, in vitro assays have provided, and continue to provide, valuable insight into progenitor cell function in the murine system. The short-term methylcellulose and long-term, stroma-dependent liquid cultures (Dexter cultures) have been the mainstays of hematopoietic analysis in humans (99–103). Quantitative in vitro assays provide valuable data on the enrichment of lymphoid and myeloerythroid progenitor cell function (25, 26, 68, 69); however, the ultimate proof of stem-cell activity resides in in vivo assays, such as the CFU-S, CFU-T, and long-term reconstitution of all blood cell lineages (25, 31–33). It can be argued that the only "proof" of stem-cell activity depends on the rescue of lethally irradiated animals and their subsequent long-term reconstitution in all hematopoietic lineages. The existence of long-term repopulating progenitors and stem cells has been shown in humans after allogeneic BMTs, which resulted in full reconstitution of the marrow recipient by donor-derived hematopoietic cells (see Chapter 12). Furthermore, insight into in vivo human hematopoietic cell function has been gained by recent negative selection or purging trials, as well as by a limited number of positive selection trials (104,105). Unfortunately, the majority of clinical trials using positive or negative selection have been performed in autologous BMTs, which preclude proof that the infused, selected cell population is responsible for the survival of the patient and long-term hematopoietic reconstitution. Therefore, the challenge facing investigations into isolation and characterization of human HSCs continues to be the lack of definitive assay systems.

In Vitro Studies of Human Hematopoietic Progenitors

In vitro assay systems developed using murine cells have been modified over the years for use with human marrow cells. The methylcellulose assay developed by Bradley and Metcalf (99) and Pluznik and Sachs (100), which utilizes exogenous growth factors and serum to support cell growth in a semisolid matrix, supports the growth and differentiation of committed progenitors of the erythroid, granulocytic, macrophage, and megakaryocytic lineages (106). The methylcellulose cultures support growth and differentiation of single lineage–committed progenitors as well as multilineage "mixed colonies," wherein a single cell gives rise to erythroid, granulocytic, macrophage, and megakaryocytic (myeloerythroid) lineages. These "mixed colonies" are believed to represent multipotent progenitors, which are more mature than stem cells. Large colonies formed in methylcellulose in response to purified factors enriched in 5-FU–treated marrow have been termed *high proliferative potential* (HPP) and may represent an earlier progenitor than the "mixed colony" (107). Progenitors that are believed to be even more primitive give rise to "blast cells" in the methylcellulose assay (108). These colonies maintain limited self-renewal capacity, indicated by their ability to be replated into methylcellulose, where they may generate more blast cell colonies as well as multipotent (myeloerythroid) and differentiated colony types (108).

In vitro growth and differentiation of human hematopoietic progenitors also occur in long-term (4–8 wk) liquid culture systems, which utilize mixed stromal cell layers derived from marrow to support hematopoiesis. Dexter cultures support growth and differentiation of granulocytic, monocytic, erythrocytic, and megakaryocytic progenitors for several weeks (102,103). In mice, Dexter cultures are able to support some maintenance of CFU-S and long-term reconstituting cells for variable times (68,69). Whitlock-Witte stromal cultures also support a brief burst of myeloerythropoiesis in mice, but then B-lineage differentiation takes over. With the loss of myelopoiesis, there is a concomitant loss of CFU-S and long-term reconstituting cells (25). To our knowledge, there have been no reports of long-term culture systems that support growth and differentiation of human B-cell progenitors analogous to the mouse Whitlock-Witte culture system. However, progress has been made in human B-lymphopoiesis using either an agar support matrix or a stromal cell–based liquid culture system (109–111).

CD34 Is Expressed by Human Hematopoietic Progenitors

A notable advance in the purification of human hematopoietic progenitors came with the discovery of the CD34 antigen (112–116). Previous attempts to purify cells based on density and size produced significant enrichments but were insufficient to purify progenitors or candidate HSCs to homogeneity (116–119).

The CD34 antigen is expressed by 1 to 5% of normal human adult marrow cells (112–114) and by 2 to 10% of normal fetal liver and marrow cells (120). Morphologically, these cells are a mixture of immature blastic cells and a small percentage of mature lineage-committed cells of the myeloid, erythroid, and lymphoid series (112–114). Virtually all colonies detected in the methylcellulose assay are derived from cells that express the CD34 antigen. Furthermore, CD34-positive cells are able to establish long-term, stromal cell–dependent cultures in vitro, in contrast to cells that lack CD34 (112–114,121,122). Despite the 10- to 100-fold enrichment for hematopoietic progenitors, the CD34 cell subset is by no means a pure progenitor or HSC population. Analysis of the cell-surface phenotype of CD34-positive cells suggests that the majority are committed to a particular lineage. Fully 90 to 95% of the CD34-positive cells express antigens indicative of commitment to the lymphoid or the myeloerythroid lineages (112–115). By definition, those cells committed to a particular lineage as indicated by morphology, cell-surface phenotype, or colony formation ability are not true HSCs. Therefore, one might expect that at most 0.05 to 0.25% of adult marrow, or 0.1 to 0.5% of fetal marrow, are HSCs. In the mouse system, 1/2,000 (0.05%) or fewer marrow cells are HSCs, as shown by their ability to reconstitute lethally irradiated animals in all lineages.

Advantage has been taken of the observation that murine HSCs lack many of the cell-surface antigens expressed by committed progenitors and mature blood cell types. Several investigators have shown that depletion of cells that express markers indicative of lymphoid development in humans does not impact significantly on results in methylcellulose or long-term culture assays (123–125). In contrast, depletion of all cells expressing antigens indicative of myeloid or erythroid development results in a significant decrease in the frequency of colonies in the methylcellulose assay (126–131), suggesting that the majority of colonies formed in methylcellulose are the result of proliferation of committed progenitors. The CD33 antigen, which is coexpressed with CD34 by the majority of progenitors detectable in the methylcellulose assay, is absent from the cells that initiate long-term, stroma-dependent liquid cultures (126–128). These long-term culture-initiating cells (LTC-IC) respond poorly in the methylcellulose assay, although their daughter cells may express CD33 and give rise to differentiated colony types in methylcellulose. Furthermore, virtually all blast cell colonies arise from the $CD34^+$ $CD33^-$ population (127).

Several investigators have implicated HLA class II (DR) antigens as useful markers of human hematopoietic cells. Those cells that express CD34 but lack detectable levels of HLA-DR are enriched for cells which give rise to long-term cultures (132–134), as well as blast-cell colonies (135). The majority (97%) of these cells are in the G0/G1 phase of the cell cycle and are therefore considered to be resting cells (136). In mice, radioprotective $Thy\text{-}1.1^{lo}Lin^-$ cells do not express detectable levels of MHC class II $I\text{-}A^b$ antigens (Uchida N, Weissman IL. Unpublished data).

Other cell surface molecules that appear to be useful in selecting against mature hematopoietic cells and committed progenitors include CD38 (a widely expressed antigen with unknown function) and CD71 (the transferrin receptor) (137,138). It has been shown that more than 90% of cells that express CD34 also express CD38 (139). The $CD34^+CD38^-$ cells are predominantly blast cells morphologically, and liquid cultures in the absence of stromal cells with added IL-3, IL-6, GM-CSF, and G-CSF showed that serial transfer of $CD34^+CD38^-$ cells was possible over a 120-day period (139). It has also been shown that $CD34^+CD71^-$ cells are enriched for cells that support the initiation of long-term cultures (131,138).

In addition to CD34, other molecules have been used to identify human progenitor cells. As described, Rh123, a mitochondrial dye, and antibodies to the c-kit receptor have been used in the murine system to characterize purified populations of HSCs (7,18,19, 41,42). The most primitive hematopoietic progenitors stain poorly with Rh123, whereas more committed progenitors retain higher levels of Rh123 (19,42). It appears that the P-glycoprotein is responsible for transporting the Rh123 out of cells and may itself serve as a marker of HSCs (140). Cells that are $CD34^+$Rh123-dull are responsible for virtually all (94%) of the long-term stroma culture-initiating activity of human marrow cells (120,141,142). In contrast, the $CD34^+$Rh123-bright cell fraction is depleted of long-term culture activity but is enriched for clonogenic-committed progenitors detected in the methylcellulose assay (120,141). More than half of human marrow cells that express CD34 also express the c-kit receptor and are enriched for each of the colony-forming cells in clonogenic assays (143–145). Furthermore, subfractionations using CD34, HLA-DR, and c-kit receptor antibodies have shown that the $CD34^+DR^-c\text{-}kitR^+$ cells are enriched for high proliferative potential as well as long-term culture initiating cells (146). Lansdorp and colleagues (138,147) reported that the CD45 RO isoform is expressed preferentially on primitive hematopoietic progenitors.

Murine marrow stromal cell lines are able to support long-term human hematopoiesis of fetal human marrow cells (120). Marrow stromal cell lines derived from murine Whitlock-Witte cultures support the growth and differentiation of human B-cell and myeloerythroid progenitors from whole fetal human marrow (120). The derived B cells express CD19; the majority are positive for CD10, and a small percentage express CD20, indicating that the majority of the B cells are immature. The myeloerythroid cells are detected either by their expression of CD15 and CD33 or by their ability to form clonal colonies in methylcellulose. These cultures can be replated and continuously produce cells for up to 4 months. The availability of a cloned stromal cell line allowed the establishment of reproducible limiting dilution and single-cell assays of purified hematopoietic progenitors (Table 6-1). Limiting dilution analysis showed that more than 99% of the cells initiating these long-term cultures express CD34. Further analysis indi-

Table 6-1.
Differentiation Potential of Various Human Fetal BM Cell Populations From Limit Dilution or Single-cell Analysis[a]

Population (% total)	*Growth-positive*	*% With B and Myeloid Cells*
Whole BM (100%)[a]	>1/3,000	ND
$CD34^+$ (2–10%)[a]	1/200	ND
$CD34^-$ (90–98%)[a]	>1/50,000	ND
$Thy\text{-}1^+$ $CD34^+$ (0.01–0.5%)	1/20	66
$Thy\text{-}1^-$ $CD34^+$ (2–10%)	1/323	0
$Thy\text{-}1^+$ Lin^- (0.1–0.5%)	1/21	60
$Thy\text{-}1^+$ Lin^+ (0.3–2%)	0/288	0
Lin^- $CD34^+$ (0.1–0.5%)	1/27	47
Lin^+ $CD34^+$ (2–10%)	1/80	25
$Thy\text{-}1^+$ $CD34^+$ $Rh\text{-}123^{lo}$ (0.03–0.15%)	1/25	ND
$Thy\text{-}1^+$ $CD34^+$ $Rh\text{-}123^{hi}$ (0.03–0.15%)	0/1,483	ND

[a]The frequency of wells containing B-lymphoid and myeloid cells is determined by analyzing the growth-positive wells for the presence of B cells ($CD10^+$, $CD19^+$) and myeloid cells ($CD15^+$, $CD33^+$) by FACS analysis. Numbers represent the mean value of three to six experiments.
ND = not determined.
(From Baum CM, Weissman IL, Tsukamoto AS, Buckle AM, Peault B. Isolation of a candidate human hematopoietic stem-cell population. Proc Natl Acad Sci USA 1992;89:2804–2808; reprinted with permission from the National Academy of Sciences.)

cated that the initiating cells reside in the CD34-positive population depleted of CD3-, 4-, 8-, 10-, 14-, 15-, 19-, 20-, 33-, 38-, and 71-expressing cells (Lin^-). Furthermore, the stromal culture–initiating cells from human fetal marrow express low levels of the human Thy-1 antigen (120,121).

The ability of $CD34^+Thy\text{-}1^+$ cells to establish long-term cultures was enriched 10- to 20-fold over unseparated $CD34^+$ cells, consistent with the fact that Thy-1 is detectable on approximately 5% of human fetal marrow $CD34^+$ cells (121). Individual cells of the $CD34^+Thy\text{-}1^+$ phenotype are able to differentiate into B cells ($CD19^+$), myeloid cells ($CD15^+$,$CD33^+$), and erythroid cells (BFU-e) in stromal-dependent cell cultures. Up to 100,000 cells could be derived from a single input cell over the 4- to 6-week culture period, and single cells could give rise to hundreds of colonies (e.g., CFU-GM, BFU-e) in the methylcellulose assay. Furthermore, these single-cell cultures could be retransferred up to 4 times over a 14-week period. In contrast, the $CD34^+Thy\text{-}1^+$ and $CD34^+Thy\text{-}1^-$ populations were about equally effective in the methylcellulose clonogenic assay. Similar results were obtained for $CD34^+Lin^-$, $CD34^+Rho123^{lo}$, and $CD34^+Thy\text{-}1^+Lin^-$ populations. These in vitro data support and extend the observations of others. Taken together, the data suggest that human HSCs are contained within the $CD34^+$, the $Thy\text{-}1^+$, the $Rho123^{lo}$, the c-kit R^+, the DR^-, the CD45 RO^+, and the Lin^- subsets. Studies that combine all of these markers are now underway.

In Vivo Studies of Human Hematopoietic Cell Function

Mouse HSCs are defined by their ability to permanently reconstitute a lethally irradiated animal in all hematopoietic lineages and to renew HSCs, thereby preventing "hematopoietic death." Allogeneic BMT in humans after myeloablative therapy shows that within donor marrow there is a population of cells which can constitute all lineages and results in long-term engraftment. Enriched populations of marrow cells have been used in primate BMT studies because the CD34 marker is highly conserved and therefore can be recognized by some of the same antibodies that recognize the human CD34 antigen (148). A fraction of the baboons were shown to survive autologous BMT of a crude population of $CD34^+$ cells and to have sustained hematopoiesis thereafter (148). Unfortunately, the contribution of the $CD34^+$ cells to survival is obscured by the fact that there is no marker to determine if the cells that resulted in long-term hematopoiesis were the baboon's own residual marrow cells or the added $CD34^+$ fraction, which also contained committed progenitors that may provide sufficient marrow function to prevent death until endogenous HSCs take over. Studies are now underway to evaluate $CD34^+$ cells in primates in allogeneic BMT to test whether they are responsible for sustained engraftment.

Experimental protocols using purified marrow progenitor populations are now underway in humans at several centers (105,149). In one of these studies, $CD34^+$ cells from patients undergoing BMT for breast cancer are being used to help purge the marrow of breast carcinoma cells, because the cancer cells in these populations do not express detectable levels of CD34 (105,149). Patients transplanted with $CD34^+$ cells have shown hematopoietic recovery, which is likely due to the $CD34^+$ cells, although reconstitution by endogenous cells not depleted by the myeloablative regimen or cells contaminating the $CD34^+$ population cannot be ruled out (105,146). Recent studies have shown that human marrow depleted of $CD33^+$ cells to remove leukemic cells can result in long-term hematopoietic recovery (104). Although preliminary, the results of both the CD34-positive selection and the CD33 depletion suggest that engraftment is delayed significantly when compared to historic control subjects given unfractionated BMTs (104,105). This finding is in contrast to the mouse system, in which purified HSCs exhibited similar kinetics to unfractionated marrow in reconstituting hematopoietic function. This discrepancy is as yet unexplained and may be due to a number of factors, including mouse HSCs are isolated from healthy animals rather than chemotherapy-treated autologous donors; experimental marrow ablation in mice is more likely to be complete than most myeloablative regimens in humans; and mouse HSCs may be inherently different than human HSCs.

In an alternative approach to an animal model of

human hematopoiesis, fetal human marrow was transplanted into fetal sheep in utero (150). Engraftment of human cells as shown by karyotype, methylcellulose colony formation in vitro, and cell-surface phenotype was found in 8 of 11 fetal sheep killed before birth and in 5 of 22 analyzed at birth. Some of the animals showed evidence of engraftment for at least 2 years. Furthermore, the sheep exhibited responses to exogenously added human growth factors (i.e., IL-3, GM-CSF). This system offers an interesting model of human hematopoiesis in vivo that may provide sufficient cells for further studies of human cell function, although the time and effort involved may limit the utility of this approach.

Obviously, current approaches to evaluating human HSCs are insufficient. On the one hand, systems use primate rather than human cells, and on the other hand, in autologous BMTs, evaluating engraftment is complicated by a lack of genetic markers to distinguish donor from host cell populations. The SCID/human (SCID-hu) model system has been utilized to evaluate the differentiation potential of human marrow subpopulations (151). Fetal human thymic fragments can be implanted surgically in C.B.17 scid/scid (SCID) mice, in which T-lymphopoiesis can be maintained for 1 to 3 months in the absence of added progenitor cells (151). During this period, the immature cortical cells differentiate into mature medullary T cells, with concomitant depletion of the immature thymocytes. Human thymopoiesis can be sustained long term in the SCID-hu mouse if a source of T-cell progenitors is provided (151). Fetal thymus lobules have been injected with purified fractions of human marrow in vitro, then transplanted into SCID mice. The T-cell progenitors injected are class I HLA mismatched to the recipient thymic lobule to allow determination of donor or host origin of the resultant T cells (Figure 6-6). Cell sorting experiments have shown that the $CD34^+$ marrow cells are able to repopulate the full range of T cells in the implanted SCID-hu thymus (152,153). Further subfractionation of fetal marrow showed that virtually all of the cells capable of long-term reconstitution of the SCID-hu thymus are contained in the $CD34^+Thy\text{-}1^+$ cell subset (see Figure 6-6) (120). In contrast, the $CD34^+Thy\text{-}1^-$ cells were capable of only transient T-cell repopulation in some cases (120). These data are particularly important in that they show that the $CD34^+Thy\text{-}1^+$ cell population contains not only virtually all of the long-term culture repopulating activity for B cells and myeloerythroid cells, but also thymus-repopulating cells.

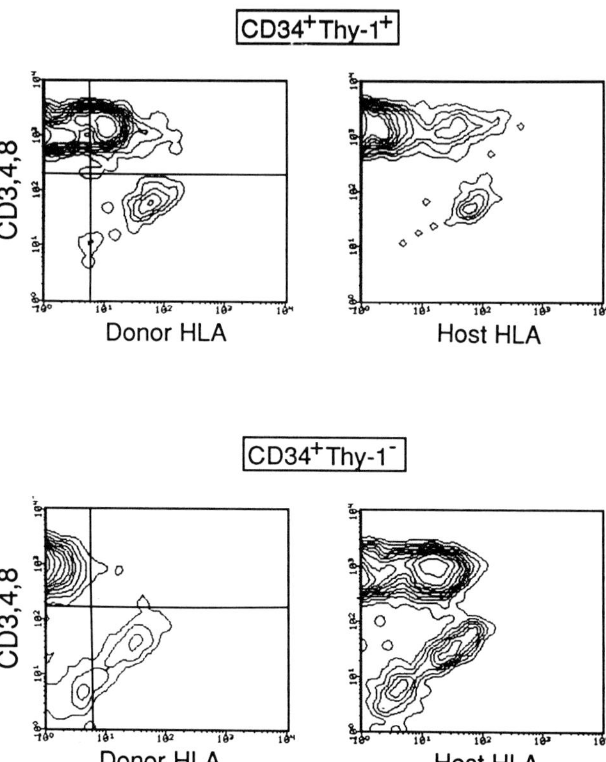

Figure 6-6. Intrathymic T-cell development of allogeneic $CD34^+$ fetal precursor cells. Human fetal thymus lobules (20 weeks' gestation) were cultured at 25°C for 7 days, then microinjected with 2,500 donor cells sorted from an HLA-dissimilar, 21-week fetal marrow. Thymus pieces were then engrafted under the kidney capsule of SCID mice for 2.5 months. Graft cell suspensions were antibody-stained as described and run on the FACScan analyzer. Chimerism was quantitatively evaluated by calculating the percentage of T cells expressing detectable levels of donor-specific HLA C1 I antigens, located in the upper right quadrant (50% in the experiment shown here). (From Baum CM, Weissman IL, Tsukamoto AS, Buckle AM, Peault B. Isolation of a candidate human hematopoietic stem-cell population. Proc Natl Acad Sci USA 1992;89:2804–2808; reprinted with permission from the National Academy of Sciences.)

In addition to allowing development of thymic lobules, the SCID mouse can support surgically implanted fragments of human fetal bone that contain cells sustaining the growth of hematopoietic marrow for up to 18 weeks (154). Each of the differentiated myeloerythroid cell lineages can be identified morphologically as well as by expression of cell-surface antigens in these bone marrow fragments. In addition, progenitors of the myeloerythroid lineages can be demonstrated in the clonogenic methylcellulose assay (154). These fragments also contain B cells, as shown by the presence of cells expressing CD19. The marrow fragments can provide the host environment for transplanted human fetal marrow progenitors. FACS-sorted human hematopoietic progenitor populations were microinjected into HLA-disparate human fetal marrow transplanted into SCID mice. The $CD34^+Thy\text{-}1^+$ cell population reconstituted the B-lymphoid ($CD19^+$) and myeloid ($CD33^+$) compartments of the host marrow (Table 6-2). In contrast, the $CD34^+Thy\text{-}1^-$ cell population, which makes up 90 to 95% of the CD34-positive subset, was unable to give rise to B cells or myeloid cells (154). The SCID-hu chimeric system is

Table 6-2.
Percentage of Donor-derived Hematopoietic Cells in Human Fetal Bone Segments Injected with 10^4 Donor Cells[a]

	2 Months		3 Months	
Population	*% Myeloid*	*%B*	*% Myeloid*	*%B*
Thy1$^+$CD34$^+$	36	47	45	86
	13	20	6	1
	19	25	0	0
	ND	6	21	29
Thy-1$^-$CD34$^+$	0	0	0	0
	0	0	1	0
	0	0	0	0

[a]The frequency of B-lymphoid cells is determined by CD19 and CD20 expression, whereas myeloid cells are determined by CD33 expression.
ND = not determined.
(From Baum CM, Weissman IL, Tsukamoto AS, Buckle AM, Peault B. Isolation of a candidate human hematopoietic stem-cell population. Proc Natl Acad Sci USA 1992;89:2804–2808; reprinted with permission from National Academy of Sciences.)

a model for BMT that is amenable to experimental manipulation. Studies are now underway to evaluate other populations of cells that are likely to harbor stem cells such as CD34$^+$Thy-1$^+$Lin$^-$, CD34$^+$Rho123^{lo}, CD34$^+$c-kitR$^+$, as well as others.

Clinical Applications of Human Hematopoietic Progenitors and Stem Cells

In the mouse model, many studies have shown that isolated HSC populations of various purities can fully reconstitute all hematopoietic lineages for the lifetime of the animal. These studies have also shown that certain characteristics of HSCs exhibited in vitro are reliable, although not infallible, indicators of a cell population's ability to reconstitute an animal in vivo. The most reliable indicator of HSC function in vitro appears to be the ability of a cell population to initiate and maintain hematopoiesis in long-term, stroma-dependent culture systems (68,69). The majority of human studies have relied on extrapolation of these data to human hematopoietic cells. Many groups have shown that isolated cell populations that constitute from 0.05 to 1% of the whole marrow contain virtually all of the long-term, culture-initiating activity and thus presumably contain HSCs. As mentioned, autologous BMT studies in primates and humans indicate that the CD34$^+$ cells contain all detectable long-term reconstituting activity of human marrow. Additional preclinical and clinical studies are required to show that this cell population contains HSCs as demonstrated by full donor-derived reconstitution of humans and other primates following allogeneic BMT.

Further subfractionation of the CD34$^+$ population into purified HSCs would be useful clinically in the isolation of normal stem cells from leukemic cells in the marrow of patients. The majority of acute leukemias express the CD34 antigen as well as other markers, which indicates that they are immature but committed to a particular lineage. Thus, lineage-specific antigens can be used in conjunction with CD34 to remove at least a subset of leukemic blasts from marrow (112–114). It has been shown that chronic myeloid leukemia (CML) is a malignancy that affects either a pluripotent progenitor or the HSC (155) (see Chapters 44 and 56). Most notably, the studies of Fialkow and colleagues (155,156) and Le Bien and associates (157) have shown that the Philadelphia chromosome, which is the result of a chromosomal translocation, t(9;22), is expressed by myeloid, erythroid, and B-lymphoid lineages. A recent report indicates that T lymphocytes may also be involved in this disease (158).

However, some patients with CML transplanted with treated autologous marrow have achieved complete remission, indicating that normal HSCs at least coexist with leukemic multipotent progenitors (159, 160). Furthermore, studies with interferon (IFN)-alpha treatment have shown that remission can be achieved (161). The BMT studies and the IFN results suggest that HSCs may not be involved, but rather the disease derives in large part from a malignant pluripotent progenitor population that expands to dominate hematopoiesis. Several groups have indicated that purified subsets of CD34$^+$ cells express less or none of the bcr/abl messenger RNA (mRNA) (162). The CD34$^+$DR$^-$ cell fraction appears to be depleted of bcr/abl mRNA relative to the CD34$^+$DR$^+$ fraction (162). However, these studies are complicated by the fact that cells were evaluated for bcr/abl mRNA levels after an in vitro culture step, a technique which has been shown by Turhan and co-workers (163) to lead to decreased Ph$^+$ cells in the culture relative to normal hematopoiesis (see Chapter 56). Consequently, these investigators have begun clinical studies utilizing cultured marrow as a means of removing malignant clones from the marrow of patients with CML (163). Cells with the CD34$^+$Thy-1$^+$Lin$^-$ phenotype have also been shown to express very low or undetectable levels of bcr/abl mRNA (Negrin RS, Baum CM. Unpublished data). It will be critical to determine whether there is a defect in transcription of translocated bcr/abl genes or if the translocation does not exist in HSCs.

Purified HSCs would provide an excellent population of cells for the introduction of genes to correct hematopoietic and metabolic deficiencies, as well as to endow HSCs and their progeny with beneficial properties for particular disease or therapy conditions (164) (see Chapter 7). Introduction of genes into purified HSCs would increase efficiency compared with whole marrow, in which less than 1/1,000 cells are HSCs. Direct introduction of genes into HSCs should also provide long-term and possibly life-long production of the desired gene product in hematolymphoid cells. For example, HSCs expressing high levels of adenosine deaminase (ADA) gene products could be curative for patients lacking the enzyme who have severe combined immunodeficiency. HSCs could also bear introduced genes that, when expressed, confer resistance to human immunodeficiency virus infection or its pathogenic effects leading to therapies for patients with acquired immune deficiency syndrome.

Obviously, the utility of HSC isolation would be increased dramatically by improvements in the ability to expand them in vitro before in vivo infusion. Advances in hematopoietic growth factor research over the past decade have provided the basis for beginning in vitro stem-cell expansion (144,165,166). However, more work remains, because current results indicate that none of the known growth factors leads to significant HSC expansion in the absence of differentiation (66,138). It is likely that within the near future, HSC and progenitor cell expansion in vitro will expand the clinical utility of purified HSCs for BMT, postchemotherapy hematopoietic supplements, and gene therapy.

Conclusions

Dramatic advances have been made in the identification, characterization and isolation of HSCs. Results in the mouse have shown that HSCs stain poorly with Rho123; express SCA-1, Thy-1, and c-kit receptor; and lack expression of antigens indicative of commitment to any of the mature blood cell lineages. Cells with this phenotype can reconstitute animals in all blood cell lineages for long periods and appear to be capable of self-renewal. In humans, candidate HSCs also appear to stain poorly with Rho123; express CD34, Thy-1, and c-kit receptor; and lack expression of HLA-DR, as well as antigens present on committed progenitors of mature blood cell lineages. The parallels between the two species are striking, including the fact that very similar in vitro culture systems can be used to study both human and mouse HSCs. Most of the findings in the mouse have been extrapolated to humans, which is particularly interesting in view of the fact that mouse HSCs give reconstitution on the same relative time scale as whole marrow. Current studies using crude preparations of purified human progenitors have suggested that engraftment is delayed. Further studies in humans or other primates using allogeneic BMT models may help address the kinetics of engraftment, as well as the relative contributions of purified progenitors and residual host marrow.

It is likely that purified populations of human marrow will have utility in BMT. In addition, these studies should help answer central scientific issues concerning stem cell self-renewal, as well as differentiation and commitment to the varied hematopoietic cell lineages.

References

1. Till JE, McCulloch EA. A direct measurement of the radiation sensitivity of normal mouse bone marrow cells. Radiat Res 1961;14:213–222.
2. Becker AJ, McCulloch EA, Till JE. Cytological demonstration of the clonal nature of spleen colonies derived from transplanted mouse marrow cells. Nature 1963; 197:452–454.
3. Siminovitch L, McCulloch EA, Till JE. The distribution of colony-forming cells among spleen colonies. J Cell Comp Physiol 1963;62:327–336.
4. Wu AM, Till JE, Siminovitch L, McCulloch EA. Cytological evidence for a relationship between normal hematopoietic colony-forming cells and cells of the lymphoid system. J Exp Med 1968;127:455–464.
5. Abramson S, Miller RG, Phillips RA. The identification in adult bone marrow of pluripotent and restricted stem cells of the myeloid and lymphoid systems. J Exp Med 1977;145:1567–1579.
6. Spangrude GJ, Smith LG, Uchida N, et al. A perspective on mouse hematopoietic stem cells. Blood 1991;78: 1395–1402.
7. Ploemacher RE, Brons RHC. Separation of CFU-S from primitive cells responsible for reconstitution of the bone marrow hematopoietic stem cell compartment following irradiation: evidence for a pre-CFU-S cells. Exp Hematol 1989;17:263–266.
8. Visser, JWM, Van Bekkum DW. Purification of pluripotent hematopoietic stem cells. Exp Hematol 1990;18: 284–256.
9. Sprangrude GJ. Hematopoietic stem-cell differentiation. Curr Opin Immunol 1991;3:171–178.
10. Jones RJ, Wagner JE, Celano P, Zicha MS, Sharkis SJ. Separation of pluripotent hematopoietic stem cells from spleen colony-forming cells. Nature 1990;347: 188–189.
11. Keller G. Hematopoietic stem cells. Curr Opin Immunol 1992;4:133–139.
12. Nakahata T, Ogawa M. Identification in culture of a class of hematopoietic colony-forming units with extensive capability to self-renew and generate multipotential hematopoietic colonies. Proc Natl Acad Sci USA 1982;79:3843–3847.
13. Metcalf D. Hematopoietic colony stimulating factors. Amsterdam: Elsevier, 1984:167.
14. Magli MC, Iscove NN, Odartchenko N. Transient nature of early hematopoietic spleen colonies. Nature 1982; 295:527–529.
15. Molineux G, Schofied R, Testa N. Development of spleen CFU-S colonies from day 8 to day 11: relationship to self-renewal capacity. Exp Hematol 1986;14: 710–713.
16. Hodgson GS, Bradley TR. Properties of hematopoietic stem cells surviving 5-luorouracil treatment: evidence for a pre-CFU-S cell? Nature 1979;281:381–382.
17. Ploemacher RE, Brons NHC. Isolation of hematopoietic stem cell subsets from murine bone marrow: II. Evidence for an early precursor of day-12 CFU-S and cells associated with radioprotective ability. Exp Hematol 1988;16:27–32.
18. Bertoncello I, Hodgson GS, Bradley TR. Multiparameter analysis of transplantable hematopoietic stem cell. II. Stem cells of long-term marrow-reconstituted recipients. Exp Hematol 1988;16:245–249.
19. Sprangrude GJ, Johnson GR. Resting and activated subsets of mouse multipotent hematopoietic stem cells. Proc Natl Acad Sci USA 1990;87:7433–7437.
20. Visser JWM, Gauman JGJ, Mulder AH, Eliason JF, Leeuw AWD. Isolation of murine pluripotent hematopoietic stem cells. J Exp Med 1984;59:1576–1590.
21. Spangrude GJ, Heimfeld S, Weissman IL. Purification

and characterization of mouse hematopoietic stem cells. Science 1988;241:58–62.

22. Visser JWM, Van Bekkum DW. Purification of pluripotent hematopoietic stem cells: past and present. Exp Hematol 1990;18:248–256.
23. Smith LG, Weissman IL, Heimfeld S. Clonal analysis of hematopoietic stem-cell differentiation in vivo. Proc Natl Acad Sci USA 1991;88:2788–2792.
24. Uchida N. Characterization of mouse hematopoietic stem cells. PhD Thesis. Stanford University, 1992.
25. Muller-Sieburg CE, Whitlock CA, Weissman IL. Isolation of two early B lymphocyte progenitors from mouse marrow: a committed pre-B cell and a clonogenic Thy-1^{lo} hematopoietic stem cell. Cell 1986;44:653–662.
26. Whitlock CA, Tidmarsh GF, Muller-Sieburg C, Weissman IL. Bone marrow stromal cell lines with lymphopoietic activity express high levels of pre-B neoplasia-associated molecules. Cell 1987;48:1009–1021.
27. Whitlock CA, Witte ON. Long-term culture of B lymphocytes and their precursors from murine bone marrow. Proc Natl Acad Sci USA 1982;79:3608–3612.
28. Lord BI. The relationship between spleen colony production and spleen cellularity. Cell Tissue Kinet 1971;4:211–216.
29. Hendry JH. The f number of primary transplanted splenic colony-forming cells. Cell Tissue Kinet 1971;4: 217–223.
30. Till JE, McCulloch EA. The 'f-Factor' of the spleen-colony assay for hematopoietic stem cells. Ser Heamatol 1972;5:15–21.
31. Ezine S, Weissman IL, Rouse R. Bone marrow cells give rise to distinct cell clones within the thymus. Nature 1984;309:629–631.
32. Spangrude GJ, Muller-Sieburg CE, Heimfeld S, Weissman IL. Two rare populations of mouse Thy-1^{lo} bone marrow cells repopulate the thymus. J Exp Med 1988;167:1671–1683.
33. Spangrude GJ, Weissman IL. Mature T cells generated from single thymic clones are not phenotypically and functionally heterogeneous. J Immunol 1988;14:1877–1890.
34. Aihara Y, Buhring J, Aihara M, Klein J. An attempt to produce "pre-T" cell hybridomas and to identify their antigens. Eur J Immunol 1986;16:1391–1399.
35. Scheid MP, Triglia D. Further description of the LY-5 system. Immunogenetics 1979;9:423–433.
36. Uchida N, Weissman IL. Searching for hematopoietic stem cells: evidence that Thy-1.1^{lo} Lin^- Sca-1^+ cells are the only stem cells in C57BL/Ka-Thy-1.1 bone marrow. J Exp Med 1992;175:175–184.
37. Dick JE, Magli MC, Huszar D, Phillips RA, Bernstein A. Introduction of a selectable gene into primitive stem cells capable of long-term reconstitution of the hematopoietic system of W/W^v mice. Cell 1985;42:71–79.
38. Keller G, Paige C, Gilboa E, Wagner EF. Expression of a foreign gene in myeloid and lymphoid cells derived from multipotent hematopoietic precursors. Nature 1985;318:149–154.
39. Lemischka IR, Raulet DH, Mulligan RC. Developmental potential and dynamic behavior of hematopoietic stem cells. Cell 1986;45:917–927.
40. Jordan CT, Lemischka IR. Clonal and systemic analysis of long term hematopoiesis in the mouse. Genes Dev 1990;4:220–232.
41. Bertoncello I, Hodgson GS, Bradley TR. Multiparameter analysis of transplantable hematopoietic stem cells: I. The separation and enrichment of stem cells homing to marrow and spleen on the basis of rhodamine-123 fluorescence. Exp Hematol 1985;13: 999–1006.
42. Li CL, Johnson GR. Rhodamine123 reveals heterogeneity within murine Lin^-, Sca-1^+ hematopoietic stem cells. J Exp Med 1992;175:1443–1447.
43. Worton RG, McCullock EA, Till JE. Physical separation of hematopoietic stem cells differing in their capacity for self renewal. J Exp Med 1969;130:91.
44. Siminovitch L, Till JE, McCulloch EA. Decline and colony-forming ability of marrow cells subjected to serial transplantation into irradiated mice. J Cell Comp Physiol 1964;64:23–32.
45. Raulet DH, Spencer DM, Hsiang YH, et al. Control of $\gamma\delta$ T-cell development. Immunol Rev 1991;120:185–204.
46. Allison JP, Havran WL. The immunobiology of T cells with invariant $\gamma\delta$ antigen receptors. Annu Rev Immunol 1991;9:679–705.
47. Ikuta K, Uchida N, Friedman J, Weissman IL. Lymphocyte development from stem cells. Annu Rev Immunol 1992;10:759–768.
48. Fantoni A, Bank A, Marks PA. Globin composition and synthesis of hemoglobins in developing fetal mice erythroid cells. Science 1967;157:1327–1329.
49. Forrester WC, Takegawa S, Papayannopoulou T, Stamatoyannopopulos G, Grousinw M. Evidence for a locus activator region. Nucleic Acids Res 1987;15:10159–10177.
50. Grosveld F, Blom van Assendelft G, Greaves DR, Kollias G. Position-independent high level expression of the human β-globin gene in transgenic mice. Cell 1987;51: 975–985.
51. Hanscombe O, Whyatt D, Fraser P, et al. Importance of globin gene order for correct developmental expression. Genes Dev 1991;5:1387–1389.
52. Hayakawa K, Hardy RR, Herzenberg, LA. Progenitors for Ly-1 B cells are distinct from progenitors for other B cells. J Exp Med 1985;161:1554–1568.
53. Solvason N, Lehuen A, Kearney JF. An embryonic source of Ly1 but not conventional B cells. Int Immunol 1991;3:543–550.
54. Havran WL, Allison JP. Developmentally ordered appearance of thymocytes expressing different T-cell antigen receptors. Nature 1988;335:443–445.
55. Ikuta K, Kina T, MacNeil I, et al. A developmental switch in thymic lymphocyte maturation potential occurs at the level of hematopoietic stem cells. Cell 1990;62:863–874.
56. Havran WL, Allison JP. Origin of Thy-1^+ dendritic epidermal cells of adult mice from fetal thymic precursors. Nature 1990;344:60–62.
57. Alt FW, Baltimore D. Joining of immunoglobulin heavy chain gene segments: implications from a chromosome with evidence of three D-J_H fusions. Proc Natl Acad Sci USA 1982;79:4118–4122.
58. Desiderio SV, Yancopoulos GD, Paskind M, et al. Insertion of N regions into heavy-chain genes is correlated with expression of terminal deoxytransferase in B cells. Nature 1984;311:752–755.
59. Sorger SB, Paterson Y, Fink PJ, Hedrick SM. T-cell receptor junctional regions and the MHC molecule affect the recognition of antigenic peptides by T cell clones. J Immunol 1990;144:1127–1135.
60. Ikuta K, Weissman IL. The junctional modifications of a T cell receptor g chain are determined at the level of thymic precursors. J Exp Med 1991;174:1279–1282.
61. Born W, Hall L, Dallas A, et al. Recognition of peptide

antigen by heat shock—reactive gamma delta T lymphocytes. Science 1990;249:67–69.
62. Havran WL, Chien Y-H, Allison JP. Recognition of self antigens by skin-derived T cells with invariant $\gamma\delta$ antigen receptors. Science 1991;252:1430–1432.
63. Young RA. Stress proteins and immunology. Annu Rev Immunol 1990;8:401–420.
64. Heimfeld S, Holzmann B, Guidos C, Palmer E, Weissman IL. Developmental analysis of the mouse hematolymphoid system. Cold Spring Harbor Symp Quant Biol 1989;54:75–85.
65. Tidmarsh GF, Heimfeld S, Whitlock CA, Weissman IL, Muller-Sieburg CE. Identification of a novel bone marrow-derived B-cell progenitor population that coexpresses B220 and Thy-1 and is highly enriched for Abelson Leukemia Virus targets. Mol Cell Biol 1989;9: 2665–2671.
66. Heimfeld S, Hudak S, Weissman IL, Rennick D. The in vitro response of phenotypically defined mouse stem cells and myeloerythroid progenitors to single or multiple growth factors. Proc Natl Acad Sci USA 1991; 88:9902–9906.
67. Muller-Sieburg CE, Townsend K, Weissman IL, Rennick D. Proliferation and differentiation of highly enriched mouse hematopoietic stem cells and progenitor cells in response to defined growth factors. J Exp Med 1988;167:1825–1840.
68. Weilbaecher K, Weissman IL, Blume K, Heimfeld S. An in vitro assay for hematopoietic stem cells: long-term colony formation in micro-Dexter cultures. Blood 1991;78:945–952.
69. van der Sluijs JP, de Jong JP, Brons NHC, Ploemacher RE. Marrow repopulating cells, but not CFU-S, establish long-term in vitro hematopoiesis on a marrow-derived stromal layer. Exp Hematol 1990;18:893.
70. Sarvella PA, Russel LB. Steel, a new dominant gene in the house mouse. J Hered 1956;47:123–128.
71. Russell ES. Hereditary anemias of the mouse: a review for geneticists. Adv Genet 1979;20:357–349.
72. McCulloch EA, Siminovitch L, Till JE, Russell ES, Bernstein SE. The cellular basis of the genetically determined hematopoietic defect in anemic mice of genotype Sl/Sl^d. Blood 1965;26:399–410.
73. Seller MJ. Donor haemoglobin in anaemic mice of the W-series transplanted with hematopoietic tissue from an unrelated donor. Nature 1966;212;81–82.
74. Bernstein SE, Russell ES, Keighley G. Two hereditary mouse anemias (Sl/Sl^d and W/W^v) deficient in response to erythropoietin. Ann NY Acad Sci 1968;149: 475–485.
75. Seller MJ. Transplantation of anaemic mice of the W-series with hematopoietic tissue bearing marker chromosomes. Nature 1968;220:300–301.
76. Qiu F, Ray P, Brown K, et al. Primary structure of *c-kit:* relationship with the CSF-1/PDGF receptor kinase family-oncogene activation of *v-kit* involves deletion of extracellular domain and C terminus. EMBO J 1988;7: 1003–1011.
77. Yarden Y, Kuang WJ, Yang-Feng T, et al. Human proto-oncogene *c-kit:* a new cell surface receptor tyrosine kinase for an unidentified ligand. EMBO J 1987;6:3341–3351.
78. Chabot B, Stepheson DA, Chapman VM, Besmer P, Bernstein A. The proto-oncogene *c-kit* encoding a transmembrane tyrosine kinase receptor maps to the mouse W locus. Nature 1988;335:88–89.
79. Geissler EN, Ryan MA, Houseman DE. The dominant-white spotting (W) locus of the mouse encodes the *c-kit* proto-oncogene. Cell 1988;55:185–192.
80. Williams DE, Eisenman J, Baird A, et al. Identification of a ligand for the *c-kit* proto-oncogene. Cell 1990;63: 167–174.
81. Copeland NG, Gilberd DJ, Cho BC, et al. Mast cell growth factor maps near the steel locus on mouse chromosome 10 and is deleted in a number of steel alleles. Cell 1990;63:175–183.
82. Martin FH, Suggs SV, Langley KE, et al. Primary structure and functional expression of rat and human cell factor DNAs. Cell 1990;63:203–211.
83. Zsebo KM, Williams DA, Geissler EN, et al. Stem cell factor is encoded at the S1 locus of the mouse and its the ligand for the *c-kit* tyrosine receptor. Cell 1990;63: 213–224.
84. Huang E, Nocka K, Beier DR, et al. The hematopoietic growth factor KL is encoded by the S1 locus and is the ligand of the *c-kit* receptor, the gene product of W locus. Cell 1990;63:225–233.
85. Anderson DM, Lyman SD, Baird A, et al. Molecular cloning of mast cell growth factor, a hematopoietin that is active in both membrane bound and soluble forms. Cell 1990;63:235–243.
86. Flanagan JG, Chan DC, Leder P. Transmembrane form of the *kit* ligand growth factor is determined by alternative splicing and is missing in the Sl^d mutant. Cell 1991;64:1025–1035.
87. Ikuta K, Weissman IL. Evidence that hematopoietic stem cells express mouse *c-kit* but do not depend on steel factor for their generation. Proc Natl Acad Sci USA 1992;89:1502–1506.
88. Okada S, Nakauchi H, Nagayoshi K, et al. Enrichment and characterization of murine hematopoietic stem cells that express *c-kit* molecule. Blood 1991;78:1706–1712.
89. Fleming WH, Alpern C, Uchida N, Ikuta K, Weissman IL. Steel factor influences the distribution and activity of murine hematopoietic stem cells in vivo. Proc Natl Acad Sci USA 1993;90:3760–3764.
90. Andrews RG, Bartelmez SH, Knitter GH, et al. A c-kit ligand, recombinant human stem cell factor, mediates reversible expansion of multiple $CD34^+$ colony-forming cell types in blood and marrow of baboons. Blood 1992;80:920–927.
91. Mathews W, Jordan CT, Wiegand GW, Pardoll D, Lemischka IR. A receptor tyrosine kinase specific to hematopoietic stem and progenitor cell-enriched populations. Cell 1991;65:1143–1152.
92. Cudkowicz G, Stimpfling JH. Deficient growth of C57BL marrow cells transplanted in F1 hybrid mice. Association with the histocompatibility-2 locus. Immunology 1964;7:291–306.
93. McCulloch EA, Till JE. Repression of colony-forming ability of C57BL hematopoietic cells transplanted into non-isologous hosts. J Cell Comp Physiol 1963;61:301–308.
94. Cudkowicz G. Genetic control of bone marrow graft rejection. I. Determinant-specific difference of reactivity in a pair of inbred mouse strains. J Exp Med 1971;134:281–293.
95. Yu YYL, Kumar V, Bennet M. Murine natural killer cells and marrow graft rejection. Annu Rev Immunol 1992;10:189–213.
96. Lotzova E, Cudkowicz G. Abrogation of resistance to bone marrow grafts by silica particles. Prevention of the silica effect by the macrophage stabilizer poly-2-vinylpyridine N-oxide. J Immunol 1974;113:798–803.

97. Lotzova E, Savary CA, Pollack SB. Prevention of rejection of allogeneic bone marrow transplants by NK1.1 antiserum. Transplantation 1983;35:490–494.
98. Sentman CL, Hackett JJ, Kumar V, Bennett M. Identification of a subset of murine natural killer cells that mediates rejection of Hh-1^d but not Hh-1^b bone marrow grafts. J Exp Med 1989;170:191–202.
99. Bradley TR, Metcalf D. The growth of mouse bone marrow cells in vitro. Aust J Exp Biol Med Sci 1966;44:287–300.
100. Pluznik DH, Sachs L. The cloning of normal "mast" cells in tissue culture. J Cell Comp Physiol 1965;66: 319–324.
101. Dexter TM, Lajtha LG. Proliferation of hematopoietic stem cells in vitro. Br J Haematol 1974;28:525–530.
102. Dexter TM, Moore MAS, Sheridan PAS. Maintenance of hematopoietic stem cells and production of differentiated progeny in allogeneic and semiallogeneic bone marrow chimeras in vitro. J Exp Med 1977;145:1612.
103. Toogood IRG, Dexter TM, Allen TD, Suda T, Lijtha LG. The development of a liquid culture system for the growth of human bone marrow cultures. Leuk Res 1980;4:449.
104. Robertson MJ, Soiffer RJ, Freedman, et al. Human bone marrow depleted of CD33-positive cells mediates delayed but durable reconstitution of hematopoiesis: clinical trial of MY9 monoclonal antibody-purged autografts for the treatment of acute myeloid leukemia. Blood 1992;79:2229–2236.
105. Berenson RJ, Bensinger WI, Hill RS, et al. Engraftment after infusion of $CD34^+$ marrow cells in patients with breast cancer or neuroblastoma. Blood 1991;77: 1717–1722.
106. Metcalf D. The hematopoietic stem and progenitor cells demonstrable using in vitro cloning techniques. In: Metcalf D, ed. The hematopoietic colony stimulating factors. New York: Elsevier, 1984;27–54.
107. McNiece IK, Stewart FM, Deacon DM, et al. Detection of human CFC with high proliferative potential. Blood 1989;74:609–612.
108. Leary AG, Ogawa M. Blast cell colony assay for umbilical cord blood and adult bone marrow progenitors. Blood 1987;69:953.
109. McGinnes K, Keystone E, Bogoch E, et al. Growth and detection of human bone marrow B-lineage colonies. Blood 1990;76:896–905.
110. McGinnes K, Quesniaux V, Hitzler J, Paige C. Human B-lymphopoiesis is supported by bone marrow-derived stromal cells. Exp Hematol 1991;19:294–303.
111. Villablanca JG, Anderson JM, Moseley M, et al. Differentiation of normal human pre-B-cells in vitro. J Exp Med 1990;172:325–334.
112. Civin CI, Strauss LC, Brovall C, Fackler MJ, Schwartz JF, Sharper JH. Antigenic analysis of hematopoiesis. III. A hematopoietic progenitor cell surface antigen defined by a monoclonal antibody raised against KG-1a cells. J Immunol 1984;133:157–165.
113. Strauss LC, Rowley SD, LaRussa VF, Sharkis SJ, Stuart RK, Civin CI. Antigenic analysis of hematopoiesis V. Characterization of My-10 antigen expression by normal lymphohematopoietic progenitor cells. Exp Hematol 1986;14:878.
114. Civin CI, Banquerigo ML, Strauss LC, Loken MR. Antigenic analysis of hematopoiesis. VI. Flow cytometric characterization of My-10-positive progenitor cells in normal human bone marrow. Exp Hematol 1987;15:10.
115. Bindle RW, Nichols RAB, Chou L, Campana D, Catousky D, Birnie GD. A novel monoclonal antibody B1-3C5 recognizes myeloblasts and non-B non-T lymphoblasts in acute leukemia, CGL in blast crisis, and reacts with immature cells in normal marrow. Leuk Res 1985;9:1–9.
116. Andrews RG, Singer JW, Bernstein ID. Monoclonal antibody 12-8 recognizes a 115-kd molecule present on both unipotent and multipotent hematopoietic colony-forming cells and their precursors. Blood 1986;67: 842–845.
117. Thomas TE, Abraham SJR, Phillips GL, Lansdorp PM. A simple procedure for large scale density separation of bone marrow cells for transplantation. Transplantation 1992;53:1163–1165.
118. Frickhofen N, Heit W, Heimpel H. Enrichment of hematopoietic progenitor cells from human bone marrow on Percoll density gradients. Blut 1982;44: 101.
119. Atzpodien J, Gulati SC, Kwon JH, Wachter M, Fried J, Clarkson BD. Human bone marrow CFU-GM and BFU-E localized by light scatter cell sorting. Exp Cell Biol 1987;55:265.
120. Baum CM, Weissman IL, Tsukamoto AS, Buckle AM, Peault B. Isolation of a candidate human hematopoietic stem-cell population. Proc Natl Acad Sci USA 1992;89:2804–2808.
121. Craig W, Kay R, Cutler RL, Lansdorp PM. Expression of Thy-1 on human hematopoietic progenitor cells. J Exp Med 1993;177:1331–1342.
122. Sutherland HJ, Lansdorp PM, Henkelman DH, Eaves AC, Eaves CJ. Functional characterization of individual human hematopoietic stem cells cultured at limiting dilution on supportive marrow stromal layers. Proc Natl Acad Sci USA 1990;87:3584.
123. Schmitt C, Eaves CJ, Lansdorp PM. Expression of CD34 on human B-cell precursors. Clin Exp Immunol 1991;85:168.
124. Loken MR, Shah VO, Dattilio KL, Civin CI. Flow cytometric analysis of human bone marrow. II. Normal B-lymphocyte development. Blood 1987;70:1316.
125. Andrews RG, Singer JW, Bernstein ID. Human hematopoietic precursors in long term culture: single $CD34^+$ cells that lack detectable T-cell, B-cell and myeloid antigens produced multiple colony forming cells when cultured with marrow stromal cells. J Exp Med 1990;172:355.
126. Andrews RG, Takahashi M, Segal GM, Powell JS, Bernstein ID, Singer JW. The L4F3 antigen is expressed by unipotent and multipotent colony-forming cells but not by their precursors. Blood 1986;68:1030.
127. Bernstein ID, Leary AG, Andrews RG, Ogawa M. Blast colony-forming cells and precursors of colony-forming cells detectable in long-term marrow culture express the same phenotype ($CD33^-CD34^+$). Exp Hematol 1991;19:680–682.
128. Andrews RG, Singer JW, Bernstein ID. Precursors of colony-forming cells in humans can be distinguished from colony-forming cells by expression of the CD33 and CD34 antigens and light scatter properties. J Exp Med 1989;169:1721–1731.
129. Sutherland HJ, Eaves CJ, Eaves AC, Dragowsks W, Lansdorp PM. Characterization and partial purification of human marrow cells capable of initiating long-term hematopoiesis in vitro. Blood 1989;74: 1563–1570.
130. Litzow MR, Brashem-Stein C, Andrews RG, Bernstein

ID. Proliferative responses to IL-3 and granulocyte colony-stimulating factor distinguish a minor subpopulation of CD34-positive marrow progenitors that do not express CD33 and a novel antigen, 7B9. Blood 1991;77:2354–2359.
131. Brandt J, Stour EF, Van Besien K, Briddell RA, Hoffman R. Cytokine-dependent long-term culture of highly enriched precursors of hematopoietic progenitor cells from human bone marrow. J Clin Invest 1990;86:932–941.
132. Moore MAS, Broxmeyer HE, Sheridan APC, Meyers PA, Jacobsen N, Winchester RJ. Continuous human bone marrow culture: Ia antigen characterization of probable pluripotential stem cells. Blood 1980;55:682.
133. Keating A, Power J, Takahashi M, Singer JW. The generation of human long-term marrow cultures from marrow depleted of Ia (HLA-DR) positive cells. Blood 1984;64:1159.
134. Lu L, Walker D, Broxmeyer HE, Hoffman R, Hu W, Walker E. Characterization of adult human marrow hematopoietic progenitors highly enriched by two-color cell sorting with My10 and major histocompatibility class II monoclonal antibodies. J Immunol 1987;139:1823–1829.
135. Brandt J, Baird N, Lu L, Srour E, Hoffman R. Characterization of a human hematopoietic progenitor cell capable of forming blast cell containing colonies in vitro. J Clin Invest 1988;82:1017–1027.
136. Srour EF, Brandt JE, Leemhuis T, Ballas CB, Hoffman R. Relationship between cytokine-dependent cell cycle progression and MHC class II antigen expression by $CD34^+$ HLA-DR-bone marrow cells. J Immunol 1992; 148:815–820.
137. Sutherland HC, Eaves CJ, Eaves AC, Lansdorp PM. Differential expression of antigens on cells that initiate hematopoiesis in long-term human marrow culture. In: Knapp W, Dorken B, Gilks WR, et al, eds. Leucocyte typing IV. White cell differentiation antigens. Oxford: Oxford University Press, 1989;910–912.
138. Lansdorp PM, Dragowska W. Long-term erythropoiesis from constant numbers of $CD34^+$ cells in serum-free cultures initiated with highly purified progenitor cells from human bone marrow. J Exp Med 1992;175:1501–1509.
139. Terstappen LWMM, Huang S, Safford M, Lansdorp PM, Loken MR. Sequential generations of hematopoietic colonies derived from single nonlineage-committed $CD34^+CD38^-$ progenitor cells. Blood 1991; 77:1218–1227.
140. Chaudhary PM, Roninson IB. Expression and activity of p-glycoprotein. A multidrug afflux pump on human hematopoietic stem cells. Cell 1991;66:85–94.
141. Udomsakdi C, Eaves CJ, Sutherland HJ, Lansdorp PM. Separation of functionally distinct subpopulations of primitive human hematopoietic cells using rhodamine-123. Exp Hematol 1991;19:338–342.
142. Srour EF, Leemhuis T, Brandt JE, Vanbesien K, Hoffman R. Simultaneous use of Rhodamine123, phycoerythrin, Texas Red, and allophycocyanin for the isolation of human hematopoietic progenitor cells. Cytometry 1991;12:179–183.
143. Papayannopoulou T, Brice M, Broudy VC, Zsebo KM. Isolation of c-kit receptor expressing cells from bone marrow, peripheral blood, and fetal liver: functional properties and composite antigenic profile. Blood 1991;78:1403–1412.
144. Ashman LK, Cambareri AC, Levinsky RJ, Juttner CA. Expression of the YB5, B8 antigen (*c-kit* proto-oncogene product) in normal human bone marrow. Blood 1991;78:30.
145. Broudy VC, Lin N, Zsebo KB, et al. Isolation of a monoclonal antibody that recognizes the human c-kit receptor. Blood 1992;79:338–346.
146. Briddell RA, Broudy VC, Bruno E, Brandt JE, Srour EF, Hoffman R. Further phenotypic characterization and isolation of human hematopoietic progenitor cells using a monoclonal antibody to the c-kit receptor. Blood 1992;79:3159–3167.
147. Lansdorp PM, Sutherland HJ, Eaves CJ. Selective expression of CD45 isoforms on functional subpopulations of $CD34^+$ hematopoietic cells from human bone marrow. J Exp Med 1990;172:363.
148. Berenson RJ, Andrews RG, Bensinger W, et al. Antigen $CD34^+$ marrow cells engraft lethally irradiated baboons. J Clin Invest 1988;81:951–955.
149. Berenson RJ, Bensinger WI, Hill R, et al. Stem cell selection—clinical experience. Prog Clin Biol Res 1991;333:403.
150. Srour EF, Zanjani ED, Brandt JE, et al. Sustained human hematopoiesis in sheep transplanted in utero during early gestation with fractionated adult human bone marrow cells. Blood 1992;79:1404–1412.
151. McCune JM, Namikawa R, Kaneshima H, Shultz LD, Lieberman M, Weissman IL. The SCID-hu mouse: murine model for the analysis of human hematolymphoid differentiation and function. Science 1988; 241:1632–1639.
152. Peault B, Weissman IL, Baum C, McCune JM, Tsukamoto A. Lymphoid reconstitution of the human fetal thymus in SCID mice with $CD34^+$ precursor cells. J Exp Med 1991;174:1283–1286.
153. Peault B, Namikawa R, Krowka J, McCune JM. Experimental human hematopoiesis in immunodeficient SCID mice engrafted with fetal blood-forming organs. In: Edwards RG, ed. Fetal tissue transplants in medicine. Cambridge, UK: Cambridge University Press, 1992:77–95.
154. Kyoizumi S, Baum CM, Kaneshima H, McCune JM, Yee EJ, Namikawa R. Implantation and maintenance of functional human bone marrow in SCID-hu mice. Blood 1992;79:1704–1711.
155. Fialkow PJ, Jacobson RJ, Panayannopoulou T. Chronic myelocytic leukemia: clonal origin in a stem cell common to the granulocyte, erythrocyte, platelet, and monocyte/macrophage. Am J Med 1977;63:125.
156. Martin PJ, Najfeld V, Hansen JA, Penfold GK, Jacobsen RJ, Fialkow PJ. Involvement of the B-lymphoid system in chronic myelogenous leukaemia. Nature 1980;287: 49.
157. Le Bien TW, Hozier J, Minowada J, Kersey HJ. Origin of chronic myelocytic leukemia in a precursor of pre-B lymphocytes. N Engl J Med 1979;301:144.
158. Jonas D, Lubbert M, Kawasaki ES. Clonal analysis of bcr-abl rearrangements in T lymphocytes from patients with chronic myelogenous leukemia. Blood 1992;79:1017–1023.
159. Thomas ED, Clift RA. Indications for marrow transplantation in chronic myelocytic leukemia. Blood 1989;73:861.
160. Hughes TP, Brito-Babapulle F, Tollit, et al. Induction of Philadelphia-negative hematopoiesis and prolongation of chronic phase in patients with chronic myeloid leukemia treated with high dose chemotherapy and transfusion of peripheral blood stem cells. In: Dicke K,

Armitage JO, Dicke-Evinger MJ, eds. Autologous bone marrow transplantation: proceedings of the Fifth International Symposium. Omaha: University of Nebraska Medical Center, 1991:219.

161. Talpaz M, Kantarjian H, Kurzrock R, Trujillo JM, Gutterman JU. Interferon-alpha produces sustained cytogenetic responses in chronic myelogenous leukemia. Ann Intern Med 1991;114:532.

162. Verfailli CM, Miller WJ, Boylan K, McGlave PB. Selection of benign primitive hematopoietic progenitors in chronic myelogenous leukemia on the basis of HLA-DR antigen expression. Blood 1992;79:1003.

163. Turhan AG, Humphries RK, Eaves CS, et al. Detection of breakpoint cluster region-negative and nonclonal hematopoiesis in vitro and in vivo after transplantation of cells selected in culture of chronic myeloid leukemia. Blood 1990;76:2404–2410.

164. Nienhuis AW, McDonagh KT, Bodine DM. Gene transfer into hematopoietic stem cells. Cancer 1991;67:2700.

165. Bernstein ID, Andrews RG, Zsebo KM. Recombinant human stem cell factor enhances the formation of colonies by $CD34^+$ and $CD34^+$ lin^- cells and the generation of colony-forming cell progeny from $CD34^+$ lin^- cells cultured with interleukin-3, granulocyte colony-stimulating factor, or granulocyte-macrophage colony-stimulating factor. Blood 1991;77:2316–2321.

166. Moore MAS. Clinical implications of positive and negative hematopoietic stem cell regulators. Blood 1991;78:1.

Chapter 7
Genetic Manipulation of Hematopoietic Stem Cells

A. Dusty Miller

This chapter focuses on the methods and applications of gene transfer into hematopoietic stem cells. Genetic modification of stem cells has many applications of both scientific and clinical relevance. First, because transferred DNA that integrates into the stem-cell genome provides a unique marker for each recipient cell and all of its progeny, the added DNA can be used as a tag to follow the differentiation of the marked cells. Second, it is possible to study the effects of specific genes on hematopoietic cells, especially those that lead to hematopoietic dysfunction, such as oncogenes. Third, the ability to transfer genes into stem cells will lead to methods to treat both hereditary and acquired disease, in particular the large number of diseases that are manifest in hematopoietic cells.

Definition of the Stem Cell

An outline of hematopoietic differentiation is shown in Figure 7-1. Hematopoiesis is initiated by a small set of cells that are capable of differentiating into the large numbers of circulating myeloid, erythroid, and lymphoid cells. A hematopoietic stem cell is defined as a cell that is capable of providing long-term hematopoiesis in recipient animals and that is capable of differentiating into all of the hematopoietic lineages. Proof of the existence of the hematopoietic stem cell comes from genetic marking studies in mice using retroviral vectors, in which long-term persistence and differentiation of single clonally marked cells into all hematopoietic lineages has been documented (1,2). In mice, a generally accepted time for "long-term" reconstitution is 4 months or more. More stringent criteria for stem cells can also be imposed, such as the ability of stem cells to reconstitute animals serially (i.e., after reconstitution of one animal for at least 4 months, the marrow can be harvested and used to reconstitute hematopoiesis in another animal for another 4 months or more). These serially transplantable cells are more primitive than cells capable of reconstituting only one animal.

Below the level of the stem cells are the more differentiated cells that are incapable of long-term persistence in animals, are committed to further differentiation along specific hematopoietic lineages, or both. In this group are the colony forming or burst forming cells that give rise to colonies in in vitro hematopoietic cell assays, such as the burst forming unit-erythroid (BFU-E) or the colony forming unit-granulocyte macrophage (CFU-GM). Also, below the stem cell level is the cell that gives rise to macroscopic colonies in the spleen of recipient animals, the colony forming unit-spleen (CFU-S). For many years it was assumed that CFU-S arose directly from hematopoietic stem cells, but evidence continues to accumulate that stem cells and CFU-S are not identical. Most importantly, cells that give rise to CFU-S can be separated from cells that provide long-term reconstitution in animals (3). Thus, the only available assay for stem cells involves demonstration that these cells can provide long-term reconstitution in animals.

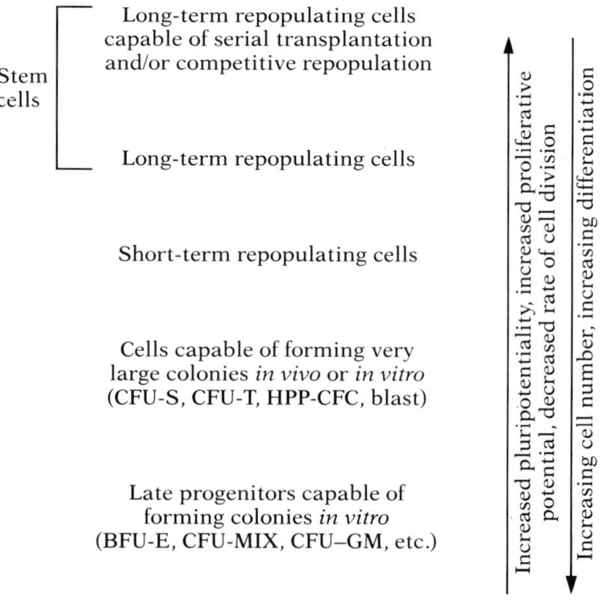

Figure 7-1. Hematopoietic cell differentiation. CFU-S = colony-forming unit-spleen; CFU-T = colony-forming unit-thymus; HPP-CFC = high proliferative potential colony-forming cell; CFU-MIX = colony-forming unit-mixed.

Methods for Genetic Modification of Stem Cells

Methods for transfer of genetic material into stem cells must contend with the fact that stem cells replicate slowly, cannot currently be expanded in number in cell culture to any practical extent, and are present in very low numbers in bone marrow, the typical source for hematopoietic stem cells. Retroviral vectors provide the principal method for gene transfer in this system because of their highly efficient gene transfer ability.

The design of the retroviral vector system is depicted in Figure 7-2. Normal replication competent retroviruses (see Figure 7-2, left panel) exist as DNA proviral forms in cells. RNAs transcribed from these proviruses encode the viral proteins. In addition to serving as the template for *gag-pol* protein synthesis, the full-length RNA is encapsidated into virions and serves as the viral genome. After entry into target cells, the viral RNA genome is reverse-transcribed and integrated into the host cell DNA to form the provirus, and the cycle begins again.

Retroviral vectors utilize the efficient gene transfer capability that retroviruses have evolved by splitting the viral life cycle into two components. First, a variety of retrovirus packaging cell lines (4) have been developed that synthesize all of the retroviral proteins without releasing infectious virus (see Figure 7-2, middle panel). This synthesis is accomplished by altering the viral genome so that the RNAs that encode viral proteins cannot be incorporated into virions, and even if incorporated, cannot be reverse-transcribed or integrated into the genome of a recipient cell. The second component of the system is the retroviral vector (5). A retroviral vector is a deleted retrovirus that cannot synthesize viral proteins but encodes an RNA that can be encapsidated into virions, reverse-transcribed, and integrated into the genome of infected cells. Introduction of the retroviral vector into retrovirus packaging cells results in the production of the vector in the absence of replication-competent retrovirus (see Figure 7-2, right panel). A variety of genes and other genetic elements can be incorporated into a retroviral vector and transmitted to recipient cells. Infection with a retroviral vector does not result in production of replicating virus because the vector cannot synthesize viral proteins. This process is often referred to as transduction rather than infection to emphasize this difference from the normal virus infection process.

A disadvantage of the use of retroviral vectors for hematopoietic stem-cell transduction is their random integration into the genome, which may cause inactivation or activation of cellular genes. Of particular concern is the possible activation of oncogenes, although the frequency of such events is expected to be very low when using these nonreplicating vectors. Problems caused by random integration are shared with all methods for introducing DNA into the genome of the transduced cell, with the possible exception of adeno-associated virus (AAV), which preferentially integrates into a specific region of human chromosome 19 (6,7), as well as methods for homologous recombination, which are currently too inefficient for use in hematopoietic stem cells. Other viral and nonviral methods for transfer of DNA that would persist in an extrachromosomal form, and thus avoid issues of random integration, must deal with potential DNA loss and unequal segregation during cell replication.

Another potential problem with the use of retroviral vectors is the potential for production of replication-competent "helper" virus. Recombinant helper virus is capable of causing proliferative disease in monkeys (8) and may have the potential to do so in humans. However, state-of-the-art techniques for retroviral vector production have apparently eliminated this problem. Helper virus has not been found in any of the vector preparations intended for use in humans or in human gene therapy subjects to date.

An early and controversial attempt to transfer DNA into human hematopoietic stem cells by the physical method of incubation of marrow cells with calcium phosphate-DNA complexes, or transfection, was not successful (9). The difficulty with this procedure and more recent attempts to use other physical methods for DNA transfer, such as encapsulation of DNA in liposomes, is that stable DNA transfer efficiencies are very low. Retroviral vectors have remained the stan-

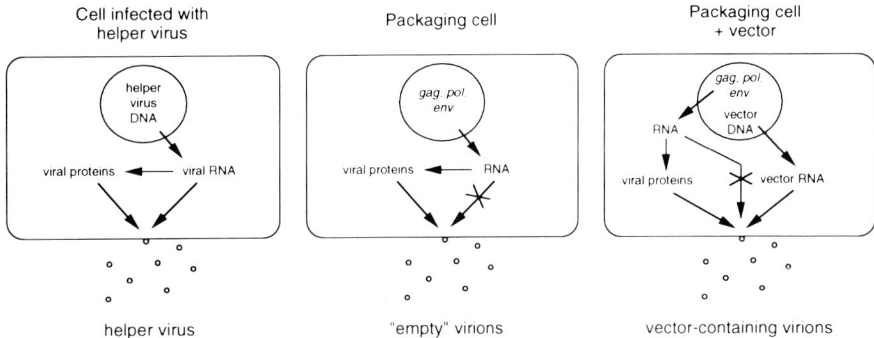

Figure 7-2. Design of the retroviral vector system.

dard tool for gene transfer into hematopoietic stem cells; however, retroviral vectors are only a partial solution to the problem, and although gene transfer into stem cells of mice has been accomplished by several research groups, results in larger animals such as dogs or monkeys have been disappointing. There is certainly room for improvement in gene transfer efficiency and long-term gene expression, which may be provided by alternative viral or physical gene transfer techniques.

Gene Transfer into Hematopoietic Stem Cells of Mice

Gene transfer into hematopoietic stem cells of mice has been demonstrated by many research groups. In the most general approach to mouse stem-cell transduction (1,2,10) (Figure 7-3), donor animals are treated with 5-fluorouracil for approximately 4 days to kill differentiated cells and presumably to induce replication of normally nondividing stem cells, because retroviral vectors promote gene transfer only in replicating cells. Bone marrow from leg bones is then removed and transduced by cocultivation with virus-producing fibroblasts for 1 to 5 days in the presence of hematopoietic growth factors. When the vector carries a selectable marker, the marrow is then exposed to the selective agent for 2 days to kill untransduced cells. This procedure results in a greater percentage of the repopulating cells having the transferred gene. The marrow is then injected into lethally irradiated recipient animals or W/W^v mutant mice that can be reconstituted in the absence of irradiation due to a stem-cell defect. Stem-cell transduction has been documented by the observation of unique retroviral markers in a variety of hematopoietic lineages for more than 4 months in primary recipient animals and after serial transplantation of marrow to secondary recipients.

Experiments designed to achieve long-term expression of genes introduced into mouse stem cells have produced more consistent results with time, although

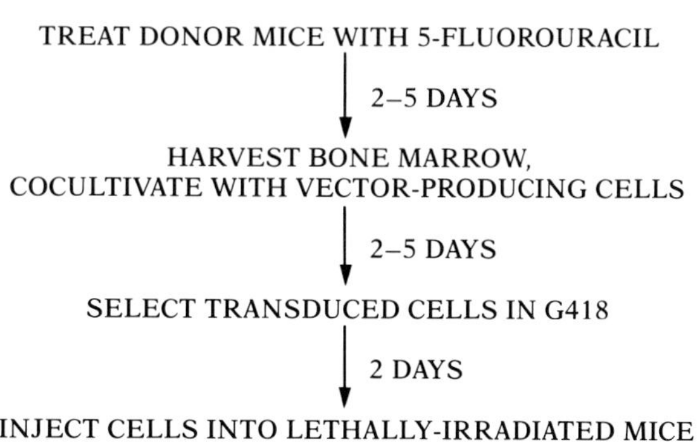

Figure 7-3. General approach to mouse hematopoietic stem cell transduction.

poorly understood factors in vector design have an important influence on long-term expression. Many of these experiments have used retroviral vectors that express human adenosine deaminase (ADA) as a reporter gene (11–15). ADA expression has been documented in bone marrow, spleen, thymus, lymph nodes, erythrocytes, and peripheral blood mononuclear cells of recipient animals at levels that can exceed endogenous mouse ADA activities in some tissues.

A more complex situation has been found for expression of the human β-globin gene, in which high-level tissue-specific expression is required for treatment of hemoglobinopathies involving β-globin. Unlike vectors carrying ADA, in which the use of an ADA complementary DNA allows useful levels of ADA protein production, the second intron of the β-globin gene cannot be removed without adverse effects on β-globin expression (16). This requirement necessitates a reverse orientation of the β-globin gene within a retroviral vector (to avoid intron removal during replication of the retroviral vector), which results in less efficient production of the vector and a concomitant reduction in gene transfer efficiency. In addition, when such vectors are used to transduce hematopoietic stem cells of mice, the expression of human β-globin in mouse erythrocytes is only approximately 1 to 2% of endogenous mouse β-globin expression (17,18). Studies have shown that additional gene regulatory elements that flank the globin locus are required for normal levels of β-globin expression. Attempts to include trimmed-down versions of these elements into retroviral vectors show that these elements are incompatible with the retroviral life cycle and are often deleted or cause a reduction in vector titer to levels that are probably insufficient for stem-cell transduction (19). Thus, although it is possible to construct a β-globin expression cassette that allows production of transgenic mice that produce normal levels of β-globin from the transgene in circulating erythrocytes, this technology has not been successfully applied to gene transfer into hematopoietic stem cells.

Although transduction of mouse stem cells and expression of therapeutically relevant proteins have been demonstrated, there are still problems with this technique. In general, only a few transduced stem cells engraft recipient animals, as revealed by the small number of different virus integration sites in hematopoietic tissues from reconstituted animals. In addition, much of the repopulating ability of marrow is lost during the transduction procedure, especially if the cells are selected for the presence of the vector prior to transplantation. These phenomena can be explained both by a loss of stem cells during transduction and by inefficient stem cell-transduction. Although these losses are acceptable in the inbred mouse model, where syngeneic donor animals are not limited in number, they may prove a considerable obstacle to gene therapy in humans.

An issue in the use of retroviral vectors for gene

transfer into animals is the possibility that replication-competent retrovirus, or helper virus, may be present in vector preparations or in the test animals and might lead to spread of the vector in vivo. Many early vector preparations were contaminated with replication-competent retrovirus, and mice have many endogenous retroviruses that can be activated and replicate, especially after irradiation used to prepare recipient animals for bone marrow transplantation (13). Such replication-competent virus could spread the vector in vivo and invalidate the assumption that vector transfer occurs in vitro before bone marrow transplantation. However, the presence of helper virus in the vector preparation seems to have little effect on expression of the transferred genes in animals in experiments performed with or without helper virus, but does increase the titer of the retroviral vector considerably.

Gene Transfer into Hematopoietic Stem Cells of Large Animals

Attempts have been made to demonstrate stem-cell transduction and long-term gene expression in large outbred animals as a prelude to application of these techniques to humans. Gene transfer into stem cells of such animals is more difficult to achieve than in mice because of the larger scale of the procedure and the fact that marrow is available only from the recipient individual, as would be true in human applications.

In utero transfer of the *neo* gene into hematopoietic stem cells of fetal sheep has been accomplished (20) by removing circulating cells 7 weeks prior to birth, transducing these cells in vitro, and returning the transduced cells to the fetus. Persistence of the transduced cells after birth was demonstrated by detection of *neo* sequences in blood, bone marrow, spleen, and thymus samples from some animals one week after birth; detection of neomycin phosphotransferase in bone marrow of one animal 6 weeks after birth; and by the presence of G418-resistant hematopoietic colony forming cells in marrow for more than 2 years after birth. However, the same transduction procedure was not successful with marrow cells from adult sheep instead of fetal cells. This difference is most likely due to the high replication rate of fetal hematopoietic cells, which would make them more susceptible to transduction by the retroviral vector.

Early gene transfer experiments into canine hematopoietic cells resulted in only transient presence of vector function in hematopoietic cells (21). Recent improvements in the vector transduction protocol have resulted in persistence of vector sequences in both lymphoid and myeloid cells in several dogs for more than 2 years, indicating successful transduction of hematopoietic stem cells (22). The vectors used carry the human *ADA* and bacterial *neo* genes, and drug resistance due to expression of the *neo* gene has been observed intermittently in up to 10% of hematopoietic colonies (CFU-GM) grown from bone marrow for 2 years. Although these results are encouraging, the level of *neo* expression was low, and expression of the ADA gene was not detected. No helper virus was detected in the vector-producing cell lines, in vector preparations, or in recipient animals.

Several retroviral vectors have been used to transduce bone marrow in cats (23). Vector sequences and drug-resistant hematopoietic cell colonies were observed in some of these animals for more than 2 years. Expression of human ADA in cats transduced with a vector that carried the *ADA* gene was not detected. All vector preparations used were contaminated with helper virus, and helper virus was detected in the experimental animals. Diabetes mellitus developed in 2 of the 4 animals 90 days after receiving transduced marrow, most likely due to the presence of helper virus.

Gene transfer experiments in monkeys have documented short-term persistence and expression of genes at low levels after transplantation of retroviral vector-transduced bone marrow (24,25), but proof of stem-cell transduction has not yet been provided. This finding is presumably a reflection of the expense and difficulty of working with primates, because there appears to be no fundamental reason that primate stem cells cannot be transduced with retroviral vectors. These experiments were complicated by the presence of helper virus in the vector preparations used for transduction. Significantly, the presence of helper virus appears to have led to development of lymphoma in several animals (8), a side effect of gene transfer that has not been observed with helper-free vectors.

Given the difficulty of showing long-term gene transfer and expression in the hematopoietic system of large adult animals, new approaches have been pursued to improve gene transfer rates. Evidence exists that marrow kept in long-term bone marrow cultures can be used to reconstitute humans (26), and methods to transduce cells efficiently in long-term culture are being developed. Techniques for purification of hematopoietic stem cells may also lead to improvements in stem-cell transduction rates. A high rate of transduction of purified pluripotential stem cells has been shown in the mouse (27). The advantages of working with purified stem cells include the practical advantage of needing to transduce fewer cells, and the possibility that culture conditions, including growth factors, can be controlled more precisely to improve stem-cell transduction and survival. Several hematopoietic growth factors have been found to improve stem-cell transduction rates, and use of these or other as yet unidentified factors may improve stem cell gene transfer rates to useful levels in large animals.

Transfer of Chemotherapy Resistance Genes

An exciting use of techniques for genetic modification of stem cells is the transfer of drug resistance genes that protect transplanted marrow from agents used in cancer chemotherapy, which would allow higher doses of drugs to be used for treatment of residual cancer after transplantation. An example of this approach is the use of a mutant dihydrofolate reductase gene (*dhfr**) to render mouse bone marrow resistant to methotrexate in vivo (28). The multidrug resistance (*mdr*) gene confers resistance to a variety of antineoplastic drugs (29), and this gene has also been shown to render mouse bone marrow resistant to the cytotoxic drug taxol in vivo (30).

The ability to select transduced hematopoietic cells in vivo should reduce the requirement for high-efficiency gene transduction into bone marrow cells for the treatment of genetic and acquired diseases. For example, a therapeutic gene might be cotransduced into bone marrow cells with one of these selectable marker genes by insertion of both genes into one retroviral vector. Drug selection after transplantation of transduced marrow cells would thus select for cells carrying the therapeutic gene by virtue of its linkage to the selectable marker gene.

Effects of Transduced Genes on Hematopoietic Cells

Retrovirus-mediated gene transfer has been used to study the effects of specific genes on hematopoietic cells. In particular, the effects of several oncogenes and hematopoietic cytokines on hematopoiesis have been evaluated after gene transfer into hematopoietic stem cells. The *bcr/abl*, viral *src*, and viral *ras* oncogenes (31–33); and the cytokines granulocyte colony stimulating factor (G-CSF), granulocyte-macrophage colony stimulating factor (GM-CSF), interleukin 3 (IL-3), and IL-6 (34–38) have all been shown to induce myeloproliferative disease in mice. The specific disease phenotypes in mice help explain the biology of these genes. In the case of the P210 *bcr/abl* gene, the disease induced in mice resembles chronic myeloid leukemia in humans and thus provides a murine model system for further study of this disease.

Gene Transfer in Hematopoietic Lineage Analysis

Because retroviral vectors provide a unique marker for each transduced cell due to their random integration into the target-cell genome, they provide an extremely useful tool for lineage analysis both in culture (39,40) and in animals (41–44). All descendants of the genetically marked cell carry the same unique marker, allowing inferences about the properties of the original marked cell that are difficult if not impossible to make by other techniques. An early example of the utility of this technique was the proof that a single cell could give rise to both myeloid and lymphoid cells by virtue of the unique retroviral marker carried by both types of cells after transplantation of mice with retroviral vector-transduced bone marrow (1,2).

Unique retroviral markers have allowed demonstration of stem-cell division in mouse long-term bone marrow cultures (40). Although the general trend in long-term marrow culture is toward reduced reconstituting ability, as measured by competitive repopulation assay, unique retroviral markers have been used to show that descendants arising in culture from a single marked cell can provide long-term hematopoiesis in several recipient animals.

In a variation of the use of retroviral vectors in lineage analysis, several vectors with different characteristics can be used to mark different pools of hematopoietic cells that can then be mixed and studied simultaneously during reconstitution (41). For example, one can use vectors carrying the same marker but with different lengths; a restriction enzyme that cuts in both ends of the vectors releases a fragment with a characteristic size for each of the different vectors. Southern analysis with a single probe can then reveal the contribution of each marked pool to a given tissue sample. Alternatively, one can use vectors with different marker genes and different probes to follow several marked hematopoietic cell populations simultaneously. However, the fact that cell marking is not 100% effective and retroviral marking may be more effective in some subpopulations of cells (particularly those that are rapidly dividing) should be considered in the analysis of the results of these experiments.

Unique retroviral marking has been used in several elegant studies to examine clonal fluctuations during hematopoietic engraftment (41–44). The general conclusion from these studies is that there is relative instability in clonal contribution early after transplantation, presumably due to the turnover of more differentiated hematopoietic cells that contribute only to short-term hematopoiesis, but contribute to stability of clonal contribution long after transplantation. These studies are complicated by losses of stem cells during retroviral transduction; only a few marked stem-cell clones contribute to hematopoiesis long after transplantation. This finding is in contrast to the situation following transplantation of unmanipulated marrow, which apparently is highly polyclonal.

Genetic Modification of Stem Cells in Humans

Experiments designed to transfer genes into hematopoietic stem cells of large animals indicate that more research should be done to improve gene transfer techniques before use in humans. However, it is likely that these techniques will be used in humans before the problems are resolved in animals in situations in which genetic modification of the stem cells is expected to present little risk for the patient. For example, an ongoing gene therapy trial involves treatment of severe combined immunodeficiency due to defective ADA production. T cells are removed from the patient, modified to produce ADA by transduction with a retroviral vector that encodes human ADA, grown to large numbers, and reinfused (45). Preliminary indications are that this therapy is effective (46), but the treatment may be transient because the modified T cells should ultimately disappear. Transfer of the vector into hematopoietic stem cells might provide long-term persistence of ADA in lymphoid cells, and because the patients are already receiving genetically modified T cells with no ill effects, it is argued that an attempt to transfer the ADA gene into stem cells from these patients would pose little additional risk.

Several approved trials of gene transfer into humans are designed to detect cancerous cells that may be present in marrow used for autologous transplantation in the treatment of cancer (47). Marrow is incubated with a retroviral vector to mark replicating cancer cells that may be present. In the case of disease recurrence, the presence of marked cells would indicate the presence of cancerous cells in the infused bone marrow. In addition to marking cancerous cells, the vector may also mark hematopoietic stem cells in the infused marrow. Thus it may be possible to study stem-cell marking and reconstitution in humans as an incidental effect of these approved studies intended to study cancer relapse (48).

Another situation in which it has been argued that gene transfer into hematopoietic stem cells of humans should be attempted, because the risks appear low based on current gene therapy trials, is in studies of engraftment for which it would be useful to know if the transplanted cells include stem cells that contribute to long-term engraftment. For example, in autologous transplantation, no markers exist to distinguish engraftment by introduced cells versus endogenous cells. Addition of a marker to the transplanted cells is the only way to address the question of exogenous versus endogenous reconstitution.

Development of techniques for gene transfer to human hematopoietic stem cells should ultimately lead to treatments for a range of genetic and acquired diseases. Data from these initial trials in humans will help determine how quickly this field will progress. Currently, however, predicted low gene transfer efficiencies in human stem cells stimulate continued research on improved gene transfer methods and on important issues of hematopoietic stem-cell biology.

References

1. Dick JE, Magli MC, Huszar D, Phillips RA, Bernstein A. Introduction of a selectable gene into primitive stem cells capable of long-term reconstitution of the hemopoietic system of W/Wv mice. Cell 1985;42:71–79.
2. Keller G, Paige C, Gilboa E, Wagner EF. Expression of a foreign gene in myeloid and lymphoid cells derived from multipotent haematopoietic precursors. Nature 1985;318:149–154.
3. Jones RJ, Wagner JE, Celano P, Zicha MS, Sharkis SJ. Separation of pluripotent haematopoietic stem cells from spleen colony-forming cells. Nature 1990;347: 188–189.
4. Miller AD. Retrovirus packaging cells. Hum Gene Therapy 1990;1:5–14.
5. Miller AD. Retroviral vectors. Curr Topics Microbiol Immunol 1992;158:1–24.
6. Kotin RM, Siniscalco M, Samulski RJ, et al. Site-specific integration of adeno-associated virus. Proc Natl Acad Sci USA 1990;87:2211–2215.
7. Samulski RJ, Zhu X, Xiao X, et al. Targeted integration of adeno-associated virus (AAV) into human chromosome 19. EMBO J 1991;10:3941–3950.
8. Kolberg RJ. Gene-transfer virus contaminant linked to monkeys' cancer. NIH Res 1992;4(2):43–44.
9. Cline MJ. Perspectives for gene therapy: inserting new genetic information into mammalian cells by physical techniques and viral vectors. Pharmacol Ther 1985;29: 69–92.
10. Bowtell DD, Johnson GR, Kelso A, Cory S. Expression of genes transferred to haemopoietic stem cells by recombinant retroviruses. Mol Biol Med 1987;4:229–250.
11. Lim B, Apperley JF, Orkin SH, Williams DA. Long-term expression of human adenosine deaminase in mice transplanted with retrovirus-infected hematopoietic stem cells. Proc Natl Acad Sci USA 1989;86:8892–8896.
12. Wilson JM, Danos O, Grossman M, Raulet DH, Mulligan RC. Expression of human adenosine deaminase in mice reconstituted with retrovirus-transduced hematopoietic stem cells. Proc Natl Acad Sci USA 1990;87:439–443.
13. Kaleko M, Garcia JV, Osborne WRA, Miller AD. Expression of human adenosine deaminase in mice after transplantation of genetically-modified bone marrow. Blood 1990;75:1733–1741.
14. Moore KA, Fletcher FA, Villalon DK, Utter AE, Belmont JW. Human adenosine deaminase expression in mice. Blood 1990;75:2085–2092.
15. van Beusechem VW, Kukler A, Einerhand MP, et al. Expression of human adenosine deaminase in mice transplanted with hemopoietic stem cells infected with amphotropic retroviruses. J Exp Med 1990;172:729–736.
16. Miller AD, Bender MA, Harris EAS, Kaleko M, Gelinas RE. Design of retroviral vectors for transfer and expression of the human β-globin gene. J Virol 1988; 62:4337–4345.
17. Dzierzak EA, Papayannopoulou T, Mulligan RC. Lineage-specific expression of a human beta-globin gene in murine bone marrow transplant recipients reconstituted with retrovirus-transduced stem cells. Nature 1988;331:35–41.
18. Bender MA, Gelinas RE, Miller AD. A majority of mice show long-term expression of a human beta-globin gene after retrovirus transfer into hematopoietic stem cells. Mol Cell Biol 1989;9:1426–1434.
19. Novak U, Harris EAS, Forrester W, Groudine M, Gelinas R. High level beta-globin expression from virally-transferred locus activation region-human beta-globin genes in MEL cells. Proc Natl Acad Sci USA 1990;87: 3386–3390.
20. Kantoff PW, Flake AW, Eglitis MA, et al. In utero gene transfer and expression: a sheep transplantation model. Blood 1989;73:1066–1073.
21. Stead RB, Kwok WW, Storb R, Miller AD. Canine model for gene therapy: inefficient gene expression in dogs reconstituted with autologous marrow infected with retroviral vectors. Blood 1988;71:742–747.
22. Schuening FG, Kawahara K, Miller AD, et al. Retrovirus-mediated gene transduction into long-term re-

populating marrow cells of dogs. Blood 1991;78:2568–2576.
23. Lothrop CD Jr, al-Lebban ZS, Niemeyer GP, et al. Expression of a foreign gene in cats reconstituted with retroviral vector infected autologous bone marrow. Blood 1991;78:237–245.
24. Kantoff PW, Gillio AP, McLachlin JR, et al. Expression of human adenosine deaminase in nonhuman primates after retrovirus-mediated gene transfer. J Exp Med 1987;166:219–234.
25. Bodine DM, McDonagh KT, Brandt SJ, et al. Development of a high titer retrovirus producer cell line capable of gene transfer into rhesus monkey hematopoietic stem cells. Proc Natl Acad Sci USA 1990;87:3738–3742.
26. Chang J, Morgenstern GR, Coutinho LH, et al. The use of bone marrow cells grown in long-term culture for autologous bone marrow transplantation in acute myeloid leukaemia: an update. Bone Marrow Transplantation 1989;4:5–9.
27. Szilvassy SJ, Fraser CC, Eaves CJ, Lansdorp PM, Eaves AC, Humphries RK. Retrovirus-mediated gene transfer to purified hemopoietic stem cells with long-term lympho-myelopoietic repopulating ability. Proc Natl Acad Sci USA 1989;86:8798–8802.
28. Corey CA, DeSilva AD, Holland CA, Williams DA. Serial transplantation of methotrexate-resistant bone marrow: protection of murine recipients from drug toxicity by progeny of transduced stem cells. Blood 1990;75:337–343.
29. McLachlin JR, Eglitis MA, Ueda K, et al. Expression of a human complementary DNA for the multidrug resistance gene in murine hematopoietic precursor cells with the use of retroviral gene transfer. J Natl Cancer Inst 1990;82:1260–1263.
30. Sorrentino BP, Brandt SJ, Bodine D, et al. Selection of drug-resistant bone marrow cells in vivo after retroviral transfer of human *MDR*1. Science 1992;257:99–103.
31. Keller G, Wagner EF. Expression of v-src induces a myeloproliferative disease in bone-marrow-reconstituted mice. Genes Dev 1989;3:827–837.
32. Daley GQ, Van Etten RA, Baltimore D. Induction of chronic myelogenous leukemia in mice by the P210bcr/abl gene of the Philadelphia chromosome. Science 1990;247:824–830.
33. Dunbar CE, Crosier PS, Nienhuis AW. Introduction of an activated RAS oncogene into murine bone marrow lymphoid progenitors via retroviral gene transfer results in thymic lymphomas. Oncogene Res 1991;6:39–51.
34. Johnson GR, Gonda TJ, Metcalf D, Hariharan IK, Cory S. A lethal myeloproliferative syndrome in mice transplanted with bone marrow cells infected with a retrovirus expressing granulocyte-macrophage colony stimulating factor. EMBO J 1989;8:441–448.
35. Chang JM, Metcalf D, Gonda TJ, Johnson GR. Long-term exposure to retrovirally expressed granulocyte-colony-stimulating factor induces a nonneoplastic granulocytic and progenitor cell hyperplasia without tissue damage in mice. J Clin Invest 1989;84:1488–1496.
36. Chang JM, Metcalf D, Lang RA, Gonda TJ, Johnson GR. Nonneoplastic hematopoietic myeloproliferative syndrome induced by dysregulated multi-CSF (IL-3) expression. Blood 1989;73:1487–1497.
37. Wong PM, Chung SW, Dunbar CE, Bodine DM, Ruscetti S, Nienhuis AW. Retrovirus-mediated transfer and expression of the interleukin-3 gene in mouse hematopoietic cells result in a myeloproliferative disorder. Mol Cell Biol 1989;9:798–808.
38. Brandt SJ, Bodine DM, Dunbar CE, Nienhuis AW. Retroviral-mediated transfer of interleukin-6 into hematopoietic cells of mice results in a syndrome resembling Castleman's disease. Curr Topics Microbiol Immunol 1990;166:37–41.
39. Hughes PF, Eaves CJ, Hogge DE, Humphries RK. High-efficiency gene transfer to human hematopoietic cells maintained in long-term marrow culture. Blood 1989;74:1915–1922.
40. Fraser CC, Szilvassy SJ, Eaves CJ, Humphries RK. Proliferation of totipotent hematopoietic stem cells in vitro with retention of long-term competitive in vivo reconstituting ability. Proc Natl Acad Sci USA 1992;89:1968–1972.
41. Jordan CT, McKearn JP, Lemischka IR. Cellular and developmental properties of fetal hematopoietic stem cells. Cell 1990;61:953–963.
42. Jordan CT, Lemischka IR. Clonal and systemic analysis of long-term hematopoiesis in the mouse. Genes Dev 1990;4:220–232.
43. Keller G, Snodgrass R. Life span of multipotential hematopoietic stem cells in vivo. J Exp Med 1990;171:1407–1418.
44. Snodgrass R, Keller G. Clonal fluctuation within the haematopoietic system of mice reconstituted with retrovirus infected stem cells. EMBO J 1987;6:3955–3960.
45. Culver KW, Anderson WF, Blaese RM. Lymphocyte gene therapy. Hum Gene Therapy 1991;2:107–109.
46. Culver KW, Berger M, Miller AD, Anderson WF, Blaese RM. Lymphocyte gene therapy for adenosine deaminase deficiency (abstract). Pediatr Res 1992;31:149a.
47. Miller AD. Human gene therapy comes of age. Nature 1992;357:455–460.
48. Rill DR, Moen RC, Buschle M, et al. An approach for the analysis of relapse and marrow reconstitution after autologous marrow transplantation using retrovirus-mediated gene transfer. Blood 1992;79:2694–2700.

Chapter 8
Preparative Regimens and Their Toxicity

Finn B. Petersen and S. I. Bearman

The ideal preparative regimen for marrow transplantation of patients with malignant diseases should be capable of eradicating malignancy, have tolerable morbidity without mortality, and have sufficient immunosuppressive effect in allogeneic marrow recipients to avoid graft rejection. "Toxicity" describes all the undesirable effects due to the preparative regimen itself. No ideal preparative regimen currently exists, and recurrence of the original disease still accounts for a significant number of treatment failures. The search for an ideal preparative regimen serving all three purposes described has been a major focus of most marrow transplant groups over the past 20 years. As a result, a large number of different preparative regimens are currently in use. This chapter covers the development and current status of preparative regimens used in marrow transplantation of patients with malignancies and explores the relationship between specific preparative regimens and organ toxicity.

Transplant-related Morbidity and Mortality

The first study to suggest a broader applicability of clinical marrow transplantation was published by Thomas and colleagues in 1977 (1). In that study, 100 patients with end-stage leukemia were transplanted with human leukocyte antigen (HLA)–identical marrow after preparation with cyclophosphamide (CY) and total body irradiation (TBI). This study represented a major advance in the treatment of this disease: 13% of the patients, all of whom would have died otherwise, became long-term, event-free survivors, even though 57% of the patients died from transplant-related complications and 30% from recurrence of the original disease after transplant. This mortality was considered a necessary concession to achieve any long-term, event-free survival. As a result, subsequent studies were designed with an inherent acceptance of a transplant-related mortality that would be considered unacceptable in anything other than a research setting. The results of transplanting patients with end-stage leukemia have not improved since the publication of Thomas and colleagues' original publication (2), and most transplant groups acknowledge that if new preparative regimens are to be effective, regimen-related deaths of some patients may be unavoidable.

There is no consensus on the degree of acceptable transplant-related mortality. In general, few deaths are accepted in studies of patients with disease that is not advanced, has a low relapse potential, or has a long natural history. In contrast, higher transplant-related mortality may be accepted in studies of patients with disease that is advanced, has high relapse potential, or has a short natural history. Thus, determination of acceptable dose levels for new preparative regimens will depend on what the investigators consider to be an acceptable balance between transplant-related mortality and disease recurrence for the specific patient population studied.

Regimen-related Toxicity

The distinction between "regimen-related toxicity" and "transplant- related morbidity" is not always clear when reviewing the literature. Transplant-related morbidity can be defined as (1) toxicity related to the preparative regimen (regimen-related toxicity [RRT]), (2) toxicity from prophylactic modalities and treatment procedures for side effects and complications, (3) pancytopenic complications, and (4) immunological conflicts between patient and donor cells (i.e., graft-versus-host-disease [GVHD] and graft rejection). Defining RRT as a distinct entity from other transplant-related morbidity is important when trying to evaluate new preparative regimens.

Grading of Regimen-related Toxicity

If RRT used to evaluate new preparative regimens in phase I trials is graded according to the system developed by the World Health Organization for reporting results of cancer treatments, all patients would experience grade IV hematological toxicity and most would also experience grade III toxicities in several organs. Thus, an alternative grading system must be employed to differentiate between acceptable and unacceptable toxicity when evaluating new preparative regimens (3).

In 1984, this issue was addressed in preparation for

developing a systematic evaluation of new preparative regimens at the Fred Hutchinson Cancer Research Center (FHCRC). First, RRT was defined as a distinct entity apart from other transplant-related morbidity (3). Next, an empiric grading system, employing the following general outline when evaluating specific organs, was devised.

Grade I toxicity is defined as mild symptoms or abnormalities that are always reversible without treatment.

Grade II toxicity is defined as moderate symptoms or abnormalities that may represent measurable target organ damage but usually require medical intervention and may interfere with other therapy.

Grade III toxicity is defined as major clinical symptoms representing life-threatening toxicity. Development of grade III toxicity cannot be tolerated on a routine basis. Grade III toxicity often requires intensive supportive care, such as hemodialysis or intubation with mechanical ventilation.

Grade IV toxicity is defined as fatal toxicity in which the organ damage resulting from toxicity is the direct cause of death.

In this schema, RRT is graded in 8 individual organs (Table 8-1) on the day of transplantation and 7, 14, 28, and 100 days after transplantation. The grading of RRT can be made prospectively (4–7) or retrospectively (8,9). These studies have demonstrated that the probability of surviving the first 100 days after transplant is dependent in part not only on the severity of RRT in any one organ system, but also on the cumulative toxicity in multiple organs (8,9). In studies from the FHCRC and the Vancouver Bone Marrow Transplant team, transplant-related mortality was 10 to 25% in patients whose cumulative RRT score from each of the 8 organs tested was less than 6, whereas mortality exceeded 70% for those whose cumulative RRT score was 7 or greater (Figure 8-1). Severe RRT also tends to occur in patients who are considered to be at high risk for relapse or who have compromised clinical performance prior to starting the preparative regimen (8) (Figure 8-2).

An effort should be made to exclude toxicity attributable to causes such as GVHD, infection, bleeding, or toxicity from agents or procedures not included in the preparative regimen.

This schema has been employed in a number of phase I trials of new preparative regimens and has facilitated determination of the maximum tolerated dose level of most (5–7) but not all regimens investigated (4). Despite careful attempts to differentiate between RRT and other contributing causes of toxicity, such as GVHD or drugs used in GVHD prophylaxis, the distinction is not always possible. Thus, it has been observed that less grade III to IV RRT develops in patients undergoing autologous marrow transplant than in patients undergoing allogeneic marrow transplant despite treatment with the same preparative regimens (3,7). This finding suggests that it may be appropriate to conduct separate dose-escalation trials in autologous and allogeneic marrow recipients.

Organ System Toxicity

The following section covers the spectrum and pathophysiology of RRT in several different organs and prophylactic or therapeutic strategies. Neurological toxicity is discussed in Chapter 34, whereas gastrointestinal toxicity, including venoclusive disease, is discussed in Chapter 33.

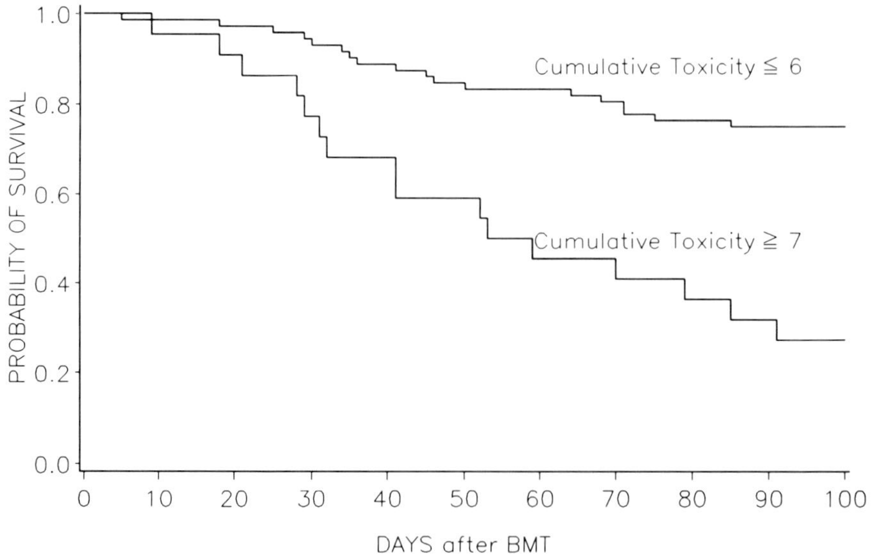

Figure 8.1. Actuarial probability of survival 100 days after transplant for patients with cumulative toxicity (p = 0.0001). (Reproduced by permission from Bearman SI, Appelbaum FR, Back A, et al. Regimen-related toxicity and early posttransplant survival in patients undergoing marrow transplantation for lymphoma. J Clin Oncol 1989;7:1288–1294.)

Table 8-1.
Regimen-related Toxicity According to Organ Systems

	Grade I	*Grade II*	*Grade III*[a]
Cardiac toxicity	Mild EKG abnormality, not requiring medical intervention; or noted heart enlargement on chest radiograph, with no clinical symptoms	Moderate EKG abnormalities requiring and responding to medical intervention; requiring continuous monitoring without treatment; or congestive heart failure responsive to digitalis or diuretics	Severe EKG abnormalities with no or only partial response to medical intervention; heart failure with no or only minor response to intervention; or decrease in voltage by more than 50%
Bladder toxicity	Macroscopic hematuria after 2 days from last chemotherapy dose, with no subjective symptoms of cystitis and not caused by infection	Macroscopic hematuria after 7 days from last chemotherapy dose not caused by infection; or hematuria after 2 days, with subjective symptoms of cystitis not caused by infection	Hemorrhagic cystitis with frank blood, necessitating invasive local intervention with installation of sclerosing agents, nephrostomy, or other surgical procedure
Renal toxicity	Increase in creatinine up to twice the baseline value (usually the last recorded before the start of conditioning)	Increase in creatinine above twice baseline but not requiring dialysis	Requirement of dialysis
Pulmonary toxicity	Dyspnea, without chest radiographic changes, not caused by infection or congestive heart failure; or chest radiographs showing isolated infiltrate or mild interstitial changes without symptoms not caused by infection or congestive heart failure	Chest radiograph with extensive localized infiltrate or moderate interstitial changes combined with dyspnea and not caused by infection or congestive heart failure; decrease of PO_2 (>10% from baseline), not requiring mechanical ventilation, or >50% oxygen on mask, and not caused by infection or congestive heart failure	Interstitial changes requiring mechanical ventilatory support or >50% oxygen on mask, and not caused by infection or congestive heart failure
Hepatic toxicity	Mild hepatic dysfunction with bilirubin ≥ 2.0 mg% and ≤6.0 mg%; weight gain >2.5% and <5% from baseline, of noncardiac origin; or SGOT increase more than two-fold but less than five-fold from lowest preconditioning	Moderate hepatic dysfunction with bilirubin >6 mg% <20 mg%; SGOT increase >five-fold from preconditioning; clinical ascites or image-documented ascites >100 mL; or weight gain >5% from baseline of noncardiac origin	Severe hepatic dysfunction with bilirubin >20 mg%; hepatic encephalopathy; or ascites compromising respiratory function
CNS toxicity	Somnolence, but patient is easily arousable and is oriented after arousal	Somnolence with confusion after arousal; or other new objective CNS symptoms with no loss of consciousness not more easily explained by other medication, bleeding, or CNS infection	Seizures or coma not explained (documented) by other medication, CNS infection, or bleeding
Stomatitis	Pain or ulceration not requiring a continuous IV narcotic drug	Pain or ulceration requiring a continuous IV narcotic drug (morphine drip)	Severe ulceration or mucositis requiring preventive intubation; or resulting in documented aspiration pneumonia with or without intubation
Gastrointestinal toxicity	Watery stools >500 mL but <2,000 mL every day not related to infection	Watery stools >2,000 mL every day not related to infection; macroscopic hemorrhagic stools with no effect on cardiovascular status not caused by infection; or subileus not related to infection	Ileus requiring nasogastric suction or surgery and not related to infection; or hemorrhagic enterocolitis affecting cardiovascular status and requiring transfusion

[a]Grade IV regimen-related toxicity is defined as fatal toxicity.
SGOT=serum glutamic oxaloacetic transaminase.

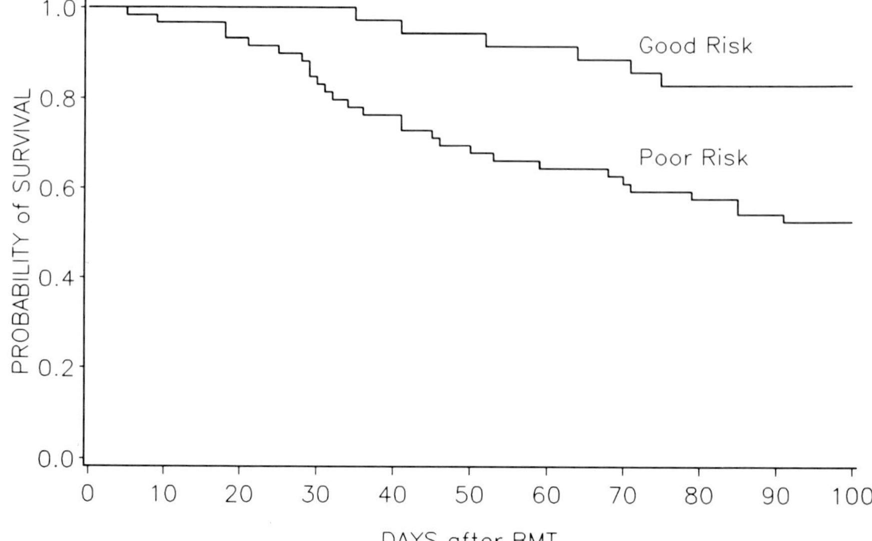

Figure 8.2. Actuarial probability of survival 100 days after transplant for good-risk and poor-risk lymphoma ($p = 0.003$). (Reproduced by permission from Bearman SI, Appelbaum FR, Back A, et al. Regimen-related toxicity and early posttransplant survival in patients undergoing marrow transplantation for lymphoma. J Clin Oncol 1989;7:1288–1294.)

Cardiac Toxicity

Life-threatening cardiac toxicity after marrow transplantation occurs in 5 to 10% of patients who receive CY-containing preparative regimens (3,10–13). Severe cardiac toxicity is characterized by electrocardiographic (ECG) voltage loss, progressive cardiac failure, or pericarditis with or without tamponade occurring within several weeks of CY administration. Minor ECG changes, such as ST-T wave segment changes, supraventricular arrhythmias, or pericarditis without hemodynamically significant efffusion (13,14), develop in up to 90% of patients receiving CY-containing preparative regimens. The degree of ECG voltage loss appears to be the same for patients in whom clinical congestive heart failure develops as for those in whom it does not. In all patients surviving the transplant procedure, ECG voltage returned to pre-CY values. Anecdotal reports of subendocardial myocardial ischemia or infarction have also been reported (13–15). On postmortem examination, patients with severe cardiac toxicity have hemorrhagic myocardial necrosis (16).

In a study of 40 children undergoing high-dose CY for solid tumors or as preparation for marrow transplantation, serial echocardiograms showed that one or more echocardiographic changes developed approximately one week after CY administration in 52% of patients and lasted for several days to weeks. The most common echocardiographic abnormality was development of pericardial effusion. A small number of patients had evidence of left ventricular dysfunction, as determined by decreased fractional shortening, increased end-diastolic volume, and increased pre-ejection period/ejection time.

The contribution of prior anthracycline therapy to development of cardiac dysfunction after high-dose CY is unclear. One study found that the pretransplant cumulative anthracycline dose was not a significant predictor for decreased pretransplant ejection fraction or for development of severe cardiac toxicity (13).

Several studies suggest that the dose of CY is a critical factor in the development of cardiac toxicity. Early reports describe fatal hemorrhagic myocardial necrosis in patients who received 240 mg/kg or more CY; however, a number of reports have showed that cardiac toxicity can occur after doses of less than 200 mg/kg (10,12,13,16). When the CY dose was calculated by body surface area, cardiac toxicity developed in 3% of patients who received less than 1.55 gm/m^2/day and in 25% of patients who received more than 1.55 gm/m^2/day; cardiac death occurred in 0 and 12% in each group, respectively (11). The contribution to cardiac toxicity of prior mediastinal radiotherapy or of TBI is unclear. No difference was reported in the incidence of grade III or IV cardiac toxicity among patients who received less than 1,950 cGy versus more than 1,950 cGy mediastinal radiotherapy prior to transplantation (8,17). However, the contribution of cardiac dysfunction prior to start of the preparative regimen is also unclear. Several transplant centers exclude patients from transplantation whose resting radionuclide ejection fraction is less than 50%. The number of patients referred for transplantation to the FHCRC with an ejection fraction of less than 50% was approximately 10% and this value was not an absolute contraindication to transplantation (13). Grades III or IV cardiac toxicity developed in 20% of patients with a pretransplant ejection fraction of less than 50%, compared with 4% of patients whose pretransplant ejection fraction was more than 50%.

There are no studies of prophylaxis against CY-induced cardiac toxicity. 2-Mercaptoethylene sulfonate (Mesna), an agent most commonly used to prevent hemorrhagic cystitis caused by CY, has been studied in the preclinical setting in rats receiving 350 to 500 mg/kg CY, which results in acute respiratory distress and death within 16 hours. Mesna administered intraperitoneally prior to and one hour after high-dose CY prevents early death in most animals. When killed 8 to 12 hours after administration of CY, the characteristic signs of lung and heart injury were absent in animals who received Mesna. The mechanism of protection is unclear but might include uptake of Mesna into cardiac cells or enhancing levels of free sulfhydryl levels in tissue. The clinical role of Mesna as prophylaxis against cardiac RRT has not been determined.

Carmustine (BCNU) is another chemotherapeutic agent that is increasingly used in transplant preparative regimens and that has been reported to be associated with cardiac toxicity (18).

Treatment of severe CY-induced cardiac toxicity consists of symptomatic pharmacological support and fluid management. Pericardiocentesis or placement of a pericardial window may be necessary for hemodynamically significant pericardial effusions.

Bladder Toxicity

Urothelial toxicity is one of the most common complications of high-dose CY. CY is hydroxylated by the hepatic microsomal P-450 system to 4-hydroperoxycyclophosphamide (4-HC). 4-HC is transported to peripheral tissues, where it is converted intracellularly to aldophosphamide and to the final active metabolites, acrolein and phosphoramide mustard. Phosphoramide mustard, the active tumorcidal metabolite, is not urotoxic (19); however, exposure of urothelium to acrolein results in mucosal hyperemia and ulceration, with hemorrhage and focal necrosis. The bladder is the most common site of CY-induced urotoxicity, but toxicity can occur elsewhere in the collecting system. One case of fatal hemorrhagic pyelitis, ureteritis, and cystitis has been reported after administration of 4.8 gm/m^2 CY (20).

Hemorrhagic cystitis after high-dose CY administration for marrow transplantation may occur in up to 70% of patients (21). Hematuria has been reported as early as immediately after termination of the CY infusion to as late as 3 months after transplantation (20–23). With adequate prophylaxis, hemorrhagic cystitis is mild in most patients with self-limited microscopic or macroscopic hematuria; however, persistent or gross hematuria may develop in a small percentage of patients, which may result in retention of clots and obstructive uropathy and require invasive therapy.

Hemorrhagic cystitis may be worse in patients who receive busulfan (BU). In one study, hemorrhagic cystitis developed in 30% of patients receiving BU and CY compared with 14% of patients receiving CY and TBI (23).

Strategies to prevent hemorrhagic cystitis include forced diuresis, continuous bladder irrigation, and systemic administration of Mesna, or combinations thereof. Mesna rapidly dimerizes to dimesna in plasma. Both Mesna and dimesna are hydrophilic and only cross lipid membranes with difficulty, which may explain why Mesna does not reduce the cytotoxic effect of chemotherapeutic agents (24). When excreted into the urine, dimesna is reduced to Mesna, which, by virtue of its free sulfhydryl group, is capable of forming thioester bonds with acrolein and minimizing bladder toxicity. Forced diuresis and continuous bladder irrigation prevent hemorrhagic cystitis by diluting the urine and minimizing exposure of the urothelium to acrolein.

Comparative studies of Mesna versus forced diuresis or bladder irrigation have been carried out at several transplant centers with mixed results. In one study, 61 patients were randomized to Mesna or forced diuresis without bladder irrigation (25). The incidence of macroscopic hematuria was 35% in the forced diuresis arm and 13% in the Mesna arm ($p < 0.05$). In another similar study, 100 patients were randomized to Mesna or hyperhydration without bladder irrigation (21). In that study, severe hematuria occurred in 12% of the Mesna group and 7% of the hyperhydration group. In a randomized study comparing Mesna with continuous bladder irrigation, hematuria was more common in the bladder irrigation group, but severe hematuria was the same in both groups (26).

Severe grade III hemorrhagic cystitis is rare. In two separate studies from FHCRC, where all patients are treated with forced saline diuresis and bladder irrigation, the incidence of severe hemorrhagic cystitis was less than 1% (3,8).

Treatment of severe hemorrhagic cystitis requires correction of thrombocytopenia, vigorous hydration, and bladder irrigation. A variety of invasive procedures, such as electrocoagulation, intravesicular silver nitrate, alum, or prostaglandin E have been reported as potentially effective treatment modalities (27). Arterial ligation and embolization, cystectomy, and urinary diversion have also been attempted (28–30).

Renal Toxicity

Renal insufficiency and renal failure are frequent complications of marrow transplantation for malignancy. Renal dysfunction after marrow transplantation may be the result of direct nephrotoxicity from irradiation (i.e., TBI) or chemotherapeutic agents. These agents include cisplatinum, CY, and ifosfamide (31,32). In addition, tumor lysis, intravascular volume depletion, and other nephrotoxic medications, such as cyclosporine, amphotericin B, and aminoglycosides can cause renal dysfunction. Patients with renal dysfunction requiring hemodialysis after marrow transplantation have a particularly poor prognosis, with a mortality rate as high as 84% (31).

Clinically significant renal RRT with commonly used preparative regimens is rare. The reported incidence of grades III or IV kidney RRT is 2 to 5% (3,8,9). Most of the patients in whom severe kidney RRT developed also had grade III or IV toxicity of another organ (3). This association between renal toxicity and toxicity in other organs has been found in a prospective analysis of risk factors for early liver toxicity and multiorgan failure (33). Renal insufficiency occurred in 11% of patients in whom liver toxicity did not develop, in 38% of patients in whom mild or moderate liver toxicity developed, and in 84% of patients in whom severe liver toxicity developed. All patients in whom renal failure developed had concurrent liver toxicity. These data suggest an intimate relationship between liver and renal dysfunction.

Preparative regimens containing cisplatinum, carboplatinum, or ifosfamide are more often associated with renal dysfunction. In a phase I study of CY, cisplatinum, and BCNU, renal insufficiency developed in 29% of patients. Addition of melphalan to that regimen increased the fraction of patients in whom renal insufficiency developed to 71%, resulting in renal failure in 29% (34). Renal failure developed in only 3% of patients treated with CY, carboplatinum, and thiotepa (35).

Clinically significant renal dysfunction after marrow transplantation is usually the result of multiple insults to the kidney. In a study of 272 consecutive patients who underwent marrow transplantation at the FHCRC, 53% of patients had doubling of the baseline serum creatinine level, and 24% required hemodialysis. Risk factors for development of renal failure requiring dialysis included hyperbilirubinemia, significant fluid retention, amphotericin administration, and a pretransplant serum creatinine level greater than 0.7 mg/dL. Other nephrotoxic agents, such as aminoglycoside antibiotics, vancomycin, and cyclosporine, and development of acute GVHD were not associated with hemodialysis-requiring renal failure. Septicemia or hypotension developed in the majority of patients with hemodialysis-requiring renal failure in the 48 hours prior to the doubling of the creatinine level. It is therefore possible that the major cause of renal failure in these patients was of hemodynamic origin.

Combinations of nephrotoxic drugs can contribute significantly to renal dysfunction. Thus, acute renal dysfunction has been shown to be more common among patients who receive cyclosporine and intravenous amphotericin B than in patients who received methotrexate and intravenous amphotericin B (36).

Treatment of renal RRT is symptomatic. Most renal RRT is reversible with strict fluid and electrolyte management and adjustment or omission of nephrotoxic drugs.

Pulmonary Toxicity

Regimen-related or noninfectious pneumonia occurs in 8 to 18% of patients who undergo marrow transplantation (3,37–39). The incidence of noninfectious pneumonia appears to be similar in recipients of allogeneic, syngeneic, or autologous marrow (3,8,38,40). Patients typically present with dyspnea, diffuse pulmonary infiltrates, a nonproductive cough, and hypoxemia. Noninfectious pneumonias are the most common cause of diffuse pulmonary infiltrates during the first 4 weeks after transplantation (37,38) and are usually characterized as diffuse alveolar damage (Plate XIII) or interstitial pneumonia (41). Noninfectious pneumonia is more common in patients who undergo transplantation for hematological malignancy compared with patients who undergo transplantation for aplastic anemia and in older patients (>40 years of age) (37,38,42). This finding may be due to toxicity from TBI, because noninfectious pneumonia is more likely to develop in patients who undergo transplantation for aplastic anemia who receive a TBI-containing regimen than those who received CY alone.

The mechanism of lung injury after marrow transplantation is only partially known. Radiation therapy and a variety of chemotherapeutic agents, such as CY, BU, and BCNU, are directly toxic to the lungs. Metabolites of BCNU, acrolein and chloroethylisocyanate, respectively, can directly deplete glutathione stores or inactivate glutathione reductase associated with lung injury (43).

Radiation therapy to the lung is associated with characteristic inflammatory interstitial and alveolar changes. Several animal and clinical studies have shown that the dose and dose rate of TBI are directly correlated with the development of interstitial pneumonia (44). Several phase I studies of escalating doses of TBI have found interstitial pneumonia to be the dose-limiting toxicity (6,45). Cytokine levels after marrow transplantation may also have an important role in the pathogenesis of lung injury. Levels of tumor necrosis factor/alpha (TNF-α) have been shown to be elevated in patients in whom idiopathic pneumonia develops after marrow transplantation (46).

Bronchoalveolar lavage and open lung biopsy are the major diagnostic studies for patients in whom diffuse infiltrates develop after marrow transplantation. Bronchoalveolar lavage has become the predominant diagnostic procedure to differentiate between noninfectious pneumonias and pneumonia due to cytomegalovirus (41). If bronchoalveolar lavage is nondiagnostic, open lung biopsy may be indicated even though it only rarely adds information when bronchoalveolar lavage is nondiagnostic (41).

Several patients have been reported with a condition that is pathologically consistent with pulmonary veno-occlusive disease (VOD) (47,48) (Plate XIV). Dyspnea, hypoxemia, and pulmonary hypertension developed in 2 children at the FHCRC 6 to 8 weeks after high-dose CY, etoposide (VP16), BCNU, and allogeneic marrow transplantation (48). Both patients responded favorably to corticosteroids. A relationship to hepatic VOD is unclear.

Despite a lack of pulmonary symptoms early after marrow transplantation, late (>1 year posttransplant) progressive decline in pulmonary function develops in some patients (49,50). Thirty-four patients without respiratory symptoms early after marrow transplantation were followed for 2 years with serial pulmonary function tests. Diffusing capacity decreased by a mean of 12% each year. This effect was most prevalent in patients who underwent transplantation for chronic myelogenous leukemia (CML), but could not be ascribed to a BU-containing preparative regimen for transplantation or to pretransplant BU therapy. Obstructive ventilatory defects after transplantation have also been observed after marrow transplantations, particularly in patients with chronic GVHD (49). It remains unclear whether such patients will progress to bronchiolitis obliterans (Plate LIX), a syndrome of severe obstructive pulmonary disease caused by bronchiolar fibrosis described in patients with chronic GVHD (51).

Treatment for pulmonary RRT includes symptomatic oxygen and ventilatory support, including mechanical ventilation (39,41). Treatment with high-dose glucocorticoids or pharmacological TNF-α blockade has been reported, but the efficacy of these approaches has not been established (52,53).

Patients with pulmonary complications requiring mechanical ventilatory support for more than 24 hours have a very poor, but not hopeless prognosis (54). In one study of 343 posttransplant patients requiring intubation and mechanical ventilation for more than 24 hours, 21% improved to the point where they were extubated. Ten of the 343 patients (3%) became long-term survivors (55).

Oral Mucositis (Stomatitis)

Several studies of transplant-related toxicity have reported the incidence of oral mucositis to exceed 90% (3,8,56). Xerostomia usually develops in patients during administration of the preparative regimen, followed by ulcerative mucosal lesions around the time of marrow infusion (Plates III and IV). Severe pain requiring narcotic analgesics is the most common manifestation of oral mucositis and often lasts until the marrow graft produces a measurable peripheral absolute granulocyte count. The development and severity of oral mucositis is dependent on the antitumor agents employed and their doses. Regimens containing TBI, BU, VP16, and thiotepa are very frequently associated with oral mucositis (3,5,35, 56,57). Significant mucositis is uncommon in the CY, cisplatinum, BCNU regimen used in many centers for autologous marrow transplantation in patients with advanced and high-risk breast cancer (34). Patients who receive 15.75 Gy TBI are more likely to require narcotic analgesics for mouth pain than patients who receive 12.0 Gy TBI (70 vs 40%) (3). In addition, prophylaxis of GVHD with methotrexate results in increased mucositis, compared with cyclosporine (58).

Life-threatening mucositis develops in very few patients (3). Occasionally, however, oral mucositis is severe enough to warrant prophylactic or emergency intubation to protect the airway (5).

Development of oral mucositis coincides with development of neutropenia after myeloablative therapy (56). Superinfection of the oral mucosa with fungus, bacteria, or virus is common and may influence the severity and duration of oral mucositis. *Candida* species and herpes simplex virus (HSV) are the most common pathogens isolated from patients with ulcerative oral lesions, and the presence of HSV prolonged the duration of mucositis (56). It has been reported that the severity of oral mucositis may be predictive of the incidence and severity of hepatic VOD (59).

Patients undergoing marrow transplantation typically perform oral care several times a day with peroxide and antifungal rinses and nontraumatic cleaning of teeth and gums. In a randomized trial to determine whether the broad spectrum antimicrobial chlorhexidine digluconate versus placebo diminished mucositis, it was found that patients randomized to receive chlorhexidine had fewer oral plaques than patients who received placebo, but the degree of mucosal ulceration was similar in the two groups (60). Other studies have demonstrated that incidence, duration, and severity of oral mucositis was reduced in chlorhexidine-treated patients (61).

It has been suggested that growth-factor and anti-TNF-α therapy may reduce the severity of oral mucositis, although the clinical significance of this effect is controversial (53,62,63).

Skin

TBI and most of the cytotoxic drugs used in preparative regimens can cause cutaneous toxicity (Plates I and II). Generalized erythema and hyperpigmentation of the skin is common in patients receiving a high dose (>12 Gy) of TBI. The erythema in most cases is self-limiting and rarely associated with skin breakdown unless the patient is obese or has cutaneous mycosis. Cytotoxic drugs that have been reported to result in significant skin toxicity include cytosine arabinoside (ARAC), thiotepa, BCNU, BU, and VP16; skin biopsies show a variety of inflammatory changes (64–67).

Metabolites from thiotepa are concentrated in perspiration and can accumulate on dressings and in skin-folds, thus increasing irritation and toxicity in these locations. Frequent dressing changes and, if possible, a shower after finishing the thiotepa infusion are generally recommended for patients receiving thiotepa doses greater than 700 mg/m^2.

Skin changes from erythema to generalized maculopapular rash can occur during infusion of the cytotoxic drug or weeks later. Because most skin biopsies in the first 3 weeks following marrow transplantation show nonspecific inflammatory changes regardless of the cause, skin biopsies are of little help during this period to make a differential diagnosis between RRT, early acute skin GVHD, folliculitis, or drug allergies. A diagnosis of skin rashes in these first 3 weeks after transplantation most often has to be made based solely on a careful clinical evaluation.

Significant skin RRT has been reported infrequently. A cutaneous syndrome, characterized by painful and generalized nonpruritic erythema and edema followed by bullae formation and epidermal detachment and desquamation, developed in several patients transplanted after regimens containing VP16, BCNU and thiotepa (64). Stevens-Johnson syndrome has also been reported after VP16 therapy (65). Desquamation followed by hyperpigmentation has been reported in several children who received autologous marrow transplants after preparation with BU and CY (67). In such severe cases, systemic glucocorticoids may be indicated to obtain anti-inflammatory control. There is some suggestion that high-dose BCNU (>300 mg/m^2) may cause particularly severe skin changes in areas exposed to previous radiotherapy (recall dermatitis).

Prophylaxis and Treatment of Regimen-related Toxicity

Hepatic Veno-occlusive Disease

The pathogenesis and risk factors for development of VOD after marrow transplantation are discussed in detail in Chapter 33. In this section, strategies to prevent or treat VOD are discussed.

Heparin

VOD is characterized histologically by deposition of clotting material within subendothelial zones of affected liver venules and sinusoids (68) (Plate VII). In an effort to prevent VOD, several groups have studied the use of intravenous heparin. Two groups studied heparin in nonrandomized trials and concluded that it protected against VOD (69). A prospective randomized trial of heparin in 161 patients undergoing marrow transplantation showed the incidence of VOD to be 14% in patients who did not receive heparin and 3% in those who did (70); however, only 10% of patients in that study were at high risk for development of VOD. A study from the FHCRC of continuous infusion heparin in 28 patients who were at high risk for development of VOD found that the overall incidence of VOD was 71%; severe VOD developed in 14% of patients (71). Thus, it remains unclear whether the potential benefits of administering heparin to patients at risk for severe VOD outweighs the potential risks.

Prostaglandin E_1

In a controlled but nonrandomized trial of 109 patients undergoing marrow transplantation for leukemia, 50 patients received prostaglandin E_1 (PGE_1) (500 μg/day for adults, 250 μg/day for children) by continuous infusion from day −8 to day 30 (72). VOD occurred in 13% of patients who received PGE_1 and in 26% of those who did not. Patients with previous hepatitis treated with PGE_1 had an incidence of VOD of 16%, compared with 63% for those who did not receive PGE_1. Toxicity limiting administration of PGE_1 was not observed. At the FHCRC, 24 patients at high risk for VOD were treated with PGE_1 at doses ranging from 1.25 to 10 ng/kg/minute, beginning on the day prior to the start of the preparative regimen and continuing until day 15 after transplantation (G. McDonald, unpublished observation). In that study, toxicities limiting PGE_1 administration were common and included postural hypotension (8%), erythema and desquamation with bullae formation (29%), pain in dependent extremities (21%), or weight gain more than 16% from baseline (13%). In a separate report, bilateral symmetrical arthritis, with or without painful extremity edema and paresthesia, developed in 24% of patients who received PGE_1 for prevention of VOD, prompting a reduction in dose or cessation of therapy in 11 and 7% of patients, respectively (73). Thus, it remains unclear whether PGE_1 is a safe and effective prophylaxis for patients at high risk for VOD.

Tissue Plasminogen Activator

The use of tissue plasminogen activator (tPA) for treatment of VOD has been reported in a single patient in whom VOD with ascites, encephalopathy, and elevated total serum bilirubin and transaminase developed. Recombinant human tPA was started on day 30 at a dose of 50 mg/day for 4 days by 3-hour infusion. Within 48 hours of starting tPA, signs and symptoms of VOD started to resolve and the patient was discharged from the hospital 7 days later (74). A pilot study of tPA plus heparin for treatment of established severe VOD was conducted at the FHCRC (75). Seven patients received 10 mg tPA by 4-hour infusion for 2 consecutive days and heparin (1,000 U IV bolus) followed by constant infusion (150 U/kg/day) for 10 days. The median total serum bilirubin level at the start of tPA therapy was 19.4 mg/dL. Five of the 7 patients had prompt decreases in total serum bilirubin levels and improvement in signs and symptoms of VOD. Three patients are alive 180 to 380 days after transplantation, with complete resolution of hyperbilirubinemia and fluid retention. Two patients failed to respond to tPA and died of progressive liver failure. None of the 7 patients experienced bleeding episodes with the treatment; however, it remains to be established whether tPA can be used safely in a majority of patients in whom severe VOD develops.

The Role of Anti-TNF-α Therapy in Reducing Regimen-related Toxicity

Recent reports have indicated that inflammatory cytokines may have an important role in the expression of RRT (53,46). Plasma levels of measured TNF-α have been correlated with the development and severity of GVHD, VOD, and posttransplant diffuse noninfectious pneumonia (46).

TNF-α is synthesized by various activated phagocytic and nonphagocytic cells, including macrophages/monocytes, lymphocytes, natural killer cells, endothelial cells, and fibroblasts. In addition to an active secreted form of TNF-α that appears in the circulation, some newly synthesized TNF-α remains cell-associated as a transmembrane form (76). The diverse biological nonspecific effects of TNF-α make it a prime suspect in either initiation or amplification of tissue injury associated with chemoradiotherapy damage in VOD, pneumonitis, or oral mucositis. TNF-α upregulates adhesion receptor expression on effector cells (monocytes, neutrophils, and vascular endothelium), leading to a procoagulant state that facilitates thrombosis thought to be important in the pathogenesis of VOD. Also, its stimulation of inflammatory eicosanoid production (i.e., inflammatory prostaglandins) and its generation of superoxide radicals leads to tissue damage (77). Recent data also suggest that high levels of TNF-α may be a potent inhibitor of hematopoiesis and as such may contribute to delayed engraftment or even graft failure following marrow transplantation (78).

Pentoxifylline (PTX) (3,7-dimethyl-1-[5-oxo-hexyl]-xanthine) is a synthetic xanthine derivative. In animal models of septicemia, adult respiratory distress syndrome (ARDS), and radiation-induced lung injury, PTX administration was associated with significantly lower TNF-α levels than in control subjects and with improved survival (79). PTX has been shown to have a marked effect on cellular mediators of inflammation and tissue injury. In addition, PTX has a pronounced effect on vascular endothelial production of noninflammatory prostaglandins of the E and I series (PG_I, PGE_2), thus further enhancing local-regional blood flow and enhancing thrombolysis (79).

In an uncontrolled pilot study, marrow transplant recipients received PTX prophylactically at doses up to 2,000 mg/day. In patients treated with PTX, transplant-related complications were significantly reduced, and plasma TNF-α levels were significantly lower when compared with transplant recipients not receiving PTX (53). However, plasma TNF-α levels in patients treated with PTX were still higher when compared with normal volunteers not undergoing BMT. Because the induction of TNF-α synthesis may occur via several signaling pathways (80), selective inhibition of different parts of that pathway may be achieved through the use of several distinct agents. It is known that glucocorticoids block the biosynthesis of TNF-α by markedly depressing the translation of the messenger RNA (mRNA) that is produced (80). It has recently been shown that ciprofloxacin (CIPRO), a flouroquinolone antibiotic, also inhibits accumulation of TNF-α mRNA and thus may act synergistically with PTX and glucocorticoids in blocking alternate pathways for TNF-α synthesis (80). In addition to its effects on TNF-α, CIPRO also may increase PTX levels up to 50% higher than those that can be achieved with PTX alone (81). Thus, a combination of PTX, glucocorticoids, and CIPRO may be more effective in reducing the serum TNF-α levels (82). Studies are currently ongoing to determine whether this reduction translates into a clinical advantage.

One potential drawback of more effective blockade of inflammatory mediator release may be a similar protective effect of tumor tissue associated with a higher incidence of disease persistence and posttransplant relapse. To distinguish such an effect in patients at high risk for posttransplant relapse would require large numbers of patients. Without improvements in posttransplant relapse rates, it is unlikely that this question can be addressed in such a patient population. However, an adverse effect on relapse may be demonstrated in patients at low risk for disease recurrence, such as patients undergoing transplantation for chronic-phase CML. Eleven patients who underwent transplantation for chronic-phase CML received prophylactic PTX in a phase I to II pilot study. Two patients died from infectious complications on days 124 and 154 after transplant. Of the remaining 9 patients, 7 have returned for their one-year follow-up. Cytogenetic and typing data confirm donor status and lack of the Ph^1 -chromosome in all 7 patients (53). If combination pharmacological modulation of inflammatory pathways does in fact lower RRT in patients undergoing BMT without increasing the probability of posttransplant relapse, lower transplant-related morbidity may permit the use of posttransplant "consolidation" either with chemoradiotherapy or immunotherapy, such as interleukin-2, interferon, and Roquinimex (Linomide). Also, it may be possible to escalate the dose level of a preparative regimen previously determined to be the maximum tolerated without TNF-α blockade. Several studies, some of which are placebo-controlled and randomized, are ongoing; it is too early to determine what role anti-TNF-α therapy will have in marrow transplantation.

Pharmacological Issues of Preparative Regimens

Normal tissue toxicity from cytotoxic drugs is a result of the interaction between pharmacokinetic and pharmacodynamic parameters and the unique properties of tissue susceptibility. Pharmacokinetic properties of most cytotoxic drugs used in preparative regimens have been shown to exhibit great variability from patient to patient, resulting in substantial differences in drug blood levels when the same dose of a drug is administered. However, knowledge of the in vivo consequences of this variability as it affects antitumor efficacy and overall toxicity to normal tissues is very limited for most drugs used in current preparative regimens. Few clinical studies of preparative regimens in marrow transplantation have taken into consideration the interpatient differences in pharmacokinetic handling of the cytotoxic drugs when determining a maximum tolerated dose of the drug or drug combination. Due to patient accrual problems, the composition of patient characteristics such as gender, age, ethnic origin, and other potential important differences most often is heterogenous and only partially reported. Thus, a maximum tolerated dose level of a drug combination determined in a particular patient population may not always be appropriate for a patient population with totally different characteristics.

When several cytotoxic drugs are used in preparative regimens, the potential for unanticipated drug interactions adds further complexity and can result in detrimental consequences. Studies have shown that very high doses of ARAC plus CY may be combined with 12 Gy TBI when the two drugs are given sequentially (83). However, if the two drugs are given simultaneously, at even a fraction of the dose shown to be tolerated when given sequentially, the results can be devastating. In one study utilizing simultaneous administration of these two drugs, hyperacute fatal toxicity (cardiovascular) developed in some patients, whereas others given the same regimen and dosing experienced development of virtually no toxicity at all (4).

Only a minority of phase I trials list any pharmacokinetic data from the cytotoxic drugs used in the preparative regimen or details of patient characteristics that could potentially influence the pharmacokinetics of the tested drugs. Access to adequately homogeneous patient populations is limited, and application of pharmacokinetic principles to clinical medicine is complex. These are the most likely reasons that almost all preparative regimens have been tested in phase I trials with fixed drug dosing rather than with doses tailored to each individual patient's unique biological properties. However, because all preparative regimens currently used are associated with significant morbidity and inefficiency at destroying all in vivo tumor, attempts to apply pharmacokinetic principles may be required if improvements are to be achieved.

Improving efficacy by applying pharmacokinetic principles may be particularly necessary for preparative regimens containing BU, a widely used alkylating agent. It is usually administered in 16 doses over 4 days (84,85). This drug is unique because it is available only in an oral formulation. It has been shown that absorption rates vary widely, leading to 2- to 3-fold interpatient differences in plasma BU concentrations on identical dosing (86,87). This variability may contribute to serious toxic effects as well as to the difficulty of defining therapeutically optimal BU dosing schedules. Furthermore, in children less than 5 years of age who receive the same BU regimen, systemic BU clearance and distribution volume have been reported to be twice as high as those reported in adults, with consequently lower steady-state plasma concentrations of BU (88).

After it became possible to determine plasma BU concentrations, several studies showed a correlation between high plasma BU concentrations and the incidence and severity of RRT, especially VOD of the liver (86). The pharmacokinetics of BU are linear across dose levels and appear stable over time, making it possible to predict the steady-state plasma concentration from an initial dose (86,87). This predictability opens the possibility of achieving a given target dose for a group of patients by adjusting subsequent BU doses once the pharmacokinetics of the first dose have been established (87). Whether this approach will improve the clinical outcome in patients treated with BU-containing regimens has yet to be established.

Studies of the pharmacokinetics of other drugs, such as thiotepa, melphalan, and carboplatinum, have been published (89–91) although the clinical consequences of these findings need to be investigated further.

Preparative Regimens

Combining one Cytotoxic Drug with Total Body Irradiation

Early preparative regimens contained TBI as the only or the primary component used in patients undergoing marrow transplantation for hematological malignancies (92). This approach was based on observations demonstrating that marrow transplantation could salvage animals exposed to otherwise lethal radiation injury and on the knowledge that irradiation could be used as effective cell-cycle nonspecific antitumor therapy. CY was added to this regimen because it was found to be an effective antineoplastic agent, which in animal experiments appeared to have dose-limiting marrow toxicity and few extrahematopoietic toxicities that overlapped with those of TBI. Also, it was found that when CY preceded a single dose of TBI, it reduced the risk of tumor lysis in patients undergoing transplantation for relapsed leukemia (93). Subsequent studies were aimed at increasing the effectiveness of the TBI delivery, as described in Chapter 9. Studies also looked at the feasibility of replacing CY with an alternative cytotoxic drug in combination with TBI. ARAC, VP16, and melphalan all could be successfully used as a single drug in place of CY

Table 8-2.
Preparative Regimens with a Single Cytotoxic Drug Combined with Total Body Irradiation

Drug	*Total Dose*	*Before or After TBI*	*Total TBI dose*[a]	*Autologous/ Allogeneic*	*Reference*
Cyclophosphamide	120 mg/kg	Both	8–16 Gy	Both	7,45,92,97
Etoposide	60 mg/kg	Both	12–13.2 Gy	Allogeneic	57
Cytosine arabinoside	36 g/m^2	Before	10–12 Gy	Both	83,94,96,100
Melphalan	110 mg/m^2	Before	9.5–14.85 Gy	Both	95,99

[a] Dose rates and shielding of lungs vary.
TBI = total body iradiation.

(57,94,95). Changing the sequencing of the cytotoxic drug in relation to the TBI was also explored (57,96–98). The changes were made, in part, to avoid the discomfort and inconvenience that patients experienced when linear accelerator treatments were given in close proximity to high-dose chemotherapy, related to multiple sedatives and antiemetic medications.

Dose escalation studies of TBI preceded by a standard CY dose of 60 mg/kg for 2 days have shown that the maximum tolerated dose of TBI is 10 Gy when given in a single dose, 14.4 Gy when given in 1.2-Gy fractions 3 times a day, 16 Gy when given in 2-Gy fractions twice a day, and 15.75 Gy when given in 2.25/Gy fractions once a day (6,7,45). In these studies, interstitial pneumonitis was found to be the dose-limiting toxicity. In dose escalation studies of VP16 combined with 12 or 13.2 Gy fractionated TBI, 60 mg/kg VP16 was found to be the maximum tolerated dose; stomatitis and hepatic tolerance were the dose-limiting toxicities (57). Also, it was shown that 110 to 180 mg/m^2 melphalan could be combined with 9.5 to 14.85 Gy TBI (95,99) and that 36 gm/m^2 ARAC could be combined with 10 to 12 Gy TBI (83,94,96,100). Dose-limiting toxicities were stomatitis and VOD for melphalan plus TBI, and central nervous system and skin toxicity for ARAC plus TBI.

Combining More Than One Cytotoxic Drug with Total Body Irradiation

Even though preparative regimens combining a single cytotoxic drug with TBI were shown to result in long-term, event-free survival of a majority of patients undergoing transplantation for acute myeloid leukemia (AML) in first remission or chronic-phase CML, posttransplant recurrent disease remained a major reason for treatment failure when used in patients undergoing transplantation for advanced hematological malignancies. This finding led to studies of preparative regimens utilizing combinations of cytotoxic drugs given with TBI. The rationale for this approach was that in settings other than marrow transplantation, combinations of cytotoxic drugs had been shown to be more effective against malignancies than treatments utilizing single agents (i.e., malignant lymphoma, testicular carcinoma). Theoretically, when using a combination of agents, greater dose escalations would be possible without significant overlapping in toxicity.

The FHCRC systematically explored new preparative regimens containing 2 cytotoxic drugs given with a standard regimen of 12 Gy fractionated TBI. It was found that 50 mg/kg CY combined with 7 mg/kg BU or 103 mg/kg CY combined with 44 mg/kg VP16 were the maximum tolerated dose levels that could be given with 12 Gy fractionated TBI (5,7). Phase II trials to evaluate both regimens are in progress. Other investigators determined the maximum tolerated dose levels of combined CY and VP16, CY and ARAC, and BU and VP16, all in combination with TBI (83,100–103).

Some of the studies evaluating similar drug and TBI combinations appear to come to different conclusions regarding the maximum tolerated dose level (7,101); however, differences in patient selection, drug sequencing, drug delivery, and TBI delivery all varied in these studies, and thus meaningful comparisons are difficult.

Combining Cytotoxic Drugs without Total Body Irradiation

A preparative regimen without TBI is used for two major reasons. First, several transplant centers lack access to an adequate radiation facility (84). Second, some patients in need of a marrow transplantation have already received maximum tolerated doses of radiation to critical organs (104). Initial trials with combinations of BCNU, ARAC, CY, and 6-thioguanine (BACT) evolved into regimens that combined CY, BCNU, and VP16 with or without ARAC (Table 8-4). The BEAM and BCV regimens are mostly used in preparation of patients undergoing transplantation for "lymphoid" diseases, such as malignant lymphoma or acute lymphoblastic leukemia (see Table 8-4) (105–108). The TCC, TC, BCC, MVT VU, and ICE regimens are mostly used in marrow transplantation of patients with breast cancer and other solid tumors (defined in Table 8-4) (34,35,109–114).

Clinical use of BU plus CY (BU-CY) was introduced by Santos and colleagues (84). In the initial phase I trial, 16 mg/kg BU plus 200 mg/kg CY ("big" BU-CY) was found to be the maximum tolerated dose level, with VOD as the dose-limiting toxicity. Compared with historical control subjects, survival in patients with AML prepared for transplant with "big" BU-CY appeared equivalent to the survival of similar patients prepared with CY plus TBI (84). Subsequent studies led to the development of a modified regimen with 16 mg/kg BU plus 120 mg/kg CY ("small" or "little" BU-CY)

Table 8-3
Preparative Regimens with a Second Cytotoxic Drug Combined with Cyclophosphamide and Total Body Irradiation

Drug	*Total Dose*	*CY dose*	*Total TBI dose*[a]	*Autologous/ Allogeneic*	*Reference*
Cytosine arabinoside	3 g/m^2 × 2–12	60–120 mg/kg	5–12 Gy	Both	83,100
Busulfan	7 mg/kg	50 mg/kg	12 Gy	Both	5
Etoposide	40–60 mg/kg	80–100 mg/kg	12 Gy	Autologous	7,101,103

[a]Dose rates and shielding of lungs vary.
CY = cyclophopshamide; TBI = total body irradiation.

Table 8-4.
Preparative Regimens without Total Body Irradiation

Combination	*Drugs*	*Total Dose*	*Autologous/Allogeneic*	*Reference*
BUCY	Busulfan	14–16 mg/kg		
	Cyclophosphamide	120–200 mg/kg	Both	84,85
BCV	Carmustine	300–600 mg/m^2		
	Cyclophosphamide	6–7.2 g/m^2		
	Etoposide	600–2,400 mg/m^2	Both	106,107,108
BEAM	Carmustine (BCNU)	300 mg/m^2		
	Etoposide	400–800 mg/m^2		
	Cytosine arabinoside	800–1,600 mg/m^2		
	Melphalan	140 mg/mg/m^2	Autologous	105
TCC	Thiotepa	500 mg/m^2		
	Cyclophosphamide	6,000 mg/m^2		
	Carboplatinum	800 mg/m^2	Autologous	109
TC	Thiotepa	800 mg/m^2		
	Cyclophosphamide	6,000 mg/m^2	Autologous	110
BCC	Carmustine	600 mg/m^2		
	Cisplatinum	165 mg/m^2		
	Cyclophosphamide	5,625 mg/m^2	Autologous	34
MVT	Mitoxantrone	30 mg/m^2		
	Etoposide (VP16)	1,200 mg/m^2		
	Thiotepa	750 mg/m^2	Autologous	111,112
ICE	Ifosfamide	1,500 mg/m^2		
	Carboplatinum	1,000 mg/m^2		
	Etoposide	1,250 mg/m^2	Autologous	113,129

(85). Uncontrolled comparisons to patients treated with "big" BU-CY suggested that "little" BU-CY was associated with less RRT, without a demonstrable difference in antileukemic activity (85). Further attempts to reduce the CY dose are ongoing, because the relative contribution of CY to antileukemic efficacy in the BU-CY regimen is questionable (115).

BU-CY has gained wide acceptance as a preparative regimen mainly because TBI is avoided and because available data suggest that BU-CY is as effective as TBI-containing regimens in the treatment of patients with AML and CML. However, its efficacy as a preparative regimen in patients undergoing transplantation for acute lymphoblastic leukemia (ALL) and malignant lymphoma is controversial (116–118). It has also been suggested that subgroups of patients with AML (FAB-M4 and M5) may respond poorly to a BU-CY regimen (D. Blaise, unpublished observations). Other studies are evaluating the possibility of reducing the dose of BU in patients at high risk for severe RRT while retaining the antitumor efficacy. It has also been shown that a third drug may be added to BU-CY: thiotepa, VP16, or melphalan (102,119,120). The effect on event-free survival when comparing these combinations with BU-CY alone has not been determined.

TBI is known to be associated with a significant risk of potentially severe long-term side effects, such as chronic pulmonary disease, leukoencephalopathy, cataracts, secondary malignancy, and hormonal impairments, including sterility and growth retardation in children. Thus, it is hoped that equipotent preparative regimens without TBI would avoid these long-term sequelae. Due to limited follow-up, relatively few patients have achieved long-term survival following marrow transplantation with a preparative regimen without TBI, and it is currently unknown whether such benefits exist.

Preliminary studies of long-term consequences of BU-CY are not encouraging, suggesting that the incidence of long-term difficulties, especially in children, are similar in incidence and nature to those seen in patients who received CY and TBI (122,123). Some reports have also suggested that there may be a high incidence of late (>5 years after treatment) severe pulmonary fibrosis in patients who have received high doses of BCNU (50). The final determination of the relative contribution to long-term morbidity of TBI-containing regimens and regimens without TBI will come from careful long-term follow-up of patients entered into randomized trials.

Designing Trials of New Preparative Regimens

When considering a phase I trial of a new preparative regimen, the following considerations need to be assessed: (1) patients are at a very high risk of death over the short term with standard therapy, (2) the proposed new therapy may result in unacceptable and fatal RRT, (3) only modest antitumor efficacy can be expected at low doses, and (4) relatively little is known about the appropriate dose range for acceptable efficacy with tolerable toxicity. In a classic phase I trial, the initial dose level of the preparative regimen is intentionally low and is only slowly escalated until the dose level at which unacceptable toxicity is observed. The dose level just below that at which toxicity is unacceptable is defined as the maximum tolerated dose. Because such starting dose levels often have little antitumor efficacy, a slow dose escalation in the classic design may put early patients at risk of receiving ineffective therapy.

This potential shortcoming was addressed in a systematic evaluation of new preparative regimens initiated at FHCRC in 1984. First, RRT was defined as described previously. Next, incidence and severity of RRT was determined in patients who had undergone transplantation for advanced leukemia after a preparative regimen combining 120 mg/kg CY with 15.75 Gy fractionated TBI. At that time, this was the standard regimen for patients transplanted for advanced leukemia. It was determined that severe toxicity developed in 20% of patients, most often leading to death. Therefore, an acceptable maximum tolerated dose level for a new preparative regimen was defined as one with a less than 20% incidence of severe (grade III or IV) RRT. Dose levels of a new drug and radiation combination were designed according to a modification of a method described by Tsutakawa (123). According to this method, prior experience with the cytotoxic drugs to be tested was used by the investigators to estimate a minimum and maximum dose level that would be associated with a 20% or greater incidence of unacceptable toxicity. The calculated mean estimated dose level was determined to be the starting dose level, and the standard deviation was used to construct higher and lower dose levels. A modification of a method described by Hsi (124) was used to determine whether this estimated dose level was appropriate. If the observed incidence of unacceptable RRT was less than 20%, subsequent patients were treated on a higher dose level, but if the observed incidence of unacceptable RRT was higher than 20%, subsequent patients were treated on a lower dose level. Patients were treated in groups of 4. Development of grades III or IV RRT (see Table 8-1) in any organ system was defined as severe (unacceptable) toxicity. The dose level into which subsequent groups of 4 patients were entered depended on the actual observed toxicity (Table 8-5).

Subsequent patients would not be escalated to a higher dose level if they had already been treated at that level and if estimates indicated a greater than 80% probability that the incidence of unacceptable RRT at that dose level would exceed 20%. With this schema, a maximum of 20 patients would be required to determine the maximum tolerated dose of the tested treatment regimen. Furthermore, patients entered early in the trial would most likely receive a dose level close to the observed maximum tolerated.

This design has been used in several phase I trials carried out at the FHCRC (4–7). The experience is that the estimated maximum tolerated starting dose level has been no more than 2 dose levels above (6,7) or 1 dose level below (5) the observed maximum tolerated.

Attempts have been made to develop similar statistically based schemes aimed at determining the maximum tolerated dose level of a chemotherapy treatment with the lowest possible number of patients exposed to unacceptable toxicity (125).

Table 8-5.
Plan for Dose Determination

No. Patients with Unacceptable RRT / Total No. Entered on the Dose Level	*Dose Level for the Next 4 Patients*
0/4	Next higher dose level
1/4	Same dose level
2/2, 2/3, or 2/4	Next lower dose level

Summary

None of the preparative regimens currently in use can overcome all in vivo malignant disease and also result in only minimum toxicity to normal tissues. It is uncertain whether one single preparative regimen will ever achieve this goal. Most preparative regimens have been developed empirically and are often tailored to the unique circumstances of the investigating center. Although most new preparative regimens have been tested in phase I trials and some of the most promising have been evaluated in phase II trials, only a fraction have reached comparative phase III trials. Consequently, it is difficult if not impossible to assess the relative merits of most preparative regimens in use, and no single regimen stands out as preferable over all others in every transplant situation. Future developments will center on delivering the cytotoxic effect in a more targeted fashion to the tumor tissue. This targeting may be achieved by sensitizing tumor tissue to the cytotoxic effect of the preparative regimen while protecting normal tissues from the damaging effects of the regimen. Understanding the pharmacokinetics of the drugs used in preparative regimens and individualizing drug doses accordingly may also lead to increased efficacy. Because inducing a transient state of residual minimal disease may be the best that can be done for most patients undergoing transplantation for advanced disease, combining a standard preparative regimen with in vivo cytotoxic (radiolabeled or immunotoxin-conjugated) monoclonal antibodies or posttransplant immunotherapy may be needed to achieve goals.

Final comparative efficacy testing of promising preparative regimens or combinations of tumor-destroying modalities most likely will have to be done on a national or international level. Despite major progress in many fields of clinical marrow transplantation, the outcome of transplanting patients with advanced hematological malignancies has advanced only marginally, if at all, since Thomas' (1) 1977 report of the first 100 marrow transplants in Seattle. Due to the difficulties in conducting informative clinical studies of preparative regimens discussed in this chapter, improvements most likely will be incremental and difficult to interpret. However, progress has been made in improving the outcome of marrow transplantation for selected patients with less advanced hematological malignancies (i.e., CML). The challenge and hope is that current and future approaches will lead to similar improvements for patients with more higher risk malignant diseases.

References

1. Thomas ED, Buckner CD, Banaji M, et al. One hundred patients with acute leukemia treated by chemotherapy, total body irradiation and allogeneic marrow transplantation. Blood 1977;49:511–533.
2. Buckner CD, Clift RA, Appelbaum FR, et al. Effects of treatment regimens on post marrow transplant relapse. Semin Hematol 1991;28:32–34.
3. Bearman SI, Appelbaum FR, Buckner CD, et al. Regimen-related toxicity in patients undergoing bone marrow transplantation. J Clin Oncol 1988;6:1562–1568.
4. Petersen FB, Appelbaum FR, Buckner CD, et al. Simultaneous infusion of high-dose cytosine arabinoside with cyclophosphamide followed by total body irradiation and marrow infusion for the treatment of patients with advanced hematological malignancy. Bone Marrow Transplant 1988;3:619–624.
5. Petersen FB, Buckner CD, Appelbaum FR, et al. Busulfan, cyclophosphamide and fractionated total body irradiation as a preparatory regimen for marrow transplantation in patients with advanced hematological malignancies: a phase I study. Bone Marrow Transplant 1989;4:617–623.
6. Petersen FB, Deeg HJ, Buckner CD, et al. Marrow transplantation following escalating doses of fractionated total body irradiation and cyclophosphamide—a phase I trial. Int J Radiat Oncol Biol Phys 1992;23(5): 1027–1032.
7. Petersen FB, Buckner CD, Appelbaum FR, et al. Etoposide, cyclophosphamide and fractionated total body irradiation as a preparatory regimen for marrow transplantation in patients with advanced hematological malignancies: a phase I Study. Bone Marrow Transplant 1992;10:83–88.
8. Bearman SI, Appelbaum FR, Back A, et al. Regimen-related toxicity and early posttransplant survival in patients undergoing marrow transplantation for lymphoma. J Clin Oncol 1989;7:1288–1294.
9. Nevill TJ, Barnett MJ, Klingemann H-G, et al. Regimen-related toxicity of a busulfan-cyclophosphamide conditioning regimen in 70 patients undergoing allogeneic bone marrow transplantation. J Clin Oncol 1991; 9:1224–1232.
10. Steinherz LJ, Steinherz PG, Mangiacasale D, et al. Cardiac changes with cyclophosphamide. Med Pediatr Oncol 1981;9:417–422.
11. Goldberg MA, Antin JH, Guinan EC, et al. Cyclophosphamide cardiotoxicity: an analysis of dosing as a risk factor. Blood 1986;68:1114–1118.
12. Kupari M, Volin L, Suokas A, et al. Cardiac involvement in bone marrow transplantation: serial changes in left ventricular size, mass and performance. J Intern Med 1990;227:259–266.
13. Bearman SI, Petersen FB, Schor RA, et al. Radionuclide ejection fractions in the evaluation of patients being considered for bone marrow transplantation: risk for cardiac toxicity. Bone Marrow Transplant 1990;5:173–177.
14. Kupari M, Volin L, Suokas A, et al. Cardiac involvement in bone marrow transplantation: electrocardiographic changes, arrhythmias, heart failure and autopsy findings. Bone Marrow Transplant 1990;5:91–98.
15. Sugarman J, Bashore TM, Ohman EM, et al. Hypertension and reversible myocardial depression associated with autologous bone marrow transplantation. Am J Med 1990;88:52N–55N.
16. Gottdiener JS, Appelbaum FR, Ferrans VJ, et al. Cardiotoxicity associated with high-dose cyclophosphamide therapy. Arch Intern Med 1981;141:758–763.
17. Braverman AC, Antin JH, Plapert MT, et al. Cyclophosphamide cardiotoxicity in bone marrow transplantation: a prospective evaluation of new dosing regimens. J Clin Oncol 1991;9:1215–1223.
18. Kanj SS, Sharara AI, Shpall EJ, et al. Myocardial ischemia associated with high-dose carmustine infusion. Cancer 1991;68:1910–1912.
19. Cox PJ. Cyclophosphamide cystitis—identification of acrolein as the causative agent. Biochem Pharmacol 1979;28:2045–2049.
20. Efros M, Ahmed T, Choudhury M. Cyclophosphamide-induced hemorrhagic pyelitis and ureteritis associated with cystitis in marrow transplantation. J Urol 1990; 144:1231–1232.
21. Shepherd JD, Pringle LE, Barnett MJ, et al. Mesna versus hyperhydration for the prevention of cyclophosphamide-induced hemorrhagic cystitis in bone marrow transplantation. J Clin Oncol 1991;9:2016–2020.
22. Atkinson K, Biggs JC, Golovsky D, et al. Bladder irrigation does not prevent haemorrhagic cystitis in bone marrow transplant recipients. Bone Marrow Transplant 1991;7:351–354.
23. Morgan M, Dodds A, Atkinson K, et al. The toxicity of busulphan and cyclophosphamide as the preparative regimen for bone marrow transplantation. Br J Haematol 1991;77:529–534.
24. Shaw IC, Graham MI. Mesna—a short review. Cancer Treat Rev 1987;14:67–86.
25. Hows JM, Mehta A, Ward L, et al. Comparison of mesna with forced diuresis to prevent cyclophosphamide-induced haemorrhagic cystitis in marrow transplantation: a prospective randomised study. Br J Cancer 1984;50:753–756.
26. Vose JM, Pipert G, Reed EC, et al. Randomized trial comparing mesna to bladder irrigation for prevention of hemorrhagic cystitis following high-dose cyclophosphamide and bone marrow transplantation. Blood 1991;78(suppl 1):977.
27. Trigg ME, O'Reilly J, Rumelhart S, et al. Prostaglandin E1 bladder instillations to control severe hemorrhagic cystitis. J Urol 1990;143:92–94.
28. Shrom SH, Donaldson MH, Duckett JW, et al. Formalin treatment for intractable hemorrhagic cystitis. A review of the literature with 16 additional cases. Cancer 1976;38:1785–1789.
29. Lapides J. Treatment of delayed intractable hemorrhagic cystitis following radiation or chemotherapy. J Urol 1970;104:707–708.
30. Golin AL, Benson RC. Cyclophosphamide hemorrhagic cystitis requiring urinary diversion. J Urol 1977;118: 110–111.
31. Zager RA, O'Quigley J, Zager BK, et al. Acute renal failure following bone marrow transplantation: a retrospective study of 272 patients. Am J Kidney Dis 1989;13:210–216.
32. Tarbell NJ, Guinan EC, Chin L, et al. Renal insufficiency

after total body irradiation for pediatric bone marrow transplantation. Radiother Oncol 1990;18(suppl 1): 139–142.

33. McDonald GB, Hinds MS, Fisher LD. Liver disease in marrow transplant patients leads to multi organ failure: a prospective study of 355 patients. Hepatology 1991;14:163A.
34. Peters WP, Shpall EJ, Jones RB. High-dose combination alkylating agents with bone marrow support as initial treatment for metastatic breast cancer. J Clin Oncol 1990;6:1368–1376.
35. Eder JP, Elias A, Shea TC, et al. A phase I–II study of cyclophosphamide, thiotepa, and carboplatin with autologous bone marrow transplantation in solid tumor patients. J Clin Oncol 1990;8:1239–1245.
36. Kennedy MS, Deeg HJ, Siegel M, et al. Acute renal toxicity with combined use of amphotericin B and cyclosporine after marrow transplantation. Transplantation 1983;35:211–215.
37. Wingard JR, Mellits ED, Sostrin MB, et al. Interstitial pneumonitis after allogeneic bone marrow transplantation. Nine year experience at a single institution. Medicine 1988;67:175–186.
38. Meyers JD, Flournoy N, Thomas ED, et al. Nonbacterial pneumonia after allogeneic marrow transplantation: a review of ten years' experience. Rev Infect Dis 1982;4:1119–1132.
39. Chan CK, Hyland RH, Hutcheon MA. Pulmonary complications following bone marrow transplantation. Clin Chest Med 1990;11:323–332.
40. Pecego R, Hill RS, Appelbaum FR, et al. Interstitial pneumonitis following autologous bone marrow transplantation. Transplantation 1986;42:515–517.
41. Crawford SW, Hackman RC, Clark JG. Open lung biopsy diagnosis of diffuse pulmonary infiltrates after marrow transplantation. Chest 1988;94:949–953.
42. Weiner RS, Bortin MM, Gale RP. Interstitial pneumonitis after bone marrow transplantation. Assessment of risk factors. Ann Intern Med 1986;104:168–175.
43. Smith AC, Boyd MR. Preferential effects of 1,3-bis(2-chloroethyl)-1-nitrosourea (carmustine) on pulmonary glutathione reductase and glutathione/glutathione disulfide ratios: possible implications for lung toxicity. J Pharmacol Exp Ther 1984;229:658–663.
44. Keane TJ, Van Dyk J, Rider WD. Idiopathic interstitial pneumonia following bone marrow transplantation: the relationship with total body irradiation. Int J Radiat Oncol Biol Phys 1981;7:1365–1370.
45. Clift RA, Buckner CD, Thomas ED, et al. Allogeneic marrow transplantation using fractionated total body irradiation in patients with acute lymphoblastic leukemia in relapse. Leuk Res 1982;6:401–407.
46. Holler E, Kolb HJ, Moller A, et al. Increased serum levels of tumor necrosis factor α precede major complications of bone marrow transplantation. Blood 1990; 75:1011–1016.
47. Troussard X, Bernaudin JF, Cordonnier C, et al. Pulmonary venoocclusive disease after bone marrow transplantation. Thorax 1984;39:956–957.
48. Hackman RC, Madtes DK, Petersen FB. Pulmonary venoocclusive disease following bone marrow transplantation. Transplantation 1989;47:989–992.
49. Clark JG, Schwartz DA, Flournoy N, et al. Risk factors for airflow obstruction in recipients of bone marrow transplants. Ann Intern Med 1987;107:648–656.
50. O'Driscoll BR, Hasleton PS, Taylor PM, et al. Active lung fibrosis up to 17 years after chemotherapy with carmustine (BCNU) in childhood. New Engl J Med 1990;323:378–382.
51. Ralph DD, Springmeyer SC, Sullivan KM, et al. Rapidly progressive air-flow obstruction in marrow transplant recipients. Am Rev Respir Dis 1984;129:641–644.
52. Chao NJ, Duncan SR, Long GD, et al. Corticosteroid therapy for diffuse alveolar hemorrhage in autologous bone marrow transplant recipients. Ann Intern Med 1991;114:145–146.
53. Bianco JA, Appelbaum FR, Nemunaitis J, et al. Phase I–II trial of pentoxifylline for the prevention of transplant related toxicities following bone marrow transplantation. Blood 1991;78:1205–1211.
54. Crawford SW, Schwartz DA, Petersen FB, et al. Mechanical ventilation after marrow transplantation: risk factors and clinical outcome. Am Rev Respir Dis 1988; 137:682–687.
55. Crawford SW, Petersen FB. Long-term survival from respiratory failure after marrow transplantation for malignancy. Am Rev Respir Dis 1992;145:510–514; 508–509.
56. Seto BG, Kim M, Wolinsky L, et al. Oral mucositis in patients undergoing marrow transplantation. Oral Surg Oral Med Oral Pathol 1985;60:493–497.
57. Blume KG, Forman SJ, O'Donell MR, et al. Total body irradiation and high-dose etoposide: a new preparatory regimen for bone marrow transplantation in patients with advanced hematologic malignancies. Blood 1987; 69:1015–1020.
58. Storb R, Deeg HJ, Thomas ED, et al. Marrow transplantation for chronic myelocytic leukemia: a controlled trial of cyclosporine versus methotrexate for prophylaxis of graft-versus-host disease. Blood 1985;66:698–702.
59. Wingard JR, Niehaus CS, Peterson DE, et al. Oral mucositis after bone marrow transplantation. A marker of treatment toxicity and predictor of hepatic venoocclusive disease. Oral Surg Oral Med Oral Pathol 1991;72:419–424.
60. Weisdorf DJ, Bostrom B, Raether D, et al. Oropharyngeal mucositis complicating bone marrow transplantation: prognostic factors and the effect of chlorhexidine mouth rinse. Bone Marrow Transplant 1989;4:89–95.
61. Ferretti GA, Ash RC, Brown AT, et al. Control of oral mucositis and candidiasis in marrow transplantation: a prospective, double-blind trial of chlorhexidine digluconante oral rinse. Bone Marrow Transplant 1988; 3:483–493.
62. Nemunitis J, Rabinowe SN, Singer JW, et al. Recombinant granulocyte-macrophage colony-stimulating factor after autologous bone marrow transplantation for lymphoid cancer. N Engl J Med 1991;324:1773–1778.
63. Atkinson K, Biggs JC, Downs K, et al. GM-CSF after allogeneic bone marrow transplantation: accelerated recovery of neutrophils, monocytes, and lymphocytes. Aust NZ J Med 1991;21:686–692.
64. Linassier C, Colombat P, Reisenleiter M, et al. Cutaneous toxicity of autologous bone marrow transplantation in nonseminomatous germ cell tumors. Cancer 1990; 65:1143–1145.
65. Jameson CH, Solanki DL. Stevens-Johnson syndrome associated with etoposide therapy. Cancer Treat Rep 1983;67:1050–1051.
66. Herzig RH, Fay JW, Herzig GP, et al. Phase I–II studies with high-dose thiotepa and autologous marrow transplantation in patients with refractory malignancies. In: Herzig GP, ed. High-dose thiotepa and autologous

marrow transplantation. Dallas: Proceedings Advances in Cancer Chemotherapy Symposium, 1986:17–23.

67. Hartmann O, Beaujean F, Pico JL. High-dose busulfan and cyclophosphamide in advanced childhood cancers. A phase II study of 30 patients. In: Dicke KA, Spitzer G, Jagannath S, eds. Autologous bone marrow transplantation. Houston: Proceedings of the Third International Symposium, 1986:581–588.
68. Shulman HM, Luk K, Deeg HJ, et al. Induction of hepatic veno-occlusive disease in dogs. Am J Pathol 1987;126:114–125.
69. Rio B, Lamy T, Zittoun R. Preventive role of heparin for liver venoocclusive disease (VOD). Bone Marrow Transplant 1989;3(suppl 1):266.
70. Attal M, Huguet F, Rubie H, et al. Prevention of hepatic veno-occlusive disease after bone marrow transplantation by continuous infusion of low-dose heparin: a prospective, randomized trial. Blood 1992; 79:2834–2840.
71. Bearman SI, Hinds MS, Wolford JL, et al. A pilot study of continuous infusion heparin for the prevention of hepatic veno-occlusive disease after bone marrow transplantation. Bone Marrow Transplant 1990;5:407–411.
72. Gluckman E, Jolivet I, Scrobohaci ML, et al. Use of prostaglandin E1 for prevention of liver veno-occlusive disease in leukaemic patients treated by allogeneic bone marrow transplantation. Br J Haematol 1990; 74:277–281.
73. Bordigoni P, Witz F, Von Bueltzingsloewen A, et al. Prostaglandin E1 (PGE1) induced arthritis following bone marrow transplantation. Br J Haematol 1991; 78:138–139.
74. Baglin TP, Harper P, Marcus RE. Veno-occlusive disease of the liver complicating ABMT successfully treated with recombinant tissue plasminogen activator. Bone Marrow Transplant 1990;5:439–441.
75. Bearman SI, Shuhart MC, Hinds MS, et al. A pilot study of recombinant human tissue plasminogen activator for the treatment of established severe hepatic venocclusive disease after marrow transplantation (abstract). Proc ASCO 1992;11:263.
76. Kriegler M, Perez C, DeFay K, et al. A novel form of TNF/cahcectin is a cell surface cytotoxic transmembrane protein: ramifications for the complex physiology of TNF. Cell 1988;53:45–53.
77. Bevilacqua MP, Pober JS, Majeau GR, et al. Recombinant tumor necrosis factor induces procoagulant activity in cultured human vascular endothelium. Characterization and comparison with the actions of interleukin-1. Proc Natl Acad Sci USA 1986;83:4533–4537.
78. Linderman A, Ludwig WD, Oster W, et al. High-level secretion of tumor necrosis factor alpha contributes to hematopoietic failure in hairy cell leukemia. Blood 1989;73:880–884.
79. Matzky R, Darius H, Schaor K. The release of prostacyclin by pentoxifylline from human vascular tissue. Arzneimittel forschung 1982;32:1315–1318.
80. Han J, Thompson P, Beutler B. Dexamethasone and pentoxifylline inhibit endotoxin-induced cahectin/tumor necrosis factor synthesis at separate points in the signaling pathway. J Exp Med 1990;172:391–394.
81. Bailly S, Fay M, Roche Y. Effects of quinolones on tumor necrosis factor production by human monocytes. Int J Immunopharmacol 1990;12:31–36.
82. Bianco JA, Nemunaitis J, Andrews DF, et al. Combined therapy with pentoxifylline (PTX), ciprofloxacin (CIPRO) and prednisone (PD) reduces regimen related toxicity (RRT) and accelerates engraftment in patients undergoing bone marrow transplantation (BMT) (abstract). Blood 1991;78(suppl 1):237a.
83. Ridell S, Appelbaum FR, Buckner CD, et al. High-dose cytarabine and total body irradiation with or without cyclophosphamide as a preparative regimen for marrow transplantation for acute leukemia. J Clin Oncol 1988;6:576–582.
84. Santos GW, Tutschka PJ, Brookmeyer R, et al. Marrow transplantation for acute nonlymphocytic leukemia after treatment with busulfan and cyclophosphamide. New Engl J Med 1983;309:1347–1353.
85. Tutschka PJ, Copelan EA, Klein JP. Bone marrow transplantation for leukemia following a new busulfan and cyclophosphamide regimen. Blood 1987;70:1382–1388.
86. Grochow LB, Jones RJ, Brundrett RB, et al. Pharmacokinetics of busulfan: correlation with veno-occlusive disease in patients undergoing bone marrow transplantation. Cancer Chemother Pharmacol 1989;25:55–61.
87. Hill H, Sander JE, Langer F, et al. Initial-dose pharmacokinetics allow accurate prediction of average steady-state busulfan concentrations in marrow transplant patients (abstract). Blood 1991;78(suppl 1):243a.
88. Grochow LB, Krivit W, Whitley CB, et al. Busulfan disposition in children. Blood 1990;75:1723–1727.
89. Mulder PO, de-Vries EG, Uges DR, et al. Pharmacokinetics of carboplatin at a dose of 750 mg m-2 divided over three consecutive days. Br J Cancer 1990;6:460–464.
90. Boros L, Peng YM, Alberts DS, et al. Pharmacokinetics of very high-dose oral melphalan in cancer patients. Am J Clin Oncol 1990;13:19–22.
91. Ackland SP, Choi KE, Ratain MJ, et al. Human plasma pharmacokinetics of thiotepa following administration of high-dose thiotepa and cyclophosphamide. J Clin Oncol 1988;6:1192–1196.
92. Thomas ED, Storb R, Buckner CD. Total-body irradiation in preparation for marrow engraftment. Transplant Proc 1976;8:591–594.
93. Buckner CD, Rudolp RH, Fefer A, et al. High-dose cyclophosphamide therapy for malignant disease. Cancer 1972;29:357–365.
94. Coccia PF, Strandjord SE, Warkentin PI, et al. High-dose cytosine arabinoside and fractionated total-body irradiation: an improved preparative regimen for bone marrow transplantation of children with acute lymphoblastic leukemia in remission. Blood 1988;71: 888–893.
95. Powles RL, Milliken S, Helenglass G. The use of melphalan in conjunction with total body irradiation as treatment for leukemia. Transplant Proc 1989;21:2955–2957.
96. Woods WG, Ramsay NK, Weisdorf DJ, et al. Bone marrow transplantation for acute lymphocytic leukemia utilizing total body irradiation followed by high doses of cytosine arabinoside: lack of superiority over cyclophosphamide-containing conditioning regimens. Bone Marrow Transplant 1990;6:9–16.
97. Shank B, Chu FCH, Dinsmore R, et al. Hyperfractionated total body irradiation for bone marrow transplantation. Int J Radiat Oncol Biol Phys 1981;7:1109–1115.
98. Looney WB, Hopkins HA, Tubiana M. Experimental and clinical studies alternating chemotherapy and radiotherapy. Cancer Metastasis Rev 1989;8:53–79.
99. Gandola L, Lombardi F, Siena S, et al. Total body irradiation and high-dose melphalan with bone mar-

row transplantation at Istituto Nazionale Tumori, Milan, Italy. Radiother Oncol 1990;18(supp l):105–109.
100. Petersen FB, Appelbaum FR, Bigelow CL, et al. High-dose cytosine arabinoside, total body irradiation and marrow transplantation for advanced malignant lymphoma. Bone Marrow Transplant 1989;4:483–488.
101. Horning SJ, Chao NJ, Negrin RS, et al. Preliminary analysis of high dose etoposide cytoreductive regimens and autologous bone marrow transplantation in intermediate and high grade non-Hodgkin's lymphoma. In: Dicke KA, Armitage JO, Dicke MJ, eds. Autologous bone marrow transplantation. Houston: Proceedings of the Fifth International Symposium, 1990:445–452.
102. Spitzer TR, Cottler-Fox M, Torristi J, et al. Escalating doses of etoposide with cyclophosphamide and fractionated total body irradiation or busulfan as conditioning for bone marrow transplantation. Bone Marrow Transplant 1989;4:559–565.
103. Bostrom B, Weisdorf DJ, Kim T, et al. Bone marrow transplantation for advanced acute leukemia: a pilot study of high-energy total body irradiation, cyclophosphamide and continuous infusion etoposide. Bone Marrow Transplant 1990;5:83–89.
104. Appelbaum FR, Sullivan KM, Buckner CD, et al. Treatment of malignant lymphoma in 100 patients with chemotherapy, total body irradiation, and marrow transplantation. J Clin Oncol 1987;5:1340–1347.
105. Gaspard MH, Maraninchi D, Stoppa AM, et al. Intensive chemotherapy with high doses of BCNU, etoposide, cytosine arabinoside, and melphalan (BEAM) followed by autologous bone marrow transplantation: toxicity and antitumor activity in 26 patients with poor-risk malignancies. Cancer Chemother Pharmacol 1988;22:256–262.
106. Reece DE, Barnett MJ, Connors JM, et al. Intensive chemotherapy with cyclophosphamide, carmustine, and etoposide followed by autologous bone marrow transplantation for relapsed Hodgkin's disease. J Clin Oncol 1991;9:1871–1879.
107. Zander AR, Culbert S, Jagannath S, et al. High dose cyclophosphamide, BCNU, and VP-16 (CBV) as a conditioning regimen for allogeneic bone marrow transplantation for patients with acute leukemia. Cancer 1987;59:1083–1086.
108. Wheeler C, Antin JH, Churchill WH, et al. Cyclophosphamide, carmustine, and etoposide with autologous bone marrow transplantation in refractory Hodgkin's disease and non-Hodgkin's lymphoma: a dose-finding study. J Clin Oncol 1990;8:648–656.
109. Antman K, Ayash L, Elias A, et al. A phase II study of high-dose cyclophosphamide, thiotepa, and carboplatin with autologous marrow support in women with measurable advanced breast cancer responding to standard-dose therapy. J Clin Oncol 1992;10:102–110.
110. Eder JP, Antman K, Elias A, et al. Cyclophosphamide and thiotepa with autologous bone marrow transplantation in patients with solid tumors. J Natl Cancer Inst 1988;80:1221–1226.
111. Wallerstein R Jr, Spitzer G, Dunphy F, et al. A phase II study of mitoxantrone, etoposide, and thiotepa with autologous marrow support for patients with relapsed breast cancer. J Clin Oncol 1990;8:1782–1788.
112. Ellis ED, Williams SF, Moormeier JAA, et al. A phase I–II study of high-dose cyclophosphamide, thiotepa and escalating doses of mitoxantrone with autologous stem cell rescue in patients with refractory malignancies. Bone Marrow Transplant 1990;6:439–442.
113. Lotz JP, Machover D, Malassagne B, et al. Phase I–II study of two consecutive courses of high-dose epipodophyllotoxin, ifosfamide, and carboplatin with autologous bone marrow transplantation for treatment of adult patients with solid tumors. J Clin Oncol 1991; 9:1860–1870.
114. Rosenfeld CS, Przepiorka D, Schwinghammer TL, et al. Autologous bone marrow transplantation following high-dose busulfan and VP-16 for advanced non-Hodgkin's lymphoma and Hodgkin's disease. Exp Hematol 1991;19:317–321.
115. Tutschka PJ, Kapoor N, Copelean EA, et al. Early experience with 16 mg/kg of busulfan and low dose cyclophosphamide of 90 mg/kg as conditioning for allogeneic marrow grafting in leukemia (abstract). Exp Hematol 1991;19:570.
116. van der Jagt RHC, Appelbaum FR, Petersen FB, et al. Busulfan and cyclophosphamide as a preparative regimen for bone marrow transplantation in patients with prior chest radiotherapy. Bone Marrow Transplant 1991;8:211–215.
117. Petersen FB, Appelbaum FR, Hill R, et al. Autologous marrow transplantation for malignant lymphoma. A report of 101 cases from Seattle. J Clin Oncol 1990;8:638–647.
118. Copelan EA, Kapoor N, Gibbins B, et al. Allogeneic marrow transplantation in non-Hodgkin's lymphoma. Bone Marrow Transplant 1990;5:47–50.
119. Dimopopulos M, Przepiorka D, Ippoliti C, et al. High-dose thiotepa, busulfan and cyclophosphamide with autologous marrow transplantation: toxicities of three different dose schedules (abstract). Proc ASCO 1992; 11:359.
120. Phillips GL, Shepherd JD, Barnett MJ, et al. Busulfan, cyclophosphamide, and melphalan conditioning for autologous bone marrow transplantation in hematologic malignancy. J Clin Oncol 1991;9:1880–1888.
121. Sanders J, Sullivan K, Witherspoon R, et al. Long term effects and quality of life in children and adults after marrow transplantation. Bone Marrow Transplant 1989;4(suppl 4):27–29.
122. Wingard JR, Plotnick LP, Freemer CS, et al. Growth in children after bone marrow transplantation: busulfan plus cyclophosphamide versus cyclophosphamide plus total body irradiation. Blood 1992;79:1068–1073.
123. Tsutakawa RK. Selection of dose levels for estimating a percentage point of a logistic response curve. Appl Stat 1980;29:25–33.
124. Hsi BP. The multiple sample up-and-down method in bioassay. J Am Stat Ass 1969;64:147–162.
125. O'Quigley J, Pepe M, Fisher L. A practical design for phase I clinical trials in cancer. Biometrics 1990; 46:33–48.

Chapter 9
Radiotherapeutic Principles of Bone Marrow Transplantation

Brenda Shank

For bone marrow transplantation (BMT), irradiation is used in the form of total body irradiation (TBI), total lymphoid irradiation (TLI), or total abdominal irradiation (TAI). In addition, localized irradiation may be used ("boost" treatment) for areas of presumed higher concentrations of malignant cells. The main roles for irradiation as a systemic agent are immunosuppression and malignant cell eradication. For diseases such as aplastic anemia, the only role is immunosuppression to allow engraftment. In other diseases, such as the leukemias and lymphomas, both immunosuppression and malignant cell kill are important. An additional smaller role of irradiation may be to provide space in the marrow for engraftment.

There are many advantages of irradiation as a systemic agent when compared with chemotherapy: (1) it is non-cross-reactive with any other agent; (2) a given dose of irradiation may be quite homogeneous regardless of blood supply; (3) there is no sanctuary sparing, such as of the testes; (4) after the radiation is given, there is no detoxification or excretion required; and (5) the dose distribution may be tailored in the body by means of shielding of areas of greater sensitivity or "boosting" areas that may contain more than microscopic malignant cells.

Irradiation, however, does have deleterious effects on normal tissues, as does chemotherapy. For example, the gastrointestinal tract is particularly sensitive to radiation acutely; lung and lens are at risk for late complications.

The delivery of radiation may be optimized by varying the time, dose, and fractionation to minimize toxicity to normal tissues, to increase malignant cell kill, and to increase immunosuppression by greater lymphocyte destruction. Radiation delivery may also be optimized by manipulating physical parameters such as beam energy, dose rate, and patient position, which will increase accuracy, dose homogeneity, and comfort of the patient. I explain the radiobiological principles involved in magnafield irradiation with TBI as the prototype, then review the physical principles, and finally, examine the clinical evidence favoring various TBI regimens. Following this discussion, use of TLI and TAI is briefly discussed.

Radiobiological Principles

Basic Principles

All of radiotherapy is considered to be based on what has been described as the 4 Rs (1): repair, reoxygenation, redistribution, and repopulation. Repair is the process during which cells are able to repair at least a portion of the damage of irradiation. Whatever amount of repair that is going to occur is usually thought to be complete in a period of 6 hours in most cells. Reoxygenation has been considered important in solid tumors that have become anoxic through growth beyond their blood supply, but probably is not important in well-oxygenated leukemic cells. Reoxygenation occurs as tumor cells are destroyed by irradiation and dead cells are lost from the tumor, so that the remaining tumor cells become closer to the blood supply in capillaries. Redistribution is the process whereby cells become distributed nonhomogeneously throughout the cell cycle as a result of irradiation, which can destroy more cells in mitosis or S-phase than in the other phases of the cell cycle. During an interval between two radiation fractions, cells may advance through the cell cycle to be in a more or less sensitive phase of the cell cycle by the time the second dose is given (2). Repopulation is the process whereby cells continue to grow if the interval of time between two doses of irradiation is large relative to the cell cycle time. As cells divide, there appears to be less cell kill from two widely spaced doses of irradiation than there would have been had they been given a short time apart. The radiation sensitivity of any given cell type is described by a survival curve (Figure 9-1), which is a plot of the percentage of cell survival versus the dose of irradiation. This may be a straight line when plotted on logarithmic paper (exponential cell kill) if there is no repair. In contrast, if repair takes place, there is a shoulder to the survival curve reflecting the extent of repair.

There are two formulations to describe these cell survival curves. One is the multi-hit multi-target model, which allows description of the fraction of cells surviving, S, as a function of the dose per fraction, D,

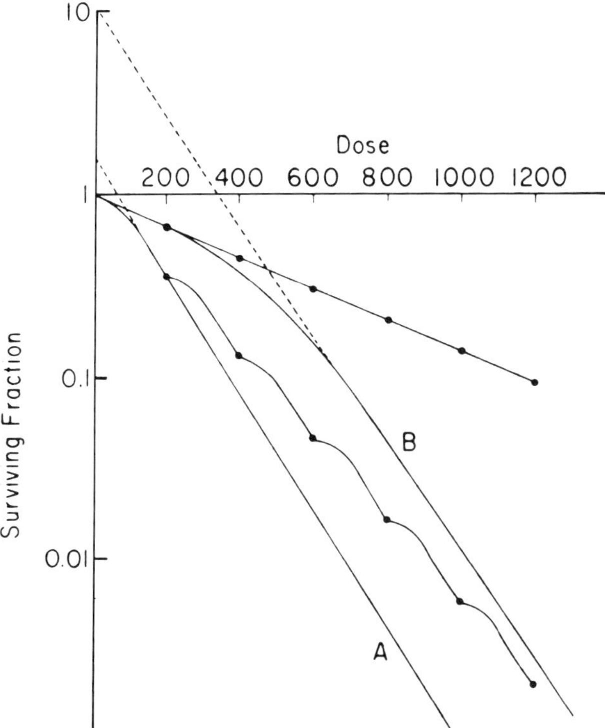

Figure 9-1. Representation of the effect of fractionation on survival of two cell populations, using 2 Gy fractions. Cell population A has only a minimal capacity to repair radiation injury (typical of many leukemic cells) compared with population B, which has a large repair capacity (similar to many normal tissues, such as lung). (Reprinted by permission from Peters LJ, Withers HR, Cundiff JH, Dicke KA. Radiobiological considerations in the use of total-body irradiation for bone marrow transplantation. Radiology 1979;131:243–247.)

in terms of D_0, which represents the slope of the survival curve beyond the initial shoulder and n, the extrapolation number, which is the fraction on the y-axis through which the straight line portion of the survival curve can be extrapolated (see Figure 9-1). This relationship is:

$$S = [1 - (1 - e^{-D/D_0})^n]^f$$

where f is the number of fractions of irradiation.

Another formulation that has come into increasing use is the linear-quadratic or LQ model (3). This formulation is simply an expression of S as a function of two terms, a linear function of D, and a function of D^2:

$$-ln\, S = f(\alpha D + \beta D^2)$$

By dividing this equation through by α, one has a term, α/β, which is characteristic of the type of effects in either tumor or normal tissue. There is a consistent finding of low values of α/β (<5 Gy) for late effects and higher values (10 Gy), for early reactions. Tumor effects generally fall in the range of early reactions with an α/β of approximately 10 Gy.

For radiation to be of benefit in treating any malignancy, there must be a therapeutic gain factor greater than 1. This therapeutic gain factor is the dose required to achieve a given effect (cell kill) in normal tissue divided by the dose required to achieve the same effect (cell kill) in the malignancy. With TBI, there is a multiplicity of normal tissues to consider that are likely to be affected by irradiation. The remainder of this section on radiobiology describes what is known about the effect of radiation on lymphocytes (the target tissue for immunosuppression), leukemic cells (the malignancy most frequently treated with TBI), and the normal tissue of most concern, lung.

Immunosuppression (Normal Lymphocytes)

It has been argued (4) that the most important benefit of TBI is immunosuppression, but this theory is not widely accepted. It has been shown in dogs (5,6) that increasing doses of radiation allowed increasing engraftment. Storb and colleagues (6) also showed that single-dose irradiation was more immunosuppressive than the same total doses when fractionated. Other data from animal studies in dogs, rats, and monkeys have shown similarly that there is a dose fractionation relationship with rejection (4). When treatment is split into multiple fractions given over several days, higher doses of irradiation (e.g., 15 Gy in 4–5 days) are necessary for engraftment in these animals, compared with only 8 Gy in a single dose.

Down and colleagues (7), in a mouse marrow chimera model, showed a steep increase in engraftment of allogeneic marrow with increasing TBI dose (with no cyclophosphamide) when given as a single dose at a high dose rate (1 Gy/min). Low dose rate (0.05 Gy/min) and fractionated TBI required higher total doses for equivalent engraftment, and increasing the interval between fractions from 6 to 24 hours required a further increase in dose. These data were consistent with appreciable sublethal damage repair in the self-renewing stem-cell population of the host. In a murine study from the Institut Gustave-Roussy (8), a fractionated schedule of 1.25 Gy three times a day to a total dose of 7.5 Gy (0.25 Gy/min) had the same effect on the hemopoietic system as 7.5 Gy in a single dose at a low dose rate (0.04 Gy/min). There was no significant repopulation with the fractionated course.

In humans undergoing allogeneic BMT using non-T-cell–depleted marrow, none of the TBI regimens have shown any difference in engraftment; essentially there is 100% engraftment with all. However, when allogeneic bone marrow is given that has been depleted of T lymphocytes to prevent graft-versus-host disease (GVHD), there have been difficulties in sustaining engraftment. Studies in animals (9) and humans (10–

14) have shown that it is possible to increase engraftment by either increasing the TBI dose or by adding TLI to TBI. TLI irradiates the sites along the central axis, in which there is a higher concentration of T lymphocytes in lymph nodes and the thoracic duct. Many studies have shown the importance of T lymphocytes in the process of graft rejection (15,16). It has been calculated by one author (17) that the addition of a single 2-Gy TBI fraction should be sufficient to decrease host T cells by one log, which could be enough to prevent graft failures in T-cell–depleted transplants, but this has not been proven experimentally.

When looking at either cell culture or lymphocyte survival in vivo, it would appear that lymphocytes have either no, or a very small, shoulder to the survival curve (see curve A in Figure 9-1). In a study from the Institut Gustave-Roussy (18), it was found that the D_0 of lymphocytes was 1.2 Gy, and there was a half time for cell loss of 30 hours after a single fraction of TBI. During fractionated irradiation, the half time also appeared to be 30 hours. When lymphocyte subsets were examined, there did not appear to be a different radiosensitivity either in vivo or with the same patient cells in vitro between B and T cells or between helper (OKT4) and suppressor/cytotoxic (OKT8) T cells.

A later study by the same group (19), of a patient who received only 3.85 Gy in three TBI fractions without a BMT due to patient refusal to continue, showed similar radiosensitivities again between T lymphocytes, B lymphocytes, and T-cell subsets (CD4 and CD8). Lymphocytes reached their nadir 48 hours after the last fraction of irradiation, and although the lymphocytes increased again at approximately 2 months, there was still a lymphopenia 3 months later. The D_0 obtained in this patient from the multi-hit multi-target equation was 1.75 Gy. In a study from the Memorial Sloan-Kettering Cancer Center (MSKCC), two patients who received only a single dose of TBI out of a planned hyperfractionated course (1.25 Gy) were studied (20) and were found to have similar lymphocyte decrements, yielding a D_0 of 1.35 Gy for one patient and 1.75 Gy for the other.

Leukemic Cells

For the purposes of this discussion, the only malignant cells considered will be leukemic cells because the majority of cytoreductive procedures utilizing TBI are for patients with leukemia. Leukemic cells, like normal lymphocytes, have generally been considered to have either no shoulder or a very minimal shoulder on the cell survival curve. Most analyses have utilized the multi-hit multi-target model and have cited D_0 and n values. Many authors have studied the radiation survival curve parameters for leukemic cells in vitro (21–25). It is clear from these studies that D_0 and n values vary considerably for different cell types and different cell lines from the same type of leukemia. In some of these cell lines there appears to be no repair whatsoever, whereas in others there does appear to be a repair component (26,27).

In one leukemic line (Reh) from a patient with acute lymphocytic leukemia (ALL) studied in detail (28), it was clear that cell survival fit the LQ model, with a continuously downward curving cell survival plot. Repair between fractions of a hyperfractionation TBI regimen (3 times/day) could explain completely the overall cell survival curve obtained when these cells were irradiated on that schedule. However, because of the relatively small amount of repair in most leukemic cells and the large amount of repair seen in most normal tissues, fractionation of TBI should have a better therapeutic gain factor, with little effect on leukemic cell kill, provided there is no or minimal cell growth between fractions.

Normal Tissues

Many normal tissues are affected by TBI (Figure 9-2); the most critical are lung, gastrointestinal tract, and lens. We will focus on lung in this section, because lung has been the dose-limiting tissue of concern in TBI. Within some early single-dose series (29–31), some form of interstitial pneumonitis (IP) developed in 50 to 100% of patients; approximately two thirds of

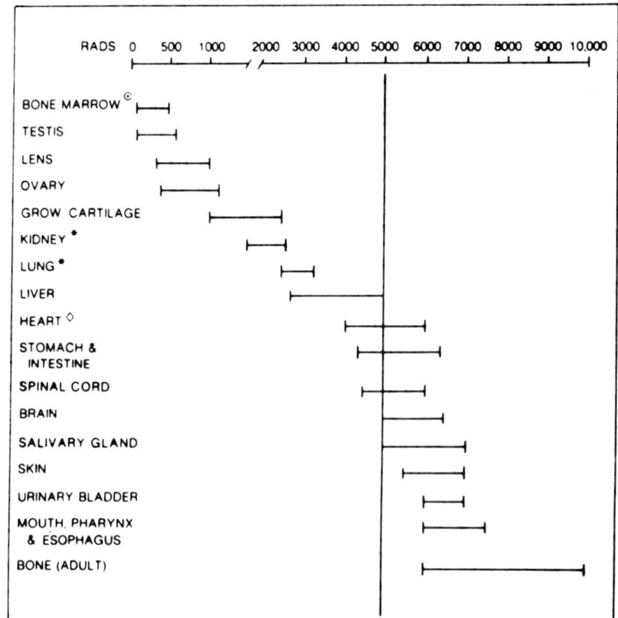

Figure 9-2. Sensitivity of various organs to radiation complications, expressed as a range (|———|), from the dose (rad = cGy) that causes 5% complications to the dose that causes 50% complications within 5 years, assuming 2 Gy fractions, 5 days/wk. *Asterisk* indicates only partial organ irradiation; whole organ irradiation causes complications at lower doses and would shift these bars to the left. (Reprinted by permission from Fajardo L-G. Pathology of radiation injury. New York: Raven, 1982:4)

the patients in whom IP developed have died from this complication (31). Wara and colleagues (32) determined, from the concept of effective dose (ED) to lung, that increasing the number of fractions contributed more to reducing the damage to lung than increasing the overall treatment time.

Thus, use of hyperfractionated regimens, in which small doses per fraction are given 2 to 3 times a day over a few days to minimize leukemic regrowth, may be of great value in reducing lung toxicity. This type of schedule would allow achievement of a higher total dose, thereby increasing leukemic cell kill. Peters and associates (33,34) suggested in 1979 that use of fractionated irradiation would be better than single-dose irradiation in reducing toxicity to normal tissue.

Various clinical studies have shown that a fractionated regimen, either daily fractionation or hyperfractionation (multiple fractions/day), have decreased overall lung toxicity. These studies are discussed in the "Clinical Results" section.

Vriesendorp (4,35) took the approach of modeling the surviving fraction of cells, which determines normal tissue damage and organ function for various fractionation schemes of TBI. He used published clinical data from different fractionation regimens to attempt to determine which values of D_0 and n best fit the ultimate clinical results. Dose rates were those published for each regimen. Using clinical TBI data in humans for lung, he suggested that the data best fit an n of 6 and a D_0 of 1.35 Gy. However, in his surviving fraction curves plotted as a function of n and D_0, the solutions of n and D_0 are not unique; any fractionation considered (i.e., 2–4 fractions varying in total dose from 8–12 Gy) was better than a single dose fraction of 8 Gy. Using values of n and D_0 he deduced for different tissues, Vriesendorp (4,35) created a table of surviving target cells (lung, intestines, bone marrow, and immune system [i.e., lymphocytes]) for a variety of different TBI schedules in the literature. These calculated results show the impressive sparing of lung and intestines to be expected with more fractionated regimens. The immune system survival results suggested that immunosuppression would be poor in highly fractionated (low dose/fraction) regimens; however, the calculated numbers published for this tissue are in error. The corrected immune system values as well as values for lung are shown in Table 9-1, with the addition of two other hyperfractionated regimens. It can be seen that immunosuppression is predicted to be excellent with these high total dose (15 Gy) hyperfractionated regimens. Malignant lymphocytes may be expected to respond similarly, because they have similar cell survival parameters.

Evans (36) performed some mouse experiments that also support the concept that increasing fractionation was very important in decreasing lung toxicity, as measured by the dose that would be lethal for 50% of the animals in 30 days ($LD_{50/30}$). He obtained a 21% increase in the $LD_{50/30}$ after increasing from one to 6 fractions, with a dose rate of 0.25 Gy/minute. With a lower dose rate (0.08 Gy/min), there was still an effect of fractionation, but the $LD_{50/30}$ was increased by only 14% for development of pneumonitis in mice studies. Many investigators have now attempted to do some form of modeling of the impact of fractionation and dose rate to predict an optimum TBI regimen.

Vitale and co-workers (37) performed calculations for 4 fractionation regimens varying from 10 Gy in a single dose to 15 Gy in 12 fractions in 4 days, the regimen initiated at MSKCC (Table 9-2). They used the concept of biologically effective dose (BED) based on the LQ model of cell survival. Tissues considered were lung and leukemic cells. They compared the relative effectiveness of these different fractionation schemes for lung and leukemia based on the reference value of their own regimen of 9.9 Gy in 3 fractions at a dose rate of 0.05 Gy/minute. The dose rate effect is more pronounced in lung than in leukemic cells in their model, but becomes insignificant in highly fractionated schemes, such as 15 Gy in 12 fractions. At any dose rate, the antileukemic effect relative to the effect on lung is greatest with the fractionation regimen that

Table 9-1.
Surviving Target Cells after Different TBI Schedules[a]

n	D_0	
1.25	1.5	Lymphocytes
6	1.35	Lung

	A	*B*	*C*	*D*	*E*	*F*	*G*	*H*	*I*	*J*	*K*
	1 × 9.0[b]	*2 × 5.0*	*5 × 2.25*	*2 × 6.0*	*3 × 4.0*	*4 × 3.0*	*6 × 2.0*	*11 × 1.2*	*8 × 1.8*	*12 × 1.25*	*10 × 1.5*
Lung	**7.61×10^{-3}**	19.3×10^{-3}	187×10^{-3}	**4.68×10^{-3}**	20.3×10^{-3}	61.3×10^{-3}	238×10^{-3}	626×10^{-3}	249×10^{-3}	551×10^{-3}	385×10^{-3}
	(100)[c]	(254)	(2460)	**(61)**	(267)	(806)	(3130)	(8230)	(3270)	(7240)	(5060)
Immune	**3.10×10^{-3}**	**1.97×10^{-3}**	1.45×10^{-3}	0.522×10^{-3}	0.638×10^{-3}	0.763×10^{-3}	1.03×10^{-3}	0.846×10^{-3}	0.289×10^{-3}	0.308×10^{-3}	0.25×10^{-3}
system	**(100)**	**(64)**	(48)	(17)	(21)	(25)	(33)	(27)	(9)	(10)	(8)

[a]Model (see text): $S = [1 - (1-e^{-D/D0})^n]^f$

[b]No. fractions (f) × dose/fraction (D), in Grays.

[c]Surviving fraction (*S* for indicated schedule as a percentage of *S* for Schedule *A*). Numbers in bold type are considered unacceptable.

TBI = total body irradiation.

Adapted by permission from Vriesendorp HM. Radiobiological speculations on therapeutic total body irradiation. Crit Rev Oncol Hematol 1990;10:211–224; and Vriesendorp HM. Prediction of effects of therapeutic total body irradiation in man. Radiother Oncol 1990; (suppl 1):37–50.

Table 9-2.
Relative Effectiveness of Different Dose Rates and Fractionation Schemes for Lung and Leukemia

Total Dose (Gy/No. Fractions)	Tissue Type	Dose Rate (Gy/min) 0.01	0.05	0.1	0.25
9.9/3	Lung	0.80	1[a]	1.04	1.06
	Leukemia	0.94	1[a]	1.01	1.02
10/1	Lung	0.91	1.62	1.89	2.09
	Leukemia	0.98	1.21	1.29	1.36
12/6	Lung	0.89	1.00	1.02	1.03
	Leukemia	1.11	1.14	1.15	1.15
15/12	Lung	1.02	1.09	1.10	1.10
	Leukemia	1.35	1.38	1.38	1.38

[a]Reference values.
Reproduced by permission from Vitale V, Scarpati D, Frassoni F, Corvo R. Total body irradiation: single dose, fractions, dose rate. Bone Marrow Transplant 1989;4(suppl 1):233–235.

allows a greater total dose to be given. In their model, when tumor proliferation was taken into account, the relative effectiveness of fractionated regimens for leukemic cell kill was reduced. In fact, 10 Gy given in one fraction would have an advantage for leukemic cell kill; however, when comparing leukemic cell destruction with the enhanced damage to lung in that single-dose regimen, the therapeutic gain factor is not enhanced.

O'Donoghue and colleagues (38) also used a mathematical model for optimal scheduling of TBI. They suggested that TBI schedules of the "accelerated hyperfractionation" type are optimal when they compared schedules that were considered isoeffective for lung damage. They recognized in their calculations that, in a hyperfractionated regimen, there is a requirement for at least 6 hours between fractions to get maximum repair of normal tissues between fractions. Therefore, they suggested that 2 fractions per day would be the most practical approach for most centers. With this constraint, they looked at leukemic cell kill as a function of dose per fraction for twice daily schedules assuming no treatment over the weekend (reality in most radiation oncology departments). They concluded that a schedule of 10 fractions (in 5 days) of 1.37 Gy would be close to optimal for presumed doubling of leukemic cells of 2 or 4 days (Figure 9-3). For longer doubling times, a smaller fraction size would be optimal, but doubling times of 2 to 4 days are probably most appropriate for leukemias (39). They suggest that a practical schedule of 10 fractions of between 1.3 and 1.5 Gy in 5 days would be worth considering and should be tested clinically. This schedule (1.5 Gy twice a day for 5 days) has been piloted at Mt Sinai Medical Center in 16 patients with no untoward acute toxicity, but no randomized trial has been done to evaluate this regimen.

Another publication by O'Donoghue (40) suggested that, with the appropriate choice of dose rate, single-dose, low-dose rate TBI in principle could be equivalent radiobiologically to fractionated TBI. However, he noted that such low dose rates would necessitate extremely long treatment times (on the order of 24 hours), which would be impractical for most centers, although this was the approach originally used in the first successful marrow grafts in humans (41). Therefore, they again concluded that fractionated TBI (with high dose rates) is preferable to low dose rate therapy for leukemias and other rapidly growing tumors, such as neuroblastomas.

Studies on sequencing of cyclophosphamide (CY) and TBI in mice have shown that there is less lung damage when CY is given 12 to 24 hours after TBI than when given 24 to 48 hours before TBI (42,43). In contrast, bone marrow damage is greater when TBI is given first (42). Other studies have indicated that CY may actually be marrow-protective when given prior to TBI (44). This finding suggests that TBI should be given prior to CY for normal tissue protection and perhaps to aid in creating bone marrow space for engraftment. In contrast, Okunewick and associates (45) showed that in mice, when the bulk of radiation was given before chemotherapy, there was a high incidence of early deaths due to regimen toxicity. In humans, TBI has been given either before or after CY, at different institutions. No obvious differences have been noted other than anecdotal evidence of improved acute

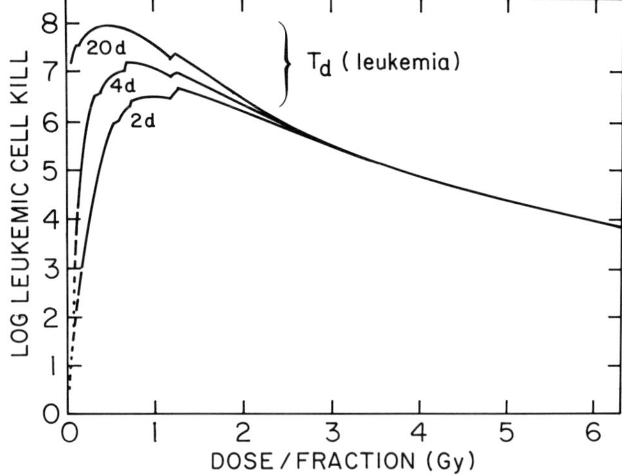

Figure 9-3. Leukemic cell kill as a function of dose/fraction, assuming two fractions/day, no weekend treatments, and total doses that would yield lung damage equivalent (isoeffective) to six fractions of 2 Gy. Curves are shown for three possible cell doubling times (T_d). (Reprinted, with minor changes, by permission from O'Donoghue JA, Wheldon TE, Gregor A. The implications of in-vitro radiation-survival curves for the optimal scheduling of total-body irradiation with bone marrow rescue in the treatment of leukemia. Br J Radiol 1987;60:279–283.)

tolerance of irradiation when CY was given after TBI; however, no randomized studies have been done. There was a nonsignificant trend toward a shorter half-life of CY after TBI (and etoposide) in humans in one study (46) when compared with the half-life when given prior to TBI in a separate study by the same authors.

Physical Considerations

When TBI or any other magna-field irradiation is performed, physical parameters to be selected include energy, total dose, number of fractions, dose per fraction, total treatment time, dose rate, patient position, distance of the patient from the source, dose homogeneity, shielding (deliberate inhomogeneity), and "boost" irradiation. Many of these parameters, such as those dealing with dose, time, and fractionation, depend on radiobiology and have already been considered in the section on "Radiobiological Principles." For an overall discussion of these technical factors at various centers, readers are directed to 2 clinical reviews (47,48). For discussions of dose measurements (dosimetry) and dose calibration, which are outside of the range of this chapter, there are several good references (49–52). Large fields have very special problems associated with dosimetry because of the large amount of internal scatter within the patient, the scatter of the wall behind the patient, the angled gantry over large treatment distances, among others; the references cited are particularly informative sources with regard to these problems.

Energy

Centers in this country primarily have used energies ranging from that of Cobalt-60 (1.25 mV) to 10 mV using a linear accelerator. Occasionally, higher energies up to 25 mV have been used, especially in Europe. When energies higher than Cobalt-60 energy are used, one must be careful to use a screen in front of the patient made of some tissue-equivalent material (beam spoiler) such as 1 cm of Lexan for 10 mV photons. This technique allows for adequate build-up of dose at the patient's surface and prevents skin underdosage. Examples of typical techniques are shown in Figure 9-4. The technique from MSKCC (lower right in Figure 9-4) demonstrates the use of a beam spoiler in front of the patient.

Dose Rate and Distance from the Source

For high-dose TBI (10 Gy) in a single dose, a low dose rate is needed (≤ 0.05 Gy/min) to prevent IP, according to both animal (53–55) and human data (56,57). Low dose rates may still be needed for fractionated irradiation schemes that employ ≥2 Gy per fraction, because mouse experiments (58) have shown that fractionation regimens that employ 2-Gy fractions still have a dose rate effect. When a high dose rate has been used, total dose has been limited (59,60), and one group (60) reported a high relapse rate (62%) in patients with other than first remission ALL or AML, or first chronic phase of CML, when 5 Gy total dose was used at a dose rate of 0.4 to 0.9 Gy/minute.

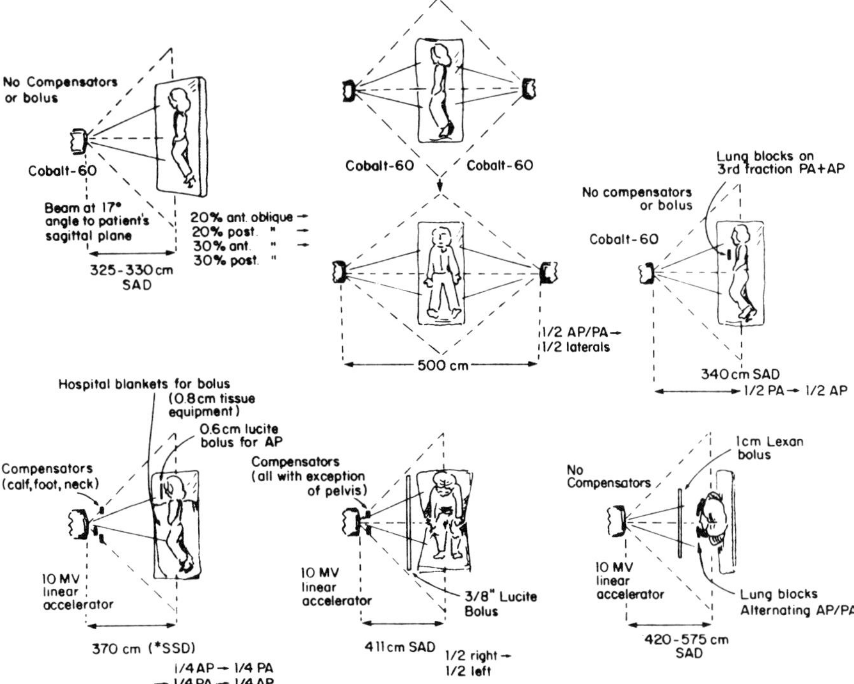

Figure 9-4. Diagram of six different patient set-ups for TBI from different institutions. Bolus or compensators are indicated, as well as source-axis-distance (SAD) or source-skin-distance (SSD). The lower right example shows the lung blocks used at Memorial Sloan-Kettering Cancer Center. (Reprinted by permission from Shank B. Techniques of magna-field irradiation. Int J Radiat Oncol Biol Phys 1983; 9:1925–1931.)

To fit the entire body in the TBI field with minimum contortion of the patient, it is necessary to increase the distance from the source because the field size increases linearly with the distance from the source. The necessary distance to allow the patient to stand or lie in an unflexed position is a function of the patient's height and the collimator opening of the particular machine used. This collimator opening differs on machines made by different manufacturers. Some treatment rooms are not long enough to allow extended distances sufficient to fit a fully extended patient within the field. Rotating the collimator to the diagonal of the square field can help, provided there is not a primary circular collimator, which limits this diagonal length.

Patient Position

The many patient positions that have been used are shown in Figure 9-4. Patient positioning at various centers has been a function of the room size and the resultant distance achievable from the source, the type of lung shielding desired, concerns over reproducibility, and attempts to achieve homogeneity and patient comfort.

If the patient is sitting and or lying down and is treated laterally, the patient is comfortable, but inhomogeneity becomes a problem and lung shielding is difficult. Better homogeneity is achieved and lung shielding is easier with the patient lying on his or her side using anterior-posterior/posterior-anterior fields, but accurate positioning is difficult and time-consuming (61). Many centers have treated patients in the standing position utilizing special treatment stands. An example of this is the stand used at MSKCC, which evolved over several years of use (Figure 9-5), and incorporates a bicycle seat for patient comfort. The patient is still in the standing position; special port film holders and supporting devices, which can be adjusted accurately day to day, are part of the device. Such stands are of great value in terms of accuracy and reproducibility from treatment to treatment.

Some of the special stands that have been used have been described in the literature (62,63). Another treatment device includes a plaster vest used as a lung block support (64).

Shielding

Many institutions have used lung shielding either (1) on all fractions whether anterior or posterior, (2) on some fractions, or (3) on only one lung. An example of these are the one-half-value-layer lung blocks used at MSKCC (31), which have been incorporated into techniques of many other centers. Some institutions have treated patients laterally and used the patient's arms to shield the lungs partially. This technique may be simple, but it is inaccurate on a day-to-day basis.

One institution has used shielding of the liver (65) with a 10% block in an attempt to decrease the incidence of veno-occlusive disease (VOD) of the liver. The same institution also used partial renal shielding. Liver shielding could create a problem of potential leukemic relapse, but long-term results are not yet available. Furthermore, VOD has been more frequently correlated with patient age, GVHD, prior hepatitis, and chemotherapy agents (e.g., busulfan) than with TBI per se (66,67).

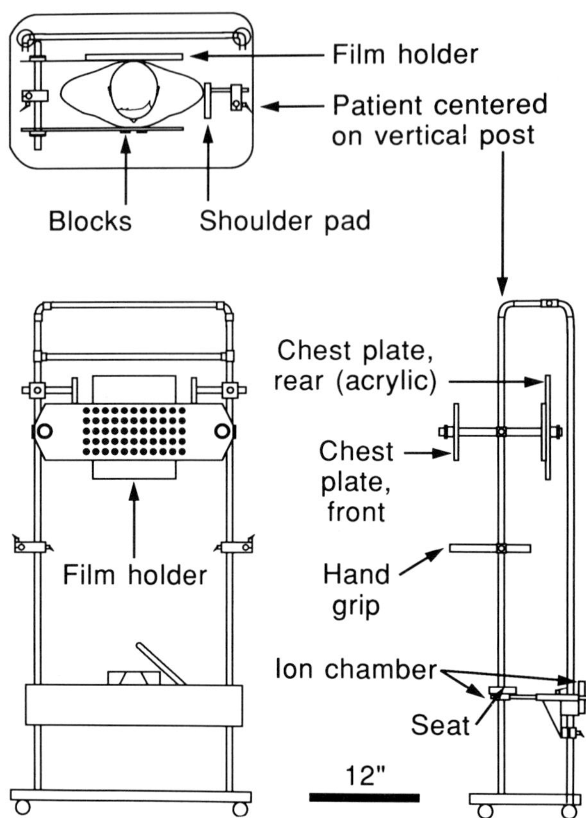

Figure 9-5. Example of TBI stand originally constructed at Memorial Sloan-Kettering Cancer Center. Top: superior view; bottom left: anterior view; bottom right: lateral view.

In protocols for some diseases, it is possible to use eye shielding; for example at MSKCC (68), when TBI was used for cytoreduction in patients with aplastic anemia, the eyes were shielded on the anterior treatment. Regimens for these benign diseases frequently utilize TLI or TAI instead of TBI so that the eyes are outside of the field and such blocking becomes unnecessary. Eye shields should not be used for leukemic patients due to the potential for recurrence in the eye or orbit.

Homogeneity

The use of a tissue equivalent screen for homogeneity at the skin surface has been discussed. Some centers have also used compensators in very thin body areas such as the neck or calf and foot. Some institutions have even used tissue compensators for the entire patient, with thinner areas having a larger amount of compensation than somewhat thicker areas, such as the head or the thigh. When questioned (47), seven investigators at major transplant institutions indicated that there was a 30% variation in different areas of the patient when compensators were not used (i.e., doses varied either from 80 to 110% or from 90 to 120%). When compensators and bolus were used, there was only an 8% variation in dose throughout the patient (from 94 to 102%). Generally, a variation in dose throughout the body of ±5% is considered excellent, and ±10% is acceptable (49).

"Boosting"

Chest Wall Boost

Boosting is the term used by radiation oncologists to describe the process of giving an additional dose of radiation by means of smaller fields to a local region considered to have residual malignant cells. This dose is given before or after a larger volume of radiation encompassing the "boost" area (e.g., TBI) has been given.

Many areas of the body have received boosted doses of radiation as part of various treatment regimens. The MSKCC regimen has used lung shields. The chest wall in the areas of the lung blocks are boosted with an electron beam, which does not penetrate deeply into lung (31), to deliver to the marrow in the ribs a radiation dose equivalent to that in marrow in other sites of the body. Results from the Institut Gustave-Roussy (Cosset JM. Personal communication), without chest wall boosts, suggested no increased leukemic relapse when these boosts were not given as part of a similar hyperfractionated regimen (14.85 Gy in 11 fractions).

Testicular Boost

After an initial high relapse rate in the testes in patients with leukemia, an electron boost to the testes (4 Gy) was added by Shank and colleagues (69). Following the addition of this boost, there were no further relapses in the testes in more than 300 male patients subsequently treated.

Boosts to Gross Disease

For some diseases, it has been considered desirable to boost sites of residual gross disease. In lymphoma, for example, 12 to 20 Gy boost treatments have been added to TBI chemotherapy regimens (62,70). In other transplant regimens that do not use TBI as part of cytoreduction, localized treatment of sites at great risk for relapse may be used, such as in breast carcinoma, where local treatment of the primary site and lymph node draining areas have been done (71).

Clinical Results

Total Body Irradiation

Acute Side Effects

In all TBI regimens, nausea and vomiting have been the most noticeable acute side effects. The hyperfractionated regimen instituted at MSKCC was found to be considerably more tolerable for the patient when compared with the original single-dose regimen (20). A recent report (72) showed that emesis was universal after one dose of 1.2 Gy in a fractionated regimen, but it also showed a statistically significant decline over the 4 days of a hyperfractionated course of irradiation ($p = 0.046$). The investigators found that metoclopramide and promethazine were better at controlling emesis than droperidol.

Other acute side effects include occasional syncope in some patients when treated in the standing position; this side effect has been found to be aggravated by the use of phenothiazines (orthostatic hypotension) or by a low hemoglobin concentration in patients with aplastic anemia. Another problem has been salivary gland swelling and discomfort, which is usually transient at the end of the TBI course, lasting a few days. One study (73) found that when fractionated irradiation was used (12 Gy in 6 fractions), there was no parotiditis, compared with single-dose irradiation (10 Gy), in which a 40% incidence of parotiditis was seen. Many patients experience increasing fatigue throughout the course of a TBI regimen.

Immunosuppression

With conventional allografts (i.e., without T-cell depletion), graft failures have rarely occurred regardless of the TBI regimen used. However, when T-cell–depleted marrow transplants are used, graft failures are frequent. It has been suggested that there are more graft failures with fractionated irradiation than with single-dose irradiation. Many reports have indicated that higher doses of TBI (10–12) or the addition of TLI (13,14,74–77) may prevent such rejection in a large proportion of patients. However, decreased graft failures have not been consistently found with either increased TBI dose (78,79) or with the addition of TLI (80).

Leukemic Relapse

Leukemic relapse as a function of dose, dose rate, or fractionation has been studied in several institutions. An early twin BMT study (41) with solely irradiation for cytoreduction demonstrated that 10 Gy single-dose TBI was insufficient in itself to destroy all leukemic cells; relapses occurred within 3 months in both patients transplanted. TBI regimens now are combined with CY or other chemotherapeutic agents.

In combination with CY, there have been 3 randomized studies of different TBI schemes reported in the literature (81–85). In 2 studies from Seattle, 2 fractionation schemes were used (12 Gy in 2 Gy fractions for 6 days versus 15.75 Gy in 2.25 Gy fractions for 7 days) for conventional marrow grafts. In the study involving patients with CML (82,83), relapse was less in the regimen in which patients received the higher dose of 15.75 Gy; however, there was an increase in nonrelapse mortality, which resulted in a decreased overall survival with the higher dose regimen. Patients with CML are older in contrast to patients with AML, who are younger and have a somewhat different experience. In the study in patients with AML (81), there again was a decrease in relapses in the higher total dose regimen. Although there was a slight increase in nonrelapse mortality, it was not significant and did not translate into a lower survival.

An earlier randomized trial from Seattle (84,85) compared single-dose irradiation (10 Gy) with fractionated irradiation (12 Gy in 6 daily fractions) in patients with AML. In this study, there was a higher relapse rate (22%) in the single-dose regimen than in the fractionated regimen (12%). One recent trial (86), with patients receiving single-dose or hyperfractionated TBI according to physician preference, randomized patients to a high or low instantaneous dose rate within the fractionation groups. There was no difference in relapse between any of the groups.

Other studies have either been single-arm studies or comparisons within institutions in different eras of an institution's experience as they shifted from one regimen to another. In many of the studies, it is difficult to separate the effects of fractionation from that of total dose because both changed in the regimens used.

In another study from Italy, which is a good comparison of total dose, Frassoni and associates (87) reported on patients with AML and CML who were ostensibly treated on a regimen of 3 fractions of 3.3 Gy each, to 9.9 Gy total dose. However, this was only a nominal dose; the actual doses received were retrospectively calculated based on detailed physics measurements. They found that the incidence of relapse at 7 years was 55% in patients who received less than 9.9 Gy compared with only 11% in patients who received more than 9.9 Gy ($p = 0.0005$). This difference ultimately had a major impact on survival: 74% at 8 years for the group receiving more than 9.9 Gy, compared with only 38% for the group receiving less than 9.9 Gy ($p = 0.005$). Further analysis of these patients by Scarpati and associates (88) showed that total dose was the most significant factor affecting relapse. They also looked at relapse as a function of dose rate (>4 cGy/min vs <4 cGy/min; range, 2.7–7.25 cGy/min), but this effect was of borderline significance.

Two nonrandomized studies have looked at the single dose regimen of 10 Gy compared with a hyperfractionated regimen of 13.2 Gy in 11 fractions over 4 days (89,90). Although there was a trend to a slightly greater relapse rate in the hyperfractionated groups, this trend was not significant because there were small numbers of patients in each study. In another study (91) using the same hyperfractionated regimen in children, with either 13.2 or 14.4 Gy (dose/fraction: 1.2–1.25 Gy), there was a very low relapse rate in patients with either ALL or AML. At 5 years, children with ALL in second remission had only a 13% relapse rate, and children with AML had a 0% relapse rate in first remission, 13% in second remission (91). This low relapse rate, unconfirmed by other investigators at this time, was attributed to the high TBI dose, the addition of a 4-Gy testes boost, and the sequencing of TBI before CY. A recent publication from France (92) described a large nonrandomized multi-institutional study in which there was an increase in relapse rate with fractionated TBI (10–13.2 Gy) when compared with a single-dose regimen (10 Gy). The 126 patients in the single-dose group had a relapse rate of 16%, whereas the 54 patients in the fractionated group had a relapse rate of 29%. In contrast, the results from a study in children with AML from the Children's Cancer Study Group (93) showed that there was an increased relapse rate in the single-dose regimens (7.5–10 Gy) given at different institutions when compared with fractionated regimens at other institutions (2 Gy × 6 fractions over 6 days or 1.2 Gy 3 times a day for 4 days for a total dose of 13.2 Gy). The 2-year relapse risk was 23% (10 of 51) in the single-dose groups versus 0% (0 of 15) in the fractionated groups ($p = 0.07$).

Another sequential study from the University of Minnesota (94) showed no significant difference in relapse rate at 3 years between a single-dose regimen of 7.5 Gy at a high dose rate (0.26 Gy/min) and a hyperfractionated regimen (1.65 Gy twice daily for 4 days, at a dose rate of 0.1 Gy/min). The relapse rate in the single-dose regimen was 19 versus 10% in the hyperfractionated regimen. The numbers were small; there were only 36 patients in the single-dose regimen and 48 patients in the hyperfractionated regimen. These authors concluded that there were no differences between these regimens, but every parameter they studied favored the hyperfractionated regimen; none, however, was significantly different in this small study.

In summary, in non-T-cell–depleted marrow transplants, leukemic relapse is generally less with higher total doses of TBI when various fractionated regimens are compared. This gain is made at the expense of a higher morbidity in patients with CML, who are an older group than patients with AML. Comparisons of single-dose regimens with fractionated regimens show no consistent difference with regard to relapse.

In T-cell–depleted BMT, however, there have been several studies (95–98) that have described an increase in relapse rate in patients with CML when fractionated schedules were used in comparison with single-dose fractionation schedules. Shank and colleagues (20) reported early results from pilot studies at MSKCC in which there was no difference in relapse rate in patients with AML with T-cell–depleted marrow grafts compared with conventional grafts. There was an increase in relapse with T-cell–depleted grafts in patients with ALL compared with conventional transplants. MSKCC performed a study randomizing 45 patients with ALL and AML to either T-cell–depleted or conventional transplants; there was no difference in relapse, using 15 Gy TBI and cyclophosphamide for preparation (99). Other authors have reported increased relapses with T-cell–depleted transplants (80,100,101).

Champlin and associates (61) found a decrease in relapse rate in recipients of T-cell–depleted transplants when switching from a protocol of 11.25 Gy in 5 fractions to a protocol with 13.5 Gy in 6 fractions. In the latter protocol, they also added one treatment with TLI (2.25 Gy). Their actuarial relapse rate dropped from 82 to 15%.

Normal Tissue Toxicity

There are many normal tissue toxicities to consider when TBI is administered. Some investigators analyzed factors of transplantation that affect all of the toxicities grouped together, termed *regimen-related toxicity* (102). One major factor was TBI dose. Two regimens were used: 12 Gy in 6 daily fractions of 2 Gy and 15.75 Gy in 7 daily fractions of 2.25 Gy. The only factor among the allogeneic marrow recipients that was significantly associated with less toxicity was the lower TBI dose. The results are somewhat confounded by the probability that other variables act in concert. For example, the higher dose TBI was more commonly administered to relapsed patients and to those patients receiving mismatched grafts. However, even in the multivariate analysis, patients receiving a higher TBI dose had a higher incidence of severe toxicity. Whether the marrow was autologous or allogeneic was the only other significant variable that emerged in this multivariate analysis.

Lung

Comparison between institutions of the incidence of any pneumonitis or fatal pneumonitis has been difficult because often the definition of IP differs; some authors include IP of known infectious etiology and others consider it to be only idiopathic IP. There is good reason to report both in studies that examine IP. Although idiopathic IP is most likely attributable to irradiation, other factors may have a role, such as chemotherapy and GVHD, and the incidence depends on how aggressively one pursues other causes. Furthermore, although infectious IP may not be directly attributable to irradiation, TBI may have a role (e.g., in increased intestinal toxicity allowing a port of entry to infectious agents).

The time frame between studies in different institutions has often been quite different; some institutions have considered only IP developing within 100 days of the transplant, whereas others may consider IP as long as 1 or 2 years following BMT. There are a few comparison studies within institutions, but they are generally comparisons between sequential methods of treatment.

IP was one of the end points examined in the randomized study from Seattle (84,85) comparing single-dose with fractionated irradiation in patients with AML in first remission. Single-dose TBI (10 Gy) or TBI fractionated daily with 2 Gy fractions for 6 days were the regimens used. The incidence of IP was less in the fractionated regimen (15%) when compared with the single-dose regimen (26%). In this study, in which patients have now been followed for 9 years, there is a significant survival difference overall between the two regimens: 30% in the single-dose group compared with 54% in the fractionated group (83). The difference in the survival curves is primarily a result of the difference in early mortality, suggesting that the improvement with fractionation is primarily a result of reduced toxicity, not decreased relapse.

A recent French study (86) with single-dose (10 Gy) and hyperfractionated TBI (2 Gy twice daily for 3 days), randomized patients to either a high or low instantaneous dose rate TBI within each group. Instantaneous dose rate means the dose rate while the beam is on (i.e., not averaging in any interruptions in treatment). Although the high dose rate single-dose group had a 45% incidence of IP, compared with only 25% in the low dose rate group, only 57 patients received single-dose TBI; this difference was therefore not significant ($p = 0.18$).

Other studies within single institutions are listed, along with the mentioned studies, in Table 9-3, and it can be seen that almost any fractionated regimen has both a lower incidence and fewer fatalities of IP when compared with single-dose regimens. Differences are often striking; for example, there was only an 18% incidence of fatal IP when the dose was hyperfractionated, compared with a 50% incidence of fatal IP in the single-dose group at MSKCC. However, lung blocks were also utilized in the fractionated group but not in the single-dose group, which confounds the effect of fractionation. However, when comparisons were made between single-dose and hyperfractionated groups at an institution where blocks were used in both regimens and the lung dose was basically similar, there was still a decrease in IP, as seen in the data from the Institut Gustave-Roussy (89). They found a 45% incidence of IP (26% fatal) in the single-dose group, but only a 13% incidence of IP (4% fatal) in the fractionated group.

With single-dose TBI, very low dose rates (0.025 Gy/min) led to a low incidence of IP (10%) and fatal IP (5%), but treatment times were up to 7 hours (103). In contrast, a study from Montreal (104) showed that, with single-dose TBI (9 Gy), a high instantaneous dose rate with a sweeping beam technique (0.21–0.235 Gy/min) resulted in a high incidence of severe IP (8 of 11, with 4 fatal), compared with the same dose given with Cobalt-60 at a constant dose rate of 0.047 to 0.063 Gy (6 of 11 IP cases, mild in 3 and fatal in none). A summary of the experience from several institutions that used low dose rate single-dose TBI demonstrated that the crude incidence of idiopathic IP increased with absolute dose to lung (105). The best fit curve was

Table 9-3.
Comparison of Interstitial Pneumonitis in Single Dose and Fractionated Regimens

Study	*Single Dose* Total Dose (Gy)	*Single Dose* %IP (%Fatal IP)	*Fractionated* Total Dose (Gy)/No. Fractions	*Fractionated* %IP (% Fatal IP)
MSKCC (69)	10	70 (50)	13.2/11 B	24 (18)
Seattle (85) (randomized study)	10	26 (26)	12/6	15 (15)
Hôpital Tenon, Paris (86)	10 B (0.15 Gy/min)	45	12/6 B (0.06 Gy/min)	29
(Randomized Dose Rate Study)	10 B (0.06 Gy/min)	25	12/6 B (0.03 Gy/min)	31
Institute Gustave-Roussy (89)	10 B	45 (26)	13.2/11 B	13 (4)
City of Hope (90)	10	28	13.2/11 B	10
Johns Hopkins (29)	8–10	70	8–12/2–4 B	37
French Multi-institute Study (92)	10 B	38[a](26)	12–13.2/3–11 B	18[a](11)
University of Minnesota (94)	7.5	25 (8)	13.2/8	23 (13)
Genoa (37)	10	60	9.9/3	5
Royal Marsden Hospital (103)	9.5–10.5[b]	10 (5)	. . .	. . .
Montreal (104)	7.5–9	56 (41)	12/6	25 (21)
Perugia (106,107)	. . .	. . .	14.4/12±B	4
			15–15.6/12–13±B	18

[a]Five-year actuarial projected incidence.
[b]Lung dose; nominal dose rate: 0.025 Gy/min.
IP = interstitial pneumonitis; B = lung blocks also used.

sigmoidal (probit regression analysis); a 50% incidence of IP occurred at approximately 11.5 Gy.

All these studies were reported in patients who received conventional transplants, with the exception of the study from Perugia (106,107), which was done in patients who received T-cell–depleted marrow transplants. When comparing this study with the others, there is an even lower incidence of IP with T-cell depletion, presumably as a result of the abrogation of GVHD. Only fractionated regimens were used, but total doses differed. IP was only 4% in the group receiving 14.4 Gy and 18% when the dose was increased by one fraction to 15.6 Gy, but patient numbers were low in each group.

At MSKCC (20), in 67 T-cell–depleted transplants in adult patients with CML, a group which historically had had a high incidence of GVHD and IP, there were only 11 of 67 (16%) IP cases; 5 of 67 (7%) were fatal. IP in 7 of these 11 patients was related to CMV and was treated with ganciclovir and immune globulin (108); 3 of 7 survived. In an adult CML conventional transplant group, there were 6 of 15 (40%) cases of fatal IP. IP was associated with a 73% incidence of GVHD, which has been practically abolished with T-cell–depleted transplants (20,78).

A study from Glasgow (109) looked at two types of regimens with lung shields with respect to their effect on pulmonary function tests at various times after BMT. One was a single-dose regimen of 9.5 Gy with a lung dose of 8 Gy, and the others were fractionated regimens, which varied from 12 to 14.4 Gy in 6 to 8 fractions, and lung doses from 11 to 13.5 Gy. In all instances, there was impairment of pulmonary function tests after the transplant, which gradually returned to normal. The most significantly altered tests were those for gas exchange: diffusion capacity (DLCO) and transfer coefficient (KCO). With the fractionated regimens, they found a significantly less marked impairment of gas exchange compared with the single-dose regimen. Furthermore, patients who had received single-dose TBI had a slower and less complete recovery of gas exchange than those who had the fractionated regimens.

Lens

Many studies have now reported a decrease in the incidence of cataract development by use of fractionated courses of irradiation compared with single-dose irradiation. The first study to report this finding was that of Deeg and colleagues (110) in 1984. They found only an 18% incidence of cataract development in the group of patients who received a fractionated course of irradiation (either 12 Gy in 6 fractions or 15.75 Gy in 7 fractions), compared with an incidence of 80% in patients who received 10 Gy single-dose TBI. In the single-dose group, half the patients required surgery for their cataracts, whereas only 20% required surgery in the fractionated group. They also noted that steroids and GVHD enhanced the development of cataracts.

Since then, Livesy and associates (111) reported an 83% incidence of the development of cataracts in a single-dose group compared with none in a fractionated group. Calissendorff and colleagues (112) compared children who had received 10 Gy TBI in a single dose for hematological malignancies with children with severe aplastic anemia who received no TBI or only 8 Gy TBI plus eyeshielding. In the single-dose group, all lens opacification developed in all children after 3 years, whereas none developed in the group with no TBI or eyeshielded TBI.

Kim and associates (94) also noted a decreased incidence of cataracts with hyperfractionated irradiation (1.65 Gy twice daily × 4 days at a dose rate of 0.1 Gy/min) when compared with high dose rate (0.26 Gy/min) single-dose irradiation of 7.5 Gy. Although the difference was not significant, the 3-year estimated incidence of cataracts with single-dose TBI was 27% and only 12% in the fractionated group. The single-dose group median age was 15 years, compared with 25 years in the fractionated group. Because risk for cataract development increases with age (113), a higher incidence in the fractionated group on the basis of age would have been expected.

In a recent randomized study (86), which compared high and low dose rates in single-dose (10 Gy) and hyperfractionated irradiation (2 Gy/fraction twice daily for 3 days), there was a statistically significant difference ($p = 0.049$) only in the single-dose groups. In the low dose rate group (6 cGy/min), cataracts developed in 1 of 28 patients (3.5%) compared with 4 of 29 (14%) in the high dose rate group (15 cGy/min). There was no significant difference in the hyperfractionated groups with dose rates of 3 and 6 cGy/min (2 vs 5.8% cataracts, respectively). Finally, Bray and colleagues (114) demonstrated that, in patients with malignancies who were treated with rapid fractionated TBI regimens (10.5–12 Gy in 3–6 fractions over 36 hours to 3 days), there was a 63% incidence of cataracts compared with patients who received no TBI (only melphalan), who had only a 9% incidence of cataracts.

Other Tissues

There are many more normal tissues and physiological functions of importance, including the endocrine system, bone growth, and fertility. Decreased morbidity has been noted with fractionated courses of irradiation compared with single-dose irradiation. Good reviews of this subject have been written by several authors (115,116). In addition, excellent reviews of endocrine problems and effects on growth and development have been published by Sanders and colleagues (117). In the studies from Seattle (115), after 10 Gy single-dose TBI, there was a much higher incidence of compensated hypothyroidism as well as overt hypothyroidism in children when compared with fractionated TBI (12–15.75 Gy over 4–7 days).

One other important area that should be studied in more detail after TBI is brain function. Children with ALL who have more than one course of cranial irradiation have increasing toxicity, with larger decrements in IQ and achievement (118). A case report (119) described somnolence syndrome 8 weeks after irradiation in an adult with AML who received CY and a rapid course of TBI (2.2 Gy twice daily for 3 days, for a total dose of 13.2 Gy).

One study of TBI patients (120) demonstrated an increasing cognitive dysfunction with increasing dose of TBI, by both univariate and multivariate analysis. The role of fractionation or prior cranial irradiation was not studied, only total dose. It would be of value to study cognitive function using the same total doses with different fractionation and to compare patients who have had TBI with and without prior prophylactic cranial irradiation.

From the studies on normal tissue toxicity, it is clear that fractionation allows higher doses of irradiation to be given with less toxicity than a much lower dose of single-dose irradiation.

Busulfan—Can It Replace TBI?

It has been suggested that TBI may be completely replaced with busulfan (BU) as part of the conditioning regimen of patients with leukemia for allogeneic marrow transplantation (121). However, the alternative of BU-CY is not without risk (122–125).

The toxicity of the BU-CY regimen was compared with TBI-CY in sequential patient populations by Morgan and associates (126). They found a high incidence of VOD in the BU-CY group (19%) compared with only 1% in the TBI-CY group. Hemorrhagic cystitis developed in 30% of patients with BU-CY compared with 14% in the group with TBI-CY. IP incidence and fatalities were similar in both groups.

Most importantly, we now have the results of a randomized trial of BU-CY versus CY-TBI (127). The French multi-institution Group for the Study of Bone Marrow Transplantation (GEGMO) has found that, in patients with AML in first remission, CY-TBI had a statistically significant improvement in disease-free survival (72 vs 47%; $p < 0.01$) and survival (75 vs 51%; $p < 0.02$). Relapse was less in the CY-TBI group (14 vs 34%; $p < 0.04$), as was transplant-related mortality (8 vs 27%; $p < 0.06$). Such comparisons of BU-CY and CY-TBI should also be done in other patient groups to clearly resolve this issue.

Total Lymphoid Irradiation

In marrow transplantation, TLI has been used alone when only immunosuppression is needed (e.g., in patients with aplastic anemia). It has been used in either a single dose, as at the University of Minnesota (128,129), or in a fractionated regimen, as at MSKCC (68). The fields that are treated are similar to those used for Hodgkin's disease (Figure 9-6); they evolved from the information derived from studies in patients with Hodgkin's disease, which demonstrated the extensive immunosuppression attained with TLI (130). For transplantation, the mantle and inverted-Y fields, which cover the entire central lymphoid axis, are treated in the same treatment session. The advantage of using TLI for immunosuppression is that one can spare many normal tissues outside of the field, such as brain and eye, kidneys, much of the small bowel, and lungs. In planning TLI regimens for immunosuppression purposes, Shank and colleagues (68) determined the relative dose equivalence of TLI to

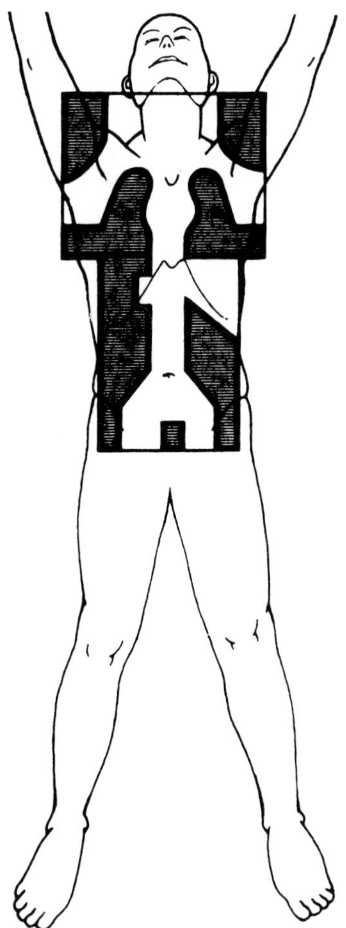

Figure 9-6. Illustration of TLI fields. The upper portion (mantle) is junctioned with a gap to the lower field (inverted Y) so as not to overlap the fields at depth in the patient. *Shaded areas* are shielded areas. (Reprinted by permission from Shank B, Brochstein JA, Castro-Malaspina H, Yahalom J, Bonfiglio P, O'Reilly RJ. Immunosuppression prior to marrow transplantation for sensitized aplastic anemia patients: comparison of TLI with TBI. Int J Radiat Oncol Biol Phys 1988;14:1133–1141.)

TBI for immunosuppression as measured by the percent of lymphocytes remaining after each technique. For one-log lymphocyte loss, 6 Gy TBI is equivalent to 10 Gy TLI when fractionated, as done at MSKCC in patients with aplastic anemia: TBI given in 2 Gy daily fractions and TLI given in 1 Gy fractions 3 times a day for 2 days. To prevent rejection in patients with aplastic anemia receiving T-cell–depleted grafts, Slavin and associates (13,14) increased the TLI dose to 18 Gy with twice daily fractionation for T-cell–depleted marrow transplants in patients with aplastic anemia. Early reports showed no GVHD and no rejection, with a relatively short follow-up.

The uses of TLI in BMT include the addition of TLI to TBI regimens, which increases engraftment when T-cell–depleted marrows are utilized (as described in the Engraftment section under "Clinical Results"). TLI combined with etoposide and CY has also been used successfully for autologous BMT in patients with relapsed and refractory Hodgkin's disease (131).

Total Abdominal Irradiation

TAI in combination with CY has been used successfully primarily for transplantation of patients with Fanconi's anemia and also severe aplastic anemia (132,133). These fields treat more than just the abdomen (Figure 9-7), but they spare the brain, eyes, and lung. It is a somewhat easier regimen to use in

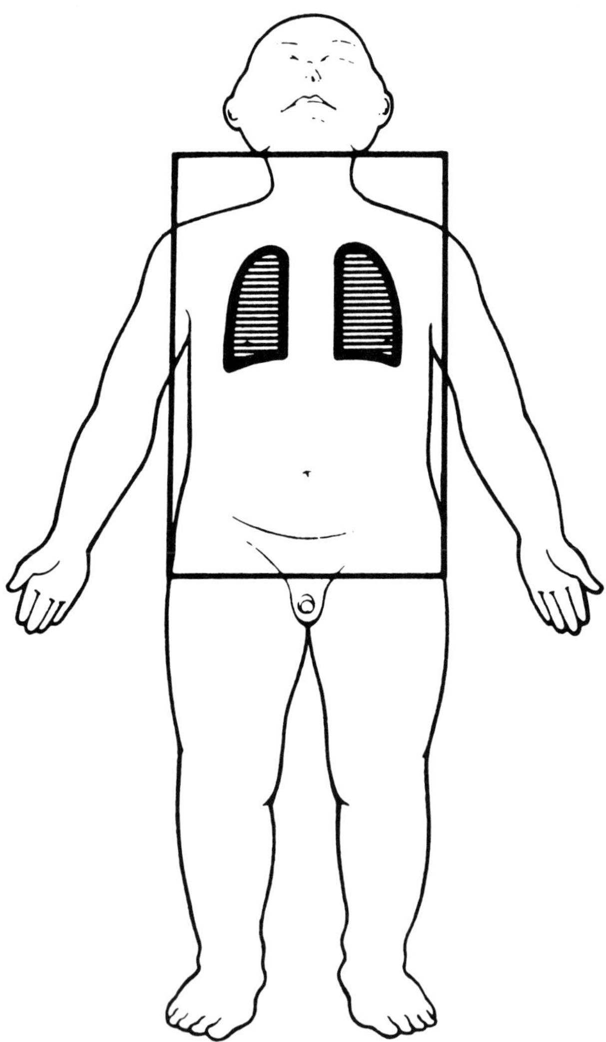

Figure 9-7. Illustration of TAI field. *Shaded areas* are lung blocks. (Reprinted by permission from Shank B, Brochstein JA, Castro-Malaspina H, Yahalom J, Bonfiglio P, O'Reilly RJ. Immunosuppression prior to marrow transplantation for sensitized aplastic anemia patients: comparison of TLI with TBI. Int J Radiat Oncol Biol Phys 1988;14:1133–1141.)

small children, because the field does not have as complicated a block arrangement as the more complex TLI fields (68). There are no data available that directly compare TLI with TAI for aplastic anemia. TAI has been implicated in one study (134) to have a high rate of secondary malignancies (22% at 8 years) in patients with aplastic anemia and Fanconi's anemia, which was not found in another study (135) when CY was used alone, with ATG or other chemotherapeutic agents. There is an association of squamous-cell carcinomas in patients with Fanconi's anemia, even without irradiation (136).

References

1. Withers HR. The four R's of radiotherapy. Adv Radiat Biol 1975;5:241–271.
2. Caldwell WL, Lamerton LF. Increased sensitivity of in vitro murine leukaemia cells to fractionated x-rays and fast neutrons. Nature 1965;208:168–170.
3. Fowler JF. The linear-quadratic formula and progress in fractionated radiotherapy. Br J Radiol 1989;62:679–694.
4. Vriesendorp HM. Radiobiological speculations on therapeutic total body irradiation. Crit Rev Oncol Hematol 1990;10:211–224.
5. Vriesendorp HM, Johnson PM, Fey TA, McDonough CM, Zoetelief J, van Bekkum DW. Optimal dose of total body irradiation for allogeneic bone marrow transplantation. Transplant Proc 1985;17:517–520.
6. Storb R, Raff RF, Appelbaum FR, et al. Comparison of fractionated to single-dose total body irradiation in conditioning canine littermates for DLA-identical marrow grafts. Blood 1989;74:1139–1143.
7. Down JD, Tarbell NJ, Thames HD, Mauch PM. Syngeneic and allogeneic bone marrow engraftment after total body irradiation: dependence on dose, dose rate, and fractionation. Blood 1991;77:661–669.
8. Girinski T, Socie G, Cosset JM, Dutreix J, Chassagne D. Similar effects on murine haemopoietic compartment of low dose rate single dose and high dose rate fractionated total body irradiation. Preliminary results after a unique dose of 750 cGy. Br J Radiol 1990;61:797–800.
9. Soderling CCB, Song CH, Blazar BR, Vallera DA. A correlation between conditioning and engraftment in recipients of MHC-mismatched T cell-depleted murine bone marrow transplants. J Immunol 1985;135:941–946.
10. Burnett AK, Robertson AG, Hann IM, Alcorn M, Gibson BE, McKinnon S. In vitro T-depletion of allogeneic bone marrow: prevention of rejection in HLA-matched transplants by increased TBI. Bone Marrow Transplant 1986;1(suppl 1):121.
11. Martin PJ, Hansen JA, Buckner CD, et al. Effects of in vitro depletion of T cells in HLA-identical allogeneic marrow grafts. Blood 1985;66:664–672.
12. Racadot E, Herve P, Beaujean F, et al. Prevention of graft-versus-host disease in HLA-matched bone marrow transplantation for malignant diseases: multicentric study of 62 patients using 3-pan-T monoclonal antibodies and rabbit complement. J Clin Oncol 1987;5:426–435.
13. Slavin S, Or R, Naparstek E, et al. New approaches for the prevention of rejection and graft-versus-host disease in clinical bone marrow transplantation. Israel J Med Sci 1992;22:264–267.
14. Slavin S, Or R, Weshler Z, Hale G, Waldmann H. The use of total lymphoid irradiation for abrogation of host resistance to T-cell depleted marrow allografts. Bone Marrow Transplant 1986;1(suppl 1):98.
15. Bordignon C, Kernan NA, Keever CA, et al. The role of residual host immunity in graft failures following T-cell-depleted marrow transplants for leukemia. Ann NY Acad Sci 1987;511:442–446.
16. Kernan NA, Bordignon C, Keever CA, et al. Graft failures after T cell depleted marrow transplants for leukemia: clinical and in vitro characteristics. Transplant Proc 1987;19(suppl 7):29–32.
17. van Bekkum DW, Wielenga JJ, van Gils F, Wagemaker G. Factors influencing reconstitution by bone marrow transplantation. In: Dainiak N, Cronkite EP, McCaffrey R, Shadduck RK, eds. The biology of hematopoiesis. New York: Wiley-Liss, 1990:479–491.
18. Dutreix J, Girinski T, Cosset JM, et al. Blood cell kinetics and total body irradiation. Radiother Oncol 1987;9:119–129.
19. Girinsky T, Baume D, Socie G, Pico JL, Malaise E, Cosset JM. Blood cell kinetics after a 385 cGy total body irradiation given to a CML patient for bone marrow transplantation. Bone Marrow Transplant 1991;7:317–320.
20. Shank B, O'Reilly RJ, Cunningham I, et al. Total body irradiation for bone marrow transplantation: the Memorial Sloan-Kettering Cancer Center experience. Radiother Oncol 1990;18(suppl 1):68–81.
21. Weichselbaum RR, Greenberger JS, Schmidt A, Karpas A, Moloney WC, Little JB. In vitro radiosensitivity of human leukemia cell lines. Radiology 1981;139:485–487.
22. Kimler BF, Park CH, Yakar D, Mies RM. Radiation response of human normal and leukemic hemopoietic cells assayed by in vitro colony formation. Int J Radiat Oncol Biol Phys 1985;11:809–816.
23. Ozawa K, Miura Y, Suda T, Motoyoshi K, Takaku F. Radiation sensitivity of leukemic progenitor cells in acute nonlymphocytic leukemia. Clin Radiol 1983;43:2339–2341.
24. Fitzgerald TJ, McKenna M, Kase K, Daugherty C, Rothstein L, Greenberger JS. Effect of X-irradiation dose rate on the clonagenic survival of human and experimental animal hematopoietic tumor cell lines: evidence for heterogeneity. Int J Radiat Oncol Biol Phys 1986;12:69–73.
25. Lehnert S, Rybka WB, Suissa S, Giambattisto D. Radiation response of haematopoietic cell lines of human origin. Int J Radiat Biol 1986;49:423–431.
26. Song CW, Kim TH, Khan FM, Kersey JH, Levitt SH. Radiobiological basis of total body irradiation with different dose rate and fractionation: repair capacity of hemopoietic cells. Int J Radiat Oncol Biol Phys 1981;7:1695–1701.
27. Rhee JG, Song CW, Kim TH, Levitt SH. Effect of fractionation and rate of radiation dose on human leukemic cells, HL-60. Radiat Res 1985;101:519–527.
28. Shank B. Hyperfractionation (T.I.D.) vs. single dose irradiation in human acute lymphocytic leukemia cells: application to TBI for marrow transplantation. Int J Radiat Oncol Biol Phys 1990;19(suppl 1):173.
29. Pino y Torres JL, Bross DS, Lam W-C, Wharam MD, Santos GW, Order SE. Risk factors in interstitial pneumonitis following allogenic bone marrow transplantation. Int J Radiat Oncol Biol Phys 1982;8:1301–1307.
30. Lichter AS, Tracy D, Lam W-C, Order SE. Total body

irradiation in bone marrow transplantation: the influence of fractionation and delay of marrow infusion. Int J Radiat Oncol Biol Phys 1980;6:301–309.

31. Shank B, Hopfan S, Kim JH, et al. Hyperfractionated total body irradiation for bone marrow transplantation: I. Early results in leukemia patients. Int J Radiat Oncol Biol Phys 1981;7:1109–1115.
32. Wara WM, Phillips TL, Margolis LW, Smith V. Radiation pneumonitis: a new approach to the derivation of time-dose factors. Cancer 1973;32:547–552.
33. Peters LJ, Withers HR, Cundiff JH, Dicke KA. Radiobiological considerations in the use of total-body irradiation for bone-marrow transplantation. Radiology 1979;131:243–247.
34. Peters L. Discussion: the radiobiological bases of TBI. Int J Radiat Oncol Biol Phys 1980;6:785–787.
35. Vriesendorp HM. Prediction of effects of therapeutic total body irradiation in man. Radiother Oncol 1990;18 (suppl 1):37–50.
36. Evans RG. Radiobiological considerations in magnafield irradiation. Int J Radiat Oncol Biol Phys 1983; 9:1907–1911.
37. Vitale V, Scarpati D, Frassoni F, Corvo R. Total body irradiation: single dose, fractions, dose rate. Bone Marrow Transplant 1989;4(suppl 1):233–235.
38. O'Donoghue JA, Wheldon TE, Gregor A. The implications of in-vitro radiation-survival curves for the optimal scheduling of total-body irradiation with bone marrow rescue in the treatment of leukaemia. Br J Radiol 1987;60:279–283.
39. Steel GG. Growth kinetics of tumours. Oxford: Clarendon Press, 1977:417–421.
40. O'Donoghue JA. Fractionated versus low dose-rate total body irradiation. Radiobiological considerations in the selection of regimes. Radiother Oncol 1986;7:241–247.
41. Thomas ED, Lochte JL Jr, Cannon JH, Sahler OD, Ferrebee JW. Supralethal whole body irradiation and isologous marrow transplantation in man. J Clin Invest 1959;38:1709–1716.
42. Yan R, Peters LJ, Travis EL. Cyclophosphamide 24 hours before or after total body irradiation: effects on lung and bone marrow. Radiother Oncol 1991;21:149–156.
43. Collis CH, Steel GG. Lung damage in mice from cyclophosphamide and thoracic irradiation: the effect of timing. Int J Radiat Oncol Biol Phys 1983;9:685–689.
44. Blackett NM, Aguado M. The enhancement of haemopoietic stem cell recovery in irradiated mice by prior treatment with cyclophosphamide. Cell Tissue Kinet 1979;12:291–298.
45. Okunewick JP, Kociban DL, Young CK, Buffo MJ. Effect of radiation and drug order in preparatory regimens for bone marrow transplantation (abstract). Proceedings of the 36th Annual meeting of the Radiation Research Society, April 17–21, 1988: 157.
46. Schueler U, Waidelich P, Kolb H, Wagner T, Ehninger G. Pharmacokinetics and metabolism of cyclophosphamide administered after total body irradiation of bone marrow transplant recipients. Eur J Clin Pharmacol 1991;40:521–523.
47. Shank B. Techniques of magna-field irradiation. Int J Radiat Oncol Biol Phys 1983;9:1925–1931.
48. Kim TH, Khan FM, Galvin JM. A report of the work party: comparison of total body irradiation techniques for bone marrow transplantation. Int J Radiat Oncol Biol Phys 1980;6:779–784.
49. Rider WD, Van Dyk J. Total and partial body irradiation. In: Bleehen NM, Glatstein E, Haybittle JL, eds. Radiation therapy planning. New York: Marcel Dekker, 1983:559–594.
50. Briot E, Dutreix A, Bridier A. Dosimetry for total body irradiation. Radiother Oncol 1990;18(suppl 1):16–29.
51. Van Dyk J. Dosimetry for total body irradiation. Radiother Oncol 1987;9:107–118.
52. Van Dyk J, Galvin JM, Glasgow GP, Podgorsak EB. The physical aspects of total and half body photon irradiation (AAPM Report No. 17). New York: American Institute of Physics, 1986.
53. Sherman DM, Carabell SC, Belli JA, Hellman S. The effect of dose rate and adriamycin on the tolerance of thoracic radiation in mice. Int J Radiat Oncol Biol Phys 1982;8:45–51.
54. Travis EL, Peters LJ, McNeill J, Thames HD Jr, Karolis C. Effect of dose-rate on total body irradiation: lethality and pathologic findings. Radiother Oncol 1985; 4:341–351.
55. Down JD, Easton DF, Steel GG. Repair in the mouse lung during low dose-rate irradiation. Radiother Oncol 1986;6:29–42.
56. Bortin MM. Pathogenesis of interstitial pneumonitis following allogeneic bone marrow transplantation for acute leukemia. In: Gale RP, ed. Recent advances in bone marrow transplantation. New York: Alan R. Liss, 1983:445–460.
57. Fryer CJH, Fitzpatrick PJ, Rider WD, Poon P. Radiation pneumonitis: experience following a large single dose of radiation. Int J Radiat Oncol Biol Phys 1978;4:931–936.
58. Tarbell NJ, Amato DA, Down JD, Mauch P, Hellman S. Fractionation and dose rate effects in mice: a model for bone marrow transplantation in man. Int J Radiat Oncol Biol Phys 1987;13:1065–1069.
59. Kim TH, Kersey JH, Sewchand W, Nesbit ME, Krivit W, Levitt SH. Total body irradiation with a high-dose-rate linear accelerator for bone-marrow transplantation in aplastic anemia and neoplastic disease. Radiology 1977;122:523–525.
60. Fyles GM, Messner HA, Lockwood G, et al. Long-term results of bone marrow transplantation for patients with AML, ALL, and CML prepared with single dose total body irradiation of 500 cGy delivered with a high dose rate. Bone Marrow Transplant 1991;8:453–463.
61. Leer JWH, Broerse JJ, DeVroome H, Chin A, Noordijk EM, Dutreix A. Techniques applied for total body irradiation. Radiother Oncol 1990;18(suppl 1):10–15.
62. Glasgow GP, Wang S, Stanton J. A total body irradiation stand for bone marrow transplant patients. Int J Radiat Oncol Biol Phys 1989;16:875–877.
63. Kutcher GJ, Bonfiglio P, Shank B, Masterson ME. Combined photon and electron technique for total body irradiation (abstract). ASTRO 1988; 31.
64. Breneman JC, Elson HR, Little R, Lamba M, Foster AE, Aron BS. A technique for delivery of total body irradiation for bone marrow transplantation in adults and adolescents. Int J Radiat Oncol Biol Phys 1990; 18:1233–1236.
65. Lawton CA, Barber-Derus S, Murray KJ, et al. Technical modifications in hyperfractionated total body irradiation for T-lymphocyte depleted bone marrow transplant. Int J Radiat Oncol Biol Phys 1989;17:319–322.
66. Berk PD, Popper H, Krueger GRF, Decter J, Herzig G, Graw RG Jr. Veno-occlusive disease of the liver after allogeneic bone marrow transplantation. Ann Intern Med 1979;90:158–164.
67. McDonald GB, Sharma P, Matthews DE, Shulman HM,

Thomas ED. Venocclusive disease of the liver after bone marrow transplantation: diagnosis, incidence, and predisposing factors. Hepatology 1984;4:116–122.
68. Shank B, Brochstein JA, Castro-Malaspina H, Yahalom J, Bonfiglio P, O'Reilly RJ. Immunosuppression prior to marrow transplantation for sensitized aplastic anemia patients: comparison of TLI with TBI. Int J Radiat Oncol Biol Phys 1988;14:1133–1141.
69. Shank B, Chu FCH, Dinsmore R, et al. Hyperfractionated total body irradiation for bone marrow transplantation. Results in seventy leukemia patients with allogeneic transplants. Int J Radiat Oncol Biol Phys 1983;9:1607–1611.
70. Chadha M, Shank B, Fuks Z, et al. Improved survival of poor prognosis diffuse histiocytic (large cell) lymphoma managed with sequential induction chemotherapy, "boost" radiation therapy, and autologous bone marrow transplantation. Int J Radiat Oncol Biol Phys 1988;14: 407–415.
71. Peters WP. Dose intensification using combination alkylating agents and autologous bone marrow support in the treatment of primary and metastatic breast cancer: a review of the Duke Bone Marrow Transplantation Program experience. Prog Clin Biol Res 1990;354B: 185–194.
72. Spitzer TR, Deeg HJ, Torrisi J, et al. Total body irradiation (TBI) induced emesis is universal after small dose fractions (120 cGy) and is not cumulative dose related (abstract). Proc Am Soc Clin Oncol 1990;9:14.
73. Valls A, Granena A, Carreras E, Ferrer E, Algara M. Total body irradiation in bone marrow transplantation: fractionated vs single dose. Acute toxicity and preliminary results. Bull Cancer 1989;76:797–804.
74. Soiffer RJ, Mauch P, Tarbell NJ, et al. Total lymphoid irradiation to prevent graft rejection in recipients of HLA non-identical T cell-depleted allogeneic marrow. Bone Marrow Transplant 1991;7:23–33.
75. Pipard G, Stepanian E, Chapuis B, et al. Total lymphoid irradiation (TLI), chemotherapy (CT) and total body irradiation (TBI) before T-cell depleted bone marrow allografts (abstract). ASTRO 1988;36.
76. Champlin R, Ho WG, Mitsuyasu R, et al. Graft failure and leukemia relapse following T-lymphocyte depleted bone marrow transplantation; effect of intensification of immunosuppressive conditioning. Transplant Proc 1987;19:2616–2619.
77. James ND, Apperley JF, Kam KC, et al. Total lymphoid irradiation preceding bone marrow transplantation for chronic myeloid leukaemia. Clin Radiol 1989;40:195–198.
78. Kernan NA, Bordignon C, Heller G, et al. Graft failure after T-cell-depleted human leukocyte antigen identical marrow transplants for leukemia: I. Analysis of risk factors and results of secondary transplants. Blood 1989;74:2227–2236.
79. Poynton CH, MacDonald D, Byrom NA, Barrett AJ. Rejection after T cell depletion of donor bone marrow. Bone Marrow Transplant 1987;2(suppl 1):153.
80. Ganem G, Kuentz M, Beaujean F, LeBourgeois JP, Cordonnier C, Vernant JP. Additional total lymphoid irradiation (TLI) in preventing graft failure of T cell depleted bone marrow transplantation (BMT) from HLA identical siblings: results of a prospective randomized study. Bone Marrow Transplant 1987;2(suppl 1):156.
81. Clift RA, Buckner CD, Applebaum FR, et al. Allogeneic marrow transplantation in patients with acute myeloid leukemia in first remission: a randomized trial of two irradiation regimens. Blood 1990;76:1867–1871.
82. Clift RA, Buckner CD, Applebaum FR, et al. Allogeneic marrow transplantation in patients with chronic myeloid leukemia in the chronic phase: a randomized trial of two irradiation regimens. Blood 1991;77:1660–1665.
83. Thomas ED. Total body irradiation regimens for marrow grafting. Int J Radiat Oncol Biol Phys 1990;19: 1285–1288.
84. Deeg HJ, Sullivan KM, Buckner CD, et al. Marrow transplantation for acute non lymphoblastic leukemia in first remission: toxicity and long-term follow-up of patients conditioned with single dose or fractionated total body irradiation. Bone Marrow Transplant 1986;1: 151–157.
85. Thomas ED, Clift RA, Hersman J, et al. Marrow transplantation for acute nonlymphoblastic leukemia in first remission using fractionated or single-dose irradiation. Int J Radiat Oncol Biol Phys 1982;8:817–821.
86. Ozsahin M, Pene F, Touboul E, et al. Total-body irradiation before bone marrow transplantation: results of two randomized instantaneous dose rates in 157 patients. Cancer 1992;69:2853–2865.
87. Frassoni F, Scarpati D, Bacigalupo A, et al. The effect of total body irradiation dose and chronic graft-versus-host disease on leukaemic relapse after allogeneic bone marrow transplantation. Br J Haematol 1989;73:211–216.
88. Scarpati D, Frassoni F, Vitale V, et al. Total body irradiation in acute myeloid leukemia and chronic myelogenous leukemia: influence of dose and dose-rate on leukemia relapse. Int J Radiat Oncol Biol Phys 1989;17:547–552.
89. Cosset JM, Baume D, Pico JL, et al. Single dose versus hyperfractionated total body irradiation before allogeneic bone marrow transplantation: a non-randomized comparative study of 54 patients at the Institut Gustave-Roussy. Radiother Oncol 1989;15:151–160.
90. Blume KG, Forman SJ, Snyder DS, et al. Allogeneic bone marrow transplantation for acute lymphoblastic leukemia during first complete remission. Transplantation 1987;43:389–392.
91. Brochstein JA, Kernan NA, Groshen S, et al. Allogeneic bone marrow transplantation after hyperfractionated total-body irradiation and cyclophosphamide in children with acute leukemia. N Engl J Med 1987;317: 1618–1624.
92. Socie G, Devergie A, Girinsky T, et al. Influence of the fractionation of total body irradiation on complications and relapse rate for chronic myelogenous leukemia. Int J Radiat Oncol Biol Phys 1991;20:397–404.
93. Feig SA, Nesbit ME, Buckley J, et al. Bone marrow transplantation for acute non-lymphocytic leukemia: a report from the Childrens Cancer Study Group of sixty-seven children transplanted in first remission. Bone Marrow Transplant 1987;2:365–374.
94. Kim TH, McGlave PB, Ramsay N, et al. Comparison of two total body irradiation regimes in allogeneic bone marrow transplantation for acute non-lymphoblastic leukemia in first remission. Int J Radiat Oncol Biol Phys 1990;19:889–897.
95. Apperley JF, Arthur C, Jones L, et al. Risk factors for relapse after T cell depleted allogeneic BMT for CML in chronic phase. Bone Marrow Transplant 1987;2(suppl 1):140.
96. Devergie A, Gluckman E, Reiffers J, et al. Bone marrow

transplantation for patients with chronic granulocytic leukaemia in France 1979–1986. Bone Marrow Transplant 1987;2(suppl 1):24.

97. Papa G, Arcese W, Bianchi A, et al. T cell depleted bone marrow transplantation in Ph+ myeloid leukaemia. Bone Marrow Transplant 1987;2(suppl 1):39.

98. Goldman JM, Gale RP, Horowitz MM, et al. Bone marrow transplantation for chronic myelogenous leukemia in chronic phase. Ann Intern Med 1988; 108:806–814.

99. Childs B, Castro-Malaspina H, Kernan N, et al. Conventional versus T-cell depleted allogeneic bone marrow transplantation for early remission acute leukemia (abstract). J Cell Biochem 1992;16A(suppl): 194.

100. Marmont A, Bacigalupo A, van Lint MT, et al. T cell depletion in allogeneic BMT for leukaemia: the Genoa experience. Bone Marrow Transplant 1987;2(suppl 1):139.

101. Mitsuyasu RT, Champlin RE, Gale RP, et al. Treatment of donor marrow with monoclonal anti-T-cell antibody and complement for the prevention of graft-versus-host disease: a prospective, randomized double-blind trial. Ann Intern Med 1986;105:20–26.

102. Bearman SI, Appelbaum FR, Buckner CD, et al. Regimen-related toxicity in patients undergoing bone marrow transplantation. J Clin Oncol 1988;6:1562–1568.

103. Barrett A, Depledge MH, Powles RL. Interstitial pneumonitis following bone marrow transplantation after low dose rate total body irradiation. Int J Radiat Oncol Biol Phys 1983;9:1029–1033.

104. Kim TH, Rybka WB, Lehnert S, Podgorsak EB, Freeman CR. Interstitial pneumonitis following total body irradiation for bone marrow transplantation using two different dose rates. Int J Radiat Oncol Biol Phys 1985;11:1285–1291.

105. Keane TJ, Van Dyk J, Rider WD. Idiopathic interstitial pneumonia following bone marrow transplantation: the relationship with total body irradiation. Int J Radiat Oncol Biol Phys 1981;7:1365–1370.

106. Latini P, Aristei C, Aversa F, et al. Lung damage following bone marrow transplantation after hyperfractionated total body irradiation. Radiother Oncol 1991;22:127–132.

107. Latini P, Aristei C, Aversa F, et al. Interstitial pneumonitis after hyperfractionated total body irradiation in HLA-matched T-depleted bone marrow transplantation. Int J Radiat Oncol Biol Phys 1992;23: 401–405.

108. Emanuel D, Cunningham I, Jules-Elysee K, et al. Cytomegalovirus pneumonia after bone marrow transplantation successfully treated with the combination of ganciclovir and high-dose intravenous immune globulin. Ann Intern Med 1988;109:777–782.

109. Tait RC, Burnett AK, Robertson AG, et al. Subclinical pulmonary function defects following autologous and allogeneic bone marrow transplantation: relationship to total body irradiation and graft-versus-host disease. Int J Radiat Oncol Biol Phys 1991;20:1219–1227.

110. Deeg HJ, Flournoy N, Sullivan KM, et al. Cataracts after total body irradiation and marrow transplantation: a sparing effect of dose fractionation. Int J Radiat Oncol Biol Phys 1984;10:957–964.

111. Livesey SJ, Holmes JA, Whittaker JA. Ocular complications of bone marrow transplantation. Eye 1989;3: 271–276.

112. Calissendorff B, Bolme P, el Azazi M. The development of cataract in children as a late side-effect of bone marrow transplantation. Bone Marrow Transplant 1991;7:427–429.

113. Choshi K, Takaku I, Mishima H, et al. Opthalmologic changes related to radiation exposure and age in adult health study sample, Hiroshima and Nagasaki. Radiat Res 1983;96:560–579.

114. Bray LC, Carey PJ, Proctor SJ, Evans RGB, Hamilton PJ. Ocular complications of bone marrow transplantation. Br J Ophthalmol 1991;75:611–614.

115. Sanders JE. Late effects in children receiving total body irradiation for bone marrow transplantation. Radiother Oncol 1990;18(suppl 1):82–87.

116. Deeg HJ. Delayed complications and long-term effects after bone marrow transplantation. Bone Marrow Transplant 1990;4:641–657.

117. Sanders JE, Long-term Follow-up Team. Endocrine problems in children after bone marrow transplant for hematologic malignancies. Bone Marrow Transplant 1991;8(suppl 1):2–4.

118. Mulhern RK, Ochs J, Fairclough D, Wasserman AL, Davis KS, Williams JM. Intellectual and academic achievement status after CNS relapse: a retrospective analysis of 40 children treated for acute lymphoblastic leukemia. J Clin Oncol 1987;5:933–940.

119. Goldberg SL, Tefferi A, Rummans TA, Chen MG, Solberg LA, Noel P. Post-irradiation somnolence syndrome in an adult patient following allogeneic bone marrow transplantation. Bone Marrow Transplant 1992;9:499–501.

120. Andrykowski MA, Altmaier EM, Barnett RL, Burish TG, Gingrich R, Henslee-Downey PJ. Cognitive dysfunction in adult survivors of allogeneic marrow transplantation: relationship to dose of total body irradiation. Bone Marrow Transplant 1990;6:269–276.

121. Tutschka PJ, Copelan EA, Kapoor N. Replacing total body irradiation with busulfan as conditioning of patients with leukemia for allogeneic marrow transplantation. Transplant Proc 1989;21:2952–2954.

122. Nevill TJ, Barnett MJ, Klingemann H-G, Reece DE, Shepherd JD, Phillips GL. Regimen-related toxicity of a busulfan-cyclophosphamide conditioning regimen in 70 patients undergoing allogeneic bone marrow transplantation. J Clin Oncol 1991;9:1224–1232.

123. Ozkaynak MF, Weinberg K, Kohn D, Sender L, Parkman R, Lenarsky C. Hepatic veno-occlusive disease post-bone marrow transplantation in children conditioned with busulfan and cyclophosphamide: incidence, risk factors, and clinical outcome. Bone Marrow Transplant 1991;7:467–474.

124. DeLaCamara R, Tomas JF, Figuera A, Berberana M, Fernandez-Ranada JM. High dose busulfan and seizures. Bone Marrow Transplant 1991;7:363–364.

125. Santos GW. Busulfan and cyclophosphamide for marrow transplantation. Bone Marrow Transplant 1989; 4(suppl 1):236–239.

126. Morgan M, Dodds A, Atkinson K, Szer J, Downs K, Biggs J. The toxicity of busulphan and cyclophosphamide as the preparative regimen for bone marrow transplantation. Br J Haematol 1991;77:529–534.

127. Blaise D, Maraninchi D, Archimbaud E, et al. Allogeneic bone marrow transplantation for acute myeloid leukemia in first remission: a randomized trial of a busulfan-Cytoxan versus Cytoxan-total body irradiation as preparative regimen: a report from the GEGMO. Blood 1993;79:2578–2582.

128. Ramsay NKC, Kim TH, McGlave P, et al. Bone marrow transplantation for severe aplastic anemia following preparation with cyclophosphamide and total lymphoid irradiation. In: Young NS, Levine AS, Humphries RK, eds. Aplastic anemia: stem cell biology and advances in treatment. New York: Alan R. Liss, 1984:315–324.
129. Kim TH, Kersey JH, Khan FM, et al. Single dose total lymphoid irradiation combined with cyclophosphamide as immunosuppression for human marrow transplantation in aplastic anemia. Int J Radiat Oncol Biol Phys 1979;5:993–996.
130. Fuks Z, Strober S, Bobrove AM, Sasazuki T, McMichael A, Kaplan HS. Long term effects of radiation of T and B lymphocytes in peripheral blood of patients with Hodgkin's disease. J Clin Invest 1976;58:803–814.
131. Yahalom J, Gulati S, Shank B, Clarkson B, Fuks Z. Total lymphoid irradiation, high-dose chemotherapy and autologous bone marrow transplantation for chemotherapy-resistant Hodgkin's disease. Int J Radiat Oncol Biol Phys 1989;17:915–922.
132. Vitale V, Barra S, Corvo R, Bacigalupo A, van Lint MT, Locatelli F. The role of thoraco-abdominal irradiation before marrow transplantation. Bone Marrow Transplant 1991;7(suppl 3):35–36.
133. Gluckman E. Radiosensitivity in Fanconi anemia: application to the conditioning for bone marrow transplantation. Radiother Oncol 1990;18(suppl 1):88–93.
134. Socie G, Henry-Amar M, Cosset JM, Devergie A, Girinsky T, Gluckman E. Increased incidence of solid malignant tumors after bone marrow transplantation for severe aplastic anemia. Blood 1991;78:277–279.
135. Witherspoon RP, Storb R, Pepe M, Longton G, Sullivan KM. Cumulative incidence of secondary solid malignant tumors in aplastic anemia. Blood 1992;79:289–290.
136. Reed K, Ravikumar TS, Gifford RRM, Grage TB. The association of Fanconi's anemia and squamous cell carcinoma. Cancer 1983;52:926–928.

Chapter 10

Pharmacology and Use of Immunosuppressive Agents After Bone Marrow Transplantation

Georgia Vogelsang

The mechanism of action of commonly utilized immunosuppressive agents, as well as their pharmacokinetics in the bone marrow transplant (BMT) setting, are discussed. Cyclosporine (CSP) is reviewed extensively. Several newer agents likely to come into mainstream clinical practice within the next few years are covered (i.e., XomaZyme, thalidomide, and FK 506). The clinical results from use of immunosuppressive agents are discussed in Chapter 26.

Methotrexate

The report by Farber and colleagues (1) that aminopterin could induce remissions in childhood acute lymphoid leukemia marked the beginning of chemotherapy of malignant disease and initiated numerous studies of antifolate drugs. The early reports by Uphoff (2) and by Lochte and associates (3) showed that methotrexate (MTX) could reduce the incidence and severity of graft-versus-host disease (GVHD) in mice. These studies were followed by studies in the canine model, which demonstrated that the administration of MTX after grafting markedly improved the survival of canine recipients of DLA-matched marrow grafts (4). MTX was the drug used for amelioration of GVHD in the first series of human patients with leukemia (5).

Pharmacokinetics

MTX is readily absorbed after oral administration (6). After intravenous administration, MTX is rapidly distributed into the extracellular space, with a half-life of a little less than one hour. There is then a second half-life of approximately 2 to 3 hours and a terminal half-life of 10 to 11 hours. Distribution into and out of the central nervous system and the pleural and ascitic fluid is very slow. Most of the drug is excreted through the kidney, with small fraction excreted in the bile.

Mechanism of Action

The principal mechanism of action is the competitive binding of dihydrofolate reductase, with consequent disruption of reduced folate, which is important in a number of intracellular processes requiring transfer of 1-carbon units, leading to failure of purine and pyrimidine synthesis affecting DNA and RNA synthesis. However, there are thought to be other effects of MTX, including those on membrane transport (6).

Clinical Pharmacology

The therapeutic and toxic effects of MTX are a function of concentration and duration of drug exposure (7). The consequences of MTX exposure can be reversed by leucovorin if it is administered before irreversible changes leading to cell death. Because of the complex inter-relationships of drug concentration, duration of exposure, renal excretion, and trapping in third spaces, clinical management of MTX can be difficult. Many regimens for MTX administration were worked out empirically, but currently available methods for rapid measurement of MTX levels permit a more rational approach to the use of the drug.

Toxicity

The principal toxicities of MTX given in the post-grafting period are myelosuppression, mucositis, and hepatic toxicity. Plasma level of the drug and duration of the exposure beyond a critical time of approximately 24 hours are the major determinants of drug toxicity and perhaps also of therapeutic effect.

Effect on Immunity

Some 40 years ago, the observation was made that folic acid deficiency resulted in impaired antibody production, often before other signs of vitamin deficiency could be recognized. It was then shown that folic acid antagonists could profoundly affect the production of circulating antibody and the homograft reaction and that a form of tolerance to the virus of murine lymphocytic choriomeningitis could be induced (reviewed in 8). Although death of cells involved in immunity is undoubtedly involved, the mechanism by which antifolic drugs affect immune function is still not fully understood.

Administration of MTX After Marrow Grafting

Animal studies demonstrated the toxicity of daily MTX due to duration of drug exposure (9). Therefore, most regimens for prevention of acute GVHD have employed administration of the drug on alternate days or with longer intervals. Lochte and colleagues (3), in studies in the mouse, showed that the critical time for MTX administration after allogeneic grafting was within the first 2 weeks. The administration of MTX on days 1, 3, 6, and 11 after allogeneic grafting was shown to ameliorate acute GVHD in the dog, with some further benefit by continuing the drug over the first 100 days (10). This regimen was employed in allografts in human patients in the 1970s (11,12).

When CSP became available, the Seattle team carried out a randomized comparison of postgraft MTX or CSP and found the two drugs to be equivalent (13). In additional randomized studies, it was found that a combination of MTX on days 1, 3, 6, and 11 and CSP given over the first 6 months was superior to either drug alone (14, 15). No other regimen has proven superior to the combination of MTX and CSP.

Prevention of Toxicity

Standard doses of MTX in patients with good renal function, a bilirubin level less than 10 mg% and without pleural effusions or ascites are not likely to produce serious toxicity. However, if there is any reason for concern, measurement of plasma levels 24 hours after the last dose is indicated. Bleyer (7) found that levels below 4×10^{-8} do not require administration of leucovorin. Above that level, leucovorin must be administered with a dose of 10 mg/m^2 every 6 hours up to 100 mg every 6 hours if the MTX level is above 10^{-6} molar (7). A recent report indicates that recombinant carboxypeptidase-G2, a bacterial enzyme that rapidly hydrolyzes MTX, may be useful as an alternate to leucovorin (16).

Trimetrexate

Failure of the regimen of combined MTX and CSP is related in part to an inability to administer full doses of the drugs early after marrow transplantation. Trimetrexate is a folate antagonist similar to MTX, except it is metabolized by the liver (17). This drug is of interest because it can be given to patients with impaired renal function or patients on drugs that may jeopardize renal function. Phase I to II trials are currently underway to evaluate trimetrexate following marrow grafting.

Cyclosporine

Although CSP has made possible the modern era of solid organ transplantation, its effects in marrow transplantation have been less spectacular. Nevertheless, CSP forms a basis for most immunosuppressive regimens now given after BMT.

CSP is a cyclic undecapeptide isolated from the fungus *Tolypocladium inglatum gams.* The three-dimensional configuration of CSP been determined (18). The active site of the molecule is in a cleft; modifications within this cleft result in inactivation of the molecule. The drug is highly lipophilic, which accounts for many of its observed clinical properties.

Effects of CSP on Cells

The cellular effects of CSP have been fairly well characterized (19,20). CSP suppresses lymphocyte proliferative responses to mitogens and alloantigens in a dose-dependent fashion. Primary responses are much more sensitive to the effects of CSP than secondary responses. CSP effects are not due to a direct lethal effect on lymphocytes (i.e., CSP is not lymphocytotoxic). The effects of CSP are very time-dependent. To inhibit in vitro stimulation by mitogens or alloantigens CSP must be added within the first few hours of initiation of cultures. The effects of CSP seem to be concentrated on T cells. For example, inhibition of B-lymphocyte stimulation appears to be due to inhibition of T-helper cells.

There was a great deal of seemingly conflicting data published initially about the effects of CSP on cytotoxic T cells. Studies by Wagner (21) using a limiting dilution assay system have shown that CSP will prevent naive precursor cytotoxic T-cell activation and the subsequent development of interleukin-2 (IL-2) responsiveness. However, the effects of CSP on proliferative responses seem to be different than its effects on cytotoxic T-cell responses. Studies by Hess (22) have shown that adding exogenous IL-2 to a mixed lymphocyte reaction containing graded doses of CSP restores a proliferative response to alloantigen. The effect of exogenous IL-2 on the induction of cytotoxic T-cell responses in a primary mixed lymphocyte reaction was completely dose-dependent on CSP. Exogenous IL-2 was unable to overcome the effects of CSP at high concentrations; however, at lower doses of CSP, IL-2 restored cytotoxic T-cell responses that had been inhibited completely by CSP. These same studies show that precursor cytotoxic T cells acquired functional IL-2 responsiveness within the first 18 hours of culture after alloantigen stimulation. Thus, to prevent sensitization of a precursor cytotoxic T cell, adequate levels of CSP must be achieved early. Moreover, IL-4 may have a role in maturation and amplification of cytotoxic T cells. Heeg and colleagues (23) have shown that both IL-2 and IL-4 are required for proper maturation of cytotoxic T cells.

Effects of CSP on Lymphokine Production

One of the earliest described effects of CSP was its inhibition of production of IL-2 when cells were exposed to alloantigen (24,25). The inhibition of IL-2 production is very sensitive to CSP; essentially 100% suppression occurs at levels of 50 ng/mL. Many of the other effects of CSP occur at much higher concentrations of the drug. Thus, the immunomodulatory effects observed will be different at different CSP concentrations. The inhibition of IL-2 production seems to be due to an inhibition of the induction of IL-2 messenger RNA (mRNA) (26). This effect is selective in that total protein synthesis was not affected by CSP. The mechanism accounting for the down-regulation of IL-2 mRNA transcription is the ablation of a calcium-dependent, intracellular signal transmitted from the cell membrane after interaction of the T-cell receptor with its ligand (27). This intracellular activation signal is required for continued lymphokine production. CSP blocks delivery of this antigen-dependent signal.

Laboratory studies as well as clinical observation suggest that some lymphocytes are not affected by CSP. Lymphokine production can occur despite the presence of CSP if an alternate activation cascade is utilized. June and colleagues (28) identified an activation cascade with subsequent IL-2 gene expression that is resistant to the effects of CSP. Stimulation of resting T lymphocytes via the CD28 cell surface determinant, a cell surface glycoprotein found on T cells, in conjunction with phorbol ester results in IL-2 gene transcription and IL-2 production. T cells activated via this alternative cascade are not sensitive to the effects of CSP. Other investigators have utilized other alternative activation cascades whereby they are able to show IL-2 production in T cells in the presence of CSP (29). These data suggest that CSP does not have a direct effect on transcription. This is supporting evidence of the calcium-dependent cytoplasmic activation signal that occurs distal to the interaction of the T-cell receptor with specific antigen and leads to lymphokine gene activation.

There are conflicting data on the effects of CSP IL-2 receptor formation. The apparently conflicting results may be related to the type of stimulus and to the dose of CSP utilized in the experiments. It appears that much higher doses of CSP are needed to prevent IL-2 receptor expression on mitogen-stimulated T lymphocytes, compared with lymphocytes stimulated with alloantigen. Data by Foxwell and associates (30) showed that CSP inhibited the expression of both the p55 and p75 chains of the high-affinity IL-2 receptor on human T lymphocytes at concentrations of 10 ng/mL. Exogenous IL-2 overcomes the block of expression of the IL-2 receptor; however, when much higher concentrations of CSP were used, exogenous IL-2 was ineffective in upregulating the IL-2 receptor. Thus, it appears that the effects of CSP on IL-2 are different at different doses. IL-2 production is extremely sensitive to CSP, whereas inhibition of IL-2 receptor expression requires at least a log higher concentration of drug.

The molecular mechanism of action of CSP is still incompletely understood. Two major CSP binding proteins have been described. CSP also binds to calmodulin, a 19-kd acidic protein, which has many calcium-dependent functions in the cell (31). Cyclophilin is a 17-kd basic protein found ubiquitously in nature that avidly binds to CSP (32).

Cyclophillin was recently found to be a peptidyl-prolyl-cis-trans isomerase that catalyzes the isomerization of proline imido peptide bonds (33). This function of cyclophilin seems to be irrelevant in the immunomodulatory effects of CSP. Elegant work by Sigal and colleagues (34) showed that analogues capable of inhibiting cyclophillin had no immunosuppressive effects on the cells. This work has been confirmed using FK506 and FK506 binding proteins. Blockage of the isomerization did not result in immunosuppressive activity (35).

The other known CSP binding protein, calmodulin, has many important, well established cellular functions. Multiple calmodulin-dependent protein kinases, phosphorylases, phosphatases, and enzymes involved in many pathways in the cell have been reported (36). However, the particular pathways affected by CSP have not been elucidated clearly. Thus, the exact mechanism of action of CSP remains to be clarified, as does the interaction between cyclophilin and calmodulin.

Pharmacokinetics

One of the major difficulties in using CSP clinically is the complex pharmacokinetics of this drug. The drug level of CSP obtained systemically is dependent on many factors; as these factors change over time, the drug level will be influenced. Adding difficulty to this whole situation is that there is no clear therapeutic window with CSP.

CSP absorption after oral administration is a good example of the difficulties encountered in its pharmacokinetics (37–41). There are large variations between patients and in the same patients over time in the absorption of CSP. CSP is slowly and incompletely absorbed from the upper small bowel. The amount absorbed varies from individual to individual and generally only one fourth of the administered dose is actually absorbed. Factors reported to affect CSP absorption include eating, diarrhea, poor liver function, intestinal dysfunction due to radiation or GVHD, any other intestinal disease, gastric emptying, and the vehicle in which CSP is delivered (42). Once CSP is absorbed, it is widely distributed in many body tissues due to its high lipid solubility. The volume of distribution has been reported to be 5 to 35 L/kg (42–44). The volume of distribution is dependent on the age of the patient (43,45). The volume of distribution and clearance decreases with increasing age. Surprisingly, obesity does not affect the volume of distribution, implying that dosing should be based on ideal rather than actual body weight (44–47). The higher concentrations observed in tissue are found in the fat, the kidney, the pancreas, the adrenal glands, and the liver. Very low levels of CSP are detected in the brain, probably due to poor passage across the blood-brain barrier. Once CSP is discontinued, it takes months for it to leach slowly from its tissue deposits.

In the blood, CSP is concentrated in erythrocytes; up to 70% is found in red cells (48). Because of erythrocyte binding, CSP levels measured in whole blood are always higher than those measured in plasma. The binding of CSP is temperature-dependent; more CSP enters the red cells as the sample cools to room temperature (49,50). These factors make CSP monitoring more difficult, because they may influence the level obtained.

CSP is metabolized extensively in the liver by the cytochrome P-450 system (49). Metabolism of CSP may be affected by age of the patient, liver disease, or by drugs that also interact with the enzymes responsible for CSP oxidation (49). For example, infants and young children have a much more rapid clearance of CSP than older patients. The multiple medications that patients receive after BMT may inhibit or induce the P-450 system. Likewise, some of these medications may modify absorption, excretion, or enterohepatic recycling of CSP. For example, ketoconazole and erythromycin cause an elevation of CSP blood levels by competition for the P-450 system (50). Other drugs, such as rifampin and phenobarbital, lower CSP concentrations by inducing the same microsomal metabolism (52,53). Phenytoin has been reported to decrease CSP drug levels either by interfering with absorption of the drug from the gastrointestinal tract or through its influence on the P-450 system (54,55). In patients receiving steroids, normal, increased, and decreased metabolism of CSP have been reported (56–58).

CSP excretion and metabolism are primarily intrahepatic. In humans, more than 90% of the intervenous doses of CSP is excreted in bile (59). Because of the importance of the liver in metabolism and elimination of CSP, hepatic dysfunction may influence CSP and may also influence accumulation of potentially immunosuppressive metabolites.

It is clear that monitoring of whole blood or plasma levels of CSP may be influenced by many factors. It is not surprising that most studies have failed to show a correlation between CSP levels and the development of GVHD in the complex BMT setting because the patient's medical condition and the medications given are constantly changing. On a theoretical basis, one may actually predict that this correlation would be difficult to establish without regard to the technical difficulties involved in ascertaining CSP levels. Thus, one log or more CSP is needed in some patients to prevent allostimulation (60). Thus, for any population there would be varying sensitivities and varying concentrations of CSP necessary to prevent allostimulation.

Several studies have addressed and found a correlation between CSP levels and the risk of GVHD. Gluckman and associates (60) reported that patients in whom GVHD developed had a lower mean CSP level measured by polyclonal radioimmunoassay (RIA) than patients in whom GVHD did not develop. Santos and colleagues (61) reported that only CSP concentrations during the first week after transplant correlated with the risk of GVHD. Yee and co-workers (62), in an extensive study involving 179 BMT recipients, studied the relationship between serum CSP concentration and the risk for development of acute GVHD. In this study, serum trough CSP concentrations were measured by polyclonal RIA. The study also used a multivariant relative risk regression model, in which weekly trough CSP concentration was modeled as a time-dependent covariate. The average CSP concentration for the week prior to development of GVHD was lower in 66 patients in whom grade II to IV GVHD developed than in those patients in whom acute GVHD did not develop. The study showed that this was a very complex interaction, with multiple factors influencing the risk for GVHD, including older age, method of delivery of CSP, and degree of human leukocyte antigen (HLA) disparity. Also confusing in this study was that the increased risk of GVHD from a low concentration of CSP was only seen after the median time of development of acute GVHD—that is, for the immediate post-transplant course, when GVHD developed in most patients, the CSP concentration did not seem to influence their risk. The study further demonstrated the complexities involved in CSP drug monitoring and the difficulties in interpreting levels in these patients.

Likewise, trying to prevent renal dysfunction utilizing CSP levels has proved difficult. Nephrotoxicity appears to be dose-dependent and to be characterized by an acute and chronic phase (63). Acute toxicity appears to be due to renal vasoconstriction and ischemia (64,65). The acute toxicity is associated with reduced glomerular filtration, increased proximal tubular reabsorption, oliguria, and hyperkalemia (63,66). It is generally reversible. Chronic toxicity is usually not reversible and causes interstitial fibrosis and loss of nephrons. Patients receiving marrow transplants have multiple causes of renal dysfunction. The effects of amphotericin and aminoglycosides cannot be separated from the nephrotoxicity due to CSP. There are data indicating that higher CSP levels were associated with more rapid development of renal dysfunction (67); however, even in groups of patients with low mean trough CSP levels, renal dysfunction will develop in the majority of patients. Thus, although CSP levels may be used as a guide to try to prevent renal toxicity, some evidence of renal dysfunction will still develop in the majority of patients even though their CSP levels are kept low. Again, adding confusion to this picture is that the same investigators were unable to reproduce these data when using high-pressure liquid chromatography (HPLC) analysis of CSP concentrations as compared with polyclonal RIA measurements. Thus, HPLC blood levels of CSP had no predictive value for subsequent development of renal toxicity. Likewise, the levels found relatively to preserve renal function were lower than those found to protect from GVHD.

A discussion of the techniques used to measure CSP is beyond the limitations of this chapter; however, there are considerable differences in the levels obtained depending on the technique used, partially due to measurement of metabolites when polyclonal RIA techniques are used. However, because some of these metabolites may be immunosuppressive properties, they may actually be a valuable addition. It is important to know the technique used at each center to interpret reported results and to compare results obtained from one to another. It is also important to understand that results obtained using one technique will not directly translate into levels using other techniques. More importantly, the polyclonal RIA used for the majority of studies discussed is no longer available. The correlations found with the polyclonal assay have not always been reproducible with either monoclonal RIA or HPLC techniques. Thus, in making clinical recommendations, it is very important to keep all these limitations in mind.

CSP monitoring thus is relatively limited but is important in documenting adequate oral absorption. It is also important when changing the route of administration while trying to give roughly equivalent doses. It may be helpful also in treatment of patients with rapidly fluctuating hepatic or renal dysfunction. In patients on dialysis with severe acute GVHD, it may also be useful in monitoring infrequent pulses of CSP. When drugs known to interfere with CSP are added, CSP monitoring may also be useful to try to prevent significant elevations or decreases in CSP levels. CSP levels are not useful in protecting patients from renal toxicity, and CSP cannot be advocated as a 100% protective measure in prevention of GVHD.

XomaZyme

Recently, a new immunotoxin has been studied in Phase I/II and subsequent Phase III trials for both treatment and prophylaxis of acute GVHD (68). XomaZyme is the first drug of this type introduced for clinical immunosuppression; however, there are multiple other compounds undergoing both preclinical and clinical studies that utilize different conjugants. Thus, XomaZyme represents a prototype for other drugs.

Mechanism of Action

The basic idea of an immunotoxin is that half the molecule is used for targeting of the therapy and half the molecule is used for its lytic activity. Commonly, monoclonal antibodies have been chosen to target particular cell populations. In the case of XomaZyme, a monoclonal antibody to the CD5 determinant is used as the recognition part of the molecule. The toxin in this case is ricin A, although other toxins, such as diphtheria toxin, are currently being studied. Ricin is derived from castor beans and is composed of two polypeptide chains linked by a disulfide bond. The ricin B chain recognizes and attaches to cell membranes indiscriminantly. The ricin A chain provides the cytotoxicity. By utilizing purified ricin A chain, which is nontoxic because of its inability to enter a cell, linked to a monoclonal antibody, directive therapy is possible.

The CD5 monoclonal antibody chosen is an antibody that is noncomplement-fixing and is of the immunoglobulin G1 (IgG1) subclass (68). CD5 recognizes T cells and a small population of B cells. The functional significance of this B-cell recognition is unknown but is an area of great interest. Ricin A catalytically inactivates ribosomes, preventing protein synthesis and causing cell death.

Pharmacokinetics

The pharmacokinetics of XomaZyme have been studied utilizing the intact conjugate, the ricin A chain, and the CD5 monoclonal antibodies (68). Each component showed biexponential pharmacokinetics. The immunoconjugate had an alpha-phase half-life of 1.3 hours and a beta-phase half-life of 52 hours. The serum pharmacokinetics of the conjugate were intermediate between those of the antibodies and the ricin A chain. When radiolabeled immunoconjugate was administered, the liver accumulated the greatest amount of radioactivity, suggesting that the liver may be the primary site of immunoconjugate metabolism.

The phase I/II study was conducted using this compound (68). A dose escalation was included; patients were treated at doses of 0.05 mg/kg, 0.1 mg/kg, 0.2 mg/kg, and 0.33 mg/kg per day for 14 days. After the initial dose escalation, 14 additional patients were treated at the intermediate doses of 0.1 mg/kg and 0.2 mg/kg for 14 days to gain additional data. Pharmacokinetic studies were also measured in 13 of these patients. Peak serum levels were obtained within 5 minutes after the end of the infusion. There was a rapid decrease in the plasma levels for the following 2 hours. Reliable terminal half-lives were calculated for patients receiving 0.1 and 0.2 mg/kg and were in the range of 1.5 to 3.9 hours. Peak serum levels range between 0.95 and 5.1 mg/mL. The peak serum level obtained correlated with the dose.

Twenty patients were followed for the development of antibodies to the immunotoxin. Antibodies did develop in 26% of patients. In none of the patients did the antibodies block binding of the monoclonal antibody to CD5. There was no correlation between immunotoxin dose and clinical response, side effects, or clearance of CD5-positive cells. A dose of 0.1 mg/kg was selected because the levels obtained with the drug given at this dose were predicted to saturate peripheral blood mononuclear cells.

Thalidomide

Thalidomide is a drug that was initially marketed as a sedative, but it has gained increasing interest as an immunosuppressant. Reports from a Phase II trial of high risk and steroid-refractory chronic GVHD showed that thalidomide had activity against this complication (69). The ultimate utility of this drug is unknown. A planned randomized trial in patients with standard risk chronic GVHD should help define what role this drug will have in the armamentarium against GVHD.

Pharmacokinetics

Despite being a very old drug, only a few pharmacokinetic studies of thalidomide have been done. The initial study in humans utilized a colorimetric assay (70). Other studies employed laboratory animals (71–75). Although it was appreciated that the pharmacokinetics were variable due to differences in intestinal absorption, further work on kinetics were delayed due to lack of a reproducible method for measuring thalidomide. An HPLC assay was developed and was used both to examine dose (level)/response curves and to examine pharmacokinetics in healthy volunteers (76,77). Initial studies showed that at levels above 5μg/mL animals had a fairly prompt response when receiving thalidomide for treatment of GVHD (78–80). Further increases in the blood level did not appear to correlate with more rapid responses.

On the basis of data generated from the old literature utilizing colorimetric assays a dose of 100 mg 4 times a day was chosen for initial clinical trials using thalidomide. This dose was also based on the usual dose given in erythema nodosum leprosum. Initial patients treated with thalidomide had plasma levels much below the predicted levels. Because of the multiple potential causes of poor absorption in patients after a BMT, a pharmacokinetic study was undertaken in normal volunteers (76). This study confirmed the variability seen in absorption and emphasized the need to assure absorption by measuring blood levels. The mean (± standard deviation) peak concentration was 1.15 ± 0.2 mg/mL in 8 healthy male volunteers receiving a single oral dose of 200 mg thalidomide. The peak concentration was 4.39 ± 1.27 hours. Absorption and elimination half-lives were 1.7 ± 1.05 hour and 8.7 ± 4.11 hours, respectively. The apparent volume of distribution and total body clearance rate, based on assumed complete bioavailability, were 120.69 ± 45.36 L/hour and 10.41 ± 2.04 L/hour. The urinary excretion of thalidomide accounted for only 0.6 ± 0.22% of total body administration over 24 hours. These data suggested that the primary route of elimination of thalidomide was nonrenal. On the basis of these data, the dose of thalidomide was increased to 200 mg 4 times a day, and plasma levels have continued to be used to indicate absorption. The side effects of thalidomide, notably the associated sedation, have not correlated well with the plasma level and cannot be used as a surrogate for assuring absorption.

Other than the studies reviewed herein, little is known of the fate of thalidomide in vivo. Most studies indicate that the drug is not metabolized but hydrolyzed spontaneously (71–82). Unfortunately, these studies are all relatively old and did not utilize up-to-date technology. Currently, studies are underway to confirm these older studies. Likewise, it is unknown whether any of the hydrolysis products are immunosuppressive or, indeed, if these products are the actual active drug. This is an area of ongoing research.

Mechanism of Action

The mechanism of action of thalidomide remains obscure. Work on thalidomide has been hampered by its rapid hydrolysis in water and the poor solubility of the native drug in water. On the basis of transplantation models, it appears that thalidomide allows for induction of antigen-specific suppressor cells (78–80). Lymphocytes from thalidomide-treated chimeras are able to suppress GVHD when transplanted with fresh donor marrow into the same recipient strain. However, these same lymphocytes are unable to prevent GVHD when fresh donor strain is transplanted into a third-party recipient strain. The drug appears to have little effect on the reconstitution of the thymus. The thymus in a thalidomide-treated animal is of normal size and cell number when compared with syngeneic untreated control animals. Cell phenotypes in the thymus are also normal. Although one group reported on the direct immunosuppressive effects of thalidomide at a cellular level, many groups have been frustrated by difficulty obtaining reproducible assays with this compound (83). An intriguing report found that thalidomide decreased tumor necrosis factor-alpha production from monocytes (82). Although this action may account for some of the effects of thalidomide and may be its primary mode of action in patients with erythema leprosum neucrosum, it is unlikely to explain all of the effects of this drug in a BMT setting. Thus, the main effects of this compound at both a cellular and a molecular level remain to be elucidated.

FK506

FK506 is a drug that has been introduced into clinical transplantation and has primarily been found useful in patients receiving hepatic allografts. Large-scale trials in human BMT have not taken place, so it is difficult to know the eventual role of this drug. However, on the basis of extensive preclinical work, it is unlikely to have a major impact in BMT because the mechanism of action of FK506 appears to be identical to CSP. Although FK506 is more potent on a gram-per-gram basis, the toxicity seen so far suggests that there will be little advantage over CSP. The one possible exception is its use in patients with hepatic GVHD. Because of the high concentrations obtained in the liver during metabolism of the drug, there may be an opportunity to dose-escalate intrahepatically without increasing systemic toxicity. Further clinical trials will determine which patients will benefit from receiving FK506 compared with other forms of therapy.

Mechanism of Action

The mechanism of action of this drug has been extensively investigated (35). At a cellular level and at a whole animal level, there is little to distinguish FK506 from CSP. At a cellular level, FK506 appears to bind to a family of unique intracellular proteins, which have been termed *FK506 binding proteins*. Despite the fact that many of these proteins have been identified, once FK506 has bound to its immunophilin, the effects of the drug seem to be identical within the cell as the CSP/cyclophilin conjugant. Thus the effects on IL-2 and IL-2 receptor, among other factors reviewed herein, are the same for FK506.

Pharmacokinetics

One of the hoped-for advantages of FK506 was less toxicity than seen with CSP. It appears that many of the toxicities reported with CSP have also been encountered with FK506 (84). These toxicities include renal impairment, neurotoxic effects, hemolytic-uremic syndrome, and hypertension. In a study performed by the Pittsburgh Liver Transplant Group, there were no substantive differences in the rate and severity of side effects (save a possible reduction in hypertension) seen in patients receiving FK506 versus those receiving CSP (84). Thus, the desired improvement in therapeutic ratio was not attained with FK506.

Pharmacokinetic studies have also been carried out by the Pittsburgh Liver Transplantation Group (85). Plasma samples following intravenous continuous infusion, short-term intravenous infusion, or oral administration of FK506 have been analyzed using enzyme-linked immunosorbent assay (ELISA). Following intravenous infusion, the peak plasma concentration was reached at the end of the infusion, with a rapid decline at the completion of the infusion, thought to indicate rapid distribution of the drug outside the plasma compartment. Once equilibrium with this outside compartment was reached, FK506 concentrations declined at a slower rate. The behavior of the drug can be described by a two compartment model. On the basis of plasma concentrations, the half-life of FK506 ranges from 3.5 to 40.5 hours, and clearance ranges from 7 to 103 mL/min/kg. The volume of distribution at steady state is equally variable, ranging from 5.6 to 65 L/kg. Thus, like many of the other drugs discussed in this chapter, there are large individual variations in the pharmacokinetics of FK506.

After oral administration, FK506 is absorbed in a variable fashion (85). Some patients have very rapid absorption, whereas others seem to have slow continuous absorption. The reasons for this variability are poorly understood. The oral bioavailability of FK506 is approximately 27%, but ranges from 5 to 67%.

FK506 is bound to red blood cells (85). In the plasma, FK506 is associated with alpha$_1$ acid glycoprotein. Outside the blood, FK506 seems to be distributed in heart, lungs, spleen, kidneys, and pancreas. Similar to CSP, no FK506 has been detected in the cerebrospinal fluid of patients. Similar to CSP, FK506 is metabolized in the liver. Most of the metabolites are excreted in the bile (86). FK506 undergoes demethylation and hydroxylation as it is metabolized.

There have been some preliminary studies on factors that may affect FK506 metabolism (87). Food does not seem to alter the extent of absorption. Patients with hepatic dysfunction have higher levels than patients with normal liver function. FK506 tends to have a longer half-life and smaller clearance values in patients with liver dysfunction (88). Many of the same medicines known to affect CSP metabolism (e.g., ketoconazole, erythromycin, fluconazole, cimetidine) also affect FK506 metabolism in a similar fashion (85). Perhaps the most important toxic synergism is that of CSP with FK506. Nephrotoxicity is greatly enhanced when these two agents are administered together (89,90).

Antithymocyte Globulin

Antithymocyte globulin (ATG) is an immune globulin prepared from animals immunized with human thymocytes. The commercially available product is prepared from horse serum. ATG made from other animals is available from investigators at several academic treatment centers for patients who are allergic to horse sera. All patients should be tested before receiving any ATG preparation to ensure they are not allergic to the sera of the animal used.

The pharmacokinetics of ATG are difficult to characterize for a variety of reasons. Moreover, there is a lot-to-lot and species-to-species variability. It is impossible to know accurately the bioactivity of each batch of ATG. The functional half-life of the active antibodies within the serum is also unknown. Nonetheless, the plasma half-life of horse IgG is approximately 6 days (92). The disposition of horse IgG in humans is not known but is believed to be catabolized and extensively bound to most body tissues. As stated, the significant variability of this biological product among lots makes a comparison between studies extremely difficult.

References

1. Farber S, Diamond LK, Mercer RD, Sylvester RF Jr, Wolff JA. Temporary remissions in acute leukemia in children produced by folic acid antagonist, 4-aminopteroyl-glutamic acid (aminopterin). N Engl J Med 1948;238:787–791.
2. Uphoff DE. Alteration of homograft reaction by A-methopterin in lethally irradiated mice treated with homologous marrow. Proc Soc Exp Biol Med 1958;99: 651–653.
3. Lochte HL Jr, Levy AS, Guenther DM, Thomas ED, Ferrebee JW. Prevention of delayed foreign marrow reaction in lethally irradiated mice by early administration of methotrexate. Nature 1962;196:1110–1111.
4. Storb R, Rudolph RH, Kolb HJ, et al. Marrow grafts

between DL-A-matched canine littermates. Transplantation 1973;15:92–100.

5. Thomas ED, Storb R, Clift RA, et al. Bone-marrow transplantation. N Engl J Med 1975;292:832–843,895–902.
6. Wiemann MC, Calabresi P. Pharmacology of antineoplastic agents. In: Calabresi P, Schein PS, Rosenberg SA, eds. Medical oncology. Basic principles and clinical management of cancer. New York: Macmillan, 1985:309–314.
7. Bleyer WA. The clinical pharmacology of methotrexate. New applications of an old drug. Cancer 1978;31:36–51.
8. Thomas ED, Storb R. The effect of amethopterin on the immune response. Ann NY Acad Sci 1971;186: 467–474.
9. Thomas ED, Collins JA, Herman EC Jr, Ferrebee JW. Marrow transplants in lethally irradiated dogs given methotrexate. Blood 1962;19:217–228.
10. Storb R, Epstein RB, Graham TC, Thomas ED. Methotrexate regimens for control of graft-versus-host disease in dogs with allogeneic marrow grafts. Transplantation 1970;9:240–246.
11. Thomas ED, Buckner CD, Banaji M, et al. One hundred patients with acute leukemia treated by chemotherapy, total body irradiation, and allogeneic marrow transplantation. Blood 1977;49:511–533.
12. Thomas ED, Sanders JE, Flournoy N, et al. Marrow transplantation for patients with acute lymphoblastic leukemia in remission. Blood 1979;54:468–476.
13. Storb R, Deeg HJ, Fisher LD, et al. Cyclosporine v methotrexate for graft-v-host disease prevention in patients given marrow grafts for leukemia: long-term follow-up of three controlled trials. Blood 1988;71: 293–298.
14. Storb R, Deeg HJ, Farewell V, et al. Marrow transplantation for severe aplastic anemia: methotrexate alone compared with a combination of methotrexate and cyclosporine for prevention of acute graft-versus-host disease. Blood 1986;68:119–125.
15. Storb R, Deeg HJ, Whitehead J, et al. Methotrexate and cyclosporine compared with cyclosporine alone for prophylaxis of acute graft-versus-host disease after marrow transplantation for leukemia. N Engl J Med 1986;314:729–735.
16. Adamson PC, Balis FM, McCully CL, Godwin KS, Poplack DG. Methotrexate pharmacokinetics following administration of recombinant carboxypeptidase-G[22] in rhesus monkeys. J Clin Oncol 1992;10:1359–1364.
17. Lin JT, Bertino JR. Trimetrexate. A second generation folate antagonist in clinical trial. J Clin Oncol 1987;5:2032–2040.
18. Wenger RM. Structure of cyclosporine and its metabolites. Transplant Proc 1990;22:1104–1108.
19. Di Padova FE. Pharmacology of cyclosporine V. Pharmacological effects on immune function: in vitro studies. Pharmacol Rev 1989;41:373–405.
20. Hess AD, Esa AN, Colombani PM. Mechanisms of action of cyclosporine: effect on cells of the immune system and on subcellular events in T cell activation. Transplant Proc 1988;20(suppl 2):29–40.
21. Wagner H. Cyclosporine A: mechanism of action. Transplant Proc 1983;15:523–526.
22. Hess AD. Effect of interleukin 2 on the immunosuppressive action of cyclosporine. Transplantation 1985;39: 62–68.
23. Heeg K, Gillis S, Wagner H. IL-4 bypassed the immune suppressive effect of cyclosporin A during the in vitro induction of immune cytotoxic T lymphocytes. J Immunol 1988;141:2330–2337.
24. Bunjes D, Hardt C, Rollinghoff M, Wagner H. Cyclosporin A mediates immunosuppression of primary cytotoxic T cell responses by impairing the release of interleukin 1 and interleukin 2. Eur J Immunol 1981; 8:657–662.
25. Hess AD, Tutschka PJ, Pu Z, Santos GW. Effect of cyclosporine A on human lymphocyte responses in vitro. IV. Production of T cell stimulatory growth factors and development of responsiveness to these growth factors in CsA-treated primary MLR cultures. J Immunol 1982;128:360–365.
26. Elliott JF, Lin Y, Mizel SB, Bleackley RC, Harnish DG, Paetkau V. Induction of interleukin 2 messenger RNA inhibited by cyclosporin A. Science 1984;226:1439–1441.
27. Hodgin PD, Hapel AJ, Johnson RM, et al. Blocking of the delivery of the antigen-mediated signal to the nucleus of T-cells by cyclosporine. Transplantation 1987;43: 685–691.
28. June CH, Ledbetter JA, Gellespie MM, Lindtsen T, Thompson CB. T cell proliferation involving the CD28 pathway is associated with cyclosporine-resistant interleukin 2 gene expression. Mol Cell Biol 1987;7: 4472–4481.
29. Reed JC, Prystowsky MB, Nowell PC. Regulation of gene expression in lectin-stimulated or lymphokine-stimulated T lymphocytes. Transplantation 1988;26 (suppl):85–91.
30. Foxwell BMJ, Siman J, Herrero IJ, Taylor D, Woerly G, Cantrell D, Ryffel B. Anti-CD3 antibody induced expression of both p55 and p75 chains of the high affinity IL-2 receptor on human T lymphocytes is inhibited by cyclosporin A. Immunology 1990;69:104–109.
31. Colombani PM, Robb A, Hess AD. Cyclosporin A binding to calmodulin: a possible site of action on T-lymphocytes. Science 1985;228:337–339.
32. Handschumacher RE, Harding MW, Rice J, Drugge RJ. Cyclophillin: a specific cytosolic binding protein for cyclosporin A. Science 1984;226:544–546.
33. Fischer G, Wittman, Liebold B, Lanf K, Kiefhaber T, Schmid FX. Cyclophillin and peptidyl-prolyl-cis-trans isomerase are probably identical proteins. Nature 1989;337:476–479.
34. Sigal NH, Dumont F, Siekierka JJ, et al. Is cyclophillin involved in the immunosuppressive and nephrotoxic mechanism of action of cyclosporin A? J Exp Med 1991;173:619–628.
35. Beirer BE, Somers PK, Wandless TJ, Burakoff SJ, Schreiber SL. Probing immunosuppressant action with a nonnatural immunophilin ligand. Science 1990;250: 556–559.
36. Hess AD, Esa AN, Colombani PM. Mechanisms of action of cyclosporine: effect on cells of the immune system and on subcellular events in T cell activation. Transplant Proc 1988;20(suppl 2):29–40.
37. Wood AJ, Maurer G, Neiderberger W, Beveridge T. CsA: pharmacokinetics, metabolism and drug interactions. Transplant Proc 1983;15:2409–2412.
38. Lokiec F, Devergie A, Poirier O, Gluckman E. Pharmacologic monitoring and clinical use of CsA. Transplant Proc 1983;15:2422–2425.
39. Yee GC, Kennedy MS, Storb R, Thomas ED. Pharmacokinetics in intravenous CsA in BMT patients. Transplant 1984;38:511–513.
40. Yee GC, Lennon TP, Gmur DG, Carlin J, Shaffer RL,

Kennedy MS, Deeg HJ. Clinical pharmacology of CsA in patients undergoing BMT. Transplant Proc 1986;28: 153–159.
41. Grevel J. Significance of CsA pharmacokinetics. Transplant Proc 1988;20:428–434.
42. Yee GC. Pharmacologic monitoring of immunosuppressive therapy. In: Burakoff SJ, Deeg HJ, Ferrara J, Atkinson K, eds. Graft-vs-host disease: immunology, pathophysiology, and treatment, vol 12. New York: Marcel Dekker, 1990:499–524.
43. Yee GC, Lennon TP, Gmur DJ, Kennedy MS, Deeg HJ. Age-dependent cyclosporine pharmacokinetics in marrow transplant recipients. Clin Pharmacol Ther 1986; 40:438–443.
44. Yee GC, McGuire TR, Gmur DJ, Lennon TP, Deeg HJ. Blood cyclosporine pharmacokinetics in patients undergoing marrow transplantation: influence of age, obesity, and hematocrit. Transplantation 1988;467:399–402.
45. Yee GC, Lennon TP, Gmur DJ, Cheney CL, Deeg HJ. Effect of obesity on cyclosporine disposition. Transplantation 1988;45:649–651.
46. Lemaire M, Tillement JP. Role of lipoproteins and erythrocytes in the in vitro binding and distribution of cyclosporine A in the blood. J Pharm Pharmacol 1982;34:715–718.
47. Niederberger W, Lemaire M, Maurer G, Nussbaumer K, Wagner O. Distribution and binding of cyclosporine in blood and tissues. Transplant Proc 1983;15:2419–2421.
48. Atkinson K, Britton K, Biggs J. Distribution and concentration of cyclosporin in human blood. J Clin Pathol 1984;37:1167–1171.
49. Quesniaux VF. Pharmacology of cyclosporine (sandimmune):immunochemistry and monitoring. Pharmacol Rev 1989;41:249–258.
50. Smith JM, Hows JM, Gordon-Smith EC, Baughan A, Goldman JM. Interaction of CyA and ketoconazole. Clin Sci 1983;64:67P–68P.
51. Cassidy MJD, van Zyl-Smit R, Pascoe MD, Swanepoel CR, Jacobson JZ. Effect of rifampicin on cyclosporin A blood levels in a renal transplant recipient. Nephron 1985;41:207–208.
52. Carstensen H, Jacobsen N, Dieperink H. Interaction between cyclosporin A and phenobarbitone. Br J Clin Pharmacol 1986;21:550–551.
53. Rowland M, Gupta SK. Cyclosporin-phenytoin interaction: re-evaluation using metabolite data. Br J Clin Pharmacol 1987;24:329–334.
54. Keown PA, Laupacis A, Carruthers G, et al. Interaction between phenytoin and cyclosporine following organ transplantation. Transplantation (Baltimore) 1984;38: 304–306.
55. Ptachcinski RJ, Venkataramanan R, Burckart GJ. Clinical pharmacokinetics of cyclosporin. Clin Pharmacokinet 1986;11:107–132.
56. Ptachcinski RJ, Venkataramanan R, Burckart GJ, Hakala TR, Rosenthal JT. Cyclosporine: high dose steroid interaction in renal transplant recipients: assessment by HPLC. Transplant Proc 1987;19(suppl 1):1728–1729.
57. Frey FJ, Schnetzer A, Horber FF, Frey BM. Evidence that cyclosporine does not affect the metabolism of prednisolone after renal transplantation. Transplantation (Baltimore) 1987;43:494–498.
58. Maurer G. Metabolism of cyclosporine. Transplant Proc 1985;17:19–26.
59. Scovza R, Vanoli M, Cigognine A, Fabro G, DeBernardo B. In vitro effects of cyclosporine A on allogeneic and autologous lymphocyte stimulation: influence of HLA phenotypes. Transplant Proc 1980;20:122–130.
60. Gluckman E, Lokeic F, Devergie A. Pharmacokinetic monitoring of cyclosporine in allogeneic bone marrow transplants. Transplant Proc 1984;17:500–501.
61. Santos GW, Tutschka PJ, Brookmeyer R, et al. Cyclosporine plus methylprednisolone versus cyclophosphamide plus methylprednisolone as prophylaxis for graft-versus-host disease: a randomized double-blind study in patients undergoing allogeneic marrow transplantation. Clin Transplant 1987;1:21–28.
62. Yee GC, Self SG, McGuire TR, Carlin J, Sanders JE, Deeg HJ. Serum cyclosporine concentration and risk of acute graft-versus-host disease after allogeneic marrow transplantation. N Engl J Med 1988;319:60–65.
63. Bennett WM, Pulliam JP. Cyclosporine nephrotoxicity. Ann Intern Med 1983;99:851–854.
64. Petric R, Freeman DJ, Wallace C, McDonald J, Stiller C, Keown P. Effect of cyclosporine on urinary prostanoic excretion, renal blood flow and glomulotubular function. Transplantation 1988;45:883–889.
65. Teraoka S, Takahashi K, Tanabe K, et al. Improvement in renal blood flow and kidney function by modulation of prostaglandin metabolism in cyclosporin treated animals. Transplant Proc 1989;21:937–940.
66. Keown PA, Stiller CR, Wallace AC. The nephrotoxicity of cyclosporine. In: Williams GM, Bardick JF, Solex K, eds. Kidney transplant rejection: current issues in diagnosis and treatment. New York: Marcel Dekker, 1986:423–457.
67. Kennedy MS, Yee GC, McGuire TR, Leonard TM, Crowley JJ, Deeg HJ. Correlation of serum cyclosporine concentration with renal dysfunction in marrow transplant recipients. Transplantation 1985;40:249–253.
68. Byers VS, Henslee PJ, Kernan NA, et al. Use of an anti-pan T-lymphocyte ricin A chain immunotoxin in steroid-resistant acute graft-versus-host disease. Blood 1990;75:1426–1432.
69. Vogelsang GB, Farmer ER, Hess AD, et al. Thalidomide therapy of chronic graft-versus-host disease. N Engl J Med 1992;326:1055–1058.
70. Bechmann VR, Kampf HH. Zur quantitativen bestimmung und zum qualitativen nachweis von n-phthalylglutaminsaureimid (thalidomide). Arzneimittel-Forsch 1961;11:45–47.
71. Fabro S, Smith RL, Williams TR. The fate of [^{14}C] thalidomide in the pregnant rabbit. J Biochem 1967; 104:565–569.
72. Hague DE, Fabro S, Smith RL. The fate of [^{14}C] thalidomide in the pregnant hamster. J Pharm Pharmacol 1967;19:603–607.
73. Nicholls PJ. A note on the absorption and excretion of ^{14}C-labeled thalidomide in pregnant mice. J Pharm Pharmacol 1966;18:46–48.
74. Schumacher HJ, Wilson JG, Terapane JF, Rosedale SL. Thalidomide: disposition in rhesus monkey and studies of its hydrolysis in tissue of this and other species. Pharmacol Exp Ther 1970;173:265–269.
75. Schumacher H, Blake DA, Gillette JR. Disposition of thalidomide in rabbits and rats. J Pharmacol Exp Ther 1968;160:201–211.
76. Chen TL, Vogelsang GB, Petty BG, et al. Plasma pharmacokinetics and urinary excretion of thalidomide after oral dosing in healthy male volunteers. Drug Metab Dispos 1988;17:402–405.
77. Czejka MJ, Koch HP. Determination of thalidomide and

its major metabolites by high-performance liquid chromatography. J Chromatogr 1987;413:181–187.
78. Vogelsang GB, Hess AD, Gordon G, Brundrett R, Santos GW. Thalidomide induction of bone marrow transplantation tolerance. Transplant Proc 1987;19:658–661.
79. Vogelsang GB, Santos GW, Colvin OM, Chen T. Thalidomide for graft-versus-host disease. Lancet 1988;1:827.
80. Vogelsang GB, Wells MC, Santos GW, Hess AD. Combination low dose thalidomide and cyclosporine prophylaxis for acute graft-versus-host disease. Transplant Proc 1988;10:226–228.
81. Schumacher H, Smith RL, Williams RT. The metabolism of thalidomide: the fate of thalidomide and some of its hydrolysis products in various species. Br J Pharmacol 1965;25:338–351.
82. Samparo EP, Sarno EN, Galilly R, Cohn ZA, Kaplan G. Thalidomide selectively inhibits tumor necrosis factor alpha production by stimulated human monocytes. J Exp Med 1991;173:699–703.
83. Schumacher H, Smith RL, Williams RT. The metabolism of thalidomide: the spontaneous hydrolysis of thalidomide in solution. Br J Pharmacol 1965;25:324–337.
84. Keenan RJ, Eiras G, Burckart GJ, et al. Immunosuppressive properties of thalidomide: inhibition of in vitro lymphocyte proliferation alone and in combination with cyclosporine or FK506. Transplantation 1991;52: 908–910.
85. Fung JJ, Alessiani M, Abu-Elmagd K, et al. Adverse effects associated with the use of FK506. Transplant Proc 1991;23:3105–3108.
86. Venkataramanan R, Jain A, Warty VS, et al. Pharmacokinetics of FK506 in transplant patients. Transplant Proc 1991;23:2736–2740.
87. Venkataramanan R, Jain A, Cadoff E, Warty V. Pharmacokinetics of FK 506: preclinical and clinical studies. Transplant Proc 1990;22:52–56.
88. Shah A, Whiting PH, Omar G, Thomson AW, Burke MD. Effects of FK506 on human hepatic microsomal cytochrome P-450-dependent drug metabolism in vitro. Transplant Proc 1991;23:2783–2785.
89. Jain AB, Venkataramanan R, Cadoff E, Fung J. Effect of hepatic dysfunction and T tube clamping on FK506 pharmacokinetics and trough concentration. Transplant Proc 1990;22:57–59.
90. Pichard L, Fabre I, Domergue J, Joyeux H, Maurel P. Effect of FK506 on human hepatic cytochromes P-450: interaction with CyA. Transplant Proc 1991;23:2791–2793.
91. Christians U, Braun F, Sattler M, Almeidal VMF, Linck A, Sewing K-Fr. Interactions of FK506 and cyclosporine metabolism. Transplant Proc 1991;23:2794–2796.
92. The Upjohn Company. Drug Reference: Atgam. Kalamazoo, MI: 1981.

Chapter 11
T-cell Depletion for Prevention of Graft-versus-Host Disease

Nancy A. Kernan

Despite improvements in immunosuppressive regimens used after transplantation, acute and chronic graft-versus-host disease (GVHD) continue to be major causes of morbidity and mortality after allogeneic bone marrow transplantation (BMT) (1–3), especially in older patients and in patients in whom donor marrow has been obtained from closely human leukocyte antigen (HLA)–matched nonsibling donors (4,5). In the late 1950s and 1960s, experiments performed in animals demonstrated that GVHD could be prevented by infusions of fetal hematopoietic tissue devoid of mature T cells (6,7). These observations suggested that in vitro elimination of immunocompetent T lymphocytes from the donor marrow with preservation of hematopoietic precursors prior to infusion might prevent development of GVHD. Demonstration that this was possible occurred with the development of antisera to mature murine T cells (8–10) and the observation that the plant lectin soybean agglutinin binds differentially to hematopoietic precursors and T cells in the marrow and the spleen of the mouse (11). In each of these models, such transplants resulted in stable long-term chimeras without GVHD. The knowledge that in vitro removal of donor T cells from the marrow could prevent development of GVHD in animal models, coupled with the development of methods for depletion of T cells in human marrow, provided the rationale for the initial clinical trials of T-cell depletion for prevention of GVHD in humans.

Attempts to prevent GVHD using antilymphocyte sera alone were unsuccessful (12). However, Reisner and colleagues (13,14) demonstrated that removal of T lymphocytes using sheep erythrocytes followed by selection of hematopoietic precursors with soybean agglutinin reduced the incidence and severity of GVHD in recipients of HLA-incompatible parental marrow for treatment of leukemia or severe combined immunodeficiency disease. Because this method is technically cumbersome, it was not until the availability of antihuman T-cell monoclonal antibodies that in vitro T-cell depletion was widely adopted as an approach to control development of GVHD. With its widespread use, however, it rapidly became clear that the results observed depended not only on the method of T-cell depletion, but also on the clinical setting, with respect to the degree of HLA identity present between the donor and the recipient, the diagnosis and stage of disease, and the intensity of the preparative cytoreduction administered prior to and immediately after transplantation. T-cell depletion alone or in combination with posttransplant immunosuppression was associated with a decrease in GVHD, but was also associated with an increase in graft failure, especially among recipients of HLA-nonidentical marrow (15–22), and an increased risk of leukemic relapse, most markedly among patients with chronic myeloid leukemia (CML) (23). The cumulative results underscored the importance of quantifying and characterizing the absolute numbers of residual T cells, T-cell subsets, progenitor cells, and accessory cells necessary for protection from GVHD, while at the same time preserving engraftment potential and a graft-versus-leukemia effect.

Laboratory Considerations and Methods of T-cell Depletion

Unmodified marrow obtained for human transplantation usually contains approximately 1 to 2 $\times$ 10^{10} nucleated cells with up to 10 to 15% mature T lymphocytes (24). Thus, recipients of unmodified marrow receive 1 to 2 $\times$ 10^7 T cells/kg recipient body weight. With this number of T cells and no prophylactic posttransplant immunosuppression, the incidence of grade II to IV GVHD among recipients of HLA-identical sibling marrow is approximately 80% (25). Enumerating the number of residual T cells in a graft following T-cell depletion proved to be problematic and required the development of new assay systems (26–30). The standard T-cell assays, including the E-rosette assay and immunofluorescence, are not sufficiently sensitive for evaluating marrows pretreated with antibodies that bind to and thus block the E-rosette or the T-cell receptors. High background proliferation of marrow progenitor cells reduces the sensitivity of mitogen-stimulated proliferation as measured by ^{3}H-thymidine incorporation. To date, limiting dilution analysis represents the most sensitive method for detecting and quantitating functional T cells remaining after marrow treatment (27–30). These assays quantify cells capable of responding to allostimulation in the presence of a mitogen and interleukin-2 (IL-2) as measured by cell proliferation (27,28), by production of IL-2 (29), or by generation of cytotoxic activity (30). With these methods, it has been demonstrated that recipients of HLA-identical T-cell–depleted marrow and no posttransplant immunosuppression are protected from clinically significant acute GVHD with marrow that contains less than 1 x 10^5 T cells/kg recipient body weight or a two-log depletion of T cells (31–33). These assays, however, have been used only to quantify the total number of clonogenic T cells infused and not specific T-cell subsets or natural killer (NK) cells that might respond in vivo to allostimulation or IL-2. In rodent models of transplantation, GVHD has been shown to be eliminated with the depletion of the $CD8^+$ cytotoxic/suppressor subset of T lymphocytes in some, but not all, donor-recipient strain combinations that are identical for the major murine histocompatibility loci but mismatched for minor histocompatibility antigens. However, most donor-recipient strains require depletion of both CD4 and CD8 T-cell subsets (34–36). The relative role of residual T-cell subsets and NK cells has not been determined in human recipients of T-cell–depleted marrow transplants.

A variety of immunological and physical techniques have been used to deplete marrow of T cells (Table 11-1). Immunological methods have relied on rodent (mostly murine) monoclonal antibodies directed against antigens with a restricted pattern of expression (37–40): CD2 present on T and NK cells, CD3 present on mature T cells, CD5 present on 95% of mature T cells and a small population of B lymphocytes, CD6 specific for mature T cells, and CD7 present on some but not all mature T and NK cells. In addition, antibodies directed against T-cell subsets, such as helper/inducer (CD4) and cytotoxic/suppressor (CD8) cells have been employed. Although there has been substantial experience with monoclonal antibodies directed against these T-cell antigens, the most widely used monoclonal antibody is a rat immunoglobulin M (IgM) monoclonal antibody, CAMPATH-1, which recognizes a heterogeneous 23 to 30 kd glycoprotein expressed by all lymphocytes (T, B, and NK) and monocytes (15).

Table 11-1.
Methods of T-cell Depletion

Monoclonal antibody–based methods
Complement mediated lysis
Immunotoxins
Immunomagnetic beads
Physical methods
Albumin gradient fractionation
E-rosette depletion alone
Soybean lectin agglutination plus E-rosette depletion
Counter flow elutriation
Combination of physical and monoclonal antibody method
Soybean agglutination plus monoclonal antibody

Because it had been demonstrated that protection of mice against GVHD could be achieved by treatment of donor marrow with anti-ø sera (8) or with an anti Thy-1 monoclonal antibody (10) alone, pilot clinical trials were performed with marrow treated with monoclonal antibodies alone (41–43). In these studies, antibodies were used to coat or opsonize T lymphocytes before infusion into the recipient, with the anticipation that T cells would be removed from the circulation in vivo by reticuloendothelial clearance of opsonized antibody-coated cells. In subsequent clinical trials, in vitro antibody treatments were performed in the presence of homologous or heterologous (rabbit) complement (17,19,44–50). Because lots of rabbit complement are variable in efficacy and toxicity to hematopoietic precursors, the use of complement in human trials requires careful screening of each batch of complement. In an effort to avoid the use of complement, investigators have explored the use of antibodies covalently bound to the plant toxin ricin (18,51,52) or its active component, ricin-A-chain (33,53,54), for prevention of GVHD. Alternatively, antibodies bound to polystyrene microspheres for removal of the coated T cells with samarium cobalt magnets have been utilized (55).

Physical methods that do not rely on antibodies for T-cell depletion include discontinuous albumin gradient fractionation (56), E-rosette depletion alone (57), soybean lectin agglutination followed by rosetting with sheep erythrocytes (13,14,20,21), and counterflow centrifugation elutriation (58–60). With physical separation methods, cell populations are not altered during the procedure and are therefore available for further manipulation or refined selection and add-back techniques. In clinical trials, a physical method coupled with an immunological technique has also been explored. Soybean agglutinin–negative cells enriched for progenitor cells were depleted of residual T cells by reaction with monoclonal antibodies bound to polystyrene-coated flasks (61).

With expertise, most antibody-mediated techniques that utilize a single antibody with complement, toxin, or magnetic beads achieve at least a two-log depletion of T cells, whereas methods that utilize multiple antibodies or physical methods alone or in combination with antibody achieve a 2.5- to 3.0-log depletion of T cells (33,62–64). Depending on the antibodies used for depletion and the method employed, cell populations other than T cells may also be depleted to differing degrees. For example, in one study, a cocktail of monoclonal antibodies (CD2–6,CD8,CD28) plus complement depleted more T and NK cells than treatment with a single antibody (CD6) plus complement (64). In another study, successive fractions obtained throughout the soybean agglutininE-rosette method were evaluated for NK and lymphokine activated killer (LAK) cell activity and IL-2 production. Although there was no endogenous NK or LAK cell activity in the final fraction (SBA-E-), incubation with IL-2 or IL-2 plus IL-1 resulted in generation of cytolytic activity against the NK-sensitive K562 cell line and the NK-resistant Daudi cell line, indicating that precursors for both NK and LAK cells are present in the final fraction given to the patient (65,66). In parallel studies, this fraction (SBA-E-) was shown to produce either low or undetectable levels of IL-2 (67). Similar studies have not been published for other methods of T-cell depletion.

Clinical Trials

Although early clinical trials examined T-cell depletion for its effect in preventing acute and chronic GVHD, with widespread use it soon became apparent that full assessment of any method of T-cell depletion also requires evaluation of outcome with respect to the probability of attaining durable engraftment and, in patients with leukemia, the probability of relapse (Table 11-2). Most investigators have defined engraftment as attainment of an absolute neutrophil count greater than or equal to 500 neutrophils/mm^3 for 3 consecutive days without considering the donor/host origin of these cells. The presence of clinically acute GVHD was assessed by standard criteria (68); significant acute GVHD was considered to be greater than or equal to grade II disease.

Graft-versus-Host Disease

Clinical trials performed with in vitro treatment of marrow with monoclonal antibodies alone, either singly (CD3) (41,42) or in combination (CD2–6, CD8, CD28) (43), demonstrated that reliance on in vivo opsonization after marrow infusion was not sufficient for prevention of GVHD, even in recipients of HLA-identical marrow transplants. Since then, immunological and physical methods that achieve a 2-$\log_{10}$ depletion of T cells in vitro have been demonstrated to protect most patients from acute GVHD such that the incidence of clinically significant grade II to IV GVHD was reduced to approximately 10% among durably engrafted patients transplanted with HLA-identical marrow. This is true for the pilot series that involved 8 to 20 patients reported between 1982 and 1988 (17–19,44–51,54), as well as the more recently published phase II trials involving larger cohorts of patients including older patients at high risk for acute GVHD (15,33,69–72). Additional posttransplant immunosuppression was not required for prevention of acute GVHD because no posttransplant immunosuppressive agent was used in three of the studies (33,69,70). Although each of the methods of T-cell depletion that achieves a reproducible 2-$\log_{10}$ depletion of donor T cells has been shown to protect HLA-matched patients from acute GVHD, not all methods have been equally effective in preventing chronic GVHD. The incidence is substantially lower than that observed in recipients of unmodified marrow (73). Among recipients of marrow depleted of T cells with CAMPATH-1M and autologous human serum or an anti-CD5 monoclonal antibody and rabbit complement or bound to ricin-A-chain, chronic GVHD was seen in 18% of patients (33,74), whereas the incidence of chronic GVHD was 0 to 5% among recipients of marrow depleted of T cells by soybean agglutinin and sheep erythrocytes, counterflow centrifugal elutriation, or anti-CD6 antibody plus complement (69,70,72).

Table 11-2.
Issues to be Considered When Evaluating Clinical Outcome of T-cell Depletion Protocols

Acute graft-versus-host disease
Chronic graft-versus-host disease
Graft rejection/failure
Immune reconstitution
B-cell lymphoproliferative disorders
Relapse (leukemia patients)
Disease-free survival

Multiple factors are known to affect the risk of development of acute GVHD after transplantation (75). However, an increase in the level of HLA genetic disparity between the donor and the recipient is probably the single most important factor: Among recipients of family member grafts, the incidence of acute GVHD is higher among recipients of 2 of 3 HLA loci—disparate grafts as compared with that observed among recipients of HLA-identical or a single locus–disparate marrow (5,50,76–84). Similarly, use of marrow derived from closely HLA-matched unrelated donors indicates that the incidence and severity of acute and chronic GVHD is increased for these patients (80,85–92).

The results observed in recipients of T-cell–depleted HLA-nonidentical marrow for treatment of congenital severe combined immunodeficiency (SCID) in patients who are at low risk for graft rejection indicate that methods of T-cell depletion that achieve a 3-$\log_{10}$ depletion of T cells can consistently prevent severe acute and chronic GVHD and provide long-term, disease-free survival (93,94). However, when these same methods for T-cell depletion are employed for patients with genetic immunodeficiencies other than SCID, 50% of patients fail to engraft despite pretransplant conditioning with busulfan (BU) and cyclophosphamide (CY) (95). Few of the initial pilot studies that evaluated the use of T-cell depletion for prevention of GVHD in leukemic recipients included patients with HLA-nonidentical donors (21,41,47). These few studies yielded results similar to those in patients with genetic immunodeficiencies other than SCID. Up to 50% of patients failed to engraft (21), and among those patients who did engraft the incidence of GVHD was reduced but not eliminated (47).

Graft Failure

Prior to the introduction of T-cell depletion, graft failure in recipients of HLA-identical marrow was almost exclusively limited to patients undergoing transplantation for treatment of aplastic anemia with a history of repeated transfusions (96–98). Among patients with leukemia who have received total body irradiation (TBI) and CY, the incidence of graft failure following a non T-cell–depleted transplant is less than 1% for recipients of HLA-matched marrow and 5% for recipients of marrow from an HLA-mismatched family member (5,76). In contrast, graft failures have been observed following every method of T-cell depletion, and the incidence ranges from 10 to 30% among recipients of HLA-identical marrow to as high as 50 to 75% among recipients of HLA-nonidentical marrow (15–21,77).

Retrospective analyses of recipients of T-cell–depleted HLA-identical marrow suggested several factors associated with graft failure: total dose of TBI, diagnosis, donor sex, donor/recipient sex match, and patient age. Three reports demonstrated an inverse relationship between the risk of graft failure and the amount of TBI (99–101). In contrast to the clear effect of dose of irradiation on engraftment, there are conflicting reports concerning the other factors. Whereas one report indicated that patients with CML were more likely to fail to engraft than patients with acute leukemia (99), another report indicated that the underlying diagnosis did not influence the rate of engraftment (102). The latter study also demonstrated a markedly increased risk of graft failure for recipients of marrow derived from male donors and for patients over the age of 25 years. Although pretransplant blood transfusions confer an increased risk of graft rejection in patients with aplastic anemia transplanted with non-T-cell–depleted marrow (103), a similar association has not been found among recipients of T-cell–depleted grafts (19,99,102).

At least three different hematopoietic patterns of graft failure have been observed (102,104): (1) failure to achieve an absolute neutrophil count of greater than or equal to 500/mm^3 for 3 consecutive days at any time after transplant associated with (Figure 11-1C) or without a lymphocytosis (Figure 11-1A); (2) initial engraftment with subsequent development of pancytopenia and marrow aplasia (Figure 11-1B); and (3) late graft failure with or without autologous marrow reconstitution (Figure 11-1D). Patterns 2 and 3 have been observed at the time of relapse in patients treated for leukemia, and such occurrences should not be considered true graft failures, but rather recurrence of disease. Each of the three patterns has been observed following HLA-identical, HLA-nonidentical, and closely HLA-matched unrelated donor marrow transplants. Although marrow manipulation could be responsible for graft failure, considerable experimental and clinical evidence suggests it is unlikely that stem-cell damage represents the predominant cause of graft failure. Rather, evidence suggests that failure to achieve initial engraftment results from immunological graft rejection that may be mediated by either cellular or humoral mechanisms (78,105–107).

It has been demonstrated in several studies that following marrow transplantation, NK cells are the first lymphoid population to recover in durably engrafted patients (108,109). In marked contrast, circulating peripheral blood cells found at the time of graft failure lack NK surface markers and function. Rather, surface phenotype analysis has revealed CD3$^+$, CD8$^+$, HLA-DR$^+$ T cells (78,110–112). At the time of lymphocytosis, T cells of host origin detected in the peripheral blood and marrow not only survived the cytoreduction regimen, but also have been shown to be functionally capable of responding in vitro when exposed to donor peripheral blood or marrow cells. For example, peripheral blood mononuclear cells obtained from a recipient of an HLA-D–mismatched marrow demonstrated a selective proliferative re-

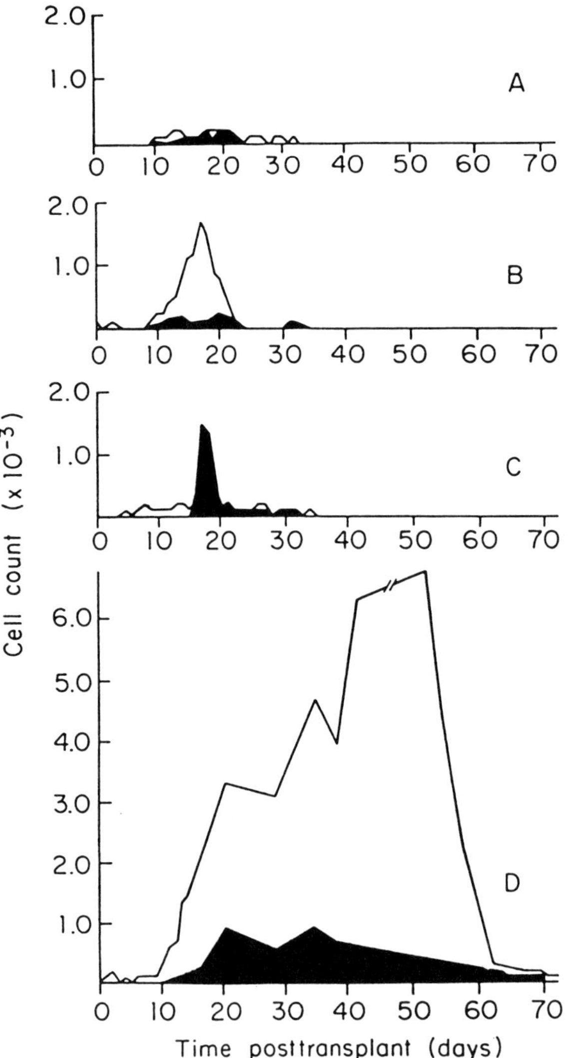

Figure 11-1. Patterns of leukocyte recovery following transplantation. *Solid lines* indicate total WBC count/mm^3; *shaded portions* indicate absolute lymphocyte count/mm^3.

sponse against donor cells in mixed lymphocyte culture, with a kinetic pattern suggesting a secondary response similar to that seen in an in vitro primed lymphocyte testing (82).

The correlation noted between the degree of HLA disparity unique to the marrow donor and the incidence of graft rejection (21) suggested that this complication may reflect immunological rejection with HLA antigen disparities serving as target antigens for host cytotoxic cells or antibodies. In one study, host T lymphocytes isolated at the time of graft failure following an HLA-nonidentical BMT demonstrated cell-mediated cytotoxicity against donor target cells, and peripheral blood lymphocytes from one patient exhibited allospecific cytotoxic reactivity directed against a single class I (HLA-B7) disparity unique to the donor (78). A similar study performed at the time of lymphocytosis in a patient treated with an HLA phenotypically matched unrelated donor demonstrated the emergence of host T lymphocytes; the target antigen for graft rejection was a variant at the HLA-B locus detectable by one-dimensional isoelectric focusing (110). The donor was HLA-B44.1 and the patient was HLA-B44.2. Of note, these two molecules differ from each other by only a single amino acid substitution (113).

Although a similar pattern of primary nonengraftment in association with T-cell lymphocytosis has been observed following infusion of T-cell–depleted HLA-identical marrow, these lymphocytes have not been shown to be cytotoxic toward donor peripheral blood targets in chromium release assays. However, a role for these cells in the pathogenesis of graft failure has been suggested by their ability to inhibit specifically donor marrow colony forming units in vitro (114,115) and, after in vitro expansion, to lyse donor-derived peripheral blood targets (116). The latter study suggested that minor histocompatibility antigen disparities between the patient and the donor triggered the rejection episode.

It is currently not clear whether the pathogenesis of secondary graft failure is the same as that for primary nonengraftment. Studies similar to those described suggest that the pathogenesis is different. Whereas primary nonengraftment appears to result from a host-mediated graft rejection, late graft failures have not necessarily been associated with an abrupt host-type lymphocytosis. Rather, grafts fail with a steady decline in the absolute neutrophil count (102). In addition, the circulating populations of cells are more likely to be a mixture of donor and host cells rather than only of host origin. In patients with viral infections, virus can infect marrow fibroblasts (117), and following T-cell–depleted transplants, cytomegalovirus (CMV)-associated failure has been observed (118). However, a viral etiology has not been identified in most instances of secondary or late graft failure.

Two unique cases of graft failure in association with acute GVHD have been described (119,120). Patients received T-cell–depleted marrow, showed signs of early engraftment, and then experienced lymphocytosis and pancytopenia with a rash and diarrhea, consistent with GVHD. With molecular techniques, lymphocytes derived from a third-party individual were identified.

All genetic studies performed on patients following a T-cell–depleted BMT have demonstrated a higher incidence of mixed chimerism in both hematopoietic and lymphoid cell populations as compared with that seen in recipients of non-T-cell–depleted grafts (121–125). The high incidence of mixed chimerism suggests that host hematopoietic and lymphoid cells are targets for and are eliminated by donor T cells. Thus, one approach to avoid graft rejection following a T-cell–depleted transplant is to utilize a method of T-cell–depletion that provides for a less complete removal of T cells (i.e., 2-$\log_{10}$ depletion rather than 3-$\log_{10}$ depletion). Using this approach, a method shown to eliminate acute GVHD among recipients of HLA-identical marrow and provide for engraftment of HLA-nonidentical marrow failed to protect these patients from severe acute or chronic GVHD (33). None of these patients received posttransplant immunosuppression. Two reports suggest that methods of T-cell depletion that provide for a 2-$\log_{10}$ depletion coupled with additional pretransplant immunosuppression (Ara-C) and posttransplant immunosuppression with cyclosporine (CSP) or antithymocyte globulin (ATG) and steroids allow for engraftment of haploidentical marrow or marrow from a closely HLA-matched unrelated donor, with a significant reduction in the incidence of acute GVHD to 20% and disease-free survival of up to 45% in individuals with leukemia (86,126). However, in these two studies, significant chronic GVHD developed in a high proportion of patients.

An alternate approach is possible with the physical methods of T-cell depletion. That is, a fixed number of lymphocytes obtained during the procedure can be added back to the final T-cell–depleted marrow. Using counterflow centrifugal elutriation, Wagner and associates (72) demonstrated that durable engraftment without the development of significant acute or chronic GVHD can be achieved with the addition of 0.5×10^6 lymphocytes/kg ideal body weight in recipients of HLA-identical marrow transplants. This approach has not yet been tested for recipients of HLA-mismatched or unrelated donor-recipient pairs.

With the possibility that donor T cells promote engraftment by elaborating specific cytokines, investigators are beginning to utilize cytokine infusions in the posttransplant period. Unfortunately, however, an initial trial with granulocyte-macrophage colony stimulating factor did not have an impact on the incidence of durable engraftment of T-cell–depleted marrow obtained by counterflow centrifugation elutriation (127). Clinical trials with other cytokines have yet to be reported.

Because host T cells have been identified at the time of immunological graft rejection and murine models of graft rejection suggested that elimination of residual host T cells with monoclonal antibodies in vivo promotes engraftment (36), the use of monoclonal antibodies has been explored (128–130). Thus far, the approach has been used successfully to promote engraftment without the development of GVHD in patients treated for immune disorders, but not in patients with leukemia.

Leukemic Relapse and Survival

Initial trials of transplantation of T-cell–depleted marrow included heterogenous groups of patients with varying diagnoses and stages of disease. When these uncontrolled trials suggested that the risk and severity of acute GVHD might be reduced following a T-cell–depleted marrow transplant, the UCLA group undertook a prospective randomized study to assess the effects of T-cell depletion of donor marrow using a monoclonal anti-T-cell antibody (CD2) and complement (17). Forty patients with acute leukemia in remission or CML in chronic or accelerated phase were randomized. Although recipients of T-cell–depleted marrow had a lower incidence of acute GVHD than control patients, they also had a higher incidence of graft failure and an apparent higher incidence of leukemic relapse. The latter observation, although not statistically significant, forced investigators to consider the possibility of an increased relapse rate among recipients of T-cell–depleted marrow and to perform T-cell depletion studies on carefully selected patient groups.

In 6 studies of T-cell depletion, 4 using an antibody-mediated method (33,71,74,131) and 2 using a physical method (70,72), the risk of hematological relapse was assessed for patients with acute leukemia undergoing transplantation in first remission. In each of these studies, the probability of relapse was less than 25%, an incidence comparable to that observed among recipients of unmodified marrow transplants for acute leukemia in early remission (132–134). Multivariate analysis indicated that neither acute nor chronic GVHD independently affected the probability of relapse of acute myelogenous leukemia (AML) when patients underwent transplantation in primary remission. Furthermore, in the report from the International Bone Marrow Transplant Registry (IBMTR) it was observed that in patients with AML in first CR, unmodified allograft recipients without GVHD had a significantly lower relapse rate than recipients of syngeneic grafts and that an antileukemic effect of an allograft for AML in primary CR was not abrogated by T-cell depletion (133).

Following standard preparatory regimens and infusion of an unmodified marrow transplant for acute leukemia, relapse rates between 15 and 75% have been reported for patients who received transplants in second or subsequent remission or in relapse. Because too few patients with advanced acute leukemia have been included in reported T-cell depletion trials, it is not possible to determine whether the use of T-cell depletion would adversely affect the probability of relapse in these patients.

In contrast to the results observed among recipients of T-cell–depleted marrow for acute leukemia, most such studies of patients with CML reported an increased risk of relapse. An increase in the rate of relapse following BMT for CML was first reported by Apperley and colleagues (135), who noted a higher rate of relapse among recipients of marrow depleted of T cells using the rat monoclonal CAMPATH-1M and autologous human serum as a source of complement for ex vivo treatment of marrow as compared with historical control subjects. This observation has been confirmed by additional investigators, as well as in a review from the IBMTR in which the relative risk (5.4) for relapse was significantly higher ($p < 0.0001$) for recipients of T-cell–depleted marrow compared with recipients of non-T-cell–depleted marrow (15,23). Separate analyses of patients with and without clinical evidence of acute or chronic GVHD confirmed an increased risk of relapse associated with T-cell depletion in all subgroups of patients. The latter observation suggested that the decreased GVHD produced by T-cell depletion does not entirely account for the increased relapse rate, and the mechanism by which T-cell depletion predisposes to relapse remains unclear. The finding is most consistent with a graft-versus-leukemia (GVL) effect that is independent of GVHD. The mechanism may be similar to that which accounts for a higher incidence of mixed chimerism in both hematopoietic and lymphoid cell populations as compared with that seen in recipients of non-T-cell–depleted grafts (121–125). That is, donor T cells (or NK cells) may eliminate residual leukemic cells as well as normal host hematopoietic and lymphoid cells (see Chapter 19). Despite its impact on the probability of relapse, T-cell depletion did not significantly affect overall probability of survival or leukemia-free survival in these studies because use of T-cell depletion offset the morbidity associated with acute and chronic GVHD (17,23,136).

Those investigators who have continued to utilize T-cell depletion for prevention of GVHD have aimed to overcome the loss of the GVL effect with approaches similar to those described for improving the rate of durable engraftment (i.e., utilization of a method of T-cell depletion that provides for a less complete removal of T cells or intensification of the pretransplant regimen). Notably, one approach utilized by Champlin and associates (71) demonstrated that with selective depletion of CD8-positive T cells and posttransplant immunosuppression with CSP, the incidence of GVHD could be reduced without a concomitant increase in relapse in patients with CML. Alternatively, addition of Ara-C or thiotepa to standard TBI and CY has been associated with a decrease in the rate of relapse (33,86,137). Although these results are promising, they are preliminary and await follow-up to evaluate the long-term impact on disease-free survival.

In the same manner that investigators are exploring the use of hematopoietic growth factors to promote engraftment, the use of in vivo administration of immunomodulatory cytokines to stimulate the GVL effect may decrease the relapse rate. IL-2 activates T and NK cells, both of which are believed to have a role in the GVL effect. In vitro studies have demonstrated that IL-2 can induce GVL activity in peripheral blood lymphocytes after transplantation against autologous cryopreserved CML cells (138,139). In animal models, IL-2 has been utilized to promote the antineoplastic effect of GVL following receipt of T-cell–depleted marrow (140). Furthermore, a pilot clinical trial with infusions of low-dose recombinant IL-2 following autologous or T-cell–depleted allogeneic BMT demonstrated that the number of NK cells can be expanded and the GVL activity in vitro can be stimulated without inducing GVHD (141). What impact posttransplant infusions of IL-2 will have on disease relapse remains to be determined.

Immunological Reconstitution

Following BMT, all patients experience a period of profound immunodeficiency (see Chapter 36). GVHD and its treatment further delay immune recovery. By reducing the incidence and severity of GVHD, T-cell depletion might benefit immune reconstitution. Such a benefit may be counteracted by the removal of functionally mature cells from the treated marrow graft. The few published studies demonstrate that there are modest quantitative and temporal differences in the reconstitution of some but not all immune functions following T-cell–depleted BMT as compared with non-T-cell–depleted marrow recipients (142–154). However, in most studies, the minimal effect on the kinetics of immune reconstitution did not appear to result in significant differences in the incidence or types of posttransplant infectious complications.

B-cell Lymphoproliferative Disorders

Although there is little reported evidence of an increased risk of infectious complications in durably engrafted recipients of T-cell–depleted marrow, there is some evidence that the incidence of Epstein-Barr virus (EBV)–associated B-cell lymphoproliferative disorders may be increased (33,155,156). This life-threatening complication of BMT occurs primarily but not exclusively in recipients of HLA-nonidentical T-cell–depleted marrow. Among 87 recipients of marrow depleted of T cells with anti-CD5, the actuarial probability for development of a lymphoproliferative disorder was 12% at 7 years (33), which is substantially higher than that observed among recipients of non-T-cell–depleted marrow (0.6%) (156). EBV has been implicated in virtually all cases of posttransplant lymphoma, usually of donor-cell origin. Because EBV-specific cytotoxic T lymphocytes are believed to be the primary mechanism for controlling the proliferation of EBV-infected lymphocytes (157), the increased incidence of this complication may reflect an impaired reconstitution of cytotoxic precursor cells noted during the first 6 months following infusion of T-cell–depleted marrow (154).

Conclusions

T-cell depletion has been shown to be the most effective approach for reducing or eliminating GVHD. Patients with congenital disorders have benefitted the most from these procedures (see Chapter 64). However, for patients with leukemia, the benefits of less GVHD and no posttransplant immunosuppression have been offset by an increase in the incidence of graft failure and relapse in patients with CML. Clinical trials have not provided insight into whether the T lymphocytes responsible for initiating GVHD are the same as or distinct from those that promote engraftment or are required for antileukemic activity. However, several investigators are pursuing studies to evaluate the effect of depletion of selected T-cell subsets. Additional immunosuppressive and antileukemic agents, whose toxicity may be tolerated when methotrexate and CSP are not utilized in the posttransplant period, are being evaluated. Infusions of hematopoietic growth factors as well as immunomodulatory agents with antileukemic potential are also being studied.

References

1. Storb R, Deeg HJ, Fisher L, et al. Cyclosporine versus methotrexate for graft-versus-host disease prevention in patients given marrow grafts for leukemia: long-term follow-up of three controlled trials. Blood 1988; 71:293–298.
2. Bross DS, Tutschka PJ, Farmer ER, et al. Predictive factors for acute GvHD in patients transplanted with HLA-identical bone marrow. Blood 1984;63:1265–1270.
3. Sullivan KM, Deeg HJ, Sanders JE, et al. Late complications after marrow transplantation. Semin Hematol 1984;21:53–63.
4. Ringden O, Nilsson B. Death by graft-versus-host disease associated with HLA mismatch, high recipient age, low marrow cell dose, and splenectomy. Transplantation 1985;40:39–44.
5. Beatty PG, Clift RA, Mickelson EM, et al. Marrow transplantation from related donors other than HLA-identical siblings. N Engl J Med 1985;313:765–771.
6. Uphoff D. Preclusion of secondary phase of irradiation syndrome by inoculation of fetal hematopoietic tissue following lethal total body x-irradiation. J Natl Cancer Inst 1958;20:625.
7. Bortin MM, Saltzstein EC. Graft versus host inhibition: fetal liver and thymus cells minimize secondary disease. Science 1969;164:316–318.
8. Rodt H, Thierfelder S, Eulitz M. Anti-lymphocyte antibodies and marrow transplantation. III. Effect of heterologous anti-brain antibodies in acute secondary disease in mice. J Immunol 1974;4:25–29.
9. Kolb HJ, Rieder I, Rodt H, et al. Anti-lymphocyte antibodies and bone marrow transplantation. VI. Graft versus host tolerance in DLA-incompatible dogs following in vitro treatment of bone marrow with absorbed anti-thymocyte globulin. Transplantation 1979;27: 242–245.

10. Vallera DA, Soderling CCR, Carlson GJ, Kersey JH. Bone marrow transplantation across major histocompatibility barriers in mice. Effects of elimination of T cells from donor grafts by pretreatment with monoclonal thy1-2 plus complement or antibody alone. Transplantation 1981;31:218–222.
11. Reisner Y, Itsicovitch L, Meshorer A, Sharon N. Hematopoietic stem cell transplantation using mouse bone marrow and spleen cells fractionated by lectins. Proc Natl Acad Sci USA 1978;75:2933.
12. Rodt H, Kolb HJ, Netzel B, et al. Effect of anti-T-cell globulin on graft-versus-host disease in leukemia patients treated with BMT. Transplant Proc 1981;13:257–261.
13. Reisner Y, Kirkpatrick D, Dupont B, Kapoor N, Pollack MS, Good RA. Transplantation for acute leukemia with HLA-A and B nonidentical parental marrow cells fractionated with soybean agglutinin and sheep red blood cells. Lancet 1981;2:327–331.
14. Reisner Y, Kapoor N, Kirkpatrick D, et al. Transplantation for severe combined immunodeficiency with HLA-A, B, D, DR incompatible parental marrow cells fractionated by soybean agglutinin and sheep red blood cells. Blood 1983;61:341–348.
15. Hale G, Cobbold S, Waldmann H. T cell depletion with Campath-1 in allogeneic bone marrow transplantation. Transplantation 1988;45:753–759.
16. Patterson J, Prentice HG, Brenner MK, et al. Graft rejection following HLA matched T-lymphocyte depleted bone marrow transplantation. Br J Haematol 1986;63:221–230.
17. Mitsuyasu RT, Champlin RE, Gale RP, et al. Treatment of donor bone marrow with monoclonal anti-T-cell antibody and complement for the prevention of graft-versus-host disease: a prospective, randomized, double-blind trial. Ann Intern Med 1986;105:20–26.
18. Filipovich AH, Vallera DA, Youle RJ, et al. Graft-versus-host disease prevention in allogeneic bone marrow transplantation from histocompatible siblings. Transplantation 1987;44:62–69.
19. Martin PJ, Hansen JA, Buckner CD, et al. Effects of in vitro depletion of T cells in HLA-identical allogeneic marrow grafts. Blood 1985;66:664–672.
20. O'Reilly RJ, Collins NH, Brochstein J, et al. Soybean lectin agglutination and E rosette depletion for removal of T cells from HLA identical marrow grafts: results in 60 consecutive patients transplanted for hematopoietic malignancy. In: Hagenbeck A, Lowenberg B, eds. Minimal residual disease in acute leukemia. The Netherlands: Martinus Nijhoff, 1986:337–433.
21. O'Reilly RJ, Collins NH, Kernan NA, et al. Transplantation of marrow depleted of T cells by soybean lectin agglutination and E rosette depletion: major histocompatibility complex-related graft resistance in leukemic transplant recipients. Transplant Proc 1985;17: 455–459.
22. Kantoff PW, Gillio A, McLachlin JR, et al. Expression of human adenosine deaminase in non-human primates after retroviral mediated gene transfer. J Exp Med 1987;166:219–234.
23. Goldman JM, Gale RP, Horowitz MM, et al. Bone marrow transplantation for chronic myelogenous leukemia in chronic phase. Ann Intern Med 1988;108:806–814.
24. Thomas ED. Marrow transplantation for malignant diseases. J Clin Oncol 1983;1:517–531.
25. Sullivan KM, Deeg HJ, Sanders J, et al. Hyperacute GVHD in patients not given immunosuppression after allogeneic marrow transplantation. Blood 1986;67: 1172–1175.
26. Knott LJ, Levinsky RJ, Newland A, Jones HM, Linch DC. Bone marrow T-cell colony forming cells: studies of their origin and use in monitoring T cell depleted bone marrow grafts. Clin Exp Immunol 1985;62:561–569.
27. Kernan NA, Flomenberg N, Collins NH, O'Reilly RJ, Dupont B. Quantitation of T-lymphocytes in human bone marrow by a limiting dilution assay. Transplantation 1985;40:317–322.
28. Martin PJ, Hansen JA. Quantitative assays for detection of residual T cells in T-depleted human marrow. Blood 1985;65:1134–1140.
29. Rozans MK, Smith BR, Emerson S, et al. Functional assessment of T cell depletion from bone marrow prior to therapeutic transplantation using limiting dilution culture methods. Transplantation 1986;42:380–386.
30. Irle C, Kaetli M, Aapro M, Chapins B, Jeannet M. Quantity and nature of residual bone marrow T-cells after treatment of the marrow with Campath-1. Exp Hematol 1987;15:163–170.
31. Kernan NA, Collins NH, Juliano L, Cartagena BS, Dupont B, O'Reilly RJ. Clonable T lymphocytes in T-cell depleted bone marrow transplants correlate with development of graft versus host disease. Blood 1986;68:770–773.
32. Atkinson K, Farrelly H, Cooley M, O'Flaherty E, Downs K, Biggs J. Human marrow T cell dose correlates with severity of subsequent acute graft-versus-host disease. Bone Marrow Transplant 1987;2:51–57.
33. Antin JH, Bierer BE, Smith BR, et al. Selective depletion of bone marrow T lymphocytes with anti-CD5 monoclonal antibodies: effective prophylaxis for graft-versus-host disease in patients with hematologic malignancies. Blood 1991;78:2139–2149.
34. Korngold R, Sprent J. T cell subsets and graft-versus-host disease. Transplantation 1987;44:335–339.
35. Korngold R, Sprent J. Variable capacity of L3T4+ T cells to cause lethal graft-versus-host disease across minor histocompatibility barriers in mice. J Exp Med 1987;165:1552–1564.
36. Cobbold SP, Martin G, Qin S, Waldmann H. Monoclonal antibodies to promote marrow engraftment and tissue graft tolerance. Nature 1986;323:164–166.
37. Bernard A, Boumsell L, Hill C. Joint report of the First International Workshop on human leucocyte differentiation antigens by the investigators of the participating laboratories. In: Bernard A, Boumsell L, Dausset J, Milstein C, Schlossman SF, eds. Leucocyte typing. New York: Springer-Verlag, 1984:9–142.
38. Haynes BF. Summary of T cell studies performed during the Second International Workshop and conference on human leukocyte differentiation antigens. In: Reinherz EL, Haynes BF, Nadler LM, Bernstein ID, eds. Leucocyte typing. New York: Springer-Verlag, 1986:3–20.
39. McMichael AJ, Gotch FM. T-cell antigens: new and previously defined clusters. In: McMichael AJ, ed. Leucocyte typing III, white cell differentiation antigens. Oxford: Oxford University Press, 1987:31–62.
40. Parkman R. The application of bone marrow transplantation to the treatment of genetic diseases. Science 1986;232:1373–1378.
41. Prentice HG, Janossy G, Skeggs D, Blacklock HA, Bradstock KF, Goldstein G. Use of anti-T-cell monoclonal antibody OKT3 to prevent acute graft-versus-host disease in allogeneic bone marrow transplantation for acute leukemia. Lancet 1982;1:700–703.

42. Filipovich AH, McGlave PB, Ramsay NKC, Goldstein G, Warkentin PI, Kersey JH. Pretreatment of donor bone marrow with monoclonal antibody OKT3 for prevention of acute graft-versus-host disease in allogeneic histocompatible bone marrow transplantation. Lancet 1982;1:1266–1269.
43. Martin PJ, Hansen JA, Thomas ED. Preincubation of donor bone marrow cells with a combination of murine monoclonal anti-T-cell antibodies without complement does not prevent graft-versus-host disease after allogeneic marrow transplantation. J Clin Immunol 1984;4:18–22.
44. Prentice HG, Janossy G, Price-Jones L, et al. Depletion of T lymphocytes in donor marrow prevents significant graft-versus-host disease in matched allogeneic leukemic marrow transplant recipients. Lancet 1984;1:472–475.
45. Waldmann HG, Hale G, Cividalli G, et al. Elimination of graft-versus-host disease by in vitro depletion of alloreactive lymphocytes with a monoclonal rat anti-human lymphocyte antibody (Campath-1). Lancet 1984;2:483–486.
46. Herve P, Flesch M, Cahn JY, et al. Removal of marrow T cells with OKT3-OKT11 monoclonal antibodies and complement to prevent graft-versus-host disease. Transplantation 1985;39:138–143.
47. Trigg ME, Billing R, Sondel PM, et al. Clinical trial depleting T lymphocytes from donor marrow for matched and mismatched allogeneic bone marrow transplants. Cancer Treat Rep 1985;69:377–386.
48. Maraninchi D, Mawas C, Guyotat D, et al. Selective depletion of marrow T cytotoxic lymphocytes (CD8) in the prevention of graft-versus-host disease after allogeneic bone marrow transplantation. Transplant Int 1988;1:91–94.
49. Gilmore MJML, Prentice HG, Price-Jones E, et al. Allogeneic bone marrow transplantation: the monitoring of granulocyte macrophage colonies following the collection of bone marrow mononuclear cells and after the subsequent in-vitro cytolysis of OKT3 lymphocytes. Br J Haematol 1983;55:587–593.
50. Cahn JY, Herve P, Flesch M, et al. Marrow transplantation from HLA non-identical family donors for the treatment of leukemia: a pilot study of 15 patients using additional immunosuppression and T-cell depletion. Br J Haematol 1988;69:345–349.
51. Filipovich AH, Youle RJ, Neville DM, Vallera DA, Quinones RR, Kersey JH. Ex-vivo treatment of donor bone marrow with anti-T-cell immunotoxins for prevention of graft-versus-host-disease. Lancet 1984;1: 469–472.
52. Filipovich AH, Vallera D, McGlave P, et al. T cell depletion with anti-CD5 immunotoxin in histocompatible bone marrow transplantation. Transplantation 1990;50:410–415.
53. Laurent G, Maraninchi D, Gluckman E, et al. Donor bone marrow treatment with T101 Fab fragment-ricin A-chain immunotoxin prevents graft-versus-host disease. Bone Marrow Transplant 1989;4:367–371.
54. Martin PJ, Hansen JA, Torok-Storb B, et al. Effects of treating marrow with a CD3-specific immunotoxin for prevention of acute graft-versus-host disease. Bone Marrow Transplant 1988;3:437–444.
55. Vartdal F, Albrechtsen D, Ringden O, et al. Immunomagnetic treatment of bone marrow allografts. Bone Marrow Transplant 1987;2:94–98.
56. Kernan NA, Henslee J, Blazar B, et al. Evaluation of an anti-T-cell immunotoxin in treatment of chronic graft-versus-host disease (abstract). Third International Conference on Monoclonal Antibody Immunoconjugates for Cancer, San Diego, CA, February 4–6, 1988.
57. Byers V, Henslee P, Kernan NA, et al. Therapeutic response to a pan-T-lymphocyte monoclonal antibody-ricin A chain immunotoxin in steroid refractory graft versus host disease (GvHD) (abstract). Blood 1987; 70:304a.
58. Noga SJ, Donnenberg AD, Schwartz CL, Strauss LC, Civin CI, Santos GW. Development of a simplified counterflow centrifugation elutriation procedure for depletion of lymphocytes from human bone marrow. Transplantation 1986;41:220–229.
59. Wagner JE, Donnenberg AD, Noga SJ, et al. Lymphocyte depletion of donor bone marrow by counterflow centrifugal elutriation: results of a Phase I clinical trial. Blood 1988;72:1168–1176.
60. De Witte T, Raymakers R, Plas A, Koekman E, Wessels H, Haanen C. Bone marrow repopulation capacity after transplantation of lymphocyte-depleted allogeneic bone marrow using counterflow centrifugation. Transplantation 1984;37:151–155.
61. Collins NH, Kernan NA, Bleau SA, O'Reilly RJ. T cell depletion of allogeneic human bone marrow grafts by soybean lectin agglutination and either sheep red blood cell rosetting or adherence on the CD5/CD8 collector. In: Gee A, ed. Bone marrow processing and purging. Florida: CRC Press, 1991:201–212.
62. Frame JN, Collins NH, Cartagena T, Waldmann H, O'Reilly RJ, Kernan NA. T cell depletion of human bone marrow: comparison of Campath-1 plus complement, anti-T cell ricin A chain immunotoxin, and soybean agglutinin alone or in combination with sheep erythrocytes or immunomagnetic beads. Transplantation 1989; 47:984–988.
63. Lowenberg B, Wagemaker E, van Bekkum DW, et al. Graft-versus-host disease following transplantation of "one log" versus "two log" T-lymphocyte depleted bone marrow from HLA-identical donors. Bone Marrow Transplant 1986;1:133–140.
64. Voltarelli JC, Corpuz S, Martin PJ. In vitro comparison of two methods of T cell depletion associated with different rate of graft failure after allogeneic marrow transplantation. Bone Marrow Transplant 1990;6:419–423.
65. Keever CA, Pekle K, Gazzola MV, Collins NH, Gillio A. NK and LAK activities from human marrow progenitors. I. The effect of interleukin-1 and interleukin-2. Cell Immunol 1990;126:211.
66. Keever CA, Pekle K, Gazzola MV, Collins NH, Bourhis NH, Gillio A. Natural killer and lymphokine-activated killer cell activities from human marrow precursors. II. The effect of IL-3 and IL-4. J Immunol 1989;143: 3241.
67. Welte K, Ciobanu N, Moore MAS, Gulati S, O'Reilly RJ, Mertelsmann R. Defective interleukin-2 production in patients after bone marrow transplantation and in vitro restoration of defective T lymphocyte proliferation by highly purified interleukin-2. Blood 1984;64:380.
68. Glucksberg H, Storb R, Fefer A, et al. Clinical manifestations of graft-versus-host disease in human recipients of marrow from HLA matched sibling donors. Transplantation 1974;18:295–304.
69. Soiffer RJ, Murray C, Mauch P, et al. Prevention of graft-versus-host disease by selective depletion of CD6-positive T lymphocytes from donor bone marrow. J Clin Oncol 1992;10:1191–1200.

70. Young JW, Papadopoulos EB, Cunningham I, et al. T-cell-depleted allogeneic bone marrow transplantation in adults with acute nonlymphocytic leukemia in first remission. Blood 1992;79:3380–3387.
71. Champlin R, Ho W, Gajewski J, et al. Selective depletion of CD8+ T lymphocytes for prevention of graft-versus-host disease after allogeneic bone marrow transplantation. Blood 1990;76:418–423.
72. Wagner JE, Santos GW, Noga SJ, et al. Bone marrow graft engineering by counterflow centrifugal elutriation: results of a phase I-II clinical trial. Blood 1990;75:1370–1377.
73. Atkinson K, Horowitz MM, Gale RP, et al. Risk factors for chronic graft-versus-host disease after HLA-identical sibling bone marrow transplantation. Blood 1990;75: 2459–2464.
74. Hale G, Waldmann H. Campath-1 for prevention of graft-versus-host disease and graft rejection. Summary of results from a multi-centre study. Bone Marrow Transplant 1988;3:11–14.
75. Gale RP, Bortin MM, van Bekkum DW, et al. Risk factors for acute graft-versus-host disease. Br J Haematol 1987;65:397–406.
76. Powles RL, Kay HEM, Clink HM, et al. Mismatched family donor for bone marrow transplantation as treatment for acute leukemia. Lancet 1983;1: 612–615.
77. Bozdech MJ, Sondel PM, Trigg ME, et al. Transplantation of HLA-haploidentical T-cell-depleted marrow for leukemia: addition of cytosine arabinoside to the pretransplant conditioning prevents rejection. Exp Hematol 1985;13:1201–1210.
78. Kernan NA, Flomenberg N, Dupont B, O'Reilly RJ. Graft rejection in recipients of T cell depleted HLA non-identical transplants for leukemia: identification of host derived anti-donor allocytotoxic T-lymphocytes. Transplantation 1987;43:482–487.
79. Anasetti C, Amos D, Beatty PG, et al. Effect of HLA compatibility on engraftment of bone marrow transplants in patients with leukemia or lymphoma. N Engl J Med 1989;320:197–204.
80. Camitta B, Ash R, Menitove J, Murray K, Lawton C, Casper J. Bone marrow transplantation for children with severe aplastic anemia: use of donors other than HLA-identical siblings. Blood 1989;74:1852–1857.
81. Shapiro RS. Epstein-Barr virus associated B-cell lymphoproliferative disorders in immunodeficiency: meeting the challenge. J Clin Oncol 1990;8:371–373.
82. Sondel PM, Hank JA, Trigg ME, et al. Transplantation of HLA-haploidentical T-cell-depleted marrow for leukemia: autologous marrow recovery with specific immune sensitization to donor antigens. Exp Hematol 1986;14:278–286.
83. Atkinson K, Farewell V, Storb R, et al. Analysis of late infections after human bone marrow transplantation: role of genotypic nonidentity between marrow donor and recipient and of nonspecific suppressor cells in patients with chronic graft-versus-host disease. Blood 1982;60:714–720.
84. Bunin NJ, Casper JT, Chitambar C, et al. Partially matched bone marrow transplantation in patients with myelodysplastic syndromes. J Clin Oncol 1988;6: 1851–1855.
85. Mackinnon S, Hows JM, Goldman JM, et al. Bone marrow transplantation for chronic myeloid leukemia: the use of histocompatible unrelated volunteer donors. Exp Hematol 1990;18:421–425.
86. Ash RC, Casper JT, Chitambar CR, et al. Successful allogeneic transplantation of T-cell depleted bone marrow from closely HLA-matched unrelated donors. N Engl J Med 1990;322:485–494.
87. Beatty PG, Hansen JA, Longton GM, et al. Marrow transplantation from HLA-matched unrelated donors for treatment of hematologic malignancies. Transplantation 1991;51:443–447.
88. Gajewski JL, Ho WG, Feig SA, Hunt L, Kaufman N, Champlin RE. Bone marrow transplantation using unrelated donors for patients with advanced leukemia or bone marrow failure. Transplantation 1990;50:244–249.
89. Gingrich RD, Ginder GD, Goeken NE, et al. Allogenic marrow grafting with partially mismatched, unrelated marrow donors. Blood 1988;71:1375–1381.
90. Howard MR, Hows JM, Gore SM, et al. Unrelated donor marrow transplantation between 1977 and 1987 at four centers in the United Kingdom. Transplantation 1990;49:547–553.
91. Hows JM, Yin JL, Marsh J, et al. Histocompatible unrelated volunteer donors compared with HLA nonidentical family donors in marrow transplantation for aplastic anemia and leukemia. Blood 1986;68:1322–1328.
92. McGlave PB, Beatty P, Ash R, Hows JM. Therapy for chronic myelogenous leukemia with unrelated donor bone marrow transplantation: results in 102 cases. Blood 1990;75:1728–1732.
93. Fischer A, Durandy A, de Villartay JP, et al. HLA-haploidentical bone marrow transplantation for severe combined immunodeficiency using E rosette fractionation and cyclosporine. Blood 1986;67:444–449.
94. O'Reilly RJ, Keever CA, Small TN, Brochstein J. The use of HLA-non-identical T-cell-depleted marrow transplants for correction of severe combined immunodeficiency disease. Immunodeficiency Rev 1989;1:273–309.
95. Fischer A, Griscelli C, Friedrich W, et al. Bone marrow transplantation for immunodeficiencies and osteopetrosis: European survey, 1968–1985. Lancet 1986;2:1080–1083.
96. Storb R, Prentice RL, Thomas ED, et al. Factors associated with graft rejection after HLA-identical marrow transplantation for aplastic anemia. Br J Haematol 1983;55:573.
97. Champlin RE, Feig SA, Ho WG, Gale RP. Graft failure following bone marrow transplantation: its biology and treatment. Exp Hematol 1984;12:728.
98. Deeg HJ, Self S, Storb R, et al. Decreased incidence of marrow graft rejection in patients with severe aplastic anemia: changing impact of risk factors. Blood 1986;68:1363–1368.
99. Martin PJ, Hansen JA, Torok-Storb B, et al. Graft failure in patients receiving T cell depleted HLA-identical allogeneic marrow transplants. Bone Marrow Transplant 1988;3:445.
100. Patterson J, Prentice HG, Brenner MK, et al. Graft rejection following HLA matched T lymphocyte depleted bone marrow transplantation. Br J Haematol 1986;63:221–230.
101. Guyotat D, Dutou L, Erhsam A, Campos L, Archimbaud E, Fiere D. Graft rejection after T cell-depleted marrow transplantation. Br J Haematol 1987;65:499–507.
102. Kernan NA, Bordignon C, Heller G, et al. Graft failure following T cell depleted HLA-identical marrow transplants for leukemia: analysis of risk factors and results of secondary transplants. Blood 1989;74:2227–2236.

103. Champlin RE, Horowitz MM, van Bekkum DW, et al. Graft failure following bone marrow transplantation for severe aplastic anemia: risk factors and treatment results. Blood 1989;73:606–613.
104. Kernan NA, Flomenberg N, Dupont B, O'Reilly RJ. Identification of cytotoxic T lymphocytes in patients rejecting T cell depleted bone marrow transplants for leukemia (abstract). Blood 1984;64:208a.
105. Bordignon C, Kernan NA, Keever CA, et al. Graft failures following T-cell depleted grafts for leukemia: emergence of host T-lymphocytes (CD3 CD8+) with donor-specific reactivity (abstract). Blood 1987;70: 303a.
106. Speck B, Zwaan FE, van Rood JJ, Eernisse JG. Allogeneic bone marrow transplantation in a patient with aplastic anemia using a phenotypically HLA-A-identical unrelated donor. Transplantation 1973;16: 24–28.
107. Barge AJ, Johnson G, Witherspoon R, Torok-Storb B. Antibody-mediated marrow failure after allogeneic bone marrow transplantation. Blood 1989;74:1477–1480.
108. Keever CA, Welte K, Small T, et al. Interleukin 2-activated killer cells in patients following transplants of soybean lectin separated and E rosette depleted bone marrow. Blood 1987;70:1893–1903.
109. Brenner MK, Reittie JE, Grob J-P, et al. The contribution of large granular lymphocytes to B cell activation and differentiation after T-cell-depleted allogeneic bone marrow transplantation. Transplantation 1986;42:257–261.
110. Fleischhauer K, Kernan NA, O'Reilly RJ, Dupont B, Yang SY. Bone marrow allograft rejection by host-derived allocytotoxic T lymphocytes recognizes a single amino acid at position 156 of the HLA-B44 class I antigen. N Engl J Med 1990;323:1818–1822.
111. Kernan NA, Bordignon C, Keever CA, et al. Graft failure after T cell depleted marrow transplants for leukemia: clinical and in vitro characteristics. Transplant Proc 1987;19:29–32.
112. Sandell L, Johnson G, Przepiorka D, Torok-Storb B. Phenotype and function of T-cells associated with marrow graft failure and rejection. In: Martelli MF, Grignani F, Reisner Y, eds. T-cell depletion in allogeneic bone marrow transplantation. Rome, Italy: Ares-Serono Symposia, 1988:49–56.
113. Fleischhauer K, Kernan NA, Dupont B, Yang SY. The two major subtypes of HLA-B44 differ for a single amino acid in codon 156. Tissue Antigens 1991;37: 133–137.
114. Bordignon C, Keever CA, Small T, Dupont B, O'Reilly RJ, Kernan NA. Graft failure following T cell depleted HLA-identical marrow transplants for leukemia: in vitro analyses of host effector mechanisms. Blood 1989;74:2237–2243.
115. Bunjes D, Heit W, Arnold R, et al. Evidence of the involvement of host-derived OKT8-positive T cells in the rejection of T-depleted, HLA-identical bone marrow grafts. Transplantation 1987;43:501–505.
116. Marijt WAF, Falkenburg JHF, Diaz-Barrientos T, et al. Multiple minor histocompatibility (mH) antigen specificities recognized by cytotoxic T lymphocyte (CTL) clones, mediating graft rejection (GR) after HLA-genotypically identical (HLA-GID) bone marrow transplantation (BMT) (abstract). Blood 1991;78:401a.
117. Torok-Storb B, Simmons P, Przepiorka D. Impairment of hemopoiesis in human allografts. Transplant Proc 1987;19:33–37.
118. Emanuel D, Kernan NA, Castro-Malaspina H, et al. Cytomegalovirus-associated bone marrow failure after allogeneic bone marrow transplantation successfully treated with combination of gancyclovir and high dose CMV immune globulin (abstract). Blood 1989;74:905a.
119. Sproul AM, Chalmers EA, Mills KI, Burnett AK, Simpson E. Third party mediated graft rejection despite irradiation of blood products. Br J Haematol 1992;80:251–262.
120. Drobyski W, Thibodeau S, Truitt RL, et al. Third party-mediated graft rejection and graft-versus-host disease after T-cell-depleted bone marrow transplantation, as demonstrated by hypervariable DNA probes and HLA-DR polymorphism. Blood 1989;74:2285–2294.
121. Bretagne S, Vidaud M, Kuentz M, et al. Mixed blood chimerism in T cell-depleted bone marrow transplant recipients: evaluation using DNA polymorphisms. Blood 1987;70:1692–1695.
122. Lawler SD, Harris H, Millar J, Barrett-Powles RL. Cytogenetic follow-up studies of recipients of T-cell depleted allogeneic bone marrow. Br J Haematol 1987;65:143.
123. Bertheas MF, Maraninchi D, Lafage M, et al. Partial chimerism after T-cell depleted allogeneic bone marrow transplantation in leukemic HLA-matched patients: a cytogenetic documentation. Blood 1988;72:89–93.
124. Schouten HC, Sizoo W, van't Veer MB, Hagenbeek A, Lowenberg B. Incomplete chimerism in erythroid, myeloid and B lymphocyte lineage after T cell-depleted allogeneic bone marrow transplantation. Bone Marrow Transplant 1988;3:407–412.
125. Offit K, Burns JP, Cunningham I, et al. Cytogenetic analysis of chimerism and leukemia relapse in chronic myelogenous leukemia patients following T cell depleted bone marrow transplantation. Blood 1990;75:1346–1355.
126. Trigg ME, Gingrich R, Goeken N, et al. Low rejection rate when using unrelated or haploidentical donors for children with leukemia undergoing marrow transplantation. Bone Marrow Transplant 1989;89:431–437.
127. De Witte T, Gratwohl A, Van Der Lely N, et al. Recombinant human granulocyte-macrophage colony-stimulating factor accelerates neutrophil and monocyte recovery after allogeneic T-cell-depleted bone marrow transplantation. Blood 1992;79:1359–1365.
128. Fischer A, Friedrich W, Fasth A, et al. Reduction of graft failure by a monoclonal antibody (anti-LFA-1 CD11a) after HLA nonidentical bone marrow transplantation in children with immunodeficiencies, osteopetrosis, and Fanconi's anemia: a European group for immunodeficiency/European group for bone marrow transplantation report. Blood 1991;77:249–256.
129. Baume D, Kuentz M, Pico JL, et al. Failure of a CD18/anti-LFA1 monoclonal antibody infusion to prevent graft rejection in leukemic patients receiving T-depleted allogeneic bone marrow transplantation. Transplantation 1989;47:472–474.
130. Willemze R, Richel DJ, Falkenburg JHF, et al. In vivo use of Campath-1G to prevent graft-versus-host disease and graft rejection after bone marrow transplantation. Bone Marrow Transplant 1992;9:255–261.
131. Prentice HG, Brenner MK. Donor marrow T cell depletion for prevention of GvHD without loss of the GvL effect. Current results in acute myeloblastic

leukaemia and future directions. In: Gale RP, Champlin RE, eds. Bone marrow transplantation: current controversies. New York: Alan R. Liss, 1989:117.

132. McGlave PB, Haake RJ, Bostron BC, et al. Allogeneic bone marrow transplantation for acute nonlymphocytic leukemia in first remission. Blood 1988;72:1512–1517.

133. Horowitz MM, Gale RP, Sondel PM, et al. Graft-versus-leukemia reactions after bone marrow transplantation. Blood 1990;75:555–562.

134. Sullivan KM, Weiden PL, Storb R, et al. Influence of acute and chronic graft-versus-host disease on relapse and survival after bone marrow transplantation from HLA-identical siblings as treatment of acute and chronic leukemia. Blood 1989;73:1720–1728.

135. Apperley JF, Jones L, Hale G, et al. Bone marrow transplantation for patients with chronic myeloid leukemia: T-cell depletion with Campath-1 reduces the incidence of graft-versus-host disease but may increase the risk of leukemic relapse. Bone Marrow Transplant 1986;1:53–66.

136. Ash RC, Horowitz MM, Gale RP, et al. Bone marrow transplantation from related donors other than HLA-identical siblings: effect of T cell depletion. Bone Marrow Transplant 1991;7:443–452.

137. Aversa F, Pelicci PG, Terenzi A, et al. Results of T-depleted BMT in chronic myelogenous leukaemia after a conditioning regimen that included thiotepa. Bone Marrow Transplant 1991;7:24.

138. Hauch M, Gazzola MV, Small T, et al. Anti-leukemia potential of interleukin-2 activated natural killer cells after bone marrow transplantation for chronic myelogenous leukemia. Blood 1990;75:2250–2262.

139. Mackinnon S, Hows JM, Goldman JM. Induction of in vitro graft-versus-leukemia activity following bone marrow transplantation for chronic myeloid leukemia. Blood 1992;76:2037–2041.

140. Brochstein JA, Kernan NA, Laver J, Emanuel D, Rabelinno E, O'Reilly RJ. Bone marrow transplantation for thrombocytopenia-absent radii (TAR) syndrome (abstract). Proceedings of the XXI Congress of the International Society of Hematology, Sydney, Australia, May 11–16, 1986.

141. Soiffer RJ, Murray C, Cochran K, et al. Clinical and immunologic effects of prolonged infusion of low-dose recombinant interleukin-2 after autologous and T-cell-depleted allogeneic bone marrow transplantation. Blood 1992;79:517–526.

142. Keever CA, Small TN, Flomenberg N, et al. Immune reconstitution following bone marrow transplantation: comparison of recipients of T cell depleted marrow with recipients of conventional marrow grafts. Blood 1989;73:1340–1350.

143. Small TN, Keever CA, Weiner-Fedus S, Heller G, O'Reilly RJ, Flomenberg N. B-cell differentiation following autologous, conventional, or T-cell depleted bone marrow transplantation: a recapitulation of normal B-cell ontogeny. Blood 1990;76:1647–1656.

144. Welte K, Keever CA, Levick J, et al. Interleukin-2 production and response to interleukin-2 by peripheral blood mononuclear cells from patients after bone marrow transplantation: II. Patients receiving soybean lectin-separated and T cell-depleted bone marrow. Blood 1987;70:1595–1603.

145. Drobyski WR, Piaskowski V, Ash RC, Casper JT, Truitt RL. Preservation of lymphokine-activated killer activity following T cell depletion of human bone marrow. Transplantation 1990;50:625–632.

146. Gast GC, Gratama JW, Verdonck LF, et al. The influence of T cell depletion on recovery of T-cell proliferation to herpes viruses and *Candida* after allogeneic bone marrow transplantation. Transplantation 1989;48:111–115.

147. Ault KA, Antin JH, Ginsberg D, et al. Phenotype of recovering lymphoid cell populations after marrow transplantation. J Exp Med 1985;161:1483–1502.

148. Janossy G, Prentice HG, Grob JP, et al. T lymphocyte regeneration after transplantation of T cell depleted allogeneic bone marrow. Clin Exp Immunol 1986;63:577–586.

149. Rooney CM, Wimperis JZ, Brenner MK, Patterson J, Hoffbrand AV, Prentice HG. Natural killer cell activity following T-cell depleted allogeneic bone marrow transplantation. Br J Haematol 1986;62:413–420.

150. Wimperis JZ, Prentice HG, Karayiannis P, et al. Transfer of a functioning humoral immune system in transplantation of T-lymphocyte depleted bone marrow. Lancet 1986;1:339–343.

151. Parreira A, Smith J, Hows JM, et al. Immunological reconstitution after bone marrow transplant with Campath-1 treated bone marrow. Clin Exp Immunol 1987;67:142–150.

152. Wimperis JZ, Brenner MK, Prentice HG, Thompson EJ, Hoffbrand AV. B cell development and regulation after T-cell depleted marrow transplantation. J Immunol 1987;138:2445–2450.

153. Brenner MK, Wimperis JZ, Reittie JE, et al. Recovery of immunoglobulin isotypes following T cell depleted allogeneic bone marrow transplantation. Br J Haematol 1986;64:125–132.

154. Daley JP, Rozans MK, Smith BR, Burakoff SJ, Rappeport JM, Miller RA. Retarded recovery of functional T cell frequencies in T cell-depleted bone marrow transplant recipients. Blood 1987;70:960–964.

155. Shapiro RS, McClain K, Frizzera G, et al. Epstein-Barr virus associated B cell lymphoproliferative disorders following bone marrow transplantation. Blood 1988;71:1234–1243.

156. Zutter MM, Martin PJ, Sale GE, et al. Epstein-Barr virus lymphoproliferation after bone marrow transplantation. Blood 1988;72:520–529.

157. Rickinson AB. Cellular immunological responses to the virus infection. In: Epstein MA, Achong BG, eds. The Epstein-Barr virus: recent advances. New York: Wiley, 1986:75–126.

Chapter 12

Documentation of Engraftment and Characterization of Chimerism Following Marrow Transplantation

Lawrence D. Petz

The modern era of bone marrow transplantation (BMT) was ushered in by the experiments of Jacobson, Lorenz, and their colleagues (1,2), who showed that mice could be protected against otherwise lethal irradiation by shielding of the spleen or by intravenous infusion of marrow. At first it was thought that this protective effect was due to a humoral factor. By 1956, however, several laboratories, using a variety of genetic markers, demonstrated that the protective effect against lethal irradiation was due to the colonization of the recipient marrow by donor cells (3–6). Thus, after successful allogeneic BMT, the recipients are chimeras (i.e., they have cell populations derived from different individuals).

Some patients have mixtures of hematopoietic cells of donor and recipient origins for varying lengths of time following BMT. The term *mixed chimera* is frequently used to distinguish these individuals from *complete chimeras* (only cells of donor origin detectable) and from those unusual patients in whom entirely autologous marrow recovery develops.

A large number of methods have been used to document and characterize chimerism after BMT. Although originally used primarily to document engraftment of the donor marrow, studies of chimerism following BMT also have the potential to (1) better our understanding of mechanisms of graft rejection and marrow failure, (2) detect the recurrence of leukemia and evaluate whether recurrent leukemia occurs in donor or recipient cells, (3) determine the clinical significance of mixed chimerism, (4) provide insights regarding the mechanisms of tolerance and graft-versus-host disease (GVHD), (5) provide information concerning the kinetics of engraftment in various disease states or after different preparative regimens, and (6) determine the origin of tissue macrophages and the cells of the marrow microenvironment.

More recently, with the development of markers of clonality that allow identification of small numbers of malignant cells, studies of chimerism after BMT have evolved to include efforts to detect and determine the significance of minimal residual disease.

Genetic Markers in Human Marrow Transplantation

Although engraftment of donor marrow is often inferred on the basis of an increase in peripheral blood counts at the expected time after BMT (7,8), numerous genetic markers have been used to document and characterize chimerism following BMT. These genetic markers vary with regard to the frequency with which they are informative and their sensitivity in detecting a minor population of cells.

Cytogenetic Markers

Cytogenetic analysis has been the diagnostic mainstay for documentation of engraftment. Evaluation of marrow cells is accomplished by taking a small aliquot of the aspirated cells, exposing them for 1 to 2 hours to colchicine, followed by analysis. Leukemic cells circulating in the peripheral blood can be evaluated by use of short-term blood culture, usually 24 hours, without added mitogenic stimulant. With this type of culture, only abnormal cells, such as leukemic cells, will be dividing. A 72-hour blood culture with mitogenic stimulant is used to study lymphocytes in the peripheral blood.

If the donor and the recipient are of different sex, successful engraftment can be confirmed during the first 2 weeks after BMT by the appearance of cells with the donor's sex chromosome (9–11). Successful engraftment may be characterized by the appearance of dividing donor cells in marrow within 2 weeks of grafting and in mitogen-stimulated blood cultures by 3 weeks (12).

Even when the sex of donor and recipient are the same, polymorphic differences revealed by various banding techniques (11) or constitutional chromosomal abnormalities may be useful in determining the source of cells.

In the case of a sex-mismatched BMT (or when there is another distinctive chromosome marker in donor or recipient), the origin of T- and B-lymphocyte populations in the engrafted marrow may be determined by taking advantage of the fact that the Epstein-Barr virus and phytohemagglutinin are specific human B- and T-cell mitogens, respectively (13). In an alternative approach, T and B lymphocytes are marked at the surface with specific (red fluorescent) fluorochromes, and the interphase nuclei are colored afterwards with (green fluorescent) quinicrine for detection of Y-chromatin (14). Using the latter method, some posttransplant patients were shown to have circulating T and B lymphocytes that were entirely of donor origin, whereas other patients had various combinations of mixtures (i.e., T-lineage of donor origin and B-lineage of recipient origin, or T- or B-lineage of donor and recipient origin) (14).

Also, if chromosome abnormalities are present that are markers of the malignant clone, such as the Philadelphia chromosome (Ph) in chronic myeloid leukemia, the remission status of the patient can be monitored (15–19). However, a cytogenetic relapse does not necessarily predict a clinical relapse, as was first demonstrated by Thomas and colleagues (15) in 6 patients, 3 of whom subsequently had no detectable Ph chromosomes even without therapeutic intervention. Cytogenetic studies have also documented that eradication of the Ph chromosome is generally unsuccessful following intensive combination chemotherapy but is frequently accomplished with BMT (19).

Chromosome analyses have also been used to document leukemic transformation of engrafted human marrow cells. This technique was first demonstrated by Fialkow and associates (20), who reported a 16-year-old girl with acute lymphoblastic leukemia who was transplanted with marrow from her brother. Leukemia recurred 62 days after the marrow graft, and the great majority of marrow and blood-cells were lymphoblasts, yet only XY cells were found. Subsequent studies have indicated that the recurrence of leukemia in donor cells is rare, although it has been reported in both acute (21–29) and chronic (30,31) leukemias. Immunoblastic sarcomas occurring in donor-derived cells have also been described following allogeneic BMT (32,33). More recently, recombinant DNA techniques, usually in conjunction with cytogenetic methods, have been used to document the origin of malignant cells in patients following BMT.

Unique cytogenetic markers in malignant cells make it possible to distinguish between normal, presumably healthy cells and chromosomally abnormal cells of the leukemic clone. In sex-mismatched transplants, a number of investigators have identified persisting host cells after BMT that lacked any cytogenetic abnormalities, suggesting that they were members of residual normal clones not involved in the leukemic process (18,34–37).

The sensitivity of chromosomal analysis depends on the number of metaphases examined. One must examine 30 metaphases to exclude 10% chimerism with 95% confidence, and 59 metaphases to exclude 5% chimerism with 95% confidence (38). Occasionally, it is difficult in the posttransplant period to obtain enough metaphases for a high degree of statistical power to exclude mixed chimerism. Also, it is possible that there may be a proliferative advantage of donor or host cells in posttransplant cytogenetic studies that are based on cultured cells, which would give misleading results. In addition, there may be differences in the mitogenic responsiveness of donor and recipient cells after transplantation. Indeed, Blazar and associates (39) reported that peripheral blood mononuclear cells stimulated with phytohemagglutinin were entirely of donor origin, but, when stimulated with a different mitogenic agent (lipopolysaccharide or pokeweed mitogen), they were noted to be of mixed donor and recipient origins.

Red Blood Cell Antigens

Red blood cell (RBC) phenotypes are highly informative genetic markers. Several antigen systems are frequently found to be different between donor and recipient (MNSs, Duffy, Rh, ABO), whereas others are of less value (Lutheran, Kp, Kell, P) (40) (Table 12-1). Typing for the following antigens may conveniently be performed: A_1, B, A, D, C, E, c, e, K, k, Fy^a, Fy^b, Jk^a, Jk^b, P_1, M, N, S, and s. In a study of 275 donor/recipient pairs, typing for these antigens revealed donor and recipient markers in 201 pairs (73%), only recipient-specific markers in 37 pairs (13%), only donor-specific markers in 29 pairs (11%), and no markers in 8 pairs (3%) (41). A minor population of RBCs can generally be detected by standard hemagglutination methods when their percentage is as low as 1 to 5% of the total.

Red cell phenotyping is easy to perform and is highly informative, but the method analyzes only one cell lineage and the pretransplant phenotype may be difficult to determine if the patient has had transfusions. Posttransplant transfusions usually make the exclusion of mixed chimerism impossible for 4 to 6 months following BMT because some transfused RBCs are detectable for as long as 150 days (42).

A method to circumvent the problem posed by

Table 12-1.
Red Cell Antigen Differences Between Sibling Pairs

Antigen System	*No. Pairs Tested*	*No. Pairs Different*	*% Different*
MNSs	56	35	62
Duffy	56	32	57
Rh	56	27	48
ABH	56	20	36
Kidd	45	13	29
Lewis	56	13	23
P	56	10	18
Kell	56	6	11
Kp	55	3	5
Lutheran	56	0	0

(Reprinted by permission from Sparkes MC, Crist ML, Sparkes RS, Gale RP, Feig SA, the UCLA Transplantation Group. From Sparkes et al. Gene markers in human bone marrow transplantation. Vox Sang 1977;33:202.)

transfusions was described by Thomas and colleagues (43), who determined the red cell phenotype of the donor and recipient to detect antigens present in the donor but lacking in the recipient. Following transplantation, the patient was transfused only with blood that lacked a donor-specific antigen. For example, a patient who was type O C(−) was transplanted with marrow from a donor who was type O (C+). After the first week following BMT, all transfusions were C(−) and the increase in the number of C(+) cells was used as an indication of engraftment. This approach was subsequently modified by Van Dijk and associates (44). They obtained a sample of patient red cells when a diagnosis was made of a disorder that might be treated with BMT. The cells were kept in a frozen state until a decision to transplant was made, at which time a correct red blood antigen profile was made undisturbed by transfused cells. Beginning 4 months preceding BMT, patients were transfused only with marker antigen-negative blood. Red cell typing was performed using standard hemagglutination techniques or using a fluorescent microsphere method (45), in which the RBCs are first incubated with an immunoglobulin G (IgG) antibody directed against the marker antigen and then incubated with anti-human IgG-coated fluorescent microspheres. The sensitivity level of this assay is one positive cell per 10,000 negative cells.

Immunoglobulin Allotypes

Immunoglobulin allotypes can be used as a genetic marker for the engraftment of B lymphocytes (41,46–48). Immunoglobulin allotyping in 75 sibling donor/recipient pairs revealed a recipient-specific marker or both donor-specific and recipient-specific markers in 37 pairs (49%), only donor-specific markers in 12 pairs (16%), and no markers in 26 pairs (35%) (41). Immunoglobulin allotypes can be detected to a level of approximately 3% of normal.

Results of immunoglobulin allotyping in a series of 10 BMT patients was reported by Sparkes and colleagues (48). Donor immunoglobulin type was found in 9 recipients, but it was usually not possible to determine whether the recipient's type persisted after transplantation. In one informative case, recipient type was not evident 51 days after BMT, whereas in another patient, there was persistence of recipient type up to 2.5 years after transplantation. Petz and associates (41) evaluated 29 mixed chimeras, including 10 patients in whom immunoglobulin allotyping was performed, using several genetic markers. Mixed chimerism was indicated by immunoglobulin allotyping in all 10 patients. In three of these patients, immunoglobulin allotypes ultimately became the only indication of the presence of host-type cells, whereas earlier in these patients' courses other genetic markers had also indicated mixed chimerism. These data suggest that a small number of persisting host B cells is sufficient to produce trace amounts of immunoglobulins of host type that can be detected by immunoglobulin allotyping (49). However, the procedure cannot be performed if the patient has been transfused recently, and the antisera needed for performing the tests are not readily available. Recipient-specific markers are present in only approximately 50% of sibling pairs.

Cell Enzyme Markers

Difference in erythrocyte isozyme pattern may also allow confirmation of marrow engraftment provided that one waits 3 to 5 months following the most recent red cell transfusion (10,40,50,51). Also, in a patient with inherited deficiency of adenosine deaminase (ADA) associated with severe combined immune deficiency, a partial engraftment of donor lymphocytes was associated with a reduction of dATP and dADP to normal values within the patient's erythrocytes (52).

Leukocyte isozyme patterns can be analyzed soon after BMT (51,53–55). Various leukocyte populations may be separated and subjected to enzyme electrophoresis.

Although use of such genetic markers is informative and practical, their use has largely been replaced by newer methods.

Other Methods

HLA Typing, Persisting RBC Antibodies, and In Situ Hybridization

A number of other methods for documenting and characterizing posttransplant chimerism have been reported. H-2 phenotyping has commonly been used for assessment of donor cell engraftment in studies of BMT in murine models. Human leukocyte antigen (HLA) typing has limited applicability following BMT in humans because most transplants have been carried out using HLA-matched sibling donors. However, with an increasing number of transplants performed using donors mismatched for at least one HLA locus (56), HLA typing for documentation of chimerism may be appropriate more frequently.

The persistence of red cell antibodies longer than 6 months after transplantation has been used as an indication of persistence of the recipient's B lymphocytes (41). Antibodies of the ABO blood group system may be used when there is a blood group incompatibility between donor and recipient. A 6-month period seems appropriate because studies have indicated that patients' RBC alloantibodies ordinarily persist for no longer than 120 days after BMT (46). Immunoglobulin allotyping was performed in 2 patients with persistent red cell antibodies and confirmed mixed chimerism of B lymphocytes (41). In 2 other patients, red cell alloantibodies persisted even though cytogenetic analyses failed to reveal recipient-type karyotypes. Occasionally, Rh antibodies or red cell autoantibodies may be present and may serve as markers.

In situ hybridization for the Y chromosome has been used to monitor engraftment (57–61), and a Y-chromosome–specific DNA probe has been used for

Southern hybridization or dot blot analysis of DNA (62).

DNA Polymorphisms

Use of DNA sequence polymorphisms is an informative and versatile method of distinguishing patient and donor cells (49,63). Following digestion with restriction endonucleases, variations in DNA sequences among individuals result in DNA fragments of differing lengths known as restriction fragment length polymorphisms (RFLPs). "Conventional" RFLP may be created by either loss or gain of a restriction enzyme cleavage site or by insertion or deletion of DNA between restriction sites. RFLPs are inherited as codominant Mendelian traits and can be identified in Southern transfer hybridizations using cloned DNA probes (63). RFLP analysis is applicable to all hematopoietic cells except fully differentiated erythrocytes, in aggregate, or in sorted cell fractions.

The applicability of genotypic analysis depends on the availability of informative DNA polymorphisms (i.e., distinguishable alleles in the marrow donor and recipient). The likelihood that a particular probe will reveal distinct alleles in recipient and donor depends on the number of alleles and their distribution in the population. Because the donor and the recipient are frequently siblings, even a highly polymorphic DNA sequence cannot guarantee that the two cell types can be distinguished. Indeed, siblings will be indistinguishable by any single genetic marker in at least 25% of cases. Probes for more than one highly polymorphic locus are therefore necessary to ensure detection of distinguishable patient and donor alleles. Using a set of 5 cloned DNA probes for highly polymorphic loci, the probability of the existence of a difference in RFLP patterns between 2 siblings was 99.7% (49,63). However, for the detection of cells of host origin, it is necessary to have a recipient-specific restriction fragment marker. Using the 5 probes, the probability of the presence of a marker was 98.7%, based on observed results of restriction fragment analysis in 30 sibling pairs (49). The sensitivity of the method using Southern transfer hybridizations is such that a minor population of DNA may be detected when it is approximately 1 to 10% of the total (49,63,64). As few as 10^6 cells yield sufficient DNA for analysis (39,64).

In addition to "conventional" RFLP, DNA polymorphisms also occur as a result of variation in the number of tandemly repeated sequences in different alleles at hypervariable regions in the human genome. These are called minisatellite or variable number of tandem repeat loci. The length variation can be detected using any restriction endonuclease that does not cleave the repeat unit, thus giving rise to a set of stable, inherited genetic markers in such loci (65). DNA polymorphisms due to variation in the number of short tandem repeats are defined by probes to the repeated DNA and not by the restriction enzyme. Complementary synthetic oligonucleotide probes may be synthesized (66,67), which under appropriate conditions display essentially absolute hybridization specificity (67). Using Southern blot analysis or in-gel hybridization, oligonucleotide probes are capable of detecting mixed chimerism when the minor population of DNA is present at 1 to 2% of the total leukocyte DNA (68).

A number of reports document the feasibility of using DNA RFLP to study marrow engraftment (39,49,63,64). Yam and colleagues (49) reported results in 27 patients and compared the results with those obtained using other genetic markers. They demonstrated marrow engraftment in the early posttransplant period (Figure 12-1), documented stable chronic

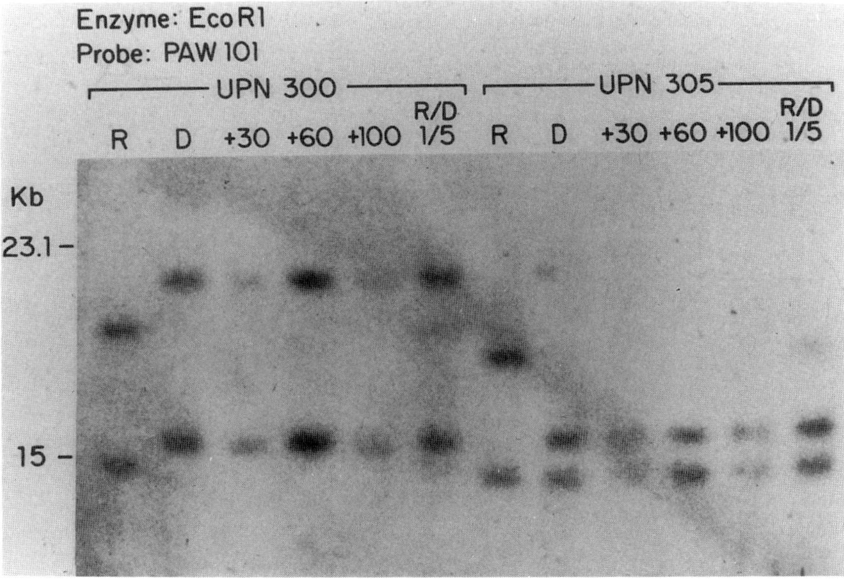

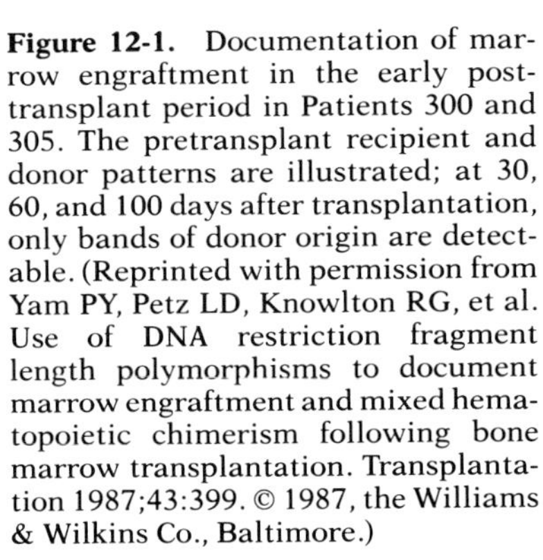

Figure 12-1. Documentation of marrow engraftment in the early posttransplant period in Patients 300 and 305. The pretransplant recipient and donor patterns are illustrated; at 30, 60, and 100 days after transplantation, only bands of donor origin are detectable. (Reprinted with permission from Yam PY, Petz LD, Knowlton RG, et al. Use of DNA restriction fragment length polymorphisms to document marrow engraftment and mixed hematopoietic chimerism following bone marrow transplantation. Transplantation 1987;43:399. © 1987, the Williams & Wilkins Co., Baltimore.)

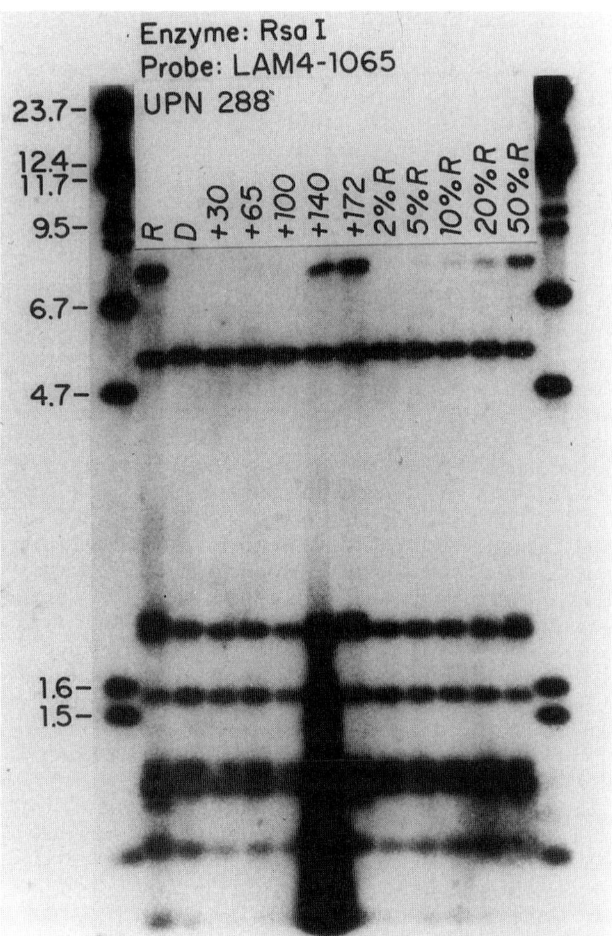

Figure 12-2. Recurrent leukemia in Patient 288 was associated with a recurrence of a recipient-specific restriction fragment. On days 30, 65, and 100 after transplantation, the recipient-specific band is not detectable, but an increasing concentration of DNA of recipient type is evident on days 140 and 172. This increase correlated with a recurrence of leukemia and suggests that the recurrence took place in cells of host origin. (Reprinted with permission from Yam PY, Petz LD, Knowlton RG, et al. Use of DNA restriction fragment length polymorphisms to document marrow engraftment and mixed hematopoietic chimerism following bone marrow transplantation. Transplantation 1987;43:399. © 1987, the Williams & Wilkins Co., Baltimore.)

mixed hematopoietic chimerism, identified transient mixed chimeras, and excluded mixed chimerism with high probability in retrospective studies even when a pretransplant DNA sample was not available.

Schubach and associates (69) demonstrated that RFLP analysis could be used to prove the origin (donor or host) of neoplastic relapse following allogeneic marrow grafting. Their patient underwent marrow grafting for acute lymphoblastic leukemia (ALL), and a widely disseminated immunoblastic sarcoma subsequently developed.

Changes in relative concentration of donor and recipient cells can be assessed in serial studies (49,63), and an increasing concentration of DNA of recipient origin associated with a recurrence of leukemia suggests that the recurrence is in cells of host origin (49) (Figure 12-2). This finding can be documented more definitively by demonstrating only recipient-type DNA in purified blast cell preparations (64,70,71).

More recently, Browne and colleagues (72) used recombinant DNA techniques, which corroborated cytogenetic results in their description of the first instance of leukemia originating in donor cells after BMT for severe aplastic anemia (SAA).

In contrast, both Biondi and associates (70) and Stein and co-workers (29) reported conflicting results when both cytogenetics and molecular techniques were used to identify the origin of the leukemic relapse in patients with ALL. These cases demonstrate that caution must be exercised when assigning the leukemic cell lineage in relapse following BMT (29). Cytogenetic analyses alone may not always detect the transformed cell line, and interpretation of molecular analyses may be difficult if the DNA probes used do not detect both donor-specific and recipient-specific markers. In addition, molecular analyses may be confounded by the loss of specific chromosomes or by the reemergence of nonleukemic cells of recipient origin (29).

By fractionating peripheral blood cells into granulocyte-, T lymphocyte-, and B lymphocyte-, and monocyte-enriched populations, it is possible to characterize further chimerism. Ginsburg and colleagues (64) demonstrated that a patient with a severe combined immunodeficiency syndrome (SCIDS) who received a BMT from his mother had T cells exclusively of donor origin, whereas granulocytes and B cells were of patient origin. In a patient who was a chronic mixed chimera in continuous complete remission 41 months after BMT for acute leukemia, Yam and colleagues (49) demonstrated that very few T cells were of recipient origin, whereas B cells of recipient origin were prominently represented (Figure 12-3).

Amplification by the Polymerase Chain Reaction of Hypervariable Regions of the Human Genome

Introduction of the polymerase chain reaction (PCR) as a method for rapid amplification of DNA in vitro has provided a powerful tool for analysis of human polymorphisms (73–75). The PCR technique allows selective amplification of a particular DNA region while it is still incorporated in total genomic DNA. The availability of the precise nucleotide sequences that flank the DNA region of interest is a prerequisite for the PCR technique. On the basis of this information, two synthetic oligonucleotides are prepared, which can hybridize to the flanking sequences of opposite strands. These two oligonucleotides serve as primers for the *Taq* polymerase, which enables an exponential amplification of the intervening DNA

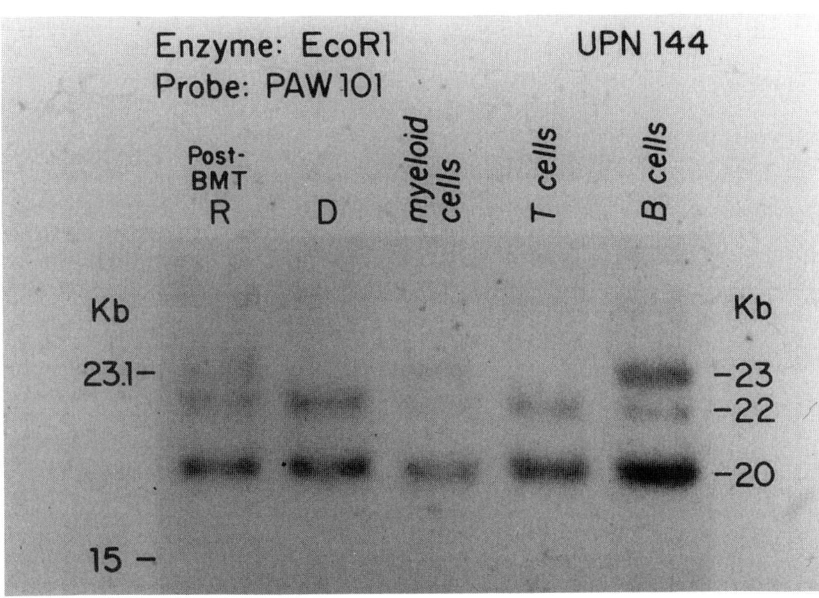

Figure 12-3. Comparison of restriction fragments of a known mixed hematopoietic chimera, UPN 144 (R) and his marrow donor (D). The study was done approximately 3.5 years after transplantation. The additional 23-kb band of nondonor origin in lane 1 is indicative of mixed chimerism. DNA isolated from various cell fractions indicates that very few T cells are of recipient origin, whereas the prominent 23-kb band in the right lane indicates that B cells of recipient origin are prominently represented. (Reprinted with permission from Yam PY, Petz LD, Knowlton RG, et al. Use of DNA restriction fragment length polymorphisms to document marrow engraftment and mixed hematopoietic chimerism following bone marrow transplantation. Transplantation 1987;43:399. © 1987, the William & Wilkins Co., Baltimore.)

region in a series of temperature-regulated cycles. Continuation of the PCR for 20 to 30 cycles theoretically results in 2^{20} to 2^{30} times amplification of the DNA region of interest. The obtained PCR products can be detected easily in a dot blot or Southern blot by the use of a probe, which specifically hybridizes to the amplified DNA fragment. Also, messenger RNA (mRNA) can be used as a target for the PCR technique, after the mRNA has been transcribed into complementary DNA (cDNA) by reverse transcriptase (76).

The major advantage of using a PCR-based analysis is increased sensitivity (i.e., it is possible to detect a very small proportion of DNA of donor or recipient origin). In addition, only small amounts of DNA are required, there is no need for restriction enzyme digestion, and the analysis can be performed more rapidly than traditional RFLP analysis (77).

PCR primers have been synthesized for the amplification of a Y chromosome–expressed sequence (57,78) and for a number of highly polymorphic loci (79–84), including variable number of tandem repeat loci (77,80,85). After amplification, the amplified products are fractionated by gel electrophoresis in agarose or polyacrylamide gel. The products may be visualized by ethidium bromide staining (57,85,86), but greater sensitivity and specificity are assured by hybridization with specific probes (66,77,81).

Ugozzoli and associates (77) designed locus-specific oligonucleotides for hybridization probes that were complementary to tandem repeat sequences and were highly informative. Using a set of 6 PCR primer pairs and locus-specific oligonucleotide probes, all 13 patients studied had recipient-specific and donor-specific fragments. A minor population of DNA could be detected even when its concentration was as low as 0.1% of the total. They demonstrated the utility of the method for detecting mixed chimerism, complete chimerism, recurrent leukemia, and endogenous repopulation of marrow (Figure 12-4).

Significance of Mixed Chimerism Following BMT

The study of mixed hematopoietic chimerism has led to improved but still incomplete knowledge concerning the significance of this phenomenon after allogeneic BMT.

Leukemic Relapse

There are conflicting data in the literature concerning the influence of mixed chimerism on the risk of leukemic relapse (12,41,42,58,87–98), and this question is currently being further evaluated using specific markers of clonality.

Using various genetic markers, several early reports indicated that mixed chimerism following BMT for hematological malignancy may exist even in patients in continuous complete remission (87–89). Singer and colleagues (87) reported a patient who had stable mixed hematopoietic chimerism in both lymphoid and myeloid cell lines but remained in complete remission for more than 5 years following BMT for ALL. Reports by Branch and associates (88) and Petz and co-workers (89) described 8 patients transplanted for acute leukemia who were mixed chimeras but who were in continuous complete remission for periods of 673 to 1,499 days following BMT (89).

A study of 172 patients treated with radiochemotherapy and BMT for hematological malignancies

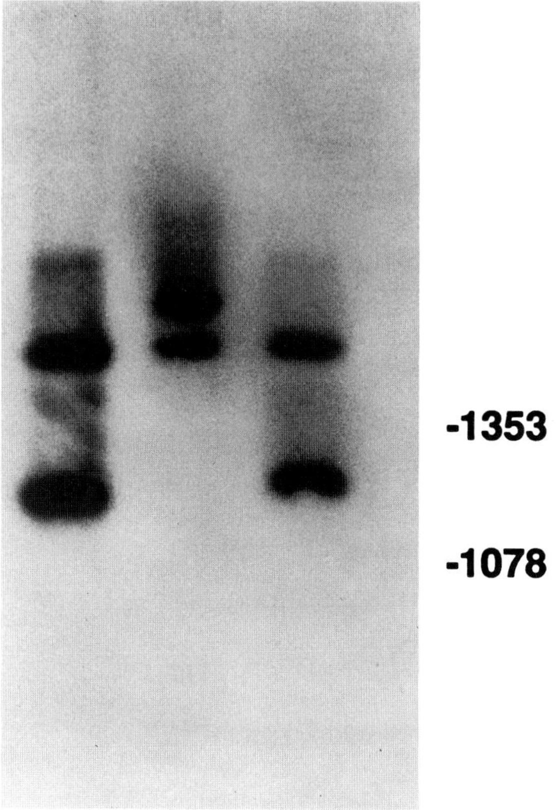

Figure 12-4. Endogenous hematopoietic cell repopulation. DNA was isolated from recipient UPN 605U (R) and the marrow donor (D) before BMT for aplastic anemia. Analyses performed on days 30, 52, and 88 following transplantation indicated that all DNA detected was of recipient origin. Only the analysis for day 88 is shown. (Reprinted with permission from Ugozzoli L, Yam P, Petz LD, et al. Amplification by the polymerase chain reaction of hypervariable regions of the human genome for evaluation of chimerism after bone marrow transplantation. Blood 1991;77:1607.)

indicated that 29 (17%) became mixed hematopoietic chimeras; 12 were stable mixed chimeras for 2 or more years following BMT. Twenty four of the 29 mixed chimeras remained in continuous complete remission for up to 116 months (>9 years) following BMT (41).

Bourhis and associates (90) used fluorescent in situ hybridization on peripheral blood cells or bone marrow cells to study 45 recipients of sex-mismatched T-cell–depleted marrow grafts for hematological malignancies (AML/ALL: 23; CML: 19; myelodysplastic syndrome: 2; non-Hodgkin's lymphoma: 1). The probability of disease-free survival was 62.5% for patients with 5% or less host cells and 28.8% for patients with more than 5% host cells. However, the follow-up time of the study was too short to draw a definite conclusion regarding the relationship of mixed chimerism to relapse.

Lawler and colleagues (91) used PCR with 7 microsatellite markers as well as cytogenetics and Y chromosome–specific PCR to evaluate mixed chimerism in 32 transplant patients, most of whom had hematological malignancies. Twelve patients received T-cell–depleted marrow and showed a high incidence of mixed chimerism as revealed by PCR (>80%). The incidence of mixed chimerism in patients who received unmanipulated marrow was lower (44%), although this was a high percentage when compared with other studies. Once mixed chimerism was detected, the percentages of recipient cells tended to increase; however, in patients exhibiting mixed chimerism who subsequently relapsed, this increase was relatively sudden. The overall level of recipient cells in the group of mixed chimerism patients who subsequently relapsed was higher than in those who exhibited stable mixed chimerism. The authors concluded that, although the occurrence of mixed chimerism was not indicative of a poor prognosis per se, sudden increases in the proportions of recipient cells may be a prelude to graft rejection or relapse.

Offit and associates (94) used the Y chromosome and autosomal heteromorphisms to distinguish between donor and host cells in 64 patients with CML after T-cell–depleted allogeneic BMT. Although mixed chimerism per se did not predict imminent graft failure or clinical relapse, mixed chimeras with greater than 25% normal host cells in the marrow at any time after transplantation had a significantly lower probability of disease-free survival and a higher probability of clinical relapse.

Durnam and colleagues (58) and Przepiorka and associates (61), using in situ hybridization for the Y chromosome, found no statistical correlation between retention of host cells in the first few weeks after BMT and the development of relapse. Only one of the 19 patients studied one year after BMT showed detectable numbers of host cells with this sensitive technique.

Similarly, Roy and co-workers (93) studied mixed hematopoietic chimerism in 43 patients with hematological malignancies who received a T-cell–depleted allogeneic BMT. RFLP studies indicated mixed chimerism in 53% of patients. The probability of relapse, survival, and disease-free survival was identical in patients with mixed chimerism and complete chimerism.

Using a sensitive method for red cell phenotyping involving the use of antibody-coated fluorescent microspheres, Bar and associates (42) reported that the incidence of mixed chimerism was 50 to 71% when tested at various times 6 to more than 24 months following BMT using marrow from sibling donors, which was depleted of 98% of lymphocytes using counterflow centrifugation. Often, only a very low percentage of patient red cells was detected; the median percentage during the first 12 months after BMT was 0.06%. No clinical evidence for leukemic recurrence was found in stable mixed chimeras with low percentages of autologous red cells (<1%) or mixed chimeras who converted to complete donor chimeras. However, 4 mixed chimeras relapsed: 2 had repeatedly high percentages of autologous red cells, and in the other 2 patients, the autologous erythrocytes increased markedly in the period before relapse. However, mixed chimeras with high percentages of autologous cells (>10%), sometimes even gradually increasing, did not necessarily relapse.

Bertheas and colleagues (92,97) reported results of cytogenetic studies performed on 60 patients with acute or chronic leukemias who were prepared by high doses of alkylating agents and fractionated TBI. Forty-three patients were recipients of untreated BMT and 17 were recipients of T-cell–depleted BMT. In the group of patients receiving T-cell–depleted marrow, mixed chimeras were significantly more frequent and prolonged in both peripheral blood and bone marrow cultures. The probability of relapse and survival was identical in patients with mixed chimerism and complete donor chimerism, except in patients with CML, in whom mixed chimerism was significantly associated with an increased risk of relapse.

Graft-versus-Host Disease

A number of investigators have found, in agreement with results in animal models (99), that there is an increased incidence of GVHD in patients with complete chimerism compared with mixed chimeras (93,96,97,100,101). Thus, the absence of GVHD (i.e., tolerance) may be responsible for the persistence of host hematopoietic cells (100,101) or, alternatively, mixed chimerism may have a role in the development of tolerance. In accord with the latter possibility, some investigators have studied mixed allogeneic chimerism in animal models as an approach to transplantation tolerance (102,103).

The Effect of T-cell Depletion on the Incidence of Mixed Chimerism

A number of reports indicate that recipients of T-cell–depleted transplants have a high incidence of mixed chimerism after BMT for leukemia (58,92–94,104, 105). The high percentage of mixed chimeras in the study of Bar and colleagues (42) was probably the result of lymphocyte depletion of the marrow graft and the high sensitivity of their method of red cell phenotyping for the demonstration of minor cell populations (as low as 0.01%).

Severe Aplastic Anemia

Mixed chimerism following allogeneic BMT for severe aplastic anemia (SAA) has been studied by several groups of investigators. Hill and colleagues (101) evaluated 96 patients with sequential cytogenetic analyses and reported that 56 patients (58.3%) were mixed chimeras when studied 14 days or more after BMT, and 40 patients (41.7%) were complete chimeras. Mixed chimerism persisted for up to 395 days after BMT; either the first graft was rejected or, more commonly, hematopoiesis reverted to 100% donor-type cells. The rejection rate was significantly increased in the mixed chimeric group, particularly in patients not receiving buffy coat; 14 of 36 patients rejected. Patients with mixed chimerism who maintained their first grafts had a significantly reduced incidence of grade II through IV acute GVHD. The probability of survival for all patients, including those who rejected their first graft, was not significantly different between mixed and complete chimeric patients.

Keable and colleagues (106) studied long-term engraftment at one to 12 years (median, 4.3 y) following BMT for SAA. Patients were conditioned with cyclophosphamide (150 mg/kg) and 6 GY thoracoabdominal irradiation and did not have ex vivo T-cell depletion of donor marrow. Chimerism was evaluated by Southern blotting using probes to variable numbers of tandem repeat regions or a probe detecting a male-specific repeated sequence on the Y chromosome. Long-term engraftment appeared complete for all patients. In contrast, Weitzel and associates (107) found in a cohort of 24 patients with SAA a 21% incidence of either partial engraftment or autologous reconstitution. Their patients and the patients of Hill and colleagues (101) did not receive irradiation in the conditioning regimen, which may account for the difference in results compared with those of Keable and associates (106). This is in agreement with the report of Champlin and co-workers (108), suggesting that the addition of irradiation increases the rate of complete engraftment.

Socie and colleagues (109) studied short-term chimerism 2 weeks to 3 months after BMT. For 14 patients grafted from a genotypically identical sibling donor, the DNA profile as determined by Southern blotting matched the respective donor profile. In contrast, the results indicated autologous marrow recovery in a patient who received marrow from an HLA-mismatched related donor and in 2 of 2 who received marrow from matched unrelated donors. The 15 patients with circulating cells of donor origin were then studied by PCR using amplification of a Y chromosome–specific sequence (sensitivity, 1 cell in 10^4) or amplification of the 33.6.3 minisatellite sequence (sensitivity, 1 cell in 10^2). All 3 patients studied with the more sensitive technique had detectable cells of host origin, whereas no residual cells of host origin were found in the 12 remaining patients, in whom the less sensitive method was used. The authors point out that the true incidence of persisting residual recipient cells will require the use of the most sensitive techniques.

Determining the Origin of the Hematopoietic Microenvironment, Hepatic Macrophages, and Alveolar Macrophages Following Allogeneic BMT

An intact hematopoietic microenvironment is required for successful engraftment of donor hematopoietic stem cells. Conflicting conclusions have been reached regarding the origin of the hematopoietic microenvironment following allogeneic BMT; most investigators suggest a host origin (110–113) rather than a donor origin (114). Simmons and associates (112) used in situ hybridization to discriminate donor cells from host in blood and bone marrow samples obtained from patients with functioning sex-mismatched but HLA-identical allografts. Without exception, marrow-derived stromal cells that proliferated in long-term cultures were found to be of host genotype, whereas the macrophage component of the adherent layer in these cultures originated from the donor. Similarly, Laver and colleagues (113) used chromosomal analysis to demonstrate the host origin of cultured marrow stromal cells obtained from patients successfully transplanted with allogeneic grafts whose hematopoietic cells were of donor origin. Eight of their study patients received conventional grafts and 10 received marrows depleted of stromal progenitors and T cells by soybean agglutination and E-rosetting. The results, with stromal-depleted marrow grafts showing engraftment with donor hematopoietic cells without the emergence of donor stromal cells, indicate that stromal and hematopoietic cells do not share a common progenitor.

Thomas and associates (115) obtained alveolar macrophages from 23 patients who had received marrow transplants for hematological disorders. The presence of a Y body in macrophages of male origin was demonstrated by fluorescence microscopy. In those patients with a marrow donor of opposite sex, the alveolar macrophages were shown to be of donor origin.

Gale and colleagues (116) obtained hepatic macrophages (Kupffer cells) from two male recipients of bone marrow from females and studied them for fluorescent Y-body staining and sex chromatin (Barr body). After transplantation, macrophages had the sex karyotype of the donor, indicating that human hepatic macrophages originate in bone marrow.

Characterization of Chimerism Using Markers of Clonality

Evaluation of chimerism following BMT has evolved to emphasize the use of sensitive recombinant DNA or immunological methods for the specific detection of individual clones of cells (76) rather than methods that are merely markers of cells of host or donor origin. This approach may be accomplished using a tumor-specific marker such as the *BCR-ABL* translocation, immunoglobulin or T-cell receptor gene rearrangements, or immunological marker analysis (76), which identify individual clones of cells. An enormous effort is being made to understand the significance of the detection of small numbers of residual malignant cells after treatment of patients for hematological malignancies. The detection of minimal residual disease may be of value not only to predict relapse and therefore to continue to treat the patient, but also to monitor the effectiveness of therapy and conceivably reduce treatment needs in patients who may already be cured. The most challenging question is whether modification of treatment according to the information provided by such methods can improve the cure rate.

These techniques have also been applied to study the effectiveness of ex vivo tumor-cell purging, the detection of malignant cells in peripheral blood stem-cell harvests, and to gain insights regarding the mechanism of graft failure. These topics are considered elsewhere in this text (see Chapters 13, 14, and 15).

Summary

To document engraftment of donor marrow after allogeneic BMT, numerous genetic markers have been utilized, including chromosomes, RBC antigens, immunoglobulin allotypes, cell enzymes, HLA typing, persisting RBC antibodies, in situ hybridization, and DNA polymorphisms. Use of these methods not only has allowed documentation of engraftment but also has resulted in a better understanding of the biology of BMT and of the diseases for which marrow transplantation is utilized. Genetic markers have been used to identify and characterize mixed chimerism, have documented the origin of recurrent leukemia as being in cells of donor or recipient origin, and have provided insights regarding GVHD, tolerance, and graft failure.

More recently, sensitive recombinant DNA and immunological techniques have been developed that allow for specific detection of clonal populations of cells as a marker of a malignant disorder. The potential of these procedures has just begun to be realized. Thus, use of genetic markers for documentation of engraftment following allogeneic BMT has provided critical information regarding numerous aspects of marrow transplantation and can be expected to provide even greater understanding in the future.

References

1. Jacobson LO, Simmons EL, Marks EK, et al. The role of the spleen in radiation injury and recovery. J Lab Clin Med 1950;35:746–770.
2. Lorenz E, Uphoff D, Reid TR, et al. Modification of irradiation injury in mice and guinea pigs by bone marrow injections. J Natl Cancer Inst 1951;12:197–201.
3. Lindsley DL, Odell TT Jr, Tausche FG. Implantation of functional erythropoietic elements following total-body irradiation. Proc Soc Exp Biol Med 1955;90:512–515.
4. Nowell PC, Cole LJ, Habermeyer JG, et al. Growth and continued function of rat marrow cells in X-radiated mice. Cancer Res 1956;16:258–261.
5. Ford CE, Hameron JL, Barnes DWH, et al. Cytological

identification of radiation-chimaeras. Nature 1956;177: 452–454.
6. Mitchison NA. The colonization of irradiated tissue by transplanted spleen cells. Br J Exp Pathol 1956;37: 239–247.
7. Thomas ED, Storb R, Clift RA, et al. Bone-marrow transplantation. New Engl J Med 1975;292:832–843, 895–902.
8. Buckner CD, Clift RA, Fefer A, Neiman P, Storb R, Thomas ED. Human marrow transplantation—current status. Prog Hematol 1973;8:299–324.
9. Thomas ED, Buckner CD, Storb R, et al. Aplastic anaemia treated by marrow transplantation. Lancet 1972;1:284–289.
10. Blume KG, Beutler E, Bross KJ, Schmidt GM, Spruce WE, Teplitz RL. Genetic markers in human bone marrow transplantation. Am J Hum Genet 1980;32: 414–419.
11. Sparkes RS. Cytogenetic analysis in human bone marrow transplantation. Cancer Genet Cytogenet 1981; 4:345–352.
12. Lawler SD, Baker MC, Harris H, Morgenstern GR. Cytogenetic studies on recipients of allogeneic bone marrow using the sex chromosomes as markers of cellular origin. Br J Haematol 1984;56:431–443.
13. Sadamori N, Ozer H, Higby DJ, Sandberg AA. Chromosomal evidence of donor B-lymphocyte engraftment after bone-marrow transplantation in a patient with multiple myeloma. N Engl J Med 1983;308: 1423–1424.
14. Korver K, DeLange GG, van den Bergh RL, Schellekens PTHA. Lymphoid chimerism after allogeneic bone marrow transplantation, Y-chromatin staining of peripheral T and B lymphocytes and allotyping of serum immunoglobulins. Transplantation 1987;44:643–650.
15. Thomas ED, Clift RA, Fefer A, et al. Marrow transplantation for the treatment of chronic myelogenous leukemia. Ann Intern Med 1986;104:155–163.
16. Grahm DL, Tefferi A, Letendre L, Gastineau DA, Hoagland HC, Noel P. Cytogenetic and molecular detection of residual leukemic cells after allogeneic bone marrow transplantation in chronic granulocytic leukemia. Mayo Clin Proc 1992;67:123–127.
17. Arthur CK, Apperley JF, Guo AP, Rassool F, Gao LM, Goldman JM. Cytogenetic events after bone marrow transplantation for chronic myeloid leukemia in chronic phase. Blood 1988;71:1179–1186.
18. Alimena G, De Cuia MR, Mecucci C, et al. Cytogenetic follow-up after allogeneic bone-marrow transplantation for Ph[1]-positive chronic myelogenous leukemia. Bone Marrow Transplant 1990;5:119–127.
19. Sessarego M, Frassoni F, Defferrari R, et al. Cytogenetic follow-up after bone marrow transplantation for Philadelphia-positive chronic myeloid leukemia. Cancer Genet Cytogenet 1989;42:253–261.
20. Fiaklow PJ, Thomas ED, Bryant JI, Neiman PE. Leukaemic transformation of engrafted human marrow cells in vivo. Lancet 1971;1:251–255.
21. Thomas ED, Bryant JI, Buckner CD, et al. Leukaemic transformation of engrafted human marrow cells in vivo. Lancet 1972;1:1310–1313.
22. Goh K, Klemperer MR. In vivo leukemic transformation: cytogenetic evidence of in vivo leukemic transformation of engrafted marrow cells. Am J Hematol 1977;2:283–290.
23. Elfenbein GJ, Brogaonkar DS, Bias WB, et al. Cytogenetic evidence for recurrence of acute myelogenous leukemia after allogeneic bone marrow transplantation in donor hematopoietic cells. Blood 1978;52:627–636.
24. Newburger PE, Latt SA, Pesando JM, et al. Leukemic relapse in donor cells after allogeneic bone-marrow transplantation. N Engl J Med 1981;304:712–714.
25. Boyd CN, Ramberg RC, Thomas ED. The incidence of recurrence of leukemia in donor cells after allogeneic bone marrow transplantation. Leuk Res 1982;6:833–837.
26. Witherspoon RP, Schubach W, Neiman P, Martin P, Thomas ED. Donor cell leukemia developing six years after marrow grafting for acute leukemia. Blood 1985;65:1172–1174.
27. Schmitz N, Johannson W, Schmidt G, von der Helm K, Loffler H. Recurrence of acute lymphoblastic leukemia in donor cells after allogeneic marrow transplantation associated with a deletion of the long arm of chromosome 6. Blood 1987;70:1099–1104.
28. Feig SA, Dreazen O, Simon M, Witey F, Schreck R, Gale RP. B cell acute lymphoblastic leukemia (ALL) in donor cells following bone marrow transplantation for T cell ALL. Bone Marrow Transplant 1988;3:331–337.
29. Stein J, Zimmerman PA, Kochera M, et al. Origin of leukemic relapse after bone marrow transplantation: comparison of cytogenetic and molecular analyses. Blood 1989;73:2033–2040.
30. Marmont A, Frassoni F, Bacigalupo A, et al. Recurrence of Ph[1]-positive leukemia in donor cells after marrow transplantation for chronic granulocytic leukemia. N Engl J Med 1984;310:903–906.
31. Smith JL, Heerema NA, Provisor AJ. Leukaemic transformation of engrafted bone marrow cells. Br J Hematol 1985;60:415–422.
32. Gossett TC, Gale RP, Fleischman H, et al. Immunoblastic sarcoma in donor cells after bone-marrow transplantation. N Engl J Med 1979;300:904–907.
33. Martin PJ, Shulman HM, Schubach WH, et al. Fatal Epstein-Barr-virus associated proliferation of donor B cells after treatment of acute graft-versus-host disease with a murine anti-T-cell antibody. Ann Intern Med 1984;101:310–315.
34. Schmitz N, Godde-Salz E, Loffler H. Cytogenetic studies on recipients of allogeneic bone marrow transplants after fractionated total body irradiation. Br J Haematol 1985;60:239–244.
35. Vincent PC, Young GAR, Singh S, Atkinson K, Biggs JC. Ph[1] negative haematological chimaerism after marrow transplantation in Ph[1] positive chronic granulocytic leukaemia. Br J Haematol 1986;63:181–185.
36. Williams SV, Williams J, Barnard DL, Mason MK. Appearance of Ph negative recipient clones in chronic myeloid leukemia patients following bone marrow transplantation. Cancer Genet Cytogenet 1992;58:143–151.
37. Becher R, Beelen DW, Graeven U, Schaefer U, Schmidt CG. Case report: triple chimaerism after allogeneic bone marrow transplantation for Philadelphia chromosome positive chronic granulocytic leukaemia. Br J Haematol 1987;67:373–374.
38. Hook EB. Exclusion of chromosomal mosaicism: tables of 90%, 95%, and 99% confidence limits and comments on use. Am J Hum Genet 1977;29:94–97.
39. Blazer BR, Orr HT, Arthur DC, Kersey JH, Filipovich AH. Restriction fragment length polymorphisms as markers of engraftment in allogeneic marrow transplantation. Blood 1985;66:1436–1444.
40. Sparkes MC, Crist ML, Sparkes RS, Gale RP, Feig SA,

the UCLA Transplantation Group. Gene markers in human bone marrow transplantation. Vox Sang 1977; 33:202–205.
41. Petz LD, Yam P, Wallace RB, et al. Mixed hematopoietic chimerism following bone marrow transplantation for hematologic malignancies. Blood 1987;70:1331–1337.
42. Bar BMAM, Schattenberg A, Van Dijk BA, De Man AJM, Kunst VAJM, De Witte T. Host and donor erythrocyte repopulation patterns after allogeneic bone marrow transplantation analyzed with antibody-coated fluorescent microspheres. Br J Haematol 1989;72:239–245.
43. Thomas ED, Lochte HL, Lu WC, Ferrebee JW. Intravenous infusion of bone marrow in patients receiving radiation and chemotherapy. N Engl J Med 1957;257: 491–496.
44. Van Dijk BA, Drenthe-Schonk AM, Bloo A, Kunst VAJM, Janssen JTP, De Witte TJM. Erythrocyte repopulation after allogeneic bone marrow transplantation, analysis using erythrocyte antigens. Transplantation 1987;44: 650–654.
45. De Man AJM, Foolen WJG, Van Dijk BA, Kunst VAJM, De Witte TM. A fluorescent microsphere method for the investigation of erythrocyte chimaerism after allogenic bone marrow transplantation using antigenic differences. Vox Sang 1988;55:37–41.
46. Witherspoon RP, Rainer S, Ochs HD, et al. Recovery of antibody production in human allogenic marrow graft recipients: influence of time posttransplantation, the presence or absence of chronic graft-versus-host disease, and antithymocyte globulin treatment. Blood 1981;58:360–368.
47. Gengozian N, Edwards CL, Vodopick HA, Hubner KF. Bone marrow transplantation in a leukemic patient following immunosuppression with antithymocyte globulin and total body irradiation. Transplantation 1973; 15:446–454.
48. Sparkes RF, Sparkes MC, Gale RP. Immunoglobulin synthesis following allogeneic bone marrow transplantation in man. Conversion to donor allotype. Transplantation 1979;27:212–213.
49. Yam PY, Petz LD, Knowlton RG, et al. Use of DNA restriction fragment length polymorphisms to document marrow engraftment and mixed hematopoietic chimerism following bone marrow transplantation. Transplantation 1987;43:399–407.
50. Storb R, Thomas ED, Buckner RA, et al. Allogeneic marrow grafting for treatment of aplastic anemia. Blood 1974;43:157–180.
51. Meera Khan P, Wijnen JT, Hagenbeek A, Vossen JM. Isozymes as host-donor blood cell "tracers" in bone marrow transplantation. In: Isozymes: current topics in biological and medical research, vol. 16. New York: Alan R. Liss, 1987:125–144.
52. Chen SH, Ochs HD, Scott CR. Adenosine deaminase deficiency. Disappearance of adenine deoxynucleotides from a patient's erythrocytes after successful marrow transplantation. J Clin Invest 1978;62:1386–1389.
53. Schmidt GM, Blume KG, Bross KJ, Spruce WE, Staatz CG, Turner MA. The use of lymphocyte phosphoglucomutase as a genetic marker in bone marrow transplant recipients. Blut 1979;38:135–137.
54. Grahovac B, Labar B, Stavljenic A. Subtyping of erythrocyte phosphoglucomutase-1 as a genetic marker for bone marrow engraftment and hematopoietic chimerism after allogeneic bone marrow transplantation in a patient with acute lymphoblastic leukemia. Clin Chem 1988;34:2586–2588.
55. Vives-Corrons JL, Merino A, Pujades A, et al. Combined study of lymphocyte phosphoglucomutase (PGM) and adenylate kinase (AK) isoenzymes in the early characterization of bone marrow engraftment. Scand J Haematol 1985;35:469–473.
56. Stroncek DF. Results of bone marrow transplants from unrelated donors. Transfusion 1992;32:180–189.
57. Hutchinson RM, Pringle JH, Potter L, Patel I, Jeffreys AJ. Rapid identification of donor and recipient cells after allogeneic bone marrow transplantation using specific genetic markers. Br J Haematol 1989;72:133–140.
58. Durnam DM, Anders KR, Fisher L, O'Quigley J, Bryant EM, Thomas ED. Analysis of the origin of marrow cells in bone marrow transplant recipients using a Y-chromosome-specific in situ hybridization assay. Blood 1989;74:2220–2226.
59. Przepiorka D, Ramberg R, Thomas ED. Host metaphases after chemoradiotherapy and allogeneic bone marrow transplantation for acute nonlymphoblastic leukemia. Leuk Res 1989;13:661–665.
60. Przepiorka D, Gonzales-Chambers R, Winkelstein A, Rosenfeld C, Shadduck RK. Chimerism studies using in situ hybridization for the Y chromosome after T cell-depleted bone marrow transplantation. Bone Marrow Transplant 1990;5:253–257.
61. Przepiorka D, Thomas ED, Durnam DM, Fisher L. Use of a probe to repeat sequence of the Y chromosome for detection of host cells in peripheral blood of bone marrow transplant recipients. Am J Clin Pathol 1991;95:201–206.
62. Morisaki H, Morisaki T, Nakahori Y, et al. Genotypic analysis using a Y-chromosome-specific probe following bone marrow transplantation. Am J Hematol 1988;27:30–33.
63. Knowlton RG, Brown VA, Braman JC, et al. Use of highly polymorphic DNA probes for genotypic analysis following bone marrow transplantation. Blood 1986;68: 378–385.
64. Ginsburg D, Antin JH, Smith BR, Orkin SH, Rappeport JM. Origin of cell populations after bone marrow transplantation, analysis using DNA sequence polymorphisms. J Clin Invest 1985;75:596–603.
65. Jeffreys AJ, Wilson V, Thein SL. Hypervariable "minisatellite" regions in human DNA. Nature 1985;314:67–73.
66. Ali S, Wallace RB. Enzymatic synthesis of DNA probes complementary to a human variable number tandem repeat locus. Anal Biochem 1989;179:280–283.
67. Wallace RB, Petz LD, Yam PY. Application of synthetic DNA probes to the analysis of DNA sequence variants in man. Cold Spring Harbor Symposia on Quantitative Biology 1986;51:257–261.
68. Yam P, Petz LD, Ali S, Stock AD, Wallace RB. Development of a single probe for documentation of chimerism following bone marrow transplantation. Am J Hum Genet 1987;41:867–881.
69. Schubach WH, Hackman R, Neiman PE, Miller G, Thomas ED. A monoclonal immunoblastic sarcoma in donor cells bearing Epstein-Barr virus genomes following allogeneic marrow grafting for acute lymphoblastic leukemia. Blood 1982;60:180–187.
70. Biondi A, Norman C, Messner HA, Minden MD. Restriction fragment length polymorphism analysis of hematopoietic cells following successful treatment of relapsed acute lymphoblastic leukemia following bone marrow transplantation. Bone Marrow Transplant 1989;4:705–709.
71. Minden MD, Messner HA, Belch A. Origin of leukemic

relapse after bone marrow transplantation detected by restriction fragment length polymorphism. J Clin Invest 1985;75:91–93.
72. Browne PV, Lawler M, Humphries P, McCann SR. Donor-cell leukemia after bone marrow transplantation for severe aplastic anemia. N Engl J Med 1991; 325:710–713.
73. Saiki RK, Scharf SJ, Faloona F, et al. Enzymatic amplification of β-globin genomic sequences and restriction site analysis for diagnosis of sickle cell anaemia. Science 1985;230:1350–1354.
74. Macintyre EA. The use of the polymerase chain reaction in haematology. Blood 1989;3:201–210.
75. Sklar J. Polymerase chain reaction: the molecular microscope of residual disease. J Clin Oncol 1991;9: 1521–1524.
76. van Dongen JJM, Breit TM, Adriaansen HJ, Beishuizen A, Hooijkaas H. Detection of minimal residual disease in acute leukemia by immunological marker analysis and polymerase chain reaction. Leukemia 1992;6(suppl 1):47–59.
77. Ugozzoli L, Yam P, Petz LD, et al. Amplification by the polymerase chain reaction of hypervariable regions of the human genome for evaluation of chimerism after bone marrow transplantation. Blood 1991;77:1607–1615.
78. Lawler M, McCann SR, Conneally E, Humphries P. Chimerism following allogeneic bone marrow transplantation: detection of residual host cells using the polymerase chain reaction. Br J Haematol 1989;73: 205–210.
79. Chalmers EA, Sproul AM, Mills KI, Gibson BES, Burnett AK. Use of the polymerase chain reaction to monitor engraftment following allogeneic bone marrow transplantation. Bone Marrow Transplant 1990;6:399–403.
80. Roth MS, Antin JH, Bingham EL, Ginsburg D. Use of polymerase chain reaction-detected sequence polymorphisms to document engraftment following allogeneic bone marrow transplantation. Transplantation 1990;49:714–720.
81. Jeffreys AJ, Wilson V, Neumann R, Keylte J. Amplification of human minisatellites by the polymerase chain reaction: towards DNA fingerprinting of single cells. Nucleic Acids Res 1988;16:10953–10971.
82. Boerwinkle E, Xiong WJ, Fourest E, Chan L. Rapid typing of tandemly repeated hypervariable loci by the polymerase chain reaction: application to the apolipoprotein B 3′ hypervariable region. Proc Natl Acad Sci USA 1989;86:212–216.
83. Bowcock AM, Ray A, Erlich H, Sehgal PB. Rapid detection and sequencing of alleles in the 3′ flanking region of the interleukin-6 gene. Nucleic Acids Res 1989;17:6855–6864.
84. Horn GT, Richards B, Klinger KW. Amplification of a highly polymorphic VNTR segment by the polymerase chain reaction. Nucleic Acids Res 1989;17:2140.
85. Nakao S, Nakatsumi T, Chuhjo T, et al. Analysis of late graft failure after allogeneic bone marrow transplantation: detection of residual host cells using amplification of variable number of tandem repeats loci. Bone Marrow Transplant 1992;9:107–111.
86. Decorte R, Cuppens H, Marynen P, Cassiman JJ. Rapid detection of hypervariable regions by the polymerase chain reaction technique. DNA Cell Biol 1990;9:461–469.
87. Singer JW, Keating A, Ramberg R, et al. Long term stable hematopoietic chimerism following marrow transplantation for acute lymphoblastic leukemia: a case report with in vitro marrow culture studies. Blood 1983;62:869–872.
88. Branch DR, Gallagher MT, Forman SJ, Winkler KJ, Petz LD, Blume KG. Endogenous stem cell repopulation resulting in mixed hematopoietic chimerism following total body irradiation and marrow transplantation for acute leukemia. Transplantation 1982; 34:226–228.
89. Petz LD, Branch RD, Stock AD, et al. Endogenous stem cell repopulation after high-dose pretransplant radiochemotherapy. Transplant Proc 1985;27:432–433.
90. Bourhis JH, Jagiello CA, Black P, O'Reilly RJ, Gerritsen WR. Mixed chimerism predicts an unfavorable determining outcome for T-cell depleted allogeneic bone marrow transplantation. Blood 1991;78(suppl 1):224a.
91. Lawler M, Humphries P, McCann SR. Evaluation of mixed chimerism by in vitro amplification of dinucleotide repeat sequences using the polymerase chain reaction. Blood 1991;77:2504–2514.
92. Bertheas MF, Maraninchi D, Lafage M, et al. Partial chimerism after T-cell depleted allogeneic bone marrow transplantation in leukemic HLA matched patients: a cytogenetic documentation. Blood 1988;72: 89–93.
93. Roy DC, Tantravahi R, Murray C, et al. Natural history of mixed chimerism after bone marrow transplantation with CD6-depleted allogeneic marrow: a stable equilibrium. Blood 1990;75:296–304.
94. Offit K, Burns JP, Cunningham I, et al. Cytogenetic analysis of chimerism and leukemia relapse in chronic myelogenous leukemia patients after T-cell depleted bone marrow transplantation. Blood 1990; 75:1346–1355.
95. Suttorp M, Schmitz N, Prange E, Gassmann W, Schaub J. Evaluation of hematopoietic chimerism following allogeneic bone marrow transplantation (BMT). Exp Hematol 1990;18:679.
96. Schattenberg A, De Witte T, Salden M, et al. Mixed hematopoietic chimerism after allogeneic bone marrow transplantation with lymphocyte-depleted bone marrow is not associated with a higher incidence of relapse. Blood 1989;73:1367–1372.
97. Bertheas MF, Lafage M, Levy P, et al. Influence of mixed chimerism on the results of allogeneic bone marrow transplantation for leukemia. Blood 1991;78: 3103–3106.
98. de Witte T, Schattenberg A, Salden M, Wessels J, Haanen C. Mixed chimerism and the relation with leukaemic relapse after allogeneic bone marrow transplantation. Bone Marrow Transplant 1987;2(suppl 1):11–12.
99. Ildstadt ST, Sachs DH. Reconstitution with syngeneic plus allogeneic or xenogeneic bone marrow leads to specific acceptance of allografts or xenografts. Nature 1984;307:168–170.
100. Frassoni F, Strada P, Sessarego M, et al. Mixed chimerism after allogeneic marrow transplantation for leukaemia: correlation with dose of total body irradiation and graft-versus-host disease. Bone Marrow Transplant 1990;5:235–240.
101. Hill RS, Peterson FB, Storb R, et al. Mixed hematologic chimerism after allogeneic marrow transplantation for severe aplastic anemia is associated with a higher risk of graft rejection and a lessened incidence of acute graft-versus-host disease. Blood 1986;67:811–816.
102. Sykes M, Sachs DH. Mixed allogeneic chimerism as an

approach to transplantation tolerance. Immunol Today 1988;9:23–27.

103. Sharabi Y, Sachs DH. Mixed chimerism and permanent specific transplantation tolerance induced by a nonlethal preparation regimen. J Exp Med 1989;169: 493–502.

104. Bretagne S, Vidaud M, Kuentz M, et al. Mixed blood chimerism in T cell depleted bone marrow transplant recipients: evaluation using DNA polymorphisms. Blood 1987;70:1692–1695.

105. Arthur CK, Apperly JF, Guo R, Rassool F, Gao LM, Goldman JM. Cytogenetics events after bone marrow transplantation for chronic myeloid leukemia in chronic phase. Blood 1988;71:1179–1186.

106. Keable H, Bourhis JH, Brison O, et al. Long-term study of chimaerism in bone marrow transplantation recipients for severe aplastic anaemia. Br J Haematol 1989;71:525–533.

107. Weitzel JN, Hows JM, Jeffreys AJ, Minn GL, Goldman JM. Use of a hypervariable minisatellite DNA probe (33×15) for evaluating engraftment two or more years after bone marrow transplantation for aplastic anaemia. Br J Haematol 1988;70:91–97.

108. Champlin RE, Horowitz MM, Van Beckum DW, et al. Severe aplastic anemia: a prospective study on the effect of early marrow transplantation on acute mortality. Blood 1989;73:606–613.

109. Socié G, Landman J, Gluckman E, et al. Short-term study of chimaerism after bone marrow transplantation for severe aplastic anaemia. Br J Haematol 1992;80:391–398.

110. Golde DW, Hocking WG, Quan SG, Sparber RS, Gale RP. Origin of human bone marrow fibroblasts. Br J Haematol 1980;44:183–187.

111. Lim B, Izaguirre CA, Aye MT, et al. Characterization of reticulofibroblastoid colonies (CFU-RF) derived from bone marrow and long term marrow culture monolayers. J Cell Physiol 1986;127:45–54.

112. Simmons PJ, Przepiorka D, Thomas ED, Torok-Storb B. Host origin of marrow stromal cells following allogeneic bone marrow transplantation. Nature 1987; 328:429–432.

113. Laver J, Jhanwar SC, O'Reilly RJ, Castro-Malaspina H. Host origin of the human hematopoietic microenvironment following allogeneic bone marrow transplantation. Blood 1987;70:1966–1968.

114. Keating A, Singer JW, Killen PD, et al. Donor origin in the in vitro haematopoietic microenvironment after marrow transplantation in man. Nature 1982;298: 280–283.

115. Thomas ED, Ramberg RE, Sale GE. Direct evidence for a bone marrow origin of the alvelor macrophage in man. Science 1976;192:1016–1018.

116. Gale RP, Sparkes RS, Golde DW. Bone marrow origin of hepatic macrophages (Kupffer cells) in humans. Science 1978;201:937–938.

Chapter 13
Antibody-mediated Purging

John G. Gribben and Lee M. Nadler

High-dose therapy with resulting myeloablation rescued by infusion of autologous bone marrow has become a major treatment option for an increasing number of patients with hematological and solid tumors (1–10). Autologous bone marrow transplantation (BMT) has several potential advantages over allogeneic transplantation. There is no need for histocompatibility testing and no risk of graft-versus-host disease (GVHD). Autologous BMT can therefore be performed in patients with no histocompatible donor or in older patients. However, the major obstacle to the use of autologous bone marrow after high-dose myeloablative therapy is that the presence of occult tumor cells harbored within the remission marrow may result in more rapid relapse of disease after infusion of these cells. To minimize the effects of the infusion of significant numbers of malignant cells, most centers secure marrow for autologous BMT when the patient is either in complete remission or when there is no evidence by histological examination of bone marrow infiltration of disease. In addition, a variety of methods have been developed to "purge" malignant cells from the marrow. The aim of purging is to eliminate any contaminating malignant cells and to leave intact the hematopoietic stem cells that are necessary for engraftment. Several approaches to eliminate malignant cells have been attempted and are summarized in Table 13-1.

Because of their specificity, monoclonal antibodies (MABs) are ideal agents for selective elimination of malignant cells. A large number of preclinical and clinical studies have now been performed in patients with no evidence of overt marrow involvement. The development of purging techniques has led subsequently to a number of studies of autologous BMT in patients with either a previous history of bone marrow infiltration or even overt marrow involvement at the time of bone marrow harvest. These studies have demonstrated that immunological purging can deplete malignant cells in vitro without significantly impairing hematological engraftment. Although the rationale for removing any contaminating cells from the autologous marrow appears compelling, the issue of purging remains highly controversial. Intense argument persists as to whether attempts to remove residual tumor cells from the harvested bone marrow have contributed to improving disease-free survival in these patients. To date, there have been no clinical trials testing the efficacy of purging by comparison of infusion of purged versus unpurged autologous bone marrow, due primarily to the large number of patients that would be required for such studies. In addition, the finding that the majority of patients who relapse after autologous BMT do so at sites of prior disease has led to the widespread view that purging of autologous marrow could contribute little to subsequent outcome after autologous BMT.

This chapter reviews the scientific rationale for the use of immunological purging, primarily in hematological malignancies. The use of MABs with specificity for lineage-restricted antigens on malignant cells, how these cells may be identified, and some of the pitfalls that are likely using this approach are discussed. Finally, preclinical and clinical experience of in vitro immunological purging are reviewed.

Rationale for Marrow Purging

The likelihood of bone marrow infiltration with tumor is determined by a number of clinical variables, such as tumor type and stage of disease. Bone marrow involvement is extremely rare in some tumors, such as testicular or ovarian cancers, but

Table 13-1.
Methods to "Purge" Tumor Cells from Marrow or Blood

Physical
Osmotic shock
Density gradient or elutriation
Size
Cytotoxic therapy in vitro
4-Hydroperoxycyclophosphamide
Asta-Z
Binding to molecules other than antibodies
Lectins
Cytokines
Synthetic molecules or solid-phase matrices
Immunological purging
Uncoupled
Conjugated to chemotherapeutic agent
Conjugated to toxin
Conjugated to magnetic bead
Conjugated to radionucleide

Table 13-2.
Sensitivity of Tumor Cell Detection in Marrow

Method of Detection	*No. Tumor Cells Detected in 10^{10} Total Marrow Cells*
Morphological analysis	
Aspirate	5×10^8
Biopsy	5×10^8
Flow cytometric analysis	$1–5 \times 10^8$
Southern blot analysis	1×10^8
Immunohistochemistry of cytospins	1×10^6
Clonogenic assay	1×10^5
Polymerase chain reaction	1×10^4

occurs less rarely in breast cancer. However, it is common in other solid tumors, such as small-cell lung cancer, neuroblastomas, and non-Hodgkin's lymphomas, and by definition is invariable in the leukemias. In general, the higher the stage of the tumor, the more likely the bone marrow is to be involved. However, in some tumors, such as the follicular non-Hodgkin's lymphomas, bone marrow involvement is almost invariable.

The ability to detect residual malignant cells within the bone marrow is clearly determined by the sensitivity of the assay used to detect these cells (Table 13-2). Because the limit of detectability of marrow infiltration by histological examination is 5%, a bone marrow judged to be histologically normal may still be infiltrated with malignant cells comprising up to 5% of the cellularity. Over the past decade, development of more sensitive techniques has allowed the detection of such occult residual disease. In particular, identification of specific gene rearrangements and chromosomal translocations in neoplastic cells has permitted development of molecular techniques that can now detect minimal residual disease within the bone marrow. Development of these newer techniques, such as flow cytometric analysis, clonal excess, and Southern blot analysis, has resulted in an increase in the sensitivity of detection of malignant cells, up to 1% of the cellularity. Use of sensitive cell culture techniques and recent application of the polymerase chain reaction (PCR) have resulted in a greatly increased sensitivity of detection of minimal residual disease within the bone marrow and are theoretically capable of detecting up to one tumor cell in one million normal cells.

Detection of Occult Residual Disease in the Bone Marrow

Cell Culture Techniques

Until recently, clonogenic assays were the most sensitive technique available to detect residual disease. In addition, these assays have the great advantage of detecting not only the presence of a malignant cell, but of evaluating whether the cell has clonogenic capacity and has the capacity to proliferate in the patient. A number of studies have used sensitive culture techniques to demonstrate that clonogenic malignant cells could be grown from morphologically normal bone marrow. In an early study, lymphoma cell lines were detected from the morphologically normal marrow of 17% of patients with undifferentiated lymphoma (11). Using a more sensitive liquid culture technique, it was shown subsequently that up to half the patients with Burkitt's lymphoma and morphologically normal marrow still had occult marrow involvement (12). Recently it has been demonstrated that up to one third of patients with intermediate and high-grade non-Hodgkin's lymphoma had clonogenic lymphoma cells in morphologically normal marrow at the time of bone marrow harvest (13). Similarly, residual leukemia cells were detected by culture techniques from the clinical complete remission bone marrows of children with acute lymphoblastic leukemia (14).

Molecular Biological Techniques

The underlying principle for the application of molecular biological techniques to the diagnosis of human malignancies lies in the detection of clonal proliferation of tumor-specific chromosomal translocations or gene rearrangements. These factors have been studied most widely in the lymphoproliferative malignancies because of the specific nature of gene rearrangements occurring at the antigen receptor. During early lymphoid development, the genes that encode the antigen receptors undergo rearrangements that join a variable coding segment to the joining segments. Also, there are additions of N insertions and a high rate of point mutations within the complementarity determining regions. In normal B cells and in B-cell malignancies, the immunoglobulin genes rearrange. Developmentally, the immunoglobulin heavy chain genes appear to rearrange first, followed by the κ light chain genes. If the κ light chains rearrange nonproductively, then λ light chain gene rearrangement occurs. In T cells, rearrangements of the T-cell receptor genes have been used to demonstrate the clonal origin of malignancies and to provide a sensitive assay for the presence of malignant cells.

Like their normal cellular counterparts, B- and T-cell malignancies undergo antigen receptor gene rearrangements. The clonal progeny of clonogenic lymphoproliferative malignancies will therefore exhibit the identical antigen receptor rearrangement. The most widely used molecular biological technique has been DNA restriction fragment analysis with Southern blot hybridization. Using this technique, up to 1% contamination of normal cells with a clonal malignancy can be detected (15). Assessment of clonality can also be demonstrated by the surface expression of immunoglobulin light chains, and detection of clonal excess also allows sensitive detection of neoplastic cells (11). These techniques have shown clearly that malignant cells can be detected in marrow judged normal by morphological assessment.

More recently, development of PCR has greatly increased the sensitivity of detection of malignant cells. Cloning of the t(14;18) breakpoints involving the bcl-2 proto-oncogene on chromosome 18 and the immunoglobulin heavy chain locus on chromosome 14 (16–18) has made it possible to use PCR amplification to detect lymphoma cells containing this translocation (19–21). This extremely sensitive technique permits detection of one lymphoma cell in one million normal cells (20). The t(14;18) occurs in approximately 85% of patients with follicular lymphomas and in 30% with diffuse non-Hodgkin's lymphomas (22–27). Using this technique, it has been demonstrated that the bone marrows of all patients with advanced stage non-Hodgkin's lymphomas containing the bcl-2 translocation were infiltrated with lymphoma cells both at the time of initial assessment and following induction or salvage therapy (28,29). However, it is not possible using this technique to determine whether the residual lymphoma cells in the marrow were truly clonogenic, because PCR amplification will detect DNA from cells that have been killed by the purging procedure.

Immunological Purging of Tumor Cells from Bone Marrow

Identification of residual malignant cells within the bone marrow has led to the development of methods to attempt to deplete these contaminating cells without impairing hematopoietic progenitors. Monoclonal antibodies are ideal agents to identify and specifically target such malignant cells. The majority of antibodies used have been generated by immunizing mice with human malignant cells or malignant cell membranes. A large number of mouse monoclonal antibodies have been developed with specificity for human cell surface antigens. The monoclonal antibodies that define unique cell surface antigens expressed on lymphoid and myeloid cells have been classified by cluster designation (CD) groups. Although it was hoped that unique, tumor-specific cell surface proteins would be recognized, all of the cell surface antigens identified to date on neoplastic cells of the hematopoietic or lymphoid malignancies represent normal differentiation antigens, and true leukemia- or lymphoma-specific antigens have not been identified. Because monoclonal antibodies are not toxic, they must be used in combination with other agents to kill the targeted cell. The most widely used technique has been to eliminate the antibody-coated target cells by complement-mediated lysis. More recently, increasing numbers of studies have been performed using iron-containing compounds, which bind to the MABs coating the targeted cell. The cells bound to the iron-containing compound can then be removed in a magnetic field. Most recently, there has been increasing interest in the use of MABs to target cytotoxic agents to malignant cells. These MAB-cytotoxic agent conjugates are known as immunotoxins.

Table 13-3.
Properties of Target Antigens Beneficial for Tumor Cell Purging

Lineage restriction
High density of expression
Limited heterogeneity
Expressed on clonogenic tumor cells
Depending on purging strategy—ability to modulate

Characteristics of Ideal Monoclonal Antibodies for Purging

The most important factor to be determined when using an MAB for purging is that the antibody should specifically target the malignant cell. Because no true tumor cell antigens have been recognized, the antibody chosen should be directed against those differentiation antigens present on the tumor cell but not on the surface of the hematopoietic stem cells that are necessary for marrow engraftment. The properties of target antigens beneficial for tumor cell purging are shown in Table 13-3. The targeted antigen should be present at high density on the cell surface to increase the efficiency of subsequent cell killing or removal. If the MAB is used with complement, a complement-fixing isotype of antibody must be used (the most efficient is immunoglobulin M [IgM]). For immunological purging using complement-mediated lysis or immunomagnetic bead separation, it is important that the antigen-antibody complex remains on the cell surface and is not internalized. In contrast, if immunotoxins are used, then the targeted antigen-antibody complex should be internalized to ensure intracellular delivery of the cellular toxin.

Differentiation Antigens on Human Hematological Cells

All hematopoietic cells are derived from the pluripotential stem cell. The characterization of the stem cell and the regulation of its growth and differentiation are crucial to understanding of hematopoiesis and to the malignant transformation in these cells that leads to development of hematological malignancies. The pluripotent stem cells are found in extremely low numbers in the bone marrow. Populations enriched for stem cells, first in the mouse and later in humans, have established that these cells have multilineage potential. During differentiation from stem cells to the mature progenitors, cells express specific cell surface antigens. These antigens can be used to identify distinct stages of myeloid and lymphoid differentiation. Malignant cells are also derived from clonogenic cells, and expression of distinct cell surface antigens on the clonogenic tumor cell forms the basis for the selective depletion of malignant cells from normal hematopoietic progenitors. A rational basis for the selection of appropriate MABs for the specific elimination of tumor cells is therefore dependent on an understanding of the expression of these normal cellular proteins on both malignant and normal hematopoietic cells. Expression of cell surface antigens on malignant cells is briefly outlined herein. For a more detailed outline of cell surface antigen expression of lymphoid and myeloid ontogeny and hematological malignancies, readers are referred to a recent review (30).

Cell Surface Antigen Expression of Myeloid Malignancies

A simplified outline of cell antigen expression during normal myeloid cell differentiation is illustrated in Figure 13-1. The earliest myeloid progenitor cells express CD34 but not CD33 on their surface. At a later stage of development, more committed hematopoietic progenitors coexpress both CD34 and CD33 and acquire human leukocyte antigen (HLA)-DR and CD13. CD34 is lost subsequently, and more mature progenitors express CD11b and CD15; in addition, cells of the monocytic lineage acquire CD14. Although immunophenotyping is less widely used in the acute myeloid leukemias than in the lymphoblastic leukemias, the expression of myeloid-restricted antigens can be used to differentiate myeloid from lymphoid leukemias.

The vast majority of acute myeloid leukemias express CDw65, and more than 80% express the myeloid restricted antigens CD33, CD13, and CD15. A number of previous studies have investigated the association between particular French American British (FAB) Classification subtypes and cell surface phenotype (31–33). The immature myeloid-specific types M1 and M2 express CD34, CD33, CD13, and HLA-DR. The promyelocytic leukemias, in contrast, do not express HLA-DR. The monocytic leukemias M4 and M5 also express antigens expressed by the more mature granulocytes and monocytes, including CD11a/CD18, CD11c, CD14, and CD15. The erythroleukemias, M6, generally express CD71 and have variable expression of CD15 and HLA-DR. The megakaryocytic leukemias, M7, have been shown to express HLA-DR and platelet glycoproteins, in addition to CD34 and CD33, but not CD14. The chronic myeloid leukemias in chronic phase are characterized by mature granulocytes and their more mature precursors. The majority of chronic myeloid leukemias in blast crisis are heterogeneous, although phenotypically they express markers of acute myeloid leukemia (34). In up to one third of patients, the blast crisis is characterized by the appearance of lymphoblasts that express CD10 and HLA-DR.

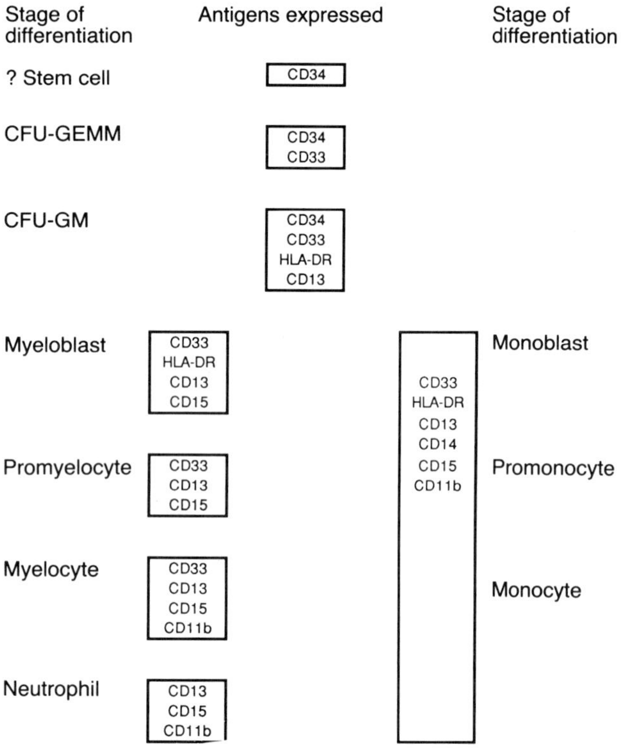

Stage of differentiation	Antigens expressed		Stage of differentiation
? Stem cell	CD34		
CFU-GEMM	CD34, CD33		
CFU-GM	CD34, CD33, HLA-DR, CD13		
Myeloblast	CD33, HLA-DR, CD13, CD15	CD33, HLA-DR, CD13, CD14, CD15, CD11b	Monoblast
Promyelocyte	CD33, CD13, CD15		Promonocyte
Myelocyte	CD33, CD13, CD15, CD11b		Monocyte
Neutrophil	CD13, CD15, CD11b		

Figure 13-1. Antigen expression during myeloid differentiation.

Cell Surface Antigen Expression of B-cell Malignancies

The stages of normal B-cell differentiation are shown in Figure 13-2. B-cell acute lymphoblastic leukemias are the malignant counterpart of cells from the earliest stages of B-cell differentiation. These cells express HLA-DR, CD9, CD10, CD24, and CD34 (35). The vast majority of B cell acute lymphoblastic leukemias also express CD19, and approximately half also express CD20. Almost one third of acute lymphoblastic leukemias express the myeloid-restricted antigens CD13 and

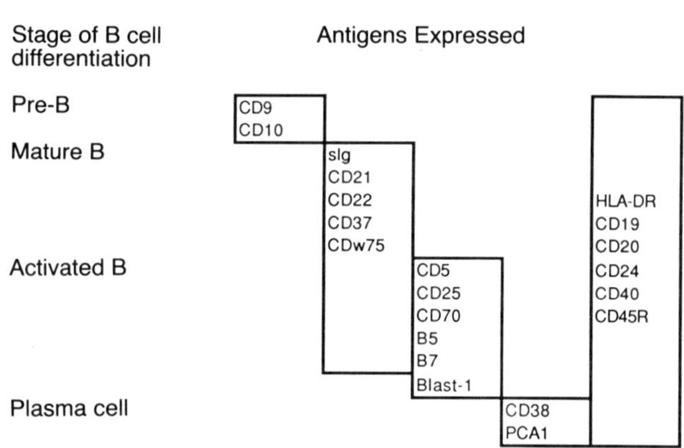

Figure 13-2. Antigen expression during B-cell differentiation.

CD33 (36). More than half the myeloid antigen-positive acute lymphoblastic leukemias also express B-cell–restricted antigens, and 20% express T-cell–restricted antigens. Rarely, acute lymphoblastic leukemias are reported to coexpress the T-cell antigen CD2 and the B-cell antigens CD19, CD10, and CD34.

The B cell non-Hodgkin's lymphomas are the malignant counterpart of cells corresponding to later stages of B-cell differentiation (37). Virtually all non-Hodgkin's lymphomas express HLA-DR, CD19, CD20, CD22, CD24, and CD45RA. In addition to these antigens, different histological subtypes of non-Hodgkin's lymphoma have characteristic cell surface antigen expression. The diffuse small lymphocytic lymphomas express CD11c/18 and CD44 and are therefore similar in antigen expression to the chronic lymphocytic leukemias. The majority of follicular lymphomas express surface immunoglobulin, CD10, CD21, and the B cell activation antigen B5. The diffuse small cleaved cell lymphomas resemble the small lymphocytic lymphomas but do not express CD5. Diffuse large-cell lymphomas are more heterogeneous in expression, but usually express the activation antigens B5 and B7. Non-cleaved small-cell non-Hodgkin's lymphomas express CD10.

Cell Surface Antigen Expression of T-cell Malignancies

The stages of normal T-cell development are briefly outlined in Figure 13-3. The majority of T cell acute lymphoblastic leukemias correspond to cells of the earliest stages of T-cell differentiation and express CD2, CD38, and CD7 (38,39). Infrequently, T cell acute lymphoblastic leukemias express CD1a, CD4, and CD8. Although many patients have cytoplasmic CD3, only rarely do they express surface CD3; less than 10% express CD10. The T cell lymphoblastic lymphomas correspond to the next stages of T-cell differentiation. The vast majority express CD2. Most also lack CD3 but express CD1, CD5, CD7, CD38, and the high-affinity subunit of the interleukin-2 (IL-2) receptor (40–42). A major difference between T cell acute lymphoblastic leukemias and lymphoblastic lymphomas is that the majority of these lymphomas express CD10 (43). The T cell non-Hodgkin's lymphomas of the diffuse small- and large-cell histological subtypes generally express the phenotype of mature peripheral blood T cells and express CD2, CD3, CD5, and CD7. The majority express CD4, and a minority express CD8, coexpress CD4 and CD8, or lack both CD4 and CD8 (44–46).

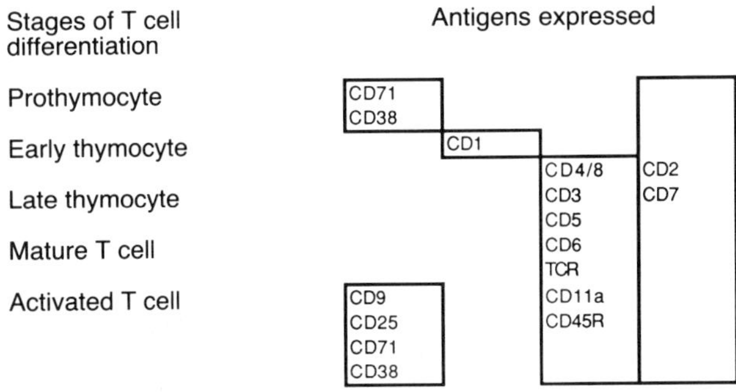

Figure 13-3. Antigen expression during T-cell differentiation.

Do Clonogenic Tumor Cells Express Targeted Antigens?

Although normal cell surface differentiation MABs have been used to eradicate cells bearing these antigens from the marrow, it is possible that the majority of tumor cells bearing these antigens are derived from more immature clonogenic cells that may lack these targeted antigens. Therefore, the surface antigen expression of the clonogenic cell of origin may be different from that expressed on the majority of the neoplastic cells.

Evidence for the existence of immature clonogenic cells has come from earlier studies of females heterozygous for glucose-6-phosphate dehydrogenase (G6PD) deficiency. Because this gene is on the X chromosome and one chromosome is randomly inactivated in each cell, a clonogenic tumor cell and all subsequent progeny will express only one G6PD type. In chronic myeloid leukemia, each of the myeloid lineage cells, including neutrophils, monocytes, red cell precursors, and megakaryoctes, express a single G6PD type, demonstrating the clonal origin of these cells (47). Subsequently, lymphocytes were also demonstrated to arise from the same clones as the leukemia (48,49). This finding demonstrates that the clonogenic cell must be an undifferentiated multilineage progenitor cell.

The stage of differentiation of the clonogenic cell in acute myeloid leukemia is less clear. In some patients, a single G6PD type is seen in the blasts, but both types are seen in erythrocytes and platelets, suggesting that the leukemia arose in a committed progenitor. However, other predominantly older patients demonstrate a single G6PD type in all lineages, suggesting that the leukemic blast cell arose in an immature stem cell (50). Because the less committed hematopoietic progenitors express CD34 but do not express CD33, whereas committed progenitors express CD33, the surface expression of CD34 and CD33 can be used to determine whether the more immature CD34+CD33-progenitors express either a clonal pattern of G6PD, and are therefore involved in the malignant process, or express both forms of G6PD and that the leukemic precursors are derived from a later stage of differentiation. The success of immunological purging techniques in the myeloid leukemias will be dependent on our understanding of the surface antigen expression of the leukemic progenitors and the hematopoietic stem cells required for the reestablishment of hematopoiesis.

Phenotypic characterization of patient samples has also provided evidence of an undifferentiated multilineage clonogenic cell in a number of patients. A small number of acute myeloid leukemias and myeloid blast crisis of chronic myelogenous leukemia (CML) also express the early T-cell antigen CD7. Recent studies have shown that almost one third of acute lymphoblastic leukemias express the myeloid antigens CD13 and CD33 (36). Up to 60% of the myeloid antigen–positive acute lymphoblastic leukemias coexpress B-cell antigens, and 20% express T-cell antigens. Rarely, acute lymphoblastic leukemias are reported to coexpress the T-cell antigen CD2 and the B-cell antigens CD19, CD10, and CD34. The nature of these biphenotypic leukemias is unclear. They may represent leukemias with inappropriate expression of genes from a different lineage. Alternatively, they could represent leukemias derived from a clonogenic cell, in which the transforming event had occurred in a progenitor cell that was not yet lineage-committed. A subset of acute leukemias fails to express cell surface antigens of either myeloid or lymphoid lineage. It is postulated that these acute undifferentiated leukemias arise from an even more primitive uncommitted progenitor cell. Unlike chronic myeloid leukemias that retain the ability to differentiate so that progeny cells express differentiation antigens, acute undifferentiated leukemias may represent leukemic expansion of clonogenic cells close to the stem cell itself. Studies in myeloma have suggested that the clonogenic cell of origin may be a pre-B cell (51). Similarly, there is some evidence that the clonogenic follicular lymphoma cell may be of bone marrow origin (52).

Preclinical Studies of Immunological Purging

Most studies have focused on the hematopoietic malignancies. The critical issues that must be addressed in marrow purging are outlined in Table 13-4. A number of these issues have already been discussed, but should be borne in mind when evaluating these studies. There are also a number of obstacles to tumor-cell purging that must be addressed. These problems are outlined in Table 13-5.

Most clinical studies have attempted to target antigens present on early progenitors in addition to the antigens expressed on the mature neoplastic cells to eradicate the clonogenic tumor cells in addition to any more mature progeny cells. In the B-cell leukemias and lymphomas, the most widely used MABs have been directed against CD9, CD10, CD19, CD20, CD24, CD37, CDw75, and the unclustered B-cell activation antigen B5. Most studies of patients with non-Hodgkin's lymphomas and myeloma also target the early antigen, CD10. For the T-cell malignancies, MABs directed against CD3, CD4, CD5, CD6, and CD7 are most widely used. In acute myeloid leukemias, MABs against CD33, CD13, CD14, CD15, and CDw65 have been investigated. CD33 is the earliest antigen expressed that is not present on the myeloid progenitors necessary for engraftment.

Table 13-4.
Critical Issues in Marrow Purging

How do we define tumor-involved bone marrow?
Are detectable marrow tumor cells clonogenic?
How much marrow involvement can be purged?
What are the most efficient methods of tumor cell purging?
How do we assess the efficacy of purging?
How do we determine which patients will benefit from marrow purging?

Table 13-5.
Obstacles to Tumor Cell Purging

Identification of clonogenic tumor cell phenotype
Heterogeneity of clonogenic tumor cells
"Polyclonal" tumors
Resistance of tumor cell to
Complement-mediated lysis
Immunotoxin cytotoxicity

More recently, it has been recognized that a large number of monoclonal antibodies have specificity for determinants on solid tumors. These antibodies have been investigated as potential purging agents in a variety of solid tumors, including breast carcinoma (53), small-cell lung cancer (54), neuroblastoma (55,56), and retinoblastoma (57).

Assessment of the Efficacy of Purging

Because MABs alone are not toxic, they must be used with agents such as complement or magnetic beads to eliminate the targeted tumor cells. Culture systems were used to examine the efficacy of different complement sources (58). Immunofluorescence and clonogenic assays were also used to assess the efficiency of different types of immunomagnetic beads (59). Similarly, using a model system, the addition of chemotherapeutic agents was shown to be more efficient than MABs and complement–mediated lysis alone (60).

Clonogenic assays were used to assess the efficacy of multiple MABs and complement-mediated lysis in cell line models (61). Multiple treatments were more efficient than single treatments, and the combination of two or more antibodies was more efficient than a single MAB to eliminate tumor cells. Using a culture assay in clinical samples, LeBien and colleagues (62) also showed that multiple MABs were superior to single MABs in combination with complement-mediated lysis to eliminate residual leukemia cells. In this study, two rounds of treatment were more efficient than a single treatment (62). In a more recent study, the ability to purge tumor cells from normal bone marrow cells using MABs and complement was also shown in an in vitro tumor-cell line model (29). In clonogenic assays using the cell line Raji in serial dilutions in irradiated normal bone marrow mononuclear cells, the growth of clonogenic lymphoma cells was reduced using three rounds of treatment with a single anti-B-cell MAB alone followed by complement-mediated lysis. A single MAB plus complement was capable of approximately three logs of tumor cell kill; however, the addition of multiple antibodies and complement appears to be much more efficient, and use of 3 MABs and complement appeared to be capable of up to 6 logs of tumor cell kill.

PCR is an extremely sensitive technique to detect residual malignant cells and has been utilized most extensively in non-Hodgkin's lymphomas. PCR has been used to assess the efficacy of immunological purging both in models using cell lines (63) and in patient samples (29).

Selection of Purging Methods

The most widely studied methods of immunological purging are complement-mediated lysis, immunomagnetic bead depletion, and immunotoxins. The advantages and disadvantages of each of these methods are shown in Table 13-6.

Complement-mediated Lysis

The earliest preclinical studies involved the addition of complement to the MAB-coated cells, which were then eliminated by complement-mediated cytotoxicity. Complement-mediated cytolysis is the most commonly employed method for immunological purging, due in part to its efficiency and specificity. In most studies, rabbit complement has been used because it circumvents the problem of homologous species restriction (the process whereby cells are generally resistant to lysis by complement from the same species). The ideal complement source must be toxic to cells coated with MAB but not toxic to cells not coated with antibody. However, there are major disadvantages of using complement. These include cost, variability of different lots so that each new lot must be tested for nonspecific toxicity, loss of cells because of washing, and inadequate lysis of neoplastic cells that only weakly express the targeted antigen. Among the factors that may influence the efficiency of complement-mediated lysis are the density of surface antigen expression, antigen modulation, and resistance to complement lysis. Therefore, the failure of immunological purging using complement-mediated lysis could be attributed to three possible mechanisms. First, the clonogenic tumor cells might not express, or only express weakly, the surface antigens expressed by the majority of tumor cells. Second, modulation of one or more of the surface antigens following attachment of the MABs to its ligand might limit complement-mediated lysis. Third, a subgroup of patients may have malignancies that are intrinsically more resistant to complement-mediated lysis.

A number of these possible mechanisms for resistance of cells to the lytic effects of complement have been investigated. Antigen expression on clonogenic cells is discussed in more detail later. Tumor cell killing by antibody-mediated complement activation appears to result from osmotic cell lysis following disruption of the semipermeable properties of the cell membrane. However, an actively metabolizing cell is capable of turning over its cell membrane (64), which may result not only in antigen modulation but also in neutralization of the lytic effects of the complement. Previous studies have shown associations between biochemical events in the cell and sensitivity to complement-mediated lysis (65). In addition, an anti-complementary factor has been described in normal bone marrow cells that limits the activation of complement, not only on the cells that produce the factor, but also on antibody-coated cells within the normal marrow (66). These anti-complementary effects may be overcome by repeated treatments with complement, and previous studies have suggested that the use of repeated treatment cycles is more efficient in removing contaminating tumor cells than single treatment cycles (67). This approach, however, is time-consuming, increases the expense of the proce-

Table 13-6.
Selection of Purging Method

Method	*Advantages*	*Disadvantages*
Complement-mediated lysis	Simple technology Relatively inexpensive 2–3 log kill	Only IgM and IgG2a efficiently fix complement Lots must be screened for efficacy and toxicity Cytotoxicity slow, with multiple rounds of treatment required Resistance to complement
Immunomagnetic beads	Efficient Rapid 5–6 logs	Expensive Concern about nonspecific cell loss
Immunotoxins	Can be efficient Easily standardized	Conjugate must internalize Longer exposure may increase nonspecific toxicity Few antigens are good targets Resistance may develop

dure with regard to both reagents and to laboratory staff effort, and may increase the nonspecific loss of hematopoietic progenitor cells. The continuous infusion of fresh complement while removing media containing the used complement may increase the efficiency and time taken to perform the procedure (68).

Several studies have demonstrated that the populations of cells that survive following complement-mediated lysis are more resistant to subsequent treatments with the same MAB and complement treatments. This resistance appears to be associated with the emergence of subpopulations of cells with a relative decrease in the surface expression of the targeted antigens (69). Such changes in relative expression of antigen density has also been observed following treatment with chemotherapy. Therefore, it is important to demonstrate that the tumor to be purged should express the targeted antigen, not only at the time of diagnosis, but also at the time of marrow harvest.

The combination of immunological and pharmacological purging has been shown to be significantly more efficient in eliminating clonogenic Burkitt's cell lines from human bone marrow than either agent alone (60). The effectiveness of purging small-cell lung cancer cell lines with MABs and complement-mediated lysis was also significantly increased when used in combination with pharmacological purging using the cyclophosphamide derivative, Asta-Z 7557 (70). This combination resulted in a 4- to 5-log reduction of clonogenic cell growth, although there was significant reduction in myeloid colony growth. In a novel study, a combined approach was used to attempt to eliminate multidrug-resistant leukemic cell lines from bone marrow (71). In this study, an MAB directed against the cell surface product of the multidrug resistance gene efficiently depleted cell lines from normal marrow. The addition of etoposide after the immunological purging resulted in a 4.6-log reduction of the clonogenic cell growth.

Magnetic Bead Depletion

Immunomagnetic bead depletion is used increasingly as a method of eliminating malignant cells from the bone marrow. The use of immunomagnetic beads was originally developed to facilitate depletion of neuroblastoma cells (55). The majority of clinical studies of marrow purging using immunomagnetic beads have been performed in children with neuroblastomas. More recently, a number of studies have been performed for a variety of other malignancies, including small-cell lung cancer, breast cancer, acute lymphoblastic leukemia, myeloma, and lymphoma.

The use of immunomagnetic beads has the advantage that there is no biological variability between lots, as has been observed with complement. Most studies utilize magnetic microspheres coated with affinity-purified sheep anti-mouse antibodies directed against the Fc portion of the MAB (Dynabeads, Dynal, Oslo, Norway). An alternative source of beads are BioMag particles (Advanced Magnetics, Cambridge, MA). These particles utilize goat-anti mouse antibodies bound to irregularly shaped colloidal nonionic iron oxide with a silane coating. More recently, a number of particles have been developed that are directly attached to the primary MAB used for purging. These reagents have the advantage of allowing more rapid and more simple purging procedures. Equipment to remove the immunomagnetic beads is now available commercially.

The efficacy of MABs and immunomagnetic beads in removing Burkitt's lymphoma cells from normal bone marrow has been demonstrated in a number of studies. Clonogenic lymphoma cell assays have demonstrated that different anti-B-cell MABs differ in their efficiency of depleting lymphoma cells from 1.9 to 2.8 logs in one cycle (72). When 3 MABs were used in a cocktail, the efficiency of purging increased to 3.3 logs following a single cycle of treatment and 5 logs after 2 cycles. Treatment of the bone marrow with beads alone or with the MABs did not significantly reduce the number of hematopoietic progenitors as assessed by colony assays. A cocktail of two MABs was used to assess the relative efficiency of purging of two different immunomagnetic particles (59). The efficacy of purging the cell line Nalm 6 was assessed using immunofluorescence or colony assays. Log tumor cell kill was significantly better using BioMag particles (3.1 logs) versus Dynabeads (1.8 logs) following a single cycle treatment. However, there was no significant difference in the efficiency of purging after 2 treatment cycles, and greater than 4.5 logs of tumor-cell depletion was obtained using either immunomagnetic bead. A combination of the peanut agglutinin-binding lectin and anti-CD19 MABs was used to remove myeloma cells from the harvested marrow using the immunomagnetic bead method (73). This technique was applied to a number of samples of myeloma bone marrow and cell line models, and in all cases removed all detectable leukemia cells.

Treatment of harvested bone marrow samples from lymphoma patients with either a 3- or a 4-MAB cocktail followed by immunomagnetic bead depletion resulted in the loss of all PCR-detectable cells after 3 cycles of treatment in all patients studied (74). After 2 treatment cycles of immunomagnetic bead depletion, 4 MABs were more efficient than 3 MABs for purging. In these same patient samples, treatment with 3 MABs and complement depleted all PCR-detectable lymphoma cells in only 44% of samples. The addition of a fourth MAB to this cocktail followed by complement lysis successfully purged the marrows of only 64% of marrow samples. In this study, immunomagnetic bead depletion had no significant effect on myeloid colony forming assays, suggesting that repeated cycles of immunomagnetic bead depletion might be performed safely. The results of this study suggest that immunomagnetic bead depletion is significantly more efficient than complement-mediated lysis in depleting lymphoma cells and that 4 MABs are more efficient than 3.

The results also demonstrate that multiple cycles of immunomagnetic bead depletion may still be required to remove PCR-detectable lymphoma cells. The increased efficiency of immunomagnetic bead depletion compared with complement-mediated lysis may be due to the presence of anticomplementary factors described. Because, theoretically, attachment of a single magnetic particle may be sufficient to allow removal of the targeted cell in a magnetic field, some lymphoma cells may have sufficiently low density of expression of the targeted antigens to allow elimination with immunomagnetic beads but not to allow complement-mediated lysis.

Using a single cycle of treatment with multiple monoclonal antibodies and beads, approximately 2.5 logs of small-cell lung cancer lines could be depleted, although there was variability in the efficiency of purging different cell lines (75). In parallel studies, there was no significant toxicity noted to myeloid progenitors. The CD15 monoclonal antibody, expressed on a variety of human cancer cell lines, was capable of depleting up to 3 logs of breast cancer cells from normal marrow using immunomagnetic bead depletion but minimally affected normal hematopoietic progenitors (53). Using two small-cell lung cancer lines, immunomagnetic bead depletion was shown to result in a 4- to 5-log reduction of cancer cells and did not adversely affect bone marrow colony growth (54). The combination of 4-hydroperoxycyclophosphamide and immunomagnetic bead depletion has been shown to remove 4 to 5 logs of clonogenic breast cancer cells (76).

Immunotoxins

Purging of autologous marrow in vitro using immunotoxins is a particularly promising approach. Several candidate toxins have been identified that are exquisitely toxic when delivered to a cell. These plant and bacterial toxins have cytotoxic function by inhibiting cellular protein synthesis. Because the mechanism of killing of toxins is different from that of chemotherapeutic agents, they are capable of killing cells that are resistant to chemotherapy (77). However, they are cytotoxic to both normal and malignant cells. The combination of these toxins with an MAB to target delivery to specific neoplastic cells is therefore a theoretically attractive proposition. For a more comprehensive overview of this field, readers are referred to a recent review by Grossbard and Nadler (78).

If native toxins were to be conjugated to MABs, the resultant immunotoxin would still be capable of binding to nonspecific targets by binding to the toxin binding site on normal cells. This nonspecific binding is overcome by modification to the toxin moiety to delete the binding site but to leave the toxin domains intact. The most widely studied toxins have been ricin, *Pseudomonas* exotoxin, and diphtheria toxin. Most experience of in vitro marrow purging has been with ricin. Strong and colleagues (79) reported the use of multiple anti-T cell intact ricin immunotoxins evaluated as potential purging agents. The cocktail containing all 4 immunotoxins in equimolar concentrations eliminated greater than 4 logs of clonogenic leukemic cells at a dose that spared more than 70% of the pluripotent hematopoietic progenitors. Evaluation of the purging efficiency of an immunotoxin prepared by conjugating anti-CD7 with pokeweed antiviral protein revealed that approximately 3 logs of clonogenic T cells could be eliminated, but that the addition of 2'deoxycoformycin and deoxyadenosine to the immunotoxin resulted in the elimination of up to 6 logs of the T-cell line, but also resulted in decreased myeloid progenitor colony assay growth (80).

Clinical Studies of Immunological Purging

A large number of clinical studies have been performed using MAB and complement-mediated lysis to purge residual neoplastic cells from autologous marrow in patients with non-Hodgkin's lymphoma, myeloma, acute lymphoblastic leukemia, acute myeloid leukemia, breast cancer, small-cell lung cancer, neuroblastoma, and retinoblastoma, among others. The results obtained in the larger reported trials using immunological purging are shown in Table 13-7. These studies have confirmed that immunological purging using MABs and complement-mediated lysis can be performed safely and that subsequent hematopoietic engraftment is not significantly delayed. However, evaluating the efficacy of purging from the results of these clinical trials is fraught with difficulties. No randomized or prospective study has been performed that could demonstrate whether the removal of occult or overt neoplastic cells resulted in improved disease-free survival. In addition, it is clear that in most malignancies, there is a need for a more effective ablative regimen to eradicate endogenous disease. Until these regimens are developed, the relative contribution, if any, of reinfused disease may be difficult to determine.

Complement-mediated Lysis

In a clinical trial of 30 patients with acute myeloid leukemia, bone marrow purging was performed using 2 MABs and complement-mediated lysis (6). All patients were in complete remission (CR) at the time of transplantation (6 in first CR, 18 in second CR, and 6 in third CR). Median recovery of colony forming unit–granulocyte macrophage (CFU-GM) was 36% for the first CR group and 47% for the patients in subsequent CR. Engraftment was prompt in most patients, and only one very heavily pretreated patient in third CR failed to engraft. Engraftment was faster in those patients infused with larger numbers of CFUs. This study did not compare results obtained using purged versus unpurged marrow, but the relapse-free survival of the patients in second and third remission was encouraging and appears to be comparable to that

Table 13-7.
Clinical Studies of Immunological Purging

Disease	No. Patients	Target Antigens	MABs	In Vitro Cell Kill	CFU-GM after Purging	Time to engraftment: Granulocytes >500	Time to engraftment: Platelets > 20,000	Reference
Complement-mediated lysis								
AML	30	CD14	PM-81	NS	36% 1st CR	27 (1st CR)	38	Ball et al. (6)
		CD15	AML 2-23		47% 2nd CR	32 (Later CR)	46	
AML	7	. . .	S4-7	2 logs	< 10%	20	58	De Fabritiis et al (82)
AML	12	CD33	My9	NS	< 2%	30	45	Robertson et al. (83)
ALL	54	CD10	RFAL 3	3 logs	NS	24	40	Simonsson et al. (84)
		CD19	SB4					
		CD7	RFT2					
NHL	17	CD24	BA-1	NS	NS	24	NS	Hurd et al. (4)
		CD9	BA-2					
		CD10	BA-3					
NHL	100	CD10	B1	NS	NS	27	29	Freedman et al. (2)
		CD20	J5					
		B5	B5					
Immunomagnetic beads								
Neuroblastoma	91	. . .	UJ13A	3 logs	18–34%	28	42	Combaret et al (56)
			Thy1			23 (part 1)	21	
			UJ127.11			50 (part 2)	75	
			UJ181.4					
			5.1H11					
Neuroblastoma	32	. . .	UJ13A	NS	NS	24	39	Philip et al. (85)
			Thy1					
			UJ127.11					
			UJ181.4					
			5.1H11					
ALL	8	CD10	AL2	NS	75%	15	27	Kemshead et al. (86)
		CD9	Pl153/3					
Immunotoxins								
ALL	13	CD7	WT 1-Ricin A	NS	97%	17	40	Preijers et al. (88)
ALL	14	CD5	T101-Ricin	0.8–3.4	NS	27	NS	Uckun et al. (89)
		CD7	G3.7-Ricin					
		+ hydroperoxycyclophosphamide						

MAB=monoclonal antibody; CFU-GM=colony forming unit—granulocyte macrophage; AML=acute myeloid leukemia; ALL=acute lymphoblastic leukemia; NHL=non-Hodgkin's lymphoma; NS=not studied.

obtained following allogeneic transplantation in similar risk patients. The Cancer and Leukemia Group B has begun a study of patients with acute myeloid leukemia in second remission, based on the pilot studies from the Dartmouth group. A subsequent study from the same group suggested that the addition of neuraminidase prior to the addition of MABs and complement increased the efficiency of purging, although this technique was performed in only a single patient (81). A study from Italy of 7 patients with acute myeloid leukemia reported rapid engraftment following infusion of the purged bone marrow, with a median time of 20 days to reach a granulocyte count of 500/μL (82). In 2 patients studied, the leukemic cells at the time of relapse no longer reacted with the MAB used for purging. At the Dana-Farber Cancer Institute, anti-CD33 MAB and complement-mediated lysis were used to purge the bone marrow of 12 patients with acute myeloid leukemias (83). Patients had durable but delayed engraftment, and platelet engraftment was particularly delayed in some patients. CFU-GM colony growth was markedly reduced following purging.

In a multicenter study, purged autologous transplantation was used in 54 patients with acute lymphoblastic leukemia (84). Marrow was purged using, as appropriate, anti-CD10, anti-CD19, anti-CD7, and rabbit complement. Transplant-related mortality was 5%, and engraftment was rapid. Although the study was not designed to show efficacy, the clinical results appear promising.

One hundred patients with B cell non-Hodgkin's lymphoma were treated with purged autologous BMT when they were in CR or minimal disease state (70). Notably, 69 patients had prior history of histological bone marrow involvement, and 37 patients had overt marrow involvement at the time of bone marrow harvest. This study was associated with an encouragingly low treatment-related mortality. Engraftment was rapid in all patients.

Although no direct study has been made comparing infusion of purged versus unpurged marrow, indirect approaches can be used to assess the clinical significance of immunological purging. In a recent study at the Dana-Farber Cancer Institute, PCR amplification of the t(14;18) was used to detect residual lymphoma cells in the bone marrow before and after purging to assess whether efficient purging had any impact on disease-free survival (29). In this study, 114 patients with B cell non-Hodgkin's lymphoma and the bcl-2 translocation were studied. Residual lymphoma cells were detected in all patients in the harvested autologous bone marrow. Following 3 cycles of immunological purging using the anti-B-cell MABs J5 (anti-CD10), B1 (anti-CD20), and B5 and complement-mediated lysis, PCR amplification detected residual lymphoma cells in 57 of these patients. The incidence of relapse was significantly increased in the 57 patients who had residual detectable lymphoma cells compared with those in whom no lymphoma cells were detectable after purging. This finding was independent of the histology of the lymphoma, the degree of bone marrow infiltration at the time of bone marrow harvest, or remission status at the time of autologous BMT. Thesc findings suggest that the infusion of detectable lymphoma cells is indeed associated with subsequent relapse. A major objection to this finding is that the majority of patients who relapse do so at sites of previous disease, suggesting that the major contribution to subsequent relapse came from endogenous disease. However, PCR analysis detected residual lymphoma cells in the circulation of patients infused with marrow containing residual lymphoma cells. It is possible that these circulating lymphoma cells are capable of homing back to the sites of previous disease, which provide the microenvironmental conditions conducive for cell growth. However, an alternative hypothesis is that the ability to purge residual lymphoma cells from the marrow was an indirect measure of a biological characteristic of the lymphoma. For instance, failure to eradicate lymphoma by immunological purging might be due to an anti-complementary factor or low antigen expression on the lymphoma cells of some patients. Patients with these characteristics might have lymphoma that is intrinsically less sensitive to the high-dose chemoradiotherapy delivered. The subsequent relapse of those patients whose marrows could not be successfully purged might therefore be due to the more aggressive nature of these lymphomas. However, to date, no association has been determined between the resistance to immunological purging and sensitivity to chemotherapy or radiotherapy.

Immunomagnetic Bead Depletion

The first clinical studies of purging using immunomagnetic beads were performed in children with neuroblastoma (55). In a recent report from France, immunomagnetic bead depletion was used to purge 123 marrow samples before autologous BMT in 91 patients with neuroblastoma. In this study, 59 patients received a single graft and 32 patients received 2 sequential procedures. Although the procedure resulted in a significant loss of mononuclear cells, there was little evidence of additional toxic effects on myeloid progenitors (56). Immunomagnetic bead depletion was also used to purge the bone marrow of 32 patients with stage IV neuroblastoma without affecting engraftment (85). Immunomagnetic beads were also used to deplete leukemic cells from the marrows of patients with common acute lymphoblastic leukemia (86)..In this study, the marrows of 18 patients were purged using a cocktail of 3 MABs, although only 8 of these patients were subsequently treated with high-dose therapy and autologous BMT. Engraftment was rapid in all patients, although it was reduced compared with that observed in patients with neuroblastoma. A panel of 6 MABs and immunomagnetic bead depletion were used to purge the bone marrow of a child with metastatic retinoblastoma and resulted in a favorable outcome (57).

A novel approach for the separation of malignant

cells was reported for 16 patients with B-cell malignancies using floating immunobeads (87). Low-density polypropylene beads precoated with rat anti-mouse MABs were added to the harvested autologous bone marrow following incubation with anti-B-cell MABs. This technique resulted in a 75% recovery of mononuclear cells, with an 83% recovery of myeloid progenitors.

Immunotoxins

A number of clinical trials have been reported using immunotoxins for purging. Seven patients with high-risk acute T cell lymphoblastic leukemia and 6 patients with T-cell lymphoma were treated by autologous BMT following purging of autologous marrow with anti-CD7 ricin A immunotoxin (WT1-ricin A)(88). Incubation of the marrow with up to 10^{-8} mol/L had no significant effect on hematopoietic progenitors as assessed by colony assay growth or on subsequent engraftment. A different approach was reported in the study by Uckun and colleagues (89). In this study, the autologous marrow from 14 consecutive patients with T cell acute lymphoblastic leukemia was purged with a combination of 2 immunotoxins, anti-CD5 and anti-CD7, linked to intact ricin, plus 4-hydroperoxy-cyclophosphamide. The efficacy of purging was assessed using multiparameter flow analysis, cell sorting, and leukemic progenitor cell colony assay. Following purging, no blast colonies were observed in the marrows of 11 of 13 evaluable patients. Engraftment occurred in 13 of the 14 patients, and the median time to reach an absolute neutrophil count greater than 500/μL was 27 days. Despite the apparent efficiency of purging, 9 patients relapsed, the majority shortly after transplantation. In this study, relapse after transplantation was most likely due to failure of the high-dose therapy to ablate endogenous disease.

Future Directions

A number of approaches can be undertaken to determine whether residual lymphoma cells in autologous marrow contribute to relapse (Table 13-8). First, a randomized trial using purged versus unpurged autologous marrow would likely provide a definitive answer. This trial would require a multicenter study of several hundred patients; however, several ethical questions would have to be addressed in the design of such of a study. Although purging appears to have no significant toxicity, it is expensive and there is no definitive data that unpurged marrow contributes to relapse. Although data do not prove that purging is essential, they are consistent with the interpretation that minimal residual disease in the marrow may contribute to relapse. If patients with 5% marrow infiltration were randomized to receive unpurged marrows, then malignant cells would be infused. We would not wish to exclude patients with minimal marrow involvement from receiving autologous BMT because those patients with histological marrow involvement whose marrows purged to PCR negativity had excellent disease-free survival. Second, if a marker gene were to be transfected into clonogenic malignant cells and the majority of cells at the site of relapse expressed the marker gene, this finding would provide compelling evidence that infused malignant cells contribute to relapse. Because the efficiency of transfection is low using existing technology and because we cannot specifically label tumor cells, a negative result would still not be definitive. Finally, if purging of the autologous marrow reduces relapse, then improvements in the efficiency of purging should result in increased disease-free survival. Such approaches would be dependent on the accurate assessment of the efficacy of purging.

Most studies performed to date have utilized immunological maneuvers to remove malignant cells from the autologous marrow by a process of negative selection. An alternative and highly attractive strategy would be to select the hematopoietic stem cell positively. There are a number of MABs that recognize the human hematopoietic progenitor cell antigen CD34, and these antibodies may be used for positive selection of CD34+ cells. The CD34+ population represents less than 2% of the low-density human mononuclear marrow cells. Precursors of all human hematopoietic lineages, including B and T lymphocytes, express CD34, and studies in nonhuman primates and in small numbers of humans have shown that isolated CD34+ cells are capable of re-establishing hematopoietic engraftment (90,91). Endothelial cells appear to be the only other cell type that expresses CD34. Although a minority of acute myeloid leukemia blasts express CD34 and the malignant stem cell in CML may also express CD34, the clonogenic stem cells for the remaining hematopoietic malignancies and for solid tumors do not express CD34. The positive selection of CD34+ cells from autologous marrow with or without negative selection to purge any more mature contaminating neoplastic cells is likely to have broad applicability in clinical autologous BMT.

Table 13-8.
Approaches to Demonstrate Efficacy of Purging

Randomized trial: purged versus unpurged
Gene transfer of marker gene
Surrogate end points
Depletion of clonogenic cells
Depletion of polymerase chain reaction–detectable cells

References

1. Armitage JO. Bone marrow transplantation in the treatment of patients with lymphoma. Blood 1989;73:1749–1758.
2. Freedman AS, Takvorian T, Anderson KC, et al. Autologous bone marrow transplantation in B-cell non-Hodgkin's lymphoma: very low treatment-related mor-

tality in 100 patients in sensitive relapse. J Clin Oncol 1990;8:1–8.
3. Gribben JG, Goldstone AH, Linch DC, et al. Effectiveness of high-dose combination chemotherapy and autologous bone marrow transplantation for patients with non-Hodgkin's lymphomas who are still responsive to conventional dose therapy. J Clin Oncol 1989;7:1621–1629.
4. Hurd DD, LeBien TW, Lasky LC, et al. Autologous bone marrow transplantation in non-Hodgkin's lymphoma: monoclonal antibodies plus complement for ex vivo marrow treatment. Am J Med 1988;85:829–834.
5. Philip T, Armitage JO, Spitzer G, et al. High-dose therapy and autologous bone marrow transplantation after failure of conventional chemotherapy in adults with intermediate-grade or high-grade non-Hodgkin's lymphoma. N Engl J Med 1987;316:1493–1498.
6. Ball ED, Mills LE, Cornwell GG, et al. Autologous bone marrow transplantation for acute myeloid leukemia using monoclonal antibody-purged bone marrow. Blood 1990;75:1199–1206.
7. Gribben JG, Linch DC, Singer CRJ, McMillan AK, Jarrett M, Goldstone AH. Successful treatment of refractory Hodgkin's disease by high dose chemotherapy and autologous bone marrow transplantation. Blood 1989;73:340–344.
8. Wallerstein R, Spitzer G, Dunphy F, et al. A Phase II study of mitoxantrone, etoposide and thiotepa with autologous marrow support for patients with relapsed breast cancer. J Clin Oncol 1990;8:1782–1788.
9. Frei E, Antman K, Teicher B, Schnipper L. Bone marrow autotransplantation for solid tumors—prospects. J Clin Oncol 1989;7:515–526.
10. Peters WP, Shpall EJ, Jones RB. High dose combination alkylating agents with bone marrow support as initial treatment for metastatic breast cancer. J Clin Oncol 1988;6:1501–1515.
11. Berliner N, Ault K, Martin P, Weisberg DS. Detection of clonal excess in lymphoproliferative disease by kappa/lambda analysis: correlation with immunoglobulin gene DNA arrangements. Blood 1986;67:80–85.
12. Favrot M, Philip I, Combaret V, et al. Monoclonal antibodies and complement purged autograft in Burkitt lymphoma and lymphoblastic leukemia. Bone Marrow Transplant 1989;4:202–204.
13. Sharp JG, Joshi SS, Armitage JO, et al. Significance of detection of occult non-Hodgkin's lymphoma in histologically uninvolved bone marrow by culture technique. Blood 1992;79:1074–1080.
14. Estrov Z, Grunberger T, Dube ID. Detection of residual acute lymphoblastic leukemia cells in cultures of bone marrow obtained during remission. N Engl J Med 1986;315:538–542.
15. Cleary ML, Chao J, Wanke R, Sklar J. Immunoglobulin gene rearrangement as a diagnostic criterion of B cell lymphoma. Proc Natl Acad Sci USA 1984;81:593–597.
16. Tsujimoto Y, Gorman J, Jaffe E, Croce CM. The t(14;18) chromosome translocations involved in B-cell neoplasms result from mistakes in VDJ joining. Science 1985;229:1390–1393.
17. Bakshi A, Jensen JP, Goldman P, et al. Cloning the chromosomal breakpoint of t(14;18) human lymphomas: clustering around J_H on chromosome 14 and near a transcriptional unit on 18. Cell 1985;41:899–906.
18. Cleary ML, Sklar J. Nucleotide sequence of a t(14;18) chromosomal breakpoint in follicular lymphoma and demonstration of a breakpoint cluster region near a transcriptionally active locus on chromosome 18. Proc Natl Acad Sci USA 1985;81:593–597.
19. Crescenzi M, Seto M, Herzig GP, Weiss PD, Griffith RC, Korsmeyer SJ. Thermostable DNA polymerase chain amplification of t(14;18) chromosome breakpoints and detection of minimal residual disease. Proc Natl Acad Sci USA 1988;85:4869–4873.
20. Ngan BY, Nourse J, Cleary ML. Detection of chromosomal translocation t(14;18) within the minor cluster region of bcl-2 by polymerase chain reaction and direct genomic sequencing of the enzymatically amplified DNA in follicular lymphomas. Blood 1989;73:1759–1762.
21. Lee MS, Chang KS, Cabanillas F, Freireich EJ, Trujillo JM, Stass SA. Detection of minimal residual disease carrying the t(14;18) by DNA sequence amplification. Science 1987;237:175–178.
22. Yunis JJ, Oken MM, Kaplan ME, Theologides RR, Howe A. Distinctive chromosomal abnormalities in histological subtypes of non-Hodgkin's lymphoma. N Engl J Med 1982;307:1231–1236.
23. Weiss LM, Warnke RA, Sklar J, Cleary ML. Molecular analysis of the t(14;18) chromosomal translocation in malignant lymphomas. N Engl J Med 1987;317:1185–1189.
24. Lee MS, Blick MB, Pathak S, et al. The gene located at chromosome 18 band q21 is rearranged in uncultured diffuse lymphomas as well as follicular lymphomas. Blood 1987;70:90–95.
25. Graninger WB, Seto M, Boutain B, Goldman P, Korsmeyer SJ. Expression of Bcl-2 and Bcl-2-Ig fusion transcripts in normal and neoplastic cells. J Clin Invest 1987;80:1512–1515.
26. Aisenberg AC, Wilkes BM, Jacobson JO. The bcl-2 gene is rearranged in many diffuse B-cell lymphomas. Blood 1988;71:969–972.
27. Yunis JJ, Mayer MG, Arnesen MA, Aeppli DP, Oken MM, Frizzera G. bcl-2 and other genomic alterations in the prognosis of large-cell lymphoma. N Engl J Med 1989;320:1047–1054.
28. Gribben JG, Freedman AS, Woo SD, et al. All advanced stage non-Hodgkin's lymphomas with a polymerase chain reaction amplifiable breakpoint of bcl-2 have residual cells containing the bcl-2 rearrangement at evaluation and after treatment. Blood 1991;78:3275–3280.
29. Gribben JG, Freedman AS, Neuberg D, et al. Immunologic purging of marrow assessed by PCR before autologous bone marrow transplantation for B-cell lymphoma. N Engl J Med 1991;325:1525–1533.
30. Freedman AS. Cell surface markers in leukemia and lymphoma. In: Harris GR, ed. Blood cell biochemistry (vol 3: lymphocytes and granulocytes). New York: Plenum Press, 1992:33–71.
31. Griffin JD, Mayer RJ, Weinstein HJ, et al. Surface marker analysis of acute myeloblastic leukemia: identification of differentiation-associated phenotypes. Blood 1983;62:557–563.
32. San Miguel JF, Gonzales M, Canizo MC, et al. Surface markers analysis in AML and correlation with FAB classification. Br J Hematol 1986;64:547–560.
33. Neame PB, Soamnoonsrup P, Browman GP, et al. Classifying acute leukemia by immunophenotyping: a combined FAB-immunologic classification of AML. Blood 1986;68:1355–1362.
34. Griffin JD, Todd RF, Ritz J, et al. Differentiation patterns in the blastic phase of chronic myeloid leukemia. Blood 1983;61:85–91.

35. Nadler LM, Takvorian T, Botnick L, et al. Anti-B1 monoclonal antibody and complement treatment in autologous bone-marrow transplantation for relapsed B-cell non-Hodgkin's lymphoma. Lancet 1984;2:427–431.
36. Sobol RE, Mick R, Royston I, et al. Clinical importance of myeloid antigen expression in adult acute lymphoblastic leukemia. N Engl J Med 1987;316:1111–1117.
37. Freedman AS, Boyd AW, Berrebi A, et al. Expression of B cell activation antigens on normal and malignant B cells. Leukemia 1987;1:9–15.
38. Reinherz EL, Nadler LM, Sallen SE, Schlossman SF. Subset derivation of T-cell acute lymphoblastic leukemia in man. J Clin Invest 1979;64:392–397.
39. Nadler LM, Reinherz EL, Weinstein HJ, D'Orsi CJ, Schlossman SF. Heterogeneity of T cell lymphoblastic malignancies. Blood 1980;55:806–810.
40. Sheibani K, Nathwani BN, Winberg CD, et al. Antigenically defined subgroups of lymphoblastic lymphoma. Relationship to clinical presentation and biologic behavior. Cancer 1987;60:183–190.
41. Sheibani K, Winberg CD, Van de Velde S, Blaney DW, Rappaport H. Distribution of lymphocytes with IL-2 receptors (Tac antigen) in reactive lymphoproliferative processes, Hodgkin's disease, and non-Hodgkin's lymphoma. Am J Pathol 1987;127:27–37.
42. Weiss LM, Bindl JM, Picozzi VJ, Link MP, Warnke RA. Lymphoblastic lymphoma: an immunophenotype study of 26 cases with comparison to T cell acute lymphoblastic leukemia. Blood 1986;67:474–478.
43. Ritz J, Nadler LM, Bhan AK, Notis-McConarty J, Pesando JM, Schlossman SF. Expression of common acute lymphoblastic antigen (CALLA) by lymphomas of B cell and T cell lineage. Blood 1981;58:648–652.
44. Cossman J, Jaffe ES, Fisher RI. Immunologic phenotypes of diffuse, aggressive, non-Hodgkin's lymphomas: correlations with clinical features. Cancer 1984; 54:1310–1317.
45. Doggett RS, Wood GS, Horning S, et al. The immunologic characterization of 95 nodal and extranodal diffuse large cell lymphomas in 89 patients. Am J Pathol 1984;115:245–252.
46. Brouet JC, Rabian C, Gisselbrecht C, Flandrin G. Clinical and immunological study of non-Hodgkin T cell lymphomas (cutaneous and lymphoblastic lymphomas excluded). Br J Haematol 1984;57:315–327.
47. Fialkow PJ, Jacobson RJ, Papayannopolou T. Chronic myelogenous leukemia: clonal origin in a stem cell common to the granulocyte, erythrocyte, platelet and monocyte/macrophage. Am J Med 1977;63:125–129.
48 Fialkow PJ, Denman AM, Jacobson RJ, Lowenthal LM. Chronic myelogenous leukemia: origin of some lymphocytes from leukemia stem cells. J Clin Invest 1978; 62:815–821.
49. Martin PJ, Najfeld V, Hansen JA, Penfold GK, Jacobson RJ, Fialkow PJ. Involvement of the B-lymphoid system in chronic myelogenous leukemia. Nature 1980;287:49–51.
50. Bernstein ID, Singer JW, Smith FO, et al. Differences in the frequency of normal and clonal precursors of colony-forming cells in chronic myelogenous leukemia and acute myelogenous leukemia. Blood 1992;79: 1811–1816.
51. Caligaris-Cappio F, Bergui L, Tesio L, et al. Identification of malignant plasma cell precursors in the bone marrow of multiple myeloma. J Clin Invest 1985;76:1243–1251.
52. Bertoli LF, Kubagawa H, Borzillo GV, et al. Bone marrow origin of a B-cell lymphoma. Blood 1988;72:94–101.
53. Vredenburgh JJ, Simpson W, Memoli VA, Ball ED. Reactivity of anti-CD15 monoclonal antibody PM-81 with breast cancer and elimination of breast cancer cell lines from human bone marrow by PM-81 and immunomagnetic beads. Cancer Res 1991;51:2451–2455.
54. Vredenburgh JJ, Ball ED. Elimination of small cell carcinoma of the lung from human bone marrow by monoclonal antibodies and immunomagnetic beads. Cancer Res 1990;50:7216–7220.
55. Treleaven J, Gibson F, Udelstad J. Removal of neuroblastoma cells from bone marrow with monoclonal antibodies conjugated to magnetic microsphere. Lancet 1984;2:70–76.
56. Combaret V, Favrot MC, Chauvin F, Bouffet E, Philip I, Philip T. Immunomagnetic depletion for malignant cells from autologous bone marrow graft: from experimental models to clinical trials. J Immunogenet 1989;16:125–136.
57. Saleh RA, Gross S, Cassano W, Gee A. Metastatic retinoblastoma successfully treated with immunomagnetic purged autologous bone marrow transplantation. Cancer 1988;62:2301–2303.
58. Roy DC, Felix M, Cannady WG, Cannistra S, Ritz J. Comparative activities of rabbit complements of different ages using an in-vitro marrow purging model. Leukemia Res 1990;14:407–416.
59. Trickett AE, Ford DJ, Lam-Po-Tang PRL, Vowels MR. Immunomagnetic bone marrow purging of common acute lymphoblastic leukemia cells: suitability of BioMag particles. Bone Marrow Transplant 1991;7:199–203.
60. De Fabritiis P, Bregni M, Lipton J, et al. Elimination of clonogenic Burkitt's lymphoma cells from human bone marrow using 4-hydroperoxycyclophosphamide in combination with monoclonal antibodies and complement. Blood 1985;65:1064–1070.
61. Bast RC, De Fabritiis P, Lipton J, et al. Elimination of malignant clonogenic cells from human bone marrows using multiple monoclonal antibodies and complement. Cancer Res 1985;45:499–503.
62. LeBien TW, Stepan DE, Bartholomew RM, Strong RC, Anderson JM. Utilization of a colony assay to assess the variables influencing elimination of leukemic cells from human bone marrow with monoclonal antibodies and complement. Blood 1985;65:945–950.
63. Negrin RS, Kiem HP, Schmidt-Wolf IGH, Blume KG, Cleary M. Use of the polymerase chain reaction to monitor the effectiveness of ex vivo tumor cell purging. Blood 1991;77:654–660.
64. Schlager SI, Ohanian SH, Borsos T. Identification of lipids associated with the ability of tumor cells to resist humoral immune attack. J Immunol 1978;120:472–480.
65. Schlager SI, Boyle MDP, Ohanian SH, Borsos T. Effect of inhibiting DNA, RNA and protein synthesis of tumor cells on their susceptibility to killing by antibody and complement. Cancer Res 1977;37:1432–1437.
66. Gee AP, Bruce KM, Morris TD, Boyle MD. Evidence for an anticomplementary factor associated with human bone marrow cells. J Natl Cancer Inst 1985;75:441–445.
67. Bast RC, Ritz J, Lipton JM, et al. Elimination of leukemic cells from human bone marrow using monoclonal antibody and complement. Cancer Res 1983;43:1389–1394.
68. Howell AL, Fogg LM, Davis BH, Ball ED. Continuous infusion of complement by an automated cell processor enhances cytotoxicity of monoclonal antibody

sensitized leukemia cells. Bone Marrow Transplant 1989;4:317–322.
69. Gee AP, Boyle MDP. Purging tumor cells from bone marrows by use of antibody and complement: a critical appraisal. J Natl Cancer Inst 1988;80:154–159.
70. Humblet Y, Feyens AM, Sekhavat M, Agaliotis D, Canon JL, Symann ML. Immunological and pharmacological removal of small cell lung cancer cells from bone marrow autografts. Cancer Res 1989;49:5058–5061.
71. Aihara M, Aihara Y, Schmidt-Wolf G, et al. A combined approach for purging multidrug-resistant leukemic cell lines in bone marrow using a monoclonal antibody and chemotherapy. Blood 1991;77:2079–2084.
72. Kvalheim G, Sorensen O, Fodstad O, et al. Immunomagnetic removal of B-lymphoma cells from human bone marrow: a procedure for clinical use. Bone Marrow Transplant 1988;3:31–41.
73. Rhodes EG, Baker P, Rhodes JM, Davies JM, Cawley JC. Peanut agglutinin in combination with CD19 monoclonal antibody has potential as a purging agent in myeloma. Exp Hematol 1991;19:833–837.
74. Gribben JG, Saporito L, Barber M, et al. Bone marrows of non-Hodgkin's lymphoma patients with a bcl-2 translocation can be purged of PCR detectable lymphoma cells using monoclonal antibodies and immunomagnetic beads. Blood 1992;80:1083–1089.
75. Elias AD, Pap SA, Bernal SD. Purging of small cell lung cancer-contaminated bone marrow by monoclonal antibodies and magnetic beads. Prog Clin Biol Res 1990;333:263–275.
76. Schpall EJ, Bast RC, Joines WT, et al. Immunomagnetic purging of breast cancer from bone marrow for autologous transplantation. Bone Marrow Transplant 1991;7:145–151.
77. FitzGerald DJ, Willingham MC, Cardarelli CO, et al. A monoclonal antibody-Pseudomonas toxin conjugate that specifically kills multidrug-resistant cells. Proc Natl Acad Sci USA 1987;84:4288–4292.
78. Grossbard ML, Nadler LM. Immunotoxin therapy of malignancy. In: DeVita VT, Hellman S, Rosenberg SA, eds. Important advances in oncology. Philadelphia: JB Lippincott, 1992:111–135.
79. Strong RC, Uckun F, Youle RJ, Kersey J, Vallera DA. Use of multiple T cell-directed intact ricin immunotoxins for autologous bone marrow transplantation. Blood 1985;66:627–635.
80. Montgomery RB, Kurtzberg J, Rhinehardt-Clark A, et al. Elimination of malignant clonogenic T cells from human bone marrow using chemoimmunoseparation with 2'-deoxycoformycin, deoxyadenosine and an immunotoxin. Bone Marrow Transplant 1990;5:395–402.
81. Ball ED, Vrendenburgh JJ, Mills LE, et al. Autologous bone marrow transplantation for acute myeloid leukemia following in vitro treatment with neuraminidase and monoclonal antibodies. Bone Marrow Transplant 1990;6:277–280.
82. De Fabritiis P, Ferrero D, Sandrelli A, et al. Monoclonal antibody purging and autologous bone marrow transplantation in acute myelogenous leukemia in complete remission. Bone Marrow Transplant 1989;4:669–674.
83. Robertson MJ, Soiffer RJ, Freedman AS, et al. Human bone marrow depleted of CD33-positive cells mediates delayed but durable reconstitution of hematopoiesis: clinical trial of My9 monoclonal antibody-purged autografts for the treatment of acute myeloid leukemia. Blood 1992;79:2229–2236.
84. Simonsson B, Burnett AK, Prentice HG, et al. Autologous bone marrow transplantation with monoclonal antibody purged marrow for high risk acute lymphoblastic leukemia. Leukemia 1989;3:631–636.
85. Philip T, Bernard JL, Zucker JM, et al. High-dose chemoradiotherapy with bone marrow transplantation as consolidation treatment in neuroblastoma: an unselected group of stage IV patients over 1 year of age. J Clin Oncol 1987;5:266–271.
86. Kemshead JT, Treleaven J, Heath L, Meara AO, Gee A, Ugelstad J. Monoclonal antibodies and magnetic microspheres for the depletion of leukemic cells from bone marrow harvested for autologous transplantation. Bone Marrow Transplant 1987;2:133–139.
87. Stoppa AM, Hirn J, Blaise D, et al. Autologous bone marrow transplantation for B cell malignancies after in vitro purging with floating immunobeads. Bone Marrow Transplant 1990;6:301–307.
88. Preijers FWMB, De Witte T, Wessels JMC, et al. Autologous transplantation of bone marrow purged in vitro with anti-CD7-(WT1-) ricin A immunotoxin in T-cell lymphoblastic leukemia and lymphoma. Blood 1989;74:1152–1158.
89. Uckun F, Kersey JH, Vallera DA, et al. Autologous bone marrow transplantation in high risk remission T-lineage acute lymphoblastic leukemia using immunotoxins plus 4-hydroperoxycyclophosphamide for marrow purging. Blood 1990;76:1723–1733.
90. Berenson RJ, Andrews RG, Bensinger WI, et al. Antigen CD34+ marrow cells engraft lethally irradiated baboons. J Clin Invest 1988;81:951–955.
91. Berenson RJ, Bensinger WI, Hill RS, et al. Engraftment after infusion of CD34+ marrow cells in patients with breast cancer or neuroblastoma. Blood 1991;77:1717–1722.

Chapter 14
Pharmacological Purging of Malignant Cells

Scott D. Rowley

In theory, malignant cells not eliminated from a marrow inoculum may be a source for relapse after autologous bone marrow transplantation (BMT). This risk of relapse is of especial concern in autologous BMT for the treatment of tumors arising from the marrow, such as acute leukemia or multiple myeloma, or those diseases such as non-Hodgkin's lymphoma or breast cancer that frequently metastasize to the marrow during the natural history of the disease. The concern can be addressed by a number of approaches that may reduce the tumor burden in the harvested marrow and the probability of relapse after BMT. These approaches include intensive preharvest or posttransplant therapy of patients (in vivo purge) or treatment of the harvested marrow cells (ex vivo purge). Most transplant programs currently require that the marrow be free of disease by morphological examination of a recently obtained aspirate or marrow biopsy before marrow harvesting. For patients with acute leukemia, however, a "remission marrow" may contain up to 5% blast cells. Although it is unknown what proportion of morphologically identifiable malignant cells are capable of clonal growth, it may be argued that a typical harvest of more than 10^{10} cells could contain as many as 5×10^8 leukemic cells. Multiple intensive consolidation courses before marrow harvesting may reduce the tumor burden to levels at which the marrow inoculum presents little risk of causing relapse, although at possibly considerable time, expense, and morbidity. Reliable and sensitive tumor detection assays would facilitate this approach to patient management by quantifying the number of malignant cells contained in a marrow aspirate at any point in the patient's therapy. The optimal timing of marrow harvesting could then be determined for each individual patient. In the absence of clinically meaningful assays, however, many centers incorporated ex vivo marrow treatments into BMT regimens in an attempt to eliminate tumor cells possibly contaminating the marrow inoculum, and with the assumption that nontoxic purging techniques would pose little risk to the patient.

A variety of ex vivo purging methods have been developed. Techniques to remove or to destroy malignant cells in the marrow must discriminate between normal and malignant stem cells. Physical, immunological, and pharmacological techniques have been studied in preclinical or clinical studies. Physical techniques, such as density separation or cryopreservation, have not been promising in in vitro testing. Immunological techniques using monoclonal antibodies directed against antigens found on the malignant cell but not shared by the normal hematopoietic precursors are another approach, the uses and limitations of which are discussed in Chapter 13. For many malignancies, specific tumor-directed antibodies are not readily available, are expensive, or are of limited efficacy because of tumor-cell heterogeneity. For these reasons, many transplant programs are investigating pharmacologics as purging agents with broad specificity and activity for a variety of malignancies. Initial preclinical studies demonstrated the feasibility of treating marrow with pharmacologics. Subsequent clinical studies established that marrows can be treated ex vivo with concentrations of drugs not achievable in vivo while still permitting satisfactory engraftment. Much of the recent experimentation with pharmacological purge agents has focused on the development of regimens with high therapeutic ratios, such as novel purging agents or combinations of drugs.

It is currently much simpler to study the cytotoxic capability of any drug in vitro than to demonstrate safety and efficacy in clinical trials. In vitro studies using tumor-derived cell lines and hematopoietic progenitor cell cultures may be completed in weeks, in contrast to the months to years required for Phase I clinical trials. Relatively few potential agents have been studied in clinical trials. In particular, evidence supporting the efficacy of ex vivo purging for any particular regimen or for any particular group of patients is scant. Clinical experience is greatest with activated oxazaphosphorines, and these agents will be discussed in depth to illustrate the potential and limitations of pharmacological purges. Other drugs are being used for ex vivo marrow treatments. Details concerning drug metabolism and cytotoxic mechanisms can be found in general oncology texts. Also, although this section discusses only the treatment of marrow cells, similar considerations apply to the treatment of hematopoietic progenitors collected from peripheral blood.

Principles of Pharmacological Purging

The same principles that apply to the systemic treatment of cancer with chemotherapeutics also apply to their use as ex vivo purge agents. Dose, duration of exposure, drug metabolism, sensitivity patterns of normal and malignant cells, and mechanisms of cytotoxicity and resistance must all be considered in developing either systemic or ex vivo regimens. A more pertinent comparison for ex vivo purging, however, is to the local use of chemotherapy to treat sites of poor drug distribution, such as intrathecal or intraperitoneal instillation. In all three situations, very high local concentrations (with frequently small total quantities of drugs) can be achieved while systemic toxicity is minimized or eliminated.

For most antineoplastics, cytotoxicity is dependent on both the concentration of the drug achieved and the duration of exposure to the drug. In the treatment of dose-responsive malignancies such as acute leukemia, malignant lymphoma, or breast cancer, systemic administration of escalated drug dosages frequently results in improved rates of remission induction and patient survival (1). This concept is the basis of high-dose chemotherapy and autologous marrow rescue. BMT negates any concerns about toxicity to normal hematopoietic progenitors from the intensive conditioning regimen, because a source of cells is available to rescue the patient from this otherwise deleterious consequence of high-dose therapy. The rationale behind the use of pharmacologics for ex vivo purging of tumor cells from marrow (or peripheral blood stem-cell collections) is the proven cytotoxic effects of these agents when administered systemically. The advantage of the ex vivo use of pharmacologics compared with systemic administration, however, is that nonhematological (extramedullary) toxicities are of little concern if the agent can be removed or detoxified before marrow reinfusion. Thus, agents such as cyclophosphamide (CY) that have unacceptable extramedullary toxicities that limit the dose administered systemically may be used ex vivo (in derived forms) at concentrations much greater than those achievable in vivo.

Dose is important because cancer cell cytotoxicity for many chemotherapeutics follows first-order kinetics (*i.e.*, for a certain drug dose, a fixed proportion of cells [not a fixed number] will be killed). Multiple cycles of therapy may be necessary to accomplish enough tumor kill to achieve remission or cure of the patient. Alternatively, drug dose can be increased so that a greater fraction of the malignant cells are killed with each cycle. The limited maintenance of hematopoietic stem-cell viability in vitro precludes multiple cycles of marrow purging. Recovery of normal marrow function that would occur in a patient after a cycle of systemic treatment cannot be similarly accomplished with current cell culture techniques for marrows treated ex vivo. Thus, purging agents must achieve a high degree of tumor-cell cytotoxicity during a single exposure. Shorter duration of exposure may be offset by achieving higher concentrations of drug. The relationship between drug concentration and exposure time to cytotoxicity explains the necessity for treating cells at concentrations not achievable in vivo.

Table 14-1.
Criteria For Ideal Pharmacological Purging Agents

Agent must be cytotoxic at the concentration achieved ex vivo
Agent must be sparing of hematopoietic stem cells at concentration used ex vivo
Cytotoxicity must be achieved during a short exposure
Agent can be removed or detoxified before marrow reinfusion or is nontoxic to host at dose infused

Marrow cells are incubated with chemotherapeutics for periods of minutes to a few hours to minimize the loss of hematopoietic progenitor cells inherent in any ex vivo manipulation of marrow. Avoidance of extramedullary toxicities therefore permits possibly equivalent or even greater degrees of tumor-cell cytotoxicity than if the drugs used for purging had been administered systemically. The limited duration of exposure generally restricts ex vivo purging to agents that are cell-cycle nonspecific. For this reason, alkylating agents are probably of greater efficacy for this use than other classes of chemotherapeutics.

Pharmacological agents used in this manner must be active in vitro. CY, for example, is a prodrug requiring initial hepatic metabolism to 4-hydroxycyclophosphamide. Thus, this drug is of no value for ex vivo purging (or for intrathecal or intraperitoneal instillation). 4-Hydroperoxycyclophosphamide (4-HC) and mafosfamide are also prodrugs, but they spontaneously and rapidly hydrolyze in the presence of water, also forming 4-hydroxycyclophosphamide. Much of the preclinical evaluation of pharmacological purging was directed at showing drug cytotoxicity under the conditions used during ex vivo incubation of marrow cells.

The important properties of purge agents are summarized in Table 14-1. These criteria are vital to the design of any purging technique, regardless of cytotoxic mechanism.

1. The drug must be both effective ex vivo and highly cytotoxic to the malignancy being treated. Clinical experience with use of a drug may suggest diseases for which this drug may also be effective as a purging agent. The extremely high concentrations that are achievable for most drugs ex vivo may also permit efficacious use of an agent in the treatment of diseases for which the drug has little obvious clinical efficacy.
2. The drug must also spare hematopoietic stem and progenitor cells at the concentrations achieved ex vivo. Toxicity to hematopoietic cells results in prolongation of aplasia and possibly in marrow failure. Agents that are relatively sparing of hema-

topoietic cells when used in vivo may be extremely damaging at the concentrations achieved during purging. Agents that are marrow-toxic may be ineffective purging agents because of similar magnitudes of toxicity for both normal marrow and malignant stem cells.
3. The drug must be cytotoxic during the short exposure time used for purging of marrow. Thus, noncycle-dependant agents may be more efficacious.
4. The amounts of some drugs used for purging may be toxic if administered directly to patients. Marrow is reinfused shortly after administration of dose-intensive therapy to patients, so additional chemotherapy infused with the marrow could be more damaging than if a similar dose of the purging agent were infused alone. Also, dimethylsulfoxide (DMSO) may enhance the transfer of some drugs into cells, again increasing the toxicity of the marrow purging agent.

In Vitro Evaluation of Chemotherapeutics

A number of drugs have been tested in preclinical assays using tumor-derived cell lines and hematopoietic progenitor cell cultures to measure the effect on malignant and normal cells, respectively (Table 14-2)(2–11). These studies are important for demonstrating the in vitro activity of the drug under the conditions of incubation and for determining the incubation parameters such as duration, temperature, cell concentration, and protein concentration, among others. In contrast, dose and efficacy can be determined only in clinical studies of a defined patient population. Few of these drugs have been tested in clinical trials despite the apparent efficacy demonstrated by several logs of tumor cell kill while sparing at least some normal myeloid progenitors (e.g., colony forming unit–granulocyte macrophage [CFU-GM]).

The homogeneity of tumor-derived cell lines limits their utility for comparing the relative cytotoxicity of the various drugs for in vitro incubation, predicting clinical efficacy, or determining the dose to be used for clinical trials. Sensitive and resistant tumor-derived cell lines can be found for each drug to be tested. These cell lines are illustrated for one drug in Table 14-3, which collates reported cell kill by 4-HC for a number of tumor-derived cell lines. Cell kills ranging from less than one log to more than 3 logs (residual tumor viability of > 10 to < 0.1%) have been reported. 4-HC is active against a wide variety of tumor-derived cell lines. In one preclinical report, adriamycin was dismissed as showing inadequate tumor-cell kill compared with 4-HC when tested against 2 lymphoma-derived cell lines (7). A similar conclusion about 4-HC might have been reached if 4-HC-resistant cell lines had been tested. In particular, animal studies may be difficult to translate into clinical protocols. Jones and colleagues (12) reported that the use of vincristine (50 μg/mL) allowed engraftment in a murine model, yet a dose less than half that (20 μg/mL) destroyed almost 99.9% of human CFU-GM (11).

The culture of human CFU-GM may be valuable in demonstrating a therapeutic ratio for the drug being tested or for modifying incubation parameters. In

Table 14-2.
Preclinical Evaluation of Drug Purging Agents

Drug[a]	*Cell Line Kill (%)*	*CFU-GM Kill (%)*	*References*
4-HC	83–>99.9[b,c,d,e]	82.5–98.8	3,4,7,11
VP16	96.1–>99.9[b,d,e]	72.7–97	4,7,11
Vincristine	75–>99.9[c,d,e]	<10–76	3,7,11
Adriamycin	98.6–99.3[b,d]	50.6–83	4,7
Bleomycin	19–91.6[c,d]	50–83.5	3,7
L-Asparaginase	0[c]	73.5	3
Cisplatinum	>99.9[d]	96	7

[a]Drug concentrations, cell concentrations, and incubation durations differ for the various studies.
[b]HL-60 cell line tested.
[c]REH, KM3, LAZ 221 cell line tested.
[d]LY-16, SK-DHL-2 cell line tested.
[e]K562, CEM, REH cell line tested.

Table 14-3.
Preclinical Evaluation of 4-HC

Dose (μg/mL)	*Duration* (*min*)	*Cell Line*	*Cell Line Kill (%)*	*Marrow Cell Preparation*	*CFU-GM Kill (%)*	*Reference*
29.2	60	HL-60	99.8	Buffy-coat	82.5	4
20	60	REH	88.0	Mononuclear	93.5	3
		KM3	91.5			
		LAZ 221	83.0			
21	30	LY-16	>99.9	Mononuclear	90	7
		SK-DHL-2	>99.9			
60	30	K562	99.5	Mononuclear	98.8	11
		CEM	>99.9			
		REH	>99.9			

4-HC = 4-hydroperoxycyclophosphamide.

vitro cultures, for example, allowed the change to incubating density-gradient separated cells (instead of buffy-coat cells) with 4-HC without repeating a Phase I dose-finding study (13). The value of in vitro cultures of normal hematopoietic progenitors can be confirmed only in clinical trials. A correlation between the quantity of progenitor cells detected with the kinetics of hematological recovery must be demonstrated before these cultures can be accepted as a surrogate for clinical evaluation. For example, in vitro hematopoietic progenitor cultures for the preclinical evaluation of merocyanine-540 purging predicted little normal cell toxicity (14). Engraftment failure, however, occurred during the Phase I clinical evaluation of this agent (15).

In vitro studies of tumor-cell kill (comparing normal and malignant progenitors) can be useful in determining incubation parameters. For example, in vitro studies demonstrated increased cytotoxicity against both tumor-derived and hematopoietic progenitor cells when methylprednisolone preceded 4-HC incubation, but enhanced cytotoxicity against the tumor cells but not against normal progenitors when the order of incubation was reversed (16). We subsequently observed this effect (resulting from inadequate removal of 4-HC before the second incubation) in an unpublished clinical trial of these two drugs in combination. A similar effect of incubation order was demonstrated by Anderson and colleagues (17) in their preclinical evaluation of combined 4-HC and immunomagnetic purging of breast cancer cell lines. In studying incubation technique, it may be presumed that cultures of normal myeloid progenitors reflect the effect of the drug incubation on the cells responsible for marrow engraftment. Divergent results are conceivable but unlikely.

Although there is some evidence that the presence of detectable tumor using in vitro assays predicts diminished disease-free survival of patients in both nontransplant and transplant settings (18–22), the direct culture of tumor cells from bone marrow (CFU-L) has not replaced the use of tumor-derived cell lines for preclinical evaluation of pharmacological purging. For pharmacological purging, in which cell disintegration is not immediate as in antibody and complement purging, tumor detection techniques based on cell phenotype or genetic markers may be impossible to interpret because these markers would still be detectable even though the treated cell had been fatally injured by the pharmacological treatment. The clinical relevance of detectable tumor is uncertain because a relationship between the tumor cells detected and those clonogenic tumor cells capable of causing relapse has not been established. Thus, the culture of malignant cells from the marrow is not accepted as evidence proving the necessity for or the efficacy of purging. For these reasons, most investigators have relied on the much simpler culture of tumor-derived cell lines to demonstrate ex vivo activity of the purging regimen under study.

Chemotherapeutics

Activated Oxazaphosphorines

Mafosfamide and 4-HC are activated oxazaphosphorines—derivatives of CY with in vitro activity. Preclinical studies and Phase I and II trials have demonstrated the feasibility of ex vivo purging with these agents. These drugs are currently the pharmacologics most commonly used for ex vivo purging.

Pharmacology

CY metabolism has been recently reviewed in detail (23). CY is a prodrug that requires hepatic metabolism to 4-hydroxycyclophosphamide for activity (Figure 14-1). The activated oxazaphosphorines, 4-HC and mafosfamide, are also prodrugs that will spontaneously decompose in the presence of water to form 4-hydroxycyclophosphamide. 4-Hydroxycyclophosphamide and its tautomer, aldophosphamide, are freely diffusible into the cell, where activation to phosphoramide mustard or enzymatic oxidation to the inactive metabolite, carboxyphosphamide, occurs. For all three drugs, phosphoramide mustard is the active metabolite. Resistance to CY and its derivatives appears to result primarily from oxidation of aldophosphamide catalyzed by cellular aldehyde dehydrogenase. It is proposed that the higher cellular levels of this enzyme

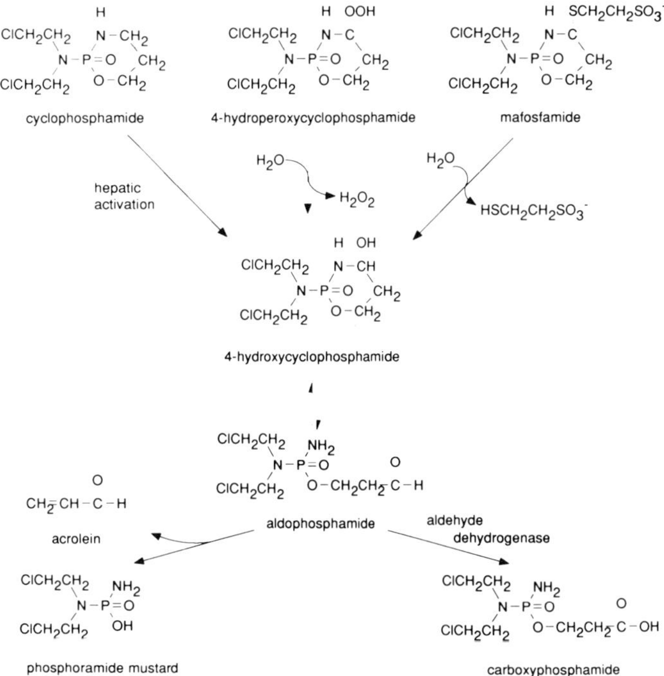

Figure 14-1. Oxazaphosphorine metabolism. Shown are the major intermediate compounds and metabolic pathways. (Adapted from Sladek NE. Metabolism of oxazaphosphorines. Pharmacol Ther 1988;37:301–355.)

account for the diminished sensitivity to CY of normal compared with malignant cells, or of primitive hematopoietic stem cells compared with the more mature, lineage-committed progenitor cells (24–29). Direct incubation of marrow cells with phosphoramide mustard abolishes this differential cytotoxicity, as can pretreatment of cells with inhibitors of aldehyde dehydrogenase, such as disulfiram (25,26).

4-Hydroxycyclophosphamide and aldophosphamide are the circulating metabolites after systemic administration of CY. These compounds are freely diffusible. Drug uptake or extrusion do not appear responsible for resistance to oxazaphosphorines. Inactivation of oxazaphosphorines is believed to be primarily from enzyme-mediated oxidation of aldophosphamide, although metabolism along glutathione-dependant pathways may also contribute (30). Depletion of intracellular glutathione increases the alkylating activity of a number of drugs, including CY, mephalan, and chlorambucil, but not phosphoramide mustard (31–33). Peripheral blood cells also contain aldehyde dehydrogenase; practically all the activity in whole blood is a result of the erythrocyte content of this enzyme (34). Therefore, greater concentrations of peripheral blood or marrow cells in the incubation mixture will increase the inactivation of 4-HC, thereby decreasing the levels of phosphoramide mustard to which the cells are exposed. Hematopoietic and tumor cells comprise a small fraction of cells in the bone marrow inoculum, so the effective concentration of phosphoramide mustard is a function of the quantity of other blood cells in the incubation mixture and the concentration of aldehyde dehydrogenase in those cells. Both the erythrocyte content (hematocrit) and the nucleated cell concentration of the 4-HC incubation mixture can modulate the cytotoxicity of these agents to normal and malignant cells, consequently affecting both the duration of post-transplant aplasia and the probability of relapse (35–37). Although red blood cells, by function of their numbers, contain the greatest amount of aldehyde dehydrogenase, other cells are also capable of inactivating these drugs, as shown by the inverse relationship between nucleated cell concentration and drug-induced cytotoxicity (35–37).

Two CY derivatives have been used in clinical trials to treat marrows before autologous BMT.

4-Hydroperoxycyclophosphamide

4-HC (molecular weight, 292.1) is a hydroperoxy-derivative of CY produced by ozonization (38). It is comparatively unstable and thus requires desiccated storage at low temperatures. 4-HC spontaneously hydrolyzes with the release of hydrogen peroxide. The half-life in Tris buffer at 37°C is 43 minutes; in the presence of phosphate buffers at alkaline pH, the half-life is considerably shorter.

Mafosfamide

Mafosfamide is a sulfoethylthio-derivative of CY formulated as both cyclohexamine (ASTA Z 7557; molecular weight, 500.4) and lysine salts (ASTA Z 7654; molecular weight, 547.5) (39). Mafosfamide spontaneously hydrolyzes with the release of 2-mercaptoethane sulfonic acid (mesna), with a half-life of approximately 8 minutes when diluted at 50 μg/mL in 70 mmol/L phosphate buffer.

The relative efficacy of these two compounds has not been tested in clinical studies. Although it has been suggested that 4-HC has greater toxicity than mafosfamide (40), equivalent molar concentrations were not used in those in vitro tests. Both these activated oxazaphosphorines are used for ex vivo purging at concentrations of 60 to 140 μg/mL, as determined by the practices of the individual transplant center (generally defined by such considerations as initial marrow preparation and incubation conditions). Different rates of hydrolysis on reconstitution of the drugs and addition to the incubation mixture may affect the relative cytotoxicity of these two agents, although adequate comparative studies have not been performed using the conditions of marrow incubation. Nevertheless, toxicity to normal hematopoietic progenitor cells is the limiting factor in purging with these agents, and the doses chosen for clinical trials were set to achieve maximal cytotoxic effect within allowable limits of normal cell toxicity. It is possible but unlikely that a difference in purging efficacy between these drugs as a result of different rates of hydrolysis would be found when both agents are used at their maximally tolerated doses.

A variety of sulfur-containing compounds, including DMSO, are able to enhance the cytotoxicity of nitrogen mustard administered in vivo (41). DMSO, used for cryopreservation of hematopoietic cells, may potentiate the uptake of various drugs, and significant neurotoxicity has been reported (e.g., with concomitant administration of DMSO and sulindac) (42). Enhanced uptake of CY metabolites (including the polar, poorly diffusible phosphoramide mustard) may account for the observation by Lopez and colleagues (43) that mafosfamide-purged marrow had lower CFU-GM survival after cryopreservation than untreated marrows (24 *vs* 79%). Halothane anesthesia (44) and inhibitors of aldehyde dehydrogenase and glutathione reductase may also increase the toxicity of CY derivatives (25,26,30,31).

Various radioprotectors protect normal cells against the toxicity of alkylating agents, including CY (45–48). The mechanism of protection has not been established. Recently, Shpall and associates (49) reported a randomized trial comparing engraftment kinetics of 4-HC-treated marrow to 4-HC-treated marrow preincubated with WR2721. Preclinical studies showed protection of CFU-GM (with 10–100 times greater recovery of CFU-GM) but no protection of breast cancer–derived cells if the compound was washed from the cell mixture before 4-HC incubation. These authors found a significant decrease in aplasia duration (mean, 26 vs 37 days; $p = 0.024$) for the latter patients. Whether this benefit is offset by less tumor cytotoxicity and greater risk of relapse is unknown but of obvious concern.

Preincubation with interleukin-1 or tumor-necrosis factor also protects hematopoietic progenitor cells against 4-HC (and irradiation), with similar increments in CFU-GM survival to that reported for WR2721 (50,51). The effect is observed after 20 hours of preincubation, suggesting that the effect results from changes in cell cycle or protein composition. Clinical evaluation of this observation has not been reported. The required lengthy preincubation is disadvantageous for clinical purging, but treatment of patients before harvesting may be feasible if a similar marrow-protective effect were found with systemic administration of these agents.

Coincubation with chemotherapeutics such as vincristine or etoposide may also protect normal hematopoietic progenitors from 4-HC or mafosfamide toxicity (6,52). This phenomenon facilitates simultaneous treatment of marrow with several drugs, as discussed later.

Effects of Activated Oxazaphosphorines on Hematopoietic Cells

Incubation of normal hematopoietic cells with either 4-HC or mafosfamide decreases hematopoietic progenitor cell survival in a dose-dependant manner (28,53,54). A differential effect on mature compared with primitive hematopoietic progenitors has been found, possibly resulting from intracellular levels of aldehyde dehydrogenase, as discussed earlier (25,26). Primitive progenitors surviving the drug exposure can give rise to CFU-GM in long-term marrow cultures of oxazaphosphorine-treated marrow initially devoid of this mature progenitor (54–56). Ex vivo incubation with these drugs can reduce the quantity of CFU-GM in clinical marrow samples below the level of detection in in vitro assays. Hematopoietic progenitor cell cultures are the only available quality-control technique for marrow processing laboratories to quantify the drug effect on normal hematopoietic cells. Such cultures are of greater clinical utility if the quantity of progenitor cells detected predicts the duration of aplasia. Patients may still recover hematopoietic function even in the absence of detectable CFU-GM. If the assay used is predictive of engraftment kinetics, however, the period of aplasia may be exceedingly prolonged.

Clinical Use of Activated Oxazaphosphorine Purging

The first study to demonstrate the feasibility of ex vivo purging of tumor cells using a pharmacological regimen was published by Sharkis and colleagues (57). Using a rat model of leukemia, they showed that short-term incubation with 4-HC killed leukemic cells contaminating the marrow inoculum but did not destroy the ability of the normal cells to rescue the rats from marrow-lethal irradiation. They demonstrated a dose response to the drug. At low doses, survival before leukemic death was prolonged compared with recipients of untreated leukemic cells; at intermediate concentrations, some but not all rats were “cured.” Only at the highest concentrations tested was leukemic death prevented by the ex vivo treatment. They did not escalate the 4-HC concentration to marrow-ablative doses, however.

A subsequent Phase I trial at Johns Hopkins Hospital of 4-HC-purged autologous BMT for patients with leukemia and lymphoma demonstrated successful engraftment of marrows treated at 4-HC concentrations up to 100 μg/mL (58). They incubated marrow buffy-coat cells with incremental doses of this drug before cryopreservation. Small aliquots of cells, either untreated or treated with lower concentrations of 4-HC, were also cryopreserved as a backup if the primary infusion failed to engraft. All evaluable patients who received marrow treated with 100 μg/mL 4-HC or less recovered hematological function. Of the 10 patients who received marrow treated with 120 μg/mL, no evidence of engraftment after 21 days was found in 3, and the reserved bone marrows were given to rescue these patients. The speed of engraftment appeared to be related to the dose of 4-HC used. On the basis of these results, these investigators decided that 100 μg/mL was the maximally tolerated dose of this agent. They and others subsequently reported Phase II trials in the treatment of acute myeloid leukemia (AML) (Table 14-4) (59–61). Engraftment appeared delayed compared with the infusion of untreated marrow, but a number of patients achieved durable remissions not expected after treatment with non-transplant regimens. At this dose, few patients required rescue with untreated cells.

Mafosfamide is the oxazaphosphorine used primarily in Europe for ex vivo pharmacological purging (62–64). Some European centers pursued a different philosophy in ex vivo purging. Instead of a standard dose of drug, they attempted to determine a maximally tolerated dose of mafosfamide for each individual patient based on the sensitivity of that patient's myeloid progenitor cells (CFU-GM) to the drug (62,63). Small aliquots of marrow were incubated with graded concentrations of mafosfamide before harvesting, and the predicted dose of drug for the clinical purge was determined. In one trial, marrows were treated with concentrations predicted to allow a 5% CFU-GM survival (62). Doses of mafosfamide ranged from 60 to 140 μg/mL, but the other incubation parameters were held constant. These investigators demonstrated that engraftment could be achieved at even very high doses of this agent. The correlation of the preincubation test with the results of the marrow treatment was poor, however (r=0.47; $p < 0.03$). Moreover, the investigators provided no evidence suggesting a correlation between the sensitivities of normal and malignant progenitors to the pharmacological agent. Therefore, although they were able to escalate the drug dose for some patients to levels higher than those used by centers treating all patients at a set drug dosage, and thereby possibly achieved a more effective purge for those patients, they also decreased the drug dose for

Table 14-4.
Phase II Trials of Activated Oxazaphosphorine Purging for AML

Center	Diagnosis	No. Patients	Drug	Dose (μg/mL)	CFU-GM Survival Median (Range)	Median Days to Granulocytes (>500)	Median Days to Platelets (>50k)	DFS	Reference
Baltimore	AML	25	4-HC	100	ND	29	57	43%	59
Pittsburgh	AML	24	4-HC	100	0.3% (0–36)	30	91	19%	60
Los Angeles	AML	13	4-HC	100[a]	0% (0–3)	40	58	61%	61
Paris	AML,ALL	24	Mafosfamide	60–140	2% (0–47)	ND	67	27–72%[b]	62
Ulm	AML	52	Mafosfamide	60–80[a]	17% (2–100)	29	ND	45%	64

[a]Light density marrow cells were isolated before drug treatment by density-gradient separation over Ficoll-Metrizoate (Ulm) or a combination gradient of Ficoll-Hypaque layered over Percoll (Los Angeles).
[b]Patients were classified into high and low risk groups, as defined by the authors.
AML = acute myeloid leukemia; CFU-GM = colony forming unit—granulocyte macrophage; DFS = disease-free survival; 4-HC = 4-hydroperoxycyclophosphamide; ALL = acute lymphoblastic leukemia; ND = not done.

other patients below levels shown by the other groups to allow satisfactory engraftment kinetics and thereby possibly increased the risk of relapse for this group of patients.

Further analysis of the Johns Hopkins experience and reports of purging by other institutions demonstrates that engraftment kinetics after BMT of 4-HC- or mafosfamide-purged marrows are strongly related to patient diagnosis (Figure 14-2) (65,66). Patients being treated for AML engraft slowly compared with patients with other diagnoses. Thus, 4-HC and mafosfamide may be used in the treatment of other diseases at doses higher than those tolerable for most patients with AML. The dose of these drugs to be used depends on clinical decisions regarding the prolongation of aplasia tolerated. Shpall and associates (67) recently concluded a Phase I trial of 4-HC purging in the treatment of breast cancer and selected a dose of 80 μg/mL (density-gradient separated marrow cells) that gave a median aplasia duration of 28 days as the optimal dose for these patients.

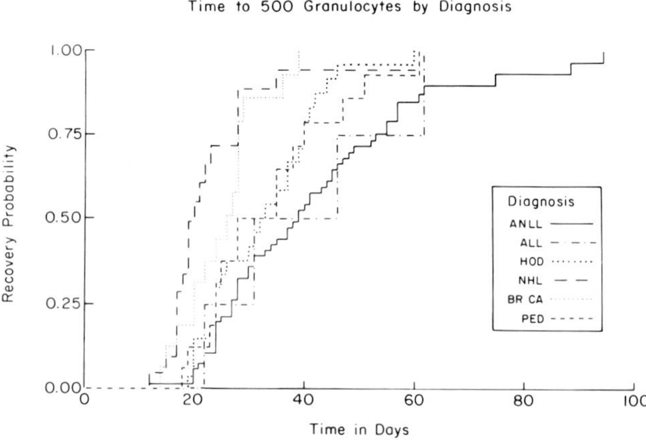

Figure 14-2. Probability of achieving a peripheral granulocyte count greater than 0.5×10^9/L after marrow reinfusion for patients classified by diagnosis. (Reprinted by permission from Macmillan Press Ltd: Rowley SD, Piantadosi S, Marcellus DC, et al. Analysis of factors predicting speed of hematologic recovery after transplantation with 4-hydroperoxycyclophosphamide-purged autologous bone marrow grafts. Bone Marrow Transplant 1991;7:183–191.)

Systemic administration of recombinant growth factors may not speed hematological recovery after BMT of 4-HC-purged marrow. In one study, none of the 7 recipients of the pharmacologically treated marrows responded to recombinant human granulocyte-macrophage colony stimulating factor (GM-CSF) (68). In another study, the response to GM-CSF appeared related to the residual quantity of CFU-GM in the marrow after ex vivo incubation (69). Patients with a significant shortening of aplasia received marrow containing a median of 17.5×10^3/kg, compared with a median of 2.0×10^3/kg for nonresponders. The quantity of nucleated cells infused did not differ for these two groups. Growth factors that preferentially stimulate the more primitive hematopoietic progenitors may have greater effect on 4-HC- or mafosfamide-purged marrow, given the differential effect of activated oxazaphosphorines on primitive compared with mature hematopoietic progenitors.

Little is known about the effect of pharmacological purging on immunological recovery after autologous transplantation. CY is immunosuppressive, as evidenced by its inclusion in conditioning regimens for allogeneic transplantation. Korbling and colleagues (70) showed a dose-dependent decrease in mixed-lymphocyte culture (MLC) reactivity for lymphocytes harvested from healthy donors and treated with 4-HC. Clinical studies of lymphocyte subpopulations and B-cell function after BMT with mafosfamide-purged marrow demonstrated abnormalities in immunological recovery (71,72), but comparison with similar patients receiving untreated marrow was not performed. Similar abnormalities in B-cell function were observed in patients who received peripheral blood stem-cell transplants without ex vivo purging (72). Whether the immunological defects described by

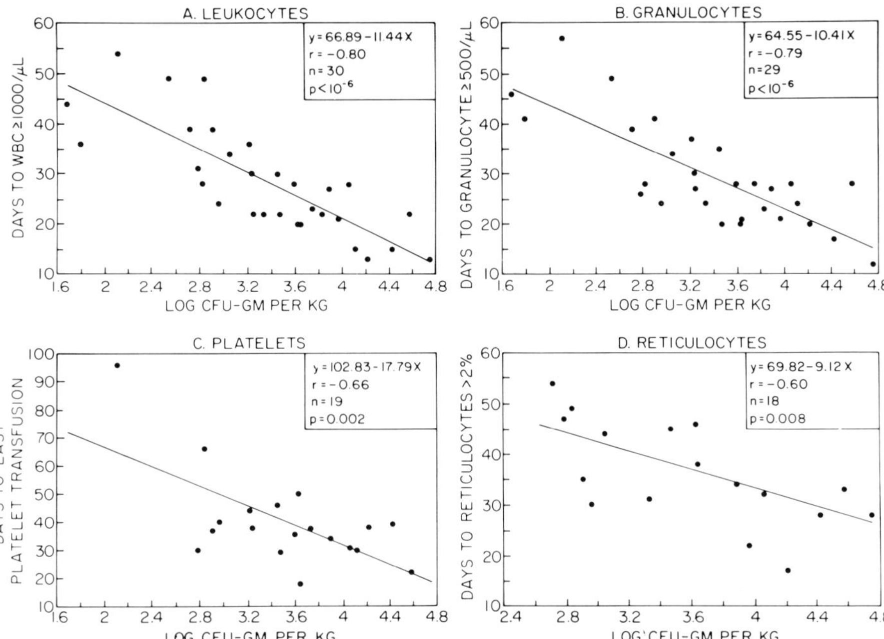

Figure 14-3. Correlation of aplasia duration with logarithm of graft CFU-GM content. Shown are numbers of days after transplantation to achieve (A) peripheral blood total leukocyte count greater than 1000/μL, (B) peripheral blood granulocyte count greater than 500/μL, (C) last platelet transfusion, and (D) peripheral blood reticulocyte concentration of greater than 2%. Correlation coefficients and linear regression equations are shown for each curve. All slopes are significantly different from 0, as shown by the *p* value for each equation. All patients received buffy coat cells treated with 100 μg/mL 4-HC. (Reprinted by permission from Grune & Stratton: Rowley SD, Zuehlsdorf M, Braine HG, et al. CFU-GM content of bone marrow graft correlates with time to hematologic reconstitution following autologous bone marrow transplantation with 4-hydroperoxycyclophosphamide-purged bone marrow. Blood 1987;70:271–275.)

these authors result from the marrow treatment or are a result of BMT cannot be determined from these reports.

Hematopoietic progenitor cell cultures were performed on the marrows for the initial Phase I trial of 4-HC purging reported by Kaizer and associates (58). These investigators were unable to correlate the quantity of myeloid progenitors (CFU-C) remaining after marrow treatment with engraftment kinetics, claiming that 4-HC uncoupled CFU-C from the engrafting cells of the marrow (58). Modifications of culture technique improved the detection of surviving myeloid progenitors and subsequently allowed correlation of these cells with the rates of leukocyte, granulocyte, platelet, and reticulocyte recoveries (Figure 14-3) (73). Assays predictive of engraftment kinetics facilitated studies of incubation technique. Herve and co-workers (37) demonstrated that increasing nucleated cell concentration in the incubation mixture moderated the toxicity to CFU-GM. Jones and associates (35) demonstrated that red cells added to the incubation mixture decreased 4-HC toxicity to both CFU-GM and tumor-derived cells (K562). The protective effects of increasing nucleated and red blood cell concentrations results from the ability of these cells to inactivate enzymatically the intermediate metabolites of these drugs, thereby decreasing the effective drug concentration to which both normal and malignant cells are exposed in the incubation mixture. A similar protective effect of red cells against mafosfamide toxicity is not unexpected, given the identical metabolism of this drug (74). Although published techniques for the treatment of buffy-coat cells with 4-HC call for adjusting the red cell concentration of the incubation mixture (75), the erythrocyte content of aldehyde dehydrogenase is not constant between patients. Density-gradient separation of marrow before 4-HC incubation improves the uniformity of the drug treatment (as measured by CFU-GM survival) by decreasing the variability of the enzyme content in the incubation mixture (13). Depletion of granulocytes and erythrocytes from the incubation mixture reduced the inactivation of 4-HC. Thus, a decrease in 4-HC dose to 60 μg/mL was required to achieve comparable 4-HC effect. Even with this reduction of dose, however, CFU-GM survival was slightly lower and duration of post-transplant aplasia was slightly longer than previously experienced with buffy-coat cells.

Efficacy of Purging With Activated Oxazaphosphorines

Mafosfamide and 4-HC have been used in the treatment of a number of malignancies, including acute and chronic leukemia (58–64,76), Hodgkin's and non-Hodgkin's lymphomas (77–79), and breast cancer (67,80). Although the feasibility of purging has been demonstrated by a number of transplant groups, evidence for the efficacy of purging has been much more elusive and limited to studies of acute leukemia. The cytotoxicity of oxazaphosphorines (and other pharmacological agents in clinical use) against malignant cells is without question. What is uncertain is primarily the necessity of ex vivo purging as a component in the treatment of any particular group of patients (defined by diagnosis, stage of disease, or other prognostic features). Only after the necessity of purging is addressed can the secondary issue of purging efficacy for the particular regimen being used in the treatment of those patients be determined.

It may be argued that the disease-free survival for patients with AML transplanted in second or subsequent remission exceeds that expected for nontransplant therapy. This comparison does not prove the value of purging in autologous BMT of this disease, however, and patient selection biases could account for some of the benefit attributed to transplantation.

Gorin and colleagues (63) reported in a multi-institutional trial of AML for the European Bone Marrow Transplant Group that purging may provide a survival advantage for patients transplanted in first remission. The advantage of purging, however (a 41% decrease in probability of relapse), was found only in those patients transplanted within 6 months of achieving remission. Purging may therefore be most important for patients at high risk of relapse.

In vitro cultures of either normal or malignant progenitors have been used in an attempt to validate the use of purging. Using the rationale that survival of CFU-GM would in general reflect the effective dose of 4-HC, and that leukemic cells respond to 4-HC in a dose-responsive manner, investigators at Johns Hopkins classified patients above and below the median CFU-GM survival of 1% found for a series of 45 patients. Patients transplanted with marrow which had lower CFU-GM survivals, presumably purged with higher effective concentrations of 4-HC, experienced a significantly greater disease-free survival than patients with less effective purges (Figure 14-4) (36). More recently, the same group reported the dose response of leukemic cells (CFU-L) cloned from harvested marrow and demonstrated this response to be predictive for disease-free survival (20). The former report is an indirect measure of purging efficacy using the survival of CFU-GM to reflect the cytotoxicity of 4-HC on the malignant cells; the latter report is inadequate proof of purging efficacy because the patients were conditioned with a CY-containing regimen, and the in vitro assay could be reflecting the in vivo sensitivity of the tumor.

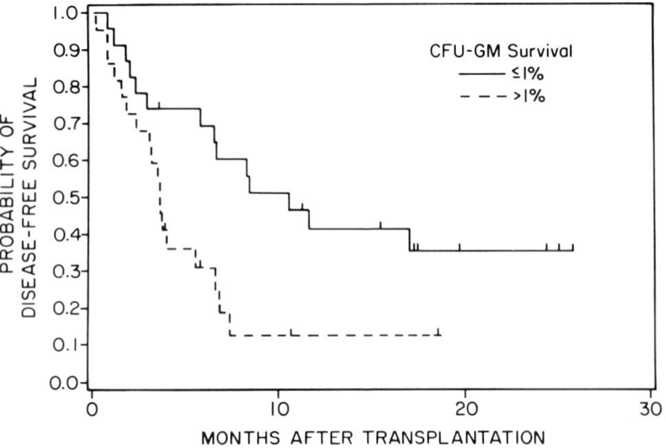

Figure 14-4. Probability of disease-free survival for patients stratified by percent CFU-GM survival. *Tick Marks* represent patients alive and disease-free at time of analysis ($p = 0.006$, log rank). (Reprinted by permission from Grune & Stratton: Rowley SD, Jones RJ, Piantadosi S, et al. Efficacy of ex vivo purging for autologous bone marrow transplantation in the treatment of acute nonlymphoblastic leukemia. Blood 1989;74:501–506.)

Toxicity of Oxazaphosphorine Purging

CY is both teratogenic and carcinogenic (81,82). The contribution of purging with CY derivatives to the development of second malignancies after autologous transplantation is uncertain. Second malignancies are not uncommon after transplantation (83). Chromosomal abnormalities after ex vivo purging with CY derivatives have been reported (84,85). Shah and associates (85) performed cytogenic analysis on 55 patients after transplantation of autologous marrow purged with 4-HC and found chromosomal abnormalities in 14. Seven of these patients had clonal abnormalities, and all were in leukemic relapse at the time of or shortly after detection. These authors were unable to detect clonal chromosomal abnormalities that were not associated with the presence of leukemic cells after BMT.

Purging with CY derivatives may produce a profound delay in engraftment kinetics (63,73). This delay is most pronounced for patients with AML (see Figure 14-2). Median time to engraftment for patients with AML receiving 4-HC- or mafosfamide-purged marrow ranged from 29 to 40 days (see Table 14-4). In one large series of 82 patients with AML undergoing autologous BMT without ex vivo purging, the median aplasia duration was only 18 days (86). Other smaller series reported aplasia durations of up to 39 days, probably reflecting patient selection or marrow processing and cryopreservation techniques (87,88). This prolongation of aplasia requires additional intensive support and may increase the risk of infectious complications. Moreover, use of mafosfamide purging was associated with a significantly increased risk of pneumonitis and hepatic venoocclusive disease in a cooperative study from Europe (63). This prolongation of aplasia, with its attendant financial and social costs and probably increased morbidity, can be justified only if these drugs improve the probability of disease-free survival for the disease being treated.

Other Pharmacologics

The occurrence of relapse and prolonged aplasia observed with oxazaphosphorine treatment of marrow has induced the investigation of other pharmacological agents for use in ex vivo purging. Clinical experience with these other agents is very limited compared with the experience accumulated with 4-HC or mafosfamide.

Vincristine

This drug has not been used clinically as a single agent for bone marrow purging. Its use in combination drug therapy is discussed later.

Methylprednisolone

This drug has been used at a concentration of 15 mg/mL to purge T cells from allogeneic marrow (89). At lower concentrations, it has been used in combinations with other pharmacologics.

Etoposide

A number of preclinical studies of etoposide (VP16) purging, either alone (90–93), or in combination with other drugs (4,5,8,52,94,95), have been published. These preclinical tests demonstrated the efficacy of VP16 against tumor-derived cell lines. This drug has also been used in clinical trials. Gulati and associates (96) reported preliminary engraftment data from a Phase I trial combining 4-HC with etoposide.

Ether Lipids

Ether lipids produce cytotoxicity by damage to the cell membrane. This effect is relatively selective for malignant cells, possibly because of the ability of normal cells to cleave the compounds. Preclinical studies documented the ability of ex vivo treatment to purge WEHI-3B cells from murine marrow while allowing marrow engraftment (97). A Phase I clinical trial documented engraftment of 23 of 24 patients receiving marrow cells treated with one ether lipid compound (98). Ether lipid–mediated cytotoxicity is temperature-dependent and may be enhanced with incubation at hyperthermic temperatures (99).

Merocyanine-540

Phototoxic lipophilic drugs will bind to the cell membrane of a variety of cell types. High-affinity binding sites are found on electrically excitable cells, such as neurons, immature blood cells, and certain malignant cells. In the presence of plasma proteins, a differential binding to leukemic cells is achieved. On exposure of the cells to light of the correct wavelength and intensity, the cytoplasmic membrane is disrupted and the leukemic cells swell and become trypan blue–positive. The rate of photolysis depends on dye and serum protein concentrations, as well as light wavelength, intensity, and exposure duration.

In preclinical testing of merocyanine-540 photolysis using either broad-spectrum or argon-laser irradiation, tumor-derived cell line kills exceeding four orders of magnitude (> 99.99%) were achieved while sparing 55% of multipotent hematopoietic progenitors (CFU-GEMM) in one study (14), and 41% of CFU-GM in another (100). Merocyanine-540 photolysis did not interfere with engraftment in a murine model but was capable of preventing leukemic death after injection of 5×10^6 cells containing 1% L1210 leukemic cells into irradiated mice.

Merocyanine-540 purging was studied in a Phase I trial at the Medical College of Wisconsin and Johns Hopkins University (15). Twenty-one patients received marrow treated ex vivo with merocyanine-540 and white light at one of three treatment levels. Toxic reactions to any residual dye in the treated marrow were not observed. Early relapse or transplant-related morbidity precluded analysis of engraftment for 9 patients. Hematological recovery was slow, requiring 23 to 67 days to achieve more than 500 granulocytes/μL; 3 patients received infusions of untreated "reserve" marrow because of engraftment delay beyond 6 weeks.

Combination Purging

An increase in the effective incubation concentration of pharmacologics such as 4-HC will achieve greater cytotoxicity, but only at the cost of increased toxicity to marrow. Combination drug purging of marrow may enhance the therapeutic ratio of the purging regimen, again emulating the systemic use of drugs. In contrast to systemic use, however, sequence and duration of exposure to multiple drugs ex vivo can be controlled more easily. Combinations of drugs or drugs with immunological agents have been studied in preclinical models using tumor-derived cell lines. Most studies included 4-HC or mafosfamide in combination with one or two other drugs. Clinical experience with these combinations is very limited.

Pharmacological Combinations

Chang and associates (52) demonstrated that the addition of etoposide to 4-HC was not only synergistic in cytotoxicity against a promyelocytic leukemic cell line, but also was antagonistic (protective) against normal myeloid progenitor cells. The contrasting effects in this model were reached at higher drug concentrations and were optimal at defined ratios of the two drugs. The authors provided no explanation for this interaction. A similar effect was described by other investigators for the combination of 4-HC with vincristine (6). Again, the protective effect was found only at higher concentrations of 4-HC. Other drugs, including methylprednisolone and cisplatin, have shown synergism with 4-HC against tumor-derived cells in preclinical testing (10,11). Similar results were found when etoposide was combined with mafosfamide (5,8).

Combinations of drugs are being studied in clinical trials. Rowley and colleagues (101) recently completed a Phase I trial of a combination of 3 drugs. They treated marrow with vincristine and 4-HC with a subsequent incubation with 10 mmol/L methylprednisolone. Despite the high concentrations of two additional drugs, they were able to treat marrow with the same concentration of 4-HC used alone. In vitro

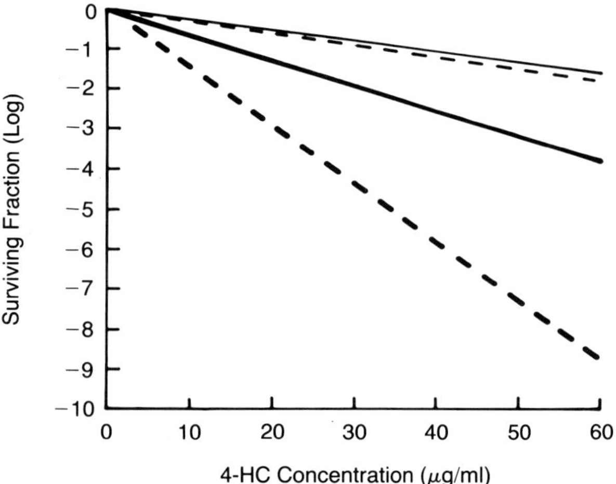

Figure 14-5. Dose-response curve of CFU-GM (—,---) and CFU-L (—,···) to 4-HC (—,—) or the drug combination (---,···). Shown is the average dose-response curve for these normal and malignant progenitors cloned in vitro from 12 patients with ALL. (Reprinted by permission from WB Saunders: Rowley SD, Miller CD, Piantadosi S, Davis JM, Santos GW, Jones RJ. Phase I study of combination drug purging for autologous bone marrow transplantation. J Clin Oncol 1991;9:2210–2218.)

assays for CFU-GM and malignant cells (CFU-L) demonstrated similar survival for normal cells but markedly enhanced cytotoxicity against the tumor cells from the combination (Figure 14-5). Engraftment failure did not occur for any of the evaluable patients. Gulati and colleagues (96) reported 30 patients who received marrow treated with 4-HC and etoposide; no patient required rescue with untreated cells.

Antibody-Pharmacological Combinations

Immunological and pharmacological purges achieve tumor-cell cytotoxicity through different mechanisms. The combination of pharmacological agents with immunological techniques circumvents possible cross-resistance that may occur with combinations of drugs or antibodies alone. For the same reason, however, cytotoxic synergism should not be expected in combining immunological and pharmacological techniques. Optimal results from combined pharmacological-immunological purges may require full-dose treatment with both methods, because the immunological treatment cannot be expected to increase the sensitivity of the malignant cells to the pharmacological agents used. One exception to this rule may be the combination of etoposide or vincristine with antibodies directed against the cell-surface P-glycoprotein responsible for resistance to these drugs (102).

Additive cytotoxicity was shown initially in preclinical studies of 4-HC and tumor-directed antibodies using lymphoma-derived cells (103). Sequence of treatment did not alter tumor-cell cytotoxicity. The addition of the immunological purge to the drug treatment did not further decrease normal hematopoietic cell survival. Similar additional tumor-cell kill was reported for other preclinical models (104), although sequence of incubation affected the survival of normal hematopoietic progenitors where this aspect was studied (17). Investigators in Minnesota combined 4-HC with either immunotoxins or antibody/complement techniques in the treatment of patients with T- and B-cell malignancies, respectively (21,22). Compared with their initial preclinical study (105), they found highly variable tumor-cell (CFU-L) survival after the purge. The dose of 4-HC used (10 μg/mL) was low, however, even for red cell–depleted marrow preparations. They did not determine the separate effects of the immunological and pharmacological treatments on the malignant cells, which would be important in deciding if the 4-HC dose was adequate, considering the recent report of relative resistance to 4-HC of lymphoid compared with myeloid malignancies (20,113).

Summary

Chemotherapeutics are effective when administered systemically and presumably when used ex vivo for the treatment of marrow. Whether the high concentrations but limited exposure of ex vivo purging are adequate to deplete tumor cells contaminating a marrow inoculum and whether this treatment contributes to the disease-free survival of autologous marrow recipients is uncertain. The toxicity of these agents to normal hematopoietic progenitor cells is obvious. Ex vivo marrow treatment increases the duration of post-transplant aplasia, thus increasing the associated morbidity of transplantation. Purging should therefore be pursued only if the expected benefits offset the known toxicities of marrow treatment.

References

1. Frei E III, Canellos GP. Dose: a critical factor in cancer chemotherapy. Am J Med 1980;69:585–594.
2. Yalowich JC, Zucali JR, Gross M, Ross WE. Effects of verapamil on etoposide, vincristine, and adriamycin activity in normal human bone marrow granulocyte-macrophage progenitors and in human K562 leukemia cells in vitro. Cancer Res 1985;45:4921–4924.
3. Blaauw A, Spitzer G, Dicke K, Drewinko B, Vellekoop L, Zander A. Potential drugs for elimination of acute lymphatic leukemia cells from autologous bone marrow. Exp Hematol 1986;14:683–688.
4. Chang TT, Gulati S, Chou T-C, Colvin M, Clarkson B. Comparative cytotoxicity of various drug combinations for human leukemic cells and normal hematopoietic precursors. Cancer Res 1987;47:119–122.
5. De Fabritiis P, Pulsoni A, Sandrelli A, et al. Efficacy of a combined treatment with ASTA-Z 7654 and VP16-213 in vitro in eradicating clonogenic tumor cells from human bone marrow. Bone Marrow Transplant 1987;2:287–298.
6. Auber ML, Horwitz LJ, Blaauw A, et al. Evaluation of drugs for elimination of leukemic cells from the bone marrow of patients with acute leukemia. Blood 1988;71:166–172.

7. Gulati S, Atzpodien J, Langleben A, et al. Comparative regimens for the ex vivo chemopurification of B cell lymphoma-contaminated marrow. Acta Haematol 1988; 80:65–70.
8. Tamayo E, Herve P. Preclinical studies of the combination of mafosfamide (Asta-Z 7654) and etoposide (VP-16-213) for purging leukemic autologous marrow. Exp Hematol 1988;16:97–101.
9. Shimazaki S, Gulati SC, Atzpodien J, Fried J, Colvin OM, Clarkson BD. Ex vivo treatment of myeloma cells by 4-hydroperoxycyclophosphamide and VP-16-213. Acta Haematol 1988;80:17–22.
10. Peters RH, Brandon CS, Avila LA, Colvin OM, Stuart RK. In vitro synergism of 4-hydroperoxycyclophosphamide and cisplatin: relevance for bone marrow purging. Cancer Chemother Pharmacol 1989;23:129–134.
11. Jones RJ, Miller CB, Zehnbauer BA, Rowley SD, Colvin OM, Sensenbrenner LL. In vitro evaluation of combination drug purging for autologous bone marrow transplantation. Bone Marrow Transplant 1990;5:301–307.
12. Jones RJ, Colvin OM, Sensenbrenner LL. Prediction of the ability to purge tumor from murine bone marrow using clonogenic assays. Cancer Res 1988;48:3394–3397.
13. Rowley SD, Davis JM, Piantadosi S, Jones RJ, Yeager AM, Santos GW. Density-gradient separation of autologous bone marrow grafts before ex vivo purging with 4-hydroperoxycyclophosphamide. Bone Marrow Transplant 1990;6:321–327.
14. Sieber F, Rao S, Rowley SD, Sieber-Blum M. Dye-mediated photolysis of human neuroblastoma cells: implications for autologous bone marrow transplantation. Blood 1986;68:32–36.
15. Sieber F. Extracorporeal purging of bone marrow grafts by dye-sensitized photoirradiation. In: Gee AP, ed. Bone marrow processing and purging. A practical guide. Boca Raton: CRC Press, 1991:263–280.
16. Zuehlsdorf M, Rowley SD, Braine HJG, Colvin OM, Sensenbrenner LL, Santos GW. Increased ratio of cytotoxicity for K562 and human CFU-GM by sequential incubations of 4-hydroperoxcyclophosphamide (4-HC) and methylprednisolone (MP) compared to 4HC alone. Blood 1986;68 (suppl 1):294a.
17. Anderson IC, Shpall EJ, Leslie DS, et al. Elimination of malignant clonogenic breast cancer cells from human bone marrow. Cancer Res 1989;49:4659–4664.
18. Estrov Z, Grunberger T, Dube ID, Wang Y-P, Freedman MH. Detection of residual acute lymphoblastic leukemia cells in cultures of bone marrow obtained during remission. N Engl J Med 1986;315:538–542.
19. Gribben JG, Freedman AS, Neuberg D, et al. Immunologic purging of marrow assessed by PCR before autologous bone marrow transplantation for B-cell lymphoma. N Engl J Med 1991;325:1525–1533.
20. Miller CB, Zehnbauer BA, Piantadosi S, Rowley SD, Jones RJ. Correlation of occult clonogenic leukemia drug sensitivity with relapse after autologous bone marrow transplantation. Blood 1991;78:1125–1131.
21. Uckun FM, Kersey JH, Vallera DA, et al. Autologous bone marrow transplantation in high risk remission T-lineage acute lymphoblastic leukemia using immunotoxins plus 4-hydroperoxycyclophosphamide for marrow purging. Blood 1990;76:1723–1733.
22. Uckun FM, Kersey JH, Haake R, Weisdorf D, Ramsay NKC. Autologous bone marrow transplantation in high-risk remission B-lineage acute lymphoblastic leukemia using a cocktail of three monoclonal antibodies (BA-1/CD24, BA-2/CD9, and BA-3/CD10) plus complement and 4-hydroperoxycyclophosphamide for ex vivo bone marrow purging. Blood 1992;79:1094–1104.
23. Sladek NE. Metabolism of oxazaphosphorines. Pharmacol Ther 1988;37:301–355.
24. Hilton J. Role of aldehyde dehydrogenase in cyclophosphamide-resistant L1210 leukemia. Cancer Res 1984; 44:5156–5160.
25. Hilton J. Deoxyribonucleic acid crosslinking by 4-hydroperoxycyclophosphamide in cyclophosphamide-sensitive and -resistant L1210 cells. Biochem Pharmacol 1984;33:1867–1872.
26. Kohn FR, Landkamer GJ, Manthey CL, Ramsay NKC, Sladek NE. Effect of aldehyde dehydrogenase inhibitors on the ex vivo sensitivity of human multipotent and committed hematopoietic progenitor cells and malignant blood cells to oxazaphosphorines. Cancer Res 1987;47:3180–3185.
27. Sahovic EA, Colvin M, Hilton J, Ogawa M. Role for aldehyde dehydrogenase in survival of progenitors for murine blast cell colonies after treatment with 4-hydroperoxycyclophosphamide in vitro. Cancer Res 1988;48:1223–1226.
28. Gordon MY, Goldman JM, Gordon-Smith EC. 4-Hydroperoxycyclophosphamide inhibits proliferation by human granulocyte-macrophage colony-forming cells (GM-CFC) but spares more primitive progenitor cells. Leuk Res 1985;9:1017–1021.
29. Kastan MB, Schlaffer E, Russo JE, Colvin OM, Civin CI, Hilton J. Direct demonstration of elevated aldehyde dehydrogenase in human hematopoietic progenitor cells. Blood 1990;75:1947–1950.
30. Lee FYF. Glutathione diminishes the anti-tumour activity of 4-hydroperoxycyclophosphamide by stabilising its spontaneous breakdown to alkylating metabolites. Br J Cancer 1991;63:45–50.
31. Crook TR, Souhami RL, Whyman GD, McLean AEM. Glutathione depletion as a determinant of sensitivity of human leukemia cells to cyclophosphamide. Cancer Res 1986;46:5035–5038.
32. Ozols RF, Louie KG, Plowman J, et al. Enhanced melphalan cytotoxicity in human ovarian cancer in vitro and in tumor-bearing nude mice by buthione sulfoximine depletion of glutathione. Biochem Pharmacol 1987;36:147–153.
33. Tew KD, Bomber AM, Hoffman SJ. Ethacrynic acid and piriprost as enhancers of cytotoxicity in drug resistant and sensitive cell lines. Cancer Res 1988;48:3622–3625.
34. Helander A, Tottmar O. Cellular distribution and properties of human blood aldehyde dehydrogenase. Clin Exp Res 1986;10:71–76.
35. Jones RJ, Zuehlsdorf M, Rowley SD, et al. Variability in 4-hydroperoxycyclophosphamide activity during clinical purging for autologous bone marrow transplantation. Blood 1987;70:1490–1494.
36. Rowley SD, Jones RJ, Piantadosi S, et al. Efficacy of ex vivo purging for autologous bone marrow transplantation in the treatment of acute nonlymphoblastic leukemia. Blood 1989;74:501–506.
37. Herve P, Tamayo E, Peters A. Autologous stem cell grafting in acute myeloid leukemia: technical approach of marrow incubation in vitro with pharmacologic agents (prerequisite for clinical applications). Br J Haematol 1983;53:683–685.
38. Takamizawa A, Matsumoto S, Iwata T, Katagiri K, Tochin Y, Yamaguchi K. Studies on cyclophosphamide metabolites and their related compounds. II. Prepara-

tion of an active species of cyclophosphamide and some related compounds. J Am Chem Soc 1973;95:985–986.
39. Sindermann H, Peukert M, Hilgard P. Bone marrow purging with mafosfamide—a critical survey. Blut 1989;59:432–441.
40. de Jong JP, Nikkels PGJ, Brockbank KGM, Ploemacher RE, Voerman JSA. Comparative in vitro effects of cyclophosphamide derivatives on murine bone marrow-derived stromal and hemopoietic progenitor cell classes. Cancer Res 1985;45:4001–4005.
41. Valeriote F, Grates HE. Potentiation of nitrogen mustard cytotoxicity to leukemia cells by sulfur-containing compounds administered in vivo. J Radiat Oncol Biol Phys 1986;12:1165–1169.
42. Swanson BN, Ferguson RK, Raskin NH, Wolf BA. Peripheral neuropathy after concomitant administration of dimethyl sulfoxide and sulindac. Arthritis Rheum 1983;26:791–793.
43. Lopez M, DuPuy-Montbrun MC, Douay L, Laporte JP, Gorin NC. Standardization and characterization of the procedure for in vitro treatment of human bone marrow with cyclophosphamide derivatives. Clin Lab Haematol 1985;7:327–334.
44. Rosenow S, Kooistra KL, Powis G, Van Dyke RA. Increased toxicity of the antitumor drug cyclophosphamide in mice in the presence of the volatile anesthetic agent halothane. Cancer Chemother Pharmacol 1986; 16:35–42.
45. Glover D, Glick JH, Hurowitz S, Kligerman MM. WR-2721 protects against the hematologic toxicity of cyclophosphamide: a controlled phase II trial. J Clin Oncol 1986;4:584–588.
46. Brown JM, Hall EJ, Hirst DG, et al. Chemical modification of radiation and chemotherapy. Am J Clin Oncol 1988;11:288–301.
47. DeNeve WJ, Everett CK, Suminski JE, Valeriote FA. Influence of WR2721 on DNA cross-linking by nitrogen mustard in normal mouse bone marrow and leukemia cells in vivo. Cancer Res 1988;48:6002–6005.
48. Grdina DJ, Sigdestad CP. Radiation protectors: the unexpected benefits. Drug Metab Rev 1989;20:13–42.
49. Shpall EJ, Jones RB, Johnston C, et al. Amifostine (WR-2721) shortens the engraftment period of 4-HC purged bone marrow in breast cancer patients receiving high-dose chemotherapy with autologous bone marrow support. Blood 1991;78 (suppl 1):192a.
50. Moreb J, Zucali JR, Gross MA, Weiner RS. Protective effects of IL-1 on human hematopoietic progenitor cells treated in vitro with 4-hydroperoxycyclophosphamide. J Immunol 1989;142:1937–1942.
51. Moreb J, Zucalli JR, Rueth S. The effects of tumor necrosis factor-α on early human hematopoietic progenitor cells treated with 4-hydroperoxycyclophosphamide. Blood 1990;76:681–689.
52. Chang TT, Gulati SC, Chou T-C, et al. Synergistic effect of 4-hydroperoxycyclophosphamide and etoposide on a human promyelocyte leukemia cell line (HL-60) demonstrated by computer analysis. Cancer Res 1985;45:2434–2439.
53. Rowley SD, Colvin OM, Stuart RK. Human multilineage progenitor cell sensitivity to 4-hydroperoxycyclophosphamide. Exp Hematol 1985;13:295–298.
54. Siena S, Castro-Malaspina H, Gulati S, et al. Effects of in vitro purging with 4-hydroperoxycyclophosphamide on the hematopoietic and microenvironmental elements of human bone marrow. Blood 1985;65:655–662.
55. Winton EF, Colenda KW. Use of long-term human marrow cultures to demonstrate progenitor cell precursors in marrow treated with 4-hydroperoxycyclophosphamide. Exp Hematol 1987;15:710–714.
56. Aglietta M, Sanavio F, Stacchini A, Piacibello W. In vitro reappearance of myeloid progenitors killed by mafosfamide. Exp Hematol 1987;15:276–279.
57. Sharkis SJ, Santos GW, Colvin M. Elimination of acute myelogenous leukemic cells from marrow and tumor suspensions in the rat with 4-hydroperoxycyclophosphamide. Blood 1980;55:521–523.
58. Kaizer H, Stuart RK, Brookmeyer R, et al. Autologous bone marrow transplantation in acute leukemia: a phase I study of in vitro treatment of marrow with 4-hydroperoxycyclophosphamide to purge tumor cells. Blood 1985;65:1504–1510.
59. Yeager AM, Kaizer H, Santos GW, et al. Autologous bone marrow transplantation in patients with acute nonlymphocytic leukemia: a study of ex vivo marrow treatment with 4-hydroperoxycyclophosphamide. N Engl J Med 1986;315:141–147.
60. Rosenfeld C, Shadduck RK, Przepiorka D, Mangan KF, Colvin M. Autologous bone marrow transplantation with 4-hydroperoxycyclophosphamide purged marrows for acute nonlymphocytic leukemia in late remission or early relapse. Blood 1989;74:1159–1164.
61. Lenarsky C, Weinberg K, Petersen J, et al. Autologous bone marrow transplantation with 4-hydroperoxycyclophosphamide purged marrows for children with acute non-lymphoblastic leukemia in second remission. Bone Marrow Transplant 1990;6:425–429.
62. Gorin NC, Douay L, Laporte JP, et al. Autologous bone marrow transplantation using marrow incubated with Asta Z 7557 in adult acute leukemia. Blood 1986; 67:1367–1376.
63. Gorin NC, Aegerter P, Auvert B, et al. Autologous bone marrow transplantation for acute myelocytic leukemia in first remission: a European survey of the role of marrow purging. Blood 1990;75:1606–1614.
64. Körbling M, Hunstein W, Fliedner TM, et al. Disease-free survival after autologous bone marrow transplantation in patients with acute myelogenous leukemia. Blood 1989;74:1898–1904.
65. Rowley SD, Piantadosi S, Marcellus DC, et al. Analysis of factors predicting speed of hematologic recovery after transplantation with 4-hydroperoxycyclophosphamide-purged autologous bone marrow grafts. Bone Marrow Transplant 1991;7:183–191.
66. Douay L, Laporte J-P, Mary J-Y, et al. Difference in kinetics of hematopoietic reconstitution between ALL and ANLL after autologous bone marrow transplantation with marrow treated in vitro with mafosfamide (ASTA Z 7557). Bone Marrow Transplant 1987;2:33–43.
67. Shpall EJ, Jones RB, Bast RC, et al. 4-Hydroperoxycyclophosphamide purging of breast cancer from the mononuclear fraction of bone marrow in patients receiving high-dose chemotherapy and autologous marrow support: A phase I trial. J Clin Oncol 1991;9:85–93.
68. Nemunaitis J, Singer JW, Buckner CD, et al. Use of recombinant human granulocyte-macrophage colony-stimulating factor in graft failure after bone marrow transplantation. Blood 1990;76:245–253.
69. Blazar BR, Kersey JH, McGlave PB, et al. In vivo administration of recombinant human granulocyte/macrophage colony-stimulating factor in acute lymphoblastic leukemia patients receiving purged autografts. Blood 1989;73:849–857.
70. Korbling M, Hess AD, Tutschka PJ, Kaizer H, Colvin

MO, Santos GW. 4-Hydroperoxycyclophosphamide: a model for eliminating residual human tumour cells and T-lymphocytes from the bone marrow graft. Br J Haematol 1982;52:89–96.

71. Le Blanc G, Douay L, Laporte J-P, et al. Evaluation of lymphocyte subsets after autologous bone marrow transplantation with marrow treated by ASTA Z 7557 in acute leukemia: incidence of the in vitro treatment. Exp Hematol 1986;14:366–371.
72. Kiesel S, Pezzutto A, Moldenhauer G, et al. B-cell proliferative and differentiative responses after autologous peripheral blood stem cell or bone marrow transplantation. Blood 1988;72:672–678.
73. Rowley SD, Zuehlsdorf M, Braine HG, et al. CFU-GM content of bone marrow graft correlates with time to hematologic reconstitution following autologous bone marrow transplantation with 4-hydroperoxycyclophosphamide-purged bone marrow. Blood 1987;70:271–275.
74. Douay L, Mary JY, Giarratana MC, Najman A, Gorin NC. Establishment of a reliable experimental procedure for bone marrow purging with mafosfamide (ASTA Z 7557). Exp Hematol 1989;17:429–432.
75. Rowley SD, Davis JM. The use of 4-HC in autologous purging. In Gee A, ed. Bone marrow processing and purging. A practical guide. Boca Raton: CRC Press, 1991:247–262.
76. Carlo-Stella C, Mangoni L, Piovani G, et al. In vitro purging in chronic myelogenous leukemia: effect of mafosfamide and recombinant granulocyte-macrophage colony-stimulating factor. Bone Marrow Transplant 1991;8:265–273.
77. Braine HG, Santos GW, Kaizer H, et al. Treatment of poor prognosis non-Hodgkin's lymphoma with cyclophosphamide and total body irradiation regimens with autologous bone marrow rescue. Bone Marrow Transplant 1987;2:7–14.
78. Jones RJ, Piantadosi S, Mann RB, et al. High dose cytotoxic therapy and bone marrow transplantation for relapsed Hodgkin's disease. J Clin Oncol 1990;8:527–537.
79. Gulati SC, Shank B, Black P, et al. Autologous bone marrow transplantation for patients with poor-prognosis lymphoma. J Clin Oncol 1988;6:1303–1313.
80. Kennedy MJ, Beveridge RA, Rowley SD, Gordon GB, Abeloff MD, Davidson NE. High-dose chemotherapy with reinfusion of purged autologous bone marrow following dose-intense induction as initial therapy for metastatic breast cancer. J Natl Cancer Inst 1991; 83:920–926.
81. Friedman OM, Myles A, Colvin M. Cyclophosphamide and related phosphoramide mustards. Current status and future prospects. Adv Cancer Chemother 1979; 1:143–204.
82. Perocco P, Pane G, Santucci A, Zannotti M. Mutagenic and toxic effects of 4-hydroperoxycyclophosphamide and of 2,4-tetrahydrocyclohexylamine (ASTA-Z-7557) on human lymphocytes cultured in vitro. Exp Hematol 1985;13:1014–1017.
83. Witherspoon RP, Fisher LD, Schoch G, et al. Secondary cancers after bone marrow transplantation for leukemia or aplastic anemia. N Engl J Med 1989;321:784–789.
84. Van Den Akker J, Gorin NC, Laporte JP, et al. Chromosomal abnormalities after autologous bone marrow transplantation with marrow treated by cyclophosphamide derivatives. Lancet 1985;1:1211–1212.
85. Shah NK, Wingard J, Piantadosi S, Rowley SD, Santos GW, Griffin CA. Chromosome abnormalities in patients treated with 4-hydroperoxycyclophosphamide-purged autologous bone marrow transplantation. Cancer Genet Cytogenet 1993;65:135–140.
86. McMillan AK, Goldstone AH, Kinch DC, et al. High-dose chemotherapy and autologous bone marrow transplantation in acute myeloid leukemia. Blood 1990;76:480–488.
87. Lowenberg B, Verdonck LJ, Dekker AW, et al. Autologous bone marrow transplantation in acute myeloid leukemia in first remission: results of a Dutch prospective study. J Clin Oncol 1990;8:287–294.
88. Stewart P, Buckner CD, Bensinger W, et al. Autologous marrow transplantation in patients with acute non-lymphocytic leukemia in first remission. Exp Hematol 1985;13:267–272.
89. Rowley S, Stuart R, Hess A, Donnenberg A, Saral R, Santos G. Prevention of acute graft versus host disease (GVHD) by methylprednisolone (MP) incubation of donor bone marrow. Blood 1985;66(suppl 1):261a.
90. Stiff PJ, Koester AR. In vitro chemoseparation of leukemic cells from murine bone marrow using VP16-213: importance of stem cell assays. Exp Hematol 1987;15:263–268.
91. Lagneaux L, Marie J-P, Delforge A, et al. Comparison of in vitro inhibition of etoposide (VP16) on leukemic and normal myeloid, erythroid clonogenic cells. Exp Hematol 1989;17:843–846.
92. Kushner BH, Kwon J-H, Gulati SC, Castro-Malaspina H. Preclinical assessment of purging with VP-16-213: key role for long-term marrow cultures. Blood 1987;69:65–71.
93. Ciabanu N, Paietta E, Andreeff M, Papenhausen P, Wiernik PH. Etoposide as an in vitro purging agent for the treatment of acute leukemias and lymphomas in conjunction with autologous bone marrow transplantation. Exp Hematol 1986;14:626–635.
94. Lemoli RM, Gulati SC. In vitro cytotoxicity of VP-16-213 and nitrogen mustard: agnostic on tumor cells but not on normal human bone marrow progenitors. Exp Hematol 1990;18:1008–1012.
95. Chao NJ, Aihara M, Blume KG, Sikic BI. Modulation of etoposide (VP-16) cytotoxicity by verapamil or cyclosporine in multidrug-resistant human leukemic cells lines and normal bone marrow. Exp Hematol 1990;18:1193–1198.
96. Gulati SC, Acaba L, Yahalom J, et al. Autologous bone marrow transplantation for acute myelogenous leukemia using 4-hydroperoxycyclophosphamide and VP-16 purged bone marrow. Bone Marrrow Transplant 1992; 10:129–134.
97. Glasser L, Somberg LB, Vogler WR. Purging murine leukemic marrow with alkyl-lysophospholipids. Blood 1984;64:1288–1291.
98. Vogler WR, Berdel WE, Olson AC, Winton EF, Heffner LT, Gordon DS. Autologous bone marrow transplantation in acute leukemia with marrow purged with alkyl-lysophospholipid. Blood 1992;80:1423–1429.
99. Okamoto S, Olson AC, Berdel WE, Vogler WR. Purging of acute myeloid leukemic cells by ether lipids and hyperthermia. Blood 1988;72:1777–1783.
100. Gulliya KS, Matthews JL, Fay JW, Dowben RM. Increased survival of normal cells during laser photodynamic therapy: implications for ex vivo autologous bone marrow purging. Life Sciences 1988;42:2651–2656.
101. Rowley SD, Miller CD, Piantadosi S, Davis JM, Santos GW, Jones RJ. Phase I study of combination drug

purging for autologous bone marrow transplantation. J Clin Oncol 1991;9:2210–2218.

102. Aihara M, Aihara Y, Schmidt-Wolf G, et al. A combined approach for purging multidrug-resistant leukemic cell lines in bone marrow using a monoclonal antibody and chemotherapy. Blood 1991;77:2079–2084.

103. De Fabritiis P, Bregni M, Lipton J, et al. Elimination of clonogenic Burkitt's lymphoma cells from human bone marrow using 4-hydroperoxycyclophosphamide in combination with monoclonal antibodies and complement. Blood 1985;65:1064–1070.

104. Lemoli RM, Gasparetto C, Scheinberg DA, Moore MAS, Clarkson BD, Gulati SC. Autologous bone marrow transplantation in acute myelogenous leukemia: in vitro treatment with myeloid-specific monoclonal antibodies and drugs in combination. Blood 1991;77:1829–1836.

105. Uckun FM, Gajl-Peczalska K, Meyers DE, et al. Marrow purging in autologous bone marrow transplantation for T-lineage acute lymphoblastic leukemia: efficacy of ex vivo treatment with immunotoxins and 4-hydroperoxycyclophosphamide against fresh leukemic marrow progenitor cells. Blood 1987;69:361–366.

106. Makrynikola V, Kabral A, Bradstock KF. Effect of mafosfamide (ASTA-Z-7654) on the clonogenic cells in precursor-B acute lymphoblastic leukemia: significance for ex vivo purging of bone marrow for autologous transplantation. Bone Marrow Transplant 1991;8:351–355.

Chapter 15

Laboratory Evaluation of Minimal Residual Disease

Robert S. Negrin and Michael L. Cleary

Detection of residual malignant cells is an important component in the management of patients with malignancies, particularly in the setting of bone marrow transplantation (BMT), where management decisions and eventual disease outcome may be influenced by quantifiable levels of minimal residual disease (MRD) in the marrow before or after BMT. Detection of MRD is a technology-driven field, and currently there are rapid developments occurring with respect to the techniques and markers employed in various disease settings. This chapter reviews the technical aspects of several promising approaches that have been used for detection of MRD, followed by a discussion of current and anticipated future uses of MRD assays in BMT.

Assays for Detection of Minimal Residual Disease

A variety of techniques has been employed to detect minimal residual malignant cells in different clinical settings. Each is specific for a given characteristic of the neoplastic cells being detected and is limited in its practical detection threshhold, as summarized in Table 15-1. Historically, detection of malignant cells based on their morphological features using light microscopy has been an important modality and continues to serve a useful clinical role for many malignancies, particularly solid tumors involving nodal and extranodal sites. Currently at our institution, bone marrow core biopsies removed at the time of marrow harvest for autologous grafting are morphologically assessed for obvious involvement by malignant disease. However, for the hematological malignancies, it is clear that this approach is quite limited in its sensitivity due primarily to the subtle morphological differences in malignant cells, which are not easily distinguished at levels below 1 to 10% in the background of normal marrow elements.

Other techniques employed for detection of MRD have not offered significant advantages in terms of overall sensitivity but provide a more objective result when analyzing complex mixtures of cells, as in bone marrow, blood, or other human tissues. For example, cytogenetic studies are routinely employed for longitudinally monitoring recipients of marrow grafts for treatment of chronic myelogenous leukemia (CML) to detect reappearance of cells carrying the Philadelphia (Ph) chromosome. The detection limit for karyotype analysis is limited by the number of metaphases examined but in practice results in detection of one Ph-positive cell out of 20 to 100 analyzable metaphases. The utility of this approach is evidenced by the occasional reappearance of Ph-positive cells prior to their detection by morphological examination in many patients, presaging eventual clinical relapse (1,2). The disadvantages of this approach concern its expense; the requirement for a detectable, stable, and cytogenetically distinct chromosomal aberration; and the necessity to arrest cells in metaphase.

Recently, refinements to standard light microscopic examination of chromosomes have been reported and may be applicable to detection of MRD. Tkachuk and colleagues (3) described the use of fluorescent-labeled DNA probes to the BCR and ABL genes flanking the sites of t(9;22) on the Ph chromosome in hybridization analyses of chromosomes from CML cells (a technique referred to as two-color FISH (Fluorescence In Situ Hybridization). In normal cells, separate signals were observed for the different-colored BCR and ABL probes hybridizing to the appropriate genes on their respective chromosomes. However, in marrow cells from patients with CML, juxtaposition of the probes due to t(9;22) resulted in a distinct "fusion" signal detectable in metaphase chromosomes and also interphase nuclei. The advantage of this approach is that it can be used on interphase nuclei, obviating the need for arresting the

Table 15-1.
Assays for Detection of MRD

Method	*Marker*	*Sensitivity*
Routine pathology	Cellular morphology	10^{-1}–10^{-2}
Cytogenetics	Chromosome morphology	10^{-1}–10^{-2}
FISH	Chromosome structure	10^{-2}
Gene rearrangement	DNA configuration	10^{-2}–10^{-3}
FACS analysis	Antigen profile	10^{-3}
Clonogenic culture	In vitro growth	10^{-5}
PCR	DNA/RNA structure	10^{-5}

FISH = fluorescence in situ hybridization; FACS = fluorescence activated cell sorting; PCR = polymerase chain reaction.

cells in metaphase. However, the technique requires finely calibrated, sophisticated instrumentation and does not offer advantages in sensitivity because the theoretical probability of random alignment of the BCR and the ABL signals has been estimated to be approximately 1%. With the advent of chromosome-painting probes specific for entire chromosomes (4) and expected refinements in technology, the combination of molecular and cytogenetic techniques may significantly impact future approaches for MRD detection in patients undergoing BMT.

DNA probes have also been used with radiolabeled detection methods on Southern blot hybridizations to assess objectively the presence of MRD. An increasing number of DNA probes are available that are specific for various chromosomal abnormalities, activated cellular oncogenes, or generic markers, such as immunoglobulin (Ig) or T-cell receptor (TCR) gene rearrangements. All of these approaches depend on detection of DNA alterations acquired during neoplastic transformation or during normal differentiation of lymphoid cells, which serve as useful clonal markers. Application of Southern blotting for detection of MRD is limited by its sensitivity (at best 1%) and the fact that it is laborious, time-consuming, and difficult to perform. In general, the polymerase chain reaction (PCR), which can detect many of the same markers as Southern blotting, has supplanted the latter for detection of MRD.

Phenotypic characteristics of malignant cells may also serve as markers for evaluation of MRD. An antigen expressed on the surface of cells may allow quantitative assessment of tumor burden by fluorescence-activated cell sorter (FACS) analysis or light microscopy of appropriately prepared cell populations. This approach is dependent on the specificity of a given antigen for the tumor population, which in practice limits its applicability due to the paucity of tumor-specific surface antigens. The feasibility of this approach has been demonstrated with anti-idiotype antibodies directed against immunoglobulin molecules produced by B-lineage leukemias and lymphomas. These antibodies have been used to detect low levels of circulating idiotype-positive lymphoma cells by a process called cytological idiotyping. Because idiotypes may be shared by different lymphomas, it may not be necessary to construct a new reagent for each lymphoma (5). However, most lymphoma idiotypes are also expressed on a small proportion of normal lymphocytes (approximately 0.01%), thereby establishing the lower limits of sensitivity for this approach. Tumor-associated proteins secreted or released by malignant cells may also be quantitated to monitor disease status. For example, MRD has been assessed in lymphoma and leukemia patients using anti-idiotype antibodies to quantitate levels of circulating idiotype protein, which was not detectable by routine serological assays (6,7). When additional tumor-specific antibodies become available (e.g., antibodies directed against unique epitopes in translocation-induced fusion proteins such as BCR-ABL), these anti-idiotype antibodies may be used with even greater sensitivity in assays for MRD similar to those discussed.

PCR has emerged as the most promising approach for detection of MRD in various clinical settings. PCR offers the advantage of very high sensitivity, with a practical detection limit of approximately 10^{-5}, which exceeds by several logs other generally applicable methods (see Table 15-1). The technique involves logarithmic amplification of specific DNA or RNA sequences present in neoplastic cells but not in normal host cells. Amplification is carried out by successive rounds of DNA synthesis specifically primed by synthetic oligonucleotides flanking the target sequences. The reaction is carried out in a programmable thermal cycler using a heat-stable DNA polymerase that can withstand the heat denaturation step required to melt newly synthesized DNA strands prior to annealing of oligonucleotides for each subsequent round of DNA synthesis.

The molecular markers in hematological malignancies that are amenable to detection by PCR are listed in Table 15-2. These markers result from alterations in genomic DNA structure that are acquired either as part of the neoplastic transformation process or during normal lymphoid differentiation. Breakage and rejoining of DNA resulting from either physiological deletions or accidental translocations create unique junctions that can be amplified by PCR. The markers listed in Table 15-2 are detected by direct amplification of DNA or amplification of complementary DNA (cDNA) copies of messenger RNA (mRNA) resulting from transcription across the unique DNA junctions (Figure 15-1). The specificity of PCR derives from the composition of the amplification primers that are constructed to be homologous to sequences flanking both sides of the DNA or RNA junctions of these various markers, resulting in their logarithmic amplification during PCR.

PCR was first used to detect molecular markers in

Table 15-2.
Molecular Markers Amenable to Detection by PCR

Molecular marker	*Cytogenetic Abnormality*	*Disease*
CDRIII	None	B-lineage ALL, NHL, MM
TCR rearrangement	None	T-lineage ALL, NHL
BCL2-IGH	t(14;18)	85% FSCL, 25% DLCL
SIL-TAL	Deletion	25% T-lineage ALL
BCR-ABL fusion	t(9;22), variants	100% CML
20% ALL		
E2A-PBX1 fusion	t(1;19)	25% pre-B ALL
PML-RARa fusion	t(15;17)	100% APL
DEK-CAN fusion	t(6;9)	AML-M2, M4
E2A-HLF fusion	t(17;19)	Rare ALL

TCR = T-cell receptor; ALL = acute lymphoblastic leukemia; NHL = non-Hodgkin's lymphoma; MM = multiple myeloma; FSCL = follicular small cleaved cell lymphoma; DLCL = diffuse large cell lymphoma; CML = chronic myeloid leukemia; APL = acute promyelocytic leukemia.

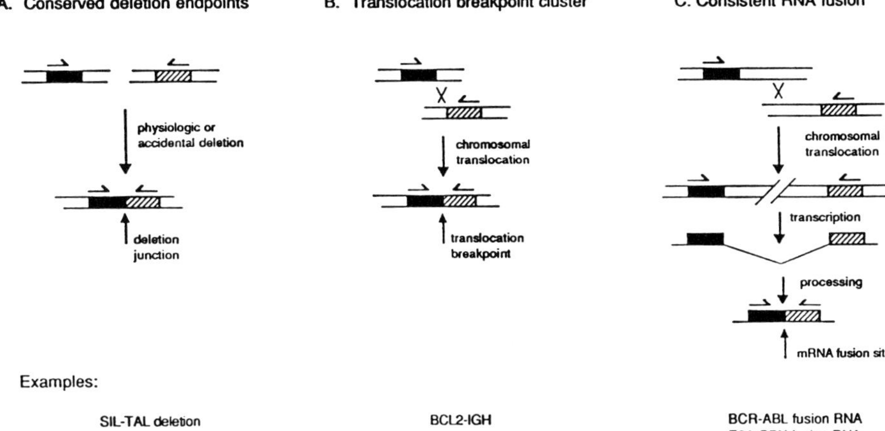

Figure 15-1. General types of genetic alterations detectable by PCR in hematological malignancies. Molecular alterations amenable to detection by PCR techniques are illustrated. Beneath each illustration are listed examples of specific molecular defects within each category that have been reported in hematolymphoid malignancies.

human malignancies by Lee and colleagues (8), who amplified the t(14;18) translocation breakpoint in neoplastic cells of patients with follicular non-Hodgkin's lymphomas. Numerous investigators have subsequently reported the utility of this approach for detecting subclinical levels of t(14;18)-carrying cells. Specific clustering of breakpoints at defined sites in the IgH gene on chromosome 14 and within or flanking the BCL2 gene on chromosome 18 allows use of generic primers to amplify and detect this marker in most but not all t(14;18) lymphomas. A small subset of t(14;18) translocations is not detectable using these methods because they occur outside the chromosome 18 breakpoint cluster sites. As described later and elsewhere in this volume, BCL2-IgH PCR has proved particularly useful for assessing the efficiency of marrow purging for autograft treatment of non-Hodgkin's lymphomas.

Unfortunately, most recurring chromosomal alterations in hematological malignancies that have been molecularly characterized to date do not demonstrate the tight genomic clustering observed for the t(14;18). One exception is a submicroscopic deletion of chromosome 1 reported to be present in up to 25% of T-lineage acute lymphoblastic leukemia (ALL; see Table 15-2). This deletion results in juxtaposition of the SIL and TAL(SCL) genes with well-defined and localized deletion end points. Therefore, generic primers homologous to sites in SIL and TAL flanking the deletion end points may be used for amplification of genomic DNA to assess MRD status in a significant proportion of T-cell ALL.

Several groups have reported PCR-based approaches for amplification of junctions within Ig (CDRIII PCR) and TCR genes created as a result of physiological rearrangement of these loci during lymphoid differentiation (9,10). Contrary to the genetic rearrangements described, these markers are not associated with the neoplastic process itself, but simply serve as useful molecular markers for individual lymphocytes and their clonal progeny. Generic primers homologous to conserved sequences in the TCR gamma or IgH variable (V) and joining (J) region genes are used to amplify the junctions of these rearranged gene segments, which are then cloned and sequenced for the purpose of constructing detection oligonucleotides. Because of the extremely high sequence diversity at these junction sites, the detection probes are tumor-specific and do not generally crossreact with junctions present in the patient's normal lymphocytes. The advantage of this approach is that it is applicable to virtually all lymphoid lineage malignancies, unlike those approaches based on specific cytogenetic abnormalities. Disadvantages concern the requirement to construct detection oligonucleotides for each patient's malignancy. It also assumes that the configurations of rearranged gene segments are stable and that there are no sequence variants within the tumor population. Exceptions to these latter requirements have been observed in subtypes of leukemia and lymphoma and may potentially limit the usefulness of this approach for assessment of MRD.

Most of the recurrent chromosomal translocations in hematopoietic malignancies do not have genomic breakpoints that are clustered tightly enough to be detected by PCR amplification of genomic DNA using a standard pair of oligonucleotide primers. However, these widely spaced genomic breakpoints frequently occur within the same transcription units on the involved chromosomes and result in synthesis of mRNA products, with conserved structural alterations that can be detected using PCR techniques (see Figure 15-1C). This detection is accomplished experimentally by converting the target mRNA to DNA with the enzyme reverse transcriptase and then amplifying the junctional sequences of interest using flanking primers. This so called reverse PCR approach was first applied to detect the BCR-ABL fusion transcript resulting from juxtaposition of the BCR and ABL genes on the Ph chromosome following t(9;22) translocation in CML and ALL cells (11).

As will be discussed, BCR-ABL PCR has been used by several groups to detect MRD in patients with CML following BMT. The advantages of BCR-ABL PCR include its inherent sensitivity and the convenience of using a standard set of primers that is capable of amplifying fusion mRNA products from all patients. Disadvantages concern the problematic quantitation, because the target is mRNA, which may be present in different amounts in various leukemias. Also, contamination remains a serious technical concern in all PCR studies of MRD.

Several other recurring translocations in leukemias have been shown to result in consistent fusion transcripts, as summarized in Table 15-2. Studies have not yet been published that report their detection as a means to monitor MRD status; however, it is anticipated that they will serve as molecular markers analogous to BCR-ABL. It is likely that in the future, additional consistent molecular abnormalities will be described in hematological malignancies, resulting in a range of disease markers for monitoring MRD status in many BMT patients using PCR or comparable techniques.

Uses of MRD Assays in BMT

Assays of MRD have a variety of potential applications in clinical BMT, including use of MRD assays to select appropriate candidates for BMT, to monitor the effectiveness of marrow purging, to predict patients at high risk for relapse, and to compare the relative efficacy of pretransplant conditioning regimens (Table 15-3). This approach assumes that the presence of malignant cells as detected by these sensitive assays has predictive value, a premise for which there is some experimental support.

Use of MRD Assays to Evaluate Potential BMT Recipients

There is considerable controversy surrounding the issue of which patients should be considered for BMT procedures. In diseases such as ALL and acute myeloid leukemia (AML), the decision to pursue BMT often hinges on clinical parameters of the patient's disease (e.g., initial white blood cell [WBC] count, cytogenetic abnormalities, presence of extramedullary disease, or response to initial chemotherapy), indicating that they are at high risk for relapse with standard chemotherapy. These decisions are rarely based on direct measurements of disease burden prior to transplant. An alternative approach may be to assess leukemic burden by MRD assays and to use this determination to guide future therapy. If effective, this approach would direct the use of BMT to those patients with persistent disease and thereby avoid some of the potential morbidity and mortality associated with this treatment.

Table 15-3.
Potential Uses of MRD Assays in Bone Marrow Transplantation (BMT)

Selection of patients at high risk of disease relapse who would be candidates for BMT
Monitoring the effectiveness of marrow purging
Predicting relapse following BMT
Comparison of the cytoreductive potentials of different preparative regimens

Currently, MRD status is not a selection criterion for BMT. However, MRD assays have shown promise in other settings to follow patients with leukemia after initial chemotherapeutic induction and throughout treatment. One approach has been to use clonogenic culture assays to detect residual tumor cells sensitivity in patients with ALL. Colonies of lymphoblasts with the same cytogenetic abnormalities and cell surface phenotype as the original tumor cells have been cultured from patients with childhood ALL (12). Thirteen patients were studied while in hematological remission, and 6 were found to be positive using this assay system. Four of these positive patients went on to relapse between 2 and 30 months from the time of the abnormal cultures, suggesting that this approach may detect those patients at high risk for relapse.

FACS analysis has been a useful method for subclassification of disease lineage. As discussed, this approach is generally not sensitive enough for detection of MRD. Modifications have been made, however, which improve the sensitivity to the level of detection of one tumor cell in 10^4 normal cells. This improvement was accomplished by combining FACS analysis with standard cytochemical or cell culture techniques. Compara and colleagues (13) utilized this approach to analyze samples obtained from patients with ALL for leukemia-associated phenotypes, such as terminal deoxynucleotidyl transferase (TdT)–positive cells, which coexpress CD13, CD33, CD37, CD2, or cytoplasmic CD3. Using this approach, 44 patients were analyzed while in hematological remission. Nineteen patients were identified with detectable minimal disease, and all patients relapsed within 4 to 25 weeks, compared with 25 patients, also in hematological remission, who were negative by these assays, 17 of whom remained in remission with a follow-up of up to 114 weeks (13).

An alternative approach has been to preselect for populations of cells likely to be enriched for malignant cells by depleting marrow of mature myeloerythroid and monocytic cells with a panel of monoclonal antibodies (MABs) and complement. The enriched cells are then analyzed for Ig or TCR gene rearrangement by Southern blotting. Using this method, a single tumor cell could be detected in 10^3 normal cells. This approach was applied to 11 patients with ALL in remission. Of the 5 patients who went on to relapse, minimal disease was detected in 4 patients 1.5 to 9 months prior to relapse (14).

PCR-based approaches have also been used to study childhood ALL. Using CDRIII PCR, a quantitative assessment of residual leukemic cells as compared with normal B lymphocytes can be made; the limit of sensitivity is 1 tumor cell in 10^5 normal cells. In one report, marrow samples obtained from patients with ALL were studied following induction chemotherapy.

In patients entering a clinical remission, there was a 3- to 4-log reduction in the number of leukemic cells as compared with a sample obtained prior to treatment. Eight patients were studied in detail. In 4 patients, residual disease could be detected in at least one follow-up marrow sample taken in remission (15). In one of these patients, a dramatic increase in the number of leukemic cells was found 3 months prior to clinical relapse.

Yokota and colleagues (16) used a somewhat different approach to monitor the presence of ALL cells following induction chemotherapy by analyzing TCR d chain rearrangements. They found that 96% of patients with T-cell ALL and 81% of patients with common ALL had TCR d chain rearrangements. In T-cell ALL, this rearrangement was predominantly of the Vd_1DJd_1 type, whereas in common ALL, the Vd_2Dd_3 rearrangement was most frequent. Twenty-seven patients with ALL were studied while in first hematological remission. In all samples, Southern blot analysis showed only germline configuration of the TCR. Eight samples were analyzed by PCR following induction chemotherapy, and all 8 samples were positive for rearrangements indicative of the presence of leukemic cells. Eleven patients were studied during maintenance chemotherapy, and 6 had amplifiable rearranged TCR sequences 7 to 19 months after diagnosis. The time interval between diagnosis and achieving PCR negativity was variable and ranged between 8 and 19 months. Relapse did not correlate with known risk factors. Two patients went on to relapse by standard criteria, both of whom were positive by PCR analysis up to 4 months prior to hematological relapse (16).

A similar approach has been used to study 6 additional patients with ALL. Four were in long-term remission 3.9 to 8.1 years following leukemic induction and all were also PCR-negative. Two additional patients were found to be PCR-positive while in hematological remission, and both patients subsequently relapsed (17).

These studies indicate the technical feasibility of analyzing patients with ALL for the presence of MRD. A central question is with what accuracy a positive result using these sensitive MRD assays predicts for relapse, or whether a small tumor burden is tolerable and possibly kept in check by immunological mechanisms. Future studies will be required, with larger numbers of patients and longer follow-up to determine whether this approach predicts for those patients who are at high risk for relapse and should therefore be treated with more aggressive therapy, such as BMT. In addition, other strategies must be developed to extend the utility of MRD assessment to other disease entities.

Use of MRD Assays to Monitor the Effectiveness of Marrow "Purging"

Autologous BMT has emerged as an important treatment option for patients with a variety of hematological malignancies and solid tumors. A central concern in the use of this approach is the possibility that the harvested marrow may be contaminated with tumor cells, which upon reinfusion may contribute to the high rate of relapse observed in these patients. A variety of techniques has been developed in an effort to "purge" marrow of these potentially contaminating tumor cells. Although the need for marrow purging has not yet been proven by a prospective clinical trial, there is accumulating evidence that contaminating tumor cells in the marrow graft could be contributing to the risk of relapse (18–20).

A major problem in the analysis of purging methods has been the lack of sensitive assays that can be used to determine the efficacy of removal of the tumor cells. Because typically during a standard autologous BMT procedure more than 10^9 cells are infused, sensitive assays are required that can detect small numbers of tumor cells in the marrow or peripheral blood mononuclear collections. There is no consensus on whether small numbers of tumor cells present in the graft are tolerated and possibly removed following reinfusion by immunological mechanisms. An additional consideration is the efficiency at which tumor cells engraft when infused intravenously. All of these factors may vary among different individual malignant cells, thus making it extremely difficult to answer the question of how effective the purging process should be.

A variety of methods has been developed, initially using animal models (21,22) and more recently human material for the purpose of bone marrow purging, some of which are listed in Table 15-4. Use of chemotherapeutic agents and MABs are covered in other areas of this book in more detail, but are discussed here in the context of their efficiency in removing residual tumor cells.

The most widely used chemotherapeutic agents for marrow purging are the cyclophosphamide derivatives 4-hydroperoxycyclophosphamide (4-HC) and mafosfamide (23), which have been widely used

Table 15-4.
Methods of Marrow Purging

- Chemotherapeutic agents
  - 4-Hydroperoxycyclophosphamide (4-HC)
  - Mafosfamide
  - Combinations of drugs such as 4-HC with etoposide, 4-HC, vincristine, and prednisone
- Monoclonal antibodies
  - Plus complement (human or rabbit)
  - Conjugated to magnetic beads
  - Conjugated to toxins or chemotherapeutic agents
- In vitro culture
- Photoactive dyes
- Immunological methods
  - Natural killer or lymphokine activated killer cells with or without interleukin-2
  - Cytotoxic T cells
- Positive stem-cell selection

clinically in patients with AML. Impressive transplant survival results have been obtained in patients with advanced disease as well as in those in first complete remission (19,24). In one study, the clinical benefits of 4-HC purging were strongly suggested in patients who underwent autologous BMT within the first 6 months of achieving their first clinical remission (19).

A central problem in the analysis of 4-HC marrow purging is determining whether the leukemic cells are adequately killed. Clearly, this agent is also toxic to normal bone marrow progenitor cells such as granulocyte-macrophage colony forming units (CFU-GMs). The efficacy of marrow purging with 4-HC was initially evaluated retrospectively by evaluating CFU-GM growth before and after 4-HC purging. Patients who eventually relapsed were compared with patients who remained in remission. In this analysis, it was found that the CFU-GM content following 4-HC purging predicted eventual patient outcome. Specifically, patients with less than 1% CFU-GM growth following 4-HC treatment had a statistically significant decreased rate of relapse as compared with patients with more than 1% CFU-GM growth (18). These data were the first to suggest that the intensity of the marrow purging procedure had some impact on eventual patient outcome. In addition, studies of this kind and other studies discussed later clearly indicate that not all purging procedures are equally effective in removing tumor cells or a surrogate marker cell population, such as CFU-GMs.

The sensitivity of myeloid leukemic cells to 4-HC was evaluated using a clonogenic assay termed *CFU-L* (colony forming units-leukemia). Using this assay, CFU-Ls were grown successfully from marrow of the majority of patients with AML in hematological remission (25). The probability of disease relapse following BMT was significantly lower in patients whose CFU-Ls were sensitive to 4-HC, as compared with those who were resistant (18 vs 77% relapse rate; $p < 0.001$). Because these patients were prepared for BMT with cyclophosphamide and their marrow was purged with 4-HC, it cannot be determined whether the improved results found in patients with sensitive disease were due to more effective preparation, purging, or both. 4-HC has also been used in combination with other chemotherapeutic drugs, including vincristine and prednisone, which resulted in greater CFU-L sensitivity in patients with ALL (26).

MABs have also been used widely for marrow purging purposes. In human systems, their efficacy was initially studied using leukemia and lymphoma cell lines. In most studies, lineage-specific rather than tumor-specific MABs have been used, which are directed against B, T, or myeloid cell surface antigens. These MABs then require activation either with complement (rabbit or human) or conjugation to either toxins or solid supports in the form of magnetic particles (27–31). Using these approaches, approximately 3 to 4 logs of tumor-cell removal was generally accomplished with minimal toxicity to normal marrow progenitor cells, as measured by CFU-GM growth. Use of MAB-based purging methods has been applied clinically in non-Hodgkin's lymphoma, AML, ALL, neuroblastoma, and breast cancer (32–34).

A major concern with the clinical use of marrow purging methods developed using tumor cell lines is the possibility that tumor-cell removal may not be as efficient with freshly harvested marrow cells. In addition, extrapolation from the generally small volumes used for these experimental studies to the large volume obtained at marrow harvest may not be valid. As discussed, the only two sensitive methods for the detection of MRD that can be used with fresh material are clonogenic and PCR-based assays. Using a clonogenic assay with T-lineage ALL blasts, it was found that the combination of ricin-conjugated anti-CD5 and anti-CD7 with 4-HC was superior to either agent alone (33). These workers also studied B-lineage ALL and used a combination of FACS and a leukemic progenitor cell clonogenic assay to monitor the effectiveness of marrow purging with MABs plus complement and 4-HC. This purging method showed variable success in effectively removing the leukemic blasts, which ranged from 0.1 to 4 logs (35).

PCR-based methods have also been used to monitor the effectiveness of marrow purging. This approach is attractive because it can be applied readily to patients with known chromosomal translocations, such as the t(14;18) translocation commonly found in non-Hodgkin's lymphomas and the t(9;22) found in CML and ALL. In addition, use of more generic PCR-based methods, as discussed, could broaden the range of patients analyzable in this fashion. Using B-lymphoma cell lines, we found that after 2 rounds of MAB-complement treatment, there was an approximately 3-log reduction in the intensity of the tumor-cell–specific PCR product (Figure 15-2). This log cell kill was confirmed using a clonogenic assay validating the use of PCR-based methods (36).

In our initial studies, the effectiveness of MABs and complement tumor-cell depletion as measured by PCR was variable depending on the tumor cell line used to contaminate the marrow specimens. A similar observation was made using a large number of clinical specimens obtained from patients with t(14;18)-positive non-Hodgkin's lymphoma (19). The significance of the presence of a positive PCR signal following marrow purging was demonstrated recently in dramatic fashion. In this study, patients whose marrow preparations were purged to PCR negativity had a much lower relapse rate, as compared with patients whose preparations remained PCR-positive (7 vs 46% relapse rates; $p < 0.00001$)(20). These data indicate that either the presence of small numbers of tumor cells that remain in the marrow following the purging procedure are a major source of eventual relapse or that sensitivity of the tumor cells to ex vivo MAB plus complement-mediated lysis in some manner predicts radiochemosensitivity of the tumor in vivo. The pattern of relapse found in this study was commonly at sites of previous disease. This finding had previously been interpretated to indicate that the

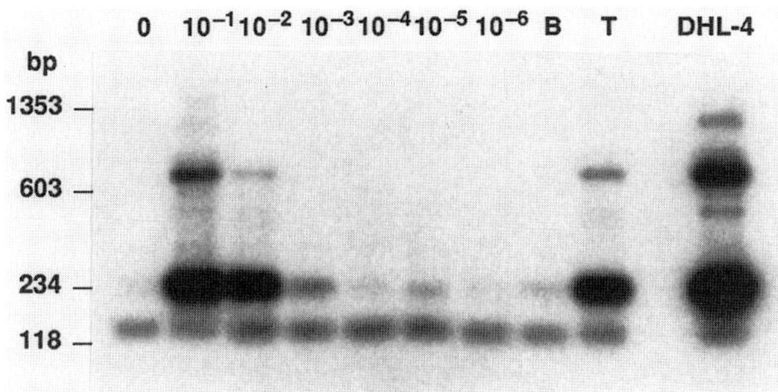

Figure 15-2. Antibody plus complement-mediated purging of the lymphoma cell line SU-DHL-4 from marrow as assayed by PCR. The B cell SU-DHL-4 tumor line harbors a t(14;18) chromosomal translocation and was added to marrow at 1% of the total cell number. This experimentally contaminated marrow specimen was treated with a panel of either B or T cell monoclonal antibodies followed by rabbit complement for two cycles. DNA was extracted and PCR was performed. The PCR products at 230 and 600 bp were visualized using a ^{32}P-labeled internal detection oligonucleotide. Ten-fold dilutions of SU-DHL-4 cells were made in normal marrow mononuclear cells and used to assess the degree of tumor cell depletion. A second pair of oligonuleotide primers was used to amplify normal β-globin (150 bp PCR product). (Reproduced by permission from Negrin RS, Kiem HP, Schmidt-Wolf IGH, Blume KG, Cleary ML. Use of the polymerase chain reaction to monitor the effectiveness of ex vivo tumor cell purging. Blood 1991;77:654–660.)

source of relapse was from inadequate eradication of the disease by the preparative regimen.

One concern with the use of PCR-based methods for analysis of marrow purging with MABs and complement is the possibility that residual DNA present from either lysed or killed but intact cells may be amplified, giving an underestimate of the true log cell kill. This misinterpretation is presumably avoided by adding DNAse to the incubation media such that any liberated DNA will be degraded immediately. By using MABs conjugated to magnetic beads or other solid supports, this problem may be avoided. Using this approach, the effective removal of tumor cells could be demonstrated (36,37). One advantage of magnetic bead–based purging methods is that DNA can be extracted from the cells removed by the MAB-conjugated magnetic beads and amplified by PCR.

Further studies with clonogenic and PCR-based methods are required to determine the optimal approach for marrow purging. One attractive alternative will be to perform positive stem-cell selection, thereby removing any contaminating tumor cells. The effectiveness of this approach can now be assessed directly using these assay systems.

Use of MRD Assays to Predict Relapse Following BMT

Relapse remains a significant clinical problem despite myeloablative therapy followed by BMT, particularly for patients who undergo autologous BMT, although patients undergoing allogeneic BMT are also at risk for relapse. For example, in patients undergoing allogeneic BMT for CML, 15 to 30% of patients in the chronic phase and 50 to 85% of patients in the accelerated phase or blast crisis will ultimately relapse (38). Therefore, predicting which patients will relapse is useful, not only for prognostic purposes, but also to attempt post-transplant therapy (e.g., with immunomodulating drugs such as interferon or interleukin-2).

The most widely studied setting for relapse prediction using MRD assays has been in patients with CML undergoing BMT. PCR-based methods to detect expression of BCR/ABL have been employed by a number of groups. To date, at least 15 articles and letters have been published that attempt to determine whether a positive PCR result following BMT predicts which patients are at risk for relapse. Unfortunately, results from the original reports are conflicting. The reasons for these disparate results are not clear; however, most studies analyzed relatively small numbers of patients at only a single time (11,39–45). This finding has raised the possibility that patient selection or sample preparation may have been important factors. Clearly, a major concern with PCR is the possibility of false-positive results from the transfer of minute amounts of genetic material from one reaction tube to the next, resulting in amplification (46,47).

A variety of studies has demonstrated that a positive result within the first 4 to 6 months following BMT does not predict eventual relapse. The reasons for this finding are not entirely clear. However, this observation may indicate that the cells detected at this point are nondividing and eventually die out or are eradicated by graft-versus-leukemia reactions. At other points, it appears that a positive result does predict an increased risk of eventual leukemic relapse.

Recently, several studies have been published analyzing larger numbers of patients with serial analysis; they demonstrate that a positive PCR result following BMT likely predicts relapse if the result is several months from the time of transplantation and if the patient is persistently PCR-positive.

In one study of 37 patients analyzed for expression of BCR/ABL following BMT while in complete hematological and cytogenetic remission, there was no correlation between a positive result within 6 months of BMT and eventual relapse (48). In 10 patients who received T-cell–depleted marrow grafts, 5 patients were PCR-positive immediately following transplant, and 3 were PCR-positive after 6 months following BMT. Two of these 3 patients who were PCR-positive at 12 months relapsed by hematological criteria at 18 and 36 months, respectively. No relapses have occurred in the patients who were PCR-positive initially and converted to PCR negativity or who were persistently negative by PCR (48).

Two larger studies shed light on this important question. In these studies, serial samples have been analyzed by PCR and three patterns of results have

Table 15-5.
PCR Analysis of Relapse Risk Following BMT For Chronic Myelogenous Leukemia

Reference	Persistent Negative	Cyto-genetic Relapse	Hemato-logical Relapse	Inter-mittent Positive	Cyto-genetic Relapse	Hemato-logical Relapse	Persistent Positive[a]	Cyto-genetic Relapse	Hemato-logical Relapse
London (48)	22	0	0	4	0	0	11	1	3
Dana-Farber (49)	4	0	0	7	0	0	13	2	6
Michigan (50)	23	0	0	23	0	5	8	0	5
UCLA (11)	15	0	0	2	0	0	2	2	0
City of Hope (52)	6	0	0	12	1	0	1	0	0
Stanford (51)	6	0	0	5	0	0	0	0	0
Totals	76	0	0	53	1	5	35	5	14
Relapse risk (%) (hematological and cytogenetic)			0			11			54

[a]Persistently positive or positive after the first 3 months from BMT.
PCR = polymerase chain reaction; BMT = bone marrow transplantation.

emerged. These patterns include patients who are persistently negative, intermittently positive, and persistently positive by PCR. In one study of 24 patients, 4 were persistently negative and 7 were intermittently positive (e.g., at least one negative result). Of these 11 patients, there have been no relapses, although 1 intermittently positive patient has had a cytogenetic relapse while being PCR-positive. Thirteen patients have been persistently positive following BMT. Of these patients, 6 have had hematological and 2 have had cytogenetic relapses (49).

Similar results were reported in another study of 64 patients. Following BMT, 23 patients have been persistently negative by PCR, and no patient has relapsed. An additional 23 patients have been positive intermittently (i.e., have had both positive and negative results), and 5 of these patients have relapsed by hematological criteria. Eight patients were persistently PCR-positive; 5 of these patients have relapsed. Cumulative actuarial relapse rates in the three groups of persistently negative, intermittently positive, and persistently positive were 0, 20, and 77%, which are statistically significantly different. In this study, the median time from the first positive PCR result to relapse was 150 days, with a range of 90 to 832 days (50).

These results are summarized in Table 15-5, along with 3 additional studies in which serial patient samples were analyzed (11,51,52). In these studies, patients with persistently positive PCR results were found to have a higher risk of relapse than those who were persistently negative. The intermittently positive group of patients are extremely interesting because the presence of small numbers of tumor cells may predict a high rate of relapse with further follow-up or may remain in check, possibly by immune-mediated mechanisms. The future challenge will be to define conditions whereby patients with a high relapse risk can be identified while the tumor burden is relatively low, and possibly to treat these patients with other approaches, such as interferon-α after BMT or to modify the preparatory regimen used.

Use of PCR to predict which patients are at risk for relapse is not limited to the analysis of CML, even though this group of patients has been the most widely studied. Ph-positive ALL has also been studied in a small number of patients; relapse was predicted in one patient (53). The use of more generic PCR-based methods clearly can be utilized for this purpose.

With the use of these sensitive molecular approaches, it is expected that patients who are likely to relapse will be identified. This analysis may also be useful to compare different preparative regimens more rapidly in patients undergoing transplant procedures with relatively indolent diseases, such as low-grade lymphomas and CML. Ultimately, it is hoped that by using these sensitive assays for the detection of minimal disease, treatment options will be based on an objective measurement of disease rather than population-based risk analyses.

References

1. Arthur CK, Apperley JF, Guo AP, Rassool F, Gao LM, Goldman JM. Cytogenetic events after bone marrow transplantation for chronic myeloid leukemias in chronic phase. Blood 1988;71:1179–1186.
2. Cooperative Study Group on Chromosomes in Transplanted Patients. Cytogenetic follow-up of 100 patients submitted to bone marrow transplantation for Philadelphia chromosome-positive chronic myeloid leukemia. Eur J Haematol 1988;40:50–57.
3. Tkachuk DC, Westbrook CA, Andreef M, et al. Detection of BCR-ABL fusion in chronic myelogenous leukemia by two-color fluorescence in situ hybridization. Science 1990;250:559–562.
4. Pinkel D, Landegent J, Collins C, et al. Fluorescence in situ hybridization with human chromosome-specific libraries: detection of trisomy 21 and translocations of chromosome 4. Proc Natl Acad Sci USA 1988;85:9138–9142.
5. Miller RA, Hart S, Samouszuk M, et al. Shared idiotypes expressed by human B cell lymphomas. N Engl J Med 1989;321:851–857.
6. Brown SL, Miller RA, Levy R. Anti-idiotype antibody therapy of B cell lymphoma. Semin Oncol 1989;16:199–210.

7. Carroll WL, Link MP, Cleary ML, et al. Anti-idiotype antibodies in childhood B cell leukemia. Blood 1988 71:1068–1073.
8. Lee MS, Chang KS, Cabanillas F, Freireich EJ, Trujillo JM, Stass SA. Detection of minimal residual cells carrying the t(14;18) by DNA sequence amplification. Science 1987;237:175–178.
9. Yamada M, Hudson S, Tournay O, et al. Detection of minimal disease in hematopoietic malignancies of the B-cell lineage by using third-complementarity-determining region (CDR-III)-specific probes. Proc Natl Acad Sci USA 1989;86:5123–5127.
10. Deane M, Norton JD. Immunoglobulin heavy chain variable region family usage is independent of tumor cell phenotype in human B lineage leukemias. Eur J Immunol 1990;20:2209–2217.
11. Sawyers CCL, Timson L, Kawasaki ES, Clark SG, Witte ON, Champlin R. Molecular relapse in chronic myelogenous leukemia patients after bone marrow transplantation detected by polymerase chain reaction. Proc Natl Acad Sci USA 1990;87:563–567.
12. Estrov Z, Grunberger T, Dube ID, Wang YP, Freedman MH. Detection of residual acute lymphoblastic leukemia cells in culture of bone marrow obtained during remission. N Engl J Med 1986;315:538–542.
13. Compara D, Coustan-Smith E, Janossy G. The immunologic detection of minimal residual disease in acute leukemia. Blood 1990;76:163–171.
14. Bregni M, Siena S, Neri A, et al. Minimal residual disease in acute lymphoblastic leukemia detected by immune selection and gene rearrangement analysis. J Clin Oncol 1989;7:338–343.
15. Yamada M, Wasserman R, Lange B, Reichard BA, Womer RB, Rovera G. Minimal residual disease in childhood B-lineage lymphoblastic leukemia. Persistence of leukemia cells during the first 18 months of treatment. N Engl J Med 1990;323:448–455.
16. Yokota S, Hansen-Hagge TE, Ludwig WD, et al. Use of polymerase chain reactions to monitor minimal residual disease in acute lymphoblastic leukemia patients. Blood 1991;77:331–339.
17. Neale GAM, Menarguwz J, Kitchingman GR, et al. Detection of minimal residual disease in T-cell acute lymphoblastic leukemia using polymerase chain reaction predicts impending relapse. Blood 1991;78:739–747.
18. Rowley SD, Jones RJ, Piantadosi S, et al. Efficacy of ex vivo purging for autologous bone marrow transplantation in the treatment of acute nonlymphoblastic leukemia. Blood 1989;74:501–506.
19. Gorin NC, Aegerter P, Auvert B, et al. Autologous bone marrow transplantation for acute myelocytic leukemia in first remission: a European survey of the role of marrow purging. Blood 1990;75:1606–1614.
20. Gribben JG, Freedman AS, Neuberg D, et al. Immunologic purging of marrow assessed by PCR before autologous bone marrow transplantation for B-cell lymphoma. N Engl J Med 1991;325:1525–1533.
21. Teeney M, Knapp RC, Greenberger JS, Bast RC Jr. Elimination of leukemic cells from rat bone marrow using antibody and complement. Cancer Res 1981; 41:3331–3335.
22. Trigg ME, Poplack DG. Transplantation of leukemic bone marrow treated with cytotoxic antileukemia antibodies and complement. Science 1982;217:259–260.
23. Sharklis SJ, Santos GW, Colvin M. Elimination of acute myelogenous leukemic cells from marrow and tumor suspensions in the rat with 4-hydroperoxycyclophosphamide. Blood 1980;55:521–523.
24. Yeager AM, Kaizer H, Santos G, et al. Autologous bone marrow transplantation in patients with acute nonlymphoblastic leukemia, using ex vivo marrow treatment with 4-hydroperoxycyclophosphamide. N Engl J Med 1986;315:141–147.
25. Miller CB, Zehnbauer BA, Piantadosi R, Rowley SD, Jones RJ. Correlation of occult clonogenic leukemia drug sensitivity with relapse after autologous bone marrow transplantation. Blood 1991;78:1125–1131.
26. Rowley SD, Miller CB, Piantadosi S, Davis JM, Santos GW, Jones RJ. Phase I study of combination drug purging for autologous bone marrow transplantation. J Clin Oncol 1991;9:2210–2218.
27. Bast RC, Ritz J, Lipton JM, et al. Elimination of leukemic cells from human bone marrow using monoclonal antibody and complement. Cancer Res 1983;43:1389–1394.
28. Treleaven JG, Ugelstad J, Philip T, et al. Removal of neuroblastoma cells from bone marrow with monoclonal antibodies conjugated to magnetic microspheres. Lancet 1984;1:70–73.
29. Bast RC, DeFabritis P, Lipton J, et al. Elimination of malignant clonogenic cells from human bone marrow using multiple monoclonal antibodies and complement. Cancer Res 1985;45:499–503.
30. Uckun FM, Ramakrishnan S, Houston LL. Immunotoxin-mediated elimination of clonogenic tumor cells in the presence of human bone marrow. J Immunol 1985;134:2010–2016.
31. Ball ED, Mills LE, Coughlin CT, Beck RJ, Cornwell GG. Autologous bone marrow transplantation in acute myelogenous leukemia: in vitro treatment with myeloid cell-specific monoclonal antibodies. Blood 1986; 68:1311–1315.
32. Nadler LM, Botnick L, Finberg R, et al. Anti-B1 monoclonal antibody and complement treatment in autologous bone marrow transplantation for relapsed B-cell non-Hodgkin's lymphoma. Lancet 1984;1:427–431.
33. Uckun FM, Gajl-Peczalska K, Meyers D, et al. Marrow purging in autologous bone marrow transplantation for T-lineage acute lymphoblastic leukemia: efficacy of ex vivo treatment with immunotoxins and 4 hydroperoxycyclophosphamide against fresh leukemic marrow progenitor cells. Blood 1987;69:361–366.
34. Ball ED, Mills LE, Cornwell GG. Autologous bone marrow transplantation for acute myeloid leukemia using monoclonal antibody-purged bone marrow. Blood 1990;75:1199–1206.
35. Uckun FM, Kersey JH, Haake R, Weisdorf D, Ramsay NKC. Autologous bone marrow transplantation in high-risk remission B-lineage acute lymphoblastic leukemia using a cocktail of three monoclonal antibodies (BA-1/CD24, BA-2/CD9, and BA-3/CD10) plus complement and 4-hydroperoxycyclophosphamide for ex vivo bone marrow purging. Blood 1992;79:1094–1104.
36. Negrin RS, Kiem HP, Schmidt-Wolf IGH, Blume KG, Cleary ML. Use of the polymerase chain reaction to monitor the effectiveness of ex vivo tumor cell purging. Blood 1991;77:654–660.
37. Gribben JG, Barber M, Blake KW, Coral F, Freedman AS, Nadler LM. Magnetic bead depletion is superior to complement mediated lysis in purging lymphoma cells from bone marrow (abstract). Blood 1991;78:247a.
38. McGlave P. Bone marrow transplants in chronic

myelogenous leukemia: an overview of determinants of survival. Semin Hematol 1990;27:23–30.
39. Lee MS, Chang KS, Freireich EJ, et al. Detection of minimal residual bcr/abl transcripts by a modified polymerase chain reaction. Blood 1988;72:893–897.
40. Gabert J, Lafage M, Maraninchi D, Thuret I, Carcassone Y, Mannoni P. Detection of residual bcr/abl translocation by polymerase chain reaction in chronic myeloid leukemia patients after bone marrow transplantation. Lancet 1989;2:1125–1127.
41. Bartram CR, Janssen JWG, Schmidberger M, Lyons J, Arnold R. Minimal residual leukemia in chronic myeloid leukemia patients after T-cell depleted bone marrow transplantation (letter). Lancet 1989;1:1260.
42. Morgan GJ, Janssen JWG, Guo A, et al. Polymerase chain reaction for detection of residual leukemia. Lancet 1989;1:928–929.
43. Roth MS, Antin JH, Bingham EL, Ginsburg D. Detection of Philadelphia chromosome-positive cells by the polymerase chain reaction following bone marrow transplant for chronic myelogenous leukemia. Blood 1989;74:882–885.
44. Lange W, Snyder DS, Castro R, Rossi JJ, Blume KG. Detection of enzymatic amplification of bcr-abl mRNA in peripheral blood and bone marrow cells of patients with chronic myelogenous leukemia. Blood 1989; 73:1735–1741.
45. Delfau MH, Kerckaert JP, d'Hasghe MC, et al. Detection of minimal residual disease in chronic myeloid leukemia patients after bone marrow transplantation by polymerase chain reaction. Leukemia 1990;4:1–5.
46. Kwok S, Higuchi R. Avoiding false positives with PCR. Nature 1989;339:237–238.
47. Hughes T, Janssen JWG, Morgan G, et al. False-positive results with PCR to detect leukaemia-specific transcripts (letter). Lancet 1990;335:1037.
48. Hughes TP, Morgan GJ, Martiat P, Goldman JM. Detection of residual leukemia after bone marrow transplant for chronic myeloid leukemia: role of the polymerase chain reaction in predicting relapse. Blood 1991;77:874–878.
49. Delage R, Soiffer RJ, Dear K, Ritz J. Clinical significance of bcr-abl gene rearrangements detected by polymerase chain reaction after allogeneic bone marrow transplantation in chronic myelogenous leukemia. Blood 1991;78:2759–2767.
50. Roth MS, Antin JH, Ash R, et al. Prognostic significance of Philadelphia chromosome-positive cells detected by the polymerase chain reaction after allogeneic bone marrow transplant for chronic myelogenous leukemia. Blood 1992;79:276–282.
51. Kohler S, Galili N, Sklar JL, Donlon TA, Blume KG, Cleary ML. Expression of bcr-abl fusion transcripts following bone marrow transplantation for Philadelphia chromosome-positive leukemia. Leukemia 1990;4:541–547.
52. Snyder DS, Rossi JJ, Wang JL, et al. Persistence of bcr-abl gene expression following bone marrow transplantation for chronic myelogenous leukemia in chronic phase. Transplantation 1991;51:1033–1040.
53. Gehly GB, Bryant EM, Lee AM, Kidd PG, Thomas ED. Chimeric BCR-abl messenger RNA as a marker for minimal residual disease in patients transplanted for Philadelphia chromosome-positive acute lymphoblastic leukemia. Blood 1991;78:458–465.

Chapter 16
Pathology of Bone Marrow Transplantation

George E. Sale, Howard M. Shulman, and Robert C. Hackman

Three major groups of complications are encountered in the course of bone marrow transplantation (BMT): chemoradiation toxicity, immunological problems (rejection or graft-versus-host disease [GVHD]), and infections (1). The early post-BMT period is one of high risk for infection and bleeding. The later period incurs the risk of GVHD, relapse, late infections, and late complications of radiation and chemotherapy. It is a mark of progress in this field that the primary patient population for pathologists has shifted from high morbidity and early mortality to a mix of acute problems with relatively subtle long-term problems.

Pretransplant Evaluation

The referral evaluation for BMT is crucial and complex, especially as indications for BMT have broadened. Primary diagnostic material, relapse and remission data, and knowledge of recent treatment all are needed for accurate appraisal (2). For leukemia, primarily morphology and phenotypic, cytogenetic, and cytochemical data must be reviewed, and a current marrow aspiration must be examined for relapse. Myelodysplastic syndromes require careful study for important distinctions (e.g., between refractory anemia and refractory anemia with excess blasts [RAEB], which require different preparative regimens). Aplastic anemia requires very precise evaluation of marrow to classify severity and also to rule out myelodysplasia or disorders such as hairy-cell leukemia insidiously simulating aplasia. Speed is necessary in patients with aplastic anemia because of clinically dangerous thrombocytopenia and the need to defer transfusions before allogeneic BMT to avoid presensitization and rejection. Lymphomas require careful simultaneous review of previous diagnostic nodal and current marrow material, because tumor cells in the marrow might preclude autologous BMT. A lengthening list of solid tumors, such as Ewing's sarcoma, neuroblastoma, and breast cancer, are now being treated with BMT and require precise pretransplant staging, often including immunohistochemistry. Evaluation of myelofibrosis is important in chronic myeloid leukemia (CML), acute myelofibrosis, myelodysplastic syndromes, and metastatic disease and may require repeated biopsies with reticulin and trichrome staining. Liver biopsy may be necessary, not only to evaluate metastases, but also to decide on the risk of veno-occlusive disease (VOD) early after BMT. Active hepatitis (especially with bridging fibrosis) and cirrhosis are both potent predictors of severe liver toxicity caused by preparative regimens. (See Chapter 33.)

Post-transplant Evaluation

Massive destruction of the host marrow by radiation or chemotherapy produces acute marrow damage with features of acute serous myelitis. These features include edema, hemorrhage into the interstitium, loss of most marrow elements except plasma cells, and relative predominance of damaged fat and iron-rich macrophages. An appearance of fat necrosis is frequent. This damage gradually resolves over the first 4 to 6 weeks as the donor marrow engrafts in the form of colonies of myeloid, megakaryocytic, and erythroid precursors and their progeny. Lymphoid cells are usually diffuse and sparse. Engraftment is usually simultaneous in the three major cell lines, but the peripheral blood platelet count is usually the last to normalize. Failure to engraft is diagnosed by the absence of both peripheral and marrow myeloid, erythroid, and thrombocytic cells. Rare cases may show apparent lymphoid engraftment only (in some instances associated with GVHD). Graft rejection has no specific histological features but may be defined as transient engraftment with regeneration of at least one cell line followed by its loss. Rejection occasionally is heralded by loss of a single line, such as pure red cell aplasia. Its elusive mechanisms are discussed elsewhere in this book. Relapse of leukemia is infrequent before day 100 unless the patient has shown persistence of marrow tumor cells 7 to 21 days after BMT. In CML, cytogenetic evidence of relapse may predate morphological evidence by many months. Cytogenetics, restriction fragment length polymorphism analysis, and Y chromosome DNA detection may help greatly to assess chimerism and relapse status. Second tumors other than Epstein-Barr virus (EBV)–induced lymphoma usually occur late. EBV-associated lymphoma should be suspected in the setting of worsening gut GVHD despite treatment. A search for peripheral immunoblasts and aggressive biopsy may provide the chance for early intervention (3).

Toxicity from Pretransplant Cytoreductive Therapy

The cytoreductive therapy given for treatment of underlying malignancy, marrow ablation and immunosuppression, may cause widespread multiorgan dysfunction (4). The histopathology within some affected organs, such as the heart, may be "nonspecific" (i.e., edema, hemorrhage, necrosis of myocytes, interstitial fibrosis) (Figure 16-1), yet the associated clinicopathological entity may be highly characteristic of toxicity. Other changes due to toxicity, particularly those in the mucous membranes, skin, and gastrointestinal tract, may cause diagnostic difficulties because of their clinical or histological overlap with GVHD. Several studies of these organs demonstrate the diffuseness of conditioning injury and marked lessening of these changes with time (5) (Figure 16-2). Cytological features, including atypia and inflammation, do not clearly separate immunologically mediated versus toxic injury to the epithelium.

The most frequent serious regimen-related toxicity involves the liver, with a clinical syndrome of jaundice, weight gain, ascites, and painful hepatomegaly. Previously, this syndrome was called hepatic veno-occlusive disease (VOD), referring specifically to the occlusive lesions within the small hepatic venules and the small endothelial-lined pores that connect the sinusoids to the small hepatic venules (6). These changes, seen best with trichrome-stained sections of liver, consist of venular luminal narrowing by trapped subendothelial red cells and matrix eventually leading to fibrous obliteration of the venules, damage to the surrounding hepatocytes, and fibrosis in the sinusoids adjacent to the terminal hepatic venules, in the center of the liver acinus (zone 3)

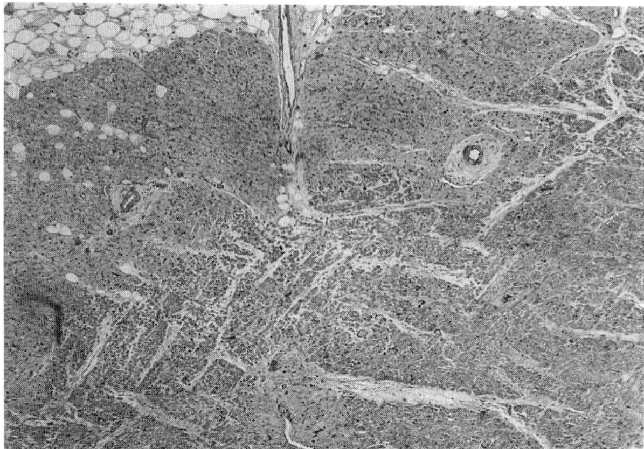

Figure 16-1. Heart, fatal cardiotoxicity, day 5. Within both ventricles were patchy transmural foci of hemorrhage admixed with necrotic myocytes. (H&E, ×32)

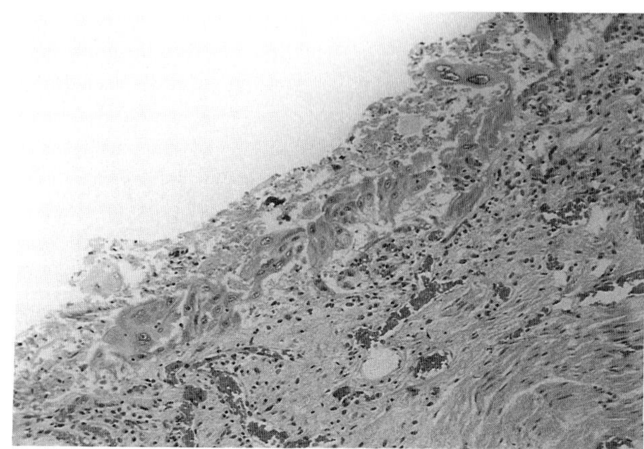

Figure 16-2. Esophagus, conditioning toxicity, day 5. The squamous mucosa displays widespread dyspolarity and ulceration. Nuclei are enlarged, irregular, and hyperchromatic. (H&E, ×80)

(Figure 16-3). Epidemiological and pathological studies suggest that the genesis of VOD is multifactorial (7,8). Conditioning injury to the zone 3 sinusoidal endothelium and hepatocytes is the proximate cause, but factors that promote coagulation, especially release of tumor necrosis factor-alpha (TNF-α) may also have a role in producing the deposition of fibrosis and Factor VIII that is seen in immunohistochemical staining of VOD lesions (9).

Recently, McDonald (8) suggested using the broader clinicopathological term *liver toxicity syndrome* rather than VOD for several reasons. First, it encompasses several zone 3 lesions that are associated with the clinical syndrome. Two studies have demonstrated that zone 3 sinusoidal fibrosis and phlebosclerosis, a nonocclusive perivenular fibrosis, are also associated with the same clinical features as VOD (6,10,11). Another zone 3 lesion reported to produce symptoms that resemble those of VOD is nodular regenerative hyperplasia, a change best seen on reticulin stains as atrophy of hepatocytes in zone 3, with compression of central venules and regeneration and expansion of hepatocyte cords in the periportal regions, creating a nonfibrotic nodularity. Snover and associates (12) reported nodular regenerative hyperplasia in 33% of their autopsies, including several patients with late-onset ascites but without VOD lesions. In a histological study of liver disease at our institution, we found nodular transformation in only 8% of all autopsies from patients transplanted in a one-year period and no association between nodular regenerative hyperplasia and symptoms of early liver toxicity (11). Nodular regenerative hyperplasia appears to be an infrequent lesion that develops later after BMT, secondary to disturbances in hemodynamics (13), and likely serves as an indicator of compensatory repair and regeneration of hepatocytes in different zones of the liver acinus.

Other reasons for using the term *liver toxicity syndrome* include the fact that up to 40% of cases with

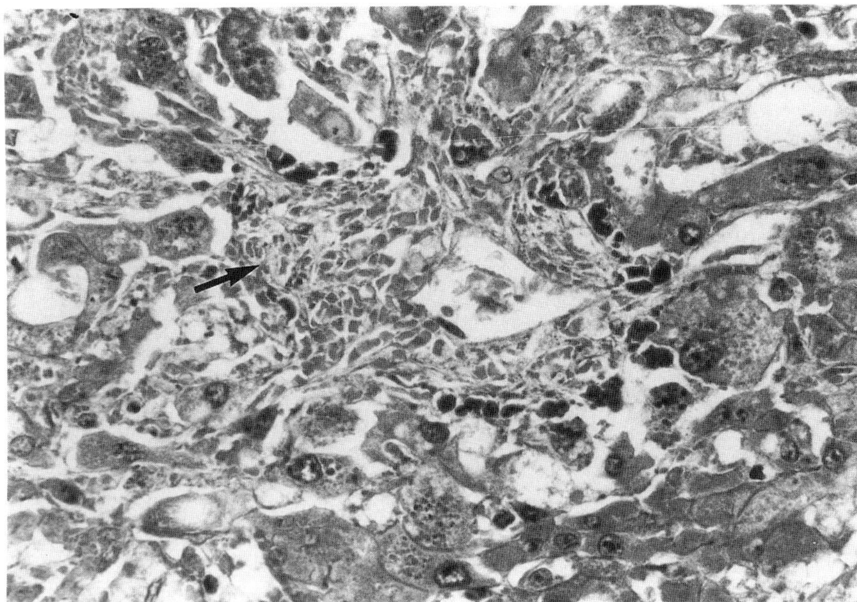

Figure 16-3. Liver, veno-occlusive disease, day 34. Sublobular vein has nearly complete lumenal obliteration by a mixture of connective tissue and entrapped blood cells *(arrow)*. Surrounding the vein is extensive hepatocyte damage and sinusoidal congestion. (Trichrome, ×80)

VOD lesions may be clinically silent (6,11,14). Problems can also arise with uniformity of histochemical stains and reproducibility of pathologists' interpretations. These problems are compounded when the histological lesions are infrequent, the luminal narrowing is mild, or there is autolysis or crush artifact. A previous limitation was that use of percutaneous needle liver biopsy was generally contraindicated with ascites or when platelets are below 60×10^9/L, a common situation in the early post-transplant period (15). This limitation has been circumvented in part by the use of transvenous liver biopsy, which includes measurement of the pressure gradient between the wedged and free hepatic venous pressures. A pressure gradient of more or less than 10 mm Hg has about an 80% predictive value (positive or negative) for biopsy diagnosis of VOD (16,17). The complication rates associated with transvenous liver biopsy vary greatly in different centers and appear connected to the experience of the radiologist and the type of biopsy instrument. Modified endomyocardial needles are more likely to cause capsule perforation than forceps biopsies. Multiple forceps biopsy samples taken during one procedure greatly improve the quantity of the specimen for histological evaluation without incurring additional bleeding risks. In our experience, all types of biopsies are satisfactory for the diagnosis of VOD, whereas samples obtained from either a percutaneous or an endomyocardial transvenous needle biopsy are more likely to produce better samples for the evaluation of GVHD.

Graft-versus-host Disease

Pathogenetically, GVHD is usually divided into afferent and efferent stages. The afferent stage involves recognition of minor or major histoincompatibilities, presumably by donor T cells (18). A classic concept for the efferent stage in GVHD is that donor cytotoxic lymphocytes attack host cells, including some epithelial cells of skin, intrahepatic bile ducts, and gut. Electron microscopic and immunohistological data demonstrate lymphocyte epithelial attachments and activation of infiltrating cytotoxic lymphocytes in human biopsy material. CD8-positive T cells with cytotoxic marking by TIA-1 antigen (19) have been found in skin and lip lesions. Natural killer (NK) cells have been found less consistently in some animal and human studies. Soluble mediators, such as TNF-α, have been implicated late in the effector arm of GVHD (20). Target cells seem to be in subregions of epithelium, where epithelial stem cells or their early progeny are located (e.g., rete ridges of skin, crypt cells of gut, and the parafollicular bulge of the hair follicle). The precise combination of surface expression of proliferation markers or of human leukocyte antigen (HLA) class I or II expression that makes these cells targets has not yet been clarified.

Skin GVHD

Histopathological interpretation of skin early after BMT is a difficult differential diagnostic exercise because of competing causes of the reactions and controversy in the field (1,21,22). The histological grading system of Lerner and colleagues (21,22) is a useful descriptor; grade I is epidermal basal-cell vacuolization, grade II is epidermal basal-cell death or apoptosis with lymphoid infiltration and satellitosis, grade III is bulla formation, and grade IV is ulceration of the skin. In practice, the useful dividing line is at grade II, and both lymphocytes and basal apoptosis should be required for this classification (Figure 16-4). Timing of the biopsy heavily influences interpretation, because direct cytotoxic effects of radiation and chemotherapy occur primarily in the first 3 weeks after BMT and produce epidermal damage overlapping with that of GVHD (21). The central feature of a lichenoid reaction with necrosis of basal cells has to be interpreted in the context of the time after chemoradiation, the presence of a marrow graft, the degree of HLA match, and the drugs used to prevent or to treat GVHD. The effects of chemoradiotherapy usually wear off in 3 to 4 weeks. At that point, the difficulties are fewer, the probability of true GVHD is higher, and epithelial atypia is less. Therefore, diagnostic confidence may be somewhat greater. The diagnostic threshold may also be lower in early chronic GVHD (e.g., day 80–100), which may be subtle and focal. Serial skin biopsies are often helpful to interpret the early skin changes and to provide a guide to clinical management.

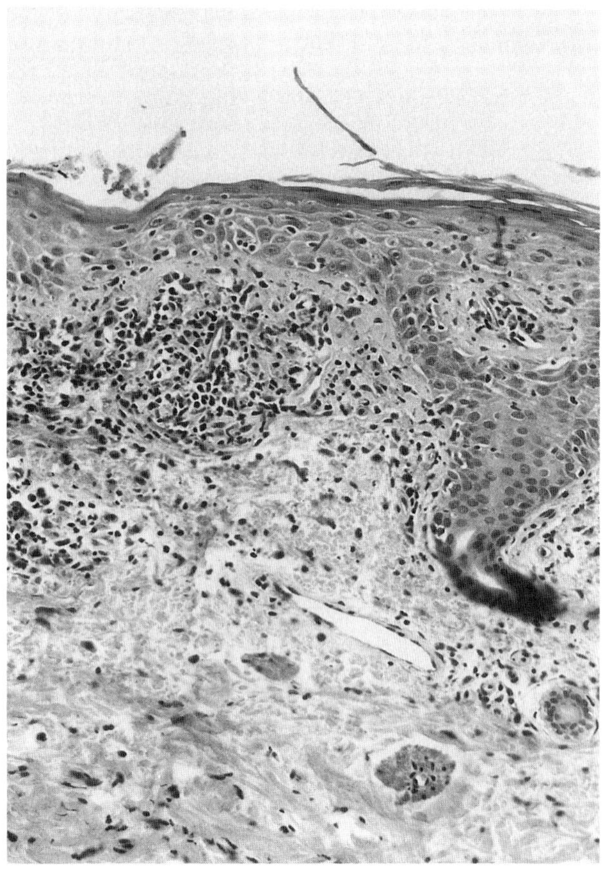

Figure 16-4. Skin, acute GVHD, day 30. Marked lichenoid reaction involving the epidermis and acrosyringium, with intraepidermal lymphocytes, apoptosis, and destruction of rete ridges. (H&E, ×51)

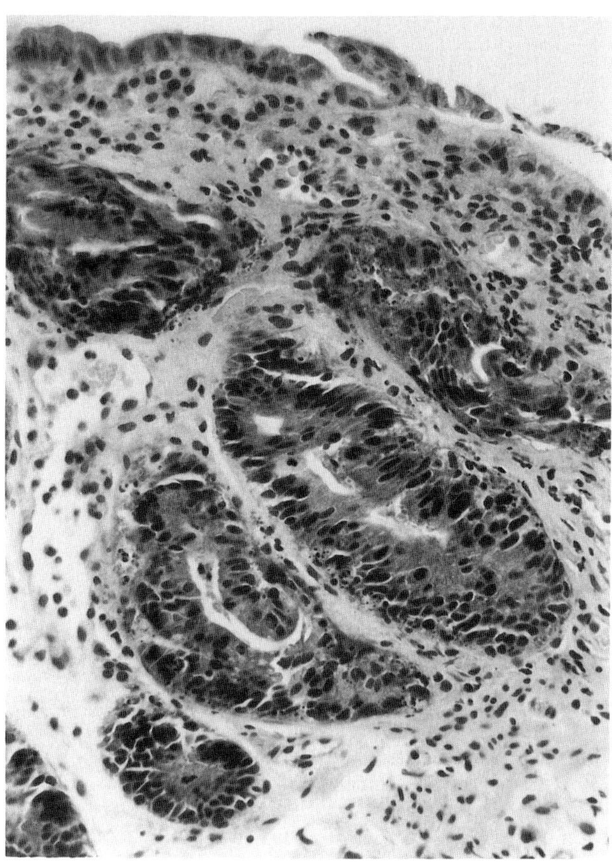

Figure 16-5. Colonic GVHD, day 36. Extensive apoptosis of enterocytes seen as nuclear dust along periphery of crypts. (H&E, ×80)

Gastrointestinal GVHD

As in skin, gastrointestinal biopsy is not very useful before day 21. After that, diarrhea volume correlates well with rectal biopsy histology. Rectal biopsy is usually reserved for difficult cases. The sequence of damage appears at four levels: grade I—individual cell necrosis in basal and lateral crypts, with *sparse lymphocytic* infiltrate (Figure 16-5); grade II—crypt abscess, in which polymorphonuclear leukocytes and eosinophils may participate; grade III—crypt loss; and grade IV—mucosal denudation.

The initial sites of injury in the gut are focused on the regenerative or stem-cell areas (i.e., the neck region of the gastric glands, the basal layer of esophagus, and the lower portion of the crypts in the small and large bowel). Two sets of data suggest that the disease in humans involves the gut diffusely. First, our autopsy study of gastrointestinal GVHD (23) showed that sections from the ileal and the rectal regions were within one histological grade of each other in most patients, and that stomach and duodenum were frequently involved. Second, gross and radiographic studies of gastrointestinal GVHD show that the diffuse changes of mucosal edema with effacement of the normal mucosal folds involve the entire small and large bowel simultaneously and sometimes include the stomach (24). Snover and associates (25) studied the role of upper gastrointestinal endoscopic biopsies in the diagnosis of acute GVHD in 16 patients with symptoms. Those biopsies showing epithelial necrosis and crypt abscesses from the small intestines were always associated with diarrhea and usually with similar histological changes in the rectal biopsy. In contrast, some patients with positive gastric biopsies may present with only nausea and vomiting (26). This study again emphasizes that a diagnosis of GVHD often requires both clinical and histopathological confirmation. This is particularly true when there is (1) an isolated positive gastric biopsy, (2) the finding of only rare grade I apoptotic bodies seen on high magnification in a small bowel biopsy, or (3) evidence of upper gastrointestinal infection with cytomegalovirus (CMV) associated with crypt abscesses or apoptotic bodies. In related studies, Nakhleh and colleagues (27) found that CMV colitis and severe T-cell deficiency can produce mucosal damage that simulates GVHD.

Aggressive surgical management of obstruction may save some patients (28). Histologically, these patients show diffuse intestinal ulceration with mucosal granulation tissue and fibrosis confined to the mucosa and the submucosa but do not have granulomas or transmural fibrosis, as in Crohn's disease. Patients with a more protracted course of GVHD of the gut over many weeks to months may develop segmental ulceration and submucosal fibrosis.

Like most squamous epithelia, that of the esophagus is involved in GVHD. The diagnosis of acute GVHD presents considerable diagnostic difficulty because esophagitis is common early after grafting and may also be due to fungal infection, herpes simplex virus (HSV), CMV, reflux, or any combination thereof. Accurate diagnosis requires histology and complete cultures for bacterial, viral, and fungal organisms, as well as special stains and immunocytochemistry studies because infectious agents are often not identified by histology alone. It is difficult to diagnose GVHD on endoscopic biopsy even if strict histological criteria similar to those for skin are used because of the frequency of nonspecific and infectious esophagitis. Increasing experience using upper gastrointestinal endoscopy with biopsy of esophagus, stomach, and duodenum shows considerable diagnostic value for distinguishing GVHD from infection by herpes viruses and fungi (29).

Pathogenetic mechanisms resulting in the destruction of enteric mucosa after BMT and GVHD have been reviewed by Beschorner (30). Cell-mediated cytotoxicity with close contact to target enterocytes has been described in ultrastructural studies of human rectal biopsies of GVHD (31). The ulcerated gut is a prime target for superinfection by CMV, gram-negative bacteria, and, less frequently, herpes simplex virus, adenovirus, and fungi such as *Candida, Aspergillus*, or *Torula* (29). Beschorner and colleagues (32), by using the immunoperoxidase technique on sections of intestine and colon, found a marked reduction in immunoglobulin A (IgA)- and IgM-bearing plasma cells in the lamina propria of patients with GVHD. This finding implies a local immunodeficiency to infection by enteric flora. The summation of these different injuries may result in depletion or loss of the mucosal stem cells, with a chronically ulcerated and fibrotic gut.

Liver GVHD

The liver is a major target of both acute and chronic GVHD. Histopathological and ultrastructural studies strongly suggest that the small interlobular and the marginal bile ducts at the periphery of the portal spaces are the preferential target of the alloimmune reaction (Figure 16-6). Experimental GVHD studies in congenic mice indicate that the cells penetrating the damaged bile ducts are T cells, that these T cells are specific for bile duct antigens, and that bile duct destruction does not require concurrent injury to the endothelium of the peribiliary capillary plexus that surrounds the ducts (33). The consequences of this reaction are (1) variable degrees of inflammation and later fibrosis, primarily within the portal zone; (2) nonspecific inflammatory and reactive changes in the hepatocyte lobules; and (3) cholestatic changes, often striking, that affect the zone around the central venule and the periportal cholangioles (Figure 16-7). Cholestasis and bile ductule proliferation, features often seen in longstanding GVHD, may reflect the consequences of the alloimmune segmental destruction of marginal bile ducts, an area of ductal progenitor cells (34). Ductule proliferation may also result from the coexisting influence of gut GVHD, which results in showering the liver with endotoxin (35), which in turn stimulates TNF-α, a promoter of bile ductule proliferation (36).

Over the years, pathologists have developed thresholds for classifying inflammatory liver disease as likely to be caused by GVHD. In both controlled experimental studies (37) and coded histopathological studies (38,39), the histological criteria that are most useful in discriminating between the etiological possibilities involve cytological and destructive changes in the bile ducts. These changes may progress from early cytotoxic lymphocyte attack on the ducts to a picture of bizarre dilated periportal pseudocholangioles seen in protracted acute GVHD of some weeks duration. Later, marked loss of bile ducts may occur. The bile duct changes that typify GVHD are seen in Figure 16-6. The bile ducts are irregular in outline. Individual or segments of epithelial cells are flattened and missing nuclei, creating a hypereosinophilic cytoplasmic syncytium. Remaining nuclei are often enlarged, hyperchromatic, irregular in outline, and pseudostratified.

Bile duct epithelial apoptosis, a presumptive sign for GVHD, is usually difficult to demonstrate. Another

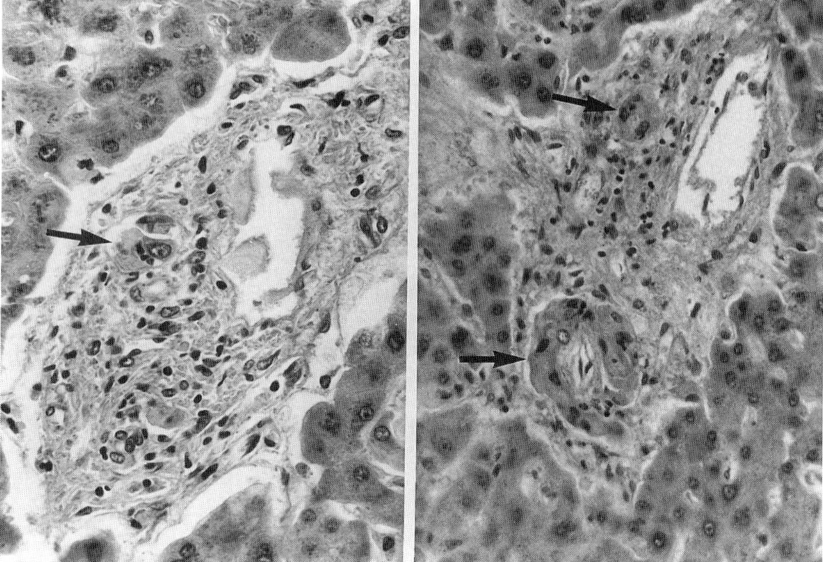

Figure 16-6. Hepatic GVHD, day 53. Despite the minimal inflammation within the portal space, the bile ducts *(arrow)* are reduced to degenerative cytoplasmic masses with a few remaining hyperchromatic nuclei. (H&E, ×128)

feature said to be relatively specific for GVHD is endothelialitis characterized by lymphocytic adhesion or transmural migration through the walls of hepatic and portal veins (39). Although this feature appears to be quite useful in the unrelated donor setting of orthotopic liver allografting, encoded histopathological studies of matched sibling marrow allogeneic BMT recipients with GVHD indicate that endothelialitis is so infrequent (and subtle) as to be of little practical use. Additional interpretive points include the fact that the duration of active GVHD influences histology. Biopsies taken early after the onset of liver dysfunction may not show the obvious bile duct changes. Also, biopsies taken during immunosuppressive treatment may show less inflammation. The distinction between chronic and acute GVHD may be difficult because flares of chronic GVHD resemble early acute GVHD. Yet, acute GVHD of 4 to 6 weeks' duration may have stellate portal fibrosis, bridging collapse, or fibrosis (see Figure 16-7) Dense portal fibrosis and loss of bile ducts, however, do correlate with chronicity (Figure 16-8) (38).

In histological terms, the primary differential diagnosis of liver GVHD is viral hepatitis or drug-liver injury. The BMT experience with chronic carriers of hepatitis B virus infection indicates little evidence of active hepatitis after BMT (40,41). The situation with hepatitis C virus (HCV) infection, the primary cause of non-A

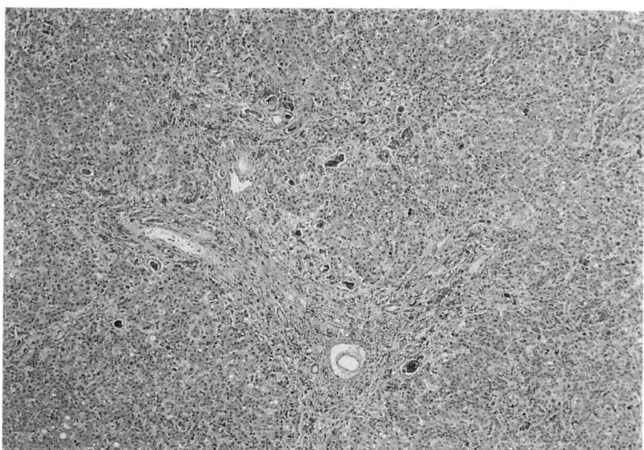

Figure 16-7. Hepatic GVHD, day 56. Pronounced hepatocellular and cholangiolar cholestasis with portal-to-portal bridging collapse. Proliferation of cholangioles along limiting plate. (H&E, ×19)

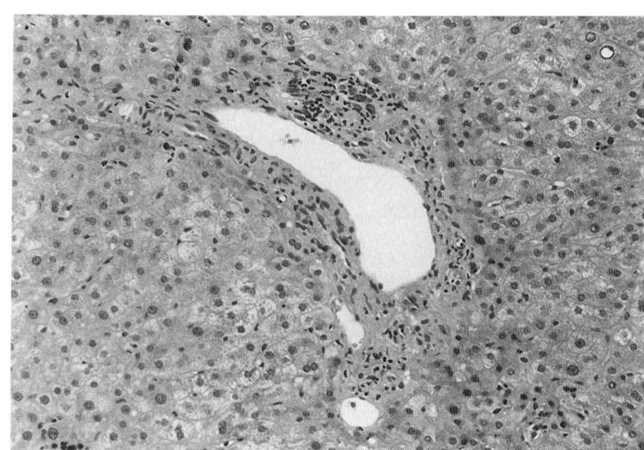

Figure 16-8. Chronic hepatic GVHD, 11 months. Destruction of small bile duct and some portal space fibrosis, with bridging or piecemeal necrosis. (H&E, ×32)

non-B hepatitis, is more complex. Two studies indicate that post-BMT seroconversion from negative to positive serology for HCV was often accompanied by abnormal liver tests and histological features of chronic hepatitis (42,43). Using the polymerase chain reaction (PCR), we followed the development of post-BMT HCV infection in 2 HCV-negative recipients who received marrow from hepatitis C viremic donors. The clinical course in their first 2 months after BMT indicated acquisition of hepatitis C viremia, but clinical and histological features did not overlap with those of acute GVHD (Myerson D and McDonald GB. Unpublished data). Unfortunately, we previously found that the distinction between chronic GVHD and chronic non-A non-B viral hepatitis (presumably HCV) was difficult when periportal inflammation and bile ductule proliferation were the predominant features (38). Furthermore, the difficulty is compounded by the fact that 90% of liver biopsy samples from patients with chronic HCV have nondestructive reactive bile duct changes (44,45) that might raise the possibility of liver GVHD. A means of resolving this histological distinction of liver GVHD from HCV may be provided by the observation that liver GVHD causes facultative expression of major histocompatibility complex (MHC) class II antigens on bile ducts (46), whereas HCV apparently does not (45). Identification of HCV in liver tissue sections by immunohistology may also allow a distinction between bile duct lesions caused by GVHD and those caused by HCV.

Immunohistology

A number of immunohistological studies have provided useful data on GVHD pathogenesis. In general, T-cell infiltrates, usually CD8 predominating, have been found in immunohistological studies of skin biopsies. Those few studies that have studied blood and tissue ratios of T-cell subsets simultaneously found parallel CD4/8 ratios (47–49). The routine diagnostic value of such studies seems somewhat limited, but the clear demonstration of T lymphocytes in epidermis can be helpful in deciding a borderline case. The pan-T-cell antibody UCHL-1 may be useful in paraffin-embedded tissues for this purpose. Similarly, DR positivity in the keratinocytes of a lesion tends to favor GVHD, although, as is well demonstrated in the literature, it is by no means specific (50–52).

Chronic GVHD

Clinical and histopathological manifestations of late-onset or persistent GVHD are so different from those of the earlier acute period that they are separated as a group into chronic GVHD. However, the histological changes may not always correspond to the operational definition of chronic GVHD using day-100 screening (53). From the pathologist's viewpoint, chronic GVHD is a multiorgan inflammatory disorder that resembles a mixture of GVHD and several autoimmune diseases. Histopathological studies of chronic GVHD have been useful for several reasons. (1) Practically, they are used to indicate disease activity and to grade therapy. (2) Prognostically, certain histological changes or involvement of certain organs are representative of extensive chronic GVHD (53–54). (3) Histological studies of chronic GVHD have provided observations that suggest some of the immunological targets and mechanisms regarding generalized fibrosis (43).

Most of the tissue sampled for assessment of chronic GVHD comes from skin, lip, and liver biopsies. Pathologists should be mindful of several caveats pertinent to the histopathology of chronic GVHD. (1) Histopathology changes over time. In the early phase, the predominant features are lymphoplasmacytic infiltration involving the epithelium and the glands (Figure 16-9). (2) These early inflammatory changes may in time cause widespread fibrosis, stenosis, obliteration, or atrophy of the involved tissues (Figures 16-10, 16-11, 16-12). (3) Following a flare of

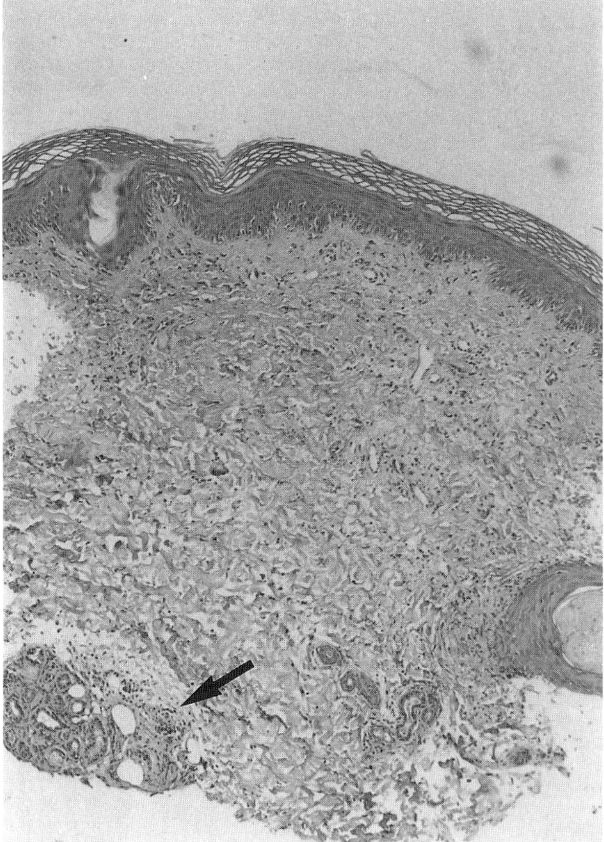

Figure 16-9. Skin, early chronic GVHD, day 314. Extensive or generalized type. The so called lichen planus-like chronic GVHD refers to the acanthotic and hyperkeratotic epidermis, which has inflammatory and destructive changes along the dermal-epidermal junction. An eccrine unit at the base of the dermis *(arrow)* and a follicle deep in the dermis are also being destroyed. The dermal collagen is unaltered. (H&E, ×8)

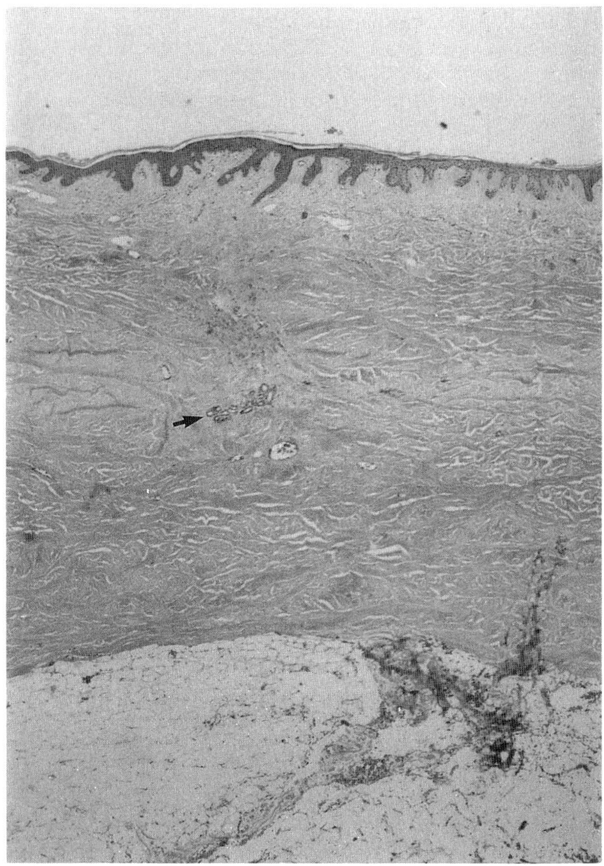

Figure 16-10. Late sclerodermatous chronic GVHD, day 910. The epidermis is atrophic. The dermal collagen is diffusely sclerotic with homogenization of the collagen, and the dermal-subcutis border is straightened. The dermis below the entrapped eccrine unit *(arrow)* represents acquired fibrous tissue resulting from chronic GVHD. (H&E, ×8)

chronic GVHD, the histological changes, particularly those in the epidermis and the liver, may be more closely akin to those of acute GVHD. Furthermore, in the absence of chronic inflammation, it may not be possible to distinguish active disease from residual late fibrotic damage (see Figure 16-12). (4) Unlike acute GVHD, chronic GVHD shows a rather extensive destruction of tubuloalveolar glands and ducts and a corresponding clinical sicca syndrome (see Figure 16-11). (5) Several infrequent manifestations of chronic GVHD mimic the naturally occurring autoimmune collagen vascular diseases, such as myositis, serositis, and arthritis. (6) Some changes of chronic GVHD appear to be largely the consequence of damage incurred during acute GVHD, such as segmental intestinal ulceration, fibrosis, and stenosis. Persistent liver test abnormalities, such as elevations of alkaline phosphatase and hyperbilirubinemia, may also reflect damage to small bile ducts incurred mainly during acute rather than chronic GVHD (7). The etiology of some late changes has not been fully resolved; GVHD, inflammation, infection, or true autoimmunity are all possibilities (see the obliterative small airway lesions in the pulmonary section). (8) The overall Karnofsky score or number of organ systems involved by chronic GVHD has proven a more useful barometer of clinical outcome than grading the histological lesions.

Generalized chronic GVHD of the skin is an inflammatory dermatitis that histologically resembles a combination of lichen planus and lupus profundus in its early stages (see Figure 16-9). When untreated or refractory, it resembles diffuse scleroderma (see Figure 16-10). The criterion for skin involvement is focal lichenoid inflammation, as in acute GVHD. This "lichenoid" pattern of hyperkeratosis, hypergranulosis, irregular acanthosis, and basal layer injury with apoptosis is associated with a decreased survival, (hazard ratio, 2.2; 95% CI = 1.1–4.3) (55) The irregular epidermal acanthosis in the early chronic phase is presumably a reflection of local secretion of growth factors, such as interleukin-3 (55). Additional criteria based on serial biopsies show progressive homogenization and reorganization of the dermal collagen (see Figure 16-10), fibrous straightening of the dermal-epidermal border, inflammation about eccrine coils, and occasionally deep panniculitis. Full-thickness biopsies from recently dyspigmented or hyperkeratotic areas should be chosen for biopsies because chronic GVHD is not uniform in its progression or involvement. Practically speaking, the most important job of the pathologist is to distinguish residual or past damage from ongoing disease activity. Because patients often are receiving or have recently finished with immunosuppressive treatment, the inflammatory changes may be quite minimal to absent. Evidence of epithelial vacuolar degeneration or apoptosis in the basilar layers of the skin and its appendages, the oral mucosa or minor salivary glands of the lip, or the bile ducts constitutes evidence of ongoing activity.

Limited or localized chronic GVHD of the skin begins as innocent-looking, dyspigmented macules with variable degrees of induration. Sampling of such areas demonstrates fibrous remodeling in the deeper reticular dermis. A small amount of epidermal degeneration or apoptosis may be present. The difference between the two types of GVHD involvement may simply depend on where in the dermis the fibrosis begins, deep with the limited form versus subepithelial in the extensive form. Hence, it is important that biopsies be of adequate size and full thickness to include the dermis and even some subcutaneous fat.

Oral chronic GVHD has epithelial changes of GVHD in both the mucosa and the minor salivary ducts, as well as a fibrosing sialadenitis. The oral biopsies often have a background of mild inflammatory change in the mucosa and the periductal interstitium of the minor salivary glands. The grading system we use distinguishes between grade I inflammation, which has a 50% specificity, and grade II inflammation (with

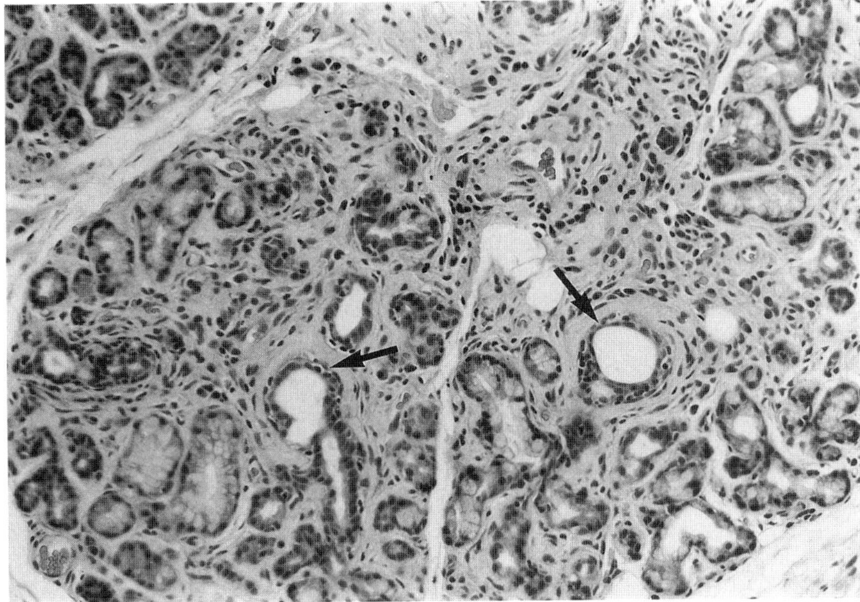

Figure 16-11. Lip biopsy, minor salivary gland. The lymphoplasmacytic inflammatory cells are centered around small ducts. Signs of ductal epithelial cell destruction, irregularity of outline nuclear stratification and hyperchromatism, and apoptosis *(arrow)* are similar to GVHD changes in small bile ducts. The glandular interstitium is becoming fibrotic and the acini are becoming atrophic, resulting in a sicca syndrome. (H&E, ×80)

apoptosis), which has a 75% specificity (56). Nakhleh and colleagues (27) suggested a modification of this threshold grading system by requiring 3 or more apoptotic bodies in the mucosa and at least a 10% loss of acinar tissue by inflammation before biopsies are considered positive for GVHD. This approach would increase specificity but decrease sensitivity (57).

Infection

Infection is a frequent complication of BMT, and the involvement of specific microorganisms has been extensively discussed in other chapters. Here we shall consider briefly the role of histological studies not only in providing the rapid and specific diagnoses required for effective treatment, but also in carrying out retrospective searches for new organisms in archival tissue.

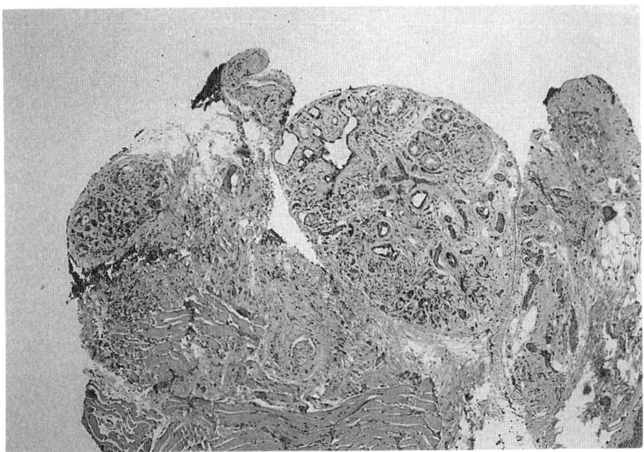

Figure 16-12. Lip biopsy, day 376. Fibrotic and destroyed minor salivary gland contains only ectatic ducts. These changes reflect previous chronic GVHD damage. Unless they are accompanied by some inflammatory component in other glands or in the mucosa, they should not be taken as a sign of active chronic GVHD. (H&E, ×32)

The histological demonstration of fungi in tissue is often crucial to the diagnosis of invasive infection because culture isolation is slow and insensitive, fungemia is sporadic, and dependable assays for antigenemia are not generally available. *Toxoplasma gondii*, *Pneumocystis carinii*, mycobacteria, and legionella are also organisms identified frequently by histological or immunocytochemical staining.

Because conditioning regimens largely ablate virus-specific immunity and because GVHD as well as its prophylaxis and treatment are broadly immunosuppressive, there is a very high rate of reactivation of latent viruses, especially members of the herpes and adenovirus groups (58,59). Occasionally, viral infection of a single organ will produce an ambiguous clinical presentation best resolved by prompt biopsy and rapid tissue evaluation. For instance, severe abdominal pain may suggest impending bowel infarction from reactivation of gut GVHD, but may actually represent acute HSV, varicella zoster virus (VZV), or adenovirus hepatitis, which can be diagnosed within a few hours by histological and immunocytochemical studies of a transjugular hepatic biopsy. Hematuria and costovertebral angle tenderness may result from adenovirus nephritis (59) (Figure 16-13).

The recent development of more effective antiviral therapy increases the need for rapid and specific viral diagnosis. Demonstration of CMV by culture, cytology, immunocytochemistry (Figures 16-14 to 16-16), hybridization, or PCR techniques in bronchoalveolar lavage (BAL) material from a patient with pneumonia

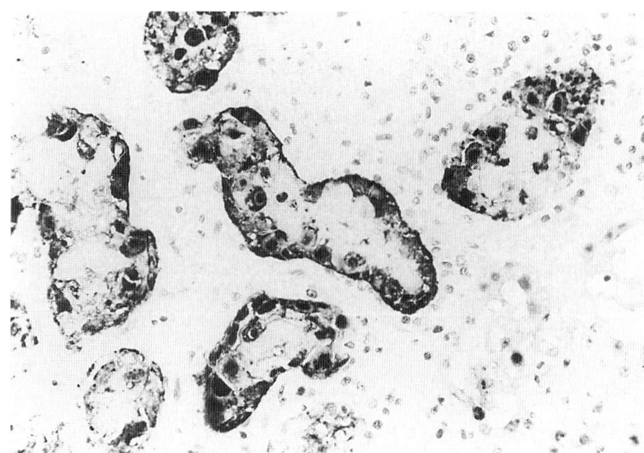

Figure 16-13. Kidney, adenovirus nephritis, day 77. Tubules lined by degenerating epithelial cells are strongly reactive for adenovirus antigen by indirect immunoperoxidase staining using a monoclonal antibody to the adenovirus hexon protein (Chemicon International, Inc, Temecula, CA). Adenovirus species 11 was isolated in culture. (×128)

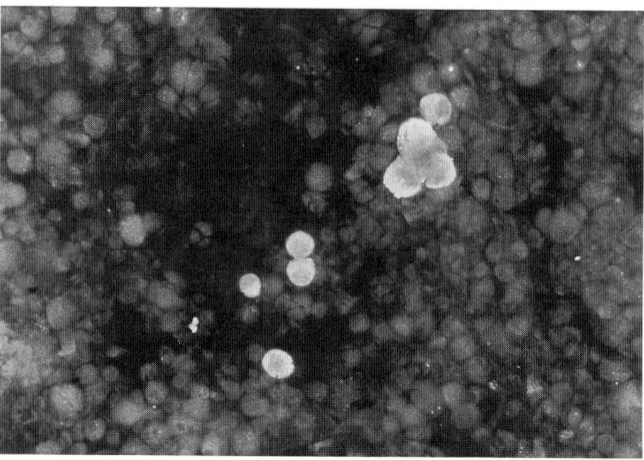

Figure 16-14. Bronchoalveolar lavage cytospin, cytomegalovirus (CMV), day 64. Late CMV antigen is demonstrated in 8 cells by indirect immunofluorescence with a monoclonal antibody primary (Genetic Systems, Seattle, WA; Syva Corp, Palo Alto, CA) (×128).

is now adequate for institution of anti-CMV therapy. Lung biopsy may still be necessary, however, when knowledge of the histological pattern is needed or if the interpretation of the lavage culture is uncertain (60).

Pulmonary Disease

The lung is susceptible to damage by varied mechanisms, including infection, chemical toxicity, irradiation damage, immune reaction, and malignant infiltration. Pathologists are appropriately reluctant to classify pneumonia in an immunocompromised patient as definitely noninfectious because microorganisms in any of the following categories may be present:

1. Previously uncharacterized (as were Legionella and human herpes virus 6).
2. Capable of causing pneumonia but usually requiring special detection techniques (*Mycoplasma*, *Chlamydia* spp).

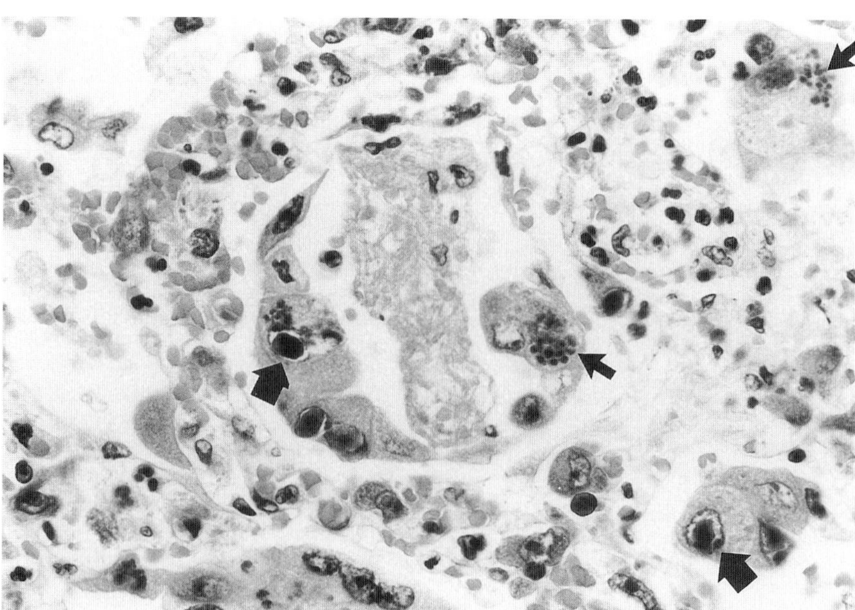

Figure 16-15. Lung, cytomegalovirus (CMV) pneumonia, day 68. Several large cells contain Cowdry type A nuclear inclusion bodies *(large arrows)*, as well as 6 to 12 smaller cytoplasmic inclusion bodies *(small arrows)* diagnostic for CMV infection. (H&E, ×128)

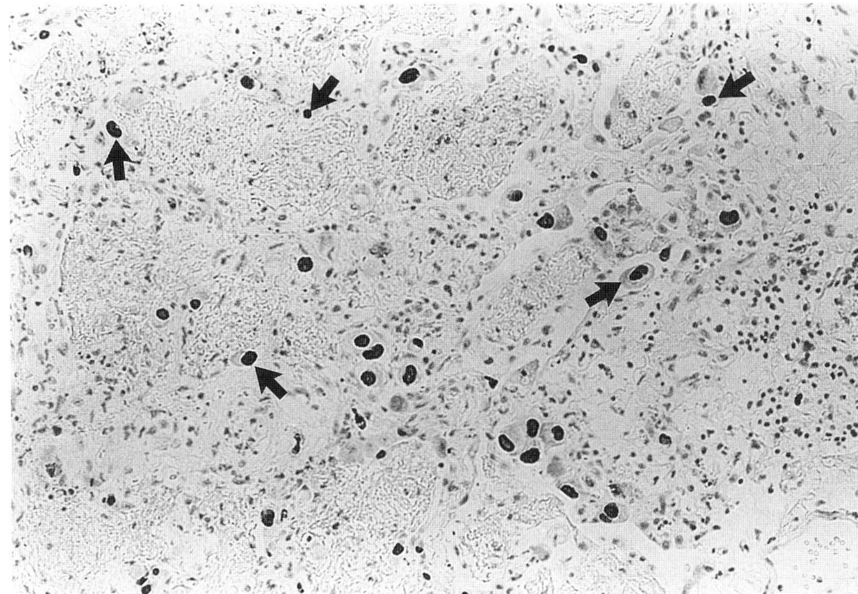

Figure 16-16. Lung, cytomegalovirus (CMV) pneumonia, day 54. Large numbers of infected cells display nuclear reactivity (some positive cells marked by *arrows*) for an early CMV antigen by monoclonal antibody indirect immunoperoxidase staining (Genetic Systems, Seattle, WA; Syva Corp, Palo Alto, CA). (×80)

3. Present in other organs but of uncertain significance as a pulmonary pathogen (*Cryptosporidia, Campylobacter* spp).
4. Visible by routine histology but subtle and not likely to be cultured (*Toxoplasma* spp).

In contrast, the mere presence of an infectious agent is not always sufficient evidence that it is the sole or even the major cause of pulmonary disease. Damage from chemotherapy, irradiation, or GVHD may also be present but manifest only by nonspecific inflammatory alterations.

Nonbacterial pneumonia, a clinical syndrome loosely referred to as "interstitial pneumonia," develops in approximately 35% of patients receiving allogeneic BMT for leukemia (58). This is a generally severe, acute process, in contrast to the insidious chronic course of disorders such as usual interstitial pneumonia (UIP) of Liebow.

Slightly fewer than half these pneumonias have been associated with CMV, 8% with other viruses (e.g., HSV, VZV, adenovirus, respiratory syncytial virus (61), and 4% with *Pneumocystis carinii. Pneumocystis* is now much less common; it usually develops in the absence of prophylactic therapy.

The remainder of interstitial pneumonias, approximately one third of the total, are idiopathic (IIP). These pneumonias probably have a multifactorial etiology, with toxicity from chemotherapy and irradiation high on the list (62).

The presence of GVHD does not increase the risk for idiopathic IP (48). IIP has not been ascribed to an allogeneic reaction in humans, although there is evidence in mice that nonbacterial pneumonia is a combined effect of GVHD and radiation (63). There is now preliminary data suggesting that reactivation of HHV-6 may have a significant role in the etiology of IIP (64).

The spectrum of severity of interstitial pneumonia varies from barely perceptible abnormalities to end-stage honeycomb lung. Although the pattern and severity are influenced by the timing of the biopsy, the degree of hypoxic damage, and the extent of toxicity secondary to oxygen therapy, these factors cannot be separated from one another morphologically. Some patients progress to diffuse consolidation in a few days, and fibrosis sufficient to produce an endstage honeycomb picture may develop in as little as 2 weeks. Thrombocytopenia may lead to intrapulmonary oozing and a variable degree of hemorrhage associated with iron-laden macrophages. Pulmonary hemorrhage is usually present in association with other characteristics of diffuse alveolar damage, such as hyaline membranes.

Pulmonary Veno-occlusive Disease

We identified 2 patients with symptomatic pulmonary hypertension documented by right heart catheterization. An open lung biopsy of one patient demonstrated pulmonary VOD (Figure 16-17). Both patients had acute lymphoblastic leukemia (ALL) and had been conditioned for BMT with high-dose bis-chloroethyl-nitrosourea (BCNU), etoposide (VP-16), and cyclophosphamide (CY) (65). This rare pulmonary disorder has been described after chemotherapy in several settings (66–68). Early identification of pulmonary VOD appears to be clinically important, because there was complete pulmonary resolution following treatment of our patients with high-dose methylprednisolone (65).

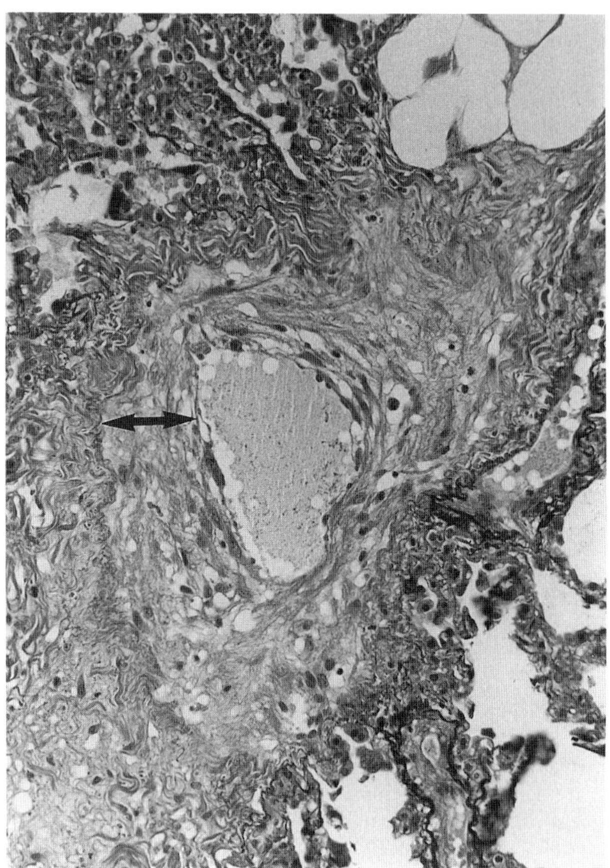

Figure 16-17. Lung, pulmonary veno-occlusive disease, day 48 after second allograft. An interlobular pulmonary vein is partially occluded by a zone of loose intimal fibrosis spanned by the double arrow. (Verhoff-Van Gieson, ×32) (Reproduced by Hackman RC, Madtes DK, Petersen FB, Clark JG. Pulmonary veno-occlusive disease following bone marrow transplantation. Transplantation 1989;47:989–992.)

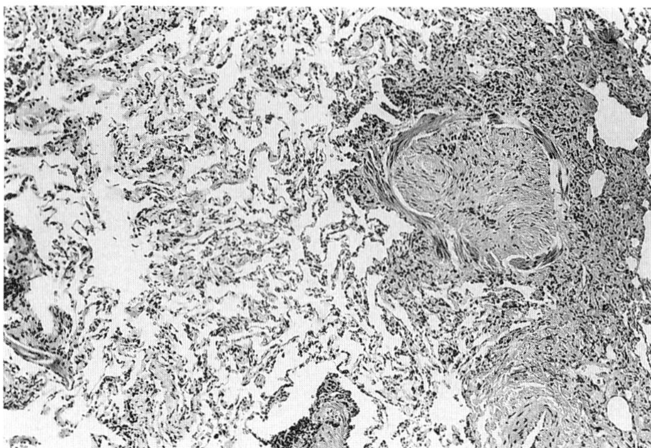

Figure 16-18. Lung, bronchiolitis obliterans, day 395. A bronchiole displays fibrous obliteration of the lumen associated with a mild peribronchial lymphocytic infiltrate. The patient had chronic GVHD and experienced severe pulmonary obstruction. (H&E, ×50)

Pulmonary Graft-versus-host Disease

Although the existence of an acute pulmonary GVH reaction is conceptually appealing, its histological appearance is unclear. Where open lung biopsies are used to study the pulmonary decompensation that sometimes coincides temporally with acute GVHD in skin, liver, and gut, the histological alterations are nonspecific and can usually be classified as diffuse alveolar damage or idiopathic IP. Occasionally, CMV pneumonia is present. It is possible that acute GVHD of the lung cannot be recognized in this setting because the repertoire of pulmonary responses is limited.

On the basis of a histological study of the large airways in a selected group of human autopsies, Beschorner (69) reported a strong correlation between "lymphocytic bronchitis" (i.e., mononuclear inflammatory infiltration of bronchial mucosa associated with necrosis of individual epithelial cells) and acute GVHD in other organs. Because most open lung biopsies do not sample bronchi with cartilage, and because studies of bronchial biopsies at several centers produced largely negative results, the entity has remained an autopsy diagnosis. Another conceptual problem is that this large airway inflammation was said to produce bronchopneumonia through impairment of the bronchociliary escalator, a pathogenetic mechanism not readily applicable to the vast majority of post-BMT pneumonias, which are interstitial. The major obstacle to acceptance of lymphocytic bronchitis as acute pulmonary GVHD for us and others has been its lack of association with GVHD in the classic target organs of skin, liver, and gut, either in humans or in the canine BMT model (70). An additional problem is that lymphocytic bronchitis is a nonspecific entity; it is present in untransplanted children dying with viral infections, in trauma victims, and in autologous BMT recipients.

In contrast to the difficulty in establishing lymphocytic bronchitis as an acute pulmonary GVH reaction is the increasing evidence that direct pulmonary GVH activity is a major contributor to bronchiolar inflammation culminating in bronchiolitis obliterans (Figure 16-18). Support of this hypothesis includes the fact that reports of more than 30 patients with chronic GVHD have been published (71), airflow obstruction is strongly associated with chronic GVHD (72), and symptoms may respond to immunosuppressive therapy. Furthermore, bronchiolitis obliterans is strongly associated with lung allograft rejection in both humans (73) and animals (74). Secondary infection may have a major role in chronic GVHD because patients have important deficiencies of immunoglobulin (75–77).

Summary

Marrow transplantation has ushered in a new group of complications, particularly GVHD, and has produced new combinations of previous complications of radiation, chemotherapy, immune deficiency, and transplantation immunopathology. Several problems remain to be solved by better immunosuppression based on newer understanding of the pathogenesis of alloimmune reactions, whereas others may be circumvented by molecular and genetic engineering.

References

1. Sale GE. Pathology of bone marrow and thymic transplantation. In: Sale GE, ed. The pathology of organ transplantation. Stoneham, London: Butterworth, 1990:229–259.
2. Sale GE, Buckner CD. Pathology of bone marrow in transplant recipients. Hematol Oncol Clin North Am 1988;2:735–756.
3. Zutter MM, Martin PJ, Sale GE, et al. Epstein-Barr virus lymphoproliferation after bone marrow transplantation. Blood 1988;72:520–529.
4. Bearman SI, Appelbaum FR, Buckner CD, et al. Regimen-related toxicity in patients undergoing bone marrow transplantation. J Clin Oncol 1988;6:1562–1568.
5. Epstein RJ, McDonald GB, Sale GE, Shulman HM, Thomas ED. The diagnostic accuracy of the rectal biopsy in acute graft-versus-host disease: a prospective study of thirteen patients. Gastroenterology 1980;78:764–771.
6. Shulman HM, McDonald GB, Matthews D, et al. An analysis of hepatic venocclusive disease and centrilobular hepatic degeneration following bone marrow transplantation. Gastroenterology 1980;79:1178–1191.
7. McDonald GB, Shulman HM, Wolford JL, Spencer GD. Liver disease after human marrow transplantation. Semin Liver Dis 1987;7:210–229.
8. McDonald GB. Liver disease after bone marrow transplantation. In: Hoofnagle JH, Goodman Z, eds. Liver biopsy interpretation for the 1990's. Clinicopathologic correlations in liver disease. Thorofare, NJ: American Association for the Study of Liver Disease, 1991:167–181.
9. Shulman HM, Gown AM, Nugent DJ. Hepatic venoocclusive disease after bone marrow transplantation. Immunohistochemical identification of the material within occluded central venules. Am J Pathol 1987; 127:549–558.
10. Jones RJ, Lee KSK, Beschorner WF, et al. Venoocclusive disease of the liver following bone marrow transplantation. Transplantation 1987;44:778–783.
11. Shulman HM, Hinds M, Schoch HG, McDonald GB. Liver toxicity after marrow transplantation: correlation between coded autopsy histology and clinical features. Lab Invest 1992;66:586 (99A).
12. Snover DC, Weisdorf S, Bloomer J, McGlave P, Weisdorf D. Nodular regenerative hyperplasia of the liver following bone marrow transplantation. Hepatology 1989; 9:443–448.
13. Wanless IR. Micronodular transformation (nodular regenerative hyperplasia) of the liver: a report of 64 cases among 2,500 autopsies and a new classification of benign hepatocellular nodules. Hepatology 1990; 11:787–797.
14. McDonald GB, Sharma P, Matthews DE, Shulman HM, Thomas ED. Venocclusive disease of the liver after bone marrow transplantation: diagnosis, incidence, and predisposing factors. Hepatology 1984;4:116–122.
15. Sharma P, McDonald GB, Banaji M. The risk of bleeding after percutaneous liver biopsy: relation to platelet count. J Clin Gastroenterol 1982;4:451–453.
16. Carreras E, Grañena A, Sierra J, et al. Transjugular liver study in bone marrow transplantation. Exp Hematol 1990;18:699.
17. Shulman HM, McDonald GB. Utility of transvenous liver biopsy and hepatic venous pressure measurements in Seattle marrow transplant recipients. Exp Hematol 1990;18:699.
18. Martin PJ. Increased disparity for minor histocompatibility antigens as a potential cause of increased GVHD risk in marrow transplantation from unrelated donors compared with related donors. Bone Marrow Transplant 1991;8:217–223.
19. Sale GE, Anderson P, Browne M, Myerson D. Evidence of cytotoxic T-cell destruction of epidermal cells in human graft-versus-host disease: immunohistology with monoclonal antibody TIA-1. Arch Pathol Lab Med 1992;116:622–625.
20. Piguet PF. Tumor necrosis factor and graft-versus-host disease. In: Burakoff S, Deeg HJ, eds. Graft-versus-host disease. New York and Basel: Marcel Dekker, 1990;255–276.
21. Sale GE, Lerner KG, Barker EA, Shulman HM, Thomas ED. The skin biopsy in the diagnosis of acute graft-versus-host disease in man. Am J Pathol 1977;89:621–635.
22. Lerner KG, Kao GF, Storb R, Buckner CD, Clift RA, Thomas ED. Histopathology of graft-versus-host reaction (GVHR) in human recipients of marrow from HLA matched sibling donors. Transplant Proc 1974;6:389–393.
23. Sale GE, Shulman HM, McDonald GB, Thomas ED. Gastrointestinal graft-versus-host disease in man. A clinicopathologic study of the rectal biopsy. Am J Surg Pathol 1979;3:291–299.
24. Fisk JD, Shulman HM, Greening RR, McDonald GB, Sale GE, Thomas ED. Gastro-intestinal radiographic features of human graft-versus-host disease. Am J Roentgenol 1981;136:329–336.
25. Snover DC, Weisdorf SA, Vercellotti GM, et al. A histopathologic study of gastric and small intestinal graft-versus-host disease following allogeneic bone marrow transplantation. Hum Pathol 1985;16:387–392.
26. Spencer GD, Hackman RC, McDonald GB, Amos DE, Cunningham BA, Meyers JD, Thomas ED. A prospective study of unexplained nausea and vomiting after marrow transplantation. Transplantation 1986;42: 602–607.
27. Nakhleh RE, Miller W, Snover DC. Significance of mucosal versus salivary gland changes in lip biopsies in the diagnosis of chronic graft-versus-host disease. Arch Pathol Lab Med 1989;113:932–934.
28. Spencer GD, Shulman HM, Myerson D, Thomas ED, McDonald GB. Diffuse intestinal ulceration after marrow transplantation: a clinicopathological study of 13 patients. Hum Pathol 1986;17:621–633.
29. McDonald GB, Shulman HM, Sullivan KM, Spencer GD. Intestinal and hepatic complications of human bone marrow transplantation. Gastroenterology 1986; 90:460–467, 770–784.
30. Beschorner WE. Destruction of the intestinal mucosa

after bone marrow transplantation and graft-versus-host disease. Surv Synth Pathol Res 1984;3:264–274.
31. Gallucci BB, Sale GE, McDonald GB, Epstein R, Shulman HM, Thomas ED. The fine structure of human rectal epithelium in acute graft-versus-host disease. Am J Surg Pathol 1982;6:293–305.
32. Beschorner WE, Yardley JH, Tutschka P, et al. Deficiency of intestinal immunity with graft-versus-host disease in humans. J Infect Dis 1981;144:38–46.
33. Peters M, Vierling J, Gershwin ME, et al. Immunology and the liver. Hepatology 1991;13:977–993.
34. Fausto N, Mead JE. Biology of disease. Regulation of liver growth: protooncogenes and transforming growth factors. Lab Invest 1989;60:4–13.
35. Fox ES, Broitman SA, Thomas P. Biology of disease. Bacterial endotoxins and the liver. Lab Invest 1990; 63:733–741.
36. Tracey KJ, Wei H, Manogue KR, et al. Cachectin/tumor necrosis factor induces cachexia, anemia and inflammation. J Exp Med 1988;167:1211–1227.
37. Sale GE, Storb R, Kolb H. Histopathology of hepatic acute graft-versus-host disease in the dog. A double blind study confirms the specificity of small bile duct lesions. Transplantation 1978;26:103–106.
38. Shulman HM, Sharma P, Amos D, Fenster LF, McDonald GB. A coded histologic study of hepatic graft-versus-host disease after human bone marrow transplantation. Hepatology 1988;8:463–470.
39. Snover DC, Weisdorf SA, Ramsay NK, McGlave P, Kersey JH. Hepatic graft-versus-host disease: a study of the predictive value of liver biopsy in diagnosis. Hepatology 1984;4:123–130.
40. Reed EC, Myerson D, Corey L, Meyers JD. Allogeneic marrow transplantation in patients positive for hepatitis B surface antigen. Blood 1991;77:195–200.
41. Locasciulli A, Bacigalupo A, Van Lint MT, et al. Hepatitis B virus (HBV) infection and liver disease after allogeneic bone marrow transplantation: a report of 30 cases. Bone Marrow Transplant 1990;6:25–29.
42. Locasciulli A, Bacigalupo A, Van Lint MT, et al. Hepatitis C virus infection in patients undergoing allogeneic bone marrow transplantation. Transplantation 1991;52:315–318.
43. Ljungman P, Duraj V, Magnius L, et al. Hepatitis C infection in allogeneic bone marrow transplant recipients. Clin Transplant 1991;5:283–286.
44. Bach N, Thung SN, Schaffner F. The histological features of chronic hepatitis C and autoimmune chronic hepatitis: a comparative analysis. Hepatology 1991;15:572–577.
45. Danque POV, Bach N, Shaffner F, Gerber MA, Thung SN. Bile duct injury in chronic hepatitis C. Lab Invest 1992;66:96a.
46. Miglio F, Mazzeo V, Baraldini M, et al. Graft versus host of the liver: clinical, morphological and immunological aspects. In: Buckner CD, Gale RP, Lucarelli G, eds. Advances and controversies in thalassemia therapy: bone marrow transplantation and other approaches. New York: Alan R. Liss, 1989:239–247.
47. Atkinson K, Munro V, Vasak E, Biggs J. Mononuclear cell subpopulation in the skin defined by monoclonal antibodies after HLA-identical sibling marrow transplantation. Br J Dermatol 1986;114:145–160.
48. Sviland L, Pearson ADJ, Green MA, et al. Immunopathology of early graft-versus-host disease—a prospective study of skin, rectum, and peripheral blood in allogeneic and autologous bone marrow transplant recipients. Transplantation 1991;52:1029–1036.
49. Synovec MS, Braddock SW, Jones J, Linder J. LN-3: a diagnostic adjunct in cutaneous graft-versus-host disease. Mod Pathol 1990;3:643–647.
50. Beschorner WE, Farmer ER, Saral R, Stirling WL, Santos GW. Epithelial class II antigen expression in cutaneous graft-versus-host disease. Transplantation 1987;44:237.
51. Loughran TP, Sullivan KM, Morton T, et al. Value of day 100 screening studies for predicting the development of chronic graft-versus-host disease after allogeneic bone marrow transplantation. Blood 1990;76:228–234.
52. Sviland L, Pearson ADJ, Eastham EJ, et al. Class II antigen by keratinocytes and enterocytes—an early feature of graft-versus-host disease. Transplantation 1988;46:402.
53. Shulman HM. Pathology of chronic graft-vs.-host disease. In: Burakoff SJ, Deeg HJ, Ferrara J, Atkinson K, eds. Graft-vs.-host disease: immunology, pathophysiology, and treatment. New York: Marcel Dekker, 1990:587–614.
54. Wingard JR, Piantadosi S, Vogelsang GB, et al. Predictors of death from chronic graft-versus-host disease after bone marrow transplantation. Blood 1989;74:1428–1435.
55. Volc-Platzer B, Valent P, Radaszkiewicz T, Mayer P, Bettelheim P, Wolff K. Recombinant human interleukin 3 induces proliferation of inflammatory cells and keratinocytes in vivo. Lab Invest 1991;64:557–566.
56. Sale GE, Shulman HM, Schubert MM, et al. Oral and ophthalmic pathology of graft-versus-host disease in man: predictive value of the lip biopsy. Hum Pathol 1981;12:1022-1030.
57. Sale GE. Pathology and recent pathogenetic studies in human graft-versus-host disease. Surv Synth Pathol Res 1984;3:235–253.
58. Meyers JD, Flournoy N, Thomas ED. Nonbacterial pneumonia after allogeneic marrow transplantation: a review of ten years' experience. Rev Infect Dis 1982;4:1119–1132.
59. Shields AF, Hackman RC, Fife KH, Corey L, Meyers JD. Adenovirus infections in patients undergoing bone marrow transplantation. N Engl J Med 1985;312:529–533.
60. Ruutu P, Ruutu T, Volin L, et al. Cytomegalovirus is frequently isolated in bronchoalveolar lavage fluid of bone marrow transplant recipients without pneumonia. Ann Intern Med 1990;112:913–916.
61. Harrington RD, Hooton TM, Hackman RC, et al. An outbreak of respiratory syncytial virus in a bone marrow transplant center. J Infect Dis 1992;165:987–993.
62. Appelbaum FR, Meyers JD, Fefer A, et al. Nonbacterial nonfungal pneumonia following marrow transplantation in 100 identical twins. Transplantation 1982; 33:265–268.
63. Lehnert S, Rybka WB, Seemayer TA. Amplification of the graft-versus-host reaction by partial body irradiation. Transplantation 1986;41:675–679.
64. Cone RE, Hackman RC, Huang M-L, et al. Human herpesvirus 6 in lung tissue from bone marrow transplant patients with pneumonia. N Engl J Med 1993 (in press).
65. Hackman RC, Madtes DK, Petersen FB, Clark JG. Pulmonary veno-occlusive disease following bone marrow transplantation. Transplantation 1989;47:989–992.
66. Lombard CM, Churg A, Winokur S. Pulmonary veno-occlusive disease following therapy for malignant neoplasms. Chest 1987;92:871.
67. Troussard X, Bernaudin JF, Cordonnier C, et al. Pulmonary veno-occlusive disease after bone marrow transplantation. Thorax 1984;39:956–957.

68. Wingard JR, Mellits ED, Jones RJ, et al. Association of hepatic veno-occlusive disease with interstitial pneumonitis in bone marrow transplant recipients. Bone Marrow Transplant 1989;4:129–130.
69. Beschorner WE, Saral R, Hutchins GM, Tutschka PJ, Santos GW. Lymphocytic bronchitis associated with graft-versus-host disease in recipients of bone marrow transplants. N Engl J Med 1978;299:1030–1036.
70. O'Brien KD, Hackman RC, Sale GE, Prentice R, Deeg J, Thomas ED, Storb R. Lymphocytic bronchitis unrelated to acute graft-versus-host disease in canine marrow graft recipients. Transplantation 1984;37:233–238.
71. Urbanski SJ, Kossakowska AE, Curtis J, et al. Idiopathic small airways pathology in patients with graft-versus-host disease following allogeneic bone marrow transplantation. Am J Surg Pathol 1987;11:965–971.
72. Clark JG, Crawford SW. Diagnostic approaches to pulmonary complications of marrow transplantation. Chest 1987;91:477–479.
73. Yousem SA, Burke CM, Billingham ME. Pathologic pulmonary alterations in long-term human heart-lung transplantation. Hum Pathol 1985;16:911–923.
74. Tazelaar HD, Prop J, Nieuwenhuis P, et al. Airway pathology in the transplanted rat lung. Transplantation 1988;45:864–869.
75. Sullivan KM. Intravenous immune globulin prophylaxis in recipients of a marrow transplant. J Allergy Clin Immunol 1989;84:632–639.
76. Sheridan JF, Tutschka PJ, Sedmak DD, Copelan EA. Immunoglobulin G subclass deficiency and pneumococcal infection after allogeneic bone marrow transplantation. Blood 1990;75:1583–1586.
77. Hackman RC. Lower respiratory tract. In: Sale GE, Shulman HM, eds. The pathology of bone marrow transplantation, vol 9. New York: Masson, 1984:156–170.

Chapter 17
Mechanisms of Tolerance

Megan Sykes, David H. Sachs, and Samuel Strober

Unlike solid organ transplant recipients, allogeneic bone marrow transplant (BMT) recipients do not receive chronic immunosuppressive therapy; instead, after completing a course of graft-versus-host disease (GVHD) prophylaxis for a limited period after BMT, persistent graft survival and the absence of GVHD depend on a state of mutual tolerance of the donor to the host (graft-vs-host, or GVH tolerance) and of the host to the donor (host-vs-graft, or HVG tolerance). Unfortunately, this state is not always achieved, and failure of engraftment or GVHD ensues. Development of tolerance in the HVG direction requires host conditioning to eliminate mature host immune cells, so that a "clean slate" is encountered by the transplanted donor marrow. Newly developing T and B lymphocytes learn to recognize the donor and host as "self," and a state of donor- and host-specific tolerance results. Numerous experimental methods of inducing lymphohematopoietic chimerism to produce a state of specific transplantation tolerance have been developed since the original studies of Owen (1), extending our knowledge of the mechanisms by which tolerance can be induced to alloantigens, and, by inference, to self antigens in normal animals. A state of donor-specific tolerance is central to successful BMT for any application, because tolerance is required for permanent marrow graft survival. In addition, the ability of BMT to induce a state of donor-specific tolerance suggests an additional potential application: induction of organ allograft acceptance without the need for chronic immunosuppressive therapy. Reliable, nontoxic methods of achieving allogeneic BMT across major histocompatibility complex (MHC) barriers will be required before this application becomes clinically feasible.

This chapter first provides a general discussion of the mechanisms of tolerance and then discusses these mechanisms in the context of specific models associated with induction of HVG tolerance. The mechanisms by which both mature T-cells preexisting in allogeneic marrow inocula and T cells developing de novo from donor marrow can be made tolerant to host antigens are reviewed.

Mechanisms of T-cell Tolerance

Three major mechanisms have been proposed to explain induction or maintenance of T-cell tolerance to self or alloantigens: clonal deletion, clonal anergy, and active suppression.

Clonal Deletion

Clonal deletion refers to the elimination of those clones of cells that can recognize a specific antigen by virtue of antigen receptor molecules on their cell surface. In this instance, a clone refers to those cells in vivo that share an identical receptor molecule. Evidence for clonal deletion as a mechanism of tolerance has been obtained using monoclonal antibodies (MABs), which are specific for certain V-gene products contributing to the β chain of the $\alpha\beta$ T-cell receptor ($\alpha\beta$TCR) (2). $\alpha\beta$TCR are the T cell surface heterodimers that recognize complexes of MHC antigens plus peptide. Certain Vβ gene products are sufficient to recognize particular antigens, termed *superantigens* (3), regardless of the composition of the remainder of the $\alpha\beta$TCR heterodimer. T cells bearing TCR that include these Vβ regions are deleted from mice which express those superantigens (e.g., I-E plus an unknown peptide; minor lymphocyte stimulatory locus [Mls] antigens) (2,4,5). Therefore, expression of these Vβ regions is a marker for the presence of T-cell clones that recognize superantigens. However, recognition of antigen/MHC complexes by most TCR is dependent on components of the TCR in addition to Vβ. The association of particular Vβ with antigen recognition has not been described for alloantigens known to function as transplantation antigens. Mls antigens have not been shown to behave as transplantation antigens (6), and I-E antigens alone are incapable of inducing skin graft rejection (7). Thus, conclusions drawn from such data on the mechanism of tolerance to transplantation antigens are somewhat inferential. However, data supporting clonal deletion as a major mechanism for induction of self-tolerance have also been obtained from studies of mice expressing a transgenic TCR specific for a "self" class I MHC-restricted peptide (H-Y plus D^b) or for a class I MHC antigen (L^d). These animals show marked depletion of $CD8^+$ T cells bearing the self-reactive TCR, consistent with the existence of similar mechanisms for the deletion during normal development of T cells recognizing self determinants that can act as conventional transplantation antigens (8,9).

In the mouse, the thymus has a critical role in the development of tolerance by a clonal deletion mechanism. Antigens expressed on marrow-derived cells that populate the thymus are extremely effective at eliminating T-cell clones with strong reactivity toward them (10). It is perhaps for this reason that BMT and the induction of chimerism is such an effective way of producing a state of systemic T-cell tolerance to alloantigen. Although it is generally thought that antigen expressed on marrow-derived dendritic cells is most important at inducing clonal deletion in the thymus (11,12), thymic B cells have also been reported to induce clonal deletion (13), and T-cell progenitors may induce tolerance among class I–specific T cells (14).

T-cell Anergy

Anergy is the phenomenon whereby engagement of TCR is associated with unresponsiveness instead of activation of T cells. Studies on mechanisms of tolerance often include functional data, such as limiting dilution analyses to quantify cytotoxic T lymphocytes, helper T cells, or T cells proliferating in response to antigen. The failure to detect T cells with a particular specificity using this approach, however, does not distinguish between clonal deletion and anergy. In vitro evidence suggests that antigen can render T cells unresponsive if the appropriate costimulatory signals are not provided by antigen-presenting cells (APC) (15). Although these costimulatory signals have not been defined fully, the B7/CD28 pathway may have an important role (16,17). T-cell anergy has been demonstrated in vivo in several murine models, including some that involve BMT. The ability of nonmarrow-derived cells to induce T-cell anergy is important to the development of tolerance to the host among developing donor T cells in fully allogeneic marrow chimeras. In these chimeras, all marrow-derived cells are of donor origin, so clonal deletion of T cells recognizing host-specific antigens is incomplete (18,19). T cells bearing these host-reactive TCR can be anergized by thymic epithelial cells (20) or by extrathymic antigen (21–23). Studies have shown clearly that T-cell clones with specificity for particular alloantigens can exist without causing destruction of tissue bearing those antigens (10,18,20,21,23,24). In some instances, T cells with receptors specific for the in vivo tolerated antigen can be stimulated to respond to the antigen in vitro (20,21,25), whereas in others, the T cells cannot be triggered through their TCR (18,21,24).

Apparently, several different mechanisms can account for the failure of T cells with self-reactive or donor-reactive TCR to cause rejection in vivo. However, the term *anergy* should be reserved for situations in which T cells can be shown not to respond when triggered through their TCR. Overall, results of these studies suggest that antigen expressed extrathymically or intrathymically on nonhematopoietic tissue induces T-cell unresponsiveness primarily by nondeletional mechanisms. In addition, resting peripheral B cells also have the capacity to induce T-cell anergy when they present antigen (26).

Suppression

A third mechanism, active suppression of T-cell responses by suppressor cells, has also been implicated in the maintenance of self- or allotolerance. Suppressive activity has been attributed to both T cells and non-T cells, and may be antigen-specific or nonspecific. In general, the models in which suppressor T-cells have been implicated involve exposure to antigen in the presence of a pre-existing immune response to the antigen. When, in contrast, antigen encounters a "clean slate" (i.e., all mature lymphocytes are eliminated prior to administration of the antigen), tolerance may be due mainly to clonal deletion or anergy mechanisms and not to active suppression.

Specific Suppression

Although functional evidence for the existence of specific suppressor cells has been obtained in several transplantation models (27–33), it has been difficult to clone these cells or to identify suppressor cell-specific surface markers. Mechanisms of specific suppression of alloreactivity have generally not been well defined. In many instances, anti-idiotypic recognition has been implicated (27,30,33). Class I MHC-restricted human T cells with specificity for the idiotype of alloreactive $CD4^+$ T cells have been cloned, and these T-suppressor cells were shown to express CD3, CD8, CD2, and CD11b surface markers, but did not express CD28 or CD16. Blocking studies suggested that the TCR, CD8, and CD2 molecules are involved in signalling to these suppressor cells. These suppressor cells are noncytotoxic (34). Although mechanisms of anti-idiotypic recognition and the mechanism of suppressive effector function have not been characterized fully in this system, results in another (rat) model suggest that cytolytic T lymphocytes (CTL) with specificity for TCR determinants on responding T cells can down-regulate the immune response (33). Some "suppressive" phenomena could be explained by competition from anergic T cells (25). If most T cells specific for a particular antigen are unable to mediate helper or effector function because they are anergic, these cells could appear to suppress a cocultured naive cell population simply by binding to antigen and therefore blocking recognition by the naive T cells. Several in vitro phenomena usually attributed to suppressor cells could be explained in this way. It has been hypothesized that anergic cells, by blocking helper T cells, could prevent the release of lymphokines needed to costimulate naive responding T cells, resulting in anergy of these naive T cells (25). Alternatively, recognition of antigen on antigen-presenting cells (APC) by anergic T cells could block APC activation and production of signals needed to costimulate naive T cells, also resulting in anergy of the naive T cells.

Evidence that suppressor cells may be involved in maintaining self-tolerance has recently been obtained from rodent models involving lethal total body irradiation (TBI), reconstitution with T-cell–depleted syngeneic marrow, and treatment with cyclosporine (CSP) during the post-BMT period of T-cell recovery. An autoimmune syndrome resembling GVHD develops in these animals when CSP is withdrawn (33,35). Both $CD4^+$ T cells (36) and $CD8^+$ cells with reactivity to common determinants on class II MHC molecules (37,38) have been implicated in this syndrome. A mixture of $CD4^+$ and $CD8^+$ cells from normal animals can protect against syngeneic GVHD (39), suggesting that suppressor cells normally exist to protect against autoimmunity and that such suppressive cells fail to develop in the presence of CSP. These phenomena may be due to CSP-induced abnormalities of the thymic environment (36,40).

Veto Cells

Another cell-mediated function down-regulating alloresponses is "veto" activity. Veto cells inactivate T cells recognizing antigens expressed on the veto cell surface (41), resulting in a pattern of apparent suppression that affects only T cells responding to those antigens. Several types of cells have been reported to have veto activity, including Thy1-negative cells in fresh marrow (42), Thy1-positive cell colonies derived from Thy1-negative marrow cells (42), CTL (43,44), and bone marrow cells with characteristics of natural killer (NK) or lymphokine-activated killer (LAK) cells (45). Veto cells have been implicated in the induction of GVH tolerance (46) and in facilitating marrow engraftment (46,47) in murine BMT models. Murine studies also suggest that veto cells might be responsible for the donor-specific transfusion effect (48,49), wherein prior administration of donor-specific transfusions induces subsequent hyporesponsiveness to that donor. Recent data have suggested at least one mechanism for the veto effect: Triggering of a CTL through a surface class I MHC molecule, while it is also triggered through its TCR, results in programmed cell death (apoptosis) of the responding CTL (50). This class I–mediated signal could result from binding of a T cell's class I molecules to CD8 molecules on the veto cell (51). A similar mechanism may also down-regulate human T-cell responses (51,52).

Natural Suppressor Cells

Another type of suppressive activity is mediated by natural suppressor (NS) cells, which suppress in an antigen-nonspecific, non-MHC–restricted manner (53–58). These cells have been detected in sites of active hematopoiesis (54,55,59–64) and in the setting of GVHD (65). NS cells have been detected in normal marrow of several species (59,62–64,66), including humans (67). These suppressive cells are found in the low density cell population and copurify with hematopoietic progenitors (64), but do not express the Sca-1 pluripotent hematopoietic stem-cell marker in mice (63). They have been reported to suppress mitogen responses (64,65), antibody responses (60,67), and T-cell responses (54,56,58,61–63,68). NS cells have a "null" surface phenotype (i.e., do not express surface markers of T cells, B cells, or macrophages) (54, 58,62,63). Although they resemble NK cells morphologically, NS cells can be distinguished by their lack of NK cell surface markers (54,55) and their lack of cytotoxic activity (53,55,58). A subset of T cells that has suppressive activity similar to NS cells has a markedly different phenotype. These cells express the Thy1 T-cell marker, NK cell surface markers, and $\alpha\beta$TCR, but do not express CD4 or CD8 (53,69–71). Interleukin-2 (IL-2) appears to be critical for the propagation of these cells in vitro (53,69,70).

Soluble factors with widely varying physical characteristics have been reported to mediate NS activity (59,72–76). The apparently different characteristics of cells with NS activity could indicate that there are several distinct cell types with NS activity, or alternatively, that NS cells vary their characteristics under different conditions, as their state of differentiation changes. NS activity has been reported to be gamma interferon–dependent (77), as well as IL-2–responsive (78). Some studies have shown that NS cells inhibit IL-2 secretion (75,79) and that suppression can be overcome by IL-2 (75). Other studies show that the capacity of IL-2 to overcome suppression is extremely limited (79,80). These variable results could indicate that NS cells respond to IL-2, but that their mechanism of action includes inhibition of helper T-cell activity, resulting in decreased IL-2 production. The opposing effects of exogenous IL-2 on NS cells and other lymphocytes that respond to IL-2 could account for the variable effects observed after addition of exogenous IL-2 (80). The role that NS cells might have in inducing tolerance in BMT recipients is discussed below.

Mechanisms of HVG Tolerance in BMT Models

Resistance to Alloengraftment

Two major factors influence the engraftment of allogeneic marrow. The first is often referred to as "space" in the lymphohematopoietic system. Although this concept is poorly understood, optimal engraftment of even syngeneic marrow transplants cannot be achieved without first eliminating some hematopoietic elements in the recipient (81,82). Destruction of recipient hematopoietic cells might create physical space in the marrow microenvironment or, more likely, could induce the production of cytokines, which up-regulate hematopoiesis.

The second factor limiting alloengraftment is the host immune system. Because of this immune resistance, allogeneic BMT can be performed successfully only in immunoincompetent recipients. T cells resist engraftment of allogeneic marrow cells in animals and humans (82–87). NK cells recognizing hematopoietic histocompatibility determinants (88), which might also be triggered by the absence of self-MHC molecules on allogeneic marrow cells (89,90), also resist allogeneic marrow engraftment in mice (88,91, 92). A definite role for NK cells in resisting alloengraftment has not been established for large animals or humans. Humoral mechanisms also mediate alloresistance. Antibodies that inhibit engraftment can occur naturally (so called natural antibodies, such as those directed against ABO blood group determinants) (93–95) or can develop as a result of presensitization, usually from blood products. Animal studies suggest that the effect of natural antibodies on marrow engraftment can be overcome by administration of large numbers of marrow cells (96). In humans, natural antibodies against ABO determinants do not present a major barrier to BMT. However, the presence of antibodies resulting from prior sensitization to determinants shared by the donor is associated with a high incidence of graft failure (97).

A permissive environment for engraftment of allogeneic marrow can exist under several physiological and artificially induced conditions. The mechanisms by which BMT induces tolerance in each of these models is discussed.

Hematopoietic Stem-cell Transfer to Developmentally or Congenitally Immunodeficient Recipients

Billingham and colleagues (98) first induced donor-specific tolerance by inoculating fetal mice with allogeneic lymphohematopoietic cells. These results demonstrated that early exposure to alloantigens could induce the immune system to regard that specific set of alloantigens as self, rather than as nonself. Mice remain susceptible to tolerance induction by the administration of allogeneic cells during the first few days of life, before T-cell immunity has fully matured. Low percentages of donor cells (a state of "microchimerism") have been detected among lymphoid populations and thymic dendritic cells of such animals when they become tolerant adults (27, 99,100).

The ability to achieve allogeneic marrow engraftment in congenitally or developmentally immunoincompetent recipients has been exploited clinically. BMT is widely used for the treatment of severe combined immunodeficiency disease, and fetal liver cell transplantation has been used recently with encouraging results for the in utero treatment of congenital immunodeficiencies (101).

In animals rendered tolerant in the neonatal period, several mechanisms have been invoked to explain the observed HVG tolerance. Specific suppressor T cells (27,102–104), which may be anti-idiotypic in specificity (27,102,103), have been detected. One prerequisite for the development of anti-idiotypic reactivity is that idiotype be present. This condition may prevail in animals rendered tolerant in the neonatal period, because some mature T cells are already present in the periphery at the time of birth. The results of studies implicating T-suppressor cells do not, however, rule out the alternative possibility that anergic T cells suppress the naive alloresponse by a "blocking" mechanism, as discussed.

Evidence for clonal deletion of donor-reactive T cells in neonatally tolerized mice was obtained in functional assays (105,106) and at the structural level using Vβ-specific MABs (107). Clonal deletion may result from the presence of marrow-derived cells of donor origin in the thymuses of such mice.

In neonatal tolerization models, lymphohematopoietic chimerism is essential for the maintenance of tolerance (27,99,100,108). The available data on mechanisms of neonatal tolerance seem consistent with the following synthesis: (1) engrafted donor-type hematopoietic progenitors provide a continuous source of donor cells in the thymus, which cause clonal deletion of newly developing donor-reactive T-cell precursors; and (2) donor-reactive T-cell precursors already existing in small numbers in the peripheral lymphoid organs of neonatal animals at the time of BMT provide a source of idiotype that stimulates the expansion of T cells with anti-idiotypic TCR, or themselves become anergized, resulting in blocking that mimics idiotype-specific suppression. This approach to the induction of tolerance may not succeed in untreated adult animals because of the larger number of donor-reactive T cells present in adults. Similar mechanisms may apply, however, in adults in whom the existing T-cell compartment is partially reduced by use of sublethal irradiation, cyclophosphamide (CY), or MABs.

BMT in Adult Recipients Following Myeloablative Conditioning

Marrow chimerism and tolerance can be achieved in otherwise normal, adult animals if immunodeficiency and "space" are artificially created by lethal TBI. Hematopoietic rescue is achieved with allogeneic marrow cells. In murine recipients of T-cell–depleted allogeneic marrow transplants, lymphoid repopulation is largely (95–99%) allogeneic; a small population of host-type cells survives permanently in such animals (109). If T-cell–depleted allogeneic and T-cell–depleted syngeneic marrow are coadministered, mixed allogeneic chimerism ensues (i.e., lymphohematopoietic cells of both donor and recipient type coexist permanently in the survivors) (109–111). These mixed chimeras show no evidence for GVHD and show specific tolerance, both in vivo and in vitro, to donor antigens (110,111).

Animals reconstituted with T-cell–depleted allogeneic marrow alone demonstrate a similar pattern of specific unresponsiveness to donor and host observed in mixed allogeneic chimeras, but tend to show poorer immunocompetence both in vivo (111–113) and in vitro (114). Immunoincompetence is probably due to a mismatch between the class II MHC restriction imposed by the host thymus and the MHC of donor-type APC (114). MHC antigens of the host thymus determine the restriction specificity of class II–restricted T cells in murine (115) and human (116–118) chimeras (Table 17-1). In fully MHC-mismatched allogeneic chimeras, peripheral APC are eventually replaced by cells from the donor marrow, which cannot provide the restriction elements necessary for recognition of antigen by T cells educated in the host thymus. This problem is avoided in mixed allogeneic chimeras, in which a continuous source of host-type APC is provided by the syngeneic component of the mixed marrow inoculum (see Table 17-1) (114). Indeed, in vitro (114) and in vivo studies (111,119) have demonstrated improved antigen responsiveness in such animals compared with conventional allogeneic chimeras prepared across full MHC barriers (112,113). For this reason, production of mixed chimeras rather than fully allogeneic chimeras may be desirable if marrow transplantation is to be utilized as a means of inducing tolerance across full MHC barriers.

Another potential advantage of mixed chimerism over allogeneic chimerism is that marrow-derived cells are most efficient at inducing clonal deletion of T cells in the thymus (10); thus, a continuous source of host-type lymphohematopoietic cells provides additional assurance that host-reactive T-cell clones will not emerge from the thymus, as can occur in animals reconstituted with T-cell–depleted allogeneic marrow alone (18) (see Table 17-1).

Clonal deletion may be the predominant mechanism of HVG tolerance in lethal TBI-treated recipients of T-cell–depleted allogeneic marrow transplants. Using Vβ-specific MABs, evidence for clonal deletion has been obtained by several groups (10,18). In vivo evidence suggests that suppressor cells are not involved in the maintenance of tolerance to donor antigens, regardless of whether T-cell–depleted allogeneic marrow is given alone or with T-cell–depleted syngeneic marrow. Tolerance can be broken readily in such chimeras by administering a relatively small number of nontolerant recipient-type spleen cells (120), providing no evidence for potent suppressive activity. Results of in vitro coculture studies support this conclusion (121). One important difference between TBI/BMT recipients and animals rendered tolerant at birth is that TBI leads to elimination of most pre-existing T cells. Thus, the number of alloreactive idiotype-bearing T cells may be too small to provide an adequate stimulus for the expansion of suppressor T cells.

In contrast to chimeras reconstituted with T-cell–depleted allogeneic marrow, animals receiving non-T-cell–depleted allogeneic marrow cells were highly resistant to the breaking of tolerance by administration of nontolerant host-type lymphocytes (120). This resistance was not due to a suppressive mechanism, but instead was due to GVH reactivity of T cells in the original marrow inoculum. Although they did not cause clinically apparent GVHD, this small number of

Table 17-1.
Comparison of the Immunological Status of Murine Mixed Chimeras Versus Fully Allogeneic Chimeras

Animal	*MHC Restriction*[a]	*Marrow-derived APC*[b]	*Immuno-competence?*[c]	*Deletion of TCR*[d]
B	B	B	+	Anti-B
A→B[e]	B	A	−	Anti-A
A+B→B[f]	B	A+B	+	Anti-A, Anti-B

[a] The MHC type able to present peptide antigen to T-lymphocytes. This restriction pattern is generally determined by the MHC of epithelial cells in the thymus, and peptide antigen is therefore usually recognized in association with host MHC antigens, regardless of the MHC phenotype of marrow-derived cells.
[b] Because thymic dendritic cells and peripheral tissue APC are marrow-derived, the APC in both sites share the same MHC type as the marrow that repopulates the animal.
[c] This column only applies to fully MHC-mismatched BMT, in which MHC antigens are not shared by the allogeneic marrow donor "A" and the host "B." Full immunocompetence is achieved only when the host-type MHC antigens that serve as restricting elements are also expressed on APC in the peripheral tissues, because these APC must present antigen for induction of T-cell responses. This is the situation in mixed chimeras shown in line 3, because some of the marrow-derived APC in the periphery are of host type B. In contrast, fully allogeneic chimeras shown in line 2 suffer a disparity between the MHC type of their peripheral APC (bearing "A" MHC antigens) and their requirements (host MHC "B") for antigen recognition by T cells.
[d] T cells with TCR specific for the indicated antigens are deleted in the thymus due to negative selection by marrow-derived APC that populate the thymus. Therefore, clonal deletion occurs for T cells recognizing antigens expressed on marrow-derived cells. As discussed in the text, host thymic epithelial cells also have some capacity to delete T cells recognizing antigens on the epithelial cells, but this deletion is incomplete.
[e] This line describes the immune reactivity in fully allogeneic chimeras (donor of strain "A" and recipient of strain "B"), in which all lymphohematopoietic cells are of donor type.
[f] This line describes the immune reactivity in mixed allogeneic chimeras, in which lymphohematopoietic cells are of both allogeneic donor ("A") and host ("B") type. Mixed chimerism can be induced in mice using several different protocols, as described in the text.
MHC = major histocompatibility complex; APC = antigen-presenting cells; TCR = T-cell receptor; BMT = bone marrow transplantation.

GVH-reactive T cells probably persisted long term and eliminated the nontolerant host-type lymphocytes that were administered later, thus preventing these host-type T cells from breaking tolerance (120). Therefore, GVH-reactive donor T cells can overcome the alloresistance mediated by nontolerant host T cells without causing GVHD.

Studies in animal models have addressed the possibility that, following lethal irradiation and reconstitution with exhaustively T-cell–depleted autologous marrow cells, tolerance might be induced by expression of antigen on nonhematopoietic organs grafted simultaneously with the T-cell–depleted autologous marrow. This approach met with some limited success (122) but was insufficient to induce tolerance to MHC-mismatched skin allografts in rodents (123) or to MHC-mismatched vascularized grafts in large animal studies (124). Similarly, in vivo treatment with MABs that deplete host T cells does not permit induction of skin allograft tolerance across MHC barriers in mice (83). Thus, alloantigen seems to be required within the lymphohematopoietic system for the most complete induction of tolerance among newly developing T cells, probably reflecting the unique ability of alloantigen expressed on marrow-derived cells to induce clonal deletion in the thymus. Murine radiation chimeras, in which the host is thymectomized prior to allogeneic BMT and transplantation of an allogeneic thymus, do not demonstrate in vitro tolerance toward host antigens (125), also suggesting that extrathymic nonhematopoietic cells are incapable of anergizing T cells. In transgenic mice, in contrast, T cells demonstrate anergy toward antigens that appear to be expressed exclusively on peripheral nonhematopoietic organs (21,126). Anergy was observed even in mice carrying two transgenes, so that most T cells expressed a transgenic TCR specific for a transgenic class I MHC molecule expressed only on pancreatic β cells (23). It is unclear why T cells can be anergized by extrathymic nonhematopoietic antigens in some experimental systems but not in others. Perhaps T cells are only susceptible to anergy induction by these antigens during early development of the animal.

The discussion so far would suggest that induction of mixed chimerism may be an optimal way of inducing donor-specific tolerance across MHC barriers. Unfortunately, however, the conventional method of producing mixed allogeneic chimeras in mice is not directly applicable to humans because of the toxicity of lethal TBI (127,128) and the high risk of GVHD (129) and graft failure (97) encountered when BMT is attempted across human leukocyte antigen (HLA) barriers. BMT following lethal TBI would not be justifiable as a means of inducing tolerance for the purpose of organ transplantation, for which less toxic chronic immunosuppressive therapy is available.

If BMT, therefore, is to be used as means of inducing donor-specific organ allograft tolerance, it will be essential to develop methods of rendering recipients immunoincompetent that are less toxic and more effective in eliminating alloresistance than those currently available. This could be achieved by developing conditioning regimens that specifically eliminate the host elements which resist alloengraftment, without producing generalized toxic effects. Such regimens might permit the engraftment of T-cell–depleted allogeneic marrow, or host resistance to GVHD might be preserved in recipients of non-T-cell–depleted allogeneic marrow. Some new approaches to achieve this goal are discussed. Another approach would involve identification of donor marrow cell subpopulations distinct from GVHD-producing T cells, which could improve alloengraftment. The existence of such cell types has been suggested by several murine studies (109,130–133).

BMT in Adult Recipients Following Conditioning with Immunosuppressive but Nonmyeloablative Protocols

Recently, several BMT protocols have been developed that involve myelotoxic or immunosuppressive, but not myeloablative, conditioning regimens. Because host hematopoietic stem cells survive, mixed chimerism often develops when allogeneic marrow is administered. Such regimens include total lymphoid irradiation (TLI) (134), sublethal TBI (135), administration of cyclophosphamide (CY) following sensitization with allogeneic donor antigens (136,137), and use of MABs against host T cells in combination with other modalities (137). Perhaps because they do not eliminate host T cells completely, however, relatively large numbers of allogeneic cells, including donor T cells, are often required to achieve engraftment (134,135,138,139). However, some of these regimens, particularly those that specifically target host T cells with MABs, show considerable promise.

TLI

TLI, which involves extensive, fractionated irradiation of lymphoid organs with shielding of hematopoietic tissue, has been used for induction of chimerism in rodent models (140,141). Large numbers of allogeneic T-cell–containing marrow cells, which can produce GVHD, are usually required to achieve engraftment (134,142,143). Host T cells that survive irradiation due to shielding of bones probably mediate resistance to marrow engraftment in such animals. In general, experiments utilizing TLI in large animals as the sole preparative modality prior to allogeneic BMT and organ transplantation have met with, at best, modest success (144–147), and chimerism was not clearly demonstrated in cases in which tolerance was documented. TLI combined with anti-T-cell antibodies is more effective in inducing tolerance to organ allografts in large outbred animals (148). This combination has been documented to induce donor-specific tolerance without BMT in patients given cadaveric renal allografts (149). Natural suppressor cells, which are abundant following conditioning with TLI (68), may have a role in the initial inactivation of residual host T cells reactive to the graft (134). Unfortunately, the long period over which pretransplant TLI must be administered limits the practical utility of this approach for cadaveric organ transplantation (149), unless regimens are developed in which TLI is administered for a brief period after transplantation. The feasibility of using post-transplant TLI with anti-T-cell antibodies to induce organ allograft acceptance has recently been reported in a primate model (150).

Fractionated Sublethal TBI

Induction of mixed chimerism using fractionated sublethal TBI and allogeneic BMT has been shown to be associated with donor-specific tolerance across complete MHC barriers in mice (135,151). Donor T cells that need not have alloreactivity against the recipient help to promote alloengraftment in this model (131,135,151). Donor-type Thy1-positive cells can transfer donor-specific tolerance from the original BMT recipients to secondary recipients. Possible mechanisms to explain this property of donor-type T cells include suppression, vetoing of recipient T cells reacting against them, or induction of clonal anergy among donor-reactive recipient T cells.

Cyclophosphamide

High doses of CY administered 2 or 3 days following inoculation with large numbers of allogeneic marrow or spleen cells induce donor-specific tolerance across multiple minor histoincompatibilities and selected MHC disparities (28,136,152). Additional host treatment with monoclonal anti-T-cell antibody permits induction of tolerance across complete MHC barriers (137). Several mechanisms may be involved in this model. Sensitization followed by administration of CY is thought to cause selective destruction of host T cells induced to proliferate in response to alloantigen, so that pre-existing donor-reactive T-cell clones are eliminated (137) and newly developing T cells can mature in the presence of donor marrow–derived antigen in the thymus. CY is more potent as an immunosuppressive than as a myeloablative agent, and only very low levels of chimerism can be demonstrated in these animals, probably reflecting the fact that CY does not create substantial marrow "space" (153). In the model involving tolerance across minor histocompatibility barriers, evidence was obtained for intrathymic clonal deletion of T cells bearing TCR that contain Vβ6, which binds to Mls superantigens expressed by the donor and not the host (136). Deletion of peripheral Vβ6-bearing $CD4^+$ cells was observed early after BMT, probably due to sensitization followed by CY administration (136). In a congenic, MHC-mismatched strain combination, chimerism was shown to disappear with time, and clonal deletion was replaced by anergy as a mechanism of tolerance (152).

Anti-T-cell Antibodies

A recent approach to the use of BMT for tolerance induction involves in vivo administration of antibodies against T cells to specifically eliminate or block the function of host cells that mediate alloresistance. Wood and colleagues (154) showed several years ago that some mice pretreated with anti-lymphocyte serum and grafted with donor-type skin several days prior to administration of allogeneic marrow cells could be rendered specifically tolerant of donor antigens. Antigen-specific suppressor cells of donor origin have been implicated in the skin graft prolongation observed in these mice (31,32). The cells in allogeneic BM inocula that could induce tolerance (133) resembled natural suppressor cells in many respects (63). Use of this protocol has been associated with the development of long-lasting, low levels of chimerism (155). A similar approach has been reported to prolong renal allograft survival in large animals (156,157). In primate studies, a $CD2^+CD8^+CD16^+CD3^-DR^-$ cell population with veto activity has been implicated in tolerance induction (158).

More recent refinements of this approach have involved in vivo administration of MABs against recipient T cell subsets (82,83). In vivo depletion of host $CD4^+$ and $CD8^+$ T cells along with TBI (at least 6 Gy) permitted engraftment of allogeneic marrow and induction of skin graft tolerance across complete MHC barriers (83). Adding a high dose of thymic irradiation (7 Gy) to the regimen permitted engraftment of fully MHC-mismatched allogeneic marrow in animals receiving only 3 Gy TBI (82). Thymic irradiation is needed because MAB treatment results in coating of thymocytes with MAB but not their elimination (82). The low dose (3 Gy) of TBI is necessary for the creation of marrow "space" (82). Permanent mixed chimerism and donor- and host-specific tolerance are reliably induced across complete MHC barriers using this regimen (Figure 17-1). Although the mechanism of tolerance in this model has not been established fully, the continuous presence of donor antigen on marrow-derived cells is required for maintenance of tolerance. Elimination of donor-type lymphohematopoietic cells using MAB against donor H-2 leads to loss of skin graft tolerance (159) (Figure 17-2). Preliminary data suggest that this loss of tolerance is due to the differentiation of new T cells in the thymus after chimerism is lost, resulting in the export of nontolerant T cells from the

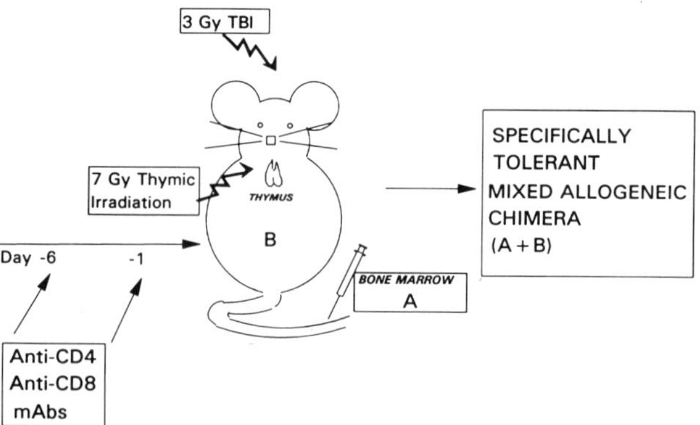

Figure 17-1. Nonmyeloablative conditioning regimen allowing the induction of mixed allogeneic chimerism and specific transplantation tolerance across complete MHC barriers in mice.

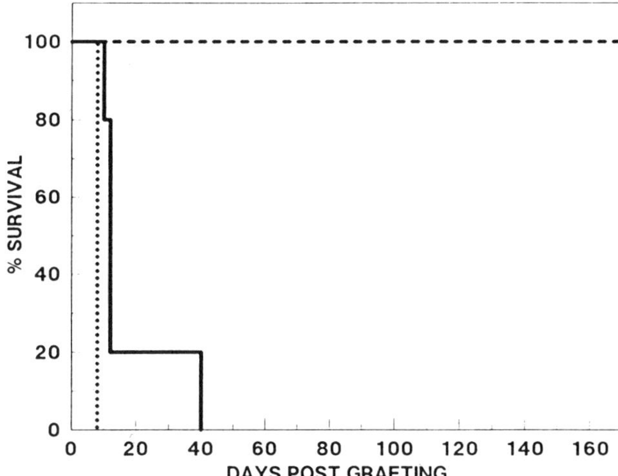

Figure 17-2. Tolerance can be broken by eliminating donor lymphohematopoietic cells using MABs specific for donor class I MHC antigens. Mixed allogeneic chimeras were prepared in the B10.D2→B10 (H-2^d→H-2^b) strain combination using the regimen shown in Figure 17-1. Between 4 and 5 months after BMT, the animals received 4 injections of anti-D^d MAB, which led to loss of chimerism and repopulation by host cells. Survival of donor-type B10.D2 skin grafted 4 months after administration of anti-D^d MAB is shown. Mixed chimeras that did not receive anti-D^d MAB (- - -) showed permanent acceptance of donor-type skin grafts, confirming their tolerant state. Animals in which chimerism was eliminated by treatment with anti-D^d MAB (——), in contrast, rejected donor-type B10.D2 skin grafts. Rejection of B10.D2 skin grafts is also shown for B10 mice in which chimerism was never induced (. . . .). All groups rejected third-party B10.BR skin grafts with a similar time course (not shown). (Reproduced by permission from Bone Marrow Transplant, 1992;9:191–197.)

thymus (Abraham VS, Sachs DH, Sykes M. Unpublished data).

The mechanisms of T-cell elimination using MABs are not entirely clear. Animals treated with T-cell–depleting MABs after thymectomy show a significant recovery of $CD4^+$ and $CD8^+$ T cells over a period of several weeks (160), suggesting that sequestration rather than destruction may actually account for some of the observed T-cell depletion. T-cell subset depletion using MABs does not appear to be dependent on the activity of complement or on antibody-dependent, cell-mediated cytotoxicity (160).

In addition to MABs that deplete their targets, anti-CD4 and anti-CD8 MABs that do not deplete their target cells in vivo can also be used to induce tolerance across minor histocompatibility barriers, probably by inducing T-cell anergy rather than clonal deletion (24). Recently, nondepleting anti-T-cell MABs have been used following a course of MABs that deplete T cells to induce skin graft tolerance across MHC barriers without BMT (25).

Mechanisms Inducing Tolerance of the Donor to the Host (GVH tolerance) in BMT

To avoid GVHD, the de novo development of host-reactive T cells from progenitors in the marrow must be prevented, and the GVH reactivity of pre-existing mature T cells in the marrow inoculum must be inhibited. Mechanisms producing both phenomena are discussed.

Tolerization of Mature GVH-reactive T Cells Present in the Marrow at the Time of BMT

A goal of research in BMT is to develop ways of administering mature allogeneic T cells within the marrow while avoiding GVHD, because GVH-reactive T cells can mediate several beneficial effects, including graft-versus-leukemia (GVL) effects (161,162) and promotion of alloengraftment (163). Results in several animal models and in humans suggest that this goal could be achieved. Some of these models and the mechanisms involved in induction of GVH tolerance are discussed.

Down-regulatory Cells in Marrow Inocula

A subset of T cells found in the marrow of normal mice that expresses the $\alpha\beta$TCR without CD4 or CD8 accessory molecules ("double-negative" T cells) shares functional activity similar to that of natural suppressor cells (164). Both the NS cells and these T cells are able to inhibit alloreactivity in vitro without antigen specificity or MHC restriction. NS cells derived from several sources have been implicated in the suppression of GVHD. Spleen cells from both neonatal mice and adult mice recovering from TLI are rich in NS cells (57) and are able to suppress GVHD when they are coinjected with non-T-cell–depleted marrow cells into lethally irradiated allogeneic recipients (57,68). Natural suppressor cells may be responsible for the protection against GVHD provided by administering T-cell–depleted syngeneic (host-type) marrow cells simultaneously with (165) or several days prior to (166) allogeneic BMT. Similar to NS cells, cloned lines of $CD4^-CD8^-\alpha\beta TCR^+$ T cells show suppressive activity in vitro and are able to inhibit acute, lethal GVHD (69,70,167). The cloned lines can be activated in vitro to secrete a cytokine that inhibits the function of APCs, and thus suppresses T-cell responses without antigen specificity (168). However, the precise relationship between NS cells and suppressive $CD4^-CD8^-\alpha\beta TCR^+$ cells, and the mechanisms by which they induce tolerance, remain to be elucidated.

Use of Interleukin-2 to Inhibit GVHD

Recent studies demonstrated that administration of a high dose of IL-2 for 2.5 days beginning on the day of BMT provides marked protection against GVHD mortality in completely MHC-mismatched mice. This

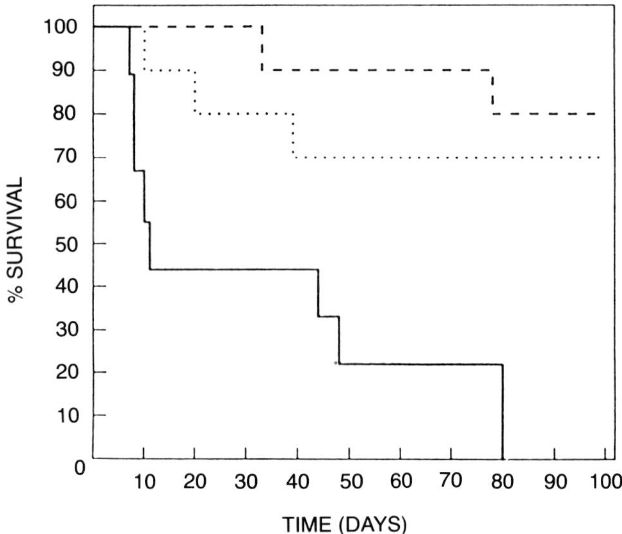

Figure 17-3. Protection from GVHD mortality using treatment with IL-2 and T-cell–depleted syngeneic bone marrow. B10 mice were lethally irradiated and received an intravenous inoculum containing fully allogeneic A/J marrow and spleen cells (——). Animals receiving similar inocula, but treated with human rIL-2 (50,000 Cetus U twice daily for 2.5 days) (. . . .) showed a marked improvement in survival. Animals receiving similar IL-2 treatment, but which also received T-cell–depleted host-type (B10) bone marrow along with A/J bone marrow and spleen cells (- - -), demonstrated even greater protection from GVHD. These animals reconstitute as completely allogeneic chimeras.

effect is enhanced when T-cell–depleted host-type marrow is coadministered (169) (Figure 17-3). Remarkably, complete allogeneic reconstitution results (169), and the GVL effect of donor T cells against a host-type T-cell leukemia/lymphoma, EL4, is completely preserved (170). This striking dissociation of the beneficial from the deleterious effects of donor T cells can be explained by the observation that different T-cell subsets are required for each effect. In most fully MHC-plus-minor-antigen disparate strain combinations examined, GVHD is mediated by both $CD4^+$ and $CD8^+$ T cells. However, $CD4^+$ cells are often necessary for the induction of acute GVHD (171–174). In contrast, $CD8^+$ T cells appear to be solely responsible for GVL effects against the host-type EL4 tumor in this model. Thus, elimination of $CD4^+$ T cells from donor inocula is sufficient to inhibit GVHD without attenuating GVL, which is entirely CD8-mediated (175). These results explain the dissociation of GVHD and GVL observed in this model.

The ability of IL-2 to protect against GVHD is paradoxical, and its mechanism is unclear. Although $NK1^+$ cells with LAK activity can protect against GVHD in adoptive transfer studies (46,70), the protective effect of IL-2 occurs independently of NK cells, LAK cells, or their precursors (176). Furthermore, the protective effect does not require the presence of host T cells (Abraham VS, Sykes M. Unpublished observations). IL-2 treatment markedly reduces the number of donor T cells present in spleens of mice receiving allogeneic T-cell–containing inocula when examined in the first week following BMT (177). These spleens contain an increased percentage of $CD3^+CD4^-CD8^-$ T cells (176), which express $\alpha\beta$TCR (Sykes M. Unpublished data). These cells may be similar to the double negative suppressor cells described, which have been shown to have an anti-GVHD effect in adoptive transfer studies.

IL-2-activated Killer Cells for Prevention of GVHD

Recent studies have demonstrated that LAK cells can inhibit GVHD (46). These cells, which are derived from the host strain, may inhibit GVHD by eliminating alloreactive donor T cells by the veto mechanism discussed (45,46). Unusual $\alpha\beta TCR^+$, $NK1.1^+$ cells with LAK activity that are cultured from marrow in high concentrations of IL-2 can delay the onset of GVHD when transferred to syngeneic hosts receiving allogeneic marrow (70).

Induction of Anergy in GVH-reactive T Lymphocytes

GVH-reactive cytotoxic T-lymphocyte precursors were not detected in limiting dilution analyses of lymphocytes from long-term TLI-treated strain A x B F_1 hybrid hosts given non-T-cell–depleted strain A marrow cells (178). Removal of the tolerant cells from the F_1 hosts by adoptive transfer into supralethally irradiated A hosts led to the rapid reappearance of B-reactive cytotoxic T lymphocytes (179). Therefore, maintenance of these cells in the original B-antigen–expressing environment of the F_1 host had maintained tolerance in B-reactive cytotoxic T lymphocytes, presumably by inducing anergy.

Induction of Tolerance Among T Cells Developing from Progenitors in the Marrow

The mechanism of GVH tolerance in lethally irradiated recipients of T-cell–depleted allogeneic marrow inocula appears mainly to involve T-cell anergy rather than clonal deletion (18). Because most host hematopoietic cells are eliminated by lethal irradiation, and bone marrow-derived cells are most effective at inducing clonal deletion in the thymus, extensive deletion of host-reactive T cells would not be expected in these animals. However, partial clonal deletion of host-reactive T cells has been described in mice receiving allogeneic BMT (4,180). This partial deletion may reflect a weak capacity of non-marrow-derived thymic stromal elements to cause deletion or, alternatively, may reflect the influence of a small percentage of residual host-type lymphohematopoietic cells (109).

A failure to delete self-reactive T-cell clones has

been observed in the thymuses of CSP-treated, irradiated rodents (181,182). A failure to induce T-cell tolerance toward self class II MHC antigens has also been observed in both murine (183) and human (184,185) GVHD directed against minor histoincompatibilities. Thymic epithelial injury (186,187) may contribute to defective T-cell maturation in GVHD, and defective production of suppressor T cells has been implicated in unmasking the activity of autoreactive T cells in human chronic GVHD (185). Thus, several mechanisms may contribute to failure of tolerance among newly developing T-cell clones in recipients with thymic injury due to GVHD or CSP treatment.

The importance of antigen expression on marrow-derived cells for the induction of tolerance among newly developing T cells in humans is illustrated by studies in patients with severe combined immunodeficiency (SCID) receiving HLA-mismatched BMT, and in whom donor T-cell but not B-cell or myeloid engraftment develops initially. Newly developing donor T cells from these patients exhibit reactivity toward donor class II MHC antigens. This reactivity disappears if engraftment of donor class II–bearing cells later occurs (188).

In murine BMT into recipients conditioned with lethal TBI, no in vitro evidence for active suppression of GVH reactivity was obtained using cells from long-term recipients of T-cell–depleted allogeneic marrow alone (189), but cells with the ability to suppress alloreactive cytotoxic T lymphocytes were detected in spleens from long-term chimeras originally reconstituted with mixed T-cell–depleted allogeneic plus syngeneic (host-type) marrow (121). These non-T-suppressor cells may consist of a mixture of veto cells and NS cells (121). Cells specifically suppressing GVH reactions have also been described in long-term rat chimeras originally reconstituted with non-T-cell–depleted allogeneic marrow (29) and in human BMT recipients in whom GVHD does not develop (190).

Mixed chimeras show excellent clonal deletion of T cells reacting against host antigens (19). This improved deletion of host-reactive T cells in recipients of mixed marrow over that achieved in recipients of T-cell–depleted allogeneic marrow alone is undoubtedly due to the intrathymic presence of host-type marrow-derived cells in mixed chimeras (see Table 17-1). In vivo administration of nontolerant donor-type spleen cells to long-term chimeras originally reconstituted with T-cell–depleted mixed allogeneic plus syngeneic marrow inocula does not induce GVHD but does convert mixed chimeras to completely allogeneic chimeras (191). The mechanisms resisting GVHD in such animals are undefined. Long-term human BMT recipients may also be more resistant to GVHD than freshly irradiated individuals; this possibility has been exploited in studies involving administration of donor lymphocytes to relapsed leukemic patients. Results were encouraging, because these cells induced remissions and produced, at most, moderate GVHD (192).

Future Directions in BMT

Although the mechanisms involved may be multiple and are not yet completely understood, it is clear that BMT offers a means for achieving long-lasting and specific transplantation tolerance across MHC barriers. To date, the majority of data demonstrating the induction of such tolerance have been obtained in rodent models. Unfortunately, although rodent models are extremely important in basic transplantation research, there are several major differences between rodents and large animals that must be considered before results can be applied to clinical problems. Of particular importance in the case of BMT is the fact that the preparative regimens by which chimerism is routinely achieved in mice involve TBI delivered at high dose rates (approximately 1.0 Gy/min), which may be too toxic to be used in large animals (Smith CV, Suzuki T, Guzetta PC, et al. Unpublished observations). This difference in preparative regimens may explain why T-cell–depleted marrow engrafts readily in lethally irradiated rodents even across MHC barriers, whereas much greater difficulty has been encountered in achieving MHC-mismatched marrow engraftment in large animals (Smith CV, Suzuki T, Guzetta PC, et al. Unpublished observations) and humans (97).

A major goal of transplant immunologists will be to extend results from experimental rodent models, first to additional preclinical models in large animals and then to clinical protocols. In addition, it will be important to continue basic research into the mechanisms by which tolerance is induced and maintained in rodent model systems, so that these mechanisms can be further exploited. For example, it now appears that it may be possible to isolate and characterize the individual cell populations responsible for induction of tolerance among donor T cells (i.e., avoidance of GVHD). It may similarly be possible to determine the nature of cells responsible for inducing and maintaining tolerance in the host immune system (i.e., avoidance of rejection). Characterization of such populations could lead to strategies for augmenting their effects, including use of specific cytokines and growth factors, as well as procedures for isolation and propagation. Specific cellular therapy for the induction of tolerance could provide a valuable adjunct in clinical BMT and potentially in clinical solid organ transplantation.

With specific reference to the use of BMT for inducing tolerance to organ transplants, it may be possible to utilize genetic engineering to achieve the same goal without the potential for inducing GVHD. One such experimental approach is based on retrovirus-mediated gene transfer of donor-type MHC genes into bone marrow hemopoietic stem cells, and studies in a murine model support its feasibility (193) (see Chapter 9). In these studies, reconstitution of recipients with autologous marrow cells expressing an allogeneic class I gene was found to confer tolerance to the product of that gene, as evidenced by prolonged survival of a corresponding skin graft. Studies are already in progress in an attempt to utilize a similar approach to induce tolerance across a class II barrier in miniature swine (194). If specific marrow cell populations are determined to be particularly effective in inducing tolerance, and if these populations can be isolated and propagated from autologous marrow or peripheral blood, application of genetic engineering to the routine induction of tolerance across MHC barriers may be possible.

References

1. Owen RD. Immunogenetic consequences of vascular anastomoses between bovine twins. Science 1945; 102:400–401.
2. Kappler JW, Roehm N, Marrack P. T-cell tolerance by clonal elimination in the thymus. Cell 1987;49:273–280.
3. Marrack P, Kappler J. The staphylococcal enterotoxins and their relatives. Science 1990;248:705–711.
4. Blackman M, Kappler J, Marrack P. The role of the T-cell receptor in positive and negative selection of developing T-cells. Science 1990;248:1335–1341.
5. Pullen AM, Kappler JW, Marrack P. Tolerance to self antigens shapes the T-cell repertoire. Immunol Rev 1989;107:125–139.
6. Korngold R, Sprent J. Lethal graft-versus-host disease after bone marrow transplantation across minor histocompatibility barriers in mice. J Exp Med 1978; 148:1687–1694.
7. Sachs DH, Cone JL, Humphrey GW. The humoral response to an Ia antigen and skin graft rejection: mechanistic possibilities. Transplant Proc 1976;8:413–416.
8. Sha WC, Nelson CA, Newberry RD, Kranz DM, Russell JH, Loh DY. Positive and negative selection of an antigen receptor on T-cells in transgenic mice. Nature 1988;336:73–76.
9. Von Boehmer H, Kisielow P. Self-nonself discrimination by T-cells. Science 1990;248:1369–1373.
10. Marrack P, Lo D, Brinster R, et al. The effect of thymus environment on T-cell development and tolerance. Cell 1988;53:627–634.
11. van Ewijk W, Ron Y, Monaco J, et al. Compartmentalization of MHC class II gene expression in transgenic mice. Cell 1988;53:357–370.
12. Ramsdell F, Fowlkes BJ. Clonal deletion versus clonal anergy: the role of the thymus in inducing self tolerance. Science 1990;248:1342–1348.
13. Inaba M, Inaba KI, Hosono M, et al. Distinct mechanisms of neonatal tolerance induced by dendritic cells and thymic B-cells. J Exp Med 1991;173:549–559.
14. Shimonkevitz RP, Bevan MJ. Split tolerance induced by the intrathymic adoptive transfer of thymocyte stem cells. J Exp Med 1988;168:143–156.
15. Schwartz RH. A cell culture model for T-lymphocyte clonal anergy. Science 1990;248:1349–1356.
16. Linsley PS, Brady W, Grosmaire L, Aruffo A, Damle NK, Ledbetter JA. Binding of the B-cell activation antigen B7 to CD28 costimulates T-cell proliferation and interleukin 2 mRNA accumulation. J Exp Med 1991;173: 721–725.
17. Gimmi CD, Freeman GJ, Gribben JG, et al. B-cell surface antigen B7 provides a costimulatory signal that induces T-cells to proliferate and secrete interleukin 2. Proc Natl Acad Sci USA 1991;88:6575–6578.
18. Ramsdell F, Lantz T, Fowlkes BJ. A nondeletional mechanism of thymic self tolerance. Science 1989; 246:1038–1041.
19. Gao EK, Lo D, Sprent J. Strong T-cell tolerance in parent→F1 bone marrow chimeras prepared with supralethal irradiation. J Exp Med 1990;171:1101–1121.
20. Salaun J, Bandeira A, Khazaal I, et al. Thymic epithelium tolerizes for histocompatibility antigens. Science 1990;247:1471–1474.
21. Burkly LC, Lo D, Flavell RA. Tolerance in transgenic mice expressing major histocompatibility molecules extrathymically on pancreatic cells. Science 1990;248: 1364–1368.
22. Morahan G, Allison J, Miller JFAP. Tolerance of class I histocompatibility antigens expressed extrathymically. Nature 1989;339:622–624.
23. Morahan G, Hoffman MW, Miller JFAP. A nondeletional mechanism of peripheral tolerance in T-cell receptor transgenic mice. Proc Natl Acad Sci USA 1991;88: 11421–11425.
24. Qin S, Cobbold S, Benjamin R, Waldmann H. Induction of classical transplantation tolerance in the adult. J Exp Med 1989;169:779–794.
25. Cobbold SP, Qin S, Waldmann H. Reprogramming the immune system for tolerance with monoclonal antibodies. Semin Immunol 1990;2:377–387.
26. Eynon EE, Parker DC. Small B-cells as antigen-presenting cells in the induction of tolerance to soluble protein antigens. J Exp Med 1992;175:131–138.
27. Roser BJ. Cellular mechanisms in neonatal and adult tolerance. Immunol Rev 1989;107:179–202.
28. Tomita Y, Mayumi H, Eto M, Nomoto K. Importance of suppressor T-cells in cyclophosphamide-induced tolerance to the non-H-2-encoded alloantigens. Is mixed chimerism really required in maintaining a skin allograft tolerance? J Immunol 1990;144:463–473.
29. Tutschka PJ, Ki PF, Beschorner WE, Hess AD, Santos GW. Suppressor cells in transplantation tolerance. II. Maturation of suppressor cells in the bone marrow chimera. Transplantation 1981;32:321–325.
30. Lancaster F, Chui YL, Batchelor JR. Anti-idiotypic T-cells suppress rejection of renal allografts in rats. Nature 1985;315:336–337.
31. Maki T, Gottshalk R, Wood ML, Monaco AP. Specific unresponsiveness to skin allografts in anti-lymphocyte serum-treated, marrow-injected mice: participation of donor marrow-derived suppressor T-cells. J Immunol 1981;127:1433–1437.
32. Wood ML, Monaco AP. Suppressor cells in specific unresponsiveness to skin allografts in ALS-treated, marrow-injected mice. Transplantation 1980;29:196–200.
33. Wilson DB. Idiotypic regulation of T-cells in graft-versus-host disease and autoimmunity. Immunol Rev 1989;107:159–176.
34. Koide J, Engleman EG. Differences in surface phenotype and mechanism of action between alloantigen-specific $CD8^+$ cytotoxic and suppressor T-cell clones. J Immunol 1990;144:32–40.
35. Beschorner WE, Shinn CA, Fischer AC, Santos GW, Hess AD. Cyclosporine-induced pseudo-graft-versus-host disease in the early post- cyclosporine period. Transplantation 1988;46:112S-117S.
36. Sorokin R, Kimura H, Schroder K, Wilson DH, Wilson DB. Cyclosporine-induced autoimmunity. Conditions for expressing disease, requirement for intact thymus, and potency estimates of autoimmune lymphocytes in drug-treated rats. J Exp Med 1986;164:1615–1625.

37. Hess AD, Horwitz L, Beschorner WE, Santos GW. Development of graft-versus-host disease-like syndrome in cyclosporine-treated rats after syngeneic bone marrow transplantation. I. Development of cytotoxic T-lymphocytes with apparent polyclonal anti-Ia specificity, including autoreactivity. J Exp Med 1985;161:718–724.
38. Hess AD, Fischer AC, Beschorner WE. Effector mechanisms in cyclosporine A-induced syngeneic graft-versus-host disease. J Immunol 1990;145:526–533.
39. Fischer AC, Laulis MK, Horwitz L, Beschorner WE, Hess AD. Host resistance to cyclosporine induced syngeneic graft-versus-host disease. J Immunol 1989; 143:827–832.
40. Beschorner WE, Namnoum JD, Hess AD. Cyclosporin A and the thymus. Am J Pathol 1987;126:487–491.
41. Miller RG. The veto phenomenon and T-cell regulation. Immunol Today 1986;7:112–114.
42. Muraoka S, Miller RG. Cells in bone marrow and in T-cell colonies grown from bone marrow can suppress generation of cytotoxic T-lymphocytes directed against their self antigens. J Exp Med 1980;152:54-71.
43. Claesson MH, Miller RG. Functional heterogeneity in allospecific cytotoxic T-lymphocyte clones I. CTL clones express strong anti-self suppressive activity. J Exp Med 1984;160:1702–1716.
44. Fink PJ, Rammensee HG, Bevan MJ. Cloned cytotoxic T-cells can suppress primary cytotoxic responses directed against them. J Immunol 1984;133:1775–1779.
45. Azuma E, Kaplan J. Role of lymphokine-activated killer cells as mediators of veto and natural suppression. J Immunol 1988;141:2601-2606.
46. Azuma E, Yamamoto H, Kaplan J. Use of lymphokine-activated killer cells to prevent bone marrow graft rejection and lethal graft-vs-host disease. J Immunol 1989;143:1524–1529.
47. Nakamura H, Gress RE. Interleukin 2 enhancement of veto suppressor cell function in T-cell–depleted bone marrow in vitro and in vivo. Transplantation 1990; 49:931–937.
48. Kast WM, Twuyver WM, Mooijaart RJD, Verveld M, Kamphuis AGA, Melief CJM, Waal LPD. Mechanism of skin allograft enhancement across an H-2 class I mutant difference. Evidence for involvement of veto cells. Eur J Immunol 1988;18:2105–2110.
49. Heeg K, Wagner H. Induction of peripheral tolerance to class I major histocompatibility complex (MHC) alloantigens in adult mice: transfused class I MHC-incompatible splenocytes veto clonal response of antigen-reactive Lyt-2+ T-cells. J Exp Med 1990; 172:719–725.
50. Sambhara SR, Miller RG. Programmed cell death of T-cells signaled by the T-cell receptor and the alpha-3 domain of class I MHC. Science 1991;252:1424–1427.
51. Hambor JE, Kaplan DR, Tykocinski ML. CD8 functions as an inhibitory ligand in mediating the immunoregulatory activity of $CD8^+$ cells. J Immunol 1990; 145:1646–1652.
52. Kaplan DR, Hambor JE, Tykocinski ML. An immunoregulatory function for the CD8 molecule. Proc Natl Acad Sci USA 1989;86:8512–8514.
53. Hertel-Wulff B, Okada S, Oseroff A, Strober S. In vitro propagation and cloning of murine natural suppressor (NS) cells. J Immunol 1984;133:2791–2796.
54. Sykes M, Eisenthal A, Sachs DH. Mechanism of protection from graft-vs-host disease in murine mixed allogeneic chimeras. I. Development of a null cell population suppressive of cell-mediated lympholysis responses and derived from the syngeneic bone marrow component. J Immunol 1988;140:2903–2911.
55. Maier T, Holda JH, Claman HN. Natural suppressor (NS) cells. Members of the LGL regulatory family. Immunol Today 1986;7:312–315.
56. Argyris BF. Suppressor activity in the spleen of neonatal mice. Cell Immunol 1978;36:354–362.
57. Strober S. Natural suppressor (NS) cells, neonatal tolerance, and total lymphoid irradiation: exploring obscure relationships. Ann Rev Immunol 1984;2:219–231.
58. Oseroff A, Okada S, Strober S. Natural suppressor (NS) cells found in the spleen of neonatal mice and adult mice given total lymphoid irradiation (TLI) express the null surface phenotype. J Immunol 1984;132:101–110.
59. Maes LY, York JL, Soderberg LSF. A soluble factor produced by bone marrow natural suppressor cells blocks interleukin 2 production and activity. Cell Immuol 1988;116:35–43.
60. Merluzzi VJ, Levy EM, Kumar V, Bennett N, Cooperband SR. In vitro activation of suppressor cells from spleens of mice treated with radioactive strontium. J Immunol 1978;121:505–508.
61. McIntosh KR, Segre M, Segre D. Characterization of cyclophosphamide-induced suppressor cells. Immunopharmacology 1982;4:279–289.
62. Dorshkind K, Rosse C. Physical, biologic, and phenotypic properties of natural regulatory cells in murine bone marrow. Am J Anat 1982;164:1–17.
63. Sykes M, Sharabi Y, Sachs DH. Natural suppressor cells in spleens of irradiated, bone marrow reconstituted mice and normal bone marrow: lack of Sca-1 expression and enrichment by depletion of Mac1-positive cells. Cell Immunol 1990;127:260–274.
64. Sugiura K, Ikehara S, Gengozian N, et al. Enrichment of natural suppressor activity in a wheat germ agglutinin positive hematopoietic progenitor-enriched fraction of monkey bone marrow. Blood 1990;75:1125–1131.
65. Holda JH, Maier T, Claman HN. Murine graft-versus-host disease across minor barriers: immunosuppressive aspects of natural suppressor cells. Immunol Rev 1985;88:87–105.
66. Noga SJ, Wagner JE, Horwitz LR, Donnenberg AD, Santos GW, Hess AD. Characterization of the natural suppressor cell population in adult rat bone marrow. J Leukocyte Biol 1988;43:279–287.
67. Mortari F, Bains MA, Singhal SK. Immunoregulatory activity of human bone marrow. Identification of suppressor cells possessing OKM1, SSEA-1, and HNK-1 antigens. J Immunol 1986;137:1133–1137.
68. King DP, Strober S, Kaplan HS. Suppression of the mixed leukocyte response and graft-vs.-host disease by spleen cells following total lymphoid irradiation (TLI). J Immunol 1981;126:1140–1144.
69. Strober S, Dejbachsh-Jones S, Van Vlassalaer P, Duwe G, Salimi S, Allison JP. Cloned natural suppressor cell lines express the CD3+CD4-CD8- surface phenotype and the α, β heterodimer of the T-cell antigen receptor. J Immunol 1989;143:1118–1122.
70. Sykes M, Hoyles KA, Romick ML, Sachs DH. In vitro and in vivo analysis of bone marrow derived CD3+, CD4−, CD8−, NK1.1+ cell lines. Cell Immunol 1990; 1290:478–493.
71. Hertel-Wulff B, Lindsten T, Schwadron R, Gilbert DM, Davis MM, Strober S. Rearrangement and expression of

T-cell receptor genes in cloned murine natural suppressor cell lines. J Exp Med 1987;166:1168-1173.
72. Hertel-Wulff B, Strober S. Immunosuppressive lymphokine derived from natural suppressor cells. J Immunol 1988;140:2633–2638.
73. Knaan-Shanzer S, Van Bekkum DW. Soluble factors secreted by naturally occurring suppressor cells that interfere with in vivo graft-vs.-host disease and with T-cell responsiveness in vitro. Eur J Immunol 1987;17: 827–834.
74. Choi KL, Maier T, Holda JH, Claman HN. Suppression of cytotoxic T-cell generation by natural suppressor cells from mice with GVHD is partially reversed by indomethacin. Cell Immunol 1988;112:271–278.
75. Saffran DC, Singhal SK. Suppression of mixed lymphocyte reactivity by murine bone marrow-derived suppressor factor-inhibition of proliferation due to a deficit in IL-2 production. Transplantation 1991;52:685–690.
76. Weingust RW, McCain GA, Singhal SK. Regulation of autoimmunity in normal and rheumatoid individuals by bone marrow-derived natural suppressor cells and their suppressor factor: BDSF. Cell Immunol 1989; 122:154–163.
77. Holda JH, Maier T, Claman HN. Evidence that IFN-γ is responsible for natural suppressor activity in GVHD spleen and normal bone marrow. Transplantation 1988;45:772–777.
78. Holda JH, Maier T, Claman HN. Natural suppressor activity in graft-vs-host spleen and normal bone marrow is augmented by IL-2 and interferon-γ. J Immunol 1986;137:3538–3543.
79. Field EH, Becker GC. Blocking of mixed lymphocyte reaction by spleen cells from total lymphoid-irradiated mice involves interruption of the IL-2 pathway. J Immunol 1992;148:354–359.
80. Sykes M, Sachs DH. Mechanisms of suppression in mixed allogeneic chimeras. Transplantation 1988; 46:135S-142S.
81. Voralia M, Semeluk A, Wegmann TG. Facilitation of syngeneic stem cell engraftment by anti-class I monoclonal antibody pretreatment of unirradiated recipients. Transplantation 1987;44:487–494.
82. Sharabi Y, Sachs DH. Mixed chimerism and permanent specific transplantation tolerance induced by a non-lethal preparative regimen. J Exp Med 1989; 169:493–502.
83. Cobbold SP, Martin G, Qin S, Waldmann H. Monoclonal antibodies to promote marrow engraftment and tissue graft tolerance. Nature 1986;323:164–165.
84. Schwartz E, Lapidot T, Gozes D, Singer TS, Reisner Y. Abrogation of bone marrow allograft resistance in mice by increased total body irradiation correlates with eradication of host clonable T-cells and alloreactive cytotoxic precursors. J Immunol 1987;138:460–465.
85. Reisner Y, Ben-Bassat I, Douer D, Kaploon A, Schwartz E, Ramot B. Demonstration of clonable alloreactive host T-cells in a primate model for bone marrow transplantation. Proc Natl Acad Sci USA1986;83:4012–4015.
86. Bordignon C, Keever CA, Small TN, et al. Graft failure after T-cell-depleted human leukocyte antigen identical marrow transplants for leukemia: II. In vitro analyses of host effector mechanisms. Blood 1989;74:2237–2243.
87. Kernan NA, Flomenberg N, Dupont B, O'Reilly RJ. Graft rejection in recipients of T-cell-depleted HLA-nonidentical marrow transplants for leukemia. Transplantation 1987;43:842–847.
88. Kiessling R, Hochman PS, Haller O, Shearer GM, Wigzell H, Cudkowicz G. Evidence for a similar or common mechanism for natural killer activity and resistance to hemopoietic grafts. Eur J Immunol 1977;7:655–663.
89. Hoglund P, Glas R, Ohlen C, Ljunggren HG, Karre K. Alteration of the natural killer repertoire in H-2 transgenic mice: specificity of rapid lymphoma cell clearance determined by the H-2 phenotype of the target. J Exp Med 1991;174:327–334.
90. Ljunggren HG, Karre K. Host resistance directed selectively against H-2-deficient lymphoma variants. J Exp Med 1985;162:1745–1759.
91. Murphy WJ, Kumar V, Bennett M. Rejection of bone marrow allografts by mice with severe combined immune deficiency (SCID). Evidence that natural killer cells can mediate the specificity of marrow graft rejection. J Exp Med 1987;165:1212–1217.
92. Ferrara JLM, Mauch P, van Dijken PJ, Crosier KE, Michaelson J, Burakoff SJ. Evidence that anti-asialo GM1 in vivo improves engraftment of T-cell-depleted bone marrow in hybrid recipients. Transplantation 1990;49:134–137.
93. Gale RP, Feig S, Ho W, Falk P, Rippee C, Sparkes R. ABO blood group system and bone marrow transplantation. Blood 1977;2:185–194.
94. Bensinger WI, Dean Buckner C, Donnall Thomas E, Clift RA. ABO-incompatible marrow transplants. Transplantation 1982;33:427–429.
95. Barge AJ, Johnson G, Witherspoon R, Torok-Storb B. Antibody-mediated marrow failure after allogeneic bone marrow transplantation. Blood 1989;74:1477–1480.
96. Aksentijevich I, Sachs DH, Sykes M. Natural antibodies can inhibit bone marrow engraftment in the rat→mouse species combination. J Immunol 1991;147: 4140–4146.
97. Anasetti C, Amos D, Beatty PG, et al. Effect of HLA compatibility on engraftment of bone marrow transplants in patients with leukemia or lymphoma. N Engl J Med 1989;320:197–204.
98. Billingham RE, Brent L, Medawar PB. "Actively acquired tolerance" of foreign cells. Nature 1953;172: 603–606.
99. Lubaroff DM, Silvers WK. The importance of chimerism in maintaining tolerance of skin allografts in mice. J Immunol 1973;111:65–71.
100. Abramowicz D, Bruyns C, Goldman M. Chimerism and cytotoxic T-lymphocyte unresponsiveness after neonatal injection of spleen cells in mice. Transplantation 1987;44:696–701.
101. Touraine JL. In utero transplantation of stem cells in humans. Nouv Rev Fr Hematol 1990;32:441–444.
102. Heeg K, Wagner H. Analysis of immunological tolerance to major histocompatibility complex antigens. I. High frequencies of tolerogen-specific cytotoxic T-lymphocyte precursors in mice neonatally tolerized to class I major histocompatibility complex antigens. Eur J Immunol 1985;15:25–30.
103. Stockinger B. Cytotoxic T-cell precursors revealed in neonatally tolerant mice. Proc Natl Acad Sci USA 1984;81:220–223.
104. Streilein JW, Gruchalla RS. Analysis of neonatally induced tolerance of H-2 alloantigens: I. Adoptive transfer indicates that tolerance of class I and class II antigens is maintained by distinct mechanisms. Immunogenetics 1981;12:161–165.
105. Nossal GJV, Pike BL. Functional clonal deletion in

immunological tolerance to major histocompatibility complex antigens. Proc Natl Acad Sci USA 1981;78: 3844–3847.
106. McCarthy SA, Bach FH. The cellular mechanism of maintenance of neonatally induced tolerance to H-2 class I antigens. J Immunol 1983;131:1676–1681.
107. Speiser DE, Schneider R, Hengartner H, Macdonald HR, Zinkernagel RM. Clonal deletion of self-reactive T-cells in irradiation bone marrow chimeras and neonatally tolerant mice. Evidence for intercellular transfer of Mls[a]. J Exp Med 1989;170:595–600.
108. Lubaroff DM, Silvers WK. The abolition of tolerance of skin homografts in rats with isoantiserum. J Immunol 1970;104:1236–1241.
109. Sykes M, Sheard M, Sachs DH. Effects of T-cell depletion in radiation bone marrow chimeras. I. Evidence for a donor cell population which increases allogeneic chimerism but which lacks the potential to produce GVHD. J Immunol 1988;141:2282–2288.
110. Ildstad ST, Sachs DH. Reconstitution with syngeneic plus allogeneic or xenogeneic bone marrow leads to specific acceptance of allografts or xenografts. Nature 1984;307:168–170.
111. Ildstad ST, Wren SM, Bluestone JA, Barbieri SA, Sachs DH. Characterization of mixed allogeneic chimeras. Immunocompetence, in vitro reactivity, and genetic specificity of tolerance. J Exp Med 1985;162:231–244.
112. Zinkernagel RM, Callahan GN, Althage A, Cooper S, Klein PA, Klein J. On the thymus in the differentiation of "H-2 self-recognition" by T-cells: evidence for dual recognition? J Exp Med 1978;147:882–896.
113. Zinkernagel RM, Althage A, Callahan G, Welsh RM Jr. On the immunocompetence of H-2 incompatible irradiation bone marrow chimeras. J Immunol 1980;124: 2356–2365.
114. Singer A, Hathcock KS, Hodes RJ. Self recognition in allogeneic radiation chimeras. A radiation host element dictates the self specificity and immune response gene phenotype of T-helper cells. J Exp Med 1981;153: 1286–1301.
115. Bradley SM, Kruisbeek AM, Singer A. Cytotoxic T-lymphocyte response in allogeneic radiation bone marrow chimeras. The chimeric host strictly dictates the self-repertoire of Ia-restricted T-cells but not K/D-restricted T-cells. J Exp Med 1982;156:1650–1656.
116. Geha RS, Rosen FS. The evolution of MHC restrictions in antigen recognition by T-cells in a haploidentical bone marrow transplant recipient. J Immunol 1989; 143:84–88.
117. Chu E, Umetsu D, Rosen FS, Geha RS. Major histocompatibility restriction of antigen recognition by T-cells in a recipient of haplotype mismatched human bone marrow transplantation. J Clin Invest 1983;72:1124–1129.
118. Roncarolo MG, Yssel H, Touraine JL, et al. Antigen recognition by MHC-incompatible cells of a human mismatched chimera. J Exp Med 1988;168:2139–2152.
119. Ruedi E, Sykes M, Ildstad ST, et al. Antiviral T-cell competence and restriction specificity of mixed allogeneic (P1+P2→P1) irradiation chimeras. Cell Immuol 1989;121:185–195.
120. Sykes M, Sheard MA, Sachs DH. Effects of T-cell depletion in radiation bone marrow chimeras II. Requirement for allogeneic T-cells in the reconstituting bone marrow inoculum for subsequent resistance to breaking of tolerance. J Exp Med 1988;168:661–673.
121. Sachs DH, Sharabi Y, Sykes M. Mixed chimerism and transplantation tolerance. In: Melchers F, Albert ED, von Boehmer H, eds. Progress in immunology, vol. VII. Berlin, Heidelberg: Springer-Verlag, 1989:1171.
122. Rapaport FT, Bachvaroff RJ, Akiyama N, Sato T, Ferrebee JW. Specific allogeneic unresponsiveness in irradiated dogs reconstituted with autologous bone marrow. Transplantation 1980;30:23–30.
123. Norin AJ, Emeson EE. Effects of restoring lethally irradiated mice with anti-Thy1.2-treated bone marrow:graft-vs-host, host-vs-graft, and mitogen reactivity. J Immunol 1978;120:754–758.
124. Moses RD, Orr KS, Bacher JD, Sachs DH, Clark RE, Gress RE. Cardiac allograft survival across major histocompatibility barriers in the rhesus monkey following T-cell-depleted autologous marrow transplantation: II. Prolonged allograft survival with extensive marrow T-cell depletion. Transplantation 1989; 47:435–438.
125. Gao EK, Kosaka H, Surh CD, Sprent J. T-cell contact with Ia antigens on nonhematopoietic cells in vivo can lead to immunity rather than tolerance. J Exp Med 1991;174:435–446.
126. Lo D, Burkly LC, Flavell RA, Palmiter RD, Brinster RL. Tolerance in transgenic mice expressing class II major histocompatibility complex on pancreatic acinar cells. J Exp Med 1989;170:87–104.
127. Deeg HJ, Storb R, Thomas ED. Bone marrow transplantation: a review of delayed complications. Br J Haematol 1984;57:185–189.
128. Travis EL, Peters LJ, McNeill J, Thames ED, Karolis C. Effect of dose-rate on total body irradiation: lethality and pathologic findings. Radiother Oncol 1985;4:341–345.
129. Clift RA, Storb R. Histoincompatible bone marrow transplants in humans. Ann Rev Immunol 1987;5:43–64.
130. Sykes M, Chester CH, Sundt TM, Romick ML, Hoyles KA, Sachs DH. Effects of T-cell depletion in radiation bone marrow chimeras: III. Characterization of allogeneic bone marrow cell populations that increase allogeneic chimerism independently of graft-vs-host disease in mixed marrow recipients. J Immunol 1989;143:3503–3511.
131. Pierce GE, Watts LM. Effects of Thy-1+ cell depletion on the capacity of donor lymphoid cells to induce tolerance across an entire MHC disparity in sublethally irradiated adult hosts. Transplantation 1989;48: 289–296.
132. Lapidot T, Lubin I, Terenzi A, Faktorowich Y, Erlich P, Reisner Y. Enhancement of bone marrow allografts from nude mice into mismatched recipients by T-cells void of graft-versus-host activity. Proc Natl Acad Sci USA 1990;87:4595–4599.
133. de Fazio S, Hartner WC, Monaco AP, Gozzo JJ. Mouse skin graft prolongation with donor strain bone marrow and anti-lymphocyte serum: surface markers of the active bone marrow cells. J Immunol 1985;135: 3034–3038.
134. Slavin S. Total lymphoid irradiation. Immunol Today 1987;3:88–92.
135. Pierce GE. Allogeneic versus semiallogeneic F1 bone marrow transplantation into sublethally irradiated MHC-disparate hosts. Effects on mixed lymphoid chimerism, skin graft tolerance, host survival, and alloreactivity. Transplantation 1990;49:138–144.
136. Eto M, Mayumi H, Tomita Y, Yoshikai Y, Nomoto K. Intrathymic clonal deletion of V beta 6+ T-cells in

cyclophosphamide-induced tolerance to H-2-compatible, Mls-disparate antigens. J Exp Med 1990;171:97–113.

137. Mayumi H, Good RA. Long-lasting skin allograft tolerance in adult mice induced across fully allogeneic (multimajor H-2 plus multiminor histocompatibility) antigen barriers by a tolerance-inducing method using cyclophosphamide. J Exp Med 1989;169:213–238.
138. Soderling CCB, Song CW, Blazar BR, Vallera DA. A correlation between conditioning and engraftment in recipients of MHC-mismatched T-cell-depleted murine bone marrow transplants. J Immunol 1985;135: 941–945.
139. Vallera DA, Soderling CCB, Carlson GJ, Kersey JH. Bone marrow transplantation across major histocompatibility barriers in mice. II. T-cell requirement for engraftment in total lymphoid irradiation-conditioned recipients. Transplantation 1982;33:243–248.
140. Slavin S, Strober S, Fuks Z, Kaplan HS. Induction of specific tissue transplantation tolerance using fractionated total lymphoid irradiation in adult mice: long-term survival of allogeneic bone marrow and skin grafts. J Exp Med 1977;146:34–39.
141. Slavin S, Reitz B, Bieber CP, Kaplan HS, Strober S. Transplantation tolerance in adult rats using total lymphoid irradiation: permanent survival of skin, heart, and marrow allografts. J Exp Med 1978;147: 700–707.
142. Sykes M, Sachs DH. Mixed allogeneic chimerism as an approach to transplantation tolerance. Immunol Today 1988;9:23–27.
143. Slavin S, Fuks Z, Kaplan HS, Strober S. Transplantation of allogeneic bone marrow without graft-versus-host disease using total lymphoid irradiation. J Exp Med 1978;147:963–972.
144. Raaf J, Bryan C, Monden M, et al. Bone marrow and renal transplantation in canine recipients prepared by total lymphoid irradiation. Transplant Proc 1981;13: 429–433.
145. Myburgh JA, Smit JA, Hill RRH, Browde S. Transplantation tolerance in primates following total lymphoid irradiation and allogeneic bone marrow injection. II. Renal allografts. Transplantation 1980;29:405–408.
146. Myburgh JA, Smit JA, Hill RRH. Transplantation tolerance in primates following total lymphoid irradiation and allogeneic bone marrow injection. I. Orthotopic liver allografts. Transplantation 1980;29: 401–404.
147. Myburgh JA, Smit JA, Browde S. Transplantation tolerance in the primate following total lymphoid irradiation (TLI) and bone marrow (BM) injection. Transplant Proc 1981;13:434–438.
148. Strober S, Modry DL, Moppe RT, et al. Induction of specific unresponsiveness to heart allografts in mongrel dogs treated with total lymphoid irradiation and anti-thymocyte globulin. J Immunol 1984;132:1013–1018.
149. Strober S, Dhillon M, Schubert M, et al. Acquired immune tolerance to cadaveric renal allografts. A study of three patients treated with total lymphoid irradiation. N Engl J Med 1989;321:28–33.
150. Thomas J, Alqaisi M, Cunningham P, et al. The development of a post-transplant TLI treatment strategy that promotes organ allograft acceptance without chronic immunosuppression. Transplantation 1992; 53:247–258.
151. Pierce GE, Watts LM. The role of donor lymphoid cells in the transfer of allograft tolerance. Transplantation 1985;40:702–707.
152. Tomita Y, Nishimura Y, Harada N, et al. Evidence for involvement of clonal anergy in MHC class I and class II disparate skin allograft tolerance after the termination of intrathymic clonal deletion. J Immunol 1990;145:4026–4036.
153. Lapidot T, Terenzi A, Singer TS, Salomon O, Reisner Y. Enhancement by dimethyl myleran of donor type chimerism in murine recipients of bone marrow allografts. Blood 1989;73:2025–2032.
154. Wood ML, Monaco AP, Gozzo JJ, Liegois A. Use of homozygous allogeneic bone marrow for induction of tolerance with anti-lymphocyte serum: dose and timing. Transplant Proc 1970;3:676–678.
155. Liegeois A, Escourrou J, Ouvre E, Charriere J. Microchimerism: a stable state of low-ratio proliferation of allogeneic bone marrow. Transplant Proc 1977;9: 273–276.
156. Thomas J, Carver FM, Cunningham P, Park K, Gonder J, Thomas F. Promotion of incompatible allograft acceptance in rhesus monkeys given posttransplant antithymocyte globulin and donor bone marrow. Transplantation 1987;43:332–338.
157. Hartner WC, De Fazio SR, Maki T, Markees TG, Monaco AP, Gozzo JJ. Prolongation of renal allograft survival in antilymphocyte-serum-treated dogs by postoperative injection of density-gradient-fractionated bone marrow. Transplantation 1986;42:593–597.
158. Thomas JM, Carver FM, Cunningham PRG, Olson LC, Thomas FT. Kidney allograft tolerance in primates without chronic immunosuppression: the role of veto cells. Transplantation 1991;51:198–207.
159. Sharabi Y, Abraham VS, Sykes M, Sachs DH. Mixed allogeneic chimeras prepared by a non-myeloablative regimen: requirement for chimerism to maintain tolerance. Bone Marrow Transplant 1992:9:191–199.
160. Ghobrial RR, Boublik M, Winn HJ, Auchincloss H Jr. In vivo use of monoclonal antibodies against murine T-cell antigens. Clin Immunol Immunopathol 1989;52: 486–506.
161. Poynton CH. T-cell depletion in bone marrow transplantation. Bone Marrow Transplant 1988;3: 265–279.
162. Butturini A, Gale RP. T-cell depletion in bone marrow transplantation for leukemia: current results and future directions. Bone Marrow Transplant 1988;3: 265–279.
163. Martin PJ, Hansen JA, Torok-Storb B, et al. Graft failure in patients receiving T-cell-depleted HLA-identical allogeneic marrow transplants. Bone Marrow Transplant 1988;3:445–456.
164. Palathumpat V, Dejbakhsh-Jones S, Holm B, Strober S. Studies of CD4- CD8- alpha-beta bone marrow T-cells with suppressor activity. J Immunol 1992;148: 373–379.
165. Ildstad ST, Wren SM, Bluestone JA, Barbieri SA, Stephany D, Sachs DH. Effect of selective T-cell depletion of host and/or donor bone marrow on lymphopoietic repopulation, tolerance, and graft-vs-host disease in mixed allogeneic chimeras (B10 + B10.D2→B10). J Immunol 1986;136:28–33.
166. Sykes M, Chester CH, Sachs DH. Protection from graft-versus-host disease in fully allogeneic chimeras by prior administration of T-cell-depleted syngeneic bone marrow. Transplantation 1988;46:327–330.
167. Strober S, Palathumpat V, Schwadron R, Hertel-Wulff

B. Cloned natural suppressor cells prevent lethal graft-vs-host disease. J Immunol 1987;138:699–703.
168. Van Vlasselaer P, Niki T, Strober S. Identification of a factor(s) from cloned murine natural suppressor cells that inhibits IL-2 secretion during antigen driven T-cell activation. Cell Immunol 1991;138:326.
169. Sykes M, Romick ML, Hoyles KA, Sachs DH. In vivo administration of interleukin 2 plus T-cell-depleted syngeneic marrow prevents graft-versus-host disease mortality and permits alloengraftment. J Exp Med 1990;171:645–658.
170. Sykes M, Romick ML, Sachs DH. Interleukin 2 prevents graft-vs-host disease without diminishing the graft-vs-leukemia effect of allogeneic lymphocytes. Proc Natl Acad Sci USA 1990;87:5633–5637.
171. Pietryga D, Blazar BR, Soderling CB, Vallera DA. The effect of T subset depletion on the incidence of lethal graft-versus-host disease in a murine major histocompatibility complex-mismatched transplantation system. Transplantation 1987;43:442–445.
172. Korngold R, Sprent J. Surface markers of T-cells causing lethal graft-vs-host disease to class I vs class II H-2 differences. J Immunol 1985;135:3004–3010.
173. Vallera DA, Soderling CCB, Kersey JH, et al. Bone marrow transplantation across major histocompatibility barriers in mice. III. Treatment of donor grafts with monoclonal antibodies directed against Lyt determinants. J Immunol 1982;128:871–875.
174. Uenaka A, Mieno M, Kuribayashi K, Shiku H, Nakayama E. Effector cells of lethal graft-versus-host disease (GVHD) in nude mice. Transplant Proc 1989;21:3031–3032.
175. Sykes M, Abraham VS, Harty MW, Pearson DA. IL-2 reduces graft-versus-host disease and preserves a graft-versus leukemia effect by selectively inhibiting $CD4^+$ T cell activity. J Immunol 1993;150:197–205.
176. Sykes M, Abraham VS. Mechanism of IL-2-mediated protection against GVHD in mice: II. Protection occurs independently of NK/LAK cells. Transplantation 1992; 53:1063–1070.
177. Abraham VS, Sachs DH, Sykes M. The mechanism of protection from GVHD mortality by IL-2: III. Early reductions in donor T-cell subsets and expansion of a CD3+CD4−CD8− cell population. J Immunol 1992; 148:3746–3752.
178. Morecki S, Leshem B, Weigensberg M, Bar S, Slavin S. Functional clonal deletion versus active suppression in transplantation tolerance induced by total lymphoid irradiation. Transplantation 1985;40:201–210.
179. Morecki S, Leshem B, Eid A, Slavin S. Alloantigen persistence in induction and maintenance of transplantation tolerance. J Exp Med 1987;165:1468–1480.
180. Sprent J, Gao E-K, Webb SR. T-cell reactivity to MHC molecules: immunity versus tolerance. Science 1990; 248:1357–1363.
181. Gao E-K, Lo D, Cheney R, Kanagawa O, Sprent J. Abnormal differentiation of thymocytes in mice treated with cyclosporin A. Nature 1988;336:176–179.
182. Beschorner WE, Hess AD, Shinn CA, Santos GW. Transfer of cyclosporine-associated syngeneic graft-versus-host disease by thymocytes. Resemblance to chronic graft-versus-host disease. Transplantation 1988;45:209–215.
183. Parkman R. Clonal analysis of murine graft-vs-host disease. I. Phenotypic and functional analysis of T-lymphocyte clones. J Immunol 1986;136:3543–3548.
184. Parkman R. Graft-versus-host disease: an alternative hypothesis. Immunol Today 1989;10:362–364.
185. Rosenkrantz K, Keever C, Kirsch J, et al. In vitro correlates of graft-host tolerance after HLA-matched and mismatched marrow transplants: suggestions from limiting dilution analysis. Transplant Proc 1987;19(suppl 7):98–103.
186. Lapp WS, Ghayur T, Mendes M, Seddik M, Seemayer TA. The functional and histological basis for graft-versus-host-induced immunosuppression. Immunol Rev 1985;88:107–131.
187. Seddick M, Seemayer TA, Lapp WS. T-cell functional defect associated with thymic epithelial injury induced by a graft-versus-host reaction. Transplantation 1980;129:61–66.
188. De Villartay J-P, Griscelli C, Fischer A. Self-tolerance to host and donor following HLA-mismatched bone marrow transplantation. Eur J Immunol 1986;16:117–122.
189. Auchincloss H Jr, Sachs DH. Mechanism of tolerance in murine radiation bone marrow chimeras. Transplantation 1983;36:436–441.
190. Tsoi M-S, Storb R, Dobbs S, Thomas ED. Specific suppressor cells in graft-host tolerance of HLA-identical marrow transplantation. Nature 1981;292: 355–357.
191. Sykes M, Sheard MA, Sachs DH. Graft-versus-host-related immunosuppression is induced in mixed chimeras by alloresponses against either host or donor lymphohematopoietic cells. J Exp Med 1988;168: 2391–2396.
192. Kolb HJ, Mittrmuller J, Clemm CH, et al. Donor leukocyte transfusions for treatment of recurrent chronic myelogenous leukemia in marrow transplant patients. Blood 1990;76:2462–2465.
193. Sykes M, Sachs DH, Nienhuis AW, Pearson DA, Moulton AD, Bodine DM. Specific prolongation of skin graft survival following retroviral transduction of bone marrow with an allogeneic major histocompatibility complex gene. Transplantation 1993;55:197–202.
194. Shafer GW, Emery DW, Gustafsson K, et al. Expression of a swine class II gene in murine bone marrow hematopoietic stem cells by retroviral-mediated gene transfer. Proc Natl Acad Sci USA 1991;88:9760–9764.

Chapter 18
Murine Models for Graft-versus-Host Disease

Jonathan Sprent and Robert Korngold

Graft-versus-host disease (GVHD) is a manifestation of alloreactivity and occurs when mature T cells are transferred to hosts expressing histocompatibility (H) differences (1–3). Before discussing the pathogenesis of GVHD and the cell types involved, it is important to consider the essential features of T-cell specificity and T-effector function.

The specificity of typical T cells expressing $\alpha\beta$ T-cell receptor (TCR) molecules is directed to peptide fragments of antigen bound to major histocompatibility complex (MHC) molecules, human leukocyte antigen (HLA) molecules in humans, and H-2 molecules in the mouse (4–9). As the result of a complex process of selection in the thymus, $\alpha\beta^+$ T cells are rendered tolerant to "self" MHC molecules (plus the various endogenous peptides bound to these molecules) but display reactivity to self MHC molecules complexed to foreign peptides (8,9). Minor H antigens—one of the principal targets for GVHD—fall into this category. T-cell specificity also encompasses reactivity to allo- (foreign, non-self) MHC molecules (4). GVHD to MHC alloantigens is intense and reflects that the precursor frequency of T cells for allo-MHC antigens is very high, far higher than for typical foreign peptide antigens complexed to self MHC molecules. Although both classes of antigens can be recognized by the same TCR molecule, the biological significance of MHC alloreactivity is poorly understood. In particular, it is still unclear whether alloreactivity is directed to MHC epitopes, MHC-associated peptides, or both.

There are two classes of MHC molecules, termed class I and class II (4,7). Class I molecules are expressed on virtually all cells and are recognized by the $CD8^+$ subset of T cells. Class II molecules show a more restricted tissue distribution and are recognized by $CD4^+$ T cells. The CD4 and CD8 molecules, which define the two major subsets of T cells, act as adhesion molecules and bind to nonpolymorphic regions of MHC class II and class I molecules, respectively (6). Such binding increases the avidity of TCR/MHC interaction and causes each T-cell subset to display MHC class specificity. Thus, the $CD8^+$ subset of T cells reacts much more effectively with class I than class II MHC molecules, whereas $CD4^+$ cells show the reverse specificity. As discussed later, this MHC class specificity of $CD4^+$ and $CD8^+$ cells applies to GVHD.

In the case of unprimed cells, T-cell activation depends on contact with MHC-associated peptides (or MHC alloantigens) expressed on specialized antigen-presenting cells (APCs) such as macrophages and dendritic cells (4,8); these cells reside in the T-dependent areas of the lymphoid tissues (i.e., the periarteriolar lymphocyte sheaths of the splenic white pulp and the paracortical areas of lymph nodes). Recognition of antigen in these sites also applies when T cells are transferred to allogeneic hosts, where the T cells encounter host alloantigens expressed constitutively on host APCs in the T-dependent areas of the recipient. After contact with antigen on APCs, T cells proliferate extensively, release various lymphokines, and differentiate into T-effector cells; in allogeneic hosts, this chain of events constitutes a GVH reaction (which may or may not progress to overt GVHD). Whereas resting T cells are confined to the recirculating lymphocyte pool (blood, lymphoid tissues, and lymph), antigen-activated T cells have the capacity to penetrate the walls of capillary blood vessels and can thus disseminate throughout the body. Activated T cells show a particular propensity for homing to the gut, liver, lung, and skin; as discussed later, these sites are commonly affected by GVHD. When activated T cells re-encounter antigen in these sites, the cells express various effector functions.

The effector functions of T cells are complex and difficult to categorize (4). Direct destruction of target cells by cytotoxic T lymphocytes (CTLs) is the simplest type of effector function and is probably a major cause of the protean pathology seen in GVHD. Other T cells have limited CTL activity but, after re-encountering antigen on local APCs in the tissue concerned, are able to release large quantities of various lymphokines. By attracting a spectrum of mononuclear cells from the blood and also by causing direct tissue destruction (in the case of toxic lymphokines such as tumor necrosis factor-alpha [TNF-α]), these lymphokines elicit the typical lesions seen in delayed-type hypersensitivity (DTH). In many textbooks it is stated that the effector functions of $CD4^+$ and $CD8^+$ cells are quite distinct, with $CD8^+$ cells functioning as CTL and $CD4^+$ cells accounting for DTH. This is an oversimplification, however, because some $CD8^+$ cells can release lymphokines and cause DTH and some $CD4^+$ cells exhibit CTL activity (4).

Target Antigens for GVHD

As mentioned earlier, GVHD is directed to two broad categories of histocompatibility alloantigens: major (MHC) antigens and minor antigens. These antigens also provide the main targets for allograft rejection. Because of the availability of congeneic strains, mice are the species of choice for studying GVHD directed to major versus minor histocompatibility antigens and for determining the relative contributions of $CD4^+$ and $CD8^+$ cells to GVHD. Before discussing the various models for murine GVHD, it is important to consider the issue of host resistance to GVHD.

Susceptibility to GVHD: the Problem of Host-versus-Graft Reactions

GVHD is not an inevitable consequence of transferring T cells across histocompatibility barriers. Thus, injecting normal adult mice with even large doses of allogeneic lymphoid cells generally causes no pathology; the host mouse mounts a powerful response to the donor alloantigens and the injected T cells are rapidly destroyed. Host-versus-graft (HVG) reactions involve three cell types: T cells, B cells, and natural killer (NK) cells (10–13). HVG reactions mediated by T and B cells take several days to develop and cause graft rejection by a combination of CTL activity and production of alloantibody. In adult mice, the simplest approach for inactivating host T and B cells is to expose the host to total body irradiation (TBI), because resting T and B cells are highly radiosensitive.

HVG reactions mediated by NK cells are often intense and occur within hours of donor cell transfer (11,12). The target antigens for NK cells are still poorly defined, but there is accumulating evidence that the specificity of NK cells participating in HVG reactions is directed to cells that lack self class I molecules (13). NK-mediated HVG reactions do not apply when H-2-heterozygous $(a \times b)F_1$ cells are transferred to homozygous strain *a* mice because the host strain *a* class I molecules are fully represented on the donor cells. In this situation, HVG reactions are mediated solely by alloreactive T and B cells. A different situation applies in $a \rightarrow b$, $a \rightarrow (a \times b)F_1$ and $(a \times b)F_1 \rightarrow (a \times c)F_1$ combinations. In each of these combinations, the donor cells do not express the *complete* set of class I molecules of the host. For example, in the $a \rightarrow (a \times b)F_1$ combination, the host NK cells recognize self class I^a on the donor cells but do not see self class I^b: The failure to recognize self class I^b on the donor cells causes the F_1 hosts to display "hybrid resistance," and their NK cells reject the parental strain cells. Similar lack of self class I recognition applies in $a \rightarrow b$ and $(a \times b)F_1 \rightarrow (a \times c)F_1$ combinations; the GVH reaction by the host NK cells is termed *allogeneic resistance* (14). In the case of parent $\rightarrow F_1$ combinations, the intensity of hybrid resistance varies considerably according to the particular class I disparity involved. In practice, hybrid resistance is only a problem when there is heterozygosity for the H-$2D^b$ class I molecule (e.g., when C57BL [K^bD^b] cells are transferred to [C57BL × CBA (K^kD^k)]F_1 hosts).

NK-mediated HVG reactions are especially strong in H-2 different $a \rightarrow b$ combinations. Inactivation of NK cells in situ is not easy because these cells are highly radioresistant; injection of anti-NK antibodies can be effective, but this is a cumbersome and expensive procedure. In practice, there are a number of ways to work around the problem of NK-mediated HVG reactions. For example, if it is essential to use fully H-2-different $a \rightarrow b$ combinations, the activity of host NK cells can usually be overcome simply by injecting the donor lymphoid cells in large doses. The easiest solution, however, is to use $a \rightarrow (a \times b)F_1$ combinations; as mentioned, hybrid resistance in parent $\rightarrow F_1$ combinations is generally insignificant unless H-$2D^b$ heterozygosity is involved. NK-mediated HVG reactions do not operate in minor histocompatibility-different combinations; the donor and the host are H-2–identical.

In a clinical setting, the GVHD seen after bone marrow transplantation (BMT) is often complicated by concomitant HVG reactions, especially if the host has been presensitized to the donor as the result of blood transfusion. In the case of MHC-incompatible strain combinations, the mouse models outlined herein are deliberately designed to avoid the problem of HVG reactions by (1) using nonimmunized F_1 hybrid mice as hosts for parental strain T cells, (2) avoiding H-$2D^b$ heterozygosity, and (3) exposing the host mice to TBI. With this protocol, one can examine "pure" GVHD with little or no interference from host T, B, or NK cells. All the models discussed involve intravenous transfer of cells.

GVHD Directed to MHC Antigens

Because of the high precursor frequency of T cells for allo-MHC antigens, these antigens elicit a very intense form of GVHD (3,15–20). Thus, transfer of even small numbers of parental strain T cells ($<10^5$) into irradiated F_1 mice leads to a high incidence of lethal GVHD. GVHD is especially severe when the host expresses combined H-2 class I and II differences. GVHD directed to whole H-2 differences involves both $CD4^+$ and $CD8^+$ cells, and either population alone is able to induce lethal GVHD (16–19). Assessing the relative importance of class I versus class II antigens as targets for GVHD necessitates using donor/host combinations differing solely at class I or II loci.

GVHD to H-2 Class II Antigens

Most mouse strains express two types of class II molecules: I-A and I-E. These molecules are the homologues of HLA-DQ and HLA-DR molecules, respectively. I-E alloantigens are much less immunogenic than I-A antigens, and GVHD directed selectively to I-E antigens tends to be weak and is generally nonlethal. I-A antigens, in contrast, are highly potent inducers of lethal GVHD. To study GVHD directed selectively to I-A antigens, the most convenient combination is C57BL/6 (B6) and B6.C-H-2^{bm12} (bm12) (17). These two strains are identical except for three amino acid differences in the β-chain of the I-A molecule. Although seemingly small, this mutation is highly immunogenic for T cells. Indeed, the response of B6 T cells to bm12 and vice versa is as strong as with an allelic (nonmutant) I-A difference (21).

The key feature of GVHD developing in the B6/bm12 combination is that GVHD induction is strictly controlled by $CD4^+$ cells, with little or no contribution from $CD8^+$ cells (17,22). Thus, whereas small numbers of B6 (or bm12) $CD4^+$ cells cause close to 100% mortality in irradiated (B6 × bm12)F_1 hosts under defined conditions, even high doses of B6 (or bm12) $CD8^+$ cells cause no mortality (provided that the $CD8^+$ cells are thoroughly depleted of $CD4^+$ cells). The failure of $CD8^+$ cells to mediate anti-class II GVHD is to be expected because, as mentioned earlier, the specificity of $CD8^+$ cells is strongly skewed to recognition of class I antigens. Proliferative responses of purified B6 $CD8^+$ cells to bm12 APCs are extremely weak, both in vivo and in vitro (21).

When B6 $CD4^+$ cells are transferred to irradiated (B6 × bm12)F_1 mice, the donor T cells initially home to the T-dependent areas of the spleen and the lymph nodes. The T cells respond to host class II antigens expressed on host APCs (typical APCs are highly radioresistant) and then mount a powerful proliferative response (17). Large numbers of donor-derived blast cells enter the circulation and then percolate throughout the body to reach the skin, gut, liver, among other sites, where the cells mediate their effector functions. The type of GVHD that results from this GVH reaction depends critically on a number of different factors, including (1) the dose of TBI used to condition the host, (2) the dose of $CD4^+$ cells injected, and (3) the source of marrow cells (donor or host) used for reconstitution (22).

Donor Marrow Plus Donor $CD4^+$ Cells

The simplest model for GVHD is to inject the F_1 host mice with a mixture of donor $CD4^+$ cells and donor marrow cells (22); under these conditions, the donor $CD4^+$ cells selectively attack the host and do not impair stem-cell reconstitution. The severity of GVHD in this situation is quite variable and seems to be a reflection of the general health of the animal colony. If the mice are in excellent health and free from infection, GVHD tends to be quite mild when the conditioning dose of TBI is not more than 800 cGy (Table 18-1). Mortality rates are low and, except for transient splenomegaly, the mice show minimal pathology. Raising the dose of TBI to 1,000 cGy, however, leads to acute GVHD and heavy mortality; most deaths occur within 2 weeks of T-cell injection (see Table 18-1). This acute pattern of GVHD is characterized by marked weight loss, mild atrophy of the lymphohemopoietic system, and a distended small intestine. Exudative enteropathy is apparent, and death is probably largely a reflection of gut damage leading to dehydration and acute infection (20,23,24). Toxic lymphokines have a key role in gut damage, which is apparent from the finding that mice can be protected against gut damage (and death) by injecting anti-TNF-α antibodies (25).

Induction of acute lethal GVHD in heavily irradiated recipients requires surprisingly few $CD4^+$ cells (see Table 18-1). Doses of 1×10^5 $CD4^+$ cells elicit close to 100% mortality and even 1×10^4 cells cause significant mortality. This effect applies to "clean" mice. If the health of the colony is suboptimal, acute lethal GVHD is seen with much lower doses of TBI (e.g., 700 cGy).

Chronic GVHD tends to be sporadic in this model and is generally seen only when very low numbers of $CD4^+$ cells are transferred. With higher numbers of

Table 18-1.
Mortality in Irradiated (B6 × bm12)F_1 Mice Given B6 Marrow Cells Plus Varying Doses of B6 $CD4^+$ cells[a]

Cells Transferred with B6 Marrow	*No. Cells*	*No. Mice*	*% Mortality*	*MST (days)*
		Hosts given 1,000 cGy		
B6 $CD4^+$	2×10^7	29	38	>100
	5×10^6	8	63	25
	3×10^6	15	93	13
	1×10^6	40	100	9
	3×10^5	20	95	13
	1×10^5	15	100	16
	1×10^4	13	54	77
	1×10^3	7	29	>100
	BM only	24	4	>100
B6 $CD8^+$	1×10^7	15	0	>100
	1×10^6	10	5	>100
B6 spleen	1×10^8	45	10	>100
		Hosts given 800 cGy		
B6 $CD4^+$	1×10^7	8	0	>100
	5×10^6	16	0	>100
	3×10^6	13	38	>100
	1×10^6	8	13	>100
	3×10^5	24	8	>100

[a]The data show pooled results of 9 separate experiments (6 for mice given 1,000 cGy and 3 for mice given 800 cGy). Cells were injected intravenously together with 2×10^6 T-cell–depleted B6 BM cells (except for spleen cells where marrow cells were omitted). T-cell subsets were purified from pooled lymph node cells. To prevent unnecessary suffering, mice unable to take food or water were killed.
MST = median survival time.
Data from Sprent J, Schaefer M, Korngold R. Role of T-cell subsets in lethal graft-versus-host disease (GVHD) directed to class I versus class II H-2 differences. II. Protective effects of L3T4+ cells in anti-class II H-2 differences. J Immunol 1990;144:2946–2954.

$CD4^+$ cells, the few mice that survive acute GVHD generally show rapid recovery. When chronic GVHD is seen, the hosts show prolonged weight loss, lymphoid atrophy, and evidence of infection. Skin lesions are rare.

Donor Marrow Plus High Doses of Donor $CD4^+$ Cells

The acute lethal GVHD seen in heavily irradiated recipients applies when the donor $CD4^+$ cells are injected in the range of 3×10^6 cells to 1×10^4 cells (22). Injection of higher doses of $CD4^+$ cells paradoxically leads to protection. Thus, whereas doses of 1×10^6 $CD4^+$ cells generally cause close to 100% mortality, increasing the number of $CD4^+$ cells to 2×10^7 reduces the mortality rate to less than 40% (22) (see Table 18-1). Even lower mortality rates occur when bulk populations of $CD4^+$ cells and B cells are injected. Thus, if 1,000 cGy–irradiated (B6 × bm12)F_1 mice are injected with a dose of 1×10^8 unseparated B6 spleen cells (a mixture of $CD4^+$ cells, $CD8^+$ cells, B cells, and stem cells), mortality rates are less than 10% (see Table 18-1). In considering the mechanism of this protection, it should be pointed out that mice kept under "germ-free" conditions are relatively resistant to lethal GVHD (26). It is quite likely therefore that lethal GVHD is largely a consequence of infection; the tissue damage elicited by the GVH reaction makes the host susceptible to invasion by pathogens. The capacity of large doses of $CD4^+$ cells and B cells to protect against mortality could thus be attributed to restoration of immunocompetence. Cellular and humoral immunity are restored, and the host repels pathogens entering through damaged mucosal surfaces. According to this interpretation, bulk populations of donor lymphoid cells do not limit the *intensity* of the initial GVH reaction but merely counteract the *consequences* of this reaction. The bm12 F_1 recipients of bulk populations of donor B6 lymphoid cells do go through a "crisis" approximately 2 weeks after transfer (hunched posture and lethargy) but then progress to full recovery.

Host Marrow and Donor $CD4^+$ Cells

A very different pattern of GVHD occurs when donor $CD4^+$ cells are transferred with host rather than donor marrow cells (20,22) (Table 18-2). In this situation, the donor $CD4^+$ cells attack the F_1 host stem cells and cause death from hemopoietic failure within 3 weeks; stem-cell engraftment is apparent one week after transfer, but by day 14 the entire lymphohemopoietic system, including the marrow, shows near-total aplasia. Mortality rates approach 100% and are little influenced by either the dose of $CD4^+$ cells injected (1×10^5 to 2×10^7) or the conditioning dose of TBI used (600–1,000 cGy). Even with a low dose of 600 cGy, as few as 10^5 $CD4^+$ cells cause close to 100% mortality.

It should be emphasized that the above syndrome of lethal marrow aplasia does not occur when the donor $CD4^+$ cells are transferred with a *mixture* of donor and host BM because the $CD4^+$ cells attack the host stem cells but do not prevent engraftment of the donor cells. Because semipurified $CD4^+$ cells are often contaminated with stem cells, especially when derived from spleen cells, demonstrating marrow aplasia mediated by $CD4^+$ cells depends critically on using a highly purified population of these cells. Lymph nodes are the best starting population for preparing stem-cell-free $CD4^+$ cells.

Table 18-2.
Death from Marrow Aplasia in Lightly Irradiated (B6 × bm12)F_1 Mice Given B6 $CD4^+$ Cells Plus Host Marrow Cells[a]

Origin of Marrow Cells Transferred with 2×10^6 B6 $CD4^+$ Cells	*Irradiation (cGy)*	*No. Mice*	*% Mortality*	*MST (days)*	*Aplasia in Host Marrow at Day 14*
B6	1,000	10	100	11	
F_1	1,000	10	100	12	
B6 + F_1	1,000	10	100	10	
B6	800	8	0	>100	+/−[b]
F_1	800	10	100	15	++++[c]
B6 + F_1	800	10	0	>100	+/−
B6	600	8	0	>100	+/−
F_1	600	10	100	18	++++
B6 + F_1	600	8	0	>100	+/−
	600	5	100	18	++++

[a]See Table 18-1; data are pooled from 2 separate experiments. Marrow cells were given in a dose of 2×10^6/mouse (or 2×10^6 of each marrow population when a mixture of marrow was injected). No deaths were observed in control groups given irradiation plus marrow alone (or in mice given 600 cGy without marrow).
[b]Minimal or no aplasia (reduction in marrow counts) in tibiae relative to mice given marrow cells alone.
[c]Marked (>90% aplasia) relative to marrow-only control animals.
MST = median survival time.
Data from Sprent J, Schaefer M, Korngold R. Role of T-cell subsets in lethal graft-versus-host disease (GVHD) directed to class I versus class II H-2 differences. II. Protective effects of $L3T4^+$ cells in anti-class II H-2 differences. J Immunol 1990;144:2946–2954.

GVHD to H-2 Class I Antigens

As for class II molecules, mice express two class I molecules, H-2K and H-2D. Both types of molecules are potent targets for lethal GVHD. Although a number of class I-different, class II-identical strain combinations are available, the simplest approach for studying anti-class I GVHD is to use class I mutant mice (e.g., the series of "bm" mutant mice) (27). On the basis of skin graft rejection, investigators have isolated more than a dozen different bm mutant strains of mice exhibiting small mutations (1–4 amino acid substitutions) of the H-2K molecules of the B6 ($H\text{-}2^b$) strain. The immunogenicity of these mutant molecules for "wild-type" B6 T cells is quite variable. Some mutants (e.g., bm1) are strongly stimulatory, whereas others (e.g., bm9) elicit only low responses (21). This finding applies to proliferative and CTL responses generated in vitro. Detailed information on the capacity of the various class I mutants to elicit GVHD is not yet available. The data discussed apply to the B6 → bm1 combination, using (B6 × bm1)F_1 mice as hosts.

Despite the dogma that $CD8^+$ cells function poorly without exogenous help, purified B6 $CD8^+$ cells give spectacularly high proliferative and CTL responses to bm1 stimulators in vitro in the absence of $CD4^+$ cells or their products (21). Helper-independent responses of $CD8^+$ cells also apply in vivo (17,21). Thus, when purified B6 $CD8^+$ cells are transferred to irradiated bm1 F_1 mice, the donor cells proliferate extensively in the lymphoid tissues in the absence of $CD4^+$ cells and then disseminate throughout the body to mediate their effector functions. The end result is GVHD. B6 $CD4^+$ cells respond very poorly to bm1, and even large doses of B6 $CD4^+$ cells fail to elicit GVHD in bm1 F_1 hosts (28).

Donor Marrow Plus Donor $CD8^+$ Cells

In the class II-different combination of B6 and bm12, as mentioned, B6 $CD4^+$ cells plus donor marrow fail to cause lethal GVHD in clean mice unless the hosts receive heavy irradiation. This is not the case with $CD8^+$ cells in the class I-different B6/bm1 combination. Injecting irradiated (B6 × bm1)F_1 hosts with B6 $CD8^+$ cells plus B6 marrow cells causes heavy mortality regardless of whether the hosts are conditioned with heavy (1,000 cGy) or light irradiation (600 cGy) (28) (Table 18-3). Mortality rates approaching 100% are seen with a wide range of T-cell numbers (i.e., from 2×10^7 to 1×10^5 cells). The striking finding is that GVHD tends to be chronic rather than acute. Except for mild weight loss, most of the recipients appear reasonably healthy for the first 3 to 4 weeks after transfer. Then, often quite suddenly, the mice become obviously ill with hunched posture, diarrhea, and marked weight loss. The condition of the mice worsens progressively and death occurs approximately 5 to 8 weeks after transfer. At autopsy, the mice show the typical signs of chronic GVHD with marked weight loss, lymphohemopoietic atrophy, and lymphocytic infiltrations in various organs. Skin lesions can be severe, although this finding is variable. Gut damage is evident, but is much less severe than in class II-different combinations (23,24).

Effects of Adding $CD4^+$ Cells

Despite the evidence that $CD8^+$ cells mediate helper-independent responses in vitro, it could be argued that GVHD elicited to class I antigens in vivo reflects help from radioresistant host $CD4^+$ cells. This does not seem to be the case, however, because purified $CD8^+$ cells cause lethal GVHD in hosts given multiple injections of anti-CD4 antibody (28). Nevertheless, supplementing the injected $CD8^+$ cells with small doses of donor $CD4^+$ cells causes a marked alteration in the pattern of GVHD; instead of progressive chronic GVHD, acute GVHD develops in the hosts and they die 2 to 3 weeks after transfer. This finding implies that although $CD8^+$ cells function well in the absence of exogenous help in vivo, adding help significantly increases their potency.

The capacity of $CD4^+$ cells to augment GVHD

Table 18-3.
Mortality in Irradiated (B6 × bm1)F_1 Mice Given B6 $CD8^+$ Cells Plus B6 Marrow Cells

Cells Transferred with B6 Marrow Cells	*Dose of Irradiation (cGy)*	*No. Cells Injected*	*No. Mice*	*% Mortality*	*MST (days)*
B6 $CD8^+$	1000	1×10^7	16	100	33
	1000	1×10^6	22	100	35
	1000	1×10^5	16	88	52
	600	5×10^6	8	100	33
	600	2.5×10^5	8	100	33
B6 spleen	1000	1×10^8	30	10	>100
B6 $CD4^+$	1000	1×10^7	12	0	>100
		1×10^6	25	4	>100
Marrow only	1000	—	60	5	>100

[a]See Table 18-1; data from 12 different experiments.
Data from Sprent J, Schaefer M, Gao E-K, Korngold R. Role of T-cell subsets in lethal graft-versus-host disease (GVHD) directed to class I versus class II H-2 differences. I. $L3T4^+$ cells can either augment or retard GVHD elicited by lyt-2^+ cells in class I-different hosts. J Exp Med 1988;167:556–569. MST = median survival time.

elicited by $CD8^+$ cells only applies when $CD4^+$ cells are injected in small numbers ($\leq 1 \times 10^6$). When high numbers of $CD4^+$ cells are transferred, marked protection occurs (28). Thus, if an inoculum of 2×10^6 B6 $CD8^+$ cells is supplemented with 2×10^7 B6 $CD4^+$ cells, death rates in irradiated (B6 × bm1)F_1 hosts drop from 100 to 0%. Mortality rates are also very low when a large dose of 1×10^8 unseparated B6 spleen cells is transferred (see Table 18-3). As for the B6 → bm12 combination, the protective effects of large doses of $CD4^+$ cells in the B6 → bm1 combinations is probably a reflection of restoration of immunocompetence.

Host Marrow Plus Donor $CD8^+$ Cells

Like $CD4^+$ cells in the B6 → bm12 combination, B6 $CD8^+$ cells cause marked aplasia in bm1 hosts when transferred with host rather than donor marrow cells (28). In the absence of donor marrow, profound marrow aplasia rapidly develops—presumably reflecting direct stem-cell attack by CTL—and the mice die within 2 weeks. With a mixture of donor and host marrow cells, hemopoietic failure is avoided and the hosts show the typical pattern of progressive chronic GVHD discussed.

GVHD in Nonirradiated Hosts

All of the patterns of anti-class II and anti-class I GVHD discussed refer to experiments with irradiated hosts. What happens when nonirradiated hosts are used? The results vary according to the age of the recipients.

If *neonatal* F_1 hosts are used, a lethal form of GVHD, characterized by prominent lymphocytic infiltrations in various organs, especially the liver, and enlargement of the spleen, develops in recipients of parental strain T cells (17,29). Splenomegaly is most pronounced at approximately 10 days after injection, and measuring the size of the spleen in neonates has long been a popular model for assessing the severity of GVHD (29). Induction of splenomegaly is usually attributed to the action of $CD4^+$ cells, but, at least in the B6 → bm1 combination, purified $CD8^+$ cells cause prominent spleen enlargement (17). With large doses of T cells, the host mice usually die after a period of 2 to 3 weeks; this applies to both $CD4^+$ and $CD8^+$ cells.

When nonirradiated *adult* mice are used as hosts, two distinct patterns of GVHD are seen (30,31). When GVHD is directed solely to class II MHC antigens (e.g., when purified B6 $CD4^+$ cells are transferred to nonirradiated [B6 × bm12]F_1 mice), a chronic "proliferative" form of sublethal GVHD associated with splenomegaly and prominent autoantibody production develops. In this situation, the donor $CD4^+$ cells mount a prolonged response against host class II antigens and release large quantities of lymphokines. Autoantibody production is presumed to be a reflection of aberrant T-B interaction: The donor $CD4^+$ cells respond to the alloantigens on the host B cells and drive the B cells to undergo polyclonal activation. This proliferative type of nonlethal GVHD is also seen when purified $CD4^+$ cells are transferred across whole MHC barriers (32).

A quite different type of GVHD occurs when unseparated T cells are transferred to nonirradiated hosts expressing combined class I plus II differences (e.g., when B6 T cells are transferred to [bm1 × bm12]F_1 mice) (30). The GVH reaction involves both $CD4^+$ and $CD8^+$ cells. In the early stage of this reaction, the host mice exhibit the proliferative form of GVHD discussed. After a few weeks, however, lymphoproliferation is succeeded by a phase of progressive chronic GVHD associated with lymphoid aplasia; many of the recipients eventually die. Although this aplastic form of GVHD is known to require the presence of donor $CD8^+$ cells, the chain of events that leads to aplasia is still poorly understood. Some workers argue that the $CD8^+$ cells act as suppressor cells (33,34). The simplest possibility, however, is that the $CD8^+$ cells act as CTL and cause progressive tissue damage, aided by help from the donor $CD4^+$ cells. Such exogenous help seems to be essential because only minimal disease occurs when the donor cells are depleted of $CD4^+$ cells (or unseparated T cells are transferred to hosts expressing only a class I difference rather than a combined class I/II difference). The inability of purified $CD8^+$ cells to cause lethal GVHD applies only to nonirradiated hosts. As discussed earlier, $CD8^+$ cells are highly potent at causing an aplastic form of lethal GVHD in irradiated hosts.

Although transferring unseparated T cells to hosts expressing a combined class I/II difference generally causes an aplastic form of GVHD, this is by no means an invariable finding. For example, when (B6 × DBA/2)F_1 mice (H-2^b × H-2^d) are injected with unseparated DBA/2 T cells, the proliferative type of GVHD rather than aplastic GVHD develops (34). In contrast, injecting either B6 or B10.D2 (H-2^d) T cells causes aplastic GVHD. Although the disparity in the effect mediated by B10.D2 and DBA/2 (both H-2^d) T cells has yet to be resolved, the most likely possibility is that DBA/2 mice have a quantitative and qualitative deficiency of $CD8^+$ cells (35).

GVHD to Minor Histocompatibility Antigens

Mouse models for GVHD directed to minor histocompatibility antigens are of obvious clinical relevance because BMT in humans is restricted largely to MHC (HLA)-compatible donor/host combinations. As discussed elsewhere in this volume, GVHD in HLA-compatible combinations can be very severe. This disease is probably directed largely and perhaps entirely to minor histocompatibility antigens.

The first evidence that minor histocompatibility antigens provide targets for GVHD in mice came from studies in which untreated marrow cells were transferred to irradiated H-2-compatible hosts expressing a variety of non H-2 differences (36,37). A high incidence of lethal GVHD was seen, but only when the donor and the host differed at three or more minor histocompatibility loci. Difference at other loci (e.g., Ly or Mls loci) failed to cause GVHD. Evidence that GVHD was caused by T cells came from the finding that depleting the marrow inoculum of contaminating mature T cells with anti-Thy 1 antibody plus complement abolished GVHD. In contrast to human marrow, however, mouse marrow contains only small numbers of mature T cells (1–2%).

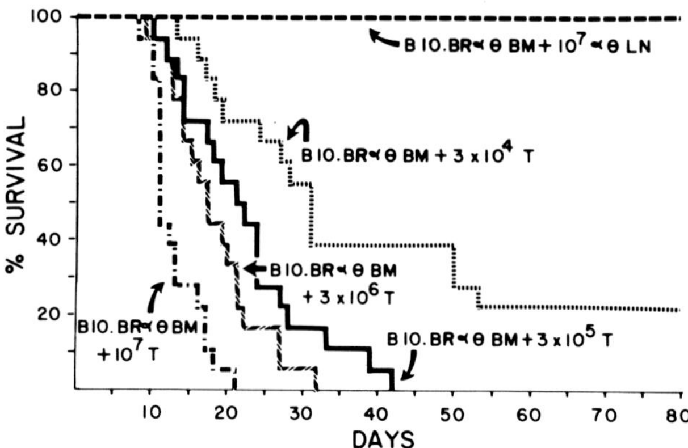

Figure 18-1. Lethal GVHD in irradiated (750 cGy) CBA/J mice given graded doses of purified B10.BR LN T cells. The data show cumulative mortality after transferring 10^7 anti-Thy 1.2-serum-treated B10.BR marrow cells (B10.BR α θ BM) supplemented with varying numbers of nylon-wool-purified B10.BR LN T cells or with anti-Thy 1.2 serum-treated B10.BR LN cells (α θ LN). Data pooled from 3 experiments involving a total of 18 mice per group. (Reproduced by permission from Korngold R, Sprent J. Lethal graft-versus-host disease after bone-marrow transplantation across minor histocompatibility barriers in mice. Prevention by removing mature T-cells from marrow. J Exp Med 1978;148:1687–1698.)

Target Antigens

Although it is clear that lethal GVHD in non-H-2-different combinations requires minor histocompatibility antigen incompatibility, which particular minor histocompatibility antigens provide the targets for GVHD is still unclear. Preliminary work with congeneic strains of mice differing selectively at defined minor histocompatibility antigens has shown that only a proportion of isolated minor histocompatibility antigen differences elicit lethal GVHD (Korngold R. Unpublished data). Why some minor histocompatibility antigens are less potent than others in inducing GVHD is unclear, although differences in tissue distribution and T-precursor frequency are obvious possibilities. The data discussed refer to strain combinations expressing multiple minor histocompatibility antigen differences.

Features of GVHD

Studies with 6 strain combinations expressing 3 or more minor histocompatibility antigen differences have shown that transferring a mixture of purified unprimed donor T cells plus T-cell–depleted donor marrow cells to mice given an intermediate dose of irradiation (750–800 cGy) causes heavy mortality in each combination (38). The most detailed information has come from the CBA⇄B10.BR combination (36,39, 40). Lethal GVHD in this combination approaches 100% and occurs with even very small numbers of T cells ($<1 \times 10^5$). On the basis of the effects of filtering the donor T cells from blood to lymph through H-2 recombinant intermediate hosts, the T cells mediating GVHD in the CBA → B10.BR combination respond to minor histocompatibility antigens presented by host class I rather than class II molecules (39,40); the cells comprise a mixture of H-2D-restricted and H-2K-restricted T cells.

The patterns of GVHD elicited by minor histocompatibility antigen depend on the dose of T cells injected: Large numbers of T cells produce acute GVHD and early deaths, whereas smaller numbers of T cells lead to a chronic form of GVHD with late mortality (36) (Figure 18-1). Histopathology is most prominent in mice with chronic GVHD and involves lymphoid atrophy, weight loss, and lymphocyte infiltration of the skin, liver, and lungs (41–45); involvement of the gut is mild, although chronic diarrhea develops in some mice. Symptoms of GVHD tend to be more severe in hosts conditioned with heavy irradiation (800–1,000 cGy) rather than light irradiation (600–800 cGy) and when the general health of the colony is suboptimal. With regard to the marrow inoculum, using host rather than donor marrow has little effect in potentiating GVHD (46). This finding contrasts with anti-H-2 GVHD, in which reconstitution with host marrow leads to marked marrow aplasia. The capacity of large doses of $CD4^+$ cells to protect against lethal GVHD does not seem to apply to GVHD directed to minor histocompatibility antigens (46). The reason for this difference is obscure.

Role of $CD8^+$ Cells

GVHD to minor histocompatibility antigens is mediated largely, although not exclusively, by $CD8^+$ cells (38,39) (Table 18-4). The critical role of $CD4^+$ cells is apparent from the finding that the effector cells in the CBA → B10.BR combination are H-2 class I–restricted. In this and other combinations, depleting the injected T cells of $CD4^+$ cells generally has little or no effect in reducing the intensity of GVHD (39); likewise injecting the host mice with anti-CD4 antibody has minimal effects (46). These findings imply that the capacity of $CD8^+$ cells to mediate GVHD to minor histocompatibility antigens does not require help from $CD4^+$ cells.

Role of $CD4^+$ Cells

In the case of the CBA → B10.BR combination and certain other combinations, $CD4^+$ cells have no obvious role in GVHD. The helper function of these cells is not required, and transferring even high doses of purified CD4$^+$ cells generally fails to cause GVHD. Nevertheless in 2 of 6 combinations tested, namely B10.D2 → BALB/c and B10.D2 → DBA/2, purified CD4$^+$ cells did cause a high incidence of lethal GVHD (39,47) (see Table 18-4). The histopathology of GVHD mediated by CD4$^+$ and CD8$^+$ cells is quite similar, although gut pathology is more prominent in recipients of CD4$^+$ cells (45). Why CD4$^+$ cells mediate GVHD in only a limited number of minor histocompatibility antigen-different combinations is obscure.

Pathogenesis

As for anti-H-2 GVHD, the effector mechanisms involved in GVHD to minor histocompatibility antigens are still not fully understood. In the case of CD8$^+$ cells, it would seem very likely that tissue damage reflects a combination of CTL activity and lymphokine release. However, studies with recombinant inbred strains have shown that the minor histocompatibility antigens that act as targets for GVHD do not necessarily evoke strong in vitro CTL responses, and vice versa (48). This finding is difficult to interpret, however, because CTL responses to minor histocompatibility antigens are subject to a curious form of immunodominance; CTL responses to weak antigens are suppressed by responses to stronger antigens. As for CD8$^+$ cells, tissue destruction by CD4$^+$ cells against minor histocompatibility antigens presumably involves both CTL activity and lymphokine release.

Syngeneic GVHD

Transferring T cells plus marrow cells to syngeneic irradiated hosts normally leads to full lymphohemopoietic reconstitution with no signs of GVHD. This effect is to be expected because T cells generally show full tolerance to self antigens (with the exception of tissue-specific self antigens, which are normally sequestered from the immune system). In certain situations, however, a syndrome of syngeneic (autologous) GVHD develops in mice and rats reconstituted with syngeneic marrow cells (49–55). This form of GVHD occurs when the irradiated recipients are given repeated injections of cyclosporine (CSA) for a period of several weeks. The recipients remain healthy during the course of the injections, but then become acutely ill with classic signs of GVHD such as lymphoid hyperplasia, lymphocyte infiltration of various organs, and severe weight loss. Mortality rates are often high during this acute form of GVHD, but chronic GVHD with lymphoid aplasia and fibrosis develops in some of the survivors. Similar patterns of disease occur when T cells from CSA-treated irradiated hosts are adoptively transferred to secondary syngeneic hosts (but only if the secondary hosts are irradiated). The most intense form of syngeneic GVHD requires the combined actions of CD4$^+$ and CD8$^+$ cells (53). As for allo-GVHD, CD4$^+$ cells cause lymphoproliferation, presumably through lymphokine release, whereas CD8$^+$ cells mediate tissue destruction and lymphoid aplasia through CTL activity; in consort, the two T-cell subsets act synergistically and cause heavy mortality.

Although easily induced in rats, CSA-mediated syngeneic GVHD tends to be sporadic in mice and shows marked strain variation (54). Some strains (e.g., DBA/2) are highly susceptible, whereas certain other strains are quite resistant. The reason for this strain variability is unclear, although strain differences in the level of incipient infection is a likely possibility. In this respect (as for allo-GVHD), syngeneic GVHD can be prevented by infusing large doses of normal T cells (52).

Table 18-4.
Lethal GVHD in 6 Minor Histocompatibility Antigen–different H-2-compatible Strain Combinations: GVHD Mediated by Purified T Cells and T-cell Subsets[a]

			% Mortality (median survival time) After Transfer of Donor T Cells Plus Donor Marrow			
Donor → Recipient	*H-2*	*Some of the Known Genetic Differences Between Donor and Host*	*Whole T*	*CD4$^+$*	*CD8$^+$*	*Marrow Alone*
C3H.SW → B6	H-2^b	H-1,-3,-7,-8,-9,-13	48	5	77	0
		Lyt-1,2, Mls^b	(58)	(>80)	(45)	(>80)
DBA/2 → B10.D2	H-2^d	H-1,-3,-4,-8,-13	26	12	73	8
		Lyt-1,2, Mls^b	(>80)	(>80)	(53)	(>80)
B10.BR → CBA/J	H-2^k	H-1,-3,-7,-8,-9,-12	96	35	96	8
		Tla, Mls^a, Lyt-1,2	(38)	(73)	(39)	(>80)
B10.S → SJL	H-2^s	H-1,-3,-7,-8,-9	88	13	88	0
		-12,-13, Tla, Mls^c	(34)	(>80)	(35)	(>80)
B10.D2 → DBA/2	H-2^d	H-1,-3,-4,-8,-13, Mls^a	92	85	42	7
		Lyt-1,2	(38)	(45)	(58)	(>80)
B10.D2 → BALB/c	H-2^d	H-1,-3,-4,-7,-8,-9,-13	93	78	75	0
		Lyt-1,2, Mls^c	(20)	(24)	(39)	(>80)

See Table 18-1. Data were pooled from more than 20 experiments, with totals of 15 to 39 mice for each strain combination. Donor marrow cells (4×10^6) were T-cell–depleted. T cells and T-cell subsets were injected in a dose of 1×10^6 cells.
Data from Korngold R, Sprent J. Variable capacity of L3T4$^+$ T-cells to cause lethal graft-versus-host disease across minor histocompatibility barriers in mice. J Exp Med 1987;165:1522–1564.

The cause of syngeneic GVHD is still unclear. There are two broad possibilities. The first possibility is that CSA treatment breaks self tolerance by interfering with clonal deletion of autoreactive T cells in the thymus (50). In support of this hypothesis it has been found that, in I-E$^+$ strains of mice, CSA treatment prevents intrathymic deletion of I-E-reactive T cells expressing Vβ11 and Vβ17 TCR molecules (55,56); the incomplete deletion of these T cells correlates with diminished expression of MHC class II molecules in the thymic medulla (50). The problem with this explanation is that the incomplete Vβ deletion mediated by CSA is strain-dependent and does not seem to correlate with susceptibility to syngeneic GVHD (57).

The second possibility is that CSA-induced syngeneic GVHD is the end result of lymphocytopenia and infection (58). In addition to impairing clonal deletion in the thymus, CSA treatment causes a marked reduction in the export of new T cells from the thymus. At the end of CSA treatment, T-cell counts in spleen and lymph nodes are 10-fold lower than in control mice given irradiation without CSA (55). Why should T lymphocytopenia cause GVHD? There are a number of situations in mice in which a syndrome of generalized autoimmunity associated with multi-organ lymphocytic infiltration spontaneously develops. This syndrome, which has many features in common with CSA-mediated syngeneic GVHD, is seen in neonatally thymectomized mice (59), nude (athymic) mice grafted with neonatal thymuses (60), and in certain TCR-transgenic mice (Sakaguchi S. Personal communication). In each situation, development of generalized autoimmunity is preceded by a prolonged period of T lymphocytopenia. As discussed elsewhere (58), one can envisage a scenario where a quantitative deficiency of T cells predisposes to chronic infection in various organs. As the result of inflammation, tissue-specific antigens, which are normally sequestered from the immune system, are released from the infected organs and reach the lymphoid tissues. Nontolerant T cells then respond to the antigens and differentiate into effector cells. These activated T cells then percolate throughout the body and find their way to the organ expressing the self antigen concerned. The end result is multi-organ autoimmunity—or "syngeneic GVHD" in the CSA model. This chain of events fails to occur when the T-cell pool is of normal size. A fully functional immune system clears infection and thereby prevents tissue-specific antigens from reaching the lymphoid organs. In this respect it is notable that for each of the discussed models, adding bulk populations of normal T cells prevents disease induction.

References

1. Möller G. Graft versus host reaction. Immunol Rev 1985;88:1–238.
2. Burakoff SJ, Deeg HJ, Ferrara J, Atkinson K, Eds. Graft-vs.-host disease: immunology, pathophysiology, and treatment. New York: Marcel Dekker, 1990:1–725.
3. Korngold R, Sprent J. Graft-versus-host disease in experimental allogeneic bone marrow transplantation. Proc Soc Exp Biol Med 1991;197:12–18.
4. Sprent J, Webb SR. Function and specificity of T-cell subsets in the mouse. Adv Immunol 1987;41:39–133.
5. Hedrick SM. T lymphocyte receptors. In: Paul WE, ed. Fundamental immunology, ed 2. New York: Raven, 1989:291–314.
6. Shevach EM. Accessory molecules. In: Paul WE, ed. Fundamental immunology, ed 2. New York: Raven, 1989:413–444.
7. Carbone FR, Bevan MJ. Major histocompatibility complex control of T-cell recognition. In: Paul WE, ed. Fundamental immunology, ed 2. New York: Raven, 1989:541–570.
8. Sprent J. T lymphocytes and the thymus. In: Paul WE, ed. Fundamental immunology, ed 2. New York: Raven, 1989:69–94.
9. von Boehmer H. Developmental biology of T-cells in T-cell receptor transgenic mice. Annu Rev Immunol 1990;8:531–556.
10. Sprent J, Korngold R. A comparison of lethal graft-versus-host disease to minor-versus-major differences in mice: implications for marrow transplantation in man. Prog Immunol 1983;5:1461–1475.
11. Bennett M. Biology and genetics of hybrid resistance. Adv Immunol 1987;41:333–445.
12. Murphy WJ, Kumar V, Bennett M. Rejection of bone marrow allografts by mice with severe combined immunodeficiency (SCID): evidence that natural killer (NK) cells can mediate the specificity of marrow graft rejection. J Exp Med 1987;165:1212–1217.
13. Bix M, Liao N-S, Zijlstra M, Loring J, Jaenisch R, Raulet D. Rejection of class I MHC-deficient haemopoietic cells by irradiated MHC-matched mice. Nature 1991;349: 329–331.
14. Möller G. Elimination of allogeneic lymphoid cells. Immunol Rev 1983;73:1–126.
15. Vallera DA, Soderling CCB, Kersey JH. Bone marrow transplantation across major histocompatibility barriers in mice: III. Treatment of donor grafts with monoclonal antibodies directed against Lyt determinants. J Immunol 1982;128:871–875.
16. Korngold R, Sprent J. Surface markers of T-cells causing lethal graft-versus-host disease to class I vs class II H-2 differences. J Immunol 1985;135:3004–3010.
17. Sprent, J, Schaefer M, Lo D, Korngold R. Properties of purified T-cell subsets. II. In vivo responses to class I vs class II H-2 differences. J Exp Med 1986;163:998–1011.
18. Korngold R, Sprent J. Purified T-cell subsets and lethal graft-versus-host disease in mice. In: Gale RP, Champlin R, eds. Progress in bone marrow transplantation. New York: Alan R. Liss, 1987:213–218.
19. Cobbold S, Martin G, Waldmann H. Monoclonal antibodies for the prevention of graft-versus-host disease and marrow graft rejection. Transplantation 1986;42: 239–247.
20. Piguet P-F. GVHR elicited by products of class I or class II loci of the MHC: analysis of the response of mouse T lymphocytes to products of class I and class II loci of the MHC in correlation with GVHR-induced mortality, medullary aplasia, and enteropathy. J Immunol 1985; 135:1637–1643.
21. Sprent J, Schaefer M, Lo D, Korngold R. Function of purified L3T4$^+$ and Lyt-2$^+$ cells in vitro and in vivo. Immunol Rev 1986;91:195–218.
22. Sprent J, Schaefer M, Korngold R. Role of T-cell subsets

in lethal graft-versus-host disease (GVHD) directed to class I versus class II H-2 differences. II. Protective effects of L3T4$^+$ cells in anti-class II H-2 differences. J Immunol 1990;144:2946–2954.
23. Guy-Grand D, Vassalli P. Gut injury in mouse graft-versus-host reactions. J Clin Invest 1986;77:1584–1595.
24. Mowat AM, Sprent J. Induction of intestinal graft-versus-host reactions across mutant major histocompatibility antigens by T lymphocyte subsets in mice. Transplantation 1989;47:857–863.
25. Piguet PF, Grau GE, Allet B, Vassalli P. Tumor necrosis factor/cachectin is an effector of skin and gut lesions of the acute phase of graft-vs.-host disease. J Exp Med 1987;166:1280–1289.
26. Vossen JM, Heidt PJ. Gnotobiotic measures for prevention of acute graft-versus-host disease. In: Burakoff SJ, Deeg HJ, Ferrara JLM, Atkinson K, eds. Graft-versus-host disease: immunology, pathophysiology, and treatment. New York: Marcel Dekker, 1990:403–413.
27. Nathenson SG, Geliebter J, Pfaffenbach GM, Zeff RA. Murine major histocompatibility complex class-I mutants: molecular analysis and structure-function implications. Ann Rev Immunol 1986;4:471–502.
28. Sprent J, Schaefer M, Gao E-K, Korngold R. Role of T-cell subsets in lethal graft-versus-host disease (GVHD) directed to class I versus class II H-2 differences. I. L3T4$^+$ cells can either augment or retard GVHD elicited by Lyt-2$^+$ cells in class I-different hosts. J Exp Med 1988;167:556–569.
29. Simonsen M. Graft-versus-host reactions. Their natural history and applicability as tools of research. Prog Allergy 1962;6;349–467.
30. Rolink AG, Pals ST, Gleichmann E. Allosuppressor and allohelper T-cells in acute and chronic graft-vs.-host disease. II. F_1 recipients carrying mutations at H-2K and/or I-A. J Exp Med 1983;157:755–771.
31. Gleichmann E, Pals ST, Rolink AG, Radaszkiewicz T, Gleichmann H. Graft-versus-host reactions: clues to the etiopathology of a spectrum of immunological diseases. Immunol Today 1984;5:324–332.
32. Rolink AG, Gleichmann E. Allosuppressor and allohelper T-cells in acute and chronic graft-vs.-host disease. III. Different Lyt subsets of donor T-cells induce different pathological syndromes. J Exp Med 1983;158:546–558.
33. Rolink AG, Radaszkiewicz T, Pals ST, van der Meer WGJ, Gleichmann E. Allosuppressor and allohelper T-cells in acute and chronic graft-vs.-host disease. I. Alloreactive suppressor cells rather than killer T-cells appear to be the decisive cells in lethal graft-vs.-host disease. J Exp Med 1982;155:1501–1522.
34. van Elven EH, Rolink AG, van der Veen F, Gleichmann E. Capacity of genetically different T lymphocytes to induce lethal graft-versus-host disease correlates with their capacity to generate suppression but not with their capacity to generate anti-F_1 killer cells. A non-H-2 locus determines the inability to induce lethal graft-versus-hosts disease. J Exp Med 1981;153:1474–1488.
35. Via CS, Sharrow SO, Shearer GM. Role of cytotoxic T lymphocytes in the prevention of lupus-like disease occurring in a murine model of graft-vs.-host disease. J Exp Med 1987;139:1840–1849.
36. Korngold R, Sprent J. Lethal graft-versus-host disease after bone-marrow transplantation across minor histocompatibility barriers in mice. Prevention by removing mature T-cells from marrow. J Exp Med 1978;148: 1687–1698.
37. Hamilton BL, Bevan MJ, Parkman R. Anti-recipient cytotoxic T lymphocyte precursors are present in the spleens of mice with acute graft-versus-host disease due to minor histocompatibility antigens. J Immunol 1981;126:621–625.
38. Korngold R, Sprent J. Variable capacity of L3T4$^+$ T-cells to cause lethal graft-versus-host disease across minor histocompatibility barriers in mice. J Exp Med 1987;165:1522–1564.
39. Korngold R, Sprent J. Lethal GVHD across minor histocompatibility barriers: nature of the effector cells and role of the H-2 complex. Immunol Rev 1983;71:5–29.
40. Korngold R, Sprent J. Features of T-cells causing H-2-restricted lethal graft-versus-host disease across minor histocompatibility barriers. J Exp Med 1982;155: 872–883.
41. Jaffee BD, Claman HN. Chronic graft-versus-host disease (GVHD) as a model for scleroderma. I. Description of model systems. Cell Immunol 1983;77:1–12.
42. Ferrara J, Guillen FJ, Sleckman B, Burakoff SJ, Murphy GF. Cutaneous acute graft-versus-host disease to minor histocompatibility antigens in a murine model: histologic analysis and correlation to clinical disease. J Invest Dermatol 1986;123:401–406.
43. Rappaport H, Khalil A, Halle-Pannenko O, Pritchard L, Dantcher D, Mathe G. Histopathologic sequence of events in adult mice undergoing lethal graft-vs-host reaction developed across H-2 and/or non H-2 histocompatibility barriers. Am J Pathol 1979;96:121–143.
44. Charley MR, Bangert JL, Hamilton BL, Gilliam JN, Sontheimer RD. Murine graft-versus-host skin disease: a chronologic and quantitative analysis of two histologic patterns. J Invest Dermatol 1983;81:412–417.
45. Murphy GF, Whitaker D, Sprent J, Korngold R. Characterization of target injury of murine acute graft-versus-host disease directed to multiple minor histocompatibility antigens elicited by either CD4$^+$ or CD8$^+$ effector cells. Am J Pathol 1991;138:983–990.
46. Korngold R. Lethal graft-versus-host disease in mice directed to multiple minor histocompatibility antigens: features of CD8$^+$ and CD4$^+$ T-cell responses. Bone Marrow Transplant 1992;9:355–364.
47. Hamilton BL. L3T4-positive T-cells participate in the induction of graft-vs-host disease in response to minor histocompatibility antigens. J Immunol 1987;139: 2511–2515.
48. Korngold R, Wettstein PJ. Immunodominance in the graft-vs-host disease T-cell response to minor histocompatibility antigen. J Immunol 1990;145:4079–4088.
49. Glazier A, Tutschka PJ, Farmer ER, Santos GW. Graft-versus-host disease in cyclosporine A treated rats after syngeneic and autologous bone marrow reconstitution. J Exp Med 1983;158:1–8.
50. Cheney RT, Sprent J. Capacity of cyclosporine to induce autograft-versus-host disease and impair intrathymic T-cell differentiation. Trans Proc 1985;17:528–530.
51. Sorokin R, Kimura H, Schroder K, Wilson DH, Wilson DB. Cyclosporine-induced autoimmunity. Conditions for expressing disease, requirement for intact thymus, and potency estimates of autoimmune lymphocytes in drug-treated rats. J Exp Med 1986;164:1615–1625.
52. Hess AD. Syngeneic graft-v-host disease. In: Burakoff SJ, Deeg HJ, Ferrara J, Atkinson K, eds. Graft-vs.-host disease. New York: Marcel Dekker, 1990:95–107.
53. Hess AD, Fischer AC, Beschorner WE. Effector mechanisms in cyclosporine A-induced syngeneic graft-

versus-host disease. Role of CD4+ and CD8+ T lymphocyte subsets. J Immunol 1990;145:526–533.

54. Bryson JS, Jennings CD, Caywood BE, Kaplan AM. Strain specificity in the induction of syngeneic graft-versus-host disease in mice. Transplantation 1991;51: 911–913.

55. Gao E-K, Lo D, Cheney R, Kanagawa O, Sprent J. Abnormal differentiation of thymocytes in mice treated with cyclosporin A. Nature 1988;366:176–179.

56. Jenkins MK, Schwartz RH, Pardoll DM. Effects of cyclosporine A on T-cell development and clonal deletion. Science 1988;241:1655–1658.

57. Bryson JS, Caywood BE, Kaplan AM. Relationship of cyclosporine A-mediated inhibition of clonal deletion and development of syngeneic graft-versus-host disease. J Immunol 1991;147:391–397.

58. Sprent J. The thymus and T-cell tolerance. In: Myasthenia gravis and related disorders: experimental and clinical aspects. Ann NY Acad 1993;681:5–15.

59. Sakaguchi S, Takahashi T, Nishizuka Y. Study on cellular events on postthymectomy autoimmune oophoritis in mice. II. Requirement of Lyt-1 cells in normal female mice for the prevention of oophoritis. J Exp Med 1982;156:1577–1586.

60. Sakaguchi S, Sakaguchi N. Thymus and autoimmunity: capacity of the normal thymus to produce pathogenic self-reactive T-cells and conditions required for the induction of autoimmune disease. J Exp Med 1990; 172:537–545.

Chapter 19

Graft-versus-tumor Responses: Adoptive Cellular Therapy in Bone Marrow Transplantation

Alexander Fefer

"Adoptive cellular therapy" refers to the use of transferred lymphocytes for cancer therapy. The lymphocyte that has been most intensively investigated and demonstrated to be most therapeutically effective in animal models has been a T lymphocyte specifically reactive to tumor-associated antigens (1–3) and used in conjunction with noncurative chemotherapy. In such "adoptive chemoimmunotherapy" models, autologous, syngeneic, or allogeneic lymphocytes must, with rare exceptions, be immune to the tumor-associated antigens, whereas allogeneic lymphocytes also can be effective therapeutically if they are sensitized to normal host histocompatibility antigens (1,4). More recently, lymphocytes—largely of non-T phenotype—with lymphokine-activated killer (LAK) activity (5) have also been reported to be effective therapeutically when used in conjunction with exogenously administered interleukin-2 (IL-2) in animal models (6) and in humans (7). The prerequisites for successful therapy with lymphocytes in animal models are reviewed elsewhere (1,4).

Normal allogeneic marrow infused into leukemic animals pretreated with very high doses of chemotherapy and supralethal doses of total body irradiation reconstitutes hemopoietic and immunological function, induces graft-versus-host disease (GVHD), and exerts an antileukemic effect, termed a *graft-versus leukemia* (GVL) effect (8). There is now strong circumstantial evidence for the existence of a GVL effect of allogeneic marrow in humans. Thus, allogeneic bone marrow transplantation (BMT) in humans may represent a form of adoptive cellular immunotherapy. Efforts to dissociate the lethal effects of GVHD from the desired antileukemic effects of allogeneic BMT continue to dominate both experimental and clinical studies.

This chapter briefly reviews (1) animal models for cellular immunotherapy using tumor-specific T cells or LAK cells; (2) preliminary results of such immunotherapy in humans; (3) induction and manipulation of GVHD and GVL in animal models; (4) evidence for the existence of a GVL effect in clinical BMT; (5) attempts to induce or enhance the GVL effect in human marrow recipients; and (6) future directions toward enhancing the graft-versus-tumor effect in human BMT recipients.

Cellular Immunotherapy Using Tumor-specific T Cells in Animal Models

A number of animal models have been developed in which disseminated antigenic tumors can be eradicated by the adoptive transfer of T cells specifically immune to the tumor associated antigens—especially as an adjunct to noncurative chemotherapy (1,2,9–11). These models have served as prototypes of what might be achieved if the host immune response to an autologous tumor could be identified, selectively amplified, and used in humans.

The most extensively studied model has involved the treatment of disseminated FBL-3, a Friend retrovirus-induced erythroleukemia, in C57B1/6 mice with cyclophosphamide (CY) and syngeneic lymphocytes (11). Untreated mice died rapidly, as did mice treated only with immune cells; treatment with CY alone, or with CY plus cells immune to unrelated antigens prolonged survival but cured no mice. In contrast, treatment with CY plus cells immune to FBL-3 cured the vast majority of leukemic mice (11).

Subsequent studies (10,12–14) in this model as well as in other similar models yielded the following observations related to successful immunotherapy: (1) donor T cells were required for therapeutic efficacy; (2) the T cells had to be immunologically specifically reactive to tumor-associated antigens and the encoded major histocompatibility complex (MHC) antigens; (3) the infused lymphocytes had to proliferate and persist in the recipient for a long period; (4) therapeutic efficacy depended directly on the number of donor T cells infused (i.e., the larger the number the greater the effect); (5) the T-cell growth factor IL-2 enhanced the growth of tumor-specific T cells in vitro, and IL-2 in vivo augmented the therapeutic efficacy of such adoptively transferred lymphocytes; (6) the generation of such cells in vitro and their therapeutic efficacy in vivo was enhanced further by restimulation in vitro with appropriate tumor antigen; and (7) both $CD8^+$ and $CD4^+$ T-cell subsets could mediate the immunological eradication of tumor. The effector mechanism, however, was different for each subset. For example, the main mechanism by which $CD4^+$ T cells can eradicate tumor is by secreting lymphokines that promote the activity of other tumoricidal effector cells, such as macrophages. In contrast, $CD8^+$ T cells recognize the tumor antigens in the context of class I MHC molecules and lyse tumors directly with class I–restricted specificity.

Cellular Immunotherapy Using LAK Cells in Animal Models

Murine lymphocytes cultured in pharmacological concentrations of IL-2 for several days acquire the ability to lyse promiscuously in a non-MHC restricted fashion in a wide variety of tumor targets with relative sparing of normal tissue (15). LAK activity is mediated by a heterogenous population of cells; most represent activated natural killer (NK) cells, but some arise from T cells. For purposes of this chapter, we refer to LAK cells; LAK precursor cells, which are cells that acquire LAK activity when cultured in IL-2; or LAK effector cells, which are cells that have direct LAK activity without requiring additional exposure to IL-2 in vitro (15).

Extensive studies have demonstrated that LAK cells cause regression of established tumors and inhibit growth of pulmonary and hepatic metastases in syngeneic mice. In a series of studies in tumor-bearing mice (6,16–18), LAK cells alone (without IL-2) had little therapeutic effect; IL-2 alone, especially if given in high doses, had a significant therapeutic effect; but a combination of LAK cells plus IL-2 was therapeutically most effective. A higher dose of IL-2 induced a greater LAK activity and anti-tumor effect in vivo. A larger number of LAK cells also exerted a greater anti-tumor effect. Although the mechanism by which IL-2 alone or IL-2 plus LAK cells mediate a therapeutic effect has not yet been identified, the effects might be mediated by LAK cells induced by IL-2 or by tumor-specific T lymphocytes augmented in number and activity by IL-2 or by secretion of other lymphokines or cytokines in response to IL-2 ± lymphocytes. The mechanism by which LAK cells recognize, bind, and selectively lyse malignant targets has also yet to be identified.

Cellular Immunotherapy Using Tumor-specific T Cells in Humans

Murine studies (10) suggest that immune T cells have several theoretical advantages over LAK cells, including (1) target specificity; (2) ability to "home" to sites of tumor and proliferate there in response to tumor; (3) ability to persist in vivo long term; (4) ability to maintain proliferative and cytolytic function in the presence of far lower IL-2 concentration; and (5) immunological memory.

Many attempts have been made to detect T cells specifically reactive to autologous tumor in humans. The most encouraging results have been reported with T cells obtained from biopsies of melanoma—designated as tumor-infiltrating lymphocytes (TIL)—and grown in IL-2. In a variable percentage of patients, such cells expressed specific or preferential cytolytic reactivity for autologous tumor (19–21). Preliminary results of the first clinical trial using CY, TIL, and high-dose IL-2 for patients with metastatic melanoma suggested that 50% of the patients exhibited a partial response (3). Under somewhat different conditions, 2 of 9 patients treated for widely metastatic melanoma with tumor-specific T cells and IL-2 exhibited an enduring complete response (22). The encouraging tumor responses represent a major impetus to further laboratory and clinical studies to confirm, extend, and improve the results. No successful T-cell therapy specifically directed at tumor antigens has yet been reported for any other cancer in humans.

Cellular Immunotherapy Using LAK Cells in Humans

Cells with LAK activity have been generated from peripheral blood lymphocytes of normal people and cancer patients. Most LAK cells have the phenotypic characteristics of activated NK cells ($CD56^+$, $CD16^+$, $CD3^-$), but some are "NK-like" T cells that coexpress CD3 and NK markers (23). LAK cells lyse fresh tumor cells obtained from patients with a variety of malignancies, including acute myeloid leukemia (AML), acute lymphoblastic leukemia (ALL), chronic myeloid leukemia (CML), or malignant lymphoma (24–27). Such susceptibility is noncell-cycle–specific and is maintained in cell lines that demonstrate pleiotropic drug resistance markers (28,29). LAK cells have little or no effect on hematological progenitors in vitro.

In Phase I/II clinical trials with a variety of IL-2 preparations and regimens ± LAK cells, objective tumor responses have been reported in 8 to 35% of patients with advanced malignancies, especially metastatic renal-cell carcinoma and melanoma (7,30–32). In the two most recent trials of IL-2 plus LAK cells for metastatic renal-cell carcinoma at the University of Washington, 14 of 42 patients had a significant and durable tumor response, with 7 complete responses of up to 3.5 years' duration (33). The treatment regimens that have included the highest response rates have tended to be the most toxic ones. However, the relationship between IL-2 dose (± LAK cells) and the immunomodulatory and anti-tumor effects in patients is not clear because of the heterogeneity of the patients treated and of the IL-2 regimens used (7,34–38).

Treatment with IL-2 ± LAK cells has induced remissions in some patients with advanced hematological malignancies. Several patients with Hodgkin's disease or non-Hodgkin's lymphoma resistant to conventional therapy have experienced a partial remission (PR) or a complete remission (CR) after receiving IL-2 ± LAK cells (30,36,39–41). Overall, 20 to 25% of patients with malignant lymphoma of various types have responded to a variety of regimens of IL-2 ± LAK cells. Some patients with acute leukemia have also responded. In one pilot study of 5 patients with acute leukemia (4 with AML, 1 with ALL) with minimal residual disease persisting after salvage chemotherapy, 4 responded to IL-2 therapy and 3 with a CR lasting as long as 24 months or more (30,36,39–43). In another ongoing Phase II study of IL-2 for patients refractory to chemotherapy, among 13 evaluable patients with AML in relapse, 2 had a CR and 2 had a PR (Maraninchi D. Personal communication).

Graft-versus-leukemia Effect of Allogeneic BMT in Animal Models

Barnes and colleagues (44) were the first to postulate that allogeneic bone marrow infused into a tumor-bearing lethally x-irradiated mouse would colonize the host and would "destroy by the action of the immunity these residual leukemia cells, . . . and perhaps the host." In their classic studies (44,45), mice with a transplanted leukemia received lethal whole body x-irradiation plus normal syngeneic or histoincompatible marrow. Recipients of syngeneic marrow died of recurrent leukemia, whereas a few of the recipients of allogeneic marrow were cured, but almost all ultimately died of GVHD. The term *graft-versus-leukemia* (GVL) was adopted much later to describe the antitumor effect and to distinguish it from the GVH reaction (8).

Mathé and associates (46) first suggested that one might use the GVH reaction against the tumor but then treat the GVHD and thereby save the cured host. Unfortunately, it is extremely difficult to control a GVH reaction once it is established (47). Another therapeutic possibility has been somehow to confer preferential anti-tumor specificity to the GVH reaction (1). This approach, which is based on the assumption that the effectors or targets for GVL are qualitatively or quantitatively different from those for GVHD, also represents a major challenge and, with rare exceptions (48–51), remains largely unrealized.

In animal models, the GVL effect may or may not be separable or distinguishable from the GVH reaction, in that the effector cells responsible for the GVL effect and for GVHD have been the same in some models but different in others (48–54).

The effector cells in GVHD have been identified as T cells. The role of T-cell subsets in murine GVHD systems has been reviewed (55). The relationship between GVL-reactive and GVH-reactive murine T cells also has been examined at a clonal level (56–58).

Effector cells that mediate the GVL effect in animals (and probably humans) may include (1) cytotoxic T lymphocytes (CTLs) specific for minor histocompatibility antigens present on both normal host tissue and leukemic cells or against antigens expressed only on or preferentially on malignant cells; (2) lymphocytes that mediate their antitumor effects via secondary lymphokine secretion; or (3) cytolytic T or non-T cells that mediate their anti-tumor effect through an MHC-unrestricted mechanism. IL-2 can stimulate the proliferation and function of all these effector cells.

In murine models, IL-2 can induce, exacerbate, or even protect against GVHD, depending on the model and the timing (59–66). Little is known about the effect of LAK cells on GVHD. In one model, lethal GVHD was prevented by the addition of recipient-type "veto" LAK cells but was exacerbated by LAK cells of donor or third-party origin (67).

The role of IL-2 or LAK in the GVL effect has received too little attention in murine models. In a syngeneic BMT model for lymphoma, IL-2 was curative (68). In another syngeneic model, BMT using marrow activated by preincubation with IL-2 and followed by systemic administration of IL-2 reduced the number of metastases of melanoma (69) and cured some leukemic mice (70). Finally, in one H-2-incompatible BMT model, IL-2 administered at the time of BMT induced a significant GVL effect against a lymphoma, without exacerbating GVHD (64,65). These results suggest a graft-versus-tumor effect induced by IL-2 ± LAK cells.

Evidence for a GVL Effect in Clinical Allogeneic BMT

Temporal Associations Between GVHD and Hematological Remission

Two patients (71,72) with ALL have been reported who relapsed early after allogeneic BMT; disease disappeared during a flare-up of GVHD and then they once again relapsed. A third patient with Burkitt's lymphoma who relapsed one month after BMT had cyclosporine (CSP) prophylaxis discontinued, developed GVHD, had a CR of the lymphoma, then received CSP and prednisone for recurrence of GVHD and suffered a relapse of the fatal lymphoma (73). Another patient with AML who relapsed after allogeneic BMT entered a CR after immunosuppression was discontinued (74).

Incidence of Leukemic Relapse is Lower after Allogeneic BMT than after Syngeneic BMT

A comparison was made between the leukemic relapse rate in recipients of syngeneic marrow—who are not at risk for GVHD—and allogeneic marrow—who are at risk for GVHD. The patients analyzed were known to be at high risk for relapse (i.e., patients transplanted for ALL and AML in second or subsequent CR or in relapse). The results (75), presented in Figure 19-1, show that leukemic relapse was significantly higher in syngeneic marrow recipients than in allogeneic marrow recipients. The two patient groups were comparable in diagnosis, age, and interval from diagnosis to BMT, and received comparable conditioning regimens.

A similar pattern was observed among patients at low risk for post-transplant relapse (i.e., those with AML in first CR, who received allogeneic vs syngeneic

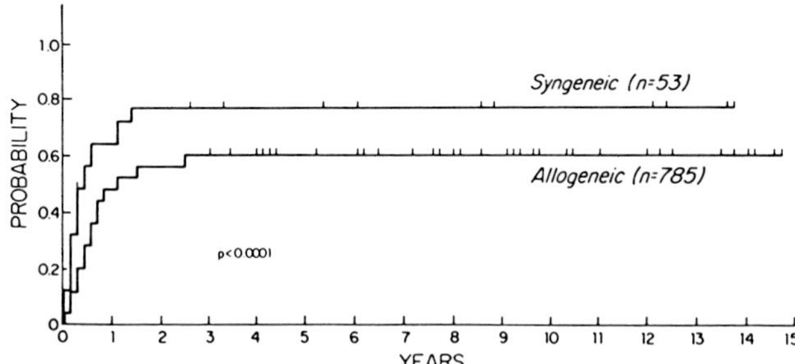

Figure 19-1. Kaplan-Meier product limit estimates of the probability of relapse of leukemia among recipients of allogeneic and syngeneic marrow (Reproduced by permission from Fefer A, et al. [75].)

marrow) (76). The results substantiate original reports from single institutions (77) and from the International Bone Marrow Transplant Registry (IBMTR) (78–80) and strongly suggest that an antileukemic effect is associated with the infusion of allogeneic marrow.

Table 19-1.
Multivariate Determinants of Relapse of Leukemia

	Proportional Hazards Analysis[a]		
Disease at Transplant	*Significant Factors*	*Relative Risk*	*p* Value
Early-stage leukemia			
AML in first remission	MTX/CSP	2.34	0.017
ALL in first remission	Acute GVHD	0.11	0.006
CML in chronic phase	None	. . .	. . .
Late-stage leukemia			
AML in relapse	A/C GVHD	0.42	0.003
	MTX	0.58	0.038
ALL in relapse	A/C GVHD	0.33	<0.001
	MTX/CSP	2.78	<0.001
CML in AP/BC	A/C GVHD	0.42	0.048

[a]Step-wise proportional hazards regression of 1,198 transplant patients using 4 time-dependent GVHD covariates.
A = acute; AP = accelerated phase; BC = blast crisis; C = chronic; CP = chronic phase; CSP = cyclosporine; MTX = methotrexate.
Reproduced by permission from Sullivan K, et al. [186].

Incidence of Leukemic Relapse is Lower in Allogeneic Marrow Recipients in whom GVHD Develops than in Allogeneic Marrow Recipients in whom GVHD does not Develop

Multivariate analyses demonstrate that GVHD is the most significant independent factor associated with a decreased relapse rate (77,79,81,82–86). Multivariate analysis of 1,198 patients with high-risk leukemia transplanted in Seattle demonstrated GVHD to be significantly associated with increased relapse-free survival (86). This effect was independent of age, sex, preparative regimen, GVHD prophylaxis, or length of follow-up. Proportional hazards regression models using acute GVHD and chronic GVHD as time-dependent covariates demonstrated a significant association of GVHD, with a decreased relative risk of relapse in patients at high risk for relapse (86) (Table 19-1).

Figure 19-2 presents the probability of relapse as a function of acute or chronic GVHD in 154 patients with ALL or AML transplanted in relapse. A two-fold reduction in recurrent leukemia was observed in patients in whom GVHD developed. A similar effect was also observed in patients transplanted for ALL in first CR (see Table 19-1). The relationship between clinical chronic GVHD and leukemic relapse was found to be dramatic in a placebo-controlled study (87). Patients with chronic GVHD that remained subclinical throughout therapy had a significantly higher (55%) probability of leukemic relapse than did patients whose chronic GVHD was or became clinically evident (87) (Figure 19-3).

Collectively, these results demonstrate that moder-

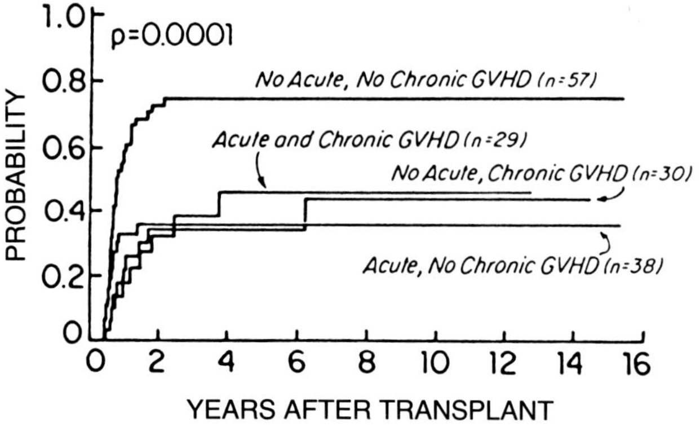

Figure 19-2. Probability of relapse in 154 patients with ALL or AML transplanted in relapse, grouped by GVHD status. All patients were alive in remission 150 days after BMT (Reproduced by permission from Sullivan K, et al. [86].)

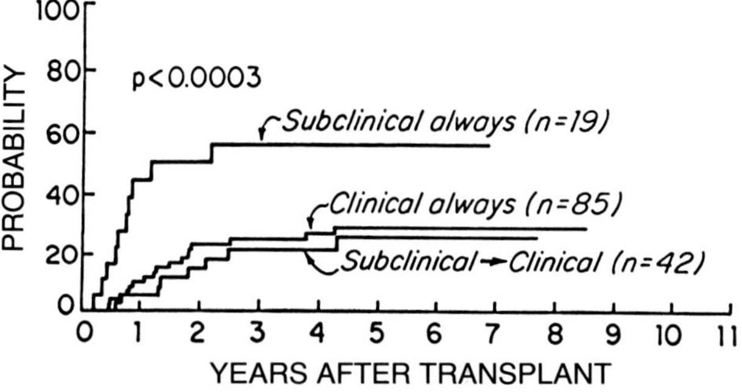

Figure 19-3. The probability of leukemic relapse after allogeneic BMT as a function of the development of clinical chronic GVHD (Reproduced by permission from Sullivan K, et al. [87].)

ate or severe clinical acute or chronic GVHD is associated with a detectable GVL effect.

Incidence of Leukemic Relapse is Lower in Recipients of Allogeneic Marrow *Without* GVHD than in Recipients of Syngeneic Marrow

The first comparative study of two patient populations (79) revealed that leukemic relapses were significantly less frequent among 79 allogeneic marrow recipients who had significant GVHD than among 117 allogeneic marrow recipients with mild or no GVHD, and that relapses in the latter group occurred with the *same* frequency as in 46 syngeneic marrow recipients. The results in a patient population heterogeneous with regard to diagnosis and phase of leukemia suggested that clinical GVHD was a prerequisite for a GVL effect.

A similar IBMTR analysis of patients with a low relapse risk (i.e., ALL and AML in first CR and chronic phase CML) (78) suggested a different conclusion. The results, summarized in Figure 19-4, show that even in recipients of allogeneic marrow who did not exhibit clinical GVHD, the relapse rate was significantly lower than in recipients of syngeneic marrow. This analysis has recently been updated (88) and evaluated for different diagnoses. Table 19-2 presents the factors that are statistically significant for influencing the relative risk (RR) of relapse. With the RR for recipients of allogeneic non-T-cell–depleted marrow without GVHD set arbitrarily at 1.00 as the reference standard, in patients transplanted for AML in first CR, the RR for allogeneic marrow recipients with acute and chronic GVHD was significantly lower than that for allogeneic marrow recipients experiencing no GVHD, but the RR for the latter group was still significantly lower than for syngeneic marrow. These results indicate that clinical GVHD is *not* a prerequisite for significant GVL (i.e., allogeneic marrow may induce a detectable GVL effect independent of clinically evident GVHD).

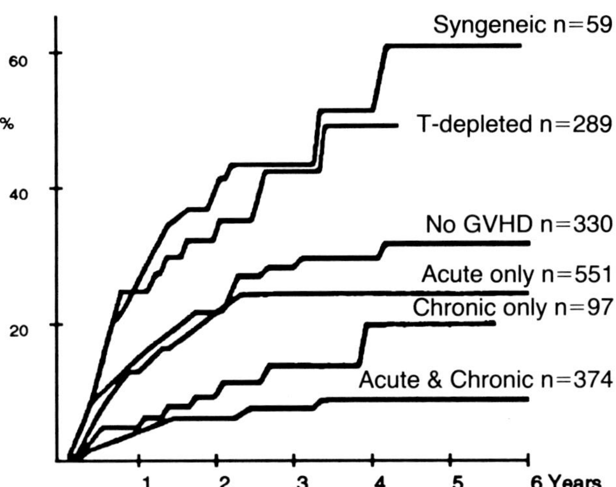

Figure 19-4. Actuarial probability of leukemic relapse after BMT for ALL in first CR, AML in first CR, and CML in chronic phase as a function of type of marrow graft and as a function of development of acute or chronic GVHD (Reproduced by permission from Horowitz MM, et al. [88].)

Incidence of Leukemic Relapse is Higher in Recipients of T-cell–depleted Allogeneic Marrow than in Recipients of Unmodified Allogeneic Marrow

The most cogent circumstantial evidence for the existence of a GVL effect in clinical BMT, and for the view that such a GVL effect is T-cell–dependent, is the finding that allogeneic recipients of unmodified marrow have a significantly lower incidence of leukemic relapse than recipients of T-cell–depleted marrow.

Table 19-2.
Relative Risk of Relapse after Bone Marrow Transplantation for Early Leukemia[a]

	ALL 1st CR		*AML 1st CR*		*CML/CP*	
Study Group	*RR*	*P*	*RR*	*P*	*RR*	*P*
Allogeneic, nondepleted						
No GVHD[b]	1.00	...	1.00	...	1.00	...
AGVHD only	0.36	0.004	...	...	...	...
AGVHD and CGHVD	0.38	0.02	0.34	0.0003	0.24	0.03
Syngeneic	...	...	2.58	0.008	...	...
Allogeneic, T-depleted						
No GVHD	...	...	...	...	6.91	0.0001
Acute and/or CGVHD	...	...	...	...	4.45	0.003

[a]Relative risks are derived from multivariate Cox regression adjusting for leukocyte count at diagnosis, recipient age, organ impairment pretransplant, donor-recipient sex-match, and drug used to prevent GVHD.
[b]Reference group.
RR = relative risk in comparison to reference group; ALL = acute lymphoblastic leukemia; AML = acute myeloid leukemia; CML = chronic myeloid leukemia; CR = complete remission; CP = chronic phase; GVHD = graft-versus-host disease.
(Reproduced by permission from Horowitz MM, et al. [88].)

This effect has been documented most dramatically in patients transplanted for chronic-phase CML. For example, in a study of 405 such patients from 82 centers in 27 countries (89), the incidence of relapse was 10% in recipients of non-T-cell–depleted marrow who had moderate to severe acute GVHD and 50% in recipients of T-cell–depleted marrow who had no or mild acute GVHD. Similarly, among recipients of non-T-cell–depleted marrow who had mild to severe chronic GVHD, only 10% relapsed, whereas among recipients of T-cell–depleted marrow who had no chronic GVHD, 55% relapsed. Confirmatory findings (90) have been reported. Similar findings have also been observed in patients transplanted for CML in the accelerated phase (91).

Detailed results of allogeneic BMT for the largest number of patients with CML in chronic phase as a function of T-cell depletion have been reported from the IBMTR and are presented in Table 19-2 (88). Recipients of unmodified marrow who exhibited acute and chronic GVHD had a significantly lower RR of relapse, as compared with recipients of unmodified marrow who experienced no GVHD—consistent with the view that GVHD is associated with a GVL effect. However, even recipients of T-cell–depleted marrow who experienced no GVHD had a far higher RR of relapse than did recipients of unmodified allogeneic marrow who had no GVHD, suggesting that in the absence of clinical GVHD, unmodified allogeneic marrow exerted an antileukemic effect (consistent with data summarized herein) but that this effect depended on the presence of T cells and was abrogated by T-cell depletion. Among recipients of T-cell–depleted marrow, the RR of relapse was not significantly different for those with GVHD and those without. The most dramatic result, however, was the observation that the RR of relapse for recipients of *T-cell–depleted* marrow with GVHD was still significantly higher than that of recipients of *unmodified* marrow without GVHD. The results support the existence of a GVL effect independent of clinical GVHD but dependent somehow on the presence of T cells in the infused marrow. The results suggest that T cells may be the direct effectors for GVL, or that other cells that cross-react with T cells are also required for the GVL effect but are eliminated in the course of T-cell depletion. Alternatively, T cells may not be the effectors but are required as intermediaries (e.g., for cytokine generation), to enable other effector cells such as LAK cells or NK cells to exert their antileukemic effect.

Collectively, the clinical data presented suggest three antitumor responses after BMT: (1) antileukemic activity associated with clinically evident GVHD, (2) antileukemic activity that can operate in the absence of GVHD, and (3) antileukemic activity independent of GVHD and diminished or abrogated by T-cell depletion. Different effector populations may contribute to GVL/GVH reactions depending on the nature of and setting for the transplant.

Effector Cells and Targets for Clinical GVL Effect

In humans, as in mice (57), different immune effector cells may act independently or in association with GVHD to mediate the GVL effect. CTL and LAK cells with reactivity to leukemic cells have been identified in marrow transplant recipients. van Rood and associates (92) described CTL, specific for class I molecules encoded telomeric to HLA-A, in the peripheral blood of allogeneic marrow recipients and hypothesized that such cells have a role in chronic GVHD and the associated GVL effect.

Some GVL antileukemic clones have been reported to have characteristics of natural killer cells (93–95). Activated NK/LAK cells, some of which lyse autologous leukemia, have been isolated from the peripheral blood following autologous or allogeneic BMT (93,95–98), leading to speculation that such cells might exert a direct GVL effect in vivo. The antitumor effect exerted by GVL effector cells derived from T- or NK-lineage may be mediated not only by their lytic activity but also by release of lymphokines, such as IL-2, tumor necrosis factor, and gamma interferon (95,99).

In allogeneic BMT, potential targets for GVL are normal host alloantigens and putative tumor-specific or tumor-associated antigens. Attempts to identify tumor-specific antigens that act as targets for immune reactions in humans have met with relatively little success. Normal cellular differentiation markers, such as those encoded by the di-allelic TCA locus (100), mimic tumor-associated antigens and may provide a target for alloreactive CTL by virtue of their preferential expression on tumor cells. In a limiting dilution analysis (101), cytotoxic CTL responses against fresh allogeneic leukemia cells were detected at a clonal level and were directed against histocompatibility antigens. In addition, there was a low frequency of CTL that were putatively leukemia-specific.

Attempts to Influence the GVL Effect

Preliminary attempts have been made to induce or exacerbate GVHD by manipulating post-BMT immunosuppression in an effort to decrease the leukemic relapse rate. In one study, 16 leukemic patients received no GVHD prophylaxis after unmodified HLA-identical sibling BMT (102). A high frequency of severe and hyperacute GVHD was observed, without a detectable effect on the incidence of leukemic relapses (103). In another clinical trial, leukemic patients received CY, total body irradiation (TBI), and unmodified HLA-identical sibling marrow and were then randomly assigned to one of three regimens for GVHD prophylaxis: a standard course of methotrexate (MTX) for 102 days after BMT; an 11-day course of MTX; or standard course of MTX plus viable buffy-coat cells from the peripheral blood of the marrow donor (104). The frequency of grade II to IV acute GVHD was 25, 59, and 82% in the three groups, respectively ($p =$

0.0001). However, the probability of leukemic relapse did not differ significantly. Thus, abbreviation of the MTX course or addition of donor buffy-coat cells increased the incidence of acute GVHD without altering the incidence of chronic GVHD, and no effect on the leukemic relapse rate was detected—partially because of a marked increase in the fatal complications associated with GVHD.

Evidence for a GVL effect exerted by *allogeneic* marrow, which can be documented only by using recipients of *syngeneic* marrow as controls, does not rule out the possibility that syngeneic or even autologous marrow also exerts some GVL effect. This effect, however, cannot be documented because appropriate controls do not exist. Indeed, GVHD can be induced in animal models (105) using either syngeneic or autologous marrow, cyclosporine, and thymic radiation (105). The pathogenesis appears to represent an imbalance of T-cell regulation, with generation of T-cells reacting against autologous Ia antigen. Accordingly, an attempt has been made to induce a GVH reaction (for a possible GVL effect) in 5 patients with lymphoma by administering cyclosporine (1 mg/kg/day) for 28 days after autologous BMT (106). Grade II acute GVHD of the skin developed in all patients by day 9 to 13, which resolved. No data were reported regarding relapse or survival.

Thus, to date, the major limitation of BMT for patients with refractory hematological malignancies continues to be a very high relapse rate after BMT (107–109). Another way to induce or augment a GVL effect is by using IL-2 ± lymphocytes as consolidative immunotherapy after BMT. Systemic administration of IL-2 with or without infusion of ex vivo-generated LAK cells (30,110) represents a new potentially noncross-resistant treatment modality for use as consolidative cellular immunotherapy after BMT as a way to induce or amplify a graft-versus-tumor response and thereby eradicate the minimal residual disease and prevent or delay relapses. This possibility is suggested by the following observations: (1) human leukemia and lymphoma cells are lysable by LAK cells in vitro (24,26,111); (2) IL-2/LAK therapy has induced remissions in some patients with leukemia and lymphoma (30,36,39–43); and (3) a state of minimal residual disease (i.e., complete remission) is readily attainable with present pretransplant conditioning regimens. Although the rationale for using IL-2 ± LAK cells after BMT applies to both allogeneic and autologous BMT, initial attention focused on studies after autologous BMT because it represents a simpler clinical setting without the complications potentially posed by immunological barriers between marrow donor and recipient. Moreover, immunotherapy after autologous BMT, if effective, should theoretically, be able to eradicate whatever clonogenic malignant cells might be present and infused with the stored marrow, thereby obviating the need for purging marrow of tumor cells.

Because relapses most often occur within the first year after autologous BMT (107–109), IL-2 ± LAK cells would have to be administered early after autologous BMT, after the patients have recovered from transplant-related toxicities and at a time when the tumor burden is still minimal but before relapses are likely to occur. In fact, IL-2-responsive LAK precursor cells have been demonstrated to be present in the circulation of patients as early as 17 days after autologous BMT (96).

Several Phase Ib clinical trials with IL-2 alone have been reported after autologous BMT to identify the maximum tolerated dose of IL-2 and to document its immunomodulatory effects, if any (112–114). The dose-limiting toxicities have been hypotension and thrombocytopenia. All toxicities reversed quickly after stopping IL-2. Neutrophil counts tended to increase throughout the course of IL-2 treatment.

Patients usually exhibited transient early lymphopenia followed by a rebound lymphocytosis 24 hours after finishing the IL-2 course. This increase reflected variable increases in the number of cells expressing CD3, CD4, CD8, and CD25. IL-2 therapy increased the percentage of circulating lymphocytes expressing CD16 and CD56 surface markers, which are associated with NK and LAK activities.

Thus, the Phase I trials of post-autologous BMT for hematological malignancies have identified an IL-2 regimen that can be tolerated safely during the first few weeks after autologous BMT and which induced immunomodulatory effects (112–114). Moreover, a trial has just been completed that demonstrated autologous LAK cells can be generated and infused with the maximum tolerated dose of IL-2 in patients with lymphoma early after autologous BMT (115). The preliminary clinical results obtained with IL-2 after autologous BMT for patients with AML at high risk for relapse and with IL-2/LAK for patients with high-risk lymphoma are encouraging and have stimulated the initiation of several randomized trials of such consolidative immunotherapy versus no immunotherapy after autologous BMT in such patients to definitely determine the effect, if any, on the relapse rate.

Future Directions

Future clinical trials directed at inducing or amplifying a graft-versus-tumor effect are likely to involve combinations of lymphokines and other biological response modifiers that might manipulate the GVL effector mechanisms to the benefit of the host. Moreover, they are likely to involve the use of lymphocytes rendered by modern molecular techniques exquisitely specific and reactive against the malignant cells. Thus, although most of the data generated to date with tumor-specific T cells have involved lymphocytes against malignant melanoma, some of the principles to be derived might be applicable to patients with other malignancies. For example, T cells might be generated that are reactive strictly to the idiotype of a particular B-cell lymphoma. Moreover, T-cell recognition of transforming proteins encoding by mutated *ras* proto-oncogenes has already been reported (116), as has T-cell immunity to the joining region of p210 *bcr-abl* protein (117). It is therefore conceivable that such specific T cells might be generated, identified, expanded, cloned, and eventually infused for therapy—similar to the way $CD8^+$ T-cell clones specific for cytomegalovirus have been generated, expanded, and infused into marrow recipients (118). Such an approach is most likely to be attempted against minimal residual disease (e.g., after BMT). Progress in molecular immunology and gene transfer technology suggests the possibility that eventually such antitumor responses may be induced preferentially or enhanced in BMT and that BMT approaches will be designed that will rely on less noxious but specific antitumor lymphocytes and lymphokines and less on the aggressive nonspecific chemoradiotherapy regimens currently used.

References

1. Fefer A, Cheever M, Greenberg P. Lymphocyte transfer as potential cancer immunotherapy. In: Mihich E ed. Immunological approaches to cancer therapeutics. New York: John Wiley & Sons, 1982:299–332.
2. Fefer A, Cheever M, Greenberg P. Overview of prospects and problems of lymphocyte transfer for cancer therapy. In: Fefer A, Goldstein AL, eds. Progress in cancer research and therapy: the potential role of T cells in cancer therapy, vol **22.** New York: Raven, 1982:1–6.
3. Rosenberg S, Packard B, Aebersold P, et al. Use of tumor-infiltrating lymphocytes and interleukin-2 in the immunotherapy of patients with metastatic melanoma: a preliminary report. N Engl J Med 1988;319:1676–1680.
4. Cheever M, Greenberg P, Fefer A. Potential for specific cancer therapy with immune T lymphocytes. J Biol Reponse Mod 1984;3:113–127.
5. Grimm E, Mazumder A, Zhand H, Rosenberg S. The lymphokine-activated killer cell phenomenon: lysis of NK resistant fresh solid tumor cells by IL-2-activated autologous human peripheral blood lymphocytes. J Exp Med 1982;155:1823–1841.
6. Mulé J, Shu S, Rosenberg S. The anti-tumor efficacy of lymphokine-activated killer cells and recombinant Interleuekin 2 in vivo. J Immunol 1985;135:646–652.
7. Rosenberg SA, Lotze MT, Muul LM, et al. A progress report on the treatment of 157 patients with advanced cancer using lymphokine-activated killer cells and interleukin-2 or high-dose interleukin-2 alone. N Engl J Med 1987;316:889–897.
8. Bortin M, Rimm A, Saltzstein E. Graft versus leukemia: quantification of adoptive immunotherapy in murine leukemia. Science 1973;179:811–813.
9. Fefer A, Einstein A Jr, Cheever M, Berenson J. Models for syngeneic adoptive chemoimmunotherapy of murine leukemias. Ann NY Acad Sci 1976;276:573–583.
10. Greenberg P. Adoptive T cell therapy of tumors: mechanisms operative in the recognition and elimination of tumor cells. In: Dixon F ed. Advances in immunology, vol **49.** Orlando, FL: Academic Press, 1991:281.
11. Fass L, Fefer A. Studies of adoptive chemoimmunotherapy of a Friend virus-induced lymphoma. Cancer Res 1972;32:997–1001.
12. Greenberg P, Cheever M, Fefer A. Eradication of disseminated murine leukemia by chemo-immunotherapy with cyclophosphamide and adoptively transferred immune syngeneic Lyt-1^+2^-T lymphocytes. J Exp Med 1981;154: 952–963.
13. Greenberg P. Therapy of murine leukemia with cyclophosphamide and immune Lyt-2^+ cells: cytolytic T cells can mediate eradication of disseminated leukemia. J Immunol 1986;136:1917–1922.
14. Cheever M, Greenberg P, Fefer A, Gillis S. Augmentation of the anti-tumor therapeutic efficacy of long-term cultured T lymphocytes by in vivo administration of purified interleukin-2. J Exp Med 1982;155:968.
15. Ortaldo JR, Mason A, Overton R. Lymphokine-activated killer cells. J Exp Med 1986;164:1193–1205.
16. Rosenberg S, Mulé J, Spiess P, Reichert CM, Schwartz SL. Regression of established pulmonary metastases and subcutaneous tumor mediated by the systemic administration of high-dose recombinant Interleukin 2. J Exp Med 1985;161:1169–1188.
17. Lafreniere R, Rosenberg S. Successful immunotherapy of experimental hepatic metastases with lymphokine-activated killer cells and recombinant interleukin-2. Cancer Res 1985;161:1169–1188.
18. Mazumder A, Rosenberg S. Successful immunotherapy of natural killer-resistant established pulmonary melanoma metastases by the intravenous adoptive transfer of syngeneic lymphocytes activated in vitro by interleukin 2. J Exp Med 1984;159:495–507.
19. Topalian S, Solomon D, Rosenberg S. Tumor-specific cytolysis by lymphocytes infiltrating human melanoma. J Immunol 1989;142:3714–3725.
20. Itoh K, Platsoucas C, Balch C. Autologous tumor-specific cytotoxic T lymphocytes in the infiltrate of human metastatic melanomas: activation by interleukin-2 and autologous tumor cells, and involvement of the T cell receptor. J Exp Med 1988;168:1419–1441.
21. Higuchi C, Triesman J, Thompson J, Lindgren C, Fefer A. Cytolytic T-lymphocytes infiltrating human melanoma expanded by culture with interleukin-2. (abstract). Proc Am Assoc Cancer Res 1990;31:269.
22. Thompson J, Lindgren C, Benz L, Benyunes M, Fefer A. Tumor-infiltrating lymphocytes (TIL) for the treatment of malignant melanoma (MM): a pilot trial (abstract). Proc Am Assoc Cancer Res 1991;82:1609.
23. Lotzová E, Ades E. Natural killer cells: definition, heterogeneity, lytic mechanism, functions and clinical application. Natl Immunol Cell Growth Regul 1989;8: 1–9.
24. Lotzová E, Savary CA, Herberman RB. Induction of NK cell activity against fresh human leukemia in culture with Interleukin 2. J Immunol 1987;138:2718–2727.
25. Mackinnon S, Hows JM, Goldman JM. Induction of in vitro graft-versus-leukemia activity following bone marrow transplantation for chronic myeloid leukemia. Blood 1990;76:2037–2045.
26. Oshimi K, Oshimi Y, Akutsu M, et al. Cytotoxicity of Interleukin 2-activated lymphocytes for leukemia and lymphoma cells. Blood 1986;68:938–948.
27. Dawson MM, Johnston D, Taylor GM, Moore M. Lymphokine activated killing of fresh human leukemias. Leuk Res 1986;10:683–688.
28. Landay AL, Zarcone D, Grossi CE, Bauer K. Relationship between target cell cycle and susceptibility to natural killer lysis. Cancer Res 1987;47:2767–2770.
29. Allavena P, Damia G, Colombo T, Maggioni D, D'Incalci M, Mantovani A. Lymphokine-activated killer (LAK)

and monocyte-mediated cytotoxicity on tumor cell lines resistant to antitumor agents. Cell Immunol 1989;120:250–258.
30. West WH, Tauer KW, Yannelli JR, et al. Constant-infusion recombinant interleukin-2 in adoptive immunotherapy of advanced cancer. N Engl J Med 1987;316: 898–905.
31. Thompson JA, Lee DJ, Lindgren CG, et al. Influence of schedule of interleukin 2 administration on therapy with interleukin 2 and lymphokine activated killer cells. Cancer Res 1989;49:235–240.
32. Thompson J, Collins C, Higuchi C, et al. High-dose continuous intravenous infusion Interleukin-2 and lymphokine-activated killer cell therapy for renal cell carcinoma. Abstr. 1606. Proc Am Assoc Cancer Res 1990;31:271.
33. Thompson J, Shulman K, Benyunes M, et al. Prolonged continuous intravenous infusion interleukin-2 and lymphokine-activated killer cell therapy for metastatic renal cell carcinoma. J Clin Oncol 1992;10:960–968.
34. Thompson JA, Lee DJ, Cox WW, et al. Recombinant Interleukin 2 toxicity, pharmacokinetics, and immunomodulatory effects in a phase I trial. Cancer Res 1987;47:4202–4207.
35. Thompson JA, Lee DJ, Lindgren CG, et al. Influence of dose and duration of infusion of Interleukin-2 on toxicity and immunomodulation. J Clin Oncol 1988;6: 669–678.
36. Rosenberg SA, Lotze MT, Yang JC, et al. Experience with the use of high-dose interleukin-2 in the treatment of 652 cancer patients. Ann Surg 1989;210:474–485.
37. Parkinson D. Interleukin 2 in cancer therapy. Semin Oncol 1988;15:10–26.
38. Rosenberg S. Immunotherapy of cancer by systemic administration of lymphoid cells and IL-2. Biol Resp Mod 1984;3:501.
39. Paciucci PA, Holland JF, Glidewell O, Odchimar R. Recombinant interleukin-2 by continuous infusion and adoptive transfer of recombinant interleukin-2-activated cells in patients with advanced cancer. J Clin Oncol 1989;7:869–878.
40. Schoof DD, Gramolini BA, Davidson DL, Massaro AF, Wilson RE, Eberlein TJ. Adoptive immunotherapy of human cancer using low-dose recombinant interleukin-2 and lymphokine-activated killer cells. Cancer Res 1988;48:5007–5010.
41. Bernstein ZP, Vaickus L, Friedman N, et al. IL-2 LAK therapy of non-Hodgkin's lymphoma and Hodgkin's disease. J Immunother 1991;10:141–146.
42. Foa R, Meloni G, Tosti S, et al. Treatment of residual disease in acute leukemia patients with recombinant interleukin 2 (IL2): clinical and biological findings. Bone Marrow Transplant 1990;6:98–102.
43. Foa R, Meloni G, Tosti S, et al. Treatment of acute myeloid leukemia patients with recombinant IL2: clinical and biological findings. ASH Abstr. 1071. Blood 1990;76:270a.
44. Barnes D, Loutit J, Neal F. Treatment of murine leukemia with X-rays and homologous bone marrow. Br Med J 1956;2:626–630.
45. Barnes D, Loutit J. Treatment of murine leukemia with X-rays and homologous bone marrow. Br J Haematol 1957;3:241–252.
46. Mathé G, Amiel J, Niemetz J. Greffe de moelle osseuse après irradiation totale chez des souris leucémiques suivie de l'administration d'un antimitotique pour réduire la fréquence du syndrome secondaire et ajouter à l'effet antileucémique. CR Acad Sci (Paris) 1962;254:3603–3605.
47. Glucksberg H, Fefer A. Chemotherapy of established graft-versus-host (GVH) disease in mice. Transplantation 1972;13:300–305.
48. Truitt R, LeFever A, Shih C-Y. Graft-versus-leukemia reactions: experimental models and clinical trials. In: Gale RP, Champlin R, eds. Progress in bone marrow transplantation. New York: Alan R. Liss, 1987:219–232.
49. Truitt R, Shih C-Y, LeFever A. Manipulation of graft-versus-host disease for a graft-versus-leukemia effect after allogeneic bone marrow transplantation in AKR mice with spontaneous leukemia/lymphoma. Transplantation 1986;41:301–310.
50. Truitt R, Pollard M, Srivastava K. Allogeneic bone marrow chimerism in germfree state. III. Therapy of leukemic AKR mice. Proc Soc Exp Biol Med 1974;146: 153–158.
51. Slavin S, Weiss L, Morecki S, Weigensberg M. Eradication of murine leukemia with histoincompatible marrow grafts in mice conditioned with total lymphoid irradiation (TLI). Cancer Immunol Immunother 1981; 11:155–158.
52. Denham S, Attridge S, Barfoot R, Alexander P. Effect of cyclosporin A on the anti-leukaemia action associated with graft-versus-host disease. Br J Cancer 1983; 47:791–795.
53. Meredith R, O'Kunewick J. Possibility of graft-versus-leukemia determinants independent of the major histocompatibility complex in allogeneic marrow transplantation. Transplantation 1983;35:378–385.
54. Bortin M, Rimm A, Salzstein E, Rodey G. Graft versus leukemia. III. Apparent independent antihost and antileukemia activity of transplanted immunocompetent cells. Transplantation 1973;16:182–188.
55. Korngold R, Sprent J. T cell subsets and graft-versus-host disease. Transplantation 1987;44:335–339.
56. Truitt R, LeFever A, Shih C-Y. Analysis of effector cells in the graft-versus-leukemia reaction and their relation to graft-versus-host disease. In: Martelli, Grignani, Reisner eds. T-cell depletion in allogeneic bone marrow transplantation. Rome: Ares-Serono Symposia, 1988:73–85.
57. Truitt R, LeFever A, Shih C-Y, Jeske J, Martin T. Graft-vs-leukemia effects. In: Burakoff, Deeg, Ferrara, Atkinson eds. Graft-vs-host disease. New York: Marcel Dekker, 1990.
58. LeFever A, Truitt R, Shih C-Y. Reactivity of in vitro-expanded alloimmune cytotoxic T lymphocytes and Qa-1-specific cytotoxic T lymphocytes against AKR leukemia in vivo. Transplantation 1985;40:531–537.
59. Clancy JJ, Goral J, Kovacs E, Ellis T. Role of recombinant interleukin-2 (rIL-2) and large granular lymphocytes (LGLs) in acute rat graft-versus-host disease (GVHD). Transplant Proc 1989;21:88–89.
60. Ghayur T, Seemayer T, Kongshavn P, Cartner J, and Lapp W. Graft-versus host reactions in the beige mouse: an investigation of the role of host and donor natural killer cells in the pathogenesis of graft-versus-host disease. Transplantation 1987;44:261–266.
61. Malkovsk'y M, Brenner MK, Hunt R, et al. T-cell depletion of allogeneic bone marrow prevents acceleration of graft-versus-host disease induced by exogenous interleukin 2. Cell Immunol 1986;103:476–480.
62. Merluzzi VJ, Welte K, Last-Barney K, et al. Production and response to Interleukin 2 in vitro and in vivo after bone marrow transplantation in mice. J Immunol 1985;134:2426–2430.

63. Toshitani A, Taniguchi K, Himeno K, Kawani Y-I, Nonoto K. Adoptive transfer of H-2-incompatible lymphokine-activated killer (LAK) cells: an approach for successful cancer immunotherapy free from graft-versus-host disease (GVHD) using murine models. Cell Immunol 1988;115:373–382.
64. Sykes M, Romick ML, Sachs DH. Interleukin 2 prevents graft-versus-host disease while preserving the graft-versus-leukemia effect of allogeneic T cells. Proc Natl Acad Sci USA 1990;87:5633–5637.
65. Sykes M, Romick ML, Hoyles KA, Sachs DH. In vivo administration of interleukin 2 plus T cell-depleted syngeneic marrow prevents graft-versus-host disease mortality and permits alloengraftment. J Exp Med 1990;171:645–658.
66. Sprent J, Schaefer M, Gao E-K, Korngold R. Role of T cell subsets in lethal graft-versus-host disease (GVHD) directed to class I versus class II H-2 differences. J Exp Med 1988;167:556–569.
67. Azuma E, Yamamoto H, Kaplan J. Use of lymphokine-activated killer cells to prevent bone marrow graft rejection and lethal graft-vs-host disease. J Immunol 1989;143:1524–1529.
68. Slavin S, Eckerstein A, Weiss L. Adoptive immunotherapy in conjunction with bone marrow transplantation—amplification of natural host defence mechanisms against cancer by recombinant IL-2. Natl Immunol Cell Growth Regul 1988;7:180–184.
69. Agah R, Malloy B, Kerner M, et al. Potent graft antitumor effect in natural killer-resistant disseminated tumors by transplantation of Interleukin 2-activated syngeneic bone marrow in mice. Cancer Res 1989;49:5959–5963.
70. Charak BS, Brynes RK, Groshen S, Chen S-C, Mazumder A. Bone marrow transplantation with interleukin-2-activated bone marrow followed by interleukin-2 therapy for acute myeloid leukemia in mice. Blood 1990;76:2187–2190.
71. Odom L, August C, Githens J, Humbert J. "Graft-versus-leukemia" reaction following bone marrow transplantation for acute lymphoblastic leukemia. In: O'Kunewick P, Meredith J eds. Graft-versus-leukemia in man and animal models. Boca Raton, FL: CRC Press, 1981:25–43.
72. Odom L, August C, Githens J, et al. Remission of relapsed leukaemia during a graft-versus-host reaction: a "graft-versus leukaemia reaction" in man? Lancet 1978;2:537–540.
73. Sullivan K, Shulman H. Chronic graft-versus-host disease, obliterative bronchiolitis, and graft-versus-leukemia effect: case histories. Transplant Proc 1989; 21:51–62.
74. Higano C, Brixey M, Bryant E, et al. Durable complete remission of acute non-lymphocytic leukemia associated with discontinuation of immunosuppression following relapse after allogeneic bone marrow transplantation: a case report of a graft-versus-leukemia effect. Transplantation 1990;50:175–177.
75. Fefer A, Sullivan K, Weiden P, et al. Graft versus leukemia effect in man: the relapse rate of acute leukemia is lower after allogeneic than after syngeneic marrow transplantation. In: Truitt R, Gale RP, Bortin MM, eds. Cellular immunotherapy of cancer. New York: Alan R. Liss, 1987:401–408.
76. Gale R, Champlin R. How does bone-marrow transplantation cure leukaemia? Lancet. 1984;2:28–30.
77. Weiden PL, Sullivan KM, Flournoy N, Storb R, Thomas ED. Antileukemic effect of chronic graft-versus-host disease. N Engl J Med 1981;304:1529–1533.
78. Ringdén O, Horowitz M. Graft-versus-leukemia reactions in humans. Transplant Proc 1989;21:2989–2992.
79. Weiden P, Flournoy N, Thomas ED, et al. Antileukemic effect of graft-versus-host disease in human recipients of allogeneic-marrow grafts. N Engl J Med 1979;300: 1068–1073.
80. Butturini A, Bortin M, Gale R. Graft-versus-leukemia following bone marrow transplantation. Bone Marrow Transplant 1987;2:233–242.
81. Bacigalupo A, Lint VMT, Frassoni F, Marmont A. Graft-versus-leukaemia effect following allogeneic bone marrow transplantation. Br J Haematol 1985;61:749–750.
82. Sanders J, Flournoy N, Thomas ED, et al. Marrow transplant experience in children with acute lymphoblastic leukemia: an analysis of factors associated with survival, relapse, and graft-versus-host disease. Med Pediatr Oncol 1985;13:165–172.
83. Weisdorf D, Nesbit M, Ramsay N, et al. Allogeneic bone marrow transplantation for acute lymphoblastic leukemia in remission: prolonged survival associated with acute graft-versus-host disease. J Clin Oncol 1987;5:1348–1355.
84. Kersey J, Weisdorf D, Nesbit M, et al. Comparison of autologous and allogeneic bone marrow transplantation for treatment of high-risk refractory acute lymphoblastic leukemia. N Engl J Med 1987;317:461–467.
85. Sullivan K, Fefer A, Witherspoon R, et al. Graft-versus-leukemia in man: relationship of acute and chronic graft-versus-host disease to relapse of acute leukemia following allogeneic bone marrow transplantation. In: Truitt R, Gale RP, Bortin MM, eds. Cellular immunotherapy of cancer. New York: Alan R. Liss, 1987:391–399.
86. Sullivan K, Weiden P, Storb R, et al. Influence of acute and chronic graft-versus-host disease on relapse and survival after bone marrow transplantation from HLA-identical siblings as treatment of acute and chronic leukemia. Blood 1989;73:1720–1728.
87. Sullivan K, Witherspoon R, Storb R, et al. Prednisone and azathioprine compared with prednisone and placebo for treatment of chronic graft-v-host disease: prognostic influence of prolonged thrombocytopenia after allogeneic marrow transplantation. Blood 1988; 72:546–554.
88. Horowitz MM, Gale RP, Sondel PM, et al. Graft-versus-leukemia reactions following bone marrow transplantation in humans. Blood 1990;75:555–562.
89. Goldman JM, Gale RP, Horowitz MM, et al. Bone marrow transplantation for chronic myelogenous leukemia in chronic phase: increased risk for relapse associated with T-cell depletion. Ann Intern Med 1988;108:806–814.
90. Apperley J, Mauro F, Goldman J, et al. Bone marrow transplantation for chronic myeloid leukaemia in first chronic phase: importance of a graft-versus-leukaemia effect. Br J Haematol. 1988;69:239–245.
91. Martin P, Clift R, Fisher L, et al. HLA-identical marrow transplantation during accelerated-phase chronic myelogenous leukemia: analysis of survival and remission duration. Blood 1988;72:1978–1984.
92. van Rood JJ, Goulmy E, Leeuwen VA. The immunogenetics of chronic graft versus host disease and its relevance to the graft versus leukemia effect. In: Truitt R, Gale RP, Bortin MM, eds. Cellular immunotherapy of cancer. New York: Alan R. Liss, 1987:433–438.
93. Hercend T, Takvorian T, Nowill A, et al. Characteriza-

tion of natural killer cells with antileukemia activity following allogeneic bone marrow transplantation. Blood 1986;67:722–726.

94. Delmon L, Ythier A, Moingeon P, et al. Characterization of antileukemia cells' cytotoxic effector function. Transplantation 1986;42:252–256.
95. Reittie JE, Gottlieb D, Heslop HE, et al. Endogenously generated activated killer cells circulate after autologous and allogeneic marrow transplantation but not after chemotherapy. Blood 1989;73:1351–1358.
96. Higuchi C, Thompson J, Cox T, Lindgren C, Buckner C, Fefer A. Lymphokine-activated killer function following autologous bone marrow transplantation for refractory hematologic malignancies. Cancer Res 1989;49: 5509–5513.
97. Keever CA, Welte K, Small T, et al. Interleukin 2-activated killer cells in patients following transplants of soybean lectin-separated and E rosette-depleted bone marrow. Blood 1987;70:1893–1903.
98. Rooney CM, Wimperis JZ, Brenner MK, Patterson J, Hoffbrand AV, Prentice HG. Natural killer cell activity following T-cell depleted allogeneic bone marrow transplantation. Br J Haematol 1986;62:413–420.
99. Heslop HE, Gottlieb DJ, Reittie JE, et al. Spontaneous and interleukin 2 induced secretion of tumour necrosis factor and gamma interferon following autologous marrow transplantation or chemotherapy. Br J Haematol 1989;72:122–126.
100. van Leeuwen A, Schrier P, Giphart M, et al. TCA: a polymorphic genetic marker in leukemias and melanoma cell lines. Blood 1986;67:1139–1142.
101. Sosman J, Oetel K, Hank H, Fisch P, Sondel P. Specific recognition of human leukemic cells by allogeneic T cell lines. Transplantation 1989;48:486–495.
102. Sullivan K, Deeg H, Sanders J, et al. Hyperacute graft-v-host disease in patients not given immunosuppression after allogeneic marrow transplantation. Blood 1986;67:1172–1175.
103. Sullivan K, Storb R, Witherspoon R, et al. Deletion of immunosuppressive prophylaxis after marrow transplantation increases hyperacute graft-versus-host disease but does not influence chronic graft-versus-host disease or relapse in patients with advanced leukemia. Clin Transplant 1989;3:5–11.
104. Sullivan KM, Storb R, Buckner CD, et al. Graft-versus-host disease as adoptive immunotherapy in patients with advanced hematologic neoplasms. N Engl J Med 1989;320:828–834.
105. Santos G. Syngeneic or autologous graft-versus-host disease. Int J Cell Cloning 1989;7:92–99.
106. Jones R, Vogelsang G, Hess A, et al. Induction of graft-versus-host disease after autologous bone marrow transplantation. Lancet 1989;1:754–757.
107. Philip T, Armitage JO, Spitzer G, et al. High dose therapy and autologous bone marrow transplantation after failure of conventional chemotherapy in adults with intermediate grade or high grade non-Hodgkin's lymphoma. N Engl J Med 1987;316:1493–1498.
108. Takvorian T, Canellos G, Ritz J, et al. Prolonged disease-free survival after autologous bone marrow transplantation in patients with non-Hodgkin's lymphoma with a poor prognosis. N Engl J Med 1987;316: 1499–1505.
109. Petersen F, Appelbaum F, Hill R, et al. Autologous marrow transplantation for malignant lymphoma: a report of 101 cases from Seattle. J Clin Oncol 1990;8:638–647.
110. Rosenberg S, Lotze M, Muul L, et al. Observations on the systemic administration of autologous lymphokine-activated killer cells and recombinant interleukin-2 to patients with metastatic cancer. N Engl J Med 1985;313:1485–1492.
111. Adler A, Chervenick PA, Whiteside TL, Lotzova E, Herberman R. Interleukin-2 induction of lymphokine-activated killer (LAK) activity in the peripheral blood and bone marrow of acute leukemia patients. I. Feasibility of LAK generation in adult patients with active disease and in remission. Blood 1988;71:709–716.
112. Higuchi CM, Thompson JA, Petersen FB, Buckner CD, Fefer A. Toxicity and immunomodulatory effects of interleukin 2 after autologous bone marrow transplantation for hematologic malignancies. Blood 1991;77: 2561–2568.
113. Blaise D, Olive D, Stoppa AM, et al. Hematologic and immunologic effects of the systemic administration of recombinant interleukin-2 after autologous bone marrow transplantation. Blood 1990;76:1092–1097.
114. Gottlieb DJ, Brenner MK, Heslop HE, et al. A phase I clinical trial of recombinant interleukin 2 following high dose chemoradiotherapy for haematological malignancy: applicability to the elimination of minimal residual disease. Br J Cancer 1989;60:610–615.
115. Benyunes M, York A, Lindgren C, et al. IL-2 ± LAK cells as consolidative therapy after autologous BMT for hematologic malignancies: a feasibility trial (abstract). Proc Am Soc Clin Oncol 1992;11:319.
116. Peace D, Chen W, Nelson H, Cheever M. T cell recognition of transforming proteins encoded by mutated ras proto-oncogenes. J Immunol 1991;146:2059–2065.
117. Chen W, Peace D, Rovira D, You S-G, Cheever M. T cell immunity to the joining region of p210 bcr-abl protein. Proc Natl Acad Sci USA 1992;89:1468–1472.
118. Riddell S, Watanabe K, Goodrich J, Li C-R, Agha M, Greenberg P. Reconstitution of viral immunity in immunocompromised humans by the adoptive transfer of T cell clones. Science 1992;257:238–241.

Chapter 20
Biostatistical Methods in Marrow Transplantation

Joyce C. Niland and Lloyd D. Fisher

It is impossible to cover the ideas and methods of statistics needed for analyses of bone marrow transplant (BMT) data in one chapter. This chapter, designed for a clinical audience, concentrates on the methodology most often used in BMT studies. We focus on the general concepts, procedures, and interpretations of specific study designs and statistical analyses, with particular emphasis on clinical trials (i.e., planned experiments to assess the efficacy of treatments in humans). It is assumed that the reader is acquainted with the usual concepts of a beginning course in statistics: probability, estimation of parameters, hypothesis testing, and confidence intervals; if not, there are texts for an introduction to biostatistics (1–3) and clinical trials (4–6). The mathematics will not be presented herein, although references will be given.

The first section of this chapter focuses on the successive phases of a clinical trial, with mention of some recent advances in this area (7). The last section describes selected statistical techniques often used in the analysis of marrow transplantation data and gives examples of their use in BMT.

Phases of Clinical Trials in BMT

In this section we present the three main phases of a clinical trial: rationale, study design, and some currently accepted procedures for trial conduct. We present cautionary notes regarding study conduct and interpretation, and illustrate each phase with a recent BMT investigation. We end each phase with recent developments and future directions in clinical trials.

Phase I Clinical Trials

The primary aim of a *Phase I clinical trial* is to determine the *maximal tolerated dose* (MTD) for a new drug, biologic, new drug combination, radiation therapy, or other dose variable strategy, under the assumption that a larger dose is more likely to give therapeutic benefit to patients as well as an increase in adverse events. Because the adverse events associated with large doses may be life-threatening, the concept of the MTD is a relative one that depends on the acceptable level of toxicity weighed against possible clinical gain. When contrasted with Phase I studies of patients with solid tumors, Phase I trials in acute leukemia are often more aggressive and the MTD frequently higher with respect to hematological toxicities because it is generally accepted that antileukemic activity will be accompanied by myelosuppressive activity (6). If the mortality rate in a subset of patients is quite high using an existing therapy (e.g., a conditioning regimen with 20% treatment-related mortality), then even with high levels of toxicity the potential gain is enormous.

Standard Procedure to Conduct a Phase I Trial

Although the emphasis of a Phase I trial is defining toxicity and determining a suitable dose for future efficacy testing, there is at least hope that the treatment will benefit the individual patients. Thus, Phase I trials in BMT are often performed on selected homogeneous subsets of high-risk patients. This approach contrasts with that of a typical Phase I solid tumor study, in which the sample consists of a heterogeneous group of volunteers with advanced cancer no longer responsive to standard therapy.

Requirements for entry into a Phase I study typically include (1) minimum estimated life expectancy of at least 8 to 12 weeks; (2) a reasonably good performance status (e.g., a minimum Karnofsky Performance Status [KPS] of 80); (3) cessation of all prior experimental therapy for a minimum of 2 to 6 weeks; and (4) adequate major organ function to allow normal metabolism of the new agent. Protocol elements specified in a standard Phase I trial include patient selection and diagnosis, drug description, types of adverse events to be evaluated (although any observed adverse events should be recorded), and criteria for response (8). Although potential benefit must also be considered, a safe starting dose should be selected based on preclinical pharmacology, animal toxicity, or use in other types of patients (9). Typically, one tenth of the mouse equivalent dose lethal to 10% of nontumor-bearing animals (MELD 10) is considered a safe starting dose in humans. Guarino and colleagues (10) discussed in some detail the problems of arriving at a precise number for the MELD 10. The level of toxicity considered unacceptable, which will therefore determine the MTD, should be defined in advance.

The usual procedure in a Phase I trial is to gradually

increase the dose in successive groups of patients until the predetermined level of unacceptable toxicity occurs. A number of dose escalation schemes are available. One widely used approach is the "*modified Fibonacci*" scheme, in which the starting dose is doubled (100% greater) to obtain the second level, the third level is 67% greater than the second level, the fourth level is 50% greater than the third level, and each subsequent level is 33% greater than the preceding dose level. Alternative dose escalation schemes include doubling the dose at each step; the constant step-size scheme, in which each dose is increased by a constant increment (c) over the previous dose; and the unit step-size scheme, in which the constant step-size scheme is applied, with c equal to the initial dose (8). In the process of dose escalation, care must be taken to avoid overaccrual to subtherapeutic dose levels and overexposure of patients to unacceptably high toxicity levels (11). The typical number of doses in our experience is 6; 25 is the usual number of patients accrued. Often in trials involving BMT patients, the study therapy will have been used in other types of patients and a crude estimate of the toxicity may exist. However, the patterns of toxicity can change markedly in the BMT population, so that caution is still needed.

One dose escalation procedure commonly used (Figure 20-1) is to accrue 3 patients to a given dose level, allowing sufficient time to observe adverse reactions before moving to the next dose level. If no grade III or IV toxicity is observed in the 3 patients after one complete course, doses are escalated one level. If a single patient experiences grade III toxicity, 3 additional patients are treated at the same dose level; drug doses may continue to be escalated only if no additional grade III or IV toxicity is observed. However, if a second grade III toxicity is observed or any grade IV toxicity is seen, the MTD is established to be the next lower dose level. In some situations it is recommended that 6 patients be accrued at the MTD dose level, with the occurrence of no grade IV and at most one grade III toxicity, before the trial is considered complete. This approach will provide evidence that this dose results in acceptable toxicity before an ensuing Phase II trial.

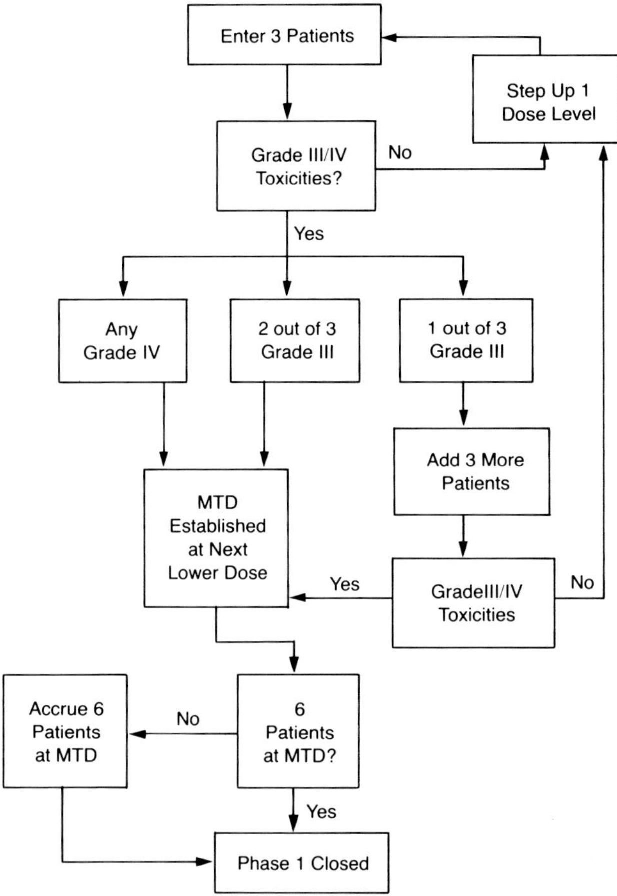

Figure 20-1. Flow chart for conduct of a standard Phase I trial.

Cautions in the Conduct of a Phase I Trial

Some investigators see an ethical dilemma in enrolling patients in a Phase I trial because responses are not the primary objective. Although the probability of therapeutic benefit is unknown, the possibility of a response does exist, and a Phase I trial is often a good means of continuing active therapy. Some efficacy data will accrue from Phase I studies; however, the information is limited because only the highest doses are of interest. Although response rates should be examined at the close of a Phase I trial, a lack of response should not necessarily deter the investigator from performing a Phase II trial. Conversely, responses observed during the uncontrolled Phase I trial should not be used as a substitute for performing a full Phase II or III study.

A recent criticism of Phase I trials is that ". . . the recommended dose has no interpretation as an estimate of the dose which yields a specified rate of severe [side effects]" (12). In the opinion of these authors, the uncertainty in the dose selected is not generally appreciated. Often only 3 patients are observed with the usual scheme; who would think of using an estimate and a confidence interval based on only 3 patients? This issue is especially severe when one desires a dose with a specified amount of severe toxicity (e.g., because a favorable risk/benefit ratio may result) (12,13). The uncertainty in dose based on Phase I trials implies that investigators should be alert to the possibility of considering other doses as more information accumulates.

Example of a Phase I Trial in BMT

A Phase I trial was conducted to test a new preparatory regimen for BMT in patients with advanced hematological malignancies (14). Patients were treated with fractionated total body irradiation (TBI) combined with high doses of etoposide (VP-16) prior to BMT. A constant step-size dose escalation scheme was used, with VP-16 dose levels set at 30, 40, 50, 60, and 70 mg/kg. Thirty-one patients were treated on this Phase I trial; the dose-limiting toxicity of VP-16, used in combination with a fixed dose of radiation, was found to be severe stomatitis (grade III–IV) at 70 mg/kg. Therefore, 60 mg/kg was established as the MTD; 16 additional subjects received this dose in a subsequent Phase II trial to examine efficacy.

Recent Developments and Future Directions for Phase I Trials

In an attempt to reconcile the needs of dose-finding experimentation with the ethical demands of established medical practice, new Phase I designs have been explored. One approach, the "continual reassessment method" (12), has been found to compare favorably to the traditional Phase I design. This method concentrates experimentation at the dose that is estimated to produce a targeted, acceptable toxicity level, based on all available evidence at the time. Other approaches to Phase I trials have been suggested and may prove valuable (12,13).

Phase II Clinical Trials

Once the appropriate Phase I dose level has been established, a *Phase II clinical trial* is conducted to determine whether the new therapy has sufficient evidence of biological activity to warrant further investigation. Phase II trials in BMT are performed not only for antitumor activity, but also to prevent relapse, for prophylaxis and treatment of graft-versus-host disease (GVHD), for treatment of symptoms of other therapies (e.g., pain relief), and for prophylaxis against and treatment of infections.

Standard Procedures to Conduct a Phase II Trial

Phase II trials are typically conducted in patients most likely to respond favorably, so that activity is not missed. Therefore, subjects with maximum performance status and a minimum amount of prior therapy should be chosen when ethically possible. In addition, all patients in a Phase II trial must demonstrate measurable disease, so that the drug's activity can be assessed.

The *one sample group sequential design* of Fleming (15) is a commonly employed approach for Phase II trials. The initial sample size is dependent on the desired minimum response rate. Gehan and Schneiderman (16) described the number of consecutive non-responding patients that must be observed to terminate a trial early with the assurance (with 95 or 90% power) that the true response rate will not be higher than a predetermined level. As an example from Table 20-1, if a new therapy must yield at least a 20% response rate, then 14 patients would be enrolled initially; if no responses were seen in this first group of patients, the investigator could conclude with 95% certainty that the true response in similar patients is less than 20%. However, if at least one response was observed, an additional 11 patients would be accrued, yielding a total sample size of 25 patients. This number allows estimation of the response rate with a maximum standard error of 10% (occurring when the probability of response is equal to 50%). It may be desirable to use a larger sample size than 25 to obtain a smaller standard error of the response estimate (and a narrower confidence interval); in this case, it makes sense to increase the first accrual stage beyond 14 patients.

Table 20-1.
Number of Patients Required for Phase II Trial of an Agent for Given Levels of Therapeutic Effectiveness and Type II Error

Rejection Error (β)(%)	*Therapeutic Effectiveness (%)*									
	5	*10*	*15*	*20*	*25*	*30*	*35*	*40*	*45*	*50*
5	59	29	19	14	11	9	7	6	6	5
10	45	22	15	11	9	7	6	5	4	4

Reproduced by permission from Gehan EA, Schneiderman MA. Experimental design of clinical trials. In: Holland JF, Frei E III, eds. Cancer Medicine, ed.2. Philadelphia: Lea and Febiger, 1982: 531–555.

The Optimized Two-stage Phase II Design

Sample sizes for an *optimized two-stage Phase II* design have been developed by Simon (17). As with the designs of Fleming (15) and Gehan and Schneiderman (16), early termination of the study is permitted only when rejecting a therapy due to a low response rate. Early acceptance of a promising drug might be desirable in certain instances (e.g., if a limited number of patients were available, or if a drug were very expensive); Fleming (15) and Chang and O'Brien (18) described designs that include this option. However, even if substantial drug activity is present in the first stage, accruing additional patients in the second stage allows better estimation of the proportion, extent, and durability of response.

Simon's optimal design (17) ensures that the sample size for the first stage will be as small as possible, which is particularly desirable when studying a homogeneous BMT population. In optimizing the sample size, two possible types of errors are important: (1) alpha—the probability of failing to reject the treatment even though the true response rate is less than the minimum required response rate; and (2) beta—the probability of rejecting the treatment even though the true response rate is greater than or equal to the response rate of interest. Alpha is the less serious error for drug discovery, but is more serious with respect to the unnecessary cost of a follow-up Phase III trial for a drug that actually should have been rejected. Table 20-2, based on the article by Simon (17), shows the optimal sample sizes when

Table 20-2.
Sample Sizes for Optimal Two-stage Phase II Designs

		Sample Sizes for Optimal Phase II Design[a]					
		First Stage of Accrual			*Second Stage of Accrual*		
Drug Not of Interest if True Response Rate ≤	*Desirable True Response Rate*	*Accrue n_1 Patients (n_1)*	*Reject if ≤ r_1 Responses (r_1)*	*Otherwise*	*Add n_2 Patients (n_2)*	*Reject if ≤ r Total Responses ($r = r_1 + r_2$)*	*Maximum Sample Size (n)*
0.05	0.20	10	0		19	3	29
	0.25	9	0		8	2	17
0.10	0.25	18	2		25	7	43
	0.30	10	1		19	5	29
0.20	0.35	22	5		50	19	72
	0.40	13	3		30	12	43
0.30	0.45	27	9		54	30	81
	0.50	15	5		31	18	46
0.40	0.55	26	11		58	40	84
	0.60	16	7		30	23	46
0.50	0.65	28	15		55	48	83
	0.70	15	8		28	26	43
0.60	0.75	27	17		40	46	67
	0.80	11	7		32	30	43
0.70	0.85	19	14		40	46	59
	0.90	6	4		21	22	27
0.80	0.95	9	7		20	26	29

[a]Assuming alpha = 0.05 and beta = 0.20.

alpha is set at 0.05 and beta at 0.20, reasonable values for most Phase II studies. In the table, the difference between the response rate below which the drug is uninteresting, and above which it is definitely of interest, ranges from 0.15 to 0.20. Smaller differences would require sample sizes too large to be practical, and results would be difficult to interpret due to the lack of concurrent controls. For Phase II studies in BMT, the minimum response rate of interest will often be in the range of 50 to 60%, whereas the desirable response rate to be achieved will often be 65 to 70%.

Cautions in the Conduct of a Phase II Trial

Phase II trials are sometimes performed to accumulate experience with a therapy before deciding whether to embark on a Phase III trial. Another commonly employed design is to conduct a fixed sample size Phase II trial, and to compare the results to historical control subjects. Because of the difficulties of choosing appropriate control subjects, Phase II trials are usually considered to be hypothesis-generating rather than definitive proof of efficacy. The decision to terminate a Phase II trial early (i.e., after stage 1) for a treatment with poor activity in a well-defined homogeneous group of patients is usually less difficult than the decision to halt a Phase III trial prior to its full accrual. However, caution is still needed, and other factors, such as secondary end points or activity level of the drug in selected subsets of patients, need to be considered.

Example of a Phase II Trial in BMT

A Phase II trial was conducted to determine the effectiveness of thalidomide in the treatment of steroid- and cyclosporine-resistant chronic GVHD (19). Because patients in whom chronic GVHD develops after failing to respond to cyclosporine and prednisone are unlikely to respond to further standard treatments, a response rate as low as 5% would warrant continuing the trial; a response rate in the range of 25% was desired. Using these estimates and Table 20-2, the optimal first stage sample size was 9 patients. Because there were some responders among the first 9 patients, the drug was not rejected and the trial was continued to a sample size of 18 patients to obtain a more stable estimate of response. Ten responses gave an estimated response rate of 56% and an exact 95% confidence interval of 31 to 78%; further investigation of this drug was warranted because the true response rate was greater than 25% with 95% certainty.

Recent Developments and Future Directions for Phase II Trials

Certain variations on the standard Phase II design have been more recently explored, such as inclusion of a Phase II treatment arm as part of a Phase III clinical trial (20); randomized Phase II trials (which are really active-control Phase III trials) to select the most promising of several new agents (21); and "calibrated" Phase II trials, in which a subgroup of patients are randomized to a standard treatment to verify that the patient population under study is capable of responding to an active treatment (22).

Phase III Clinical Trials

A *randomized Phase III clinical trial* is an experiment in which patients are assigned to therapeutic strategies by random, or probabilistic, assignment to determine which strategy is superior. These trials can be contrasted with observational studies, which may also compare competing therapeutic strategies, but the choice of therapy received does not involve randomization. The primary rationale for the randomized clinical trial is to assure that the groups under comparison are comparable (4,23–26). Although the need to evaluate competing therapeutic strategies on comparable groups has been recognized for a long time (23), the difficulty of assuring that groups of patients treated in different manners are really comparable has often gone unrecognized. The randomized clinical trial is a relatively recent innovation in the evaluation of new and modified therapies; the first trials were published in 1931, 1938, and 1944 (27–29).

Table 20-3, adapted from Green and Byar (30), suggests a hierarchy of study designs from the most convincing to the least convincing. One reason the randomized trial is so convincing is because it statistically balances treatment groups not only with respect to known and recorded factors but also with respect to *unknown or unrecorded patient factors*. Although humans might not construct comparable groups because of unconscious biases (30) (which can run in either direction), statistical balance obeys the laws of probability. Although perfect balance is not expected, the effects of imbalances can be treated by these laws. A randomized trial is also convincing because the data may be analyzed without requiring statistical assumptions (25,31–34), whereas the assumptions needed in an observational data analysis can falsely introduce, or obscure, treatment differences. Lack of adequate variables to characterize patient prognosis is the most important problem with observational analyses; mathematical models may inadequately mirror the prognosis, and the sample size may be too small to detect this inadequacy. If prognosis does involve many variables, a very large number of patients would be needed to appropriately analyze the data.

Often historical control subjects are suggested in lieu of random concurrent control subjects. Usually historical control patients are those treated earlier at the same institutions using a different therapy from the new therapy under consideration; sometimes results from the literature are used. Although some believe that historical control subjects are convincing in certain situations (35,36), most scientists consider such comparisons to be only suggestive of benefit rather than proving benefit. A standard argument for the use of historical control subjects is the "penicillin argument": Wouldn't the advance be clear enough without a randomized trial? Although there may be a few advances so clear cut that historical control subjects would suffice, they are few and far between; furthermore, a randomized evaluation of such great leaps forward would require only a very few patients. For example, if the true probabilities of success were 100 versus 0%, it would require only 8 patients to obtain 100% statistical power for a two-sided hypothesis test. When the results of randomized trials have been compared with what would have been concluded using historical control subjects the results often differed (37,38). The scientific cogency of results from a randomized trial is so much greater than results from other designs that the United States Food and Drug Administration generally requires randomized comparisons as proof of efficacy and safety for new drugs.

Table 20-3.
Hierarchy of Strength of Evidence Concerning Efficacy of Treatment

Confirmed randomized controlled clinical trials
Single randomized controlled clinical trials
Series based on historical control groups
"Case-control" observational studies
Analyses using computer databases
Series with literature control subjects
Case series without control subjects
Anecdotal case reports

Standard Procedures to Conduct a Phase III Trial

Stratified and Adaptive Randomization

Stratified randomization (and a more technically complex version, called *adaptive randomization*) is used when there is considerable, known heterogeneity in outcome for patients. This heterogeneity may lead to worries that all "good" risk patients may end up in one treatment arm and the "bad" risk patients in the other, resulting in an unfair comparison; this is especially important in very small trials. Similarly, the variability among patients with respect to outcome makes it difficult for biostatisticians to detect true treatment differences.

This concern is most easily addressed in the experimental design phase. To make a fair comparison, patients could be divided into risk groups (or strata) based on different values of a small number of known prognostic variables. Within each stratum the randomization could balance between treatment arms for small numbers (blocks) of patients. For example, in a trial with two arms, the randomization could be blocked so that after every 4 patients, 2 would be randomized to each arm; within each stratum the difference in numbers randomized to the two therapies would not exceed 2. To remove "noise" associated with different prognoses, treatments can be compared within strata and comparisons summarized across strata. Thus, blocked randomization would closely balance on prognostic factors and would remove much variability due to the heterogeneity. Blocking can potentially lead to biased assignments if someone knows the algorithm and keeps track of patient characteristics, although this is unlikely to occur.

One problem with stratified randomization is that the number of strata can grow rapidly if the goal is to obtain balance on a large number of variables at once. If there are 10 blocking factors that take on one of two possible values (e.g., male or female, normal or abnormal), the number of strata would be 1,024. If we try to use large numbers of randomized blocks, then many blocks may have only zero or one patient, making comparison impossible. Two approaches have been used to deal with this problem. One is to use a mathematical model (e.g., based on a linear combination of variables) to predict the end point of the trial. Strata could then be defined by values of this linear combination. Alternatively, we could define a measure of balance for each factor of interest. The randomization could then be changed by increasing the probability of the outcome that promoted balance in the most unbalanced factor or in some overall measure of imbalance. Such schemes are called *adaptive randomization schemes*. We will not pursue the topic further herein, but a large body of literature is available (4,39–47).

Interim Analyses/Sequential Trials

Most trials comparing 2 therapeutic options are performed using the 0.05 significance level—the data are analyzed such that if both treatment arms have the same effect, a treatment difference will be established only 1 time in 20. If enrollment or follow-up takes place over an extended time, there are compelling ethical reasons to examine the data at interim time points, so that if one treatment arm is superior the trial may be terminated early. However, if each interim test has a significance level of 0.05, then the overall significance level will be higher than 0.05, often dramatically so (48). Methods are available for *sequential trials*, which allow *interim monitoring* while preserving the overall significance level of the trial (49–59). For a fixed statistical power, interim monitoring will increase the required sample size unless a large difference is required for early stopping.

Cautions in the Conduct of a Phase III Trial

The relative effects of therapies being compared may differ in patient subgroups. In the extreme case, one therapy may be beneficial in one subgroup and a different therapy may be beneficial in another subgroup. Such a *qualitative interaction* means that the ideal result of the trial would not be that one therapy is best, but rather that one therapy is best for some patients and the second is best for the other patients. Because there are practical, financial, ethical, and scientific reasons for designing trials with a minimal sample size, trials are not usually designed based on the sample size required to detect qualitative treatment interactions. Therefore, power to compare the relative efficacy in a subgroup of patients is more limited than the power to compare treatments in the trial as a whole. Often there are a number of possible subgroups to examine; these multiple comparisons increase the likelihood of spurious findings unless adjustment is used. Neither stratification nor adaptive randomization adequately address this concern unless strong qualitative interactions exist.

To preserve the protections of randomization, the outcomes for all randomized patients should be compared by assigned treatment, even if some patients did not receive the assigned treatment. There are exceptions: one can argue for excluding ineligible individuals if the eligibility criteria have been decided on before the trial, if these criteria are available before randomization, and if exclusion is made without knowledge of outcome. Analyses including all randomized patients in their randomization groups regardless of treatment received are known as *intent-to-treat* analyses (60,61). Intent-to-treat analysis can introduce strain between biostatisticians, who focus more on the problems of biased or unfair comparisons, and clinicians, who focus more on biology. However, if the trial is designed and performed well, the results of intent-to-treat and biological analyses should coincide.

Example of a Phase III Trial in BMT

A randomized, controlled clinical trial of prophylactic ganciclovir for cytomegalovirus (CMV) pulmonary infection in recipients of allogeneic BMTs was conducted by Schmidt and associates (62). Patients at high risk due to positivity for CMV by bronchoalveolar lavage on day 35 after transplantation were randomly assigned to ganciclovir or to observation. The randomization was stratified based on known prognostic factors for CMV pneumonia (i.e., the presence or absence of GVHD and patient's age, ≤ 25 or > 25 yr), with block size equal to 4 within each stratum.

Because CMV-associated interstitial pneumonia remains a major cause of death after allogeneic BMT, and the end point could be assessed by day 120, sequential monitoring was conducted after each patient reached death or 120-day survival. The proportions of patients with CMV pneumonia in the ganciclovir and placebo groups were compared using a *sequential probability ratio test*, maintaining an overall alpha level of 0.05 (63). Sequential monitoring allowed the trial to be terminated before the fixed sample size of 74 patients; after the first 40 patients had been randomized, a statistically significant difference was identified and further randomization was halted. When a placebo-controlled trial is terminated early due to a significant treatment effect, care should be taken to immediately switch any remaining placebo subjects to the active treatment if this might benefit them.

The primary results of this Phase III trial are shown in Table 20-4. An intent-to-treat analysis was performed with all 40 randomized patients, as well as an analysis that excluded 7 patients considered inevaluable for CMV pneumonia. As a conservative approach,

Table 20-4.
Prophylactic Effect of Ganciclovir to Prevent CMV Pneumonia

Treatment Assignment	*No. Patients*	*Patients Who Died or Had Pneumonia (%)*[a]	*Relative Risk (95% CI)*[b]	p *Value*[c]
Patients who could be evaluated				
Group 1 (ganciclovir)	18	4 (22)	0.33 (0.13–0.85)	0.015
Group 2 (observation)	15	10 (67)		
All randomized patients				
Group 1 (ganciclovir)	20	5(25)	0.36(0.16–0.80)	0.010
Group 2 (observation)	20	14(70)		

[a]Data for patients who could be evaluated include 2 with CMV pneumonia and 2 deaths in group 1, and 10 with CMV pneumonia in group 2. Data for all randomized patients include 3 with CMV pneumonia and 2 deaths in group 1, and 13 with CMV pneumonia and 1 death in group 2.
[b]Indicates the risk of CMV pneumonia or death among the patients receiving ganciclovir. as compared with those under observation. CI denotes confidence interval.
[c]By two-tailed Fisher's exact test. When stepwise logistic regression was used to adjust for severe graft-versus-host disease (≥ Grade II) at day 35, a significant treatment effect was still observed ($p < 0.001$).
CMV = cytomegalovirus.
Reprinted, by permission of the New England Journal of Medicine, from Schmidt GM, Horak DA, Niland JC, et al. A randomized controlled trial of prophylactic ganciclovir for cytomegalovirus pulmonary infection in recipients of allogeneic bone marrow transplants. N Engl J Med 1991; 324: 1005–1011.

either pneumonia or early death due to any cause were considered failures in this analysis. Both the reduced sample size and the intent-to-treat analyses showed that the risk of CMV pneumonia or death before day 120 in the ganciclovir group was one third that in the observation group (relative risk = 0.33 or 0.36); both analyses were statistically significant ($p = 0.01$).

Recent Developments and Future Directions in Phase III Trials

With the growing availability of efficacious treatments in BMT, the aim of clinical trials is shifting from *efficacy trials* to studies designed to demonstrate that a new treatment is therapeutically equivalent to some standard treatment (*equivalency trials*) (64). This may be the goal when the new treatment confers some advantages over the standard treatment (e.g., less toxicity, lower cost, better quality of life). For example, prophylactic intravenous ganciclovir prevents the development of CMV interstitial pneumonia in high-risk BMT patients (62); however, the intravenous preparation involves considerable expense, toxicity, and extended hospitalization. If an oral ganciclovir preparation could be shown to differ from the standard therapy by less than some small, clinically acceptable amount, it would be the therapy of choice. Of course, it is possible that the new therapy could be proven to be *superior* to the standard.

Although equivalency studies are now being reported, relatively few employ the appropriate design required to demonstrate a nonsignificant difference in efficacy. Often the classic test of significance is inappropriately employed; there is a danger of incorrectly accepting the null hypothesis of no difference solely due to inadequate sample size. If one wishes to use significance testing, the appropriate "null" hypothesis is that the standard therapy is *more* effective than the experimental therapy, by at least some specified amount (64,65). Because interpretation of significance tests depends heavily on sample size, and because statistical significance is often inappropriately used as a binary decision rule (66), some investigators conduct equivalency trials using confidence intervals (67). We focus on this approach because it is also more intuitively appealing and allows for sequential monitoring using repeat confidence intervals.

It is impossible to demonstrate that a new treatment is exactly equivalent to a standard treatment. Therefore, to examine therapeutic equivalence, a maximum "acceptable" difference (delta) in the effectiveness of two treatments must be specified in advance. With a fatal outcome, the new treatment can only be considered equivalent to the standard if no more than a very small decline in efficacy is allowed; with less toxic outcomes, larger differences may be acceptable. Other parameters that must be specified are the confidence level (alpha) for the upper limit of the true difference between the new and the standard treatment, and the probability (1-beta) that the confidence limit for the true difference will not exceed the specified value of delta (66).

Because the acceptable difference between two equivalent treatments is usually small (especially in contrast to the larger differences in demonstrating superior therapeutic efficacy), the required sample sizes tend to be large. Estimated sample sizes for equivalency testing are given in Table 20-5, assuming a true common response rate between the two treatments (ranging from 70 to 90%) and values of the acceptable difference in these response rates between 5 and 15%. Typical values for alpha and (1-beta) in this setting (0.10 and 0.80, respectively) are assumed. The sample sizes for equivalency testing are seen to be lower than those required if the same trial were to be (inappropriately) conducted using the traditional significance testing approach. This will be the case

Table 20-5.
Samples Sizes Required for Efficacy Versus Equivalency Testing for Differences in the Range of 5 to 15%

True Response Rate[a]	Acceptable Delta (%)	Required Sample Size Per Group[b] — Efficacy Testing[c]	Required Sample Size Per Group[b] — Equivalency Testing
70%	5	790	756
	10	204	189
	15	93	84
80%	5	628	576
	10	168	144
	15	79	64
90%	5	394	324
	10	114	81
	15	57	36

[a]Assuming true response rates are equal in the two groups.
[b]Assuming alpha = 0.10 and (1-beta) = 0.80.
[c]Using the chi-square test of proportions, without Yates continuity correction.

whenever the common response rate is greater than the quantity (1 + delta)/2 (66). This inequality will frequently hold true, because if the response rate is too low (e.g., less than 50%), investigators are more likely to conduct efficacy trials in an attempt to identify better treatments; equivalency tests become of paramount importance only when response rates are satisfactorily high. If the assumption of a true common response rate does not hold (e.g., one therapy is actually slightly better), the required sample size may be greatly increased.

Selected Modern Statistical Analyses

In this section, we focus on two areas of statistical methodology frequently used in BMT research: (1) analysis of times to an event (e.g., survival analysis) and (2) modeling via regression (e.g., Cox and logistic). Table 20-6 presents an overview of these methods. The complexity of applying these techniques appropriately is often not appreciated, leading to their misuse or misinterpretation. For each type of statistical technique, we present the rationale, general procedures, cautionary notes, and an example in BMT research.

Analyses of Time to an Event

Survival analysis is one of the most frequently used statistical techniques in trials of BMT patients. We present the standard techniques for estimating overall survival, procedures for handling extensions to special cases, and methods for graphical presentation of time-to-event data.

The Product-Limit Estimate for All Cause Mortality

Consider a randomized clinical trial in which patients are enrolled uniformly in time over a period of 2 years and followed for another year. Suppose we want to estimate the probability of surviving 2 years; only half the patients (those enrolled in the first year) could have been observed for 2 full years. A reasonable estimate of 2-year survival would be the proportion of first year enrollees that actually survived 2 years; yet the survival information of those enrolled in the second year should also be useful in estimating the 2-year survival, even though those patients have not been in the study for 2 full years. Furthermore, we do not know the true survival time for patients who have not died at the time of our analysis; we know they lived at least some length of time (to the last follow-up), but we do not know when their death will occur. In this case, the time of death is said to be *censored.* An estimate of survival that efficiently makes use of censored observations is called by two names: the *product-limit* or the *Kaplan-Meier estimate* (68,69).

Although in the preceding paragraph we used death as the event of interest, any event occurring over time (e.g., onset of clinical GVHD or relapse) may be used as the end point of interest. For these other end points, events that censor the event of interest *confound* the interpretation.

The *log rank statistic* is one method of testing the null hypothesis that the true survival times in the treatment arms of a trial are the same. The test compares the expected number of deaths in each treatment arm with the observed number (under the null hypothesis of no difference). Because this test puts equal weight on each of the time points observed, this statistic is most efficient where survival differences follow a *proportional hazards risk* (see section on Cox regression).

Cautions in Using the Product-Limit Estimate

Before considering an example it is important to note that an assumption of the product-limit curve is that censoring must be independent of the outcome of interest. "*Statistical independence*" means that for the several outcomes, measurements, or events under consideration, the occurrence or value of one event has no influence on the other events. For example, if we consider survival, the survival experience of one patient should not influence the survival experience of another patient under most circumstances. However, consider the situation in which half the patients were killed in one earthquake; then the events of death would no longer be statistically independent. Similarly, if patients are enrolled over time, then censoring could be related to survival time if the highest risk patients were enrolled first; using this estimate, the survival experience of later patients would then be too pessimistic. Alternatively, if much of the censoring came from patients who were lost to follow-up, this fact could represent a preponderance of lower risk patients (e.g., if they felt healthy enough to move), higher risk patients (e.g., if they were lost because they died and this cannot be ascertained), or anything in between. The assumption that censoring time and the time of death are statistically independent is usually

Table 20-6.
Summary of Time to Event Analyses and Modeling via Regression

Technique	*Objective*	*Assumptions*	*Interpretive Subtleties*
Time to Event Analyses			
Product-limit (Kaplan-Meier) curve	Estimate and display overall survival experience for the whole group	1. Censoring time is statistically independent of length of survival	1. Loss to follow-up must be unrelated to prognosis
Product-limit curve with competing risks	Estimate and display overall survival experience assuming that only one cause of death is operative	1. Censoring time is statistically independent of the likelihood of any cause-specific event occurring 2. Individuals at higher risk for one cause are not at changed risk for other causes	1. The independence of the risk of death from different causes cannot be checked from the data 2. Specification of failure rates given removal of certain failure types will be sensible only in very special cases
Cumulative incidence curve	Estimate the mortality experience due to one particular type of death (among a variety of competing risks)	1. Censoring time is statistically independent of the likelihood of any cause-specific event occurring	1. A change in the probability of any of the competing risks would change the cumulative incidence experience of the event of interest as well
Prevalence curve	Estimate the proportion that have experienced the event of interest among those alive at time t	1. Censoring time is statistically independent of the likelihood of the event of interest occurring	1. The prevalence curve can drop if the event decreases, or if individuals die (possibly due to the event) 2. The curve can rise due to an increase in the event, or if those without the event die due to other causes
Modeling via Regression			
Cox proportional hazards regression	Model the influence of a set of variables on survival time	1. Censoring time is statistically independent of length of survival 2. The hazard for any individual is proportional to some common base-hazard	1. Interpretation of the relative risk is more straightforward for dichotomous variables, more complex for categorical variables with >2 values or continuous variables 2. Confounding and effect modification can alter the final model (see text)
Logistic regression	Model the influence of a set of variables on a binary event	If the binary event can occur at varying time points: 1. Censoring time is statistically independent of the binary outcome 2. Subjects have all been followed for the same length of time	1. Interpretation of the odds ratio is more straightforward for dichotomous variables, more complex for categorical variables with >2 values or continuous variables 2. Confounding and effect modification can alter the final model (see text) 3. Care must be taken that the model is not purely "data-driven" when using logistic regression for prediction

reasonable in a clinical trial because the censoring time is typically due to both the time of last follow-up and the time at which the patient is enrolled in the trial; enrollment time is not usually related to patient risk.

A final cautionary note is that the product-limit estimate of median survival, or survival at any specified time point, is commonly reported in the BMT literature without any indication of the accuracy of this estimate (i.e., the standard error or the confidence interval). This can be misleading, particularly in studies with small sample sizes. A number of authors have addressed the topic of calculating confidence intervals for product-limit survival estimates (70–73), which should be included routinely when reporting estimates based on a limited number of patients.

Example of the Product-Limit Estimate of Survival

The method is illustrated with data from a randomized clinical trial that studied the addition of prednisone to a methotrexate-cyclosporine regimen used for prophy-

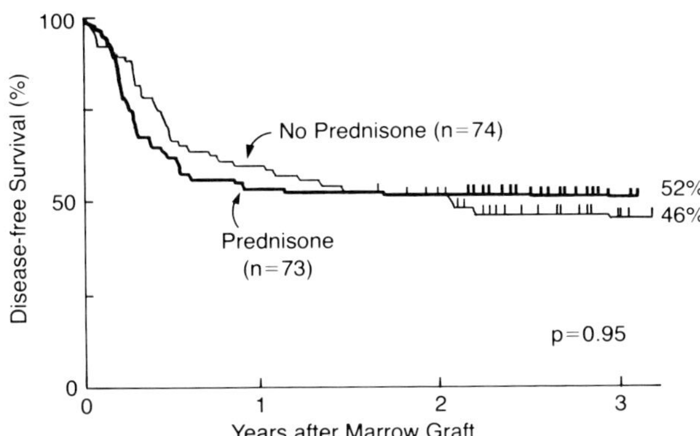

Figure 20-2. Disease-free survival curves for two randomized groups with and without prednisone. *Tic marks* indicate patients alive at last follow-up. (Reproduced by permission from Storb R, Pepe MS, Appelbaum FR, et al. What role for prednisone in prevention of acute graft-versus-host disease in patients undergoing marrow transplants? Blood 1990; 76: 1037–1045.)

laxis of acute GVHD (74). Figure 20-2 shows the disease-free survival curve for 147 consecutive patients with leukemia, myelodysplastic syndrome, or aplastic anemia treated by marrow grafts from matched siblings or family members. In estimating disease-free survival, the event is occurrence of the first of either relapse or death. Disease-free survival is often the best statistic for comparison between two transplant groups, because it ignores the effect of second-line therapies used subsequent to relapse and appropriately considers BMT patients who die in remission (e.g., due to GVHD or pneumonia) as treatment failures (75). It can be seen that disease-free survival in this study was not different in the groups with and without prednisone; the projected values 2 years after transplantation were 51% in both groups ($p = 0.95$).

Time to Event Analysis with Competing Risks

One of the features of BMT research is the ability to reasonably accurately determine causes of death or other events. Thus, deaths attributable to conditioning regimen, disease relapse, GVHD, engraftment failure, or infection (with engraftment) may be separately identified with some degree of certainty. Furthermore, therapies can be designed that might increase the risk of death from one cause (e.g., conditioning regimen) in the hopes of gaining more by reducing the risk of death from another cause (e.g., relapse). The presence of these *competing risks* imposes certain limitations on the interpretation of BMT data, limitations which must be understood if appropriate inferences are to be made (76). Some methods for handling analyses involving competing risks follow.

Product-Limit Estimate with Competing Risks

Suppose we could eliminate all causes of death other than relapse. What is the probability that a patient would experience a relapse-related death by time t? It is impossible to answer this question without making some assumptions because the different causes of death may be related in two ways: (1) the modification of one cause (e.g., conditioning) may increase or decrease the risk from another cause (e.g., relapse mortality); and (2) patients at highest risk from one cause of death may also be at increased risk for another cause (e.g., advanced age may increase risk from several different causes). Worse yet, it can be shown that we cannot determine from the data how the risks are related. Thus, it is necessary to assume that the competing risks of death are statistically independent, meaning that patients who are removed from observation because of a competing risk are at the same risk for the cause of interest as those remaining. If this assumption is correct and losses to follow-up are also statistically independent of any cause of death, then we can use the product-limit estimate with censoring both for other causes of death and for limited follow-up. This curve estimates the impact on the event of interest if all other competing causes of death are removed.

Cautions in Estimating Survival with Competing Risks

The assumptions described are usually not totally tenable, although they may not be too unreasonable—specification of failure rates given removal of certain failure types will be sensible only in very special cases. In a limited number of circumstances, data may exist to help answer the question of the risk of death due to a particular cause if other causes could be eliminated. For example, if one were interested in knowing the risk of death due to relapse if the risk from GVHD could be eliminated, survival estimates from syngeneic transplants could be utilized because the competing risk of GVHD-related death has been removed naturally in this setting.

The Cumulative Incidence Curve

Summarization and presentation of clinical trial relapse data depend on which question is being asked. Suppose we wish to know how many patients in the trial will relapse by a given time. An appropriate method of graphically presenting this is the cumulative incidence curve. This curve estimates the proportion of patients who have relapsed by each point in time. Of course, if all the patients in a trial have been observed for that length of time, the proportion is simply the ratio of those who relapsed to the number in the trial (or on one treatment arm if only one arm is being considered). Often because of censoring due to enrollment over time, the curve would be estimated in a more complex manner (68).

Cautions in Using the Cumulative Incidence Curve

As with the standard product-limit estimate of survival, the assumption that length of follow-up is statistically independent of the probability of any cause-specific event must hold. Also, a change in the probability of any of the competing risks would change the cumulative incidence experience of the event of interest.

Example of the Cumulative Incidence Curve
Figure 20-3 is from the article by Storb and colleagues (74). The factor being presented is incidence of acute GVHD. The estimate of acute GVHD at day 100 was 36% for patients who were not administered prednisone compared with 45% for patients who received prednisone. The estimate of cumulative incidence of day 100 acute GVHD was even lower (25%) among human leukocyte antigen (HLA)-identical patients who did not receive prednisone.

Analysis of Time to Events that May Stop and Reoccur

Additional summarization and analysis issues occur with events that are not necessarily fatal and that may come and go. Examples are the occurrence of clinically important acute GVHD, chronic GVHD, and infection. If we are interested in the time to the first occurrence only, then the analyses described may be used. However, other approaches are necessary if we wish to examine the issue in more depth.

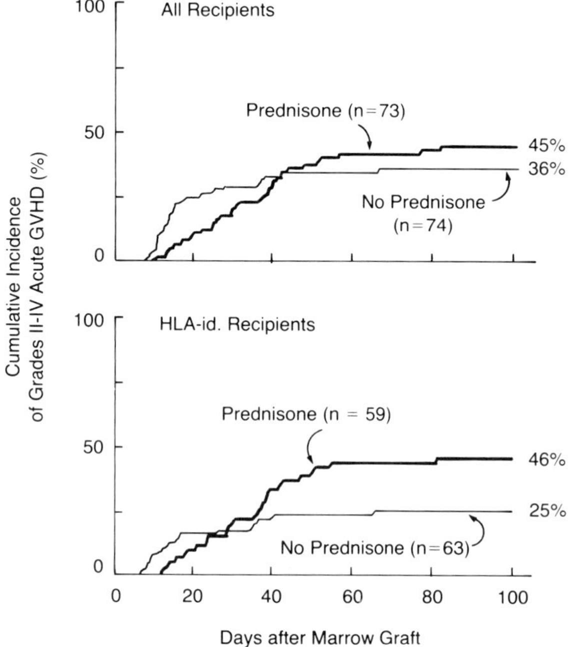

Figure 20-3. Cumulative incidence curves of acute grade II through IV GVHD in patients with HLA-identical donor or one mismatch. (Top) All patients. (Bottom) HLA-identical patients. (Reproduced by permission from Storb R, Pepe MS, Appelbaum FR, et al. What role for prednisone in prevention of acute graft-versus-host disease in patients undergoing marrow transplants? Blood 1990; 76: 1037–1045.)

The Prevalence Curve
We focus on chronic GVHD as the event of interest. One measure of the importance of this event at any point in time is the proportion of patients with chronic GVHD among those at risk; this proportion can be estimated by a prevalence curve (77). Such a curve gives some idea of the importance of GVHD risk over time for the remaining patients alive after transplantation.

Cautions in Using the Prevalence Curve. The usual assumption of statistical independence of censoring times and the likelihood of the event of interest occurring must be true to estimate the prevalence curve. In addition, it is important to understand that the prevalence curve can drop over time either due to individuals losing the state being considered (e.g., no longer having clinically evident chronic GVHD), or by dying from the state being considered (e.g., infection secondary to chronic GVHD treatment) or from another cause. For example, if relapse was the outcome of interest, for some leukemias, patients would probably either die relatively rapidly or no longer be in relapse (e.g., due to a successful second transplant). In this case, the prevalence curve would be at a low level at most time points. For CML, however, patients might well remain in chronic-phase relapse for an extended period, and the prevalence curve would be higher.

Example of the Prevalence Curve. Continuing the graphical presentations from Storb and colleagues (74), Figure 20-4 illustrates the prevalence curve for active chronic GVHD among patients free of leukemic relapse, stratified by whether the patients had experienced acute GVHD. It can be seen that chronic GVHD is a more significant problem among disease-free surviving patients who received prednisone than among those who did not, and that chronic GVHD is higher among those patients in whom acute GVHD developed.

Modeling via Regression

Cox Proportional Hazards Regression Model

In BMT studies, the time to an event is often influenced by several variables, which requires a more complex form of survival analysis than that discussed in the previous sections. *Proportional hazards regression* (or *Cox regression*) is a technique that models the influence of a set of variables on the "survival" time (a term used generically to indicate the time to any event of interest) (78). The goal is the same as in the more familiar linear regression model: to find the most parsimonious and biologically plausible model that best describes the relationship between the response variable and one or more independent variables. A set of regression coefficients is estimated to relate the effect of each factor on the time to the event, whether this might be death or some other important event, such as development of GVHD, infection, or relapse.

As with product-limit curves, there must exist a

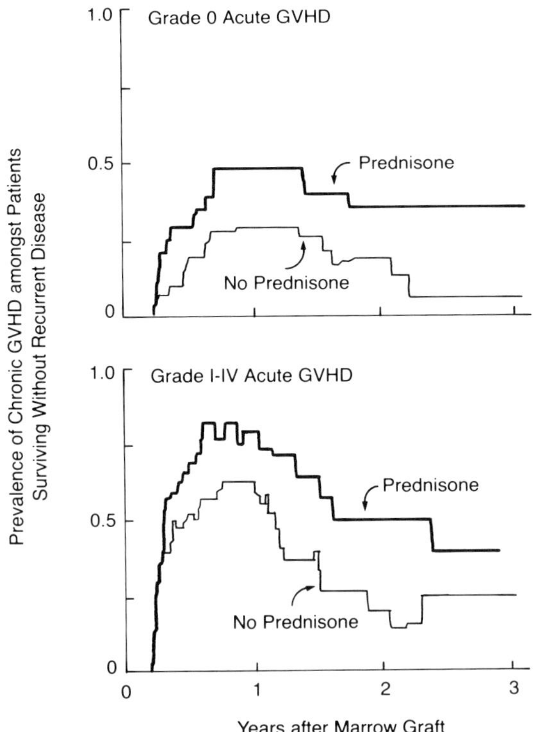

Figure 20-4. Prevalence curves for active chronic GVHD. (Top) Patients with Grade 0 acute GVHD. (Bottom) Patients with Grade I to IV acute GVHD. (Reproduced by permission from Storb R, Pepe MS, Appelbaum FR, et al. What role for prednisone in prevention of acute graft-versus-host disease in patients undergoing marrow transplants? Blood 1990; 76: 1037–1045.)

well-defined starting point from which the occurrence of the event can be measured; this is usually the date of transplantation. The data may be censored as before. The independent, or predictor, variables (called covariates) in Cox regression can be either categorical (e.g., sex, diagnosis, or treatment arm) or continuous (e.g., age at transplant, or length of time from diagnosis to transplant). The technique can be used as a univariate model with a single covariate, or a multivariate model with many covariates.

The model is named "proportional hazards" because it is based on the assumption that the hazards (e.g., the instantaneous probability of the event occurring at each time point) for any two individuals are proportional. The *hazard rate* for an individual is equal to the product of a common baseline hazard for all individuals (requiring no distributional assumptions) and the relative risk function based on some function of regression coefficients (estimated parametrically) and covariates in the model. This assumption allows calculation of the *hazard ratio* (or *relative risk*) at each time point between individuals with and without a given characteristic, or with differing values of a covariate. The relative risk is a measure of the association between significant variables in the model and time to the event of interest; its interpretation will depend on how a covariate is coded and the particular units of the covariate. Interpretation of the relative risk is more straightforward for a dichotomous independent variable and becomes more complex for categorical variables, which take on more than two possible values, and for continuous covariates.

In Cox regression, confidence intervals can be calculated for the coefficients of the covariates and the estimated survival probabilities, and hypothesis tests can be performed. One goal of a multivariate Cox regression analysis is to test for treatment effects while controlling for patient characteristics. This analysis *statistically adjusts* the estimated effects of each variable in the model for associations with other covariates to allow for appropriate descriptions of relationships between a primary risk factor and outcome when other covariates (potential confounders) are present. A prognostic index for patients with a particular set of covariate values can be defined (79). One can also define a therapeutic index, which represents the difference in the prognostic index between patients who share the same covariates but who have been given different treatments; this index can be applied to help determine the best treatment on a case-by-case basis (80).

Another important step in modeling a set of data is to determine whether there is evidence of *interaction* in the data, meaning that the association between a risk factor and the outcome variable differs or depends in some way on the level of a given covariate. The covariate that modifies the effect of another risk factor on the outcome of interest is called an *effect modifier.* An effect modifier is established by observing statistical significance of an interaction term when added to the model, provided this interaction is also biologically plausible. If effect modification is identified, then analyses must be carried out separately within each level of the effect modifier.

Extensions of the Proportional Hazards Regression Model

The previous discussion assumes that the covariates do not vary over time, such as diagnosis or age at transplant. Many covariates that can influence survival change over time (*time-dependent*), such as CMV positivity or presence of GVHD. With modern software packages it is possible to include such time-dependent covariates in the model; however, all covariates must be known for all individuals at risk at every failure time, and the interpretation of the results becomes less obvious. Prediction of future survival is not immediate, because we may not know the future values of time-dependent covariates for a given patient. The computational time also increases greatly when time-dependent covariates are incorporated into the model. For these reasons, this extension of Cox regression has not been as widely used as might be warranted in past BMT research, although the advent of high-speed personal computers has now made this option more viable with respect to computational time.

Other extensions of proportional hazards regression are inclusion of patients with delayed entry (81) (although this approach is more applicable to natural history studies of disease, rather than BMT trials, in which day of transplantation is usually the starting point); multistate models, in which there are several events of interest (82); and transitions between healthy and disease states, in which there are different "death" rates, or a patient may experience the same event more than one time (e.g., infections, GVHD) (83).

Cautions in using Cox Regression

The reporting of Cox regression results in the literature is often deficient in major features (84). First, the purpose of the analysis (e.g., to test a new treatment against a standard, vs to separate patients by their prognosis) should be clearly stated. The variables that were included in the analysis (not just those remaining in the final model) should be listed to allow readers to see whether the number of variables being modeled grossly outweighs the available data, both in terms of number of patients and number of events of interest. The values of each variable and any interaction terms tested should be clearly spelled out. The table for the final model should include the estimate of the effect for each variable (regression coefficients or relative risks) and a measure of the uncertainty of these estimates (standard errors or confidence intervals). The "goodness-of-fit" of the model should be investigated to determine the validity of the proportional hazards assumption and the appropriateness of the scoring of the covariates (85); some simple computational and graphical methods exist to perform such tests (68,86–88). Discussion of goodness-of-fit of the model is uncommon, perhaps reflecting the infrequency with which this assumption is investigated. Finally, it may be pertinent to specify intermediate results for important hypotheses, as well as the predictive ability of the final model.

Example of Cox Regression in BMT

A retrospective study was conducted to compare disease-free survival rates between 24 allogeneic and 24 autologous BMT patients, with adjustment for other factors. Univariate, multivariate, and step-wise Cox regression analyses were performed to determine whether differences in survival observed between allograft and autograft recipients were influenced by other risk factors (i.e., age, time from diagnosis to BMT, KPS at BMT, remission status at BMT, dose of TBI, prior chest radiation, and acute GVHD) and whether there were any significant interactions between type of marrow graft and these factors. Model goodness-of-fit was tested using a covariate-time interaction term (68), as well as by graphical inspection, and the proportional hazards assumption was found to be appropriate. The results from the final Cox regression model are presented in Table 20-7. Because a significant interaction was seen between marrow graft and prior chest radiation, separate step-wise Cox regression analyses were performed within strata

Table 20-7.
Results of Stepwise Cox Regression to Test for Differences in Disease-free Survival by Prior Chest Radiation

Stratum	*Variable*	*Relative Risk*	*95% Confidence Interval*	*p Value*
Prior chest radiation	KPS	0.61	(0.38, 0.99)	0.04
No prior chest radiation	Allograft	5.08	(1.70, 15.22)	0.004

KPS = Karnofsky Performance Score.

based on this variable. For patients with prior chest radiation, KPS was the only significant predictor of disease-free survival ($p = 0.04$), with a relative risk of 0.61. However, among those without prior chest radiation, allograft recipients had a significantly lower disease-free survival rate ($p = 0.004$), with a relative risk of death or relapse of 5.08, when compared with recipients of autologous transplants. No other variables were found to be significantly associated with this outcome.

Logistic Regression

Another regression model frequently used in BMT analysis is *logistic regression* (89). This model has a similar goal as Cox regression, namely to find the best fitting model to explain the relationship between independent and dependent variables. However, in logistic regression, the dependent (outcome) variable is a binary event (e.g., success or failure, response or no response) rather than the time to an event, as with Cox regression. One of the earliest uses of this technique was in 1967 in the landmark article by Truett and colleagues (90), in which they applied logistic regression to analyze the well known Framingham study data to model the probability of a coronary event in a multivariate fashion. Since that time, logistic regression has become a standard method for analysis of binary outcomes in health research.

The covariates in logistic regression can be either categorical or continuous. The technique is similar to other regression methods; namely estimating coefficients for each model covariate, assessing statistical significance of these covariates to predict outcome, and developing parsimonious models by only adding variables with statistically significant predictive ability in the presence of the other covariates. Interpretation of the meaning of model coefficients is given through the *odds ratio,* a measure of association that represents how much more likely (or unlikely) it is for the response to be present among those with a given value of the explanatory variable. As with Cox regression, interpretation of the odds ratio is more straightforward for a dichotomous independent variable and becomes more complex for categorical variables with more than two possible values, or for continuous covariates. The comments with respect to effect modification given under Cox regression apply here as well.

Extensions of Logistic Regression to Special Cases

A specialized version of logistic regression can be applied in the situation of *matched case-control data* (91). In addition, a technique called *partial logistic regression* allows biostatisticians to estimate hazard rates and survival curves from censored data in a flexible way that provides both estimates and standard errors and which may be more efficient than the nonparametric Kaplan-Meier (product-limit) estimates of survival (92).

Logistic regression can also be used for modeling *prognostic prediction* (93). The critical aspect of sample size is usually not the total number of patients in the analysis, but rather the number with the end point of interest. Losses to follow-up should be minimal and unrelated to outcome, or the prognostic estimates may be biased. If the data used to fit the model are used to evaluate predictive ability, the estimates will be biased in a favorable direction. Therefore, one standard procedure is to split the dataset into a "*training*" dataset for the purpose of developing the model and a "*test*" dataset for validating this model and assessing the predictive accuracy in an unbiased model. An alternative is to perform what is known as a "jackknife" procedure (94)—iteratively estimating the coefficients, excluding a fixed number of observations at a time.

Cautions in using Logistic Regression

As with other techniques, reporting of the results from logistic regression is often deficient, and goodness-of-fit assessment is infrequently mentioned (95–97). Unlike the earlier techniques, which are specifically designed to handle varying lengths of follow-up, if the end point being examined via logistic regression is one that can occur at varying time points for each patient, the patients should all be followed for approximately the same length so that each has the same opportunity to experience the outcome of interest.

Example of Logistic Regression in BMT

As a follow-up to the ganciclovir prophylaxis study of Schmidt and associates (62), a prognostic study was conducted using data from the same patients to determine the value of pulmonary function tests in predicting the development of CMV pneumonia (98). Univariate logistical regression revealed significant associations between development of CMV pneumonia and percent predicted forced expiratory volume at one second (FEV_1), forced vital capacity (FVC), and total lung capacity (TLC) on day 13 prior to transplant ($p < 0.01$). Stepwise logistic regression analysis yielded significant independent predictors for pneumonia: CMV positivity on day 35 by bronchoalveolar lavage (BAL) (odds ratio (OR) = 4.8; $p = 0.0002$), and day-13 percent predicted FEV_1 (OR = 0.92; $p = 0.0004$). A jackknife estimate showed that 82% of

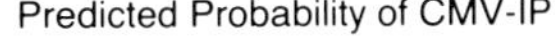

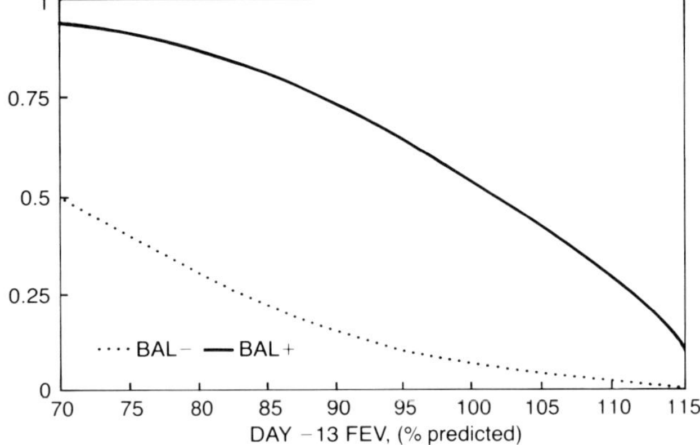

Figure 20-5. Prediction of the probability of development of CMV pneumonia based on the fitted logistic regression model using both BAL status and FEV_1. (Reproduced by permission from Horak DA, Schmidt GM, Zaia JA, et al. Pretransplant pulmonary function predicts cytomegalovirus-associated interstitial pneumonia following bone marrow transplantation. Chest 1993; 102: 1484–1490.

study patients were correctly classified with respect to development of pneumonia. The relationship between these variables and prediction of CMV pneumonia is depicted in Figure 20-5. Although not intended for clinical use, this graph demonstrates the independent contributions of both FEV_1 and BAL positivity toward the risk of CMV pneumonia.

Summary

Many of the statistical methods commonly in use in BMT trials currently can be quite complex, involving subtleties in the appropriate choice of study design, analytic programming, and interpretation of the results. With the increasing popularity and availability of personal computers and statistical software packages, many physicians are beginning to explore their own data and to perform some of their own analyses. This is to be encouraged, because it often helps to identify errors in data, and may lead to useful analyses or generation of interesting hypotheses; however, the conduct of such analyses during an ongoing trial is to be discouraged unless they are part of a formal interim monitoring plan with safeguards to prevent adverse effects on the completion of the trial. We recommend that unless the statistical analyses are straightforward (e.g., descriptive displays or statistical tests involving two variables only) a biostatistician should be involved to assure that appropriate techniques are applied, underlying assumptions have been met, and more complex analyses are being correctly carried out. "Expert" computer systems cannot currently evaluate whether these conditions are present or not. The availability of quick answers from programming a few commands in a software package can be dangerous and can lead to erroneous results with no warning message. A number of the newer software packages (and even textbooks) have been written by nonstatisticians and can contain erroneous statements or results. A general rule of thumb to guide investigators is that once an analysis simultaneously involves 3 or more variables, it becomes advisable to collaborate with a biostatistician.

References

1. Fisher LD, van Belle G. Biostatistics: a methodology for the health sciences. New York: John Wiley and Sons, 1993.
2. Brown BW, Hollander M. Statistics: a biomedical introduction. New York: John Wiley and Sons, 1971.
3. Zar JH. Biostatistical analysis, ed 2. New Jersey: Prentice Hall, 1984.
4. Friedman LM, Furberg CD, DeMets DL. Fundamentals of clinical trials. Boston: John Wright, PSG Inc, 1981.
5. Meinert CL. Clinical trials: design, conduct, and analysis. New York: Oxford University Press, 1986.
6. Leventhal BG, Wittes RE. Research methods in clinical oncology. New York: Raven, 1988.
7. Simon R. A decade of progress in statistical methodology for clinical trials. Stat Med 1991;10:1789–1817.
8. Louis J. Coordinated phase I studies for cooperative chemotherapy groups. Cancer Chemother Rep 1962;16: 99–105.
9. Woolley PV, Schein PS. Clinical pharmacology and phase I trial design. In: DeVita VT Jr, Busch H, eds. Methods in cancer research. vol XVII. New York: Acedemic Press, 1979:177–198.
10. Guarino AM, Rozencweig M, Kline I, et al. Adequacies and inadequacies in assessing murine toxicity data with antineoplastic agents. Cancer Res 1979;39:2204–2210.
11. Collins JM, Zaharko DS, Dedrick RL, Chabner BA. Potential roles for preclinical pharmacology in phase I clinical trials. Cancer Treat Rep 1986;70:73–80.
12. O'Quigley J, Pepe M, Fisher L. Continual reassessment method: a practical design for phase I clinical trials in cancer. Biometrics 1990;46:33–48.
13. Storer BE. Design and analysis of phase I clinical trials. Biometrics 1989;45:925–937.
14. Blume KG, Forman SJ, O'Donnell MR, et al. Total body irradiation and high-dose etoposide: a new preparatory regimen for bone marrow transplantation in patients with advanced hematologic malignancies. Blood 1987;69:1015–1020.
15. Fleming TR. One-sample multiple testing procedures for phase II clinical trials. Biometrics 1982;38:143–151.
16. Gehan EA, Schneiderman MA. Experimental design of clinical trials. In: Holland JF, Frei E III, eds. Cancer Medicine, ed 2. Philadelphia: Lea and Febiger, 1982: 531–553.
17. Simon R. Optimal two-stage designs for phase II clinical trials. Controlled Clin Trials 1989;10:1–10.
18. Chang MN, O'Brien PC. Confidence intervals following group sequential tests. Controlled Clin Trials 1986;7: 18–26.
19. Parker PM, Fahey JL, Schmidt GM, et al. Thalidomide for the treatment of chronic graft-versus-host disease (GVHD) (abstract) Blood 1989;74(suppl 1):123a.
20. Schaid DJ, Ingle JN, Wieand S, Ahmann DL. A design for phase II testing of anticancer agents within a phase III clinical trial. Controlled Clin Trials 1988;9:107–118.
21. Simon R, Wittes RE, Ellenberg SS. Randomized phase II clinical trials. Cancer Treat Rep 1985;69:1375–1381.
22. Herson J, Carter SK. Calibrated phase II clinical trials in oncology. Stat Med 1986;5:441–447.
23. Gehan EA. Progress of therapy in acute leukemia 1948–1981: randomized versus nonrandomized clinical trials. Controlled Clin Trials 1982;3:199–207.
24. Bull JP. The historical development of clinical therapeutic trials. J Chronic Dis 1959;10:218–248.
25. Ederer F. Why do we need controls? Why do we need to randomize? Am J Ophthalmol 1975;76:758–762.
26. Green SB. Patient heterogeneity and the randomized clinical trials. Controlled Clin Trials 1982;3:189–198.
27. Amberson JB Jr, McMahon BT, Pinner M. A clinical trial of sanocrysin in pulmonary tuberculosis. Am Rev Tuberculosis 1931;24:401–435.
28. Diehl HS, Baker AB, Cowan DW. Cold vaccines: an evaluation based on a controlled study. JAMA 1938; 111:1168–1173.
29. Patulin Clinical Trials Committee (of the Medical Research Council). Clinical trial of Patulin in the common cold. Lancet 1944;2:373–375.
30. Green SB, Byar DP. Using observational data from registries to compare treatments: the fallacy of omnimetrics. State Med 1984;3:361–370.
31. Green SB. Patient heterogeneity and the need for randomized clinical trials. Controlled Clin Trials 1982;3:189–198.
32. Bradley JV. Distribution-free statistical tests. Englewood Cliffs: Prentice Hall, 1968:68–145.
33. Hoeffding W. The large-sample power of tests based on permutations of observations. Ann Math Stat 1952;23: 169–192.
34. Kempthorne O. The randomization theory of experimental inference. J Am Stat Assoc 1955;50:946–967.
35. Gehan EA, Freireich EJ. Non-randomized controls in cancer clinical trials. N Engl J Med 1974;290:198–203.
36. Gehan EA. Design of controlled clinical trials: use of historical controls. Cancer Treat Rep 1982;66:1089–1093.
37. Micciolo R, Valagussa P, Marubini E. The use of historical controls in breast cancer: an assessment of three consecutive studies. Controlled Clin Trials 1985; 6:259–270.
38. Sacks H, Chalmers TC, Smith H Jr. Randomized versus historical controls for clinical trials. Am J Med 1982;72:233–240.
39. Begg CD, Iglewicz B. A treatment allocation procedure for sequential clinical trials. Biometrics 1980;36:81–90.
40. Efron B. Forcing a sequential experiment to be balanced. Biometrika 1971;58:403–417.
41. Freedman LS, White SJ. On the use of Pocock and Simon's method for balancing treatment numbers and prognostic factors in the controlled clinical trial. Biometrics 1976;32:691–694.
42. Matts JP, McHugh RB. Analysis of accrual randomized clinical trials with balanced groups in strata. J Chronic Dis 1978;31:725–740.
43. Pocock SJ. Allocation of patients to treatments in clinical trials. Biometrics 1979;35:183–197.
44. Pocock SJ, Simon R. Sequential treatment assignment with balancing for prognostic factors in the controlled clinical trial. Biometrics 1975;31:103–115.
45. Simon R. Adaptive treatment assignment methods and clinical trials. Biometrics 1977;33:743–749.
46. Taves DR. Minimization: a new method of assigning patients to treatment and control groups. Clin Pharmacol Ther 1974;15:443–453.

47. Zelen M. The randomization and stratification of patients to clinical trials. J Chronic Dis 1974;27:365–375.
48. Armitage P, McPherson CK, Rowe BC. Repeated significance tests on accumulating data. J R Stat Soc 1969;132:235–244.
49. DeMets DL, Gail MH. Use of logrank tests and group sequential methods at fixed calendar times. Biometrics 1985;41:1039–1044.
50. Fleming TR, Harrington DP, O'Brien PC. Designs for group sequential tests. Controlled Clin Trials 1984;5: 348–361.
51. Jennison C, Turnbull BW. Statistical approaches to interim monitoring of medical trials: a review and commentary. Statistical Sci 1990;5:299–317.
52. Johnson MF. Issues in planning interim analyses. Drug Inf J 1990;24:361–370.
53. Lan KKG, DeMets DL. Discrete sequential boundaries for clinical trials. Biometrika 1983;70:659–663.
54. Lan KKG, DeMets DL. Changing frequency of interim analysis in sequential monitoring. Biometrics 1989;45: 1017–1020.
55. O'Brien PC, Fleming TR. A multiple testing procedure for clinical trials. Biometrics 1979;35:549–556.
56. Pocock SJ. Group sequential methods in the design and analysis of clinical trials. Biometrika 1977;64:191–199.
57. Pocock SJ. Interim analyses for randomized clinical trials: the group sequential approach. Biometrics 1982;38:153–162.
58. Slud E, Wei LJ. Two-sample repeated significance tests based on the modified Wilcoxon statistic. J Am Stat Assoc 1982;77:862–868.
59. Tsiatis AA. Repeated significance testing for a general class of statistics used in censored survival analysis. J Am Stat Assoc 1982;77:855–861.
60. Fisher LD, Dixon, DO, Herson J, Frankowski RF. Analysis of randomized clinical trials: intention to treat. In: Peace KE, ed. Statistical issues in drug research and development. New York: Marcel Dekker, 1990:331–344, 349–350.
61. Peto R, Pike MC, Armitage P, et al. Design and analysis of randomized clinical trials requiring prolonged observation of each patient: I. Introduction and design. Br J Cancer 1976;34:585–612.
62. Schmidt GM, Horak DA, Niland JC, et al. A randomized, controlled trial of prophylactic ganciclovir for cytomegalovirus pulmonary infection in recipients of allogeneic bone marrow transplants. N Engl J Med 1991;324:1005–1011.
63. Whitehead J. Design and analysis of sequential clinical trials. West Suffix, England: Howrood, 1983:47–67.
64. Dunnett CW, Gent M. Significance testing to establish equivalence between treatments, with special reference to data in the form of 2 × 2 tables. Biometrics 1977;33:593–602.
65. Blackwelder WC. "Proving the null hypothesis" in clinical trials. Controlled Clin Trials 1982;3:345–353.
66. Makuch R, Simon R. Sample size requirements for evaluating a conservative therapy. Cancer Treat Rep 1978;62:1037–1040.
67. Durrleman S, Simon R. Planning and monitoring of equivalence studies. Biometrics 1990;46:329–336.
68. Kalbfleisch JD, Prentice RL. The statistical analysis of failure time data. New York: John Wiley and Sons, 1980.
69. Kaplan EL, Meier P. Nonparametric estimation from incomplete observations. J Am Stat Assoc 1958;53: 457–481.
70. Simon R, Lee YJ. Nonparametric confidence limits for survival probabilities and median survival time. Cancer Treat Rep 1982;66:37–42.
71. Emerson JD. Nonparametric confidence intervals for the median in the presence of right censoring. Biometrics 1982;38:17–27.
72. Anderson JR, Bernstein L, Pike MC. Approximate confidence intervals for probabilities of survival and quantiles in life-table analysis. Biometrics 1982;38:407–416.
73. Slud EV, Byar DP, Green SB. A comparison of reflected versus test-based confidence intervals for the median survival time, based on censored data. Biometrics 1984;40:587–600.
74. Storb R, Pepe MS, Appelbaum FR, et al. What role for prednisone in prevention of acute graft-versus-host disease in patients undergoing marrow transplants? Blood 1990;76:1037–1045.
75. Begg CB, McGlave PB, Bennett JM, Cassileth PA, Oken MM. A critical comparison of allogeneic bone marrow transplantation and conventional chemotherapy as treatment for acute nonlymphocytic leukemia. J Clin Oncol 1984;2:369–378.
76. Kalbfleisch JD, Prentice RL. The statistical analysis of failure time data. New York: Wiley, 1980.
77. Pepe MS, Longton G, Thornquist M. A qualifier Q for the survival function to describe the prevalence of a transient condition. Stat Med 1991;10:413–421.
78. Cox DR. Regression models and life tables (with discussion). J R Stat Soc [B] 1972;34:187–220.
79. Schlichting P, Christensen E, Andersen PK, et al. Prognostic factors in cirrhosis identified by Cox's regression model. Hepatology 1983;3:889–895.
80. Christensen E, Schlichting P, Andersen PK, et al. A therapeutic index that predicts individual effect of prednisone in patients with cirrhosis. Gastroenterology 1985;88:156–165.
81. Cnaan A, Ryan L. Survival analysis in natural history studies of disease. Stat Med 1989;8:1255–1268.
82. Clayton D. The analysis of event history data: a review of progress and outstanding problems. Stat Med 1988;7:819–841.
83. Andersen PK. Multistate models in survival analysis: a study of nephropathy and mortality in diabetes. Stat Med 1988;7:661–670.
84. Anderson PK. Survival analysis 1982–1991: the second decade of the proportional hazards regression model. Stat Med 1991;10:1931–1941.
85. Gill R, Schumacher M. A simple test of the proportional hazards assumption. Biometrika 1987;2:289–300.
86. Andersen PK. Testing goodness-of-fit of Cox's regression and life model. Biometrics 1982;38:67–77.
87. Nagelkerke NJD, Oosting J, Hart AAM. A simple test for goodness-of-fit of Cox's proportional hazards model. Biometrics 1984;40:483–486.
88. Arjas E. A graphical method for assessing goodness-of-fit in Cox's proportional hazards model. J Am Stat Assoc 1988;83:204–212.
89. Hosmer DW, Lemeshow S. Applied logistic regression. New York: John Wiley and Sons, 1989.
90. Truett J, Cornfield J, Kannel W. A multivariate analysis of the risk of coronary heart disease in Framingham. J Chronic Dis 1967;20:511–524.
91. Breslow NE, Day NE. Statistical methods in cancer research, vol. 1: the analysis of case-control studies. Lyon, France: International Agency on Cancer, 1980.
92. Efron B. Logistic regression, survival analysis, and the Kaplan-Meier curve. J Am Stat Assoc 1988;38:414–425.
93. Harell FE, Lee KL, Matchar DB, Reichert TA. Regression models for prognostic prediction: advantages,

problems, and suggested solutions. Cancer Treat Rep 1985;69:1071–1077.

94. Efron B. The jackknife, the bootstrap and other resampling plans. Society for Industrial and Applied Mathematics, 1982.

95. Brown CC. On a goodness-of-fit test for the logistic model based on score statistics. Communications in Statistics 1982;11:1087–1105.

96. Hosmer DW, Lemeshow S. A goodness-of-fit test for the multiple logistic regression model. Communications in Statistics 1980;A10:1043–1069.

97. Hosmer DW, Lemeshow S. Goodness-of-fit testing for multiple logistic regression analysis when the estimated probabilities are small. Biometrical J 1988;30: 911–924.

98. Horak DA, Schmidt GM, Zaia JA, Niland JC, Ahn C, Forman SJ. Pretransplant pulmonary function predicts cytomegalovirus-associated interstitial pneumonia following bone marrow transplantation. Chest 1993;102: 1484–1490. (in press).

Chapter 21
Bone Marrow Donors

C. D. Buckner, F. B. Petersen, and B. A. Bolonesi

Most human marrow donors have been human leukocyte antigen (HLA)-identical siblings, but improving results of bone marrow transplantation (BMT) have encouraged expansion of the donor pool to include less than perfectly HLA-matched family members and HLA-matched and partially matched unrelated donors. Patients with malignancy can also serve as their own source of hematopoietic stem cells for BMT.

The decision to perform an allogeneic BMT involves weighing the benefits to the patient against the risks to the normal donor. In general, marrow donation is considered a safe procedure, although one death following marrow harvesting has been reported (1). Marrow harvesting involves the inherent risks of general or regional anesthesia, blood loss, and trauma to skin, blood vessels, nerves, muscle, and bone at aspiration sites. What is known about marrow donation and its complications is discussed in this chapter.

Evaluation of Donors

Psychological Aspects of Marrow Donation

Marrow donation in adults involves giving voluntary informed consent to an operative procedure that entails significant morbidity and the risk of death without any benefit to the donor. Although refusals by relatives of ill patients to donate marrow are rare, it is important to keep in mind that there are considerable cultural and societal pressures on the donor. It would be very difficult for a family member to refuse to donate marrow that would potentially save the life of a relative even if he or she did not want to undergo the procedure.

Donor attitudes and perceptions toward marrow donation and the BMT procedure need to be assessed. Donors often have a distorted concept of the procedure, which can usually be remedied by thorough counselling. It is important to identify donors who need psychiatric evaluation. Allogeneic BMT involves administration of lethal doses of drugs or drugs and irradiation from which the recipient is unlikely to recover without the infusion of marrow. It is therefore crucial that the donor be fully committed to donating marrow prior to beginning the preparative regimen. Whenever there is a serious question about the reliability of a donor, consideration should be given to cryopreserving marrow (2) before initiating the pretreatment regimen.

Detailed discussion of the psychological and social aspects of family member marrow donation is beyond the scope of this review, but these subjects have been evaluated in adults (3–5) and children (6–8).

For unrelated volunteer donors there are no psychological pressures involved, and individuals donate out of pure altruism. In fact, direct contact between an unrelated marrow donor and the marrow recipient is prohibited by the National Marrow Donor Program in the United States. However, this is not universal policy, and there is still debate on this issue. There has been one study of the attitudes of unrelated marrow donors after donation (9). Twenty unrelated marrow donors were evaluated after marrow harvest, and no serious emotional or physical effects were observed. However, many more individuals will need to be evaluated to define the impact of marrow harvest on volunteer marrow donors.

Ethical and Legal Aspects of Marrow Donation

For adults donating marrow to relatives there are no significant legal issues involved in marrow donation as long as enough information is provided to obtain truly informed consent. However, marrow donation from unrelated volunteers creates ethical and legal issues (10). Children are routinely used as donors in the United States with parental consent, which creates ethical and legal problems (11–15). The legality of giving such consent is not straightforward. The laws involved and the interpretation of these laws differ from state to state and from country to country (15). For example, in the State of Washington, parents do not have the legal prerogative to give consent for marrow donation by their children because the procedure has no medical benefit and can potentially be harmful. Initially, all minor donors in Washington were made wards of the court, limited guardians ad litem were appointed, and court approval was then obtained for harvesting. The rationale used to convince the court to allow minors to donate marrow was that the child would suffer psychological harm if not allowed to provide marrow for a sick sibling, especially if the sibling died as a consequence. Because the number of marrow transplants performed in the State of Washington was large, the local court indicated that approval was not necessary after the precedent had been established. However, in some states and foreign countries, a court hearing is necessary for each individual minor child to donate marrow.

The ability to perform prenatal diagnosis and to determine the HLA type of the fetus has created another potential ethical and legal problem. Parents with a child who needs an allogeneic BMT could theoretically conceive a succession of fetuses until a compatible one is identified, with the mismatched fetuses being aborted (16).

Assessing Risks to the Marrow Donor

One thousand five hundred forty-nine individuals donated marrow to a related recipient at the Fred Hutchinson Cancer Research Center between 1983 and 1990. The characteristics and complications observed in these donors are shown in Tables 21-1 through 21-5 (17).

All potential marrow donors undergo thorough medical evaluation to determine suitability for marrow donation (18,19). In addition to a thorough physical examination, all donors have screening laboratory tests performed, which include complete blood counts, biochemistry profile, hepatitis screen, cytomegalovirus (CMV) antibody status, human immunodeficiency virus (HIV) antibody status, serological test for syphilis, electrocardiogram, and chest radiographs. All donors with medical problems are evaluated by an appropriate subspecialist physician, and further laboratory evaluations are performed as required. It is difficult to define rigid criteria for the acceptability or nonacceptability of a donor with medical problems because individuals not in perfect health may wish to accept increased risk to donate marrow to a relative.

Table 21-1.
Marrow Donor Characteristics[a]

	All Donors	*Normal Donors[b] (Age 18–55 yr)*
Number of Donors	1,549	701
Sex		
Women	740 (47%)	314 (44%)
Men	809 (53%)	387 (56%)
Age, median (range)	30 (0.5–70)	31 (18–50)
<18 yr	337 (22%)	0
>17 yr	1212 (78%)	701
Anesthesia		
General	1457 (94%)	652 (93%)
Spinal	92 (6%)	49 (7%)
Autologous blood stored		
Yes	1282 (82%)	701 (100%)
No	267 (18%)	0
Donors with adverse medical risk factors	167 (11%)	0

[a]Donors harvested at Fred Hutchinson Cancer Research Center, 1983–1990.
[b]Excludes the following donors: age < 17 or > 55; with risk factors for anesthesia; with no autologous blood stored; who weigh <55 kg; women who weigh > 90 kg; and men who weigh > 100 kg.

Table 21-2.
Medical Problems in Marrow Donors Detected Prior To Harvest[a]

Hypertension requiring pharmacological control	20%
Obesity (body weight >125% of ideal weight)	19%
Cardiac problems requiring pharmacological control or history of myocardial infarction	18%
Asthma requiring daily pharmacological control	10%
Active pulmonary problems (chronic obstruction pulmonary disease or active infiltrates)	5%
Diabetes mellitus requiring pharmacological control	4%
Active infections requiring antibiotics	3%
Seizure and other neurological problems requiring pharmacological control	3%
Alcoholism	3%
Gastrointestinal diseases requiring systemic pharmacological control	3%
Active vertebral disc disease or status postlumbar spine surgery	2%
Liver function abnormalities	2%
Renal abnormalities or status postrenal transplant	2%
Other	6%

[a]Donors harvested at Fred Hutchinson Cancer Research Center, 1983–1990. Number of donors evaluated = 1,549; number of preexisting medical problems observed = 206; number of donors with preexisting medical problems = 167.

Two hundred and six medical problems believed to increase the risk of anesthesia or the marrow harvest procedure were identified in 167 (11%) of 1,549 donors (Table 21-1), and 39 had more than one identifiable medical problem. The types of preharvest medical problems are listed in Table 21-2. The incidence of medical problems was higher in older individuals; 26 of 58 donors (45%) older than 55 years of age had adverse risk factors for undergoing anesthesia. In addition to common medical problems, asymptomatic neuroblastoma was detected in one infant donor, whose sibling had neuroblastoma, which led to early effective treatment (20).

In the case of volunteer unrelated donors, only normal individuals between the ages of 18 and 55 are allowed to donate marrow under the auspices of the National Marrow Donor Program, with health requirements similar to those applied to normal blood donors (21).

Assessing Risks for Transmitting Disease to the Recipient

In general, marrow donors are subjected to the same testing as blood donors and are screened for transmissible infectious diseases such as HIV and hepatitis B and C. Donors with evidence of active hepatitis or HIV are excluded from marrow donation. However, donors who are hepatitis B surface or core antibody–positive but surface antigen–negative are not excluded and do not pose a risk to the recipient (22). In fact, there is suggestive evidence that marrow from a donor immune to hepatitis B could have an antiviral effect in marrow recipients who are surface antigen–positive (22,23).

Potential donors who have antibodies to hepatitis C virus (HCV) should have serum analyzed by polymerase chain reaction for HCV RNA. Exclusion of donors with evidence of HCV (HCV RNA–positive) is controversial, but it is very likely that recipients of HCV-positive marrow will become infected (24). The course of patients with pre-existing HCV who undergo BMT suggests that the risk of serious hepatitis in the first 100 days is low, but that the frequency of chronic hepatitis and cirrhosis is high (25,26). There are few available data concerning the course of acute HCV infection transmitted by donor marrow. Recipients of HCV-positive marrow became viremic shortly after BMT (McDonald GM. Unpublished observations), but the long-term consequences are unknown. It is certain that many marrow transplant recipients were exposed to HCV before the screening test was available. There is one report of non-A non-B hepatitis being spread to platelet donors and marrow transplant recipients by an infected platelet donor. One marrow recipient involved in this epidemic died of fulminant hepatic failure (27,28). It is unknown whether this represented infection due to HCV.

CMV in the donor can be transmitted to recipients who are CMV-negative, with the potential for fatal consequences (29). Recipients who are CMV-positive can theoretically be infected with a different strain of virus from a CMV-positive donor, but the frequency and consequences of this phenomenon are unknown. In instances where the recipient is seronegative for CMV antibody and there is a choice of donors, the seronegative donor should be selected. Other infections that can potentially be transmitted with marrow include toxoplasmosis, malaria, *Yersinia*, *Leishmania*, syphilis, and gonorrhea (30). Donors with infections due to Epstein-Barr virus, adenovirus, and respiratory syncytial virus should not be used as donors while symptomatic to avoid complications of anesthesia and the possibility of disease transmission.

Noninfectious diseases such as myasthenia gravis (31) and autoimmune thrombocytopenic purpura (32) have possibly been transferred by marrow transplantation. Donors with a familial history of inherited diseases such as Fanconi's anemia (33) and monosomy 7 preleukemic syndrome (34) should undergo marrow and cytogenetic examination, and if affected, they should not be used as marrow donors. Donors who are heterozygous for sickle-cell anemia and thalassemia are acceptable marrow donors (35).

Marrow donors in the early 1970s, especially twins, were subjected to marrow aspiration to rule out malignancy. This practice was abandoned because of the absence of observed abnormalities in donors with normal peripheral blood counts. However, there has been one case of leukemia transmitted from a marrow donor to a sibling (36). This donor had normal peripheral blood counts prior to marrow aspiration for the BMT, but had acute myeloid leukemia, which was transferred to a sibling transplanted for chronic myeloid leukemia.

There is evidence that more graft-versus-host disease develops in recipients of marrow from multiparous women than in recipients of marrow from men or from women who have not been pregnant (37). This finding is presumed to be related to immunization of the mother by the fetus. Marrow donors who have been recipients of blood transfusions should also be presumed to be immunized. When there is a choice of equally HLA-matched donors, preference should be given to men, nulliparous women, and previously untransfused individuals.

Technique

Hospitalization

Marrow donors without significant medical problems are admitted to the hospital on the morning of harvest. The aspiration procedure is carried out in the operating room under sterile conditions. The aspiration team most often consists of an anesthesiologist, one physician, an assistant who aspirates the marrow, two surgical assistants who pass the instruments and take care of the aspirated marrow, and a cirulating nurse. The median duration of 1,549 procedures was 1 hour and 15 minutes for obtaining a median of 750 mL marrow volume (Table 21-3). Procedure time was significantly prolonged if both the anterior and the posterior crests were aspirated due to the time needed to turn the donor and to perform skin preparation. In most centers, donors without complications remain in the hospital overnight and are discharged within 24 to 36 hours of marrow aspiration. In one center, aspiration of autologous marrow has been performed on an out-patient basis (38).

Table 21-3.
Marrow Harvest Characteristics[a]

Volume of marrow aspirated, median mL (range)	750 (55–1750)
Time of marrow aspiration, median minutes (range)	75 (10–205)
Marrow cells × 10^8/kg donor weight, median (range)	2.5 (0.3–12.0)
Volume of marrow, mL/kg of donor weight, median (range)	11.9 (0.8–27.5)
Marrow cells × 10^8/kg recipient weight, median (range)	2.6 (0.1–22.4)
Volume of marrow, mL/kg of recipient weight, median (range)	11.4 (1.2–51.1)

[a]Donors harvested at Fred Hutchinson Cancer Research Center, 1983–1990. Donors harvested = 1,549.

Anesthesia

Most transplant centers utilize general anesthesia (39); however, the procedure can be performed under caudal or spinal anesthesia. There are no studies evaluating the relative safety of different methods of anesthesia for marrow harvesting. In Seattle, the majority of donors (94%) elected, after consultations with the anesthesiologist, to have the aspirations performed under general anesthesia. This selection probably has a high personal bias on the part of the patient or anesthesiologist. However, for specific donors with adverse risk factors, the type of anesthesia should be more specifically selected (40).

Anatomical Considerations

Most of the marrow used for transplantation is aspirated from the posterior iliac crests (41). Some transplant teams aspirate the anterior crests as well, but most centers only aspirate the anterior crests when the yield from the posterior crests is small or when large cell yields are needed because of size differences between the donor and the recipient. The sternum can be used, but this approach is rarely necessary (41,42). Five percent of 1,549 donors had the anterior crests aspirated, and only 3 donors had the sternum aspirated. The tibia could also be used as a source of marrow in infants, but this technique is not advised because of risk of damaging the nutrient artery supplying the tibia and the potential for damaging the long bone.

Marrow can also be obtained from surgically resected bone, usually from the iliac crests and ribs (43). One potential advantage to this approach is the lack of peripheral blood contamination resulting in a lower number of T cells. However, the most practical use of this approach is for obtaining cadaver marrow (44–48).

Collection, Processing, and Infusion of Marrow

Characteristics of the marrow harvest for 1,549 marrow donors are shown in Table 21-3. The technique for human marrow aspiration and processing widely used currently was originally described by Thomas and Storb in 1970 (43). However, individual transplant centers have modified this procedure to fit their own needs (49–51).

Marrow is aspirated with large-bore needles through multiple punctures of the bone through skin sites. The total number of skin puncture sites can be as low as 6 to 8, but to aspirate the entire posterior crest, more skin punctures are usually necessary. Approximately 200 to 300 separate aspirations through different bone sites are made. The usual volume aspirated is kept below 10 mL from any one bone puncture to decrease the amount of blood contamination (52). All syringes are rinsed with tissue culture media containing heparin, and marrow is placed in an open beaker (42) or a closed system (53) containing tissue culture medium and preservative-free heparin. A closed system theoretically decreases the probability of airborne bacterial contamination of the marrow, but the practical implications of this technique have not been documented. In one center, the incidence of bacterial contamination was 17%; the predominant organisms were skin flora, but there were no adverse consequences of this contamination (54). Presumably, the greater the delay between aspiration and infusion, the more likely it is that the infusion of contaminated marrow will have clinical significance.

Collected marrow is usually filtered in the operating room using 200 to 300 μm square stainless steel screens (42). Filtration can also be accomplished by gravity using manufactured kits (53) or at the bedside using platelet filtration sets (Buckner CD, personal observations).

When filtered in the operating room, whole marrow is infused intravenously without further filtration. However, marrow can be centrifuged to remove fat, plasma, or red cells (55), and buffy-coat preparations can also be prepared using a variety of techniques (56–58). All manipulations may potentially damage or deplete the marrow of hematopoietic stem cells. Marrow is usually infused immediately after harvesting because hematopoietic stem-cell viability will decline with time (59–61). However, there may be no adverse consequences of delay if the marrow is infused within 12 to 24 hours of harvesting. Unrelated donor marrow is routinely transported at room temperature between centers, often involving transcontinental shipment, and delays between aspiration and infusion are often 12 to 24 hours without apparent deleterious effects on engraftment (62,63). Autologous marrow has been stored for 48 hours at 4°C with successful engraftment (64). Although there are no precise data concerning the optimal conditions for marrow storage during delays in infusion, additional anticoagulation is generally added, usually in the form of ACD or CPD-A1 in concentrations ordinarily used for anticoagulation and preservation of blood.

Volume of Marrow Aspirated

The target volume for BMT purposes is considered to be 10 to 15 mL/kg recipient or donor body weight, depending on the smaller individual. This volume of marrow yields approximately 3×10^8 nucleated marrow cells/kg (Table 21-3). These volumes and numbers were arrived at empirically but represent realistic target volumes that usually yield sufficient hematopoietic stem cells for allogeneic engraftment of unmanipulated marrow. The maximum volume aspirated from a given donor depends on body size and restrictions placed on allogeneic blood transfusions. Persistent aspiration from the same marrow sites yields mostly peripheral blood; at some point in the procedure there is little benefit to collecting further volume (52).

There is suggestive evidence that marrow from children, especially infants, has a higher concentration of nucleated cells and probably a higher percentage of marrow repopulating cells than marrow from adult donors (20,42). A successful marrow transplant was achieved in a 36-kg recipient from a 6-kg donor (20). Thus, there should be little hesitation to using younger, smaller children as donors for larger, older individuals. The youngest marrow donor in Seattle was 4 months of age.

Blood Transfusion Policies

The general policy in most centers is to store one or more units of autologous blood 1 to 3 weeks prior to marrow harvest. The stored blood is infused during or immediately following the aspiration procedure. Storage of autologous blood is not routinely carried out in children under 30 kg in body weight. In some centers, marrow is centrifuged, and plasma and red cells are returned to the donor. Oral iron (ferrous gluconate or sulfate) is given for 2 to 3 weeks prior to and for 30 days following marrow donation to compensate for blood loss.

Table 21-5.
Life-Threatening Complications[a]

Age	*Sex*	*Risk Factor*	*Complications*	*Hospital Days*
52	M	Hypertension	Severe hypotension in OR[b]	2
50	M	Hypertension	Cardiac arrest in OR	2
7	M	None	Severe hypoxemia in OR	1
43	M	Obese/smoker	Cardiac arrest during intubation	1
52	M	Cardiac	Severe hypotension in OR[b]	5
34	M	None	*Staphylococcus aureus* septicemia and osteomyelitis	17

[a]Donors harvested at Fred Hutchinson Cancer Research Center, 1983–1990. Donors at risk = 1,549.
[b]Severe hypotension = diastolic < 50% of baseline.
OR = operating room.

Complications of Marrow Donation

Morbidity

Morbid events following marrow aspiration of 1,549 marrow donations are summarized in Table 21-4. Forty-five (3%) of 1,549 marrow donors experienced major complications, defined as receiving more than 5 units of blood (n = 5), more than 21 days of hip pain requiring orthopedic follow-up (n = 8), orthostatic blood pressure decrements after aspiration with syncope (n = 16), and life-threatening complications (n = 6). Table 21-4 also summarizes the complications observed in 701 marrow donors, ages 18 through 55, without adverse risk factors. These donors represent the population of patients meeting the requirements for unrelated marrow donation under the auspices of the National Marrow Donor Program.

A total of 167 of 1,549 donors had pre-existing medical problems deemed to be adverse risk factors for undergoing anesthesia or the harvest procedure. Thirty-four of these 167 donors (20%) had complications from the marrow harvest, 4 (2.4%) of which were classified as major. Post harvest complications developed in 259 (19%) of 1,382 donors without preharvest medical risk factors, 41 (3%) of which were classified as major. However, 4 of 6 life-threatening complications occurred in the 167 donors with pre-existing medical problems.

Table 21-4.
Complications Following Marrow Donation[a]

	All Donors	*Normal Donors[b] (Age 18–55 yr)*
Total number of donors	1,549	701
Number of complications	599	200
Number of donors with complications	426 (27%)	152 (22%)
Postaspiration hypotension or weakness requiring >1 day in hospital	134 (9%)	54 (8%)
Bleeding or allogeneic blood transfusions	221 (14%)	47 (7%)
Excess pain	123 (8%)	57 (8%)
Fever	71 (5%)	25 (4%)
Other complications	50 (3%)	59 (8%)
Life-threatening complications	6 (.4%)	1 (.1%)

[a]Donors harvested at Fred Hutchinson Cancer Research Center, 1983–1990.
[b]Excludes the following donors: age < 17 or > 55; with risk factors for anesthesia; with no autologous blood stored; who weigh < 55 kg; women who weigh > 90 kg; and men who weigh > 100 kg.

Hospitalization

In the original report from Seattle, marrow donors were hospitalized from 2 to 14 days (41). The policy at that time was to admit donors to the hospital the night before the operation and to keep them in the hospital overnight after the harvest. Thus, 81% of marrow donations involved 2 days of hospitalization. More recently, donors without adverse risk factors for donation have been admitted to the hospital on the morning of the harvest, and 89% of such donors were discharged within 36 hours of marrow donation. The remaining 11% of donors were hospitalized a median of 2 days (range, 2–18 days), and the causes of additional hospitalization are shown in Tables 21-4 and 21-5.

It may be possible to reduce hospitalization time further by performing the marrow harvest on an outpatient basis. A trial of autologous marrow aspiration on an out-patient basis has been reported; 36 of 39 patients with malignancy had marrow aspirated and were discharged later on the same day (38). Two patients had overnight admissions for hypotension and one for fever. Whether this approach is appropriate for normal marrow donors remains to be determined.

Pain

Multiple marrow aspirations result in trauma to the iliac bones, and postoperative pain and discomfort are universal. In a study of postdonation pain, it was found that donors used analgesia (codeine with acetaminophen) for a mean of 3.3 days (range, 1–13) after marrow harvest, and men reported more pain than women (65). Approximately 8% of marrow donors have "excessive pain," which is probably due to hematomas at the aspiration sites causing pressure neuropathies. Sciatic pain lasting 18 months and hip pain due to displaced cortical fractures have also been described (41).

Fever and Infection

Postoperative fever, usually unexplained, occurs in 5 to 10% of donors, with resolution within 24 to 48 hours (1,41). Local infections developed in 5 of 1,549 donors (0.3%), one of whom had concurrent septicemia. An additional 5 donors received empiric antibiotics for suspected but not documented infection.

Allogeneic Blood Transfusions

There have been no reports of disease transmission to normal marrow donors from allogeneic blood transfusions; however, this statistic may reflect inadequate follow-up, because many marrow donors received allogeneic blood transfusions prior to the availability of screening tests for HIV and hepatitis C. Any allogeneic blood transfusion is a potential risk to the marrow donor and should be avoided if possible.

All allogeneic blood given intraoperatively to marrow donors is irradiated to prevent graft-versus-host disease from third-party lymphocytes transferred from the transfused blood to the aspirated marrow (20).

In an earlier publication, 19% of adult men and 31% of adult women donors received allogeneic blood despite the fact that the majority had an autologous unit of blood stored (41). Fifty percent of all children and 85% of infants under the age of 2 received allogeneic blood transfusions following marrow donation (20,41). Buisson and colleagues (66) reported that 18 of 28 children (ages, 13 mo to 17 yr) received allogeneic blood transfusions following marrow donation. Attempts have been made to reduce the number of donors exposed to allogeneic blood. In a more recent analysis, 1,126 of 1,212 (93%) adult donors had autologous blood stored prior to marrow harvest, whereas 86 (7%) did not for various reasons. One hundred twenty-three (10%) of the 1,212 adult donors who had autologous blood stored and reinfused also received allogeneic blood during or shortly after the harvest procedure. Ninety-six transfused donors were women and 27 were men. Thus, 4% of adult men and 17% of adult women who had an autologous unit of blood stored required allogeneic blood transfusions after the harvest procedure.

In most instances, the need for allogeneic blood in adults could not be predicted from the initial hematocrit or the intraoperative blood loss. However, preoperative hematocrit levels (after drawing blood for laboratory studies and an autologous unit of blood) were lower in donors subsequently receiving transfusions than in those not receiving allogeneic blood. Presumably, a minority of donors, usually women, have an inordinate amount of periosteal and soft-tissue bleeding, leading to excessive blood loss requiring replacement.

Thompson and McCullough (67) found that the volume of marrow harvested correlated closely with the volume of blood transfused. Their data indicate that the amount of blood needed for transfusion could be estimated prior to harvest by knowing the amount of marrow required (67). This calculation may prove true for the majority of marrow donors, but these calculations would not affect those donors with unexpected large volume periosteal and soft-tissue bleeding who have to be transfused postoperatively.

One hundred fifty-six (56%) of 337 donors aged 17 or less had autologous blood stored. The youngest marrow donor who had blood stored was 7 years of age; the lowest weight was 21 kg. Five of 156 (3%) children who had one unit of blood stored received allogeneic blood, as compared with 91 of 181 (50%) children who had no autologous blood stored.

Administration of recombinant human erythropoietin (rh-Epo) and iron to patients undergoing elective surgery has increased the number of units of blood that can be stored in a 3-week period (68). Theoretically, administration of rh-Epo plus iron to marrow donors for 2 to 3 weeks prior to marrow donation could decrease the need for allogeneic blood transfusions by accelerating recovery from the obligate blood loss of laboratory testing and the storage of an autologous unit of blood, particularly for children. In selected patients, use of rh-Epo might facilitate the storage of more than one unit of autologous blood.

In Seattle, 10 normal marrow donors were given rh-Epo (100 U/kg/day) for 2 to 3 weeks prior to marrow harvest (69). In control donors, the average changes in hematocrit values between the initial out-patient visit and the preoperative and postoperative values were −4.5 and −11.1%, respectively. In the donors receiving rh-Epo, the comparable values for preoperative and postoperative hematocrit values were +5.5% and −3.0%. Despite the small numbers, these differences were statistically significant, indicating that the 2- to 3-week administration of rh-Epo increased red cell production, as compared with control donors. However, further trials will be necessary to define donor populations that will benefit from this approach. Also, due to the time-frame involved, it may be desirable to give rh-Epo to donors prior to arrival at the transplant center. Some transplant centers coordinate storage of up to 3 units of donor blood over a 5-week period. If done locally at an approved blood bank, such blood can be shipped to the marrow transplant center.

Other Effects

Foldes and associates (70) reported increased serum osteocalcin and alkaline phosphatase levels after marrow donation, suggesting a systemic osteogenic response. The significance of these findings is unknown.

Life-Threatening Complications

The incidence of life-threatening complications from marrow harvesting was 0.21% following 2,027 marrow donations from normal individuals (1,42). In this group of donors, life-threatening complications were noted in 9; septicemia developed in 3, and one each had pulmonary embolism, aspiration pneumonia, cardiopulmonary arrest, ventricular tachycardia, carotid artery occlusion, and femoral artery occlusion. Five of these 9 life-threatening complications reported could be attributed to anesthesia.

Life-threatening complications in 1,549 additional marrow donors from Seattle are summarized in Table 21-5. Six patients (0.4%) had life-threatening complications, 4 of which occurred in donors who had adverse preoperative risk factors. Five of the 6 complications could be attributed to anesthesia.

Seven hundred and one of the 1,549 marrow donors were ages 18 through 55 and without adverse risk factors for anesthesia. In this group of donors, who would have been eligible to be unrelated volunteer donors, there was only 1 life-threatening complication (0.1%).

Infant Marrow Donation

Uncomplicated marrow donation has been reported from 23 donors less than 2 years and as young as 4 months of age (20); however, 22 of 23 received allogeneic blood transfusions. There has been one report of marrow donation from a premature 7-week-old baby girl (71). This was a 3.95-kg child who donated 200 mL marrow, which represented two-thirds of the blood volume and essentially required exchange transfusions with irradiated blood. In most instances it is advised that transplantation be delayed, if possible, until the infant is 3 to 4 months of age before being used as a marrow donor. Umbilical cord blood is rich in hematopoietic stem cells and can be used for transplantation purposes (72–74).

Older Age and Marrow Donation

There is some evidence that the volume of marrow aspirated and the concentration of nucleated cells declines with age, but the consequences of these changes on outcome of BMT is unknown (41). There have been no published data concerning the effects of increasing age on donor complications. The overwhelming majority of marrow donors have been under the age of 55. In the original report from Seattle, only 14 of 1,160 donors were over the age of 59 and there was no apparent increase in complications (41). In the subsequent 1,549 marrow donations, there were 58 donors over the age of 55, and 57% experienced an event-free donation, as compared with 72% of the total group. Twenty-six (45%) of the 58 older donors did not have adverse risk factors for donation, and 10 (38%) experienced complications from the aspiration procedure; 7 required more than one day of hospitalization. This may not be different than the 22% incidence of postaspiration complications observed in healthy donors between 18 to 55 years of age who would have qualified for unrelated marrow donation (See Table 21-4). A reasonable approach for related family member donors is not to have an age limit but to evaluate the anesthetic and operative risks based on the health of the individual donor and to weigh the risks of donation against the potential benefits to the recipient.

Peripheral Blood Hematopoietic Stem Cells

Peripheral blood contains hematopoietic stem cells capable of complete hematopoietic repopulation. However, in the normal steady state, the concentration of these cells is too low for practical use for allogeneic BMT. Multiple collections by apheresis are required to obtain sufficient cells, even for autologous BMT. There has been one attempt to utilize peripheral blood stem cells for allografting in humans (75). The allogeneic donor underwent 10 apheresis procedures to collect buffy-coat cells, which were depleted of T cells and cryopreserved. After the patient received cytoreductive treatment, these cells were thawed and infused into the recipient. Successful early engraftment was achieved, but the patient died on day 32 of causes unrelated to engraftment.

There are situations in which hematopoietic stem cells are increased in the peripheral blood. Umbilical cord blood is a rich source of hematopoietic stem cells, and successful allogeneic engraftment has been achieved using unfractionated cord blood (72–74). Theoretically, cord blood could be HLA-typed, cryopreserved, and serve as a source of hematopoietic stem cells for HLA-matched unrelated individuals. However, the effect of recipient weight in relation to a relatively small amount of cord blood may render such an approach impractical except for infants and small children.

The absolute number of circulating hematopoietic cells in the peripheral blood is increased during recovery from cytotoxic therapy, but this is clearly an inappropriate manipulation of normal donors. However, the use of recombinant growth factors to increase the number of circulating peripheral blood hematopoietic precursors is a very promising approach to harvesting hematopoietic stem cells from allogeneic donors. Recombinant growth factors, including granulocyte colony stimulating factor (76), granulocyte-macrophage colony stimulating factor (77), and interleukin-3 (78), increase the number of peripheral blood progenitor cells. Other recombinant growth factors, such as stem-cell factor (c-kit ligand), may be even more effective in mobilizing such cells but have not been evaluated in humans (79). Theoretically, the optimal recombinant growth factor or combination of growth factors could be administered to normal donors to increase the number of hematopoietic precursors in the peripheral blood. These cells could be collected during 1 to 3 apheresis procedures, T-cell–depleted, and used as a source of hematopoietic stem cells for allogeneic engraftment. It will have to be determined whether consistent and enduring engraftment can be achieved with this approach and if the morbidity associated with growth factor administration and the apheresis procedures is less than that observed following multiple marrow aspirations in the operating room.

Cryopreservation of Allogeneic Marrow

There is extensive experience with cryopreservation of marrow for autologous marrow transplantation; however, experience with use of cryopreserved allogeneic marrow in humans is limited (2). In Seattle, 6 patients received cryopreserved allogeneic marrow; 2 experienced graft failure and both had relatively low marrow cell doses collected. These data suggest the feasibility of cryopreserving allogeneic marrow with the caveat that relatively large cell doses should be collected to compensate for the inevitable cell loss from marrow processing, cryopreservation, and thawing.

The Potential Use of Cadaver Marrow

Ferrebee and colleagues (44), in 1959, demonstrated that cadaver marrow could be collected and cryopreserved with retention of viability, as measured by in vitro assays, after thawing. These studies were confirmed in 1985 by Mugishima and co-workers (45), who found that surgically removed cadaver marrow contained less T cells than aspirated marrow. They also demonstrated that surgically obtained cadaver marrow could be depleted of T cells, cryopreserved, and thawed with retention of viability, as measured by more sophisticated in vitro assays than were available to the original investigators. These findings have subsequently been confirmed by others (46,47). In 1957, cryopreserved cadaver marrow from an unrelated donor was infused following total body irradiation without complications and with evidence of engraftment of red cells (80). More recently, marrow was obtained from a cadaver who was HLA-matched with his son, who had acute lymphoblastic leukemia. The marrow was cryopreserved and subsequently infused following intensive chemotherapy. Engraftment was achieved, but the patient died of graft-versus-host disease (48). There are also a number of reports in the Russian language concerning the use of cadaver marrow for transplantation purposes; however, evaluation of these reports is beyond the scope of this chapter.

Although the use of cadaver marrow is a logical approach to increasing the number of marrows available for unrelated transplants, the logistical difficulties make it unlikely that cadaver marrow will supplant that from living donors in the near future.

Autologous Marrow Harvesting

In general, complications following harvesting for autologous BMT have been similar to those observed in normal donors. Jin and associates (81) reported two life-threatening events following 224 marrow harvests: (1) postoperative pneumonia that resolved after 5 days of antibiotic therapy, (2) postoperative bradycardia with a nodal rhythm that reversed after atropine administration.

Kessinger and Armitage (82) compared the complication rate following normal versus autologous marrow harvesting and concluded that autologous patients with malignancies had more unexplained fever and infection than normal donors donating for allogeneic BMT. In their study of 170 marrow harvests, bacterial septicemia developed in 2 patients, and local aspiration site cellulitis developed in one. Cairo and associates (83) reported one life-threatening complication (pulmonary embolus related to venous stasis from tumor obstruction) following 65 autologous marrow harvests.

Summary

Marrow harvesting from normal donors for BMT is obviously a practical procedure, as attested to by the increasing number of transplants being performed. However, marrow donation is not a completely benign procedure; all donors will experience some degree of discomfort, and approximately 3% will have prolonged morbidity. Life-threatening complications due to anesthesia or the procedure itself occur in a 0.10 to 0.41% of donors. Although use of allogeneic blood transfusions is diminishing, further efforts, such as administration of rh-Epo to donors and storage of more than one unit of blood where the need can be predicted, should be carried out to eliminate such transfusions. Extreme diligence is required of transplant teams to prevent and treat complications in donors. It is also important for various marrow transplant teams and transplant registries to evaluate and publish the details of donor complications to identify and hopefully to prevent such complications in the future.

References

1. Bortin MM, Buckner CD. Major complications of marrow harvesting for transplantation. Exp Hematol 1983;11:916–921.
2. Lasky LC, Van Baren N, Weisdorf DJ, et al. Successful allogeneic cryopreserved marrow transplantation. Transfusion 1980;29:182–184.
3. Lesko LM, Hawkins DR. Psychological aspects of transplantation medicine. In: Akhtar S, ed. New psychiatric

syndromes: DSM-III and beyond. New York: Jason Aronson, 1983:265–309.
4. Wolcott DL, Wellisch DK, Fawzy FI, Landsverk J. Psychological adjustment of adult bone marrow transplant donors whose recipient survives. Transplantation 1986;41:484–488.
5. Freund BL, Siegel K. Problems in transition following bone marrow transplantation: psychosocial aspects. Am J Orthopsychiatry 1986;56:244–252.
6. Patenaude A, Szymanski L, Rappeport J. Psychological costs of bone marrow transplantation in children. Am J Orthopsychiatry 1979;49:409–422.
7. Wiley FM, Lindamood MM, Pfefferbaum-Levine B. Donor-patient relationship in pediatric bone marrow transplantation. J Assoc Pediatr Oncol Nurses 1984;1: 8–14.
8. Pasquier N, Pujol M, Souillet G, Philippe N. The child receiving a graft, the child donating the graft and their family, a year later. Revue Medicale de la Suisse Romande 1988;108:121–122.
9. Stroncek D, Strand R, Scott E, et al. Attitudes and physical condition of unrelated bone marrow donors immediately after donation. Transfusion 1989;29:317–322.
10. McCullough J. Bone marrow transplantation from unrelated volunteer donors: summary of a conference on scientific, ethical, legal, financial, and other practical issues. Transfusion 1982;22:78–81.
11. Levine MD, Camitta BM, Nathan D, et al. The medical ethics of bone marrow transplantation in childhood. J Pediatr 1975;86:145–150.
12. Serota FT, August CS, O'Shea AT, et al. Role of a child advocate in the selection of donors for pediatric bone marrow transplantation. J Pediatr 1981;98:847–850.
13. Brant J. Legal issues involving bone marrow transplants to minors. Am J Pediatr Hematol Oncol 1984;6:89–91.
14. Williams TE. Legal issues and ethical dilemmas surrounding bone marrow transplantation in children. Am J Pediatr Hematol Oncol 1984;6:83–88.
15. Masini B, Guidi S, Maurri M. Minor donor of bone marrow graft: medico-legal aspects. Recenti Progressi In Medicina 1991;82:500–504.
16. Moreau C. Conceiving a fetus for bone marrow donation: an ethical problem in prenatal diagnosis. Prenat Diagn 1989;9:329–334.
17. Petersen FB, Buckner CD, Bolonesi B, et al. Marrow harvesting from normal donors (abstract). Exp Hematol 1990;18:676.
18. Ruggiero MR. The donor in bone marrow transplantation. Semin Oncol Nurs 1988;4:9–14.
19. Dannie E. Assessment of bone marrow donors. Nursing Standard 1992;5:3–6.
20. Sanders J, Buckner CD, Bensinger WI, Levy W, Chard R, Thomas ED. Experience with marrow harvesting from donors less than two years of age. Bone Marrow Transplant 1987;2:45–50.
21. Standards for Blood Banks and Transfusion Services. Arlington, VA: American Association of Blood Banks, 1992:95.
22. Chen P-M, Fan S, Liu C-J, et al. Changing of hepatitis B virus markers in patients with bone marrow transplantation. Transplantation. 1990;49:708–713.
23. Ilan Y, Nagler A, Adler R, Deparstek E, Slavin S, Shouval D. Adoptive transfer of immunity to hepatitis B in humans following T-depleted bone marrow transplantation from immune donors. Hepatology 1991;14:130A.
24. Locasciulli A, Bacigalupo A, Alberti A, et al. Predictability before transplant of hepatic complications following allogeneic bone marrow transplantation. Transplantation 1989;48:68–72.
25. Ljungman P, Duraj V, Magnius L, Aschan J, Lönnqvist B, Ringden O. Hepatitis C infection in allogeneic bone marrow transplant recipients. Transplant 1991;5:283–286.
26. Locasciulli A, Bacigalupo A, Vanlint MT, et al. Hepatitis C virus infection in patients undergoing allogeneic bone marrow transplantation. Transplantation 1991;52:315–318.
27. Meyers JD, Huff JC, Homes KK, Thomas ED, Bryan JA. Parenterally transmitted hepatitis A associated with platelet transfusions. Epidemiologic study of an outbreak in a marrow transplantation center. Ann Intern Med 1974;81:145–151.
28. Meyers JD, Dienstag JL, Purcell RH, Thomas ED, Holmes KK. Parenterally transmitted non-A, non-B hepatitis. An epidemic reassessed. Ann Intern Med 1977;87:57–59.
29. Meyers JD, Flournoy N, Thomas ED. Risk factors for cytomegalovirus infection after human marrow transplantation. J Infect Dis 1986;153:478–488.
30. Rossi EC, Simon TL, Moss GS, eds. Principles of transfusion medicine. San Francisco: Williams & Wilkins, 1991.
31. Smith CIE, Aarli JA, Biberfeld P, et al. Myasthenia gravis after bone-marrow transplantation. Evidence for a donor origin. N Engl J Med 1983;309:1565–1568.
32. Waters AH, Metcalfe P, Minchinton RM, et al. Autoimmune thrombocytopenia acquired from allogeneic bone marrow graft: compensated thrombocytopenia in bone marrow donor and recipient. Lancet 1983;2:1430.
33. Deeg HJ, Storb R, Thomas ED, et al. Fanconi's anemia treated by allogeneic marrow transplantation. Blood 1983;61:954–959.
34. Paul B, Reid MM, Davison EV, et al. Familial myelodysplasia: progressive disease associated with emergence of monosomy 7. Br J Haematol 1987;65:321–323.
35. Lucarelli G, Galimberti M, Polchi P, et al. Bone marrow transplantation in patients with thalassemia. N Engl J Med 1990;322:417–421.
36. Niederwieser DW, Appelbaum FR, Gastl G, et al. Inadvertent transmission of a donor's acute myeloid leukemia in bone marrow transplantation for chronic myelocytic leukemia. N Engl J Med 1990;322:1794–1796.
37. Flowers MED, Pepe MS, Longton G, et al. Previous donor pregnancy as a risk factor for acute graft-versus-host disease in patients with aplastic anemia treated by allogeneic marrow transplantation. Br J Haematol 1990;74:492–496.
38. Brandwein JM, Callum J, Rubinger M, Scott JG, Keating A. An evaluation of outpatient bone marrow harvesting. J Clin Oncol 1989;7:648–650.
39. Filshie J, Pollock AN, Hughes RG, Omar YA. The anesthetic management of bone marrow harvest for transplantation. Anaesthesia 1984;39:480–485.
40. Hirsh RA. An approach to assessing perioperative risk. In: Goldmann DR, Brown FH, Levy WK, Slap GB, Sussman EJ, eds. Medical care of the surgical patient: a problem-oriented approach to management. Philadelphia: J.B. Lippincott, 1982:31–39.
41. Buckner CD, Clift RA, Sanders JE, et al. Marrow harvesting from normal donors. Blood 1984;64:630–634.
42. Thomas ED, Storb R. Technique for human marrow grafting. Blood 1970;36:507–515.

43. Sharp TG, Sachs DH, Matthews JG, Maples J, Woody JN, Rosenberg SA. Harvest of human bone marrow directly from bone. J Immunol Methods 1984;69:187–195.
44. Ferrebee JW, Atkins L, Lochte HL Jr., et al. The collection, storage and preparation of viable cadaver marrow for intravenous use. Blood 1959;14:140–147.
45. Mugishima H, Terasaki P, Sueyoshi A. Bone marrow from cadaver donors for transplantation. Blood 1985; 65:392–396.
46. Blazar BR, Lasky LC, Perentesis JP, et al. Successful donor cell engraftment in a recipient of bone marrow from a cadaveric donor. Blood 1986;67:1655–1660.
47. Lucas PJ, Quinones RR, Moses RD, Nakamura H, Gress RE. Alternative donor sources in HLA-mismatched marrow transplantation: T cell depletion of surgically resected cadaveric marrow. Bone Marrow Transplant 1988;3:211–220.
48. Gress RE, Bare C, Lucas PJ, et al. Efficacy of T cell depletion of surgically resected cadaveric marrows by monoclonal antibodies: considerations in HLA-mismatched marrow transplantation. Prog Clin Biol Res 1990;333:471–488.
49. Treleaven JG. Bone marrow harvesting and reinfusion. In: Gee AP, ed. Bone marrow processing and purging. A practical guide. Boca Raton: CRC Press, 1991:31–38.
50. Pflieger H, Wiesneth M, Schmeiser T, Kubanek B. A simple technique for processing of bone marrow for human marrow transplantation. Blut 1982;45:411–414.
51. Shinohara Y. Technology of bone marrow transplantation—harvest and manipulation of bone marrow cells. J Clin Med 1990;48:2023–2027.
52. Batinic D, Marusic M, Pavletic Z, et al. Relationship between differing volumes of bone marrow aspirates and their cellular composition. Bone Marrow Transplant 1990;6:103–107.
53. Lin A, Carr T, Herzig R, Rowley S, Buchholz D. Evaluation of a disposable bone marrow collection and filtration kit (abstract). Transfusion 1987;27:529.
54. Davis J, Rowley S, Dick J, et al. Bacterial contamination of bone marrow grafts: incidence and clinical significance. In: Gee AP, Gross S, eds. Bone marrow transplantation. New York: Macmillan Press, 1987:125.
55. Jin N-R, Hill R, Segal G, et al. Preparation of red-blood-cell-depleted marrow for ABO-incompatible marrow transplantation by density-gradient separation using the IBM 2991 cell processor. Exp Hematol 1987;15:93–98.
56. McMannis JD. Use of the Cobe 2991™ cell processor for bone marrow processing. In: Gee AP, ed. Bone marrow processing and purging. A practical guide. Boca Raton: CRC Press, 1991:73–84.
57. Cullis HM, Areman E, Carter CS. Nucleated cell separation using the Fenwal CS 3000™. In: Gee AP, ed. Bone marrow processing and purging. A practical guide. Boca Raton: CRC Press, 1991:54–70.
58. Hartl ML. Bone marrow processing with the Haemonetics V50 plus™. In: Gee AP, ed. Bone marrow processing and purging. A practical guide. Boca Raton: CRC Press, 1991:87–103.
59. Mangalik A, Robinson WA, Drebing C, Hartmann D, Joshi JH. Liquid storage of bone marrow. Exp Hematol 1979;7:76–94.
60. Mannick JA, Lochte HL Jr, Thomas ED, Ferrebee JW. In vitro and in vivo assessment of the viability of dog marrow after storage. Blood 1960;15:517–524.
61. Lasky LC, McCullough J, Zanjani ED. Liquid storage of unseparated human bone marrow. Transfusion 1986; 26:331–334.
62. Petersen FB, Weinberg P, Hansen JA, Thomas ED. Collection and transplantation of human bone marrow cells from unrelated donors. Transfusion Sci 1991;12: 155–159.
63. Janssen WE, Lee C. Transportation of bone marrow for in vitro processing and transplantation. In: Gee AP, ed. Bone marrow processing and purging. A practical guide. Boca Raton: CRC Press, 1991:40–51.
64. Burnett AK, Tansey P, Hills C, et al. Haematological reconstitution following high dose and supralethal chemoradiotherapy using stored, non-cryopreserved autologous bone marrow. Br J Haematol 1983;54:309–316.
65. Hill HF, Chapman CR, Jackson T, Sullivan KM. Assessment and management of donor pain following marrow harvest for allogeneic bone marrow transplantation. Bone Marrow Transplant 1989;4:157–161.
66. Buisson C, Attia J, Barrier G. Anesthesia and bone marrow harvesting in children. Annales Francaises d'Anesthesia et de Reanimation 1989;8:90–102.
67. Thompson HW, McCullough J. Use of blood components containing red cells by donors of allogeneic bone marrow. Transfusion 1986;26:98–100.
68. Goodnough LT, Rudnick S, Price TH, et al. Increased preoperative collection of autologous blood with recombinant human erythropoietin therapy. N Engl J Med 1989;321:1163–1168.
69. York A, Clift RA, Sanders JE, Buckner CD. Recombinant human erythropoietin (rh-Epo) administration to normal marrow donors. Bone Marrow Transplant 1992;10: 415–417.
70. Foldes J, Naparstek E, Statter M, Menczel J, Bab I. Osteogenic response to marrow aspiration: increased serum osteocalcin and alkaline phosphatase in human bone marrow donors. Bone Mineral Res 1989;4:643–646.
71. Urban C, Weber G, Slavc I, Kerbl R. Anesthetic management of marrow harvesting from a 7 week-old premature baby. Bone Marrow Transplant 1990;6:443–444.
72. Gluckman E, Broxmeyer HE, Auerbach AD, et al. Hematopoietic reconstitution in a patient with Fanconi's anemia by means of umbilical-cord blood from an HLA-identical sibling. N Engl J Med 1989;321: 1174–1178.
73. Broxmeyer HE, Kurtzberg J, Gluckman E, et al. Umbilical cord blood hematopoietic stem and repopulating cells in human clinical transplantation. Blood Cells 1991;17:313–329.
74. Broxmeyer HE, Gluckman E, Auerbach A, et al. Human umbilical cord blood: a clinically useful source of transplantable hematopoietic stem/progenitor cells. Int J Cell Cloning 1990;1:76–89.
75. Kessinger A, Smith DM, Strandjord SE, et al. Allogeneic transplantation of blood-derived, T cell-depleted hemopoietic stem cells after myeloablative treatment in a patient with acute lymphoblastic leukemia. Bone Marrow Transplant 1989;4:643–646.
76. Demetri GD, Griffin JD. Granulocyte colony stimulating factor and its receptor. Blood 1991;78:2791–2808.
77. Monroy RL, Davis TA, MacVittie TJ. Short analytical review: granulocyte-macrophage colony-stimulating factor: more than a hemopoietin. Clin Immunol Immunopathol 1990;54:333–346.
78. Alter R, Welnick LA, Jackson JD, et al. In vitro clonigenic monitoring of peripheral stem cell growth

before and during interleukin 3 administration (abstract). J Cell Biochem 1991;D101:181.
79. Andrews RG, Knitter GH, Bartelmez SH, et al. Recombinant human SCF, a c-kit ligand, stimulates hematopoiesis in primates. Blood 1991;78:1975–1980.
80. Thomas ED, Lochte HL Jr, Lu WC, Ferrebee JW. Intravenous infusion of bone marrow in patients receiving radiation and chemotherapy. N Engl J Med 1957;257:491–496.
81. Jin NR, Hill RS, Petersen FB, et al. Marrow harvesting for autologous marrow transplantation. Exp Hematol 1985;13:879–884.
82. Kessinger A, Armitage JO. Harvesting marrow for autologous transplantation from patients with malignancies. Bone Marrow Transplant 1987;2:15–18.
83. Cairo MS, VandeVen C, Toy C, Sender L. Clinical and laboratory experience in marrow harvesting in children for autologous bone marrow transplantation. Bone Marrow Transplant 1989;4:305–308.

Part II
Supportive Care

Chapter 22
Principles of Transfusion Support Before and After Bone Marrow Transplantation

Sherrill J. Slichter

The impact of bone marrow transplantation (BMT) on transfusion services is substantial. Most patients who are candidates for BMT have diseases that require transfusions prior to transplant. Furthermore, the marrow-ablative procedures given to ensure a successful graft result in a prolonged period of aplasia necessitating transfusion support until the transplanted marrow produces new blood cells.

Pretransplant Transfusions

Prevention of Graft Rejection

Prior blood product transfusions given to either normal animals (1,2) or patients with aplastic anemia (3) result in a higher incidence of graft rejection than in untransfused marrow graft recipients. However, in transfused patients with acute leukemia, the incidence of marrow graft rejection is less than 1%. Because leukemic patients are usually transfused while receiving chemotherapy, it has been postulated that the chemotherapy produces enough immunosuppression either to prevent transfusion-induced sensitization or to contribute to the overall immunosuppressive effect required for sustained engraftment.

Effect of Prior Blood Product Transfusions on Marrow Engraftment in a Canine Model

A comprehensive series of transfusion experiments over two decades has produced clear evidence that prior blood transfusions can affect marrow engraftment, and these experiments have also identified how these adverse effects can be prevented. In nontransfused dogs, the rate of engraftment is 76 of 83 (91%) from an unrelated, DLA-mismatched donor; it is 59 of 60 (98%) with a DLA-matched littermate donor (4–6). DLA-typing is used to identify DLA-lymphocyte antigens in the dog analogous to the human leukocyte antigens [HLA]. However, less than 10% of the recipients of mismatched marrow show sustained engraftment, compared with 50% of the recipients of matched marrow (5).

With 3 transfusions of whole blood 24, 17, and 10 days prior to BMT, the rate of engraftment from DLA-matched littermate donors is reduced to 73% if the whole blood donor is a nonmatched unrelated donor (7), and is further reduced to 0% if the blood is from the DLA-matched littermate marrow donor (2,6). These data indicate that the minor histocompatibility antigens that are not detected by matching littermates for the DLA-A and D locus antigens are present on cells in whole blood and that these antigens are highly immunogenic and able to sensitize the marrow recipient to these antigens, leading to graft rejection. The sensitizing antigens are also present in the general canine population, as indicated by a reduced rate of engraftment in recipients who received only blood transfusions from nonmatched, unrelated donors (6).

Evaluation of Techniques to Reduce or Eliminate Transfusion-induced Graft-Rejection

Having established a transfusion program that resulted in a 100% incidence of graft rejection in the dog (2,6), it was then possible to explore systematically methods of preventing transfusion-induced graft-rejection. Three major methods were evaluated: (1) identification and removal of the immunizing cell (WBC depletion); (2) modification of the transfused blood products to reduce their immunogenicity (ultraviolet [UV] irradiation, heat inactivation, or γ-irradiation); and (3) immunosuppression of the transfused recipient.

Leukocyte-Poor Platelets or RBCs. To evaluate the effects of leukocyte reduction on transfusion-induced graft-rejection, 15 dogs were transfused with leukocyte-poor platelets and 8 engrafted (53%). Similarly, 9 of 14 (64%) dogs given leukocyte-poor RBCs engrafted (6). The median residual leukocyte dose transfused was 6.7×10^3 WBC/kg (99.9% depletion), with a range of 0 to 27 for the transfused platelets, and was 1.7×10^4 WBC/kg (99.8% depletion) with a range of 0 to 100 for the transfused RBCs. It was concluded that either some, but not all, of the minor histocompatibility antigens that result in graft rejection are expressed on platelets and RBCs, or, more likely, that there were still enough residual contaminating WBCs to induce graft rejection.

Experiments were then performed to identify the type of transfused WBC that induced graft rejection. All 6 dogs transfused with granulocytes at a dose of approximately 12.5 × 10^3/kg (97±1% granulocytes and 2±2% mononuclear cells) harvested from Ficoll-Hypaque–separated blood engrafted (8). Similarly, all 7 dogs transfused with a Ficoll-Hypaque–separated and cotton-wool nonadherent WBC fraction that contained 97±3% lymphocytes, 0.5±0.8% monocytes, and 2±2% neutrophils engrafted (8). Because this preparation also had very low numbers of Ia-positive dendritic cells (a type of small lymphocyte that adheres to cotton wool), it was concluded that they were likely to be the sensitizing cells.

UV Irradiation. UV irradiation inactivates antigen-presenting cells (APC), the majority of which are dendritic cells. The role of UV irradiation of blood prior to transfusion as a means of preventing graft rejection was then evaluated (9). None of the 10 dogs given UV-irradiated blood rejected their marrow grafts (10). Following UV exposure, lymphocytes from whole blood can neither respond nor stimulate in mixed lymphocyte culture (MLC). When stimulatory activity is eliminated, dendritic cells are considered to have been inactivated.

Further evidence that dendritic cells are immunogenic was obtained from experiments in which non-UV–irradiated dendritic cells were added back to UV-irradiated whole blood; 4 of 4 transfused dogs rejected the marrow graft (11).

Heat Inactivation Similar to UV irradiation, heating blood to 45°C for 45 minutes results in abrogation of mononuclear cell stimulatory activity in MLC (12). Because of the difficulty of achieving blood layers thin enough to permit adequate penetration of UV irradiation, heat-inactivated blood was tested; however, only 1 of 4 (25%) of the transfused marrow graft-recipient dogs engrafted (13).

Gamma Irradiation Unexpectedly, 2 Gy of γ-irradiation prevented transfusion-induced graft failure (i.e., 9 of 10 [90%] of the transfused dogs engrafted) (13). It is postulated that either minor non-DLA histocompatibility antigens expressed on the transfused cells are modified by low dose γ-irradiation or some type of minor APC is inactivated.

Immunosuppression of Transplant Recipient. There was no evidence that methotrexate (MTX)(14), procarbazine (15), anti-thymocyte serum (ATS) (15), or anti-Ia monoclonal antibodies (16) prevented transfusion-induced graft rejection in the dog model. However, a combined program of ATS *plus* procarbazine did facilitate engraftment; only 10 to 20 % of the treated recipients rejected their grafts, compared with 70 to 73% of untreated recipients ($p < 0.01$) (15,17). Unfortunately, the beneficial effects of this treatment were abrogated if transfusions were continued during the course of the treatment; all continuously transfused recipients rejected their grafts (15). This may be an important issue for those patients who require continuous transfusion support prior to BMT. The only other successful treatment program was with cyclosporine (CSP); only 2 of 9 transfused dogs rejected their grafts, compared with 19 of 19 untreated control dogs (18). However, this treatment program was not tested for efficacy when continuous transfusions were given prior to BMT.

Effect Of Prior Blood Product Transfusions On Marrow Engraftment In Patients With Aplastic Anemia

For patients with aplastic anemia transplanted between 1970 and 1975, graft rejection was a serious problem. Twenty-one of Seattle's first 73 patients with aplastic anemia (29%) rejected their grafts (19). In 30 patients with aplastic anemia undergoing allogeneic BMT who had received either no previous transfusions or transfusions only within 3 days of receiving immunosuppressive cyclophosphamide (CY) as their pre-BMT conditioning therapy, 27 (90%) had sustained marrow engraftment, compared with engraftment rates of 41 to 75% in transfused patients (20). This study was extended to include a total of 50 untransfused patients, and 42 were still living, with an actuarial survival rate of 82% at 10 years (21).

Later studies demonstrated a reduction in the incidence of graft rejection in multiply transfused patients to less than 15% (3,22), compared with the rejection rate seen in untransfused aplastics (10%) (21). Accounting for this reduction may be more liberal use of marrow donor buffy-coat infusions, use of more aggressive immunosuppressive treatment programs to abrogate transfusion-induced sensitization, or changes in transfusion practice (see Chapter 43). One change in transfusion practice is avoiding pre-BMT family member transfusions. Because the minor histocompatibility antigens that cause family member transfusion-induced rejection are inherited but are not on the same chromosome as the major histocompatibility locus, any family member transfusions could lead to a higher probability of exposure to the relevant antigens, compared with the more diffuse distribution of these antigens and, therefore, a lower sensitization risk associated with random donor transfusions. Although family member transfusions given to 18 patients with leukemia prior to BMT did not result in any instances of graft rejection (23), certainly in patients with aplastic anemia and probably even in patients with leukemia, pre-BMT family member transfusions should be avoided. The only exception to this policy is for thrombocytopenic patients with life-threatening bleeding who are refractory to both random donor and HLA-matched community donor platelets and for whom HLA-matched family member platelet tranfusions may be life-saving.

Indications for Platelet Transfusions and Prevention of Platelet Alloimmunization

Although transfusion-induced graft rejection rates in patients with aplastic anemia have clearly improved over time, there are still transfusion-transmitted infections, a lack of compatible platelet donors for some alloimmunized patients, and the cost of unnecessary or ineffective transfusions that need to be considered when planning for long-term transfusion needs of patients being considered for BMT. Thus, there continue to be compelling reasons for minimizing transfusion therapy—both before and after BMT. Even though patients usually require both RBC and platelet support pre-BMT because of disease or therapy-induced marrow aplasia, this discussion is limited to platelet transfusions.

Indications For Platelet Transfusion

The appropriate prophylactic platelet transfusion level that will prevent bleeding in patients with hypoproliferative thrombocytopenia remains controversial. Although most clinicians use a 20×10^9/L platelet count as the indication for prophylactic platelet transfusions in patients with decreased platelet production and a recent National Institutes of Health (NIH) Consensus Conference Statement reaffirmed this level (24), there is little direct evidence to substantiate this practice. For example, in one of the earliest studies published on platelet transfusion therapy, in 1962 (25), the authors indicated that they could not determine a threshold platelet level that was required to prevent bleeding in 92 children with acute leukemia. Serious bleeding was present during 10 to 30% of the thrombocytopenic days at platelet counts less than 5×10^9/L. At platelet counts between 5 and 100×10^9/L, there was little difference in the frequency of serious bleeding episodes. In addition, this study was performed before it was recognized that aspirin causes platelet dysfunction. Because many of these children were undoubtedly febrile and thus receiving aspirin, the actual bleeding risk at any given platelet level is probably less than this study indicates.

Additional evidence for the occurrence of spontaneous bleeding only at very low platelet counts comes from observations of chromium-labeled stool blood loss measurements in 20 patients with aplastic thrombocytopenia (26). In these patients, stool blood loss was less than 5 mL/day (within the normal range) at platelet counts greater than 10×10^9/L. At platelet counts between 5 and 10×10^9/L, blood loss averaged 9 ± 7 mL/day. At levels less than 5×10^9/L, blood loss was markedly elevated to 50 ± 20 mL/day.

In another study of 62 leukemic children in which the relationship between bleeding manifestations and platelet count was assessed, serious bleeding occurred in 26% of the patients with platelet counts between 0 and 10×10^9/L, in 10% of patients with platelet counts between 10 and 20×10^9/L, and in 4 to 5% of patients with platelet counts between 20 and 40×10^9/L (27). Minor bleeding into skin or mucous membranes, microscopic hematuria, guaiac-positive stools, and epistaxis were found in approximately 50% of patients with platelet counts between 0 and 40×10^9/L, but there was no correlation between bleeding and platelet count.

In a retrospective study, bleeding manifestations were evaluated in 64 leukemic patients with platelet counts of either less than 10×10^9/L or between 10 and 20×10^9/L (28). There was a clear increase in bleeding risk for patients with platelet counts less than 10×10^9/L, whereas at higher platelet counts, the risk of severe bleeding was only 3%. In general, for all types of bleeding, the risk was increased for leukemic versus chemotherapy-induced thrombocytopenia, for patients with decreasing rather than stable or increasing platelet counts, and for febrile versus afebrile patients. This study also indicated that the bleeding risk was greater in patients under 18 years of age and in those with acute lymphoblastic leukemia (ALL) versus those with acute myeloid leukemia (AML).

The practicality of a more restrictive platelet transfusion policy was prospectively assessed in 102 patients being treated for acute leukemia (29). The indications for platelet transfusions in this study were any one of the following: (1) a platelet count of less than 5×10^9/L; (2) a platelet count of 6 to 10×10^9/L and temperature >38°C or fresh minor hemorrhages; (3) a platelet count of 11 to 20×10^9/L and other coagulation factor deficiencies, or heparin therapy, or a planned marrow biopsy or lumbar puncture; or (4) a platelet count of $>20 \times 10^9$/L and major bleeding or a surgical procedure. Bleeding risk by platelet count is shown in Figure 22-1. There were 3 hemorrhagic deaths—one patient with a platelet count of 1×10^9/L who was alloimmunized and did not have a compati-

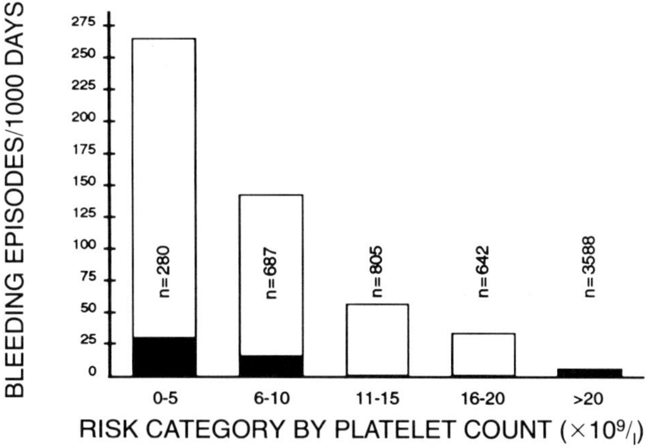

Figure 22-1. Relation of bleeding risk to platelet counts, computed per 1,000 days at risk. *Open bars* indicate minor bleeding complications; *solid bars* indicate major bleeding complications. *Numbers in bars* are numbers of observed days at risk in a given class. The correlation coefficient between the four lowest platelet count categories and the incidence of bleeding is $r = 0.963$, $p < 0.01$. Patients with platelet counts greater than 20×10^9/L were not included in the correlation coefficient determination because the few bleeding complications in this group were related to factors other than solely the platelet count, and because of the broad range of counts in this category. (*Reproduced by permission* from Gmur J, Burger J, Schanz U, Fehr J, Schaffner A. Safety of stringent prophylactic platelet transfusion policy for patients with acute leukaemia. Lancet 1991;338:1223–1226.)

ble donor and two on low doses of heparin with platelet counts of 35×10^9/L and 55×10^9/L at the time of bleeding.

Two other studies in patients with acute leukemia compared prophylactic platelet transfusions with those given for active bleeding and found no difference in RBC requirements or bleeding deaths (30,31). Those patients in the prophylactic arm required twice as many platelets.

In summary, patients with production-related thrombocytopenia and platelet counts less than 5×10^9/L should be given prophylactic platelet transfusions to avoid the risk of substantial bleeding. At platelet counts between 5 and 20×10^9/L, clinical judgment should be used to assess the severity of bleeding and the need for platelet therapy. When a patient has significant bleeding at a platelet count higher than 10×10^9/L, platelet dysfunction is present (as evidenced by a longer-than-expected bleeding time for the platelet count) (32), the vascular system has been disrupted, or there are additional coagulation factor deficiencies. In these situations, platelets should be given only to control significant bleeding until the underlying problem can be resolved.

Prevention of Platelet Alloimmunization

Between 30 to 70% of multiply transfused patients become refractory to pooled random donor platelet concentrates (33). Criteria for platelet refractoriness are usually based on a combination of post-transfusion platelet increments and antibody testing.

The patient's disease and its treatment have major effects on alloimmunization rates. Patients with aplastic anemia have much higher immunization rates than patients with malignant disorders. In one study, alloantibodies developed in 7 of 8 (88%) patients with aplastic anemia compared with 20 of 65 (31%) transfused patients with AML (34). Overall, in a series of studies (34–40), alloantibodies developed in 380 of 944 (40%) patients with malignant disorders receiving chemotherapy. Unfortunately, there are neither laboratory tests nor clinical characteristics that can be used to predict which patients will become alloimmunized.

A high percentage of BMT patients require HLA-matched single-donor platelets—either because they are refractory to random donor platelets at the time of BMT or they become so following BMT. The issue of platelet alloimmunization may become even more critical as the number of BMTs from partially HLA-matched family members, unrelated donors, and autologous BMTs increase. These patients do not have HLA-matched siblings for platelet support. Although HLA-typed platelet apheresis programs are increasing in number and size, the complexity of the HLA system means that HLA-compatible donors will not be available for every patient.

Analogous to the strategies available to prevent graft rejection, there are 3 basic approaches to preventing platelet alloimmunization: (1) immunosuppression of the transfused recipient, (2) limit exposure to incompatible donor antigens, or (3) reduce the immunogenicity of the transfused blood products.

Immunosuppression of the Transfusion Recipient

Animal platelet transfusion studies have shown that several different types of immunosuppressive therapy may prevent platelet alloimmunization. In a dog platelet transfusion model, none of the 9 recipients given CSP therapy became refractory to platelets from a single random-donor dog, even after 8 weekly transfusions (41). Furthermore, 6 of 9 recipients (67%) remained responsive to an additional 8 weekly transfusions, even after CSP was discontinued. In 6 of 7 baboons (86%) given either prednisone, antithymocyte globulin (ATG), or a combination of these two agents, platelet refractoriness did not occur after repeated weekly platelet transfusions from a single random-donor baboon (42).

It is unlikely that immunosuppressive therapy given specifically to prevent platelet alloimmunization will be acceptable because of the risks that might result from such therapy.

Limit Exposure to Incompatible Donor Antigens

There are basically three approaches to limiting exposure to incompatible donor antigens: (1) reduce transfusion frequency, (2) administer single-donor apheresis platelets instead of pooled random donor platelets and (3) administer antigen-compatible donor platelets.

Reduce Transfusion Frequency. Unfortunately, this is not a very practical approach because the patients in whom platelet alloantibodies develop are also those who have prolonged periods of thrombocytopenia requiring multiple platelet transfusions. The best way to reduce transfusion frequency is to avoid unnecessary transfusions.

Provide Single-donor Apheresis Platelets. There have been 3 prospective randomized trials to determine the relative benefits of providing single random-donor apheresis platelets compared with pooled random-donor platelet transfusions to prevent platelet alloimmunization (43–45). Patients in the pooled random donor arm of these studies received up to 10 times the number of donor exposures as those in the single donor arm. Despite these large differences in donor exposures, only one of these studies showed a significant decrease in rates of platelet refractoriness and lymphocytotoxic antibody formation in the patients receiving single-donor platelets (45). Furthermore, the number of transfusion events for both platelets and RBCs was the same in both arms in all the studies.

In a dog platelet transfusion model, recipient dogs were given either repeated transfusions of a pool of platelets obtained from the same 6 random-donor dogs, or they received transfusions from any one of 6 random donors until they became platelet refractory, and then a new donor was used (46). There was no difference in the frequency of platelet refractoriness for either transfusion program; 17 of 22 (77%) of the recipients of pooled random-donor platelets became refractory to all 6 donors, compared with 6 of 10 (60%) of the dogs who received platelets sequentially ($p >$ 0.05). However, it required significantly fewer pooled random-donor transfusions (5.5 ± 1.0), compared with single random-donor transfusions (14.0 ± 5.0), to develop refractoriness ($p < 0.01$). Thus, single random-donor platelet transfusions in the dog delay, but do not prevent, platelet refractoriness.

Because only approximately 40% of chronically transfused patients with malignant disorders become alloimmunized (33), it may not be worthwhile to provide all chronically thrombocytopenic patients with the more expensive single random-donor apheresis transfusions when, at best, alloimmunization is likely to be only delayed rather than prevented.

Select Compatible Donors. ABO-compatible. A and B antigens are expressed on the surface of platelets (47). To determine the effect of ABO-mismatching on platelet alloimmunization, 49 leukemic patients undergoing induction chemotherapy were assigned randomly to receive two sets of paired transfusions of ABO-compatible or ABO-incompatible pooled random-donor platelet transfusions (48). Although there were no differences in post-transfusion platelet responses after the first set of transfusions, the corrected count increment (CCI) after the second ABO-compatible transfusion averaged 14.9×10^9/L, compared with 9.5×10^9/L for the second ABO-incompatible transfusion ($p <$ 0.0007). Platelet survivals were similar in both groups.

In another study of 26 patients undergoing treatment for acute leukemia or autografting for relapsed Hodgkin's disease who were randomly assigned to receive either ABO-compatible or ABO-incompatible platelets, platelet refractoriness was significantly lower in the group receiving ABO-compatible platelets—not only because patients did not increase their anti-A or anti-B isohemagglutinin titers, but also because the ABO-compatible recipients had a much lower incidence of lymphocytotoxic and platelet-specific alloantibody formation (49). Nine of the 13 patients (69%) who were given ABO-mismatched platelet transfusions became platelet-refractory, compared with only 1 of 13 patients (8%) who received ABO-compatible platelets ($p <$ 0.0014). The repeated administration of ABO-mismatched platelets produced a significant increase in anti-A/B titers in 7 of 13 patients (54%) that were generally correlated with poor platelet increments. In addition, lymphocytotoxic antibodies developed in 5 of 13 of these recipients (38%), and platelet-specific alloantibodies developed in 4 of 13 (31%), compared with only 1 of 13 (8%) and 1 of 13 (8%), respectively, of the recipients of ABO-compatible platelets. The close temporal association between the development of HLA- and platelet-specific alloantibodies and increases in anti-A/B titers suggests that, in the process of responding to the ABO-incompatible antigens, recognition of other incompatible antigens also occurred.

Data from these two studies (48,49) suggest that provision of ABO-compatible platelets may be a simple method of reducing the incidence of alloimmune platelet refractoriness.

HLA-compatible. Because HLA antigens are the predominant immunogens expressed on the surface of platelets, two transfusion trials evaluated the benefits of HLA-matched compared with random single-donor apheresis platelet transfusions (50,51). In neither of these two studies was there evidence that provision of HLA-matched apheresis platelets provided an additional benefit over that achieved with single random-donor apheresis transfusions.

Modify the Transfused Platelets and RBCs to Reduce their Immunogenicity. In some of the investigations discussed, only the transfused platelets were modified and evaluated. However, transfusion studies modifying both RBCs and platelets are needed to determine the efficacy of any of these methods in preventing platelet alloimmunization.

Leukocyte Reduction. It has been well documented that alloantigen recognition requires the expression of both class I and class II HLA antigens on the surface of the transfused cells (52,53). Because platelets, in contrast to white blood cells, express only class I but not class II antigens and RBCs do not express HLA antigens, the question of whether leukocyte-poor blood components will prevent platelet alloimmunization has been investigated. Animal studies in both rats (52) and mice (54) demonstrate that leukocyte-depleted platelets do not cause alloimmunization.

In humans, administration of less than 5×10^6 leukocytes did not result in lymphocytotoxic antibody formation following a limited number of injections (55,56). Although centrifugation techniques can be used to produce leukocyte-poor blood products, a number of very efficient leukocyte reduction filters are now available (57), requiring new techniques to count accurately the very low number of WBCs remaining in the filtered products (58).

To date, there have been 6 prospective randomized clinical trials involving 299 patients evaluating the efficacy of leukocyte-poor RBCs and platelets compared with unmodified RBCs and platelets in preventing platelet alloimmunization (Table 22-1) (51,59–63). There was substantial variability in patient selection, methods of leukocyte reduction, end point criteria, leukocyte concentration of control and leukocyte-poor blood products, and trial results. Four of the 6 studies showed significant reductions in development of lymphocytotoxic antibodies in patients given leukocyte-poor products (51,60,61,63). However, in the 3 studies that tested for platelet-specific alloantibodies, there were no differences between the control and the leukocyte-poor arms (51,60,62). The incidence of clinical platelet refractoriness was reduced by leukocyte-poor blood products in only 3 of the trials (46,60,61).

Two recent editorials have suggested caution in interpreting the data from these leukocyte-poor transfusion trials because of the small numbers of patients

Table 22-1.
Leukocyte-poor Transfusion Trials[a]

		Control		Leukocyte-poor		Antibody-positive				Clinically Platelet-refractory	
						Lymphocytotoxic		Platelet			
Author, Year, Ref	No. Patients	Platelets (WBC × 10^6)	RBC (WBC × 10^8)	Platelets (WBC × 10^5)	RBC (WBC × 10^6)	Control	Leuko-poor	Control	Leuko-poor	Control	Leuko-Poor
Schiffer *et al*, 1983, (59)	56	65	Frozen,[b] washed	12	Frozen[b], washed	42%	20%	N T		19%	16%
						($p = 0.07$)				N S	
Murphy *et al*, 1986, (51)	50	5,380[c]	NI	90–220[c]	<8	48%	16%	10%	11%	23%	5%
						($p < 0.02$)		N S		N S	
Sniecinski *et al*, 1988, (60)	40	530	3900	6	50	50%	15%	35%	15%	50%	15%
						($p < 0.01$)		N S		($p < 0.01$)	
Andreu *et al*, 1988, (61)	69	477–678	2300	47–151	61	31%	12%	N T		47%	21%
						($p < 0.05$)				($p < 0.05$)	
Oksanen *et al*, 1991, (62)	31	800	1000	0.2	0.1	26%	13%	33%	31%	26%	13%
						N S		N S		N S	
van Marwijk Kooy *et al*, 1991, (63)	53	35[d]	<5[d]	<5	<5	42%	7%	N T		46%	11%
						($p < 0.004$)				($p < 0.005$)	

[a]Leukocyte data is reported as average number or range of residual WBCs per transfusion event for platelets or per unit of RBCs transfused.
[b]Frozen washed RBCs have no identifiable intact white cells.
[c]Single random donor apheresis transfusions were given rather than the pooled random donor transfusions used in all other studies, except for Andreu *et al*, where 1 of 4 trial sites used single random donor apheresis transfusions.
[d]Control platelets leukocyte-reduced by centrifugation and RBCs made leukocyte-poor by filtration.
NI = no information; NT = not tested; NS = difference not significant between control and leukocyte-poor data.

and the conflicting data on the levels of leukocytes that either produce or prevent platelet alloimmunization or platelet refractoriness (64,65). In another study of patients receiving leukocyte-poor RBC and platelet products, the rate of platelet refractoriness was significantly higher in previously pregnant women (15 of 71, 21%), compared with nonpresensitized patients (16/264, 6%; $p < 0.001$) (66). These findings suggest that patients with prior antigenic exposure through pregnancy, or probably by transfusions, may not benefit from filtered blood products.

UV Irradiation. Instead of removing WBCs from the transfused blood products, another approach would be to alter the transfusions to eliminate their immunogenicity. In a dog platelet transfusion model, 11 of 12 recipients (92%) of UV-irradiated donor platelets did not become platelet-refractory after 8 weekly single random-donor transfusions, compared with 3 of 21 recipients (14%) who were given platelets not exposed to UV ($p < 0.01$). Furthermore, in the dogs given UV-irradiated platelets, tolerance to unmodified platelets from the same or other random donors was observed in 73 and 43% of the dogs, respectively.

The in vivo viability and function of human platelets remain intact after the platelets have been UV-irradiated in special plastic bags that permit adequate UV penetration (67–70). Furthermore, platelets could be UV-irradiated and stored with no adverse effects on poststorage platelet viability.

A large multi-institutional trial sponsored by the National Heart, Lung, and Blood Institute was recently initiated in the United States to explore the relative merits of leukocyte reduction or UV irradiation in the prevention of platelet alloimmunization (71). Certainly either of these 2 approaches, which require only a manipulation of the product prior to transfusion, is to be preferred over the other approaches that would involve either some type of immunosuppression of the recipient or require selected donor transfusions.

Prevention of Transfusion-associated CMV Infection

Infections due to CMV remain a major cause of morbidity and mortality in patients undergoing BMT (see Chapter 28) (72). In CMV-seronegative BMT recipients, the major source of CMV transmission is from either CMV-seropositive blood or marrow donors. The majority of CMV-seropositive patients appear to have reactivation of latent virus as the source of their infection. Evidence of active CMV infection following BMT developed in 69% of 258 patients who were seropositive at the time of BMT, compared with 28% in 208 seronegative patients with seronegative marrow donors ($p < 0.00005$), emphasizing the significance of the patient's baseline CMV status on post-BMT CMV infection (73). All of these patients received blood products from donors not screened for their CMV status. The ease of transmitting CMV infection by transfusion in a susceptible population was illustrated in 47 patients who were seronegative before starting unscreened transfusions; 11 (23%) seroconverted 28 to 275 days after beginning transfusion support (74). These studies emphasize the need to control the transfusion support of BMT candidates to prevent CMV transmission.

Identify and Avoid Transfusions From CMV-seropositive Donors

Individuals infected with CMV remain latently infected (75) and manifest persistent immunoglobulin G (IgG) antibodies that can be detected reliably by a variety of techniques. However, of the donors who are CMV antibody–positive, only 5 to 12% are infectious (76). Despite the fact that many individuals who are not infectious will be eliminated as donors, provision of blood from CMV-seronegative donors is the only technique of donor selection that reliably prevents CMV transmission by transfusion (77–79).

There are no data to show that patients who are CMV-seropositive derive benefit from the provision of CMV-seronegative blood products (77,80). Several factors make it difficult to prove whether the current infection is reactivation of the existing virus or a new infection, because the virus cannot be grown from seropositive blood donors. However, transfusion studies in a mouse model are of some interest and suggest that the mere act of transfusion of blood from either an isogeneic or an allogeneic noninfected donor may activate a latent virus infection (81). In non-CMV–infected animals transfused from mice carrying a latent CMV virus, infections occur in allogeneic but not in syngeneic recipients, indicating that an associated antigen response may be required for CMV infection.

Although the possibility of acquiring a new strain of CMV cannot be excluded when CMV-seropositive blood is given to a CMV-seropositive recipient, the frequency with which this occurs does not justify giving CMV-seronegative blood to BMT candidates who are already CMV-seropositive.

Provide Leukocyte-poor Blood Products

Leukocytes are thought to harbor latent CMV viruses. In acutely infected patients, CMV is routinely isolated from both mononuclear and polymorphonuclear leukocytes (82,83). The short life expectancy of the granulocyte makes it unlikely to be the site of long-term latency.

Additional evidence for localization of the virus to the WBC fraction comes from transfusion studies demonstrating a reduction in CMV transmission with washed RBCs (84,85), or frozen deglycerolized RBCs (86–89). Furthermore, fresh frozen plasma (90) cryoprecipitate, gamma globulin, or clotting factor concentrates do not transmit CMV (76).

Unfortunately, the amount of leukocyte reduction required to prevent CMV transmission is unknown. Frozen-washed deglycerolized blood, which does not transmit CMV, has residual leukocyte counts of 1 to 25 $\times$ 10^6/U (91,92). There is evidence that the level of leukocyte reduction achieved by centrifugation or by using filters is enough to prevent CMV infection by transfusion in the majority of patients (93–96).

In summary, the data look promising that CMV transmission can be prevented by leukocyte depletion. Because donor populations vary in terms of CMV positivity by geographic region, ranging between 40 to 100% (97), the availability of a method of consistently preventing CMV transmission by transfusion that does not require CMV antibody screening will be very helpful.

Postmarrow Grafting Transfusion Support

Prevention of Transfusion-induced Graft-versus-host Disease

In the latest cumulative literature survey, transfusion induced graft-versus-host disease (T-GVHD) has now been reported in 131 patients, with an overall mortality rate of 90% (98). Although T-GVHD has been reported in recipients who received as few as 8 $\times$ 10^4 lymphocytes/kg body weight (99,100), most authors have calculated that the minimum transfusion dose required is 10^7 viable lymphocytes/kg (101,102), and all fatalities have occurred above this dose. On the basis of the lymphocyte contamination of most cellular blood products, one unit of platelets, RBCs, or granulocytes may be enough to cause T-GVHD (103).

T-GVHD has been reported after transfusion of all cellular blood products. Acellular blood products, such as fresh frozen plasma and cryoprecipitate, do not initiate GVHD (98). Although frozen, reconstituted RBCs have never been documented to transmit GVHD, there is still a theoretical risk with this product, because freezing removes only 94% of the lymphocytes, and 40% of the residual lymphocytes will still undergo blast transformation when stimulated with mitogens (104). Although WBC reduction filters are now capable of removing more than 99% of the WBCs, the residual leukocyte load may still result in T-GVHD in susceptible recipients (105).

The susceptible host must lack the ability to reject histoincompatible cells; therefore, individuals with defective cell-mediated immune function are at risk, whereas those with defective humoral immunity are not (106). T-GVHD is characterized by high fever, a scaly maculopapular erythematous rash, diarrhea, hepatocellular damage with marked elevations of liver function tests, and pancytopenia. Because of the high-dose chemoradiation therapy given to BMT patients, BMT recipients are at risk for the development of T-GVHD (103).

Gamma Irradiation

Gamma (γ)-irradiation of cellular blood products has long been recognized as an effective method of preventing T-GVHD (107). The only remaining controversy is the dose required to achieve this effect and whether the selected dose has any adverse effect on the viability or function of the RBCs, granulocytes, or platelets being transfused.

Dose Required

The dose of γ-irradiation required to eliminate the lymphocyte proliferative response in an allogeneic MLC assay is 0.5 Gy (108), whereas the dose required to decrease the lymphocyte response to a mitogen is 5 Gy (109). Because the allogeneic MLC reactivity most closely reflects the induction of T-GVHD, the lower radiation dose is likely to be sufficient. To account for differences in radiation exposure based on the irradiation source used (usually a self-contained, commercially available cesium^{137} irradiator), bag geometry, or product volume, most transfusion services have used a dose 3-fold higher than the postulated effective minimum dose, or 1.5 Gy (110). At the NIH Transfusion Service, there have been no documented cases of T-GVHD in 8,300 recipients given blood products irradiated with 1.5 Gy (111). The majority of the patients had hematological malignancies or were receiving BMT. However, T-GVHD and graft rejection in a BMT patient whose blood products were irradiated with 2.0 Gy has been reported (112). In addition, an institutional survey of 1,444 blood banks or transfusion services' γ-irradiation usage documented development of T-GVHD in 2 other BMT patients who were receiving γ-irradiated blood products (110). Thus, there may be some argument for increasing the radiation dose to prevent T-GVHD. Using a limiting dilution method of analysis, which is a more sensitive measurement of T-lymphocyte growth than MLC, it was shown that T-lymphocyte function was still intact after 1.5 Gy, and, thus, for some immunosuppressed recipients, a dose of 3 to 4 Gy may be more appropriate (112). Surprisingly, in the institutional review of irradiation usage, 12 and 18.6% of institutions did not irradiate cellular blood products for recipients of allogeneic or autologous BMT (110). This practice may reflect the fact that only 12% of the surveyed institutions had irradiation facilities. BMT should not be done in locations that do not have the resources to irradiate donor blood products.

Effects of γ-Irradiation on Viability and Function of RBCs, Granulocytes, and Platelets

RBCs, stored for 21 days and then exposed to γ-irradiation doses of 5, 10, or 20 Gy, showed no differences in any in vitro measure of RBC viability when compared with similarly stored nonirradiated RBCs (109). Chromium-labeled survivals in normal volunteers demonstrated no loss of in vivo viability when RBCs were stored for 21 days and irradiated with doses up to 20 Gy, compared with the viability of similarly stored nonirradiated RBCs. However, there are no data on the viability of RBCs that have been irradiated and then stored. Until such data are available, RBCs should be irradiated only just before transfusion.

Casein-stimulated chemotactic activity decreases linearly with increasing doses of irradiation from 0.5 Gy to 120 Gy but is clinically significant only with doses of more than 10 Gy (108). In two instances, granulocytes irradiated with 5 Gy were identified in Rebuck skin windows after transfusion into neutropenic patients (109). At doses up to 10 Gy, leukocytes showed normal bacterial ingestion and killing (109).

When platelets were stored for up to 5 days and then γ-irradiated with 5 Gy, there was no evidence of platelet dysfunction as measured by a variety of in vitro parameters (113,114). In a paired control study where normal volunteers donated platelets on two different occasions, there were no differences in in vivo platelet viability between the irradiated and the nonirradiated radiochromium-labeled platelets. On one occasion the platelets were irradiated with 3 Gy prior to storage for 5 days and, on the other occasion, the platelets were similarly stored without irradiation (115). Furthermore, in 36 thrombocytopenic patients who received 98 nonirradiated or 51 platelet transfusions irradiated just prior to transfusion, there was no difference in CCIs either 1 or 24 hours after transfusion (116).

UV Irradiation

UV irradiation may represent an alternative technique of preventing T-GVHD. To explore this possibility, 10 dogs were given 9.2 Gy of TBI and an autologous BMT (117). Following BMT, the dogs were given 10 daily leukocyte transfusions from histoincompatible dogs. T-GVHD developed in all 4 dogs given nonirradiated leukocytes, as well as in 2 of 3 dogs given leukocytes irradiated with 20 mJ/cm^2 UV-B exposure. However, T-GVHD developed in none of the 3 dogs given 1,000 mJ/cm^2 UV-B irradiation. Transfusion experiments are needed in humans before this treatment can be adapted.

Treatment of T-GVHD

Treatment of T-GVHD with a variety of agents, including steroids, ATG, CY, anti-T cell monoclonal antibody CD7, and anti-T lymphoblastic monoclonal antibody, has generally been unsuccessful (98). The very high morbidity and mortality associated with T-GVHD emphasizes the need for effective prevention by setting up stringent controls to ensure that all cellular blood products are γ-irradiated before transfusion.

Prevention of CMV Infection by Transfusion

Granulocyte transfusions from CMV-seropositive donors have been identified as a major source of CMV transmission (118,119). During a prospective randomized trial of prophylactic granulocyte transfusions given during BMT, CMV infection was significantly more common in CMV-seronegative recipients who were receiving prophylactic granulocytes from CMV-unscreened donors (9 of 13 [69%] vs only 3 of 13 [23%] in the untransfused control group) (120). There was no effect of granulocyte transfusions in patients who were already CMV-seropositive before BMT. No mention was made of the CMV status of the marrow donor in this study. In a subsequent study of CMV-seronegative patients with CMV-seronegative marrow donors, the infection rate was 33% if they received no granulocyte transfusions, 77% if granulocytes were provided from CMV-seropositive donors ($p < 0.005$), but only 32% if granulocytes were from CMV-seronegative donors, which is no different from those not receiving granulocytes (121). If the marrow donor was CMV-seropositive, granulocyte transfusions from CMV-seropositive donors had no additional effect on CMV infection rates in either CMV-seropositive or CMV-seronegative recipients.

CMV infection was 28% among CMV-seronegative patients with a seronegative marrow donor and increased to 57% when the donor was CMV-seropositive (122). CMV infection was significantly more common among seropositive patients (69%) and not further affected by the serology of the marrow donor.

CMV-seronegative Blood Products

The effectiveness of CMV-seronegative blood products in preventing CMV infection in seronegative patients receiving allogeneic BMTs has been documented in 2 randomized prospective trials (Table 22-2) (123,124). Overall, among recipients with a CMV-seronegative marrow donor, only 3 of 75 (4%) recipients of CMV-seronegative blood seroconverted versus 22 of 69 (32%) who received CMV-unscreened blood products. If the marrow donor was CMV-seropositive, the provision of CMV-seronegative blood products was not helpful.

Follow-up data were provided from one of these studies on a total of 104 seronegative patients who had been assigned to receive seronegative blood products (125). Data from these patients were analyzed to determine how often they did not receive their assigned seronegative blood products. Eleven of the 104 patients (11%) did not receive exclusively CMV-seronegative blood products because the blood center or nursing personnel erred. Three other patients were knowingly given CMV-unscreened blood products; 2 because of massive bleeding and one because of platelet refractoriness. Only 4 of 104 patients had a primary CMV infection within 100 days of BMT, and only one of these infections occurred in a patient who had been given exclusively CMV-seronegative blood products. Thus, despite the fact that there were 15 to 35 CMV-seronegative patients/month who required an average of 19 units of RBCs and 105 units of platelets from a base of approximately 9,000 monthly donations (of whom 51% of the donors were CMV-seropositive), the blood center was quite effective in meeting the transfusion needs of these patients.

Leukocyte-poor Blood Products

Four studies in BMT patients have now evaluated leukocyte-poor blood products to prevent CMV infection in CMV-seronegative patients who received either an autologous or an allogeneic BMT from a CMV-seronegative donor (Table 22-3) (126–129). These studies used a variety of combinations of leukocyte reduction or CMV-seronegative donors. Only 1 of the 124 patients given leukocyte-poor transfusions had any evidence of CMV infection. However, only one of the trials was a prospective randomized trial, and, in this study, CMV infection developed in none of the 35 patients in the leukocyte-poor arm, compared with 7 of 30 patients (23%) in the control arm who received CMV-unscreened, unmodified blood products ($p < 0.001$) (129). The patients in this study were protected despite receiving an average of 25 units of RBCs (range, 4–97) and 165 platelet concentrates (range, 6–428).

Blood Product Requirements

The period of marrow aplasia for all BMT patients usually lasts 2 to 6 weeks, or sometimes longer. Even though marrow cellularity progressively increases over time after BMT, with a normal complement of identifiable precursor cells by 3 to 6 months (130), the number of committed progenitor cells (CFU-GM, CFU-E, and BFU-E) in both blood and marrow remain abnormally low for longer periods (131,132). Therefore, any adverse effect on hematopoiesis is usually

Table 22-2.
Use of CMV-seronegative Blood Products in the Prevention of CMV Infection[a]

	Seronegative Marrow Donor			*Seropositive Marrow Donor*		
	Blood Products			*Blood Products*		
Author, Ref	*CMV-negative*	*CMV Unscreened*	*p* Value	*CMV-Negative*	*CMV Unscreened*	*p* Value
Bowden *et al* (123)	1/32 (3%)	8/25 (32%)	<0.007	3/12 (25%)	5/16 (31%)	N S
Miller *et al* (124)	2/45 (4%)	14/44 (32%)	<0.0006	6/19 (32%)	7/17 (41%)	N S
Total	3/75 (4%)	22/69 (32%)		9/31 (29%)	12/33 (36%)	

[a]Data reported as number infected/number in group (percent infected).
CMV = cytomegalovirus.

Table 22-3.
Use of Leukocyte-poor Blood Products in the Prevention of CMV Infection

	Leukocyte-poor Blood Products					
	RBC		*Platelet*		*CMV Infection*[a]	
	Method[b]	*Total WBCs × 10⁶*	*Method*[b]	*Total WBCs × 10⁶*	*Control*	*Leukocyte-poor*
Verdonck *et al* (126)	Filtered	<1	Seronegative	...	...	0/29
Bowden *et al* (127)	Filtered[c]	...	Filtered[c]	...	...	1/32 (3%)
De Witte *et al* (128)	Filtered	<50	Centrifugation	<100	...	0/28
Bowden *et al* (129)	Seronegative	...	Centrifugation	<10	7/30 (23%) ($p < 0.001$)	0/35

[a]Data reported as number infected/number in group.
[b]Methods evaluated to prevent CMV transmission were filtration to remove WBCs, centrifugation with removal of the buffy coat, or administration of CMV-seronegative blood products.
[c]Filtered at bedside; no counts available.
CMV = cytomegalovirus.

immediately reflected in a decrease in peripheral blood counts.

Almost all patients require RBC and platelet transfusions, and a variable number may require WBC transfusions or plasma coagulation factor replacement (133,134). These transfusion requirements place a substantial demand on blood centers. An average of 16 RBC transfusions and 37 platelet transfusion events, with the equivalent of 4 to 6 units of platelet concentrates per transfusion (median, 24; range, 1–223), were required to support the 390 patients transplanted by the Seattle team in 1990.

Factors That Affect Hematopoietic Recovery Following BMT

Patient Factors

Diagnosis. An analysis of leukocyte recovery rates in 164 patients transplanted with marrow from an HLA-identical sibling showed the fastest rates in those with aplastic anemia, AML, ALL, CML, respectively (135).

Spleen Size. In patients with CML, the effects of splenectomy (20 patients), palpable splenomegaly (21 patients), or nonpalpable spleens (26 patients) on rates of marrow engraftment were evaluated (136). Time to achieve a WBC count of 0.5×10^9/L was 13 days for the splenectomized patients versus 22 days for the nonsplenectomized patients; time to achieve platelet independence was day 16 versus 28, respectively ($p < 0.005$). Evidence for early engraftment in splenectomized versus nonsplenectomized patients was confirmed in 2 additional studies (137,138).

In another study in nonsplenectomized CML patients, there was a statistically significantly higher rate of graft failure (7 of 19, 37%) in patients with palpable spleens, compared with 2 of 23 (9%) in those with nonpalpable spleens ($p < 0.05$)(139).

Conditioning Program. Addition of a continuous 6-day infusion of anthracyclines to the standard regimen of CY and TBI prior to BMT delayed marrow engraftment by 7 to 9 days in 26 patients compared with 20 who received only the standard program (140). Higher doses of TBI had a modest effect on preventing or delaying platelet engraftment (141,142).

Postgrafting GVHD Prophylaxis. Several controlled randomized prospective trials in patients with a variety of malignant and nonmalignant disorders demonstrated that when CSP rather than MTX is used as post-BMT GVHD prophylaxis, there is earlier engraftment (141,143–145). These differences were attributed to the known myelotoxic effects of MTX. When a short course of MTX combined with CSP was prospectively compared with CSP alone (146,147), median day to granulocyte count greater than 1×10^9/L was 24 for the combined treatments, compared with 19 for patients treated with CSP only ($p = 0.003$) (147). Patients who received GVHD prophylaxis with MTX had a 2.6-times greater likelihood of achieving RBC-independence than those receiving CSP with or without short-term MTX (141). Erythropoietin levels were significantly lower in patients treated with MTX *plus* CSP, compared with those given no GVHD prophylaxis because they were receiving T-cell–depleted marrow (148). It was postulated that the CSP depressed renal-cell function, leading to lower erythropoietin levels and more RBC transfusion.

CMV Infection. There is substantial evidence that viral infection may adversely affect hematopoiesis in general, and megakaryocytopoiesis in particular (149). The mechanisms for this effect on megakaryocytopoiesis are being pursued actively and may include direct infection of megakaryocytes resulting in cytotoxic damage (150), or stromal cells may be infected, leading to reduced production of stimulatory cytokines (151–154).

Three relatively large studies have evaluated the effects of CMV infection on granulocyte and platelet recovery rates following BMT (142,155,156). In a study of 159 patients undergoing autologous BMT, there was no effect of CMV status at the time of BMT (CMV-seropositive vs CMV-seronegative) nor of active infection on granulocyte or platelet recovery rates (142). In contrast, the 2 other studies did show an effect, particularly on platelet recovery rates, in specific subsets of patients. Of the 36 seronegative patients undergoing autologous BMT, 18 (50%) became infected, and there was no effect of infection on either granulocyte or platelet recovery rates (155). However, among the 81 initially seropositive autologous BMT recipients, infection developed in 27 (33%) after BMT. In these patients with reactivated CMV, the median time to platelet recovery was 97 days, compared with 35 days in the noninfected group ($p = 0.003$). Neutrophil recovery was also slightly longer (median, 31 vs 24 days, respectively; $p = 0.02$).

In the other study, 87 patients underwent autologous BMT, and 56 underwent allogeneic BMT (156). These patients received leukocyte-poor RBCs and platelets from CMV-seronegative donors if they were seronegative. In the allogeneic BMT patients (all of whom received T-cell–depleted marrow grafts), platelet recovery to 50×10^9/L in the 24 CMV-seropositive patients was 41 days (median) compared with 27 days in the 32 CMV-seronegative patients ($p = 0.007$). There was no effect on granulocyte recovery. The delayed platelet recovery was considered to be related to the reactivation of CMV infection that occurred in 9 of 21 CMV-seropositive patients versus no CMV infections in the CMV-seronegative patients. In the autologous BMT patients, platelet recovery was so delayed in the patients transplanted for leukemia that an effect of CMV status was not observed. However, among the 33 seropositive lymphoma patients, platelet recovery was delayed to a median of 36 versus 24 days in the seronegative patients ($p = 0.0002$).

Medications. Ganciclovir is being evaluated for its potential benefit in BMT patients either to prevent CMV infection or as treatment (157). There is evidence from in vitro measurements of CFU-GM growth that ganciclovir is myelosuppressive (158), and it delayed neutrophil and platelet engraftment in a dog model (159) and in humans (160).

In addition, there may be several other drugs that are associated with either delayed engraftment or depressed hematopoiesis after engraftment. These drugs may include trimethoprim-sulfamethoxazole (TMP-SMX) (161,162), acyclovir (163), cotrimoxazole (164), and beta-lactam antibiotics (165).

Acute GVHD. Development of severe acute GVHD and its treatment may have a significant effect on hematopoiesis after marrow grafting. In 303 patients with AML who received marrow grafts from predominantly HLA-matched donors (270 patients), the rate of engraftment was significantly affected by the development of severe GVHD (141). Patients with mild GVHD (grades 0–II) were 1.3 times more likely to achieve granulocyte counts of 200×10^6/L on any given day than those with severe GVHD (grades III, IV) ($p = 0.05$), 4.4 times more likely to become RBC transfusion–independent ($p = 0.000$), and 2.3 times more likely to become platelet transfusion–independent ($p = 0.000$).

If a patient had chronic thrombocytopenia following BMT (i.e., failure to generate a platelet count $\geq 10 \times 10^9$/L by day 40 post-BMT), they were much more likely to have severe GVHD (8 of 15, 53%), compared with nonthrombocytopenic patients (8 of 41, 20%; $p < 0.05$) (162).

Cytokines. In contrast to the previous sections, which have discussed the adverse effects of a variety of factors on hematopoietic engraftment, the availability of several different cytokines that can accelerate hematopoietic reconstitution—as well as effectively restore hematopoiesis in some patients with graft failure—is an exciting advance in BMT. Data on the ability of these cytokines to facilitate early recovery of both neutrophils and platelets and to manage patients with graft failure are extensively reviewed in Chapter 24. These studies have shown a much more consistent effect of the two major cytokines thus far evaluated extensively—G-CSF and GM-CSF—on neutrophil recovery rather than platelets, as would be predicted from their known biological effects. However, it is anticipated that other cytokines currently being evaluated in Phase I/II clinical trials—such as IL-1, IL-3, IL-6, and leukemia inhibitory factor (LIF)—may accelerate platelet recovery rates.

Graft Factors

ABO and Rh-incompatible Transplants. The inital concerns about ABO-incompatible BMTs were whether the rates of graft rejection or GVHD would be increased. Graft rejection might be anticipated if there were ABO antigens in the donor but not in the recipient (i.e., a major mismatched BMT). However, several investigators have documented that donor-recipient ABO-incompatibility does not increase the incidence of either graft rejection or GVHD (see Chapter 35) (166–168).

Source of Stem Cells. There are substantial differences in rates of marrow engraftment depending on whether the graft consists of allogeneic or autologous marrow or peripheral blood stem cells that have been obtained either in a steady state, after cytokine administration, or in the recovery phase following chemotherapy (see Chapter 21).

Over a 4.5-year period, all patients admitted to a single institution for BMT were evaluated (169). Thirty-eight patients underwent autologous peripheral blood stem-cell transplant (APBSCT), with the cells harvested during the recovery phase following high-dose chemotherapy; 13 underwent autologous BMT, and 14 underwent allogeneic BMT. Time to reach neutrophil counts of 0.5×10^9/L were a median of 11 days (range, 9–17) for APBSCT, 22 days (range, 12–35) for autologous BMT, and 24.5 days (range, 17–30) for allogeneic BMT. Similar values for reaching platelet counts of 50×10^9/L were 14 (9, not reached), 32 (21, not reached), and 33 days (18, not reached), respectively.

Comparisons of allografts versus autografts were

performed in 33 and 20 patients with AML in first complete remission, respectively (170). Four of the autografts were purged with mafosfamide. The median interval for granulocyte recovery to 0.5×10^9/L was 24 days in the allo-BMT patients and 30 days in the auto-BMT patients ($p = 0.0001$). To recover platelet counts to 50×10^9/L required 27 and 62 days, respectively ($p < 0.0001$).

Because of an unusual pattern of late decline in WBC and platelet counts between 26 to 40 days after BMT in some patients with APBSCT (171), there has been interest in combining auto-BMT with APBSC harvests. This approach would have the advantages of early peripheral blood reconstruction from the mobilized committed progenitor cells in the APBSCT and greater numbers of pluripotent stem cells present in the marrow. Using this approach in 20 patients with advanced malignant diseases compared with another 20 patients who underwent auto-BMT without chemotherapy-mobilized APBSCT, the time to achieve 0.5×10^9/L granulocytes was reduced from a median of 25 to 10 days ($p < 0.02$), and to achieve a platelet count of 50×10^9/L was reduced from 34 to 21 days ($p < 0.05$) (172). However, no benefit of adding APBSC was seen if the APBSC were collected when the patient was in a steady state (173).

The value of colony-stimulating factors in mobilizing progenitor cells into the blood for harvesting and, indeed, the role of PBSCT, are still evolving (174–176). However, there is no question that the use of cytokines may greatly reduce transfusion requirements for BMT patients.

Recipient HLA-compatibility with Marrow Donor. Because of the success of BMT from genetically HLA-identical donors, the question of whether similar results could be achieved with phenotypically HLA-matched related and unrelated donors or family donors with varying degrees of HLA-incompatibility is being evaluated. The results of BMT from 105 consecutive patients with hematological malignancies who underwent BMTs with marrow from related donors other than HLA-identical siblings were compared with those of a concurrent group of 728 patients who underwent BMT with marrow from an HLA-matched sibling (177). The median day on which the granulocyte count first reached 1×10^9/L did not differ between the two groups; however, 19% of the study group compared with only 9% of the matched sibling donor group failed to achieve a granulocyte count of 1×10^9/L after 40 days ($p < 0.005$); 15% required a second marrow infusion because of graft failure compared with 7% ($p < 0.005$); 5% compared with 0.1% had graft rejection ($p = 0.001$); and 70% compared with 42% ($p < 0.001$) had GVHD, respectively.

In an analysis of 270 patients who received HLA-identical sibling BMTs for treatment of AML in first remission compared with 33 patients who received a related but 1-antigen–mismatched marrow graft, those receiving an HLA-matched BMT had a 1.8-times greater chance of achieving a granulocyte count of 0.2×10^9/L on any given day, a 1.4 times greater chance of achieving platelet independence, and a 1.8 times greater chance of becoming RBC transfusion–independent than did recipients of a mismatched graft (141).

In a retrospective analysis, data from 52 patients who received a phenotypically HLA-matched BMT from an unrelated donor for hematological malignancies were compared with data from a similar group of 104 patients who received a BMT from an HLA-matched sibling. The median time to myeloid engraftment was 25 days for both groups (178).

Summary

There are a variety of factors that can delay engraftment or result in graft rejection. All of these factors have a determining role in the type and amount of blood product support required after BMT.

RBC Transfusions

Most BMT programs suggest maintaining hematocrit levels of 25 to 30%, and the majority of the RBCs transfused are required in the first 4 weeks following BMT. Most increases in RBC transfusion requirements are due to ABO-incompatible transplants, which often result in delayed engraftment (see Chapter 35). In a multivariate statistical analysis of 22 determinants evaluated in 82 patients transplanted for aplastic anemia, the only factor in addition to ABO-incompatibility that increased RBC transfusion requirements was advanced recipient age (179).

Mixed hematopoietic chimerism, discussed in Chapter 12 (180–183), may be reflected as a "mixed" field reaction when performing blood typing after BMT if donor and recipient are of different RBC phenotypes. To determine the explanation for a "mixed" field reaction, it is important to perform full phenotype analysis on both marrow donor and recipient before BMT.

Granulocyte Transfusions

There is a direct relationship between granulocyte count and infection (184). A critical level of 0.2×10^9 granulocytes/L for a prolonged period is associated with a marked increase in infections. Although it is expected that granulocyte transfusion would prevent infections in such patients, there are several problems associated with granulocyte transfusions: (1) the short intravascular survival of granulocytes (approximately 6 hr) suggests that the usual daily administration of this product is too infrequent to provide adequate coverage; (2) the low dose and infrequent transfusion schedule make it difficult to document efficacy by following post-transfusion granulocyte increments—except in the limited blood volume of children; (3) prior RBC or platelet transfusions in granulocytopenic patients may lead to alloantibodies that limit granulocyte donors to HLA-matched or at least HLA partially matched individuals; and (4) because of the low concentration of circulating granulocytes, it is difficult to harvest enough of these cells from a normal donor to provide an effective transfusion dose. However, the administration of granulocyte colony stimulating factor (G-CSF) to leukocyte donors may substantially increase granulocyte yields (185).

G-CSF was given to 8 normal granulocyte donors undergoing leukapheresis, and there was a 10-fold increase in the donor's circulating granulocyte count, which resulted in a 6-fold increase in the number of granulocytes harvested compared with historical control data. Despite these difficulties, granulocyte transfusions may be beneficial in patients with documented infections who are unresponsive to antibiotics and for whom marrow granulocyte recovery will be delayed. On the negative side, granulocyte transfusions are associated with an increased incidence of alloimmunization to platelets (186) and to the transmission of CMV infection when seropositive donors are used (121).

Because there is a defined period of severe granulocytopenia in BMT patients and usually the ready availability of HLA-compatible donors, this setting represents an opportunity to assess directly the efficacy of granulocyte transfusions. In 69 patients receiving allogeneic BMT for hematological malignancy or aplasia, daily prophylactic administration of granulocyte transfusions from an HLA-matched or haploidentical family member into patients whose granulocyte counts were less than 0.2×10^9/L significantly reduced the incidence of septicemia (0 of 29 septicemic episodes in the granulocyte transfusion group vs 10 of 40 [25%] in the untreated group; $p <$ 0.005) (187). Although there were no infection-related deaths in the granulocyte-treated patients versus a 10% incidence in the untreated control group, overall mortality was not improved due to comparable death rates in both groups from leukemic relapse, interstitial pneumonia, GVHD, and graft rejection. In addition, improvements in infection control with laminar air flow isolation and prophylactic broad-spectrum antibiotics (188), combined with an increased incidence of CMV infections following granulocyte transfusions (120,121), has markedly reduced the use of granulocyte transfusions in BMT patients. Furthermore, more rapid WBC engraftment rates with the use of GM-CSF and G-CSF should further reduce the period of granulocytopenia (see Chapter 24).

Currently, documented bacterial or fungal infections that do not respond rapidly to appropriate antibiotic therapy in a BMT recipient with fewer than 0.2×10^9 granulocytes/L is regarded as an indication for therapeutic granulocyte transfusions. Persistent high fever unresponsive to antibacterial and antifungal therapy and without culture-proof of infection is also an indication for therapeutic granulocyte transfusions, particularly if accompanied by clinical deterioration. Once initiated, therapeutic granulocyte transfusions should be continued until the marrow graft sustains the granulocyte count at greater than 0.2×10^9/L (189).

Several reports have documented an apparent autoimmune granulocytopenia following either allogeneic or autologous BMT (190–192). Often these are isolated cases of neutropenia, but they may occur in conjunction with other immune-mediated cytopenias. The differential diagnosis includes graft failure, graft rejection, drug-induced suppression, and transient neutropenia related to GM-CSF or G-CSF withdrawal. Patients often respond to conventional treatment, such as steroids or splenectomy.

Platelet Transfusions

Providing adequate platelet support after BMT represents a substantial challenge both to the physician managing the patient and to the blood center providing the platelets. Meeting platelet transfusion needs is difficult because of the duration of thrombocytopenia, the short lifespan of transfused platelets, and the development of platelet refractoriness. Determining why patients are refractory to transfused platelets and then finding effective ways to deal with the problem is often a frustrating process.

Megakaryocyte Colony Stimulating Activity (Meg-CSA) or Growth-promoting Activity (Meg-GPA) After BMT

Meg-CSA or Meg-GPA after BMT have been measured to determine their relationship to megakaryocyte engraftment and platelet count after BMT (193–195). There is a biphasic increase in Meg-CSA after BMT, starting with an initial peak following the marrow conditioning program, a gradual decline, and then a second peak approximately 2 weeks after BMT (194). The initial peak was seen in all 23 study patients and was postulated to be due to tissue injury from the conditioning program with release of stored Meg-CSA. However, the second peak was seen only in patients who engrafted. There were substantial differences in Meg-CSA levels in the 12 patients who received T-cell–depleted compared with unmodified allogeneic (5 patients) or autologous grafts (6 patients) (195). The peak Meg-CSA activity was not only higher in those patients who received T-cell–depleted grafts, but it occurred 30 days rather than 20 days after BMT, as was seen in the other two groups. In both humans (194) and rats (196), there is evidence that the level of Meg-GPA is not influenced directly by the platelet count, because maintaining varying peripheral platelet counts with platelet transfusions was not reflected in any changes in the amount of measurable Meg-GPA. Overall, these data suggest that the megakaryocyte pool rather than the circulating platelet count is the negative feedback regulator of Meg-GPA (194).

Causes Of Persistent or Recurrent Thrombocytopenia

Discussed in this section are those factors that only affect platelet counts, and they can generally be divided into immune- and nonimmune-mediated causes.

Isolated Autoimmune Thrombocytopenia In a prospective study of 14 autograft and 32 allograft recipients, 52% demonstrated antibodies to their marrow donor's platelets in the early postgrafting period (197). By immunoglobulin allotyping, the antibodies were shown to be of donor type and were therefore autoantibodies. The majority of these antibodies were IgG, but IgM autoantibodies developed in 3 patients after day 200. The occurrence of these autoantibodies did not necessarily predict whether the patient would become thrombocytopenic, suggesting that in some of the patients the newly engrafted marrow was able to compensate by increasing platelet production.

Serial platelet-associated IgG (PAIgG) tests were performed in 41 patients receiving an allogeneic BMT for AML (198). Of the 34 patients tested before BMT, 2 had increased levels of PAIgG. At day 36 post-BMT, 36 patients were evaluated. In 21 patients, autoantibody tests or crossmatch tests with the marrow donor's platelets were negative, and 13 of these patients (62%) had self-sustaining platelet counts greater than 30×10^9/L. In contrast, in the 15 patients with elevated PAIgG levels, only 4 (27%) had self-sustaining platelet counts ($p < 0.05$). Prolonged elevated PAIgG levels after BMT were also correlated with delayed megakaryocyte engraftment ($p < 0.01$).

In another prospective study, platelet IgM autoantibodies were found in 5 of 10 patients who underwent allogeneic BMT, and in 1 of 1 who underwent syngeneic BMT (199). These antibodies either caused delayed normalization of platelet counts or were associated with late, mostly transient episodes of thrombocytopenia. Several other isolated case reports of autoimmune thrombocytopenia (ATP) have been reported following allogeneic, autologous, or syngeneic BMT (200–203). The target platelet antigen in one patient was directed against glycoproteins IIb/IIIa (204). This is the same glycoprotein that binds the majority of autoantibodies in patients with ATP (205). In addition, there have been two reported cases of autoimmune-mediated pancytopenia (206,207).

In general, these patients undergoing BMT have responded to therapy similar to that given to other patients with ATP (e.g., steroids, intravenous IgG, vincristine, or splenectomy).

ATP and Associated Viral Infections. ATP in association with viral illnesses is a relatively common finding (208); therefore, its occurrence in virally infected patients after BMT is not unexpected. Thirty-nine BMT patients (14 autologous and 25 allogeneic) were prospectively evaluated for development of PAIgG (209). Seventeen became thrombocytopenic (43%); 9 had persistent thrombocytopenia, and recurrent thrombocytopenia developed in 8 after having had platelet counts greater than 100×10^9/L. All thrombocytopenic patients, except 2 with late-onset thrombocytopenia, had increased amounts of PAIgG. Sixteen (94%) had an associated viral infection ($p = 0.005$), 11 of which were due to CMV.

Secondary thrombocytopenia occurring after an interval of self-sustaining platelet counts was found in 7 of 26 viremic patients with CMV (27%) after allogeneic BMT (210). Two of these patients had absent megakaryocytes in the marrow, and the other 5 with megakaryocytes had increased levels of PAIgG.

ATP and Associated GVHD. Thrombocytopenia in the context of GVHD is associated with a poor prognosis (211,212). Because hematopoietic progenitor cells are usually decreased in patients with GVHD, it is not surprising that these patients would become thrombocytopenic, with the development of autoantibodies (213).

Isolated thrombocytopenia developed in 24 of 65 fully engrafted allogeneic BMT patients (37%) who survived at least 60 days after BMT (162). Fifteen patients (23%) had persistent thrombocytopenia with platelet counts less than 100×10^9/L for the first 4 months after BMT, and 79% of these patients died compared with 33% of the nonthrombocytopenic or transiently thrombocytopenic patients ($p < 0.01$). Patients with persistent thrombocytopenia demonstrated a higher incidence of grade III to IV acute GVHD (53 vs 20%; $p < 0.05$) and a significantly higher incidence of chronic GVHD (92 vs 39%; $p < 0.01$). Three of 6 thrombocytopenic patients tested for autoantibodies were positive. Survival studies using radiolabeled platelets from the marrow donor were very short for 4 thrombocytopenic patients. Six patients with chronic GVHD were treated with prednisone and azathioprine, with no improvement in their platelet counts.

Persistent thrombocytopenia ($<100 \times 10^9$/L) was found in 20 patients 60 days after BMT (214). Twelve had autoantibody assays performed. Five of the patients (42%) had autoantibodies, and these patients represented 5 of 6 (83%) of the study patients who had grade II to IV acute or chronic GVHD, whereas 6 antibody-negative patients had no evidence of GVHD ($p < 0.01$). Patients with autoantibodies had lower platelet counts (30 ± 10 vs $49 \pm 29 \times 10^9$/L; $p < 0.05$) and shorter either radiolabeled auto or marrow donor platelet survivals (1.3 ± 0.9 vs 3.6 ± 2.0 days; $p < 0.05$). Four of the 6 patients with ATP and GVHD showed improvements in their platelet counts after treatment of their GVHD with prednisone, azathioprine, or procarbazine.

Other Immune-mediated Thrombocytopenias. One case of antibodies directed against the PL^{A1} antigen (215) and several drug-related immune thrombocytopenias (216) have been reported.

Nonimmune-mediated Thrombocytopenia. In most of the studies discussed in this section, platelet antibody testing was not performed. Therefore, in the absence of antibody tests, an immune-mediated mechanism cannot be excluded for some of these patients.

Transient thrombocytopenia that resolved with either discontinuation of the drug or reduction in the dose have been described for TMX-SMX (162) and CSP (217), respectively. In addition to delayed engraftment described with CMV infections, a variety of other infections have been associated with either persistent or recurrent thrombocytopenia (214,218). Finally, development of veno-occlusive disease (VOD), hemolytic uremia syndrome, or thrombotic thrombocytopenic purpura after BMT may be associated with delayed platelet engraftment or recurrent thrombocytopenia (217,219–225).

Principles of Platelet Support and Platelet Requirements

Principles of Platelet Support. In Seattle, prophylactic pooled random donor platelet transfusions are given whenever a patient's platelet count falls to 15 to 20 × 10^9/L. Transfusions at levels higher than 20 × 10^9/L are given only with evidence of significant bleeding that is often related to GVHD-induced gastrointestinal ulcerations or cyclophosphamide-mediated hemorrhagic cystitis. Although there are data to suggest that significant spontaneous bleeding may not occur until platelet counts are 5 to 10 × 10^9/L (see previous section on pre-BMT platelet support), the frequency of drug- or disease-induced mucous membrane defects that are likely to bleed, *plus* treatment with numerous drugs that may increase the chances of drug-induced platelet dysfunction may justify the higher transfusion level in selected BMT patients. However, platelet transfusion trials in BMT patients to determine appropriate platelet transfusion levels have never been performed. Also, it has never been determined if BMT patients, who are heavily immunosuppressed, would benefit from approaches to preventing platelet alloimmunization.

Platelet Transfusion Requirements. Platelet and RBC transfusion requirements in 303 patients with AML, transplanted in first complete remission with either HLA-identical or one antigen mismatched donors, are illustrated in Table 22-4 (141). This table illustrates the effects of some of the factors previously discussed that prevent or delay engraftment.

In addition to the multiple factors that can adversely influence platelet transfusion needs, there are two that decrease platelet requirements. Only 1 of 17 patients (6%) with CML in chronic phase who had been splenectomized versus 23 of 38 (61%) who had not been splenectomized became refractory to random donor platelets after BMT ($p < 0.0001$) (136). Thus, the requirements for both random donor and HLA-matched apheresis donor platelet support were significantly less in the splenectomized group.

In a prospective study, 382 BMT patients were randomly assigned to receive intravenous (IV) IgG or not (226). Because of significant reductions in interstitial pneumonia, gram-negative septicemia, local infection, and acute GVHD, the median day of the last platelet transfusion was 31 compared with 52 for the treated versus the untreated group, respectively ($p < 0.055$). Although the median units of platelets transfused per thrombocytopenic day was the same (2.7 vs 2.6, respectively), the treated group required 51 less platelet concentrates than the untreated group because of the earlier development of platelet transfusion independence.

Mechanisms and Management of Platelet Refractoriness

In an analysis of 264 patients with aplastic anemia, 71 of 210 (34%) of the transfused patients were already platelet-refractory on admission, whereas none of the 54 previously untransfused patients were refractory to

Table 22-4.
Several Factors Affecting Transfusion Requirements After BMT

Variable	*No. Patients*	*Mean (Median) Units* Platelets		*p* Value	Red Cells		*p* Value
GVHD prophylaxis							
MTX	151	167	(106)	0.001	18	(13)	0.02
CSP	68	99	(44)		21	(16)	
MTX + CSP	76	98	(64)		18	(16)	
Acute GVHD							
0–2	228	91	(60)	0.0001	14	(12)	0.0001
3–4	74	271	(217)		31	(28)	
Infection Prophylaxis							
Laminar air flow	98	177	(94)	0.01	22	(15)	0.02
Others[a]	205	116	(72)		16	(14)	
ABO							
Compatible	207	138	(82)	0.08	17	(14)	0.003
Incompatible[b]	45	155	(80)		24	(22)	

[a]Patients in this group had either no treatment, granulocyte transfusions, systemic antibiotics, or laminar air flow *plus* systemic antibiotics.
[b]Includes only patients with major ABO incompatibility.
GVHD = graft-versus-host disease; MTX = methotrexate; CSP = cyclosporine A.
Reproduced by permission from Bensinger W, Petersen FB, Banaji M, et al. Engraftment and transfusion requirements after allogeneic marrow transplantation for patients with acute non-lymphocytic leukemia in first complete remission. Bone Marrow Transplant 1989;4:409–414.

pooled random donor platelets (227). Among many variables analyzed for their effects on platelet refractoriness using a binary logistical regression model, only the presence of lymphocytotoxic antibodies ($p <$ 0.001) and the number of platelet units transfused before admission correlated with refractoriness ($p <$ 0.02).

In an analysis of 186 patients with AML in remission or 67 patients with CML in chronic phase, only 6% of the former and 17% of the latter were refractory to random donor platelets on admission (136). However, an additional 35 to 44% of these patients became refractory to platelets following BMT. In general, platelet refractoriness can be separated into immune and nonimmune mechanisms.

Management of Alloimmunized Patients. To diagnose alloimmunization, platelet or lymphocytotoxic antibodies must be demonstrated against homologous platelets or lymphocytes. Unfortunately, the presence of an alloantibody does not necessarily mean that a poor response to platelet therapy is due to immunization. However, if the antibody reacts with the majority of donor platelets tested and an autoantibody can be excluded, the patient probably has been broadly immunized and is likely to be alloimmune-refractory to random donor platelets. For alloimmunized patients, finding a compatible platelet donor requires identifying the specificity of the antibody and selecting a donor who does not carry the incompatible antigen, selecting donors based on matching for the patient's antigens, or using crossmatch tests to identify compatible donors. In the early post-BMT period, one would expect existing antibodies, determined by the patient's ABO, HLA, and platelet-specific antigen specificities, to be important, whereas late developing alloantibodies will usually reflect donor antigen types. Therefore, repeat antibody testing to monitor any changes in antibody specificities may be necessary.

Determine Antibody Specificity Using Cell Panels. Platelet alloimmunization due to minor RBC antigens has not been described, even though some of these antigens are expressed on platelets (228–230). Therefore, it is not necessary to identify antibodies to these antigens. However, significant information can often be gained by testing patients' sera for antibody reactivity with selected lymphocyte panels. If HLA antibody specificity is determined, then HLA-typed donors can be selected to avoid the offending antigen. Avoiding a limited number of incompatible antigens rather than matching for antigens will greatly expand the available donor pool for some patients.

ABO Matching. The relevance of ABH antigens to platelet transfusion therapy was first reported in 1965 (231). Radiolabeled A_1 platelets, when given to group O normal recipients, resulted in recoveries of 19% compared with 63% observed with ABO-compatible platelets. However, when group B platelets were given to incompatible recipients, average recovery was maintained at 57%. When group A_1B platelets were given to group O recipients, average recovery was only 8%. ABO-incompatible platelet recovery was inversely related to the isohemagglutination titers of the transfused recipient.

Several large platelet transfusion studies have established the transfusion relevance of donor-recipient ABO antigen compatibility. The effects of ABO compatibility on transfusion responses have been documented in 91 platelet-refractory patients who received 389 HLA-selected apheresis platelet transfusions (232). For the ABO-compatible platelets, recoveries averaged 73±4% compared with 55±5% for ABO-mismatched transfusions at one hour ($p < 0.01$), and recoveries were 37±3 versus 29±4%, respectively, 24 hours after transfusion ($p < 0.05$). In a second, similar study in 51 platelet-refractory patients given 316 HLA-selected donor apheresis transfusions, ABO-compatible platelet transfusions gave average CCIs of 10×10^9/L, compared with 5.9×10^9/L for ABO-incompatible platelets ($p < 0.01$)(233).

Although these studies showed no effect of ABO incompatibility on platelet survival but only on recovery, a recent report has demonstrated rapid platelet destruction when ABO-incompatible platelets were given to 2 group O recipients with high titers of immune (IgG) anti-A or anti-B antibodies (234). Thus, there may be certain situations in which survival, as well as recovery, is compromised with the transfusion of ABO-incompatible platelets.

HLA Matching. HLA-A and HLA-B antigens are the major immunogens expressed on the surface of platelets (235). HLA-C, HLA-D, and HLA-DR antigens are either not present or only weakly expressed on the platelet surface; incompatibility for these antigens has not been documented to cause refractoriness to platelet transfusions (236,237). Although HLA-matched donors may cause compatible transfusion responses in patients who have become refractory to pooled random donor platelets (238,239), the complexity of the HLA system makes it difficult to find HLA-matched donors. Therefore, the effectiveness of donor platelets mismatched for crossreactive HLA antigens was evaluated (240). Four hundred twenty-one single-donor apheresis transfusions were administered to 59 alloimmunized platelet-refractory patients. Partially matched single-donor platelets were effective when the mismatch at one or two loci involved crossreactive groups only. However, approximately 30% of even the best matched donors did not provide good post-transfusion platelet increments. Possible immunological explanations for these incompatible transfusion results are the presence of platelet-specific antibodies or antibodies against crossreactive HLA antigens.

Platelet-specific Antigen Matching. Patients with platelet-specific alloantibodies are most often highly refractory to all platelet donors and, more specifically, even HLA well-matched donors (241). Antisera from such patients were screened by Western blot and radioimmunoprecipitation procedures to identify antibodies that bound to platelet membrane glycoproteins. Of 39 platelet-reactive antisera screened against platelet membranes, 9 (23%) showed a reaction with one or more platelet membrane glycoproteins.

Additional evidence that such platelet-specific antibodies may produce platelet refractoriness comes from transfusion studies using HLA-fully matched family or unrelated donors. Seven studies reported a failure rate of HLA-A-matched platelets from either family members or unrelated donors of 6 to 39%, with an average of 19% (41 of 212) (242). Because all the platelet-specific antigens described to date have a relatively high gene frequency for one of the alleles, alloimmunization rates to platelet-specific antigens should be low.

Unfortunately, there are not enough platelet-specific antisera available to type community donor platelet apheresis panels for these antigens. Therefore, the best approach to finding compatible donors for patients alloimmunized to platelet-specific antigens is to evaluate family members. Either platelet antigen typing, platelet crossmatch testing, or transfusion trials with family members can be used to select compatible donors. Such patients are also likely to have formed HLA antibodies as well as platelet-specific alloantibodies; therefore, family members may also have to be HLA-compatible to obtain platelet increments.

Platelet Crossmatch Testing. In clinically stable patients, the predictability of the crossmatch tests is greater than 80%, whereas in unselected patients who may have factors other than alloimmunization that can affect transfusion responses, predictability is between 60 to 85% (243–248). From a cost-effectiveness standpoint, it has been suggested that crossmatching random donor platelet concentrates and pooling compatible units to constitute a transfusion dose is an appropriate approach (249). Except for highly alloimmunized patients with antibodies to almost all members of a screening panel, a pool of compatible donors usually can be found in a random population. However, for highly immunized patients, only 4 to 5% of the screened donors will be compatible (246–248). Therefore, screening the large number of donors required to find matches for the latter patients may not be cost-effective.

One of the biggest problems with platelet crossmatch testing is the lack of a uniform test procedure. Until some standardization is reached in the field, it will remain difficult to interpret results achieved in different laboratories.

Strategies for Managing Persistently Platelet-refractory Patients. For some alloimmunized patients, compatible platelet donors cannot be identified. For these patients, procedures that may reverse an already established immune response or that may improve hemostasis should be sought.

IVIgG Administration. The effectiveness of IVIgG in managing patients with alloimmune platelet destruction is unclear. Some studies have shown improved platelet responses in some treated patients (250–253), whereas other patients have shown no response (254–256). One study suggested that higher doses of IVIgG and use of HLA-compatible platelets after IVIgG may improve results (253). In the only randomized placebo-controlled trial in which platelets from the same donor were given before and after treatment, a significant increase in platelet counts in the treated group compared with the untreated group one hour after transfusion was documented (8,413 vs 1,050 × 10^9/L CCI, respectively; $p < 0.007$) (251). Although platelet increments were improved, platelet survival was increased in only one of the treated patients. Considering the high cost of IVIgG and the very transient improvement, the authors did not consider this to be a cost-effective therapy. Currently, IVIgG infusions should be given only to patients who are refractory to all forms of platelet therapy and who have severe bleeding problems.

Plasma Exchange. In theory, it is possible to remove alloantibodies by plasma exchange. However, because most alloantibodies are IgG, which are distributed within both the intravascular and the extravascular spaces, complete removal is extremely difficult. In addition, unless concurrent immunosuppressive therapy is used to at least impair—if not prevent—additional antibody formation, the therapy will at best be only transiently successful.

Eighteen patients with aplastic anemia or acute leukemia who were refractory to pooled random donor platelets underwent a plasma exchange procedure either before or after BMT (257). Improved postexchange platelet responses were directly related to the volume of plasma removed. Those patients who had the best postexchange platelet responses had 3 daily, 10-liter plasma exchanges. Overall, 11 of the 18 patients (61%) showed improved responses to platelets from random or related donors. As with IVIgG therapy, this approach is an expensive, time-consuming procedure and should be used only for patients who have evidence of alloantibodies, who are not otherwise supportable by platelet transfusions, and who have life-threatening bleeding problems.

Control of Bleeding with Fibrinolytic Inhibitors: Epsilon-Aminocaproic Acid (EACA). For patients with life-threatening bleeding, a trial of therapy with EACA may be indicated. In limited, uncontrolled clinical studies, a total of 40 patients with thrombocytopenia due to marrow failure who were refractory to platelet therapy, as well as some patients with autoimmune thrombocytopenic purpura, have been given EACA (258–260). Bleeding was controlled in 36 of the 40 patients (90%). However, in the only controlled prospective clinical trial conducted in 18 patients with acute leukemia randomized to receive either platelet therapy or platelet therapy *plus* EACA, there were no differences in capillary bleeding, major vessel bleeding, or number of platelet transfusions required per day (261). Thus, the efficacy of EACA therapy remains unproven.

Identification and Management of Nonimmune Causes of Platelet Refractoriness. If platelet antibody screening tests are negative, the presumption is that the patient has nonimmune causes of platelet refractoriness.

Table 22-5.
Transfusion Responses to Fresh or Stored Platelet Concentrates in Thrombocytopenic Patients

			Corrected Platelet Count Increment (× $10^9/L$)[a]			
Author, Ref	*No. Recipients*	*Storage Time (days)*	*1-Hour*	*p* Value	*18–48 Hours*	*p* Value
Snyder et al. (263)	13	5	13.6 ± 10.4			
	8	5	15.6 ± 12.2			
Hogge et al. (264)	16	Fresh	20.1 ± 8.4	0.02	10.8 ± 4.4	0.0001
	16	3	12.2 ± 8.1		7.5 ± 5.6	
	16	7	10.0 ± 7.2		7.0 ± 5.5	
Schiffer et al. (262)[b]	135	1	15.5 ± 6.3		10.9 ± 5.3	
	81	2	16.1 ± 5.9		10.5 ± 5.5	
	53	3	13.6 ± 5.5		10.0 ± 5.2	
	60	4	13.0 ± 5.0		8.5 ± 4.4	
	33	5	13.2 ± 6.0		8.9 ± 5.0	
Lazarus et al. (265)	15	<1	9.5 (5.0–18.0)	0.01		
	15	1–2	7.2 (5.4–14.5)			
	15	2–3	1.0 (0.0–4.8)			
Peter-Salonen et al. (266)	51	Fresh	9.5 ± 7.0	0.014	4.7 ± 2.8	0.004
	20	1–4	5.6 ± 4.9		2.4 ± 2.8	

[a]Corrected platelet count increment = absolute platelet increment × body surface area (m^2)/number of platelets transfused × 10^{11}.
[b]Data from nonsplenectomized patients.

Stored Platelets. Although the platelet increments in one study (262) did not differ based on a storage time of 1 to 5 days, in every instance in which stored platelets were compared with fresh platelets, there was a statistically significant decrease in platelet increments one and then 18 to 48 hours after transfusion (Table 22-5) (263–266). Thus, one cause of poor responses to platelet transfusions may be use of stored platelets. On a practical level, the easiest adverse factor to test for in platelet-refractory patients and one that may produce a high yield of improved responses is to give "fresh" platelets. Of 108 patients who were both refractory to pooled random donor platelets and had no evidence of antibodies, only 3 (3%) did not show improved platelet responses when they were given single random apheresis platelets that had been stored for 36 hours or less (267). If giving fresher platelets is unsuccessful, then other potential causes of platelet refractoriness should be addressed.

Clinical Factors. Two recent studies have used multiple linear regression analysis to evaluate platelet transfusion response data in conjunction with the patient's medical status. Although many of these clinical factors cannot be modified to improve platelet responses, it is important to know which factors are usually associated with poor platelet responses so that any possible changes can be made.

When 941 pooled random donor platelet transfusions were given to 133 patients with marrow failure, splenectomy was the only factor that improved post-transfusion platelet responses; patients transfused after a BMT had the poorest transfusion increments (268,269). Other adverse factors affecting CCIs were disseminated intravascular coagulation, amphotericin B, a palpable spleen, and HLA-lymphocytotoxic antibodies. In another study, 334 HLA-selected apheresis transfusions were given to 29 platelet-refractory patients (243). Fever and splenomegaly significantly reduced platelet recoveries, whereas sepsis/infection and donors poorly matched for HLA-antigens reduced platelet survivals. In addition to the observed general increase in poor platelet responses seen in BMT patients (268,269), patients in whom liver disease and, more specifically, VOD of the liver develop have an extremely high rate of platelet refractoriness (220,270,271).

References

1. van Putten LM, van Bekkum DW, de Vries MJ, Balner H. The effect of preceding blood transfusions on the fate of homologous bone marrow grafts in lethally irradiated monkeys. Blood 1967;30:749–757.
2. Weiden PL, Storb R, Thomas ED, et al. Preceding transfusions and marrow graft rejection in dogs and man. Transplant Proc 1976;8:551–554.
3. Storb R, Thomas ED, Buckner CD, et al. Marrow transplantation for aplastic anemia. Semin Hematol 1984;21:27–35.
4. Weiden PL, Storb R, Kolb HJ, Graham TC, Kao G, Thomas ED. Effect of time on sensitization to hemopoietic grafts by preceding blood transfusion. Transplantation 1975;19:240–244.
5. Deeg HJ, Storb R, Thomas ED. The dog as a pre-clinical model of marrow transplantation. In: Gale RP, ed. Recent advances in bone marrow transplantation. New York: Alan R. Liss, 1983:527–546.
6. Storb R, Weiden PL, Deeg HJ, et al. Rejection of marrow from DLA-identical canine littermates given transfusions before grafting: antigens involved are expressed on leukocytes and skin epithelial cells but not on platelets and red blood cells. Blood 1979;54:477–483.
7. Storb R, Rudolph RH, Graham TC, Thomas ED. The influence of transfusions from unrelated donors upon marrow grafts between histocompatible canine siblings. J Immunol 1971;107:409–413.
8. Deeg HJ, Torok-Storb B, Storb R, et al. Rejection of DLA-

identical canine litter-mate marrow after transfusion-induced sensitization: Antigens involved are expressed on cotton-wool adherent but not on nonadherent mononuclear cells, granulocytes, or thoracic duct lymphocytes. In: Baum SJ, Ledney GD, Khan A, eds. Experimental hematology today 1981. New York: Karger, 1981:31–37.
9. Lindahl-Kiessling K, Safwenberg J. Inability of UV-irradiated lymphocytes to stimulate allogeneic cells in mixed lymphocyte culture. Int Arch Allergy 1971;41: 670–678.
10. Deeg HJ, Aprile J, Graham TC, Appelbaum FR, Storb R. Ultraviolet irradiation of blood prevents transfusion-induced sensitization and marrow graft rejection in dogs. Blood 1986;67:537–539.
11. Deeg HJ, Aprile J, Storb R, et al. Functional dendritic cells are required for transfusion-induced sensitization in canine marrow graft recipients. Blood 1988;71:1138–1140.
12. Loertscher R, Abbud-Filho M, Leichtman AB, et al. Differential effect of gamma-irradiation and heat-treated lymphocytes on T cell activation, and interleukin-2 and interleukin-3 release in the human mixed lymphocyte reaction. Transplantation 1987;44:673–680.
13. Bean MA, Storb R, Graham T. Prevention of transfusion-induced sensitization to minor histocompatibility antigens on DLA-identical canine marrow grafts by gamma irradiation of marrow donor blood. Transplantation 1991;52:956–960.
14. Storb R, Kolb HJ, Graham TC, Kane PJ, Thomas ED. The effect of prior blood transfusions on hemopoietic grafts from histoincompatible canine littermates. Transplantation 1972;14:248–252.
15. Storb R, Floersheim GL, Weiden PL, et al. Effect of prior blood transfusions on marrow grafts: abrogation of sensitization by procarbazine and antithymocyte serum. J Immunol 1974;112:1508–1516.
16. Storb R, Deeg HJ, Appelbaum FR, Schuening R, Sandmaier B, Raff RF. Failure of anti-Ia monoclonal antibody to abrogate transfusion-induced sensitization and prevent marrow graft rejection in DLA-identical canine littermates. Transplantation 1988;45:505–506.
17. Weiden PL, Storb R, Slichter SJ, Warren RP, Sale GE. Effect of six weekly transfusions on canine marrow grafts: tests for sensitization and abrogation of sensitization by procarbazine and antithymocyte serum. J Immunol 1976;117:143–150.
18. Storb R, Deeg HJ, Atkinson K, et al. Cyclosporin-A abrogates transfusion-induced sensitization and prevents marrow graft rejection in DLA-identical canine littermates. Blood 1982;60:524–526.
19. Storb R, Prentice RL, Thomas ED. Marrow transplantation for treatment of aplastic anemia: an analysis of factors associated with graft rejection. N Engl J Med 1977;296:61–66.
20. Storb R, Thomas ED, Buckner CD, et al. Marrow transplantation in thirty "untransfused" patients with severe aplastic anemia. Ann Intern Med 1980;92:30–36.
21. Anasetti C, Doney KC, Storb R, et al. Marrow transplantation for severe aplastic anemia: long term outcome in fifty "untransfused" patients. Ann Intern Med 1986;104:461–466.
22. Feig SA, Champlin R, Arenson E, et al. Improved survival following bone marrow transplantation for aplastic anaemia. Br J Haematol 1983;54:509–517.
23. Ho WG, Champlin RE, Winston DJ, Feig SA, Gale RP. Bone marrow transplantation in patients with leukaemia previously transfused with blood products from family members. Br J Haematol 1987;67:67–70.
24. National Institutes Of Health. Consensus development conference on platelet transfusion therapy. JAMA 1987;257:1777–1780.
25. Gaydos LA, Freireich EJ, Mantel N. The quantitative relation between platelet count and hemorrhage in patients with acute leukemia. N Engl J Med 1962;266: 905–909.
26. Slichter SJ, Harker LA. Thrombocytopenia: mechanisms and management of defects in platelet production. Clin Haematol 1978;7:523–539.
27. Roy AJ, Jaffe N, Djerassi I. Prophylactic platelet transfusions in children with acute leukemia: a dose response study. Transfusion 1973;13:283–290.
28. Aderka D, Praff G, Santo M, Weinberger A, Pinkhas J. Bleeding due to thrombocytopenia in acute leukemias and re-evaluation of the prophylactic platelet transfusion policy. Am J Med Sci 1986;291:147–151.
29. Gmur J, Burger J, Schanz U, Fehr J, Schaffner A. Safety of stringent prophylactic platelet transfusion policy for patients with acute leukaemia. Lancet 1991;338:1223–1226.
30. Solomon J, Bofenkamp T, Fahey JL, Chillar RK, Beutler E. Platelet prophylaxis in acute non-lymphocytic leukemia (letter). Lancet 1978;1:267.
31. Murphy S, Litwin S, Herring LM, et al. The indications for platelet transfusion in children with acute leukemia. Am J Hematol 1982;12:347–356.
32. Harker LA, Slichter SJ. The bleeding time as a screening test for evaluating platelet function. N Engl J Med 1972;287:155–159.
33. Slichter SJ. Prevention of platelet alloimmunization. In: Murawski K, Peetoom F, eds. Transfusion medicine: recent technological advances. New York: Alan R. Liss, 1986:83–116.
34. Holohan W, Terasaki PI, Diesseroth AB. Suppression of transfusion-related alloimmunization in intensively treated cancer patients. Blood 1981;58:122–128.
35. Lee EJ, Schiffer CA. Serial measurement of lymphocytotoxic antibody and response to nonmatched platelet transfusions in alloimmunized patients. Blood 1987;70:1727–1729.
36. Pamphilon DH, Farrell DH, Donaldson C, Raymond PA, Brady CA, Bradley BA. Development of lymphocytotoxic and platelet reactive antibodies: a prospective study in patients with acute leukemia. Vox Sang 1989;57:177–181.
37. Tejada F, Bias WB, Santos GW, Zieve PD. Immunologic response of patients with acute leukemia to platelet transfusions. Blood 1973;42:405–412.
38. Howard JE, Perkins HA. The natural history of alloimmunization to platelets. Transfusion 1978;18: 496–503.
39. Murphy MF, Metcalfe P, Ord J, et al. Disappearance of HLA and platelet-specific antibodies in acute leukaemia patients alloimmunized by multiple transfusions. Br J Haematol 1987;67:255–260.
40. McGrath K, Wolf M, Bishop J, et al. Transient platelet and HLA antibody formation in multitransfused patients with malignancy. Br Haematol 1988;68:345–350.
41. Slichter SJ, Deeg HJ, Kennedy MS. Prevention of platelet alloimmunization in dogs with systemic cyclosporine and by UV-irradiation or cyclosporine-loading of donor platelets. Blood 1987;69:414–418.
42. Slichter SJ, Weiden PL, Kane PJ, Storb RF. Approaches to preventing or reversing platelet alloimmunization using animal models. Transfusion 1988;28:103–108.

43. Sintnicolaas K, Vriesendorp HM, Sizoo W, et al. Delayed alloimmunization by random single donor platelet transfusions. Lancet 1981;1:750–754.
44. Kakaiya RM, Hezzey AJ, Bove JR, et al. Alloimmunization following apheresis platelets vs pooled platelet concentrate transfusion—a prospective randomized study (abstract). Transfusion 1981;21:600.
45. Gmur J, von Felten A, Osterwalder B, Scali G, Sauter Chr, Frick P. Delayed alloimmunization using random single donor platelet transfusions: a prospective study in thrombocytopenic patients with acute leukemia. Blood 1983;61:473–479.
46. Slichter SJ, O'Donnell MR, Weiden PL, Storb R, Schroeder ML. Canine platelet alloimmunization: the role of donor selection. Br J Haematol 1986;63:713–727.
47. Dunstan RA, Simpson MB, Knowles RW, Rosse WF. The origin of ABH antigens on human platelets. Blood 1985;65:615–619.
48. Lee EJ, Schiffer CA. ABO compatibility can influence the results of platelet transfusion. Results of a randomized trial. Transfusion 1989;29:384–389.
49. Carr R, Hutton JL, Jenkins JA, Lucas GF, Amphlett NW. Transfusion of ABO-mismatched platelets leads to early platelet refractoriness. Br J Haematol 1990;75:408–413.
50. Messerschmidt G, Makuch R, Appelbaum F, et al. A prospective randomized trial of HLA-matched versus mismatched single-donor platelet transfusions in cancer patients. Cancer 1988;62:795–801.
51. Murphy MF, Metcalfe P, Thomas H, et al. Use of leukocyte-poor blood components and HLA-matched-platelet donors to prevent HLA alloimmunization. Br J Haematol 1986;62:529–534.
52. Welsh KI, Burgos H, Batchelor JR. The immune response to allogeneic rat platelets: Ag-B antigens in matrix lacking Ia. Eur J Immunology 1977;7:267–272.
53. Batchelor JR, Welsh KI, Burgos H. Transplantation antigens per se are poor immunogens within a species. Nature 1978;273:54–56.
54. Claas FHJ, Smeenk RJT, Schmidt R, van Steenbrugge GJ, Eernisse JG. Alloimmunization against the MHC antigens after platelet transfusions is due to contaminating leukocytes in the platelet suspension. Exp Hematol 1981;9:84–89.
55. Fisher M, Chapman JR, Ting A, Morris PJ. Alloimmunization to HLA antigens following transfusion with leukocyte-poor and purified platelet suspensions. Vox Sang 1985;49:331–335.
56. Petranyi GG, Padanyi A, Horuzsko A, et al. Mixed lymphocyte culture-evidence that pretransplant transfusion with platelets induces FcR and blocking antibody production similar to that induced by leukocyte transfusion. Transplantation 1988;45:823–824.
57. Chambers LA, Garcia LW. White blood cell content of transfusion components. Lab Med 1991;22:857.
58. Friedman LI, Sadoff BJ, Stromberg RR. White cell counting in red cells and platelets: How few can we count? (editorial). Transfusion 1990;30:387–389.
59. Schiffer CA, Dutcher JP, Aisner J, Hogge D, Wiernik PH, Reilly JP. A randomized trial of leukocyte-depleted platelet transfusions to modify alloimmunization in patients with leukemia. Blood 1983;62:815–820.
60. Sniecinski I, O'Donnell MR, Nowicki B, Hill LR. Prevention of refractoriness and HLA-alloimmunization using filtered blood products. Blood 1988;71:1402–1407.
61. Andreu G, Dewailly J, Leberre C, et al. Prevention of HLA immunization with leukocyte-poor packed red cells and platelet concentrates obtained by filtration. Blood 1988;72:964–969.
62. Oksanen K, Kekomaki R, Ruutu T, Koskimies S, Myllyla G. Prevention of alloimmunization in patients with acute leukemia by use of white cell-reduced blood components—a randomized trial. Transfusion 1991;31:588–594.
63. van Marwijk Kooy M, van Prooijen HC, Moes M, Bosma-Stants I, Akkerman JWN. Use of Leukocyte-depleted platelet concentrates for the prevention of refractoriness and primary HLA alloimmunization: a prospective, randomized trial. Blood 1991;77:201–205.
64. Schiffer CA. Prevention of platelet alloimmunization (editorial). Blood 1991;77:1–4.
65. Snyder EL. Clinical use of white cell-poor blood components. Transfusion 1989;29:568–571.
66. Brand A, Claas FHJ, Voogt PJ, Wasser MNJM, Eernisse JG. Alloimmunization after leukocyte-depleted multiple random donor platelet transfusions. Vox Sang 1988;54:160–166.
67. Slichter SJ. UV irradiation: effects on the immune system and on platelet function, viability, and alloimmunization, In: Sibinga CTS, Kater L, eds. Advances in haemapheresis. Proceedings of the Third International Congress of the World Apheresis Association. Dordrecht, The Netherlands: Kluwer Academic Publishers, 1991:205–228.
68. Pamphilon DH, Potter M, Cutts M, et al. Platelet concentrates irradiated with ultraviolet light retain satisfactory in vitro storage characteristics and in vivo survival. Br J Haematol 1990;75:240–244.
69. Andreu G, Boccaccio C, Lecrubier C, et al. Ultraviolet irradiation of platelet concentrates: feasibility in transfusion practice. Transfusion 1990;30:401–406.
70. Buchholz DH, Miripol J, Aster RH, et al. Ultraviolet irradiation of platelets to prevent recipient alloimmunization (abstract). Transfusion 1988;28:26S.
71. Nemo GJ, McCurdy PR. Prevention of platelet alloimmunization (editorial). Transfusion 1991;31:584–586.
72. Reusser P. Cytomegalovirus infection and disease after bone marrow transplantation: epidemiology, prevention, and treatment. Bone Marrow Transplant 1991;7:52–56.
73. Meyers JD, Flournoy N, Thomas ED. Risk factors for cytomegalovirus infection after human marrow transplantation. J Infect Dis 1986;153:478–488.
74. Kelsey SM, Newland AC. Cytomegalovirus seroconversion in patients receiving intensive induction therapy prior to allogeneic bone marrow transplantation. Bone Marrow Transplant 1989;4:543–546.
75. Ho M. Observations from transplantation contributing to the understanding of pathogenesis of CMV infection. Transplant Proc 1991;23(suppl 3):104–109.
76. Bowden RA, Meyers JD. Transfusion-associated cytomegalovirus infection. In: Dutcher JP, ed. Modern transfusion therapy, vol. 2. Boca Raton, FL: CRC Press, 1990:269–282.
77. Yeager AS, Grumet FC, Hafleigh EB, Arvin AM, Bradley JS, Prober CG. Prevention of transfusion-acquired cytomegalovirus infections in newborn infants. J Pediatr 1981;98:281–287.
78. Benson JWT, Bodden SJ, Tobin JO'H. Cytomegalovirus and blood transfusion in neonates. Arch Dis Child 1979;54:538–541.
79. Kurtz JB, Thompson JF, Tinf A, Apinto DJ. The problem of cytomegalovirus infection in renal allograft recipients. J Med 1984;53:341–349.

80. Adler SP, Baggett J, McVoy M. Transfusion-associated cytomegalovirus infections in seropositive cardiac surgery patients. Lancet 1985;1:743–746.
81. Cheung KS, Lang DJ. Transmission and activation of cytomegalovirus with blood transfusion: a mouse model. J Infect Dis 1977;135:841–845.
82. Jordan MC. Latent infection and the elusive cytomegalovirus. Rev Infect Dis 1983;5:205–215.
83. Howell CL, Miller MJ, Martin WJ. Comparison of rates of virus isolation from leukocyte populations separated from blood by conventional and Ficoll-Hypaque/Macrodex methods. J Clin Microbiol 1979;10:533–537.
84. Lang DJ, Ebert PA, Rodgers BM, et al. Reduction of postperfusion cytomegalovirus-infections following the use of leukocyte depleted blood. Transfusion 1977;17:391–395.
85. Luban NLC, Williams AE, MacDonald MG, Mikesell GT, Williams KM, Sacher RA. Low incidence of acquired cytomegalovirus infection in neonates transfused with washed red blood cells. Am J Dis Child 1987;141:416–419.
86. Tolkoff-Rubin NE, Rubin RH, Keller EE, et al. Cytomegalovirus infection in dialysis patients and personnel. Ann Intern Med 1978;89:625–628.
87. Adler SP, Lawrence LT, Baggett J, Biro V, Sharp DE. Prevention of transfusion-associated cytomegalovirus infection in very low-birthweight infants using frozen blood and donors seronegative for cytomegalovirus. Transfusion 1984;24:333–335.
88. Taylor BJ, Jacobs RF, Baker RL, Moses EB, McSwain BE, Shulman G. Frozen deglycerolized blood prevents transfusion-acquired cytomegalovirus infections in neonates. Pediatr Infect Dis 1986;5:188–191.
89. Brady MT, Milam JD, Anderson DC, et al. Use of deglycerolized red blood cells to prevent posttransfusion infection with cytomegalovirus in neonates. J Infect Dis 1984;150:334–339.
90. Bowden RA, Sayers M. The risk of transmitting cytomegalovirus infection by fresh frozen plasma. Transfusion 1990;30:762–763.
91. Angue M, Chatelain P, Richaud P, et al. Deleucocytation en systeme clos des concentres de globules rouges humaines. Rev Fr Transfus Hemobiol 1989;32:265–276.
92. Beaujean, F, Segier JM, Leforestier C, et al. Comparison of leukocyte and platelet contamination in red cell concentrates prepared either by filtration or by cryopreservation. ISBT/AABB Joint Meeting, Los Angeles, CA, Nov 10–15, 1990, p. 11.
93. Murphy MF, Grint PCA, Hardiman AE, Lister TA, Waters AH. Use of leucocyte-poor blood components to prevent primary cytomegalovirus (CMV) infection in patients with acute leukaemia (letter). Br J Haematol 1988;70:253–254.
94. de Graan-Hentzen YCE, Gratama JW, Mudde GC, et al. Prevention of primary cytomegalovirus infection in patients with hematologic malignancies by intensive white cell depletion of blood products. Transfusion 1989;29:757–760.
95. Gilbert GL, Hayes K, Hudson IL, James J, The Neonatal Cytomegalovirus Infection Study Group. Prevention of transfusion-acquired cytomegalovirus infection in infants by blood filtration to remove leucocytes. Lancet 1989;1:1228–1231.
96. Andreu G. Rolc of leukocyte depletion in the prevention of transfusion-induced cytomegalovirus infection. Semin Hematol 1991;28(suppl 5):26–31.
97. Adler SP. Cytomegalovirus and transfusions. Transfusion Med Rev 1988;2:235–244.
98. Greenbaum BH. Transfusion-associated graft-versus-host disease: historical perspectives, incidence, and current use of irradiated blood products. J Clin Oncol 1991;9:1889–1902.
99. Huang SW, Amman AJ, Levy RL, et al. Treatment of severe combined immunodeficiency by a small number of pretreated nonmatched marrow cells. Transplantation 1973;15:174–176.
100. Rubinstein A, Radl J, Cottier H. Unusual combined immunodeficiency syndrome exhibiting kappa-lgD paraproteinemia. Residual gut immunity and graft versus host reaction after plasma infusion. Acta Pediatr Scand 1973;62:365–372.
101. Brubaker DB. Human posttransfusion graft-versus-host disease. Vox Sang 1983;45:401–420.
102. von Fliedner V, Higby DJ, Kim U. Graft-versus-host reaction following blood product transfusion. Am J Med 1982;72:951–961.
103. Leitman SF, Holland PV. Irradiation of blood products. Indications and guidelines. Transfusion 1985;25:293–300.
104. Crowley JP, Skrabut EM, Valeri CR. Immunocompetent lymphocytes in previously frozen washed red cells. Vox Sang 1974;26:513–517.
105. Akahoshi M, Takanashi M, Masuda M, et al. A case of transfusion-associated graft-versus-host disease not prevented by white cell-reduction filters. Transfusion 1992;32:169–172.
106. Brubaker DB. Human posttransfusion graft-versus-host disease. Vox Sang 1983;45:401–420.
107. Thomas ED, Storb R, Clift RA, et al. Bone marrow transplantation. N Engl J Med 1975;292:832–843.
108. Valerius NH, Johansen KS, Nielsen OS, Platz P, Rosenkvist J, Sorensen H. Effect of in vitro x-irradiation on lymphocyte and granulocyte function. Scand J Hematol 1981;27:9–18.
109. Button LN, DeWolf WC, Newburger PE, Jacobson MS, Kevy SV. The effects of irradiation on blood components. Transfusion 1981;21:419–426.
110. Anderson KC, Goodnough LT, Sayers M, et al. Variation in blood component irradiation practice: implications for prevention of transfusion-associated graft-versus-host disease. Blood 1991;77:2096–2102.
111. Leitman SF, Holland PV. Irradiation of blood products (letter). Transfusion 1986;26:543.
112. Drobyski W, Thibodeau S, Truitt RL, et al. Third-party-mediated graft rejection and graft-versus-host disease after T-cell-depleted bone marrow transplantation, as demonstrated by hypervariable DNA probes and HLA-DR polymorphism. Blood 1989;74:2285–2294.
113. Moroff G, George VM, Siegl AM, Luban NLC. The influence of irradiation on stored platelets. Transfusion 1986;26:453–456.
114. Rock G, Adams GA, Labow RS. The effects of irradiation on platelet function. Transfusion 1988;28:451–455.
115. Read EJ, Kodis C, Carter CS, Leitman SF. Viability of platelets following storage in the irradiated state. A pair-controlled study. Transfusion 1988;28:446–450.
116. Duguid JKM, Carr R, Jenkins JA, Hutton JL, Lucas GF, Davies JM. Clinical evaluation of the effects of storage time and irradiation on transfused platelets. Vox Sang 1991;60:151–154.
117. Deeg HJ, Graham TC, Gerhard-Miller L. Appelbaum

FR, Schuening F, Storb R. Prevention of transfusion-induced graft-versus-host disease in dogs by ultraviolet irradiation. Blood 1989;74:2592–2595.
118. Appelbaum FR, Meyers JD, Fefer A, et al. Nonbacterial nonfungal pneumonia following marrow transplantation in 100 identical twins. Transplantion 1982;33:265–268.
119. Pecego R, Hill R, Appelbaum FR, et al. Interstitial pneumonitis following autologous bone marrow transplantation. Transplantation 1986;42:515–517.
120. Winston DJ, Ho WG, Young LS, Gale RP. Prophylactic granulocyte transfusions during human bone marrow transplantation. Am J Med 1980;68:893–897.
121. Hersman J, Meyers JD, Thomas ED, Buckner CD, Clift R. The effect of granulocyte transfusions on the incidence of cytomegalovirus infection after allogeneic marrow transplantation. Ann Intern Med 1982; 96:149–152.
122. Meyers JD. Prevention and treatment of cytomegalovirus infection after marrow transplantation. Bone Marrow Transplant 1988;3:95–104.
123. Bowden RA, Sayers M, Flournoy N, et al. Cytomegalovirus immune globulin and seronegative blood products to prevent primary cytomegalovirus infection after marrow transplantation. N Engl J Med 1986; 314:1006–1010.
124. Miller WJ, McCullough J, Balfour HH, et al. Prevention of cytomegalovirus infection following bone marrow transplantation: a randomized trial of blood product screening. Bone Marrow Transplant 1991;7:227–234.
125. Bowden RA, Sayers M, Gleaves CA, Banaji M, Newton B, Meyers JD. Cytomegalovirus-seronegative blood components for the prevention of primary cytomegalovirus infection after marrow transplantation. Considerations for blood banks. Transfusion 1987;27:478–481.
126. Verdonck LF, de Graan-Hentzen YCE, Dekker AW, Mudde GC, de Gast GC. Cytomegalovirus seronegative platelets and leukocyte-poor red blood cells from random donors can prevent primary cytomegalovirus infection after bone marrow transplantation. Bone Marrow Transplant 1987;2:73–78.
127. Bowden RA, Sayers MH, Cays M, Slichter SJ. The role of blood product filtration in the prevention of transfusion associated cytomegalovirus infection after marrow transplant (abstract). Transfusion 1989;29 (suppl):57S.
128. De Witte T, Schattenberg A, van Dijk BA, et al. Prevention of primary cytomegalovirus infection after allogeneic bone marrow transplantation by using leukocyte-poor random blood products from cytomegalovirus-unscreened blood-bank donors. Transplantation 1990;50:964–968.
129. Bowden RA, Slichter SJ, Sayers MH, Mori M, Cays MJ, Meyers JD. Use of leukocyte-depleted platelets and cytomegalovirus-seronegative red blood cells for prevention of primary cytomegalovirus infection after marrow transplant. Blood 1991;78:246–250.
130. Atkinson K. Reconstruction of the haemopoietic and immune systems after marrow transplantation. Bone Marrow Transplant 1990;5:209–226.
131. Atkinson K, Norrie S, Chan P, Zehnwirth B, Downs K, Biggs J. Haemopoietic progenitor cell function after HLA-identical sibling bone marrow transplantation: influence of chronic graft-versus-host disease. Int J Cell Cloning 1986;4:203–220.
132. Arnold R, Schmeiser T, Heit W, et al. Hemopoietic reconstitution after bone marrow transplantation. Exp Hematol 1986;14:271–277.
133. Warkentin PI. Transfusion of patients undergoing bone marrow transplantation. Hum Pathol 1983;14:261–266.
134. Weiden PL, Storb R. Transfusion problems associated with transplantation. Semin Hematol 1981;18:163–176.
135. Atkinson K, Downs K, Ashby M, Dodds A, Concannon A, Biggs J. Recipients of HLA-identical sibling marrow transplants with severe aplastic anemia engraft more quickly, and those with chronic myeloid leukemia more slowly, than those with acute leukemia. Bone Marrow Transplant 1989;4:23–27.
136. Banaji M, Bearman SI, Buckner CD, et al. The effects of splenectomy on engraftment and platelet transfusion requirements in patients with chronic meylogenous leukemia undergoing marrow transplantation. Am J Hematol 1986;22:275–283.
137. Goldman JM, Johnson SA, Anwarul I, Catovsky D, Galton DAG. Haematological reconstitution after autografting for chronic granulocytic leukaemia in transformation: the influence of previous splenectomy. Br J Haematol 1980;45:223–231.
138. Baughn ASJ, Worsley AM, McCarthy DM, et al. Haematological reconstitution and severity of graft-versus-host disease after bone marrow transplantation for chronic-granulocytic leukaemia: the influence of previous splenectomy. Br J Haematol 1984;56:445–454.
139. Helenglass G, Treleaven J, Parikh P, Aboud H, Smith C, Powles R. Delayed engraftment associated with splenomegaly in patients undergoing bone marrow transplantation for chronic myeloid leukaemia. Bone Marrow Transplant 1990;5:247–251.
140. Van Der Lely N, De Witte T, Raemaekers J, Schattenberg A, Haanen C. Anthracyclines added to the conditioning regimen for allogeneic bone marrow transplantation are associated with a slower haematopoietic recovery. Bone Marrow Transplant 1989;4:163–166.
141. Bensinger W, Petersen FB, Banaji M, et al. Engraftment and transfusion requirements after allogeneic marrow transplantation for patients with acute nonlymphocytic leukemia in first complete remission. Bone Marrow Transplant 1989;4:409–414.
142. Reusser P, Fisher LD, Buckner CD, Thomas ED, Meyers JD. Cytomegalovirus infection after autologous bone marrow transplantation: occurrence of cytomegalovirus disease and effect on engraftment. Blood 1990;75:1888–1894.
143. Deeg HJ, Storb R, Thomas ED, et al. Cyclosporine as prophylaxis for graft-versus-host disease: a randomized study in patients undergoing marrow transplantation for acute nonlymphoblastic leukemia. Blood 1985;65:1325–1334.
144. Ringden O, Backman L, Lonnqvist B, et al. A randomized trial comparing use of cyclosporin and methotrexate for graft-versus-host disease prophylaxis on bone marrow transplant recipients with haematological malignancies. Bone Marrow Transplant 1986;1:41–51.
145. Atkinson K, Biggs JC, Ting A, Concannon AJ, Dodds AJ, Pun A. Cyclosporin A is associated with faster engraftment and less mucositis than methotrexate after allogeneic bone marrow transplantation. Br J Haematol 1983;53:265–270.
146. Storb R, Deeg HJ, Farewell V, et al. Marrow transplantation for severe aplastic anemia: methotrexate alone

compared with a combination of methotrexate and cyclosporine for prevention of acute graft-versus-host disease. Blood 1986;68:119–125.
147. Storb R, Deeg HJ, Whitehead, J, et al. Methotrexate and cyclosporine compared with cyclosporine alone for prophylaxis of acute graft versus host disease after marrow transplantation for leukemia. N Engl J Med 1986;314:729–735.
148. Abedi MR, Backman L, Bostrom L, Lindback B, Ringden O. Markedly increased serum erythropoietin levels following conditioning for allogeneic bone marrow transplantation. Bone Marrow Transplant 1990;6:121–126.
149. Young N, Mortimer P. Viruses and bone marrow failure. Blood 1984;63:729–737.
150. Petursson SR, Chervenick PA, Wu B. Megakaryocytopoiesis and granulopoiesis after murine cytomegalovirus infection. J Lab Clin Med 1984;104:381–390.
151. Duncombe AS, Grundy JE, Prentice HG, Brenner MK. IL2 activated killer cells may contribute to cytomegalovirus induced marrow hypoplasia after bone marrow transplantation. Bone Marrow Transplant 1991;7:81–87.
152. Dilloo D, Josting A, Burdach S. CMV infection modulates interleukin-6 production in human bone marrow stroma cells. Bone Marrow Transplant 1991;7(suppl 2):152.
153. Simmons P, Kaushansky K, Torok-Storb B. Mechanisms of cytomegalovirus-mediated myelosuppression: Perturbation of stromal cell function versus direct infection of myeloid cells. Proc Natl Acad Sci USA 1990;87:1386–1390.
154. Sing GK, Ruscetti FW. Preferential suppression of myelopoiesis in normal human bone marrow cells after in vitro challenge with human cytomegalovirus. Blood 1990;75:1965–1973.
155. Wingard JR, Chen DYH, Burns DWH, et al. Cytomegalovirus infection after autologous bone marrow transplantation with comparison to infection after allogeneic bone marrow transplantation. Blood 1988; 71:1432–1437.
156. Verdonck LF, de Gast GC, van Heugten HG, Nieuwenhuis HK, Dekker AW. Cytomegalovirus infection causes delayed platelet recovery after bone marrow transplantation. Blood 1991;78:844–848.
157. Winston DJ, Ho WG, Champlin RE. Ganciclovir and intravenous immunoglobulin in bone marrow transplants. In: Champlin RE, Gale RP, eds. New strategies in bone marrow transplantation. New York: Wiley-Liss, 1991:337–348.
158. Somadossi JP, Carlisle R. Toxicity of 3′-azido-3′-deoxythymidine and 9-(1,3-dihydroxy-2-propoxymethyl)guanine for normal human hematopoietic progenitor cells in vitro. Antimicrob Agents Chemother 1987;31:452–454.
159. Appelbaum FR, Meyer JD, Deeg JC, Graham T, Schuening F, Storb R. Prophylactic 9-[2-hydroxy-1-(hydroxymethyl)ethoxymethyl]guanine (ganciclovir) following marrow transplantation in dogs: a toxicity trial. Antimicrob Agents Chemother 1988;32:271–273.
160. Shepp DH, Dandliker PS, De Miranda P, et al. Activity of 9-[2-hydroxy-1-(hydroxymethyl)ethoxymethyl]-guanine (BW 759U) in the treatment of cytomegalovirus pneumonia. Ann Intern Med 1985;103:368–373.
161. Deeg HJ, Meyers JD, Storb R, Graham TC, Weiden PL. Effect of trimethoprimsulfamethoxazole on hematological recovery after total body irradiation and autologous marrow infusion in dogs. Transplantation 1979;28:243–246.
162. First LR, Smith BR, Lipton J, Nathan DG, Parkman R, Rappeport JM. Isolated thrombocytopenia after allogeneic bone marrow transplantation: existence of transient and chronic thrombocytopenic syndromes. Blood 1985;65:368–374.
163. Meyers JD, Wade JC, Mitchell CD, et al. Multicenter collaborative trial of intravenous acyclovir for the treatment of mucocutaneous herpes simplex virus infection in the immunocompromised host. Am J Med 1982;73:229–235.
164. Schey SA, Kay HEM. Myelosuppression complicating cotrimoxazole prophylaxis after bone marrow transplantation. Br J Haematol 1984;56:179–180.
165. Neftel KA, Hauser SP, Muller MR. Inhibition of granulopoiesis in vivo and in vitro by beta-lactam antibiotics. J Infect Dis 1985;152:90–98.
166. McCullough J, Lasky LC, Warkentin PI. Role of the blood bank in bone marrow transplantation. In: McCullough J, Sandler SF, eds. Advances in immunobiology: blood cell antigens and bone marrow transplantation. New York: Alan R. Liss, 1984:379–412.
167. Hershko C, Gale RP, Ho W, Fitchen J. ABH antigens and bone marrow transplantation. Br J Haematol 1980;44:65–73.
168. Buckner CD, Clift RA, Sanders JE, et al. ABO incompatible marrow transplants. Transplantation 1978;26:233–238.
169. To LB, Roberts MM, Haylock DN, et al. Comparison of haematological recovery times and supportive care requirements of autologous recovery phase peripheral blood stem cell transplants, autologous bone marrow transplants, and allogeneic bone marrow transplants. Bone Marrow Transplant 1992;9:277–284.
170. Ferrant A, Doyen C, Delannoy A, et al. Allogeneic or autologous bone marrow transplantation for acute non-lymphocytic leukemia in first remission. Bone Marrow Transplant 1991;7:303–309.
171. To LB, Haylock DN, Dyson PG, Thorp D, Roberts MM, Juttner CA. An unusual pattern of hemopoietic reconstitution in patients with acute myeloid leukemia transplanted with autologous recovery phase peripheral blood. Bone Marrow Transplant 1990;6: 109–114.
172. Lopez M, Mortel O, Pouillart P, et al. Acceleration of hemopoietic recovery after autologous bone marrow transplantation by low doses of peripheral blood stem cells. Bone Marrow Transplant 1991;7:173–181.
173. Lobo F, Kessinger A, Landmark JD, et al. Addition of peripheral blood stem cells collected without mobilization techniques to transplanted autologous bone marrow did not hasten marrow recovery following myeloablative therapy. Bone Marrow Transplant 1991;8: 389–392.
174. Sheridan WP. The role of colony-stimulating factors in bone marrow transplantation. Cancer Invest 1991; 9:221–228.
175. Inwards D, Kessinger A. Peripheral blood stem cell transplantation: historical perspective, current status, and prospects for the future. Transfus Med Rev 1992;6:183–190.
176. Kessinger A, Armitage JO. The evolving role of autologous peripheral stem cell transplantation following high-dose therapy for malignancies. Blood 1991;77: 211–213.
177. Beatty PG, Clift RA, Mickelson EM, et al. Marrow

transplantation from related donors other than HLA-identical siblings. N Engl J Med 1985;313:765–771.

178. Beatty PG, Hansen JA, Longton GM, et al. Marrow transplantation from HLA-matched unrelated donors for treatment of hematologic malignancies. Transplantation 1991;51:443–447.

179. Wulff JC, Santner TJ, Storb R, et al. Transfusion requirements after HLA-identical marrow transplantation in 82 patients with aplastic anemia. Vox Sang 1983;44:366–374.

180. Petz LD, Yam P, Wallace RB, et al. Mixed hematopoietic chimerism following bone marrow transplantation for hematologic malignancies: incidence, characterization, and implications for GVHD and leukemia relapse. In: Gale RP, Champlin R, eds. Progress in bone marrow transplantation. New York: Alan R. Liss, 1987:121–134.

181. Ginsburg D, Antin JH, Smith BR, et al. Origin of cell populations after bone marrow transplantation. Analysis using DNA sequence polymorphisms. J Clin Invest 1985;75:596–603.

182. Hill RS, Peterson FB, Storb R, et al. Mixed hematologic chimerism after allogeneic marrow transplantation for severe aplastic anemia is associated with a higher risk of graft rejection and a lessened incidence of acute graft-versus-host disease. Blood 1986;67:811–816.

183. Walker H, Singer CRJ, Patterson J, et al. The significance of host haemapoietic cells detected by cytogenetic analysis of bone marrow from recipients of bone marrow transplants. Br J Haematol 1986;62: 385–391.

184. Buckner CD, Clift RA. Prophylaxis and treatment of infection of the immunocompromised host by granulocyte transfusions. Clin Hematol 1984;13:557–572.

185. Bensinger WI, Price TH, Dale DC, et al. Daily G-CSF administration in normal granulocyte donors undergoing leukapheresis (abstract). Blood 1992;80(suppl 1):291a.

186. Schiffer CA, Aisner J, Daly PA, Schimpff SC, Wiernik PH. Alloimmunization following prophylactic granulocyte transfusion. Blood 1979;54:766–774.

187. Clift RA, Sanders JE, Thomas ED, et al. Granulocyte transfusions for the prevention of infection in patients receiving bone marrow transplants. N Engl J Med 1978;298:1052–1057.

188. Petersen FB, Buckner CD, Clift RA, et al. Laminar air flow isolation and decontamination: a prospective randomized study of the effects of prophylactic systemic antibiotics in bone marrow transplant patients. Infection 1986;14:115–121.

189. Storb R, Weiden PL. Transfusion problems associated with transplantation. Semin Hematol 1981;18:163–176.

190. Klumpp TR. Immunohematologic complications of bone marrow transplantation. Bone Marrow Transplant 1991;8:159–170.

191. Minchinton RM, Waters AH. The occurrence and significance of neutrophil antibodies. Br J Haematol 1984;56:521–528.

192. Koeppler H, Goldman JM. 'Auto'-immune neutropenia after allogeneic bone marrow transplantation unresponsive to conventional immunosuppression but resolving promptly after splenectomy. Eur J Haematol 1988;41:182–185.

193. Adams JA, Gordon AA, Jiang YZ, et al. Thrombocytopenia after bone marrow transplantation for leukaemia: changes in megakaryocyte growth and growth-promoting activity. Br J Haematol 1990;75:195–201.

194. de Alarcon PA, Schmieder JA, Gingrich R, Klugman MP. Pattern of response of megakaryocyte colony-stimulating activity in the serum of patients undergoing bone marrow transplantation. Exp Hematol 1988;16:316–319.

195. Fauser AA, Kanz L. Spurll GM, Lohr GW. Megakaryocytic colony-stimulating activity in patients receiving a marrow transplant during hematopoietic reconstitution. Transplantation 1988;46:543–547.

196. Miura M, Jackson CW, Steward SA. Increase in circulating megakaryocyte growth-promiting activity (Meg-GPA) following sublethal irradiation is not related to decreased platelets. Exp Hematol 1988;16:139–144.

197. Minchinton RM, Waters AH. Autoimmune thrombocytopenia and neutropenia after bone marrow transplantation (letter). Blood 1985;66:752.

198. Bierling P, Vernant JP, Cordonnier C, et al. Platelet associated IgG after BMT for acute leukaemia (abstract). Exp Hem 1983;11(suppl 13):15.

199. Gmur J, Burger J, von Felten A. Autoimmune thrombocytopenia following allogeneic bone marrow transplantation: a pilot study. Bone Marrow Transplant 1986;1(suppl 1):171–172.

200. Minchinton RM, Waters AH, Malpas JS, Gordon-Smith EC, Barrett AJ. Selective thrombocytopenia and neutropenia occurring after bone marrow transplantation—evidence of an auto-immune basis. Clin Lab Haematol 1984;6:157–163.

201. Katayama N, Oda K, Furuta I, et al. Autoimmune thrombocytopenia after allogeneic bone marrow transplantation: a case report. Acta Haematol Jpn 1988;51: 137–141.

202. Spruce W, Forman S, McMillan R, Farbstein M, Turner M, Blume K. Idiopathic thrombocytopenic purpura following bone marrow transplantation. Acta Haematol 1983;69:47–51.

203. Bierling P, Cordonnier C, Fromont P, et al. Acquired autoimmune thrombocytopenia after allogeneic bone marrow transplantation. Br J Haematol 1985;59:643–646.

204. Benda H, Panzer S, Kiefel V, et al. Identification of the target platelet glycoprotein in autoimmune thrombocytopenia occurring after allogeneic bone marrow transplantation. Blut 1989;58:151–153.

205. McMillan R, Tani P, Millard F, Berchtold P, Renshard L, Woods VL. Platelet-associated and plasma anti-glycoprotein autoantibodies in chronic ITP. Blood 1987;70:1040–1045.

206. Bashey A, Owen I, Lucas GF, et al. Late onset immune pancytopenia following bone marrow transplantation. Br J Haematol 1991;78:268–274.

207. Klumpp TR, Caliguri MA, Rabinowe SN, Soiffer RJ, Murray C, Ritz J. Autoimmune pancytopenia following allogeneic bone marrow transplantation. Bone Marrow Transplant 1990;6:445–447.

208. Kaplan C, Morinet F, Cartron J. Virus-induced autoimmune thrombocytopenia and neutropenia. Semin Hematol 1992;29:34–44.

209. Cahn JY, Chabot J, Esperou H, Flesch M, Plouvier E, Herve P. Autoimmune-like thrombocytopenia after bone marrow transplantation (letter). Blood 1989;74: 2771.

210. Vilmer E, Mazeron MC, Rabian C, et al. Clinical significance of cytomegalovirus viremia in bone marrow transplantation. Transplantation 1985;40:30–35.

211. Sullivan KM. Acute and chronic graft-versus-host disease in man. Int J Cell Cloning 1986;4(suppl 1): 42–93.

212. Sullivan KM, Witherspoon RP, Storb R, et al. Alternating-day cyclosporine and prednisone for treatment of high risk chronic graft-versus-host disease. Blood 1988;72:555–561.
213. Atkinson K, Norrie S, Chan P, Zehnwirth B, Downs K, Biggs JC. Hemopoietic progenitor cell function after HLA-identical sibling bone marrow transplantation: influence of chronic graft-versus-host disease. Int J Cell Cloning 1986;4:203–220.
214. Anasetti C, Rybka W, Sullivan M, Banaji M, Slichter SJ. Graft-*v*-host disease is associated with autoimmune-like thrombocytopenia. Blood 1989;73:1054–1058.
215. Panzer S, Kiefel V, Bartram CR, et al. Immune thrombocytopenia more than a year after allogeneic marrow transplantation due to antibodies against donor platelets with anti-PL^{A1} specificity: evidence for a host-derived immune reaction. Br J Haematol 1989;71:259–264.
216. Brand A, Claas FHJ, Falkenburg JHF, van Rood JJ, Eernisse JG. Blood component therapy in bone marrow transplantation. Semin Hematol 1984;21:141–155.
217. Avalos BR, Copelan EA, Tutschka PJ. Consumptive coagulopathy in cyclosporine treated recipients of HLA matched bone marrow grafts (abstract). Blood 1984;64(suppl1):209a.
218. Torok-Storb B, Simmons P, Volterelli J, Przepiorka D, Sandell L, Johnson G. Mechanisms of marrow graft failure. Bone Marrow Transplant 1988;3(suppl 1):15–17.
219. Shulman H, Striker G, Deeg HJ, Kennedy M, Storb R, Thomas ED. Nephrotoxicity of cyclosporin A after allogeneic marrow transplantation. Glomerular thromboses and tubular injury. N Engl J Med 1981;305: 1392–1395.
220. Marsa-Vila L, Gorin NC, Laporte JP, et al. Prophylactic heparin does not prevent liver veno-occlusive disease following autologous bone marrow transplantation. Eur J Haematol 1991;47:346–354.
221. Atkinson K, Biggs JC, Hayes J, et al. Cyclosporin A associated nephrotoxicity in the first 100 days after allogeneic bone marrow transplantation: three distinct syndromes. Br J Haematol 1983;54:59–67.
222. Chappell ME, Keeling DM, Prentice HG, Sweny P. Haemolytic uraemic syndrome after bone marrow transplantation: an adverse effect of total body irradiation? Bone Marrow Transplant 1988;3:339–347.
223. Holler E, Kolb HJ, Hiller E, et al. Microangiopathy in patients on cyclosporine prophylaxis who developed acute graft-versus-host disease after HLA-identical bone marrow transplantation. Blood 1989;73:2018–2024.
224. Juckett M, Perry EH, Daniels BS, Weisdorf DJ. Hemolytic uremic syndrome following bone marrow transplantation. Bone Marrow Transplant 1991;7:405–409.
225. Silva VA, Frei-Lahr D, Brown RA, Herzig GP. Plasma exchange and vincristine in the treatment of hemolytic uremic syndrome/thrombotic thrombocytopenic purpura associated with bone marrow transplantation. J Clin Apheresis 1991;6:16–20.
226. Sullivan KM, Kopecky KJ, Jocom J, et al. Immunodulatory and antimicrobial efficacy of intravenous immunoglobulin in bone marrow transplantation. N Engl J Med 1990;323:705–712.
227. Klingemann HG, Self S, Banaji M, et al. Refractoriness to random donor platelet transfusions in patients with aplastic anaemia: a multivariate analysis of data from 264 cases. Br J Haematol 1987;66:115–121.
228. Dunstan RA, Simpson MB, Rosse WF. Le^a blood group antigen on human platelets. Am J Clin Pathol 1985;83:90–94.
229. Dunstan RA, Simpson MB, Rosse WF. Presence of I/i antigen system on human platelets. Am J Clin Pathol 1984;82:74–77.
230. Dunstan RA, Simpson MB, Rosse WF. Presence of P blood group antigens on human platelets. Am J Clin Pathol 1985;83:731–735.
231. Aster RH. Effect of anticoagulant and ABO incompatibility on recovery of transfused human platelets. Blood 1965;26:732–743.
232. Duquesnoy RJ, Anderson AJ, Tomasulo PA, Aster RH. ABO compatibility and platelet transfusions of alloimmunized thrombocytopenic patients. Blood 1979;54: 595–599.
233. Heal JM, Blumberg N, Masel D. An evaluation of crossmatching, HLA, and ABO matching for platelet transfusions to refractory patients. Blood 1987;70:23–30.
234. Brand A, Sintnicolaas K, Claas FHJ, Eernisse JG. ABH antibodies causing platelet transfusion refractoriness. Transfusion 1986;26:463–466.
235. Svejgaard A, Kissmeyer-Nielsen F, Thorsby E. HL-A typing of platelets. In: Terasaki PI, ed. Histocompatibility testing 1970. Copenhagen, The Netherlands: Munksgaard, 1970:153–164.
236. Duquesnoy RJ, Filip DJ, Tomasulo PA, et al. Role of HLA-C matching in histocompatible platelet transfusion therapy of alloimmunized thrombocytopenic patients. Transplant Proc 1977;9:1827–1828.
237. van Rood JJ, van Leeuwen A, Keuning JJ, et al. The serological recognition of the human MLC determinants using a modified cytotoxicity technique. Tissue Antigens 1975;5:73–79.
238. Yankee RA, Grumet FC, Rogentine GN. Platelet transfusion therapy. The selection of compatible donors for refractory patients by lymphocyte HLA typing. N Engl J Med 1969;281:1208–1212.
239. Yankee RA, Graff KS, Dowling R, et al. Selection of unrelated compatible platelet donors by lymphocyte HL-A matching. N Engl J Med 1973;288:760–764.
240. Duquesnoy RJ, Filip DJ, Rodey GE, Rimm AA, Aster RH. Successful transfusion of platelets "mismatched" for HLA antigens to alloimmunized thrombocytopenic patients. Am J Hematol 1977;2:219–226.
241. Slichter SJ, Teramura G. Frequency of platelet-specific alloantibodies in platelet refractory thrombocytopenic patients (abstract). Blood 1988;72(suppl 1):286a.
242. Schiffer CA. Management of patients refractory to platelet transfusion—an evaluation of methods of donor selection. Prog Hematol 1987;15:91–113.
243. McFarland JG, Anderson AJ, Slichter SJ. Factors influencing the transfusion response to HLA-selected apheresis donor platelets in patients refractory to random platelet concentrates. Br J Haematol 1989;73:380–386.
244. Kickler TS, Nedd PM, Braine HG. Platelet crossmatching. A direct approach to the selection of platelet transfusions for the alloimmunized thrombocytopenic patient. Am J Clin Pathol 1988;90:69–72.
245. Rachel JM, Summers TC, Sinor LT, Plapp FV. Use of a solid phase red blood cell adherence method for pretransfusion platelet compatibility testing. Am J Clin Pathol 1988;90:63–68.
246. Freedman J, Hooi C, Garvey MB. Prospective platelet crossmatching for selection of compatible random donors. Br J Haematol 1984;56:9–18.
247. Freedman J, Garvey MB, Salomon de Friedberg Z, et

al. Random donor platelet crossmatching: comparison of four platelet antibody detection methods. Am J Hematol 1988;28:1–7.

248. O'Connell BA, Schiffer CA. Donor selection for alloimmunized patients by platelet crossmatching of random-donor platelet concentrates. Transfusion 1990; 30:314–317.

249. Freedman J, Gafni A, Garvey MB, Blanchette V. A cost-effectiveness evaluation of platelet crossmatching and HLA matching in the management of alloimmunized thrombocytopenic patients. Transfusion 1989;29:201–207.

250. Kekomaki R, Elfenbein G, Gardner R, Graham-Pole J, Mehta P, Gross S. Improved response of patients refractory to random-donor platelet transfusions by intravenous gamma globulin. Am J Med 1984;76:199–203.

251. Kickler T, Braine HG, Piantadosi S, et al. A randomized, placebo-controlled trial of intravenous gammaglobulin in alloimmunized thrombocytopenic patients. Blood 1990;75:313–316.

252. Ziegler ZR, Shadduck RK, Rosenfeld CS, et al. High-dose intravenous gamma globulin improves responses to single-donor platelets in patients refractory to platelet transfusion. Blood 1987;70:1433–1436.

253. Zeigler ZR, Shadduck RK, Rosenfeld CS, et al. Intravenous gamma globulin decreases platelet-associated IgG and improves transfusion responses in platelet refractory states. Am J Hematol 1991;38:15–23.

254. Knupp C, Chamberlain JK, Raab SO. High-dose intravenous gamma globulin in alloimmunized platelet transfusion recipients (letter). Blood 1985;65:776.

255. Lee EJ, Norris D, Schiffer CA. Intravenous immune globulin for patients alloimmunized to random donor platelet transfusion. Transfusion 1987;27:245.

256. Schiffer CA, Hogge DE, Aisner J, et al. High-dose intravenous gammaglobulin in alloimmunized platelet transfusion recipients. Blood 1984;64:937–940.

257. Bensinger WI, Buckner CD, Clift RA, et al. Plasma exchange for platelet alloimmunization. Transplantation 1986;41:602–605.

258. Bartholomew JR, Salgia R, Bell WR. Control of bleeding in patients with immune and nonimmune thrombocytopenia with aminocaproic acid. Arch Intern Med 1989;149:1959–1961.

259. Gardner FH, Helmer RE. Aminocaproic acid. Use in control of hemorrhage in patients with amegakaryocytic thrombocytopenia. JAMA 1980;243:35–37.

260. Garewal HS, Durie BGM. Anti-fibrinolytic therapy with aminocaproic acid for the control of bleeding in thrombocytopenic patients. Scand J Haematol 1985; 35:497–500.

261. Gallardo RL, Gardner FH. Antifibrinolytic therapy for bleeding control during remission induction for acute leukemia (abstract). Blood 1983;62(suppl 1):202a.

262. Schiffer CA, Lee EJ, Ness PM, Reilly J. Clinical evaluation of platelet concentrates stored for one to five days. Blood 1986;67:1591–1594.

263. Snyder EL, Ezekowitz M, Aster R, et al. Extended storage of platelets in a new plastic container. II. In vivo response to infusion of platelets stored for 5 days. Transfusion 1985;25:209–214.

264. Hogge DE, Thompson BW, Schiffer CA. Platelet storage for 7 days in second-generation blood bags. Transfusion 1986;26:131–135.

265. Lazarus HM, Herzig RH, Warm SE, Fishman DJ. Transfusion experience with platelet concentrates stored for 24 to 72 hours at 22°C. Transfusion 1982;22:39–43.

266. Peter-Salonen K, Bucher U, Nydegger UE. Comparison of posttransfusion recoveries achieved with either fresh or stored platelet concentrates. Blut 1987;54: 207–212.

267. Skodlar J, Bolgiano D, Teramura G, Slichter SJ. Distinguishing between mechanisms of platelet refractoriness: abnormal post-storage platelet viability vs immune destruction (abstract). Blood 1992;80 (suppl 1):260a.

268. Bishop JF, McGrath K, Wolf MM, et al. Clinical factors influencing the efficacy of pooled platelet transfusions. Blood 1988;71:383–387.

269. Bishop JF, Matthews JP, McGrath K, Yuen K, Wolf MM, Szer J. Factors influencing 20-hour increments after platelet transfusion. Transfusion 1991;31:392–396.

270. Rio B, Andreu G. Nicod A, et al. Thrombocytopenia in venocclusive disease after bone marrow transplantation or chemotherapy. Blood 1986;67:1773–1776.

271. Brugieres L, Hartmann O, Benhamou E, et al. Veno-occlusive disease of the liver following high-dose chemotherapy and autologous bone marrow transplantation in children with solid tumors: incidence, clinical course and outcome. Bone Marrow Transplant 1988;3:53–58.

Chapter 23
Cryopreservation of Hematopoietic Stem Cells

Patrick J. Stiff

The ability to cryopreserve living tissues successfully was first reported in 1949 (1), with the recovery of viable sperm frozen in glycerol. Shortly thereafter, red cells were successfully cryopreserved (2) and, in 1955, hematopoietic stem cells (3). These studies led to the first autologous bone marrow transplantation (BMT) trials, which were reported in 1958 (4). Although cryopreservation methods were easily adapted to human marrow, these early trials did not verify the ability to cryopreserve and store hematopoietic stem cells successfully because the pretransplant preparative regimens used were not sufficiently myeloablative (4–8). It was not until the late 1970s that the cryobiological techniques developed 20 years earlier were finally proven to be effective (9,10). Since then, very little has changed in basic marrow cryopreservation storage and thawing techniques, although refinements have made them less cumbersome and thus more widely available. Collection, cryopreservation, storage, and reinfusion of sufficient hematopoietic stem cells to re-establish hematopoiesis following lethal marrow injury now permits curative therapy for patients with hematological malignancies, as well as Hodgkin's disease and non-Hodgkin's lymphoma. The only limitations of autologous BMT are that the marrow be collected at a time when there is little or no risk of tumor contamination and prior to excessive damage to normal stem cells by previous marrow-toxic therapy. With more effective preparative regimens, the list of indications for autologous BMT continues to grow and now includes selected patients with solid tumors.

Cryobiological Fundamentals

Cryopreservation of hematopoietic stem cells allows long-term preservation of these cells by suspending the biochemical processes that are critical for their growth and differentiation. The adverse factors associated with cryopreservation—the physical damage caused by intracellular ice crystal formation and the toxic effects of a high intracellular solute concentration that develops during freezing—must be overcome to assure that the thawed cells will be capable of restoring hematopoiesis.

The exact sequence of events during freezing and thawing of cells and the precise mechanism of action of cryoprotectants remain somewhat controversial(11–14). Cells in a suspension should begin to freeze at the freezing point of water that contains physiological concentrations of solutes, −0.6°C. Freezing of cells in suspension begins initially in the extracellular space, however, only when the temperature reaches −10°C, which is the temperature that ice crystal nidus formation begins (15). The suspension between these temperatures is thus "supercooled." Intracellular freezing does not begin until the temperatures are lowered further, possibly even below −40°C (16). This difference in intracellular versus extracellular freezing point temperature is presumably due to multiple factors, including the ability of the cell wall to withstand penetration by extracellular ice crystals; the increasing intracellular solute load that occurs during extracellular freezing, which lowers the freezing point; and the very small intracellular fluid volume. If the temperatures are lowered either extremely rapidly or slowly, irreversible damage to the cells occurs by different mechanisms (11).

The rate at which cells in suspension are frozen appears to be critical to the survival of the cells when thawed. If the suspension is frozen rapidly, intracellular ice crystals form, which damage organelles and penetrate the cell wall, causing lysis and subsequently death of the cell when thawed (17). Conversely, if the cell suspension is frozen too slowly, the freezing of the water in the extracellular compartment leads to an increase in extracellular fluid osmolarity, causing an osmotic efflux of water from the "supercooled" cell. As the extracellular water continues to freeze, the cell becomes progressively more dehydrated, increasing its solute load. If this increase in intracellular osmolarity occurs before the cell freezes, it can be lethal, due to acid-based and biochemical disturbances as well as cell wall damage caused by excessive cell shrinkage (18).

In addition to cellular damage due to ice and high solute concentrations, during the transition of the extracellular fluid space from liquid to solid, heat is released (heat of fusion), which is also capable of producing cellular damage. This release of heat leads to a disruption of the freezing curve that persists until the entire extracellular fluid space is completely frozen. A one-minute duration for the phase change appears optimal for cryopreservation of hematopoietic stem cells (19,20). However, prolongation of this transitional phase from one to as long as 16 minutes appears to be tolerable, as measured by pluripotent stem-cell assays and the ability of hematopoietic stem cells to reconstitute hematopoiesis after lethal marrow injury (19,21–24).

For every cell type there is an "ideal" cooling rate, as depicted by an inverted "U" diagram, which is somewhere between the two freezing rate extremes (Figure 23-1). At this ideal rate, and usually with the aid of a cryoprotective agent, intracellular contents become only mildly dehydrated, such that when intracellular ice crystals do eventually form, they are not of sufficient size to cause organelle or cell-wall damage. In addition, freezing at this rate is fast enough to prevent damage from lethal intracellular osmolality. This optimal cooling rate is dependent on cell size and water permeability, which function as independent factors (15,24). Smaller very permeable cells, such as human mature red cells, are most viable when frozen at fast rates, and larger and less permeable cells, such as lymphocytes and hematopoietic stem cells, are optimally frozen at slower freezing rates. Overall hematopoietic stem-cell viability appears optimal when freezing rates are relatively slow and controlled at a constant rate—1°C/minute (controlled-rate freezing) (25–27)—although rates that approximate 3°C/minute without the use of a controlled rate freezer by simple immersion in a −70 to −80°C freezer have been shown to be adequate in clinical trials that use this method (23,28). The cryoprotectant used to preserve the cells, however, may be important in this regard (22,23).

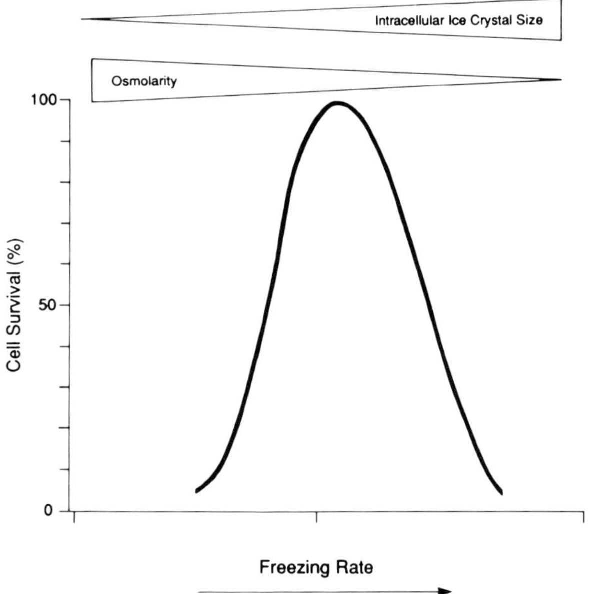

Figure 23-1. Ideal inverted "U" freezing curve. The optimal freezing rate for hematopoietic stem cells is 1°C/min in a cryoprotectant solution. At this rate, intracellular ice crystals are small and cellular dehydration is not damaging.

If the freezing technique is successful in inhibiting all intracellular biochemical processes, storage times appear not to be relevant to stem-cell viability. Storage in the liquid phase of liquid nitrogen (−196°C) appears to maintain viability for up to 10 years (29–32). Storage at higher temperatures, including the vapor phase of liquid nitrogen, has been associated in some studies with a decreased viability for storage periods as short as 9 months (33–35). In animal studies, however, storage temperatures appear to be most important when the marrow dose for transplantation is at or near the minimum required to reconstitute hematopoiesis after lethal marrow damage (29,33,35). Marrow viability as measured by stem-cell assays and by the ability to restore hematopoiesis after lethal marrow injury can be maintained for at least 2 years at temperatures as high as −80°C when the number of cells stored is above the minimum number needed to reconstitute hematopoiesis (23,33,36,37).

As cells are warmed, the intracellular crystals formed during optimal freezing conditions actually increase in size (recrystallization)(38). The growth of these crystals and thus their ability to cause cell damage has been shown to be minimal at rapid rewarming rates (16,25,27). In addition, the damaging high intracellular solute load that develops during the slow 1°C/minute freezing rate is rapidly decreased by this rapid rewarming rate, because dilution of the intracellular contents also occurs at a fast rate.

Cryoprotective Agents

Cryoprotective agents are required to protect most living cells during the freezing process. They act to minimize both the intracellular ice formation and the cellular dehydration that occur during freezing (16,26,39–41). Two classes of drugs provide cryoprotection: low molecular weight molecules, which have the capability to diffuse rapidly into the cell; and high molecular weight molecules, which provide extracellular protection. The first group of agents are the most widely used and include glycerol and dimethylsulfoxide (DMSO). They diffuse into the cell prior to freezing, increasing the intracellular osmolality. For rapid cooling rates, this increased osmolality limits the size and thus the damage caused by intracellular ice crystals. These agents also lead to narrowing of the difference between intracellular and extracellular solute concentrations during slow cooling. This effect decreases the amount of intracellular dehydration that occurs at these slow rates, which protects the intracellular contents from dehydration injury.

For red cells, the first and still most widely used cryoprotectant agent is glycerol (2). It equilibrates rapidly in the red cell and at clinically used concentrations of 40% provides excellent cryoprotection. Although this agent also successfully cryopreserved hematopoietic stem cells in early studies (19,25,34, 35,41–46), it has been replaced by DMSO, which has the advantages of diffusing more rapidly into nucleated marrow cells and does not need to be washed from cell suspensions before infusion (47–53). At concentrations used clinically (10%), DMSO is not toxic to normal stem cells when they are exposed for short periods, and, when infused with unwashed thawed marrow, it usually produces only mild side effects.

Since publication of the early studies using glycerol and DMSO, a number of different classes of drugs have been shown to function as cryoprotective agents, including alcohols, glycols, amides, and high molecular weight polysaccharides. The second main class of cryoprotective agents that has been explored for marrow cryopreservation includes hydroxyethyl starch (HES), polyvinylpyrrolidone (PVP), and dextran, which, unlike DMSO and glycerol, do not cross cell membranes (16,22,54). The exact mechanism by which these extracellular cryoprotectants act is unknown, but it is thought that they form a tight barrier around the cell during freezing, thereby decreasing the amount of cellular dehydration that occurs with the clinically used slow freezing rates (55).

Several studies have demonstrated the utility of using both an extracellular and an intracellular cryoprotectant in combination, and one such method used clinically at many centers involves the use of both DMSO and HES (22,23,56–60). A 5% DMSO, 6% HES mixture was developed initially to cryopreserve granulocytes for transfusion during neutropenic periods (61–63). This combination was shown to cryopreserve granulocytes effectively, with post-thaw recovery rates of 72 to 101% and Trypan blue dye exclusion rates of 72 to 89% in these studies (64). DMSO used alone is not satisfactory for cryopreservation of granulocytes, as the membranes lyse during thawing, releasing nucleoproteins into the surrounding media, which causes agglutination with surrounding cells. These clumps can cause clinical symptoms when infused, including substernal tightness and occasionally some shortness of breath. To prevent this agglutination, most centers that cryopreserve marrow using 10% DMSO alone freeze in 100-mL aliquots and reinfuse rapidly over 10 minutes. Others remove these cells prior to freezing by density centrifugation (65) or add DNAse to the post-thaw suspensions to dissolve the clumps (66). Initial in vitro studies using human unfractionated marrow cryopreserved in 5% DMSO, 6% HES reported a nucleated cell recovery post-thaw of 90 to 100% and Trypan Blue dye exclusion of 80% for cells stored for up to 16 months, demonstrating the recovery of intact granulocytes (22). In addition, there was no macroscopic clumping seen after thaw. Subsequent clinical trials have verified the utility of this cryoprotectant combination (23,60). No visible clumping is seen after thawing, and hematopoietic reconstitution occurs as rapidly as it does for marrow cryopreserved in 10% DMSO alone.

For all cryopreservation methods it appears critical to have a source of protein in the freezing solution (67,68). This protein usually takes the form of residual or added plasma or albumin, which is added prior to the mixing of the cells with the cryoprotectant. Although the exact mechanism for the protein requirement is unknown, it may act by stabilizing cell membranes after thawing (68).

Although DMSO and other nonpolar compounds are effective cryoprotectants, concentrations of DMSO exceeding 1% are toxic to stem cells at temperatures above the freezing point both before and after freezing (69). The mechanism for the efficacy of DMSO at low temperatures appears to be that it is excluded from the hydration shell of proteins at temperatures below the freezing point, which leads to their stabilization. However, at higher temperatures, it interacts with the hydrophobic residues in the proteins, acting to denature or destroy them (70). Therefore, exposure times to DMSO must be brief, with initiation of the freezing process within 10 minutes of the exposure to DMSO, and infusion into patients or dilution to concentrations less than 1% within 10 minutes after thawing.

Cyropreservation Procedure

After collection in a manner identical to that for allogeneic transplantation, marrow that is to be cryopreserved is depleted of red cells either by sedimentation or centrifugation. Red cells are not preserved by current methods, and the hemoglobin load if excessive can cause renal tubular damage. The cells are then generally frozen using one of two methods: the standard method wherein cells are frozen in 10% DMSO, using controlled-rate freezing at 1°C/minute, and stored in liquid nitrogen (9,10,50–52,57,66,71); or a simplified method with cells frozen in 5% DMSO, 6% HES without controlled-rate freezing by placement in a −80°C freezer and storage at −80°C (23).

For the standard method, marrow is often initially centrifuged using a cell separator to eliminate red blood cells. Such processing is not toxic to the stem-cell pool and does not lead to delayed engraftment of any cell line. Most centers adjust cell concentrations to a final concentration of 30 to 40 × 10^6 cells/mL, because concentrations higher than 50 × 10^6 cells/mL seem to be associated with increased cell clumping after thawing. Prior to adding DMSO, the cells are chilled to 4°C to minimize the toxicity of DMSO, which itself can cause denaturation of proteins and cell death if the cells are not cryopreserved within one hour. The cells and the cryoprotectant are mixed at this temperature over a 10-minute period, and the cell/cryoprotectant mixture is placed in 100-mL aliquots into 300-mL polyolefin bags, which are then placed into metal frames. The marrow suspension is frozen as a sheet in the bags with a thickness of less than 5 mm. The frames are placed into the programmed rate-controlled freezer, where the cells are frozen at 1°C/minute until they reach −80 to −100°C, at which point they are transferred to the vapor or liquid phase of liquid nitrogen. Cells are cryopreserved in small aliquots to diffuse the heat of fusion more quickly and to minimize the clinical effects of post-thaw granulocyte clumping and gel formation. A 70-kg patient would have approximately 5 to 8 aliquots of marrow frozen. Polyolefin bags are routinely used, because standard polyvinyl chloride blood bags shatter when thawed after exposure to liquid nitrogen temperatures.

At the time of infusion, the 100-mL aliquots are rapidly warmed by placement into a 37°C water bath and then infused without filtering, not longer than 10 minutes per bag, because visible clumping begins to appear for unfractionated marrow after 20 minutes. Removal of the DMSO prior to infusion is unnecessary; in fact, if granulocytes have not been depleted prior to cryopreservation, washing the cells can actually dramatically increase the degree of cell clumping.

The current practice of rate-controlled freezing is based on early data which used the recovery of murine spleen colony forming units (CFU-S) in 12% glycerol as the determinant of efficacy (19). Although the optimum rate appeared to be 1°C/minute in these studies, increasing the cooling rates after the phase change from 1 to 3°C/minute decreased the CFU-S recovery by only 8%. In addition, increasing the duration of the phase change to 4 and 16 minutes decreased the CFU-S recovery only 16 and 28%. Subsequent studies have demonstrated successful cryopreservation of granulocytes, lymphocytes, and platelets by simple immersion of the cell suspension in a −80°C freezer (i.e., not at a carefully controlled rate of 1°C/min) (61–64,72). This "dump" method of cryopreservation was tested initially for marrow suspensions cryopreserved in 5% DMSO, 6% HES in 1983 (22) and has been shown to be as successful as the rate-controlled method. As shown in Figure 23-2, the average freezing rate for the "dump" method to −80°C is approximately 2 to 3°C/minute. Recently, this nonrate-controlled method was evaluated using only 10% DMSO as the cryoprotectant (28). By keeping the cell volume in the freezing bags at 60 to 70 mL, cell viabilities have been maintained that are equivalent to that for control samples frozen using the traditional method.

Using both DMSO and HES as cryoprotectants permits cryopreservation of larger quantities of marrow per bag because granulocytes are preserved successfully. Marrow cryopreserved in this mixture is depleted of red cells as in the standard method, and the cells reconstituted to a final volume of 300 mL regardless of cell concentration. After chilling to 4°C, an equal volume of the cryoprotectant mixture (10% DMSO, 12% HES, 8% human albumin in a balanced salt solution) is admixed with the cells over a 10-minute period; 300 mL cell/cryoprotectant mixture are then placed into polyolefin bags, which are placed horizontally in freezing frames with a thickness of 1 cm in a −80°C freezer. For long-term storage, after an overnight storage period at −80°, the cells can be placed into a liquid nitrogen freezer.

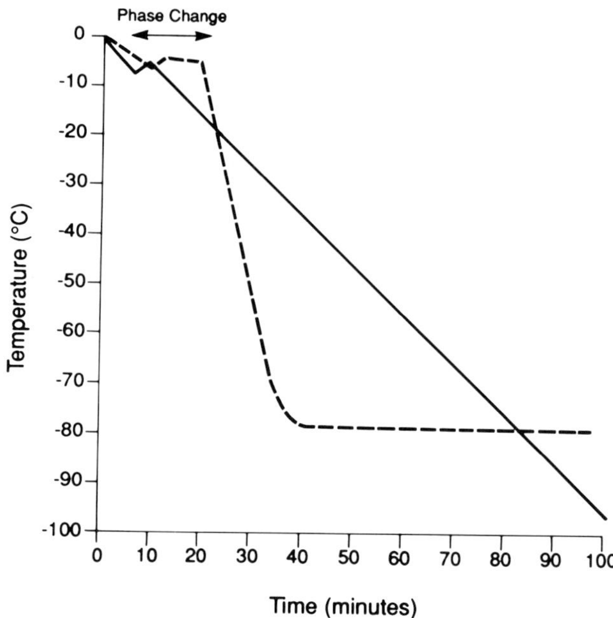

Figure 23-2. Freezing curves for human marrow suspensions: rate-controlled freezing at 1°C/minute (————), and freezing by immersion in a −80°C freezer (-----), with its longer phase change plateau and faster freezing rate.

Although stem-cell recovery after long-term storage in many preclinical studies was shown to be optimal for marrow held at liquid nitrogen temperatures, early animal studies suggested that storage at −79°C for periods up to 6 months did not significantly damage the stem-cell pool. Stem-cell assays have verified that marrow stored at −80°C for at least as long as 2 years has the ability to reconstitute hematopoiesis (73). Longer term storage at this temperature remains untested, largely because the vast majority of patients undergoing autologous BMT do so within 2 years of marrow collection. A comparison of the two methods used clinically to cryopreserve bone marrow for autologous BMT is shown in Table 23-1.

Assessment of Viability of Cryopreserved Marrow

Prior to initiation of large-scale clinical trials, the viability of cryopreserved marrow was assessed using in vitro stem-cell assays and autologous transplants in animals using graded doses of nucleated marrow cells. Unlike for allogeneic BMT, there is currently no biological marker for the engraftment of cryopreserved human marrow. Thus, except for hematopoietic reconstitution after proven lethal marrow injury, there is no good way to demonstrate the viability of cryopreserved marrow. Because the goal is to preserve stem cells that occur at frequencies less than $1/10^4$ in marrow, assays such as histological

Table 23-1.
Comparison of the Two Cryopreservation Methods Used Clinically for Autologous BMT

Cryoprotectant	*10% DMSO*	*5% DMSO/ 6% HES/ 8% HSA*
Freezing rate	1°C/min	Placement in −80°C freezer
Volume/bag	100 mL	300 mL
#of Bags	4–8	2
Storage temperature	−120 to −196°C	−80° or −120 to −196°C
Cell concentrations	30–40 × 10^6	Volume-based[a]
Processing time	4 hr	1.5 hr
Infusion time	10 min	30 min
Advantages	Optimal freezing rate based on in vitro studies Storage for years at −196°C	Quick No clumping Inexpensive
Disadvantages	Time-consuming Expensive Cell clumping	Long-term storage at −80°C not tested

[a]Final volume of 600 mL regardless of cell count.
DMSO = dimethylsulfoxide; HES = hydroxyethyl starch; HSA = human serum albumin.

evaluation or crude assays of viability such as dye exclusion tests are of no value in assessing the efficacy of stem-cell viability.

Initial animal studies focused on the minimum number of nucleated cells needed to reconstitute animals and included studies in rodent, canine, and monkey models (33,36,44,48,74). These studies established that the minimum number of cryopreserved cells needed to reconstitute animals after lethal radiation was 0.25 to 0.5 × 10^8 cells/kg, which was the same as noncryopreserved marrow cells. At these minimum cell doses, engraftment correlated with nucleated cell dose. For human studies, however, the number of nucleated cells routinely autotransplanted does not correlate with engraftment, primarily because most centers have set a minimum of 1.5 to 2.0 × 10^8 cells/kg, or approximately four-fold higher than the minimum in animal studies, as the minimum acceptable for clinical trials. Thus, the loss of up to 75% of the harvested nucleated cells could still lead to consistent engraftment.

Recovery of committed stem cells following cryopreservation has also been studied extensively. In most studies, 50 to 70% of CFU-GM and erythroid burst forming units (BFU-E) are recovered post-thaw (9,36,38,65,66,75–77). Most studies fail to correlate the recovery of these cells with engraftment because these assays do not measure the pluripotent stem-cell pool, and because, as for nucleated cells, a four-fold excess of these cells is usually harvested. In fact, for drug-purged marrow, engraftment still occurs with recoveries of CFU-GM as low as 1 to 5% post-thaw (78). Recoveries may also be artificially low due to technical difficulties in the in vitro assays of thawed cells. For example, concentrations of DMSO greater than 1% are toxic to stem cells assayed using in vitro assays (69), and certain soluble growth factors do not seem to stimulate thawed marrow as well as white cell underlayers. Nevertheless, it is believed that for quality control purposes, these assays should be done both before freezing and after thawing. If CFU-GM and BFU-E recoveries are below 50% for unpurged marrow, or if there are fewer than 10^4 CFU-GM harvested per kg body weight, there may be a problem with the cryopreservation technique that could lead to very slow engraftment after BMT (71).

Several studies have suggested that more primitive stem cells, as measured by various assays, may be useful in predicting engraftment. For example, chemopurged marrow generates the same number of committed stem cells as unpurged bone marrow in long-term marrow cultures using the method developed by Dexter (79). Correlation between engraftment and CFU-GEMM and CFU-D, which measure a more primitive stem-cell pool, has also been described (80,81). With the recent advent of cell surface markers for the multipotential stem-cell population as marked for by CD34, it may be possible to correlate the number of CD34-positive cells with engraftment. Such studies have not been reported.

The only reliable method to determine the viability of cryopreserved human marrow is to evaluate engraftment following BMT. Because this approach is unacceptable in evaluating prospective patients, most transplantation teams use indirect measures of marrow viability in their patient selection, such as a normal preharvest white blood cell (WBC) and platelet counts and a normal preharvest marrow cellularity; they will proceed to transplantation only if they have harvested more than 1.5 × 10^8 nucleated marrow cells/kg, or, as demonstrated in one study, a minimum of 1 × 10^3 CFU-GM/kg (71).

Noncryopreserved Stem-cell Preservation

Due to the expenses in setting up a cryopreservation laboratory and to the fact that long-term storage is not needed for many patients undergoing autologous BMT, several groups have investigated the use of a noncryopreserved, refrigerated technique to store the marrow until the time of infusion (82–86). These studies are based on preclinical evidence that committed stem cells remain viable up to 9 days when held at 4°C (87–89). Several studies report higher CFU-GM recovery after refrigeration for short periods than that typically obtained after cryopreservation (90). Marrow has been stored and infused after refrigeration at 4 to 10°C for periods up to 5 days with evidence of successful engraftment. Times to both WBC and platelet recovery are similar to those of cryopreserved marrow (86). Standard blood collection bags containing either heparin alone or heparin combined with acid citrate dextrose adenine (ACDA) or citrate phosphate dextrose adenine (CPDA) anticoagulants are used to hold the marrow, which is kept in a blood bank refrigerator, until the time of infusion (90,91). Infusions are performed as they would be for fresh marrow. Longer periods are untested; however, preclinical data show a rapid decline in viability after these short periods.

Toxicity of Cryopreserved Stem-cell Infusions

The clinical toxicity related to the infusion of cryopreserved marrow is generally transient and mild. The side effects appear to be related to several factors. The most common side effect in most studies is nausea during the infusion that appears to be related to the infusion of DMSO, which in the nontransplant setting causes nausea related to the taste of the sulfur-containing nature of the drug. Lightheadedness has been reported occasionally (92). Chills, fever, hypertension, bradycardia, shortness of breath, and transient substernal chest tightness are also described and appear to be related to the infusion of lysed mature WBC which were successfully cryopreserved in DMSO alone and formed microaggregates or gels (93,94). These symptoms may also be related to the infusion of bacteria that contaminate the marrow during collection in approximately 15% of patients (94). The number of patients experiencing these side effects varies at different transplant centers; reactions are seen less frequently when marrow is depleted of mature WBC prior to processing (93), or when the marrow is cryopreserved using DMSO/HES (23), which preserves these terminally differentiated cells.

Engraftment Following Cryopreserved Autologous BMT

The only way to determine if any cryopreservation method is successful is to verify its ability to re-establish hematopoiesis following lethal marrow injury. This ability is often difficult because only a few preparative regimens have been proven to be marrow-lethal, and many patients have received marrow-damaging therapy prior to autologous BMT. Engraftment times should approximate those for syngeneic transplants. Engraftment following syngeneic BMT, defined as a granulocyte count greater than 500/μL, is 16 days, and a platelet count greater than 20,000/μL is 19 days (95). Many early autologous BMT studies report engraftment times similar to these syngenic studies; however, the autologous preparative regimens, which did not incorporate radiation, were not completely myeloablative. With the advent of marrow-lethal total body irradiation (TBI)–based regimens, as first reported in 1977 by Dicke and colleagues (96), autologous marrow engraftment times are usually slightly longer than those for syngeneic transplants, presumably due to the fact that most patients undergoing autologous BMT have received significant amounts of prior myelotoxic therapy. Most studies report median recovery times following autologous BMT of 18 to 25 days for granulocyte counts to reach 500/μL and 20 to 35 days for platelets to reach 20,000/μL.

Table 23-2.
Predictors of Delayed Engraftment Following Autologous BMT: Neutrophil Recovery

Factor	*p Value*	*Reference*
CFU-GM < 10^3/kg	<0.05	71
CFU-GEMM <1.4 × 10^4	0.007	81
CFU-D[a]	0.0013	80
Prior platinum chemotherapy	0.002	104
Platinum/mitoxantrone–based preparation regimen	0.014	104
Increasing number of radiotherapy courses	0.045	104

[a]When BCNU or TBI-based preparation regimens were used.

Engraftment times following unpurged autologous BMT vary widely, with a 5 to 10% fatality rate prior to engraftment and a small percentage with delayed engraftment despite the fact that preharvest assays of marrow viability are within normal limits. Platelet engraftment is usually more of a problem than granulocytic recovery. This disproportionate delay in platelet count recovery may be due in part to the smaller percentage of megakaryocytic as compared with myeloid and erythroid progenitor cells surviving following cryopreservation by standard methods (97). However, prior therapy appears to be the most significant factor in delayed engraftment.

Several analyses looking for predictive factors for delayed engraftment following autologous BMT have been completed and are sumarized in Tables 23-2 and 23-3 for granulocytic and platelet recoveries, respectively. Not surprisingly, prior myelosuppressive therapy and its intensity appears to be the most important factor (98–104). Several of these analyses have implicated platinum analogs to be the most important of these agents (102,104). In a recent multivariate analysis of 121 consecutive patients undergoing autologous BMT at a single center, numerous variables were evaluated for delayed engraftment (104). The variables evaluated included nucleated, CFU-GM, and BFU-E cell dose infused; different preparative regimens; the number of prior conventional chemother-

Table 23-3.
Predictors of Delayed Engraftment Following Autologous BMT: Platelet Recovery

Factor	*p Value*	*Reference*
BFU-E < 3 × 10^3	<0.05	71
CFU-GEMM < 8 × 10^3	0.004	81
MNC/kg	0.002	102
Pretreatment albumin level	0.003	102
BM involvement by tumor	0.006	102
Prior cis-platin	0.025	102
Hodgkin's disease	0.003	104
Prior platinum chemotherapy	0.039	104

MNC = mononuclear cells.

apy regimens and duration of prior chemotherapy; prior radiation therapy; prior therapy with platinum compounds; and the percent recovery of committed stem cells after thawing. Engraftment was evaluated 28 and 35 days after transplantation. Factors predicting failure of granulocyte engraftment (count < 500/μL) were prior platinum therapy, and a carboplatinum, mitoxantrone, and cyclophosphamide preparative regimen (relative risk, 12.0 and 17.5, respectively). The latter may have been due to the persistence in vivo of a low yet potentially myelosuppressive concentration of mitoxantrone, which is known to have a long terminal half-life. Predictors of delayed platelet engraftment (count < 20,000/μL) at these time points were also prior platinum therapy, as well as patients undergoing transplantation for Hodgkin's disease, all of whom had received at least mustargen, vincristine, prednisone, procarbazine (MOPP) chemotherapy (relative risk, 3.8 and 14.8, respectively). As in most other studies in which univariate analyses were performed, cell, CFU-GM, and BFU-E doses, as well as percent recovery of committed stem cells post-thaw were not risk factors for delayed engraftment.

There has been no significant difference in the recovery rates of patients whose marrow was cryopreserved using 5% DMSO, 6% HES in single institution studies as compared with 10% DMSO alone (23,60). In a recent trial, of 123 patients there was no difference in engraftment times for 5% DMSO, 6% HES for either granulocytes (16 days) or platelets (17 days) compared to prior patients for 10% DMSO alone (60).

Effect of Cryopreservation on Immune Function and Leukemic Cells

There appears to be no difference in the reconstitution of immune function following autologous versus syngeneic BMT, suggesting that lymphocytes are successfully cryopreserved by current methods. Although cryopreservation of lymphocytes is done mainly for in vitro testing purposes, with the advent of lymphocyte cytokine therapy, cryopreservation of these cells may become important (e.g., to reduce relapses following autologous BMT).

Lymphocytes are usually cryopreserved in 7.5 to 10% DMSO using controlled-rate freezing at 1°C/min (105–107). This method preserves 70 to 80% of the prefreeze cells. These cells can be used in stimulation assays without a significant decrease in function, as compared with fresh cells. The relative number of lymphocyte subsets, including T and B cells, and the response to phytohemagglutin and concanavalin A are little affected by cryopreservation (108–109). Most studies demonstrate a decrease in natural killer (NK) cell function as well as mixed lymphocyte responses for cryopreserved lymphocytes. NK cell recovery is 50 to 70%, as compared with fresh cells; however, this recovery improves if the cells are incubated after thawing for 18 hours prior to assay (109,110). Lymphocyte-activated killer (LAK) cell activity is also reduced in some studies, ranging from 33 to 87% recovery (110,111). Their effectiveness improves to the level of fresh lymphocytes if the cells are incubated with interleukin-2 (IL-2) for several days after thawing. Whereas LAK activity is decreased, IL-2 production appears to be normal or increased for cryopreserved monocyte-depleted mononuclear cells (112).

Leukemic stem-cell viability appears to be decreased after cryopreservation, as compared with CFU-GM and BFU-E (113). The clinical significance of this phenomenon for purging remains to be determined because the assays used to determine leukemic cell viability may only represent a committed stem-cell pool as the CFU-GM/BFU-E pool represents. In addition, only approximately one log of these leukemic clonogenic cells are lost in cryopreservation, which is insufficient in animal models to decrease relapse rates after BMT.

References

1. Polge C, Smith AU, Parkes AS. Revival of spermatozoa after vitrification and dehydration at low temperature. Nature 1949;164:666.
2. Smith AU. Prevention of hemolysis during freezing and thawing of red blood cells. Lancet 1950;2:910.
3. Barnes DWH, Loutit JF. The radiation recovery factor. Preservation by the Polge-Smith-Parkes technique. J Natl Cancer Inst 1954;15:901–905.
4. Kurnick NB, Montano A, Gerdes JC, Feder BH. Preliminary observations on the treatment of postirradiation hematopoietic depression in man by the infusion of stored autogenous bone marrow. Ann Intern Med 1958;49:973–986.
5. Westbury G, Humble JG, Newton KA, Skinner MEG, Pegg DE. Disseminated malignant melanoma. Response to treatment by massive dosage of a cytotoxic agent combined with autogenous marrow replacement. Lancet 1959;1:968–969.
6. McFarland WF, Granville NB, Dameshek W. Autologous bone marrow infusion as an adjunct in therapy of malignant disease. Blood 1959;14:503–521.
7. Clifford P, Clift RA, Duff JK. Nitrogen mustard therapy combined with autologous marrow infusion. Lancet 1961;1:687–690.
8. Meyer LM, Fliedner TD, Cronkite EP. Autologous bone-marrow transfusion following chemotherapy. Ann NY Acad Sci 1964;114:499–509.
9. Dicke KA, McCredie KB, Spitzer G, et al. Autologous bone marrow transplantation in patients with adult acute leukemia in relapse. Transplantation 1978;26: 169–173.
10. Appelbaum FR, Herzig GP, Ziegler JL, Graw RG, Levine AS, Deisseroth AB. Successful engraftment of cryopreserved autologous bone marrow in patients with malignant lymphoma. Blood 1978;52: 85–95.
11. Mazur P. Cryobiology: the freezing of biological systems. Science 1970;168:939–949.
12. Pegg DE. Long term preservation of cells and tissues: a review. J Clin Pathol 1976:29:271–275.
13. Merryman HT. Freezing of living cells: biophysical considerations. NCI Monograph 1961;7:7–15.
14. Merryman HT. Preservation of living cells. Fed Proc 1963;22:81–89.

15. Mazur P. The role of cell membranes in the freezing of yeast and other single cells. Ann NY Acad Sci 1965;124:658–676.
16. Leibo SP, Farrant J, Mazur P, Hanna MG Jr, Smith LH. Effect of freezing on marrow stem cell suspensions: interactions of cooling and warming rates in the presence of PVP, sucrose or glycerol. Cryobiology 1970;6:315–321.
17. Mazur P. The role of intracellular freezing in the death of cells cooled at supraoptimal rates. Cryobiology 1977;14:251–272.
18. Bank H, Mazur P. Relation between ultrastructure and viability of frozen-thawed Chinese hamster tissue-culture cells. Exp Cell Res 1972:71:441–454.
19. Lewis JP, Passovoy M, Trobaugh FE. The effect of cooling regimens on the transplantation potential of marrow. Transfusion 1967;7:17–32.
20. Rowe AW. Biochemical aspect of cryoprotective agents in freezing and thawing. Cryobiology 1966;3:12–18.
21. Foreman J, Pegg DE. Cell preservation in a programmed cooling machine: the effect of variations in supercooling. Cryobiology 1979;16:315–321.
22. Stiff PJ, Murgo AJ, Zaroulis CG, DeRisi MF, Clarkson BD. Unfractionated marrow cell cryopreservation using dimethylsulfoxide and hydroxyethyl starch. Cryobiology 1983;21:17–21.
23. Stiff PJ, Koester AR, Weidner MK, Dvorak K, Fisher RI. Autologous bone marrow transplantation using unfractionated cells cryopreserved in dimethylsulfoxide and hydroxyethyl starch without controlled-rate freezing. Blood 1987;70:974–978.
24. Mazur P. Kinetics of water loss from cells at subzero temperatures and the likelihood of intracellular freezing. J Gen Physiol 1962;47:347–369.
25. Bender MA, Phan TT, Smith LH. Preservation of viable bone marrow cells by freezing. J Appl Physiol 1960; 15:520–524.
26. Leibo SP, Mazur P. The role of cooling rates in low-temperature preservation. Cryobiology 1971;8:447–452.
27. Mazur P. Theoretical and experimental effects of cooling and warming velocity on the survival of frozen and thawed cells. Cryobiology 1966;2:181–192.
28. Clark J, Pati A, McCarthy D. Successful cryopreservation of human bone marrow does not require a controlled rate freezer. Bone Marrow Transplant 1991; 7:121–125.
29. Malinin TI, Pegg DE, Perry VP, Brodine VP. Long term storage of bone marrow cells at liquid nitrogen and dry ice temperatures. Cryobiology 1970;7:65–69.
30. Smith LH, Phan TT. Long term preservation of bone marrow. Nature 1965;205:503–504.
31. O'Grady LF, Lewis JP. The long term preservation of bone marrow. Transfusion 1972;12:312–316.
32. Ashwood-Smith MJ, Friedman GB. Lethal and chromosomal effects of freezing, thawing, storage time and X-irradiation on mammalian cells preserved at −196°C in DMSO. Cryobiology 1979;16:132–140.
33. Appelbaum FR, Herzig GP, Graw RG, Bull MI, Bowles C, Gorin NC, Deisseroth A. Study of cell dose and storage time on engraftment of cryopreserved autologous bone marrow in a canine model. Transplantation 1978;26:245–248.
34. Pegg DE. Cytology of human bone marrow subjected to prolonged storage at −79°C. J Appl Physiol 1964; 19:301–309.
35. Phan TT, Bender MA. Factors affecting survival of mouse bone marrow cells during freezing and thawing in glycerol. J Appl Physiol 1960;15:939–942.
36. Gorin NC, Herzig G, Bull MI, Graw RG Jr. Long-term preservation of bone marrow and stem cell pool in dogs. Blood 1978;51:257–261.
37. Thomas ED, Ferrebee JW. Prolonged storage of marrow and its use in the treatment of radiation injury, short communication. Transfusion 1962;2:115–117.
38. Luyet BJ, Rapatz G. Patterns of ice formation in some aqueous solutions. Biodynamica 1958;8:1–6.
39. Lovelock JE. The mechanism of the protective action of glycerol against haemolysis by freezing and thawing. Biochim Biophys Acta 1953;11:28.
40. Farrant J. Mechanism of cell damage during freezing and thawing and its prevention. Nature 1965;205: 1284–1287.
41. Merryman HT. Cryoprotective agents. Cryobiology 1971;8:173–183.
42. Ferrebee JW, Billen D, Urso IM, Lu WC, Thomas ED, Congdon CC. Preservation of radiation recovery factor in frozen marrow. Blood 1957;12:1096–1105.
43. Kurnick NB, Nokay N, Hamptom B. Survival of frozen stored human and mouse bone marrow cells. Radiat Res 1967;32:706–722.
44. Lewis JP, Trobaugh FE Jr. The assay of the transplantation potential of fresh and stored bone marrow by two in-vivo systems. Ann NY Acad Sci 1964;114: 677–685.
45. O'Grady LF, Lewis JP. Stem cell renewal in frozen bone marrow. Cryobiology 1969;5:250–253.
46. Porter KA, Murray JE. Successful homotransplantation of rabbit bone marrow after preservation in glycerol at −70°C. Cancer Res 1958;18:117–119.
47. Ashwood-Smith MJ. Preservation of mouse bone marrow at −79°C with dimethyl sulfoxide. Nature 1961; 190:1204–1205.
48. Buckner CD, Storb R, Dillingham LA, Thomas ED. Low temperature preservation of monkey marrow in dimethyl sulfoxide. Cryobiology 1970;7:136–140.
49. Storb R, Epstein RB, LeBlond RF, Rudolph RH, Thomas ED. Transplantation of allogeneic canine bone marrow stored at −80°C in dimethyl sulfoxide. Blood 1969;33:918–923.
50. Wells JR, Sullivan A, Cline MJ. A technique for the separation and cryopreservation of myeloid stem cells from human bone marrow. Cryobiology 1979;16:201–215.
51. Weiner RS, Richman CM, Yankee RA. Dilution techniques for optimum recovery of cryopreserved bone marrow cells. Exp Hematol 1979;7:1–7.
52. Parker LM, Binder N, Celman R, Richman CM, Weiner RS, Yankee RA. Prolonged cryopreservation of human bone marrow. Transplantation 1981;31:454–457.
53. Mannick JA, Lochte HL, Thomas ED, Ferrebee JW. In vitro and in vivo assessment of the viability of dog marrow after storage. Blood 1960;15:517–524.
54. Ashwood-Smith MJ, Warby C, Connor KW, Becker G. Low-temperature preservation of mammalian cells in tissue culture with polyvinylpyrrolidone (PVP), dextrans and hydroxyethyl starch (HES). Cryobiology 1972;9:441–449.
55. Takahashi T, Hirsh A, Erbe E, Williams RJ. Mechanisms of cryoprotection by extracellular polymeric solutes. Biophys J 1988;54:509–518.
56. van Putten LM. Quantitative aspects of the storage of bone marrow cells for transplantation. Eur J Cancer 1965;1:15–22.

57. Areman EM, Sacher RA, Deeg HJ. Processing and storage of human bone marrow: a survey of current practices in North America. Bone Marrow Transplant 1990;6:203–209.
58. Gulati SC, Shank B, Blank P, et al. Autologous bone marrow transplantation for patients with poor prognosis lymphoma. J Clin Oncol 1988;6:1303–1313.
59. Makino S, Harada M, Akashi K, et al. A simplified method for cryopreservation of peripheral blood stem cells at −80 degrees C without rate-controlled freezing. Bone Marrow Transplant 1991;8:239–244.
60. Nademanee A, Schmidt GM, Sniecinski I, Forman SJ. Storage of unfractionated bone marrow (BM) without rate-controlled freezing is equivalent to standard technique for short-term storage. Blood 1991;78:251a.
61. Lionetti FJ, Hunt SM, Gore JM, Curby WA. Cryopreservation of human granulocytes. Cryobiology 1975; 12:181–191.
62. Lionetti FJ, Hunt SM, Mattaliano RJ, Valeri CR. In vitro studies of cryopreserved baboon granulocytes. Transfusion 1978;18:685–692.
63. Lionetti FJ, Luscinskas FW, Hunt SM, Valeri CR, Callahan AB. Factors affecting the stability of cryogenically preserved granulocytes. Cryobiology 1980;17: 297–310.
64. Zaroulis CG, Liederman I. Successful freeze-preservation of human granulocytes. Cryobiology 1980; 17:311–317.
65. Wells JR, Sullivan A, Cline MJ. A technique for the separation and cryopreservation of myeloid stem cells from human bone marrow. Cryobiology 1979;16:201–210.
66. Spitzer G, Dicke KA, Litam J, et al. High-dose combination chemotherapy with autologous bone marrow transplantation in adult solid tumors. Cancer 1980;45:3075–3085.
67. Ragab AH, Gilkerson E, Myers M. Factors in the cryopreservation of bone marrow cells from children with acute lymphocytic leukemia. Cryobiology 1977; 14:125–134.
68. Grilli G, Porcellili A, Lucarelli G. Role of serum cryopreservation and subsequent viability of mouse bone marrow hematopoietic stem cells. Cryobiology 1980;17:516–520.
69. Goldman JM, Th'ng KH, Pack DS, Spiers SD, Lowenthal RN, Ruutu T. Collection, cryopreservation and subsequent viability of hematopoietic stem cells intended for the treatment of chronic granulocytic leukemia in blast-cell transition. Br J Hematol 1978;40:185–195.
70. Arakawa T, Carpenter JF, Kita YA, Crowe JH. The basis for toxicity of certain cryoprotectants: a hypothesis. Cryobiology 1990;27:401–415.
71. Gorin NC. Collection, manipulation and freezing of hematopoietic stem cells. Clin Hematol 1986;15:19–48.
72. Schiffer CA, Aisner J, Weirnik PH. Frozen autologous platelets for patients with leukemia. N Engl J Med 1978;299:7–12.
73. Stiff PJ, Dvorak K, Schulz W. A simplified bone marrow cryopreservation method. Blood 1988;71:1102–1103.
74. Gorin NC, Bull MI, Herzig GP, Graw RG. Long term preservation of bone marrow for autologous bone marrow transplantation. Clin Res 1975;23:338a.
75. Grande M, Berthier R, Hollard D. Frozen human bone marrow from normal individuals: a possible control for the culture of human bone marrow in agar. Exp Hematol 1977;5:436–442.
76. Gray JL, Robinson WA. In vitro colony formation by human bone marrow cells after freezing. J Lab Clin Med 1973;81:317–322.
77. Douay L, Gorin NC, David R, et al. Study of granulocyte progenitor (CFUc) preservation after slow freezing of bone marrow in the gas phase of liquid nitrogen. Exp Hematol 1982;10:360–366.
78. Rowley SD, Zuehlsdorf M, Braine HG, et al. CFU-GM content of bone marrow graft correlates with time to hematologic reconstitution following autologous bone marrow transplantation with 4-hydroperoxycyclophosphamide purged bone marrow. Blood 1987;70:271–275.
79. Stiff PJ, Schulz WC, Bishop M, Marks L. Anti-CD33 monoclonal antibody and etoposide/cytosine arabinoside combinations for the ex vivo purification of bone marrow in acute non-lymphocytic leukemia. Blood 1991;77:352–362.
80. Stewart FM, Kaiser DL, Ishitani KP, Pirsch GW, Niskanen E. Progenitor cell numbers (CFU-GM, CFU-D, and CFU-Mix) and hematopoietic recovery following autologous bone marrow transplantation. Exp Hematol 1989;17:974–980.
81. Roodman GD, LeMaistre CF, Clark GM, et al. CFU-GEMM correlate with neutrophil and platelet recovery in patients receiving autologous marrow transplantation after high dose melphalan chemotherapy. Bone Marrow Transplant 1987;2:165–173.
82. Robinson WA, Hartmann DW, Mangalik A, Morton N, Joshi JH. Autologous nonfrozen bone marrow transplantation after intensive chemotherapy: a pilot study. Acta Haematol 1981;66:145–153.
83. Burnett AK, Tansey P, Hills C, et al. Hematological reconstitution following high-dose and supralethal chemo-radiotherapy using stored non-cryopreserved autologous bone marrow. Br J Hematol 1982;54:309–316.
84. Carella AM, Santini G, Santoro A, et al. Massive chemotherapy with non-frozen autologous bone marrow transplantation in 13 cases of refractory Hodgkin's disease. Eur J Cancer Clin Oncol 1985;21:607–613.
85. Cornblut MA, Corringham RET, Prentice HG, Boesen EM, McElwain TJ. Treatment of Ewing's sarcoma with high dose melphalan and autologous bone marrow transplantation. Cancer Treat Rep 1981;65:241–244.
86. Ahmed T, Wuest D, Ciavarella D, et al. Marrow storage techniques: a clinical comparison of refrigeration versus cryopreservation. Acta Hematol 1991;85:173–178.
87. Billen D. Recovery of lethally irradiated mice by treatment with bone marrow cells maintained in vitro. Nature 1957;179:574–575.
88. Wells JR, Cline MJ. Preservation of granulocytic precursors in non-frozen, stored human bone marrow. Transplantation 1976;22:568–571.
89. Kohsaki M, Yanes B, Ungerleider JS, Murphy MJ. Nonfrozen preservation of committed hematopoietic stem cells from normal human bone marrow. Cells 1981; 1:111–123.
90. Delforge A, Ronge-Collard E, Stryckmans P, Spiro T, Malasame MA. Granulocyte-macrophage progenitor cell preservation at 4°C. Br J Haematol 1983;53:49–54.
91. Takahashi M, Singer JW. Effects of marrow storage at 4°C on the subsequent generation of long term cultures. Exp Hematol 1985;13:691–695.
92. Brobyn RD. The human toxicity of dimethyl sulfoxide. Ann NY Acad Sci 1975;243:497–506.
93. Davis JM, Rowley SD, Braine HG, Piantadosi S, Santos GW. Clinical toxicity of cryopreserved bone marrow graft infusion. Blood 1990;75:781–786.

94. Stroncek DF, Fautsch SK, Lasky LC, Hurd DD, Ramsay NKC, McCullough J. Adverse reactions in patients transfused with cryopreserved marrow. Transfusion 1991;31:521–526.
95. Fefer A, Einstein AB, Thomas ED, et al. Bone marrow transplantation for hematologic neoplasia in 16 patients with identical twins. N Engl J Med 1974; 290:1389–1393.
96. Dicke KA, Zander AR, Spitzer G, et al. Autologous bone marrow transplantation in relapsed acute leukemia. Exp Hematol 1979;7(suppl 5):170–187.
97. Fabian I, Douer D, Wells JR, Cline MJ. Cryopreservation of human multipotential stem cell. Exp Hematol 1982;10:119–122.
98. Hartmann O, Beaujean F, Bayet S, et al. Hematopoietic recovery following autologous bone marrow transplantation: role of cryopreservation, number of cells infused and nature of high dose chemotherapy. Eur J Cancer Clin Oncol 1985;21:53–60.
99. Douay L, Gorin NC, Mary JY, et al. Recovery of CFU-GM from cryopreserved marrow and in vivo evaluation after autologous bone marrow transplantation are predictive of engraftment. Exp Hematol 1986;14:358–365.
100. Rowley SD, Piantadosi S, Marcellus DC, et al. Analysis of factors predicting speed of hematologic recovery after transplantation with 4-hydroperoxycyclophosphamide-purged autologous bone marrow grafts. Bone Marrow Transplant 1991;7:183–191.
101. Visani G, Dinota A, Tosi P, et al. Cryopreserved autologous bone marrow transplantation in patients with acute nonlymphoid leukemia: chemotherapy before harvesting is the main factor in delaying hematological recovery. Cryobiology 1990;27:103–106.
102. Mick R, Williams SF, Bitran JD. Patients at increased risk for late engraftment after transplantation; a novel method for their identification. Bone Marrow Transplant 1990;6:185–191.
103. Spitzer G, Verma DS, Fisher R, et al. The myeloid progenitor cell. Its value in predicting hematopoietic recovery after autologous bone marrow transplantation. Blood 1980;55:317–323.
104. Stiff PJ, Fisher SG, McKenzie RS, Koch D, Oldenburg DH. A multivariate analysis of risk factors of delayed engraftment following autologous bone marrow transplantation (ABMT). Blood 1991;78:241a.
105. Goulub SH, Sulit HL, Morton D. The use of viable frozen lymphocytes for studies in human tumor immunology. Transplantation 1975;119:195–202.
106. Sears SF, Rosenberg S. Advantages of cryopreserved lymphocytes for sequential evaluation of human immune competence. 1. Mitogen stimulation. J Natl Cancer Inst 1977;58:183–187.
107. Glassman AB, Bennett CE. Cryopreservation of human lymphocytes: a brief review and evaluation of an automated liquid nitrogen freezer. Transfusion 1979; 19:178–181.
108. Venkataraman M, Westerman MP. Susceptibility of human T cells, T-cell subsets, and B cells to cryopreservation. Cryobiology 1986;23:199–208.
109. Callery CD, Golightly M, Sidell N, Golub SH. Lymphocyte surface markers and cytotoxicity following cryopreservation. J Immunol Methods 1980;35:213–223.
110. Kawai H, Komyama A, Katoh M, Yabuhara A, Miyagawa Y, Akabane T. Induction of lymphocyte-activated killer and natural killer activities from cryopreserved lymphocytes. Transfusion 1988;28:531–535.
111. Schmidt-Wolf IGH, Aihara M, Negrin RS, Blume KG, Chao NJ. Lymphocyte-activated killer cell activity after cryopreservation. J Immunol Methods 1989; 125:185–189.
112. Venkataraman M. Cryopreservation-induced enhancement of interleukin-2 production in human peripheral blood mononuclear cells. Cryobiology 1992;29:167–174.
113. Allieri MA, Lopez M, Douay L, Mary JY, NGuyen L, Gorin NC. Clonogeneic leukemic progenitor cells in acute myelocytic leukemia are highly sensitive to cryopreservation: possible purging effect for autologous bone marrow transplantation. Bone Marrow Transplant 1991;7:101–105.

Chapter 24
Use of Recombinant Growth Factors in Bone Marrow Transplantation

Jack W. Singer and John Nemunaitis

A number of glycoprotein growth regulatory factors that influence the proliferation and differentiation of hematopoietic cells have been identified and molecularly cloned (1–5). Several of these growth factors enhance the rate of marrow recovery after cytotoxic therapy. Three (erythropoietin, granulocyte colony stimulating factor [G-CSF], and granulocyte-macrophage colony stimulating factor [GM-CSF] are currently approved by the Food and Drug Administration for clinical use. Several others are in various stages of clinical trials. Experience with these novel agents in bone marrow transplantation (BMT) is limited and their optimal uses remain undefined. However, their safety profile has been excellent and there has been no data suggesting that any recombinant cytokine has led to an increase in the rates of relapse in recipients of either autologous or allogeneic marrow grafts. The goal of this chapter is to provide a background in the biology of hematopoietic growth factors, to discuss preclinical and clinical studies, and to suggest ways in which currently available and newer agents might be of benefit to patients undergoing BMT.

Regulation of Hematopoietic Cell Production

The hematopoietic system is a highly specialized organ whose primary functions are to deliver oxygen to tissues, to maintain hemostasis, and to respond to infections. Two unique features of the hematopoietic system are critical to an understanding of the biology of both cytokines and BMT: (1) derivation of mature blood cells from relatively small numbers of stem cells that have a life-time capacity for self-renewal, and (2) the ability of stem cells to home, lodge, and proliferate only in bone marrow.

Bone marrow produces approximately 10^{11} mature cells per day, including approximately 2×10^9 granulocytes/kg body weight (6). Despite the need to produce this huge volume of mature cells, the hematopoietic system closely regulates production, such that the concentrations of mature blood cells in circulation are maintained within narrow ranges under basal conditions. In response to stress, the hematopoietic system rapidly expands production of mature cells. Control of maturation of hematopoietic cells is maintained through a complex system of positive and negative regulatory factors termed *cytokines*. The stimulatory cytokines may have a role in maintaining and controlling basal hemopoiesis as well as directing the response to hematopoietic stress. Through amplification of cells produced during stem-cell maturation, the cytokine network allows the hematopoietic system to respond rapidly to perturbations produced by events such as infection or hemolysis. Production of mature cells can be increased within several days by up to 10-fold. This huge increment in output is predominantly due to cytokine-stimulated amplification during maturation of committed progenitors. These committed cells, capable of only a limited number of cell divisions, are derived from small numbers of uncommitted, self-renewing stem cells. Extrapolations from murine studies suggest that there are fewer than 10×10^6 stem cells in an adult; it is likely that fewer than 10% are actively dividing in nonstressed individuals. The remainder are quiescent and are maintained as a reserve pool. With hematopoietic stress, additional stem cells may be recruited by as yet unidentified stimuli to enter the dividing pool.

The existence of hematopoietic stem cells was suggested by the observation that bone marrow cells injected into irradiated mice formed clonal, multilineage colonies in the spleen. Cells from single spleen colonies were able to form additional colonies when injected into secondary recipients, indicating that spleen colony forming cells (CFU-S) were self-renewing (7). Confirmation of the existence of a common murine lymphohematopoietic stem cell capable of reconstituting murine hematopoiesis has come from studies using genetically marked blood cells (8). In vitro clonal assays were later developed that identified progenitor cells capable of producing multilineage colonies (CFU-Mix) or colonies consisting of cells within a single lineage, such as red blood cells (BFU-E), the granulocyte-macrophage lineage (CFU-GM), or the megakaryocyte lineage (CFU-Meg) (9). Growth of hematopoietic colonies in vitro was absolutely dependent on four glycoproteins termed *colony stimulating factors* (CSFs). These factors have been isolated, molecularly cloned, and produced in recombinant form. Their receptors have also been identified and molecularly cloned. The CSFs are granulocyte-CSF (G-CSF), which stimulates growth of granulocyte colonies; granulocyte/macrophage-CSF (GM-CSF), which induces the growth of granulocyte, macrophage, eosinophil, and erythroid colonies; interleukin-3 (IL-3), which stimulates granulocyte/macrophage, eosinophil, erythroid, and megakaryocyte colonies; and macrophage-CSF (M-CSF), which induces only macrophage colony growth. It was a logical assumption that these cytokines were responsible for the hormonal regulation of blood cell maturation in vivo and that administration of these agents in pharmacological amounts might profoundly stimulate hematopoiesis.

In vivo, hematopoietic stem cells only proliferate in a specific complex microenvironment that is present in the medullary portion of red marrow-bearing bones. The cellular components of this environment consist of specialized marrow stromal cells, endothelial cells, and macrophages. The microenvironmental cells probably express specific ligands that bind to adhesion molecules expressed by stem cells (10). These interactions are probably also responsible for "homing" of hematopoietic stem cells to the bone marrow and have obvious relevance in BMT. The long-term marrow culture system represents an in vitro model that more closely mimics physiological hematopoiesis than colony assays. In this system, an adherent cell layer is formed that is an in vitro counterpart of the hematopoietic microenvironment. These adherent stromal cells not only provide an appropriate microenvironment for adhesion of primitive cells, but also provide a constitutive source for multiple hematopoietic growth factors. This complex culture system allows semiquantitative measurements of more primitive human stem cells than can be measured in colony forming systems (11,12). Unlike colony assays, long-term marrow cultures also allow limited self-renewal of early progenitors. Adherent stromal cells in long-term marrow cultures predominantly consist of a population of smooth-muscle–like cells that produce a rich extracellular matrix of interstitial and basal lamina collagens, fibronectin, thrombospondin, and a complex proteoglycan mixture (13). The extracellular matrix provides binding sites for adhesion molecules expressed by immature hematopoietic cells (14–16) and may bind and increase the effective local concentrations of cytokines produced by stromal cells, T lymphocytes, and macrophages within the microenvironment (17,18). Stromal cells produce a number of cytokines that stimulate the growth and differentiation of primitive hematopoietic progenitor cells, including the c-kit ligand, interleukin-11, interleukin-6 (IL-6), G-CSF and interleukin-1 (IL-1) (19–24).

Studies defining the phenotype of human primitive progenitor cells that proliferate in long-term culture but not in colony assays suggest that the progenitor of colony forming cells, termed the *long-term culture initiating cell (LTCIC)*, expresses the CD34 antigen but not other myeloid or lymphoid differentiative markers, such as human leukocyte antigen-DR (HLA-DR), CD33, or CD38 (25–28). These cells are therefore characterized as CD34-positive, lineage (lin)-negative. Although these cells are likely candidates for lymphohematopoietic stem cells with repopulating ability, both characteristics await rigorous proof.

Evidence for a common lymphoid-myeloid stem cell in humans comes from studies of patients with chronic myeloid leukemia (CML) who were heterozygous for the X-linked marker, glucose-6-phosphate dehydrogenase. Fialkow and co-workers (29–31) demonstrated that CML was a clonal disorder and that platelets, red blood cells, granulocytes, monocytes, eosinophils, and some B lymphocytes were derived from a common, clonal progenitor. This finding proves the existence of a common lymphohematopoietic stem cell in humans.

Much investigation has focused on the critical question of how hematopoietic stem cells regulate lineage commitment and self-renewal. A major difficulty in these studies has been the inability of in vitro systems to allow adequate studies of stem cell self-renewal. However, the mechanisms of lineage commitment have been extensively linked. The most prevalent current opinion is that stem cells undergo lineage commitment in an apparently random fashion that is not directly influenced by growth factors. Elegant studies by Leary and co-workers (32) demonstrated that when the two daughter cells arising from the first cell division of a blast colony forming progenitor cell were separated and plated independently, there was no correlation in the lineage commitment of the daughter cells. One of the pair might produce an erythroid colony while the other formed a granulocyte-macrophage colony. Addition of growth factors did not alter the apparently random nature of commitment. These observations suggest lineage commitment is random or stochastic in nature and not subject to regulation by growth factors. Nevertheless, cytokines are essential for continued survival and differentiation of both multilineage and committed progenitor cells and can modulate the number of end-stage cells produced from a committed progenitor. These data suggest that administration of cytokines after BMT, when stem cells are actively dividing, is not likely to lead to terminal differentiation with consequent graft failure. If stem-cell commitment was directly influenced by cytokines such as G-CSF, and if there were relatively few stem cells, as is the case in patients early after BMT, then cytokine therapy might lead to graft failure. However, there is no evidence from clinical studies involving hundreds of patients that cytokines cause graft failure following BMT.

Growth Factor Receptors

Developing hematopoietic cells express several hundred receptors for each of the CSFs in addition to receptors for other cytokines, such as IL-1, tumor necrosis factor alpha (TNF-α), IL-6, and the c-kit ligand. Therefore, several growth factors can interact on a single cell. Occupancy of a small percentage of the receptors is often sufficient to induce responses. Except for the M-CSF (CSF-1) receptor, which is the product of the protooncogene c-fms (33), and c-kit (34), the receptor for c-kit ligand (stem-cell factor), the colony stimulating factor receptors do not have integral tyrosine kinase activity and are likely to associate with additional proteins with kinase activity to elicit signal transduction.

The mechanism by which cytokines elicit specific signal cascades and cellular responses are as yet unknown. It is apparent that many cytokines are polyfunctional (35) and that the response to receptor occupancy is controlled at the level of the cell. It is also likely that signals from several receptors with a common message to the cell may join in a common pathway leading to activation of a downstream regulatory molecule, such as protein kinase C. In addition to transducing signals from cytokines, receptor molecules in a soluble form may suppress the effect of cytokines by binding to the cytokine before it can bind to the membrane-associated receptor (36). Soluble receptors for inflammatory cytokines have potential uses as biological agents that suppress cytokine-mediated processes, such as inflammation and graft-versus-host disease (GVHD). Both the number of growth factor receptors and their affinity are also subject to regulation by cytokines, thus introducing an even greater degree of complexity to physiological control of intercellular signalling. For example, TNF-α, a cytokine associated with a number of adverse events after BMT, suppresses the expression of both G-CSF and GM-CSF receptors on hematopoietic progenitor cells (37–41). Thus, elevation of TNF-α from adverse events may suppress the response to both endogenous and exogenous cytokines. These findings imply that optimal responses to these cytokines may be obtained when they are used in combination with agents that suppress TNF-α.

Biological Effects of Hematopoietic Growth Factors

Hematopoietic cytokines may have either lineage-restricted or more generalized effects. For example, IL-6 has pluripotent stimulating activity. It stimulates multipotent hematopoietic progenitor cells as well as myeloid and megakaryocytic progenitor cells. It also mediates the acute phase response by hepatocytes, and stimulates lymphocyte, mesenchymal, and ectodermal cell proliferation (42–46). In contrast, erythropoietin only influences cells committed to erythroid differentiation.

Growth factors also modulate cellular activities by induction of other cytokines. For example, through its effects on cells in the granulocyte-macrophage lineage, GM-CSF may indirectly influence lymphocytes and endothelial cells by stimulating the production of polyfunctional cytokines such as IL-1, TNF-α, and IL-6 (47). Although GM-CSF upregulates TNF-α mRNA in macrophages, it is an incomplete signal for TNF-α secretion (48,49). Nevertheless, GM-CSF may enhance TNF-α production following a second stimulus such as endotoxin.

Some cytokines are polyfunctional (35); they may induce proliferation in some cells while stimulating differentiation, enhanced functional abilities, or even programmed cell death in other cells. Examples of polyfunctional molecules include TNF-α which stimulates proliferation of some fibroblastic cells and thymocytes while inhibiting proliferation of erythroid cells and causing programmed cell death in certain tumor cells (35,50,51). GM-CSF, IL-3, and G-CSF are bifunctional; they induce proliferation of early myeloid cells and activate terminally differentiated cells such as granulocytes, eosinophils, and macrophages (52). These independent effects may be mediated by multiple receptor species or by differential receptor signal coupling in cells at different stages of maturation.

In the intact organism, cytokines work in concert and not as individual growth hormones. Thus, it is not surprising that in preclinical studies, cytokines in combinations are more potent than when used individually. Synergy in both in vivo and in vitro studies has been noted between IL-1 and G-CSF, IL-3 and GM-CSF, and c-kit ligand and G-CSF or GM-CSF (23,53–57). These data suggest that combinations of cytokines eventually will prove more effective than single agents at enhancing hematopoiesis in humans.

Although some tumor cells express receptors for hematopoietic growth factors, most are not stimulated to proliferate (58), perhaps due to lack of appropriate coupling to second messenger pathways. Concern that growth factors would stimulate tumor cell growth on this basis has also been allayed by clinical studies. Even when administered to patients with acute myeloid leukemia, in which blast cells nearly always have active receptors, neither G-CSF nor GM-CSF were associated with a higher relapse rate (59–64).

Table 24-1 summarizes the relevant biological activities of hematopoietic growth factors. Agents with a multiplicity of potential clinical effects will soon be available to clinicians. It is a daunting task to define the toxicities of these agents in BMT and to determine if a newer agent or a combination of cytokines will have significant advantages over G-CSF or GM-CSF. The goal of this chapter is to summarize current clinical knowledge of hematopoietic growth factors in BMT and to suggest where newer agents may prove clinically useful.

rhG-CSF

G-CSF is an O-glycosylated, single polypeptide chain consisting of 177 amino acids (65–69). It is produced by fibroblasts, endothelial cells, and monocytes, but not by T lymphocytes, and it stimulates formation of mature neutrophils from committed progenitor cells. G-CSF weakly upregulates neutrophil function as determined by assays such as intracellular killing and

Table 24-1.
Cytokines and Their Target Cells

	Target Cells					
Cytokine	*Erythroid*	*Neutrophils*	*Monocytes*	*Eosinophils-Basophils*	*Mega-karyocytes*	*Early Myeloid Progenitor Cells*
Erythropoietin	+	−	−	−	−	−
G-CSF	−	+	−	−	−	−
GM-CSF	−	+	+	+	−	−
IL-3[a]	+	+	+	+	+	+
IL-6[a,b]	−	−	−	−	+	+
IL-1[a]	−	+	+	−	−	+
Leukemia Inhibitory Factor (LIF)	−	−	−	−	+	+
c-kit Ligand (stem-cell factor)[a]	+	+	+	+	+	+
IL-11	−	−	−	−	+	−
IL-3-GM-CSF fusion molecule (PIXY 321)	−	+	+	+	+	+

[a]May prime for response to late-acting growth factors, such as G-CSF or GM-CSF.
[b]Also stimulates B lymphocytes and hepatocytes.

production of reactive oxygen species. G-CSF is less potent as a functional activator than GM-CSF, and unlike GM-CSF, G-CSF does not affect monocyte or macrophage function (52). Administration of recombinant human G-CSF (rhG-CSF) to nonhuman primates is well tolerated and induces prompt neutrophilia (70). Cynomolgus monkeys treated with high-dose cyclophosphamide, busulfan, and total body irradiation with autologous bone marrow rescue had earlier neutrophil recovery when given rhG-CSF than control animals (71). Similar results have been observed in dogs given allogeneic bone marrow grafts (72) and in dogs allowed to recovery following otherwise lethal irradiation (73). When G-CSF is administered with IL-1 or IL-3 to mice following administration of 5-fluorouracil, synergistic marrow stimulation was observed (74).

When administered to normal humans, rhG-CSF depresses neutrophil counts within 30 minutes and then elevates the level of circulating neutrophils in a dose-dependent fashion without significant toxicities (75,76). Within 3 to 4 days, rhG-CSF also stimulates an increase in both immature and committed colony forming cells in circulation, suggesting that G-CSF can be used to mobilize peripheral blood progenitor cells (PBPC) for autologous BMT (77). Serum levels of G-CSF but not GM-CSF increase during the neutropenic period after cytotoxic therapy and decrease to low levels just preceding neutrophil count recovery (78). G-CSF levels are also elevated during infections, suggesting that it is the physiological regulatory factor responsible for neutrophilia in response to infections (79).

Clinical Studies

RhG-CSF is well tolerated over a wide range of doses. When rhG-CSF is administered following administration of cytotoxic agents, there is a dose-response relationship for a decrease in duration of neutropenia and in the rate of increase of granulocyte count attained following recovery. Although the recommended dose of rhG-CSF is 5μg/kg/day, the optimal dose may be regimen-dependent and is influenced by the amount and type of prior chemotherapy. Doses of rhG-CSF higher than 5μg/kg may be required for optimal stimulation of PBPCs for autografting. Primarily due to the high cost of rhG-CSF, the dose used should be the lowest one that produces the desired clinical effect.

When rhG-CSF was given to patients receiving multiagent chemotherapy for bladder cancer with the regimen consisting of methotrexate, vinblastine, adriamycin and cisplatin (MVAC) in a Phase II study, higher nadir neutrophil counts and decreases in mucositis were seen in cycles given with rhG-CSF. This effect allowed patients to receive more dose-intensive therapy (75). Administration of rhG-CSF in patients receiving doxorubicin as a single agent allowed doses of up to 150 mg/m^2 every 14 days for up to 3 cycles, with less neutropenia than observed in patients who received the conventional dose of 75 mg/m^2 every 3 weeks (80). In a randomized controlled trial of rhG-CSF in patients undergoing chemotherapy for small-cell lung cancer, G-CSF decreased the frequency of neutropenic fever from 57% in the control group to 28%. The frequency of severe neutropenia was reduced from 98 to 84%, and its median duration was shortened from 6 to 3 days (81).

Limited numbers of studies with rhG-CSF have been performed in patients undergoing BMT (Table 24-2). In clinical trials using historical patients for comparison, G-CSF appeared to decrease the period of neutropenia in patients undergoing autologous or allogeneic BMT (82–84). No randomized studies using rhG-CSF in BMT have been published. The clinical profile of rhG-CSF suggests that it can be used interchangeably with rhGM-CSF in autologous BMT, although conclusive data that the two are equivalent requires a prospective comparative study (85). Studies in canines (72) and in humans (86) suggest that rhG-CSF can be used safely following allogeneic BMT.

Table 24-2.
Results of Phase I/II Trials with rhG-CSF Following BMT Compared with Historical Control Patients

No. of Patients		*Day ANC > 500 × 10⁹/L*		*Day Platelet–Independent*		*% of Patients with Infection*		*Day Initial Discharge*		
G-CSF	*Control*	*G-CSF*	*Control*	*G-CSF*	*Control*	*G-CSF*	*Control*	*G-CSF*	*Control*	*Reference*
15	18	11	20	33	45	53	61	23	29	82
18	58	13	22	28	32	17	36	NR	NR	83
24	24	S[a]	S[a]	NS[a]	NS[a]	18	35	NR	NR	187,188
25[b]	NR	16	NR	NR	NR	NR	NR	NR	NR	189
9[c]	NR	13	NR	NR	NR	NR	NR	NR	NR	189

[a]S = values not given but reported as being significantly earlier in patients who received rhG-CSF; NS = values not given but reported as being not significantly different.
[b]Patients who received methotrexate and cyclosporine for GVHD prophylaxis after sibling HLA-matched BMT.
[c]Patients who received cyclosporine without methotrexate for GVHD prophylaxis after sibling HLA-matched BMT; incidence of GVHD 47%.
NR = not reported.

Substantial acceleration of engraftment was observed even in patients who received methotrexate as part of a GVHD prophylactic regimen (86).

No published data conclusively demonstrate that G-CSF is of value in treating infections that occur while patients are neutropenic from cytotoxic therapy. It is, however, likely that treating such patients with either rhG-CSF or rhGM-CSF is beneficial. Both CSFs enhance the functional activity of phagocytic cells and stimulate earlier neutrophil recovery.

Use of rhG-CSF to Mobilize Peripheral Blood Progenitor Cells for Autologous BMT

After 3 to 4 daily doses of G-CSF, there is a 10- to 100-fold increase in the number of circulating erythroid, granulocyte-macrophage, and multipotent hematopoietic progenitor cells obtainable by leukapheresis (87) (Singer JW et al. unpublished data). Preliminary studies from the Fred Hutchinson Cancer Research Center suggest that sufficient numbers of repopulating stem cells can be obtained by leukaphereses to durably engraft patients after myeloablative regimens without additional marrow cells if the patients have not received extensive prior chemotherapy (Singer JW et al. unpublished data). Use of cytokines to stimulate PBPC production may make it possible to carry out autologous transplants for patients with marrow with tumor involvement or whose marrow has been damaged by prior pelvic irradiation (88). Use of rhG-CSF-stimulated PBPC in addition to bone marrow may decrease the morbidity of autologous BMT by substantially decreasing the time for platelet and granulocyte recovery (77). Additional studies with economic analyses are needed to verify these preliminary data and to define the role and cost-effectiveness of PBPC in autologous BMT.

GM-CSF

GM-CSF is an N-glycosylated glycoprotein with a molecular weight of 22,000 daltons produced by fibroblasts, endothelial cells, and activated T lymphocytes, but not by monocytes (52,89). In vitro, GM-CSF stimulates the growth of granulocyte, monocyte, erythroid, and multilineage hematopoietic colonies and thus appears to have a broader spectrum of activity than G-CSF. In addition to stimulating proliferation of immature hematopoietic cells, GM-CSF is a potent activator of mature macrophages and granulocytes (reviewed in 52). It induces increased expression of adhesion molecules, which allows neutrophils to adhere to endothelial cells and also enhances neutrophil superoxide production, degranulation, phagocytosis, and intracellular killing (90–93). GM-CSF induces the production of cytokines from both macrophages and mature neutrophils, which amplify inflammatory responses, including IL-1, TNF-α, and IL-8 (48,94). In contrast, G-CSF does not upregulate IL-8 production in granulocytes or monocytes. IL-8 is a potent neutrophil chemoattractant and activator and may be necessary for transendothelial migration (95,96). Thus, local production of GM-CSF by cells at the site of inflammation may amplify accumulation of inflammatory cells. The ability of GM-CSF to activate phagocytic cells that are relatively resistant to cytotoxic therapy, such as tissue macrophages, suggests that GM-CSF may be a more active cytokine than G-CSF when used to treat infections that occur during neutropenia. By mechanisms such as those described, GM-CSF protects neutropenic mice against bacterial and fungal challenges (97) and improves survival in mice when administered after infusion of infectious organisms (98,99). RhG-CSF is less effective than rhGM-CSF in protecting against fungal infections (100).

Prophylactic administration of rhGM-CSF to nonhuman primates undergoing autologous BMT was well tolerated and associated with accelerated neutrophil and platelet recovery (101,102). The effect of rhGM-CSF was greatly enhanced by priming the animals with rhIL-3, suggesting a potential clinical strategy for combining early and later acting cytokines (103,104). Such a strategy may also prove useful in increasing the yields of PBPC (105,106). Animal studies of rhGM-CSF following allografting indicated that there were no adverse effects on GVHD, there was enhancement of neutrophil recovery, and survival was improved (107–109).

Clinical Studies

RhGM-CSF stimulates the production of neutrophils, eosinophils, and monocytes. In normal individuals, treatment with rhGM-CSF can elevate the white blood cell count to greater than 50,000/μL within one week. RhGM-CSF also increases the frequency and number of circulating CD34+ hematopoietic progenitor cells (110). The number of progenitor cells can be enhanced further if rhGM-CSF is administered following high-dose cyclophosphamide (111–113). The maximum tolerated dose of yeast-derived rhGM-CSF in most studies has been 250 μg/m^2, although hematopoietic stimulation is observed at doses as low as 30 μg/m^2 (114,115). At doses above 250 μg/m^2 given by 2-hour intravenous infusion, there is a substantial incidence of severe bone pain, and reversible pleural or pericardial effusions have developed in a number of patients (114,115). RhGM-CSF may also be administered subcutaneously.

RhGM-CSF reversed the neutropenia associated with acquired immune deficiency syndrome and elevated neutrophil counts in some patients with myelodysplasia (116–118). Studies of rhGM-CSF in patients receiving combination chemotherapy suggest that it accelerates neutrophil recovery and may allow an increase in dose-intensity of therapy. In a study in patients with sarcoma undergoing intensive therapy with doxorubicin, ifosfamide, and dacarbazine, rhGM-CSF decreased the duration of neutropenia and appeared to accelerate platelet recovery (119). However, stimulation of platelet recovery has not been consistently observed in other trials.

rhGM-CSF In Autologous BMT

Patients autografted for breast cancer following intensive chemotherapy with cyclophosphamide, cisplatin, and carmustine and then given rhGM-CSF by continuous infusion had earlier recovery of neutrophil counts than historical patients not given rhGM-CSF (120) (Table 24-3). A potential pitfall of stimulating neutrophils with rhGM-CSF was noted during these studies. It was observed that patients receiving rhGM-CSF by continuous infusion had depression of neutrophil migration to a skin window, suggesting that rhGM-CSF may suppress the neutrophilic response to infections (121). It is likely that continuous infusion rhGM-CSF suppressed neutrophil migration to a site of inflammation by maintaining pharmacological levels of the cytokine in blood. GM-CSF has migration-inhibiting activity. Neutrophils therefore will not migrate from the intravascular space with a high concentration to a site of injury unless the local concentration of chemoattractants, such as IL-8, can overcome the migration-inhibitory effects of rhGM-CSF. Due to its short half-life in circulation, clinically important suppression of neutrophil migration can be prevented by less prolonged administration. Using the skin window technique but administering rhGM-CSF over 4 hours, Toner and coworkers (122) were not able to demonstrate inhibition of neutrophil migration. Unlike rhGM-CSF, rhG-CSF is not associated with inhibition of neutrophil migration. Despite these theoretical concerns that rhGM-CSF might actually decrease the ability to fight local infections, clinical studies have shown this concern to be unfounded. In a randomized, placebo-controlled trial, rhGM-CSF decreased the incidence of infection (123).

In a phase I dose-finding study in patients undergoing autologous BMT for lymphoid malignancies, the maximum tolerated dose of rhGM-CSF (yeast-derived) given by daily 2-hour infusions from days 0 to 21 after the marrow infusion was 250 μg/m^2 (114). At a dose of

Table 24-3.
Results of Phase I/II Trials with rhGM-CSF Following Autologous BMT Compared with Historical Control Patients

No. of Patients		*Day ANC > 500 × 10^9/L*		*Day Platelet-Independent*		*% Patients with Infection*		*Day Initial Discharge*		
GM-CSF	*Control*	*GM-CSF*	*Control*	*GM-CSF*	*Control*	*GM-CSF*	*Control*	*GM-CSF*	*Control*	*Reference*
19	24	14	19	NS[a]	NS[a]	16	35	NR	NR	120
22	86	17	25	28	38	18	30	32	41	125
6	86	22	25	30	38	0	30	30	41	125
12	19	18	25	30	28	58	68	30	30	190
5	27	14	24	NR[b]	NR[b]	NR	52	36	47	191
15	27	28	24	NR[c]	NR[c]	NR	52	50	47	191
5	27	23	24	NR[c]	NR[c]	NR	52	43	47	191
6	NR	11	20	NR	NR	NR	NR	NR	NR	192
16	52	14	20	24	26	6	NR	NR	NR	193

[a]NS = values not shown, but reported as not significantly different.
[b]Day of platelet transfusion independence was not reported, but the number of platelet units required were significantly less during the first 28 days (81 vs 149 U) compared with historical control subjects.
[c]Number of platelet units infused from day 0–28 of all patients who received ≤ 0.45 CFU-GM/kg (n = 30) was 215 in the GM-CSF–treated patients and 149 in the control group.
NR = not reported.

Table 24-4.
Results of Phase III Trials with rhGM-CSF Following Autologous BMT

No. of Patients		*Day ANC > 500 × 10⁹/L*[a]		*Day of Platelet Independent*		*% of Patients with Infection*		*Day Initial Discharge*		
GM-CSF	*Control*	*GM-CSF*	*Control*	*GM-CSF*	*Control*	*GM-CSF*	*Control*	*GM-CSF*	*Control*	*Reference*
65	63	19	26	26	29	17	30	27	33	123
41	47	14	21	19	19	39	47	23	28	194, 195
39	40	15	28	39	31	38	70	30	31	194, 196
36	33	12	16	35	52	3	19	27	27	197
12	12	NR[b]	NR[b]	14	21	NS	NS	32	41	198

[a]Day ANC > 1,000 × 10⁹/μL was day 16 in the GM-CSF group vs day 27 in the placebo group.

500 μg/m², pleural or pericardial effusions developed in several patients. Other patients had bone pain during the infusion of sufficient severity to require narcotic analgesics. All side effects rapidly resolved following discontinuing or reducing the dosage of rhGM-CSF. Compared with historical patients, patients treated with rhGM-CSF at doses of 60 μg/m² or greater appeared to have earlier neutrophil and platelet recovery. Long-term follow-up of these patients suggested that rhGM-CSF had no effect on long-term marrow function or on the incidence of relapse (124). No additional hematological benefits were noted when rhGM-CSF was given by continuous instead of short infusions (125). In view of the potential adverse effects on neutrophil migration of continuous infusions of rhGM-CSF (121) and the greater logistical difficulties, most later studies were standardized to 2- to 4-hour infusions. The results of these trials and Phase I/II trials performed at other centers are shown in Table 24-3.

To prove the apparent benefit of rhGM-CSF observed in Phase II studies, several multicenter randomized, double-blind, placebo-controlled trials of rhGM-CSF in autologous BMT for lymphoid malignancy were performed (123) (Table 24-4). In the first trial, 128 patients were entered; 65 received rhGM-CSF and 63 were given a placebo from day 0 to 20 following marrow infusion. The number of days of severe neutropenia (<100 μL) were not different between the two groups. However, the GM-CSF patients reached neutrophil counts of 500/μL and 1,000/μL 7 days earlier than control patients (19 vs 26 days; $p < 0.001$) (Figure 24-1). rhGM-CSF–treated patients required a median of 6 fewer days of hospitalization and had fewer infectious episodes than control patients. In an analysis of the cost differences between the groups at one of the centers, the Fred Hutchinson Cancer Research Center, the mean cost per case in the rhGM-CSF group was $14,500 less than in the placebo controls (Nemunaitis J, et al. Unpublished data). Subsequent Phase III trials had similar outcomes (Table 24-4). These studies led to Federal Drug Administration (FDA) approval for rhGM-CSF as indicated adjunctive therapy in patients undergoing autologous BMT for lymphoid neoplasia. It has therefore become the benchmark against which future growth factors will be compared. rhGM-CSF may also be useful to prevent or treat neutropenia in patients receiving myelosuppressive agents such as ganciclovir after BMT (126).

rhGM-CSF Stimulation of PBPC for Autologous BMT

rhGM-CSF given either with or without cytotoxic therapy produces large increases in the numbers of circulating hematopoietic progenitor cells in humans. Preliminary data from several centers indicate that PBPC collected during the early neutrophil recovery phase in patients given high-dose cyclosphosphamide (or other cytotoxic therapy) and rhGM-CSF provides a sufficient source of stem cells to produce adequate reconstitution without bone marrow (Table 24-5). Because relatively few patients have been transplanted with cytokine-stimulated PBPC as the sole source of stem cells and because clinical follow-up is currently short, the durability of reconstitution cannot yet be evaluated.

Additional studies are also needed to determine the optimal method for collection of PBPC and to define further their role in autologous transplantation. Due

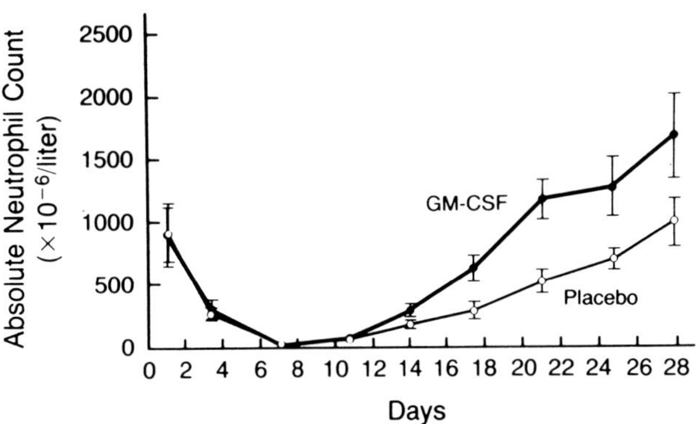

Figure 24-1. Mean daily absolute neutrophil counts in 65 patients who received rhGM-CSF and 63 patients who received placebo. The *vertical bars* denote 1 standard deviation. (Reprinted, by permission of the New England Journal of Medicine, from Nemunaitis J, et al. Recombinant granulocyte-macrophage colony-stimulating factor after autologous bone marrow transplantation for lymphoid cancer. N Engl J Med 1991;324:1773–1778.)

Table 24-5.
Phase I/II Trials with rhGM-CSF and Autologous Peripheral Blood Progenitor Cell (PBPC) Transplant

No. of Patients (Disease)[a]	*Comments*	*Reference*
13 (sarcoma)	Total PB CFU-GM mononuclear cells increased 18-fold after GM-CSF administration	110
7 (NHL)	Addition of GM-CSF to high-dose CY increased CFU-GM up to 1,000-fold. ANC > 500/μL on day 4. Platelet transfusion–independent on day 10.	113
3 (BC, NHL)	Addition of GM-CSF to high-dose CY increased CD34+ cells 5-fold	202
17 (NR)	Total PB CFU-GM increased 10-fold in patients who received GM-CSF. Days ANC < 100/μL was 8 compared with 11 days for historical control subjects	203
11 (ST)	Addition of GM-CSF to chemotherapy (adriamycin, CY) more than doubled the CFU-GM yield	204
20 (NHL, BC)	Peak CFU-GM/mL: 5,000 with CY; 24,000 with GM-CSF/CY; 149 in normal control subjects	205
6 (NHL, HD)	CFU-GM/mL increased 9-fold with rhGM-CSF. Day ANC > 500/μL day 29; day platelet transfusion–independent, day 39	206
11 (BC, NHL)	Day to achieve WBC > 1,000/μL was day 14 in patients who received GM-CSF + CY vs day 17 in patients who only received CY. CFU-GM/kg were 7 times greater in patients who received GM-CSF + CY vs CY alone.	207

NHL = non-Hodgkin's lymphoma; BC = breast cancer; NR = not reported; ST = solid tumors; HD = Hodgkin's disease; PB = peripheral blood; CFU-GM = granulocyte-macrophage colony-forming units; CY = cyclophosphamide.

to the considerable costs incurred by collection of PBPC, the benefit compared with transplants using only bone marrow needs to be evaluated from an economic as well as a medical point of view in well-controlled studies. Currently, it is apparent that PBPC collected with rhGM-CSF or rhG-CSF following cytotoxic therapy provides both an alternative and an adjunct to marrow for reconstitution. PBPC provides a potential sole source of stem cells in patients in whom marrow cannot be harvested due to tumor contamination or prior marrow radiation. If stable reconstitution can be obtained reproducibly in patients undergoing autografting using cytokine stimulated PBPC, then consideration can be given to using PBPC as a stem-cell source in allografts.

rhGM-CSF Following Allogeneic BMT from HLA-identical Siblings

The morbidity of allogeneic BMT is substantially greater than autologous BMT due to GVHD and the therapeutic interventions necessary to prevent and treat it. The one year, nonrelapse mortality of a "good risk" autograft is approximately 10%, whereas that of an HLA-identical sibling allograft in a good risk patient is 20 to 30%. In addition to the regimen-related and infectious complications associated with marrow ablation, allogeneic BMT recipients must receive non-cytotoxic immunosuppressive drugs (cyclosporine and prednisone) or cytotoxic immunosuppressive agents (methotrexate) following the marrow infusion to suppress GVHD. All of these agents contribute to regimen-related morbidity by increasing the risk of infections and the severity of mucositis compared with patients who receive autografts and require no immunosuppressive therapy. Moreover, neutrophil function and production of endogenous GM-CSF by lymphocytes are both deficient in patients after allografting (127). GM-CSF may be of benefit following allogeneic BMT by improving neutrophil function as well as by accelerating the rate of neutrophil recovery (128).

To assess the potential for rhGM-CSF to decrease the morbidity associated with allogeneic BMT, trials were performed in patients transplanted from HLA-identical sibling and from unrelated marrow donors. rhGM-CSF has a potential to increase the severity of GVHD by activating macrophages and dendritic cells. These cells, which process and present antigens to lymphoid cells, also produce inflammatory mediators such as IL-1 and TNF-α (48,49,129), which amplify T-cell responses to immune stimulation (130–134). Thus, at least theoretically, GM-CSF could lead to an increase in either the incidence or the severity of GVHD.

Two independent dose-escalation trials of rhGM-CSF were performed in patients undergoing transplants from HLA-identical sibling donors, one in patients given cyclosporine and prednisone for GVHD prophylaxis, and another in patients who received cyclosporine and methotrexate (135). In the patients who received cyclosporine and prednisone, rhGM-CSF substantially accelerated the time to achieve neutrophil engraftment compared with historical control patients. An absolute neutrophil count of 1,000/μL was achieved on a median of day 16 with rhGM-CSF versus day 21 in similarly treated historical patients. Patients treated with rhGM-CSF had a lower incidence of early infectious complications than historical patients, with an incidence of GVHD that was similar to the historical rate. In patients who received cyclosporine and methotrexate for GVHD prophylaxis, rhGM-CSF decreased the time to achieve an absolute neutrophil count (ANC) of 1,000/μL by only 3 days (from 23 days in historical patients to 20 days). Nevertheless, the incidence of infections was lower than the historical incidence, suggesting that rhGM-CSF may protect severely neutropenic patients against infection. Other trials suggest similar results (Table 24-6). A multicenter, randomized,

Table 24-6.
Results of Trials with rhGM-CSF Following Allogeneic BMT

No. of Patients		*Day ANC > 500 × 10^9/L*		*Day Platelet-Independent*		*% of Patients with Infection*		*Day Initial Discharge*			
GM-CSF	*Control*	*GM-CSF*	*Control*	*GM-CSF*	*Control*	*GM-CSF*	*Control*	*GM-CSF*	*Control*	*Comments*	*Reference*
28	50[a]	14	19	23	21	18	NR	24	31	Severity and incidence of GVHD not affected. CSP/prednisone for GVHD prophylaxis.	135
19	43[a]	20	24	23	20	22	NR	33	36	CSP/MTX for GVHD prophylaxis.	135
29	28[b]	15	18	NS[c]	NS[a,c]	NS[c,d]	NS[c,d]	NR	NR	T-cell–depleted allogeneic marrow for GVHD prophylaxis. Infection-related mortality in GM-CSF–treated patients 3 vs 21% in placebo-treated patients; relapse 22 vs 36%.	199
20	20[b]	13	19	NR	NR	NR	NR	24	24	No effect on relapse or survival. CSP for GVHD prophylaxis.	200
40	78[a]	21	21	26	31	8	27	NR	NR	Nonrelapse mortality and grade III GVHD is less in GM-CSF–treated patients. CSP + MTX for GVHD prophylaxis.	144
20	40[a]	14	18	16	23	NR	NR	20	37	Bone marrow incubated with GM-CSF and IL-3 before infusion into patient. Overall incidence of GVHD not different.	201

[a]Historical control patients.
[b]Prospective placebo control patients.
[c]NS = values not shown but reported as not significantly different.
[d]Bone marrow incubated with rhGM-CSF and rhIL-3 before infusion into patients
NR = not reported; GVHD = graft–versus–host disease; CSP = cyclosporine; MTX = methotrexate.

controlled trial is in progress to determine if rhGM-CSF is of benefit in allogeneic BMT patients who received non-methotrexate-based GVHD prophylaxis.

Protection against infection during neutropenia may be due to a GM-CSF–induced increase in the functional capacities of relatively radiation- and chemotherapy-resistant cells such as tissue macrophages. A rhGM-CSF–caused reduction in the incidence of either infections or endotoxinemia may lead to a salutary effect on GVHD. Endotoxin activates a cytokine cascade through induction of TNF-α, IL-1, IL-6, IL-8, all of which may enhance either T-cell reactivity or the inflammatory response (136–139). TNF-α appears to be a major mediator of GVHD, and blocking TNF-α with antibodies appears to decrease its severity (140,141). The levels of plasma TNF-α in patients treated with rhGM-CSF were significantly lower than those in similar patients who did not receive rhGM-CSF.

rhGM-CSF In Allogeneic BMT From Unrelated Donors

BMT from unrelated donors has a greater morbidity and mortality than transplants from matched sibling donors due to a higher incidence of severe GVHD and infections (142,143). The incidence of grade II or greater GVHD is approximately 75%, whereas life-threatening grade III to IV GVHD occurs in approximately 35% of patients. Most of the deaths of marrow transplant recipients from unrelated donor marrows are due to severe acute and chronic GVHD and infections. The day 100 nonrelapse mortality is approximately 35%, and, in a recent review of pooled data from several centers, nearly one half of good-risk patients with CML in chronic phase did not survive one year (142).

In view of the findings that rhGM-CSF decreases the incidence of infections in patients undergoing autologous BMT and the encouraging preliminary results from its use in patients transplanted from HLA-identical sibling donors, a Phase II trial of rhGM-CSF in BMT from unrelated donors was initiated (144). Patients received rhGM-CSF (yeast-derived) at a dose of 250 $\mu g/m^2$ given from day 0 to 20 or 27. After an initial group of patients received 21 doses and most had not yet reached an ANC of 500/μL before day 21, the course was lengthened to 28 doses. All patients received cyclosporine and methotrexate for GVHD prophylaxis. Compared with historical patients trans-

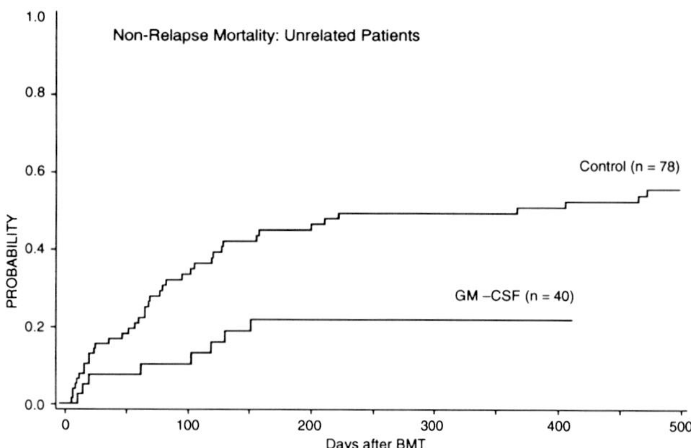

Figure 24-2. Kaplan-Meier estimate of nonrelapse mortality of 40 patients who received rhGM-CSF from day 0 through day 21 or 28 after a marrow graft from an unrelated donor, compared with 78 historical control patients.

planted from unrelated donors who did not receive rhGM-CSF, 40 patients who received rhGM-CSF had a median time to reach an ANC of 500/μL of 23 days, a value identical to that of historical patients. However, the incidence of septicemia in patients who received rhGM-CSF was only 8%, compared with an incidence of 28% in the historical patients, suggesting, as did the study in related donor transplants, that rhGM-CSF protects against infection in severely neutropenic individuals. Although the overall incidence of GVHD was similar to that in historical cases, patients receiving rhGM-CSF had a lower incidence of grade III to IV GVHD. The lower incidence of severe GVHD and infections may have led to an apparent significant improvement in nonrelapse mortality for patients who received rhGM-CSF compared with historical patients (Figure 24-2). These data, however, must be interpreted cautiously because the groups were not completely comparable for risk factors and were not concurrent. Advances such as early diagnosis and effective treatment of cytomegalovirus infection, improvement in HLA typing technology, and differences in other aspects of supportive care may also have contributed to the lower mortality in patients who received rhGM-CSF. To determine if rhGM-CSF is of benefit in unrelated donor transplantation, these findings are now being tested in a randomized, controlled trial.

rhGM-CSF in Marrow Graft Failure

Approximately 10% of patients who undergo either autologous or allogeneic BMT fail to reconstitute or late hematopoietic failure develops. In a historical review of all patients who were transplanted at the FHCRC who either failed to achieve an ANC of 100/μL by day 28 or in whom persistent, severe neutropenia (ANC <500/μL) (not associated with drugs such as ganciclovir) developed after successful engraftment, the long-term survival was only 20% (115). Except for patients with aplastic anemia who immunologically rejected their grafts and underwent a successful second transplant, most patients with graft failure die. A phase I to II trial of rhGM-CSF was instituted to determine if it could affect the outcome in graft failure. Patients who failed to achieve an ANC of 100/μL by day 28, patients who had late-onset, persistent neutropenia (<500/μL for 7 days), and patients with less than 100 neutrophils/μL at day 21 with a severe infection were offered therapy. Only patients with graft failure due to relapse were excluded. Patients with immunological rejection of their grafts or GVHD were not excluded. rhGM-CSF (yeast-derived) was administered for 14 days. If patients did not respond within 21 days, a second course was given at a higher dose. A third course was also allowed. After initial accrual at the FHCRC demonstrated the safety of rhGM-CSF in graft failure, the trial was expanded to a multicenter Phase II trial with an overall accrual of more than 100 patients (115).

Approximately 60% of patients with graft failure responded to one or two courses of rhGM-CSF, with an increase in ANC to more than 500/μL within 14 days of starting therapy. In patients who had active infections, response to rhGM-CSF was associated with resolution. Although there was no apparent immediate stimulation of platelet recovery, most patients whose granulocyte production improved eventually became platelet-independent. The overall survival of patients treated with rhGM-CSF for graft failure was significantly better as compared with historical survival rates (Figure 24-3). Due to the lack of other effective therapy, a randomized trial has not been performed. On the basis of the Phase II trial, it has been suggested that patients with graft failure receive one or more courses of rhGM-CSF in view of the otherwise dismal prognosis. The FDA has approved the use of rhGM-CSF as indicated therapy in patients

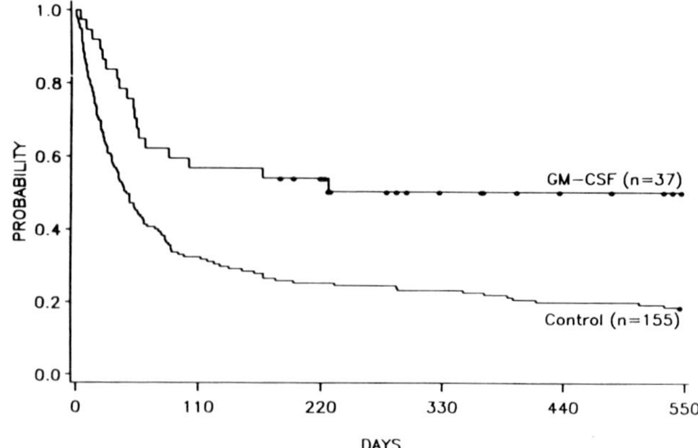

Figure 24-3. Kaplan-Meier estimates of survival for 155 historical patients with graft failure and 37 marrow graft failure patients who received rhGM-CSF. Day 0 in the control patients was the day on which they met the definition of graft failure. Day 0 in the rhGM-CSF patients was the day therapy was initiated.

in whom marrow graft failure develops. Patients who do not respond to rhGM-CSF should be enrolled in clinical trials evaluating the toxicities and possible effectiveness of newer cytokines, which may affect earlier cells than GM-CSF. Trials of the c-kit ligand (stem-cell factor), the GM-CSF-IL-3 fusion molecule (PIXY321), and IL-1 with G-CSF or GM-CSF are of particular interest in graft failure.

Cytokines Currently Under Development

M-CSF

M-CSF is a monocyte-macrophage activator and growth factor produced by nearly all cells. M-CSF increases the functional activities of monocytes and macrophages, including phagocytosis and intracellular killing of bacteria and fungi and effector cell function in antibody-dependent cytotoxity assays (145,146). Results of BMT with M-CSF in a murine model suggest that it stimulated granulopoiesis and improved survival (147). In primates, rhM-CSF had no significant toxicities other than dose-related thrombocytopenia (148).

Both purified urinary M-CSF and rhM-CSF have been given to patients after BMT to stimulate hematopoiesis with marginal effects (148–150). rhM-CSF may prove to be most useful as an adjunct in the treatment of established intracellular infections and as a biological agent to increase the host response to monoclonal antibodies directed at tumor-associated antigens. Murine studies suggest that M-CSF augments the ability to kill *Candida* both in vitro and in vivo in neutropenic hosts (146,148,151–153).

Despite aggressive use of currently available antibiotic therapy, fungal infections in marrow transplant patients are associated with a high short-term mortality (154). To examine whether a cytokine such as M-CSF, which increases the ability of phagocytic cells to kill intracellular organisms, might change the natural history of fungal infections after BMT, a single center Phase I to II trial was performed (149). Patients were eligible to receive rhM-CSF if they had either a biopsy-proven closed-space infection, at least 2 positiye blood cultures after removal of indwelling lines, or radiological evidence for fungal infections (pneumonia or abscesses) with at least one positive blood culture. rhM-CSF was given with standard antifungal therapy for 30 days. Patients were considered to have complete responses only if there was either complete radiological resolution of all lesions or if no organisms were seen on rebiopsy. rhM-CSF was well tolerated at doses up to 2,000 $\mu g/m^2$/day, when reversible thrombocytopenia became dose-limiting. Although it was not possible to evaluate efficacy in this trial, several patients who had progressive disease on amphotericin B alone resolved their infections when rhM-CSF was added. Two patients who had amphotericin B–refractory fungal infections acquired during induction therapy for acute leukemia had complete resolution of infections and were able to undergo successful allogeneic BMT without recurrences of fungal infections. When compared with historical patients in whom closed-space fungal disease developed after BMT, there appeared to be a survival advantage for patients who received rhM-CSF in addition to standard antifungal therapy (155). A multicenter randomized trial has been developed to examine the potential efficacy of rhM-CSF in the treatment of fungal disease after BMT.

Interleukin-3

IL-3 is a multipotent colony stimulating factor that stimulates the growth of granulocytes, megakaryocytes, eosinophils, and erythroid cells in vitro and stimulated both neutrophil and platelet recovery in animals (156,157). It is potentially synergistic with GM-CSF and G-CSF and may be the first cytokine available that substantially stimulates platelet recovery (157–161).

IL-3 has undergone Phase I and II trials in Europe in patients with myelodysplasia (162) and is under study in autologous BMT and following chemotherapy. Clinical data are still too preliminary to be analyzed for efficacy.

A fusion molecule (PIXY321) containing both GM-CSF and IL-3 created through genetic engineering is potentially more potent than either IL-3 or GM-CSF (163,164). GM-CSF and IL-3 administered separately are synergistic (160), and preliminary preclinical data suggest this synergism will be true for the fusion molecule as well. Animal studies indicate that the activities of both IL-3 and GM-CSF appear to be preserved without additional toxicity.

Interleukin-1

There are two genetically distinct IL-1 molecules (α and β) currently undergoing clinical trials (165,166). They activate the same receptors and have nearly identical effects. Unlike the colony stimulating factors, IL-1 affects cells in nearly all lineages and thus may have substantial numbers of undesirable side effects. IL-1 has hematopoietic stimulatory and radioprotective effects. In animal trials, IL-1 was synergistic with growth factors such as G-CSF or GM-CSF in accelerating hematopoietic recovery following cytotoxic therapy (55,167–173). rhIL-1 improved the survival of mice given allogeneic bone marrow transplants (171). IL-1, but not G-CSF or GM-CSF, improved survival in mice following high-dose 5-fluorouracil. This finding suggested that IL-1 may protect against the effects of intensive cytotoxic therapy by abrogating nonhematopoietic toxicities through induction of free-radical scavenging activity (174,175).

During Phase I trials, IL-1 was found to produce significant toxicity, including fevers, reversible hypotension, occasional hypertension, and headaches (175). Clinical data are as yet too preliminary to assess fully either the toxicity of IL-1 or its efficacy as a hematopoietic stimulant. No data are available as to the effectiveness of IL-1 when used to prime stem cells for response to a second cytokine, such as rhGM-CSF or rhG-CSF. IL-1 as a single agent had no apparent hematopoietic stimulatory effects in patients with graft failure who were refractory to rhGM-CSF.

c-kit Ligand (Also Called Steel Factor, Stem-Cell Factor, and Mast Cell Growth Factor)

The c-kit ligand is a potent cytokine that stimulates very immature hematopoietic progenitor cells and is synergistic with other growth factors in promoting the expansion and maturation of blood cells (21,176). When added to erythropoietin, the c-kit ligand produces a large increase in the size of erythroid colonies (177–179). The c-kit ligand may prove to be the most effective cytokine for stimulating an increase in PBPC. Administered as a single agent in primates, stem-cell factor increased marrow cellularity and raised neutrophil, lymphocyte, red blood cell, and platelet counts (180). When given after cytotoxic therapy in dogs, it substantially accelerated hematopoietic recovery (Schuening F. Personal communication). In addition, stem-cell factor protects dogs following otherwise supralethal doses of irradiation. (Schuening F. Personal communication). Trials in humans have begun, but no data are yet available. If c-kit ligand proves to be nontoxic, it may be the first clinically useful growth factor capable of stimulating platelet and red cell recovery in BMT patients. The c-kit ligand may also be an ideal agent to combine with a second cytokine, such as G-CSF or GM-CSF (181).

rhIL-6

rhIL-6 is a 26-kd protein that recently entered clinical trials in patients with myelodysplasia and in patients with refractory cancer. Animal studies suggest that IL-6 may have significant platelet stimulatory properties (182–184). It may therefore be of interest in BMT patients with late sustained thrombocytopenia. Due to the broad spectrum of nonhematopoietic activities of IL-6, administration is likely to affect other organ systems (184).

Other Cytokines of Interest in BMT

Two cytokines that stimulated platelet production in preclinical studies have been developed and should enter clinical trials shortly: IL-11 and leukemia inhibitory factor (LIF) (183,185,186). Both are likely to have a multiplicity of nonhematopoietic effects that may make them unsuitable for use as hemopoietins. However, this effect is speculative until Phase I trials are completed. In vitro data suggest that IL-11 may stimulate early hematopoietic progenitors in addition to megakaryocytes (23,24).

Summary

The development of recombinant cytokines has already led to the ability to decrease the morbidity and cost of autologous BMT. However, it is apparent that additional, carefully controlled clinical trials are needed to define the optimal use of these potent but expensive agents. Cytokines may decrease the cost of BMT, allow application of more intensive therapeutic regimens with lower morbidity, and lead to application of BMT earlier in the course of disease. These advances may ultimately result in the cure of a greater proportion of patients.

References

1. Clark SC, Kamen R. The human hematopoietic colony-stimulating factors. Science 1987;236:1229–1237.
2. Metcalf D. The granulocyte-macrophage colony stimulating factors. Science 1985;229:16–22.
3. Metcalf D. The molecular biology of the granulocyte/macrophage colony-stimulating factors. Blood 1986;67: 257–267.
4. Nicola NA. Hemopoietic growth factors and their receptors. Ann Rev Biochem 1989;58:45–77.
5. Metcalf D. Control of granulocytes and macrophages: molecular; cellular; and clinical aspects. Science 1991;254:529–533.
6. Boggs DR. The kinetics of neutrophilic leukocytes in health and disease. Semin Hematol 1967;4:359–374.
7. Till JE, McCulloch EA. A direct measurement of the radiation sensitivity of normal mouse bone marrow cells. Radiat Res 1961;14:213–222.
8. Lemischka IR, Raulet DH, Mulligan RC. Developmental potential and dynamic behavior of hematopoietic stem cells. Cell 1986;45:917–924.
9. Metcalf D. Clonal culture of hemopoietic cells. Amsterdam: Elsiever/North American Biomedical Press, 1984.
10. Gordon MY, Dowding CR, Riley GP, Greaves MF. Characterization of stroma-dependent blast colony-forming cells in human marrow. J Cell Physiol 1987;130:150–156.
11. Dexter TM, Allen TD, Lajtha LG. Conditions controlling the proliferation of haemopoietic stem cells in vitro. J Cell Physiol 1977;91:335–344.
12. Dexter TM. Stromal cell associated hematopoiesis. J Cell Physiol 1982;(suppl 1):87–94.
13. Singer JW, Keating A, Wight TN. The human haemopoietic microenvironment. In: Hoffbrand AV ed. Recent advances in haematology, number 4; (ed.). Edinburgh: Churchill Livingstone, 1985:1–24.
14. Gordon MY, Clarke D, Atkinson J, Greaves MF. Hemopoietic progenitor cell binding to the stromal microenvironment in vitro. Exp Hematol 1990;18:837–842.
15. Tavassoli M, Hardy CL, Aizawa S, Matsuoka T, Minguell J. Molecular mechanism of hematopoietic stem cell binding to the supportive stroma. Prog Clin Biol Res 1990;352:87–110.
16. Long MW. Blood cell cytoadhesion molecules. Exp Hematol 1992;20:288–301.
17. Gordon MY, Riley GP, Watt SM, Greaves ME. Compartmentalization of a haematopoietic growth factor (GM-CSF) by glycosaminoglycans in the bone marrow microenvironment. Nature 1987;326:403–405.
18. Roberts R, Gallagher J, Spooncer E, Allen TD, Bloomfield F, Dexter TM. Heparan sulfate-bound growth

factors: a mechanism for stromal cell-mediated haemopoiesis. Nature 1988;332:376–378.
19. Slack JL, Nemunaitis J, Andrews DF, Singer JW. Regulation of cytokine and growth factor gene expression in human bone marrow stromal cells transformed with simian virus 40. Blood 1990;75:2319–2327.
20. Nemunaitis J, Andrews DF, Crittenden C, Kaushansky K, Singer JW. Response of simian virus 40 (SV40)-transformed, cultured human marrow stromal cells to hematopoietic growth factors. J Clin Invest 1989;83: 593–601.
21. Williams DE, Eisenman J, Baird A, et al. Identification of a ligand for the c-kit proto-oncogene. Cell 1990;63: 167–174.
22. Huang E, Nocka K, Beier DR, et al. The hematopoietic growth factor KL is encoded by the *Sl* locus and is the ligand of the c-kit receptor; the gene product of the *W* locus. Cell 1990;63:225–233.
23. Musashi M, Clark SC, Sudo T, Urdal D, Ogawa M. Synergistic interaction between interleukin-11 and interleukin-4 in support of proliferation of primitive hematopoietic progenitors of mice. Blood 1991;78: 1448–1451.
24. Paul SR, Bennett F, Calvetti JA, et al. Molecular cloning of a cDNA encoding interleukin-11; a stromal cell-derived lymphopoietic and hematopoietic cytokine. Proc Natl Acad Sci USA 1990;87:7512–7516.
25. Andrews RG, Singer JW, Bernstein ID. Monoclonal antibody 12.8 recognizes a 115 kd molecule present on both unipotent and multipotent hematopoietic colony-forming cells and their progenitors. Blood 1986;67:842–845.
26. Andrews RG, Takahashi M, Segal GM, Powell JS, Singer JW, Bernstein ID. The L4F3 antigen is expressed by uni- and multipotent colony forming cells but not by their precursors. Blood 1986;68:1030–1035.
27. Andrews RG, Singer JW, Bernstein ID. Precursors of colony-forming cells in humans can be distinguished from colony-forming cells by expression of the CD33 and CD34 antigens and light scatter properties. J Exp Med 1989;169:1721–1731.
28. Andrews RG, Singer JW, Bernstein ID. Human hematopoitic precursors in long-term culture: single CD34+ cells that lack detectable T; B; and myeloid antigens produce multiple colony-forming cells when cultured with marrow stromal cells. J Exp Med 1990;172:355–364.
29. Fialkow PJ, Jacobson RJ, Papayannopoulou T. Chronic myelocytic leukemia: clonal origin in a stem cell common to the granulocyte; erythrocyte; platelet and monocyte/macrophage. Am J Med 1977;63:125–130.
30. Fialkow PJ, Denman AM, Jacobson RJ, Lowenthal MN. Chronic myelocytic leukemia. Origin of some lymphocytes from leukemic stem cells. J Clin Invest 1978;62: 815–823.
31. Martin PJ, Najfeld V, Fialkow PJ. B-lymphoid cell involvement in chronic myelogenous leukemia: implications for the pathogenesis of the disease. Cancer Genet Cytogenet 1982;6:359–368.
32. Leary AG, Strauss LC, Civin KC, Ogawa M. Disparate differentiation in hemopoietic colonies derived from human paired progenitors. Blood 1985;66:327–332.
33. Sherr CJ, Rettenmier CW, Roussel MF. Macrophage colony-stimulating factor; CSF-1; and its proto-oncogene-Encoded receptor. Cold Spring Harbor Symp Quant Biol 1988;53:521–530.
34. Geissler EN, Liao M, Brook JD, et al. Stem cell factor (SCF); a novel hematopoietic growth factor and ligand for c-kit tyrosine kinase receptor; maps on human chromosome 12 between 12q14.3 and 12qter. Somat Cell Mol Genet 1991;17:207–214.
35. Sporn MB, Roberts AB. Peptide growth factors are multifunctional. Nature 1988;332:217–219.
36. Heller RA, Song K, Onasch MA, Fischer WH, Chang D, Ringold GM. Complementary DNA cloning of a receptor for tumor necrosis factor and demonstration of a shed form of the receptor. Proc Natl Acad Sci USA 1990;87:6151–6155.
37. Shieh JH, Peterson RHF, Warren DJ, Moore MAS. Modulation of colony-stimulating factor-1 receptors on macrophages by tumor necrosis factor. J Immunol 1989;143:2534–2539.
38. Elbaz O, Budel LM, Hoogerbrugge H, et al. Tumor necrosis factor downregulates granulocyte-colony-stimulating factor receptor expression on human acute myeloid leukemia cells and granulocytes. J Clin Invest 1991;87:838–841.
39. Shieh JH, Peterson RH, Moore MA. Modulation of granulocyte colony-stimulating factor receptors on murine peritoneal exudate macrophages by tumor necrosis factor-alpha. J Immunol 1991;146:2648–2653.
40. Elbaz O, Budel LM, Hoogerbrugge H, et al. Tumor necrosis factor downregulates granulocyte-colony-stimulating factor receptor expression on human acute myeloid leukemia cells and granulocytes. J Clin Invest 1991;87:838–841.
41. Elbaz O, Budel LM, Hoogerbrugge H, et al. Tumor necrosis factor regulates the expression of granulocyte-macrophage colony-stimulating factor and interleukin-3 receptors on human acute myeloid leukemia cells. Blood 1991;77:989–995.
42. Castell JV, Gomez-Lechon MJ, David M, et al. Interleukin-6 is the major regulator of acute phase protein synthesis in adult human hepatocytes. FEBS Lett 1989;242:237–239.
43. Hirano T, Taga T, Yamasaki K, et al. A multifunctional cytokine (IL-6/BSF-2) and its receptor. Int Arch Allergy Appl Immunol 1989;88:29–33.
44. Wong G, Clark S. Multiple actions of interleukin 6 within a cytokine network. Immunol Today 1988;9:137–139.
45. Williams N, De Giorgio T, Banu N, Withy R, Hirano T, Kishimoto T. Recombinant interleukin 6 stimulates immature murine megakaryocytes. Exp Hematol 1990; 18:69–72.
46. Kishimoto T. The biology of interleukin-6. Blood 1989;74:1–10.
47. Sisson SD, Dinarello CA. Production of interleukin-1α interleukin-1β and tumor necrosis factor by human mononuclear cells stimulated with granulocyte-macrophage colony-stimulating factor. Blood 1988;72:1368–1374.
48. Cannistra SA, Rambaldi A, Spriggs DR, Kufe D, Griffin JD. Human granulocyte-macrophage colony-stimulating factor induces expression of the tumor necrosis factor gene by the U937 cell line and by normal human monocytes. J Clin Invest 1987;79:1720–1728.
49. Heidenreich S, Gong JH, Schmidt A, Nain M, Gemsa D. Macrophage activation by granulocyte/macrophage colony-stimulating factor: Priming for enhanced release of tumor necrosis factor-α and prostaglandin E_2. J Immunol 1989;143:1198–1205.
50. Haranaka K. Antiproliferative and proliferative effects of TNF on normal and tumor cells. Biotherapy 1991;3:121–125.

51. Beutler B, Cerami A. Cachectin and tumor necrosis factor as two sides of the same biological coin. Nature 1986;321:584–588.
52. Cannistra SA, Griffin JD. Regulation of the production and function of granulocytes and monocytes. Semin Hematol 1988;25:173–188.
53. Muench MO, Schneider G, Moore MAS. Interactions among colony-stimulating factors; IL-1β; IL-6; and kit ligand in the regulation of primitive hematopoietic cells. Exp Hematol 1992;20:339–349.
54. Ogawa M, Clark SC. Synergistic interaction between interleukin-6 and interleukin-3 in support of stem cell proliferation in culture. Blood Cells 1988;14:329–337.
55. Ikebuchi K, Ihle JN, Hirai Y, Wong GG, Clark SC, Ogawa M. Synergistic factors for stem cell proliferation: further studies of the target stem cells and the mechanism of stimulation by interleukin-1; interleukin-6; and granulocyte colony-stimulating factor. Blood 1988;72: 2007–2014.
56. Ikebuchi K, Wong GG, Clark SC, Ihle JN, Hirai Y, Ogawa M. Interleukin 6 enhancement of interleukin 3-dependent proliferation of multipotential hemopoietic progenitors. Proc Natl Acad Sci USA 1987;84: 9035–9039.
57. Tsuji K, Zsebo KM, Ogawa M. Murine mast cell colony formation supported by IL-3; IL-4; and recombinant rat stem cell factor; ligand for c-kit. J Cell Physiol 1991;148:362–369.
58. Foulke RS, Marshall MH, Trotta PP, Von Hoff DD. In vitro assessment of the effects of granulocyte-macrophage colony-stimulating factor on primary human tumors and derived lines. Cancer Res 1990;50:6264–6267.
59. Evans JPM, Mire-Sluis AR, Hoffbrand AV, Wickremasighe RG. Binding of G-CSF, GMS-CSF, tumor necrosis factor-α, and gamma-interferon to cell surface receptors on human myeloid leukemia cells triggers rapid tyrosine and serine phosphorylation of a 75-Kd protein. Blood 1990;75:88–95.
60. Buechner T, Hiddemann W, Koenigsmann M, et al. Recombinant human GM-CSF following chemotherapy in high-risk AML. Bone Marrow Transplant 1990;6(suppl 1):131–134.
61. Budel LM, Touw IP, Delwel R, Lowenberg B. Granulocyte colony-stimulating factor receptors in human acute myelocytic leukemia. Blood 1989;74:2668–2673.
62. Piao YF, Okabe T. Receptor binding of human granulocyte colony-stimulating factor to the blast cells of myeloid leukemia. Cancer Res 1990;50:1671–1674.
63. Teshima H, Ishikawa J, Kitayama H, et al. Clinical effects of recombinant human granulocyte colony-stimulating factor in leukemia patients: a phase I/II study. Exp Hematol 1989;17:853–858.
64. Motoji T, Watanabe M, Uzumaki H, et al. Granulocyte colony-stimulating factor (G-CSF) receptors on acute myeloblastic leukaemia cells and their relationship with the proliferative response to G-CSF in clonogenic assay. Br J Haematol 1991;77:54–59.
65. Nagata S, Tsuchiya M, Asano S, et al. The chromosomal gene structure and two mRNAs for human granulocyte colony-stimulating factor. EMBO J 1986;5:575–581.
66. Nagata S, Tschuiya M, Asano S, et al. Molecular cloning and expression of cDNA for human granulocyte colony-stimulating factor. Nature 1986;319:415–418.
67. Souza LM, Boone TC, Gabrilove J, et al. Recombinant human granulocyte colony-stimulating factor: effects on normal and leukemic myeloid cells. Science 1986; 232:61–65.
68. Metcalf D. The molecular biology of the granulocyte/macrophage colony-stimulating factors. Blood 1986;67: 257–267.
69. Nagata S. Gene structure and function of granulocyte colony-stimulating factor. BioEssays 1989;10:113–117.
70. Welte K, Bonilla MA, Gillio AP, et al. Recombinant human granulocyte colony-stimulating factor. Effects on hematopoiesis in normal and cyclophosphamide-treated primates. J Exp Med 1987;165:941–948.
71. Gillio AP, Bonilla MA, Potter GP, et al. Effects of recombinant human granulocyte colony-stimulating factor on hematopoietic reconstitution after autologous bone marrow transplantation in primates. Transplant Proc 1987;6(suppl 7):153–156.
72. Schuening FG, Storb R, Goehle S, et al. Recombinant human granulocyte colony-stimulating factor accelerates recovery after DLA-identical littermate marrow transplants in dogs. Blood 1990;76:636–640.
73. Schuening FG, Storb R, Goehle S, et al. Effect of recombinant human granulocyte colony-stimulating factor on hematopoiesis of normal dogs and on hematopoietic recovery after otherwise lethal total body irradiation. Blood 1989;74:1308–1313.
74. Moore MA, Swarren DJ, Synergy of interleukin 1 and granulocyte colony stimulating factor: in vivo stimulation of stem-cell recovery and hematopoietic regeneration following 5-fluorouracil treatment of mice. Proc Natl Acad Sci USA 1987;84:7134–7138.
75. Gabrilove JL, Jakubowski A, Scher H, et al. Effect of granulocyte colony-stimulating factor on neutropenia and associated morbidity due to chemotherapy for transitional-cell carcinoma of the urothelium. N Engl J Med 1988;318:1414–1422.
76. Morstyn G, Burgess A. Hemopoietic growth factors: a review. Cancer Res 1988;48:5624–5637.
77. Peters WP. Dose-intensive therapy in breast cancer. In: DeVita VT Jr, Hellman S, Rosenberg SA, eds. Important advances in oncology. Philadelphia: J.B. Lippincott, 1991:135–150.
78. Watari K, Asano S, Shirafuji N, et al. Serum granulocyte colony-stimulating factor levels in healthy volunteers and patients with various disorders as estimated by enzyme immunoassay. Blood 1989;73:117–122.
79. Kawakami M, Tsutumi H, Kumakawa T, et al. Levels of serum granulocyte colony-stimulating factor in patients with infection. Blood 1990;76:1962–1964.
80. Bronchud MH, Howell A, Crowther D, Hopwood P, Souza L, Dexter TM. The use of granulocyte colony-stimulating factor to increase the intensity of treatment with doxorubicin in patients with advanced breast and ovarian cancer. Br J Cancer 1989;60:121–125.
81. Crawford J, Ozer H, Stoller R, et al. Reduction by granulocyte colony-stimulating factor of fever and neutropenia induced by chemotherapy in patients with small-cell lung cancer. N Engl J Med 1991;325:164–170.
82. Sheridan WP, Morstyn G, Wolf M, et al. Granulocyte colony-stimulating factor and neutrophil recovery after high-dose chemotherapy and autologous bone marrow transplantation. Lancet 1989;2:891–895.
83. Taylor KM, Jagannath S, Spitzer G, et al. Recombinant human granulocyte colony-stimulating factor hastens granulocyte recovery after high-dose chemotherapy and autologous bone marrow transplantation in Hodgkin's disease. J Clin Oncol 1989;7:1791–1799.
84. Taylor K, Spitzer G, Jagannath S, Dicke K, Souza L. Phase II study of recombinant human granulocyte colony-stimulating factor (rG-CSF) in Hodgkin's dis-

ease after high-dose chemotherapy with ABMT (Abstract). Blood 1988;72(suppl 1):135a.

85. Peters WP, Kurtzberg I, Atwater S, et al. Comparative effects of rHuG-CSF and rHuGM-CSF on hematopoietic reconstitution and granulocyte function following high dose chemotherapy and autologous bone marrow transplantation (abstract). Blood 1988;72(suppl 1):130a.
86. Masoka T, Takaku F, Kato S, et al. Recombinant human granulocyte colony-stimulating factor in allogeneic bone marrow transplantation. Exp Hematol 1989;17:1047–1050.
87. Molineux G, Pojda Z, Hampson IN, Lord B, Dexter TM. Transplantation potential of peripheral blood stem cells induced by granulocyte colony-stimulating factor. Blood 1990;76:2153–2158.
88. Kessinger A, Armitage JO. The evolving role of autologous peripheral stem cell transplantation following high-dose therapy for malignancies. Blood 1991;77: 211–213.
89. Wong GG, Witek JS, Temple PA, et al. Human GM-CSF: molecular cloning of a complementary DNA and purification of the natural and recombinant proteins. Science 1985;228:810–815.
90. Sullivan R, Fredette JP, Socinski M, et al. Enhancement of superoxide anion release by granulocytes harvested from patients receiving granulocyte-macrophage colony-stimulating factor. Br J Haematol 1989;71:475–479.
91. Weisbart RH, Golde DW, Gasson JC. Biosynthetic human GM-CSF modulates the number and affinity of neutrophil f-met-leu-phe receptors. J Immunol 1986; 137:3584–3587.
92. Fleishman J, Golde DW, Weisbart RH, Gasson JC. Granulocyte-macrophage colony-stimulating factor enhances phagocytosis of bacteria by human neutrophils. Blood 1986;68:708–711.
93. Weisbart RH, Golde DW, Clark SC, Wong GG, Gasson JC. Human granulocyte/macrophage colony stimulating factor is a neutrophil activator. Nature 1985;314: 361–363.
94. Lindemann A, Reidel D, Oster W, Ziegler-Heitbrock HW, Mertelsmann R, Hermann F. Granulocyte-macrophage colony-stimulating factor induces cytokine secretion by human polymorphonuclear leukocytes. J Clin Invest 1989;83:1308–1312.
95. Ribeiro RA, Flores CA, Cunha F, Ferreira SH. IL-8 causes in vivo neutrophil migration by a cell-dependent mechanism. Immunology 1991;73:472–477.
96. Kunkel SL, Strieter RM, Chensue SW, et al. Tumor necrosis factor-alpha; interleukin-8 and chemotactic cytokines. Prog Clin Biol Res 1990;349:433–444.
97. Frenck RW, Sarman G, Harper TE, Buescher ES. The ability of recombinant murine granulocyte-macrophage colony-stimulating factor to protect neonatal rats from septic death due to Staphylococcus aureus. J Infect Dis 1990;162:109–114.
98. Bermudez LE, Martinelli JC, Gascon R. Protection against gram-negative bacteremia in neutropenic mice with recombinant granulocyte-macrophage colony-stimulating factor. Cytokine 1990;2:287–293.
99. Mayer P, Schultz E, Lam C. Recombinant human granulocyte-macrophage colony-stimulating factor augments neutrophil recovery and enhances resistance to infections in myelosuppressed mice. J Infect Dis 1991;163:584–590.
100. Roilides E, Walsh TJ, Pizozo PA, Rubin M. Granulocyte colony-stimulating factor enhances the phagocytic and bactericidal activity of normal and defective human neutrophils. J Infect Dis 1991;163:579–583.
101. Nienhuis AW, Donahue RE, Karlsson S, et al. Recombinant human granulocyte-macrophage colony-stimulating factor (GM-CSF) shortens the period of neutropenia after autologous bone marrow transplantation in a primate model. J Clin Invest 1987;80:572–577.
102. Monroy RL, Skelly RR, Macvittie TJ, et al. The effect of recombinant GM-CSF on the recovery of monkeys transplanted with autologous bone marrow. Blood 1987;70:1696–1699.
103. Donahue RE, Seehra J, Metzger M, et al. Human IL-3 and GM-CSF act synergistically in stimulating hematopoiesis in primates. Science 1988;241:1820–1822.
104. Krumwieh D, Seiler FR. In vivo effects of recombinant colony stimulating factors on hematopoiesis in cynomolgus monkeys. Transplant Proc 1989;21:2964–2967.
105. Geisser K, Valent TP, Mayer P, et al. Recombinant human interleukin-3 expands the pool of circulating hematopoietic progenitor cells in primates—synergism with recombinant human granulocyte-macrophage colony-stimulating factor. Blood 1990;75: 2305–2310.
106. Broxmeyer HE, Williams DE, Hangoc G, et al. Synergistic myelopoietic actions in vivo after administration to mice of combinations of purified natural murine colony-stimulating factor 1, recombinant murine interleukin 3, and recombinant murine granulocyte/macrophage colony-stimulating factor. Proc Natl Acad Sci USA 1987;84:3871–3875.
107. Blazar BR, Widmer MB, Soderling CRB, et al. Augmentation of donor bone marrow engraftment in histoincompatible murine recipients by granulocyte-macrophage colony-stimulating factor. Blood 1988; 71:320–328.
108. Blazar BR, Widmer MB, Cosman D, Sassenfeld HM, Vallera DA. Improved survival and leukocyte reconstitution without detrimental effects on engraftment in murine recipients of human recombinant granulocyte colony-stimulating factor after transplantation of T-cell-depleted histoincompatible bone marrow. Blood 1989;74:2264–2269.
109. Atkinson K, Matias C, Guiffre A, et al. In vivo administration of granulocyte colony-stimulating factor (G-CSF), granulocyte-macrophage CSF, interleukin-1 (IL-1), and IL-4, alone and in combination, after allogeneic murine hematopoietic stem cell transplantation. Blood 1991;77:1376–1382.
110. Socinski MA, Cannistra SA, Elias A, Antman KH, Schnipper L, Griffin JD. Granulocyte-macrophage colony stimulating factor expands the circulating haemopoietic progenitor cell compartment in man. Lancet 1988;21:1194–1198.
111. Siena S, Bregni M, Brandod B, Ravagnani F, Bonnadonna G, Gianni AM. Circulation of CD34+ hematopoietic stem cells in the peripheral blood of high dose cyclophosphamide-treated patients: enchancement by intravenous recombinant human granulocyte-macrophage colony-stimulating factor. Blood 1989;74: 1905–1914.
112. Tarella C, Ferrero D, Bregni M, et al. Peripheral blood expansion of early progenitor cells after high-dose cyclophosphamide and rhGM-CSF. Eur J Cancer 1991;27:22–27.
113. Gianni AM, Bregni M, Stern AC, et al. Granulocyte-macrophage colony-stimulating factor to harvest circu-

lating haemopoietic stem cells for autotransplantation. Lancet 1989;2:580–585.
114. Nemunaitis J, Singer JW, Buckner CD, et al. Use of recombinant human granulocyte/macrophage colony stimulating factor in autologous bone marrow transplantation for lymphoid malignancies. Blood 1988;72: 834–836.
115. Nemunaitis J, Singer JW, Buckner CD, et al. Use of recombinant human granulocyte-macrophage colony-stimulating factor in graft failure after bone marrow transplantation. Blood 1990;76:245–253.
116. Thompson JA, Lee DJ, Kidd P, et al. Subcutaneous granulocyte-macrophage colony-stimulating factor in patients with myelodysplastic syndrome: toxicity; pharmacokinetics; and hematological effects. J Clin Oncol 1989;7:629–637.
117. Vadhan RS, Keating M, Lemaistre A, et al. Effects of recombinant human granulocyte-macrophage colony-stimulating factor in patients with myelodysplastic syndromes. N Engl J Med 1987;317:1545–1552.
118. Glaspy JA, Golde DW. Clinical trials of myeloid growth factors. Exp Hematol 1990;18:1137–1141.
119. Antman KS, Griffin JD, Elias A, et al. Effects of recombinant human granulocyte-macrophage colony-stimulating factor on chemotherapy-induced myelosuppression. N Engl J Med 1988;319:593–598.
120. Brandt SJ, Peters WP, Atwater SK, et al. Effect of recombinant human granulocyte-macrophage colony-stimulating factor on hematopoietic reconstitution after high-dose chemotherapy and autologous bone marrow transplantation. N Engl J Med 1988;318:869–876.
121. Peters WP, Stuart A, Affronti ML, Kim CS, Coleman RE. Neutrophil migration is defective during recombinant human granulocyte-macrophage colony-stimulating factor infusion after autologous bone marrow transplantation in humans. Blood 1988;72:1310–1315.
122. Toner GC, Jakubowski AA, Crown JP, et al. Colony-stimulating factors and neutrophil migration. Ann Intern Med 1989;110:846–847.
123. Nemunaitis J, Rabinowe SN, Singer JW, et al. Recombinant granulocyte-macrophage colony-stimulating factor after autologous bone marrow transplantation for lymphoid cancer. N Engl J Med 1991;324:1773–1778.
124. Nemunaitis J, Singer JW, Buckner CD, et al. Long-term follow-up of patients who received recombinant human granulocyte-macrophage colony stimulating factor after autologous bone marrow transplantation for lymphoid malignancy. Bone Marrow Transplant 1991;7:49–52.
125. Nemunaitis J, Singer JW, Buckner CD, et al. Use of recombinant human granulocyte-macrophage colony stimulating factor (rhGM-CSF) in autologous marrow transplantation for lymphoid malignancies. In: Dicke KA, ed. Autologous bone marrow transplantation: proceedings of the third international symposium. Houston: University of Texas, 1989:631–636.
126. Fouillard L, Gorin NC, Laporte JP, et al. GM-CSF and gancyclovir for cytomegalovirus infection after autologous bone marrow transplantation. Lancet 1989;2: 1273.
127. Thomas S, Clark SC, Rappeport JM, Nathan DG, Emerson SG. Deficient T cell granulocyte-macrophage colony stimulating factor production in allogeneic bone marrow transplant recipients. Transplantation 1990;49:703–708.
128. Fabian I, Kletter Y, Bleiberg I, Gadish M, Naparsteck E, Slavin S. Effect of exogenous human granulocyte-macrophage colony-stimulating factor on neutrophil function following allogeneic bone marrow transplantation. Exp Hematol 1991;19:868–873.
129. Wing EJ, Magee DM, Whiteside TL, Kaplan SS, Shadduck RK. Recombinant human granulocyte/macrophage colony-stimulating factor enhances monocyte cytotoxicity and secretion of tumor necrosis factor α and interferon in cancer patients. Blood 1989;73:643–646.
130. Engelmann H, Holtmann H, Brakebusch C, et al. Antibodies to a soluble form of a tumor necrosis factor (TNF) receptor have TNF-like activity. J Biol Chem 1990;265:14497–14504.
131. Suda T, Murray R, Guidos C, Zlotnik A. Growth-promoting activity of IL-1 alpha; IL-6; and tumor necrosis factor-alpha in combination with IL-2; IL-4; or IL-7 on murine thymocytes. Differential effects on CD4/CD8 subsets and on CD3+/CD3− double-negative thymocytes. J Immunol 1990;144:3039–3045.
132. Houssiau FA, Coulie PG, Van Snick J. Distinct roles of IL-1 and IL-6 in human T cell activation. J Immunol 1989;143:2520–2524.
133. Falk W, Mannel DN, Darjes H, Krammer PH. IL-1 induces high affinity IL-2 receptor expression of CD4-8- thymocytes. J Immunol 1989;143:513–517.
134. Hackett RJ, Davis LS, Lipsky PE. Comparative effects of tumor necrosis factor-alpha and IL-1 beta on mitogen-induced T cell activation. J Immunol 1988; 140:2639–2644.
135. Nemunaitis J, Buckner CD, Appelbaum FR, et al. Phase I/II trial of recombinant human granulocyte-macrophage colony-stimulating factor following allogeneic bone marrow transplantation. Blood 1991;77: 2065–2071.
136. Royall JA, Berkow RL, Beckman JS, Cunningham MK, Matalon S, Freeman BA. Tumor necrosis factor and interleukin 1 increase vascular endothelial permeability. Am J Physiol 1989;257:399–410.
137. Goldfeld AE, Doyle C, Maniatis T. Human tumor necrosis factor α gene regulation by virus and lipopolysaccharide. Proc Natl Acad Sci USA 1990;87: 9769–9773.
138. Moore FD Jr. Socher SH, Davis C. Tumor necrosis factor and endotoxin can cause neutrophil activation through separate pathways. Arch Surg 1991;126:70–73.
139. Deforge LE, Remick DG. Kinetics of TNF; IL-6; and IL-8 gene expression in LPS-stimulated human whole blood. Biochem Biophys Res Commun 1991;174:18–24.
140. Piguet PF, Grau GE, Allet B, Vassalli P. Tumor necrosis factor/cachectin is an effector of skin and gut lesions of the acute phase of graft-versus-host disease. J Exp Med 1987;166:1280–1289.
141. Shalaby MR, Fendly B, Sheehan KC, Schreiber RD, Ammann AJ. Prevention of the graft-versus-host reaction in newborn mice by antibodies to tumor necrosis factor. Transplantation 1989;47:1057–1061.
142. McGlave PB, Beatty P, Ash RH, et al. Therapy for chronic myelogenous leukemia with unrelated donor bone marrow transplantation: results in 102 cases. Blood 1990;75:1728–1732.
143. Beatty PG, Hansen JA, Anasetti C. Marrow transplantation from unrelated HLA-matched volunteer donors. Transplant Proc 1989;2:2993–2994.
144. Nemunaitis J, Anasetti C, Storb R, et al. Phase II trial of recombinant human granulocyte-macrophage col-

ony stimulating factor (rhGM-CSF) in patients undergoing allogeneic bone marrow transplantation from unrelated donors. Blood 1992;79:2572–2577.

145. Ralph PW. Biological properties and molecular biology of the human macrophage growth factor; CSF-1. Immunobiology 1986;172:194–204.
146. Karbassi A, Becker JM, Foster JS, Moore RN. Enhanced killing of *Candida albicans* by murine macrophages treated with macrophage colony-stimulating factor: evidence for augmented expression of mannose receptors. J Immunol 1987;139:417–421.
147. Yanai N, Yamada M,Motoyoshi K, et al. Effect of human macrophage colony-stimulating factor on granulopoiesis and survival in bone marrow transplanted mice. Jpn J Cancer Res 1990;81:351–362.
148. Garnick NB, Stoudemier JB. Preclinical and clinical evaluation of recombinant human macrophage colony-stimulating factor (rhM-CSF). Intl J Cell Cloning 1990;8(suppl 1):356–373.
149. Nemunaitis J, Meyers JD, Buckner CD, et al. Phase I trial of recombinant human macrophage colony-stimulating factor in patients with invasive fungal infections. Blood 1991;78:907–913.
150. Masaoka T, Shibata H, Ohno R, et al. Double-blind test of human urinary macrophage colony-stimulating factor for allogeneic and syngeneic bone marrow transplantation: effectiveness of treatment and two-year followup for relapse of leukemia. Br J Haematol 1990;76:501–505.
151. Wang M, Friedman HD, Jeu JY. Enhancement of human monocyte function against *Candida albicans* by the colony-stimulating factors (CSF): IL-3; granulocyte-macrophage-CSF; and macrophage-CSF. J Immunol 1989;143:671–677.
152. Sasada M, Johnston RB. Macrophage microbiocidal activity. Correlation between phagocytosis-associated oxidative metabolism and killing of candida by macrophages. J Exp Med 1980;152:85–98.
153. Motoyoshi K, Takaku F, Maekawa T, et al. Protective effect of partially purified urinary colony-stimulating factor on granulocytopenia after antitumor chemotherapy. Exp Hematol 1986;14:1069–1075.
154. Meyers JE. Infections in bone marrow transplant recipients. Am J Med 1986;61(suppl 1A):27–35.
155. Nemunaitis J, Singer JW. Macrophage colony-stimulating factor (M-CSF). Biology and clinical applications. In: Armitage J, Antman K, eds. High-dose cancer therapy: pharmacology; hematopoietics; and stem cells. Baltimore: Williams and Wilkins, 1992: 344–361.
156. Oster W, Schulz G. Interleukin-3: biological and clinical effects. Int J Cell Cloning 1991;9:5–23.
157. Lindemann A, Ganser A, Hermann F, et al. Biologic effects of recombinant interleukin-3 in vivo. J Clin Oncol 1991;9:2120–2127.
158. Griffin JD. Hemopoietins in oncology: factoring out myelosuppression. J Clin Oncol 1989;7:151–155.
159. Yang YC, Clark SC. Interleukin-3: molecular biology and biologic activities. Hematol Oncol Clin North Am 1989;3:441–452.
160. Donahue RE, Seehra J, Metzger M, et al. Human IL-3 and GM-CSF act synergistically in stimulating hematopoiesis in primates. Science 1988;241:1820–1823.
161. Ganser A, Seipelt G, Lindemann A, et al. Effect of recombinant human interleukin-3 in patients with myelodysplastic syndromes. Blood 1990;76:455–462.
162. Wagemaker G, Van Gils F, Burger H, et al. Highly increased production of bone marrow-derived blood cells by administration of homologous interleukin-3 to rhesus monkey. Blood 1990;76:2235–2241.
163. Williams DE, Park LS. Hematopoietic effects of a granulocyte-macrophage colony-stimulating factor/interleukin-3 fusion protein. Cancer 1991;67(suppl): 2705–2707.
164. Williams DE, Park LS, Broxmeyer HE. Hybrid cytokines as hematopoietic growth factors. Int J Cell Cloning 1991;9:542–547.
165. Dinarello CA. Interleukin-1. Ann NY Acad Sci 1988; 546:122–132.
166. Dinarello CA, Cannon JG, Mier JW. Multiple biological activities of human recombinant interleukin 1. J Clin Invest 1986;77:1734–1739.
167. Williams DE, Morrissey PJ. Alterations in megakaryocyte and platelet compartments following in vivo IL-1β administration to normal mice. J Immunol 1989;142:4361–4365.
168. Gallicchio VS, Doukas MA, Hulette BC, Hughes NK, Gass C. Protection of 3′-azido-3′-deoxythymidine induced toxicity to murine hematopoietic progenitors (CFU-GM; BFU-E and CFU-MEG) with interleukin-1. Proc Soc Exp Biol Med 1989;192:201–204.
169. Schaafsma MR, Falkenburg JHF, Duinkerken N, et al. Interleukin-1 synergizes with granulocyte-macrophage colony-stimulating factor on granulocytic colony formation by intermediate production of granulocyte colony-stimulating factor. Blood 1989;74:2398–2404.
170. Schwartz GN, Patchen ML, Neta R, Macvittie TJ. Radioprotection of mice with interleukin-1: relationship to the number of erythroid and granulocyte-macrophage colony-forming cells. Radiat Res 1990;121:220–226.
171. Oppenheim JJ, Neta R, Tiberghien P, Gress R, Kenny JJ, Longo DL. Interleukin-1 enhances survival of lethally irradiated mice treated with allogeneic bone marrow cells. Blood 1989;74:2257–2263.
172. Takaue Y, Kawano Y, Reading CL, et al. Effects of recombinant human G-CSF, GM-CSF, IL-3, and IL-1α on the growth of purified peripheral blood progenitors. Blood 1990;76:330–335.
173. Iscove NN, Yan XQ. Precursors (pre-CFC_{multi}) of multilineage hemopoietic colony-forming cells quantifated in vitro: uniqueness of IL-1 requirement, partial separation from pluripotential colony-forming cells, and correlation with long term reconstituting cells in vivo. J Immunol 1990;145:190–195.
174. Moore MA, Stolfi RL, Martin DS. Hematologic effects of IL-1β; granulocyte colony-stimulating factor; and granulocyte-macrophage colony-stimulating factor in tumor-bearing mice treated with fluorouracil. J Natl Cancer Inst 1990;82:1031–1037.
175. Starnes HF, Biological effects and possible applications of interleukin-1. Semin Hematol 1991;28: 34–41.
176. Matsui Y, Zsebo KM, Hogan BLM. Embryonic expression of a haematopoietic growth factor encoded by the *Sl* locus and the ligand for c-kit. Nature 1990;347: 667–669.
177. De Vries P, Brasel KA, Eisenman JR, Alpert AR, Williams DE. The effect of recombinant mast cell growth factor on purified murine hematopoietic stem cells. J Exp Med 1991;173:1205–1211.
178. Migliaccio G, Migliaccio AR, Druzin ML, Giardina PJ, Zsebo KM, Adamson JW. Effects of recombinant human stem cell factor (SCF) on the growth of human progenitor cells in vitro. J Cell Physiol 1991;148:503–509.
179. Metcalf D, Nicola NA. Direct proliferative actions of stem cell factor on murine bone marrow cells in vitro:

effects of combination with colony-stimulating factors. Proc Natl Acad Sci USA 1991;88:6239–6243.
180. Andrews RG, Knitter GH, Bartelmez SH, et al. Recombinant human stem cell factor; a c-kit ligand; stimulates hematopoiesis in primates. Blood 1991;78:1975–1980.
181. Ulich TR, Del Castillo J, McNiece IK, et al. Stem cell factor in combination with granulocyte colony-stimulating factor (CSF) or granulocyte-macrophage CSF synergistically increases granulopoiesis in vivo. Blood 1991;78:1954–1962.
182. Ishibashi T, Kimura H, Shikama Y, et al. Interleukin-6 is a potent thrombopoietic factor in vivo in mice. Blood 1989;74:1241–1244.
183. Asano S, Okano A, Ozawa K, et al. In vivo effects of recombinant human interleukin-6 in primates: stimulated production of platelets. Blood 1990;75:1602–1605.
184. Mayer P, Gissler K, Valent P, Ceska M, Bettelheim P, Liehl E. Recombinant human interleukin 6 is a potent inducer of the acute phase response and elevates the blood platelets in nonhuman primates. Exp Hematol 1991;19:688–696.
185. Navarro S, Debili N, Le Couedic JP, et al. Interleukin-6 and its receptor are expressed by human megakaryocytes: in vitro effects on proliferation and endoreplication. Blood 1991;77:461–471.
186. Meshulam DH, Blair HE, Wong BH, Charman S, Minorada J, Rocklin RE. Purification of a lymphoid cell line product with leukocyte inhibitory factor activity. Proc Natl Acad Sci USA 1982;79:601–605.
187. Peters WP. The effect of recombinant human colony-stimulating factors on hematopoietic reconstitution following autologous bone marrow transplantation. Semin Hematol 1989;26(suppl 2):18–23.
188. Auer I, Ribas A, Gale RP. What is the role of recombinant colony-stimulating factors in bone marrow transplantation. Bone Marrow Transplant 1990;6:79–87.
189. Masaoka T, Takaku F, Kato S, et al. Recombinant human granulocyte colony-stimulating factor in allogeneic bone marrow transplantation. Exp Hematol 1989;17:1047–1050.
190. Devereaux S, Linch DC, Gribben JG, McMillan A, Patterson K, Goldstone AH. GM-CSF accelerates neutrophil recovery after autologous bone marrow transplantation for Hodgkin's disease. Bone Marrow Transplant 1989;4:49–54.
191. Blazar BR, Kersey JH, McGlave PB, et al. In vivo administration of recombinant human granulocyte/macrophage colony-stimulating factor in acute lymphoblastic leukemia patients receiving purged autografts. Blood 1989;73:849–857.
192. Link H, Freund M, Kirchner H, Stoll M, Schmid H, Bucksy P. Recombinant human granulocyte-macrophage colony-stimulating factor (rhGM-CSF) after bone marrow transplantation. Behring Inst Mitt 1988;83:313–319.
193. Lazarus HM, Coiffer B, Hyatt M, et al. Recombinant granulocyte-macrophage colony-stimulating factor after autologous bone marrow transplantation for relapsed non-Hodgkin's lymphoma: blood and bone marrow progenitor growth studies. A phase II Eastern Cooperative Oncology Group Trial. Blood 1991;78:830–837.
194. Rabinowe SN, Nemunaitis J, Armitage J, Nadler LM. The impact of myeloid growth factors on engraftment following autologous bone marrow transplantation for malignant lymphoma. Semin Hematol 1991;28(suppl 2):6–16.
195. Gorin NC, Coiffier B, Hayat M, et al. RHU GM-CSF shortens aplasia duration after ABMT in non-Hodgkin's lymphoma: a randomized placebo-controlled double-blind study. Bone Marrow Transplant 1991:7(suppl 2):82.
196. Visani G, Gamberi B, Greenberg P, et al. The use of GM-CSF as an adjunct to autologous/syngeneic bone marrow transplantation: a prospective randomized controlled trial. Bone Marrow Transplant 1991;7(suppl 2):81.
197. Advani R, Chao NJ, Horning SJ, et al. Granulocyte-macrophage colony-stimulating factor (GM-CSF) as an adjunct to autologous hematopoietic stem cell transplantation for lymphoma. Ann Intern Med 1992;116:183–189.
198. Gulati SC, Bennett CL. Granulocyte-macrophage colony-stimulating factor (GM-CSF) as adjunct therapy in relapsed Hodgkin's disease. Ann Intern Med 1992;116:177–182.
199. DeWitte T, Gratwohl A, Vanderlely N, et al. Recombinant human granulocyte-macrophage colony-stimulating factor (rhGM-CSF) reduces infection-related mortality after allogeneic T-depleted bone marrow transplantation. Bone Marrow Transplant 1991;7:83–89.
200. Powles R, Smith C, Milan S, et al. Human recombinant GM-CSF in allogeneic bone marrow transplantation for leukaemia: a double-blind; placebo-controlled trial. Lancet 1990;336:1417–1420.
201. Naparstek E, Hardogen Y, Ben-Shahar A, et al. Enhanced marrow recovery by short preincubationb of marrow allografts with human recombinant interleukin-3 and granulocyte-macrophage colony-stimulating factor. Blood 1992;80:1673–1678.
202. Siena S, Bregni M, Brando B, Ravagnani F, Bonadonna G, Gianni AM. Circulation of CD34+ hematopoietic stem cells in the peripheral blood of high-dose cyclophosphamide-treated patients: enhancement by intravenous recombinant human granulocyte-macrophage colony-stimulating factor. Blood 1989;74:1905–1914.
203. Peters WP, Kertzberg J, Kirkpatrick G, et al. GM-CSF primed peripheral blood progenitor cells (PBPC) coupled with autologous bone marrow transplantation (ABMT) will eliminate absolute leukopenia following high-dose chemotherapy (Abstract). Blood 1989;74:50.
204. Ventura GJ, Hester JP, Spitzer G, et al. Use of GM-CSF mobilized peripheral blood stem cells for hematopoietic recovery after high-dose chemotherapy in autologous bone marrow transplantation (Abstract). Blood 1989;74:425.
205. Tarella C, Ferro D, Bregni M, et al. Peripheral blood expansion of early progenitor cells after high-dose cyclophosphamide and rhGM-CSF. Eur J Cancer 1991;27:22–27.
206. Haas R, Ho AD, Bredthauer U, et al. Successful autologous transplantation of peripheral blood stem cells mobilized with recombinant human granulocyte-macrophage colony-stimulating factor. Exp Hematol 1990;18:94–98.
207. Ravagnani F, Bregni M, Siena S, et al. Role of recombinant human granulocyte-macrophage colony stimulating factor for large scale collection of peripheral blood stem cells for autologous transplantation. Hematologica 1990;75:22–25.

Chapter 25

Nutritional Support of Bone Marrow Transplantation Recipients

Sally A. S. Weisdorf and Sarah Jane Schwarzenberg

This chapter outlines the metabolic support of bone marrow transplantation (BMT) recipients through the complex progression of medical events that typically occur in the course of BMT. Provision of nutritional support to BMT recipients requires an integrated approach between physicians with expertise in nutritional and metabolic requirements of stressed patients and physicians with expertise in management of the rapidly changing physiology of patients recovering from high-dose chemotherapy and radiation. Nutritional support consultants must anticipate and avoid complications, including weight gain or loss, fluid and electrolyte imbalance, sugar and protein overload, and liver dysfunction. The overriding goal is to enable patients to recover the ability to nourish themselves normally (i.e., orally) as quickly as possible following BMT.

Physiological Changes during BMT

The course of BMT can be divided into three periods, each presenting distinct metabolic challenges (1): (1) cytoreduction and tissue damage, (2) pancytopenia and tissue repair, and (3) engraftment, which can be complicated by graft-versus-host disease (GVHD), graft rejection, or return of the primary disease process. Specific organ failure, such as of liver, kidney, heart, or lung, can confound nutritional requirements during any of these sequential periods. These organ failure syndromes can be due to veno-occlusive disease (2), biliary obstruction, recurrence of preexisting hepatitis (3), drug toxicity, and GVHD when there is hepatic dysfunction. These complications can include toxic renal insufficiency or renal failure with fluid and electrolyte imbalance (4); cardiac failure due to drug toxicity, compounded by fluid and electrolyte imbalance (5); or pulmonary failure due to drug toxicity, infection, GVHD, and fluid imbalance (6). Multiple organ failure syndrome can supervene in these settings, often temporally related to sepsis.

Cytoreduction

The first barrier to oral nutrition during cytoreduction is the central nervous system effect of chemotherapy and radiation, which causes severe vomiting. Intestinal dysmotility due to narcotic analgesics can exacerbate vomiting. Cytoreductive therapy also causes painful mucositis in the oral pharynx and the esophagus. Taste sensation is altered; both hypogeusia and dysgeusia are reported (7). The normal growth and repair of intestinal mucosa is disrupted. Histological changes attributable to cytoreductive conditioning therapy have been reported to persist up to day 21 after BMT (8). The loss of functioning intestinal epithelium results in malabsorption and reversal of salt and water absorption. The result is typically an interval of watery diarrhea in the first week following chemo/radiotherapy (9). Stool sodium transiently increases to 50–80 meq/liter. There is usually enough mucosal disruption to cause a transient increase in exudative protein loss into the feces (10), with concomitant loss of zinc and failure to absorb minerals and vitamins. At the same time that patients are unable to ingest and absorb nutrients adequately, protein breakdown is occurring, due both to direct tissue damage and to relative immobilization. Nitrogen losses have been documented in a number of studies (11–14). The massive increased waste nitrogen must be processed by the liver via the urea cycle, which increases the energy demands of the liver and consequently of the whole patient.

Neutropenia

Following cytoreduction, the patient is profoundly neutropenic for 12 to 21 days. Thus, there is a high risk for bacterial infection, treatment of which increases the risk of fungal invasion (15). The damaged intestine may serve as a portal of entry for such infection or can itself be affected with bacterial or fungal overgrowth (16). Narcotic pain therapy can cause intestinal stasis, predisposing to intestinal bacterial overgrowth, which leads to further mucosal damage. Bacterial deconjugation of bile acids promotes fat malabsorption. Passage of bile acid into the colon results in secretory diarrhea by the direct toxic effect that bile salts exert on colonic mucosa. Systemic effects of infection, such as fever, have appetite-suppressant effects as well.

Tissue damage and nitrogen mobilization from protein breakdown are exacerbated by infection, with altered nutrient utilization resulting from the cytokines and hormones elaborated during systemic infection. During the same time that neutropenia is at a maximum, tissue repair is occurring, thus increasing nutrient requirements.

Engraftment

After engraftment, mucosal lesions heal and patients are often able to resume some oral intake. The absence of enteral nutrients and the consequent lack of the neuroendocrine trophic factors that are stimulated in the intestine by nutrients may affect absorption by delaying epithelial cell regeneration. When diarrhea occurs during this time, the differential diagnosis includes GVHD and infection (1,10). Acute GVHD of the intestine can involve the entire intestinal tract (8,17,18). Intestinal GVHD is a lesion that directly damages mucosa and varies in intensity from scattered cell necrosis to complete epithelial denudation (19). Clinically, GVHD diarrhea is similar to that resulting from cytoreduction, but is more severe and prolonged. It has been characterized by massive protein loss in the stool (10) and can cause a profound decrease in nitrogen balance (20). The protein exudation is accompanied by large stool zinc losses, due to the disruption of its enteropancreatic circulation. Decreased zinc stores are reflected clinically in low levels of serum alkaline phosphatase noted even in patients whose elevated bilirubin and 5′-nucleotidase levels indicate obvious cholestasis. Stool sodium increases to approximately 70 to 100 mEq/L.

Several specific nutritional effects result from GVHD treatment with high-dose steroids. Corticosteroids promote muscle breakdown and hepatic gluconeogenesis from amino acid and thus increase urea cycle activity to dispose of nitrogen. The alteration of energy metabolism can be manifest as hyperglycemia and hypertriglyceridemia, which have also been reported as complications of cyclosporine (CSP) therapy (21). The hypoproteinemia that results can be compounded further by fluid overload from the simultaneous use of fluid resuscitation and nephrotoxic agents, including CSP and antibiotics. Renal sodium wasting is common at this time, added to fecal sodium losses. Attempts to correct serum sodium levels can result in increased total body sodium and fluid retention, leading to the use of diuretic agents that may exacerbate the nephrotoxicity. Renal magnesium wasting is caused by CSP and diuretics (22).

Nutritional Support during BMT

Prior to the general acceptance of total parenteral nutrition (TPN) to support BMT recipients, enteral intake was the mainstay of nutritional intake for patients at some centers. A retrospective analysis comparing 22 BMT recipients supported orally and given TPN *ad libitum* with 22 age- and disease-matched BMT recipients given prophylactic TPN showed that prophylactic TPN patients engrafted more rapidly but that clinical outcomes were not different (23). More recently, it was shown that with intensive dietary counseling and use of both nasogastric feedings and intravenous protein supplementation, nutritional support was maintained without a prolonged course of TPN in a majority (approximately 75%) of patients (24). However, a prospective, randomized study of 137 patients transplanted at the University of Minnesota between 1983 and 1985 showed that starting TPN during cytoreduction and continuing through the resumption of oral intake had a positive effect on overall survival (Figure 25-1). Improved survival may have been due to a nutritional effect on graft function, as suggested by murine studies (25). Normally nourished patients either received prophylactic TPN or had TPN withheld until nutritional depletion was documented. Sixty-one percent of the latter group reached this level of nutritional depletion at a median of 21 days after BMT and required longer hospitalizations. Thus, the efficacy of prophylactic TPN in BMT was documented in this study (26).

Standard TPN Therapy

Guidelines for prescription of TPN have been published in the context of studies done with varied aims. Table 25-1 lists prescriptions used in 12 of these studies in chronological order. The purpose of some of these studies was to determine optimal nutritional support for BMT recipients (26–30); other studies were aimed at determining nutritional outcomes of support (12–14, 31–33). The guidelines are similar from center to center in their prescription of energy intake for BMT recipients. The prescribed energy

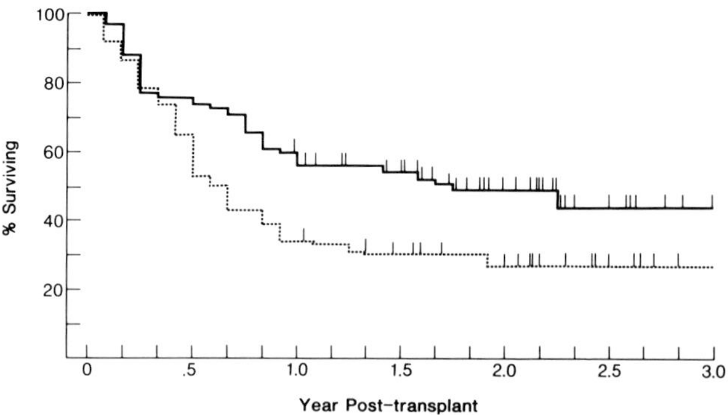

Figure 25-1. Overall survival for 71 patients given prophylactic TPN (*solid line*) versus 66 control patients not receiving prophylactic TPN (*broken line*) in a prospective, randomized trial ($p = .011$). Tick marks indicate patients surviving at the time of analysis (1986). (Reprinted with permission from Weisdorf, SA, Lysne J, Wind D, et al. Positive effect of prophylactic total parenteral nutrition on long-term outcome of bone marrow transplantation. Transplantation 1987;43:833–838. © 1987, Baltimore: Williams & Wilkins Co.)

Table 25-1.
Calorie and Protein Intake Prescribed in Studies of TPN in BMT

Institution	*N*	*Caloric Intake*	*Protein Intake*	*Lipid (% kcal)*	*NPC/N*	*Starting Day*	*Oral Intake*	*Study Duration (days)*	*Reference*
City of Hope	10	150% BEE	1.4 gm/kg	. . .	170:1	+1	Yes	28–60	12
FHCRC	7	160% BEE	1.5 gm/kg	0/25/50		−6	Yes	25	27
FHCRC	20	160% (adult)	1.5 gm/kg	0/25/50		−1	Yes	37	28
		170% (child)	2.0 gm/kg						
Johns Hopkins University	31	35 kcal/kg	1.4 gm/kg	. . .		−1	Yes	30	24
University of Minnesota	71	150% BEE	1.0 (adult)	33	150:1	−6	Yes	35	26
			2.0 (child)		200:1				
FHCRC	40	160% BEE	1.5 gm/kg	25–30		−6	Yes	35	31
Groningen University	11	3,400 kcal/d	148 gm/day	40		−3	Yes	21	29
Basel University	6	35 kcal/kg	1.8 gm/kg	33	125:1	0	No	7	32
McGill University	10	150% BEE	1.4 gm/kg	2X/wk		+1	No	24	13
	5	100% BEE	0.8 gm/kg						
Ohio State University	14	40 kcal/kg	1.1 gm/kg	. . .	120:1	−1	+/−	18	14
	14		2.2 gm/kg		100:1				
University of Milan	25	90 kcal/kg (infant)	2.5–3.0 gm/kg	. . .	150:1	−7	Yes	26	33
		68 kcal/kg (toddler)	1.5–2.5 gm/kg						
		55 kcal/kg (older)							
Brigham & Women's	45	150% BEE	1.5 gm/kg	30	165:1	+1	Yes	28	30

BEE = basal energy expenditure; NPC/N = nonprotein-calorie-to-nitrogen ratio; FHCRC = Fred Hutchison Cancer Research Center.

intake includes protein calories in some, but only nonprotein caloric intake in others. The Harris-Benedict equations (34) are used to estimate basal energy expenditure (BEE) in the majority of these reports, and ideal body weight was used in these calculations. There is a trend to lower estimation of initial energy requirements in the more recent studies, based on more accurate measurements of actual energy expenditure. Use of fat as an energy source varied, depending on the goal of the study. In the study that actually compared different levels of fat intake, lipid was shown to be helpful in maintaining energy balance without significant complications (30). Fat-free TPN can be complicated by hepatic steatosis and glycogenosis, causing increased transaminase and serum triglyceride levels; thus, a balanced caloric intake (using both fat and carbohydrate) is recommended. Electrolytes, minerals, vitamins, and trace elements are added to the TPN according to the recommended daily allowance (RDA) and individual needs. Standard trace element solutions contain chromium, zinc, copper, manganese, and often selenium.

One recent study compared two levels of energy and protein intake and found that the lower intakes supported nutritional status with fewer metabolic complications (13). In this study, nitrogen balance was not different between the groups. Although fluid intake was similar in both groups, body weight was lower, serum albumin levels were higher, and serum sodium levels were more often in the normal range in the group with the lower protein/calorie intake. All of these factors suggest less water retention in these patients. An earlier study of body composition showed that there was a fluid shift from the intracellular to the extracellular compartment (35). This study used protein and energy intakes similar to the high intake group (13). This shift may account for the apparent fluid overload, without an actual increase in total body water. In contrast, another recent study compared a standard protein prescription with a high protein prescription with the same total energy intake (14). These authors reported an improvement in nitrogen balance with this approach. They also reported that measured energy expenditure was lower than they had predicted. Other studies have examined specialized nutrition therapy (30,31).

Monitoring Nutritional Support

To individualize therapy, certain nutritional and metabolic parameters need to be monitored. It is somewhat arbitrary to distinguish between monitoring schema to follow nutrition therapy and to follow the overall medical status of a patient. Certain laboratory studies are indicated to anticipate and correct potential metabolic problems that can be caused by parenteral nutrition or metabolic problems of other causes, which can be treated with the parenteral nutrition solution. From the studies listed in Table 25-1, a consensus can be derived (Table 25-2).

Weight is followed primarily to judge hydration status, which is also reflected by electrolytes, blood urea nitrogen (BUN), creatinine, and albumin levels. Glucose tolerance can vary in this setting and needs to be monitored. There is an association between hyperglycemia and *Candida* sepsis (36); thus, awareness of changing glucose tolerance can be helpful in anticipating infectious complications as well as metabolic complications. Liver function abnormalities may result from TPN, or liver dysfunction from other causes may

Table 25-2.
Nutrition Support Monitoring Studies

Daily	*Biweekly*	*Weekly*
Weight, urine glucose, calorie/ protein intake, electrolytes, glucose, urea, creatinine (first 3 days)	Glucose, urea, creatinine, electrolytes, Ca, Mg, phosphorus transaminases, 5′nucleotidase, bilirubin, alkaline phosphatase	Triglyceride, albumin, transferrin, nitrogen balance, zinc

require modification of the TPN formula (see section on complications). A particularly difficult and as yet poorly understood occurrence in BMT patients is hyperammonemia (37). This abnormality is not common enough to require routine laboratory monitoring, but an awareness of the potential for hyperammonemia should be kept in mind when evaluating liver function, level of nutrition, and, particularly, protein support.

Parenteral and enteral protein and caloric intake are recorded daily to allow reduction of parenteral intake as enteral intake increases. Measurement of electrolytes, major minerals, and zinc is needed to adjust a patient's TPN formula. Ascribing abnormalities in serum albumin to protein nutrition does not seem to be reliable in this setting. Serum albumin is helpful in assessment of fluid status and as a guide to albumin replacement therapy for maintenance of intravascular volume. Transferrin levels seem more reflective of amino acid intake for visceral protein synthesis (26). We found that prealbumin levels reflect caloric rather than protein intake and should not be used to adjust protein intake. Although nitrogen balance is helpful, attempting to maintain positive balance is unrealistic and could result in an increased demand on the liver to process ammonia. An additional study that assists in individualizing therapy and anticipating complications is measurement of Resting Energy Expenditure (REE) and Respiratory Quotient (RQ) with a metabolic cart. The quantity and appropriate mix of energy producing substrate can be optimized with these data (14).

Adjusting TPN during BMT

For adequately nourished patients, a graded approach is recommended. From the start of cytoreduction until day 7 after BMT, a high energy formula is prescribed (140–150% BEE based on the Harris-Benedict equations). Protein calories are included in this total, and approximately 33% of total calories are given as lipid over 18 hours on a daily basis. At this time, protein is given at the RDA, 1 gm/kg in adults and 2 gm/kg in children. Because this is the period during which tissue damage is occurring, resulting in an increased endogenous nitrogen burden, exogenous nitrogen is prescribed only for maintenance of lean body mass. This maintenance formula is similar to those prescribed after surgery or trauma in patients who are unable to eat for at least one week. Seven days after transplant (the third week of TPN), the energy intake is decreased to 120 to 130% BEE, and protein intake is increased to compensate for negative nitrogen balance, hypoproteinemia, and tissue repair. This recommendation anticipates the additional protein required for tissue repair and regrowth, but decreases the amount of energy the patient utilizes to dispose of a high caloric intake. By Day 21 after BMT, recovery of enteral intake is anticipated, and the TPN caloric intake is decreased further, usually by decreasing lipid infusion from 7 to 3 times per week. Two types of patients require further therapeutic modifications of nutrition support: patients that are malnourished at the time of hospitalization for BMT, and patients in whom hypermetabolism develops as a result of stress.

Malnourished Patients

Baseline nutritional assessment will identify patients who are malnourished prior to BMT (38). Malnutrition is more likely to occur in children with multiply relapsed acute lymphoblastic leukemia, any patient on long-term steroid therapy, patients with a history of multiple infections (immunodeficiency patients), and patients with metabolic disorders associated with neurological impairment. These patients require restorative rather than maintenance nutritional therapy. Restorative therapy uses lower total energy intake and higher protein intake. Greater attention is paid to micronutrient shifts, particularly of potassium, phosphorus, magnesium, and zinc. Body stores of these elements are low in chronic malnutrition, although serum levels are initially normal. With increased nutrition, serum stores are utilized and can decrease precipitously. Fluid overload is also a frequent complication of intensive nutritional therapy in chronically undernourished patients (39).

Hypermetabolism

Hypermetabolism and multiple organ failure syndrome are parts of a clinical spectrum initiated by a severe defect in tissue perfusion or oxygenation (40). Hypermetabolism may result from sepsis, multiple trauma (41,42), acute pancreatitis (40), or other catabolic events (e.g., severe GVHD), which are characterized as metabolic stress. Sepsis is the most common stress associated with hypermetabolism in BMT recipients. Subsequent to the initial perfusion deficit, stability may be restored for 48 to 72 hours, but thereafter a hypermetabolic state develops, associated with pulmonary injury. The hypermetabolic state may resolve over 7 to 10 days or it may persist, with progressive kidney and liver dysfunction. These final stages constitute multiple organ failure syndrome, which has a mortality rate in excess of 50% (40).

Hypermetabolism is characterized by the loss of body protein, in distinction to simple starvation, in which lean body mass is preserved. Protein catabolism is accounted for, in part, by utilization of amino acids from skeletal muscle in areas of wound healing or in acute phase response protein synthesis. However, in the hypermetabolic state, amino acids are also utilized for gluconeogenesis, and branched chain amino acids may be oxidized outside the liver for energy. The net result is a dramatic shift to negative nitrogen balance and azotemia with hyperglycemia (40,43). These changes are difficult to correct with either glucose infusions or insulin. Despite hyperglycemia, glucose oxidation and uptake do not increase (43). Fat metabolism is also altered, lipid stores are mobilized, and lipid oxidation increases. In the progression from sepsis to multisystem organ failure with development of liver dysfunction, hepatic lipogenesis increases, triglyceride clearance is impaired, and utilization of lipids by peripheral tissues declines. Thus, lipid clearance becomes macrophage-dependent, possibly limiting these cells' phagocytic capacity (43).

The goals of nutritional support in hypermetabolic patients are to maintain lean body mass, to administer adequate calories, and to maintain acceptable levels of electrolytes, glucose, and BUN. Protein is administered at increased levels (up to 1.5 to 2.0 gm/kg/day in adults and up to 2.5 to 3.0 gm/kg/day in children) to compensate for urinary nitrogen loss. Glucose administration should not exceed 5.0 gm/kg/day, and fat intake should not exceed 1.0 gm/kg/day in adults. This therapy will not achieve positive caloric balance in hypermetabolism, nor will it prevent loss of lean body mass. It will, however, support the ongoing inflammation-associated protein synthesis and allow for improved nitrogen balance, which has been associated with increased survival (40,43).

Adjustments of TPN are required frequently. Transferrin levels less than 170 mg/dL and albumin levels less than 2.8 mg/dL have been associated with adverse outcomes in sepsis and indicate a need to alter nitrogen intake. Severe azotemia (BUN $>$ 80–100 mg/dL) requires decreasing protein intake or dialysis to permit increased protein support. Because stress hypermetabolism utilizes a mixed fuel source, the respiratory quotient (RQ) should range from 0.8 to 0.85. Excess carbohydrate intake is associated with increased CO_2 production and an RQ greater than 1.0. Patients with respiratory difficulty may benefit from decreasing their CO_2 production by increasing the percentage of their calories given as lipid. Indirect calorimetry can indicate if caloric intake is too high. Excess energy intake does not preserve lean body mass or restore the patient to health more quickly, but promotes hyperglycemia, lipogenesis, hypertriglyceridemia, and hepatic steatosis. Fluid overload in stressed patients is an indication to concentrate TPN, which decreases free water and corrects hyponatremia. Electrolyte supplementation can be given separately from the TPN, avoiding the need for frequent TPN reformulation. Recommended allowances of trace elements and vitamins may not be adequate in severely stressed patients, particularly for zinc, copper, and vitamin K. Patients with renal or hepatic dysfunction may require further modification of the TPN, and weekly serum trace element monitoring can anticipate chromium toxicity or excessive manganese and copper supplementation (42,43).

Transition to Enteral Feedings

Oral intake can resume when mucositis subsides, and narcotic therapy is reduced. BMT is associated with intestinal pseudo-obstruction of various causes, including radiation, drugs, and viral infections (44), but narcotics are the major factor limiting intestinal motility. Narcotic weaning as mucositis improves and pain subsides facilitates reintroduction of oral intake. The initial foods desired by BMT recipients are usually cold and very sweet. Taste sensation is altered after BMT, with a decreased threshold for sweet and salt that may last for more than one year (7). Continuing parenteral amino acid administration is often necessary, even in patients consuming adequate calories, because protein-containing foods are often refused. A dietitian trained in post-BMT management is essential to counsel patients regarding appropriate food choices and to encourage patients to keep retrying foods (45). As appetite improves, a previously rejected food may become more acceptable. The dietary kitchen must be flexible, and, if possible, a kitchen on the BMT ward or in communal family quarters should be available. Patients may respond better to familiar dishes or ethnic foods. Dietary prescriptions at some institutions include complex, highly restrictive diets, eliminating vegetables and requiring autoclaving of foods. Lactose intake should be limited in the first year after BMT, but a low-bacteria diet (46) is not necessary. Patients with intestinal GVHD may benefit from the protocol of Gauvreau and colleagues (47), which utilizes a phased dietary restoration plan. GVHD, malignant relapse, or infection may cause a temporary dependence on TPN. Some patients leave the hospital on TPN, and children are often resistant to oral intake until in familiar surroundings. If there is no organic cause of prolonged refusal of enteral intake, nasogastric or nasojejunal feedings can be used to promote intestinal recovery, thus stimulating appetite. With prolonged food refusal, food aversion is suspected and behavioral modification therapy can be sought.

Graft-versus-Host Disease

GVHD and its therapy can be a major challenge for continuing oral nutrition. If hepatic GVHD is present, cholestasis and consequent fat malabsorption may further complicate oral nutrition (3,48). In severe intestinal GVHD, the majority of a patient's calories and protein are provided parenterally. Basal caloric needs are given, in a balanced formulation, with 30% of the calories from lipid. These patients require increased protein administration, sometimes up to 3 gm/kg/day, to improve nitrogen balance and to maintain lean body mass when protein-losing enteropathy is present. Although TPN is needed to provide the majority of nutrition, in general, some enteral nutrition should be maintained. Enteral nutrition stimulates gall bladder function, thus reducing cholestatic complications, and has a trophic effect on the intestine, thus reducing bacterial translocation into the blood stream.

Complications of Nutritional Support

There are risks for complications in both parenteral and enteral nutritional support, and recent standard textbooks cover these risks in detail (49,50). Significant metabolic complications can occur using TPN. Contributing factors include the length of time TPN is given, malnutrition of the recipient prior to BMT, and the presence of organ failure during BMT, particularly hepatic or renal failure. Enteral feeding tube placement and maintenance in BMT recipients are associated with risks of formula aspiration, sinusitis, and bowel perforation. Some of the more common problems encountered in BMT recipients are reviewed briefly.

Catheter-related Complications

The availability of large bore, multiple-port, right atrial silicone catheters for venous access is a significant improvement over the less stable access systems previously used (51). Central venous access catheters remain a major source of complications in BMT recipients. The incidence of central catheter sepsis is high, despite the use of strict aseptic technique for blood draws, infusions, and tubing changes, as well as daily site cleaning and dressing changes. In a prospective study of 143 Hickman catheter placements in 111 BMT recipients, 44% of the patients had positive blood cultures during the lifetime of the catheter (52). Of these infections, 40 of 63 were coagulase-negative *Staphylococcus*, suggestive of primary line sepsis rather than catheter contamination from a blood-borne enteric source. The majority of these infections are treated with antibiotics and not catheter removal (52,53). In the prospective study, mechanical obstruction occurred in 38% of the catheters and more than once in some. Approximately half these episodes required no intervention, whereas the others responded to heparin, urokinase, or required catheter replacement. Table 25-3 outlines the protocol used at the University of Minnesota to dissolve clots in catheters (54). Other complications, including dislodgment or leakage, occurred in this study (52) in small numbers.

Hepatic Enzyme Elevations

Table 25-4 lists potential causes of cholestasis or hepatic enzyme elevations in the transplant period, of which TPN is one. Hepatic complications associated with TPN occur in only a subset of TPN recipients. The initial manifestation is an elevation of transaminase levels approximately 1 to 2 weeks after the start of TPN infusion. Bilirubin elevations and elevations of canalicular enzymes (alkaline phospha-

Table 25-3.
Protocol for Treatment of Fibrin-occluded Vascular Access Catheters

To preserve occluded central lines, urokinase clearance is attempted prior to replacement. Urokinase is utilized after evaluation of the line by the physician caring for the patient. Documentation of the presence of a clot and the position of the catheter may be done by echography or a roentgenographic dye study prior to the use of urokinase. Allergy to urokinase is the only absolute contraindication to its use, but caution should be observed in the following situations:

- Suspicion of bacterial endocarditis
- Febrile patient with less than 24 hr of intravenous antibiotic therapy
- Clinical bleeding
- Central nervous system tumors
- Surgery, trauma, or lumbar puncture in the last 10 days
- Surgery, intramuscular injection, arterial puncture, or lumbar puncture anticipated during urokinase infusion
- Prothrombin time >16 sec
- Partial thromboplastin time >60 sec
- Fibrinogen<100 mg/dL
- Fibrin degradation products >240 mg/dL
- Platelet count <30,000/μl
- Hemostatic abnormalities
- Severe hypertension

Nota Bene: Never use a tuberculin syringe to clear vascular catheters, as the force exerted by these small syringes may burst the catheter. It is recommended that any syringe be at least 3 mL in size.

I. Procedure for a totally occluded catheter (catheter will neither draw nor infuse): gentle suction is applied to the catheter, a small amount of fluid is removed from the line; then, while maintaining suction, the line is clamped. A syringe is attached containing 5000 U urokinase, the line is unclamped, and the urokinase is instilled slowly (it may not be possible to instill the full volume of urokinase). It is allowed to remain in the line for 30 min to 2 hr, then is aspirated and the line tested. If it is still occluded, the process is repeated.

II. Procedure for withdraw occlusion (catheter infuses but does not draw): If the catheter will infuse, it is important to dilute the urokinase with saline to a volume of 2.0 mL to insure that the catheter is filled. The same procedure for clearing is used as in I above, but if a second attempt is necessary, 10,000 U urokinase and a 30-min to 2-hr dwell time may be used.

III. Continuous infusion protocol: If the line remains occluded but infusion is possible, a continuous infusion of urokinase may be attempted at a physician's discretion. A roentgenographic dye study prior to the use of continuous infusion of urokinase is strongly recommended to document catheter placement and the size of the clot. Coagulation studies are obtained prior to the infusion. The infusion consists of 200 U/kg/lumen/hr for 12 hr and may be repeated once. The minimum infusion rate is 20 mL/hr/lumen, to allow adequate volume to clear the catheter.

[a]This protocol was derived from protocols of the University of Minnesota Hospital and of the Los Angeles Children's Hospital by Holly Bagnall-Reeb, RN, MN.

Table 25-4.
Causes of Hepatic Injury in BMT

Infection: bacterial, viral, fungal
Endotoxemia
Recurrence of malignancy
Veno-occlusive disease
Medications inducing cholestasis (e.g., methotrexate, furosemide)
Allergic response to medication
Graft-versus-host disease
Total parenteral nutrition

tase, 5′-nucleotidase) may occur 2 to 3 weeks into therapy. The transaminase level elevations often resolve spontaneously. Liver biopsy will show steatosis, glycogenosis, intrahepatic cholestasis, and sometimes a nonspecific portal infiltrate. This injury is associated with administration of a high nonprotein-calorie-to-nitrogen ratio (NPC/N) or lipid-free formulations. Most abnormalities resolve on discontinuation of TPN, cycling, or adjustment of the NPC/N, and there is little or no functional disability of the liver. If TPN therapy is long term, functional abnormalities may develop. Steatonecrosis and fibrosis can occur and may progress to cirrhosis, with complications of hepatic dysfunction and portal hypertension. The time course for development of this lesion is variable and can depend on the age of the patient (adults are more resistant to necrotic changes associated with TPN than children) and the presence of other hepatotoxic factors. Some studies have shown fibrosis with as little as 6 months of TPN. Finally, acalculous cholecystitis or gallstone formation can occur during administration of TPN (55).

Treatment and prevention of the hepatic complications of TPN involve both limiting other hepatotoxic or cholestatic therapies and use of specific modalities to improve hepatic function during TPN (56). Methods used for rising liver enzymes include the following:

1. Evaluation of the patient for a cause of liver disease (other than TPN) or for sepsis.
2. Cycling TPN over 12 to 18 rather than 24 hours (57,58).
3. Initiation of small enteral feeds to provide a protective effect on the liver during TPN (55).
4. Decreasing the total calorie intake empirically by 10 to 15% to reduce the NPC/N and to provide a balanced caloric intake (55).
5. Treatment with ursodeoxycholic acid, 15 to 20 mg/kg/day orally divided into four doses, to decrease cholestasis.
6. In older children and adults, a trial of enterol metronidazole to decrease endotoxin formation.

It is not appropriate to respond to enzyme elevations by stopping TPN if enteral alimentation cannot be used. Malnutrition also has adverse effects on the liver.

Other Metabolic Abnormalities

The potential disruption of normal electrolyte, mineral, and vitamin balance exists in any critically ill patient and certainly in BMT recipients. Parenteral nutrition is associated with increased episodes of hyperlipidemia and hyperglycemia, although it may be more difficult to administer adequate electrolytes and minerals to enterally alimented patients (especially magnesium). Essential fatty acid deficiency is a problem in parenterally nourished patients who do not receive lipids (59) and in enterally nourished patients with cholestasis. Hyperammonemia occurs in extremely catabolic patients (37).

Novel Therapies

There are several experimental alterations in nutritional support formulation and adjunctive therapy that may ultimately improve the ability to nourish BMT recipients safely and effectively. Moreover, the trend in nutritional support is toward specific modifications during critical illness (41). Four such therapies are being studied in BMT recipients and form the arena from which new approaches will be developed.

Glutamine

Studies have suggested that glutamine is an essential amino acid under conditions of stress and hypermetabolism. Glutamine has a crucial role in nitrogen transport as a scavenger of ammonia and is used in nucleotide synthesis. Intestinal mucosa utilizes large amounts of glutamine in nucleotide synthesis to support its rapid regeneration. In the enterocyte, metabolism of glutamine produces α-ketoglutarate, which enters the tricarboxylic acid cycle, and ammonia, citrulline, alanine, and proline. Alanine is utilized by the liver for gluconeogenesis, whereas citrulline is used in the urea cycle to synthesize arginine. Critical illness has been associated with plasma glutamine depletion, which impairs normal maintenance of intestinal mucosal integrity. Loss of the mucosal barrier can result in increased bacterial translocation with increased episodes of sepsis due to enteric organisms (60).

Glutamine in doses up to 0.57 gm/kg/day in a balanced TPN solution has been shown to be safe in humans, both in normal volunteers and in a group of BMT patients (61). Glutamine supplementation of TPN has been shown to improve nitrogen balance in normal patients in the postoperative period (60). Glutamine supplementation of TPN was recently studied in a double-blind, randomized, controlled trial of allogeneic BMT recipients. The TPN was identical in calorie and nitrogen content; one group received standard amino acids and the other group received glutamine (0.57 gm/kg/day) and standard amino acid solution to the same total nitrogen content as the control group. The group receiving glutamine demonstrated improved nitrogen balance and decreased morbidity. The number of bacterial infections and the length of hospital stay were less in the glutamine group (30). The safety of glutamine in parenteral nutrition has not been documented in patients with renal or hepatic failure or in patients with central nervous system abnormalities. Given the loss of intestinal mucosal integrity due to cytoreduction therapy and GVHD, glutamine-enriched nutritional support may prove advantageous in BMT recipients. Some animal studies have suggested that enteral glutamine is more effective than parenteral glutamine (62), a claim that is not yet substantiated in humans.

Branched Chain Amino Acids

Amino acid solutions enriched in the branched chain amino acids (BCAA) (isoleucine, leucine, and valine) have been shown to improve nitrogen balance in various critical care situations. Improvement in nitrogen balance is small in most studies, and the BCAA-enriched formulae cost significantly more than standard amino acid preparations. Despite a number of theories, it has not been clear by what metabolic pathways the increase in nitrogen retention occurs (63), although it is speculated that BCAA oxidation has a somatic protein-sparing effect.

BCAA-enriched nutritional support was studied in a group of BMT recipients. Patients were randomized in a double-blind fashion to receive TPN containing either 45 or 23% BCAA. The TPN formulations were isocaloric and isonitrogenous. BCAA did not improve nitrogen balance during the first month after BMT. Unfortunately, the number of patients studied was small (8 patients in the 45% BCAA group and 11 patients in the 23% BCAA group). The patients in the 45% BCAA group were treated more often with high-dose steroids and were more stressed (defined as the presence of one of several clinical complications) compared with the 23% BCAA group (31). This study has not settled the controversy over BCAA use in BMT. However, in BMT patients with hypermetabolism and loss of lean body mass, in whom aggressive nitrogen administration (up to 2.5–3.0 gm/kg/day with a transferrin level remaining below 100 mg/dL) does not restore nitrogen balance, BCAA can be added to the amino acid mixture (to a total of 45% BCAA) for approximately 8 to 10 days. A plasma amino acid profile is obtained before initiating BCAA-enrichment and then reviewed weekly to avoid excess accumulation of BCAA.

Growth Hormone

Growth hormone, a polypeptide produced in the pituitary gland, is a major anabolic hormone. Trials in several centers demonstrate its utility in promoting nitrogen balance after surgery (64), during sepsis or trauma (65), and after severe burns or trauma (66). In a group of volunteers receiving prednisone, growth hormone decreased the catabolism associated with prednisone therapy, preventing protein loss (67,68). These studies hold particular promise for BMT recipients, but the published trials had small numbers of patients, often normal volunteers, receiving growth hormone for short periods. More trials in critically ill populations are needed before this therapy can be used clinically.

Early Enteral Alimentation

Several groups have challenged the assumption that TPN is superior to enteral alimentation during the acute phase of many critical illnesses (e.g., head trauma, sepsis, multiple trauma). These groups have shown that an aggressive protocol for early enteral alimentation may decrease infection rates in critically ill patients (69). BMT recipients, however, are generally not good candidates for enteral alimentation by feeding tube because of mucositis, neutropenia, and vomiting associated with cytoreduction and GVHD. However, in a study addressing the use of a predominantly enteral feeding program compared with a predominantly parenteral feeding program, it was suggested that BMT recipients could be supported by a very aggressive enteral feeding program. This study randomized patients to two different nutritional support protocols during BMT; 30 to an individualized enteral program using intensive counseling and (in some patients) tube feedings, and 27 to parenteral nutrition. Of the 30 enteral patients, 73% required supplemental intravenous amino acids for adequate nutritional support and 23% were crossed over to parenteral nutrition because of failure to achieve adequate total enteral intake. The study showed that the parenterally nourished group had more days of diuretic use, more hyperglycemia, and more catheter complications, but had fewer episodes of hypomagnesemia. There was no difference between the groups in length of stay, hematopoietic recovery, or survival. The authors point out the high cost of parenteral nutrition and suggest that parenteral nutrition be utilized for patients who are enteral alimentation failures (24). This study fails to address the role of nutritional support in the most severely ill BMT patients, but it introduces an important treatment option, which is the use of combined parenteral and enteral alimentation to take advantage of both the mucosal-preserving aspects of enteral alimentation and the more physiological nutritional support of parenteral alimentation (29).

Long-term Nutritional Support Considerations

Discharge from the hospital does not end the need for nutritional care in BMT recipients. In a recent study of 192 children and adults evaluated one year after BMT, malnutrition was common (70). Approximately 16% of patients were 10% or more below their ideal body weights, and significant weight loss seemed associated with discharge from the transplant center. Oral sensitivity was seen in 23% of patients; a smaller number had stomatitis (8%). Diarrhea or steatorrhea occurred in 21%. Although many of these complications could be attributed to chronic GVHD, even patients with limited or no GVHD had significant nutritional problems. It is clear that BMT recipients require specific, intensive posthospitalization observation and long-term management of nutrition.

References

1. McDonald GB, Shulman HM, Sullivan KM, Spencer GD. Intestinal and hepatic complications of human bone marrow transplantation. Part I. Gastroenterology 1986;90:460–477.
2. McDonald GB, Sharma P, Matthews DE, Shulman HM, Thomas ED. Venocclusive disease of the liver after bone marrow transplantation: diagnosis, incidence, and predisposing factors. Hepatology 1984;4:116–122.
3. McDonald GB, Shulman HM, Sullivan KM, Spencer GD. Intestinal and hepatic complications of human bone marrow transplantation. Part II. Gastroenterology 1986;90:770–784.
4. Zager RA, O'Quigley J, Zager BK, et al. Acute renal failure following bone marrow transplantation: a retrospective study of 272 patients. Am J Kidney Dis 1989;13:210–216.
5. Kupari M, Volin L, Suokas A, Timonene T, Hekali P, Ruutu T. Cardiac involvement in bone marrow transplantation: electrocardiographic changes, arrhythmias, heart failure and autopsy findings. Bone Marrow Transplant 1990;5:91–98.
6. Buckner CD, Meyers JD, Springmeyer SC, et al. Pulmonary complications of marrow transplantation: review of the Seattle experience. Exp Hematol 1984;12(suppl 15):1–5.
7. Mattsson T, Arvidson K, Heimdahl A, Ljungman P, Dahllöf G, Ringdén O. Alterations in taste acuity associated with allogeneic bone marrow transplantation. J Oral Pathol Med 1992;21:31–37.
8. Sale GE, Shulman HM, McDonald GB, Thomas ED. Gastrointestinal graft-versus-host disease in man. A clinicopatholgic study of the rectal biopsy. Am J Surg Pathol 1979;3:291–299.
9. Bearman SI, Appelbaum FR, Buckner CD, et al. Regimen-related toxicity in patients undergoing bone marrow transplantation. J Clin Oncol 1988;6:1562–1568.
10. Weisdorf SA, Salati LM, Longsdorf JA, Ramsay NKC, Sharp HL. Graft-versus host disease of the intestine: a protein losing enteropathy characterized by fecal α_1-antitrypsin. Gastroenterology 1983;85:1076–1081.
11. Cheney CL, Lenssen P, Aker SN, et al. Sex differences in nitrogen balance following marrow grafting for leukemia. J Am Coll Nutr 1987;6:223–230.
12. Schmidt GM, Blume KG, Bross KJ, Spruce WE, Waldron JC, Levine R. Parenteral nutrition in bone marrow transplant recipients. Exp Hematol 1980;8:506–511.
13. Taveroff A, McArdle AH, Rybka WB. Reducing parenteral energy and protein intake improves metabolic homeostasis after bone marrow transplantation. Am J Clin Nutr 1991;54:1087–1092.
14. Geibig CB, Owens JP, Mirtallo JM, Bowers D, Nahikian-Nelms M, Tutschka P. Parenteral nutrition for marrow transplant recipients: evaluation of an increased nitrogen dose. JPEN 1991;15:184–188.
15. Winston DJ, Ho WG, Champlin RE. Current approaches to the management of infections in bone marrow transplants. Eur J Cancer Clin Oncol 1989;25(suppl 2):S25–35.
16. King CE, Toskes PP. Breath tests in the diagnosis of small intestine bacterial overgrowth. CRC Crit Rev Clin Lab Sci 1984;21:269–281
17. Snover DC, Weisdorf SA, Vercellotti GM, Rank B, Hutton S, McGlave P. A histopathologic study of gastric and small intestinal graft-versus-host disease following allogeneic bone marrow transplantation. Hum Pathol 1984;16:387–392.
18. Roy J, Snover D, Weisdorf S, Mulvahill A, Filipovich A, Weisdorf D. Simultaneous upper and lower endoscopic biopsy in the diagnosis of intestinal graft-versus-host disease. Transplantation 1991;51:642–646.
19. Snover DC. Graft-versus-host disease of the gastrointestinal tract. Am J Surg Pathol 1990;14(suppl 1):101–108.
20. Szeluga DJ, Stuart RK, Brookmeyer R, Untermohlen V, Santos GW. Energy requirements of parenterally fed bone marrow transplant recipients. JPEN 1985;9:139–143.
21. Carreras E, Villamor N, Reverter JC, Sierra J, Grañena A, Rozman C. Hypertriglyceridemia in bone marrow transplant recipients: another side effect of cyclosporine A. Bone Marrow Transplant 1989;4:385–388.
22. June CH, Thompson CB, Kennedy MS, Nims J, Thomas ED. Profound hypomagnesemia and renal magnesium wasting associated with the use of cyclosporine for marrow transplantation. Transplantation 1985;39:620–624.
23. Weisdorf S, Hofland C, Sharp HL, et al. Total parenteral nutrition in bone marrow transplantation: a clinical evaluation. J Pediatr Gastroenterol Nutr 1984;3:95–100.
24. Szeluga DJ, Stuart RK, Brookmeyer R, Untermohlen V, Santos GW. Nutritional support of bone marrow transplant recipients: a prospective, randomized clinical trial comparing total parenteral nutrition to an enteral feeding program. Cancer Res 1987;47:3309–3316.
25. Stuart RK, Sensenbrenner LL. Adverse effects of nutritional deprivation on transplanted hematopoietic cells. Exp Hematol 1979;7:435–442.
26. Weisdorf SA, Lysne J, Wind D, et al. Positive effect of prophylactic total parenteral nutrition on long-term outcome of bone marrow transplantation. Transplantation 1987;43:833–838.
27. Hutchinson ML, Clemans GW, Springmeyer SC, Flournoy N. Energy expenditure estimation in recipients of marrow transplants. Cancer 1984;54:1734–1738.
28. Hutchinson ML, Clemans GW. Prospective trial of liposyn® 20% in patients undergoing bone marrow transplantation. Clin Nutr 1984;3:5–9.
29. Mulder POM, Bouman JG, Gietema JA, et al. Hyperalimentation in autologous bone marrow transplantation for solid tumors: comparison of total parenteral versus partial parenteral plus enteral nutrition. Cancer 1989;64:2045–2052.
30. Ziegler TR, Young LS, Benfell K, et al. Clinical and metabolic efficacy of glutamine-supplemented parenteral nutrition after bone marrow transplantation: a randomized, double-blind, controlled study. Ann Intern Med 1992;116:821–828.
31. Lenssen P, Cheney CL, Aker SN, et al. Intravenous

branched chain amino acid in marrow transplant recipients. JPEN 1987;11:112–118.
32. Keller U, Kraenzlin ME, Gratwohl A, et al. Protein metabolism assessed by 1-^{13}C leucine infusions in patients undergoing bone marrow transplantation. JPEN 1990;14:480–484.
33. Uderzo C, Rovelli A, Bonomi M, Fomia L, Pirovano L, Masera G. Total parenteral nutrition and nutritional assessment in leukaemic children undergoing bone marrow transplantation. Eur J Cancer 1991;27:758–762.
34. Harris JA, Benedict FG. Biometric studies of basal metabolism in man. Washington, DC: Carnegie Institute of Washington, 1919 (publication no. 279).
35. Cheney CL, Abson KG, Aker SN, et al. Body composition changes in marrow transplant recipients receiving total parenteral nutrition. Cancer 1987;59:1515–1519.
36. Curry CR, Quie PG. Fungal septicemia in patients receiving parenteral hyperalimentation N Engl J Med 1971;285:1221–1225.
37. Mitchell RB, Wagner JE, Karp JE, et al. Syndrome of idiopathic hyperammonemia after high-dose chemotherapy: review of nine cases. Am J Med 1988;85:662–667.
38. Layton PB, Galluci BB, Aker SN. Nutritional assessment of allogeneic bone marrow transplant recipients. Cancer Nurs 1981;127–135.
39. Apovian CM, McMahon MM, Bistrian BR. Guidelines for refeeding the marasmic patient. Crit Care Med 1990;18:1030–1033.
40. Barton R, Cerra FB. The hypermetabolism-multiple organ failure syndrome. Chest 1989;96:1153–1160.
41. Wilmore DW. Catabolic Illness: strategies for enhancing recovery. N Engl J Med 1991;325:695–702.
42. Cochran EB, Kamper CA, Phelps SJ, Brown RO. Parenteral nutrition in the critically ill patient. Clin Pharmacol 1989;8:783–799.
43. Moore RS, Cerra FB. Sepsis. In: Fischer JE, ed. Total parenteral nutrition, ed 2. Boston: Little, Brown, 1992:347–365.
44. Krishnamurthy S, Schuffler MD. Pathology of neuromuscular disorders of the small intestine and colon. Gastroenterology 1987;93:610–639.
45. Gauvreau-Stern JM, Cheney CL, Aker SN, Lenssen P. Food intake patterns and foodservice requirements on a marrow transplant unit. J Am Diet Assoc 1989;89:367–372.
46. Driedger L, Burstall CD. Bone marrow transplantation: dietitian's experience and perspective. J Am Diet Assoc 1987;87:1387–1388.
47. Gauvreau JM, Lenssen P, Cheney CL, Aker SN, Hutchinson ML, Barale KV. Nutritional management of patients with intestinal graft-versus-host disease. J Am Diet Assoc 1981;79:673–677.
48. Wolford JL, McDonald GB. A problem-oriented approach to intestinal and liver disease after marrow transplantation. J Clin Gastroenterol 1988;10:419–433.
49. Rombeau JL, Caldwell MD, eds. Clinical nutrition: enteral and tube feeding, ed 2. Philadelphia: W.B. Saunders, 1990.
50. Fischer JE, ed. Total parenteral nutrition, ed 2. Boston: Little, Brown, 1991.
51. Aker SN, Cheney CL, Sanders JE, Lenssen PL, Hickman RO, Thomas ED. Nutritional support in marrow transplant recipients with single versus double lumen right atrial catheters. Exp Hematol 1982;10:732–737.
52. Ulz L, Petersen FB, Ford R, et al. A prospective study of complications in Hickman right-atrial catheters in marrow transplant patients. JPEN 1990;14:27–30.
53. Petersen FB, Clift RA, Hickman RO, et al. Hickman catheter complications in marrow transplant recipients. JPEN 1986;10:58–62.
54. Bagnall H, Gomperts E, Atkinson J. Continuous infusion low dose urokinase in the treatment of central venous catheter thrombosis in infants and children. Pediatrics 1989;83:963–966.
55. Fisher RL. Hepatobiliary abnormalities associated with total parenteral nutrition. Gastroenterol Clin North Am 1989;18:645–666.
56. Sax HC, Bower RH. Hepatic complications of total parenteral nutrition. JPEN 1988;12:615–618.
57. Maini B, Blackburn GL, Bistrian BR, et al. Cyclic hyperalimentation: an optimal technique for preservation of visceral protein. J Surg Res 1976;20:515–525.
58. Reed MD, Lazarus HM, Herzig RH, et al. Cyclic parenteral nutrition during bone marrow transplantation in children. Cancer 1983;51:1563–1570.
59. Clemans GW, Yamanaka W, Flournoy N, et al. Plasma fatty acid patterns of bone marrow transplant patients primarily supported by fat-free parenteral nutrition. JPEN 1981;5:221–225.
60. Souba WW. Glutamine: a key substrate for the splanchnic bed. Annu Rev Nutr 1991;11:285–308.
61. Ziegler TR, Benfell K, Smith RJ, et al. Safety and metabolic effects of L-glutamine administration in humans. JPEN 1990;14(suppl):137S–146S.
62. Alverdy JC. Effects of glutamine-supplemented diets on immunology of the gut. JPEN 1990;14(suppl):109S–113S.
63. Schlichtig R, Ayres SM. Nutritional support of the critically ill. Chicago: Year Book Medical Publishers, 1988.
64. Piccolboni D, de Vincentiis L, Guerriero G, et al. Nutritional and hormonal effects of biosynthetic human growth hormone in surgical patients on total parenteral nutrition. Nutrition 1991;7:177–184.
65. Douglas RG, Humberstone DA, Haystead A, Shaw JHF. Metabolic effects of recombinant human growth hormone: isotopic studies in the postabsorptive state and during total parenteral nutrition. Br J Surg 1990;77:785–790.
66. Ziegler TR, Young LS, Ferrari-Baliviera E, Demling RH, Wilmore DW. Use of human growth hormone combined with nutritional support in a critical care unit. JPEN 1990;14:574–581.
67. Horber FF, Haymond MW. Human growth hormone prevents the protein catabolic side effects of prednisone in humans. J Clin Invest 1990;86:265–272.
68. Bennet WM, Haymond MW. Growth hormone and lean tissue catabolism during long-term glucocorticoid treatment. Clin Endocrinol 1992;36:161–164.
69. Moore FA, Moore EE, Jones TN, McCroskey BL, Peterson VM. TEN versus TPN following major abdominal trauma-reduced septic morbidity. J Trauma 1989;29:916–923.
70. Lenssen P, Sherry ME, Cheney CL, et al. Prevalence of nutrition-related problems among long-term survivors of allogeneic marrow transplantation. J Am Diet Assoc 1990;90:835–842.

Part III
Complications and Their Management

Chapter 26
Graft-versus-Host Disease

Keith M. Sullivan

Graft-versus-host disease (GVHD) is a singularly important threat to the successful outcome of allogeneic bone marrow transplantation (BMT). Of considerable interest to cell biologists and immunologists, the prevention and treatment of GVHD are of critical importance to transplant physicians and patients. Previous chapters have described animal studies of GVHD and tolerance. This chapter details the clinical features of acute and chronic GVHD in humans.

Background

Historical Development

Terminology

A description of GVHD in animals, then known as secondary disease, was reported in 1955 by Barnes and Loutit (1). Named to differentiate it from the primary disease of radiation sickness, fatal secondary disease was observed in irradiated mice given allogeneic spleen cells but not in recipients of syngeneic cells. By the late 1950s it was apparent that the diarrhea and skin abnormalities of secondary disease and runt disease (a wasting syndrome in unirradiated newborn mice given allogeneic spleen cells) were the result of immunologically competent cells introduced into an immunoincompetent host. The term *graft-versus-host* was introduced to describe the vector of this immunological assault (2,3).

Human GVHD

Early human transplants of allogeneic marrow were complicated by GVHD (4–8). Features were remarkably similar to animal studies of GVHD (9) and to reports of GVHD developing in immunodeficient children receiving blood transfusions (10).

Because it has been difficult to separate the illness caused by immunological attack from the consequences of this attack (including immunodeficiency, organ dysfunction, and infection), both aspects have been considered a part of human GVHD. The term *acute GVHD* is used to describe a distinctive syndrome of dermatitis, hepatitis, and enteritis developing within 100 days of allogeneic BMT. Chronic GVHD is a more pleiotropic syndrome that develops after day 100.

Pathogenesis

Classic Criteria

In a remarkably perceptive summary in 1966, Billingham (11) defined the criteria for the development of GVHD.

1. "The graft must contain immunologically competent cells.
2. The host must possess important transplantation alloantigens that are lacking in the donor graft, so that the host appears foreign to the graft and is, therefore, capable of stimulating it antigenically.
3. The host itself must be incapable of mounting an effective immunological reaction against the graft, at least for sufficient time for the latter to manifest its immunological capabilities; that is, it must have the security of tenure."

These criteria require only scant modification to incorporate recent understanding of the biology of GVHD. The occurrence of autologous GVHD suggests that inappropriate recognition of host self-antigens may occur, and transfusion-associated GVHD may develop in certain immunoincompetent individuals.

Alloreactivity

As reviewed in Chapter 18, abundant animal data demonstrate that T lymphocytes contained in the donor marrow inoculum proliferate and differentiate in vivo in response to disparate histocompatibility antigens on host tissues and directly, or through secondary mechanisms, attack recipient cells, thus producing the signs and symptoms of acute GVHD (9,11–13). The afferent arm of acute GVHD consists of antigen presentation, activation of individual T cells, clonal proliferation, and differentiation (14). Cell death of host targets results from alloreactivity of donor derived T cells. In the efferent phase, release of lymphokines from activated lymphocytes contributes to cell death, either directly or through recruitment of secondary effectors, such as natural killer cells. Tumor necrosis factor (TNF) appears to be an important mediator of GVHD (15,16).

Microbial Environment

The microbial environment of the host may also influence the development of GVHD. Compared with conventionally housed irradiated mice, enteric GVHD was significantly reduced in germ-free mice given incompatible marrow (17). Microorganisms could act as triggers of GVHD, perhaps by sharing antigenic epitopes with gut epithelial cells or by reactivation of latent virus-inducing antigens on cell surfaces to become targets of alloreactivity (18).

Tolerance

Chapter 17 details the mechanisms of graft-host tolerance after allogeneic BMT. Tolerance can be achieved by elimination (clonal deletion) in the thymus of host reactive cells; therefore, thymic damage could abrogate self-tolerance (19,20). Alternatively, the presence of specific suppressor T cells may be of importance in transplantation tolerance (12,21). Alterations in this regulatory immune balance could explain the development of GVHD-like syndromes following autologous BMT.

Autologous GVHD

Animal Models

Histocompatibility differences between donor and recipient may not always be needed to produce GVHD; rather, inappropriate recognition of self-antigens may produce a GVHD-like syndrome (22–24). Apparent GVHD develops in lethally irradiated animals given cyclosporine (CSP) after syngeneic BMT when CSP is withdrawn. Autoreactive T cells are found in a damaged thymus in which class II–bearing cells are absent and clonal deletion of antiself autoreactive cells does not occur (25–27). Administration of CSP in the context of thymic damage appears to be key to permitting development of autoreactive cells and preventing development of immune regulatory cells.

Human Studies

Mild and usually self-limited episodes of dermal GVHD occasionally develop in patients after syngeneic and autologous BMT (28–30). Larger series reported these findings in 7 of 96 autologous and 2 of 19 syngeneic marrow recipients (31). Hepatic and gastrointestinal abnormalities consistent with acute GVHD have also been described (32).

Considerable controversy surrounds interpretation of these reports. Differential diagnosis from chemoradiotherapy effects, infections, and drug-related abnormalities may be difficult (33). Nevertheless, the biology of this syndrome holds considerable interest especially if clinical protocols can be derived to augment any graft-versus-leukemia (GVL) effect associated with autologous GVHD (34).

Transfusion-associated GVHD

Etiology and Incidence

Transfusion-associated GVHD was initially recognized in children with immunodeficiencies (10,35). Since these original descriptions 25 years ago, a total of 131 patients have been reported (36). In most cases, patients with congenital or acquired immunodeficiencies (including BMT) received whole blood, packed red cells, platelet or granulocyte transfusions, or fresh plasma (37–40). No cases have been observed in patients with acquired immune deficiency syndrome (AIDS) (36), and no cases have resulted from transfusion of cryoprecipitate or fresh frozen plasma (41).

This syndrome has been reported in immunocompetent individuals (42–44). In Japan, the incidence is estimated to be approximately 1 in 500 open heart operations (42). In certain inbred populations sharing common haplotypes, it is likely that blood from a donor homozygous for an extended haplotype could be transfused into a recipient heterozygous for the same extended haplotype (45,46). In this setting, donor cells would not be rejected as foreign and could precipitate GVHD.

Diagnosis and Clinical Features

Histocompatibility typing demonstrates marrow and peripheral blood cells of donor origin, and skin biopsy confirms characteristic lesions of acute GVHD. The syndrome occurs 4 to 30 days after transfusion and resembles hyperacute GVHD following allogeneic BMT. Fever, erythroderma, diarrhea, and liver abnormalities progress despite immunosuppressive therapy with corticosteroids, CSP, or antithymocyte globulin (ATG). Marrow aplasia is commonly observed and contributes to the observed 90% mortality (36). Because early mortality is so high, few patients with chronic GVHD following blood transfusion have been reported (47).

Prevention

The efficacy of blood product irradiation to prevent transfusion-associated GVHD has long been recognized, and initial clinical practice routinely employed irradiation of blood products with 1,500 cGy (48). This dose of gamma irradiation from cobalt^{60} or cesium^{137} sources effectively prevents lymphocyte proliferation without adverse effect on blood cell morphology or function (49). Although there has been individual variation, 97% of institutions surveyed in the American Association of Blood Banks employ doses of 1,500 to 3,500 cGy (50). This practice appears to be highly effective; only a single case of transfusion-associated GVHD was reported in a patient given blood components radiated with 2,000 cGy from a nonrotating cesium[137] source (51). Although the debate continues as to which patients should receive irradiated blood products, BMT recipients are universally recommended (36,50).

Acute GVHD in Allogeneic Marrow Recipients

Incidence and Predictive Factors

Donor-host Factors

Human leukocyte antigen (HLA) disparity between marrow donor and recipient is the most powerful factor governing the severity and kinetics of GVHD. As shown in Figure 26-1, acute GVHD is increased with HLA-nonidentical related marrow donors (52). As reviewed in Chapter 51, a similar high incidence of acute GVHD has been observed with marrow from HLA-matched unrelated donors (53). The importance of minor transplantation antigens not detected by current typing techniques is underscored by the low incidence of acute GVHD in populations featuring genetic homogeneity (54). Although some studies have identified certain HLA antigens associated with increased rates of GVHD (55,56), these correlations have not been observed consistently (57,58).

Sex mismatching and donor parity have been associated with an increased risk of acute GVHD (56–60). Sex-specific minor antigens could account for these findings, as could female donor T cells recognizing H-Y antigens on host Y chromosome–containing cells. Moreover, previously parous donors could have had maternal alloimmunization due to unshared minor antigens of the fetus (59).

Age is another key factor associated with the development of acute GVHD (56,57,60). Among patients under 20 years of age given standard methotrexate (MTX) as GVHD prophylaxis, the incidence of significant (grade II–IV) acute GVHD was approximately 20% (61,62); in contrast, the incidence of acute GVHD was 30% in patients 45 to 50 years old, and 79% in those 51 to 62 years old (63). In a recursive partition model of factors influencing GVHD among HLA-identical marrow recipients, the risk of GVHD varied from 19 to 66%, depending on recipient age, donor-recipient sex matching, and donor parity (56).

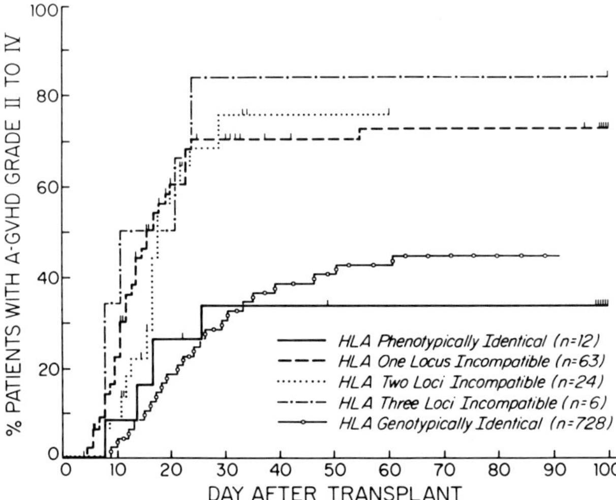

Figure 26-1. Cumulative probability of grade II-IV acute GVDH after allogeneic BMT from a genotypically HLA-identical sibling or other family members mismatched for 0-3 loci on the nonshared haplotype. (Reprinted, by permission of the New England Journal of Medicine, from Beatty PG, Clift RA, Mickelson EM, et al. Marrow transplantation from related donors other than HLA-identical siblings. N Engl J Med 1985;313:765–771.)

Immune Modulation

The incidence of acute GVHD after HLA-identical BMT also varies with the efficacy of post-transplant immunosuppressive prophylaxis. A reduction of less than 80% of the scheduled dose of MTX or CSP leads to a significant increase in the incidence of acute GVHD (58). Multivariate analysis revealed that an increased dose of total body irradiation (TBI) conditioning also predicted an increased risk of GVHD. Among HLA-identical patients receiving GVHD prophylaxis with MTX and CSP, acute GVHD developed in 48% of patients given 1,575 cGy TBI, compared with 21% of patients given 1,200 cGy TBI ($p = 0.02$) (64). One speculation is that more ablative conditioning might eliminate persisting host cells and restrict the development of mixed donor-host chimerism, which has been associated with a decreased probability of GVHD (65,66). Alternatively, more intensive conditioning could increase gut damage, modify microbial environment, release cytokine mediators, or attenuate the dose of GVHD prophylaxis that can be given safely.

Several reports suggest a role of host infection in the development of GVHD. Clinical data are inconclusive: Some studies indicate that donor or host infection (as denoted by seropositivity for herpes viruses) predicts the subsequent development of GVHD (67), whereas others find no predictive association (58,68).

Predictive Assays

In vitro assays have been developed in an attempt to predict GVHD. As described in Chapter 4, the frequencies of alloreactive cytotoxic T-lymphocyte precursors and helper T-lymphocyte precursors may have pretransplant predictive value in selecting donor-recipient pairs with a reduced risk of GVHD. Skin-explant models also have been developed in which donor lymphocytes sensitized in vitro against recipient cells are cultured with recipient skin (69,70). In other models, a mixed epidermal cell-lymphocyte reaction is used to detect incompatibility (71). Although correlations with GVHD appear to be statistically significant, individual variations have been observed.

Clinical Features

Dermal

The initial manifestation of acute GVHD is often a macropapular exanthem (72). Among the first 43 patients transplanted in Seattle from HLA-identical donors, the median day of onset of skin rash was 19 (range, 5–47) days post-transplant (73). Lesions may be pruritic or painful, red to violaceous in color, and initially involve the palms and soles (Plate XVII). The characteristic predilection for these sites appears related to concentration of stem cells in the rete ridges (74) (Plate XXII). As the rash intensifies, confluent involvement of the cheeks, ears, neck, and trunk is noted (Plate XVIII), often associated with papule formation (Plate XIX).

A hyperacute form of GVHD has been described, which includes fever, generalized erythroderma, and desquamation developing 7 to 14 days after transplantation (75). Epidermal necrosis is the most severe form of cutaneous GVHD (76), and bullae formation and epidermal separation may resemble toxic epidermal necrolysis (Plate XX).

The differential diagnosis of post-transplant skin rash includes chemoradiotherapy effects, drug allergy, and viral exanthem. Topography and review of serial skin biopsies help establish the diagnosis. Rarely, a necrolytic rash may be due to a staphylococcal scalded skin syndrome, which responds to appropriate antibiotics (77).

Hepatic

The liver is the next most frequently involved target of acute GVHD (73,78). Cholestatic jaundice is common; however, hepatic failure with encephalopathy due solely to GVHD of the liver is unusual. Hypoalbuminemia is usually not due to liver failure, but rather due to GVHD-associated intestinal protein leak and negative nitrogen balance (79).

The differential diagnosis includes hepatic veno-occlusive disease, infection, and drug toxicity (80). Hepatotoxicity due to CSP may cause isolated hyperbilirubinemia, which improves within several days as the dose of drug is modified (81). Although not usually required in patients with typical manifestations of dermal and intestinal GVHD, liver biopsy may be useful in some patients because the bile duct damage of GVHD is often characteristic (see Chapter 16; Plates XXXI and XXXVI).

Intestinal

Symptoms of acute GVHD of the distal small bowel and colon include profuse diarrhea, intestinal bleeding, crampy abdominal pain, and ileus. The diarrhea is often green, mucoid, watery, and mixed with exfoliated cells, which may form fecal casts. Even with cessation of oral intake, voluminous secretory diarrhea may persist, and stool volumes should be recorded to quantitate the severity of involvement and response to treatment. Intestinal radiographs show mucosal and submucosal edema with rapid barium transit time and loss of haustral folds (82,83). In general, signs of enteric GVHD develop as the chemoradiotherapy effects resolve in the first several weeks after transplantation. A subset of patients presenting with initial signs of GVHD after day 30 has been reported (84).

A variant of enteric GVHD has been described in 13% of patients receiving HLA-identical transplants (85). Presenting symptoms include anorexia and dyspepsia, and patients with upper gastrointestinal disease may not manifest lower tract involvement. Apparently more common in older patients, upper tract disease responds well to immunosuppressive therapy, although a high proportion (74%) of patients progress to chronic GVHD.

Differential diagnosis includes residual effects of chemoradiotherapy and intestinal infection. Endoscopic findings of enteric GVHD range from normal to extensive edema (Plate XXV) and mucosal sloughing (Plate XXVIII). Lesions may be most prominent in the cecum, the ileum, and the ascending colon, but may also involve the stomach, the duodenum, and the rectum (Plate XXX). Histology reveals crypt-cell necrosis and dropout (86) (Plate XXVI). Gastrointestinal endoscopy and biopsy are mandatory for the diagnosis of upper tract disease (85). As reviewed in Chapter 33, routine endoscopic biopsy of patients with unexplained nausea and vomiting often reveals herpes virus infection with or without associated acute GVHD (87).

Other Findings

Thrombocytopenia and anemia have been reported in GVHD (88,89), and the effects on lymphohematopoietic histology are reviewed in Chapter 16. A leaky capillary syndrome of microangiopathy, hemolysis, and thrombocytopenia has been associated with severe acute GVHD in CSP recipients (90,91).

Ocular symptoms have been described in patients with acute GVHD (92,93). Photophobia, hemorrhagic conjunctivitis, pseudomembrane formation, and lagophthalmos developed within 50 days of BMT. Patients with acute GVHD with conjunctival involvement had a poorer survival than patients with GVHD without conjunctival disease (94).

Diagnosis and Grading

Staging

Acute GVHD is a clinicopathological syndrome involving the skin, the liver, and the gut (73,95). As detailed in Chapter 16, characteristic findings in biopsies of skin (eosinophilic bodies), liver (bile duct damage), and gut (crypt-cell degeneration) early after BMT may be difficult to distinguish from the effects of chemoradiotherapy conditioning (86,96,97). Serial biopsies

Table 26-1.
Clinical Staging of Acute Graft-versus-host Disease

Stage	*Skin*	*Liver*	*Gut*
+	Maculopapular rash <25% body surface	Bilirubin, 2–3 mg/dL	Diarrhea, 500–1,000 mL/day
++	Maculopapular rash 25–50% body surface	Bilirubin, 3–6 mg/dL	Diarrhea, 1,000–1,5000 mL/day
+++	Generalized erythroderma	Bilirubin, 6–15 mg/dL	Diarrhea, >1,500 mL/day
++++	Desquamation and bullae	Bilirubin, >15 mg/dL	Pain or ileus

and observations help establish the diagnosis and severity of GVHD (98).

Grading

Tables 26-1 and 26-2 present a commonly used staging and grading system for acute GVHD (73). In general, grade I acute GVHD has a favorable prognosis and does not require treatment. Grade II is moderately severe disease requiring therapy and usually consists of multiorgan disease. Occasionally, patients with a 3+ skin rash and impaired performance will qualify for grade II severity in the absence of liver or gut disease. A recent modification of grade II disease includes symptoms of nausea, anorexia, food intolerance, or vomiting confirmed to be enteric GVHD on upper intestinal biopsy (85). Grade III disease is severe, multiorgan GVHD, and grade IV disease is life-threatening or fatal GVHD.

The overall grade of GVHD predicts the clinical course. In any early report, patients with grade O to I GVHD had a 56% survival, compared with a 14% survival in patients with grade II to IV acute GVHD (73). Survival in patients with aplastic anemia was 88 and 45%, respectively (99).

Differential Diagnosis

Upper gastrointestinal endoscopy and biopsy in patients with anorexia and vomiting may yield a variety of diagnoses, including GVHD, peptic disease, or mycotic or viral infection (87,100). Liver abnormalities may cause diagnostic dilemmas even on review of histology (101). Given differing approaches in diagnostic procedures and interpretations, it is not surprising that there is inconsistency in the grading of acute GVHD across different transplant centers (102). Thus, full descriptions of GVHD, organ toxicity, infection, survival, and transplant-related mortality should be given when reporting the effects of regimens on GVHD prevention and treatment (103).

Prevention

Donor and Host Factors

Because histocompatibility is a key determinant of the kinetics of GVHD (52,104), molecular characterization of class I and II antigens assists in selection of the best available family or unrelated donor (see Chapters 4 and 51). For cytomegalovirus (CMV)-seronegative marrow recipients, matching with seronegative donors appears to reduce the risk of both CMV infection and GVHD (56).

Laminar airflow (LAF) protective isolation with gut decontamination decreased the incidence of acute GVHD and improved survival in patients with aplastic anemia prepared with cyclophosphamide (CY) alone (99). Similar analyses in leukemic patients have not shown a reduction in GVHD, perhaps due to poorer compliance with nonabsorbable oral antibiotics in patients prepared with TBI (105). This hypothesis is supported by a recent study showing that among 63 children transplanted under conditions of strict isolation, grade II to IV acute GVHD developed in 0 of 21 patients with successful decontamination compared with a 19% cumulative incidence of GVHD in 42 children with incomplete decontamination (106).

Single Agent Immunosuppression

On the basis of animal studies outlined in Chapter 1, post-transplant immunosuppression to prevent GVHD was incorporated into initial clinical practice (8). Procarbazine, CY, and MTX were found to be effective prophylaxis in murine and canine models (107–109). Standard MTX prophylaxis was given at a dose of 15 mg/m^2 on day 1 and 10 mg/m^2 on days 3, 6, 11, and weekly thereafter to day 102. Subsequently, one study reported no apparent difference in the incidence or

Tabel 26-2.
Clinical Grading of Acute Graft-versus-host Disease[a]

Overall Grade	*Stage*			*Functional Impairment*
	Skin	*Liver*	*Gut*	
O (none)	0	0	0	0
I (mild)	+to ++	0	0	0
II (moderate)	+to +++	+	+	+
III (severe)	++to +++	++to +++	++to +++	++
IV (life-threatening)	++to ++++	++to ++++	++to ++++	+++

[a]See Table 26-1 for staging symbols.

severity of acute GVHD in young patients who did or did not receive MTX (110). However, in a subsequent report of young patients not given immunosuppression after HLA-identical BMT, hyperacute GVHD developed in all 15 patients who engrafted (75). In comparison, age-matched historic control subjects receiving standard MTX had a 25% incidence of grade II to IV acute GVHD.

Transplant registry reviews confirm an increased risk of acute GVHD when post-transplant immunosuppression is deleted (60). A prospective randomized trial comparing standard 102-day MTX prophylaxis with an abbreviated 11-day course of MTX in patients given unmodified HLA-identical marrow found a significant increase in the incidence of grade II to IV acute GVHD when immunosuppression was discontinued at day 11 (25 vs 59%; $p < 0.002$) (61).

Initial pilot studies demonstrated effective prevention of GVHD with CSP prophylaxis (111,112). Cyclosporine was given intravenously at a dose of 1.5 mg/kg every 12 hours starting the day before BMT and continued until oral dosing (6.25 mg/kg q12h) was tolerated (113). Starting at day 50, oral CSP was tapered 5% each week and discontinued by day 180. Subsequent controlled trials comparing standard MTX with a 6-month course of CSP showed no difference in the rates of acute and chronic GVHD, leukemic relapse, interstitial pneumonia, and event-free survival (113,114).

Combination Immunosuppression

Mechanisms of action of immunosuppressive drugs differ (see Chapter 10) and provide a rationale for effective use in combination regimens (Table 26-3). A randomized trial from the Minnesota group compared standard MTX with a combination of MTX, prednisone (40 mg/m^2 on days 8–20), and ATG (15 mg/kg for 7 doses between day 8 and 20). Acute GVHD developed in 48 and 21% of the patients, respectively (115). Overall survival and chronic GVHD, however, did not differ. The City of Hope team combined standard MTX with prednisone (0.5–1.0 mg/kg/day) starting at day 15 and tapering throughout the first year (116). Acute GVHD and chronic GVHD rates were 39 and 9%, respectively. In a follow-up randomized study, these investigators compared MTX and prednisone with CSP and prednisone (117). The incidence of acute GVHD in the two groups was 47 and 28%, respectively. Others have compared steroids combined with CSP or CY (118).

A combined regimen of an 11-day course of MTX and a 180-day course of CSP was found to be effective in DLA-nonidentical unrelated and haploidentical

Table 26-3.
Randomized Trials of Combination Immunosuppression after HLA-identical Marrow Transplantation

Investigator (Reference)	*Disease Groups*	*No. Patients*	*Combined Agents*	*Median Age (yr)*	*Acute GVHD*	*Chronic GVHD*	*Survival*
Ramsay (115)	Nonmalignant and malignant	32	MTX +ATG + P	16	21% (p=0.01)	6%	52% (NS)
		35	MTX	16	48%	9%	44%
Storb (120,123)	Aplastic anemia	22	MTX + CSP	23	18% (p=0.01)	58% (NS)	73% (NS)
		24	MTX	23	53%	36%	58%
Storb (121,122)	AML in CR1 and CML in CP	43	MTX + CSP	30	33% (p=0.01)	26%	65% (NS)
		50	CSP	30	54%	24%	54%
Forman (117)	Acute leukemia and CML	53	MTX + P	26	47% (p=0.05)	?	53%
		54	CSP + P	26	28%	?	57%
Santos (118)	Nonmalignant and malignant	42	CSP + MP	23	32% (p=0.005)	40% (NS)	38% (p=0.03)
		40	CY + MP	24	68%	18%	20%
Sullivan (61)	Advanced hematological malignancies	25	Long-term MTX + BC	19	82% (p=0.016)	44%	24%
		40	Short-term MTX	18	59% (p=0.0016)	51%	30%
		44	Long-term MTX	19	25%	33%	41%
Storb (126)	Nonmalignant and malignant	59	MTX + CSP + P	32	46% (p=0.02)	62% (p=0.01)	52% (NS)
		63	MTX + CSP	28	25%	40%	46%
Forman (127)	Malignant disease	63	MTX + CSP + P	?	10% (p=0.057)	30%	?
		59	CSP + P	?	22%	30%	?

AML = acute myeloid leukemia; ATG = antithymocyte globulin; BC = donor buffy-coat cells; CML = chronic myeloid leukemia; CP = chronic phase; CR = complete remission; CSP = cyclosporine; CY = cyclophosphamide; GVHD = graft-versus-host disease; MP = methylprednisolone; MTX = methotrexate; NS = not significant; P = prednisone.

littermate canine transplants (119). Subsequent controlled clinical trials comparing this regimen with standard MTX in patients with aplastic anemia and with CSP alone in patients with leukemia showed a significant reduction in acute GVHD and associated improved survival (120,121). Long-term follow-up studies confirm these findings (122–125). Attempts to enhance the efficacy of MTX and CSP prophylaxis have been reported. The addition of prednisone given from day 0 through day 21 at 1 mg/kg daily and reduced from day 22 to day 35 to 0.5 mg/kg/day was not beneficial (126). An ongoing study of prednisone given from day 7 to day 180, combined with MTX on days 1, 3, and 6, and CSP given to day 180 results in an incidence of acute GVHD of 10%, which suggests improvement when compared with a 22% incidence in patients randomized to CSP and prednisone (127).

Reducing the dose of intravenous CSP from 3.0 to 1 to 1.5 mg/kg/day during the first 14 to 20 days after BMT appears to retain the efficacy of prophylaxis and to reduce attendant toxicity (128,129). A reduction in MTX or CSP doses for a brief time early after BMT may avoid hepatic and renal toxicity and permit subsequent full dosing of GVHD prophylaxis (58,130). This approach may be especially beneficial in patients receiving intensified pretransplant conditioning, in whom doses of GVHD prophylaxis are often attenuated and rates of GVHD are amplified due to regimen-related toxicities (64).

Antibody Treatment

Polyvalent intravenous immunoglobulin (IVIg) has been beneficial in several autoimmune disorders with immunopathological features (131–133). Initial studies of IVIg in BMT were aimed at infection prophylaxis (134). More recently, IVIg was found to reduce the frequency of acute GVHD (135). This benefit was most apparent in patients ≥ 20 years or older and was associated with a reduction in transplant-related mortality (136). Figure 26-2 illustrates these findings (137). Current studies are aimed at determining the optimal dose and schedule of IVIg prophylaxis.

Two prospective studies randomly assigned patients receiving standard MTX to receive or to not receive additional ATG prophylaxis (138,139). Neither study showed an alteration in the incidence or severity of GVHD. More recently, anti T-cell monoclonal antibodies against the interleukin-2 (IL-2) receptor were given to deplete activated T cells and to prevent acute GVHD. Clinical trials of anti-IL-2 receptor antibody administration suggest some benefit in suppressing early signs of hyperacute GVHD (140,141). Murine models show reduction of GVHD and mortality with antibody inhibition of IL-1 and tumor necrosis factor-alpha (TNF-α) (15,142).

Marrow T-cell Depletion

Many techniques have been used for in vitro treatment of marrow to remove T cells and to prevent

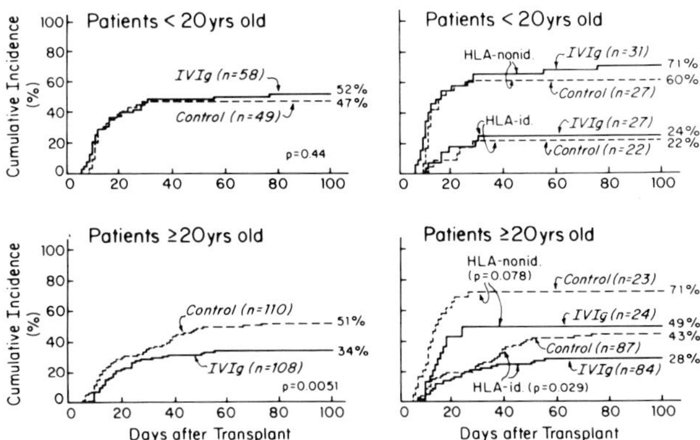

Figure 26-2. Cumulative incidence of grade II-IV acute GVHD in patients given intravenous immunoglobulin (solid lines) and in control patients not given immunoglobulin (broken lines). In the left panel, patients are grouped according to age. In the right panel, the same age groups are displayed by donor HLA-disparity. Among these 325 patients receiving allografts, 58 of 107 who were less than 20 years of age (54%) and 47 of 218 who were 20 or more years of age (22%) received marrow from HLA-nonidentical donors. (Reprinted, by permission of the New England Journal of Medicine, from Sullivan KM, Kopecky KJ, Buckner CD, Storb R. Intravenous IgG to prevent graft-versus-host disease after bone marrow transplantation (letter). N Engl J Med 1990;323:705–712.)

GVHD (143–149). Chapter 11 reviews these technologies in detail. Almost all studies show a significant reduction in the incidence and severity of acute GVHD, but results are offset by an increase in the rate of graft failure and recurrent leukemia (150–153).

Other Approaches

New immunosuppressive agents are being placed into clinical trials as single agents or in combination to prevent GVHD. Trimetrexate, succinylacetone, FK-506, rapamycin, thalidomide, and ultraviolet radiation are of interest (154–160). Chapter 10 presents mechanisms of actions, toxicities, and preliminary clinical experience with these agents.

Treatment

Primary Therapy

Cytotoxic agents and glucocorticoids have been used to treat established acute GVHD (8,108,161,162). Although responses have been observed at doses of methylprednisolone (MP) varying from 1 to 60 mg/kg/day, fatal infections have been observed with ultra high-dose regimens, and most clinicians employ a standard tapering schedule of 2 mg/kg/day MP in divided doses (163–166). Plates XXIII and XXIV illustrate the clinical response to MP treatment. Although initial pilot studies demonstrated benefit of ATG in controlling human acute GVHD (167), subsequent randomized comparisons of intravenous ATG

(15 mg/kg every other day for 6 days) and MP (2 mg/kg/day) showed no difference in efficacy or survival with the two treatments (168). Similarly, pilot data of therapy with CSP appeared encouraging (169), but subsequent randomized trials found a similar 25% survival in patients treated with either intravenous CSP (3–5 mg/kg/day) or standard MP (170). Sequential administration of ATG and CSP (with or without MP) was evaluated as primary treatment of acute GVHD (171). Long-term survival was 49% in the ATG plus CSP group but only 11% in the triple therapy group.

Response to primary therapy of acute GVHD was analyzed in 740 patients (172). Treatment failure (defined as initiation of secondary treatment or nonrelapse mortality) was increased with ATG compared with therapy with either CSP or MP. Patients given MTX and CSP prophylaxis were less likely to experience treatment failure than those given other prophylaxis regimens. Consequently, MP seems the best initial treatment for patients receiving MTX and CSP prophylaxis. However, considerable room for improvement is apparent due to the 80% nonrelapse mortality observed in patients failing initial treatment.

Secondary Therapy

Patients failing initial therapy (commonly defined as progression after 3 days, no change after 7 days, or incomplete response after 14 days of MP treatment) have been treated with a variety of salvage regimens. Treatment with OKT3 monoclonal antibody has shown some benefit (173) but was associated with toxicity and TNF release (174). Secondary therapy with a mitogenic anti-CD3 antibody was associated with a 24% incidence of Epstein-Barr virus–associated lymphoproliferative syndrome (175–178). A nonmitogenic anti-CD3 antibody appears to modulate T-cell function safely and to lessen GVHD (179). An anti-CD5 immunoconjugate also appears to modulate steroid-resistant acute GVHD (180).

In an attempt to target activated T cells, antibody therapy specific for the IL-2 receptor has been reported (181). In patients with steroid-resistant acute GVHD, 65% of patients had a complete response and 19% a partial response to treatment (182). However, a second study concluded that only 1 of 10 patients had a complete response (183). A humanized anti-Tac antibody to the IL-2 receptor has been developed (184), and clinical trials are currently in progress in BMT patients.

Monoclonal antibody therapy has also been targeted against the efferent arm of GVHD. A murine IgG_1 antibody specific for TNF-α was evaluated in 19 patients with acute GVHD refractory to MP and anti-IL-2 receptor treatment (185). Five patients had no response and 14 had a partial response to anti-TNF therapy. All responders had a return of GVHD after discontinuing treatment, and 16 of the 19 patients died of transplant-related complications.

An alternative approach includes use of ultraviolet irradiation to suppress cutaneous GVHD (186). Psoralen and ultraviolet A irradiation (PUVA) has shown benefit in 11 patients (5 complete and 6 partial responses) (187). Importantly, survival may be improved in patients treated for steroid-resistant disease (188).

Response to secondary therapy of acute GVHD has been reported in 427 patients (189). Highest rates of response were observed in patients in whom GVHD recurred during a steroid taper and for whom the dose of MP was subsequently increased.

Supportive Care

Gut rest, hyperalimentation, pain control, and antibiotic prophylaxis are routine elements of supportive care of patients with GVHD (190). Octreotide (a somatostatin analog) appears to be of benefit in controlling secretory diarrhea in some patients (191,192). Antiviral prophylaxis may be especially important in preventing interstitial pneumonia in patients with refractory GVHD (193). Similarly, new antifungal agents, such as the triazols and liposomal amphotericin, may be of benefit in preventing and treating serious mycotic infections (194).

Prognosis

Clinical Severity

Outcome is predicted by the overall grade of acute GVHD (99). Response to treatment is another key determinant of outcome (195). As shown in Figure 26-3, mortality in patients with grade II to IV acute GVHD is lowest in those achieving a complete response to initial treatment (172).

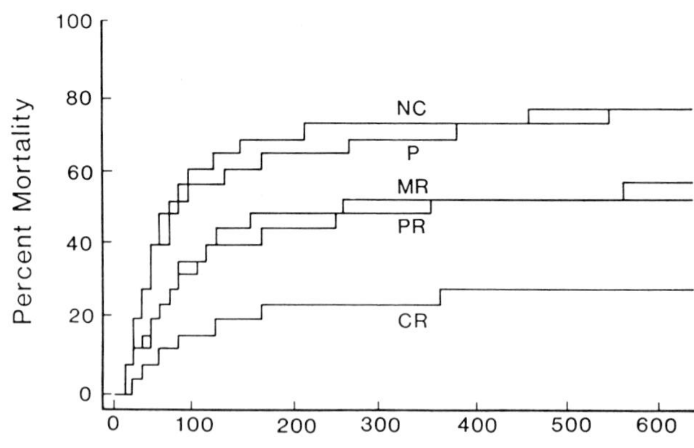

Figure 26-3. Transplant-related mortality of patients displayed by outcome to primary treatment of acute GVHD. Abbreviations include CR (complete response), PR (partial response), MR (mixed response), NC (no change) and P (progression). (Reproduced by permission from Martin PJ, Schoch G, Fisher L, et al. A retrospective analysis of therapy for acute graft-versus-host disease: initial treatment. Blood 1990; 76:1464–1472.)

Prognostic Factors

Factors associated with impaired survival include HLA-nonidentical marrow donors, liver abnormalities in addition to GVHD, and early time to onset and treatment of GVHD. Similar times to treatment failure and determinants of outcome were observed in patients receiving primary and secondary therapy (172,189). These findings support the validity of testing new immunosuppressive modalities in patients with inadequate response to primary treatment.

Chronic GVHD in Allogeneic Marrow Recipients

Pathogenesis

Alloreactivity vs Autoreactivity

Alloreactivity contributes to the pathogenesis of chronic GVHD. Some investigators consider chronic GVHD to be a late phase of acute GVHD due to minor antigen recognition. Others consider it more of an autoimmune-like process. In both experimental and clinical studies of chronic GVHD, thymic atrophy (Plate LX), lymphocyte depletion, and loss of thymic epithelial secretory function are noted (196–198). Absence of thymic function by age or injury could be responsible for autoreactivity, similar to the pathogenesis of autologous GVHD (23). This hypothesis is supported by experimental data in which T cells from animals with chronic GVHD are specific for reactivity to host class II determinants (199). Moreover, similarities of clinical features of chronic GVHD and autoimmune diseases are frequently observed.

Autoantibody Formation

Autoantibody formation has been noted in experimental models of chronic GVHD (200,201). Clinical reports parallel these findings (202–204). Antinuclear, antidouble-stranded DNA, and anti-smooth muscle autoantibodies range in frequency from 11 to 62% of patients with chronic GVHD. More recently, anticytoskeletal and antinucleolar antibodies have been detected in patients with chronic GVHD (205–207), and specific nucleolar phosphoproteins have been identified as GVHD targets (208).

Incidence and Predictive Factors

Incidence

Among patients surviving 150 days after allogeneic BMT, chronic GVHD was observed in 33% of HLA-identical sibling transplants, in 49% of HLA-nonidentical related transplants, and in 64% of matched unrelated donor transplants (209). Data from single institution and registry studies suggest that the incidence of chronic GVHD may be as high as 80% in one antigen HLA-nonidentical unrelated transplants.

Predictive Factors

In addition to HLA disparity, prior acute GVHD and increasing patient age are factors associated with an increased risk of developing chronic GVHD (210–212). As shown in Figure 26-4, among recipients of HLA-identical marrow who survived beyond day 150, the probability for development of chronic GVHD was 13% in children less than 10 years old, 28% in adolescents 10 to 19 years old, and 42 to 46% in adults over age 20 (209). In contrast, there appeared to be little reduction in GVHD in young patients given HLA-nonidentical and unrelated marrow.

Other predictive factors appear more controversial. Abbreviation or deletion of MTX prophylaxis in some reports did not influence the development of chronic GVHD (213). In contrast, other studies suggest a reduction in chronic GVHD with prolonged CSP prophylaxis (214–216). Random red cell transfusions given shortly before transplantation have been associated with a decreased risk of chronic GVHD, whereas unirradiated donor buffy coat or marrow reinfusions appear associated with an increased risk for development of GVHD (217,218). In one report, splenectomy appeared to increase the risk for development of chronic GVHD, possibly due to increased rates of infection in splenectomized patients (219).

The relationship between infection and subsequent chronic GVHD is unclear. European centers report that latent herpes virus in the marrow donor and recipient may be important for the development of acute and chronic GVHD (67,220). In other reports, no association of CMV infection with subsequent development of chronic GVHD was observed (221).

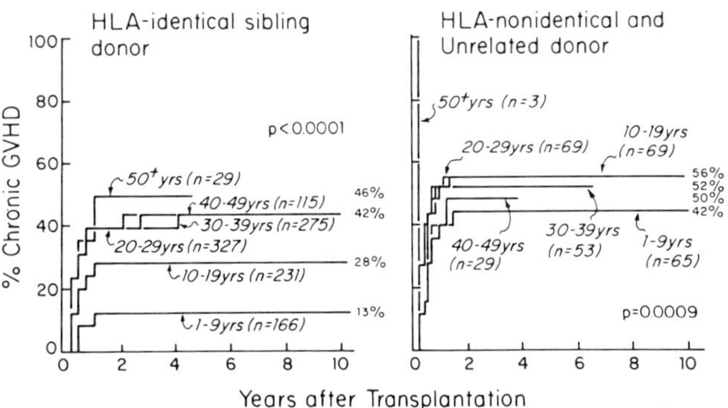

Figure 26-4. Probability of developing clinical extensive chronic GVHD in patients with hematologic malignancies who survived at least 150 days after BMT from HLA-identical siblings (left panel) or HLA-nonidentical family members or unrelated donors (right panel). (Reproduced with permission from Sullivan KM, Agura E, Anasetti C, et al. Chronic graft-versus-host disease and other late complications of bone marrow transplantation. Semin Hematol 1991;28:250–259.)

Clinical Features

Dermal

Two types of cutaneous involvement have been described (72,222). An early phase resembles lichen planus (223). Lesions may be scanty or evanescent, ranging from polygonal papules to more typical lesions (Plate XLV). Inspection with side-angle lighting more clearly defines the raised, flat-topped lesions. In a later phase, poikiloderma is observed (Plates XLVII and XLVIII). In patients with a localized type histology, epidermal atrophy and dense focal dermal fibrosis are noted in the absence of significant inflammation (Plate LI). As shown in Plate XLIX, clinical features resemble morphea (224). In other patients, a generalized type histology is noted, with inflammation in eccrine coils and pilar units resulting in fibrosis throughout the dermis and the adnexal structures (Plate L). Generalized scleroderma may lead to joint contractures and debility (225,226).

The tempo of dermal abnormalities may show wide variation. In some patients, erythema, hyperkeratosis, and desquamation develop rapidly, sometimes after solar exposure. Erythema may begin in the malar area and may resemble lupus erythematosus but soon spread to sun-exposed and sun-shielded areas. In others, the onset is insidious, with patchy hyperpigmentation, reticular mottling, perifollicular papules, and papulosquamous plaques. Guttate lesions may appear on the trunk as shiny indurated areas or be localized to areas of pressure-point trauma, prior injury, or irritation (227,228). Rarely, vesicles, bullae, or bullous pemphigoid lesions have been reported (229,230). Alopecia and nail loss are not uncommon (Plate LII). Regrowth of body hair and return of sweat gland function usually herald disease improvement.

Skin lesions are sometimes incorrectly attributed to reactions to drugs such as trimethoprim sulfamethoxazole (TMP-SMX). Skin biopsies are very useful in establishing the correct diagnosis. The differential diagnosis from dyskeratosis congenita may be difficult and should be considered in patients with aplastic anemia undergoing allogeneic BMT (231).

Hepatic

Liver function tests show predominantly cholestatic abnormalities. The degree of hyperbilirubinemia correlates less closely with clinical outcome than in patients with acute GVHD (226). Although reported, development of portal hypertension, cirrhosis, and death from hepatic failure are surprisingly rare despite years of hepatic abnormalities (232,233).

The differential diagnosis of late hepatic abnormalities is broad and includes viral infection, hepatotoxic drug reactions, gallstones, and infiltrative hepatic abnormalities, including fungal infection and neoplastic disease. Liver biopsies are helpful in establishing a diagnosis (see Chapter 16). Both naturally occurring primary biliary cirrhosis and chronic GVHD show similar bile duct damage and features of ocular and oral sicca (234).

Ocular

Ophthalmic symptoms of keratoconjunctivitis sicca include burning, irritation, photophobia, and pain. Tear function is evaluated by Schirmer's testing and fluorescein biomicroscopy of the cornea. Punctate keratopathy can range from minimal stippling to massive erosions. Even in the absence of symptoms, patients should be screened for ocular sicca and started on artificial tear replacement if indicated. Punctal ligation may be of benefit to conserve corneal wetting in the dry eye.

A more common cause of impaired visual acuity is development of cataracts following marrow transplantation (235). Use of prednisone after day 100 to treat chronic GVHD and of pretransplant TBI promote cataract formation (236). Cataract repair may be performed safely even in the presence of a severely dry eye.

Oral

Oral dryness, sensitivity to acidic or spicy foods, and increasing pain after day 100 after transplant strongly suggest development of chronic GVHD (237,238). In a prospective study of 60 long-term survivors after allogeneic BMT, oral atrophy, erythema, and lichenoid lesions of the buccal and labial mucosa were significantly correlated with development of chronic GVHD (239).

A common clinical error is to confuse lichen planus–like lesions of chronic GVHD with oral candidiasis. Lichenoid reactions range from fine white reticular striae on buccal surfaces to large plaques on the buccal surface or the lateral tongue (Plate LV). Oral herpes simplex may exacerbate the pain associated with chronic GVHD. Serial viral cultures may be needed to establish the diagnosis and to direct appropriate antiviral therapy.

Pulmonary

Bronchodilator-resistant obstructive lung disease is a clinical feature of chronic GVHD (240). Histopathology reveals characteristic lesions of obliterative bronchiolitis (241) (Plate LIX). The frequency of this complication is increased in patients with chronic GVHD who received a 102-day course of MTX as GVHD prophylaxis (240). In addition, patients with chronic GVHD and hypogammaglobulinemia or IgG subclass deficiencies appear to be at increased risk for late obstructive airway disease (242,243). The 3-year mortality in patients with chronic GVHD was increased significantly in those in whom obstructive lung disease developed compared with chronic GVHD patients with normal pulmonary function (244).

Gastrointestinal

Intestinal involvement is uncommon in chronic GVHD. Dysphagia, pain, and insidious weight loss are often presenting symptoms of chronic GVHD of the esophagus (245). Manometric studies demonstrate poor acid clearance, and motor abnormalities range from aperistalsis to high-amplitude contractions. Radiographic findings include web formation, ring-like narrowings, and tapering structures of the mid and upper esophagus (246). It was possible to distinguish esophageal involvement of chronic GVHD from that of naturally occurring progressive systemic sclerosis in a coded review of autopsy material (245). Nerve fibers and silver stains of the myenteric plexus were of normal appearance in all patients with chronic GVHD, in contrast to that of patients with scleroderma.

Neuromuscular

There is no compelling evidence for a central nervous system component of chronic GVHD (247,248). Metabolic and infectious etiologies are common causes of neurological impairment, although a recent case report suggests cerebral involvement in a patient with chronic GVHD (249). Sural nerve biopsy results and response to immunosuppressive therapy demonstrate that the peripheral nervous system may be a target of chronic GVHD (250).

Myasthenia gravis has been reported in 7 patients with chronic GVHD (248,251,252). Clinical and laboratory features mirror those of classic autoimmune myasthenia gravis, including the development of acetylcholine receptor antibodies. All patients have responded to cholinesterase inhibitors and immunosuppressive drugs. Polymyositis (Plate LVII) has also been reported in a number of patients with chronic GVHD (226,253,254). Strength improved following corticosteroid treatment.

Other Findings

Vaginitis and vaginal strictures have been noted in women with chronic GVHD (255). In a recent study of women examined 1 year after allogeneic BMT, the gynecological effects of chronic GVHD could be distinguished from those of primary ovarian failure due to TBI (256).

Less easy to dissociate were the effects of GVHD on marrow function of long-term survivors. Although a graft-versus-host stroma effect has been defined in animal models, few clinical studies have been reported (257). In one study, chronic GVHD was associated with poor growth of hematopoietic progenitor cells (258). In another, autoimmune-like thrombocytopenia with increased platelet destruction was described (89). Multiple mechanisms may have a role in the poor graft function observed in some patients with severe GVHD (88,259).

Changing Features

The protean manifestations of chronic GVHD have been likened to those of progressive systemic sclerosis, systemic lupus erythematous, lichen planus, Sjögren's syndrome, eosinophilic fasciitis, rheumatoid arthritis, and primary biliary cirrhosis (202,226,234,260,261). Correlations, however, are not exact, as evidenced by the rarity of characteristic esophageal or renal involvement common to several autoimmune diseases (245, 261,262).

The spectrum of abnormalities in chronic GVHD appears to be changing as a result of earlier diagnosis and institution of immunosuppressive therapy. Figure 26-5 presents a comparison of clinical features in patients in an initial cohort (226), compared with those more recently transplanted when earlier diagnosis and treatment were standard (263). Ocular, esophageal, pulmonary, and serosal involvement have been less frequent in recent years. Weight loss and contracture formation have also been reduced.

Diagnosis and Grading

Staging

As described in Chapter 16, clinicians rely on histological review of oral and skin biopsies to diagnose and to gauge response to therapy (264). Table 26-4 presents a summary of the clinicopathological classification of chronic GVHD (261). Patients with *limited* disease involving the skin or liver have a favorable untreated course (226). In contrast, patients with *extensive* disease involving multiple organs have an adverse natural course. This staging system is easily derived and highly reproducible when tested in an international survey (265).

Grading

In general, the grading system for acute GVHD correlates poorly with outcome in chronic GVHD.

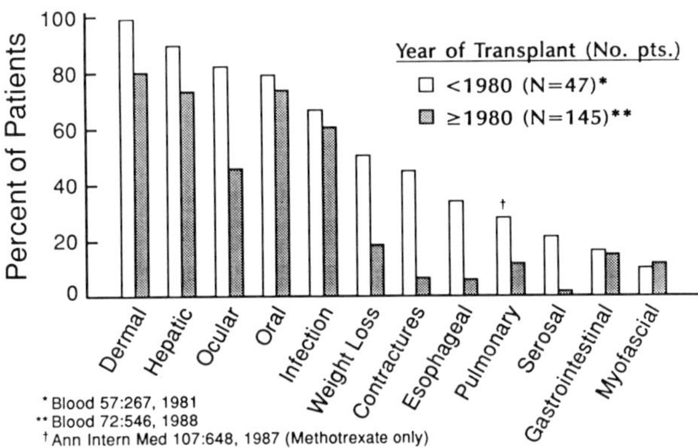

Figure 26-5. Features of clinical extensive chronic GVHD in patients transplanted before 1980 (open columns) and since 1980 (shaded columns) in Seattle (from 226, 240, 263).

Table 26-4.
Clinicopathological Classification of Chronic Graft-versus-host Disease

Limited chronic GVHD
Either or both
1. Localized skin involvement
2. Hepatic dysfunction due to chronic GVHD

Extensive chronic GVHD
Either
1. Generalized skin involvement, or
2. Localized skin involvement and/or hepatic dysfunction due to chronic GVHD

Plus
3a. Liver histology showing chronic aggressive hepatitis, bridging necrosis, or cirrhosis, or
b. Involvement of eye (Schirmer's test with less than 5 mm wetting), or
c. Involvement of minor salivary glands or oral mucosa demonstrated on labial biopsy, or
d. Involvement of any other target organ

GVHD = graft-versus-host disease.

Morbidity and mortality are highest in patients with a *progressive* onset of chronic GVHD directly following acute GVHD, intermediate in those with a *quiescent* onset following resolution of acute GVHD, and lowest in patients with a de novo onset (226). Approximately 20% of patients with chronic GVHD have a de novo onset without prior acute GVHD.

Diagnosis

The median day of diagnosis in HLA-identical sibling transplants is 201 days after transplant; in contrast, HLA-nonidentical related and unrelated donor marrow recipients have an earlier diagnosis and onset (159 and 133 days, respectively) (209). Few patients experience development of chronic GVHD beyond day 500. As shown in Table 26-5, screening studies to detect early clinical chronic GVHD are routinely conducted on all allogeneic BMT recipients 100 days after transplantation (266). Even in the absence of current signs or symptoms of chronic GVHD, a positive random skin biopsy or a history of prior acute GVHD independently predicted a 3-fold increase in the relative risk of subsequent chronic GVHD.

Prevention

Thymic Factors

On the basis of the hypothesis that impaired thymic regulation of autoreactive T cells contributes to the immunopathogenesis of chronic GVHD, attempts have been made to prevent chronic GVHD by modification of thymic function. Transplantation of thymic tissue grafts or administration of thymic factors did not reduce the incidence or severity of chronic GVHD (267,268).

T-cell Depletion

The risk of chronic GVHD was found to be reduced by approximately 50% after T-cell depletion of HLA-identical marrow (153). Overall survival, however, was not improved. Moreover, chronic GVHD was still noted in 85% of long-term survivors who received T-cell–depleted marrow from unrelated donors (146).

Intravenous Immunoglobulin

Weekly administration of IVIg through day 90 post-transplant reduced the incidence and mortality of acute GVHD (136). When the same dose of 500 mg/kg IVIg was given on a monthly schedule from day 90 to day 360 post-transplant, median serum IgG levels rapidly decreased from 1,600 to 900 mg/dL, and the cumulative incidence of chronic GVHD was not different from that of control patients randomized not to receive IVIg (269).

Prolonged Immunosuppression

Several studies suggest that the incidence of chronic GVHD may be reduced when an extended course of CSP prophylaxis is administered (214–216). These observations are supported by the fact that chronic GVHD usually develops during or shortly after the routine 6-month taper of CSP prophylaxis.

Treatment

Natural History

An initial report established the clinicopathological criteria for diagnosis and grading (261). Thirteen

Table 26-5.
Screening Studies for Chronic Graft-versus-host Disease

Organ/System	*Clinical Finding*	*Screening Study*
Dermal	Dyspigmentation, xerosis, erythema, scleroderma, onychodystrophy, alopecia	Skin biopsy—3 mm punch biopsy from posterior iliac crest and forearm areas
Oral	Lichen planus, xerostomia	Oral biospy from inner lower lip
Ocular	Sicca, keratitis	No. 1 Schirmer's test
Hepatic	Jaundice	Alkaline phosphatase, SGOT, bilirubin
Pulmonary	Obstructive/restrictive pulmonary disease	Pulmonary function studies and arterial blood gas
Vaginal	Sicca, atrophy	Gynecological evaluation
Nutritional	Protein and caloric deficiency	Weight, muscle/fat store measurement
Clinical performance	Contractures, debility	Karnofsky score or Lansky play index

SGOT = serum glutamic oxaloacetic transaminase.

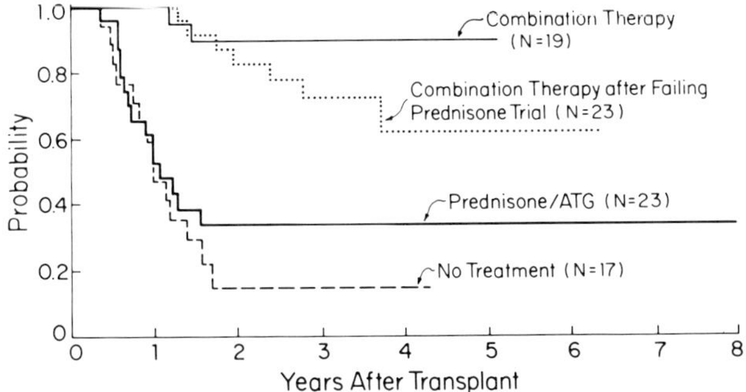

Figure 26-6. Kaplan-Meier estimates of the probability of survival without disability (i.e., Karnofsky performance) in patients with clinical extensive chronic GVHD transplanted in Seattle before 1980. (Reproduced with permission from Sullivan KM, Deeg HJ, Sanders JE, et al. Late complications after marrow transplantation. Semin Hematol 1984;21:53–56.)

patients with clinical extensive chronic GVHD were not treated and only 2 survived (Karnofsky performance ≥ 70%) (226). There appeared to be no spontaneous improvement in disabled survivors despite years of observation.

Primary Treatment

Another 13 patients received a brief course of ATG or a prolonged course of corticosteroids given late in the course of disease and only 3 survived without disability (226). Similar experience with other immunosuppressive drugs or plasmapheresis given late in the disease had little apparent benefit (202). In 21 patients with extensive chronic GVHD, prednisone (1.0 mg/kg/every other day) was given with either CY, procarbazine, or azathioprine (all 1.5 mg/kg/day) early in the course of disease before clinical deterioration (226). Procarbazine appeared to be less effective, and CY was associated with hemorrhagic cystitis. Chronic GVHD responded to a median of 13 months of combination therapy with prednisone and azathioprine (Plates LIII and LIV). Figure 26-6 presents these and additional patients treated prior to 1980 (270). Late prednisone or ATG appeared little different than no treatment. Combination therapy given as either primary or secondary treatment was associated with improved disability-free survival. Results, however, could not be compared directly because patients given combination therapy were treated in later years when treatment was given earlier in their disease.

To determine the benefit of early combination therapy, we conducted a double-blind randomized trial comparing prednisone and azathioprine with prednisone and placebo (263). Patients with persisting thrombocytopenia were not randomized due to concern about using cytotoxic drugs in cytopenic patients; instead, these patients were placed into treatment with an equivalent dose of alternate-day prednisone. All three groups received prophylaxis with TMP-SMX. As shown in Table 26-6, nonrelapse mortality was significantly higher (40 vs 21%) in standard-risk patients randomized to prednisone and azathioprine. This mortality was due to an increase in fatal infections in patients receiving cytotoxic treat-

Table 26-6.
Primary Treatment of Extensive Chronic GVHD: Studies by the Seattle Team

				3-year Kaplan-Meier estimates			
Study (ref. #)	*Primary Treatment*	*Study Year*	*No. Patients*	*Survival*	*Nonrelapse mortality*	*Bacteremial Septicemia*	*Any Pneumonia*
Standard risk patients[a]							
I (226)	None	1973–76	13	18%			
	Late pred	1973–76	13	23%			
	Early pred + Az	1977–80	21	76%			
II (263)R	Pred + Placebo	1980–83	63	61%[b] (p=0.03)	21%[c] (p=0.003)		
	Pred + Az	1980–83	63	47%	40%		
IV (290)R	Pred	1985–89	85	71%	17%	17%	26%
	CSP/Pred	1985–89	83	80%[d]	11%[e]	12%[f]	47%
High-risk patients[g]							
II (263)	Pred	1980–82	38	26%[b]	58%[c]		
III (271)	CSP/Pred	1982–85	40	52%	40%		
V (290)R	CSP	1985–89	61	35%	42%	53%	63%[f]
	CSP/Pred	1985–89	60	48%[d]	35%[e]	33%[f]	29%[f]

[a]Platelets >100,000/μL.
[b]p<0.0001.
[c]p<0.001.
[d]p<0.0001.
[e]p=0.00036.
[f]p=0.015.
[g]Platelets <100,000/μL.
Az = azathioprine; CSP = cyclosporine; Pred = prednisone; R = randomized.

ment. Survival was 61% in patients randomized to prednisone and placebo. This survival rate was significantly higher than the 26% survival observed in high-risk patients with thrombocytopenia treated with an identical prednisone regimen. The reason for the increased infectious mortality in high-risk patients was unclear because granulocyte counts were normal. It appeared that the hypomegakaryocytic thrombocytopenia was a marker for more severe chronic GVHD, often of progressive-type onset in patients with prior acute GVHD.

We next studied the addition of oral CSP (6 mg every 12 hr every other day) alternating with prednisone (1 mg/kg every other day) in patients at high risk for GVHD with thrombocytopenia (271). Renal toxicity was modest (272). As shown in Table 26-6, survival improved and infections decreased with this regimen. Functional performance of the long-term survivors was maintained near normal, and the incidence of disabling scleroderma was decreased from 43 to 6% (Figure 26-5). However, infections remained a frequent cause of morbidity and contributed to transplant-related mortality.

A report from the Baltimore team described the use of thalidomide in high-risk patients (273). The 3-year survival was 48% in 21 patients receiving primary treatment. Infections seemed to be diminished in the long-term survivors.

Secondary Treatment

Azathioprine, alternating CSP and prednisone or thalidomide give surprisingly similar survival (approximately 75%) in patients failing initial steroid therapy (269,273). Other studies explored the use of PUVA in patients with refractory cutaneous chronic GVHD (188,274,275). Dermal responses are commonly observed and some improvement has been noted at extracutaneous sites. Low dose total lymphoid irradiation was also reported to lead to partial or complete improvement in 9 patients receiving 100 cGy thoracoabdominal irradiation (276). Preliminary reports of new macrolide compounds have also shown promise in patients with steroid-refractory chronic GVHD (277,278).

Supportive Care

Dermal GVHD may benefit from burn care management to speed reepitheliazation and closure of portals of infection. Skin allografting from the marrow donor without further immunosuppression has been performed successfully (279). Neuromuscular manifestations of chronic GVHD (i.e., muscular aches, cramping, and carpal spasm) have responded to clonazepam treatment (280). Liver function abnormalities in patients with refractory hepatic chronic GVHD decreased by approximately 30% following bile acid displacement therapy with ursodeoxycholic acid (UDCA) (281). Long-term effects of UDCA therapy are being studied.

Antimicrobial prophylaxis is an important aspect of the treatment of patients with chronic GVHD. The relation of immunodeficiency, GVHD-associated immunosuppression, and infection are complex interactions of critical importance in management of patients with GVHD.

Late Infections

Immunodeficiency

As detailed in Chapter 36, multiple immune defects are observed in patients with chronic GVHD. Thymic injury, impaired mucosal defense, chemotactic defects, functional asplenia, T-cell alloreactivity, and qualitative and quantitative B-cell abnormalities contribute to the susceptibility to late infection.

Spectrum of Infection

Bacteremia and sinopulmonary infections due to *Streptococcus pneumoniae* and *Haemophilus influenzae* frequently develop in patients with chronic GVHD (263,282,283). Pulmonary infection after day 100 post-transplant developed in 50% of allograft recipients with chronic GVHD, 21% of allografts free of chronic GVHD, and 2% of autograft recipients (269). Late infections appear to be increased particularly in unrelated marrow recipients. The probability of bacteremia or septicemia after day 100 was 22% in 364 HLA-identical sibling transplant recipients and 38% in 38 unrelated transplant recipients ($p = 0.008$) (209). Chronic GVHD and HLA-nonidentity contribute to this increased rate of infection in unrelated marrow recipients, as does the frequent presence of hypogammaglobulinemia (269).

Antimicrobial Prophylaxis

Most BMT patients receive *Pneumocystis carinii* prophylaxis through day 120 post-transplant or for as long as they continue on chronic GVHD therapy with corticosteroids. Prophylaxis with TMP-SMX significantly reduced the incidence of late interstitial pneumonia from 28 to 8% in patients with chronic GVHD (284).

Immunizations

After the first year, healthy patients free of chronic GVHD are likely to respond to influenza, pneumococcal polysaccharide, inactivated poliovirus, diphtheria, pertussis, tetanus toxoid, and *Haemophilus influenzae* type b conjugate vaccines (285,286). Patients being treated for chronic GVHD who are receiving immunosuppressive therapy may or may not form an adequate antibody response (287,288). Antibody titers can be tested 2 and 4 weeks following vaccination to evaluate immune responsiveness.

Live virus vaccines such as measles, mumps, rubella (MMR), oral polio virus vaccine, oral typhoid, and Bacillus Calmette-Guerin vaccine carry risk in the

Table 26-7.
Multivariate Analysis of Relapse and Treatment Failure According to GVHD Factors*

Disease Status at transplantation	*Relapse of Leukemia*			*Treatment Failure (Relapse or Death)*		
	GVHD Factor	*Relative Risk*	*p* Value	*GVHD Factor*	*Relative Risk*	*p* Value
AML in 1st remission (n=251)	MTX/CSP	2.34	0.017	A-GVHD	2.33	<0.001
AML ≥ 2nd remission (n=55)	A-GVHD	0.21	0.42	None	. . .	. . .
AML in relapse (n=202)	A or C-GVHD	0.42	0.003	None	. . .	. . .
	MTX	0.58	0.038	. . .	. . .	. . .
ALL in 1st remission (n=56)	A-GVHD	0.11	0.006	CSP	13.85	0.024
ALL ≥ 2nd remission (n=147)	A-GVHD	0.48	0.045	None	. . .	. . .
ALL in relapse (n=202)	A or C-GVHD	0.33	<0.001	A or C-GVHD	0.70	0.033
	MTX/CSP	2.78	<0.001	MTX/CSP	1.69	0.016
CML in chronic phase (n=174)	None	. . .	. . .	A and C-GVHD	3.29	<0.001
				MTX	1.85	0.013
CML in accelerated phase (n=61)	None	. . .	. . .	MTX	0.45	0.024
				MTX/CSP	0.24	0.003
CML in blast crisis (n=50)	MTX/CSP	6.03	0.012	A or C-GVHD	0.37	0.009

*Proportional hazards regression analysis using four time-dependent GVHD covariates (acute, no chronic, n=337; chronic, no acute, n=145; either acute or chronic; n=482; both acute and chronic GVHD, n=121) and four GVHD prophylaxis regimens (CSP alone, n=178; MTX alone, n=754; MTX+CSP, n=249; other regimens, n=21). Patient age, donor/patient gender, and pretransplant preparative regimens were also included in the models but are not displayed in this table (see 294).
A = acute; ALL = acute lymphoblastic leukemia; AML = acute myeloid leukemia; C = chronic; CML = chronic myeloid leukemia; CSP = cyclosporine prophylaxis; GVHD = graft-versus-host disease; MTX = methotrexate prophylaxis.

immunocompromised host. Current studies suggest that MMR can be given safely after the second year after transplantation in patients free of chronic GVHD (289).

Prognosis

Transplant-related Mortality

As previously noted, mortality is increased in patients with extensive disease, progressive-type onset, thrombocytopenia, and HLA-nonidentical marrow donors. Multivariate analysis of 143 patients treated with alternating-day CSP and prednisone demonstrated that independent risk factors for mortality included progressive-type onset, advanced-stage malignancy, and thrombocytopenia (290). Multivariate analysis of 85 patients with chronic GVHD treated in Baltimore revealed an increased risk of death in patients with a progressive-type onset, elevated serum bilirubin levels, and lichenoid histology on skin biopsy (291). Six-year survival for all 85 patients was 42%, but survival in the 26 patients with a progressive onset was only 10% (291).

Malignancy-related Mortality

As reviewed in Chapter 19, chronic GVHD appears to be associated with a GVL effect, which contributes to improved survival in patients transplanted in advanced stages of leukemia (292). The effect appears less beneficial in patients transplanted in remission (293). Table 26-7 illustrates the prognostic influence of GVHD on treatment failure (relapse or death from any cause) following HLA-identical sibling transplantation (294).

Although immunodeficiency and chronic antigenic stimulation have been associated with lymphomagenesis in animal models, there was no clear evidence of an association of chronic GVHD with secondary malignancies in 2,246 patients undergoing marrow transplantation (177). However, of 5 patients in whom secondary neoplasms developed among 320 individuals transplanted for aplastic anemia, all 5 had chronic GVHD and were treated for extended periods with azathioprine and prednisone (295). Chapter 39 details more fully the factors related to development of secondary cancers.

Quality of Life

Chronic GVHD has a key influence on transplant-related morbidity, including growth and development of children (296), sexual satisfaction (256,297), and employment and functional status (298–300). These vital issues are further detailed in Chapters 38, 41, and 42.

Acknowledgment:
Special thanks to Dr Keiko Tanaka for her assistance in obtaining several of the photographs used in the color plates.

References

1. Barnes DWH, Loutit JF. Spleen protection: the cellular hypothesis. In: Bacq ZM, ed. Radiobiology symposium. London: Butterworth; 1955.
2. Billingham RE, Brent I. A simple method for inducing tolerance of skin homografts in mice. Transplant Bull 1957;4:67–71.
3. Simonsen M. Graft-versus-host reactions: the history

that never was, and the way things happened to happen. Immunol Rev 1985;88:5–23.
4. Mathé G, Amiel JL, Schwarzenberg L, Cattan A, Schneider M. Haematopoietic chimera in man after allogeneic (Homologous) bone-marrow transplantation (control of the secondary syndrome. Specific tolerance due to the chimerism). Br Med J 1963;2:1633–1635.
5. Graw RG, Herzig GP, Rogentine GN, et al. Graft-versus-host reaction complicating HL-A matched bone-marrow transplantation. Lancet 1970;2:1053–1055.
6. Kersey JH, Meuwissen HJ, Good RA. Graft-versus-host reactions following transplantation of allogeneic hematopoietic cells. Hum Pathol 1971;2:389–402.
7. Gatti RA, Kersey JH, Yunis EJ, Good RA. Graft-versus-host disease. Prog Clin Pathol 1973;5:1–18.
8. Thomas ED, Storb R, Clift RA, et al. Bone-marrow transplantation. N Engl J Med 1975;292:832–843,895–902.
9. Grebe SC, Streilein JW. Graft-versus-host reactions: a review. Adv Immunol 1976;22:119–221.
10. Hathaway WE, Githens JH, Blackburn WR, Fulginiti V, Kempe CH. Aplastic anemia, histiocytosis and erythrodermia in immunologically deficient children: probable human runt disease. N Engl J Med 1965;273:953–958.
11. Billingham RE. The biology of graft-versus-host reactions. In: The Harvey Lectures. New York: Academic Press, 1966;62:21–78.
12. Tsoi MS. Immunological mechanisms of graft-versus-host disease in man. Transplantation 1982;33:459–464.
13. Korngold R, Sprent J. T cell subsets and graft-versus-host disease. Transplantation 1987;44:335–339.
14. Ferrara JLM, Deeg HJ. Graft-versus-host disease. N Engl J Med 1991;324:667–674.
15. Piguet P-F, Grau GE, Allet B, Vassalli P. Tumor necrosis factor/cachectin is an effector of skin and gut lesions of the acute phase of graft-vs-host disease. J Exp Med 1987;166:1280–1289.
16. Symington FW, Pepe MS, Chen AB, Deliganis A. Serum tumor necrosis factor alpha associated with acute graft-versus-host disease in humans. Transplantation 1992;50: 518–520.
17. van Bekkum DW, Roodenburg J, Heidt PJ, van der Waaij D. Mitigation of secondary disease of allogeneic mouse radiation chimeras by modification of the intestinal microflora. J Natl Cancer Inst 1974;52:401–404.
18. Grundy JE, Shanley JD, Shearer GM. Augmentation of graft-versus-host reaction by cytomegalovirus infection resulting in interstitial pneumonitis. Transplantation 1985;39:548–553.
19. Atkinson K, Storb R, Weiden PL, Deeg HJ, Gerhard-Miller L, Thomas ED. In vitro tests correlating with presence or absence of graft-vs-host disease in DLA nonidentical canine radiation chimeras: evidence that clonal abortion maintains stable graft-host tolerance. J Immunol 1980;124:1808–1814.
20. Fukushi N, Arase H, Wang B, et al. Thymus: a direct target tissue in graft-versus-host reaction after allogeneic bone marrow transplantation that results in abrogation of induction of self-tolerance. Proc Natl Acad Sci USA 1990;87:6301–6305.
21. Rosenkrantz K, Keever C, Bhimani K, et al. Both ongoing suppression and clonal elimination contribute to graft-host tolerance after transplantation of HLA mismatched T cell-depleted marrow for severe combined immunodeficiency. J Immunol 1990;144:1721–1728.
22. Santos GW. Syngeneic or autologous graft-versus-host disease. Int J Cell Cloning 1989;7:92–99.
23. Hess AD, Horwitz L, Beschorner WE, Santos GW. Development of graft-vs.-host disease-like syndrome in cyclosporine-treated rats after syngeneic bone marrow transplantation. I. Development of cytotoxic T lymphocytes with apparent polyclonal anti-Ia specificity, including autoreactivity. J Exp Med 1985;161:718–730.
24. Hess AD, Fischer AC, Beschorner WE. Effector mechanisms in cyclosporine A-induced syngeneic graft-versus-host disease. J Immunol 1990;145:526–533.
25. Fischer AC, Beschorner WE, Hess AD. Requirements for the induction and adoptive transfer of cyclosporine-induced syngeneic graft-versus-host disease. J Exp Med 1989;169:1031–1041.
26. Shinozawa T, Beschorner WE, Hess AD. The thymus and prolonged administration of cyclosporine. Transplantation 1990;50:106–111.
27. Fischer AC, Hess AD. Age-related factors in cyclosporine-induced syngeneic graft-versus-host disease: regulatory role of marrow-derived T lymphocytes. J Exp Med 1990;172:85–95.
28. Rappeport JM, Mihm M, Reinherz EL, Lopansri S, Parkman R. Acute graft-vs.-host disease in recipients of bone marrow transplants from identical twin donors. Lancet 1979;2:717–720.
29. Gluckman E, Devergie A, Sohier J, Saurat JH. Graft-versus-host disease in recipients of syngeneic bone marrow. Lancet 1980;1:253–254.
30. Thein SL, Goldman JM, Galton DAG. Acute "graft-versus-host disease" after autografting for chronic granulocytic leukemia in transformation. Ann Intern Med 1981;94:210–211.
31. Hood AF, Vogelsang GB, Black LP, Farmer ER, Santos GW. Acute graft-vs-host disease. Development following autologous and syngeneic bone marrow transplantation. Arch Dermatol 1987;123:745–750.
32. Einsele H, Ehninger G, Schneider EM, et al. High frequency of graft-versus-host-like syndromes following syngeneic bone marrow transplantation. Transplantation 1988;45:579–585.
33. Rappeport JM. Syngeneic and autologous graft-vs.-host disease: immunology, pathology and treatment. In: Burakoff SJ, Deeg HJ, Ferrara J, Atkinson K, eds. Graft-versus-host disease. New York: Marcel Dekker, 1990: 455–466.
34. Jones RJ, Vogelsang GB, Hess AD, et al. Induction of graft-versus-host disease after autologous bone marrow transplantation. Lancet. 1990;1:754–757.
35. Hathaway WE, Fulginiti VA, Pierce CW, et al. Graft-vs-host reaction following a single blood transfusion. JAMA 1967;201:1015–1020.
36. Greenbaum BH. Transfusion-associated graft-versus-host disease: historical perspectives, incidence, and current use of irradiated blood products. J Clin Oncol 1991;9:1889–1902.
37. Parkman R, Mosier D, Umansky I, Cochran W, Carpenter CB, Rosen FS. Graft-versus-host disease after intrauterine and exchange transfusions for hemolytic disease of the newborn. N Engl J Med 1974;290:359–363.
38. Seemayer TA, Bolande RP. Thymic involution mimicing thymic dysplasia. A consequence of transfusion-induced graft versus host disease in a premature infant. Arch Pathol Lab Med 1980;104:141–145.
39. Weiden PL, Zuckerman N, Hansen JA, et al. Fatal graft-versus-host disease in a patient with lymphoblastic

leukemia following normal granulocyte transfusions. Blood 1981;57:328–332.
40. Von Fliedner V, Higby DJ, Kim U. Graft-versus-host reaction following blood product transfusion. Am J Med 1982;72:951–961.
41. Anderson KC, Weinstein HJ. Transfusion-associated graft-versus-host disease. N Engl J Med 1990;323:315–321.
42. Juji T, Takahashi K, Shibata Y, et al. Post-transfusion graft-versus-host disease in immunocompetent patients after cardiac surgery in Japan. N Engl J Med 1989;321:56.
43. Vogelsang GB. Transfusion-associated graft-versus-host disease in nonimmunocompromised hosts. Transfusion 1990;30:101–103.
44. Capon SM, DePond WD, Tyan DB, et al. Transfusion-associated graft-versus-host disease in an immunocompetent patient. Ann Intern Med 1991;114:1025–1026.
45. Kruskall MS, Alper CA, Awdeh Z, Yunis EJ. HLA-homozygous donors and transfusion-associated graft-versus-host disease. N Engl J Med 1990;322:1005–1006.
46. Thaler M, Shamiss A, Ongrad S, et al. The role of blood from HLA-homozygous donors in fatal transfusion-associated graft-versus-host disease after open-heart surgery. N Engl J Med 1989;321:25–28.
47. Siimes MA, Koskimies S. Chronic graft-versus-host disease after blood transfusion confirmed by incompatible HLA antigens in bone marrow. Lancet 1982;1:42–43.
48. Thomas ED, Herman EC Jr, Greenough WB III, et al. Irradiation and marrow infusion in leukemia. Arch Intern Med 1961;107:829–845.
49. Button LN, DeWolf WC, Newburger PE, Jacobsen MS, Kevy SV. The effects of irradiation on blood components. Transfusion 1981;21:419–426.
50. Anderson KC, Goodnough LT, Sayers M, et al. Variation in blood component irradiation practice: implications for prevention of transfusion-associated graft-versus-host disease. Blood 1991;77:2096–2102.
51. Drobyski W, Thibodeau S, Truitt RL, et al. Third-party-mediated graft rejection and graft-versus-host disease after T-cell-depleted bone marrow transplantation, as demonstrated by hypervariable DNA probes and HLA-DR polymorphism. Blood 1989;74:2285–2294.
52. Beatty PG, Clift RA, Mickelson EM, et al. Marrow transplantation from related donors other than HLA-identical siblings. N Engl J Med 1985;313:765–771.
53. Beatty PG, Hansen JA, Longton GM, et al. Marrow transplantation from HLA-matched unrelated donors for treatment of hematologic malignancies. Transplantation 1991;51:443–447.
54. Morishima Y, Morishita Y, Tanimoto M, et al. Low incidence of acute graft-versus-host disease by the administration of methotrexate and cyclosporine in Japanese leukemia patients after bone marrow transplantation from human leukocyte antigen compatible siblings; possible role of genetic homogeneity. Blood 1989;74:2252–2256.
55. Storb R, Prentice RL, Hansen JA, Thomas ED. Association between HLA-B antigens and acute graft-versus-host disease. Lancet 1983;2:816–819.
56. Weisdorf D, Hakke R, Blazar B, et al. Risk factors for acute graft-versus-host disease in histocompatible donor bone marrow transplantation. Transplantation 1991;51:1197–1203.
57. Bross DS, Tutschka PJ, Farmer ER, et al. Predictive factors for acute graft-versus-host disease in patients transplanted with HLA-identical bone marrow. Blood 1984;63:1265–1270.
58. Nash RA, Pepe MS, Storb R, et al. Acute graft-versus-host disease: analysis of risk factors after allogeneic marrow transplantation and prophylaxis with cyclosporine and methotrexate. Blood 1992;80:1838–1845.
59. Flowers MED, Pepe MS, Longton G, et al. Previous donor pregnancy as a risk factor for acute graft-versus-host disease in patients with aplastic anemia treated by allogeneic marrow transplantation. Br J Haematol 1990;74:492–496.
60. Gale RP, Bortin MM, van Bekkum DW, et al. Risk factors for acute graft-versus-host disease. Br J Haematol 1987;67:397–406.
61. Sullivan KM, Storb R, Buckner CD, et al. Graft-versus-host disease as adoptive immunotherapy in patients with advanced hematologic neoplasms. N Engl J Med 1989;320:828–834.
62. Sanders JE, Flournoy N, Thomas ED, et al. Marrow transplant experience in children with acute lymphoblastic leukemia: an analysis of factors associated with survival, relapse and graft-versus-host disease. Med Pediatr Oncol 1985;13:165–172.
63. Klingemann H-G, Storb R, Fefer A, et al. Bone marrow transplantation in patients aged 45 years and older. Blood 1986;67:770–776.
64. Clift RA, Buckner CD, Appelbaum FR, et al. Allogeneic marrow transplantation in patients with acute myeloid leukemia in first remission. A randomized trial of two irradiation regimens. Blood 1990;76:1867–1871.
65. Hill RS, Petersen FB, Storb R, et al. Mixed hematologic chimerism after allogeneic marrow transplantation for severe aplastic anemia is associated with a higher risk of graft rejection and a lessened incidence of acute graft-versus-host disease. Blood 1986;67:811–816.
66. Petz LD, Yam P, Wallace RB, et al. Mixed hematopoietic chimerism following bone marrow transplantation for hematologic malignancies. Blood 1987;70:1331.
67. Gratama JW, Zwaan FE, Stijnen T, et al. Herpes-virus immunity and acute graft-versus-host disease. Lancet 1987;1:471–473.
68. Miller W, Flynn P, McCullough J, et al. Cytomegalovirus infection after bone marrow transplantation: an association with acute graft-v-host disease. Blood 1986;67:1162–1167.
69. Vogelsang GB, Hess AD, Berkman AW, et al. An in vitro predictive test for graft versus host disease in patients with genotypic HLA-identical bone marrow transplants. N Engl J Med 1985;313:645–650.
70. Sviland L, Dickinson AM, Carey PJ, Pearson ADJ, Proctor SJ. An in vitro predictive test for clinical graft-versus-host disease in allogeneic bone marrow transplant recipients. Bone Marrow Transplant 1990;5:105–109.
71. Bagot M, Mary J-V, Heslan M, et al. The mixed epidermal cell lymphyocyte-reaction is the most predictive factor of acute graft-versus-host disease in bone marrow graft recipients. Br J Haematol 1988;70:403–409.
72. Saurat JH. Cutaneous manifestations of graft-versus-host disease. Int J Dermatol 1981;4:249–256.
73. Glucksberg H, Storb R, Fefer A, et al. Clinical manifestations of graft-versus-host disease in human recipients of marrow from HL-A-matched sibling donors. Transplantation 1974;18:295–304.
74. Sale GE, Shulman HM, Gallucci BB, Thomas ED.

Young rete ridge keratinocytes are preferred targets in cutaneous graft-versus-host disease. Am J Pathol 1985;118:278–287.

75. Sullivan KM, Deeg HJ, Sanders J, et al. Hyperacute GVHD in patients not given immunosuppression after allogeneic marrow transplantation. Blood 1986;67: 1172–1175.
76. Peck GL, Elias PM, Graw RG. Graft-versus-host reaction and toxic epidermal necrolysis. Lancet 1972; 2:1151.
77. Goldberg NS, Ahmed T, Robinson B, Ascensao J, Horowitz H. Staphylococcal scalded skin syndrome mimicking acute graft-vs-host disease in a bone marrow transplant recipient. Arch Dermatol 1989;125:85–87.
78. McDonald GB, Shulman HM, Sullivan KM, Spencer GD. Intestinal and hepatic complications of human bone marrow transplantation. Gastroenterology 1986; 90:460–477, 770–784.
79. Weisdorf SA, Salati M, Longsdorf JA, Ramsay NKC, Sharp HL. Graft-versus-host disease of the intestine: a protein losing enteropathy characterized by fecal α-antitrypsin. Gastroenterology 1983;85:1076–1081.
80. McDonald GB, Shulman HM, Wolford JL, Spencer GD. Liver disease after human marrow transplantation. Semin Liver Dis 1987;7:210–220.
81. Atkinson K, Biggs J, Dodds A, Concannon A. Cyclosporine-associated hepatotoxicity after allogeneic marrow transplantation in man: differentiation from other causes of posttransplant liver disease. Transplant Proc 1983;15:2761–2767.
82. Fisk JD, Shulman HM, Greening RR, McDonald GB, Sale GE, Thomas ED. Gastrointestinal radiographic features of human graft-vs.-host disease. Am J Roentgenol 1981;136:329–336.
83. Schimmelpenninck M, Zwaan F. Radiographic features of small intestinal injury in human graft-versus-host disease. Gastrointest Radiol 1982;7:29–33.
84. Serota FT, Rosenberg HK, Rosen J, Koch PA. Delayed onset of gastrointestinal disease in the recipients of bone marrow transplants: a variant graft-versus-host reaction. Transplantation 1982;34:60–64.
85. Weisdorf DJ, Snover DC, Haake R, et al. Acute upper gastrointestinal graft-versus-host disease: clinical significance and response to immunosuppressive therapy. Blood 1990;76:624–629.
86. Epstein RJ, McDonald GB, Sale GE, Shulman HM, Thomas ED. The diagnostic accuracy of the rectal biopsy in acute graft-versus-host disease: a prospective study of thirteen patients. Gastroenterology 1980; 78:764–771.
87. Spencer GD, Hackman RC, McDonald GB, et al. A prospective study of unexplained nausea and vomiting after marrow transplantation. Transplantation 1986;42: 602–607.
88. First LR, Smith BR, Lipton J, Nathan DG, Parkman R, Rappeport JM. Isolated thrombocytopenia after allogeneic bone marrow transplantation: existence of transient and chronic thrombocytopenic syndromes. Blood 1985;65:368–374.
89. Anasetti C, Rybka W, Sullivan KM, Banaji M, Slichter SJ. Graft-v-host disease is associated with autoimmune-like thrombocytopenia. Blood 1989;73:1054–1058.
90. Powles R, Pedrazzini A, Crofts M, et al. Mismatched family bone marrow transplantation. Semin Hematol 1984;21:182–187.
91. Holler E, Kolb HJ, Hiller E, et al. Microangiopathy in patients on cyclosporine prophylaxis who developed acute graft-versus-host disease after HLA-identical bone marrow transplantation. Blood 1989;73:2018–2024.
92. Jack MK, Jack GM, Sale GE, Shulman HM, Sullivan KM. Ocular manifestations of graft-*v*-host disease. Arch Ophthalmol 1983;101:1080–1084.
93. Franklin RM, Kenyon KR, Tutschka PJ, Saral R, Green WR, Santos GW. Ocular manifestations of graft-vs-host disease. Ophthalmology 1983;90:4–13.
94. Jabs DA, Wingard J, Green RW, Farmer ER, Vogelsang G, Saral R. The eye in bone marrow transplantation. Arch Ophthalmol 1989;107:1343–1348.
95. van Bekkum DW, DeVries MJ. Radiation chimeras. New York: Academic Press, 1967:146–155.
96. Sale GE, Lerner KG, Barker EA, Shulman HM, Thomas ED. The skin biopsy in the diagnosis of acute graft-versus-host disease in man. Am J Pathol 1977;89: 621–635.
97. Snover DC, Weisdorf SA, Ramsay NK, McGlave P, Kersey JH. Hepatic graft versus host disease: a study of the predictive value of liver biopsy in diagnosis. Hepatology 1984;4:123–130.
98. Vogelsang GB, Hess AD, Santos GW. Acute graft-versus-host disease: clinical characteristics in the cyclosporine era. Medicine 1988;67:163–174.
99. Storb R, Prentice RL, Buckner CD, et al. Graft-versus-host disease and survival in patients with aplastic anemia treated by marrow grafts from HLA-identical siblings. Beneficial effect of a protective environment. N Engl J Med 1983;308:302–307.
100. Roy J, Snover D, Weisdorf S, Mulvahill A, Filipovich A, Weisdorf D. Simultaneous upper and lower endoscopic biopsy in the diagnosis of intestinal graft-versus-host disease. Transplantation 1991;51:642–646.
101. Shulman HM, Sharma P, Amos D, Fenster LF, McDonald GB. A coded histologic study of hepatic graft-versus-host disease after human bone marrow transplantation. Hepatology 1988;8:463–470.
102. Atkinson K, Horowitz MM, Biggs JC, Gale RP, Rimm AA, Bortin MM. The clinical diagnosis of acute graft-versus-host disease: a diversity of views amongst marrow transplant centers. Bone Marrow Transplant 1988;3:5–10.
103. Clift R, Goldman J, Gratwohl A, Horowitz M. Proposals for standardized reporting of results of bone marrow transplantation for leukaemia. Bone Marrow Transplant 1989;4:445–448.
104. Anasetti C, Beatty PG, Storb R, et al. Effect of HLA incompatibility on graft-versus-host disease, relapse, and survival after marrow transplantation for patients with leukemia or lymphoma. Hum Immunol 1990; 29:79–91.
105. Petersen FB, Buckner CD, Clift RA, et al. Laminar air flow isolation and decontamination: a prospective randomized study of the effects of prophylactic systemic antibiotics in bone marrow transplant patients. Infection 1986;14:115–121.
106. Vossen JM, Heidt PJ. Gnotobiotic measures for the prevention of acute graft-vs-host disease. In: Burakoff SJ, Deeg HJ, Ferrara J, Atkinson K, eds. Graft-vs-host disease: immunology, pathology and treatment. New York: Marcel Dekker, 1990:403–414.
107. Uphoff DE. Alteration of homograft reaction by A-methopterin in lethally irradiated mice treated with homologous marrow. Proc Soc Exp Biol Med 1958; 99:651–653.

108. Santos GW, Owens AH. Production of graft-versus-host disease in the rat and its treatment with cytotoxic agents. Nature 1966;210:139–140.
109. Storb R, Epstein RB, Graham TC, Thomas ED. Methotrexate regimens for control of graft-versus-host disease in dogs with allogeneic marrow grafts. Transplantation 1970;9:240–246.
110. Lazarus HM, Coccia PF, Herzig RH, et al. Incidence of acute graft-versus-host disease with and without methotrexate prophylaxis in allogeneic bone marrow transplant patients. Blood 1984;64:215–220.
111. Powles RL, Clink HM, Spence D, et al. Cyclosporin A to prevent graft-versus-host disease in man after allogeneic bone-marrow transplantation. Lancet 1980;1: 327–329.
112. Tutschka PJ, Beschorner WE, Hess AD, Santos GW. Cyclosporin-A to prevent graft-versus-host disease: a pilot study in 22 patients receiving allogeneic marrow transplants. Blood 1983;61:318–325.
113. Deeg HJ, Storb R, Thomas ED, et al. Cyclosporine as prophylaxis for graft-versus-host disease: a randomized study in patients undergoing marrow transplantation for acute nonlymphoblastic leukemia. Blood 1985;65:1325–1334.
114. Storb R, Deeg HJ, Fisher LD, et al. Cyclosporine v methotrexate for graft-v-host disease prevention in patients given marrow grafts for leukemia: long-term follow-up of three controlled trials. Blood 1988; 71:293–298.
115. Ramsay NKC, Kersey JH, Robison LL, et al. A randomized study of the prevention of acute graft-versus-host disease. N Engl J Med 1982;306:392–397.
116. Blume KG, Beutler E, Bross KJ, et al. Bone-marrow ablation and allogeneic marrow transplantation in acute leukemia. N Engl J Med 1980;302:1041–1046.
117. Forman SJ, Blume KG, Krance RA, et al. A prospective randomized study of acute graft-v-host disease in 107 patients with leukemia: methotrexate/prednisone v cyclosporine A/prednisone. Transplant Proc 1987; 19:2605–2607.
118. Santos GW, Tutschka PJ, Brookmeyer R, et al. Cyclosporine plus methylprednisolone versus cyclophosphamide plus methylprednisolone as prophylaxis for graft-versus-host disease: a randomized double-blind study in patients undergoing allogeneic marrow transplantation. Clin Transplant 1987;1:21–28.
119. Deeg HJ, Storb R, Appelbaum FR, Kennedy MS, Graham TC, Thomas ED. Combined immunosuppression with cyclosporine and methotrexate in dogs given bone marrow grafts from DLA-haploidentical littermates. Transplantation 1984;37:62–65.
120. Storb R, Deeg HJ, Farewell V, et al. Marrow transplantation for severe aplastic anemia: methotrexate alone compared with a combination of methotrexate and cyclosporine for prevention of acute graft-versus-host disease. Blood 1986;68:119–125.
121. Storb R, Deeg HJ, Whitehead J, et al. Methotrexate and cyclosporine compared with cyclosporine alone for prophylaxis of acute graft versus host disease after marrow transplantation for leukemia. N Engl J Med 1986;314:729–735.
122. Storb R, Deeg HJ, Pepe M, et al. Methotrexate and cyclosporine versus cyclosporine alone for prophylaxis of graft-versus-host disease in patients given HLA-identical marrow grafts for leukemia: long-term follow-up of a controlled trial. Blood 1989;73:1729–1734.
123. Storb R, Deeg HJ, Pepe M, et al. Graft-versus-host disease prevention by methotrexate combined with cyclosporin compared to methotrexate alone in patients given marrow grafts for severe aplastic anaemia: long-term follow-up of a controlled trial. Br J Haematol 1989;72:567–572.
124. Storb R, Sanders JE, Pepe M, et al. Graft-versus-host disease prophylaxis with methotrexate/cyclosporine in children with severe aplastic anemia treated with cyclophosphamide and HLA-identical marrow grafts. Blood 1991;78:1144–1149.
125. Gluckman E, Horowitz MM, Champlin RE, et al. Bone marrow transplantation for severe aplastic anemia: influence of conditioning and graft-versus-host disease prophylaxis regimens on outcome. Blood 1992;79: 269–275.
126. Storb R, Pepe M, Anasetti C, et al. What role for prednisone in prevention of acute graft-versus-host disease in patients undergoing marrow transplants? Blood 1990;76:1037–1045.
127. Ringdén O, Kersey JH. Prevention and therapy of graft-versus-host disease. Report from a work-shop. Bone Marrow Transplant 1992;10(suppl 1):22–24.
128. Stockschlaeder M, Storb R, Pepe M, et al. A pilot study of low-dose cyclosporine for graft-versus-host prophylaxis in marrow transplantation. Br J Haematol 1992;80:49–54.
129. Bacigalupo A, Van Lint MT, Occhini D, et al. Increased risk of leukemia relapse with high-dose cyclosporine A after allogeneic marrow transplantation for acute leukemia. Blood 1991;77:1423–1428.
130. Deeg HJ, Spitzer TR, Cottler-Fox M, Cahill R, Pickle LW. Conditioning-related toxicity and acute graft-versus-host disease in patients given methotrexate/cyclosporine prophylaxis. Bone Marrow Transplant 1991;7:193–198.
131. Imbach P, Barandun S, d'Apuzzo V, et al. High-dose intravenous gammaglobulin for idiopathic thrombocytopenic purpura in childhood. Lancet 1981;1:1228–1231.
132. Newburger JW, Takahashi M, Burns JC, et al. The treatment of Kawasaki syndrome with intravenous gamma globulin. N Engl J Med 1986;315:341–347.
133. Dwyer JM. Manipulating the immune system with immune globulin. N Engl J Med 1992;326:107–116.
134. Sullivan KM. Immunoglobin therapy in bone marrow transplantation. Am J Med 1987;83(suppl 4A):34–45.
135. Winston DJ, Ho WG, Lin C-H, et al. Intravenous immune globulin for prevention of cytomegalovirus infection and interstitial pneumonia after bone marrow transplantation. Ann Intern Med 1987;106:12–18.
136. Sullivan KM, Kopecky KJ, Jocom J, et al. Immunomodulatory and antimicrobial efficacy of intravenous immunoglobulin in bone marrow transplantation. N Engl J Med 1990;323:705–712.
137. Sullivan KM, Kopecky KJ, Buckner CD, Storb R. Intravenous IgG to prevent graft-versus-host disease after bone marrow transplantation (letter). N Engl J Med 1991;324:631–633.
138. Weiden PL, Doney K, Storb R, Thomas ED. Antihuman thymocyte globulin for prophylaxis of graft-versus-host disease. A randomized trial in patients with leukemia treated with HLA-identical sibling marrow grafts. Transplantation 1979;27:227–230.
139. Doney KC, Weiden PL, Storb R, Thomas ED. Failure of early administration of antithymocyte globulin to lessen graft-versus-host disease in human allogeneic

marrow transplant recipients. Transplantation 1981; 31:141–143.
140. Anasetti C, Martin PJ, Storb R, et al. Prophylaxis of graft-versus-host disease by administration of the murine anti-IL-2 receptor antibody-2A3. Bone Marrow Transplant 1991;7:375–381.
141. Blaise D, Olive D, Hirn M, et al. Prevention of acute GVHD by in vivo use of anti-interleukin-2 receptor monoclonal antibody (33B3.1): a feasibility trial in 15 patients. Bone Marrow Transplant 1991;8:105–111.
142. McCarthy PL Jr, Abhyankar S, Neben S, et al. Inhibition of interleukin-1 by an interleukin-1 receptor antagonist prevents graft-versus-host disease. Blood 1991;78:1915–1918.
143. Reisner Y, Kapoor N, Kirkpatrick D, et al. Transplantation for acute leukaemia with HLA-A and B non-identical parental marrow cells fractionated with soybean agglutinin and sheep red blood cells. Lancet 1981;2:327–331.
144. Prentice HG, Blacklock HA, Janossy G, et al. Use of anti-T-cell monoclonal antibody OKT3 to prevent acute graft-versus-host disease in allogeneic bone-marrow transplantation for acute leukaemia. Lancet 1982;1:700–703.
145. Hale G, Cobbold S, Waldmann H. T cell depletion with Campath-1 in allogeneic bone marrow transplantation. Transplantation 1988;45:753–759.
146. Ash RC, Casper JT, Chitambar CR, et al. Successful allogeneic transplantation of T-cell-depleted bone marrow from closely HLA-matched unrelated donors. N Engl J Med 1990;322:485–494.
147. Wagner JE, Santos GW, Noga SJ, et al. Bone marrow graft engineering by counterflow centrifugal elutriation: results of a phase I-II clinical trial. Blood 1990;75:1370–1377.
148. Champlin R, Ho W, Gajewski J, et al. Selective depletion of CD8+ T lymphocytes for prevention of graft-versus-host disease after allogeneic bone marrow transplantation. Blood 1990;76:418–423.
149. Antin JH, Bierer BE, Smith BR, et al. Selective depletion of bone marrow T lymphocytes with anti-CD5 monoclonal antibodies: effective prophylaxis for graft-versus-host disease in patients with hematologic malignancies. Blood 1991;78:2139–2149.
150. Martin PJ, Hansen JA, Buckner CD, et al. Effects of in vitro depletion of T cells in HLA-identical allogeneic marrow grafts. Blood 1985;66:664–672.
151. Mitsuyasu RT, Champlin RE, Gale RP, et al. Treatment of donor bone marrow with monoclonal anti-T-cell antibody and complement for the prevention of graft-versus-host disease. Ann Intern Med 1986;105:20–26.
152. Goldman JM, Gale RP, Horowitz MM, et al. Bone marrow transplantation for chronic myelogenous leukemia in chronic phase: increased risk of relapse associated with T-cell depletion. Ann Intern Med 1988;108:806–814.
153. Marmont AM, Horowitz MM, Gale RP, et al. T-cell depletion of HLA-identical transplants in leukemia. Blood 1991;78:2120–2130.
154. Appelbaum FR, Raff RF, Storb R, et al. Use of trimetrexate for the prevention of graft-versus-host disease. Bone Marrow Transplant 1989;4:421–424.
155. Hess RA, Tschudy DP, Blaese RM. Immunosuppression by succinylacetone. II. Prevention of graft-vs-host disease. J Immunol 1987;139:2845–2849.
156. Metcalfe SM, Richards FM. Cyclosporine, FK506, and rapamycin. Transplantation 1990;49:798–802.
157. Dumont FJ, Staruch MJ, Koprak SL, Melino MR, Sigal NH. Distinct mechanisms of suppression of murine T cell activation by the related macrolides FK-506 and rapamycin. J Immunol 1990;144:251–258.
158. Morris RE, Meiser BM, Wu J, Shorthouse R, Wang J. Use of rapamycin for the suppression of alloimmune reactions in vivo: schedule-dependence, tolerance induction, synergy with cyclosporine and FK 506 and effect on host-versus-graft and graft-versus-host reactions. Transplant Proc 1991;23:521–524.
159. Vogelsang GB, Hess AD, Gordon G, Santos GW. Treatment and prevention of acute graft-versus-host disease with thalidomide in a rat model. Transplantation 1986;41:644–647.
160. Deeg HJ, Bazar L, Sigaroudinia M, Cottler-Fox M. Ultraviolet B light inactivates bone marrow T lymphocytes but spares hematopoietic precursor cells. Blood 1989;73:369–371.
161. Storb R, Graham TC, Shiurba R, Thomas ED. Treatment of canine graft-versus-host disease with methotrexate and cyclophosphamide following bone marrow transplantation from histoincompatible donors. Transplantation 1970;10:165–172.
162. Glucksberg H, Fefer A. Combination chemotherapy for clinically established graft-versus-host disease in mice. Cancer Res 1973;33:859–861.
163. Kendra J, Barrett AJ, Lucas C, et al. Response of graft versus host disease to high doses of methylprednisolone. Clin Lab Haematol 1981;3:19–26.
164. Bacigalupo A, Van Lint MT, Frassoni F, et al. High dose bolus methylprednisolone for the treatment of acute graft versus host disease. Blut 1983;46:125–132.
165. Kanojia MD, Anagnostou AA, Zander AR, et al. High-dose methylprednisolone treatment for acute graft-versus-host disease after bone marrow transplantation in adults. Transplantation 1984;37:246–249.
166. Deeg HJ, Henslee-Downey PJ. Management of acute graft-versus-host disease. Bone Marrow Transplant 1990;6:1–8.
167. Storb R, Gluckman E, Thomas ED, et al. Treatment of established human graft-versus-host disease by antithymocyte globulin. Blood 1974;44:57–75.
168. Doney KC, Weiden PL, Storb R, Thomas ED. Treatment of graft-versus-host disease in human allogeneic marrow graft recipients: a randomized trial comparing antithymocyte globulin and corticosteroids. Am J Hematol 1981;11:1–8.
169. Powles RL, Clink H, Sloane J, Barrett AJ, Kay HEM, McElwain TJ. Cyclosporin A for the treatment of graft-versus-host disease in man. Lancet 1978;2:1327–1331.
170. Kennedy MS, Deeg HJ, Storb R, et al. Treatment of acute graft-versus-host disease after allogeneic marrow transplantation: randomized study comparing corticosteroids and cyclosporine. Am J Med 1985; 78:978–983.
171. Deeg HJ, Loughran TP Jr, Storb R, et al. Treatment of human acute graft-versus-host disease with antithymocyte globulin and cyclosporine with or without methylprednisolone.Transplantation1985;40:162–166.
172. Martin PJ, Schoch G, Fisher L, et al. A retrospective analysis of therapy for acute graft-versus-host disease: initial treatment. Blood 1990;76:1464–1472.
173. Gratama JW, Jansen J, Lipovich RA, Tanke HJ, Goldstein G, Zwaan FE. Treatment of acute graft-versus-host disease with monoclonal antibody OKT3. Clinical results and effect on circulating T lymphocytes. Transplantation 1984;38:469–474.

174. Gleixner B, Kolb HJ, Holler E, et al. Treatment of GVHD with OKT3: clinical outcome and side-effects associated with release of TNFα. Bone Marrow Transplant 1991;8:93–98.
175. Martin PJ, Hansen JA, Anasetti C, et al. Treatment of acute graft-versus-host disease with anti-CD3 monoclonal antibodies. Am J Kidney Dis 1988;11:149–152.
176. Martin PJ, Shulman HM, Schubach WH, et al. Fatal Epstein-Barr-virus-associated proliferation of donor B cells after treatment of acute graft-versus-host disease with a murine monoclonal anti-T-cell antibody. Ann Intern Med 1984;101:310–315.
177. Witherspoon RP, Fisher LD, Schoch G, et al. Secondary cancers after bone marrow transplantation for leukemia or aplastic anemia. N Engl J Med 1989;321:784–789.
178. Zutter MM, Martin PJ, Sale GE, et al. Epstein-Barr virus lymphoproliferation after bone marrow transplantation. Blood 1988;72:520–529.
179. Anasetti C, Martin PJ, Storb R, et al. Treatment of acute graft-versus-host disease with a nonmitogenic anti-CD3 monoclonal antibody. Transplantation 1992; 54:844–851.
180. Byers VS, Henslee PJ, Kernan NA, et al. Use of an anti-pan T-lymphocyte ricin A chain immunotoxin in steroid-resistant acute graft-versus-host disease. Blood 1990;75:1426–1432.
181. Ferrara JLM, Marion A, McIntyre JF, Murphy GF, Burakoff SJ. Amelioration of acute graft vs host disease due to minor histocompatibility antigens by in vivo administration of anti-interleukin 2 receptor antibody. J Immunol 1986;137:1874–1877.
182. Hervé P, Wijdenes J, Bergerat JP, et al. Treatment of corticosteroid resistant acute graft-versus-host disease by in vivo administration of anti-interleukin-2 receptor monoclonal antibody (B-B10). Blood 1990;75: 1017–1023.
183. Anasetti C, Martin PJ, Hansen JA, et al. A phase I-II study evaluating the murine anti-IL-2 receptor antibody 2A3 for treatment of acute graft-versus-host disease. Transplantation 1990;50:49–54.
184. Brown PS Jr, Parenteau GL, Dirbas FM, et al. Anti-Tac-H, a humanized antibody to the interleukin 2 receptor, prolongs primate cardiac allograft survival. Proc Natl Acad Sci USA 1991;88:2663–2667.
185. Hervé P, Flesch M, Tiberghien J, et al. Phase I-II trial of a monoclonal anti-tumor necrosis factor α antibody for the treatment of refractory severe acute graft-versus-host disease. Blood 1992;79:3362–3368.
186. Deeg HJ. Ultraviolet irradiation in transplantation biology. Manipulation of immunity and immunogenicity. Transplantation 1988;45:845–851.
187. Eppinger T, Ehninger G, Steinert M, Niethammer D, Dopfer R. 8-Methoxypsoralen and ultraviolet A therapy for cutaneous manifestations of graft-versus-host disease. Transplantation 1990;50:807–811.
188. Deeg HJ, Erickson K, Storb R, Sullivan KM. Photoinactivation of lymphohemopoietic cells: studies in transfusion medicine and bone marrow transplantation. Blood Cells 1992;18:151–162.
189. Martin PJ, Schoch G, Fisher L, et al. A retrospective analysis of therapy for acute graft-versus-host disease: secondary treatment. Blood 1991;77:1821–1828.
190. Gauvreau JM, Lenssen P, Cheney CL, Aker SN, Hutchinson ML, Barale KV. Nutritional management of patients with acute gastrointestinal graft-versus-host disease. J Am Diet Assoc 1981;79:673–677.
191. Bianco JA, Higano C, Singer J, Appelbaum FR, McDonald GB. The somatostatin analog octreotide in the management of the secretory diarrhea of the acute intestinal graft-versus-host disease in a patient after bone marrow transplantation. Transplantation 1990; 49:1194–1195.
192. Ely P, Dunitz J, Rogosheske J. Use of a somatostatin analogue, octreotide acetate, in the management of acute gastrointestinal graft-versus-host disease. Am J Med 1991;90:707–711.
193. Goodrich JM, Mori M, Gleaves CA, et al. Early treatment with ganciclovir to prevent cytomegalovirus disease after allogeneic bone marrow transplantation. N Engl J Med 1991;325:1601–1607.
194. Goodman JL, Winston DJ, Greenfield RA, et al. A controlled trial of fluconazole to prevent fungal infections in patients undergoing bone marrow transplantation. N Engl J Med 1992;326:845–851.
195. Weisdorf D, Haake R, Blazar B, et al. Treatment of moderate/severe acute graft-versus-host disease after allogeneic bone marrow transplantation: an analysis of clinical risk features and outcome. Blood 1990;75: 1024–1030.
196. Beschorner WE, Tutschka PJ, Santos GW. Chronic graft-versus-host disease in the rat radiation chimera: I. Clinical features, hematology, histology, and immunopathology in long-term chimeras. Transplantation 1982;33:393–399.
197. Tutschka PJ, Teasdall R, Beschorner WE, Santos GW. Chronic graft-versus-host disease in the rat radiation chimera. II. Immunological evaluation in long-term chimeras. Transplantation 1982;34:289–294.
198. Atkinson K, Incefy GS, Storb R, et al. Low serum thymic hormone levels in patients with chronic graft-versus-host disease. Blood 1982;59:1073–1077.
199. Parkman R. Clonal analysis of murine graft-vs-host disease. J Immunol 1986;136:3543–3548.
200. Fialkow PJ, Gilchrist C, Allison AC. Autoimmunity in chronic graft-versus-host disease. Clin Exp Immunol 1973;13:479–486.
201. Beschorner WE, Tutschka PJ, Santos GW. Chronic graft-versus-host disease in the rat radiation chimera. III. Immunology and immunopathology in rapidly induced models. Transplantation 1983;35: 224–230.
202. Graze PR, Gale RP. Chronic graft versus host disease: a syndrome of disordered immunity. Am J Med 1979; 66:611–620.
203. Lister J, Messner H, Keystone E, Miller R, Fritzler MJ. Autoantibody analysis of patients with graft versus host disease. J Clin Lab Immunol 1987;24:19–23.
204. Rouquette-Gally AM, Boyeldieu D, Prost AC, Gluckman E. Autoimmunity after allogeneic bone marrow transplantation. Transplantation 1988;46:238–240.
205. Tazzari PL, Gobbi M, Zauli D, et al. Close association between antibodies to cytoskeletal intermediate filaments, and chronic graft-versus-host disease. Transplantation 1987;44:234–236.
206. Dighiero G, Intrator L, Cordonnier C, Tortevoye P, Vernant J-P. High levels of anti-cytoskeleton autoantibodies are frequently associated with chronic GVHD. Br J Haematol 1987;67:301–305.
207. Kier P, Penner E, Bakos S, et al. Autoantibodies in chronic GVHD: high prevalence of antinucleolar antibodies. Bone Marrow Transplant 1990;6:93–96.
208. Wesierska-Gadek J, Penner E, Hitchman E, Kier P, Sauermann G. Nucleolar proteins B23 and C23 as

target antigens in chronic graft-versus-host disease. Blood 1992;79:1081–1086.
209. Sullivan KM, Agura E, Anasetti C, et al. Chronic graft-versus-host disease and other late complications of bone marrow transplantation. Semin Hematol 1991; 28:250–259.
210. Storb R, Prentice RL, Sullivan KM, et al. Predictive factors in chronic graft-versus-host disease in patients with aplastic anemia treated by marrow transplantation from HLA-identical siblings. Ann Intern Med 1983;98:461–466.
211. Niederwieser D, Pepe M, Storb R, Witherspoon R, Longton G, Sullivan K. Factors predicting chronic graft-versus-host disease and survival after marrow transplantation for aplastic anemia. Bone Marrow Transplant 1989;4:151–156.
212. Atkinson K, Horowitz MM, Gale RP, et al. Risk factors for chronic graft-versus-host disease after HLA-identical sibling bone marrow transplantation. Blood 1990;75:2459–2464.
213. Sullivan KM, Storb R, Witherspoon RP, et al. Deletion of immunosuppressive prophylaxis after marrow transplantation increases hyperacute graft-versus-host disease but does not influence chronic graft-versus-host disease or relapse in patients with advanced leukemia. Clin Transplant 1989;3:5–11.
214. Ruutu T, Volin L, Elonen E. Low incidence of severe acute and chronic graft-versus-host disease as a result of prolonged cyclosporine prophylaxis and early aggressive treatment with corticosteroids. Transplant Proc 1988;20:491–493.
215. Lönnqvist B, Aschan J, Ljungman P, Ringdén O. Long-term cyclosporin therapy may decrease the risk of chronic graft-versus-host disease. Br J Haematol 1990;74:547–548.
216. Bacigalupo A, Maiolino A, Van Lint MT, et al. Cyclosporin A and chronic graft versus host disease. Bone Marrow Transplant 1990;6:341–344.
217. de Gast GC, Beatty PG, Amos D, et al. Transfusions shortly before HLA-matched marrow transplantation for leukemia are associated with a decrease in chronic graft-versus-host disease. Bone Marrow Transplant 1991;7:293–295.
218. Bolger GB, Sullivan KM, Storb R, et al. Second marrow infusion for poor graft function after allogeneic marrow transplantation. Bone Marrow Transplant 1986;1:21–30.
219. Boström L, Ringdén O, Jacobsen N, Zwaan F, Nilsson B. A European multicenter study of chronic graft-versus-host disease. The role of cytomegalovirus serology in recipients and donors, acute graft-versus-host disease, and splenectomy. Transplantation 1990;49: 1100–1105.
220. Boström L, Ringdén O, Sundberg B, Ljungman P, Linde A, Nilsson B. Pretransplant herpes virus serology and chronic graft-versus-host disease. Bone Marrow Transplant 1989;4:547–552.
221. Ljungman P, Niederwieser D, Pepe MS, Longton G, Storb R, Meyers JD. Cytomegalovirus infection after marrow transplantation for aplastic anemia. Bone Marrow Transplant 1990;6:295–300.
222. Shulman HM, Sale GE, Lerner KG, et al. Chronic cutaneous graft-versus-host disease in man. Am J Pathol 1978;91:545–570.
223. Saurat JH, Gluckman E, Bussel A, Didierjean L, Puissant A. The lichen planus-like eruption after bone marrow transplantation. Br J Dermatol 1975;93:675–681.
224. Van Vloten WA, Scheffer E, Dooren LJ. Localized scleroderma-like lesions after bone marrow transplantation in man. Br J Dermatol 1977;96:337–341.
225. Lawley TJ, Peck GL, Moutsopoulos HM, Gratwohl AA, Deisseroth AB. Scleroderma, Sjögren-like syndrome, and chronic graft-versus-host disease. Ann Intern Med 1977;87:707–709.
226. Sullivan KM, Shulman HM, Storb R, et al. Chronic graft-versus-host disease in 52 patients: adverse natural course and successful treatment with combination immunosuppression. Blood 1981;57:267–276.
227. Fenyk JR Jr, Warkentin PI, Goltz RW, et al. Sclerodermatous graft-versus-host disease limited to an area of measles exanthem. Lancet 1978;1:472–473.
228. Socie L, Gluckman E, Cosset JM, et al. Unusual localization of cutaneous chronic graft-versus-host disease in the irradiation fields in four cases. Bone Marrow Transplant 1989;4:133–135.
229. Hymes SR, Farmer ER, Burns WH, et al. Bullous sclerodermalike changes in chronic graft-vs-host disease. Arch Dermatol 1985;121:1189–1192.
230. Ueda M, Mori T, Shiobara S, et al. Development of bullous pemphigoid after allogeneic bone marrow transplantation. Report of a case. Transplantation 1986;42:320–322.
231. Ling NS, Fenske NA, Julius RL, Espinoza CG, Drake LA. Dyskeratosis congenita in a girl simulating chronic graft-vs-host disease. Arch Dermatol 1985; 121:1424–1428.
232. Yau JC, Zander AR, Srigley JR, et al. Chronic graft-versus-host disease complicated by micronodular cirrhosis and esophageal varices. Transplantation 1986; 41:129–130.
233. Knapp AB, Crawford JM, Rappeport JM, Gollan JL. Cirrhosis as a consequence of graft-versus-host disease. Gastroenterology 1987;92:513–519.
234. Epstein O, Thomas HC, Sherlock S. Primary biliary cirrhosis is a dry gland syndrome with features of chronic graft-versus-host disease. Lancet 1980;1:1166–1168.
235. Deeg HJ, Flournoy N, Sullivan KM, et al. Cataracts after total body irradiation and marrow transplantation: a sparing effect of dose fractionation. Int J Radiat Oncol Biol Phys 1984;10:957–964.
236. Urban RC, Cotlier E. Corticosteroid-induced cataracts. Surv Ophthalmol 1986;31:102–110.
237. Gratwhol AA, Moutsopoulous HM, Chused TM, et al. Sjögren-type syndrome after allogeneic bone-marrow transplantation. Ann Intern Med 1977;87:703–706.
238. Schubert MM, Sullivan KM. Recognition, incidence, and management of oral graft-versus-host disease. NCI Monogr 1990;9:135–143.
239. Schubert MM, Sullivan KM, Morton TH, et al. Oral manifestations of chronic graft-v-host disease. Arch Intern Med 1984;144:1591–1595.
240. Clark JG, Schwartz DA, Flournoy N, Sullivan KM, Crawford SW, Thomas ED. Risk factors for airflow obstruction in recipients of bone marrow transplants. Ann Intern Med 1987;107:648–656.
241. Sullivan KM, Shulman HM. Chronic graft-versus-host disease, obliterative bronchiolitis, and graft-versus-leukemia effect: case histories. Transplant Proc 1989; 21:51–62.
242. Holland HK, Wingard JR, Beschorner WE, Saral R, Santos GW. Bronchiolitis obliterans in bone marrow transplantation and its relationship to chronic graft-v-host disease and low serum IgG. Blood 1988;72:621–627.

243. Sullivan KM. Intravenous immune gloublin prophylaxis in recipients of a marrow transplant. J Allergy Clin Immunol 1989;84:632–639.
244. Clark JG, Crawford SW, Madtes DK, Sullivan KM. The clinical presentation and course of obstructive lung disease after allogeneic marrow transplantation. Ann Intern Med 1989;111:368–376.
245. McDonald GB, Sullivan KM, Schuffler MD, Shulman HM, Thomas ED. Esophageal abnormalities in chronic graft-versus-host disease in humans. Gastroenterology 1981;80:914–921.
246. McDonald GB, Sullivan KM, Plumley TF. Radiographic features of esophageal involvement in chronic graft-vs.-host disease. Am J Roentgenol 1984;142:501–506.
247. Patchell RA, White CL, Clark AW. Neurologic complications of bone marrow transplantation. Neurology 1985;35:300–306.
248. Nelson KR, McQuillen MP. Neurologic complications of graft-versus-host disease. Neurol Clin 1988;6:389–403.
249. Marosi C, Budka H, Grimm G, et al. Fatal encephalitis in a patient with chronic graft-versus-host disease. Bone Marrow Transplant 1990;6:53–57.
250. Greenspan A, Deeg HJ, Cottler-Fox M, Sirdofski M, Spitzer TR, Kattah J. Incapacitating peripheral neuropathy as a manifestation of chronic graft-versus-host disease. Bone Marrow Transplant 1990;5:349–352.
251. Smith CIE, Aarli JA, Biberfeld P, et al. Myasthenia gravis after bone-marrow transplantation. N Engl J Med 1983;309:1565–1568.
252. Bolger GB, Sullivan KM, Spencer AM, et al. Myasthenia gravis after allogeneic bone marrow transplantation: relationship to chronic graft-versus-host disease. Neurology 1986;36:1087–1091.
253. Reyes MG, Noronha P, Thomas W Jr, Heredia R. Myositis of chronic graft versus host disease. Neurology 1983;33:1222–1224.
254. Urbano-Márquez A, Estruch R, Grau JM, et al. Inflammatory myopathy associated with chronic graft-versus-host disease. Neurology 1986;36:1091–1093.
255. Corson SL, Sullivan K, Batzer F, August C, Storb R, Thomas ED. Gynecologic manifestations of chronic graft-versus-host disease. Obstet Gynecol 1982;60:488–492.
256. Schubert MA, Sullivan KM, Schubert MM, et al. Gynecological abnormalities following allogeneic bone marrow transplantation. Bone Marrow Transplant 1990;5:425–430.
257. Hirabayashi N. Studies on graft versus host (GvH) reactions. I. Impairment of hemopoietic stroma in mice suffering from GvH disease. Exp Hematol 1981;9:101–110.
258. Atkinson K, Norrie S, Chan P, Zehnwirth B, Downs K, Biggs J. Hemopoietic progenitor cell function after HLA-identical sibling bone marrow transplantation: influence of chronic graft-versus-host disease. Int J Cell Cloning 1986;4:203–220.
259. Peralvo J, Bacigalupo A, Pittaluga PA, et al. Poor graft function associated with graft-versus-host disease after allogeneic marrow transplantation. Bone Marrow Transplant 1987;2:279–285.
260. Furst DE, Clements PJ, Graze P, Gale R, Roberts N. A syndrome resembling progressive systemic sclerosis after bone marrow transplantation. A model for scleroderma? Arthritis Rheum 1979;22:904–910.
261. Shulman HM, Sullivan KM, Weiden PL, et al. Chronic graft-versus-host syndrome in man. A long-term clinicopathologic study of 20 Seattle patients. Am J Med 1980;69:204–217.
262. Gomez-Garcia P, Herrera-Arroyo C, Torres-Gomez A, et al. Renal involvement in chronic graft-versus-host disease: a report of two cases. Bone Marrow Transplant 1988;3:357–362.
263. Sullivan KM, Witherspoon RP, Storb R, et al. Prednisone and azathioprine compared with prednisone and placebo for treatment of chronic graft-v-host disease: prognostic influence of prolonged thrombocytopenia after allogeneic marrow transplantation. Blood 1988;72:546–554.
264. Loughran TP Jr, Sullivan KM. Early detection and monitoring of chronic graft-vs.-host disease. In: Burakoff SJ, Deeg HJ, Ferrara J, Atkinson K, eds. Graft-vs.-host disease: immunology, pathophysiology, and treatment. New York: Marcel Dekker, 1990:631–636.
265. Atkinson K, Horowitz MM, Gale RP, Lee MB, Rimm AA, Bortin MM. Consensus among bone marrow transplanters for diagnosis, grading and treatment of chronic graft-versus-host disease. Bone Marrow Transplant 1989;4:247–254.
266. Loughran TP Jr, Sullivan K, Morton T, et al. Value of day 100 screening studies for predicting the development of chronic graft-versus-host disease after allogeneic bone marrow transplantation. Blood 1990;76:228–234.
267. Atkinson K, Storb R, Ochs HD, et al. Thymus transplantation after allogeneic bone marrow graft to prevent chronic graft-versus-host disease in humans. Transplantation 1982;33:168–173.
268. Witherspoon RP, Sullivan KM, Lum LG, et al. Use of thymic grafts or thymic factors to augment immunologic recovery after bone marrow transplantation: brief report with 2 to 12 years' follow-up. Bone Marrow Transplant 1988;3:425–435.
269. Sullivan KM, Mori M, Sanders J, et al. Late complications of allogeneic and autologous marrow transplantation. Bone Marrow Transplant 1992;10(suppl 1):127–134.
270. Sullivan KM, Deeg HJ, Sanders JE, et al. Late complications after marrow transplantation. Semin Hematol 1984;21:53–63.
271. Sullivan KM, Witherspoon RP, Storb R, et al. Alternating-day cyclosporine and prednisone for treatment of high-risk chronic graft-v-host disease. Blood 1988;72:555–561.
272. Sullivan KM, Siadak MF, Witherspoon RP. Cyclosporine treatment of chronic graft-versus-host disease following allogeneic bone marrow transplantation. Transplant Proc 1990;22:1336–1338.
273. Vogelsang GB, Farmer ER, Hess AD, et al. Thalidomide for the treatment of chronic graft versus host disease. N Engl J Med 1992;326:1055–1058.
274. Hymes SR, Morison WL, Farmer ER, Walters LL, Tutschka PJ, Santos GW. Methoxsalen and ultraviolet A radiation in treatment of chronic cutaneous graft-versus-host reaction. Acad Dermatol 1985;12:30–37.
275. Atkinson K, Weller P, Ryman W, Biggs J. PUVA therapy for drug-resistant graft-versus-host disease. Bone Marrow Transplant 1986;1:227–236.
276. Socie G, Devergie A, Cosset JM, et al. Low-dose (one gray) total-lymphoid irradiation for extensive, drug-resistant chronic graft-versus-host disease. Transplantation 1990;49:657–658.
277. Tzakis AG, Abu-Elmagd K, Fung JJ, et al. FK 506 rescue in chronic graft-versus-host-disease after bone

marrow transplantation. Transplant Proc 1991;23: 3225–3227.

278. Masaoka T, Shibata H, Kakishita E, Kanamaru A, Takemoto Y, Moriyama Y. Phase II study of FK 506 for allogeneic bone marrow transplantation. Transplant Proc 1991;23:3228–3231.

279. Knobler HY, Sagher U, Peled IJ, et al. Tolerance to donor-type skin in the recipient of a bone marrow allograft. Transplantation 1985;40:223–225.

280. Adams F, Messner H. Neuropharmacologic therapy of the neuromuscular manifestations of graft-versus-host disease (abstract). Proceedings of ASCO. Leukemia 1987;6:145.

281. Fried RH, Murakami CS, Fisher LD, Willson RA, Sullivan KM, McDonald GB. Ursodeoxycholic acid treatment of refractory chronic graft-versus-host of the liver. Ann Intern Med 1992;116:624–629.

282. Atkinson K, Farewell V, Storb R, et al. Analysis of late infections after human bone marrow transplantation: role of genotypic nonidentity between marrow donor and recipient and of nonspecific suppressor cells in patients with chronic graft-versus-host disease. Blood 1982;60:714–720.

283. Winston DJ, Schiffman G, Wang DC, et al. Pneumococcal infections after human bone marrow transplantation. Ann Intern Med 1979;91:835–841.

284. Sullivan KM, Meyers JD, Flournoy N, Storb R, Thomas ED. Early and late interstitial pneumonia following human bone marrow transplantation. Int J Cell Cloning 1986;4:107–121.

285. Engelhard D, Handsher R, Naparstek E, et al. Immune response to polio vaccination in bone marrow transplant recipients. Bone Marrow Transplant 1991; 8:295–300.

286. Centers for Disease Control. Update and adult immunizations: recommendations of the Immunization Practices Advisory Committee. MMWR 1991; 40 (No.RR-12):13–15.

287. Winston DJ, Ho WG, Schiffman G, Champlin RE, Feig SA, Gale RP. Pneumococcal vaccination of recipients of bone marrow transplants. Arch Intern Med 1983; 143:1735–1737.

288. Lapp WS, Ghayur T, Mendes M, Seddik M, Seemayer TA. The functional and histological basis for graft-versus-host-induced immunosuppression. Immunol Rev 1985;88:107–133.

289. Ljungman P, Fridell E, Lönnqvist B, et al. Efficacy and safety of vaccination of marrow transplant recipients with a live attenuated measles, mumps, and rubella vaccine. J Infect Dis 1989;159:610–615.

290. Sullivan KM, Mori M, Witherspoon R, Sanders J, Appelbaum FR, Storb R. Alternating-day cyclosporine and prednisone (CSP/PRED) treatment of chronic graft-vs-host disease (GVHD): predictors of survival (abstract). Blood 1990;76(suppl 1):568a.

291. Wingard JR, Piantadosi S, Vogelsang GB, et al. Predictors of death from chronic graft versus host disease after bone marrow transplantation. Blood 1989;74:1428–1435.

292. Weiden PL, Sullivan KM, Flournoy N, Storb R, Thomas ED, the Seattle Marrow Transplant Team. Antileukemic effect of chronic graft-versus-host disease. Contribution to improved survival after allogeneic marrow transplantation. N Engl J Med 1981; 304:1529–1533.

293. Horowitz MM, Gale RP, Sondel PM, et al. Graft-versus-leukemia reactions after bone marrow transplantation. Blood 1990;75:555–562.

294. Sullivan KM, Weiden PL, Storb R, et al. Influence of acute and chronic graft-versus-host disease on relapse and survival after bone marrow transplantation from HLA-identical siblings as treatment of acute and chronic leukemia. Blood 1989;73:1720–1728.

295. Witherspoon RP, Storb R, Pepe M, Longton G, Sullivan KM. Cumulative incidence of secondary solid malignant tumors in aplastic anemia patients given marrow grafts after conditioning with chemotherapy alone (letter). Blood 1992;79:289–290.

296. Sanders JE. Effects of chronic graft-vs.-host disease on growth and development. In: Burakoff SJ, Deeg HJ, Ferrara J, Atkinson K, eds. Graft-vs.-host disease: immunology, pathophysiology, and treatment. New York: Marcel Dekker, 1990:665–680.

297. Wingard JR, Curbow B, Baker F, Zabora J, Piantadosi S. Sexual satisfaction in survivors of bone marrow transplantation. Bone Marrow Transplant 1992;9:185–190.

298. Andrykowski MA, Altmaier EM, Barnett RL, Otis ML, Gingrich R, Henslee-Downey PJ. The quality of life in adult survivors of allogeneic bone marrow transplantation. Transplantation 1990;50:399–406.

299. Wingard JR, Curbow B, Baker F, Piantadosi S. Health, functional status, and employment of adult survivors of bone marrow transplantation. Ann Intern Med 1991;114:113–118.

300. Syrjala KL, Chapko MK, Vitaliano PP, Cummings C, Sullivan KM. Recovery after allogeneic marrow transplantation: a prospective study of predictors of long-term physical and psychosocial functioning. Bone Marrow Transplant 1993;11:319–327.

Chapter 27

Prevention and Treatment of Bacterial and Fungal Infections

John R. Wingard

Susceptibility to infections has been a major problem in the clinical management of patients undergoing bone marrow transplantation (BMT). Most transplant-associated deaths have been attributable to either infection or graft-versus-host disease (GVHD), or a combination of both. Major strides have been made in the supportive care of transplant patients due to a variety of advances in infection control: an improved understanding of the pathogenesis of these infectious syndromes, introduction of new antimicrobial agents, new strategies to prevent or treat infections, and recognition of the contribution of infectious pathogens to other transplant complications, such as GVHD. However, shifts in patterns of opportunistic pathogens, changing antimicrobial susceptibility, changes in host immunodeficiency due to new immunosuppressive regimens for prevention and treatment of GVHD, introduction of new preparative regimens for use in the treatment of solid tumors, and the increasing use of matched unrelated donors continue to pose new and evolving challenges for the management of infectious complications.

Compromised Host Defenses that Underlie the Vulnerability to Bacterial and Fungal Infections

The type of deficit in host defenses following BMT varies over time (Figure 27-1)(1). Three periods have been described: (1) *early recovery*, corresponding to the first several weeks after transplant, the pre-engraftment phase; (2) *mid-recovery*, corresponding to the second and third months after transplant, the early postengraftment phase; and (3) *late recovery*, corresponding to the interval beyond 3 months. Table 27-1 lists the predominant deficits present at various periods.

Early Recovery

The cytoreductive agents used in BMT preparative regimens damage rapidly dividing cell populations, especially bone marrow progenitor cells and mucosal epithelial cells. Accordingly, for several weeks after the marrow transplant, pancytopenia and damage to mucosal barriers are prominent deficits in the host defenses against infectious pathogens.

The duration of neutropenia varies according to the number of stem cells used to effect reconstitution, the occurrence of certain viral infections, such as cytomegalovirus (CMV), the use of cytotoxic agents after transplantation as prophylaxis for GVHD, the use of agents to purge bone marrow ex vivo of potentially contaminating tumor cells, and the use of cytokines to stimulate recovery.

The degree of mucosal damage varies according to the preparative regimen; busulfan, etoposide, melphalan, cytarabine, and total body irradiation are associated with varying degrees of mucositis. Although stomatitis is readily observable, damage to the mucosa of the entire gastrointestinal tract occurs. The reactivation of herpes simplex virus (HSV) type I, which occurs in approximately 70% of seropositive patients, usually occurs during the first or second

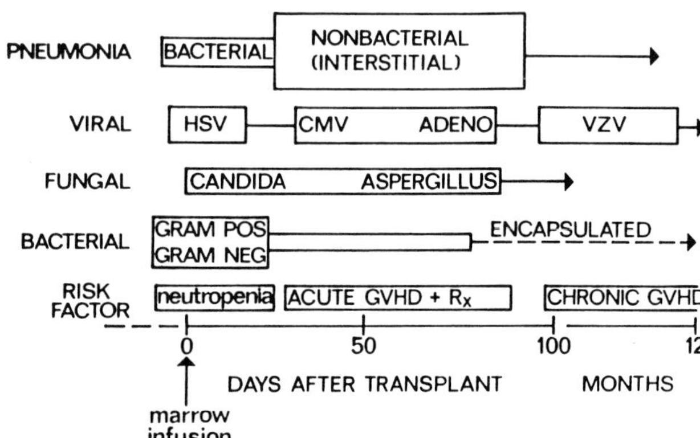

Figure 27-1. Infectious syndromes at various times after bone marrow transplantation. (Reproduced by permission from Meyers JD. Infections in marrow recipients. In: Mandell GL, Douglas RG, Bennett JE, eds. Principles and practice of infectious diseases, ed 2. New York: John Wiley and Sons, 1985: 1674–1676.)

Table 27-1.
Host Defenses Compromised by BMT that Make Patients Vulnerable to Bacterial and Fungal Infections

Early recovery
Neutropenia
Oral and gastrointestinal mucosal damage due to cytoreductive therapy
Skin barrier compromised by central venous catheters
Mid-recovery
Skin and gastrointestinal mucosal damage due to GVHD
Decreased cellular immunity due to GVHD and immunosuppressive therapy
Skin barrier compromised by central venous catheters
Decreased cellular immunity due to viral infections, especially cytomegalovirus
Late recovery
Decreased cellular immunity; persistent with chronic GVHD
Nonspecific suppressor cells with chronic GVHD
Reduced opsonization
Decreased reticuloendothelial function
Immunoglobulin G subclass deficiencies

BMT = bone marrow transplantation; GVHD = graft-versus-host disease.

week after BMT and can lead to diffuse or localized ulceration of the mucosa of the oral cavity and the lower esophagus. Use of cytotoxic agents after transplantation, such as methotrexate (MTX) or cyclophosphamide (CY) to prevent GVHD, can result in exacerbation of mucositis and delay in healing.

Frequent use of indwelling central venous catheters compromises the integrity of the integument as a physical barrier to potential pathogens residing on the skin. Bone marrow puncture sites and peripheral venous catheters can also compromise the skin barrier. Reactivation of HSV type II occurs in seropositive patients (many of whom do not recall a primary episode of genital herpes), and can result in urethral, labial, perineal, and perianal skin and mucosal breakdown.

Mid-recovery

After engraftment, patients next enter a period of profound deficiency of cell-mediated immunity. The degree and duration of cellular immunodeficiency is influenced by type of transplant, degree of donor and recipient histocompatibility, whether T lymphocytes have been eliminated from the allogeneic marrow graft, whether immunological or pharmacological purging of autologous marrow was performed, the type of post-transplant immunosuppressive treatment used as prophylaxis for GVHD, the occurrence of viral infections (especially CMV), and the occurrence and severity of GVHD. Humoral immunity is also markedly impaired during this period. The integrity of the mucosal barriers may continue to be compromised by recurrent HSV infections, use of cytotoxic agents, and intestinal involvement by GVHD. Indwelling venous catheters typically remain in place during this period, making the patient susceptible to infection from skin flora.

Late Recovery

With time, there is gradual recovery of both cellular and humoral immunity. Generally, the recovery is more rapid after autologous than allogeneic BMT. Among autograft recipients, those given myeloablative preparative regimens (as typically used for acute leukemias) are more immunodeficient and for longer intervals than those given less intensive, nonablative preparative regimens, such as those used for solid tumor therapy. Although not carefully studied yet, immune recovery after a sibling-related human leukocyte antigen (HLA)-identical transplant would be expected to be more rapid than after an HLA-disparate or HLA-matched unrelated donor transplant.

The occurrence and severity of GVHD also influences the tempo of immune recovery and can be associated with dysregulated immune responses. If chronic GVHD occurs, cellular and humoral immunodeficiency can persist for months, even years. Reticuloendothelial function can be severely impaired, especially in patients with chronic GVHD. Immunoglobulin (Ig) deficiencies can occur, and even in the face of normal levels of the isotypes, IgG subclass deficiencies can be present. By one year, immune recovery is usually complete; even then, however, responses to various immunizations can be impaired or absent in some patients.

Spectrum of Bacterial and Fungal Infections

Just as the defects in host immunity vary over time, so does the spectrum of infections. Tables 27-2 and 27-3 list common bacterial and fungal infections encountered during these periods.

Table 27-2.
Bacterial and Fungal Infectious Syndromes Encountered Early after BMT During the Pre-engraftment Phase (Early Recovery)

	Relative Frequency[a]	*Relative Life-threatening Potential*
First Fever		
Staphylococci	+++	+
Alpha-hemolytic streptococci	+	++
Gram-negative bacilli	+	+++
Subsequent fevers		
Antibiotic-resistant gram-negative bacilli	+	+++
Staphylococci	+++	+
Candida species	++	++
Aspergillus species	+	+++
Other fungal genera	+	++

[a]Increasing frequency and life-threatening potential are depicted by increased numbers of "+" signs.

Table 27-3.
Bacterial and Fungal Infections Encountered after Engraftment

	Relative Frequencies[a]		
	Allogeneic BMT with No GVHD	*Allogeneic BMT with GVHD*	*Autologous BMT*
Early (mid-recovery)			
Staphylococci	++	++	++
Candida species	++	+++	+
Aspergillus species	++	+++	+
Gram-negative bacilli	−	+	−
Encapsulated bacteria	−	+	−
Late (late recovery)			
Encapsulated bacteria	−	++	−
Candida species	−	+	−
Aspergillus species	−	+	−

[a]Increased frequency is depicted by increased numbers of "+" signs; "−" indicates uncommon infections.
BMT = bone marrow transplantation; GVHD = graft-versus-host disease.

Early Recovery

Most febrile episodes are infectious in etiology. Because the signs and symptoms of infection are obscured during neutropenia (2) and an untreated bacterial or fungal infection during neutropenia is rapidly life-threatening, all fevers should operationally be regarded as infectious until proved otherwise.

Bacterial pathogens account for more than 90% of first infections during neutropenia (see Table 27-2). Gram-negative bacteria are the most virulent bacterial pathogens in neutropenic patients and historically have been the cause of frequent morbidity and mortality. The most common Gram-negative bacteria have been *Eschericia coli*, *Klebsiella* spp., and *Pseudomonas aeruginosa*. In recent years, water-borne organisms, such as *Acinetobacter* spp. have increased. The portal of entry for these organisms generally is the damaged mucosa of the gastrointestinal tract. Perianal fissures or skin breakdown are other potential sources, especially for *P. aeruginosa* (3). Occasionally, venous catheters can also serve as an entry site for gram-negative bacteria.

In recent years, gram-positive bacteria have emerged as major pathogens, and bacteremia rates for gram-positive pathogens now exceed those for gram-negative bacteria (4–6), which is in large part attributable to the nearly universal use of indwelling central venous catheters. Occasionally, gram-positive organisms may invade the host via the gastrointestinal tract as well. *Staphylococcus epidermidis*, *S. aureus*, alpha hemolytic streptococci, and *Corynebacterium* spp. are the most common organisms.

The portal of entry for alpha hemolytic streptococci may in large part be the oral mucosa (7). Thus, patients with stomatitis due to chemotherapy, radiotherapy, or HSV-induced mucosal ulcerations are particularly at risk. Several large series have reported bacteremia rates of 15 to 20% in BMT populations (8). Where speciated, *Streptococcus mitis*, an organism that normally resides on the buccal mucosa, is the most common alpha hemolytic streptococcus. Although, in general, gram-positive bacteria are less virulent than gram-negative bacteria, approximately 10% of alpha hemolytic streptococcal bacteremias are associated with a toxic shock–like syndrome, which in many instances can be fatal despite prompt institution of appropriate antimicrobial agents (8). Corynebacterial infections are often associated with infected bone marrow needle puncture sites or infected peripheral venous catheters, often with associated thrombophlebitis.

After institution of antibiotics during first fever, the microbial flora changes. Superinfections, as manifested by recurrent or persistent fever during the second or subsequent week of neutropenia, are more heterogeneous in etiology (see Table 27-2). There are four categories commonly encountered.

First and foremost, gram-negative bacteria, especially those that are resistant to the antibiotic regimen used to treat first fever, are of paramount concern (9). These bacteria account for only roughly 10% of superinfections, but are the most virulent and have rapid life-threatening potential if appropriate antibiotic modification is not made.

The second category, and the most common etiology, is *S. epidermidis*, accounting for roughly half of infections. These organisms are less virulent than gram-negative bacteria and are quickly isolated from blood cultures of bacteremic patients. Thus, clinicians can wait until multiple blood cultures are positive to ensure that the isolate is a true pathogen rather than an innocent contaminant.

The third group, accounting for approximately one third of superinfections, are due to *Candida* species. Historically, the most common have been *Candida albicans* and *C. tropicalis*. Although *C. albicans* is the most prevalent *Candida* species, *C. tropicalis* appears to be more virulent in neutropenic patients (10). The portal of entry for this commensal organism is the damaged mucosa of the gastrointestinal tract. In recent years, less common and less virulent *Candida* species have emerged as opportunistic pathogens, including *C. lusitaniae*, *C. parapsilosis*, *Torulopsis glabrata*, and *C. krusei*. The most common manifestation of disseminated *Candida* infection is refractory fever unresponsive to antibiotics. Macronodular skin lesions, polymyalgias, polyarthralgias, and new-onset azotemia are occasional clues to diagnosis. Blood cultures are important but may be negative, even with disseminated disease. *Candida* antigen and antibody tests have not proven to be reliable. The enolase assay has been shown to document some infections missed by conventional diagnostic tests (11), but its false-negative rate of 25% and its seeming dependence on the tissue burden of organisms limit its utility in early diagnosis. Thus, accurate diagnosis early in the course of infection remains problematic. Risk factors include increased duration of neutropenia, increasing patient age, T-cell depletion, donor-recipient mismatch, use of corticosteroids, use of cytarabine or total body irradiation in the preparative regimen, and recovery of *Candida* organisms from surveillance cultures (12–14).

Aspergillus infections, especially by *A. fumigatus* and *A. flavus*, occur in 4 to 20% of patients and constitute the fourth category of superinfections (15–17). The major host risk factors include greater duration and depth of neutropenia and a prior infection by *Aspergillus*, but use of corticosteroids and presence of GVHD and CMV infection are also risk factors, especially after engraftment. The portal of entry for this airborne organism is the nasal passages, the sinuses, and the respiratory tract. Several hospital outbreaks have been described, attributable to contamination of air ventilation systems (18–22). The most common presentation is that of a pulmonary infarction. Infiltrates are often subtle and may be easily missed on a chest radiograph. Computerized tomographic (CT) scans of the chest are more sensitive and may demonstrate nodular infiltrates with a surrounding "halo" zone of decreased attenuation, and, in more advanced stages, cavitation (23). Hematogenous dissemination can occur frequently with involvement of the heart, the brain, the gastrointestinal tract, the kidney, the diaphragm, the liver, and the spleen (16). Mucormycosis can also present as a pulmonary infarction, clinically indistinguishable from *Aspergillus* infection. Although most *Aspergillus* organisms enter the host via the respiratory passages, there have been sporadic reports of primary cutaneous *Aspergillus* infection associated with insertion of central venous catheters (24).

Occasionally, *Trichosporon beigelii* and *Fusarium* spp. (Plate XLIV) are also causes of deep-seated fungal infection. The ever-expanding array of new opportunistic pathogens necessitates continuing vigilance during prolonged neutropenia.

Mid-recovery

With recovery of the neutrophil count, most bacterial and fungal infections resolve and antimicrobial agents can frequently be discontinued. A notable exception is the increasingly frequent syndrome of hepatosplenic candidiasis, sometimes known as chronic systemic candidiasis (25). This infectious syndrome may manifest primarily as new occurrence of a fever at the time of neutrophil recovery or persistence of fever despite neutrophil recovery. There may be no other clinical findings present on examination. Occasionally, alkaline phosphatase levels may be elevated, and a CT or an MRI scan of the liver and spleen is useful in showing areas of reduced attenuation in a focal distribution. Histologically, the organism may be demonstrated or granulomas may be present. This syndrome should be considered in the differential diagnosis of a fever of obscure etiology in the mid-recovery period (Table 27-4).

Another common cause of fever of obscure origin is sinusitis. Frequently sinusitis is without specific focal signs or symptoms, but it is readily detected by either radiographs or CT scans of the sinuses. Another cause of a fever of obscure origin is an occult infection of the central venous catheter. Blood cultures may be unrevealing initially, and removal of the catheter is occasionally necessary to ascertain with certainty the etiology of the fever. In general, the differential diagnosis listed in Table 27-4 has been quite useful in explaining the vast majority of fevers of obscure etiology after engraftment.

Table 27-4.
Causes of Fevers of Obscure Origin After Engraftment

Cytomegalovirus infection
Central venous catheter infections
Occult sinusitis
Hepatosplenic candidiasis
Pulmonary or disseminated *Aspergillus* infection

Patients who have undergone allogeneic BMT are more susceptible to infections during the mid-recovery period than autograft recipients, particularly if acute GVHD occurs and requires more immunosuppressive therapy. Particularly problematic are *Candida* and *Aspergillus* infections in patients on high doses of corticosteroids. Although *Cryptococcus neoformans* is rarely a pathogen during the pre-engraftment period, it is an occasional pathogen during the mid-recovery period as a cause of fungemia, pulmonary infection, or meningitis, especially in patients with GVHD or those receiving corticosteroids. Patients with intestinal GVHD are susceptible to recurrent bacteremias due to gram-negative bacteria.

Late Recovery

With gradual immune recovery, the risk for infections progressively declines. Autograft recipients have a very low risk for continuing bacterial or fungal infections during this period. Allogeneic transplant recipients in the absence of chronic GVHD have a progressively receding risk for these infections. However, patients with chronic GVHD are highly susceptible for recurrent bacterial infections, especially from encapsulated bacteria, including *S. pneumonia*, *H. influenzae*, and *Neisseria meningitidis*, due to poor reticuloendothelial function and diminished opsonizing antibodies. The continued use of immunosuppressive therapies also makes these patients susceptible to fungal infections. Generally, these tend to be mucosal fungal infections, but systemic infection can also occur.

Treatment Strategies

First Fever During Neutropenia

With the recognition that most febrile episodes during neutropenia are infectious in origin, awareness of their life-threatening potential, and the knowledge that most first infections are due to bacteria, evaluation should be prompt and thorough. Special attention should be directed to the oral cavity, catheter sites, and the perianal area. Cultures of suspected sites of infection should be obtained, and in all patients at least two sets of blood samples should be submitted for bacterial and fungal culture.

After evaluation, antibacterial agents should be instituted promptly on an empiric basis even in the absence of signs and symptoms of infection; this strategy has been found in a number of studies to reduce the morbidity and mortality associated with these infections, and this practice has become universally adopted as the standard of care for management of the initial fever during neutropenia. A variety of antibiotic regimens have been advocated, and dozens of controlled trials has compared one regimen with another. It is currently debatable as to whether one regimen is superior to another. What is generally agreed on, however, is that antibiotics should be begun promptly at the first sign of fever, without waiting for isolation of an organism in blood or other cultures, even in the absence of signs or symptoms of infection, because the classic findings associated with infection can be obscured when the host is unable to mount an inflammatory response (2).

In choosing an antibiotic regimen, efficacy is of paramount importance. Other important considerations include toxicities, the likelihood of emergence of resistance, the risk for superinfection (frequency as well as type), and cost. A consensus committee of the Infectious Diseases Society of America reviewed the available studies and attempted to provide guidelines for management of the first fever during neutropenia (26). Their suggested strategy is indicated in Figure 27-2. Four general approaches are discussed in detail (26); the advantages and disadvantages of these options are briefly reviewed.

The first strategy, and the one with longest track record, is a combination of an antipseudomonal β-lactam plus an aminoglycoside. The advantage of this combination is potential synergy against some gram-negative bacteria, coverage against anaerobes, infrequent emergence of antibiotic resistance, and low cost. This regimen should be considered for patients at high risk for *P. aeruginosa* infections. Disadvantages include nephrotoxicity, ototoxicity, the need for monitoring aminoglycoside levels to assure therapeutic levels and to minimize toxicity, and a lack of coverage against most gram-positive bacteria.

A second option is the use of a single agent, such as ceftazidime, imipenem, or cefoperazone, which

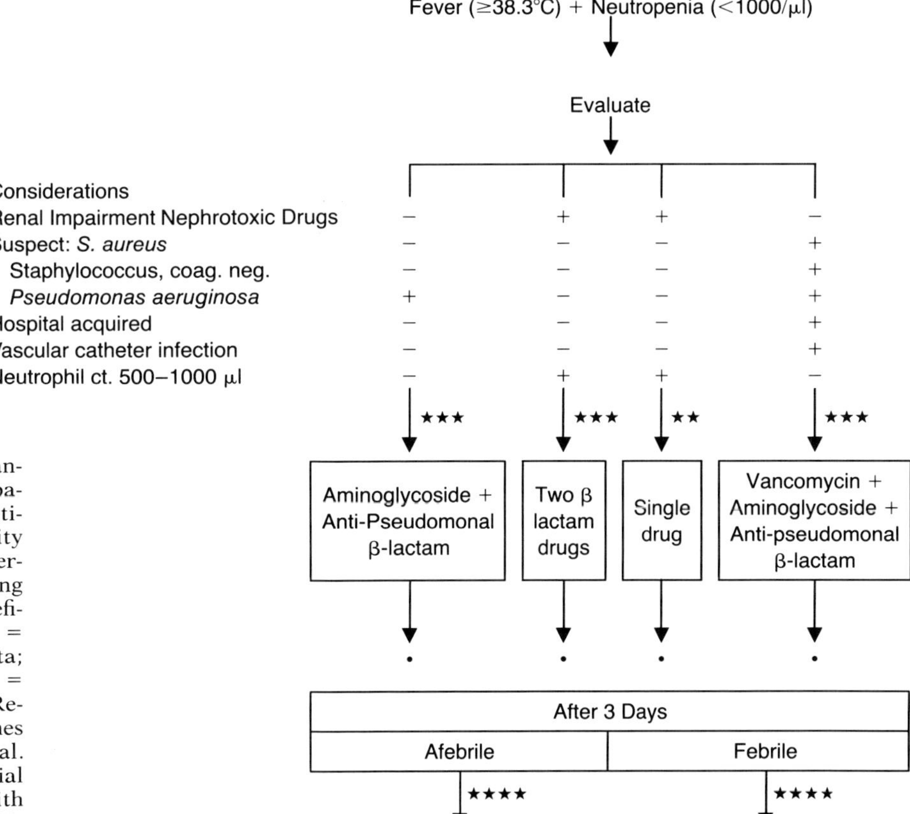

Figure 27-2. Guide to the initial management of febrile neutropenic patients. If a causative agent is identified, modify to optimal susceptibility but maintain broad-spectrum coverage. Stars indicate committee's rating of recommendations: ★★★★ = definite choice, strong support; ★★★ = choice adequate, support with data; ★★ = promising, but not proven, ★ = inadequate data to support use. (Reproduced by permission from Hughes WT, Armstrong D, Bodey GP, et al. Guidelines for the use of antimicrobial agents in neutropenic patients with unexplained fever. J Infect Dis 1990; 161:381–396.)

affords high systemic levels, broad-spectrum activity, and little toxicity (27–31). Disadvantages of this approach include little activity against most gram-positive bacteria and anaerobes (for ceftazidime or cefoperazone) and the frequent need to add additional agents, especially for documented infections.

A third option is to use two β-lactams, such as a cephalosporin, plus an ureidopenicillin, such as piperacillin or mezlocillin. This combination offers broad-spectrum activity with little toxicity and anaerobic coverage, but there is little coverage against gram-positive organisms and there is the possibility of antagonism in certain bacterial infections (32).

A fourth option is to combine vancomycin with an aminoglycoside plus an antipseudomonal β-lactam. This combination offers the advantage of excellent coverage against gram-positive bacteria in addition to the advantages and disadvantages noted in the first option. Opinion is divided as to the need for empiric vancomycin, because many gram-positive infections are easily controlled once identified (4–6, 33–35), as well as concerns as to the emergence of resistance if the agent is overused (36). Certainly, inclusion of vancomycin in first-time therapy should be considered strongly in patients with suspected staphylococcal infections or patients with infected catheters.

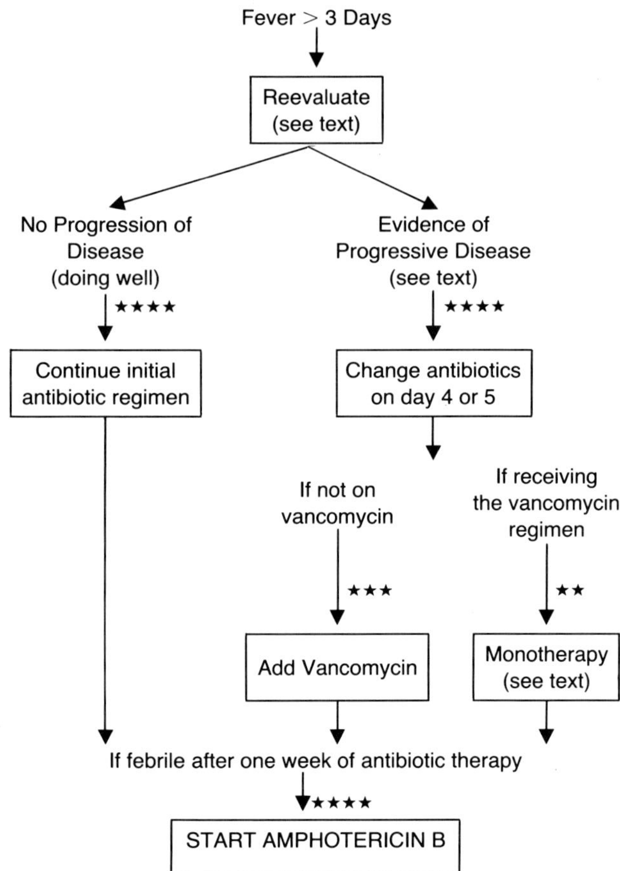

Figure 27-3. Management of patient with persistent fever after 3 days of treatment. See figure 27-2 for star rating system. (Reproduced by permission from Hughes WT, Armstrong D, Bodey GP, et al. Guidelines for the use of antimicrobial agents in neutropenic patients with unexplained fever. J Infect Dis 1990; 161:381–396.)

Subsequent Fever During Neutropenia

The response to the initial antibiotic regimen dictates subsequent management decisions. If the patient defervesces, then the initial regimen is generally continued without modification until resolution of neutropenia, regardless of whether an infection was documented. Occasionally, if the patient has defervesced and no infection has been documented, antibiotics can be discontinued prior to resolution of neutropenia. However, they should be discontinued with caution and the patient should be monitored closely to reinstitute therapy if fever should recur. Generally, it is advisable to avoid this approach if there is ongoing active oral or gastrointestinal mucositis present.

If fever persists, patients require careful monitoring (Figure 27-3). If no infection has been documented after careful evaluation and there are no signs of progressive infection, then the initial regimen can be continued without modification. If an infection has been documented, then therapy targeted against the pathogen should be instituted. If signs of progressive infection occur, modification of the initial regimen should be instituted to cover suspected pathogens not covered by the initial regimen.

If fever persists or recurs 4 to 7 or more days after initiation of antibiotics, the patient is at high risk for fungal infection. Because of the difficulties of accurate diagnosis early in the course of fungal infections, empiric antifungal therapy should be strongly considered. Empiric antifungal therapy with amphotericin B has been shown to reduce both the incidence and the morbidity of fungal infections (37,38). Unfortunately, nephrotoxicity is quite problematic in patients receiving both amphotericin B and cyclosporine, and renal function should be monitored carefully, with dose adjustments made as necessary to avoid renal failure.

Treatment of *Candida* Infections

Amphotericin B is the treatment of choice for documented *Candida* infection. Generally, amphotericin B in a dose of 0.5 mg/kg/day affords adequate therapy for *C. albicans* and *C. tropicalis* infections, the most common *Candida* pathogens. Higher doses, in the range of 1.0 to 1.5 mg/kg/day, are necessary to treat some of the less common and less susceptible *Candida* species. Some clinicians advocate the use of flucytosine, although no controlled trials have been performed (39–42). The addition of flucytosine appears to be particularly useful in the treatment of several of the less-susceptible *Candida* species other than *C. albicans*, such as *C. krusei*, *C. lusitaniae*, *C. guilliermondii*, and *C. parapsilosis*. Because of its myelosuppressive properties, serum levels of flucytosine should be monitored, with doses adjusted to achieve peak serum levels of 30 to 60 μg/ml to minimize toxicity. Furthermore, because of the rapid emergence of resistance, flucytosine should not be used alone. Animal studies suggest that adjunctive use of granulocyte colony stimulating factor (G-CSF) with amphotericin B may be beneficial (43).

Open-label trials of fluconazole, a triazole, indicate that it offers an alternative treatment for systemic *Candida* infections (44–46). Although fluconazole offers a much less toxic alternative to amphotericin B, there have been no controlled trials comparing the efficacy of amphotericin B and fluconazole. Fluconazole is fungistatic, whereas amphotericin B is fungicidal, which poses at least a theoretical disadvantage in neutropenic patients. Animal studies suggest that fluconazole may be less effective than amphotericin B as treatment of an established *Candida* infection (47).

Duration of therapy is controversial because no controlled trials have been performed. Generally, it is advisable to continue therapy until previously positive cultures become negative, infiltrates or infected lesions resolve, and, when possible, the underlying deficit in host defenses improves (e.g., restoration of neutrophils, resolution of GVHD, discontinuation of corticosteroids). Hepatosplenic candidiasis requires very prolonged courses of therapy, which makes fluconazole an attractive and less toxic alternative to amphotericin B (45,46).

Treatment of *Aspergillus* Infections

Amphotericin B is the treatment of choice for *Aspergillus* infection. Higher doses in the range of 1.0 to 1.5 mg/kg/day are generally required for control. Historically, successful treatment of *Aspergillus* in the BMT setting is rare (16). With a more aggressive diagnostic approach, earlier initiation of antifungal therapy, and more intensive treatment, the prospects for a successful outcome have improved (39,42). Addition of flucytosine has been found by some to be an important adjunct to amphotericin B, although no controlled trials have been performed (39,42). The earlier discussion regarding caution with the use of flucytosine and the appropriate duration of antifungal therapy are pertinent to *Aspergillus* infection as well. Studies evaluating the adjunctive role of M-CSF added to amphotericin B are underway (48).

There are anecdotal reports that the triazole itraconazole is efficacious in the treatment of *Aspergillus* infection (49–51). Unfortunately, there have been no controlled trials comparing its activity with amphotericin B. Its potential advantage over amphotericin B is that it appears to be less toxic and may offer an oral treatment for the usually prolonged courses of treatment necessary for adequate control.

Liposomal or lipid complexes of amphotericin B are under investigation as a treatment for *Aspergillus* and other fungal infections (52,53). Preliminary studies suggest less toxicity with comparable or perhaps increased efficacy compared with free amphotericin B.

Adjunctive Therapies

Prior to the development of effective antibiotics, granulocyte transfusions were used frequently to treat or to prevent infections in severely neutropenic patients (54–56). They have been used rarely in recent years because of the high risk for conveying CMV infection if multiple donors not screened for CMV are used, and because of their marginal benefit when added to modern antibiotic regimens. However, granulocyte transfusions can be useful in patients in whom bacterial or fungal infection progresses despite optimal antimicrobial agents or for an infection by a multiply resistant pathogen for which there is no satisfactory antimicrobial regimen. Use of granulocyte donors serologically negative for CMV avoids the risk of increased CMV infection.

Alternative approaches under current investigation are the use of growth factors such as GM-CSF, G-CSF, and M-CSF to stimulate endogenous phagocytic progenitors, as adjunctive therapy along with antimicrobial agents in the treatment of severe bacterial and fungal infections (43,48). Monoclonal antibodies against endotoxin appear promising as adjunctive treatment of gram-negative bacterial sepsis when there is a risk for septic shock (57,58). Their high cost and the difficulties in identifying the small number of patients unlikely to respond to antibiotics alone make it difficult to know how best to use these agents.

Treatment of Late Bacterial Infections

Recurrent sinopulmonary infections, which are frequently associated with chronic GVHD or Ig deficiency, can generally be treated successfully by a variety of antibiotics, including penicillin, trimethoprim-sulfamethoxazole, cefaclor, or cefuroxime. In Ig deficiency, intravenous immune globulin also can be helpful but very costly.

Preventive Strategies

The first and foremost principle of infection prophylaxis is to minimize the possibility that encounters with the health care team and exposure to the hospital environment places patients at a greater risk for acquiring infection. Accordingly, clinical procedures, especially the placement of venous and urinary catheters, should be avoided when possible. Handwashing by care providers is of paramount importance to avoid transmission of infectious agents from one patient to another, or from staff to patients. Opinion has been divided as to the need for and value of decontaminating regimens to reduce the endogenous flora and use of pathogen-free diets. However, abstinence from fresh fruits and vegetables is usually advised.

Particular attention has been placed on the need for minimizing exposure to airborne organisms. Opinion is divided as to the value of various isolation strategies (59–65). There has been only one prospective randomized trial in BMT patients (65) that compared infection rates in patients cared for in laminar airflow (LAF) rooms versus rooms without LAF. LAF patients also underwent "decontamination procedures" to reduce endogenous microbial colonization. Lower rates of septicemia and major local infections occurred in LAF patients compared with control subjects. It was not possible to distinguish the relative contributions of LAF or decontamination as both were used together, and infections caused by airborne versus endogenous organisms were not distinguished. However, the oral non-absorbable antibiotics were poorly tolerated, and the gastrointestinal flora was not suppressed in most patients. The value of isolation seems to be most compelling for *Aspergillus* as several leukemia and BMT units have encountered outbreaks when construction or contamination of air ventilation systems have occurred (18–22, 63, 66). Some centers have employed the use of LAF usually in conjunction with decontaminating procedures, whereas other centers have used high efficiency particular air (HEPA) filtration systems. The relative merits of these precautions have not been clarified.

Knowledge that most infectious pathogens originate from the endogenous flora, as well as the observations that in many instances these organisms are acquired after entry to the hospital environment, have led to investigation of the utility of bacterial and fungal surveillance cultures. Bacterial surveillance cultures have been found to be useful in detecting antibiotic-resistant bacteria (67) and certain *Candida* species (13,68), and some centers have found surveillance cultures to be of value in predicting *Aspergillus* and *Trichosporon* infections (69–71) but others have not (68,72). Such surveillance culture programs have been useful primarily in the setting of prolonged neutropenia for detecting causes of superinfection. The disadvantage of routine use of surveillance cultures is high cost and the enormous workload for the microbiology laboratories. Accordingly, routine surveillance of individual patients has not been utilized widely. Notwithstanding, there is universal agreement that ongoing hospitalwide and unit-specific infection surveillance programs need to be in place to detect shifting trends in infectious pathogens, as well as patterns of antibiotic resistance (13,67,68,71).

Bacterial Prophylaxis During Neutropenia

The frequency and severity of gram-negative bacterial infections during neutropenia with concomitant gastrointestinal mucosal damage led to an early emphasis on suppressing the intestinal flora to prevent invasive infections. Early efforts to prevent bacterial infections employed the use of oral nonabsorbable agents. Agents such as vancomycin, gentamicin, neomycin, colistin, and polymyxin B have been advocated in various combinations. A variety of controlled trials have been conducted and some have shown a beneficial effect (65, 73, 74). Unfortunately, difficulties with patient compliance, as well as concerns about the emergence of resistance and the high cost of several of these regimens have led to poor acceptance.

A more tolerable regimen that has been shown to be beneficial in controlled trials is that of trimethoprim-sulfamethoxazole, which has been found to reduce both gram-positive and gram-negative bacterial infections (75–77). These studies have been conducted in patients with a variety of hematological malignancies, but not in the BMT setting. Its broad spectrum activity against a number of gram-negative bacteria is offset by its lack of activity against *P. aeruginosa*, a major pathogen in BMT patients. Moreover, concerns have been raised about delays in engraftment, patient tolerance, and selection of resistant organisms (78, 79). Because of these concerns and the lack of data in BMT patients, this regimen has not been adopted widely.

The fluoroquinolones have been shown in controlled trials to reduce significantly gram-negative bacterial infections (80,81) and appear to be more effective than other oral antibiotic regimes (82,83). Norfloxacin and ciprofloxacin have been used most widely, but there are a number of other quinolones in various stages of clinical development. These agents under development appear to differ more in their pharmacological properties rather than antimicrobial spectra. Ciprofloxacin has a potential advantage over norfloxacin in that it achieves higher blood levels and has activity against some gram-positive organisms. However, ciprofloxacin is not active against most methicillin-resistant staphylococci that constitute the majority of staphylococcal isolates. Concerns about the emergence of quinolone resistance have been raised. In a prospectively evaluated cohort of approximately 500 patients at the Johns Hopkins Oncology Center, no quinolone resistance was detected in patients treated prophylactically with norfloxacin. These agents have very little activity against anaerobes, thus, the intestinal anaerobic flora is spared during use of these agents. Preservation of the anaerobic flora is generally regarded as being protective against more virulent pathogens and thus may be a desirable attribute.

Administration of immune globulin intravenously has been shown to reduce septicemia by gram-negative bacteria in the BMT setting (84). Although there may be other reasons to consider use of immune globulin (e.g., to reduce GVHD or CMV infection), its high cost and cheaper effective antibiotic alternatives do not make this approach attractive for prevention of bacterial infection.

Late Bacterial Prophylaxis after Engraftment

Morbidity and mortality from chronic GVHD are frequently due to infection. Antibiotic prophylaxis significantly reduces the mortality from chronic GVHD (85). Accordingly, all patients with chronic GVHD should be placed on daily antibiotic prophylaxis with either penicillin or trimethoprim-sulfamethoxazole. If penicillin is used, additional prophylaxis for *P. carinii*, with either trimethoprim-sulfamethoxazole or aerosolized pentamidine, should also be administered. Even in the absence of chronic GVHD, patients with recurrent sinopulmonary infection should be considered for prophylaxis to prevent infection from encapsulated organisms. Agents such as penicillin, cefaclor, cefuroxime, and trimethoprim-sulfamethoxazole are particularly useful. Moreover, patients who have previously undergone splenectomy should be considered strongly for antibiotic prophylaxis against encapsulated bacteria. For patients with Ig deficiencies, immune globulin is likely to be of benefit (86), but it is quite costly, and further studies are needed to compare antibiotic prophylaxis with immune globulin. The availability of pneumococcal, *H. influenzae*, and meningococcal vaccines are particularly attractive for consideration in this patient population, but patients at greatest need (patients with chronic GVHD) are very unlikely to respond to these vaccines. Prospective trials of pretransplant immunization of transplant recipients, perhaps with donor immunization, will need to be conducted to assess this approach.

Candida Prophylaxis During Neutropenia

A variety of oral agents, including nystatin, clotrimazole, miconazole, and amphotericin B have been evaluated in controlled studies. Largely, these agents have been ineffective. Moreover, patient tolerance is problematic. Unfortunately, centers in which the polyenes (nystatin and amphotericin B) have been used widely have begun to report the emergence of resistance (87). Generally, resistance to polyenes has been associated with reduced virulence, so only sporadic invasive infections by these resistant organisms have been reported (88–90).

Amphotericin B, given intravenously in low doses, has been used prophylactically but its efficacy remains uncertain (91–93). One trial conducted in autologous BMT patients using a dose of 0.1 mg/kg/day showed a trend toward a lower infection rate, but it was statistically insignificant (92). These patients were mostly transplanted for solid tumors and were given growth factors to speed engraftment. The low infection rate in the control group may have confounded the ability to detect a benefit. No polyene resistance was detected. Unfortunately, there was considerable, although not serious, toxicity, even with this low-dose regimen. In a study comparing sequential cohorts of allogeneic BMT patients receiving high-dose corticosteroids, patients given low-dose amphotericin B (0.1–0.2 mg/kg/day) had lower rates of fungal infection (*Candida* and *Aspergillus*) than those not receiving amphotericin B (93). Because of its toxicity, there has been little enthusiasm for prophylaxis using amphotericin B outside of its empiric use in persistently febrile patients, as noted.

A number of controlled trials have shown ketoconazole to be effective prophylaxis by reducing the number of mucosal *Candida* infections. However, no study has demonstrated its effectiveness in reducing systemic *Candida* infections (94). Unfortunately, most reports have not had adequate sample sizes to definitely address ketoconazole's effect on systemic infections. In one trial, 21% of patients were unable to tolerate ketoconazole given in higher-than-usual oral doses (95). A disadvantage is the necessity for gastric acidity for absorption, and it has no activity against *Aspergillus* infection. Its activity against *C. tropicalis* may also be suboptimal (96). Miconazole given intravenously has been shown to be effective in reducing the incidence and mortality from disseminated fungal infection (97). Disadvantages to the use of miconazole include its lack of activity against *Aspergillus*, toxicities such as nausea and vomiting, phlebitis, and occasional cardiac arrhythmias if administered too rapidly. The need for intravenous administration is regarded by some as a disadvantage, although it obviates the concern about bioavailability, which is a concern with ketoconazole.

The triazole class of antifungals offers a group of agents with excellent antifungal activity and little toxicity. The first such compound marketed in the United States was fluconazole. It is available in both oral and intravenous formulations, is mostly excreted in the urine, has excellent penetration into the cerebrospinal fluid, is readily absorbed after oral administration without dependance on gastric acidity (even in the BMT setting (98)), and has a long half-life (24–36 h), which permits once-daily dosing. Two controlled trials have shown it to be effective in reducing disseminated and mucosal *Candida* infections compared with placebo (99,100); in one trial in which it was compared with an oral polyene (amphotericin B or nystatin) (101), it was found to be better than an oral polyene. It interacts with other drugs that are metabolized via the cytochrome P-450 enzyme system (such as cyclosporine [CSP]), but in doses usually used (100–400 mg/day) this interaction appears to be insignificant clinically (102). Nevertheless, potentiation of CSPs effect on renal function should be monitored. It can also elevate hepatic transaminase levels, but this increase is usually subclinical. Fluconazole's major disadvantage is its lack of activity against *Aspergillus*. The controlled trials have not shown an increase in *Aspergillus* infections, but there has also been no reduction in the incidence of *Aspergillus* infections. Furthermore, there are several less common and less virulent *Candida* species, such as *C. krusei* and *Torulopsis glabrata*, that are not susceptible to fluconazole; breakthrough infections with these relatively infrequent pathogens have been reported by some but not all groups (103,104). The controlled trials of fluconazole did not find an increase in *C. krusei* or *Torulopsis glabrata* infections. There may be an association of breakthrough infections from these less susceptible *Candida* species with the use of fluoroquinolones as antibacterial prophylaxis (103). There are less data to support itraconazole as prophylaxis (105).

Aspergillus Prophylaxis

There are few data examining the prophylaxis of *Aspergillus* infection. Patients who have a prior history of *Aspergillus* infection are at high risk for subsequent reactivation during subsequent courses of chemotherapy or BMT (106). One trial used high doses of amphotericin B plus flucytosine prophylactically in patients undergoing chemotherapy for acute leukemia with an earlier history of invasive aspergillosis (41). This combination was successful in preventing reactivation of endogenous organisms in most patients, and no patients died. Although nephrotoxicity was observed, there were no instances of permanent renal failure. The availability of less toxic antifungal regimens such as itraconazole, saperconazole, or other triazoles, will permit a wider exploration of such an approach.

Because the portal of entry is usually the nasal passages, delivery of amphotericin B directly to the sinopulmonary mucosa by a nasal spray was tested in a randomized double-blind trial in patients with acute leukemia (107). Although colonization rates were reduced, there was no reduction in infection rates by *Aspergillus*.

Nonrandomized trials with sequential cohorts have compared ketoconazole with itraconazole as antifungal prophylaxis (105,108). There was a lower rate of fungal infections in patients given itraconazole, especially *Aspergillus* infections. Knowledge of itraconazole's dependence on gastric acidity for absorption and the observation that plasma levels correlated with efficacy has raised a concern about reliable bioavailability after oral administration. Furthermore, there was an apparent increase in several other fungal pathogens in one study (108). Controlled trials are needed to establish the role of this and other promising triazoles.

Immunobiological Agents

Several studies have shown that the use of immune globulin reduces bacterial, fungal, and viral infections after BMT (84, 86, 109, 110). The relative merits of it as a general antimicrobial measure versus the various specific antimicrobial agents remain unclear. Generally, immune globulin is well tolerated. Its disadvantages include its high cost, large fluid volumes associated with its administration, and occasional side effects.

Another approach is to reduce the underlying vulnerability that made the host susceptible for the infection in the first place. During the first month, neutropenia is a major factor. Use of G-CSF and GM-CSF has been shown to shorten the duration of neutropenia, to speed engraftment, and to reduce the number of infections and use of antimicrobial agents. The advantages, disadvantages, and indications for the use of these cytokines are discussed elsewhere (see Chapter 24). A variety of other cytokines are in clinical development that may offer similar or additional benefits.

After engraftment, diminished cell-mediated immunity is a major deficit. Use of less toxic immunosuppressive agents to avoid the global immunosuppression frequently associated with the use of high doses of corticosteroids as well as improvements in strategies to reduce severe GVHD should also result in a lower risk for systemic fungal infections.

Summary

The morbidity and mortality from infection have dramatically diminished in recent years as a result of an improved understanding of the deficits in host defenses and the spectrum of infections that occur at various intervals after BMT, as well as introduction of new, more effective, and less toxic antimicrobial regimens and improved strategies of using older antimicrobial agents. These advances in supportive care have facilitated enormous strides in reducing transplant-associated mortality and thereby improving the acceptability of BMT as a treatment option for an ever widening array of malignant diseases.

Variations in trends of opportunistic pathogens, the ever continuing emergence of antimicrobial resistance among micro-organisms, changes in host characteristics due to new preparative and immunosuppressive regimens, expansion of BMT to new patient populations (with older ages and different underlying diseases), and adoption of post-transplant immunoadjuvant therapies to reduce the risk for relapse require continuing vigilance and will pose new challenges to the control of infections. Newer antimicrobial agents that are safer, more effective, and have broader spectra of activity must be sought. Better diagnostic tools to detect pathogens more rapidly and to document infections more accurately, especially due to fungi, and to detect them earlier in the course of infection are needed. The expanding array of biological agents offers the opportunity to reduce host susceptibility to infection and will likely prove important adjuncts to antimicrobial agents directed against the growing repertoire of opportunistic pathogens.

References

1. Meyers JD. Infections in marrow recipients. In: Mandell GL, Douglas RG, Bennett JE, eds. Principles and practice of infectious diseases, ed 2. New York: John Wiley and Sons, 1985:1674–1676.
2. Sickles EA, Green WH, Wiernick PH. Clinical presentation of infection in granulocytopenic patients. Arch Intern Med 1975;135:715–719.
3. Schmipff SC, Moody MM, Young VM. Relationship of colonization with *Pseudomonas aeruginosa* to development of *Pseudomonas* bacteremia in cancer patients. Antimicrob Agents Chemother 1970;10:240–244.
4. Rubin M, Hathorn JW, Marshall D, et al. Gram-positive infections and the use of vancomycin in 550 episodes of fever and neutropenia. Ann Intern Med 1988;108:30–35.
5. Lowder JN, Lazarus HM, Herzig RH. Bacteremias and fungemias in oncologic patients with central venous

catheters: changing spectrum of infection. Arch Intern Med 1982;142:1456–1459.

6. Karp JE, Dick JD, Angelopulos C, et al. Empiric use of vancomycin during prolonged treatment-induced granulocytopenia. Randomized, double-blind, placebo-controlled clinical trial in patients with acute leukemia. Am J Med 1986;81:237–242.
7. Wingard JR. Infectious and noninfectious systemic consequences. Consensus development conference on oral complications of cancer therapies: diagnosis, prevention and treatment. NCI Monogr 1990;9:21–26.
8. Villablanca JG, Steiner M, Kersey J, et al. The clinical spectrum of infections with viridans streptococci in bone marrow transplant patients. Bone Marrow Transplant 1990;6:387–393.
9. Wingard JR, Santos GW, Saral R. Differences between first and subsequent fevers during prolonged neutropenia. Cancer 1987;59:844–849.
10. Wingard JR, Dick JD, Merz WG, et al. Differences in virulence of clinical isolates of *Candida tropicalis* and *Candida albicans* in mice. Infect Immun 1982;37:833–836.
11. Walsh TJ, Hathorn JW, Sobel JD, et al. Detection of circulating candida enolase by immunoassay in patients with cancer and invasive candidiasis. N Engl J Med 1991;324:1026.
12. Verfaillie C, Weisdorf D, Haake R, Hostetter M, Ramsay NKC, McGlave P. *Candida* infections in bone marrow transplant recipients. Bone Marrow Transplant 1991; 8:177–184.
13. Sandford GR, Merz WG, Wingard JR, et al. The value of fungal surveillance cultures as predictors of systemic fungal infections. J Infect Dis 1980;142:503–509.
14. Pirsch JD, Maki DG. Infectious complications in adults with bone marrow transplantation and T-Cell depletion of donor marrow. Ann Intern Med 1986;104:619–631.
15. Winston DJ, Gale RP, Meyer DV, et al. Infectious complications of human bone marrow transplantation. Medicine 1979;58:1–31.
16. Wingard JR, Beals SU, Santos GW, et al. Aspergillus infections in bone marrow transplant recipients. Bone Marrow Transplant 1987;2:175–181.
17. Peterson PK, McGlave P, Ramsay NKC, et al. A prospective study of infectious diseases following bone marrow transplantation: emergence of *Aspergillus* and cytomegalovirus as the major causes of mortality. Infect Control 1983;4:81–89.
18. Rose HD. Mechanical control of hospital ventilation and *Aspergillus* infections. Am Rev Respir Dis 1972; 105:306–307.
19. Rotstein C, Cummings KM, Tidings J, et al. An outbreak of invasive aspergillosis among allogeneic bone marrow transplants: a case-control study. Infect Control 1985; 6:347–355.
20. Mahoney DH Jr, Steuber CP, Starling KA, Barrett FF, Goldberg J, Fernbach DJ. An outbreak of aspergillosis in children with acute leukemia. J Pediatr 1979;95:70–72.
21. Lentino JR, Rosenkranz MA, Michaels JA, Kurup VP, Rose HD, Rytel MW. Nosocomial aspergillosis: a retrospective review of airborne disease secondary to road construction and contaminated air conditioners. Am J Epidemiol 1982;116:430–437.
22. Aisner J, Schimpff SC, Bennett JE, Young VM, Wiernick PH. *Aspergillus* infections in cancer patients: association with fireproofing materials in a new hospital. JAMA 1976;235:411–412.
23. Kuhlman JE, Fishman EK, Burch PA, et al. Invasive pulmonary aspergillosis in acute leukemia: the contribution of CT to early diagnosis and aggressive management. Chest 1987;92:95–99.
24. Allo MD, Miller J, Townsend T, Tan C. Primary cutaneous aspergillosis associated with Hickman intravenous catheters. N Engl J Med 1987;317:1105–1108.
25. Thaler M, Pastakia B, Shawker TH, O'Leary T, Pizzo PA. Hepatic candidiasis in cancer patients; the evolving picture of the syndrome. Ann Intern Med 1988;108:88–100.
26. Hughes WT, Armstrong D, Bodey GP, et al. Guidelines for the use of antimicrobial agents in neutropenic patients with unexplained fever. J Infect Dis 1990; 161:381–396.
27. Pizzo PA, Hathorn JW, Hiemenz J, et al. A randomized trial comparing ceftazidime alone with combination antibiotic therapy in cancer patients with fever and neutropenia. N Engl J Med 1986;315:552–558.
28. Liang R, Yung R, Chiu R, et al. Ceftazidime versus imipenem-cilastatin as initial monotherapy for febrile neutropenic patients. Antimicrob Agents Chemother 1990;34:1336–1341.
29. Schuchter L, Kaelin W, Petty B, et al. Ceftazidime (C) vs ticarcillin and gentamicin (TG) in febrile neutropenic bone marrow transplant (BMT) patients (pts): a prospective, randomized, double-blind trial. Blood 1988; 72(suppl 1):406a.
30. Granowetten L, Wells H, Lange BJ. Ceftazidime with or without vancomycin vs. cepahlothin, carbenicillin and gentamicin as initial therapy of the febrile neutropenic pediatric cancer patient. Pediatr Infect Dis J 1988; 7:165–170.
31. Rubin M, Pizzo PA. Monotherapy for empirical management of febrile neutropenic patients. NCI Monogr 1990;9:111–116.
32. Gutmann L, Williamson R, Kitzic MD, Acar JF. Synergism and antagonism in double beta-lactam antibiotic combinations. Am J Med 1986;80(suppl 5C):21–29.
33. Attal M, Schlaifer D, Rubie H, et al. Prevention of gram-positive infections after bone marrow transplantation by systemic vancomycin: a prospective, randomized trial. J Clin Oncol 1991;9:865–870.
34. Shenep J, Hughes WT, Roberson PK, et al. Vancomycin, ticarcillin, and amikacin compared with ticarcillin-clavulanate and amikacin in the empirical treatment of febrile, neutropenic children with cancer. N Engl J Med 1988;319:1053–1058.
35. EORTC International Antimicrobial Therapy Cooperative Group, NCI of Canada. Vancomycin added to empirical combination antibiotic therapy for fever in granulocytopenic cancer patients. J Infect Dis 1991; 163:951–958.
36. Schwalbe RS, Stapleton JT, Gilligan PH. Emergence of vancomycin resistance in coagulase-negative staphylococci. N Engl J Med 1988;316:927–931.
37. Pizzo PA, Robichaud RN, Gill FA, et al. Empiric antibiotic and antifungal therapy for cancer patients with prolonged fever and granulocytopenia. Am J Med 1982;72:101–110.
38. EORTC International Antimicrobial Therapy Cooperative Group. Empiric antifungal therapy in febrile granulocytopenic patients. Am J Med 1989;86:668–672.
39. Saral R. Candida and aspergillus infections in immunocompromised patients: an overview. Rev Infect Dis 1991;13:487–492.
40. Horn R, Wong B, Kiehn TE, Armstrong D. Fungemia in a cancer hospital: changing frequency, earlier onset, and results of therapy. Rev Infect Dis 1985;7:646–655.

41. Karp JE, Burch PA, Merz WG. An approach to intensive antileukemia therapy in patients with previous invasive aspergillosis. Am J Med 1988;85:203–206.
42. Burch PA, Karp JE, Merz WG, et al. Favorable outcome of invasive aspergillosis in patients with acute leukemia. J Clin Oncol 1987;5:1985–1993.
43. Polak-Wyss A. Protective effect of human granulocyte colony stimulating factor (hG-CSF) on *Candida* infections in normal and immunosuppressed mice. Mycoses 1991;34:109–118.
44. Robinson PA, Knirsch AK, Joseph JA. Flucoazole for life threatening fungal infections in patients who cannot be treated with conventional antifungal agents. Rev Infect Dis 1990;12(suppl 3):S349–S363.
45. Kauffman CA, Bradley SF, Ross SC, Weber DR. Hepatosplenic Candidiasis: successful treatment with fluconazole. Am J Med 1991;91:137–141.
46. Anaissie E, Bodey GP, Kantarjian H, et al. Fluconazole therapy for chronic disseminated candidiasis in patients with leukemia and prior amphotericin B therapy. Am J Med 1991;91:142–150.
47. Walsh TJ, Schizuko A, Mechinaud F, et al. Effects of preventive, early, and late antifungal chemotherapy with fluconazole in different granulocytopenic models of experimental disseminated candidiasis. J Infect Dis 1990;161:755–760.
48. Nemunaitis J, Meyers JD, Buckner CD, et al. Phase I trial of recombinant human macrophage colony-stimulating factor in patients with invasive fungal infections. Blood 1991;78:907–913.
49. Van't Wout JW, Novakova I, Verhagen CAH, Fibbe WE, De Pauw BE, van der Meer JWM. The efficacy of itraconazole against systemic fungal infections in neutropenic patients: a randomized comparative study with amphotericin B. J Infect 1991;22:45–52.
50. Denning DW, Tucker RM, Hanson LH, et al. Treatment of invasive aspergillosis with itraconazole. Am J Med 1989;86:791–800.
51. De Beule K, De Donker P, Cauwenbergh G, et al. The treatment of aspergillosis and aspergilloma with itraconazole, clinical results of an open international study (1982–1987). Mycoses 1988;31:476–485.
52. Lopez-Berenstein G, Bodey GP, Fainstein V, et al. Treatment of systemic fungal infections with liposomal amphotericin B. Arch Intern Med 1989;149:2533–2536.
53. Lopez-Berestein G, Bodey GP, Frankel LS, et al. Treatment of hepatosplenic candidiasis with liposomal-amphotericin B. J Clin Oncol 1987;5:310–317.
54. Clift RA, Sanders JE, Thomas ED, et al. Granulocyte transfusions for the prevention of infection in patients receiving bone marrow transfusions. N Engl J Med 1978;298:1052–1057.
55. Ruther RL, Anderson B, Cunningham BL, et al. Efficacy of granulocyte transfusions in the control of systemic candidiasis in the leukopenic host. Blood 1981;52:493–498.
56. Winston D, Ho WG, Young LS. Prophylactic granulocyte transfusions during human bone marrow transplantation. Am J Med 1980;68:893–899.
57. Bernard GR, Grossman JE, Campbell GD. Multicenter trial of a monoclonal anti-endotoxin antibody (Xomen-E5) in gram negative sepsis. Chest 1989;96:137S.
58. Ziegler EJ, Fisher CJ Jr, Sprung CL, et al. Treatment of gram-negative bacteremia and septic shock with HA-1A human monoclonal antibody against endotoxin—a randomized, double-blind, placebo-controlled trial. N Engl J Med 1991;324:429–436.
59. Armstrong D. Symposium on infectious complications of neoplastic disease (part II): protected environments are discomforting and expensive and do not offer meaningful protection. Am J Med 1984;76:685–689.
60. Bodey GP. Symposium on infectious complications of neoplastic disease (part II): current status of prophylaxis of infection with protected environments. Am J Med 1984;76:678–684.
61. Nauseef WM, Maki DG. A study of the value of simple protective isolation in patients with granulocytopenia. N Engl J Med 1981;304:448–453.
62. Navari RM, Buckner CD, Clift RA, et al. Prophylaxis of infection in patients with aplastic anemia receiving allogeneic marrow transplants. Am J Med 1984;76:564–572.
63. Sherertz RJ, Belani A, Kramer BS, et al. Impact of air filtration on nosocomial Aspergillus infections: unique risk of bone marrow transplant recipients. Am J Med 1987;83:709–718.
64. Schimpff SC, Hahn DM, Brouillet MD, Young VM, Fortner CL, Wiernik PH. Comparison of basic infection prevention techniques, with standard room reverse isolation or with reverse isolaton plus added air infiltration. Leuk Res 1978;2:231–240.
65. Buckner CD, Clift RA, Sanders JE, et al. Protective environment for marrow transplant recipients. A prospective study. Ann Intern Med 1978;89:893–901.
66. Arnow PM, Anderson RL, Mainous PD, Smith EJ. Pulmonary aspergillosis during hospital renovation. Am Rev Respir Dis 1978;118:49–53.
67. Wingard JR, Dick JD, Charache P, Saral R. Antibiotic-resistant bacteria in surveillance stool cultures of patients with prolonged neutropenia. Antimicrob Agents Chemother 1986;30:435–439.
68. Walsh TJ. Role of surveillance cultures in prevention and treatment of fungal infections. NCI Monogr 1990;9:43–45.
69. Aisner J, Murillo J, Schimpff SC, et al. Invasive aspergillosis in acute leukemia: correlation with nose cultures and antibiotic use. Ann Intern Med 1979;90:4–9.
70. Haupt HM, Merz WG, Beschorner WE, et al. Colonization and infection with *Trichosporon* species in the immunosuppressed host. J Infect Dis 1983;147:199–203.
71. Schimpff SC. Surveillance cultures. NCI Monogr 1990;9:37–42.
72. Walsh TJ, Newman KR, Moody M, et al. Trichosporonosis in patients with neoplastic disease. Medicine 1986;65:268–279.
73. Levine AS, Siegel SE, Schreiber AD, et al. Protected environments and prophylactic antibiotics: a prospective controlled study of their utility in the therapy of acute leukemia. N Engl J Med 1973;288:477–484.
74. King K. Prophylactic non-absorbant antibiotics in leukaemic patients. J Hyg (Camb) 1980;85:141–151.
75. Dekker AW, Rozenberg-Arska M, Sixma JJ, et al. Prevention of infection by trimethoprim-sulfamethoxaxole plus amphotericin B in patients with acute nonlymphocytic leukemia. Ann Intern Med 1981;95:555–559.
76. Gualtieri RJ, Donowitz GR, Kaiser DL, et al. Double-blind randomized study of prophylactic trimethoprim-sulfamethoxazole in granulocytopenic patients with hematologic malignancies. Am J Med 1983;74:934–940.
77. Gurwith MJ, Brunton JL, Lank BA, et al. A prospective controlled investigation of prophylactic trimethoprim-sulfamethoxazole in hospitalized granulocytopenic patients. Am J Med 1979;66:248–256.
78. Murray BE, Rensimer ER, DuPont HL. Emergence of high-level trimethoprim resistance in fecal Escherichia

coli during oral administration of trimethoprim or trimethoprim-sulfamethoxazole. N Engl J Med 1982; 306:130–135.
79. Wilson JM, Guiney DG. Failure of oral trimethoprim-sulfamethoxazole prophylaxis in acute leukemia. N Engl J Med 1982;306:16–20.
80. Dekker AW, Rozenberg-Arska M, Verhoef J. Infection prophylaxis in acute leukemia: a comparison of ciprofloxacin with trimethoprim-sulfamethoxazole and colistin. Ann Intern Med 1987;106:7–12.
81. Karp JE, Merz WG, Hendricksen C, et al. Oral norfloxacin for prevention of gram-negative bacterial infections in patients with acute leukemia and granulocytopenia. Ann Intern Med 1987;106:1–7.
82. Winston DJ, Ho WG, Nakao SL, Gale RP, Champlin RE. Norfloxacin versus vancomycin/polymyxin for prevention of infections in granulocytopenic patients. Am J Med 1986;80:884–889.
83. Bow EJ, Rayner E, Louie TJ. Comparison of norfloxacin with cotrimoxazole for infectious prophylaxis in acute leukemia. Am J Med 1988;84:847–854.
84. Sullivan KM, Kopecky K, Jocom J, et al. Immunomodulatory and antimicrobial efficacy of intravenous immunoglobulin in bone marrow transplantation. N Engl J Med 1990;323:705–712.
85. Sullivan KM, Dahlberg S, Storb R, et al. Infection prophylaxis with chronic graft-versus-host disease. Exp Hematol 1983;11(suppl 14);193.
86. Sullivan KM, Kopecky K, Witherspoon RP, et al. Intravenous immunoglobulin (IVIg) for prevention of late infections after bone marrow transplantation (BMT) (abstract). Exp Hematol 1990;18:689.
87. Dick JD, Merz WG, Saral R. Incidence of polyene-resistant yeasts recovered from clinical specimens. Antimicrob Agents Chemother 1980;18:158–163.
88. Merz WG, Sandford GR. Isolation and characterization of a polyene-resistant variant of *Candida tropicalis*. J Clin Microbiol 1979;9:677–680.
89. Dick JD, Rosengard BR, Merz WG, et al. Fatal disseminated Candidiasis due to amphotericin-B-resistant *Candida guilliermondii*. Ann Intern Med 1985;102:67–68.
90. Conly J, Rennie R, Johnson J, Farah S, Hellman L. Disseminated Candidiasis due to amphotericin B-resistant *Candida albicans*. J Infect Dis 1992;165:761–768.
91. Tam JY, Blume KG, Prober CG. Fluconazole and *Candida krusei* fungemia (letter). N Engl J Med 1992;325:1315.
92. Perfect JR, Klotman ME, Gilbert CC, et al. Prophylactic intravenous amphotericin B in neutropenic autologous bone marrow transplant recipients. J Infect Dis 1992;165:891–897.
93. O'Donnell MR, Schmidt GM, Tegtmeier B, et al. Prophylactic low dose amphotericin B (AM-B) decreases systemic fungal infection (SFT) in allogeneic bone marrow transplant (BMT) recipients. Blood 1990;76(Suppl 1):558.
94. Benhamou E, Hartmann O, Nogues C, Maraninchi D, Valteau D, Lemerie J. Does ketoconazole prevent fungal infections in children treated with high dose chemotherapy and bone marrow transplantation? Results of a randomized placebo-controlled trial. Bone Marrow Transplant 1991;7:127–131.
95. Walsh TJ, Rubin M, Hathorn J, et al. Amphotericin B vs high-dose ketoconazole for empirical antifungal therapy among febrile, granulocytopeinic cancer patients. Arch Intern Med 1991;151:765–770.
96. Fainstein V, Bodey GP, Elting L, et al. Amphotericin B or ketoconazole therapy of fungal infections in neutropenic cancer patients. Antimicrob Agents Chemother 1987;31:11–15.
97. Wingard JR, Vaughan WP, Braine HG, et al. Prevention of fungal sepsis in patients with prolonged neutropenia: a randomized, double-blind, placebo-controlled trial of intravenous miconazole. Am J Med 1987;83: 1103–1110.
98. Milliken S, Helenglass G, Powles R. Fluconazole pharmacokinetics following oral dosage in leukemic patients receiving autologous bone marrow transplantation. Bone Marrow Transplant 1988;3(suppl 1):324–325.
99. Goodman JL, Winston DJ, Greenfield RA. A controlled trial of fluconazole to prevent fungal infections in patients undergoing bone marrow transplantation. N Engl J Med 1992;326:845–851.
100. Winston DJ, Islam Z, Beull DN, Acute Leukemia Study Group. Fluconazole prophylaxis of fungal infections in acute leukemia patients: results of a placebo-controlled double-blind, multicenter trial. Program and Abstracts of the 31st International Conference on Antimicrobial Agents and Chemotherapy, Chicago, Sept 29–Oct 2, 1991; Washington DC: American Society of Microbiology, 1991. 99.
101. Brammer KW. Management of fungal infection in neutropenic patients with fluconazole. Hematol Bluttransfus 1990;33:546–550.
102. Kruger HU, Schuler U, Zimmerman R, Ehninger G. No severe drug interaction of fluconazole, a triazole antifungal agent, with cyclosporin. Bone Marrow Transplant 1988;3(suppl 1):271.
103. Wingard JR, Merz WG, Rinaldi MG, Johnson TR, Karp JE, Saral R. Increase in *Candida krusei* infection among patients with bone marrow transplantation and neutropenia treated prophylactically with fluconazole. N Engl J Med 1991;325:1274–1277.
104. Persons DA, Laughlin M, Tanner D, Perfect J, Gockerman JP, Hathorn JW. Fluconazole and *Candida krusei* fungemia. N Engl J Med 1991;325:1315.
105. Tricot G, Joosten E, Boogaerts MA, Pitte JV, Cauwenbergh G. Ketoconazole vs itraconazole for antifungal prophylaxis in patients with severe granulocytopenia; preliminary results of two nonrandomized studies. Rev Infect Dis 1987;9(suppl 1):S94–S99.
106. Robertson MJ, Larson RA. Recurrent fungal pneumonias in patients with acute nonlymphocytic leukemia undergoing multiple courses of intensive chemotherapy. Am J Med 1988;84:233–239.
107. Cushing D, Bustamante C, Devlin A. Finley R, Wade J. Aspergillus infection prophylaxis: amphotericin B (AB) nose spray, a double-blind trial. Program and Abstracts of the International Conference on Antimicrobial Agents and Chemotherapy, Chicago, Sept 29–Oct 2, 1991:222.
108. Boogaerts MA, Verhoef GE, Zachee P, Demuynck H, Verbist L, De Beule K. Antifungal prophylaxis with itraconazole in prolonged neutropenia: correlation with plasma levels. Mycoses 1989;32(suppl 1):103–108.
109. Graham-Pole J, Casper CJ, Elfenbein G, et al. Intravenous immunoglobulin may lessen all forms of infection in patients receiving allogeneic bone marrow transplantation for acute lymphoblastic leukemia: a pediatric oncology group study. Bone Marrow Transplant 1988;3:559–566.
110. Petersen FB, Bowden RA, Thornquist M, et al. The effect of prophylactic intravenous immune globulin on the incidence of septicemia in marrow transplant recipients. Bone Marrow Transplant 1987;2:141–148.

Chapter 28
Cytomegalovirus Infection

John A. Zaia

In memory of Joel D. Meyers, MD, who was present at the beginning, and by his labor and his intellect wrote the significant bibliography defining cytomegalovirus infection in marrow transplantation.

The sequential occurrence of different specific infections after bone marrow transplantation (BMT) is well described (1) and is the basis for certain management decisions after transplantation (2,3). Foremost among these infectious complications are those associated with human cytomegalovirus (CMV). In the setting of allogeneic BMT, CMV infection will develop in approximately 70 to 80% of recipients (4–8). The timing of this infection, in the period of 28 to 72 days after BMT, is remarkably similar among the population of persons receiving either solid organ or marrow allografts. Yet, the syndromes associated with CMV infection are principally different in the BMT setting because of the associated pulmonary disease and its high morbidity and mortality. Unlike many virus infections, which have a limited but consistent presentation of disease, CMV can target a variety of organs with infection but remain unexplainedly nonsymptomatic in some persons, whereas in others producing severe effects. Although this virus infection remains incompletely understood, there is sufficient information to recognize a complexity of biological and clinical issues that form the basis for current and future approaches to this problem. It is important for both transplant physicians managing patients and for students and other interested medical personnel involved in BMT to appreciate the various aspects of the problem posed by CMV. Thus, this chapter reviews the important virological basis for understanding CMV, the theoretical considerations relating to CMV immunology and pathogenesis, and the clinical approaches to diagnosis, prevention, and management of CMV in BMT recipients.

Virology and Epidemiology of CMV

Structure of Human CMV

CMV is classified as a beta herpesvirus, which groups it with those herpesviruses that have a restricted host range, a relatively long reproductive cycle, and a consequent slow progression of infection (9). CMV is a DNA virus that has the typical herpes virion structure consisting of (1) a core containing a linear, double-stranded DNA; (2) a delta-icosahedral capsid (approximately 150 nm diameter) containing 162 capsomeres; (3) an amorphic, asymmetrical material surrounding the capsid and designated the tegument or the matrix; and (4) an envelope containing viral glycoproteins on its surface. As shown in Figure 28-1, CMV infection in vitro is associated with intact herpesvirus particles, defective virions, and CMV-dense bodies. Only the intact virions are thought to be infectious; the defective particles and the viral dense bodies contain nucleocapsid and matrix viral proteins. The clinical significance of defective virions in the CMV-associated syndromes is unknown. The genomic size of the DNA is approximately 240 kilobase pairs, which is the largest of the known herpesviruses (10). This large genome is thought to encode nearly 200 proteins based on an analysis of open reading frames (11), but only a few of these proteins have been characterized. A more detailed virological description of CMV is beyond the scope of this chapter, and interested readers are referred to recent reviews of this subject (12,13).

Immune Response to CMV Infection

Humoral Immunity to CMV

Despite the many potential polypeptides encoded in the CMV genome, only a small number of proteins and glycoproteins are known to be recognized by the immune system (14) (Figure 28-2). Neutralizing antibody is directed toward the surface glycoproteins, principally the gB and gH herpesvirus homologs. In nature, the discrete glycoproteins noted in Figure 28-2 exist as molecular complexes gcI, gcII, and gcIII (15). In marrow recipients, the humoral immune response to CMV has been described and is the same as that observed in normal persons with predominant antibody responses to gB, gH, pp65, and the capsid proteins (16) (see Figure 28-2). In general, antibody to herpesvirus infections can prevent or significantly control primary virus infection (17), and it is likely that this is true with CMV, because intravenous immune globulin (IVIg) used in passive immunization of marrow recipient has been reported to modify the

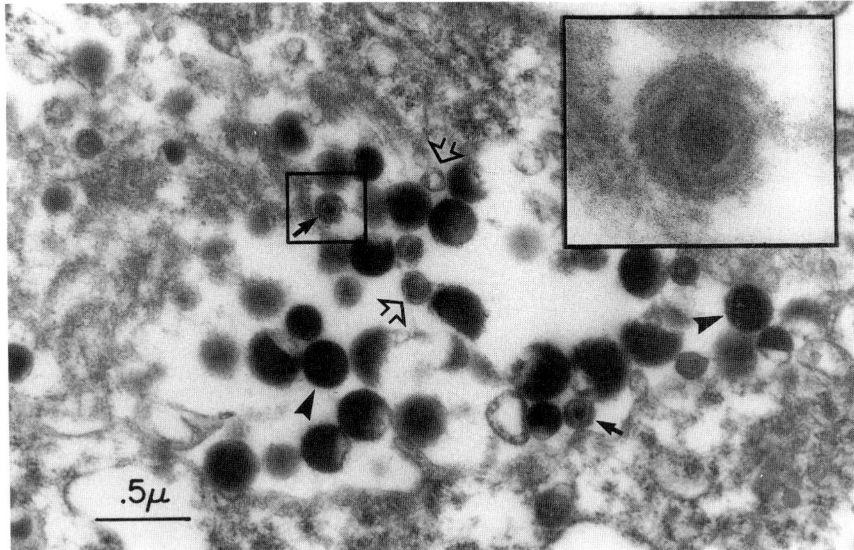

Figure 28-1. Electron micrograph of cytomegalovirus (CMV) virions and defective particles. CMV-infected human foreskin fibroblasts were subjected to glutaraldehyde and osmium tetroxide fixation and electron microscopy, revealing intact virions (*solid arrows*), defective virions (*open arrows*), and dense bodies (*arrowheads*). (×38,750; inset, ×182,500.) (Photomicrograph prepared by John Hardy, City of Hope National Medical Center.)

incidence of CMV infection in CMV-seronegative allograft recipients; however, this effect is controversial (for detailed discussion, see "Use of Immunoglobulin in BMT"). In marrow allograft recipients with CMV infection, however, there is no clear evidence that CMV-specific antibody protects from severe disease, although specific antibody production might well serve as a marker for overall immune responsiveness to this infection. In the earliest experience with CMV-associated interstitial penumonia (CMV-IP) in marrow allograft recipients, the most serious occurrence of disease was seen in the group having minimal antibody response to CMV (18). Subsequent studies of pretransplant CMV antibody levels have not substantiated a protective effect; in fact, pretransplant CMV antibody titers are generally linked to risk for subsequent CMV infection (8,19). In the analysis of polypeptide-specific CMV antibody response in marrow allograft recipients with and without CMV-IP, Zaia and colleagues (16) reported a variable response in patients. BMT recipients who reacted with a wide range of protein-specific antibody generally had an uncomplicated course of CMV infection, and several patients with severe CMV-IP had a narrow range of antibody response. However, patients with a poor polypeptide-specific antibody response had an uncomplicated course of infection, and fatal CMV-IP developed in others with antibody to multiple CMV proteins. Thus, although CMV antibody might have some role in the control of CMV infection, it has not been found to be essential for recovery.

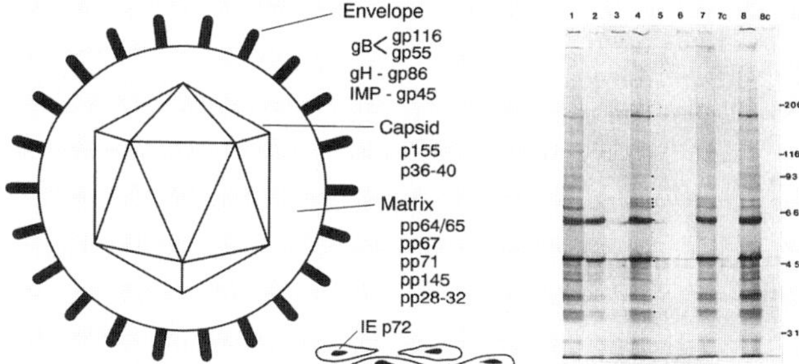

Figure 28-2. Immunologically significant proteins of cytomegalovirus (CMV). (*Left*) The CMV virion and infected cells showing the viral immediate-early protein (IEp72) and structural proteins of the viral envelope, the matrix (tegument), and the nucleocapsid. The numbers refer to the relative molecular mass for glycoproteins (gp) and phosphoproteins (pp); two herpesvirus protein homologs are represented as gB and gH; and the immediate-early membrane protein (IMP) is shown. (*Right*) Radioimmunoprecipitation using normal sera (lanes 1–8) reacted with lysate from ^{14}C-labeled, CMV-infected human fibroblasts or with uninfected control cell lysate (c). (Modified with permission from Zaia JA. Epidemiology and pathogenesis of cytomegalovirus disease. Semin Hematol 1990; 27:5–10; and Zaia JA, Forman SJ, Ting Y-P, et al. Polypeptide-specific antibody response to human cytomegalovirus after infection in bone marrow transplant recipients. J Infect Dis 1986; 153:780–787.)

Cellular Immunity of CMV

It has been shown that cytotoxic T-lymphocyte (CTL) function is most critical for protection from severe disease and mortality in the setting of BMT. It was recognized, in work by Meyers and associates (20), that CMV-specific cellular immunity was suppressed in marrow recipients with CMV infection. Quinnan and colleagues (21,22) initially demonstrated that CMV-specific, human leukocyte antigen (HLA)-restricted CTL function was associated with survival from CMV-IP in this patient population. More recently, the role of virus-specific CTLs was confirmed by Reusser and coworkers (23) in an analysis of allograft recipients with and without CMV-IP. The role of specific CMV proteins in the induction of CTL function in humans was first described by Borysiewicz and associates (24), who demonstrated that nonvirion, immediate-early proteins of CMV, as well as the virion envelope glycoprotein, gB, could induce CTL immunity. In addition, it has been shown that a cellular immune response exists to the internal matrix protein, pp65 (25), and to the gcI to III glycoprotein complexes (26). Of interest, the matrix protein induces CTL, and this CTL response can occur in the absence of active virus replication (27). Clearly, there is an immune response that recognizes structural CMV proteins that are processed and presented by CMV-infected cells without any requirement for viral gene expression (28). This response is similar in other virus infections, in which internal proteins of the virus can be processed and presented to the T-cell system (29–30). The persistence of viral antigens, in the absence of continued viral replication, could thus serve as a stimulus for cellular-mediated immunity in the human host with chronic CMV infection. This subject deserves attention, which is beyond the scope of this chapter, and interested readers are referred elsewhere (31).

Immunization for CMV

Passive immunization with antibody to CMV has been studied extensively in the marrow allograft population, and this topic is discussed later (see "Use of Immunoglobulin in BMT"). Adoptive cellular immunotherapy, utilizing CTLs that are reactive to specific CMV proteins, has recently been proposed as a method for protection of marrow allograft recipients (32). In this approach, donor CD8+ class I major histocompatibility complex (MHC)-restricted CMV-specific CTLs are cloned, expanded in the presence of CMV-antigens plus interleukin-2, and administered to the recipient. The safety and efficacy of this form of passive immunization is currently under investigation. Adoptive immunotherapy has the potential to inhibit post-transplantation virus activation in the absence of toxic antiviral agents, and for this reason it offers an exciting new preventive approach to CMV management. In addition, this method suggests an alternative approach—stimulation of CMV immunity in the donor and transfer to the recipient with the marrow at the time of BMT. It has been reported that some component of donor immunity to CMV is transferred to the recipient (33). In this study, Boland and colleagues demonstrated that among CMV-seropositive allograft recipients, those receiving marrow from CMV-seropositive donors had an earlier lymphocyte proliferative response to CMV than those with seronegative marrow donors. It is not clear whether CTL function is augmented by CMV-seropositive marrow, and clearly CMV disease occurs in this setting. Nevertheless, in the future, it will be important to determine if some degree of protection from CMV could be afforded by immunization of the donor. In this regard, CMV vaccines are under development (34), and it has been shown that a live CMV vaccine does have a clinical effect in the setting of renal transplantation (35). The use of a live vaccine in marrow recipients, or even in donors just prior to BMT, is more problematic because of the potential for virus dissemination in immunosuppressed recipients. There is evidence that subunit viral preparations can induce immune responses to CMV (36), and the development of noninfectious CMV vaccines that utilize selected viral polypeptides could be feasible.

Characteristics of Virus Growth

From a clinical standpoint, a significant aspect of viral replication is the ability of the CMV genome to exist in cells in either a quiescent or an active state of transcription. In the active state of transcription, there is a sequential expression of 3 categories of genomic elements termed *major immediate early* (mIE), *early*, or *late viral proteins* (9,37,38). The mIE transcripts are transactivated by an incoming virion protein, the 71-kd tegument protein (39), in the absence of virion DNA replication, and these mIE gene products then regulate the synthesis of the "early" proteins, which facilitate viral DNA replication and can also affect host cell transcription. By 12 to 18 hours after infection, viral DNA replication occurs, and "late" proteins, derived from transcription of the newly synthesized DNA, are generated and assembled into the structural elements of the virion. The importance of this phenomenon to clinicians is that inhibition of viral DNA replication does not stop mIE transcription and, although it would restrict new virus production, it would not affect pathological processes mediated by mIE. Virus-induced cytopathology is present in vitro at times when only IE gene expression has occurred. During these times it has also been described that certain housekeeper proteins such as fibronectin have undergone down-regulation of transcription (40). Although the actual role of mIE in the pathogenesis of CMV disease is unknown, it is possible that a component of CMV pathology is contributed by these gene products. The ineffectiveness of CMV inhibitors, which act by blocking viral DNA replication, in the treatment of advanced CMV infection suggests that this concept might have clinical relevance.

CMV Latency

The term *latency* refers to the presence of viral genome in the absence of active production of infectious virus. Whether some transcriptional/translational activity is present in the latent state will not be considered herein, but readers are referred to discussions of this topic (12). For practical purposes, the diagnostic assays establish whether the infection is active (i.e., either the conventional tissue culture assay or the rapid centrifugal culture is positive for CMV, or late viral antigens are present in a clinical specimen). If the person under study is seronegative for CMV and has no detectible infectious virus, then it is assumed that there is no latent infection present. Conversely, the person with seropositivity for CMV antibody who has no detectible evidence for infectious virus is assumed to have a latent CMV infection. The evidence for latency of CMV is based on circumstantial evidence in humans in which virus infection follows tissue or cellular transfer, but latency is more solidly established in the murine model of CMV infection (41). Lymphoid cells from previously infected mice, which show no active viral infection, undergo activation of infection when cocultivated with allogeneic fibroblasts. It is likely, although not proven conclusively, that latency is nothing more than the functional absence of sufficient cellular transcriptional factors for permissive replication. Looked at from this standpoint, virus (re)activation to the permissive state involves induction of these transcription factors (12).

One of the frustrating aspects of understanding CMV latency has been localizing the tissue source of virus latency. In humans, virus transmission is well documented in blood transfusions, solid organ transplantation, and BMT (13). In these settings, cultures from specimen aliquots are negative for virus, but the specimen is nevertheless associated with subsequent infection in the recipient. Clinical observations have noted that transmission of virus by blood is relatively inefficient compared with transmission by solid organs such as kidney and heart (13). It is currently believed that stromal elements of most if not all solid organs harbor latent CMV infection and that these cells are transferred with the organ or, less frequently, with blood transfusions and thus serve as the vehicle for transmission of virus (42). As noted, actual activation of the virus within these cells may be dependent on metabolic activation of the cell, but this is not known. In the mouse, it has been shown that acute infection in the spleen is localized to the stromal elements, and there is evidence that this region of the spleen becomes negative for infectious virus but remains positive for CMV DNA (42,43). The cellular composition of this stroma is mixed and contains endothelial cells, fibroblasts, and cells that line the splenic sinusoids. It is possible that occurrence of these cells in the blood is the vehicle for transmission of CMV with transfusions, and similar marrow stromal elements could well have a role in CMV transmission during BMT.

Epidemiology of CMV Infection in Marrow Transplantation

Changing Pattern of CMV Epidemiology

The epidemiological description of CMV infection in the BMT population is among the best described and has established that CMV infection can originate from both endogenous and exogenous sources (19). Yet, because of differences in the incidence of infection or disease at different BMT centers, there is some confusion regarding the risks for infection and disease. Contributing to this confusion is the fact that the incidence of CMV infection in this population has changed over the past decade because of the major changes in patient management. The most important of these changes has been curtailment of CMV exposure via granulocyte transfusion therapy and CMV-seropositive blood product support in susceptible recipients. In addition, acyclovir prophylactic therapy and, more recently, ganciclovir prophylaxis has been instituted to decrease CMV infection. The declining prevalence of CMV-associated disease in certain centers has been documented (8).

The prevalence of CMV infection and disease is best described by the control groups from several blinded studies that attempted to alter the occurrence of CMV infection after BMT. Thus, the incidence of CMV infection in CMV-seronegative recipients of seronegative donor marrow has dropped to nearly 0% from 60 to 70% prior to the introduction of CMV-seronegative blood support (44–46). In CMV-seropositive recipients, the incidence of this infection has also varied through the 1980s and continues to change into the 1990s with the introduction of preventive chemotherapy (for detailed discussion, see "Clinical Approaches to Management of CMV").

CMV Infection Rate in Marrow Allograft Recipients—Early Experience

The first descriptions of CMV-associated disease in marrow allograft recipients appeared in the 1970s and described a relatively new disease: CMV-IP (18,47,48). Data from 3 separate centers collected in the 1970s and early 1980s are summarized in Table 28-1. CMV infection was very common but much more prevalent in CMV-seropositive recipients than in CMV-seronegative recipients. The rate of CMV disease also followed this pattern and, in the seropositive population was 15 to 25%. The most detailed analysis of CMV infection in marrow allograft recipients was made by Meyers and associates (49) and included a prospective assessment of infection in 545 patients studied between 1979 and 1982. Because it so accurately reflects the epidemiology of CMV in the period prior to effective intervention, the details of this study are worth reviewing. Evidence of CMV infection was present in 51.4% of patients with active virus cultured from 43.1%. CMV seroconversion was noted in 30.8% of patients. Among the infected patients, approximately 40% had virus recovered without undergoing antibody seroconversion, and an additional 16%

Table 28-1.
Incidence of CMV Infection—Early BMT Experience

Source, Year, Ref	*CMV Antibody Pre-BMT*[a]	*CMV Infection (%)*	*CMV Disease (%)*
Meyers, 1986 (49)	No	102/285 (36)	30/285 (11)
	Yes	178/258 (69)	60/258 (23)
Miller, 1986 (5)	No	26/137 (19)	12/137 (9)
	Yes	28/44 (64)	11/44 (25)
Wingard, 1988 (6)	No	15/115 (13)	1/115 (1)
	Yes	97/232 (42)	37/232 (16)

[a]CMV antibody status of recipient before BMT.
CMV = cytomegalovirus; BMT = bone marrow transplantation.

underwent seroconversion without isolation of virus. The median time to infection in throat and urine was 54 and 59 days, respectively, after BMT. The excretion of virus and seroconversion was significantly associated with the serological status of recipients and donors prior to BMT. The incidence of CMV infection among seronegative patients was significantly increased by the use of a seropositive marrow donor (26 vs 53%; $p < 0.001$). This risk factor for CMV infection persisted when other seropositive blood support was used in seronegative BMT recipients. This finding underlines the importance of the donor marrow in contributing to an exogenous source of CMV infection. In seropositive BMT recipients, CMV infection was significantly more common (69 vs 28%) and was not affected by the serology of the marrow donor nor by use of CMV-seropositive blood support. Excretion of virus but not seroconversion increased significantly with increasing age. When age and serological status were considered, the age effect was observed only for CMV excretion among seronegative patients. Excretion of CMV was highest among recipients transplanted for acute myeloblastic leukemia (AML), which was again related to the increased proportion of CMV-seropositive patients in the group with AML.

The most striking differences between past and current CMV epidemiology is apparent when the attack rates are analyzed by both donor and recipient pre-BMT serology (Table 28-2). As noted, CMV-seronegative recipients of marrow from seronegative donors would now be expected to be at minimum risk for CMV infection (44–46). As noted, this is attributable to the control of exogenous CMV exposure. In the early experience, however, this group had an infection rate as high as or even higher than those with prior CMV infection. Thus, prior to 1985, CMV disease occurred at a higher rate in seronegative recipients, in marked contrast to current observations.

Table 28-2.
Incidence of CMV Infection in Marrow Allograft Recipients by Donor/Recipient CMV Serology[a]

Source, Year, Ref	*CMV Antibody In Donor*	*CMV Antibody in Recipient (%)*	
		Yes	*No*
Meyers, 1986 (49)	No	81/118 (69)	58/208 (28)
	Yes	97/140 (69)	44/77 (57)
Miller, 1986 (5)	No	15/21 (71)	20/107 (19)
	Yes	13/23 (57)	6/30 (20)

[a]CMV antibody determination prior to BMT.
CMV = cytomegalovirus; BMT = bone marrow transplantation.

CMV Infection Rates in Allograft Recipients—Recent Experience

Currently, virtually every BMT center has its own distinct patient population and management approaches, and the incidences of CMV infection and disease appear to vary considerably between centers. To determine the current true incidence of CMV infection and disease, the rates recorded in the control arms of clinical trials of various agents used in allograft populations were tabulated (Table 28-3),

Table 28-3.
Incidence of CMV Infection and Disease—Recent BMT Experience[a]

Source, Year, Ref	*CMV Antibody in Recipient Pretransplantation*	*Infection (%)*	*Time*	*Disease*	*Time*
Bowden, 1986 (50)	No	8/20 (40)	d56	3/20 (15)	d58
Winston, 1987 (51)	No	21/37 (57)	d53	17/37 (46)	d52
Sullivan, 1990[b] (46)	No	1/58 (2)	NA	0/61 (0)	NA
De Witte, 1990[c] (52)	No	0/28 (0)	NA	0/28 (0)	NA
Bowden, 1991 (53)	No	26/60 (43)	d54	12/60 (20)	d60
Bowden, 1991 (44)	No	7/30 (23)	d59	2/30 (7)	NP
Miller, 1991 (45)	No	21/61 (34)	NP	3/55 (5)	NP
Meyers, 1988 (54)	Yes	49/65 (75)	d40	20/65 (31)	NP
Sullivan, 1990 (46)	Yes	NP (50)	NP	67/308 (22)	NP
De Witte, 1990 (52)	Yes	42/48 (86)	NP	10/48 (21)	NP
Schmidt, 1991 (55)	Yes	56/104 (54)[d]	d35	30/84 (36)	d51
Goodrich, 1991 (56)	Yes	107/194 (55)	d40	15/35 (43)	NP
Goodrich, 1992 (57)	Yes	14/31 (45)	NP	9/31 (29)	NP

[a]Results include only control groups from these clinical trials, except for De Witte (1990), which was a prospective but uncontrolled study, and Schmidt (1991) and Goodrich (1991), in which CMV infection data was collected prior to therapy and hence includes all patients.
[b]Data from the subgroup of subjects who were CMV-seronegative recipients of a CMV-seronegative donor marrow and who received CMV-seronegative blood support.
[c]Study includes only CMV-seronegative recipients receiving leukocyte-poor blood support.
[d]Study includes only CMV-infection rate for bronchoalveolar lavage specimens.
CMV = cytomegalovirus; BMT = bone marrow transplantation; NA = does not apply; NP = data not provided in source document.

including data from 5 centers and separating marrow recipients into those with and without pretransplant CMV antibody. Again, rates of infection and disease were high in the 1980s (50,51) but decreased dramatically after introduction of CMV-negative blood support (46,52). Even in the latter part of the 1980s, the control groups that did not receive selected blood support had high infection rates, suggesting that other anticancer or anti-GVHD management regimen changes did not account for the decrease in CMV attack rates (44,45,51,53).

For CMV-seropositive recipients, infection rates remained as high as ever, if not higher. Attack rates ranged from 45 to 86%, and prevalence rates for CMV disease ranged from 21 to 43% (46, 52, 54–57). Clearly, the problem of CMV infection currently exists only in recipients at risk for secondary or reactive CMV. For this reason, attempts to protect this population focus on methods to inhibit reactivation of the virus, which is discussed in detail later (see "Clinical Approaches to Management of CMV").

CMV Infection Rates in Autologous/Syngeneic Recipients

Wingard and colleagues (58) reported that the incidence of CMV infection in a cohort of 143 autologous marrow recipients was 45%, which is similar to the infection rate in the allogeneic setting. However, there was a 2% rate of CMV disease occurrence, suggesting that pathogenesis is a function of alloreactivity. In this study, it was noted that the incidence of CMV-IP was not different than that of allograft recipients having no acute GVHD. Reusser and associates (59) also studied the epidemiology of CMV in autologous marrow recipients and noted a CMV disease rate of approximately 10% in this same population. Thus, although the presence of an allograft contributes to the development of CMV-IP, there remains a risk for CMV-IP even in marrow autograft recipients. In contrast, Appelbaum and co-workers (60) reported on the incidence of CMV infection and disease in 100 recipients of syngeneic transplantation, and, although the incidence of infection approached that seen in allograft recipients, the occurrence of CMV disease was rare.

Exogenous Versus Endogenous Source of CMV

A question frequently raised concerns the strain of CMV that occurs in BMT recipients: Does this CMV originate from the patient, from the donor, or from the blood product support used in patient management? It is recognized that most CMV isolates are different, based on genetic polymorphism analyses (11,12,61). These genetic polymorphisms occur throughout the entire CMV genome, and, as a result, although the restriction endonuclease profiles of various CMV strains show many similarities, no two strains are identical unless they are related epidemiologically (e.g., mother-to-infant or blood-donor-to-patient transmissions) (62–64).

Human CMV genomes are colinear and have at least 80% sequence homology (11,12); however, when specific coding regions are compared, certain strains have as little as 40% sequence identity. Despite this diversity, there have been no significant biological differences described among the human CMV strains. Of importance clinically, however, is that repeated infection can occur with different strains of CMV in one person, and, for immunodeficient persons, it has been shown that multiple strains of CMV can be present at the same time (65). In the marrow allograft setting, recipients can have multiple strains present in urine and blood simultaneously, and a strain can be present in lung tissue which is different from that in the urine (66). In this regard, the question arises whether the strain of CMV originates from donor or recipient.

The study by Winston and associates (67) demonstrated in 4 marrow allograft recipients, from whom isolates were obtained prior to BMT, that the CMV isolated subsequently was similar to the original CMV type in 2 patients and different in 2. It is likely that CMV can infect and cause serious disease from either an endogenous or an exogenous source. The experience of Miller and colleagues (45) in CMV-seronegative recipients of seropositive donor marrow, who received no other CMV-seropositive blood support yet had a similar CMV infection rate as those receiving CMV-seropositive blood support, indicates that the marrow itself is a significant source of CMV.

In summary, the source of CMV, as a problem in BMT, varies. In susceptible (i.e., CMV-seronegative) recipients, the source is either the donor marrow, the blood product support, or both. In CMV-seropositive recipients, the source of virus can be endogenous or donor marrow, although other sources such as blood product support cannot be ruled out as sources of infection.

Diagnosis of CMV Infection

Conventional Methods of CMV Detection

As its name implies, the conventional method for detection of CMV involves observation of the cytopathogenic effects in tissue culture or in tissue specimens. Interested readers are referred to technological references that describe the methods for culturing CMV from clinical specimens (68). In general, the CMV mIE proteins are used as a marker for infection, because these proteins are present within hours of culture and even in the absence of permissive virus replication. CMV mIE antigens are located in the nucleus, and detection of these gene products provides a ready means for rapid detection of infectious virus. Using this approach (Figure 28-3), the rapid centrifugal culture method has become a valuable diagnostic test for CMV infection (69–71). This method is conventionally referred to as "the shell vial" method, an allusion to the original tissue culture vials used for centrifugal inoculation of the specimen onto the

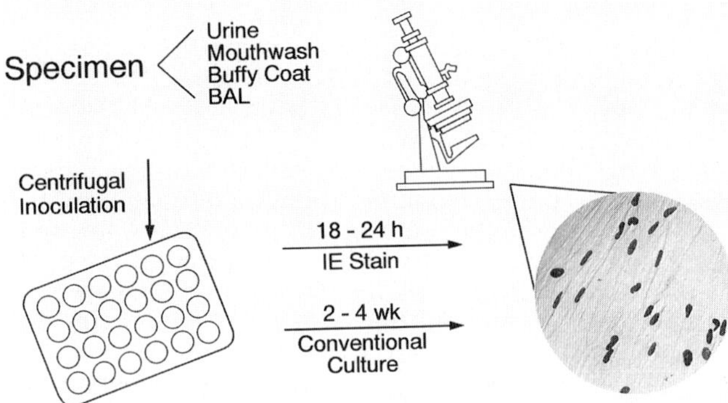

Figure 28-3. Laboratory detection of infectious cytomegalovirus (CMV). Shown are the rapid centrifugal and conventional tissue culture methods for detection of infectious CMV in clinical specimens. The photomicrograph shows MRC5 human lung fibroblasts stained with immunoperoxidase and monoclonal antibody to the major immediate early protein (mIE p72). (×640)

monolayer of tissue culture cells on the bottom of the vial. As currently applied in many laboratories, assays are performed in microtiter plates, which permits efficient processing of multiple specimens. Conventional long-term (2–4 wk) culture in human fibroblast monolayer tissue culture is used as a backup for this test and remains the standard for evaluating all other methods (68).

With regard to the comparative sensitivity of these two virus isolation methods, there are reports indicating that the rapid, centrifugal method is as good or better than conventional culture methods in terms of sensitivity (72–74), but if the specimen itself is likely to be toxic to the cell monolayer, such as occurs with white blood cell specimens, then the rapid method is less sensitive than conventional tissue culture (75–77). Thus, it is recommended that both methods be used for diagnostic evaluation of certain specimens (73). However, the longer time of performance is a major impediment to use of conventional culture in evaluation of acutely ill patients. Thus, because of its reliability in fluid specimens such as urine, mouthwash, and bronchoalveolar lavage, the rapid CMV centrifugal culture has become the mainstay of the CMV diagnostic laboratory.

Newer Methods of CMV Detection

Detection of CMV Antigen in Blood

As indicated, virus isolation takes time and can produce significant delay in diagnosis. Therefore, supplemental assays are being used that directly detect viral antigens or DNA in clinical specimens and provide more rapid methods for detection of CMV. It is recognized from in vitro studies that within 2 hours after CMV infection, an early/late matrix protein of CMV (pp65) is present in the nuclei of infected cells (12). This is believed to result from nucleotropic localization of pp65 from incoming virions. This same viral protein is found in the nuclei of peripheral blood granulocytes in association with clinical CMV infection, and detection of this antigen is used to document early CMV dissemination in immunocompromised patients (Figure 28-4). This CMV "antigenemia" method was first described by van der Bij and associates (78) and utilizes monoclonal antibody staining of peripheral blood leukocytes. The initial reports of this method referred to this antigen as an immediate-early protein, implying that it detected infection prior to the onset of permissive virus infection. However, it is now recognized that the monoclonal antisera used in this assay recognizes pp65 (79). The presence of this antigen in leukocytes means that either the phagocytes ingested viral particles or were actually infected by the virus. Gerna and colleagues (80) studied the presence of both pp65 and mIE in both polymorphonuclear leukocytes and monocyte/macrophages in an immunocompromised population, composed mainly of heart transplant recipients, and noted that 73% of pp65-positive leukocytes expressed mIE, with evidence of mIE-specific RNA in most cells. This finding would mean that the granulocytes are actually infected by CMV in the process of virus dissemination.

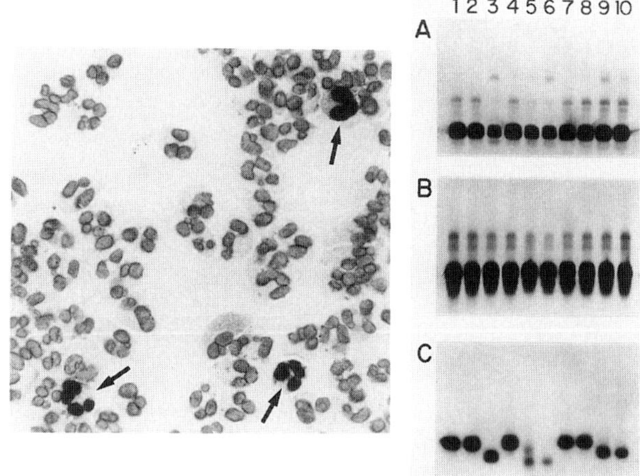

Figure 28-4. New diagnostic methods for cytomegalovirus (CMV). (Left) Photomicrograph showing three CMV antigen–positive polymorphonuclear leukocytes as detected with CMV antigenemia assay; (magnification ×640). (Reproduced by permission from Grefte JMM, van der Gun BTF, Schmolke S, et al. Cytomegalovirus antigenemia assay: identification of the viral antigen as the lower matrix protein pp 65. J Infect Dis 1992; 166:684.) (Right) Southern blot hybridization of polymerase chain reaction–amplified DNA from 10 wild isolates of CMV with amplification of genomic DNA encoding an immediate early protein (A), an early/late protein pp65 (B), or the hyper variable *a* sequence of CMV (C). (Reproduced by permission from Zaia JA, Gallez-Hawkins G, Churchill MA, et al. Comparative analysis of human cytomegalovirus *a*-sequence in multiple clinical isolates using polymerase chain reaction and restriction fragment length polymorphism assays. J Clin Microbiol 1990; 38: 2602–2607.)

The clinical experience with this assay indicates that antigenemia does in fact correlate with the subsequent development of CMV blood infection (81–83). CMV antigenemia detection in organ transplantation indicates that the onset of antigenemia precedes the detection of "infectious" CMV, using the culture-based assays. Recently, this method has been applied to BMT recipients by Boeckh and co-workers (84). In this study, the antigenemia assay was compared with the rapid centrifugal culture method in 59 CMV-seropositive marrow allograft recipients. The antigenemia assay was positive in 21 of 22 CMV culture–positive individuals (sensitivity, 95%; specificity, 91%). As important, however, was that the median time to onset of antigenemia was significantly earlier for the antigenemia assay (day 47 vs day 55; p = 0.0006), as has been described in other transplant populations (81–83). In addition, in 9 persons in whom CMV disease developed without preceding positive viral cultures, CMV was detected by antigenemia in 8. Levels of antigenemia were also significantly higher in patients in whom disease subsequently developed. This antigen assay appears to be a surrogate marker for CMV blood infection, and as such could have important application to clinical management of antiviral agents (see "Clinical Approaches to Management of CMV"). Because of the problematic nature of the assay, it has not yet been widely adopted, but in selected populations, such as evaluation of transplant populations, this test could become a primary means for detection of CMV infection.

CMV DNA Detection Methods

Methods that detect CMV DNA directly or indirectly have been used for diagnosis of CMV infection (85). *In situ* cytohybridization has been available for nearly a decade and is currently able to detect single infected cells (86–88). In a renal transplant population, this method detected CMV-infected blood cells prior to conventional assays (89). However, analysis of CMV infection, with this or other DNA-based detection assays in organs such as liver or lung, can be unreliable because of sampling error (86,90). Modification of *in situ* methods by means of polymerase chain reaction (PCR) amplification of CMV DNA has been reported and promises to improve the versatility of this assay (91). Nevertheless, *in situ* cytohybridization technology remains labor-intensive, which limits its use except in the research setting.

The PCR assay is currently being developed for more practical and sensitive application to diagnosis of CMV infection (92–94). In addition to its diagnostic potential (see Figure 28-4), PCR has been used to differentiate strains of CMV by selective amplification of hypervariable regions of the viral genome (66,95,96). With this method, strain differentiation or other CMV genomic characterization are possible without the necessity of virus isolation (96).

PCR detection of CMV has been applied to BMT recipients by Einsele and colleagues (97). In 28 patients followed at weekly intervals, PCR assay detected CMV blood infection more frequently than did the conventional culture method (83 vs 67%) and was positive in all patients with CMV-IP diagnosed by conventional means. In addition, detection of CMV infection by PCR occurred at very early times (weeks 1 and 2), compared with conventional detection (weeks 5 and 6). These results raise the question of whether the PCR assay will be too sensitive to distinguish, within the population of CMV-seropositive transplant recipients, the subgroup at high risk for progressive infection. In CMV-seropositive individuals, the sensitivity of the assay creates a potential problem of reading positive even when active virus infection is not present. Ideally, to be useful for patient management, the PCR assay should not detect all persons with CMV infection, because the antibody assay can perform this function, but only those with progressive infection. Thus, it remains to be determined whether PCR will have prospective application to management of transplant patients at risk for severe CMV infection.

In this regard, however, Einsele and associates (98) reported that PCR can be useful for evaluating recipients with CMV disease who are receiving ganciclovir therapy. Among 15 patients in this study, the PCR assay remained positive after virus clearance was documented in all patients (n = 5) who subsequently died of CMV-IP, and also in all patients (n = 3) who relapsed after therapy was stopped during early clinical and virological response to ganciclovir. In those patients with successful treatment (n = 8), the PCR assay converted to negative in all. Thus, PCR promises to be a means to evaluate antiviral management in BMT recipients. More recently, it has been shown that detection of CMV by PCR can be applied to both serum (99) and plasma (100). Ishigaki and coworkers (99) showed the presence of CMV in sera in recipients of BMT in whom CMV-IP subsequently developed, but the utility of this assay method is currently unknown. In summary, the best application of diagnostic PCR for CMV in transplantation medicine remains to be determined, but the PCR assay promises to be a useful means to guide patient management in the future.

Regarding the relative diagnostic performance of the PCR assay and the CMV antigenemia assay, there are two studies that compared these tests in prospective analyses in transplant populations (101,102). In 16 patients with CMV blood infection, Jiwa and associates (101) reported that the antigenemia assay was positive for a mean of 2.5 weeks, and the PCR assay remained positive for a mean of 4.4 weeks. In a study of 21 CMV-seropositive heart or lung transplant recipients, Boland and colleagues (102) confirmed that PCR detection of CMV occurs earlier and lasts longer than the antigenemia assay (102). Again, although the PCR assay appears to be more sensitive, it remains to be determined whether the antigenemia assay is a better clinical tool for direction of patient management.

Pathogenesis of CMV Disease

Overview

In the non-BMT setting, there is great variation in the type of symptom-complex that occurs in association with CMV infection. This can range from the extreme of severe organ dysfunction (e.g., encephalitis, retinitis, adrenalitis, enteritis, hepatitis) seen in association with profound immunological impairment such as in patients with acquired immune deficiency syndrome (AIDS) or in neonates (103,104) to mononucleosis syndromes, with malaise and fatigue, such as those that occur in adolescents and in young adults (105). The usual course of CMV infection is not associated with specific signs or symptoms of disease, which is also true with CMV infection after marrow or solid organ transplantation (106,107). In the transplantation populations, this heterogeneity of CMV-associated syndromes is most apparent. When renal, heart/lung, and marrow transplant populations are compared, the rates of infection with CMV and the incubation periods are nearly identical; however, the types of disease vary (i.e., CMV-IP is a more frequent problem for marrow allograft recipients) (13, 108–110).

It is important to appreciate this heterogeneity for what it tells us about the mechanism of disease. In AIDS and in fetuses, CMV infection is progressive and unchecked, and in these settings the virus demonstrates its neurotropism with direct tissue damage in the central nervous system (CNS). The neurotropic aspect of CMV infection is rarely ever seen in BMT recipients (4). The principal differences in presentation of CMV disease between the transplantation population and the groups in which CNS complications of CMV infection are more common is the predominance of mononucleosis-like symptoms in the transplantation patients (compare references 103–110). The cardinal features of CMV infection in transplantation recipients are fever, neutropenia, thrombocytopenia, and malaise, and these signs and symptoms are more frequently observed without other organ-specific involvement. This symptom complex has suggested an aspect of disease pathogenesis that is separate from the organ-tropic features of virus disease. Furthermore, because these symptoms have been associated with immunological abnormalities specific for transplantation populations, such as host-versus-graft disease or GVHD, the symptom complex associated with CMV could be due not so much to the virus as to the host response to infection (90,111,112). Thus, as noted (see "Epidemiology of CMV Infection in Marrow Transplantation"), the occurrence of CMV-IP in marrow allograft recipients correlates with the presence and the severity of GVHD (49). It appears, then, that acute GVHD serves as a host element that is necessary for development of CMV infection and possibly for evolution of CMV-associated clinical syndromes, although the latter remains conjectural. Thus, understanding the interaction of virus and host has a central role in understanding the pathogenesis of CMV disease. In this regard, it is recognized not only that the progression of virus infection is affected by host immune factors, but also that infectious virus can influence the function of the immune system. Understanding the pathogenesis of CMV disease in BMT therefore involves elements related (1) to progressive virus infection, (2) to the effect of this infection on general cellular function and on specific immune function, and (3) to the development of GVHD.

Role of Progressive CMV Infection

In the simplest terms, certain disease syndromes occur because of persistent virus infection, which leads to organ dysfunction, and others occur because the host is reacting to the infection, causing functional abnormalities. The fact that inhibition of CMV infection and therapeutic effect is observed with appropriate antiviral agents such as ganciclovir or foscarnet in retinitis and enteritis in patients with AIDS means that the persistant virus infection, with resultant specific tissue cytopathology, causes the disease. It is recognized that CMV infection is very active in the retina during CMV retinitis based on electron microscopic (EM) analysis (113), and inhibition of virus replication is associated with restoration of organ function (114). In contrast, antiviral agents when used alone usually fail to effect clinical improvement in CMV-associated disease in the transplantation population. This finding indicates that the pathogenesis of disease is different in BMT recipients than in patients with AIDS. For example, both CMV-IP and CMV-associated enteritis in marrow allograft recipients failed to respond to ganciclovir treatment even though the treatment effectively inhibited CMV excretion (115,116).

In the BMT population, studies have shown that the occurrence of CMV infection at sites such as kidney or throat do not correlate with incidence of subsequent CMV disease (55,56,106). However, CMV blood infection and asymptomatic pulmonary infection strongly correlate with disease (55,106). Thus, it appears that the progression of CMV from regional to disseminated infection is necessary prior to the onset of serious CMV disease in this setting. This progression is particularly well illustrated in the analysis of blood-borne infection in those with and without CMV-IP. In the study by Schmidt and colleagues (55), it was observed that both asymptomatic pulmonary and blood CMV infection strongly correlated with rates of subsequent CMV-IP (55) (Figure 28-5, Upper). In this study, a subgroup of patients with CMV-negative bronchoalveolar lavage specimens on day 35 after BMT remained at risk for CMV lung infection. As shown in the lower panel of Figure 28-5, late-onset CMV blood infection developed in these individuals in association with the later onset CMV-IP. Thus, the progression of CMV infection to the peripheral blood occurs in association with the development of CMV-IP and is a major risk for CMV-IP. An obvious implication of this observation is that interruption of

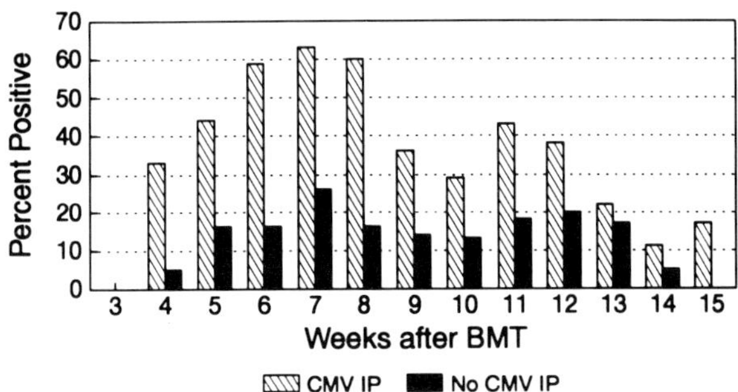

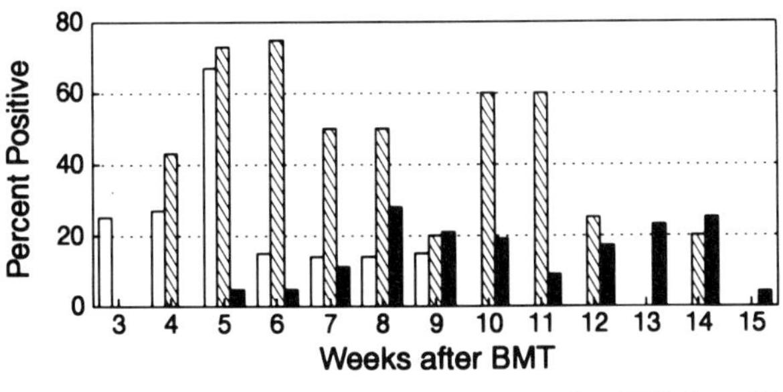

Figure 28-5. Incidence of cytomegalovirus (CMV)-positive blood cultures in relationship to CMV lung infection. (Upper) Percent of subjects positive for CMV in blood according to subsequent occurrence of CMV-IP (*hatched bars*) or no CMV-IP (*solid bars*). (Lower) Percent of subjects positive for CMV in blood according to positive CMV in lung on day 35 after bone marrow transplantation, with ganciclovir therapy (*open bars*) or without therapy (*hatched bars*), or negative for CMV in lung on day 35 (*solid bars*). Subjects were studied as described in (55).

CMV infection should provide a means to prevent this disease, and successful applications of this strategy are described in "Clinical Approaches to Management of CMV."

Effect of CMV Infection on Cellular Function

Interaction of Virus and Cell

As noted, CMV enters the host cell and expresses a cascade of proteins that leads to production of infectious viral particles (37,38). Two events happen during this time that alter cellular function. The first event is activation of the signal transduction system at the time of virus binding to the cell surface; the second event is introduction to the cytoplasm of proteins that have influence on cellular metabolism and function. Albrecht and co-workers (117) have shown that CMV infection alters the second messenger systems of the cell, with changes in diacylglycerol, inositol triphosphate, intracellular calcium, and protein kinase C. The effect of this activation is to up-regulate protein and DNA synthetic cellular pathways, resulting in oncogene expression and heightened cellular metabolic activity. Boldogh and colleagues reported that CMV infection, using either infectious or inactivated CMV inocula, up-regulates the transcription of the proto-oncogenes *c-myc, c-fos,* and *c-jun,* and such cellular perturbations undoubtedly extend to other areas of transcriptional regulation. Thus, CMV can modify cellular metabolism without entering the cell and inducing viral protein synthesis (118). Although putative binding proteins for CMV have been identified on the cell surface of susceptible cells (119–122), no receptor for signal transduction has been identified for CMV.

When the relatively large and complex CMV virion (see Figure 28-2) enters the infected cell, structural proteins of the virus having biological function enter and contribute to the regulation of mIE viral protein synthesis, which subsequently affect transcription of selective cell proteins. The exact function of this family of IE proteins is only generally understood, but it has been shown that one of these proteins (called mIE or IE1) is necessary both for further viral protein expression and for permissive virus replication (123). Another protein (IE2) is thought to repress IE viral gene expression and might well repress other cellular transcriptional events (124). In this regard, selected cellular proteins are either down- or up-regulated during CMV infection; for example, fibronectin and fibronectin-specific RNA is down-regulated immediately after infection without concomitant alteration in β-actin–specific RNA (40). The effect on housekeeper gene down-regulation might well begin the process of cell enlargement that is recognized as characteristic of CMV pathology. It is also recognized that the mIE gene products are transcriptionally activated by DNA response elements nearly identical to those present in host genes, such as IL-2 (125–127). For example, Hunninghake and associates (126) reported that the promoter/enhancer region of the mIE gene contains cyclic-AMP response elements, and Sambucetti and colleagues (127) described within this region consensus binding sites for the cellular transcription factors CREB/ATF, NF-kB, and AP-1. The biological significance of these findings is not fully appreciated, but they suggest CMV replication is facilitated by events that activate these cellular systems.

Interaction of CMV and the Immune System

It has been recognized for nearly 2 decades that the function of the immune system is altered during CMV infection, and the mechanisms involved in this immunosuppression are gradually becoming understood (128). The monocyte has been postulated to be the central site for CMV-induced interference with immune function (129–131). Human monocytes, for example, exhibit an inhibited response to concanavalin A–induced proliferation after CMV infection (130). It has been reported that CMV infection of these cells results in diminished production of IL-1 and IL-2, and it has been suggested that CMV influences these cells by impairing their ability to produce and respond to cytokines (132,133). These responses are mediated at the cellular level via protein kinase C–dependent and inositol triphosphate–dependent signal transduction pathways, and, as noted, both pathways have been shown to be altered by CMV infection (117,118). Thus, it is possible that CMV infection results in a metabolic derangement that impairs the ability of cells of the immune system to produce or react to mediators of the immune response.

The question that remains unanswered is how these in vitro observations apply to transplantation medicine. It has been reported that CMV-specific cellular immunity develops slowly after BMT (20) and that marrow recipients are deficient in IL-2 production (134). In addition, Duncombe and co-workers (135) reported that gamma-interferon and tumor necrosis factor production after BMT is enhanced in vitro by exposure of lymphocytes to marrow fibroblasts infected with CMV. Importantly, there is evidence that the specific CTL response to CMV targets is disturbed in BMT recipients by CMV infection (136). Because functional CTLs are needed for control of CMV infection in BMT recipients (21–23), CMV-induced deficiency in cellular immunity would contribute to the pathogenesis of CMV disease by permitting continued progression of CMV infection.

It has been proposed that CMV might affect the cellular immune system by influencing HLA-dependent mechanisms in cell-to-cell interaction (137). The CMV genome encodes polypeptide sequences with molecular mimicry to HLA class I and class II peptides (138,139). In addition, it was reported by Grundy and associates (140) that CMV infection in vitro could be neutralized using β_2-microglobulin, a protein component of class I HLA antigens. Thus, it has been conjectured that CMV could influence immune function either by binding to HLA molecules or by inducing differences in HLA and preventing cell-to-cell interactions necessary for CTL induction. However, it has since been shown that the interaction of CMV and β_2-microglobulin does not involve interaction with the α-chain of class I HLA antigen (141). Furthermore, when the class I homolog is functionally deleted from the CMV genome, there is no noticeable effect on in vitro virus replication (142). Hence, there is no evidence that this mechanism of CMV interaction with HLA is active in the pathogenetic processes associated with CMV infection in vivo.

CMV-induced GVHD

Because of the observation that the most serious forms of CMV infection in BMT recipients are associated with severe GVHD (49), the question has been raised regarding the contribution of this virus to the generation of alloreactive cytotoxic lymphocytes. In allogeneic marrow recipients, evidence that CMV infection is a risk factor for acute GVHD is lacking, since acute GVHD clearly appears to precede and to serve as a factor for development and severity of CMV infection (5,49). With regard to acute GVHD, CMV excretion but not seroconversion has been significantly related to grade of severity of GVHD. In the study by Meyers and associates (49), patients with grade II to IV GVHD had significantly more CMV infection than those with grade 0 to I GVHD (63 vs 42%; $p = 0.0001$). The time of onset of acute GVHD (median, day 19 after transplantation) generally preceded the onset of CMV excretion (median, day 51 and +56 for GVHD grade 0–I and II–IV, respectively). Also, the occurrence of acute GVHD has been associated with a significant increase in the probability of CMV infection among both seropositive and seronegative recipients. However, there has been no significant association observed between the usual risk factors for GVHD, such as HLA-mismatched or sex-mismatched donor/recipient pair, and subsequent CMV infection. Furthermore, attempts to find CMV in skin lesions of patients with GVHD have been unsuccessful (143). In addition, there is no evidence that CMV antigens are nonspecific inducers of mitogenesis nor that CMV serves as a superantigen that could cause general activation of the immune system.

Nevertheless, seroepidemiological data support the interaction of CMV and the pathogenesis of GVHD. Boström and co-workers (144) reported that pre-BMT CMV seropositivity in recipients and to herpes simplex antibody in donors were important risk factors for acute GVHD. Gratama and associates (145) found that pretransplant seropositivity to herpes simplex antibody in donors was associated with increased incidence of acute GVHD, and that pre-BMT seronegativity in either donors or recipients was associated with a lower incidence of GVHD. A study of the Leukemia Working Party of the European Group for Bone Marrow Transplantation (146) evaluated 379 BMT recipients and confirmed that pretransplant seropositivity to 3 or more herpesviruses in recipients was a significant risk factor for GVHD. This group further evaluated 285 BMT recipients and reported that pre-BMT seropositivity for CMV antibody in recipients and donors was a significant risk factor for the development of chronic GVHD (146). In this regard, Lönnqvist and colleagues (147) reported an association between chronic GVHD and CMV infection, and Jacobsen and associates (148) reported that the pre-BMT seropositivity to CMV antibody in donors correlated with the development of chronic GVHD.

Until there is evidence that inhibition of CMV using antiviral drugs can alter the occurrence of GVHD, the linkage between CMV and GVHD will remain circumstantial. The implication from the epidemiological data is that CMV alters the host in some way that could facilitate GVHD. In murine studies, acute murine CMV infection enhances the ability of parental spleen cells to induce GVHD in F1 hybrid mice (149). In this regard, in human BMT, CMV-seropositive donors transmit more CD8-positive T-cytotoxic cells in their grafts than do seronegative donors (150). Gratama and associates (145) speculated further that increased expression of certain antigenic markers on the CD8-positive cells could be related to the presence of latent CMV in those lymphocytes. It is also possible that the presence of virus-encoded proteins on the cell surface mediates certain immunological events that eventually result in GVHD, but there is no evidence supporting this relationship.

Clinical Approaches to Management of CMV

Natural Course of CMV Infection in BMT Recipients

General Considerations

Since the discovery of cytomegaloviruses in animals and humans more than 35 years ago, two issues are apparent in considering the management of infection. First, these viruses are frequently found in many different tissues, and second, they are not clearly associated with disease at times of active infection. As described, CMV isolates frequently can be obtained from urine, blood, and even the lung in asymptomatic individuals. In addition, these viruses are ubiquitous with different species-specific strains occurring in virtually all vertebrate animals; however, they cause no known animal diseases in nature. It has taken iatrogenic alteration of normal immune function to produce life-threatening infection by this otherwise benign virus. In addition, the mononucleosis syndromes with malaise, fatigue, thrombocytopenia, and neutropenia, and even the more organ-specific syndromes, such as hepatitis and pneumonitis, can represent a broad differential diagnosis. In most situations, the diagnostic evaluation must exclude other explanations for the symptomology before the diagnosis of CMV disease is made. In addition, in BMT recipients, contrary to the general rule that primary CMV infection is more severe than reactivation-associated disease, clinicians are more likely to be confronted with severe CMV-associated disease in persons with reactivation of the infection (1,49). This situation occurs because primary infection can currently be prevented by use of selected blood product support and because the CMV-seropositive population forms the majority of BMT recipients in most centers. The general approach to CMV-specific management of BMT recipients involves an understanding of the risks of severe disease and using this information to direct preventive interventional strategies in an effort to minimize disease.

Definitions of CMV Disease

CMV infection in BMT recipients is usually defined as either (1) the isolation of CMV in tissue culture; (2) the identification of CMV in tissue specimens by histological and histochemical means (i.e., cells having Cowdry-type A intranuclear or cytoplasmic inclusion bodies [Plate XL]; (3) specific antigen staining; or detection of specific DNA *in situ*) direct CMV DNA or CMV antigen detection; or (4) a four-fold or greater increase in CMV antibody titer. CMV pneumonia is defined as a progressive interstitial pulmonary process, as evidenced by chest radiography, with concomitant evidence of CMV infection in the lung (Plate XL) and without evidence for other etiology of pneumonitis. CMV enteritis is defined as an enteropathic syndrome with pain, nausea and vomiting, or diarrhea, and evidence of CMV infection (Plate XXXIV) at the site of an erythematous or ulcerative (Plate XXXIII) mucosal lesion. In general, other CMV-associated organ-related syndromes (e.g., hepatitis, encephalitis) are defined as syndromes with specific organ dysfunction and concomitant presence of active CMV infection. Without histological evidence of CMV infection in the involved organ, the diagnosis of CMV disease cannot be made with confidence.

Analysis of Risk for CMV Disease

Although it would appear to be obvious, the most significant risk factor for the occurrence of CMV-associated disease after allogeneic BMT is the development of CMV infection. This risk is important to note because it is a strong confirmation that the heterogeneous syndromes that can present during CMV infection are in fact due to this infection and that CMV is not merely present and masking another pathological process. In addition, it allows us to focus on management of patients by recognizing the factors that predict for CMV infection and disease. There have been many analyses of risk for CMV disease after BMT that have demonstrated risks, including (1) host factors, such as previous CMV infection, age, and diagnosis/remission disease status; 2) treatment factors, such as TBI, preparative chemotherapy, and GVHD prophylaxis; and (3) the syngeneic versus the nonsyngeneic nature of the recipient/donor match (1,4–8,49,151,152). From a practical standpoint, however, the central risks that define how patients will be managed relate only to the chances CMV infection will develop and to whether continued immunosuppression will alter the chance of resolution of the infection. When considered in this way, the only important risk factors for development of severe CMV disease are patient age, pretransplantation seropositivity for CMV antibody, HLA-mismatch recipient/donor status, and presence of acute GVHD. Thus, treatment will be different for CMV-seronegative recipients of seronegative donor marrow than for CMV-seropositive recipients, for pediatric versus adult recipients, for recipients of a marrow allograft versus an autologous BMT, and for recipients with GVHD versus those without such complications. Nevertheless, even those in lowest risk groups face some chance of CMV disease after BMT; therefore, it is important for the entire transplant team involved to be familiar with prevention, clinical course, and treatment of CMV infection.

CMV-associated Interstitial Pneumonia

As described in the epidemiology section, prior to the development of methods for prevention of CMV infection, CMV-IP occurred in 15 to 30% of marrow allograft recipients (1,4,7,152). The prevalence rates noted in Table 28-3 are the most accurate available, but institutional rates of CMV-IP will vary based on newer antiviral prophylactic regimens currently being developed. CMV-IP occurs at a median time of 50 to 60 days after BMT, with the onset of fever, nonproductive cough, tachypnea, and, occasionally, chest pain (1, 18,48). Hypoxia is the major physiological abnormality observed, and radiological abnormalities suggestive of interstitial pneumonitis are common (Figure 28-6). Although infiltrates usually become diffuse and are basilar, there is considerable variation in the radiological pattern, which can reveal segmental, lobar, or diffuse interstitial or nodular infiltrates (153,154). The differential diagnosis includes radiation-induced pulmonary disease, cytotoxic chemotherapy–induced pulmonary damage, pulmonary hemorrhage, pulmonary edema, metastatic neoplasia, and other infections of fungal, viral, or bacterial etiology. As illustrated in Figure 28-7, the histopathology of CMV-IP involves thickening of the interalveolar membranes with cellular infiltrates and edema (18,48,154) (Plate XL). CMV infections occur in an eratic distribution and are not clearly related to sites of typical CMV pathology (87,90). Zaia and colleagues (111) analyzed clinical and virological aspects of 32 consecutive autopsied cases of CMV-IP. When the group was arbitrarily subdivided into those with survival 14 days or less or more than 14 days from time of initial clinical disease (hypoxia), the mean time to death was 8.4 versus 28.5 days, indicating the variable duration of CMV-IP. The amount of CMV/gm lung, as measured by infectious titer or by amount of CMV DNA, did not significantly correlate with the duration of disease. Similarly, Slavin and associates (155) reported that quantitative assessment of infectious CMV in BAL specimens of allograft recipients could not distinguish patients in terms of disease severity, and virus burden was not predictive of outcome.

Although the diagnostic procedure of choice in the past was lung biopsy, since the mid-1980s, BAL has become the preferred method of diagnosis of CMV-IP (156,157). As noted in "Diagnosis of CMV Infection," the specimen is analyzed for infectious virus and for cytological evidence of CMV. As shown in Figure 28-7, inclusion bodies typical for CMV can often be seen in CMV-positive BAL specimens.

Clinical Course and Treatment of CMV-IP

Treatment of CMV-IP has had mixed success in immunocompromised persons, probably due to variations in patient groups (i.e., different diagnoses, different levels of immunosuppression) and to the varying contribution from host factors, known and unknown, that modify CMV infection. Overall, outcome for untreated disease has historically been very poor, with a mortality in the initial reports in the 1970s of 65% (18,48) and in the 1980s of approximately 85% (Table 28-4). Attempts to treat this disease with antiviral agents have been uniformly unsuccessful despite the fact that many of these agents have produced a dramatic antiviral effect (115,158–171). Thus, for example, use of vidarabine (158), leukocyte interferon (159), vidarabine plus interferon (160), acyclovir (161), interferon plus acyclovir (162,165), recombinant DNA-derived interferon (163,164), ganciclovir (115,166,167), ganciclovir plus corticosteroids (168), CMV immune globulin (169,170), and foscarnet (171) did not produce a significant improvement in the outcome of CMV-IP.

In the first report of ganciclovir therapy for CMV-IP in this population by Shepp and colleagues (115), ganciclovir was used at a total dose ranging from 7.5 to 15 mg/kg/day in 10 persons; only one patient

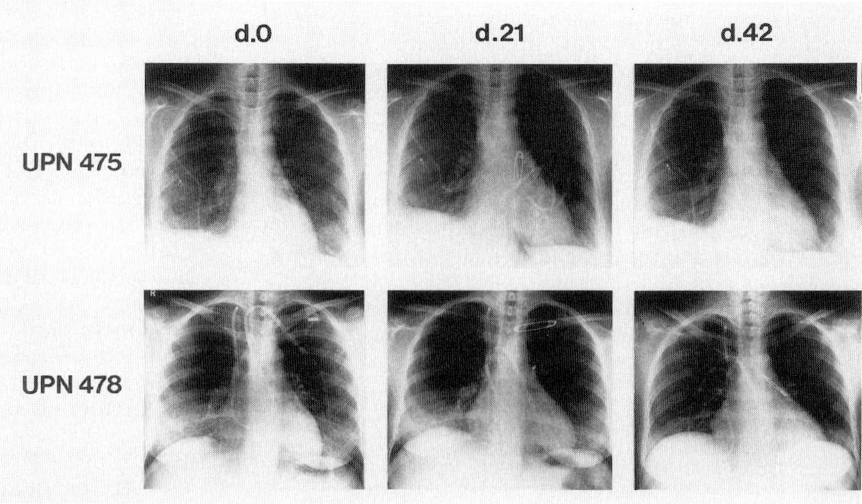

Figure 28-6. Clinical course of treated cytomegalovirus (CMV) interstitial pneumonia. Shown are a series of radiographs from 2 patients (UPN475 and UPN478) treated with ganciclovir as described in Table 28-6; radiographs are from days 0, 21, and 42 of treatment. Note the resolution of the right lower lobe pneumonitis in both patients.

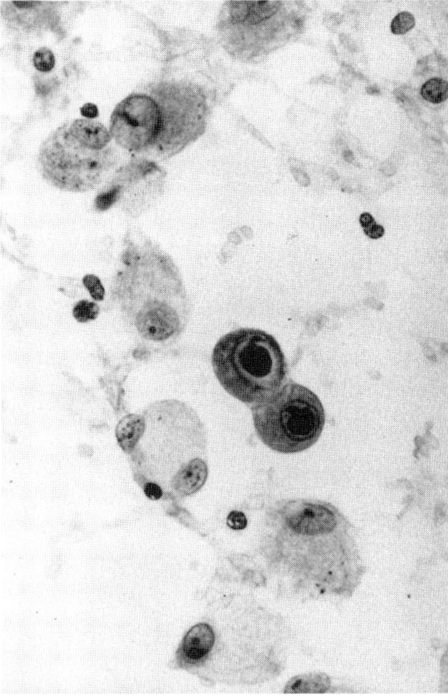

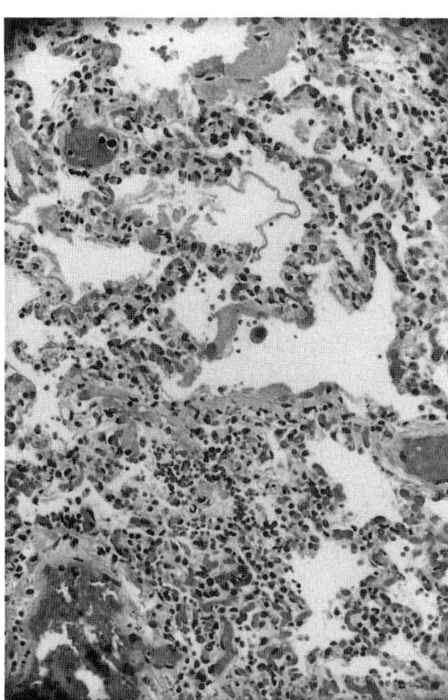

Figure 28-7. Histopathology of cytomegalovirus-associated interstitial pneumonia (CMV-IP). (*Right*) Photomicrograph of thin section of lung from a patient with CMV-IP stained with hematoxylin and eosin. Note cell in alveolar space containing Cowdry type-A intranuclear inclusion bodies typical of CMV. (×640) (*Left*) Photomicrograph of Papanicolaou-stained bronchoalveolar lavage specimen from a patient with CMV-IP. Note similar CMV-induced "owl's eye" intranuclear inclusion bodies. (×1,000)

survived. In a study reported by Winston and associates (166), ganciclovir used at a dose of 10 mg/kg/day resulted in a survival of 22% in 9 marrow recipients with CMV-IP. Erice and co-workers (167) reported that ganciclovir (7.5 mg/kg/day) was associated with a 45% survival rate in a study that included nonmarrow transplant patients. Thus, unlike initial experience in the use of ganciclovir for treatment of CMV diseases in patients with AIDS, in which prompt clinical response was the rule (172), ganciclovir alone was not able to improve the outcome of CMV-IP in BMT recipients.

As described in the "Pathogenesis of CMV Disease," the inability of agents that act only to suppress virus replication to treat CMV-IP successfully has suggested that there are additional factors contributing to pathogenesis besides virus cytopathology. Because CMV-IP could be caused by both CMV infection and the host response to infection, it was suggested that antiviral therapy be combined with immune response modification (90). The initial use of combined treatment was reported by Reed and associates (168), who described the use of ganciclovir plus methylprednisolone in 6 marrow recipients. In this study, ganciclovir was given at a dose of 7.5 mg/kg/day, and methylprednisolone was given at 16 mg/kg/day for one week and then tapered over 14 days. Only one of 6 patients survived, and severe marrow and renal toxicity were observed in 5. Clearly, this regimen produced no improvement. Use of a CMV antibody–enriched intravenous immune globulin (CMVIg) has been evaluated for treatment of CMV-IP with mixed results. In the initial study of Blacklock and colleagues (169), 9 of 18 marrow recipients survived CMV-IP, but the only other reported use of CMVIg for treatment of CMV-IP could not confirm this result (170).

Table 28-4.
Treatment of CMV-IP with Antiviral Agents

Source, Year, Ref	*Agent*	*Survival Rate (%)*
Kraemer, 1978 (158)	Vidarabine	16.6
Meyers, 1980 (159)	Leukocyte IFN	0
Meyers, 1982 (160)	IFN and vidarabine	14.2
Wade, 1982 (161)	Acyclovir	12.5
Wade, 1983 (162)	IFN and acyclovir	23
Meyers, 1983 (163)	rDNA IFN	0
Winston, 1983 (164)	rDNA IFN	60
Shepp, 1984 (165)	IFN and acyclovir	12.5
Shepp, 1985 (115)	Ganciclovir	10
Winston, 1988 (166)	Ganciclovir	22.2
Erice, 1987 (167)	Ganciclovir	45
Reed, 1986 (168)	Ganciclovir and steroid	16.6
Blacklock, 1985 (169)	CMVIg	50
Reed, 1987 (170)	CMVIg	21.4
Ringden, 1985 (171)	Foscarnet	0

CMV-IP = cytomegalovirus-associated interstitial pneumonia; IFN = interferon; rDNA IFN = recombinant interferon; CMVIg = cytomegalovirus immune globulin.

Animal studies performed at this same time deserve note because they provided additional observations relevant to the combination of ganciclovir and immune globulin. In a mouse model of CMV-IP, Shanley and co-workers (173) reported that ganciclovir, although decreasing the amount of murine CMV infection in mouse lung, failed to prevent interstitial pneumonia. However, Wilson and associates (174) demonstrated that the combination of ganciclovir and mouse immune serum would protect from a lethal challenge with murine CMV. In this study, neither ganciclovir nor immune serum alone provided protection.

These studies set the stage for regimens that combined ganciclovir and IVIg (ganciclovir/IVIg) for the treatment of CMV-IP. The initial reports of combined use of ganciclovir/IVIg and improved outcome of CMV-IP were by Reed and co-workers (175) and by Bratanow and associates (176). Subsequently, several centers published results using this type of therapeutic method, and the results are summarized in Table 28-5 (177–180). In the study reported by Reed and co-workers (177), two IVIg products were used in conjunction with ganciclovir. One product (CMV-IVIg) contained high titer CMV-specific antibody and was given at a dose of 400 mg/kg on days 1, 2, and 7, and then at half this dose on days 14 and 21. Of 50 patients in this group, 25 (50%) had at least a 6-week survival, and 16 patients (32%) were alive at 6 months, with a median follow-up of 9 months. In an additional group, patients were treated with a standard, commercially available IVIg containing a lower titer CMV-specific antibody given at 500 mg/kg every other day for 9 doses. Thirteen patients were entered into this group; 5 (38%) were alive at 6 weeks and 5 (38%) were alive at 6 months, with a median follow-up of 5 months.

In results reported by Emanuel and colleagues (178), 20 patients received a regimen of IVIg consisting of 500 mg/kg every other day for 10 doses and then every 2 weeks for 8 doses in conjunction with ganciclovir. In this study, 14 (70%) of 20 patients were alive at 6 weeks and 10 (50%) at 6 months, with a median follow-up of 24 months. In the report of Schmidt and associates (178), 40 patients were treated with therapy that included antiviral induction treatment lasting 3 weeks, or until there was documented clearing of pulmonary CMV infection, followed by a maintenance treatment lasting until significant immunosuppressive medications were stopped. In this regimen, ganciclovir was given at 10 mg/kg/day and IVIg at 500 mg/kg every other day for 21 days, followed by 5 mg/kg/day 5 days per week and IVIg at 500 mg/kg weekly until day 180 after BMT. With this treatment, 32 (80%) marrow recipients were alive 6 weeks after treatment was started, and 16 (40%) were alive at a median follow-up of 18 months. Ganciclovir/IVIg treatment of CMV-IP has met with varying success in some BMT centers, which is probably due to variations in patient populations. For example, Ljungman and co-workers (180) noted that patients who did not receive TBI compared with those who received TBI benefitted more from ganciclovir/IVIg treatment of CMV-IP (75 vs 27% survival at 30 days, respectively; $p = 0.009$).

Table 28-5.
Survival from CMV Pneumonia Treated with Ganciclovir/IVIg

Source, Year, Ref	*6 weeks*	*6 months*
Reed, 1988 (177)	48%	38%
Emanuel, 1988 (178)	65%	50%
Schmidt, 1988 (179)	85%	40%
Ljungman, 1992 (180)	31%	NP

IVIg = intravenous immunoglobulin; NP = not provided in reference.

Table 28-6.
Treatment of CMV-IP

Induction phase—21 days	
GCV[a]	5 mg/kg IV every 12 hr
IVIg	500 mg/kg IV every other day
Maintenance phase—during continued immunosuppression	
GCV[a]	5 mg/kg IV every day 5 d/wk
IVIg	500 mg/kg IV every week

[a]If the absolute neutrophil count is <1,000 mm for 2 consecutive days, then stop GCV until count recovers; consider use of growth factors G-CSF or GM-CSF.
CMV-IP = cytomegalovirus-associated interstitial pneumonia; GCV = ganciclovir; IVIg = intravenous immunoglobulin.

Thus, it was not until ganciclovir was combined with IVIg that an improvement in the outcome of this disease was observed. Although these results were derived from uncontrolled studies, ganciclovir/IVIg has become the recommended treatment for CMV-IP in BMT recipients, and a method of treatment is outlined in Table 28-6. Repeat BAL is suggested after the initial 21 days of treatment to confirm the initial response to antiviral therapy. Reactivation of CMV is the usual course when ganciclovir is stopped; therefore, it is further recommended that maintenance therapy be continued for the duration of major immunosuppressive treatment. The expected course of resolution of treated CMV-IP is shown in Figure 28-6. Fever and hypoxia usually resolve within the first week of treatment but radiographic changes persist for many weeks. Patients with a slow response to treatment prompt the consideration regarding either the presence of ganciclovir-resistant CMV or the accuracy of the original diagnosis. Both questions can be addressed by repeat BAL.

CMV infection is usually eliminated from the lavage specimen by 21 days of treatment, and deterioration of pulmonary function with continued positive CMV lung infection at this time suggests ganciclovir resistance (181), although this resistance is rare in the setting of BMT (Zaia J. Unpublished data). If ganciclovir resistance occurs, or if ganciclovir cannot be used because of marrow toxicity, then foscarnet is indicated. However, no convincing data exist that indicate foscarnet therapy is equivalent to ganciclovir in this setting. As derived from experience with treatment of retinitis in persons with AIDS, foscarnet is given at a dose of 60 mg/kg 3 times daily during an initial 7-day induction period and then maintained at a dose of 90 mg/kg/day for an extended period determined by the immunosuppression of the patient. Foscarnet is nephrotoxic, and it is recommended that calculation of the dosage be determined by concomitant creatinine clearance. There has not been a systematic evaluation of the efficacy of foscarnet plus IVIg for treatment of CMV-IP.

The major complications associated with ganciclovir treatment are neutropenia and creatinine level elevation. Neutropenia occurs in approximately 30% of patients and, based on the experience of Goodrich and colleagues (57), lasts for a median of 12 days, but it can last for up to 74 days. Therefore, in certain patients, in addition to cessation of therapy, the use of growth factors such as granulocyte colony stimulating factor (G-CSF) or GM-CSF is suggested. To minimize this problem, a stopping rule for ganciclovir use must be employed. A rule used by the author is based on the presence of an absolute neutrophil count less than 1,000 mm^3 on two consecutive days (see Table 28-6). Additional respiratory support is essential during the treatment of CMV-IP, and, based on the individual patient, steroid therapy should be considered, particularly in patients requiring intubation.

CMV-associated Enteritis

Gastrointestinal syndromes associated with CMV are an increasingly important problem in allograft recipients. Ulceration associated with CMV infection can be identified in the esophagus (Plates XXXIII and XXXIV), the stomach, the small bowel, and the large intestine (182). The diagnosis is made by the association of CMV infection with mucosal pathology and appropriate symptoms. The appropriate method for treatment of this disease is not currently known. One controlled study using ganciclovir showed that despite antiviral effect, there was no significant improvement in the clinical course (116). However, on the basis of experiences in CMV-IP, it is common practice to use the ganciclovir/IVIg combination according to the treatment regimen for CMV-IP (see Table 28-6).

Other CMV-associated Syndromes

Because CMV infection develops in nearly 80% of all transplant recipients, accurate association of other syndromes with this infection can be difficult. Nevertheless, in addition to a mononucleosis-like syndrome with fever, arthralgia, and malaise, both hepatitis and suppressed marrow function, including neutropenia and thrombocytopenia, have been associated with acute CMV infections. The course of asymptomatic CMV infection is not well described in allograft recipients, but it appears that febrile episodes are a significant part of this infection. To understand the clinical effects of asymptomatic CMV infection, Zaia and associates (111) evaluated consecutive patients with CMV infection during BMT and found a significant association of fever between days 42 to 56 in those with otherwise asymptomatic infection. There was no increased rate of neutropenia in those with CMV infection. However, neutropenia is associated with CMV infection during this same period; for example, in 66 patients examined by Meyers and colleagues (1) there was a decrease in leukocyte and platelet count compared to the control group (59 vs 36%; *p* value not significant). The anecdotal use of ganciclovir for treatment of neutropenia has been reported to reverse some cases of neutropenia.

In summary, the acute course of CMV-IP is no longer an inexorably morbid condition once feared in BMT recipients due to the availability of treatment for this disease. Treatment with ganciclovir/IVIg has made a significant change in the management of transplant recipients; however, it is clear that the problem of CMV has not been solved by this treatment. Fifty to 80% of patients will now survive the acute disease, but an important portion of patients with CMV-IP remain unresponsive to treatment. In addition, even patients surviving CMV-IP face a long-term outcome that remains less than satisfactory. For CMV-IP, 6-month survival is 30 to 50% (177–180). This percentage is not different from the survival reported in the initial description of this disease (18). Currently, mortality in these patients is related less to CMV than to complications of GVHD and to neoplastic disease recurrence. As shown by the case illustration in Figure 28-8, late onset of fungal pneumonia frequently complicates the course of these patients who have acute and chronic GVHD. Thus, short-term survival of allogeneic BMT recipients with CMV-IP has improved considerably with use of ganciclovir/IVIg therapy, but, in patients at risk for CMV disease after transplantation, prevention rather than treatment of CMV infection would undoubtedly be a better alternative.

Prevention of CMV Infection after BMT

Prevention of CMV Using Selected Blood Products

As described, CMV infection arises either from exogenous introduction of virus via blood elements and transplanted tissue or from reactivation of endogenous virus. Persons who have had CMV infection prior to BMT form the group at risk for most problems relating to CMV after BMT (see Table 28-3). Seronegative transplant recipients are at much lower risk for serious infection as long as exposure to exogenous sources of infection can be minimized. Meyers and colleagues (183), and Bowden and associates (50) provided convincing evidence that granulocytes are a major source of exogenous CMV after BMT. The exposure to CMV by contact with random blood products has been confirmed by several other studies (8,184).

Prevention of CMV with CMV-seronegative Blood Donors

Controlled comparisons of selected blood support for prevention of CMV infection in CMV seronegative marrow allograft recipients is summarized in Table 28-7. Bowden and colleagues (50) initially studied this issue and the use of immune globulin to prevent CMV infection. Passive immunization did not reduce infection, but the use of CMV-seronegative blood donor support significantly reduced both CMV infection and

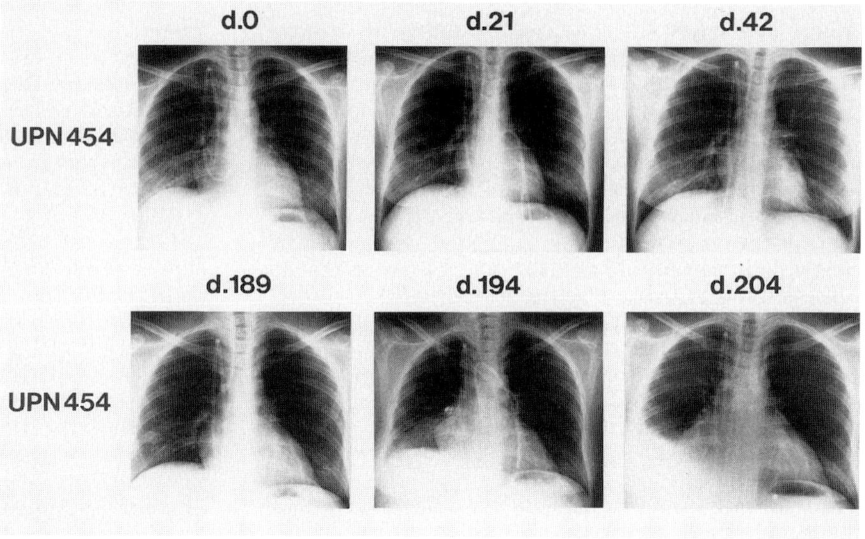

Figure 28-8. Late complication of treated cytomegalovirus-associated interstitial pneumonia (CMV-IP). Patient (UPN454) was treated on day 0 (d.0) with ganciclovir according to the regimen in Table 28-6, with resolution of pneumonitis (d.21 and d.42). Subsequently, a right lower lobe nodule developed (d.189), progressing to right lower lobe pneumonia (d.194 and d.204) and then death from *Aspergillus* infection and chronic graft-versus-host disease.

CMV disease. Subsequently, Bowden and colleagues (44) performed a randomized controlled trial comparing the use of leukocyte-depleted platelets plus CMV-seronegative red blood cells with standard unscreened blood products for prevention of primary CMV infection during the first 100 days after autologous BMT. In this study, platelets were depleted of leukocytes by centrifugation, and blood products were screened for CMV seronegativity by latex agglutination assay and enzyme immunoassay. The probability for development of CMV infection was significantly greater in patients receiving standard unscreened blood products (0 vs 23%; $p = 0.0013$); there was no infection in the 35 patients who had received the leukocyte-poor platelets and the screened CMV-seronegative red blood cells. Miller and co-workers (45) confirmed the effectiveness of screened CMV-seronegative blood products in a randomized trial of 125 patients. Among those patients receiving CMV-seronegative donor marrow, CMV infection was significantly reduced in those receiving screened blood products (6 vs 37%; $p = 0.0006$). Blood product screening was not effective prevention if the marrow donor was seropositive (62 vs 42%; $p = 0.8$). In this study, exposure to CMV infection from any blood source, either seropositive donor or unscreened blood products, resulted in statistically similar infection rates (62 vs 38%; $p = 0.5$), thus suggesting that exposure to CMV from either unscreened blood products or seropositive donor marrow is equally likely to result in eventual CMV infection. Thus, use of screened seronegative donor blood support is currently limited to those who are seronegative at the time of transplant and are receiving tissue from a seronegative donor. There is no reason to believe that use of seronegative support in seropositive recipients is beneficial. Furthermore, because the marrow is an important exogenous source of CMV, there is no recognized advantage in attempting to protect further recipients from exogenous sources of CMV if the donor is CMV-seropositive. Uncontrolled studies have also reported that the use of either CMV-seronegative or centrifuged platelets and filtered red blood cell products would minimize the exposure of patients to CMV-infected cells of blood and prevent exogenous CMV infection (185,186).

Table 28-7.
Prevention of CMV Infection Using CMV-seronegative Blood Support[a]

Source, Year, Ref	*Selected Blood (%)*	*Standard Blood (%)*	*p Value*
Bowden, 1986 (50)[b]	1/32 (3)	8/25 (32)	<0.007
Bowden, 1991 (44)[c]	0/35 (0)	7/30 (23)	0.0013
Miller, 1991 (45)[d,e]	8/64 (13)	21/61 (34)	0.002
BMT donor negative	6%	37%	0.0006
BMT donor positive	62%	42%	0.8

[a]Unless noted, marrow allograft recipients were CMV-seronegative and had a CMV-seronegative marrow donor.
[b]Combines groups receiving selected seronegative blood or no screened blood with groups receiving or not receiving CMV immune globulin.
[c]Blood product selection used CMV-seronegative donors of RBCs and leukocyte-depleted RBCs and platelets.
[d]Blood product selection used CMV-seronegative donors of blood products; marrow donor CMV serological status is indicated as negative or positive.
[e]Number of CMV-seronegative and CMV-seropositive BMT donors was not provided in source material.
CMV = cytomegalovirus; BMT = bone marrow transplantation.

Prevention of CMV with Filtered Blood Products

Use of blood filters provides a mechanism to produce leukocyte-poor blood products and has been shown to reduce the risk of CMV transmission in groups such as neonates (187) and transplant recipients (188). Additional studies are needed to more completely evaluate the strengths or limitations of this method, and studies are currently comparing donor screening versus blood product filtration.

Prevention of CMV Using Acyclovir

Initial attempts to suppress the reactivation of CMV infection in transplant recipients have used either oral or intravenous acyclovir (189–191). Both an oral regimen in renal transplant recipients, using a dose of 800 mg 4 times daily, and an intravenous regimen in BMT recipients, using a dose of 500 mg/m^2 3 times daily, significantly reduced CMV reactivation and disease. Because the mean 50% inhibitory dose of acyclovir for CMV strains is 63.1 ± 30.2 μmol/L (192), and because peak acyclovir levels in the plasma with these regimens can be expected to range from 25 to 100 μmol/L, it is a curious observation that acyclovir has apparent activity against CMV pathogenesis. Yet, clearly prophylactic administration of acyclovir in allogeneic BMT recipients and in renal allograft recipients significantly reduced the incidence of infection, decreased the occurrence of disease, and lowered patient mortality (189–191). In the report of Meyers and associates (189), the incidence of active CMV infection in BMT recipients dropped from 75% in the control patients to 59% in the acyclovir-treated group. Although the overall probability of CMV reactivation remained 0.70 in the acyclovir-treated group compared with 0.87 in the control group, there was a reduction in the infection-associated clinical syndromes, such as CMV-IP and CMV enteritis. The most striking result of this study, and the reason acyclovir prophylaxis subsequently has become widely used in BMT, was the significant reduction in mortality in the treated group (54 vs 29%; $p < 0.01$). In addition, there were fewer deaths associated with any infectious cause in the acyclovir group (45 vs 22%; $p < 0.01$). The time at which virus was first isolated was significantly increased from 40 to 62 days after BMT in the treated group, but acyclovir had no effect in patients in whom there was early reactivation of CMV. The altered time of first virus detection suggested an effect on CMV reactivation, and it appears that this change in timing of virus reactivation altered the development of disease. Thus, the important contribution of acyclovir prophylaxis for CMV is that it has demonstrated for the first time that perturbation of the natural course of CMV reactivation can have pronounced effects on clinical disease. This observation offers insight into methods for prevention of CMV disease using strategies directed toward early inhibition of virus infection. Currently, however, considering the high cost of intravenous acyclovir and the advent of more potent agents for inhibition of CMV, there is less justification for use of intravenous acyclovir in chemoprevention of CMV.

Prevention of CMV Infection with Risk-adjusted Use of Ganciclovir

Ganciclovir has been used in efforts to prevent reactivation of endogenous CMV and to modify infection in BMT. In this management strategy, antiviral chemotherapy is administered either at the time of positive culture prior to symptomatic disease (preemptive therapy) or prior to infection (prophylactic therapy). As shown in Table 28-8, risk-determined approaches to therapy have resulted in significant reductions in clinical disease (55,56). Schmidt and associates (55) used asymptomatic pulmonary CMV infection as the determinant for use of ganciclovir (5 mg/kg IV b.i.d. for 14 days and then daily until day 120 after BMT). The purpose of this study was to determine if ganciclovir could prevent the development of CMV-IP after virus reactivation occurred and after the virus had been detected in the lungs. Allogeneic BMT recipients were randomly assigned to receive ganciclovir after routine CMV-positive BAL on day 35 after BMT. Study subjects were free of pulmonary symptoms and had normal chest radiographs at the time of BAL. The end point observation was CMV-IP or death, and all follow-up radiographs were coded and reviewed by a panel of radiologists to confirm the diagnosis of IP. Of 104 patients enrolled in this study, 40 (39%) were found to have asymptomatic pulmonary CMV infection as judged by CMV culture from BAL, and 20 patients were randomized either to ganciclovir therapy or to no treatment. The occurrence of either CMV-IP or death was significantly reduced in the ganciclovir-treated group (25 vs 70%; $p = 0.01$) (Figure 28-9, upper). CMV-IP developed in no patients who completed the full course of induction and maintenance therapy with ganciclovir, yet among those patients who had negative day 35 BAL, 12 of 55 (22%) subsequently had CMV pneumonia. The antiviral effects of this regimen are shown in the lower panel of Figure 28-9. Among the 40 BAL-positive specimens obtained on day 35, 38 were positive by rapid centrifugal culture method and 2 were positive by cytological method and subsequently confirmed by conventional culture. Among the treated subjects, 33% remained CMV-positive at repeat BAL 14 days after ganciclovir was started. All untreated CMV-positive individuals remained positive at repeat BAL

Table 28-8.
Chemotherapeutic Prevention of CMV after BMT using Ganciclovir[a]

Source, Year, Ref	*Control*	*GCV*	*Untreated*
Preemptive therapy			
Schmidt, 1991 (55)	65%	15%	12%
Goodrich, 1991 (56)	43%	3%	12%
Universal therapy			
Atkinson, 1991 (194)	17%[b]	0%[c]	
Goodrich, 1993 (57)	32%	9%[d]	
Winston, 1993 (195)	24%	10%[e]	

[a]Results expressed as rate of CMV-associated disease.
[b]Historic control.
[c]$p = 0.05$.
[d]$p = 0.015$.
[e]$p = 0.09$.
CMV = cytomegalovirus; BMT = bone marrow transplantation; GCV = ganciclovir.

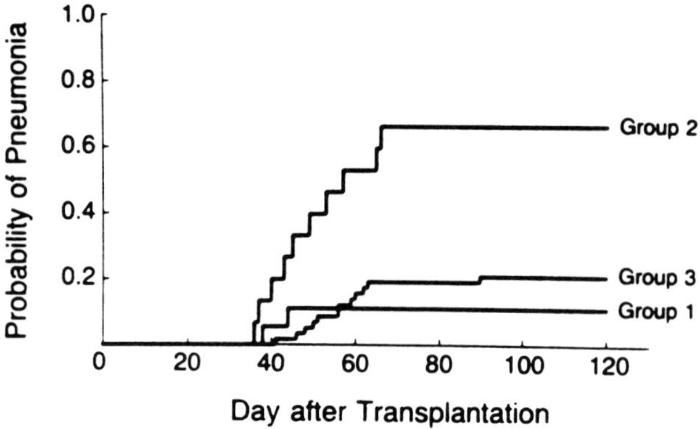

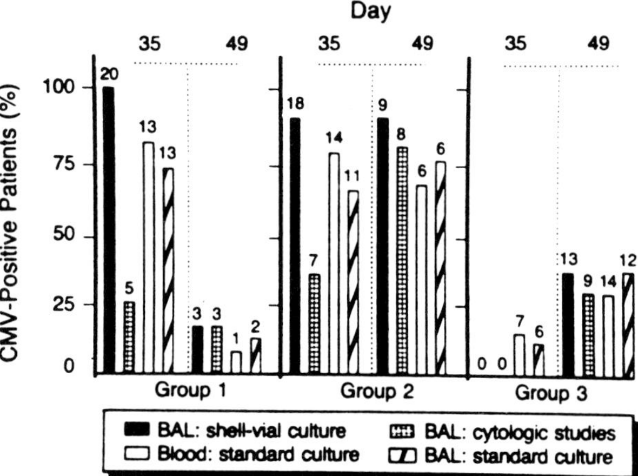

Figure 28-9. Effects of preemptive therapy for prevention of cytomegalovirus (CMV) disease. (Upper) Kaplan-Meier product limit estimates of the probability of CMV-IP in subjects with asymptomatic CMV lung infection on day 35 after bone marrow transplantation, (BMT), treated with ganciclovir (group 1), no ganciclovir (group 2), or with no detectible CMV lung infection on day 35 after BMT (group 3). (Lower) Results of CMV cultures and cytological studies of specimens obtained on days 35 and 49 according to study group. Inset legend refers to methods used to detect CMV in blood or bronchoalveolar lavage specimen. (Reproduced by permission from Schmidt GM, Horak DA, Niland JC, et al. A randomized controlled trial of prophylactic ganciclovir for cytomegalovirus pulmonary infection in recipients of allogeneic bone marrow transplants. N Engl J Med 1991; 324:1005–1011.)

on day 49. Interestingly, 52% of those who were CMV-negative at BAL on day 35 were positive at BAL on day 49, suggesting that infection, when it occurred in this group, was progressing at a different time course than that in the other group. As noted, this biphasic distribution of CMV progression among allograft recipients was confirmed by analysis of blood cultures (see "Pathogenesis of CMV Disease"; and Figure 28-5).

An alternative method for risk-based preemptive therapy is to treat at the time of first CMV infection. This method was evaluated in the study by Goodrich and co-workers (56), in which marrow recipients were treated with ganciclovir at the time of first CMV infection. In this study, patients received weekly throat, urine, and blood cultures and, based on positive cultures, were randomly assigned to treatment with placebo or ganciclovir (5 mg/kg IV b.i.d. for 7 days and then daily until day 100 after BMT). Ganciclovir treatment significantly reduced the occurrence of CMV-associated disease (3 vs 43%; $p < 0.00001$) and had a profound effect on mortality (2.7 vs 17%; $p = 0.041$). As with the BAL-based study, CMV-associated disease developed in 12% of patients because detection of CMV culture occurred either prior to or simultaneously with the development of clinical signs and symptoms.

Critique of Preemptive Therapy with Ganciclovir

As noted, use of ganciclovir for prevention of disease after the onset of infection has been termed *preemptive therapy* (55,193) to distinguish it from prophylactic therapy, which aims at preventing both infection and subsequent disease. Preemptive therapy is based on selective usage of an antiviral agent, and the specific strategies for its implementation are based on risk factors for disease. As noted, preemptive therapy with ganciclovir is an effective method for prevention of a significant amount of CMV-associated morbidity after BMT. Nevertheless, this method, as applied to date, still allows for a certain proportion of disease to continue, the reasons for which reside in the methods used for CMV detection. In the BAL-based method, certain patients had negative BAL rapid-culture results, and CMV-IP still developed. The reason for this finding is two-fold: (1) there is a false-negative rate with any CMV detection method, including the BAL method; and (2) pulmonary CMV infection developed in certain individuals later than most and after the time of the prospective BAL. Similarly, in the culture surveillance method for preemptive ganciclovir therapy, disease develops in certain patients prior to or simultaneously with the detection of positive CMV cultures (56). Nevertheless, these preemptive methods of ganciclovir use provide an effective means to reduce the incidence of CMV-associated disease in marrow allograft patients. At the City of Hope, using preemptive therapy based on BAL, in an additional 170 BMT recipients undergoing surveillance BAL culture at day 35, 36% were CMV culture–positive. No CMV disease occurred in this ganciclovir-treated group; however, CMV-IP occurred in 3% of those who were BAL culture–negative at day 35 (Schmidt GM. Personal communication).

How can this preemptive treatment method be improved? As noted, the 3 most significant risk factors for CMV-IP are GVHD (1,49), asymptomatic CMV infection of lung (55), and CMV infection of blood (49,55,56). It is possible that any of these risks could be used to determine who should receive ganciclovir treatment. In our experience, the blood culture results are only predictive when used at day 28, 35, or 42, but, for the group that is CMV-negative at day 35 BAL, later blood cultures could be useful indicators of risk for CMV-IP (see Figure 28-5). However, blood culture results are usually not available in time for intervention with ganciclovir; therefore, more rapid methods for determining blood infection are necessary. A method for efficiently sampling virus with relatively noninvasive means that is as predictive for subsequent CMV-IP as BAL analysis is currently needed. CMV antigenemia detection is one such method that has been proposed, and it has been shown by Boeckh and associates (84) to be positive prior to the onset of active infection and is a potential marker for subsequent disease, as discussed. More recently, PCR has been used to detect CMV in plasma and is currently being evaluated as a means for detecting risk of CMV disease (99,100). It is likely that other sensitive methods will be developed for the detection of CMV infection that could be used to determine therapy with ganciclovir.

Prevention of CMV by Universal Treatment with Ganciclovir

The alternative approach to prevention of CMV in high-risk patients is to treat all patients with ganciclovir (57,194,195). As shown in Table 28-8, administration of ganciclovir to all CMV-seropositive persons was performed either prior to BMT or at the time of engraftment. The early routine use of ganciclovir during BMT was assessed by Atkinson and colleagues (195) in a nonrandomized study in which ganciclovir was given (5 mg/kg IV b.i.d. from day −8 to −1 and resumed when absolute neutrophil count [ANC] = 1×10^9/L at 5 mg/kg IV 3 days/wk until day +84). This regimen was found to eliminate the occurrence of CMV-IP.

Subsequently, in a randomized, controlled trial, Goodrich and associates (57) studied the effect of ganciclovir given at a dose of 5 mg/kg IV b.i.d. for 5 days and then every day until day 100 after BMT in BMT recipients who were CMV-seropositive at the time of engraftment. This method significantly reduced CMV excretion (3 vs 45%; $p = 0.0001$) and CMV-associated disease (10 vs 29%; $p = 0.0008$). CMV-IP and CMV enteropathy occurred only in those receiving placebo or in those no longer receiving ganciclovir. Subsequent CMV disease occurred in 10% of the treated group after cessation of therapy at day 100. There was no difference between control and treated groups in terms of mortality, either during treatment (19 vs 12%, respectively; $p = 0.4$) or at day 180 (26 vs 30%, respectively). This lack of effect of ganciclovir treatment on mortality is different from the effect observed with preemptive use of ganciclovir (56). Importantly, however, the treatment was marrow-toxic and resulted in some neutropenia-associated complications. Drug-related neutropenia occurred at a significant rate in the ganciclovir group (30 vs 0%; $p = 0.0014$). The median duration of neutropenia was 12 days (range, 4–20 days) and occurred at a median time of onset of 36 days (range, 6–74 days) after starting ganciclovir. Patients on ganciclovir who became neutropenic had a significantly increased risk of bacterial infection, and there was one septic death in this group. Finally, in a study by Winston and associates (195), in which ganciclovir was given prior to BMT at a dose of 2.5 mg/kg IV q8h from day −8 to −1 pre-BMT and was resumed when the ANC was greater than 1×10^9/L at 6 mg/kg dose 5 days/week until day 120 after BMT, the group receiving ganciclovir had a significant reduction in rate of CMV infection (20 vs 56%; $p = 0.0009$) but no significant reduction of CMV disease (10 vs 24%; $p = 0.09$).

Critique of Universal Therapy with Ganciclovir

Prophylactic ganciclovir used universally in BMT recipients at risk for CMV has effectively reduced CMV infection but has not been unequivocally associated with a beneficial outcome. Progressive CMV infection will not develop in all CMV-seropositive BMT recipients during the course of transplantation, but all recipients receiving ganciclovir are at risk for the toxic side effects of the drug. The occurrence of marrow suppression in the 70% of those in whom CMV disease does not develop defeats the purpose of the therapy, which is unavoidable with the univeral-use strategy. Ganciclovir-associated neutropenia has been reported in 30 to 60% of BMT recipients (57,167), which creates a new risk for infection to substitute for the risk of CMV infection. Furthermore, the cost of treating all allogeneic marrow transplant recipients in this way is not inconsiderable. Therefore, considering the toxicity of these agents and their expense, general use of ganciclovir in all CMV-seropositive persons is currently not recommended. Rather, as noted, risk-adjusted approaches to preventive chemotherapy are being evaluated using newer diagnostic tests.

Prophylaxis of CMV Using Foscarnet

Foscarnet was evaluated by Reusser and colleagues (196) in BMT patients and was shown to reduce the occurrence of CMV infection significantly in a Phase I/II pilot study. No controlled study of the overall clinical effect of foscarnet in transplant recipients has been completed.

Use of Immunoglobulin in BMT

Overview

One of the most controversial areas in the management of transplant patients with regard to CMV infection is the use of passive immunization with IVIg. This is an expensive method for modifying the course of CMV infection, and it has had mixed success in different organ transplant settings. Nevertheless, because early experience in BMT (18) showed that favorable outcome was associated with elevated CMV antibody, the use of IVIg was evaluated in many centers. These passive immunization studies utilized either conventional IVIg or CMVIg (197). In general, this method decreased the incidence of CMV infection compared with control patients, but the effect on CMV-associated disease was variable, with no effect seen in certain studies.

Clinical Trials with CMVIG/IVIG

As noted, most CMV-associated disease in marrow recipients occurs in seropositive recipients. How, then, can Ig be effective in the prevention of CMV complications when seropositive individuals remain at risk for serious disease? To approach this question, we must review the experience with controlled use of either IVIg or CMVIg in BMT recipients. As shown in Table 28-9, 7 controlled studies provide information regarding the efficacy of prophylactic passive immunization in preventing either CMV infection or disease (46, 50,53,183,198–200). Most studies showed a decreased incidence of CMV infection with or without an effect on concomitant disease.

An initial study by Meyers and associates (183) used intramuscular CMVIg developed by the Massachusetts State Biologics Institute and given at a dose of 6 mL/m² CMVIg/IM on day −4, −2, and 0 of transplantation and then weekly until day +77. This study showed several important effects of passive therapy. The initial observation was that passive immunization actually resulted in increased CMV antibody titer in BMT recipients. The major result of this study, however, was the demonstration that CMVIg had no effect on development of CMV infection in those receiving white cell transfusions from seropositive donors. However, those patients receiving no such granulocyte support had a significant reduction in the incidence of CMV infection. The number of recipients of CMVIg and seronegative blood support was small, and there was no significant difference in disease between these two groups.

Table 28-9.
Prophylactic CMVIg/IVIg in BMT

Source, Year, Ref	*CMV Infection*	*CMV Disease*
CMVIg		
Meyers, 1983 (183)	Decreased	No change
Bowden, 1986 (50)	Decreased	Decreased
Bowden, 1991 (53)	Decreased	No change
IVIg[a]		
O'Reilly, 1983 (198)	Decreased	Decreased
Kubanek, 1985 (199)	ND	Decreased
Winston, 1987 (200)	No change	Decreased
Sullivan 1990 (46)	No change	Decreased

CMVIg = cytomegalovirus (CMV)-specific intravenous immune globulin prepared from plasma screened for high CMV antibody; IVIg = intravenous immune globulin; BMT = bone marrow transplantation; ND = not demonstrated.

This study was followed by a study by Bowden and colleagues (50), in which seronegative subjects were randomized to receive one of four different regimens: (1) CMVIg and seronegative blood support, (2) seronegative blood support alone, (3) CMVIg alone, or (4) no treatment. Those who received seronegative blood products had significantly less CMV infection than those who received standard blood products. Again, the use of seronegative blood products did not appear to prevent CMV infection in patients who had seropositive marrow donors. The incidence of infection in those receiving CMVIg alone was not different from that in those receiving screened blood products (29 vs 35%, respectively). Thus, this study did not confirm the utility of CMVIg in the prevention of CMV infection; however, it provided strong evidence that use of screened blood product support can virtually eliminate the exogenous exposure to CMV in this population.

The question then existed as to whether CMVIg could be used in seronegative recipients of seropositive donor marrow to protect from primary infection. Bowden and associates (53) completed a study in which patients were randomized to receive CMVIg at a dose of 200 mg/kg on day −8 and −6 pre-BMT, and then weekly for the first month and every 2 weeks thereafter for a completion of 10 doses or to receive no treatment. There was significantly less CMV viremia (17 vs 33%; $p = 0.01$) and overall CMV infection (32 vs 43%; $p = 0.04$) in the treated group. Nevertheless, as in the original study with intramuscular CMVIg, there was no difference in the incidence of CMV disease (17 vs 20%), including CMV-IP and CMV enteritis, nor in the incidence of CMV syndrome (15 vs 15%), including fever, leukopenia, and hepatitis. Similarly, there was no difference in the median time of onset of CMV infection or disease, the median number of hospital days, or the survival of the two groups. Thus, several clinical studies of CMVIg from the same center show consistent effects on viral infection but no significant effects on clinical outcome.

With regard to the use of ordinary IVIg from pooled plasma, a different outcome has been observed in several controlled studies with regard to the effect on clinical CMV disease in BMT recipients (46,198–200). Winston and colleagues (200) treated seronegative recipients of allogeneic BMT with IVIg (20 mL/kg before BMT and then once weekly until day 120), or with placebo, and, although there was no difference in the incidence of CMV infection in the treated compared with the untreated group, there was significant reduction in the occurrence of CMV-IP. High-dose IVIg (1,000 mg/kg) appeared to lower the incidence of CMV-associated disease with regard to symptomatic infection (52 vs 25%; $p = 0.04$) and interstitial pneumonia (52 vs 22%; $p = 0.02$) in the treated group. It was noted, in addition, that 15 of 15 control patients with CMV viremia had symptomatic disease, whereas only 7 of 12 IVIg recipients with viremia had symptomatic disease ($p = 0.01$).

The question of how IVIg exerts this influence on CMV-associated disease needs to be addressed. Although IVIg contains neutralizing antibody, its effect in transplantation is probably different from that of conventional antiviral agents, which function solely by inhibiting virus replication. Use of IVIg in transplant recipients possibly provides essential host support, but in doing this, it is acting not as an antiviral but as either a specific or a nonspecific biological response modifier. The best evidence for this effect was demonstrated by Sullivan and associates (46), who used prophylactic IVIg and demonstrated an effect on the occurrence of acute GVHD in allogeneic marrow recipients (46). In this study, patients were randomized to receive IVIg at a dose of 500 mg/kg in 15 weekly infusions from day −7 to day +90 after transplantation and thereafter at monthly infusion until completion of one year. The importance of this study is that it demonstrated several clinical effects. First, regarding CMV infection, approximately half the 240 seropositive patients had CMV infection, and there was no difference in the incidence between the two study groups. Second, there was an effect on the cumulative incidence of interstitial pneumonia in the two groups. Among the 61 seronegative patients evaluated, there was no case of CMV-IP, and among the 308 seropositive patients, there was a significant reduction in the incidence of CMV-IP (22 vs 13%; p = 0.021). Interestingly, as has been noted, there was no apparent effect on virus infections in the groups, and half the 241 seropositive patients with complete culture data had CMV infection. However, the cumulative incidence of CMV-IP was influenced by the use of IVIg despite the fact that there was no significant reduction in the CMV infection rate. Among CMV-seronegative patients less than 20 years old, there was almost no CMV infection because of the use of screened blood products, and the incidence of IP was not affected by the use of IVIg. In the older patients, the overall incidence of IP was significantly reduced (21 vs 9%; p = 0.0032) by the use of IVIg. In addition, the use of IVIg was associated with decreased transplantation-related mortality in patients 20 years or older who received HLA-identical transplants (46 vs 30%; p = 0.023).

Third, in this study, the severity of GVHD was significantly different in the group at greater risk for GVHD, namely those 20 years of age or older. This effect was observed in 220 patients receiving HLA-identical transplants (43 vs 28%; p = 0.029) and in 105 receiving HLA-nonidentical transplants (71 vs 49%; p = 0.078). Moreover, there was a significant difference between treated and untreated groups in the incidence of septicemia and local infection, and, in particular, gram-negative septicemia was significantly reduced (0.24 vs 0.08 per 100 patient-days; p = 0.0039). This protective effect was most pronounced during the period of neutropenia, but was still significantly different after the period of neutrophil recovery. It is likely that the reduced rate of acute GVHD favorably influenced the development of CMV-associated disease, bacterial infection, and fungal infection. Thus, IVIg promoted significant improvement in the course of BMT and served in a supportive role with other blood products during the post-BMT period. On the basis of these results, IVIg is now used in many centers for support of allogeneic as well as autologous BMT recipients. Although the dosage varies, IVIg is generally administered at a dose of 500 mg/kg every other week from day −8 to day 100 after BMT for allograft recipients.

Role of Monoclonal Antibody in CMV Infection

Monoclonal antibody to CMV is an experimental reagent for which there is currently little published information. A human IgG1 monoclonal antibody to CMV targeted to the gH glycoprotein, and an additional one directed to the gB glycoprotein, have been used in an open Phase 1 trial and have been shown to be safe at doses of 2 mg/kg (201). This material has been used without complication in an uncontrolled study for treatment of CMV infection in renal transplant recipients (202), but its effect on infection or on clinical disease in the marrow transplant population is currently not known.

References

1. Meyers JD, Thomas ED. Infection complicating bone marrow transplantation. In: Rubin RH, Young LS, eds. Clinical approach to infection in the compromised host, ed 2. New York: Plenum, 1981:525–556.
2. Zaia JA. Viral infections associated with bone marrow transplantation. Hematol/Oncol Clin North Am 1990;4: 603–623.
3. Winston DJ, Gale RP, Meyers DV, and Young LS. Infectious complications of human bone marrow transplantation. Medicine 1979;58:1–31.
4. Meyers JD, Fluornoy N, Thomas ED. Nonbacterial pneumonia after allogeneic marrow transplantation. A review of ten years' experience. Rev Infect Dis 1982;4:1119–1132.
5. Miller W, Flynn P, McCullough J, et al. Cytomegalovirus infection after bone marrow transplantation: an association with acute graft-v-host disease. Blood 1986;67: 1162–1167.
6. Wingard JR, Mellitis ED, Sostrin MB, et al. Interstitial pneumonitis after allogeneic bone marrow transplantation. Nine-year experience at a single institution. Medicine 1988;67:175–186.
7. Winston DJ, Ho WG, Champlin RE. Cytomegalovirus infections after allogeneic bone marrow transplantation. Rev Infect Dis 1990;12(suppl):S776–S792.
8. Wingard JR, Piantadosi S, Burns WH, Zahurak ML, Santos GW, Saral R. Cytomegalovirus infections in bone marrow transplant recipients given intensive cytoreductive therapy. Rev Infect Dis 1990;12(suppl):S793–S804.
9. Mocarski ES Jr, Abenes GB, Manning WC, Sambucetti LC, Cherrington JM. Molecular genetic analysis of cytomegalovirus gene regulation in growth, persistance, and latency. In: McDougall JK, ed. Cytomegalovirus. Curr Top Microbiol Immunol 1990;154:47–74.
10. DeMarchi JM, Blankship ML, Brown GD, Kaplan AS. Size and complexity of human cytomegalovirus DNA. Virology 1978;89:643–646.

11. Chee MA, Bankier AT, Beck S, et al. An analysis of the protein coding content of the sequence of human cytomegalovirus strain AD169. Curr Top Microbiol 1990;154:125–169.
12. Stinski MF. Cytomegalovirus and its replication. In: Fields BN, Knipe DM, eds. Virology, ed 2. New York: Raven, 1990:1959–1980.
13. Ho M. Cytomegalovirus: biology and infection, ed 2. New York: Plenum, 1991.
14. Britt WJ. Recent advances in the identification of significant human cytomegalovirus-encoded protein. Transplant Proc 1990;23(suppl 3):64–69.
15. Gretch DR, Kari B, Rasmussen L, Gehrz RC, Stinski MF. Identification and characterization of three distinct families of glycoprotein complexes in the envelopes of human cytomegalovirus. J Virol 1988;62:875–881.
16. Zaia JA, Forman SJ, Ting Y-P, Vanderwal-Urbina E, Blume KG. Polypeptide-specific antibody response to human cytomegalovirus after infection in bone marrow transplant recipients. J Infect Dis 1986;153:780–787.
17. Zaia JA, Levin MJ, Preblud SR. The status of passive immunization for herpesvirus infections. In: Alving BM, Finlayson JS, eds. Immunoglobulins: characteristics and use of intravenous preparations. DHHS Publication No. (FDA)-80–9005. Washington, DC: U.S. Government Printing Office, 1980:111–121.
18. Neiman P, Wasserman PB, Wentworth B, et al. Interstitial pneumonia and cytomegalovirus infection as complications of human marrow transplantation. Transplantation 1973;15:478–485.
19. Meyers JD. Prevention of cytomegalovirus infection after marrow transplantation. Rev Infect Dis 1989;11 (Suppl 7):S1691–S1705.
20. Meyers JD, Flournoy N, Thomas ED. Cytomegalovirus infection and specific cell-mediated immunity after marrow transplant. J Infect Dis 1980;142:816–824.
21. Quinnan GV, Kirmani N, Rook AH, et al. Cytotoxic T cells in cytomegalovirus infection: HLA-restricted T lymphocyte and non T lymphocyte cytotoxic responses correlate with recovery from cytomegalovirus in bone marrow recipients. N Engl J Med 1982;307:7–13.
22. Rook AH, Quinnan GV, Frederick WJR, et al. Importance of cytotoxic lymphocytes during cytomegalovirus infection in renal transplant recipients. Am J Med 1984;76:385–392.
23. Reusser P, Riddell SR, Meyers JD, Greenberg PD. Cytotoxic T-lymphocyte response to cytomegalovirus after human allogeneic bone marrow transplantation: pattern of recovery and correlation with cytomegalovirus infection and disease. Blood 1991;78:1373–1380.
24. Borysiewicz LK, Hickling JK, Graham S, et al. Human cytomegalovirus-specific cytotoxic T cells: relative frequency of stage-specific CTL recognizing the 72KD immediate early protein and glycoprotein B expressed by recombinant vaccina viruses. J Exp Med 1988; 168:919–931.
25. Forman SJ, Zaia JA, Clark BR, et al. In vitro cellular response to the late 64K glycoprotein of cytomegalovirus; evidence for T-cell activation. Transplant Proc 1985;1:507–509.
26. Liu Y-NC, Kari B, Gehrz RC. Human immune responses to major human cytomegalovirus glycoprotein complexes. J Virol 1988;62:1066–1070.
27. Riddell SR, Rabin M, Geballe AP, Britt WJ, Greenberg PD. Class I MHC-restricted cytotoxic T lymphocyte recognition of cells infected with human cytomegalovirus does not require endogenous viral gene expression. J Immunol 1991;146:2795–2804.
28. McLaughlin-Taylor E, Tanamachi B, Pande H, et al. Identification of the major late human cytomegalovirus matrix protein pp65 as a target antigen for CD8+ virus-specific CTL. J Med Virol 1993 (in press).
29. Moore MW, Carbone FR, Bevan MJ. Introduction of soluble protein into the class I pathway of antigen processing and presentation. Cell 1988;54:777–785.
30. Reddehase, MJ, Rothbard JB, Koszinowski UH. A pentapeptide as minimal antigenic determinant for MHC class I restricted T-lymphocytes. Nature 1989; 337:651–653.
31. Sissions JGP, Borysiewicz LK, Rodgers B, Scott D. Cytomegalovirus. Its cellular immunology and biology. Immunol Today 1986;7:57–61.
32. Riddell SR, Watanabe KS, Goodrich JM, Li CR, Agha ME, Greenberg PD. Restoration of viral immunity in immunodeficient humans by the adoptive transfer of T cell clones. Science 1992;257:238–241.
33. Boland GH, Vlieger AM, Ververs C, De Gast GC. Evidence for transfer of cellular and humoral immunity to cytomegalovirus from donor to recipient in allogeneic bone marrow transplantation. Clin Exp Immunol 1992;88:506–511.
34. Plotkin SA, Furukawa T, Zygraich N, Huygelen D. Candidate cytomegalovirus strain for human vaccination. Infect Immun 1975;12:521–527.
35. Plotkin SA. Cytomegalovirus vaccine development—past and present. Transplant Proc 1990;23(suppl 3):85–89.
36. Gönczöl E, Ianacone J, Ho W, Starr S, Meignier B, Plotkin S. The isolated gA/gB glycoprotein complex of human cytomegalovirus envelope induces humoral and cellular immune-responses in human volunteers. Vaccine 1990;8:130–136.
37. Stinski MF. Sequence of protein synthesis in cells infected with human cytomegalovirus: early and late viral-induced polypeptides. J Virol 1978;26:686–701.
38. Walthen M, Stinski M. Temporal patterns of human cytomegalovirus transcription: mapping the viral RNAs synthesized at immediate early, early, and late times after infection. J Virol 1982;41:462–477.
39. Liu B, Stinski MF. Human cytomegalovirus contains a tegument protein that enhances transcription from promoters with upstream ATF and AP-1 *cis*-acting elements. J Virol 1992;66:4434–4444.
40. Pande H, Terramani T, Churchill MA, Hawkins GG, Zaia J. Regulation of fibronectin gene expression by human cytomegalovirus. J Virol 1990;64:1366–1369.
41. Dutko FJ, Oldstone MBA. Cytomegalovirus causes a latent infection in undifferentiated cells and is activated by induction of cell differentiation. J Exp Med 1981;154:1636–1651.
42. Jordan MC, Pomeroy C. Latent CMV infection in the mouse. Transplant Proc 1990;23(suppl 3):17–21.
43. Mercer JA, Wiley CA, Spector DH. Pathogenesis of murine cytomegalovirus infection: identification of infected cells in the spleen during acute and latent infections. J Virol 1988;62:987–997.
44. Bowden RA, Slichter SJ, Sayers MH, Mori M, Cays MJ, Meyers JD. Use of leukocyte-depleted platelets and cytomegalovirus-seronegative red blood cells for prevention of primary cytomegalovirus infection after marrow transplant. Blood 1991;78:246–250.
45. Miller WJ, McCullough J, Balfour Jr HH, et al. Prevention of cytomegalovirus infection following

bone marrow transplantation: a randomized trial of blood product screening. Bone Marrow Transplant 1991;7:227–234.

46. Sullivan KM, Kopecky KJ, Jocom J, et al. Immunomodulatory and antimicrobial efficacy of intravenous immunoglobulin in bone marrow transplantation. N Engl J Med 1990;323:705–712.
47. Neiman PE, Reeves W, Ray George, et al. A prospective analysis of interstitial pneumonia and opportunistic viral infection among recipients of allogeneic bone marrow grafts. J Infect Dis 1977;136:754–767.
48. Meyers JD, Spencer HC Jr, Watts JC, et al. Cytomegalovirus pneumonia after human marrow transplantation. Ann Intern Med 1975;82:181–188.
49. Meyers JD, Flournoy N, Thomas ED. Risk factors for cytomegalovirus infection after human marrow transplantation. J Infect Dis 1986;153:478–488.
50. Bowden RA, Sayers M, Flournoy N, et al. Cytomegalovirus immune globulin and seronegative blood products to prevent primary cytomegalovirus infection after marrow transplantation. N Engl J Med 1986;314:1006–1010.
51. Winston DJ, Ho WG, Lin C-H, et al. Intravenous immune globulin for prevention of cytomegalovirus infection and interstitial pneumonia after bone marrow transplantation. Ann Intern Med 1987;106:12–18.
52. De Witte T, Schattenberg A, Van Dijk BA, Galama J, Olthuis H, Van Der Meer JWW, Kunst VAJM. Prevention of primary cytomegalovirus infection after allogeneic bone marrow transplantation by using leukocyte-poor random blood products from cytomegalovirus-unscreened blood-bank donors. Transplantation 1990;50: 964–968.
53. Bowden RA, Fisher LK, Rogers K, Cays M, Meyers JD. Cytomegalovirus (CMV)-specific intravenous immunoglobulin for the prevention of primary CMV infection and disease after marrow transplant. J Infect Dis 1991;164:483–487.
54. Meyers JD, Reed EC, Shepp DH, et al. Acyclovir for prevention of cytomegalovirus infection and disease after allogeneic marrow transplantation. N Engl J Med 1988;318:70–75.
55. Schmidt GM, Horak DA, Niland JC, et al. A randomized controlled trial of prophylactic ganciclovir for cytomegalovirus pulmonary infection in recipients of allogeneic bone marrow transplants. N Engl J Med 1991; 324:1005–1011.
56. Goodrich JM, Mori M, Gleaves CA, et al. Early treatment with ganciclovir to prevent cytomegalovirus disease after allogeneic bone marrow transplantation. N Engl J Med 1991;325:1601–1607.
57. Goodrich JM, Bowden RA, Fisher L, Keller C, Schoch BA, Meyers JD. Prevention of cytomegalovirus disease after allogeneic marrow transplant by ganciclovir prophylaxis. Ann Intern Med 1993;118:173–178.
58. Wingard JR, Chen DY-H, Burns WH, et al. Cytomegalovirus infection after autologous bone marrow transplantation with comparison to infection after allogeneic bone marrow transplantation. Blood 1988; 71:1432–1437.
59. Reusser P, Fisher LD, Buckner CD, Thomas ED, Meyers JD. Cytomegalovirus infection after autologous bone marrow transplantation: occurrence of cytomegalovirus disease and effect on engraftment. Blood 1990;75:1888–1894.
60. Appelbaum FR, Meyers JD, Fefer A, et al. Nonbacterial nonfungal pneumonia following marrow transplantation in 100 identical twins. Transplantation 1982; 33:265–268.
61. Huang E-S, Alford CA, Reynolds DW, Stagno S, Pass RF. Molecular epidemiology of cytomegalovirius infection in women and their infants. N Engl J Med 1980; 303:958–962.
62. Spector SA, Spector DH. Molecular epidemiology of cytomegalovirus infection in premature twin infants and their mother. Pediatr Infect Dis 1982;1:405–409.
63. Yow MD, Lakeman AD, Stagno S, Reynolds RB, Plavidal FJ. Use of restriction enzymes to investigate the source of a primary cytomegalovirus infection in a pediatric nurse. Pediatrics 1982;70:713–716.
64. Collier AC, Chandler SH, Handsfield HH, Corey L, McDougall JK. Identification of multiple strains of cytomegalovirus in homosexual men. J Infect Dis 1989; 159:123–126.
65. Drew WL, Sweet ES, Miner RC, Mocarski ES. Multiple infections by cytomegalovirus in patients with acquired immunodeficiency syndrome: documentation by Southern blot hybridization. J Infect Dis 1984;150:952–953.
66. Zaia JA, Gallez-Hawkins G, Churchill MA, et al. Comparative analysis of human cytomegalovirus *a*-sequence in multiple clinical isolates using polymerase chain reaction and restriction fragment length polymorphism assays. J Clin Microbiol 1990;38:2602–2607.
67. Winston DJ, Huang E-S, Miller MJ, Lin C-H, Ho WG, Gale RP, Champlin RE. Molecular epidemiology of cytomegalovirus infections associated with bone marrow transplantation. Ann Intern Med 1985;102:16–20.
68. Gregory WW, Menegus MA. Practical protocol for cytomegalovirus isolation: use of MRC-5 cell monolayers incubated for 2 weeks. J Clin Microbiol 1983; 17:605–609.
69. Gleaves CA, Smith TF, Shuster EA, Pearson GR. Rapid detection of cytomegalovirus in MRC-5 cells inoculated with urine specimens by using low-speed centrifugation and monoclonal atibody to an early antigen. J Clin Microbiol 1984;19:917–919.
70. Swenson PD, Kaplan MH. Rapid detection of cytomegalovirus in cell culture by indirect immunoperoxidase staining with monoclonal antibody to an early nuclear antigen. J Clin Microbiol 1985;21:669–673.
71. Stirk PR, Griffiths PD. Use of monoclonal antibodies for the diagnosis of cytomegalovirus infection by the detection of early antigen fluorescent foci (DEAFF) in cell culture. J Med Virol 1987;21:329–337.
72. Gleaves CA, Smith TF, Shuster EA, Pearson GR. Comparison of standard tube and shell vial cell culture techniques for the detection of cytomegalovirus in clinical specimens. J Clin Microbiol 1985;21:217–221.
73. Paya CV, Wold AD, Smith TF. Detection of cytomegalovirus infections in specimens other than urine by the shell vial assay and conventional tube cell cultures. J Clin Microbiol 1897;25:755–757.
74. Erice A, Holm MA, Gill PC, et al. Cytomegalovirus (CMV) antigenemia assay is more sensitive than shell vial cultures for rapid detection of CMV in polymorphnuclear blood leukocytes. J Clin Microbiol 1992;30:2822–2825.
75. Ashley R, Peterson E, Abbo A, Gold D, Corey L. Comparison of monoclonal antibodies for rapid detection of cytomegalovirus in spin-amplified plate cultures. J Clin Microbiol 1989;27:2858–2860.
76. Leland DS, Hansing RL, French ML. Clinical experience with cytomegalovirus isolation using conventional

cell cultures and early antigen detection in centrifugation-enhanced shell vial cultures. J Clin Microbiol 1989;27:1159–1162.
77. Rabella N, Drew WL. Comparison of conventional and shell vial cultures for detecting cytomegalovirus infection. J Clin Microbiol 1990;28:806–807.
78. van der Bij W, Torensma R, vanSon WJ, et al. Rapid immunodiagnosis of active cytomegalovirus infection by monoclonal antibody staining of blood leukocytes. J Med Virol 1988;25:179–188.
79. Grefte JMM, van der Gun BTF, Schmolke S, et al. Cytomegalovirus antigenemia assay: identification of the viral antigen as the lower matrix protein pp65. J Infect Dis 1992;166:683–684.
80. Gerna G, Zipeto D, Percivalle E, et al. Human cytomegalovirus infection of the major leukocyte subpopulations and evidence for initial viral replication in polymorphonuclear leukocytes from viremic patients. J Infect Dis 1992;166:1236–1244.
81. van den Berg AP, van der Bij W, van Son WJ, et al. Cytomegalovirus antigenemia as a useful marker of symptomatic cytomegalovirus infection after renal transplantation: a report of 130 consecutive patients. Transplantation 1989;48:991–995.
82. Revello MG, Percivalle E, Zavattoni M, Parea M, Grossi P, Gerna G. Detection of human cytomegalovirus immediate early antigen in leukocytes as a marker of viremia in immunocompromised patients. J Med Virol 1989;29:-88–93.
83. Boland GJ, de Gast GC, Hene RJ, et al. Early detection of active cytomegalovirus (CMV) infection after heart and kidney transplantation by testing for immediate early antigenemia and influence of cellular immunity on the occurrence of CMV infection. J Clin Microbiol 1990;28:2069–2075.
84. Boeckh M, Bowden RA, Goodrich JM, Pettinger M, Meyers JD. Cytomegalovirus antigen detection in peripheral blood leukocytes after allogeneic marrow transplantation. Blood 1992;80:1358–1364.
85. Spector SA, Hsia K, Denaro F, Spector DH. Use of molecular probes to detect human cytomegalovirus and human immunodeficiency virus. Clin Chem 1989;35:1581–1587.
86. Myerson D, Hackman RD, Nelson JA, Ward DC, McDougall JK. Widespread presence of histologically occult cytomegalovirus. Hum Pathol 1984;15:430–439.
87. Myerson D, Hackman RC, Meyers JD. Diagnosis of cytomegalovirus pneumonia in *in situ* hybridization. J Infect Dis 1984;150:272–277.
88. Dankner WM, McCutchan JA, Richman DD, Hirata K, Spector SA. Localization of human cytomegalovirus in peripheral blood leukocytes by *in situ* hybridization. J Infect Dis 1990;161:31–36.
89. Stöckl E, Popow-Kraupp T, Heinz FX, Hulbacher F, Balcke P, Kunz C. Potential of *in situ* hybridization for early diagnosis of productive cytomegalovirus infection. J Clin Microbiol 1988;26:2536–2540.
90. Zaia JA. The biology of human cytomegalovirus infection after bone marrow transplantation. Int J Cell Cloning 1986;4:135–154.
91. Nuovo GJ, Gallery F, MacConnell P, Becker J, Block W. An improved technique for the *in situ* detection of DNA after polymerase chain reaction amplification. Am J Pathol 1991;139:1239–1244.
92. Demmler GJ, Buffone GJ, Schimbor CM, May RA. Detection of cytomegalovirus in urine from newborns by using polymerase chain reaction DNA amplification. J Infect Dis 1988;158:1177–1184.
93. Cassol SA, Poon M-C, Pal R, et al. Primer-mediated enzymatic amplification of cytomegalovirus (CMV) DNA. J Clin Invest 1989;83:1109–1115.
94. Hsia K, Spector DH, Lawrie J, Spector SA. Enzymatic amplification of human cytomegalovirus sequences by polymerase chain reaction. J Clin Microbiol 1989;27:1802–1809.
95. Chow S. Differentiation of cytomegalovirus strains by restriction analysis of DNA sequences amplified from clinical specimens. J Infect Dis 1990;162:738–742.
96. Chou S, Dennison KM. Analysis of interstrain variation in cytomegalovirus glycoprotein B sequences encoding neutralization-related epitopes. J Infect Dis 1991;163:1229–1234.
97. Einsele H, Steidle M, Vallbracht A, Saal JG, Ehninger G, Muller CA. Early occurrence of human cytomegalovirus infection after bone marrow transplantation as demonstrated by the polymerase chain reaction technique. Blood 1991;77:1104–1110.
98. Einsele H, Ehninger G, Steidle M, et al. Polymerase chain reaction to evaluate antiviral therapy for cytomegalovirus disease. Lancet 1991;2:1170–1172.
99. Ishigaki S, Takeda M, Kura T, Ban N, Saitoh T. Cytomegalovirus DNA in the sera of patients with cytomegalovirus pneumonia. Br J Haematol 1991;79:198–204.
100. Spector SA, Merrill R, Wolf D, Dankner WM. Detection of human cytomegalovirus in plasma of AIDS patients during acute visceral disease by DNA amplification. J Clin Microbiol 1992;30:2359–2365.
101. Jiwa NM, van Gemert GW, Raap AK, et al. Rapid detection of human cytomegalovirus DNA in peripheral blood leukocytes of viremic transplant recipients by the polymerase chain reaction. Transplantation 1989;48:72–76.
102. Boland GJ, de Weger RA, Tilanus MGJ, Ververs C, Bosboom-Kalsbeek K, de Gast GC. Detection of cytomegalovirius (CMV) in granulocytes by polymerase chain reaction compared with the CMV antigen test. J Clin Microbiol 1992;30:1763–1767.
103. Jacobson MA, Mills J. Serious cytomegalovirus disease in the acquired immunodeficiency syndrome (AIDS). Ann Intern Med 1988;108:585–594.
104. Zaia JA, Lang DJ. Cytomegalovirus infection of the fetus and neonate. Neurol Clin North Am 1984;2:387–410.
105. Klemola E. Cytomegalovirus infection in previously healthy adults. Ann Intern Med 1973;79:267–268.
106. Meyers JD, Ljungman P, Fisher LD. Cytomegalovirus excretion as a predictor of cytomegalovirus disease after marrow transplantation: importance of cytomegalovirus viremia. J Infect Dis 1990;162:373–380.
107. Betts RF, Freeman RB, Douglas RG Jr, et al. Clinical manifestations of renal allograft derived primary cytomegalovirus infection. Am J Dis Child 1977;131:759–763.
108. Zaia JA, Schmidt GM. Ganciclovir treatment of bone marrow transplant recipients with cytomegalovirus disease. In: Spector SA, ed. Ganciclovir therapy for cytomegalovirus infection. New York: Marcel Dekker, 1991:155–183.
109. Dummer JS, White LT, Ho M, et al. The morbidity of cytomegalovirus infection in heart and heart-lung transplant recipients on cyclosporine. J Infect Dis 1985;152:1182–1191.
110. Rubin RH, Cosimi AB, Tolkoff-Rubin NE, Russell PS, Hirsch MS. Infectious disease syndromes attributable to cytomegalovirus and their significance among renal transplant recipients. Transplantation 1977;24:458–464.

111. Zaia JA. Understanding human cytomegalovirus infection. In: Champlin RE, Gale RP, eds. New strategies in bone marrow transplantation. UCLA symposia on molecular and cellular biology new series, vol 137. New York: Wiley-Liss, 1990:319–334.
112. Grundy JE, Shanley JD, Griffiths PD. Is cytomegalovirus interstitial pneumonitis in transplant recipients an immunopathological condition? Lancet 1987;2:996–999.
113. D'Amico DJ, Talamo JH, Felsenstein D, Hirsch MS, Albert DM, Schooley RT. Ophthalmoscopic and histologic findings in cytomegalovirus retinitis treated with BW-B759U. Arch Ophthalmol 1986;104:1788–1793.
114. AIDS Research Group. Mortality in patients with the acquired immunodeficiency syndrome treated with either foscarnet or ganciclovir for cytomegalovirus retinitis. N Engl J Med 1992;326:213–220.
115. Shepp DH, Dandliker PS, de Miranda P, et al. Activity of 9-[2-hydroxyl-1-(hydroxymethyl), ethoxymethyl] guanine in the treatment of cytomegalovirus pneumonia. Ann Intern Med 1985;103:368–373.
116. Reed EC, Wolford JL, Kopecky KJ, et al. Ganciclovir for the treatment of cytomegalovirus gastroenteritis in bone marrow transplant patients: a randomized placebo-controlled trial. Ann Intern Med 1990;112: 505–510.
117. Albrecht T, Boldogh I, Fons M, et al. Cell-activation responses to cytomegalovirus infection: relationship to the phasing of CMV replication and to the induction of cellular damage. Subcell Biochem 1989;15:157–202.
118. Boldogh I, AbuBakar S, Albrecht T. Activation of proto-oncogenes: an immediate early event in human cytomegalovirus infection. Science 1990;247: 561–564.
119. Keay S, Merigan TC, Rasmussen L. Identification of cell surface receptors for the 86-kilodalton glycoprotein of human cytomegalovirus. Proc Natl Acad Sci USA 1989;86:10100–10103.
120. Taylor HP, Cooper NRJ. The human cytomegalovirus receptor on fibroblasts is a 30-kilodalton membrane protein. Virology 1990;63:3991–3998.
121. Adlish JD, Lahijani RS, St Jeor S. Identification of a putative cell receptor for human cytomegalovirus. Virology 1990;176:337–345.
122. Söderberg C, Giugni TD, Zaia JA, Larsson S, Wahlberg JM, Möller E. CD13 (human aminopeptidase N) mediates human cytomegalovirus infection. J Virol 1993 (in press).
123. Stenberg RM, Stinski MF. Autoregulation of the human cytomegalovirus major immediate-early gene. J Virol 1985;56:676–682.
124. Pizzorno M, O'Hara P, Sha L, LaFemina RL, Hayward GS. Transactivation and autoregulation of gene expression by the immediate-early region 2 gene products of human cytomegalovirus. J Virol 1988;62:1167–1179.
125. Hennighausen L, Fleckenstein. Nuclear factor 1 interacts with five DNA elements in the promoter region of the human cytomegalovirus major immediate early gene. EMBO J 1986;5:1367–1371.
126. Hunninghake GW, Monick MM, Liu B, Stinski MF. The promoter regulatory region of the major immediate-early gene of human cytomegalovirus responds to T-lymphocyte stimulation and contains functional cyclic AMP-response elements. J Virol 1989;63:3026–3033.
127. Sambucetti LC, Cherrington JM, Wilkinson GWG, Mocarski ES. NF-kB activation of the cytomegalovirus enhancer is mediated by a viral transactivator and by T cell stimulation. EMBO J 1989;8:4251–4258.
128. Ho M. Immunology of cytomegalovirus: immunosuppressive effects during infections. Birth Defects 1984; 20:131–147.
129. Carney WP, Hirsch MS. Mechanisms of immunosuppression in CMV mononucleosis. II. Virus-monocyte interactions. J Infect Dis 1981;144:47–54.
130. Dudding LR, Garnett HM. Interaction of strain AD169 and a clinical isolates of cytomegalovirus with peripheral monocytes: the effect of lipopolysaccharide stimulation. J Infect Dis 1987;155:891–896.
131. Schrier RD, Oldstone MB. Recent clinical isolates of cytomegalovirus suppress human cytomegalovirus-specific human leukocyte antigen-restricted cytotoxic T-lymphocyte activity. J Virol 1986;59:127–131.
132. Rodgers BC, Scott DM, Mundin J, Sissons JGP. Monocyte-derived inhibitor of interleukin 1 induced by human cytomegalovirus. J Virol 1985;55:527–532.
133. Kapasi K, Rice GPA. Cytomegalovirus infection of peripheral blood mononuclear cells: effects on interleukin-1 and -2 production and responsiveness. J Virol 1988;62:3603–3607.
134. Bowden RA, Dobbs S, Amos D, Meyers JD. Comparison of interleukin 2 and gamma-interferon production by peripheral blood mononuclerar cells in response to cytomegalovirus afater marrow transplantation. Transplantation 1990;50:38–42.
135. Duncombe AS, Meager A, Prentice HG, et al. Gamma-interferon and tumor necrosis factor production after marrow transplantation is augmented by exposure to marrow fibroblasts infected with cytomegalovirus. Blood 1990;76:1046–1053.
136. Duncombe AS, Grundy JE, Oblakowski P, et al. Bone marrow transplant recipients have defective MHC-restricted cytotoxic responses against cytomegalovirus in comparison with Epstein-Barr: the importance of target cell expression. Blood 1992;79:3059–3066.
137. Griffiths PD, Grundy JE. Molecular biology and immunology of cytomegalovirus. Biochemistry 1987;241: 313–325.
138. Beck S, Barrell GB. 45kDa CMV protein with ≈50 homology to Class I MHC. Nature 1988;331: 269–272.
139. Fujinami RS, Nelson JA, Walker L, Oldstone MA. Sequence homology and immunogic cross-reactivity of human cytomegalovirus with HLA-DR β chain: a means for graft rejection and immunosuppression. J Virol 1988;62:100–105.
140. Grundy JE, McKeating JA, Ward PJ, Sanderson AR, Griffiths PD. $\beta 2$ microglobulin enhances the infectivity of cytomegalovirus and when bound to the virus enables class 1 HLA molecules to be used as a virus receptor. J Gen Virol 1987;68:793–803.
141. Rose JS, Grundy JE. Beta 2 microglobulin on the envelope of urinary cytomegalovirus is not associated with host class I human leukocyte antigen alpha chain. J Gen Virol 1992;73:507–512.
142. Browne H, Churcher M, Minson T. Construction and characterization of a human cytomegalovirus mutant with the UL18 (class I homolog) gene deleted. J Virol 1992;66:6784–6787.
143. Horn TD, Farmer ER, Vogelsang GB, Wingard JR, Santos GW. Cutaneous GVHD lacks evidence of cutaneous CMV by the immunoperoxidase technique. J Invest Dermatol 1989;93:92–95.
144. Boström L, Ringden O, Sundberg B, Linde A, Tollemar J, Nilsson B. Pretransplant herpes virus serology and

graft-versus-host disease. Transplantation 1988;46: 548–552.
145. Gratama JW, Zwaan FE, Stijnen T, et al. Herpes virus immunity and acute graft-versus-host disease. Lancet 1987;1:471–474.
146. Bostrom L, Ringden O, Gratama JW, Jacobsen N, Zawwn F, Nilsson B, for the Leukaemia Working Party of the European Group for Bone Marrow Transplantation. The impact of pretransplant herpesvirus serology on acute and chronic graft-versus-host disease. Transplant Proc 1990;22:206–207.
147. Lönnqvist B, Ringden O, Wahren B, Gahrton G, Lundgren G. Cytomegalovirus infection associated with and preceeding chronic graft-versus-host disease. Transplantation 1984;38:465–468.
148. Jacobsen N, Anderson HK, Skinhoj P, et al. Correlation between donor CMV immunity and chronic GVHD after allogeneic bone marrow transplantation. Scand J Haematol 1986;36:499–506.
149. Grundy JE, Shanley JD, Shearer GM. Augmentation of graft-versus-host reaction by cytomegalovirus infection resulting in interstitial pneumonitis. Transplantation 1985;39:548–553.
150. Gratama JW, Fibbe WE, Naipal AMIH, et al. Cytomegalovirus immunity and T lymphocytes in bone marrow donors and acute GVHD. Bone Marrow Transplant 1986;1:141–146.
151. Zaia JA. Epidemiology and pathogenesis of cytomegalovirus disease. Semin Hematol 1990;27:5–10.
152. Weiner RS, Bortin MM, Gale RP, et al. Interstitial peumonitis after bone marrow transplantation: assessment of risk factors. Ann Intern Med 1986;104:168–175.
153. Khouri NF, Saral R, Armstrong EM, et al. Pulmonary interstitial changes following bone marrow transplantation: a complex, multifactor disorder. Radiology 1979;133:587–592.
154. Beschorner WE, Hutchins GM, Burns WH, Saral R, Tutschka PJ, Santos GW. Cytomegalovirus pneumonia in bone marrow transplant recipients: miliary and diffuse patterns. Am Rev Resp Dis 1980;122:107–114.
155. Slavin MA, Gleaves CA, Schoch HG, Bowden RA. Quantification of cytomegalovirus in bronchoalveolar lavage fluid after allogeneic marrow transplantation by centrifugation culture. J Clin Microbiol 1992; 30:2776–2779.
156. Stover DE, Zaman MB, Jajdu SI, Lange M, Gold J, Armstrong D. Bronchoalveolar lavage in the diagnosis of diffuse pulmonary infiltrates in the immunosuppressed host. Ann Intern Med 1984;101:1–7.
157. Springmeyer SC, Hackman RC, Holle R, et al. Use of bronchoalveolar lavage to diagnose acute diffuse pneumonia in the immunocompromised host. J Infect Dis 1986;154:604–610.
158. Kraemer KG, Neiman PE, Reeves WC, Thomas ED. Prophylactic adenine arabinoside following marrow transplantation. Transplant Proc 1978;10:237–240.
159. Meyers JD, McGuffin RW, Neiman PE, Singer JW, Thomas ED. Toxicity and efficacy of human leukocyte interferon for treatment of cytomegalovirus pneumonia after marrow transplantation. J Infect Dis 1980;141: 555–562.
160. Meyers JD, McGuffin RW, Bryson YJ, Cantell K, Thomas ED. Treatment of cytomegalovirus pneumonia after marrow transplant with combined vidarabine and human leukocyte interferon. J Infect Dis 1982;146:80–84.
161. Wade JC, Hintz M, McGuffin RW, Springmeyer SC, Connor JD, Meyers JD. Treatment of cytomegalovirus pneumonia with high dose acyclovir. Am J Med 1982;73:249–256.
162. Wade JC, McGuffin RW, Springmeyer SC, Newton B, Singer JW, Meyers JD. Treatment of cytomegaloviral pneumonia with high-dose acyclovir and human leukocyte interferon. J Infect Dis 1983;148:557–562.
163. Meyers JD, Day LM, Lum LG, Sullivan KM. Recombinant leukocyte A interferon for the treatment of serious viral infection after marrow transplant: a phase I study. J Infect Dis 1983;148:551–556.
164. Winston DJ, Ho WG, Schroff RW, Champlin RE, Gale RP. Safety and tolerance of recombinant leukocyte A interferon in bone marrow transplant recipients. Antimicrob Agents Chemother 1983;23:846–851.
165. Shepp DH, Newton BA, Meyers JD. Intravenous lymphoblastoid interferon and acyclovir for treatment of cytomegaloviral pneumonia. J Infect Dis 1984;150: 776–777.
166. Winston DJ, Ho WG, Bartoni K, et al. Ganciclovir therapy for cytomegalovirus infections in recipients of bone marrow transplants and other immunosuppressed patients. Rev Infect Dis 1988;10(suppl 3): S547–S553.
167. Erice A, Jordan MC, Chace BA, Fletcher C, Chinnock BJ, Balfour HH Jr. Ganciclovir treatment of cytomegalovirus disease in transplant recipients and other immunocompromised hosts. J Am Med Assoc 1987;257: 3082–3087.
168. Reed EC, Dandliker PS, Meyers JD. Treatment of cytomegalovirus pneumonia with 9-[2-hydroxy-1-(hydroxymethyl)ethoxymethyl] guanine and high dose corticosteroids. Ann Intern Med 1986;105:214–216.
169. Blacklock HA, Griffiths P, Stirk P, Prentice HG. Specific hyperimmune globulin for cytomegalovirus pneumonitis. Lancet 1985;2:152–153.
170. Reed EC, Bowden RA, Dandliker PS, Gleaves CA, Meyers JD. Efficacy of cytomegalovirus immunoglobulin in marrow transplant recipients with cytomegalovirus pneumonia. J Infect Dis 1987;156:641–645.
171. Ringden O, Wilczek H, Lönnqvist, Gahrton G, Wahren AB, Lernestedt J-O. Foscarnet for cytomegalovirus infections. Lancet 1985;1:1503–1504.
172. Masur H, Lane HC, Palestine A, et al. Effect of 9-(1,3-dihydroxy-2-propoxymethyl) guanine on serious cytomegalovirus disease in eight immunosuppressed homosexual men. Ann Intern Med 1986;104:41–44.
173. Shanley JD, Pesanti EL. The relation of viral replication to interstitial pneumonitis in murine cytomegalovirus lung infection. J Infect Dis 1985;151:454–458.
174. Wilson EJ, Medearis DN Jr, Hansen LA, Rubin RH. 9-(1–3-dihydroxy-2-propoxymethyl) guanine prevents death but not immunity in murine cytomegalovirus-infected normal and immunosuppressed BALB/c mice. Antimicrob Agents Chemother 1987;31:1017–1020.
175. Reed EC, Bowden RA, Dandliker PS, Meyers JD. Treatment of cytomegalovirus (CMV) pneumonia in bone marrow transplant (BMT) patients (PTS) with ganciclovir (GCV) and CMV immunoglobulin (CMV-IG). Blood 1987;70(suppl 1):313a.
176. Bratanow N, Ash RC, Turner P, et al. The use of 9(1,3-dihydroxy-2-propoxymethyl)guanine (ganciclovir, DHPG) and intravenous immunoglobulin (IVIG) in the treatment of serious cytomegalovirus (CMV) infections in thirty-one allogeneic bone mar-

row transplant (BMT) patients. Blood 1987;70(suppl 1):302a.

177. Reed EC, Bowden RA, Dandliker PS, Lilleby KE, Meyers JD. Treatment of cytomegalovirus pneumonia with ganciclovir and intravenous cytomegalovirus immunoglobulin in patients with bone marrow transplants. Ann Intern Med 1988;109:783–788.
178. Emanuel D, Cunningham I, Jules-Elysee K, et al. Cytomegalovirus pneumonia after bone marrow transplantation succesfully treated with the combination of ganciclovir and high-dose intravenous immune globulin. Ann Intern Med 1988;109:777–782.
179. Schmidt GM, Kovacs A, Zaia JA, et al. Ganciclovir/ immunoglobulin combination therapy for the treatment of human cytomegalovirus-associated interstitial pneumonia in bone marrow allograft recipients. Transplantation 1988;46:905–907.
180. Ljungman P, Englehard D, Link H, et al. Treatment of interstitial pneumonitis due to cytomegalovirus with ganciclovir and intravenous immune globulin: experience of European Bone Marrow Transplant Group. Clin Infect Dis 1992;14:831–835.
181. Drew WL, Miner RC, Busch DF, et al. Prevalence of resistance inpatients receiving ganciclovir for serious cytomegalovirus infection. J Infect Dis 1990;163:716–719.
182. McDonald GB, Sharma P, Hackman RC, Meyers JD, Thomas ED. Esophageal infections in immunosuppressed patients after marrow transplantation. Gastroenterology 1985;88:1111–1117.
183. Meyers JD, Leszczynski J, Zaia J, et al. Prevention of cytomegalovirus infection by cytomegalovirus immune globulin after marrow transplantation. Ann Intern Med 1983;98:442–446.
184. Winston DJ, Ho WG, Howell CL, et al. Cytomegalovirus infections associated with leukocyte transfusions. Ann Intern Med 1980;93:671–675.
185. Verdonck LF, de Graan-Hentzer YCE, Dekker AW, et al. Cytomegalovirus seronegative platelets and leukocyte-poor red blood cells from random donors can prevent primary cytomegalovirus infection after bone marrow transplantation. Bone Marrow Transplant 1987;2:73.
186. de Graan-Hentzen YCE, Gratama JW, Mudde GC, et al. Prevention of primary cytomegalovirus infection in patients with hematologic malignancies by intensive white cell depletion of blood products. Transfusion 1989;29:757.
187. Gilbert GL, Hayes K, Hudson IL, James J, the Neonatal CMV Infection Study Group. Prevention of transfusion-acquired cytomegalovirus infection in infants by blood filtration to remove leukocytes. Lancet 1989;1:1228.
188. Bowden RA, Sayers MH, Cays M, Slichter SJ. The role of blood product filtration in the prevention of transfusion associated cytomegalovirus (CMV) infection after marrow transplant. Transfusion 1989;29:5205.
189. Meyers JD, Reed EC, Shepp DH, et al. Acyclovir for prevention of cytomegalovirus infection and disease after allogeneic marrow transplantation. N Engl J Med 1988;318:70–75.
190. Balfour HH Jr, Chace BA, Stapleton JT, et al. A randomized, placebo-controlled trial of oral acyclovir for the prevention of cytomegalovirus disease in recipients of renal allografts. N Engl J Med 1989;320:1381–1387.
191. Fletcher CV, Englund JA, Edelman CK, et al. Pharmacologic basis for high-dose oral acyclovir prophylaxis of cytomegalovirus disease in renal allograft recipients. Antimicrob Agents Chemother 1991;35:938–943.
192. Cole NL, Balfour HH Jr. In vitro susceptibility of cytomegalovirus isolates from immunocompromised patients to acyclovir and gancicolvir. Diagn Microbiol Infect Dis 1987;6:255–261.
193. Rubin RH. Preemptive therapy in immunocompromised hosts. N Engl J Med 1991;324:1057–1058.
194. Atkinson K, Downs K, Golenia M, et al. Prophylactic use of ganciclovir in allogeneic bone marrow transplantation; absence of clinical cytomegalovirius infection. Br J Hematol 1991;79:57–62.
195. Winston DJ, Ho WG, Bartoni K, et al. Ganciclovir prophylaxis of cytomegalovirus infection and disease in allogeneic bone marrow transplant recipients. Ann Intern Med 1993;118:179–184.
196. Reusser P, Gambertoglio JG, Lilleby K, Meyers JD. Phase I-II trial of foscarnet for prevention of cytomegalovirus infection in autologous and allogeneic marrow transplant recipients. J Infect Dis 1992;166:473–479.
197. Zaia JA, Levin MJ, Leszczynski J, Wright GG, Grady GF. Cytomegalovirus immune globulin: production from selected normal donor blood. Transplantation 1979;27:66–67.
198. O'Reilly RJ, Reich L, Gold J, et al. A randomized trial of intravenous hyperimmune globulin for the prevention of cytomegalovirus (CMV) infections following marrow transplantation: preliminary results. Transplant Proc 1983;15:1405–1411.
199. Kubanek B, Ernst P, Ostendorf P, et al. Preliminary data of a controlled trial of intravenous hyperimmune globulin in the prevention of cytomegalovirus infection in bone marrow transplant recipients. Transplant Proc 1985;17:468–469.
200. Winston DJ, Ho WG, Lin CH, et al. Intravenous immune globulin for prevention of cytomegalovirus infection and interstitial pneumonia after bone marrow transplantation. Ann Intern Med 1987;106:12–18.
201. Aulitzky WE Schulz TF, Tilg H, et al. Human monoclonal antibodies neutralizing cytomegalovirus (CMV) for prophylaxis of CMV disease: report of a phase I trial in bone marrow transplant recipients. J Infect Dis 1991;163:1344–1347.
202. Skarp-Örberg I, Hökeberg I, Olding-Stenkvist E, Tufveson G. Use of a human monoclonal anti-cytomegalovirus antibody for the treatment of severe cytomegalovirus after renal transplantation. Transplant Proc 1990;22:234.

Chapter 29
Herpes Simplex Virus

William H. Burns

The most common herpes viruses (herpes simplex virus [HSV], cytomegalovirus [CMV], and varicella-zoster virus [VZV]) have a well known temporal relationship of infections relative to the time of transplantation; most HSV infections occur during the first month after bone marrow transplantation (BMT) (1,2). HSV is a common and well recognized pathogenic herpesvirus that occurs as two basic types—type 1, which generally infects the oropharynx and typically establishes a latent infection in the trigeminal ganglia; and type 2, which generally infects the genital or perineal areas and establishes latency in the lumbosacral sensory ganglia. These viruses are distinguishable serologically, genetically, and by differential susceptibility to certain antivirals (e.g., type 2 is much less sensitive than type 1 to bromovinyl-deoxyuridine). HSV is the frequent cause of severe mucositis and esophagitis (3) and is occasionally responsible for severe morbidity or mortality from encephalitis, hepatitis (4), and pneumonia (5). The clinical introduction of acyclovir (ACV) was a milestone in our approach to the management of HSV infections.

Biology of HSV

Herpesviruses are very species-specific, and although HSV can be propagated in tissue cultures derived from many animal species, the reservoir of the virus is confined to humans. The life cycles of all herpesviruses appear to include primary infection of individuals without prior exposure to the virus, followed by the establishment of latency with subsequent reactivations. Neurons in the sensory ganglia are the site of latency for HSV. In 1905, Cushing (6) reported recrudescence of herpetic lesions following neurosurgical manipulations of the trigeminal ganglia and found that the lesions did not involve anesthetic (denervated) areas in the distribution of the nerve. He noted that his observations "point strongly toward a ganglionic origin for herpes of this type." Goodpasture (7) formulated more completely the hypothesis that sensory ganglia are the sites of latency from which virus can be reactivated and travel down axons to the epithelial surface. Carton and Kilbourne (8) demonstrated that sectioning the fifth cranial nerve proximally resulted in the appearance of herpetic lesions 48 to 96 hours later in the homolateral distribution of the affected ganglion. Attempts to grow herpes from scrapings of skin from the location of recurrent herpetic lesions during quiescent periods were uniformly negative (9), and herpetic lesions did not appear in skin grafts obtained from such areas (10). These clinical observations have been supplemented recently with direct methods, including recovery of HSV from sensory ganglia obtained at autopsies, DNA and RNA in situ hybridization studies using HSV specific probes, and the development of animal models, particularly in the mouse, that have allowed detailed investigations of the establishment of latency, the latent state, and virus reactivation (11,12).

Most of our knowledge of HSV infection at the cellular level comes from in vitro studies of infection of non-neuronal cells and is therefore most applicable to lytic infection of epidermal and other non-neuronal cells (12). After adsorption of virus to the cell membrane, the virion is de-enveloped and the virus capsid and a tegument protein of the virion, known as α-transinducing factor (α-TIF; also VP16 or Vmw65), are independently transported to the cell nucleus. There the α-TIF and a host transcription activating factor (Oct-1 or NF-III) form a complex that, along with other factors, interact and bind to specific sites present in the promoter regions of the viral immediate-early genes. Products of the immediate-early genes have an important role in activation of early viral genes, including thymidine kinase (TK) and DNA polymerase, which are involved in nucleotide metabolism or viral DNA replication. Viral DNA, which exists in a linear duplex form in the virion, is circularized upon entering the nucleus and is replicated in concatemeric forms. Late viral genes are then expressed, producing late proteins, which are primarily structural components of the virion. Among them are glycoproteins known to contain epitopes that interact with neutralizing antibodies.

The establishment by all herpesviruses of a lifelong latent state that serves as a reservoir from which infectious virus can be reactivated and passed on to uninfected individuals is the most outstanding characteristic of these viruses, and an understanding of the biological aspects and molecular basis of this phase of infection continues as a major challenge. For many of the herpesviruses, the sites of latency, particularly those that are biologically important in the life cycle of the virus, are not known with assurance. For HSV and VZV, as noted, a large number of clinical and experimental observations have established that neurons in sensory ganglia are the biologically relevant site of latency for these viruses. Virus infection in the epidermis or a mucosal surface results in adsorption of virions to nerve endings. The virus capsid containing the nucleic acid is transported via axonal flow to the neuron nucleus. It has been hypothesized that the axonal distance that must be traversed by the virion protein α-TIF may result in its being present in an ineffective concentration in the nucleus and may contribute to the virus not proceeding to a lytic cycle. The lack of Oct-1 in neurons may also curtail entry into the lytic cycle.

It is increasingly clear that viral DNA replication is not necessary for establishing latency. In animal models, virus replication can be measured in the newly infected ganglia, but this may reflect the large virus input used in these models or it may not be occurring in neurons where latency is established. Temperature-sensitive mutants of HSV unable to replicate at the body temperature of the mouse are able to establish latency and can be fully reactivated when explants of the ganglia are cultured at permissive temperatures (13). A mutation in the α-TIF gene that renders the virus incapable of replication in mouse ganglia has also been used to demonstrate that there is no requirement for viral DNA replication for latency to be established (14). Examination of the ganglia at various times after infection with this mutant indicated that latency can be established as rapidly as 12 to 48 hours after corneal infection.

Characterization of the latent state at the molecular level is still incomplete. Viral genomes appear to be present in neurons in concatemeric or circular forms, perhaps episomally (15,16). From infectious center assays in which dispersed ganglia were seeded onto susceptible cells, it was estimated that approximately 1% of ganglionic neurons harbor latent HSV (17,18). Isolation of latent viral DNA and host DNA from mouse brains indicated a surprisingly high proportion of viral DNA, and it has been concluded that there must be multiple copies of viral genomic DNA per latently infected neuron (11). It is clear that there is transcription of latency-associated transcripts (LATs) of varying lengths spliced from a sequence spanning approximately 8 kb, including overlapping of the 3′ end of the immediate early gene ICPO in an antisense manner. This transcription is under the control of a specific promoter located an unusually long distance upstream of the 5′ terminus. There is no polyadenylation of these transcripts, which remain nuclear, and protein products have not been identified. Mutants with deletions within these transcripts are still capable of establishing and maintaining latency, although their reactivation efficiency is impaired. In fact, there is no part of the HSV genome demonstrably necessary for establishment of latency, and host factors are critically important.

From the latent state, the virus may be reactivated and form progeny virus able to exit the neuron and cause lytic infection in the innervated skin or mucosa. Factors that may mediate this effect on the gross level include trauma to the neuron or its axons, exposure of the skin to ultraviolet light, toxicities of an undefined nature following chemotherapy, fever, anxiety, and hormonal changes. The molecular mechanisms underlying these reactivations are unknown. Changes in relevant nuclear transcription activating factors or loss of as yet undefined suppressive factors are probably important. The presence of TK and activation of the immediate-early gene ICPO are also important and possibly critical factors. Because the mutant lacking functional α-TIF is able to reactivate from ganglia normally, that factor seemingly so important early in lytic infections in vitro is apparently unimportant for in vivo reactivation (14,19). This finding is not surprising because α-TIF is synthesized late in lytic infections.

It is unknown whether abortive reactivations (not resulting in completely formed, infectious virions) may also occur. Possibly there is a basal or periodic reactivation producing progeny virus that is clinically undetectable. It is also unclear what the fate of the neuron in vivo is when HSV is reactivated. Upon reactivation, does a lytic infection occur in the neuron similar to that observed in neurons and non-neuronal cells in vitro? Or does a more limited process occur that allows the neuron to produce progeny virus yet survive and re-establish latency? Evidence from an animal model suggested that the neuron dies when HSV is reactivated (13). However, individuals may have recrudescence of HSV at the same site many times per year over many years. If the involved neurons were eliminated, then a large number of neurons innervating the same area must harbor the virus from the initial infection, or infection of adjacent neurons either directly within the ganglia or via infection/reinfection at the nerve endings ("round-trip" mechanism) as suggested by Klein (20) occur. It may be that a combination of these alternatives are operative.

At this point, one must distinguish between factors that result in molecular reactivation/replication of the virus and factors that allow the development of clinical lesions due to viral replication at the mucosal surface with resulting inflammation (recrudescence). Cell-mediated responses have long been recognized as important in the control of HSV infections. Progressive and fatal HSV infections may develop in patients with congenital immunodeficiencies affecting the development of T-cell immunity, whereas patients with gammaglobulin deficiencies but intact cell-mediated immunity generally handle the infection well. In the setting of BMT, the pancytopenia and the profound impairment of the immune system routinely observed allow reactivated infections to become very severe and sometimes fatal. This effect does not mean that immunosuppression per se is a stimulus to virus reactivation, but it does allow for increased severity of the infection.

HSV Infection Following Marrow Transplantation

Without antiviral prophylaxis, between 70 and 80% of BMT patients seropositive for HSV will reactivate the virus clinically and virologically a median of 17 days after initiation of the preparative regimen (1,2,21). Virtually all infection observed clinically is from virus reactivation. Approximately 85% of the infections involve the oral cavity, and 15% are genital infections. Mucocutaneous infections of the oral cavity can lead to decreased oral intake, severe pain, and can serve as portals of entry for superinfecting bacteria and fungi or as a source of virus for subsequent spread following maneuvers such as placement of an endotracheal tube. Prior to the introduction of ACV, 5% of pneumonias in BMT patients were caused by HSV, and some were fatal (5). Hepatitis caused by HSV (particularly HSV type 2) has been reported in a small number of patients and was usually fatal (4). Fever and abdominal pain were prominent presenting symptoms, and HSV was often not suspected because of the lack of cutaneous manifestations. Hepatitis occurred in the period before ACV was available or in patients for whom ACV prophylaxis had been discontinued. Early treatment with ACV appeared to be beneficial and should be instituted at doses used to treat zoster, because the presenting symptoms of HSV hepatitis may be similar to those of zoster involving the viscera.

Although vidarabine was of demonstrable value in HSV encephalitis (22), a controlled trial of the drug for mucocutaneous HSV infection in immunocompromised hosts showed little benefit (23). Following the introduction of ACV by Elion and co-workers (24), one of the first controlled clinical studies was a prophylactic study to prevent HSV infection in BMT patients (25). Although performed more than a decade ago, the conclusions of that study are still relevant today. Identification of a high-risk group of patients with an increased incidence of HSV reactivation in a highly predictable period allowed for a prospective, double-blinded, placebo-controlled trial. ACV or placebo was begun 3 days prior to BMT and was continued for 18 days. None of 10 patients receiving ACV reactivated HSV, whereas the expected 7 of 10 patients receiving placebo did. Seven of the 10 patients who received ACV went on to shed virus from 3 to 53 days later. Six of the patients who received placebo and who reactivated virus during the prophylactic period were then entered on a treatment study, and 2 were randomized to receive ACV for treatment of active infection. Both patients began to excrete TK-mutated–resistant virus shortly after stopping the ACV, but the lesions continued to heal (26).

Several conclusions were apparent from this study and its follow-up. It was clear that ACV is very effective prophylaxis for HSV in the BMT setting but that latent virus is not eliminated by such treatment. ACV had no observed toxicity and there was no delay in marrow recovery after the BMT. It was further suggested that resistant virus was more likely to emerge if ACV were given therapeutically for active infection. This effect led to the suggestion that if HSV infection in the early period after BMT is of sufficient severity in terms of morbidity and possible mortality, ACV prophylaxis should be undertaken (27). In this way, the selective pressure of the antiviral would be applied at a time when minimal numbers of viral genomes would be available and thus minimize the risk of selection of resistant virus. A further observation from the follow-up study was that the TK-deficient viruses would not result in increased clinical severity, a view supported by other early observations of infection by resistant virus (28). This finding was also supported by animal studies that indicated TK mutants had impaired growth in neural tissues and were impaired in their ability to be reactivated (29,30). However, it is now clear that resistant virus can cause serious and fatal infections in BMT patients (31,32). Results of this prophylactic study were confirmed by another study utilizing intravenous ACV (21) and by oral ACV prophylactic studies (33,34).

Drug Resistance of HSV

Resistance to ACV can result from mutations in either or both of two viral genes—the TK gene or the DNA polymerase gene. The major active metabolite of ACV is its triphosphate, which acts as a competitive inhibitor of GTP for the DNA polymerase and, when incorporated into the viral DNA, can terminate extension of the DNA strand. Initial phosphorylation of ACV to its monophosphate proceeds at a low level by host TK, and there is little accumulation in the uninfected cell. Viral-encoded TK expressed early after infection phosphorylates ACV to its monophosphate with great efficiency, and the activity of cellular enzymes then results in formation of the triphosphate. Accumulation of the drug only in infected cells is probably one reason for its low toxicity.

Studies of laboratory-derived mutants resistant to ACV formed the basis for understanding resistant clinical isolates that now encompass the predicted kinds of mutations (35–37). The vast majority of resistant isolates have TK mutations that can result in changes in substrate binding and decreased efficiency of phosphorylation, or in changes in the effective amounts of the enzyme expressed (38). Clinical isolates that maintain the ability to phosphorylate thymidine but not ACV have been reported. In one patient the isolate was not as impaired in its capacity to grow in neural tissue or to establish latency in or be reactivated from mouse ganglia as TK mutants that were unable to phosphorylate thymidine (39).

Laboratory-derived polymerase mutations resistant to ACV are located in highly-conserved regions of the polymerase gene and usually result in changes in sensitivity to other drugs that act on the DNA polymerase such as aphidicolin, vidarabine, and the pyrophosphate analogues phosphonoacetic acid (PAA) and phosphonoformic acid (PFA; also foscarnet) (40). The latter inhibit DNA chain formation by competitively inhibiting pyrophosphate exchange at the pyrophosphate binding site on the viral DNA polymerase. Polymerase mutants rarely have been isolated in the clinical setting, but one such isolate was reported to cause severe infection (41).

Source of Resistant Virus

HSV resistant to ACV occurs because of spontaneously arising mutations in the viral TK or DNA polymerase genes. Two studies have given similar estimated mutation frequencies. Parris and Harrington (42) examined 13 clinical isolates from patients previously unexposed to ACV and found 0.01% resistant variants in low passage virus pools. Fluctuation analyses for two isolates demonstrated that they must have been clonally distributed in the original virus population. Coen and associates (43) examined a laboratory strain (KOS) at low passage following plaque-purification and assayed progeny virus from each colony for ACV resistance. They found that resistant variants occurred at 0.01 to 0.2% of the progeny virus. The vast majority of mutants had TK mutations, but polymerase mutants and mutations in both genes also occurred.

Mutants resistant to ACV therefore arise at a frequency of approximately 10^{-4}, which is quite high even when it is considered that mutation in one of two genes may lead to resistance. Do these mutants establish latency or are they generated de novo after reactivation of wild-type virus in neurons or during subsequent replication in epithelial tissues? The answer to this question is currently unclear, although observations discussed later bear on it. BMT patients have been reported who initially had sensitive virus isolated followed by the development of resistant virus with ACV treatment, and who later shed or reactivated the original sensitive virus (31,44). Although the number of patients studied is small, the observations to date imply that it is rare for a TK mutant virus to establish latency and be reactivated. Whether this low incidence is due primarily to the impaired ability of most TK mutants to establish or reactivate from latency, to immunological factors, or to factors intrinsic to the neuron and the strain of latent HSV it already harbors is not known. Using the rabbit model, one study found a superinfecting virus could not establish trigeminal latency (45), but another study using the mouse model found host latency could be established by a superinfecting virus but at a diminished frequency (46). These interesting findings need to be extended and the underlying mechanisms investigated before their relevance to the natural human infection can be assessed.

Although it may be unusual, there is growing evidence that an individual (particularly patients with acquired immune deficiency syndrome [AIDS]) may be infected with multiple strains of HSV (47). Fingerprinting of viral DNAs with endonuclease restriction enzymes has shown that epidemiologically unrelated HSV isolates are distinguishable. Buchman and colleagues (48) first demonstrated that an individual can be infected under natural conditions with more than one strain of the same HSV serotype. Therefore, it was of interest to examine paired isolates of sensitive and resistant virus as such isolates became available. The only previous data on multiple strains in individual BMT patients were from a study of lung and mucosal isolates from 5 patients, each of whom had a unique restriction pattern found for isolates from both organs (5).

Comparison studies of sensitive and resistant virus are limited. Englund and associates (31) surveyed more than 200 patients consecutively admitted to a tertiary care center during a one-year period. Cultures for HSV and assays for ACV sensitivity identified 7 patients, all immunocompromised and receiving ACV, who were positive for resistant HSV. Twenty-six of 29 BMT patients shed sensitive HSV and were placed on ACV therapy (there was no prophylactic therapy). Resistant virus developed in 4 of these patients, and restriction analysis demonstrated the resistant strain to be the same as the antecedent sensitive strain. Hayward and colleagues (44) examined paired isolates of initial sensitive and post-ACV treatment–resistant virus from 6 BMT patients. In 3 of the 6, the resistant isolate appeared to be a different strain than the antecedent sensitive isolate. It is doubtful that the resistant virus represented a newly acquired strain in these 3 patients because (1) the resistant virus was cultured from the same sites as the initial virus, (2) only a few weeks separated culture of the two isolates, (3) it is extremely rare for seronegative patients to acquire HSV in the BMT setting, and (4) endonuclease restriction patterns of HSV isolates collected from consecutive BMT patients are unique for each patient. These considerations indicate that acquisition of HSV during the BMT period is extremely rare. Therefore, the most likely explanation for Hayward's findings is that in humans sensory ganglia may harbor and reactivate multiple strains of HSV. It is unknown whether genomes of more than one strain can be maintained in a single neuron. Theoretically, a genome that is not easily reactivated (e.g., possibly a TK mutant) may be complemented in a neuron also containing a wild-type or different mutant strain. More studies are needed to establish the frequency of multiple strains in individual patients, to characterize the strains present on multiple reactivations over time, and to relate these findings to the development and introduction into the neuronal reservoir of resistant viruses.

Prophylaxis Versus Treatment

There is controversy concerning whether ACV should be used prophylactically in the BMT setting or whether no antiviral treatment should be employed unless symptomatic infection occurs. The arguments revolve around two issues: development of resistant virus and economic factors. Good data are available concerning the former, but many factors complicate economic considerations and are difficult to quantify.

From August 1980 through February 1992, 702 courses of ACV prophylaxis were given to 356 allogeneic/syngeneic and 346 autologous BMT recipients at the Johns Hopkins Oncology Center. The prophylactic courses are defined as treatment with intravenous ACV beginning around the time of BMT (usually 2 or 3 days before) and continuing for at least 21 days (usually ending at time of discharge from the inpatient service). The dosing schedule varied from 1,500 to 375 mg/m^2 daily. Surveillance cultures from throat, blood, and urine were obtained weekly. Six patients (0.9%) were found to have positive throat cultures on only one occasion (preceded and followed by negative cultures) during the prophylactic period. Shedding occurred at days 8, 13, 14, 15, and 24 after starting ACV. Virus from three patients was available for testing, and all 3 isolates proved sensitive to ACV. It is probable that the other 3 isolates were also sensitive. The finding of "breakthrough" sensitive virus is in accordance with reports from Seattle and Minnesota, in which 10 of 17 BMT patients (combined studies) shed sensitive HSV during ACV therapy (28,31).

Four patients (0.6%), however, had multiple throat isolates recovered in the prophylactic period, and assays of isolates from 2 of these patients showed them to have TK mutations resulting in resistance to ACV; isolates from the other 2 patients were not available for testing. Both sets of tested isolates were also resistant to ganciclovir but remained sensitive to foscarnet. The first patient had negative cultures for 2 weeks before ACV was begun. The first positive culture occurred 6 days after beginning ACV at 500 mg/m^2 every 8 hours. He had symptomatic oral lesions and never ceased shedding virus prior to his death 6 weeks later. The second patient had a more complicated course. During intravenous ACV prophylaxis (500 mg/m^2 every 8 hours) during his first allogeneic BMT, no HSV was cultured. One week after discontinuation of prophylactic ACV, sensitive virus was cultured from his throat. After restarting ACV, resistant virus was cultured and continued to be shed for one month while on ACV therapy. One and one half years later the patient underwent a second BMT. Throat cultures were negative for HSV prior to beginning intravenous ACV prophylaxis (750 mg/m^2 every 8 hours). Sixteen days after beginning prophylaxis, multiple isolates of resistant HSV were obtained. The patient was highly symptomatic (oral and esophageal lesions). Endonuclease restriction pattern analysis of this patient's resistant virus from the first and second transplantations were identical to each other and to the antecedent sensitive virus (unpublished data). This patient demonstrates that resistant virus can be selected from reactivated virus, become latent, and be reactivated despite a TK mutation that greatly impairs its capacity to phosphorylate thymidine. If this can be considered a form of "exogenous reinfection" (47), then this phenomenon and also the finding of multiple strains present in the same individual (44,48) have important public health implications for vaccination strategies.

Thus, shedding of sensitive or resistant HSV can occur rarely during ACV prophylaxis. In contrast, during this same period, there were 120 ACV treatment episodes in 101 patients positive for HSV while not receiving ACV. In 19 patients, virus continued to be isolated more than 4 days after institution of ACV therapy and was associated with lesions; in all of 16 patients for which isolates were available, it was shown to be TK-mutated–resistant virus when compared with respective pretreatment isolates. In 2 other patients, resistant virus was isolated after ACV treatment had ceased and represented asymptomatic shedding. Thus, treatment of established HSV infections resulted in emergence of resistant virus in at least 18 patients (18%). This finding compares to previous reports of 3 of 52 (6%) and 4 of 29 (14%) BMT patients in whom resistant HSV developed during ACV treatment (28,31). These data support the contention that resistant virus often emerges in the BMT treatment setting but rarely in the BMT prophylactic setting (26,27).

Economic considerations include the cost of the drug and the cost of preparation and administration of the drug. However, they also include economic consequences of superinfection, bone marrow suppression, pain medications for painful herpetic lesions, and possible prolonged hospitalization secondary to HSV infections. Many of these economic factors are difficult to determine in the complex clinical setting of BMT. They also do not encompass the subjective factors of discomfort, pain, and decreased oral intake that may be caused in part by HSV infections, although one study concluded ACV prophylaxis did not diminish stomatitis (49).

It is clear that resistant virus is much more likely to emerge with therapeutic than with prophylactic administration of ACV. The decision of whether to treat prophylactically is an institutional one based on the observed morbidity/mortality experienced from HSV infections with the preparative regimens in use and on local economic factors. Another question is whether patients with active HSV infections should be treated. This becomes a question of clinical judgment based on the morbidity experienced by the patient and the presence of factors that might be expected to increase the risk of more serious infection (e.g., immunosuppression for GVHD, prolonged neutropenia, extent and location of lesions). Certainly there is no necessity to treat every patient with a positive culture in the period following engraftment.

Recommended Treatment Schedules

A number of prophylactic and treatment schedules for HSV in BMT patients have been used successfully

Table 29-1.
Suggested Dosage Guidelines for Acyclovir

Prophylaxis of HSV
Intravenous
250 mg/m², q12h
62.5 mg/m², q4h
5 mg/kg, q12h
Oral
200 mg, 4 times daily
800 mg, q12h
Treatment of HSV
IV
250 mg/m², q8h for 7–10 days
5–10 mg/kg, q8h for 7–10 days
Oral
200–400 mg, 5 times a day for 7–10 days
Renal Impairment
Intravenous
250 mg/m², q8h; C_{cr} (mL/min): >50
250 mg/m², q12h; C_{cr} (mL/min): 25–50
250 mg/m², q24h; C_{cr} (mL/min): 10–25
125 mg/m², q24h; C_{cr} (mL/min): 0–10
125 mg/m², q48h; C_{cr} (mL/min): anuria
Oral
200–400 mg, 5 times a day; C_{cr} (mL/min): >10
200–400 mg, 3 times a day; C_{cr} (mL/min): <10

C_{cr} = creatinine clearance.

(Table 29-1). At Johns Hopkins, from 1980 through 1987, we have used prophylaxis in all HSV-seropositive patients beginning 2 or 3 days prior to transplantation and continuing until discharge from the inpatient service, using our original intravenous schedule of 250 mg/m^2 every 8 hours (750 mg/m^2/day). In 1988 to 1989, we used 125 mg/m^2 every 6 hours (500 mg/m^2/day), and since 1990 we have used 62.5 mg/m^2 every 4 hours (375 mg/m^2/day). These changes were made because of the increased flexibility and the decreased personnel time required for drug preparation and administration after the introduction of sophisticated programmable infusion pumps. Patients who are seropositive for CMV receive prophylaxis with 500 mg/m^2 every 8 hours intravenous ACV regardless of HSV status in an attempt to diminish CMV disease (50). Although an oral prophylactic dose of ACV is given in Table 29-1, our recommendation is that intravenous prophylaxis is preferred because of poor patient compliance and unpredictable absorption with oral medications during the preparative regimen and the first month after transplantation.

The length of prophylaxis varies among different centers. Generally, prophylaxis is begun sometime during the week before transplantation and is continued for one month after transplantation or until hospital discharge. Later treatment of HSV infection would depend on the severity of the infection and the clinical situation. Treatment of mild infection in an increasingly immunocompetent patient is discouraged because such treatment may not be clinically useful and may select for resistant virus. There is also evidence that such treatment may suppress the development of immune responses to HSV by the new/recovering immune system, presumably by decreasing the amount of viral antigen produced (51).

Treatment of ACV-resistant Infections

Treatment of ACV-resistant HSV has been with an alternative antiviral, vidarabine, and more recently with foscarnet. These drugs do not depend on the viral TK for their activity, and vidarabine, because of its approved use in treatment of HSV encephalitis, was the first choice as a second-line drug for resistant HSV. However, the recent use of foscarnet in the treatment of CMV retinitis in patients with AIDS has rapidly extended our knowledge of its pharmacokinetics and toxicities. Recent studies in patients with AIDS comparing foscarnet with vidarabine for treatment of ACV-resistant HSV infections strongly indicate greater efficacy for foscarnet (52,53). In one study of 14 patients with AIDS with resistant HSV infections, 8 treated with foscarnet had complete responses, whereas all 6 patients treated with vidarabine failed and were switched to foscarnet (53). Recurrent HSV lesions retained sensitivity to foscarnet, although they often remained resistant to ACV. The known toxicities of foscarnet include hyperphosphatemia, hypocalcemia, and nephrotoxicity.

The decision to treat ACV-resistant HSV infections is a clinical judgment based on the same factors mentioned earlier—the morbidity experienced by the patient and the expected course of the patient. We discourage treatment unless these clinical factors dictate that treatment is necessary. Laboratory confirmation of loss of ACV sensitivity is desirable. If possible, foscarnet sensitivity should be ascertained, although initial sensitivity of the isolate to foscarnet can be assumed. If ACV has been administered orally or at low dose, high-dose intravenous ACV (500 mg/m^2 every 8 hours with normal renal function) may be tried. Otherwise, or if the infection is life-threatening, intravenous foscarnet is the drug of choice (40 mg/kg every 8 hours). Vidarabine has been used with only marginal success in immunocompromised hosts with mucocutaneous HSV infections (23) and with very little success in the treatment of ACV-resistant HSV infection (53).

References

1. Meyers JD, Flournoy N, Thomas ED. Infection with herpes simplex virus and cell-mediated immunity after marrow transplantation. J Infect Dis 1980;142:338–346.
2. Elfenbein GJ, Saral R. Infectious disease during immune recovery after bone marrow transplantation. In: Allen JC, ed. Infection and the compromised host. Baltimore: Williams & Wilkins, 1981:157–196.
3. McDonald GB, Sharma P, Hackman RC, et al. Esophageal infections in immunosuppressed patients after marrow transplantation. Gastroenterology 1985;88:1111–1117.
4. Johnson JR, Egaas S, Gleaves CA, Hackman R, Bowden RA. Hepatitis due to herpes simplex virus in marrow transplant recipients. Clin Infect Dis 1992;14:38–45.

5. Ramsey PG, Fife KH, Hackman RC, Meyers JD, Corey L. Herpes simplex virus pneumonia. Ann Intern Med 1982;97:813–820.
6. Cushing H. The surgical aspects of major neuralgia of the trigeminal nerve. JAMA 1905;44:1002–1008.
7. Goodpasture EW. Herpetic infection, with especial reference to involvement of the nervous system. Medicine 1929;8:223–243.
8. Carton CA, Kilbourne ED. Activation of latent herpes simplex by trigeminal sensory-root section. N Engl J Med 1952;246:172–176.
9. Rustigian R, Smulow JB, Tye M, Gibson WA, Shindell E. Studies on latent infection of skin and oral mucosa in individuals with recurrent herpes simplex. J Invest Dermatol 1966;47:218–221.
10. Nicolau S, Poincloux P. Étude clinique et exp'rimentale d'un cas d'herp's r'cidivant du doigt. Ann Inst Pasteur 1924;38:977–1001.
11. Roizman B, Sears AE. An inquiry into the mechanisms of herpes simplex virus latency. Ann Rev Microbiol 1987;41:543–571.
12. Roizman B, Sears AE. Herpes simplex viruses and their replication. In: Fields BN, ed. Virology, ed. 2. New York: Raven, 1990;1795–1841.
13. McLennan JL, Darby G. Herpes simplex virus latency: the cellular location of virus in dorsal root ganglia and the fate of the infected cell following virus activation. J Gen Virol 1980;51:233–243.
14. Steiner I, Spivack JG, Deshmane SL, Ace CI, Preston CM, Fraser NW. A herpes simplex virus type 1 mutant containing a nontransinducing Vmw65 protein establishes latent infection in vivo in the absence of viral replication and reactivates efficiently from explanted trigeminal ganglia. J Virol 1990;64:1630–1638.
15. Rock DL, Fraser NW. Detection of HSV-1 genome in central nervous system of latently infected mice. Nature 1983;302:523–525.
16. Mellerick DM, Fraser NW. Physical state of the latent herpes simplex virus genome in a mouse model system: evidence suggesting an episomal state. Virology 1987; 158:265–275.
17. Walz MA, Yamamoto H, Notkins AL. Immunologic response restricts the number of cells in sensory ganglia infected with herpes simplex. Nature 1976;264: 554–556.
18. Kennedy PGE, Al-Saadi SA, Clements GB. Reactivation of latent herpes simplex virus from dissociated identified dorsal root ganglion cells in culture. J Gen Virol 1983;64:1629–1635.
19. Sears AE, Hukkanen V, Labow MA, Levine AJ, Roizman B. Expression of the herpes simplex virus 1 α transinducing factor (VP16) does not induce reactivation of latent virus or prevent the establishment of latency in mice. J Virol 1991;65:2929–2935.
20. Klein RJ. Pathogenetic mechanisms of recurrent herpes simplex virus infections. Arch Virol 1976;51:1–13.
21. Hann IM, Prentice HG, Blacklock HA, et al. Acyclovir prophylaxis against herpes virus infections in severely immunocompromised patients: randomized double-blind trial. Br Med J 1983;287:384–388.
22. Whitley RJ, Soong S-J, Dolin R, et al. Adenine arabinoside therapy of biopsy-proved herpes simplex encephalitis. N Engl J Med 1977;297:289–294.
23. Whitley RJ, Spruance S, Hayden FG, et al. Vidarabine therapy for mucocutaneous herpes simplex virus infections in the immunocompromised host. J Infect Dis 1984;149:1–8.
24. Elion GB, Furman PA, Fyfe JA, et al. Selectivity of action of an antiherpetic agent, 9-(2-hydroxyethoxymethyl) guanine. Proc Natl Acad Sci USA 1977;74: 5716–5720.
25. Saral R, Burns WH, Laskin OL, Santos GW, Lietman PS. Acyclovir prophylaxis of herpes-simplex-virus infections. N Engl J Med 1981;305:63–67.
26. Burns WH, Saral R, Santos GW, Laskin OL, Lietman PS. Isolation and characterisation of resistant herpes simplex virus after acyclovir therapy. Lancet 1982;1: 421–424.
27. Ambinder RF, Lietman PS, Burns WH, Saral R. Prophylaxis: a strategy to minimise antiviral resistance. Lancet 1984;1:1154–1155.
28. Wade JC, McLaren C, Meyers JD. Frequency and significance of acyclovir-resistant herpes simplex virus isolated from marrow transplant patients receiving multiple courses of treatment with acyclovir. J Infect Dis 1983;148:1077–1082.
29. Field HJ, Wildy P. The pathogenicity of thymidine kinase- deficient mutants of herpes simplex virus in mice. J Hyg (Camb) 1978;81:267–277.
30. Field HJ, Darby G. Pathogenicity in mice of strains of herpes simplex virus which are resistant to acyclovir in vitro and in vivo. Antimicrob Agents Chemother 1980;17:209–216.
31. Englund JA, Zimmerman ME, Swierkosz EM, Goodman JL, Scholl DR, Balfour HH Jr. Herpes simplex virus resistant to acyclovir. Ann Intern Med 1990; 112:416–422.
32. Ljungman P, Ellis MN, Hackman RC, Shepp DH, Meyers JD. Acyclovir-resistant herpes simplex virus causing pneumonia after marrow transplantation. J Infect Dis 1990;162:244–248.
33. Wade JC, Newton B, Flournoy N, Myers JD. Oral acyclovir for the prevention of herpes simplex virus reactivation after marrow transplantation. Ann Intern Med 1984;100:823–828.
34. Gluckman E, Lotsberg J, Devergie A, et al. Prophylaxis of herpes infections after bone marrow transplantation by oral acyclovir. Lancet 1983;2:706–708.
35. Coen DM, Schaffer PA. Two distinct loci confer resistance to acycloguanosine in herpes simplex virus type 1. Proc Natl Acad Sci USA 1980;77:2265–2269.
36. Schnipper LE, Crumpacker CS. Resistance of herpes simplex virus to acycloguanosine: role of viral thymidine kinase and DNA polymerase loci. Proc Natl Acad Sci USA 1980;77:2270–2273.
37. Field HJ, Darby G, Wildy P. Isolation and characterization of acyclovir-resistant mutants of herpes simplex virus. J Gen Virol 1980;49:115–124.
38. McLaren C, Chen MS, Ghazzouli I, Saral R, Burns WH. Drug resistance patterns of herpes simplex virus isolates from patients treated with acyclovir. Antimicrob Agents Chemother 1985;28:740–744.
39. Ellis MN, Keller PM, Fyfe JA, et al. Clinical isolate of herpes simplex virus type 2 that induces a thymidine kinase with altered substrate specificity. Antimicrob Agents Chemother 1987;31:1117–1125.
40. Gibbs JS, Chiou HC, Bastow KF, Cheng Y-C, Coen DM. Identification of amino acids in herpes simplex virus DNA polymerase involved in substrate and drug recognition. Proc Natl Acad Sci USA 1988;85:6672–6676.
41. Sacks SL, Wanklin RJ, Reece DE, Hicks KA, Tyler KL, Coen DM. Progressive esophagitis from acyclovir-resistant herpes simplex. Clinical roles for DNA polymerase mutants and viral heterogeneity? Ann Intern Med 1989;111:893–899.
42. Parris DS, Harrington JE. Herpes simplex virus vari-

ants resistant to high concentrations of acyclovir exist in clinical isolates. Antimicrob Agents Chemother 1982;22:71–77.

43. Coen DM, Schaffer PA, Furman PA, Keller PM, St Clair MH. Biochemical and genetic analysis of acyclovir-resistant mutants of herpes simplex virus type 1. Am J Med 1982;73:351–360.
44. Hayward GS, Ambinder R, Ciufo D, Hayward SD, LeFemina RL. Structural organization of human herpesvirus DNA molecules. J Invest Dermatol 1984; 83:29S–41S.
45. Centifanto-Fitzgerald YM, Varnell ED, Kaufman HE. Initial herpes simplex virus type 1 infection prevents ganglionic superinfection by other strains. Infect Immun 1982;35:1125–1132.
46. Meignier B, Norrild B, Roizman B. Colonization of murine ganglia by a superinfecting strain of herpes simplex virus. Infect Immun 1983;41:702–708.
47. Whitley RJ. Herpes simplex viruses. In: Fields BN, ed. Virology. ed. 2. New York: Raven, 1990:1843–1887.
48. Buchman TG, Roizman B, Nahmias AJ. Demonstration of exogenous genital reinfection with herpes simplex virus type 2 by restriction endonuclease fingerprinting of viral DNA. J Infect Dis 1979; 140:295–304.
49. Woo SB, Sonis ST, Sonis AL. The role of herpes simplex virus in the development of oral mucositis in bone marrow transplant recipients. Cancer 1990; 66:2375–2379.
50. Meyers JD, Reed ECC, Shepp DH, et al. Acyclovir for prevention of cytomegalovirus infection and disease after allogeneic marrow transplantation. N Engl J Med 1988;318:70–75.
51. Wade JC, Day LM, Crowley JJ, Meyers JD. Recurrent infection with herpes simplex virus after marrow transplantation: role of the specific immune response and acyclovir treatment. J Infect Dis 1984;149:750–756.
52. Safrin S, Assaykeen T, Follansbee S, Mills J. Foscarnet therapy for acyclovir-resistant mucocutaneous herpes simplex virus infection in 26 AIDS patients: preliminary data. J Infect Dis 1990;161:1078–1084.
53. Safrin S, Crumpacker C, Chatis P, et al. A controlled trial comparing foscarnet with vidarabine for acyclovir-resistant mucocutaneous herpes simplex in the acquired immunodeficiency syndrome. The AIDS Clinical Trials Group. N Engl J Med 1991;325:551–555.

Chapter 30
Varicella Zoster Virus Infections

Sonia Nader and Ann M. Arvin

Varicella zoster virus (VZV), like other pathogens of the herpes virus family, can cause severe infections in bone marrow transplant (BMT) recipients (1,2). As in other immunodeficient patients, serious VZV disease after transplantation is related to the compromise of T-lymphocyte function (3,4). VZV infections are encountered in BMT recipients who are experiencing their initial contact with the virus or who have recurrent disease due to reactivation of latent virus. Primary VZV infection is manifest clinically as varicella or "chicken pox," in which exposure of a susceptible individual to the virus results in systemic symptoms of fever, malaise, and a characteristic vesicular rash. After primary infection, VZV establishes latency in cells of the dorsal root ganglia. Serum immunoglobulin G (IgG) antibodies to VZV provide evidence of a past primary infection and indicate that the individual is latently infected with the virus. Reactivation of endogenous latent VZV usually causes herpes zoster, in which the vesicular eruption appears in a localized, dermatomal distribution. Recurrent VZV infection also presents as atypical, nonlocalized herpes zoster in BMT recipients; these patients have a generalized vesicular exanthem that cannot be distinguished from varicella by its clinical manifestations.

In addition to describing the clinical presentations of VZV infection after BMT, we discuss the significant progress that has been made during the past decade toward understanding viral pathogenesis and the host response to VZV among BMT recipients. Fortunately, most disease caused by either primary or recurrent VZV infection, when recognized promptly, can now be treated effectively with antiviral therapy.

The Virus

VZV is a member of the alpha-herpes virus subgroup of the herpes virus genus. It is an enveloped virus that has a double-stranded DNA genome surrounded by an icosahedral capsid (5). VZV DNA contains approximately 125,000 base pairs, arranged as long-unique and short-unique segments, each of which contains terminal repeat sequences. The VZV genome has coding regions for at least 68 distinct genes. Although information about most of the VZV gene products is limited, putative functions for some VZV proteins have been deduced from homologies with herpes simplex virus type 1 (HSV-1), which is the prototype of the alpha-herpes virus subgroup. Like HSV, replication of VZV usually involves synthesis and activation of a viral thymidine kinase, which makes the virus susceptible to inhibition by the antiviral agent, acyclovir. However, mutant strains that do not require thymidine kinase to replicate can be selected by exposure to the drug. The viral glycoproteins and the immediate-early tegument protein encoded by gene 62 are known to be targets of the host response following VZV infection.

Epidemiology

Primary VZV Infection

Primary VZV infection, or varicella, is much less common than disease caused by VZV reactivation during the first year after BMT; primary infection accounts for only approximately 5% of VZV infections in this population. The lower incidence of varicella is due to the fact that more than 85% of individuals in the United States have had primary VZV infection by 8 years of age as a result of the annual varicella epidemics that occur in this and other temperate regions of the world. Nevertheless, if a BMT recipient is susceptible, the attack rate for varicella after close exposure to an index case will reflect the risk of transmission to any susceptible individual, which ranges from approximately 30% with classroom exposure to 90% with household contact. Direct contact with lesions is not required because, in contrast to other herpes viruses, VZV is transmissible by the respiratory route. The incidence of primary VZV infection is higher in pediatric BMT recipients, and, as expected, the risk correlates inversely with the age of the child. In one series, 10 of 54 children (19%) with VZV infections after BMT had primary VZV infection demonstrated serologically (6). Although 25 adult patients presented with a disseminated cutaneous VZV exanthem, only 2 patients had serological evidence of primary VZV infection (1).

Recurrent VZV Infection

The reported incidence of recurrent VZV infection after BMT ranges from 23 to 50% (1, 6–12) (Table 30-1). This

Table 30-1.
Incidence of Varicella-Zoster Virus (VZV) Infections Following Bone Marrow Transplantation

Year, Ref	Underlying Disease	Transplant Type	N	VZV Infection (%)	Clinical Presentation: Localized Zoster (%)	Atypical Zoster (%)	Varicella (%)
1980 (7)	Leukemia	Allogeneic	33	21	...	...	...
1982 (9)	Leukemia/aplastic anemia	Allogeneic/syngeneic	98	52	...	...	...
1985 (1)	Leukemia/aplastic anemia	Allogeneic/syngeneic	1,394	17	85	15	0
1986 (10)	Hematological malignancy	Allogeneic	73	36	91	7	2
1989 (6)	Leukemia/solid tumors	Autologous	236	23	75	13	18[a]
1989 (11)	Leukemia/lymphoma	Autologous	153	28	77	20	2
1991 (12)	Hodgkin's disease	Autologous	28	32	100	0	0
1992 (27)	Leukemia/lymphoma and others	Autologous/allogeneic	51	31	100	0	0

[a]This study evaluated pediatric transplant recipients only.

incidence is higher than that observed among organ transplant recipients, which is approximately 7%, but it is comparable to rates of VZV reactivation in patients with Hodgkin's disease receiving combined therapy. For purposes of comparison, the estimated annual incidence of herpes zoster in adults without underlying disease is 0.5% (13).

Reactivation of herpes viruses follows a predictable temporal pattern after BMT (2,14,15). HSV-1 causes clinically apparent disease approximately 2 to 3 weeks after BMT, and cytomegalovirus (CMV) disease usually occurs during the second to third months after BMT. Epstein-Barr virus (EBV) may also reactivate in the third month following transplantation, whereas VZV recurrences present at a median of 5 months after BMT. In general, the risk of VZV infection is highest between 2 to 10 months after transplantation, although cases have been reported as early as 1 week following BMT (Figure 30-1). The risk of VZV reactivation has been analyzed further in relation to the early post-transplant period and has been defined as the first 9 months. Locksley and colleagues (1) found that 80% of patients in whom VZV infection developed after BMT had disease in this early period. When options for antiviral therapy were limited, 21% of these patients had visceral dissemination of the virus and 12% died from complications of recurrent VZV.

Factors associated with higher rates of VZV reactivation following BMT include genotypic nonidentity for human leukocyte antigen (HLA) between donor and recipient and acute or chronic graft-versus-host disease (GVHD). In one series, 64% of patients whose donor was HLA-nonidentical had herpes zoster, compared with 44% of BMT recipients with matched donors and no GVHD. The risk of late VZV infection was increased four-fold. The presence of nonspecific suppressor cells associated with chronic GVHD correlated with a higher risk of recurrent VZV (9) (Table 30-2).

The cumulative evidence indicates that patients undergoing allogeneic or autologous BMT have approximately the same risk of recurrent VZV disease (see Table 30-1). In one recent study, recurrent VZV infection developed in 28% of autologous transplant recipients (11). The initial manifestation of recurrence was localized disease in 77% of these patients, whereas 23% had atypical nonlocalized zoster, which is comparable to the distribution of these clinical syndromes among allogeneic BMT recipients. In a pediatric BMT population, 23% of children given autologous BMTs had VZV disease at a median

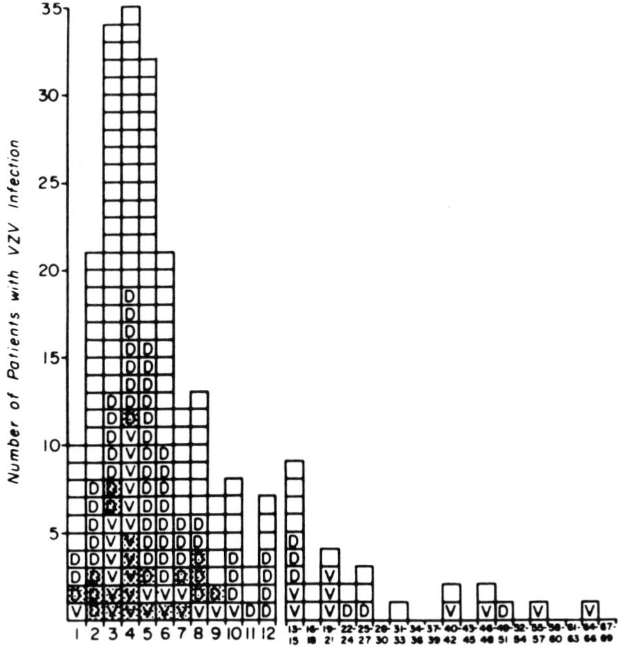

Figure 30-1. Varicella zoster virus (VZV) infections by month after marrow transplantation. *Open boxes* indicate uncomplicated herpes zoster; filled boxes indicate death. V = varicella; D = herpes zoster with subsequent dissemination. (Reproduced by permission from Locksley RM, Flournoy N, Sullivan KM, Meyers JD. Infection with varicella-zoster virus after bone marrow transplantation. J Infect Dis 1985;152:1172–1178.)

Table 30-2.
Risk of Recurrent Varicella-Zoster Virus (VZV) Infection after Bone Marrow Transplantation in Relation to HLA Matching of Recipient and Donor and the Occurrence of Graft-versus-Host Disease (GVHD) in the Recipient

	HLA-identical				
		With GVHD			
	No GVHD	*No Suppressor Cells*[a]	*With Suppressor Cells*	*HLA-nonidentical*	*Syngeneic*
No. of patients	25	21	19	14	19
Late VZ infections	24%	38%	47%	36%	11%
VZV at any time after transplant	44%	57%	79%	64%	21%

[a]Nonspecific suppressor cells were detected in cocultures with donor lymphocytes, assessing their effect on the proliferation responses to alloantigens or concanavalin-A.
Adapted from Atkinson K, Meyers J, Storb R, et al. VZV infection after marrow transplantation for aplastic anemia or leukemia. Transplantation 1980;29:47–50.

interval of 3 months after transplantation, but this series also included patients with primary VZV infection (6). Thirty-two percent of patients who received autologous BMTs for Hodgkin's lymphoma had VZV infection (12). Morbidity and mortality caused by VZV infection after autologous BMT cannot be compared with the original analyses of VZV-related disease after allogeneic BMT because antiviral therapy was available for patients in the studies of autologous BMT. In the series by Schuchter and associates (11), 15% of autologous BMT recipients had cutaneous dissemination, 5% had visceral dissemination, and 25% had morbidity, including postherpetic neuralgia and neurological dysfunction.

The underlying disease that provided the indication for BMT probably does not influence VZV reactivation. However, a history of symptomatic herpes zoster before marrow transplantation was associated with a higher risk of early post-transplant VZV disease among patients with Hodgkin's disease undergoing autologous BMT (12). VZV reactivation has not been found to predict relapse of the underlying disease in BMT recipients (6).

Reinfection with VZV

Although symptomatic reinfection with VZV is extremely rare among immunocompetent individuals, it probably occurs occasionally among severely immunocompromised patients who have had primary VZV infection. However, this hypothesis is difficult to confirm because the distinction between atypical nonlocalized herpes zoster and reinfection requires a comparison with DNA restriction enzyme analysis of the VZV isolates causing the initial infection and the new episode. On the basis of clinical criteria only, children with leukemia have been reported to have second episodes of varicella following close contact despite a past history of varicella and serological evidence of preexisting immunity. Nevertheless, anecdotal clinical experience suggests that exposure of BMT recipients who have had past primary VZV infection rarely causes any clinically apparent signs of reinfection (2).

Pathogenesis of Infection

Primary VZV Infection

Although several phases of viral replication are likely to occur during the 10- to 21-day incubation period, events during primary VZV infection have been difficult to document with laboratory methods. Epidemiological evidence suggests that infection is initiated by the inoculation of mucocutaneous sites (16,17). Infectious virus is then presumed to be transported to regional lymph nodes, possibly undergoing a phase of local replication at this site, followed by a primary viremia. Cell-associated viremia has been demonstrated later in the incubation period, which permits dissemination of infectious virus to epithelial cell sites via infected peripheral blood cells. After the initial cutaneous lesions appear, VZV can be isolated by viral culture from 24% of peripheral blood mononuclear cell (PBMC) samples taken within 24 hours (18). Cell-associated VZV viremia can be shown by in situ hybridization and was detected by polymerase chain reaction (PCR) in 67% of healthy subjects tested immediately after appearance of the rash (19,20). On the basis of these observations about pathogenesis, the efficiency with which cell-associated viremia is terminated either by the host response or by antiviral therapy is likely to influence the extent of the cutaneous exanthem and the risk of visceral dissemination.

Recurrent VZV Infection

The hypothesis that VZV becomes latent in sensory ganglia following primary infection and that herpes zoster is caused by its reactivation from latency was proved by using restriction enzyme analysis to demonstrate that a single VZV strain caused both varicella and a subsequent episode of herpes zoster in a child with Wiskott-Aldrich syndrome (21). During the primary attack, VZV is postulated to pass centripetally from the skin to the corresponding ganglia; hematological seeding of the ganglia is also possible. Once in the ganglia, VZV establishes latency, apparently without viral replication and without causing cell damage. In contrast to HSV, VZV has not been recovered from ganglion tissue using explant culture or cocultivation techniques. However, the presence of VZV nucleic acid sequences has been documented in human ganglia taken at autopsy from individuals with no evidence of recent VZV infection (22–24). Multiple VZV DNA and RNA sequences have been detected by in situ hybridization and PCR, in contrast to HSV, in which only limited gene expression has been identified in latently infected neurons (25). Latent infection appears to be more common in the trigeminal ganglion than in any of the thoracic ganglia (26). The exact cellular site of VZV latency is controversial. Hyman and colleagues (22), and Gilden and associates (23) reported detection of VZV transcripts within neurons, whereas Croen and co-workers (24) demonstrated that VZV RNA was present only in non-neuronal cells. Maintenance of VZV latency, as assessed by the prevention of symptomatic VZV reactivation, is also influenced directly by the host response to VZV, as evidenced from the high incidence of VZV reactivation after BMT. When reactivation occurs, extensive viral replication takes place in the ganglia, thus producing pathological changes, including necrosis and inflammation.

In contrast to HSV, CMV, and EBV, which can be recovered from asymptomatic patients using viral culture methods, technical problems have interfered with the detection of subclinical VZV replication. Recently, PCR was used to demonstrate episodes of subclinical VZV reactivation, detected as cell-associated viremia in BMT recipients (27) (Figure 30-2). Disseminated VZV infection has been diagnosed at autopsy in BMT recipients without cutaneous lesions (1). However, the evaluation using the VZV PCR assay provided the first virological evidence that these severely immunocompromised patients can experience VZV reactivation in the absence of clinically apparent cutaneous infection and can resolve the infection without the development of signs of visceral dissemination. Herpes zoster, like recurrent HSV, has been attributed to the spread of the reactivated virus along neural pathways from the site of latency in dorsal root ganglia. VZV viremia develops in some immunodeficient patients with localized herpes zoster, presumably because peripheral blood mononuclear cells become infected at the site of local cutaneous replication (28). Subclinical, cell-associated viremia in BMT recipients without cutaneous disease suggests that the virus may also be taken up directly by mononuclear cells at the neuronal site of viral reactivation. This mechanism for causing viremia could also account for the clinical observation of atypical, generalized herpes zoster in some BMT recipients. Because activation of T lymphocytes makes this cell population more permissive for VZV infection in vitro, cell-associated VZV viremia in BMT recipients may be potentiated by the characteristic persistence of activated lymphocytes in circulation for a prolonged period after transplantation (29).

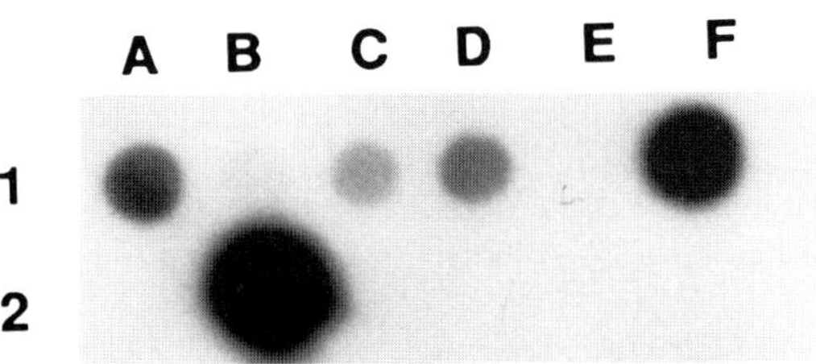

Figure 30-2. Detection of polymerase chain reaction (PCR) product after amplification of DNA from peripheral blood mononuclear cells (PBMC). Samples from 3 bone marrow transplant (BMT) recipients who had subclinical cell-associated viremia are shown in 1A, 1C, and 1D; samples from 5 BMT recipients without detectable varicella zoster virus (VZV) viremia are shown in 1B and 2C–F. Samples 1F and 2B are the VZV DNA control samples; sample 2A is PBMC from a healthy immune donor control subject. (Reproduced by permission from Wilson A, Sharp M, Koropchak CM, Ting SF, Arvin AM. Subclinical varicella-zoster virus viremia, herpes zoster and recovery of T-lymphocyte responses to varicella-zoster viral antigens after allogeneic and autologous bone marrow transplantation. J Infect Dis 1992;165:119–126.)

Host Response

Primary VZV infection is associated with development of virus-specific IgG and IgM antibodies and acquisition of cellular immunity, detectable by showing the proliferation of PBMC after in vitro stimulation with viral antigens. Although VZV IgG antibodies can neutralize virus infectivity and function in antibody-mediated cellular cytotoxicity, humoral immunity seems to be less important in the host response to VZV than cell-mediated immunity. Progressive varicella is observed in immunocompromised children despite production of VZV IgG and IgM antibodies, whereas VZV-specific T-lymphocyte proliferation fails to develop in these children (30). VZV reactivation develops in immunocompromised patients, including BMT recipients, despite circulating antibodies to VZV. No quantitative relationship between VZV antibody titers in the donor or the recipient and subsequent development of herpes zoster has been established in BMT recipients (31). However, periods of diminished VZV-specific T-lymphocyte proliferation have been correlated with an increase in susceptibility to herpes zoster among immunocompromised patient populations, including BMT recipients. In individual patients, the loss of T-cell proliferation to VZV is a necessary, but not a sufficient prerequisite for symptomatic reactivation (32). Conversely, a positive VZV-specific lymphocyte response has been correlated with a decreased risk of herpes zoster.

Previous analyses of VZV-specific cell-mediated immunity have demonstrated a gradual recovery of T-cell proliferation to VZV antigens; a larger percentage of BMT recipients have detectable responses as the interval following transplant increases (3,10,27)

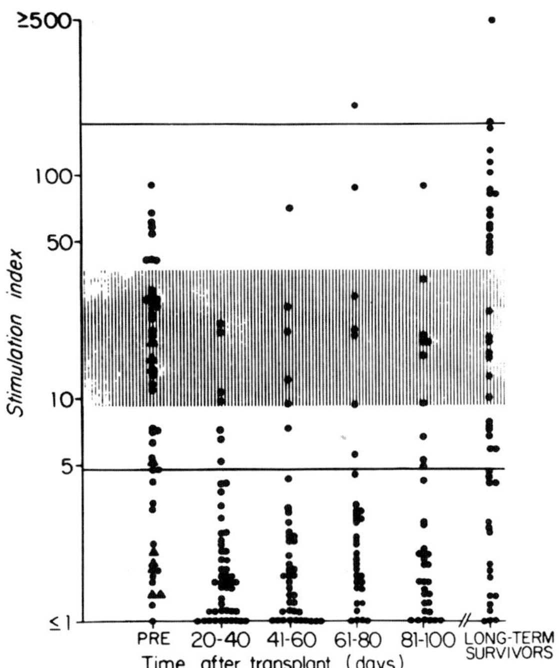

Figure 30-3. Lymphocyte transformation responses of marrow transplant recipients to varicella zoster virus (VZV) antigen. All patients and their donors had a history of VZV infection. The 9 patients who had circulating myeloblasts or lymphoblasts before transplantation are indicated by *triangles.* The 25th to 75th percentile of the normal response to VZV antigen (see Figure 1) is indicated by the *hatched area,* whereas the *horizontal lines* enclose a 95% range of normal responses. (Reproduced by permission from Meyers JD, Flournoy N, Thomas ED. Cell-mediated immunity to varicella-zoster virus after allogeneic marrow transplant. J Infect Dis 1980;141:479–487.)

Figure 30-3). The interval to recovery may be somewhat shorter in autologous BMT recipients (33). This reconstitution of cell-mediated immunity to VZV antigens is generally observed 9 to 12 months after BMT, which correlates with the time when VZV reactivation and susceptibility to severe VZV disease become less common. However, it is apparent that the recovery of virus-specific cellular immunity is delayed and often does not occur until after the patient has had an episode of herpes zoster (i.e., an *in vivo* re-exposure to VZV antigens). Meyers and colleagues (3) detected T-lymphocyte transformation to VZV in 16 of 18 patients (89%) following symptomatic recurrences of VZV, compared with 15 of 29 patients (52%) in whom herpes zoster did not develop. However, the fact that cellular immunity was reconstituted in a significant number of BMT recipients who had no preceding clinical signs of herpes zoster suggests that the subclinical episodes of viral reactivation documented by VZV PCR in BMT recipients may provide the stimulus to restore virus-specific immunity in some patients (27). Pretransplant immunity in both the donor and the recipient may also facilitate the reconstitution of VZV-specific cell-mediated immunity (34).

BMT recipients also recover cytotoxic T cells that can recognize and lyse autologous target cells that express VZV proteins (27). In recent experiments, 50% of BMT recipients showed recovery of VZV-specific cytotoxic T-lymphocyte (CTL) function when tested at a mean of 155 days after transplantation (Figure 30-4). However, the mean precursor frequency of T lymphocytes that recognized the VZV IE62 protein or glycoprotein I (gpI) was more than two-fold lower among BMT recipients than the frequency of CTL that recognized these viral proteins in PBMC from healthy, immune subjects. In these experiments, cultures from BMT recipients showed a significant reduction in the proliferation of $CD4^+$ cells when compared with the pattern of cell phenotypes in cultures from healthy subjects. The predominance of CD8+ T cells in VZV-stimulated cultures resembled the inversion of the CD4+/CD8+ T-cell ratio in peripheral blood lymphocytes that is common after BMT (35). Although CD8+ T lymphocytes have been defined as the "classic" cytotoxic effector cell, human CD4+ cells also function effectively as antiviral CTL against many viruses, including VZV (36). The diminished CD4+ T-cell response to VZV antigen may explain why the overall frequencies of CTL precursors specific for the IE62 or gp I proteins remained significantly lower after BMT than in healthy, VZV-immune individuals.

In contrast to virus-specific T-cell immunity, natural killer cell activity comparable to that observed in healthy subjects is recovered during the first few months after BMT (37). In examining cytotoxic responses after BMT, some patients were found to have a

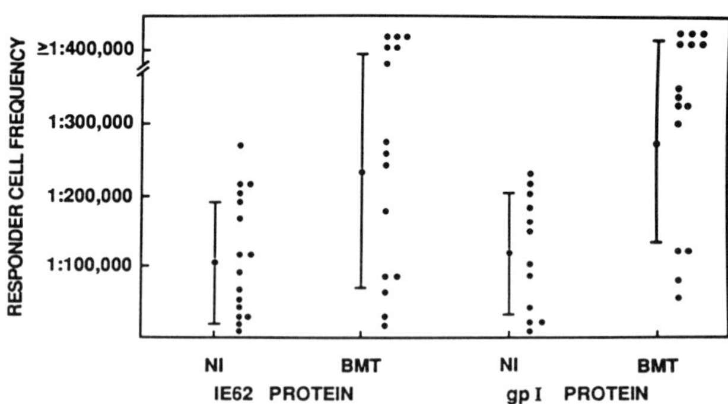

Figure 30-4. Precursor frequencies of cytotoxic T lymphocytes specific for the immediate early protein (IE62) and glycoprotein I (gpI) of varicella zoster virus (VZV) in bone marrow transplant (BMT) recipients and healthy subjects. The mean ± SD for precursor frequency estimates are indicated next to the individual data points (*dark circles*) generated by testing individual BMT recipients and healthy immune subjects. (Reproduced by permission from Wilson A, Sharp M, Koropchak CM, Ting SF, Arvin AM. Subclinical varicella-zoster virus viremia, herpes zoster and recovery of T-lymphocyte responses to varicella-zoster viral antigens after allogeneic and autologous bone marrow transplantation. J Infect Dis 1992;165:119–126.)

predominance of lymphocytes that expressed the CD16 surface antigen in culture (27). Effector cells from these cultures lysed vaccinia control targets as well as those that expressed VZV proteins, indicating natural killer (NK) cell–mediated activity. This capacity of lymphocytes from some BMT recipients to lyse targets expressing VZV proteins by a mechanism that is not antigen-specific may help to limit VZV replication prior to the recovery of virus-specific T-lymphocyte responses.

Clinical Manifestations

Primary VZV Infection

The diagnosis of varicella is usually suspected clinically in high-risk as well as in healthy children when the characteristic vesicular exanthem appears (4,38). The interval from exposure of susceptible children to appearance of the rash is approximately 14 days, with a range of 10 to 21 days; the incubation period may be somewhat shorter in immunocompromised children.

Because of its low incidence, specific descriptions of the clinical course of varicella after BMT are limited, but it is reasonable to generalize from the literature about varicella in other high-risk populations (39,40). The initial manifestations of varicella in immunocompromised children are similar to those observed in otherwise healthy children. Prodromal symptoms may precede the rash by 24 to 48 hours, usually consisting of headache, irritability, malaise, and fever. Cutaneous lesions most often appear first on the scalp, face, or trunk and are usually pruritic. Each lesion begins as a small erythematous macule that evolves into a vesicle of 1 to 4 mm in diameter, on an irregular erythematous base—the classic "dewdrop on a rose petal." In high-risk children, the vesicles may be unusually large and can involve deeper skin layers. Vesicles on mucous membranes, including the conjunctiva, the oropharynx, the rectum, or the vagina are common even among otherwise healthy children. Varicella is typically accompanied by low-grade fever, but temperature elevations may be as high as 40.5°C in high-risk patients, and fever often persists beyond the usual 3 to 4 days.

New vesicle formation typically continues for approximately 3 days (range, 1–7 days) among healthy children. This phase is often prolonged in immunocompromised children; new lesions develop in more than half for more than 7 days (40) (Figure 30-5). Although the majority of immunocompetent children with varicella have fewer than 500 lesions, it is not unusual for more than 1,500 lesions to develop in children on immunosuppressive therapy. Successive crops of varicella vesicles develop in a centrifugal pattern, appearing last on the extremities. These later crops of lesions tend to be more extensive in immunocompromised children, often involving the palms and the soles, as well as the arms and legs. In lesions that are resolving normally, the vesicle fluid rapidly becomes cloudy and the lesion may develop

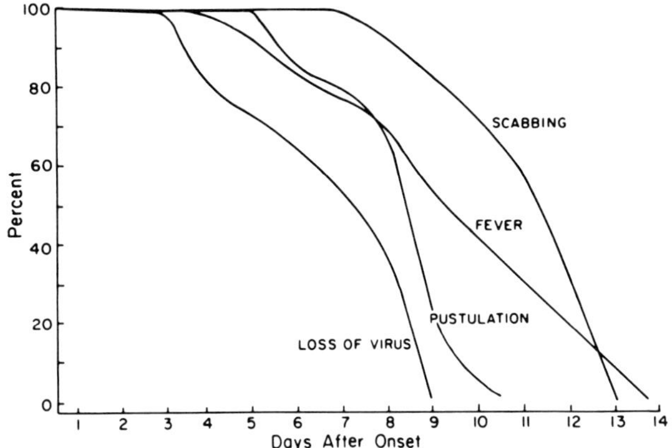

Figure 30-5. The clinical course of varicella among immunocompromised children. (Reproduced by permission from Whitley RJ. Varicella zoster virus infection. In: Galasso G, Whitley R, Merigan T, eds. Antiviral agents and viral diseases of man. New York: Raven, 1990:235–263.)

an umbilicated appearance as it becomes crusted. Among healthy children, the lesions that erupt later in the disease sometimes resolve after a maculopapular phase, but many of the late lesions also progress through the vesicular stage in immunocompromised children. In general, the time to complete crusting of lesions is prolonged in these children. Extensive hypopigmentation and scarring may be seen as the crusts resolve, presumably because of the involvement of deeper layers of the dermis in immunocompromised patients.

Patients who acquire the infection during the first 9 to 12 months after transplantation appear to be at highest risk for development of severe varicella (1). The potential complications of varicella after BMT can be anticipated from the clinical experience with primary VZV infection in other immunocompromised patient populations. BMT recipients can be compared with patients whose immunosuppression is due to treatment of lymphoproliferative malignancies or solid tumors. In one large series, visceral dissemination developed in 32% of these patients in the course of varicella, with VZV infection of the lungs, the liver, and the central nervous system (39). The mortality rate was 7% overall, with an increase to 25% in patients in whom varicella pneumonia developed. The risk for visceral involvement was significantly higher among patients whose absolute lymphocyte counts were less than 500 cells/μL, and the rate of visceral dissemination increased to 71% when the lymphocyte count declined to less than 100 cells/μL. Visceral dissemination was associated with new lesion formation for a median of 10 days in more than half the patients who were evaluated before effective antiviral therapy for VZV was available. On the basis of the analysis of placebo recipients in the original studies of antiviral treatment of varicella in high-risk children, the mortality rate was 17%; varicella pneumonia developed in 27% of the patients, 19% had hepatitis, and 6% had central nervous system disease (40).

Among the complications of primary VZV infection, varicella pneumonia is the most common cause of life-threatening illness. Respiratory symptoms, except for mild rhinitis, are unusual in uncomplicated varicella and require urgent evaluation in immunocompromised patients. Pneumonia most often develops within 3 to 7 days after the appearance of the rash and progresses rapidly to respiratory failure. Clinical signs of pneumonia may be limited to tachypnea, cough, and dyspnea, with no accompanying abnormal findings by auscultation. The degree of hypoxemia may be marked even when abnormalities on chest radiographs are minimal.

Varicella can be associated with abnormal liver function test results in immunocompetent hosts, but hepatic involvement is usually subclinical. In contrast, immunocompromised children are at risk for fulminant varicella hepatitis (Plate XLIII), with progression to hepatic failure. Severe varicella is usually accompanied by signs of coagulopathy, including epistaxis, hematuria, and gastrointestinal bleeding. Hemorrhage into the cutaneous lesions is recognized as a poor prognostic sign in high-risk patients. Bleeding is most often due to disseminated intravascular coagulopathy and hepatic failure, but isolated thrombocytopenia can occur. Vomiting and abdominal pain are uncommon in children with uncomplicated varicella, and severe abdominal or back pain should be considered a sign of life-threatening infection. Disseminated VZV infection can cause pancreatitis and disease of the gastrointestinal tract, such as esophagitis, which may account for these symptoms in some patients.

When varicella meningoencephalitis occurs in immunocompromised children, it is usually associated with other signs of visceral involvement. Symptoms of central nervous system disease usually occur between 2 to 6 days after eruption of the rash and can progress rapidly to coma. The clinical signs include vomiting, headache, altered sensorium, and seizures. The cerebrospinal fluid usually shows a mild to moderate pleocytosis and elevated protein levels. A rapidly deteriorating course progressing to death develops in some patients. Inappropriate antidiuretic hormone secretion may occur in patients who have meningoencephalitis or in patients with disseminated varicella who do not have obvious central nervous system disease (41). Adrenal cortical necrosis is noted at autopsy in patients with disseminated VZV infection.

Severe hypertension is a poor prognostic sign in immunocompromised patients with varicella. The mechanism is uncertain except in cases that are associated with nephritis.

In addition to complications directly related to viral replication, bacterial superinfections are a risk in immunocompromised patients with primary VZV infection, as in otherwise healthy children. *Staphylococcus aureus* and *Streptococcus pyogenes* (group A streptococcus) are the most common pathogens, causing cellulitis, subcutaneous abscesses, and lymphadenitis. Varicella gangrenosa, a very rare syndrome of necrotizing fascitis caused by *Streptococcus pyogenes*, is life-threatening even in intact hosts. Secondary bacterial infection of sites other than skin, including septic arthritis, osteomyelitis, and bacterial pneumonia, may follow varicella. Staphylococcal sepsis can occur, and catheter-related infections can develop in children with indwelling catheters.

Although information is limited, varicella occurring late after transplantation is usually not associated with complications. Four children who had varicella 2 years after BMT had clinical disease that resembled primary VZV in children with no immunodeficiency, and 4 children in whom varicella developed from 105 to 350 days after BMT had no complications (1,34). However, progressive varicella with severe pneumonia was reported in one child who acquired varicella 6 years after successful BMT (42).

Recurrent VZV Infection

Localized Herpes Zoster

Localized herpes zoster is the most common clinical presentation of VZV infection in BMT recipients who are seropositive at the time of transplantation; it accounted for 85% of cases in 231 BMT recipients in the study by Locksley and colleagues (1). The rash of localized herpes zoster is usually preceded by pain and parasthesias in the involved dermatome (38,43). These symptoms begin 1 to 5 days before the eruption and vary from mild sensation to very severe debilitating pain. The etiology of the initial pain is sometimes misdiagnosed as pleurisy, myocardial infarct, cholecystitis, or renal colic. In some instances, the prodrome is not followed by any skin eruption, but a typical antibody response is observed; this syndrome is referred to as "zoster sine herpete" or "silent zoster."

In healthy subjects, herpes zoster involves the thoracic dermatomes in approximately half, and cranial nerve disease occurs in 13 to 20% of patients (38). Recurrent VZV affects similar dermatomes in BMT recipients; thoracic dermatomal disease occurs in 47% and cranial nerve involvement occurs in 16% (Table 30-3).

The cutaneous lesions of localized herpes zoster appear as clusters of varicella-like vesicles in one or several sites anteriorly and posteriorly along the dermatome; typically, the lesions do not cross the midline, but some cases of bilateral dermatomal involvement have been described. Discrete vesicles often enlarge to form confluent lesions. In immunocompromised patients, including BMT recipients, the local vesicular eruption may be very extensive (evolving to occupy the whole dermatome), the lesions may become hemorrhagic, and the duration of cutaneous disease is prolonged (38). In normal hosts, new lesion formation usually continues for 3 to 7 days, followed by a phase of pustulation and crust formation; complete healing is expected by 2 to 3 weeks. In high-

Table 30-3.
Distribution of Dermatomal Involvement with Herpes Zoster in Bone Marrow Transplant Recipients and Otherwise Healthy Individuals with Recurrent Varicella Zoster Virus Infections

	Bone Marrow Transplant Recipients[a]	*Otherwise Healthy Patients*[b]
No. of patients	195	116
Dermatomes involved (%)		
Cranial	16	15
Cervical	17	22
Thoracic	47	53
Lumbar	20	18
Sacral	12	8
Dissemination (%)		
Total	36	...
Cutaneous	23	...
Visceral	13	...
Mortality (%)	7	...

[a]Adapted from Locksley RM, Flournoy N, Sullivan KM, Meyers JD. Infection with varicella-zoster virus after bone marrow transplantation. J Infect Dis 1985;152:1172–1178.
[b]Adapted from Brunell PA. Varicella zoster virus. In: Mandell GL, Douglas RG, Bennett JE, eds. Principles and practice of infectious diseases. New York: Wiley, 1985:952–960.

risk patients, the average time for cessation of new lesion formation is 8 days, and crusting is not complete until an average of 18 days. A chronic cutaneous reactivation of VZV that persists for months may occasionally develop in immunosuppressed patients (44).

When VZV reactivation involves cranial nerves, complications are more likely in both immunocompromised and immunocompetent patients (4). In one series, corneal damage, facial scarring, palsy of the seventh cranial nerve, or hearing loss occurred in 35% of patients (1). The distribution of the ophthalmic branch of the trigeminal nerve is a common site of herpes zoster. The development of vesicular lesions on the nose is a sign of involvement of the ophthalmic branch and indicates a risk for ocular complications. The clinical findings of ocular herpes zoster include conjunctivitis, keratitis, anterior uveitis, or, rarely, panophthalmitis. Although corneal lesions are common, blindness is an unusual complication of herpes zoster ophthalmicus (45). Loss of vision associated with herpes zoster is usually secondary to retrobulbar neuritis. VZV reactivation may produce facial palsy when it involves the seventh cranial nerve. Herpes zoster oticus is associated with VZV reactivation from the geniculate ganglion and produces the Ramsay Hunt syndrome with unilateral deafness and vestibular symptoms. Oral lesions of the palate may develop without any cutaneous lesions when the second branch of the fifth cranial nerve is affected.

Cerebral angiitis is a syndrome of cerebral vascular inflammation with thrombosis and microinfarcts associated with VZV reactivation at cranial nerve sites. In severe cases, massive thrombosis with contralateral hemiparesis may result (46). Infarct in the distribution of the middle cerebral artery can be demonstrated by computed tomography. Pathological findings include a granulomatous inflammatory process in the arterial wall, mononuclear cell infiltrates, vascular necrosis, and viral particles within the smooth muscle cells of the affected arteries. The syndrome is rare, and there is no evidence that BMT recipients or other immunocompromised patients are at increased risk for cerebral angiitis. However, it is important to recognize this complication in patients in whom hemiparesis develops approximately 6 to 8 weeks after the symptoms of herpes zoster.

When the anterior horn cells are involved in VZV reactivation, inflammation and necrosis may follow with resulting motor deficits. In otherwise healthy individuals, motor paralysis was present in 11.5% of those with cervical herpes zoster, 7% with lumbosacral disease, and 0.3% with thoracic zoster (47). Full recovery of the motor deficit is expected in 85 to 90% of patients. Transverse myelitis and ascending paralysis are rare neurological syndromes caused by recurrent VZV infection with or without immunosuppression.

Immunocompromised patients are at increased risk of postherpetic neuralgia, which is the most common complication of herpes zoster in all patient populations. The definition of postherpetic pain varies from any pain lasting after the crusts of the cutaneous lesions have disappeared to pain that persists more than 2 months. Estimates of the incidence of postherpetic neuralgia vary depending on the definition used. In one study of healthy individuals, postherpetic neuralgia developed in 9% of patients with herpes zoster (12), whereas Locksley and colleagues (1) observed postherpetic neuralgia in 25% of patients with herpes zoster after BMT. Postherpetic neuralgia is uncommon in children, even in those who are immunocompromised; it was noted in only 1 of 41 (2%) pediatric BMT recipients in whom herpes zoster developed (6).

Bacterial superinfection and local scarring are common in BMT recipients with herpes zoster; they occur with an incidence of 17 and 19%, respectively.

Cutaneous and Visceral Dissemination

In contrast to healthy subjects, cutaneous dissemination often develops in BMT recipients, and is defined as more than 5 vesicular lesions beyond the primary dermatome. Cutaneous dissemination occurred in 24% of BMT recipients and was equally common among those who had recurrent VZV during the early or late period after transplantation (1). BMT recipients are also at risk for visceral dissemination during episodes of VZV reactivation (see Figure 30-1). Because it is a sign of viremia, cutaneous dissemination provides a marker for the risk for visceral dissemination. However, visceral dissemination also occurs in patients whose cutaneous lesions are localized to the primary dermatome. Without antiviral therapy, visceral dissemination was observed in 13% of BMT recipients with herpes zoster. The potential sites of visceral dissemination with recurrent VZV are the same as those associated with disseminated primary VZV infection. The clinical complications that result include pneumonia, hepatitis, disseminated intravascular coagulopathy, and encephalitis. The mortality that accompanies VZV reactivation is almost always due to viral pneumonia, but fatal fulminant hepatitis and disseminated intravascular coagulopathy without VZV pneumonia have been reported (48). Acute GVHD is the only risk factor associated significantly with VZV dissemination. VZV has also been identified as the causative agent of late interstitial pneumonia in BMT recipients with chronic GVHD (49).

Occasionally, BMT recipients present with signs of visceral dissemination 24 to 96 hours before the localized cutaneous eruption of recurrent VZV becomes evident. Among these patients, the clinical presentation is characterized by abdominal pain, often midepigastric or periumbilical, with or without associated nausea, vomiting, or fever. Pancreatitis, hepatitis, gastrointestinal hemorrhage, and disseminated intravascular coagulopathy have been described in patients with abdominal symptoms preceding the rash (50). Visceral dissemination can also occur without any signs of cutaneous disease. Three BMT recipients had fatal VZV infection and no skin lesions during the course of their illness despite evidence of widespread organ infection at autopsy (1).

Immunosuppression also predisposes to central nervous system infection with recurrent VZV, although symptomatic neurological complications of herpes zoster are rare, even in these patients. In evaluating these patients clinically, abnormal cerebrospinal fluid findings are common, even in immunocompetent patients with herpes zoster. Lymphocytic pleocytosis and elevated protein levels were observed in approximately 40% of healthy individuals who had no abnormalities by neurological examination, whereas the incidence of herpes zoster–associated encephalitis is estimated to be only 0.2 to 0.5% (12,51). The clinical symptoms and signs of central nervous system disease are headache, photophobia, meningismus, and altered state of consciousness (52,53). Neurological symptoms usually appear within a few days after the exanthem. The temperature is usually normal or mildly elevated. Seizures are rare, but an electroencephalogram may show diffuse slowing or epileptiform activity.

As would be expected, the occurrence of visceral dissemination increases the mortality of recurrent VZV infection substantially, from an overall death rate of 7 to 55%. The mortality rate in immunocompromised patients in whom both pneumonia and encephalitis develop is higher than in those patients who have encephalitis only.

Atypical Nonlocalized Herpes Zoster

Atypical nonlocalized herpes zoster after BMT is sometimes categorized as varicella because the BMT recipient is presumed to lack VZV immunity, regardless of prior immune status. However, identifying the syndrome as a distinct clinical presentation is useful because the pathogenesis of infection and the timing of the host response may be affected by differences between the endogenous and the exogenous routes of infection, and residual immunity may modify the clinical course. The incidence of atypical nonlocalized herpes zoster is variable; it accounts for 0 to 25% of episodes of VZV reactivation after BMT. Clinically, patients with atypical nonlocalized herpes zoster have cutaneous vesicles that are identical to those of varicella. The number of lesions is quite variable, but the eruption is often extensive, involving face, trunk, extremities, palms, and soles. This syndrome occurs in autologous as well as allogeneic BMT recipients and accounted for 21% of episodes of recurrent VZV in one series (12). The morbidity of untreated infection is high; visceral dissemination developed in 45% of patients, resulting in a mortality rate of 28% during the period before antiviral therapy was available (1).

Second Episodes of Recurrent VZV

Second episodes of VZV reactivation after BMT are uncommon. Approximately 2% of patients had two episodes of herpes zoster, occurring an average of 25 months after transplantation (range, 4–41 months). All second episodes involved the same dermatome (1).

Subclinical Reactivation of Latent VZV

The occurrence of subclinical VZV reactivation in BMT recipients has been shown in a recent study using the PCR method to demonstrate cell-associated VZV viremia (27). Subclinical VZV reactivation was detected in 19% of 37 BMT recipients. Clinical signs of herpes zoster subsequently developed in 2 of 7 patients who had subclinical VZV viremia at intervals of 60 and 130 days later. Three patients who had subclinical VZV viremia between 17 and 85 days after BMT had cleared the cell-associated viremia when they were retested by VZV PCR; 2 patients were not re-evaluated by VZV PCR, but herpes zoster did not develop. Thus, 5 of 7 patients (71%) who had subclinical viremia did not progress to clinical infection.

Laboratory Diagnosis

Direct Detection of VZV-infected Cells by Immunofluorescence

The optimal method for rapid diagnosis of cutaneous VZV infection is to obtain epithelial cells from a fresh lesion and to stain the specimen using fluorescein-conjugated monoclonal antibodies to VZV antigens (54–56). The VZV-specific monoclonal antibodies bind to viral proteins that are synthesized within infected cells; fixing the cells prior to staining makes the cell membrane permeable, allowing the detection of VZV proteins in the cytoplasm and the nucleus, as well as on the cell surface. This method is referred to as the direct fluorescence antigen (DFA) technique. The most important step in the diagnostic procedure is to disrupt the roof of the vesicle to obtain intact cells from the base of the lesion. Cells can be recovered efficiently by rotating the blunt end of a wooden applicator stick in the uncovered lesion or by scraping with a scapel and transferring the material to a glass slide. Unless at least 5 intact cells are visible on the slide, the specimen should not be considered adequate for processing by the DFA method. It is important to include parallel staining of a portion of the specimen with reagents to detect HSV, because VZV and HSV lesions are often indistinguishable clinically and to provide a control for the specificity of the assay. Proper interpretation of DFA slides requires experience; the most common error is to identify false-positive results because of lack of expertise at distinguishing background nonspecific fluorescence. If the clinical course of the patient is not consistent with a diagnosis of VZV infection based on the DFA method, the laboratory result should be questioned.

DFA and indirect immunofluorescence or immunoperoxidase methods can also be used to demonstrate the presence of VZV in properly prepared tissue sections of lung, liver, and other organs from patients with disseminated VZV infections.

When laboratory facilities for DFA testing are not available, the Tzanck stain and other cytological methods can be used to detect multinucleated giant cells in a lesion scraping; however, false-negative results are common, and these methods do not differentiate VZV from HSV infection. Herpes viral particles can be detected by electron microscopy, but few diagnostic laboratories are equipped to perform this procedure, the method is not rapid, and the morphology of herpes viruses is too similar to distinguish these viruses by electron microscopy.

Viral Isolation in Tissue Culture Cells

VZV can be detected in clinical samples using standard tissue culture methods for viral isolation (54,57). The highest yield for viral culture depends on obtaining vesicular fluid along with infected cells from the base of the cutaneous lesion. Vesicular fluid can be collected in a tuberculin syringe or by using a cotton or a Dacron swab. Swabs should be put in viral transport medium immediately, agitated, and pressed against the side of the vial to remove absorbed fluid; the swab should be taken out of the vial before it is sent to the laboratory. If storage for more than a few hours is required, the specimen should be kept on dry ice or frozen at −70°C; storing the specimen at −20°C, in a standard refrigerator freezer, for 24 hours usually inactivates the virus.

Optimal recovery of infectious virus in tissue culture requires the use of diploid cell lines or human embryonic lung fibroblasts (57). The cytopathic effect appears within 2 to 14 days after inoculation. Because the average time to detection of the virus in tissue culture is 7 days, diagnosis by viral culture is not rapid enough to influence clinical decisions in most circumstances. The sensitivity of tissue culture for detection of VZV is also substantially less than for identification of HSV and CMV. Procedures such as centrifugation enhancement may shorten the duration required to detect cytopathic effects (58). There are some differences in the morphology of plaques produced by VZV compared with the other herpes viruses, but the identity of the virus isolate must be proved by immunofluorescence staining with virus-specific antisera. As in CMV, the shell vial culture method has been adopted by some laboratories to improve the sensitivity of VZV isolation and to permit earlier identification of positive specimens. This method combines centrifugation and staining with fluorescein-conjugated monoclonal antibodies to VZV; positive results may be available within 1 to 3 days after inoculation. In a recent study, VZV was detected in 70% of specimens by shell vial culture, compared with a 64% rate of detection by standard issue culture methods, but viral diagnosis by either tissue culture method was less sensitive than DFA, which was positive in 92% of specimens (56).

The likelihood of recovery of VZV from cutaneous lesions is directly related to the stage of the lesion; clear vesicles are much more likely to be positive than specimens from lesions that have become pustular or crusted. Varicella lesions are usually positive for 3 days, whereas virus can be recovered for one week or longer in herpes zoster lesions. VZV can be isolated from peripheral blood mononuclear cells by tissue culture inoculation of specimens from immunocompromised patients with recurrent as well as primary VZV infections (28). In contrast to meningoencephalitis associated with primary VZV infection, the virus has been isolated from the cerebrospinal fluid of patients with herpes zoster (51). Bronchial washings may yield varicella in patients with varicella pneumonia. The lungs are the most common autopsy organ from which VZV has been isolated, but the virus has been recovered from many sites, including heart, liver, pancreas, gastrointestinal tract, brain, and eyes.

Viral DNA Detection

VZV DNA sequences can be detected using radiolabeled or biotinylated nucleic acid probes for in situ hybridization or Southern blot procedures (20, 59). In situ hybridization was more sensitive than viral culture for demonstrating viremia in patients with varicella. The presence of VZV gene sequences in human ganglion tissue has been demonstrated using probe methods (22–24). PCR is a sensitive method for detecting VZV in clinical samples from patients with varicella and herpes zoster, but it is not available for routine diagnosis.

Serological Diagnosis

Serological screening of prospective BMT recipients for VZV antibodies is a valuable tool to establish immune status before transplantation. Many serological methods are available for measuring IgG antibodies to VZV (54). The most sensitive serological assays for detection of VZV antibodies are fluorescent-antibody staining of membrane antigen (FAMA) and radioimmunoassay (RIA). Other methods that are relatively reliable for establishing immune status include enzyme-linked immunosorbent (ELISA) and anticomplement immunofluorescence (ACIF). However, the commercially available ELISA kits for VZV antibodies have a high degree of specificity but are not as sensitive as research laboratory procedures such as FAMA. Although these methods do not usually yield false-positive results, 10 to 15% of immune individuals may be identified as susceptible. Complement fixation methods are not satisfactory for determining immune status. A latex agglutination method, which is sensitive as well as specific, has become available recently and is an excellent alternative for use in clinical diagnostic virology laboratories (60).

Although seroconversion can be documented with primary VZV infection and boosts in antibody titers accompany recurrent VZV, serological diagnosis of acute infection requires paired sera and is rarely useful for clinical purposes. There are no reliable commercial methods to test for VZV IgM antibodies. In addition, although VZV IgM antibodies can be detected by research methods in patients with varicella, the majority of patients with recurrent infection also produce VZV IgM (61).

Antiviral Therapy for VZV Infection

Acyclovir

Currently, acyclovir is the drug of choice for the treatment of primary and recurrent VZV infections. The antiviral activity of acyclovir (9,2 hydroxyethoxymethylguanine) against VZV follows the same pathway that mediates its interference with the replication of HSV. The metabolism of the drug to the triphosphate form by the viral thymidine kinase produces a compound that functions as a competitive inhibitor and chain terminator of viral DNA polymerase. However, although HSV-1 and HSV-2 isolates are usually inhibited in vitro by 0.125 and 0.215 μg/mL acyclovir, respectively, the mean concentrations required to inhibit VZV isolates are often 0.82 to 4.64 μg/mL, with ranges as low as 0.3 μg/mL and as high as 10.8 μg/mL (62,63).

Plasma concentrations achieved by intravenous administration of acyclovir at doses of 10 mg/kg or 250 to 500 mg/m^2 range from 15 to 25 μg/mL (64). These concentrations are several-fold above the in vitro inhibitory concentrations for most VZV isolates. In contrast, only approximately 20% of the oral dose of acyclovir is absorbed. Oral administration to pediatric patients at doses of 600 mg/m^2 given 4 times produced peak plasma concentrations of approximately 1.0 to 1.5 μg/mL (65). An oral dose of 200 mg acyclovir given 5 times a day to adults (approximately 115 μg/mL for an adult male) produces plasma concentrations of approximately 0.5 μg/mL; increasing the unit dose to 600 mg resulted in plasma concentrations of 1.3 μg/mL (66). Thus, acyclovir concentrations required to inhibit VZV isolates can be expected to be significantly above the mean peak plasma concentration achieved by oral dosing.

Antiviral Treatment of Varicella

Administration of intravenous acyclovir to immunocompromised children with varicella has the potential to terminate the cell-associated viremia that produces malignant progressive varicella in these patients and to prevent the onset of varicella pneumonitis, each of which is correlated with a high risk of fatal infection (39,67). The dosage of intravenous acyclovir for varicella in high-risk patients is 500 mg/m^2/dose every 8 hours, with administration continuing for 7 days. When this dosage was tested in placebo-controlled trials, the effect of the drug on the number of days to defervescence and resolution of cutaneous lesions was not significant, but varicella pneumonitis was prevented in the acyclovir recipients (68,69). The efficacy of acyclovir and its superiority to vidarabine in preventing the visceral dissemination of VZV was confirmed by Feldman and Lott (39), who found that varicella pneumonitis developed in none of 16 children with cancer given acyclovir, whereas 6 of 21 (29%) patients treated with vidarabine progressed to pneumonia. The clinical impact of specific antiviral therapy was illustrated by the fact that none of 37 children with varicella who received vidarabine or acyclovir had fatal infection (39).

Primary VZV infection in BMT recipients occurring within the first year after transplantation should be considered to require intravenous acylovir therapy. The goal of antiviral therapy for varicella in high-risk patients is to initiate drug treatment within 72 hours after the appearance of the cutaneous rash. Parents and patients need to be educated about the typical appearance of varicella lesions because many cases occur without any known exposure, and prompt diagnosis during the early phase of infection is important to the success of antiviral therapy. Because there are other causes of vesicular rashes in childhood and in immunocompromised patients, the clinical diagnosis should be confirmed using the DFA technique. Although most children do not have clinical signs of dissemination immediately, the interval during which preventive therapy can be initiated is very short. The progressive nature of varicella in immunocompromised patients only becomes apparent with successive crops of new lesions, but visceral dissemination also occurs during this interval. The average period to onset of varicella pneumonitis is 6 days; most cases occur within 4 to 8 days among untreated high-risk patients. In addition to preventing life-threatening dissemination, acyclovir therapy can also be expected to minimize the extent of the cutaneous disease and to shorten significantly the time to complete healing (40). More rapid resolution of the cutaneous lesions may also reduce the risk of secondary bacterial infections.

Immunocompromised children who present with signs of disseminated VZV infection, including pneumonia, hepatitis, thrombocytopenia, or encephalitis, should receive immediate treatment with intravenous acyclovir. The efficacy of acyclovir for the treatment of established varicella pneumonia or other visceral sites of infection has not been determined in a controlled trial. Five placebo recipients in the original acyclovir trial in whom pneumonitis developed were placed on the drug approximately 6 to 8 days after the appearance of the varicella rash, and all of these patients improved after initiation of the drug (68). However, in another series, 3 of 4 high-risk patients who were not treated until at least 5 days after the onset of the cutaneous lesions had evidence of visceral dissemination at initiation of treatment; all 3 patients had progressive varicella and 2 patients died (70).

Although varicella zoster immune globulin (VZIG) administration is clearly indicated for high-risk children whose exposure to VZV is identified within 96 hours, the fact that a child has received VZIG does not preclude the possibility that severe varicella will develop. The incidence of varicella despite VZIG prophylaxis is significantly higher for children with household exposures than for those who have less prolonged contact with the index case, and the attack rate is affected by the VZV IgG titer of the preparation (71). In the placebo-controlled trial of intravenous acyclovir, one of 6 (17%) placebo recipients who had received zoster immune globulin (ZIG) or zoster immune plasma (ZIP) before entry required reassignment to open drug because of progressive varicella (68). In the St. Jude experience, the risk of varicella pneumonitis was reduced significantly by passive antibody prophylaxis, but pneumonia developed in 11% of children despite receiving ZIG, ZIP, or VZIG (39). Because of these risks, BMT recipients in whom varicella develops should be treated with intravenous acyclovir even if passive antibody prophylaxis was given at the time of exposure.

At intervals beyond 9 to 12 months after BMT, it may be acceptable to monitor the clinical course of varicella without giving acyclovir, assuming that patients have no evidence of GVHD and are not receiving immunosuppressive therapy. However, given the predictable benefits of a short course of acyclovir, its administration is easily justified for the management of these patients.

Antiviral Treatment of Herpes Zoster

Acyclovir has been shown to be effective for the treatment of recurrent VZV infection in immunocompromised patients in placebo-controlled trials and through extensive clinical experience with the drug. The dose of acyclovir is 500 mg/m^2 or 10 mg/kg given every 8 hours intravenously. Therapy should be continued for 7 days or for 2 days after cessation of new lesion formation, whichever provides the longer treatment course.

In an early study of the efficacy of acyclovir, all immunocompromised patients with herpes zoster experienced improvement of symptoms within 24 hours, no new skin lesions were noted after 24 hours, and none had visceral dissemination (72). In a subsequent placebo-controlled trial, local progression and progression of cutaneous dissemination was terminated with acyclovir therapy (73). One of 52 treated patients had progressive VZV disease, compared with 11 of 42 placebo recipients. Meyers and associates (74) showed that intravenous acyclovir had clinical benefit in a study enrolling only BMT recipients with herpes zoster. Treatment resulted in a shorter time to cessation of new lesion formation, more rapid crusting and healing, and prevention of cutaneous and visceral dissemination in patients who presented with localized herpes zoster. When acyclovir was compared with vidarabine for the treatment of herpes zoster, cutaneous dissemination developed in none of 12 acyclovir recipients, compared with 5 of 10 patients given vidarabine (75). Acyclovir decreased the duration of local viral replication; viral cultures remained positive for VZV for only 4 days after initiation of treatment. On the basis of this experience, acyclovir therapy initiated within 72 hours after the onset of VZV reactivation can be expected to reduce the duration of new lesion formation in BMT recipients to approximately 3 days. On average, early antiviral treatment should cause the cessation of acute pain within 4 days, crusting of lesions by 7 days, and complete healing by 2 to 3 weeks (Figure 30-6). Although early acyclovir treatment is likely to produce the best results, clinical benefit can still occur when therapy is delayed for more than 3 days (73). None of 29 immunocompromised patients whose

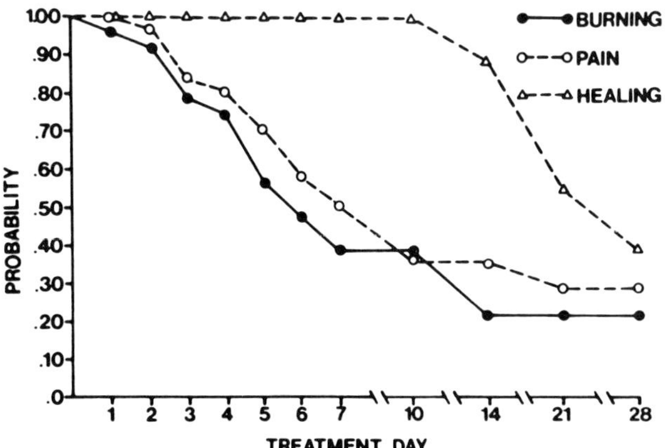

Figure 30-6. Probability of lesion burning (23 patients; ●—●); of lesion pain (31 patients; ○---○), and of no total healing (31 patients, ▲---▲) by treatment day. (Reproduced by Meyers J, Wade J, Shepp D, et al. Acyclovir treatment of VZV infection in the compromised host. Transplantation 1984;37:571–574.)

therapy was initiated more than 3 days after the onset of the rash had progressive herpes zoster, compared with 3 of 17 patients in the placebo group.

Although acyclovir eliminates the life-threatening complications of VZV reactivation in most patients, relapse of herpes zoster is a clinical problem in some BMT recipients treated with acyclovir. In one series, new lesions developed in 5 of 40 patients (13%); relapse occurred less than 4 days after treatment was stopped in 3 of the 5 patients (74). It is possible that early acyclovir therapy delays the recovery of VZV-specific immunity in some patients. Nevertheless, most patients respond to treatment with a second course of acyclovir.

Unfortunately, although acyclovir is clearly effective for the treatment of acute herpes zoster in BMT recipients, it does not appear to decrease the incidence of postherpetic neuralgia. In one series, 21% of 40 patients had recurrence of pain after cessation of therapy (74). There is no evidence that longer courses of treatment would help to reduce the risk of postherpetic neuralgia. The fact that the acute pain associated with herpes zoster is ameliorated by acyclovir suggests that a different mechanism is responsible for postherpetic pain.

The efficacy of oral acyclovir for herpes zoster in BMT recipients has not been firmly established. This route of administration should be reserved for carefully selected patients who have localized herpes zoster occurring in the late period after BMT. Because the bioavailability of oral acyclovir is low, this route of administration requires giving 800 mg/dose 5 times a day. Patients receiving oral acyclovir should be monitored for signs of progressive VZV infection and should be treated with intravenous drug if complications arise. When patients are treated with the intravenous regimen of acyclovir for herpes zoster, there is no need to provide further treatment with oral acyclovir after discharge.

Acyclovir Toxicity

The safety of acyclovir has been established in numerous clinical trials. Although BMT recipients also tolerate the drug well, the incidence of side effects is higher in this population. In one series, gastrointestinal symptoms of nausea and vomiting occurred in 40% of treated patients (75). Nephrotoxicity, defined as a 50% increase in serum creatinine levels, was also more common than in other patient populations treated with acyclovir; 10 to 25% of BMT recipients receiving acyclovir are reported to have an abnormal serum creatinine level, but these elevations may be caused by other medications given concurrently (76). Because acyclovir is excreted by glomerular filtration, other drugs that affect renal function, such as cyclosporine, can interact to cause elevated plasma concentrations of the drug. The dosage and dose interval for acyclovir administration should be adjusted based on the relative impairment of creatinine clearance. The dosage interval should be lengthened to every 12 hours for clearances of 25 to 50 mL/min and to 24 hours for clearances of 10 to 25 mL/min; if the clearance is 0 to 10 mL/min, the dosage should be reduced to 250 mg/m^2 given every 24 to 48 hours. It is also important to maintain adequate hydration in patients receiving acyclovir to avoid precipitation of the drug in renal tubules. A few cases of acute neurotoxicity have been reported in patients with deficient renal clearance who were receiving acyclovir. Abnormal liver function test results in patients being treated with acyclovir for VZV infections should be considered possible evidence of hepatitis rather than drug toxicity. Acyclovir does not have hematological toxicity and does not interfere with engraftment in BMT recipients.

Other Antiviral Compounds

Although vidarabine is no longer the drug of choice for the treatment of herpes zoster in BMT recipients, it may be used in patients who do not tolerate acyclovir. Although VZV resistance to acyclovir has not been common in BMT recipients, it has been reported in patients with the acquired immune deficiency syndrome. Vidarabine may have some clinical benefit in these circumstances. Human and recombinant leukocyte interferon have also been shown to have significant clinical efficacy in immunocompromised patients with herpes zoster and to provide an alternative to the nucleoside analogue drugs for the treatment of resistant VZV infection (76).

Several new compounds are currently under investigation for the treatment of VZV infections. Acyclovir analogues that have improved absorption after oral administration are being tested, as is 1-b-D-arabinofuranosyl-E-5-[2-bromovinyl] uracil (BVaraU), a new nucleoside analogue that is well absorbed orally (77,78). This compound is phosphorylated by the viral thymidine kinase, like acyclovir, and then requires metabolism by the viral thymidylate kinase. It resembles acyclovir in that the phosphorylated form acts as a chain terminator and a viral polymerase inhibitor, and metabolism in uninfected cells is minimal. Dihydroxypropoxymethylguanine (ganciclovir, DHPG) has in vitro activity against VZV that is equivalent to acyclovir, but clinical studies of its efficacy for the treatment of VZV infections have not been done because of its greater toxicity. However, it is theoretically possible that administration of ganciclovir to BMT recipients who have CMV infection could alter the course of concurrent VZV infection.

Prophylaxis for VZV Infection

Varicella Zoster Immune Globulin

VZIG is a passive antibody preparation containing VZV IgG antibodies prepared from high-titer immune human serum. VZIG is distributed by the American Red Cross Blood Services and can be obtained by calling the local Red Cross Blood Center. The dosage is one vial/10 kg body weight given intramuscularly.

VZIG is indicated for the prophylaxis of primary VZV infection in susceptible, VZV-seronegative, high-risk patients, including BMT recipients. Its prophylactic effect depends on administration to the patient within 96 hours, and preferably within 48 hours after exposure to an index case has occurred. Varicella exposure is defined as household contact, shared hospital room, or indoor play for at least one hour with a child who is in the contagious phase of varicella, which is the interval from 2 days before to 5 days after onset of the rash. If a patient has received any of the commercial preparations of high-dose intravenous Ig (100–400 mg/kg) for other indications within 3 weeks before the exposure, it is not necessary to administer VZIG (79). A second dose of VZIG should be given if a new exposure occurs more than 2 weeks after a dose of VZIG has been given. Although the risk of VZV transmission from an individual with herpes zoster is low, close contact between a susceptible BMT recipient and a patient with recurrent VZV lesions also justifies administration of VZIG.

There is no indication that passive antibody prophylaxis will reduce the risk of VZV reactivation after BMT in patients who have serological evidence of prior VZV infection. Passive antibody administration is not effective for the treatment of herpes zoster.

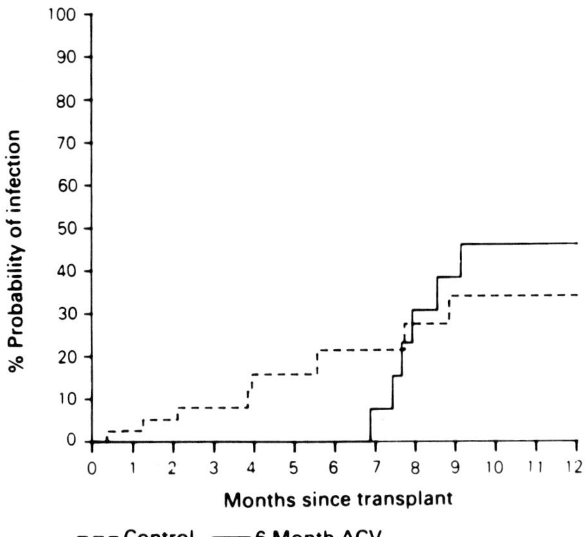

Figure 30-7. Cumulative probability of varicella zoster virus infection in patients receiving acyclovir (*solid line*) or placebo (*dotted line*). (Reproduced by permission from Selby P, Powels R, Easton D, et al. The prophylactic role of intravenous and long term oral acyclovir after allogeneic bone marrow transplantation. Br J Cancer 1989;59:434–438.)

Acyclovir Prophylaxis

The efficacy of acyclovir prophylaxis for preventing recurrent VZV infection in BMT recipients was shown in 3 placebo-controlled trials that involved a total of 202 patients (80–82). The prophylactic doses of acyclovir that have been tested were 250 mg/m^2 given intravenously twice a day for a period of 5 weeks after transplantation, followed by 400 mg orally every 8 hours for 6 months; and 5 mg/kg intravenously every 8 hours for 3 weeks followed by 800 mg orally every 6 hours for 6 months. Herpes zoster developed in none of the acyclovir recipients during the period of therapy, compared with a 15% incidence in the placebo group. The lower dose was as effective as the higher dose regimen. However, VZV reactivation occurred when acyclovir was discontinued, so that there was no overall reduction in the number of episodes by one year (Figure 30-7). Infections in the acyclovir group were concentrated in the second half of the year.

Despite the evidence that it inhibits early VZV reactivation, administration of acyclovir as prophylaxis to prevent herpes zoster in BMT recipients is not common. Although herpes zoster early after BMT has a high risk of causing disseminated disease, prompt initiation of acyclovir for the treatment of recurrent VZV infections has proved to be very effective. None of the placebo recipients in the acyclovir prophylaxis studies had fatal dissemination when given intravenous acyclovir at the onset of recurrent VZV infection (81,82). In addition, avoiding prolonged low-dose administration of acyclovir may help minimize the emergence of VZV strains that are resistant to the drug.

Varicella Vaccine

The investigational live attenuated varicella vaccine (Oka-Merck strain) has been given to children with leukemia in remission (83); however, it is not appropriate for administration to susceptible BMT recipients because it contains infectious virus. Immunizing susceptible healthy household contacts with varicella vaccine may be useful for some families to reduce the risk of household exposure of the BMT recipient to varicella in siblings (84). Some vaccine recipients become candidates for BMT, post-transplant reactivation of vaccine virus has been demonstrated in a few instances. However, evidence suggests that the vaccine virus reactivates less commonly than wild type VZV (85). If symptomatic reactivation occurs, the vaccine virus is susceptible to inhibition by acyclovir, and episodes of vaccine-related herpes zoster can be treated with this drug (86).

References

1. Locksley RM, Flournoy N, Sullivan KM, Meyers JD. Infection with varicella-zoster virus after marrow transplantation. J Infect Dis 1985;152:1172–1178.
2. Zaia J. Viral infections with bone marrow transplantation. Hematol Oncol Clin North Am 1990;4:603–623.
3. Meyers JD, Flournoy N, Thomas ED. Cell-mediated immunity to varicella-zoster virus after allogeneic marrow transplant. J Infec Dis 1980;141:479–487.

4. Arvin AM. Clinical manifestations of varicella and herpes zoster and the immune response to varicella-zoster virus. In: Hyman R, ed. The natural history of varicella zoster virus. Boca Raton: CRC Press, 1987:67–130.
5. Gelb L. Varicella-zoster virus. In: Fields BN, Knipe DM, eds. Virology. New York: Raven, 1989:2011–2054.
6. Wacker P, Hartmann O, Salloum E, Lemerle J. VZV infections after bone marrow transplantation in children. Bone Marrow Transplant 1989;4:191–194.
7. Blume K, Beutler E, Bross K, et al. Bone marrow ablation and allogeneic bone marrow transplantation in acute leukemias. N Engl J Med 1980;302:1041–1046.
8. Atkinson K, Meyers J, Storb R, et al. VZV infection after marrow transplantation for aplastic anemia or leukemia. Transplantation 1980;29:47–50.
9. Atkinson K, Farwell V, Storb R, et al. Analysis of late infections after human bone marrow transplantation: role of genotypic nonidentity between marrow donor and recipient and of nonspecific suppressor cells in patients with chronic graft versus host disease. Blood 1982;60:714–720.
10. Ljungman P, Lonnqvist B, Gahrton G, et al. Clinical and subclinical reactivation of VZV in immunocompromised patients. J Infect Dis 1986;153:840–847.
11. Schuchter L, Wingard J, Piantadosi S, et al. Herpes zoster infection after autologous bone marrow transplantation. Blood 1989;74:1424–1427.
12. Christiansen N, Haake R, Hurd D. Early herpes zoster in adult patients with Hodgkins disease undergoing bone marrow transplant. Bone Marrow Transplant 1991;7:435–437.
13. Ragozzino M, Melton L, Kurland L, et al. Population based study of herpes zoster and its sequelae. Medicine 1982;61:310–316.
14. Saral R, Burns WH, Prentice HG. Herpes virus infections: clinical manifestations and therapeutic strategies in immunocompromised patients. Clin Haematol 1984; 13:645–660.
15. Wingard JR. Management of infectious complications of bone marrow transplantation. Oncology 1990;4:69–75.
16. Grose C. Varicella zoster virus: pathogenesis of the human diseases, the virus and viral replication. In: Hyman R, ed. The natural history of varicella zoster virus. Boca Raton: CRC Press, 1987:1–66.
17. Arvin AM. Varicella-zoster viral infections in healthy and immunocompromised children. In: Feigin RD, ed. Seminars in pediatric infectious diseases, vol 2. Philadelphia: WB Saunders, 1991:1–11.
18. Asano Y, Itakura N, Hiroishi Y, et al. Viral replication and immunologic responses in children naturally infected with varicella-zoster virus and in varicella vaccine recipients. J Infect Dis 1985;152:863–868.
19. Koropchak CM, Solem S, Diaz PS, Arvin AM. Investigation of varicella-zoster virus infection of lymphocytes by in situ hybridization. J Virol 1989;63:2392–2395.
20. Koropchak CM, Graham G, Palmer J, et al. Investigation of varicella-zoster virus infection by polymerase chain reaction in the immunocompetent host with acute varicella. J Infect Dis 1991;163:1016–1022.
21. Straus S, Reinhold W, Smith H, et al. Endonuclease analysis of viral DNA from varicella and subsequent zoster in the same patient. N Engl J Med 1984; 311:1326–1328.
22. Hyman R, Ecker J, Tenser R. Varicella zoster virus RNA in human trigeminal ganglia. Lancet 1983;2:814–816.
23. Gilden D, Vafai A, Shtram Y, et al. Varicella zoster virus DNA in human sensory ganglia. Nature 1983; 306:478–480.
24. Croen K, Otrove J, Dragovic L, Straus S. Patterns of gene expression and sites of latency in human nerve ganglia are different for VZV and HSV. Proc Natl Acad Sci USA 1988;85:9773–9777.
25. Croen K, Staus S. Varicella-zoster virus latency. Annu Rev Microbiol 1991;4:265–282.
26. Mahalingam R, Wellish M, Wolf W, et al. Latent VZV DNA in human trigeminal and thoracic ganglia. N Engl J Med 1990;323:627–631.
27. Wilson A, Sharp M, Koropchak CM, Ting SF, Arvin AM. Subclinical varicella-zoster virus viremia, herpes zoster and recovery of T-lymphocyte responses to varicella-zoster viral antigens after allogeneic and autologous bone marrow transplantation. J Infect Dis 1992; 165:119–126.
28. Feldman S, Epp E. Isolation of varicella-zoster virus from blood. J Pediatr 1976;88:265–268.
29. Atkinson K, Hansen JA, Strob R, Goehle S, Goldstein G, Thomas ED. T cell subpopulations identified by monoclonal antibodies after human bone marrow transplantation. Helper-inducer and cytotoxic-suppressor subsets. Blood 1982;59:1292–1298.
30. Arvin M, Koropchak CM, Williams BR, Grumet FC, Foung SK. Early immune response in healthy and immunocompromised subjects with primary varicella-zoster virus infection. J Infect Dis 1986;154:422–429.
31. Webster A, Grint P, Brenner MK, Prentice HG, Griffiths PD. Titration of IgG antibodies against varicella zoster virus before bone marrow transplantation is not predictive of future zoster. J Med Virol 1989;27:117–119.
32. Arvin AM, Pollard RB, Rasmussen LE, Merigan TC. Cellular and humoral immunity in the pathogenesis of recurrent herpes viral infections in patients with lymphoma. J Clin Invest 1980;65:869–878.
33. Gratama JW, Verdonck LF, Van der Linden JA, et al. Cellular immunity to vaccinations and herpes virus infections after bone marrow transplantation. Transplantation 1986;41:719–724.
34. Kato S, Yabe MY, Kimura M, et al. Studies on transfer of varicella-zoster-virus specific T-cell immunity from bone marrow donor to recipient. Blood 1990;75:806–809.
35. Ault KA, Antin JH, Ginsburg D, et al. Phenotype of recovery lymphoid cell populations after marrow transplantation. J Exp Med 1985;161:1483–1501.
36. Arvin AM, Sharp MS, Smith S, et al. Equivalent recognition of a varicella-zoster virus immediate early protein (IE62) and glycoprotein I by cytotoxic T-lymphocytes of either CD4+ or CD8+ phenotype. J Immunol 1991;146:257–264.
37. Neiderwieser D, Gastl G, Rumpold H, Kraft MD, Huber C. Rapid reappearance of large granular lymphocytes (LGL) with concomitant reconstitution of natural killer (NK) activity after human bone marrow transplantation. Br J Haematol 1987;65:301–305.
38. Whitley RJ. Varicella zoster virus infections. In: Galasso G, Whitley R, Merigan T, eds. Antiviral agents and viral diseases of man. New York: Raven, 1990:235–263.
39. Feldman S, Lott L. Varicella in children with cancer. Impact of antiviral therapy and prophylaxis. Pediatrics 1987;80:465–471.
40. Whitley RJ. Chickenpox in the immunocompromised host. In: Balfour HH, ed. Advances in therapy against herpes virus infections in immunocompromised hosts. New York: Park Row Publications, 1985:25–39.

41. Ingraham J, Estes N, Bern M, De Girolami P. Disseminated varicella zoster virus infection and the syndrome of inappropriate ADH. Arch Intern Med 1983;143: 1270–1273.
42. Ballow M, Hirschhorn R. Varicella pneumonia in a bone marrow transplanted immune-reconstituted adenosine deaminase deficient patient with severe combined immunodeficiency disease. J Clin Immunol 1985;5: 180–186.
43. Brunell PA. Varicella zoster virus. In: Mandell GL, Douglas RG, Bennett JE, eds. Principles and practice of infectious diseases. New York: Wiley, 1985:952–960.
44. Gallagher J, Merigan T. Prolonged herpes zoster infection associated with immunosuppressive therapy. Ann Intern Med 1979;91:842–844.
45. Womack L, Liesegang T. Complications of herpes zoster ophthalmicus. Arch Ophthalmol 1983;101:42–51.
46. Linneman C, Alvira M. Pathogenesis of varicella-zoster angiitis in the central nervous system. Arch Neurol 1980;37:239–243.
47. Jamsek J, Greenberg S, Taber L. Herpes zoster associated encephalitis: clinicopathologic report of 12 cases and review of the literature. Medicine 1983;62:81–88.
48. Morishita K, Kodo H, Asano S, et al. Fulminant varicella hepatitis following bone marrow transplantation. JAMA 1985;253:511.
49. Sullivan K, Meyers J, Flournoy N, et al. Early and late interstitial pneumonia following human bone marrow transplantation. Int J Cell Cloning 1986;4(suppl):107–124.
50. Schiller G, Nimer S, Gajewski J, et al. Abdominal presentation of VZV infection in recipients of allogeneic bone marrow transplantation. Bone Marrow Transplant 1991;7:489–491.
51. Gold E, Robin F. Isolation of herpes zoster from the spinal fluid of a patient. Virology 1958;6:293–295.
52. McKendall R, Klawns H. Nervous system complications of varicella zoster. In: Vinken P, Bruyn G, eds. Handbook of clinical neurology. Infection of the nervous system. Amsterdam: Elsevier North Holland, 1978:161–167.
53. Reichman R. Neurologic complications of varicella zoster infections. Ann Intern Med 1978;375:89–96.
54. Gershon A, LaRussa P, Steinberg S. Varicella zoster virus. In: Lennette EH, ed. Laboratory diagnosis of viral infections. New York: Dekker Publication, 1992: 749–765.
55. Schmidt NJ, Gallo D, Devlin V, Woodie JD, Emmons RW. Direct immunofluorescence staining for detection of herpes simplex and varicella-zoster virus antigens in vesicular lesion and certain tissue specimens. J Clin Microbiol 1980;12:651–655.
56. Gleaves CA, Lee CF, Bustamante CI, Meyers JD. Use of murine monoclonal antibodies for laboratory diagnosis of varicella-zoster virus infection. J Clin Microbiol 1988;26:1623–1625.
57. Levin M, Leventhal S, Masters H. Factors influencing quantitative isolation of varicella zoster virus. J Clin Microbiol 1984;19:880–883.
58. West PG, Aldrich A, Hartwig, Haller G. Increased detection rate for varicella-zoster virus with combination of two techniques. J Clin Microbiol 1988;26: 2680–2681.
59. Forghani B, Yu G, Hurst J. Comparison of biotinylated DNA and RNA probes for rapid detection of varicella-zoster virus genome by in situ hybridization. J Clin Microbiol 1991;29:583–591.
60. Steinberg S, Gershon A. Measurement of antibodies to VZV by using a latex agglutination test. J Clin Microbiol 1991;29:1527–1530.
61. Schmidt N, Arvin AM. Sensitivity of different assay systems for immunoglobulin M, responses to varicella zoster virus in reactivated infection. J Clin Microbiol 1986;23:978–979.
62. Biron KK, Elion GB. In vitro susceptibility of varicella-zoster to acyclovir. Antimicrob Agents Chemother 1980;18:443–447.
63. Crumpacker CS, Schnipper LE, Zaia JA, Levin MJ. Growth inhibition by acycloguanosine of herpes viruses isolated from human infections. Antimicrob Agents Chemother 1979;15:642–645.
64. Bryson YJ. The use of acyclovir in children. Pediatr Infect Dis 1984;3:345–351.
65. Sullender W, Arvin AM, Diaz P, et al. Acyclovir pharmacokinetics following suspension administration to children. Antimicrob Agents Chemother 1987;31: 1722–1726.
66. de Miranda P, Blum MR. Pharmacokinetics of oral acyclovir after intravenous and oral administration. J Antimicrob Chemother 1983;12(suppl B):29–33.
67. Myers M. Viremia caused by varicella-zoster virus: association with malignant progressive varicella. J Infect Dis 1979;140:229–234.
68. Prober C, Kirk E, Keeney R. Acyclovir therapy of chickenpox in immunosuppressed children, a collaborative study. J Pediatr 1984;101:622–625.
69. Balfour HJ Jr, McMonigal K, Bean B. Acyclovir therapy of VZV infections in immunocompromised patients. J Antimicrob Chemother 1983;12(suppl B):169–179.
70. Balfour HH Jr. Intravenous acyclovir therapy for varicella in immunocompromised children. J Pediatr 1984;104:134–136.
71. Zaia JA, Levin MJ, Preblud SR, et al. Evaluation of varicella-zoster immune globulin: protection of immunosuppressed children after household exposure to varicella. J Infect Dis 1983;147:737–743.
72. Selby P, Jameson B, Watson J, et al. Parenteral acyclovir for herpes virus infections of man. Lancet 1979;1:1267–1270.
73. Balfour H, Dean B, Laskin O, et al. Acyclovir halts the progression of herpes zoster in immunocompromised patients. N Engl J Med 1983;308:1448–1453.
74. Meyers J, Wade J, Shepp D, et al. Acyclovir treatment of VZV infection in the compromised host. Transplantation 1984;37:571–574.
75. Shepp D, Dandliker P, Meyers J. Treatment of varicella zoster patients in severely immunocompromised patients. N Engl J Med 1986;314:208–212.
76. Merigan T, Rand K, Pollard R, et al. Human leukocyte interferon for the treatment of herpes zoster in patients with cancer. N Engl J Med 1978;298:981–987.
77. DeClerq E. Pyrimidine nucleoside analogues as antiviral agents. In: DeClerq E, Walker RT, eds. Targets for the design of antiviral agents. Geneva: NATO, ASI Series, 1984:203–226.
78. Selby P, Blake S, Mbidde EK, Hickmott E. Amino (hydroxyethoxymethyl) purine: a new well absorbed pro-drug of acyclovir. Lancet 1984;2:1428–1430.
79. Paryani SG, Arvin AM, Koropchak CM, et al. A comparison of varicella-zoster antibody titers in patients given intravenous immune serum globulin or varicella zoster immune globulin. J Pediatr 1984;105:201–205.
80. Ljungman P, Wilczek H, Gahrton G, et al. Long term acyclovir prophylaxis in bone marrow transplant recipi-

ents and lymphocyte proliferation responses to herpes virus in vitro. Transplant 1986;1:185–192.
81. Selby P, Powels R, Easton D, et al. The prophylactic role of intravenous and long term oral acyclovir after allogeneic bone marrow transplantation. Br J Cancer 1989;59:434–438.
82. Perren T, Powels R, Easton D, et al. Prevention of herpes zoster in patients by long term acyclovir after bone marrow transplantation. Am J Med 1988;85:S99–S101.
83. Gershon AA, Steinberg SP, Gelb L, et al. Live attenuated varicella vaccine: efficacy for children with leukemia in remission. JAMA 1984;252:355–362.
84. Diaz PS, Smith S, Hunter E, Au D, Arvin AM. Lack of transmission of the live attenuated varicella vaccine to immunocompromised children following immunization of their siblings. Pediatrics 1991;87:166–170.
85. Hardy I, Chu B, Gershon AA, Steinberg SP, LaRussa P. The incidence of zoster after immunization with live attenuated varicella vaccine. N Engl J Med 1991;325:1545–1550.
86. Shiraki K, Yamanishi K, Takahashi M. Susceptibility to acyclovir of Oka-strain varicella vaccine and vaccine-derived viruses isolated from immunocompromised patients. J Infect Dis 1984;150:306–310.

Chapter 31

Epstein-Barr Virus Infections in Bone Marrow Transplantation Recipients

Jan W. Gratama

Similar to other herpes viruses, Epstein-Barr virus (EBV) consists of a core that contains a double-stranded DNA molecule of approximately 172,000 base pairs, an icosahedral capsid, and an envelope enclosing the capsid. Primary EBV infection is followed by lifelong carrier status of the virus in "latent" form in peripheral blood B lymphocytes (1). Complete virions are produced by the oropharyngeal epithelium (2). Because it is transmitted via infected saliva in most cases, EBV has a worldwide distribution; approximately 95% of humans are infected. Most infections occur within the first years of life and are asymptomatic. In affluent populations with high standards of hygiene, primary EBV infections may not occur until late adolescence or adulthood (3,4). Approximately half of these late primary infections result in the clinical illness termed *infectious mononucleosis* (5).

Since its discovery in 1964 (6), EBV has been associated with several malignant tumors in humans. Two of these tumors are geographically restricted: Burkitt's lymphoma (6), a childhood malignancy endemic in the African malaria belt; and nasopharyngeal carcinoma (7), which is endemic in regions of southern China. Recently, EBV has been associated with Hodgkin's disease, where EBV can be detected in the Reed-Sternberg cells of up to 50% of patients (8). Finally, it has been recognized for more than 10 years that uncontrolled proliferations of EBV-carrying B lymphocytes may occur in immunodeficient individuals (9). These immunodeficiencies may be congenital, such as the X-linked lymphoproliferative disease (10), or acquired, such as in organ and bone marrow transplant (BMT) recipients (11–13) and in patients infected with the human immunodeficiency virus (14). The lesions of oral hairy leukoplakia in the latter group of patients constitute clinically apparent foci of intense EBV replication in lingual epithelium (15).

Because of the widespread distribution of EBV, most BMT recipients and their donors carry EBV at the time of transplantation. The spectrum of clinical symptoms associated with active EBV infection in BMT recipients ranges from none to the rapidly progressing, fatal lymphoproliferation of EBV-carrying B cells. An important factor in this respect is that the hemopoietic compartment, which not only carries the virus itself but also confers immunity to EBV, is the prime target and tool of therapy in BMT.

Biology of EBV Infection

EBV Infection Patterns In Vivo

In most nosocomial infections, EBV infects humans via the oropharynx (16,17) (Figure 31-1). The virus has two target tissues: the B lymphocytes, where the infection is largely nonproductive (1); and the stratified squamous epithelium, in which EBV replication occurs (2,15). EBV binds B lymphocytes through interaction of the viral membrane glycoprotein gp350/220 with the 145-kd molecule CR2 (CD21), the cell surface receptor for the C3d complement fragment (18). CD21 contains a sequence motif similar to the interferon-alpha receptor (19). Thus, expression of the interferon-alpha receptor by lymphocytes of T-lineage may render them susceptible to EBV infection (20). This expression pattern may explain the unusual detection of EBV in some patients with T-cell (21) and large granular (22) lymphoproliferations. CD21 has not been detected in stratified squamous epithelium. Recently, polymeric immunoglobulin A (IgA) specific for EBV was found to promote infection of otherwise resistant epithelial cells by binding to the secretory component, a transmembrane protein expressed by epithelial cells, and subsequent endocytosis (23).

Primary EBV infection is characterized by viral replication in oropharyngeal epithelial cells and polyclonal proliferation of EBV-infected B lymphocytes (see Figure 31-1), followed by the appearance of activated CD8+ T lymphocytes of atypical morphology. The syndrome of acute infectious mononucleosis is characterized by fever, lymphadenopathy, pharyngitis, skin rash, and splenomegaly and usually lasts for 3 to 6 weeks, with complete resolution of the symptoms thereafter. Between 0.5 and 2% of peripheral blood B lymphocytes of patients with acute infectious mononucleosis carry EBV (24). This proportion decreases after resolution of the syndrome; the frequency of EBV-

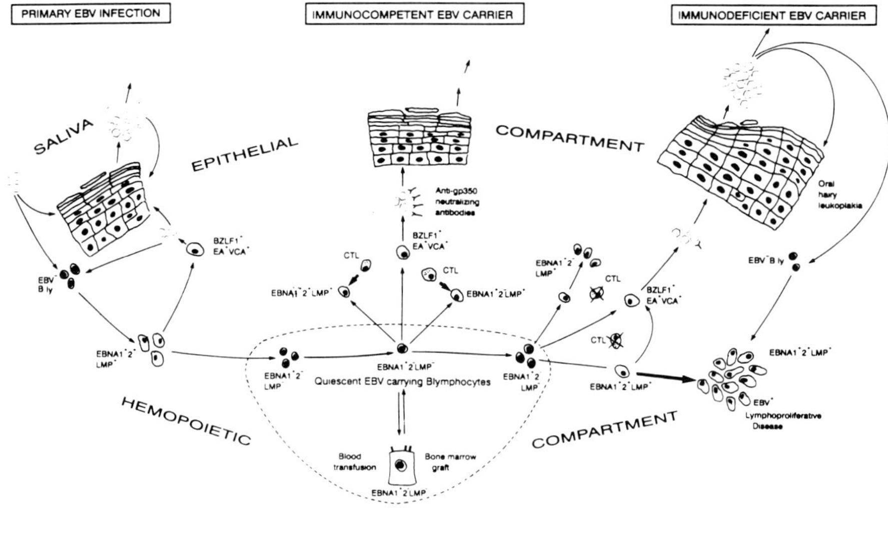

Figure 31-1. Hypothetical scheme of the interaction between Epstein-Barr virus (EBV) and its host. (Left panel) Primary infection through salivary transmission is followed by infection of B lymphocytes and oropharyngeal epithelium. EBV transforms B lymphocytes to lymphoblastoid cells expressing the full set of latent proteins (abbreviated EBNA1^{+}2^{+}LMP^{+}). Many of these cells will be eliminated by the developing EBV-specific immune response. In some B cells, EBV may enter the replicative cycle, resulting in release of virions that may infect other B cells and epithelium. In other B cells, EBV gene expression may be downregulated to the EBNA1^{+}2^{-}LMP^{-} phenotype, allowing escape from immune surveillance exerted by human leukocyte antigen (HLA)–restricted, EBV-specific cytotoxic T cells (111) (middle panel). EBNA1^{+}2^{-}LMP^{-} B cells constitute the long-term EBV reservoir and may serve as transmission vectors in blood transfusions and marrow and organ grafts. Stimulation of EBNA1^{+}2^{-}LMP^{-} B cells by cross-linking their membrane-bound immunoglobulin may activate viral genes (112). This process may lead to their entry into the replicative cycle. Virions not neutralized by antibodies may reinfect the oropharyngeal epithelium. In other EBNA1^{+}2^{-}LMP^{-} B cells, up-regulation of EBNA2 and LMP will make them prone to elimination by EBV-specific immune surveillance. (Right panel) Profound deficiency of HLA-restricted, EBV-specific cytotoxic T lymphocytes may allow uncontrolled rapid proliferation of EBNA1^{+}2^{+}LMP^{+} lymphoblasts. The gradual breakdown of EBV-specific immunity in human immunodeficiency virus carriers is associated with chronically increased viral replication leading to the development of oral hairy leukoplakia.

infected B lymphocytes in healthy carriers is estimated to be 1 in 10^6 to 10^7 mononuclear cells (25). Similarly, the rate of virus replication in the oropharynx decreases with time following primary EBV infection. In the majority of EBV-carrying individuals, infectious virus is being shed intermittently into the saliva and is the source of most primary infections (26). Occasionally, infectious mononucleosis may be caused by transmission of EBV via blood transfusion. The low incidence of seronegative individuals in the general population limits the risk of primary infection by this route (27).

The long-term cellular reservoir of EBV in its host has been a matter of debate. Also, the question of whether horizontal cell-to-cell spread of the virus occurs on an ongoing basis in immunocompetent hosts is unresolved. One view has been that the B-cell compartment is continuously or intermittently reinfected from the epithelial viral reservoir (28). Two lines of evidence argue against this view. First, in allogeneic BMT recipients, complete eradication of the recipient's pretransplant EBV strain from peripheral blood and oropharynx is associated with complete eradication of the recipient's hematopoietic system (29). Second, acyclovir therapy during one month for herpes zoster can eliminate oropharyngeal EBV shedding without reducing the numbers of circulating EBV-carrying B cells (30). Resumption of EBV replication in the oropharynx after cessation of acyclovir therapy in the latter patients would be due to reinfection of the epithelium from the B-cell compartment. Formal proof for this route of virus transfer comes, again, from the

BMT setting, in which the EBV strain of an unrelated marrow donor could be recovered from the recipient's mouthwash 60 days after BMT.

In Vitro Studies of EBV Infection

EBV-induced B-cell Transformation

Conventionally, the presence of EBV in clinical samples can be demonstrated by the establishment of B lymphoblastoid cell lines (LCL). These LCL can be obtained in two ways: (1) via in vitro infection of cord blood B lymphocytes by specimens containing EBV virions with transforming capability (31) and (2) by cocultivation of lymphocytes from EBV-carrying individuals with cord blood lymphocytes. In the latter case, the majority of EBV-carrying B cells release virus into the culture, which infects and transforms coresident B cells. A minority of the EBV-carrying B cells grow out themselves (32,33). An important limitation of these assays is their selectivity for EBV strains with B cell transforming potential. Recently, substantial differences between EBV strains were found with regard to their abilities to infect epithelial cell lines transfected with CD21, which did not correlate with their transforming potential (34). Although these assays are valuable for research purposes, they are less useful for clinical practice due to logistical problems (i.e., limited availability of biological reagents and several weeks needed to complete the assays). The polymerase chain reaction appears to be best suited for clinical detection of EBV (35).

EBV Genome and Gene Expression

The entire nucleotide acid sequence of the B95.8 laboratory strain of EBV has been determined (36). EBV DNA is present in linear form in the virion, but exists predominantly as an extrachromosomal circular molecule (i.e., episome) in the transformed B lymphocyte (37). The linear genome consists of short and long unique sequences, separated by a large internal repetitive sequence and flanked by terminal repeats (TR) at either end of the genome. The repetitive element of the large internal repeat, the 3.1-kb *Bam*HI W fragment, constitutes a useful probe for Southern blotting or in situ hybridizations because it is usually reiterated 10 times, permitting coverage of approximately 20% of an individual EBV genome (38). The formation of circular episomes is achieved by the TR, which become covalently linked during episome formation. Because both the number of TR sequences at the ends of the linear EBV genome and the extent of overlapping of TR sequences during episome formation are variable, each new circularization event leads to a differently sized TR fragment (39). Because the structure of the episome is conserved during multiplication of the EBV-infected B cell, the size of the TR fragment represents a constant clonal marker for the episome and can be used to study the clonality of EBV-transformed B-cell populations (39,40).

Two small EBV-encoded nonpolyadenylated RNA molecules (termed *EBER1* and *EBER2*) are present at very high copy numbers (up to 10^6 EBER molecules/EBV episome) in the nuclei of LCL (41,42), Burkitt's lymphoma, and nasopharyngeal carcinoma cells (Minarovits J, and Ernberg I. Personal communication). Their function is as yet unknown. Due to their abundance, EBERs are particularly suited as probes for in situ hybridization (42).

LCL, established following in vitro infection of B lymphocytes, are largely nonpermissive for virus replication ("latent" infection) and express 9 EBV-encoded proteins (43): 6 nuclear proteins (EBV nuclear antigens [EBNA] 1–6) and 3 membrane proteins (latent membrane protein [LMP], terminal protein [TP] 1, and TP 2). An alternative nomenclature for EBNA 3, 4, and 6 is EBNA 3A, 3B, and 3C, respectively; LMP, TP 1, and TP 2 are also being termed *LMP 1*, *LMP 2A*, and *LMP 2B*, respectively (43). EBNA 1, 2, 3, and 6 show considerable size variation between different EBV strains. The size of EBNA 1 varies between 65 and 97 kd in various strains as a result of differences in the length of the internal repeat sequence in the *Bam*HI K region (44). EBNA 2A varies in size from 75 to 95 kd. EBNA 3, 4, and 6 occur as differently sized molecules in the range of 130 to 180 kd. The size variation of EBNA 2, 3, and 6 is probably due to variations in the primary amino acid sequences as well. Consequently, the combined size variations can be used to "fingerprint" EBV strains for epidemiological purposes. For example, this "Ebnotyping" approach can be used to trace the spread of EBV within families (45).

The latency of EBV in LCL is under tight control. Only a minor fraction (1 in 10^2 to 10^6 cells) in LCL cultures progress from latent to replicative infection, which is associated with viral replication and release of infectious virus (46). The switch from latent to replicative infection is mediated by the transactivating, immediate-early BZLF1 protein (47). The replicative cycle is characterized by extensive transcription of the viral genome, with subsequent expression of the early and late gene products. Among the early gene products, which are resistent to inhibition of DNA synthesis (48), are the diffuse (EA-D) and restricted (EA-R) forms of the early antigen. The late gene products, (i.e., the viral capsid [VCA] and the membrane antigens [MA]) are sensitive to inhibition of viral DNA synthesis. VCA and MA are required for packaging the viral DNA and for formation of the structural components of the virion. MA are expressed in the membranes of virus-replicating cells and in the envelopes of virus particles (49). Among these MA, the gp350/220 mediates the binding of the virion to the EBV receptor (i.e., CD21) (18).

Antibody Response to EBV Infection

The antibody response to EBV in patients with acute infectious mononucleosis is preferentially directed toward viral antigens of the productive cycle. Such patients have high IgM and IgG VCA antibody titers; EA-D antibodies are detected in approximately 85% of patients (50). IgM heterophile antibodies of the Paul-Bunnell type, which are highly specific for the disease, develop in more than 90% of patients with infectious mononucleosis. During convalescence, the IgM VCA and IgG EA-D antibodies decline to nondetectable levels, whereas the heterophile antibodies decrease at a slower rate and may remain detectable for up to 18 months (51). IgG VCA antibodies decline to moderate titers, at which they are maintained usually without significant fluctuations for many decades (50). Antibodies to EA, more often to the R than to the D component, occur at low titers only in those individuals who maintain relatively high IgG VCA titers. During convalescence, a persistent antibody response to the gp350/220 MA develops; these antibodies have neutralizing capabilities (52,53). Antibodies to latent EBV antigens appear only 1 to 2 months after onset of infectious mononucleosis. Antibodies against EBNA 2 appear first to decline to nondetectable levels, whereas EBNA 1 antibodies appear later and persist at stable titers for decades (54). Thus, the antibody status of most healthy EBV carriers is characterized by stable IgG antibody titers to VCA, EBNA 1, and the gp350/220 MA (Table 31-1).

The differential kinetics of the antibody responses against replicative and latent EBV infection cycles reflect the initial predominance of virus-replicating cells after primary infection, followed by the predominance of latently infected cells during convalescence and thereafter. The turnover of latently infected B lymphocytes may provide sufficient EBNA 1–derived peptides to the immune system to maintain constant EBNA 1 antibody titers. The intermittent production of EB virions by the oropharyngeal epithelium may yield enough VCA and MA (presented in degraded form to the immune system in gastrointestinal tract lymphoid tissues) to maintain constant antibody levels against these proteins.

Table 31-1.
EBV Antibody Profiles in EBV-seropositive Bone Marrow Donors, Recipients Prior to BMT, and Recipients >360 Days After BMT[a]

EBV Antibodies	*Marrow Donors (n = 22)*	*Recipients Prior to BMT (n = 31)*	*Recipients >360 Days After BMT (n = 27)*
IgA VCA	<5 (<5, <5)	<5 (<5, <5)	<5 (<5, 640)
IgG VCA	320 (160, 1,280)	320 (80, 2,560)	1,280 (320, 10,240)
IgA EA-D	<5 (<5, <5)	<5 (<5, <5)	<5 (<5, 20)
IgG EA-D	<5 (<5, 20)	<5 (<5, 320)	20 (<5, 640)
IgG EA-R	<5 (<5, 20)	<5 (<5, <5)	<5 (<5, <5)
EBNA (Raji)	160 (10, 640)	80 (10, 640)	160 (20, 640)
EBNA 1	80 (<5, 320)	80 (<5, 640)	160 (<5, 1,280)
EBNA 2A	20 (<5, 160)	7.5 (<5, 40)	40 (<5, 320)
EBNA 2B	<5 (<5, 80)	<5 (<5, 80)	5 (<5, 160)
EBNA 6	20 (5, 160)	10 (<5, 80)	40 (5, 160)

[a]Results are expressed as median antibody titers (5th, 95th percentiles). Data are derived from (68). Antibodies against VCA (110) and the D and R varieties of EA (4) were detected using indirect immunofluorescence and those against EBNA in the Raji cell line and against EBNA subtypes in transfected cells using anticomplement immunofluorescence (106). For the detection of EBNA 1 and 6 antibodies, DG-75 cells transfected with the *Bam*HIY and *Bam*HIE fragments of B95.8 EBV were used; for the detection of EBNA 2A and 2B antibodies, RAT-2B cells transfected with the *Bam*HI Y fragment of B95.8 and Ag876 EBV, respectively, were used (68). EBV = Epstein-Barr virus; BMT = bone marrow transplantation; Ig = immunoglobulin.

Cellular Immunity to EBV Infection

Lymphocytosis during the acute phase of infectious mononucleosis is due to an expansion of activated T lymphocytes, mainly of the $CD3^+$, $CD8^+$ phenotype (55). This activation and expansion are probably the result of stimulation by EBV-infected cells. In vitro, these lymphocytes exert nonmajor histocompatibility complex (MHC)–restricted cytolysis and are even able to lyse allogeneic target cells regardless of whether these cells carry EBV (56,57). In addition, T cells from patients with infectious mononucleosis display a wide spectrum of suppressive activities that include mitogen- and antigen-induced T-cell responses (58), which may explain the depression of cell-mediated immune responses in these patients (59).

Once the acute EBV infection has subsided, homeostasis is maintained, which allows EBV to replicate and persist without damaging its host. EBV-specific memory T cells are probably critical for controlling the level of EBV-carrying B cells. Experimental support for the existence of EBV-specific memory T cells comes from the observations that in cultures of in vitro EBV-infected mononuclear cells from EBV-seropositive, but not EBV-seronegative, donors, the initial proliferation of EBV^+ B cells was followed by a complete, T-cell–dependent regression of outgrowth of LCL (60,61). Although mechanisms other than MHC-restricted cytolysis may also be important in this respect (62), three lines of evidence suggest that latent EBV gene products represent an important source of epitopes for cytotoxic T cells: (1) regression of LCL (expressing the full set of latent EBV proteins) in cultures from seropositive, but not seronegative, donors; (2) isolation of MHC-restricted, EBV-specific cytotoxic T cells from EBV carriers; and (3) the low proportion of LCL that expresses antigens of the replicative cycle. Indeed, EBNA 2, 3, 4, and 6, LMP, and TP1 were shown to provide peptides that could be recognized by MHC-restricted CTL (63,64).

EBV Infection in BMT Recipients

Clinical Signs and Symptoms

The few published studies that have addressed the question "does EBV infection cause illness in BMT recipients?" indicate that it does not (65–67). The rare syndrome of EBV-associated lymphoproliferation is an exception. Most BMT recipients and their marrow donors already carry EBV at the time of BMT. In this context, it is important to recall the limited tissue distribution of EBV: B lymphocytes and oropharyngeal epithelium. The reservoir of latent EBV, the recipient's B lymphocytes, is severely depleted by the cytoreductive therapy prior to BMT but is also present in the marrow graft itself. Oropharyngeal shedding of EBV may persist during the first months after BMT (68) without causing clinical symptoms and can be suppressed by acyclovir (30). Two patients have been reported with oral hairy leukoplakia–like lesions 100 days after BMT, but EBV was not investigated in these patients (69).

Most BMT recipients are cared for in protected environments during the first weeks after BMT, which reduces the chance of salivary transmission. The risk of EBV transmission by blood products is reduced by irradiation (Gratama JW. unpublished observations) and can be further reduced by leukocyte depletion, as has been shown for cytomegalovirus transmission (70). In addition, plasma from most blood donors, including intravenous gammaglobulin preparations, contain neutralizing anti-gp350 antibodies (71). Infectious mononucleosis has been transmitted only to susceptible (i.e., seronegative) recipients by blood transfusion if the donor happened to be in the incubation period of this disease (72,73); therefore, neutralizing antibodies may not have been present in the transfusion product. Indeed, the first report of EBV infection following BMT (74) concerned a 12-year-old EBV-seronegative recipient whose marrow donor had developed infectious mononucleosis 9 weeks prior to BMT. The full-blown infectious mononucleosis syndrome did not develop, but the patient presented with abdominal pain, vomiting, and mild hepatitis on day 21, which was followed by grade III acute graft-versus-host disease (GVHD) on day 32. The GVHD resolved as a result of steroid therapy, and no signs of uncontrolled lymphoproliferation were observed during the 13 months of follow-up.

The relationship between EBV infection and acute GVHD was studied further in two single-center studies of the interaction between pretransplant herpes virus serology and GVHD (75,76). The results were contradictory. In Leiden, The Netherlands (75), EBV-seronegative recipients of undepleted marrow from human leukocyte antigen (HLA)–identical siblings had a significantly lower risk for grades II to IV acute GVHD than EBV-seropositive recipients. Among the latter, those receiving marrow from EBV-seronegative donors had the highest risk for GVHD. In Huddinge, Sweden (76), the effects of pretransplant EBV serology on GVHD were not significant. A follow-up study by the Leiden team (77) revealed that intensification of GVHD prophylaxis (e.g., T-cell depletion of the graft or postgraft immunosuppression with combinations of drugs) abolished the effect of pretransplant EBV serology on GVHD. A stimulatory effect of EBV on GVHD would be mediated by multiple clones of T lymphocytes activated by EBV, as observed after primary EBV infection (57). Such activated T lymphocytes may be transferred with the graft (74) or generated in the recipient after stimulation by B lymphoblasts infected with EBV produced by the oropharyngeal epithelium (68); T-cell depletion of the grafts and intensification of postgraft immunosuppression would prevent their transfer and generation.

EBV-specific Immune Responses

Humoral Immunity

The pre-BMT EBV antibody profile of EBV-seropositive patients with acute leukemia in remission or chronic myeloid leukemia in the chronic phase is similar to that of healthy EBV-seropositive marrow donors. Most patients have moderate titers of IgG antibodies to VCA, and most antibody reactivity to the EBNA proteins is directed at EBNA 1 (see Table 31-1). During the peritransplant period, passive transfer of VCA and EBNA antibodies occurs through blood products. After cessation of transfusions (i.e., between 2 and 4 months after BMT), VCA titers decline to low levels and EBNA antibody titers decrease to undetectable levels in many instances (65,67,68). A minority of patients may even become completely EBV-seronegative for several years (29,78). In long-term survivors of allogeneic BMT (i.e., for 1 year or more), IgG VCA titers typically have increased to supranormal levels and are accompanied by detectable IgG EA(D) titers (65,67) (Table 31-1). Some of these patients also have IgM VCA antibodies (67). In two of these studies (65,67), EBNA titers were disproportionally low, whereas they were normal in the third study (68) (see Table 31-1). The relatively high antibody titers against antigens of the replicative cycle (VCA and EA) versus the relatively low titers against antigens of the latent cycle (EBNA) suggest a deficiency in re-establishing latent infection in B lymphocytes. This deficiency may be reflected by the inability to generate stable LCL after in vitro transformation of mononuclear cells derived from patients up to 9 months after BMT (66) and might explain in part the relatively low frequency of post-BMT EBV+ lymphoproliferations.

When irradiated and leukocyte-depleted blood products are used, most EBV-seronegative recipients of marrow from EBV-seronegative donors will remain seronegative for the first 6 months after BMT. However, frequent seroconversion followed by stable titers of IgG VCA are seen after transplantation of marrow from EBV-seropositive donors (65,67,79) (Table 31-2). Neither IgM VCA (65,67,79) nor heterophile antibodies (65,67) have been observed in any of these patients, which may be due to the transfer of EBV-specific memory cells in the graft. In contrast, an IgM VCA antibody response does occur with primary EBV infection in the absence of EBV-specific memory (12,29,74).

Cellular Immunity

According to the single study published (66), HLA-restricted, EBV-specific cytotoxic T cells could be detected in 3 of 10 patients 3 months after BMT, and in

Table 31-2.
Frequent Seroconversion of EBV-seronegative Recipients of Marrow From EBV-Seropositive Donors[a]

Marrow Donor IgG VCA Serology	*Marrow Recipient IgG VCA Seroconversion* No	Yes (%)
Negative	17	1 (6)
Positive	6	12 (67)

[a]Fisher's exact test, $p = 0.0005$.
EBV = Epstein-Barr virus; Ig = immunoglobulin; VCA = viral capsid antigen. (Reproduced by permission from Gratama JW, Oosterveer MAP, Lepoutre J, et al. Epstein-Barr virus infection in allogeneic marrow grafting: lessons for transplant physicians and virologists. Ann Hematol 1992;64:A162–A165.)

all 10 patients 6 months after BMT. These patients received unmodified marrow grafts from HLA-identical siblings and cyclosporine monotherapy for 6 months as prophylaxis for GVHD. T-cell depletion of marrow grafts, HLA-mismatching between donor and recipient, and therapy of acute GVHD using T-cell antibodies have been identified as significant risk factors for EBV$^+$ lymphoproliferations (12,13). Combined with the observation that the proliferating EBV$^+$ lymphoblasts express at least EBNA 2, 3, 6, and LMP (80,81), which constitute targets for HLA-restricted, EBV-specific CTL (63,64), the prediction that EBV$^+$ lymphoproliferations develop due to failure of HLA-restricted, EBV-specific host immunosurveillance seems justified.

Origin and Kinetics of EBV Infection in BMT Recipients

The combined size variations of EBNA 1, 2, 3, 4, and 6 in immunoblots of LCL can be used to distinguish between different EBV strains (82). We have used this "fingerprinting" or "Ebnotyping" approach to distinguish between donor and recipient virus in allogeneic BMT recipients (29,68,78). These studies, combining EBV serology with Ebnotyping, led to the following conclusions.

EBV Can Be Transferred with the Marrow Graft

This transfer is demonstrated by the following case (Figure 31-2). An EBV-seronegative patient received marrow from an HLA-identical, unrelated donor following pretreatment with cytotoxic drugs and total body irradiation as therapy for his myelodysplastic syndrome. T-cell depletion of the graft was performed ex vivo using Campath-1 monoclonal antibody. From day 60 onward, the donor's EBV strain could be recovered from the patient's mouthwash. Subsequently, severe pharyngitis with high oropharyngeal EB virus titers developed, which gradually subsided as a result of acyclovir therapy. The same EBV strain was detectable in the patient's blood 21 and 32 months after BMT and was clearly different from those obtained from his EBV-seropositive mother, father, and sister.

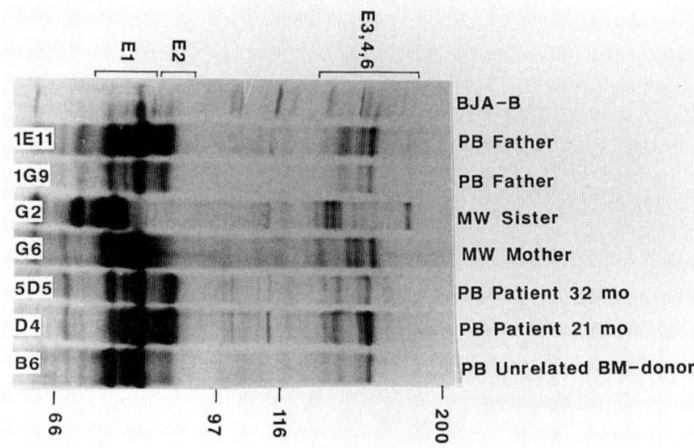

Figure 31-2. Immunoblot probed with the polyspecific serum DMJ. *Numbers on the right* indicate molecular masses in kilodaltons (kd). The BJA-B Epstein-Barr virus (EBV)–negative cell line was used to detect nonspecific reactivity. Lymphoblastic cell lines were expanded after separate harvesting of individual wells (68), of which the identification codes are given at the bottom of the lanes. EBNA 1, 2, 3, and 6 were assigned to their corresponding bands after probing with monospecific sera (29). The EBV strain of the unrelated donor is similar to that recovered from the patient 21 and 32 months after bone marrow transplantation, whereas the patient's father, mother, and sister carry different EBV strains. E = EBV nuclear antigen; MW = mouthwash; PB = peripheral blood.

EBV Can Be Eradicated from BMT Recipients

We have observed 2 patients in whom the resident EBV strain was replaced by an exogenous strain that could be traced back to the source (29). In the first patient (transplanted for acute lymphoblastic leukemia in second remission), repopulation of an EBV-seropositive recipient with marrow of a seronegative donor caused seronegativity for 4 years and made her susceptible to subsequent infection with her husband's strain. In the second patient (transplanted for acute myeloid leukemia in first remission), repopulation with marrow from his EBV-seropositive brother was followed by the disappearance of his pretransplant strain and the establishment of persistent infection with his marrow donor's strain. Grade II acute GVHD developed in both patients, followed by mild chronic GVHD in 1 patient, and both are in complete remission of their leukemia 9 and 10 years after BMT, respectively.

EBV Can Persist Following Allogeneic BMT

We have observed this pattern in 3 HLA-identical sibling transplant recipients, all transplanted for chronic myelogenous leukemia (CML) in first chronic phase; GVHD developed in none. In 2 patients, persistence of the recipient's hemopoietic cells was

Table 31-3.
Post-BMT EBV-positive Lymphoproliferations: Clinical Data on 39 Reported Patients

	Time of Onset of EBV-positive Lymphoproliferations			
Clinical Parameter	*Early (Group I) (n=26)*	*Intermediate (Group II) (n=9)*	*Late (Group III) (n=4)*	*Total (n=39) (%)*
Diagnostic indication for BMT (n=39)				
ALL	7	0	0	7 (18)
AML	5	4	0	9 (23)
CML	5	2	0	7 (18)
Other hematological malignancies	2	0	1	3 (8)
SAA	3	1	0	4 (10)
SCID	2	2	2	6 (15)
WAS	2	0	1	3 (8)
HLA match (n=39)				
Matched sibling	9	5	1	15 (38)
Mismatched family	14	4	3	21 (54)
Matched, unrelated	2	0	0	2 (5)
Autologous	1	0	0	1 (3)
T-cell depletion of graft (n=39)				
No	14	2	1	17 (44)
Yes	12	7	3	22 (56)
Sustained engraftment (n=39)				
No	0	3	4	7 (18)
Yes	26	6	0	32 (82)
Ultimate grade of acute GVHD (n=39)				
Grade 0	9	5	4	18 (46)
Grade I	2	0	0	2 (5)
Grade II	5	1	0	6 (15)
Grades III–IV	10	3	0	13 (33)
Therapy for acute GVHD (n=36)				
None	9	4	4	17 (47)
IS without anti-T Ab	2	2	0	4 (11)
IS with anti-T Ab	13	2	0	15 (42)
Status and cause of death (n=39)				
Alive	5	0	0	5 (13)
Death (other)	1	1	0	2 (5)
Death (LP)	16	4	4	24 (62)
Death (LP + other)	4	4	0	8 (21)
Recipient age (n=39)				
Years (median [range])	17 [0.7–48]	23 [0.1–36]	4 [0.3–25]	17 [0.1–48]
Time interval between onset and death (n=23)				
Days (median [range])	11 [2–45]	36 [19–44]	86 [84–109]	19 [2–109]

Data were derived from the following references: ref. 13 (n=10); ref. 12 (n=8); ref. 96 (n=4); ref. 97 (n=3); refs. 88 and 95 (n=2 each); and refs. 78, 80, 81, 87, 89, 90, 91, 92, 93, and 94 (n=1 each).
EBV = Epstein-Barr virus; BMT = bone marrow transplantation; Ab = antibodies; ALL = acute lymphoblastic leukemia; AML = acute myeloid leukemia; CML = chronic myeloid leukemia; Ig = immunoglobulin; IS = immunosuppression; LP = lymphoproliferative disease; SAA = severe aplastic anemia; SCID = severe combined immunodeficiency disease; WAS = Wiskott-Aldrich syndrome.

demonstrated, which was associated with graft failure in the first patient (78) and with cytogenetic relapse of CML in the second. The results of the Ebnotyping studies in the second patient are shown in Figure 31-3. The donor's EBV strain was predominant over the recipient's strain in the day-28 blood sample, whereas only recipient virus was obtained at day 40. The third patient received marrow from her EBV-seronegative brother. Oropharyngeal shedding of her resident strain persisted during the first month after BMT, which could also be recovered from her blood thereafter (data not shown). Although she is still in remission of her CML 2 years after BMT, residual recipient EBV-carrying B cells may have survived (83), allowing the virus to infect her oropharyngeal epithelium and the B lymphocytes originating from the marrow graft. Alternatively, donor B lymphocytes may have been infected by EBV produced by the oropharyngeal epithelium.

From these data, two factors appear to influence eradication versus persistence of resident virus following allogeneic BMT. First, EBV-carrying B lymphocytes may have been depleted proportional to the cumulative amount of cytoreductive therapy given prior to preparation for BMT. Patients with acute leukemia in remission will have received more intensive chemotherapy than patients with CML in first chronic phase. In

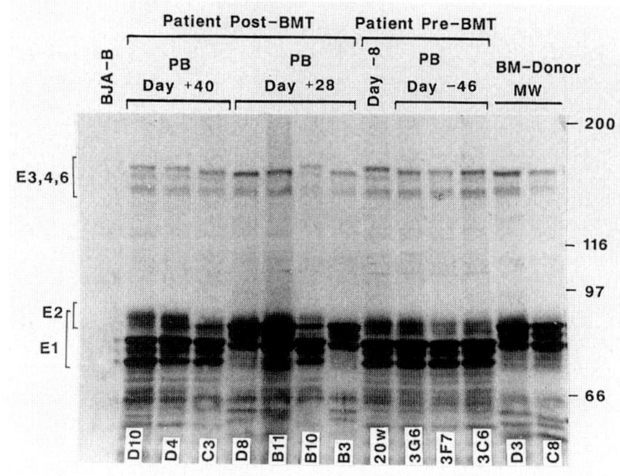

Figure 31-3. Immunoblot probed with the polyspecific serum GYS. Lymphoblastic cell lines (LCLs) were expanded after separate harvesting of individual wells (68) to detect multiple Epstein-Barr virus (EBV) strains within a single specimen, except for LCL "day −8" which was obtained after pooling of 20 wells. The EBV strains of the marrow donor and the recipient have EBNA 1 proteins of different sizes. A blood sample obtained 28 days after bone marrow transplantation revealed the donor strain in 3 wells (D8, B11, and B3) and the residual recipient strain in one well (B10). Three wells from the day 40 blood sample contained only residual recipient virus. See also Figure 31-2.

this context, isolation of transforming EBV strains from patients prior to BMT was clearly less successful than from their marrow donors (10 vs 30%) (79). Second, GVHD reactivity may have contributed to the eradication of residual EBV-carrying cells of recipient origin similar to graft-versus-leukemia reactivity (i.e., mediated via cytotoxic T lymphocytes recognizing "minor" histocompatibility antigens presented by HLA molecules) (84).

EBV-associated Lymphoproliferations (EBV^+ LP) in BMT Recipients

Risk Factors for EBV^+ LP

Uncontrolled lymphoproliferations constitute an infrequent but often fatal complication of BMT. Most lymphoproliferations carry EBV, although a few EBV-negative patients have been described (85,86). The initial sporadic reports of EBV^+ LP (87–92) were followed by two larger series from the BMT teams in Minneapolis, MN (12), and Seattle, WA (13). In the latter report (13), 15 cases of EBV^+ LP were reviewed that occurred among 2,475 allogeneic BMT recipients. The overall actuarial incidence of EBV^+ LP in this series was 0.6%. Significant risk factors for EBV+ LP were (1) treatment of acute GVHD using CD3 monoclonal antibodies, and (2) T-cell depletion of the marrow graft. The severity of acute GVHD and HLA disparity between marrow donor and recipient also contributed to the risk for EBV^+ LP. The experience of the Minneapolis BMT team (12) was in line with these observations: EBV^+ LP developed in 6 of 25 (24%) recipients of HLA-mismatched, T-cell–depleted marrow versus 0 of 47 recipients of HLA-matched T-cell–depleted marrow; 1 of 10 recipients of undepleted marrow from HLA-matched, unrelated donors; and 1 of 424 (0.2%) recipients of undepleted marrow from HLA-matched siblings.

Clinical Course of EBV^+ LP

In this and the following sections, detailed descriptions of 39 cases of EBV^+ LP are reviewed (12, 13,78,80,81,87–97). The most common clinical symptoms of EBV^+ LP on presentation were fever, lymphadenopathy, abdominal pain, hepatitis, and lethargy. Individual patients may present with hepatosplenomegaly, neurological symptoms, pharyngitis, or gastrointestinal ulcerations (Plate XXXVI). These symptoms were related to widely disseminated lymphoid infiltration of vital organs and culminated in multiple system organ failure in most patients. In 20% of the patients, EBV^+ LP was an unexpected finding at autopsy because its symptoms had been dominated by those of other complications leading to multiorgan failure, such as severe GVHD or infections.

The 39 patients were divided into three groups according to the time of onset of clinical symptoms of EBV^+ LP to summarize their clinical and laboratory data. The clinical data of these three patient groups are summarized in Table 31-3, and their virological data and tumor characteristics are summarized in Table 31-4.

Group I consisted of 26 patients with early-onset EBV^+ LP (i.e., between 30 and 77 days after BMT). All 26 patients showed sustained engraftment (see Table 31-3). Grade II or greater GVHD developed in 15 (58%), requiring treatment with multiple immunosuppressants, including anti-T-cell antibodies in 13 patients. Most of the 26 patients had rapidly progressive symptoms, which led to or contributed to death in 20 cases (77%). Time from onset of symptoms to death ranged from 2 to 45 days (median, 11 days). No treatment for EBV^+ LP was given in 9 of these patients, whereas therapeutic attempts using acyclovir, intravenous gammaglobulin, corticosteroids, interferon-gamma, or cytotoxic drugs were unsuccessful in the other 11 patients. EBV^+ LP resolved in 6 patients; 3 had disease limited to the cervical lymph nodes and were treated with excision (n = 2), local radiotherapy (n = 2), cytotoxic drugs (n = 1), or acyclovir (n = 1) (13,93). The remaining 3 patients had disseminated disease that resolved as a result of therapy with CD21 and CD24 anti-B-cell monoclonal antibodies (n = 2) and acyclovir combined with interferon-alpha (n = 1) (12,95). The initial encouraging results with anti-B-cell antibody therapy were confirmed in a subsequent open multicenter study comprising 14 BMT and 12 organ transplant recipients (98). Complete remission of EBV^+ LP was achieved in 16 patients with oligoclonal disease, but the treatment was ineffective for

Table 31-4.
Post-BMT EBV-positive Lymphoproliferations: Virological and Tumor Characteristics of 39 Reported Patients

	Time of Onset of EBV-positive Lymphoproliferations			
Clinical Parameter	*Early (Group I) (n=26)*	*Intermediate (Group II) (n=9)*	*Late (Group III) (n=4)*	*Total (n=39) (%)*
Recipient pre-BMT EBV serology (n=26)				
Negative	6	1	1	8 (31)
Positive	12	5	1	18 (69)
Donor pre-BMT EBV serology (n=24)				
Negative	1	1	1	3 (13)
Positive	15	5	1	21 (87)
Detection of clonal B-cell populations (Ig light chain staining) (n=35)				
Negative	12	3	0	15 (43)
Positive	10	6	4	17 (57)
Detection of clonal B-cell populations (Ig gene rearrangements) (n=24)				
Negative	3	1	0	4 (17)
Positive	13	6	1	20 (83)
Origin of tumor cells (n=25)				
Donor	16	3	0	19 (76)
Host	0	2	4	6 (24)

Data were derived from the following references: ref. 13 (n=10); ref. 12 (n=8); ref. 96 (n=4); ref. 97 (n=3); refs. 88 and 95 (n=2 each); and refs. 78, 80, 81, 87, 89, 90, 91, 92, 93, and 94 (n=1 each).
EBV = Epstein-Barr virus; BMT = bone marrow transplantation; Ab = antibodies; ALL = acute lymphoblastic leukemia; AML = acute myeloid leukemia; CML = chronic myeloid leukemia; Ig = immunoglobulin; IS = immunosuppression; LP = lymphoproliferative disease; SAA = severe aplastic anemia; SCID = severe combined immunodeficiency disease; WAS = Wiskott-Aldrich syndrome.

monoclonal disease or EBV$^+$ LP localized in the central nervous system.

Group II consisted of 9 patients with intermediate onset EBV$^+$ LP (i.e., between 80 and 188 days after BMT). These patients had more problems with sustained engraftment (i.e., graft failure in 3 patients; 33%), a lower frequency of grade II or greater GVHD (4 patients; 44%), and fewer therapeutic interventions of GVHD using anti-T-cell antibodies (2 patients; 22%) than the patients in group I (see Table 31-3). However, the clinical presentation of EBV$^+$ LP was similar to that observed in group I. Eight patients died from disseminated EBV$^+$ LP. Therapeutic attempts in 4 patients using acyclovir, intravenous gammaglobulin, corticosteroids, local radiotherapy, and cytotoxic drugs were unsuccessful. The disease of the ninth patient, which was restricted to the lymph nodes, remained stable as a result of therapy with acyclovir and interferon-alpha until she died 48 days later from other causes.

Group III consisted of 4 patients with late-onset EBV$^+$ LP (i.e., 440, 484, 500, and 1488 days after BMT, respectively). None had complete engraftment (see Table 31-3). Three were transplanted for congenital immunodeficiencies with marrow from HLA-mismatched donors. One patient rejected his graft, and mixed hemopoietic chimerism developed in 3. EBV$^+$ LP presented with neurological symptoms referrable to local lymphoproliferations in 2 patients (12,13). In the third patient (12), EBV$^+$ LP developed 3 months after apparently resolved infectious mononucleosis. EBV$^+$ LP developed in the fourth patient after 3 unsustained T-cell–depleted grafts from his parents, 1 year after the first transplantation and 1 month after the third. Therapeutic attempts using acyclovir, intravenous gammaglobulin, cytotoxic drugs, or antilymphocyte globulin in 2 patients were unsuccessful. All patients had disseminated EBV$^+$ LP at autopsy.

Characterization of EBV$^+$ LP

Histology

The majority of EBV$^+$ LP lesions can be classified as high-grade immunoblastic malignant lymphoma according to the Working Formulation (99). The histology of such lesions encompasses a wide spectrum of morphological characteristics, which may vary between different lesions within individual patients (13,100). The unifying feature is the presence of large pyroninophilic immunoblasts interspersed with variable numbers of plasmacytoid lymphocytes. The degree of polymorphism, the size and maturation of the individual cells, the number of plasmacytoid or atypical large cells, and the extent of necrosis may vary. The extremes are illustrated in Figure 31-4 and consist of (1) well-differentiated cells, including many small and intermediate-sized lymphocytes with distinct plasmacytoid characteristics and many interspersed mature plasma cells, closely resembling the lymphoplasmacytoid or polymorphic immunocytomas of the Kiel classification (101) (Figure 31-4A); and (2) poorly differentiated cells, including a relatively monotonous population of large transformed lymphocytes with a moderate amount of pyroninophilic cytoplasm, large nuclei, and a central discrete nucleolus (Figure 31-4B) (13).

Cytogenetics, Clonality, and Donor/Host Origin of EBV$^+$ LP cells

The proliferating lymphoblasts in EBV$^+$ LP mostly have a normal karyotype, although multiple chromosomal abnormalities in some tumors have been reported (12,87,88,90). Translocations characteristic of Burkitt's lymphoma (i.e., involving the Ig genes on chromosome 14 and less frequently on chromosomes 2 or 22, and sequences within or adjacent to the c-myc locus on chromosome 8) have not been reported.

Clonal B-cell populations were detected in the majority of patients, particularly in those with intermediate or late-onset EBV$^+$ LP, using Ig light chain staining or Ig gene rearrangement studies (see Table 31-4). Both techniques were used in 24 patients. In 6, clonal B-cell populations were identified by Ig gene

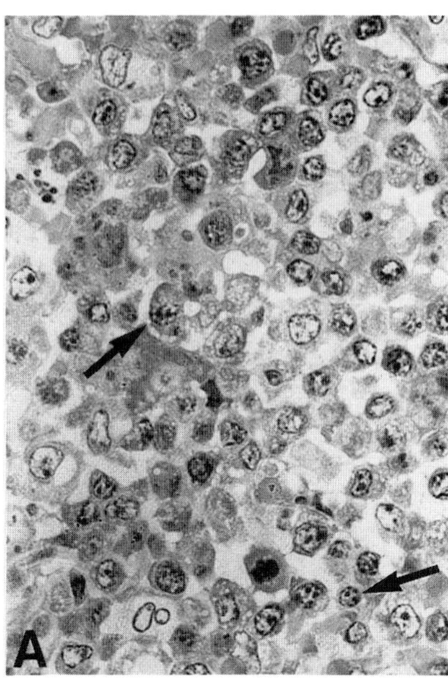

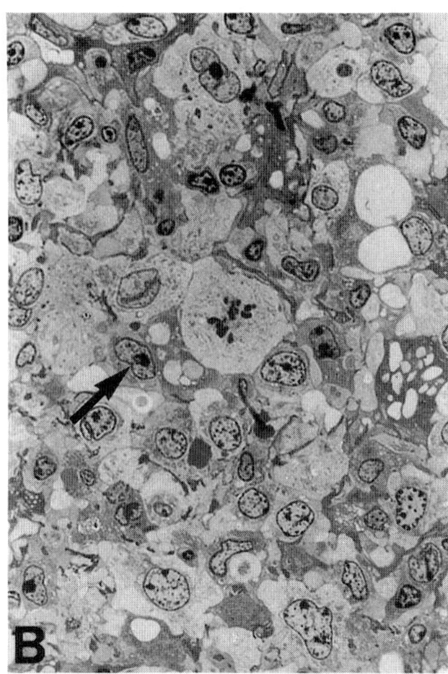

Figure 31-4. Examples of two cases of Epstein-Barr virus (EBV)–positive lymphoproliferation with differing morphology. (A) Well-differentiated immunoblastic lymphoma. Small and intermediate-sized lymphocytes with distinct plasmacytoid characteristics (*large arrow*) and mature plasma cells (*small arrow*) are common (×400). (B) Poorly differentiated immunoblastic lymphoma. A monotonous population of large transformed lymphocytes (*arrow*) with a moderate amount of pyrininophilic cytoplasm form large nodules in the splenectomy specimen (×400). (Reproduced by permission from Zutter MM, Martin PJ, Sale GE, et al. Epstein-Barr virus lymphoproliferation after bone marrow transplantation. Blood 1988;72:520–529.)

rearrangement, which could not be detected by Ig light chain staining, reflecting the greater sensitivity of the first method in detecting small clonal B-cell populations. The study of multiple lesions in individual patients (100) revealed the presence of both polyclonal and monoclonal populations in different tissues from the same patient. In some patients, the same clonal B-cell population could be detected in various lesions, whereas in other patients, distinct B-cell clones may be present in the same organ (100). These results are consistent with the hypothesis that the development of EBV$^+$ LP involves proliferation of multiple EBV-carrying B cells without the need for secondary genetic changes. The oligoclonal or monoclonal nature of the lesions may be caused by selection on the basis of cell growth rate, similar to the induction of monoclonality in cultured cell lines (102).

The cellular origin of EBV$^+$ LP is clearly correlated with the stability of engraftment and the time of onset of the disease (see Table 31-4). Data were available on 25 patients. All cases of early-onset EBV$^+$ LP occurred in patients with sustained engraftment and were of donor origin. The opposite was true for the late-onset cases, which were all of host origin and occurred in patients with significant populations of residual B lymphocytes. Tumors of both host and donor origin were reported for the intermediate onset group. Thus, rapidly growing lymphoproliferations occurring early after BMT are of donor origin, whereas more gradually developing tumors occurring late after BMT originate from residual host B cells.

EBV Serology, DNA, and Protein Expression in EBV$^+$ LP

EBV in LP may originate from 4 sources: (1) the host (B lymphocytes or epithelium), (2) the marrow graft (B lymphocytes), (3) blood transfusions (B lymphocytes), or (4) nosocomial (virions in saliva). EBV$^+$ LP developed in 8 recipients who were EBV-seronegative prior to BMT (see Table 31-4). EBV$^+$ LP developed in 7 patients between 45 and 100 days (median, 60 days) after transplantation of marrow from an EBV-seropositive donor. The eighth patient received EBV-seronegative marrow, but infectious mononucleosis developed 3 ¾ years after BMT, followed by development of EBV$^+$ LP 3 months later (12). EBV$^+$ LP developed in 2 seropositive recipients 56 and 89 days after transplantation of EBV-seronegative marrow. The lymphoma in the latter patient developed in cells of donor origin, showing that donor-derived B lymphocytes may become infected in the host. The onset of EBV$^+$ LP in seropositive patients was not accompanied by a significant increase in EBV antibody titers (12,13,78,93).

EBV was detected in the lesions of 33 of the 39 patients by hybridization of extracted DNA with probes derived from the *Bam*HI W (87,92,93,96), V (13), A, E, or H regions (12), or the *Eco*RI A (97), B, or C regions (87–89). The *Bam*HI W probe also proved useful for in situ hybridization studies (100). The average number of EBV genome copies varied between 5 and more than 50/cell (12,94). Studies in 2 patients showed that the EBV genome was present in circular, episomal form (90,92), similar to LCL and Burkitt's or acquired immune deficiency syndrome–associated lymphoma cells (103).

Detection of EBNA proteins using anticomplement immunofluorescence (104) or immunoperoxidase techniques revealed the presence of EBV in the lesions of the 6 remaining patients. Immunofluorescence and immunoblotting studies revealed that the tumor cells in most cases of EBV$^+$ LP expressed the full set of growth transformation–associated proteins (i.e.,

Table 31-5.
EBV Gene Expression and Cellular Phenotype in Various Types of EBV-carrying (Tumor) Cells

Cell Type, Ref	*B-cell Markers*	*Adhesion Molecules*	*EBV-encoded Growth Transformation–associated Proteins*
Burkitt's lymphoma (105–107)	CD10$^+$,77$^+$ CD23$^-$,39$^-$	CD11a/18$^-$, CD54$^-$,58$^-$	EBNA 1$^+$,2$^-$,3$^-$,4$^-$,6$^-$, LMP-
Nasopharyngeal carcinoma (108)			EBNA 1$^+$,2$^-$,3$^-$,4$^-$,6$^-$ (100% of patients) LMP$^+$ (65% of patients)
EBV$^+$ LP (80, 81)[a]	CD10$^-$,77$^-$, CD23$^+$,39$^+$	CD11a/18$^+$, CD54$^+$,58$^+$	EBNA 1$^+$,2$^+$,3$^+$,(4$^+$),6$^+$, LMP$^+$
In vitro LCL (105, 106)	CD10$^-$,77$^-$, CD23$^+$,39$^+$	CD11a/18$^+$, CD54$^+$,58$^+$	EBNA 1$^+$,2$^+$,3$^+$,4$^+$,6$^+$, LMP$^+$

[a]EBNA 4 expression was not confirmed using monospecific reagents (81).
EBV = Epstein-Barr virus; LP = lymphoproliferation; LCL = lymphoblastic cell line.

EBNA 1, 2, 3, 4, 6, and LMP). Hence, EBV$^+$ LP has a similar phenotype as LCL and differs clearly from other EBV-associated tumors, such as Burkitt's lymphoma or nasopharyngeal carcinoma (105–108). LCL and EBV$^+$ LP express B-cell activation markers, such as CD23 and CD39; high levels of adhesion molecules, such as CD11a/18, CD54, and CD58; and resemble activated immunoblasts (Table 31-5). Cells with this phenotype are excellent targets for HLA-restricted, EBV-specific cytotoxic T cells (106). In contrast, EBV$^+$ Burkitt's lymphoma cells resemble resting germinal center B lymphocytes (105–107); they express the CD10 and CD77 markers typical for this B-cell subset, have low or absent expression of adhesion molecules, and are not destroyed by HLA-restricted, EBV-specific cytotoxic T cells (106), which can readily be isolated from these patients (109). These combined observations are consistent with the hypothesis that EBV$^+$ LP in BMT recipients develops through failure of host immunosurveillance.

Conclusions

EBV, widespread in human populations, has two major target tissues in vivo: B lymphocytes and squamous epithelial cells. The infection status of B lymphocytes is predominantly nonproductive, whereas epithelial cells replicate EBV linked to ordered squamous epithelial cell differentiation. BMT has a significant impact on the relationship between EBV and its host. Due to the replacement of the recipient's hemopoietic tissue by that of the marrow donor, the reservoir of latent EBV will be severely depleted but may be replenished with EBV-carrying B cells transferred with the marrow graft. The same is true for HLA-restricted, EBV-specific T lymphocytes, which are believed to be pivotal in exerting immunological control over EBV infection. As a net result, clinical problems caused by EBV in the setting of autologous or allogeneic BMT are extremely rare and are confined to the often fatal syndrome caused by uncontrolled polyclonal proliferation of EBV-transformed B lymphocytes, which may ultimately result in overgrowth by a single B-cell clone. The early form of the syndrome is observed during the first months after BMT and occurs preferentially in stably engrafted recipients of HLA-mismatched, T-cell–depleted marrow after treatment with T-cell antibodies for severe acute GVHD.

Encouraging results have been achieved in treatment of oligoclonal disease by a combination of CD21 and CD24 B-cell antibodies. The late form of the disease may develop years after BMT and typically emerges from residual host B cells in incompletely engrafted recipients. At diagnosis, these lymphomas were monoclonal and ultimately fatal. Future strategies to control EBV+ LP may include early detection of increased numbers of infected B cells by quantitative polymerase chain reaction; adoptive immunotherapy using HLA-restricted, EBV-specific cytotoxic T cells to eradicate EBV-carrying cells; and vaccination to boost EBV-specific immunity in recipients with delayed immune reconstitution.

References

1. Nilsson K, Klein G, Henle W, Henle G. The establishment of lymphoblastoid cell lines from adult and from foetal human lymphoid tissue and its dependence on EBV. Int J Cancer 1971;8:443–450.
2. Sixbey JW, Nedrud JG, Raab-Traub N, Hanes RA, Pagano JS. Epstein-Barr virus replication in oropharyngeal epithelial cells. N Engl J Med 1984; 310:1225–1230.
3. Niederman JC, Evans AS, Subrahmanyan L, McCollum RW. Prevalence, incidence and persistence of EB virus antibody in young adults. N Engl J Med 1970;282:361–365.
4. Henle G, Henle W. Observations on childhood infections with the Epstein-Barr virus. J Infect Dis 1970;121:301–310.
5. Henle G, Henle W, Diehl V. Relation of Burkitt's tumor-associated herpes-type virus to infectious mononucleosis. Proc Natl Acad Sci USA 1968;59:94–101.
6. Epstein MA, Achong BG, Barr YM. Virus particles in cultured lymphoblasts from Burkitt's lymphoma. Lancet 1964;1:702–703.
7. Zur Hausen H, Schulte-Holthausen H, Klein G, et al. EBV DNA in biopsies of Burkitt tumors and anaplastic carcinomas of the nasopharynx. Nature 1970; 228: 1056–1058.
8. Herbst H, Niedobitek G, Stein H. Epstein-Barr virus infection and CD30-positive malignant lymphomas. Crit Rev Oncogenesis 1993;4:191–239.
9. Purtilo DT, Klein G. Symposium on Epstein-Barr virus-

induced lymphoproliferative disorders in immunodeficient patients. Cancer Res 1981;41:4209–4304.

10. Purtilo DT. X-linked lymphoproliferative disease as a model of Epstein-Barr virus-induced immunopathology. Springer Semin Immunopathol 1991;13:181–198.
11. Nalesnik MA. Lymphoproliferative disease in organ transplant recipients. Springer Semin Immunopathol 1991;13:199–216.
12. Shapiro RS, McClain K, Frizzera G, et al. Epstein-Barr virus associated B cell lymphoproliferative disorders following bone marrow transplantation. Blood 1988;71:1234–1243.
13. Zutter MM, Martin PJ, Sale GE, et al. Epstein-Barr virus lymphoproliferation after bone marrow transplantation. Blood 1988;72:520–529.
14. Ernberg I. Epstein-Barr virus and acquired immunodeficiency syndrome. Adv Viral Oncol 1989;8:203–217.
15. Greenspan JS, Greenspan D, Lennette ET, et al. Replication of Epstein-Barr virus within the epithelial cells of oral "hairy" leukoplakia, an AIDS-associated lesion. N Engl J Med 1985;313:1564–1571.
16. Hoagland RJ. The transmission of infectious mononucleosis. Am J Med Sci 1955;229:262–272.
17. Evans AS. Infectious mononucleosis in University of Wisconsin students: report of a 5-year investigation. Am J Hyg 1960;71:342–362.
18. Nemerow GR, Moore MD, Cooper NR. Structure and function of the B lymphocyte Epstein-Barr virus/C3d receptor. Adv Cancer Res 1990;54:273–300.
19. Delcayre AX, Salas F, Mathur S, Kovats K, Lotz M, Lernhardt W. Epstein-Barr virus/complement C3d receptor is an interferon alpha receptor. EMBO J 1991;10:919–926.
20. Watry D, Hedrick JA, Siervo S, et al. Infection of human thymocytes by Epstein-Barr virus. J Exp Med 1991; 173:971–980.
21. Jones JF, Shurin S, Abramowsky C, et al. T-cell lymphomas containing Epstein-Barr viral DNA in patients with chronic Epstein-Barr virus infections. N Engl J Med 1988;318:733–741.
22. Hart DNJ, Baker BW, Inglis MJ, et al. Epstein-Barr viral DNA in acute large granular lymphocyte (natural killer) leukemic cells. Blood 1992;79:2116–2123.
23. Sixbey JW, Yao QY. Immunoglobulin A-induced shift of Epstein-Barr virus tissue tropism. Science 1992;255:1578–1580.
24. Klein G, Svedmyr E, Jondal M, Persson P. EBV-determined nuclear antigen (EBNA)-positive cells in the peripheral blood of infectious mononucleosis patients. Int J Cancer 1976;17:21–26.
25. Rocchi G, Felici A, Ragona G, Heinz A. Quantitative evaluation of Epstein-Barr virus-infected peripheral blood leukocytes in infectious mononucleosis. N Engl J Med 1977;296:132–134.
26. Yao QY, Rickinson AB, Epstein MA. A re-examination of the Epstein-Barr virus carrier state in healthy seropositive individuals. Int J Cancer 1985;35:35–42.
27. Henle W, Henle G. Epstein-Barr virus and blood transfusions. Prog Clin Biol Res 1985;182:201–209.
28. Rickinson AB, Yao QY, Wallace LE. The Epstein-Barr virus as a model of virus-host interactions. Br Med Bull 1985;41:75–79.
29. Gratama JW, Oosterveer MA, Zwaan FE, Lepoutre J, Klein G, Ernberg I. Eradication of Epstein-Barr virus by allogeneic bone marrow transplantation: implications for sites of viral latency. Proc Natl Acad Sci USA 1988;85:8693–8696.
30. Yao QY, Ogan P, Rowe M, Wood M, Rickinson AB. Epstein-Barr virus-infected B cells persist in the circulation of acyclovir-treated virus carriers. Int J Cancer 1989;43:67–71.
31. Gerber P, Nonoyama M, Lucus S, Perlin E, Goldstein L. Oral excretion of Epstein-Barr virus by healthy subjects and patients with infectious mononucleosis. Lancet 1972;2:988–989.
32. Rickinson AB, Finerty S, Epstein M. Comparative studies on adult donor lymphocytes infected by EB virus in vitro or in vivo: origin of transformed cells arising in co-cultures with foetal lymphocytes. Int J Cancer 1977;19:775–782.
33. Lewin N, Aman P, Masucci MG, et al. Characterization of EBV-carrying B-cell populations in healthy seropositive individuals with regard to density, release of transforming virus and spontaneous outgrowth. Int J Cancer 1987;39:472–476.
34. Li QX, Young LS, Niedobitek G, et al. Epstein-Barr virus infection and replication in a human epithelial cell system. Nature 1992;356:347–350.
35. Sixbey JW, Chessney PJ, Shirley P, Buntin DM. Detection of a second widespread strain of Epstein-Barr virus. Lancet 1989; 2:761–765.
36. Baer R, Bankier AT, Biggin MD, et al. DNA sequence and expression of the B95.8 Epstein-Barr virus genome. Nature 1984;310:207–211.
37. Hurley E, Thorley-Lawson D. B cell activation and the establishment of Epstein-Barr virus latency. J Exp Med 1988;168:2059–2075.
38. Sample J, Hummel M, Braun D, Birkenbach M, Kieff E. Nucleotide sequences of mRNAs encoding Epstein-Barr virus nuclear proteins: a probable transcriptional initiation site. Proc Natl Acad Sci USA 1986;83:5096–5100.
39. Raab-Traub N, Flynn K. The structure of the termini of the Epstein-Barr virus as a marker of clonal cellular proliferation. Cell 1986;47:883–889.
40. Brown N, Liu C, Wang Y, Garcia C. B cell lymphoproliferation and lymphomagenesis are associated with clonotypic intracellular terminal regions of Epstein-Barr virus. J Virol 1988;62:962–969.
41. Jat P, Arrand JR. In vitro transcription of two Epstein-Barr virus specified small RNA molecules. Nucleic Acids Res 1982;10:3407–3425.
42. Howe JG, Steitz JA. Localization of Epstein-Barr virus-encoded small RNAs by *in situ* hybridization. Proc Natl Acad Sci USA 1986;83:9006–9010.
43. Kieff E, Liebowitz D. Epstein-Barr virus and its replication. In: Fields BN, Knipe DM, eds. Virology, ed 2. New York: Raven, 1990:1889–1920.
44. Hennessy K, Kieff E. One of two Epstein-Barr virus nuclear antigens contains a glycine-alanine copolymer domain. Proc Natl Acad Sci USA 1983;80:5665–5669.
45. Gratama JW, Oosterveer MAP, Klein G, Ernberg I. EBNA size polymorphism can be used to trace EBV spread within families. J Virol 1990;64:4703–4708.
46. Sugden B, Phelps M, Domoradzki J. Epstein-Barr virus DNA is amplified in transformed lymphocytes. J Virol 1979;31:590–595.
47. Miller G. The switch between latency and replication of Epstein-Barr virus. J Infect Dis 1990;161:833.
48. Kallin B, Luka J, Klein G. Immunochemical characterization of Epstein-Barr virus-associated early and late antigens in n-butyrate-treated P3HR1 cells. J Virol 1979;32:710–716.

49. Thorley-Lawson DA, Edson CM, Geilinger K. Epstein-Barr virus antigens—a challenge to modern biochemistry. Adv Cancer Res 1982;36:295–348.
50. Evans AS, Niederman JC, Canabre LC, West B, Richards VA. A prospective evaluation of heterophile and Epstein-Barr virus-specific IgM antibody tests in clinical and subclinical infectious mononucleosis: specificity and sensitivity of the tests and persistence of antibody. J Infect Dis 1975;132:546–554.
51. Henle W, Henle G, Horwitz CA. Epstein-Barr virus-specific diagnostic tests in infectious mononucleosis. Hum Pathol 1974;5:551–555.
52. Hoffman GJ, Lazarowits SG, Hayward SD. Monoclonal antibody against a 250,000-dalton glycoprotein of Epstein-Barr virus identifies a membrane antigen and a neutralizing antigen. Proc Natl Aacd Sci USA 1980; 77:2979–2983.
53. Thorley-Lawson DA, Geilinger K. Monoclonal antibodies against the major glycoprotein (gp350/220) of Epstein-Barr virus neutralize infectivity. Proc Natl Acad Sci USA 1980;77:5307–5311.
54. Henle W, Henle G, Andersson J, et al. Antibody responses to Epstein-Barr virus-determined nuclear antigen (EBNA)-1 and EBNA-2 in acute and chronic Epstein-Barr virus infection. Proc Natl Acad Sci USA 1987;84:570–574.
55. De Waele M, Thielemans C, Van Kamp BKG. Characterization of immunoregulatory T cells in Epstein-Barr virus-induced infectious mononucleosis by monoclonal antibodies. N Engl J Med 1981;304:460–462.
56. Klein E, Ernberg I, Masucci MG, et al. T-cell response to B-cells and Epstein-Barr virus antigens in infectious mononucleosis. Cancer Res 1981;41:4210–4215.
57. Strang G, Rickinson AB. Multiple HLA class I-dependent cytotoxicities constitute the non-HLA-restricted response in infectious mononucleosis. Eur J Immunol 1987;17:1007–1013.
58. Reinherz EL, O'Brien C, Rosenthal P, et al. The cellular basis for viral-induced immunodeficiency: analysis by monoclonal antibodies. J Immunol 1980;125:1269–1274.
59. Nikoskelainen J, Ablashi D, Isenberg RA, et al. Cellular immunity in infectious mononucleosis. II. Specific reactivity to Epstein-Barr virus antigens and correlation with clinical hematologic parameters. J Immunol 1978;121:1239–1247.
60. Moss DJ, Rickinson AB, Pope JH. Long-term T-cell mediated immunity to Epstein-Barr virus in man. I. Complete regression of virus-induced transformation in cultures of seropositive donor leukocytes. Int J Cancer 1978;22:662–668.
61. Rickinson AB, Moss DJ, Wallace LE, et al. Long-term cell-mediated immunity to Epstein-Barr virus. Cancer Res 1981;41:4216–4221.
62. Bejarano MT, Masucci MG, Ernberg I, Klein G, Klein E. Effect of cyclosporin-A (CsA) on the ability of T lymphocyte subsets to inhibit the proliferation of autologous EBV-transformed cells. Int J Cancer 1985; 35:327–333.
63. Murray RJ, Kurilla MG, Brooks JM, et al. Identification of target antigens for the human cytotoxic T cell response to Epstein-Barr virus (EBV): implications for the immune control of EBV-positive malignancies. J Exp Med 1992;176:157–168.
64. Khanna RS, Burrows SR, Kurilla MG, et al. Localization of Epstein-Barr virus cytotoxic T cell epitopes using recombinant vaccinia: implications for vaccine development. J Exp Med 1992;176:169–176.
65. Lange B, Henle W, Meyers JD, et al. Epstein-Barr virus-related serology in marrow transplant recipients. Int J Cancer 1980;26:151–157.
66. Crawford D, Mulholland N, Iliescu V, Hawkins R, Powles R. Epstein-Barr virus infection and immunity in bone marrow transplant recipients. Transplantation 1986;42:50–54.
67. Morinet F, Icart J, Ruelle C, Gluckman E, Perol Y. Epstein-Barr virus serology in bone marrow transplantation: a one-year retrospective study with detection of EBV IgM-VCA-specific antibodies. J Med Virol 1985; 18:349–360.
68. Gratama JW, Lennette ET, Lönnqvist B, et al. Detection of multiple Epstein-Barr viral strains in allogeneic bone marrow transplant recipients. J Med Virol 1992;37:39–47.
69. Epstein JB, Priddy RW, Sherlock CH. Hairy leukoplakia-like lesions in immunosuppressed patients following bone marrow transplantation. Transplantation 1988;46:462–464.
70. De Graan-Hentzen YCE, Gratama JW, Mudde GC, et al. Prevention of primary cytomegalovirus infection in patients with hematologic malignancies by intensive white cell depletion of blood products. Transfusion 1989;29:757–760.
71. Yao QY, Rowe M, Morgan AJ, et al. Salivary and serum IgA antibodies to the Epstein-Barr virus glycoprotein gp340: incidence and potential for virus neutralization. Int J Cancer 1991;48:45–50.
72. Gerber P, Walsh JH, Rosenblum EN, Purcell RH. Association of EB virus infection with the post-perfusion syndrome. Lancet 1969;1:593–596.
73. Blacklow NR, Watson BK, Miller G, Jacobson BM. Mononucleosis with heterophile antibodies and EB virus infection. Acquisition by an elderly patient in hospital. Am J Med 1971;51:549–552.
74. Sullivan JL, Wallen WC, Johnson FL. Epstein-Barr virus infection following bone-marrow transplantation. Int J Cancer 1978;22:132–135.
75. Gratama JW, Zwaan FE, Stijnen T, et al. Herpes virus immunity and acute graft-versus-host disease. Lancet 1987;1:471–474.
76. Boström L, Ringdén O, Sundberg B, Linde A, Tollemar J, Nilsson B. Pretransplant herpesvirus serology and acute graft-versus-host disease. Transplantation 1988; 46:548–552.
77. Gratama JW, Stijnen T, Weiland HT, et al. Herpes virus immunity and acute graft-versus-host disease: an update from Leiden. In: Gale RP, Champlin R, eds. New strategies in bone marrow transplantation. New York: Alan R. Liss, 1991:311–318.
78. Gratama JW, Oosterveer MAP, Lepoutre JMM, et al. Serological and molecular studies of Epstein-Barr virus infection in allogeneic marrow graft recipients. Transplantation 1990;49:725–730.
79. Gratama JW, Oosterveer MAP, Lepoutre J, et al. Epstein-Barr virus infection in allogeneic marrow grafting: lessons for transplant physicians and virologists. Ann Hematol 1992;64:A162–A165.
80. Young L, Alfieri C, Hennessy K, et al. Expression of Epstein-Barr virus transformation-associated genes in tissues of patients with EBV lymphoproliferative disease. N Engl J Med 1989;321:1080–1085.
81. Gratama JW, Zutter MM, Minarovits J, et al. Expression of Epstein-Barr virus-encoded growth transformation-associated proteins in lymphoproliferations of bone marrow transplant recipients. Int J Cancer 1991;47:188–192.

82. Kallin B, Dillner J, Ernberg I, et al. Four virally determined nuclear antigens are expressed in Epstein-Barr virus-transformed cells. Proc Natl Acad Sci USA 1986;83:1499–1503.
83. Gerhartz HH, Mittermuller J, Raghavachar A, et al. Epstein-Barr virus-positive recipient type B-cells survive in a "complete chimera" after allogeneic bone marrow transplantation. Int J Cancer 1988;42:672–676.
84. Falkenburg JHF, Goselink HM, Van der Harst D, et al. Growth inhibition of clonogenic leukemic precursor cells by minor histocompatibility antigen-specific cytotoxic T lymphocytes. J Exp Med 1991;174:27–33.
85. Fialkow PJ, Thomas ED, Bryant JJ, Neiman PE. Leukaemic transformation of engrafted human marrow cells in vivo. Lancet 1971;1:251–255.
86. Bloom RE, Brennan JK, Sullivan JL, Chiganti RSK, Dinsmore R, O'Reilly R. Lymphoma of host origin in a marrow transplant recipient in remission of acute myeloid leukemia and receiving cyclosporin A. Am J Hematol 1985;18:73–83.
87. Schubach WH, Hackman R, Neiman PE, Miller G, Thomas ED. A monoclonal immunoblastic sarcoma in donor cells bearing Epstein-Barr virus genomes following allogeneic marrow grafting for acute lymphoblastic leukemia. Blood 1982;60:180–187.
88. Martin PJ, Shulman HM, Schubach WH, et al. Fatal Epstein-Barr-virus-associated proliferation of donor B cells after treatment of acute graft-versus-host disease with a murine anti-T-cell antibody. Ann Intern Med 1984;101:310–315.
89. Shearer WT, Ritz J, Finegold MJ, et al. Epstein-Barr virus-associated B-cell proliferations of diverse clonal origins after bone marrow transplantation in a 12-year-old patient with severe combined immunodeficiency. N Engl J Med 1985;312:1151–1159.
90. Forman SJ, Sullivan JL, Wright C, Ratech H, Racklin B, Blume KG. Epstein-Barr-virus-related malignant B cell lymphoplasmacytic lymphoma following allogeneic bone marrow transplantation for aplastic anemia. Transplantation 1987;44:244–249.
91. Kapoor N, Jung LKL, Engelhard D, et al. Lymphoma in a patient with severe combined immunodeficiency with adenosine deaminase deficiency, following unsustained engraftment of histoincompatible T cell-depleted bone marrow. J Pediatr 1986;108:435–438.
92. Sullivan JL, Medveczky P, Forman SJ, et al. Epstein-Barr-virus induced lymphoproliferation: implications for antiviral chemotherapy. N Engl J Med 1984; 311:1163–1167.
93. Lyttelton MPA, Browett PJ, Brenner MK, et al. Prolonged remission of Epstein-Barr virus associated lymphoma secondary to T cell-depleted bone marrow transplantation. Bone Marrow Transplant 1988;3:641–646.
94. Skinner JC, Gildert EF, Hong R, et al. B cell lymphoproliferative disorders following T cell depleted allogeneic bone marrow transplantation. Am J Pediatr Hematol Oncol 1988;10:112–119.
95. Blanche S, Le Deist F, Veber F, et al. Treatment of severe Epstein-Barr virus-induced polyclonal B-lymphocyte proliferation by anti-B-cell monoclonal antibodies: two cases after HLA-mismatched bone marrow transplantation. Ann Intern Med 1988;108:199–203.
96. Simon M, Bartram CR, Friedrich W, et al. Fatal B-cell lymphoproliferative syndrome in allogeneic marrow graft recipients. Virchows Arch Cell Pathol [B] 1991; 60:307–319.
97. Davey DD, Kamat D, Laszewski M, et al. Epstein-Barr virus-related lymphoproliferative disorders following bone marrow transplantation: an immunologic and genotypic analysis. Mod Pathol 1989;2:27–34.
98. Fischer A, Blanche S, Le Bidois J, et al. Anti-B-cell monoclonal antibodies in the treatment of severe B-cell lymphoproliferative syndrome following bone marrow and organ transplantation. N Engl J Med 1991;324: 1451–1456.
99. The Non-Hodgkin's Lymphoma Pathologic Classification Project. National Cancer Institute sponsored study of classifications of non-Hodgkin's lymphomas: summary and description of a working formulation for clinical usage. Cancer 1982;49:2112–2135.
100. D'Amore ESG, Manivel JC, Gajl-Peczalska KJ, et al. B-cell lymphoproliferative disorders after bone marrow transplant: an analysis of ten cases with emphasis on Epstein-Barr virus detection by *in situ* hybridization. Cancer 1991;68:1285–1295.
101. Lennert K, Stein H. Histopathology of non-Hodgkin's lymphoma (based on the Kiel classification). Berlin: Springer-Verlag, 1981:45–53.
102. Nilsson K. The nature of lymphoid cell lines and their relationship to the virus. In: Epstein MA, Achong BG, eds. The Epstein-Barr virus. Berlin: Springer-Verlag, 1979:225–281.
103. Gulley ML, Raphael M, Lutz CT, Ross DW, Raab-Traub N. Epstein-Barr virus integration in human lymphomas and lymphoid cell lines. Cancer 1992;70: 185–191.
104. Reedman BM, Klein G. Cellular localization of an Epstein-Barr virus (EBV) associated complement-fixing antigen in producer and non-producer lymphoblastoid cell lines. Int J Cancer 1973;11:499–520.
105. Rowe M, Rowe DT, Gregory CD, et al. Differences in B-cell growth phenotype reflect novel patterns of Epstein-Barr virus latent gene expression in Burkitt's lymphoma cells. EMBO J 1987;6:2743–2751.
106. Gregory CD, Murray RJ, Edwards CF, Rickinson AB. Downregulation of cell adhesion molecules LFA-3 and ICAM-1 in Epstein-Barr virus-positive Burkitt's lymphoma underlies tumor cell escape from virus-specific T cell surveillance. J Exp Med 1988;187:1811–1824.
107. Gregory CD, Tursz T, Edwards CF, et al. Identification of a subset of normal B cells with a Burkitt's lymphoma (BL)-like phenotype. J Immunol 1987;139: 313–318.
108. Fahraeus R, Hu LF, Ernberg I, et al. Expression of Epstein-Barr virus-encoded proteins in nasopharyngeal carcinoma. Int J Cancer 1988;42:329–338.
109. Rooney CM, Rickinson AB, Moss DJ, Lenoir GM, Epstein MA. Cell-mediated immunosurveillance mechanisms and the pathogenesis of Burkitt's lymphoma. In: Lenoir GM, O'Conor GT, Olweny CLM, eds. Burkitt's lymphoma: a human cancer model. Lyon, France: IARC, 1985:249–264.
110. Henle G, Henle W. Immunofluorescence in cells derived from Burkitt's lymphoma. J Bacteriol 1966;91: 1248–1256.
111. Moss DJ, Misko IS, Sculley TB. Immune surveillance against Epstein-Barr virus. Semin Immunol 1992;4: 97–104.
112. Rowe M, Lear AL, Croom-Carter D, Davies AH, Rickinson AB. Three pathways of Epstein-Barr virus gene activation from EBNA1-positive latency in B lymphocytes. J Virol 1992;66:122–131.

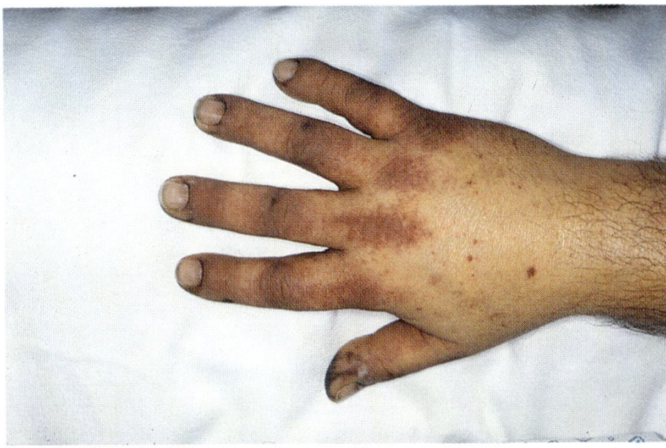

Plate I. Hand of patient who received dimethylbusulfan therapy showing bullous lesion of thumb and erythema over knuckle regions. These features are characteristic of acute cutaneous toxicity from chemoradiotherapy.

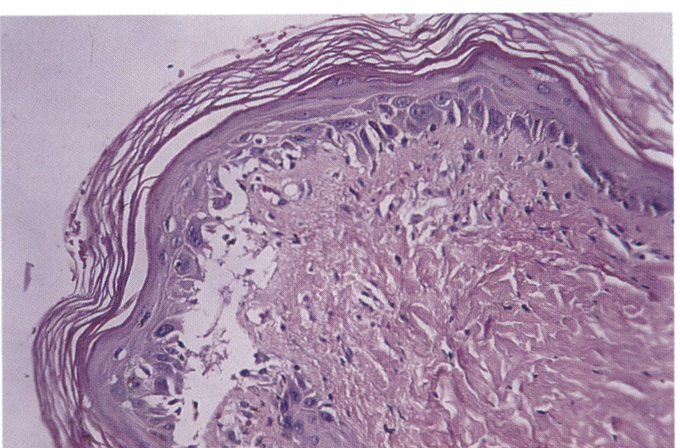

Plate II. Skin biopsy from recipient of identical twin marrow who had received a single 15 mg/kg dose of dimethylbusulfan 15 days previously. The epidermal separation, keratinocyte atypia and scanty lymphoid dermal infiltrate can also be seen in GVHD.

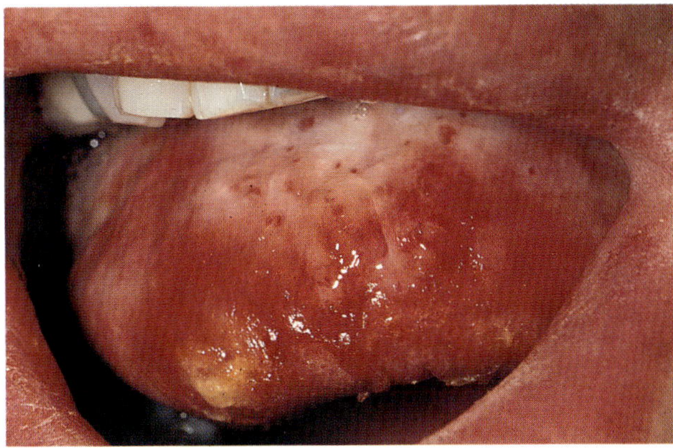

Plate III. Acute glossitis 1 day post BMT after conditioning regimen of 60 mg/kg of CY followed by 12 Gy of fractionated TBI. There is early mucosal damage with severe erythema and focal atrophy.

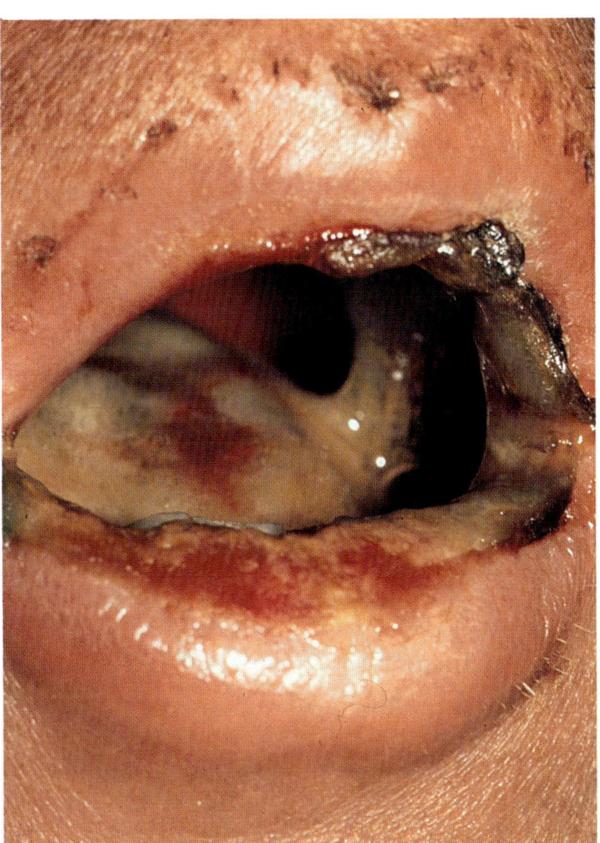

Plate IV. Severe mucositis of lips and tongue with pseudomembranous exudate 20 days after BMT following conditioning with TBI and chemotherapy. Similar changes may be present with severe acute GVHD and herpetic infection.

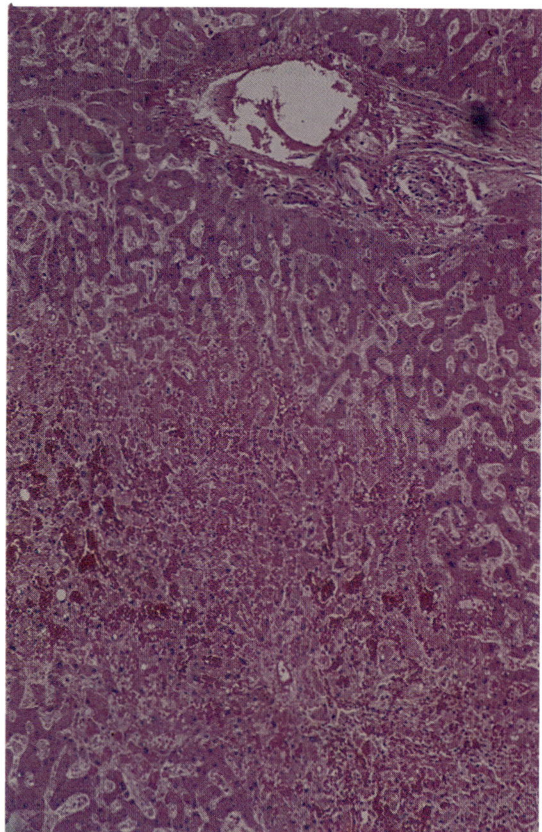

Plate V. Fatal hepatic VOD at necropsy 12 days post BMT for leukemia. At this low magnification, the H&E stained section demonstrates striking congestion, hemorrhage and hepatocyte disruption in zone 3 (centrilobular) of the liver acinus toward the bottom. The portal space and surrounding acinar zone 1 at the top are well preserved. These early severe hepatic VOD lesions at times can be identified with the H&E stain after tissue fixation with B5 or methyl Carnoy's. However, stains for connective tissue are more effective.

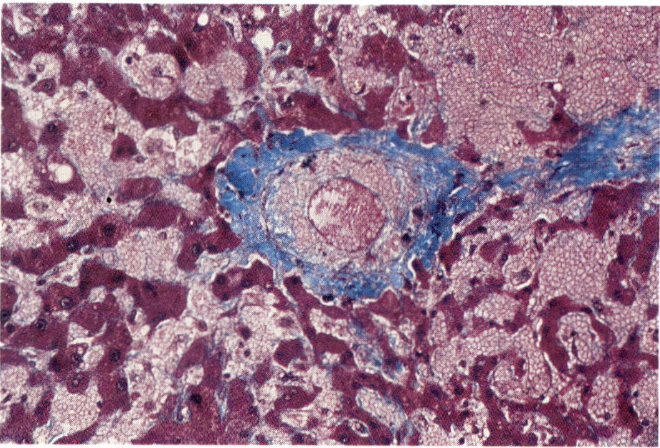

Plate VI. Hepatic VOD 95 days post BMT for malignancy. The trichrome stain shows the blue outline of an hepatic venule with marked luminal narrowing caused by subendothelial trapping of red cells. The hepatocytes of acinar zone 3 are severely disrupted. When the clinical diagnosis of hepatic VOD is uncertain, it may be confirmed by a transvenous liver biopsy with measurement of an elevated gradient between wedged and free hepatic venous pressures.

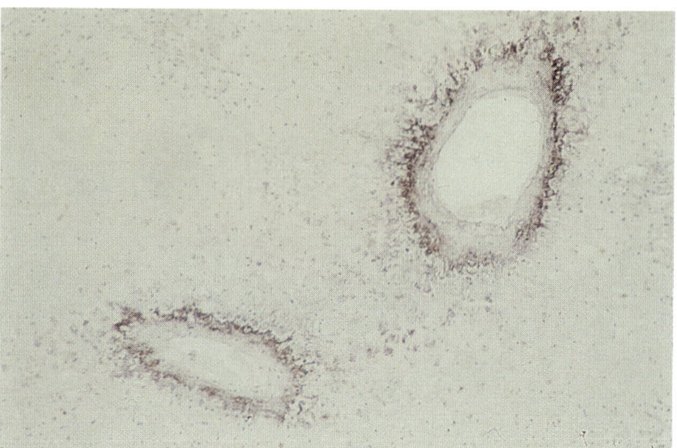

Plate VII. Early hepatic VOD showing perivenular staining for procoagulants. Immunohistochemical staining for factor VIII (von Willebrand) demonstrates post sinusoidal obstruction corresponding to the endothelium-lined pores through which the sinusoids drain into the venules. Immunostaining for fibrin localizes in the same regions. These observations provide some of the rationale for using anti-coagulation and anti-thrombotic therapy for hepatic VOD.

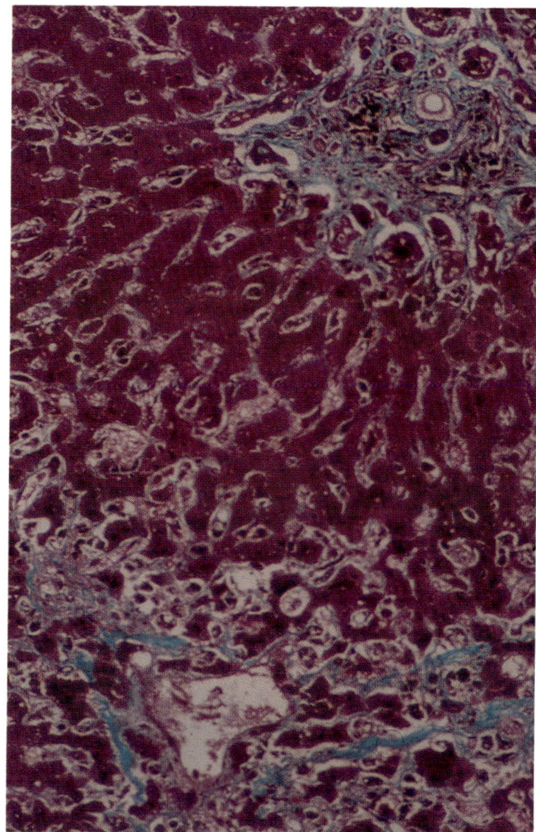

Plate VIII. Hepatic VOD and coexistent GVHD, day 26. On this trichrome stain, the two most common liver problems after BMT can be differentiated by the zone of the liver acinus they affect. The expanded portal space in the upper right demonstrates changes from GVHD including fibrosis, proliferation of atypical cholangioles along the limiting plate and destruction of small interlobular bile ducts. The VOD lesion along the lower margin shows striking collections of embolized hepatocytes beneath the endothelial basement membrane.

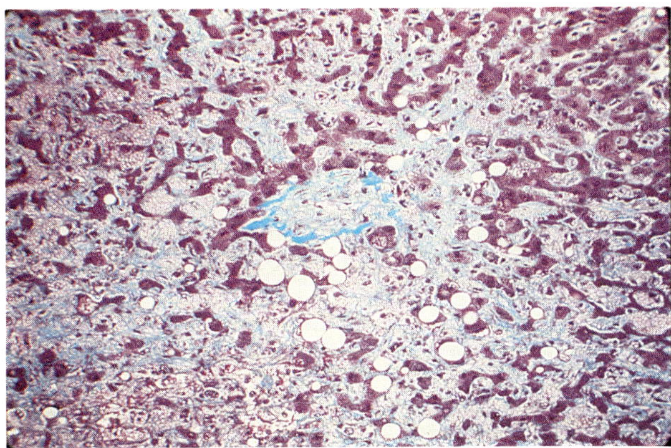

Plate IX. Late hepatic VOD, day 63. The trichrome stain demonstrates fibrotic obliteration of the venous lumen with extensive fibrosis surrounding sinusoids. The resulting vascular obstruction produced intractable ascites. Immunohistochemical stains at this time reveal extensive deposition of collagen while fibrin and other blood procoagulants are no longer identifiable.

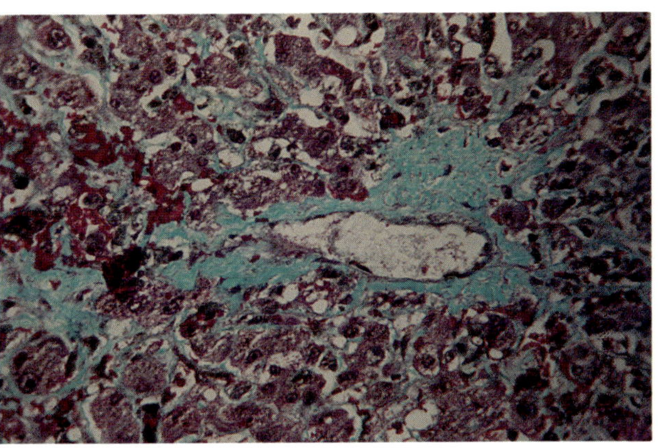

Plate X. Hepatic phlebosclerosis, day 96. Eccentric thickening of the venular wall without striking luminal narrowing was associated with an early liver toxicity syndrome. The patient had received a 5 day infusion of high dose ARAC followed by CY and TBI. Liver function abnormalities developed prior to the infusion of marrow. Changes of phlebosclerosis were widespread but there were no identifiable hepatic VOD lesions at autopsy. Trichrome stain.

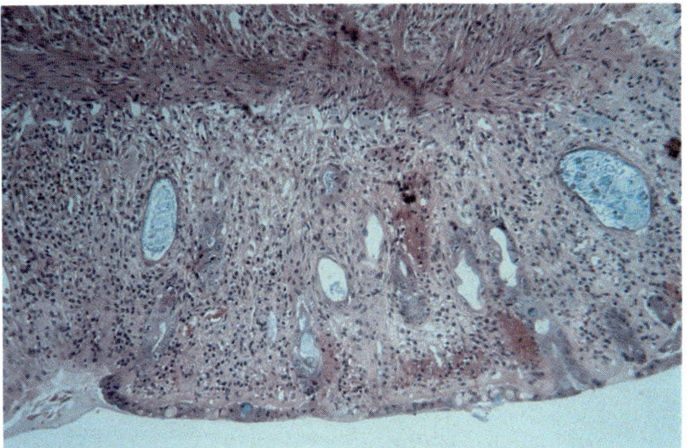

Plate XI. Effect of cytoreductive therapy on colonic mucosa, day 7. This biopsy specimen was taken following therapy with BU, CY and TBI (12 Gy). There has been obliteration of almost all epithelial cells, leaving cystic crypt remnants. H&E with alcian blue counterstain.

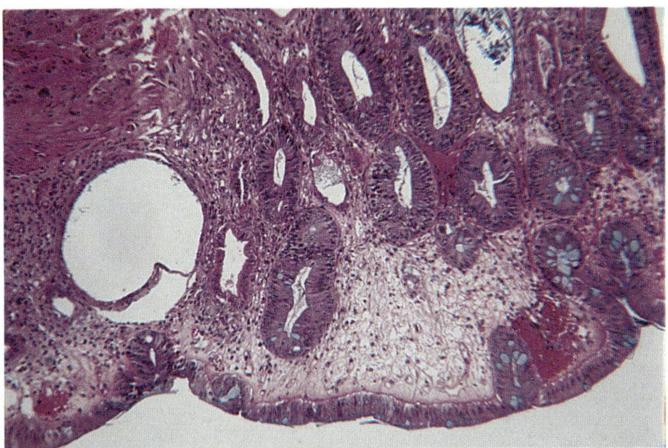

Plate XII. Recovery from the effects of cytoreductive therapy on colonic mucosa, day 16. This repeat biopsy from the same patient as in Plate XI indicates that regeneration is occurring, although some cystic crypts remain. H&E with alcian blue counterstain.

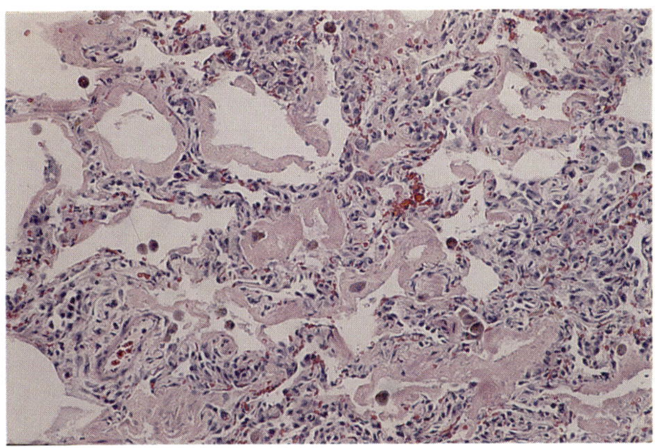

Plate XIII. Severe diffuse alveolar damage (DAD) in a lung biopsy, day 56. Alveoli and terminal bronchioles are lined by hyaline membranes composed of degenerating cells. This nonspecific pattern of severe injury may be associated with shock, infection, chemotherapy and other possible causes. DAD after BMT is often accompanied by renal and hepatic failure.

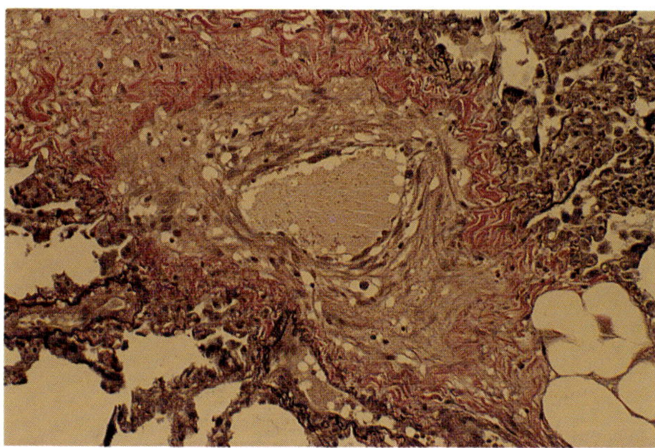

Plate XIV. Pulmonary VOD in a lung biopsy from a patient with pulmonary hypertension 48 days post second allogeneic BMT for ALL. Loose intimal fibrosis partially occludes the interlobular vein. This complication probably results from chemotherapy and may be more frequent than previously suspected. Verhoff-Van Gieson elastin stain.

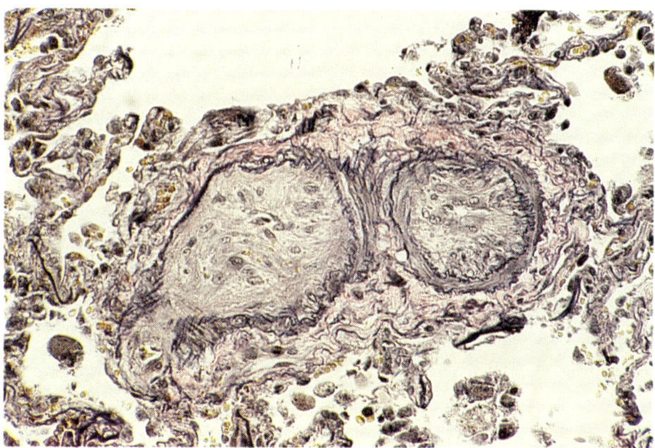

Plate XV. Pulmonary arterioles with severe concentric intimal fibrosis producing virtually complete luminal occlusion at autopsy 37 days post second allogeneic BMT for ALL. Severe hepatic VOD was also present. Verhoff-Van Gieson elastin stain.

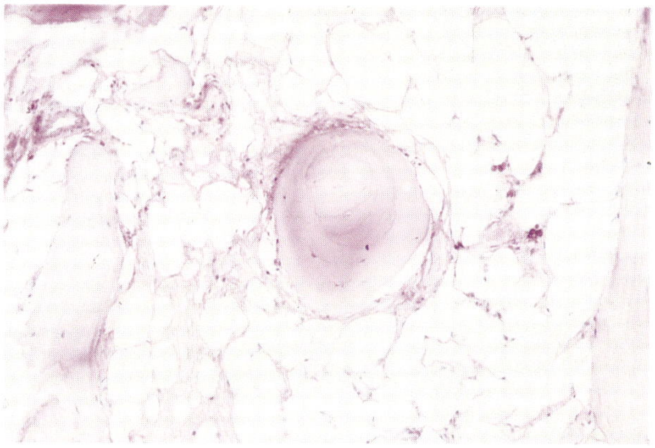

Plate XVI. Markedly hypocellular marrow without evidence of engraftment, day 7. Subtle interstitial fluid accumulation, fat necrosis and iron deposition are consistent with chemoirradiation damage.

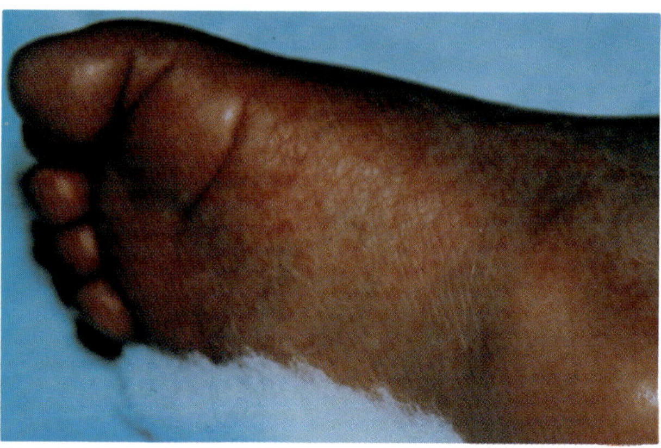

Plate XVII. Painful red to violaceous maculopapular rash consistent with acute GVHD in a 2-year-old girl involving the sole of the foot 11 days after HLA-nonidentical BMT.

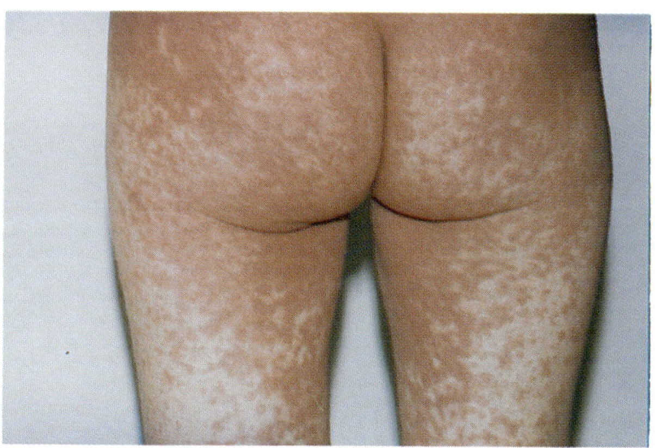

Plate XVIII. Acute GVHD with confluent erythema of the trunk and thighs in a 5-year-old boy 18 days after a 1-antigen mismatched BMT.

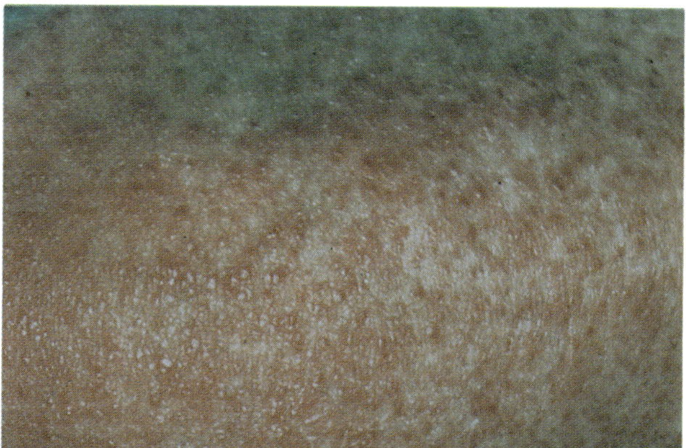

Plate XIX. Multiple red papules on the knee of a 30-year-old man with acute GVHD 40 days after a 2-antigen mismatched BMT.

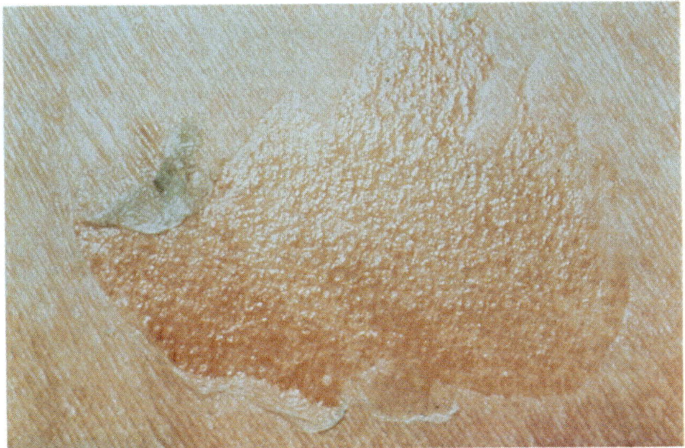

Plate XX. Epidermal separation of grade IV acute GVHD resembling toxic epidermal necrolysis, day 36 after an HLA-identical sibling BMT.

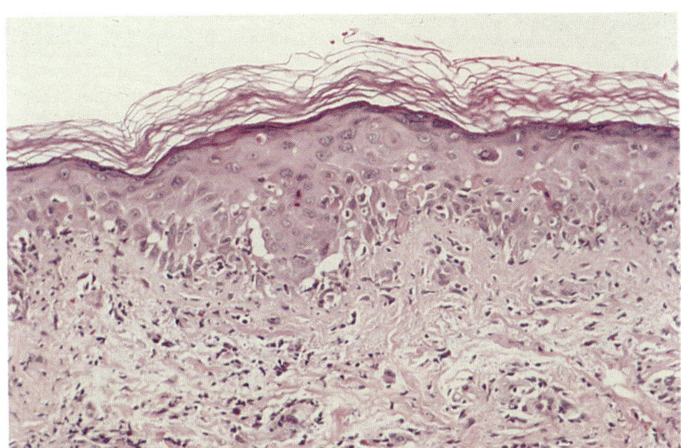

Plate XXI. Acute skin GVHD, day 28 post mismatched allogeneic BMT. The epidermis demonstrates a prominent lichenoid reaction with the tip of the rete ridge in the center of the specimen, a location of epithelial stem cells within the epidermis.

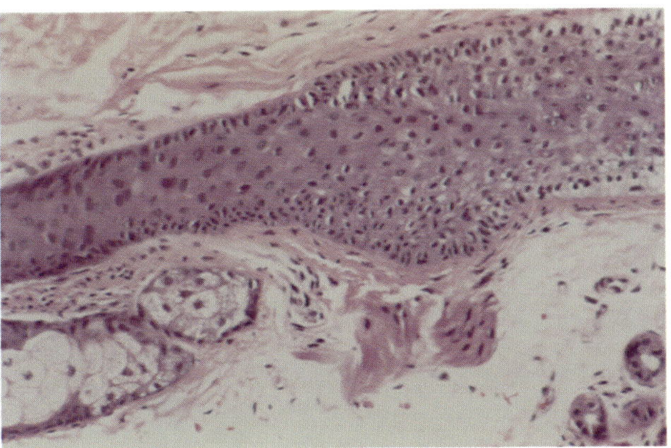

Plate XXII. Early skin GVHD involving the parafollicular bulge region of the pilar unit. Note the small numbers of mononuclear inflammatory cells which infiltrate the parafollicular bulge area near the arrector pilorum muscle in association with apoptotic bodies.

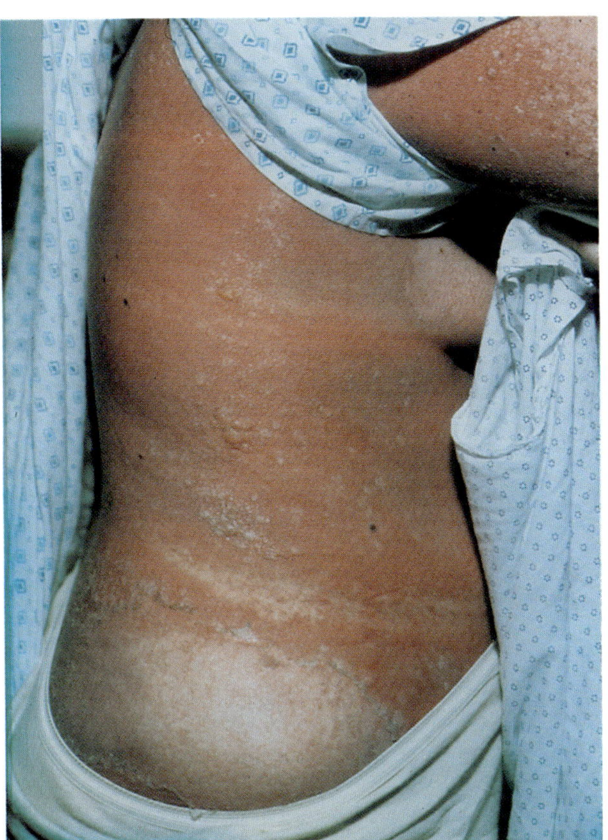

Plate XXIII. Erythema and desquamation before treatment for acute GVHD, day 27.

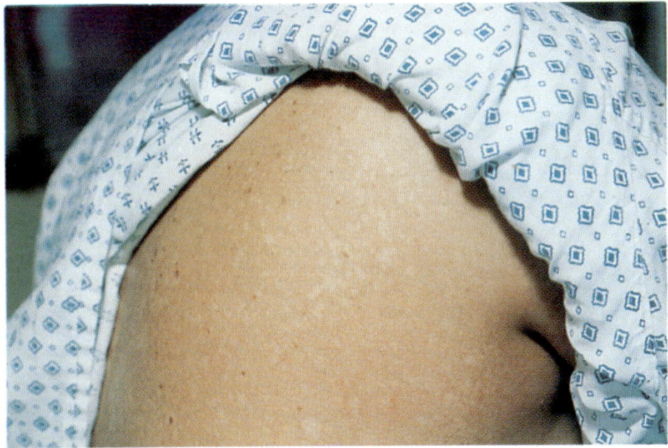

Plate XXIV. Virtually normal skin with focal depigmentation after treatment for acute GVHD, day 74 (same patient shown in Plate XXIII).

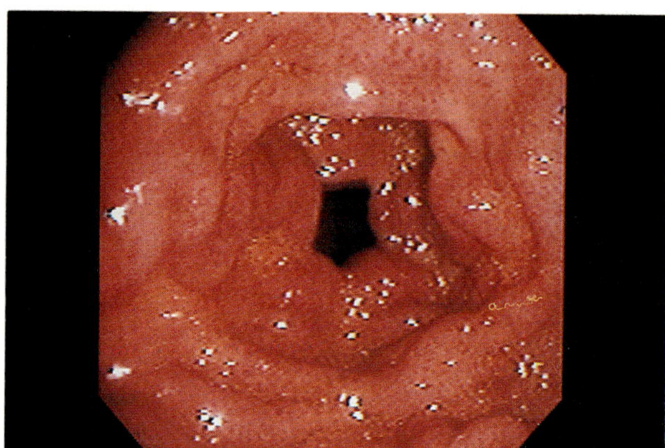

Plate XXV. Endoscopic appearance of acute GVHD in stomach, day 32. The pyloric channel is in the center of the picture. The mucosa of the gastric antrum is edematous, reddened and friable.

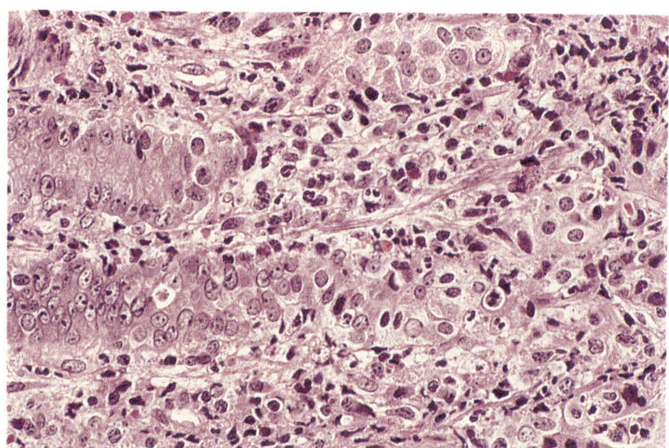

Plate XXVI. Gastric biopsy with GVHD, day 35. Of all upper endoscopic biopsy sites, that most frequently showing histologic changes of GVHD is the stomach. The gastric alterations are often focal and more subtle than those in the intestinal biopsies. Apoptotic bodies located along the basilar portion of the gastric crypts are sometimes the only diagnostic alterations. Chronic inflammation is usually spotty and may be absent. Nonetheless, the finding of apoptotic bodies in the gastric biopsy in a patient with unexplained nausea and vomiting is highly correlated with GVHD.

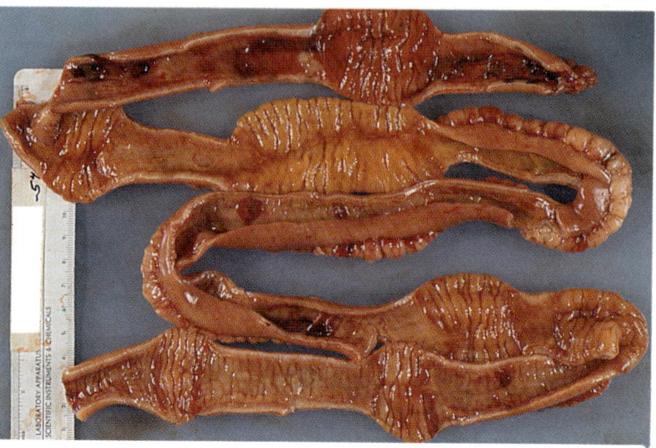

Plate XXVII. Surgical resection of severe longstanding intestinal GVHD, day 207. Scarred, ulcerated mucosa alternates with dilated areas of mucosal regeneration. The ulcerated portions demonstrate complete loss of epithelium and severe submucosal fibrosis. There is very high risk of invasive fungal or bacterial infection. Some patients have responded well to intestinal resection for localized GVHD.

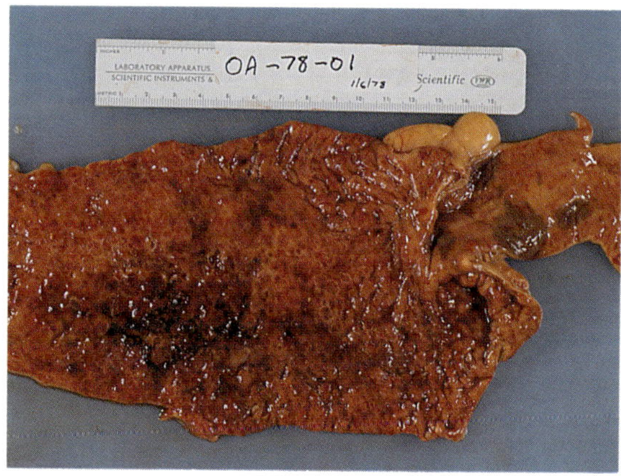

Plate XXVIII. Severe GVHD of ileum and cecum, day 80. The mucosal lining and folds are replaced by a friable beefy red diffusely ulcerated lamina propria. The numerous exposed capillaries ooze blood and serum, a major cause of morbidity from intestinal GVHD. The endothelial cells and fibroblasts within the lamina propria are often infected with CMV as was true in this patient (see Plate XLI).

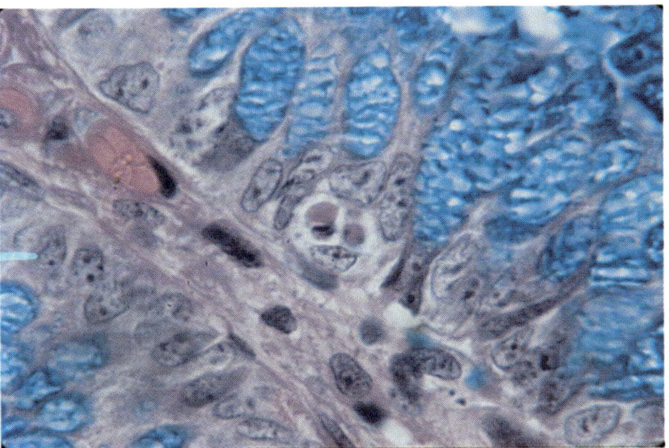

Plate XXIX. Apoptotic body typical of acute GVHD of the intestine, day 68. There is one apoptotic body, consisting of membrane-bound cellular debris lying above the basement membrane of a colonic crypt. Adjacent epithelial cells appear normal. Isolated apoptotic bodies within intact epithelium are typical of the early phase of acute GVHD. H&E with alcian blue counterstain.

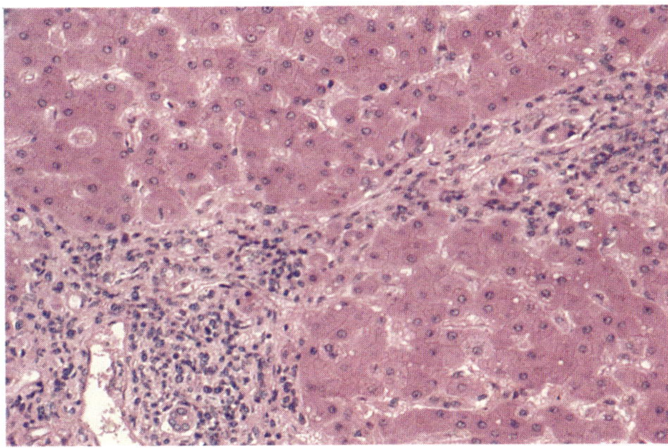

Plate XXXI. Hepatic GVHD, day 35. Portal spaces have extensively damaged bile ducts with focally necrotic epithelium, nuclei of irregular size and shape, segmental loss of nuclei, shrinkage of ductular lumen, and an eosinophilic syncytium of cytoplasm. The cellular infiltrate associated with GVHD is typically mononuclear but may include a few eosinophils and neutrophils. The amount of infiltrate is usually more sparse than shown here.

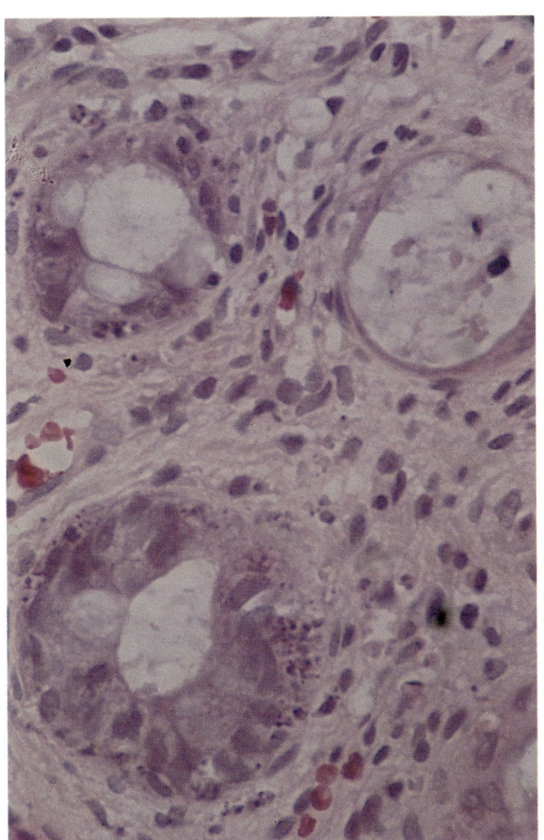

Plate XXX. Rectal biopsy with GVHD, day 53. Three mucosal crypts display varying degrees of damage. The bottom crypt shows apoptotic cells. More extensive cell damage is present in the crypt on the left. The right crypt has lost all enterocytes. Note infiltrating lymphocytes in the left crypt associated with nuclear debris characteristic of apoptosis.

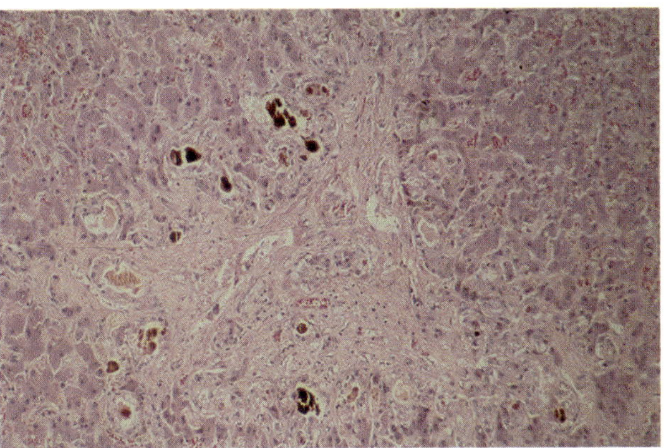

Plate XXXII. Hepatic GVHD with severe cholangiolar-hepatocellular cholestasis, day 68. Accompanying the damage to the small interlobular bile ducts are proliferations of large bile-filled cholangioles along the marginal zone of the irregularly expanded and fibrotic portal space. The full extent of this ductular proliferation is best appreciated with the use of an anticytokeratin stain. This type of cholangiolar proliferation occurs in long standing cases of GVHD.

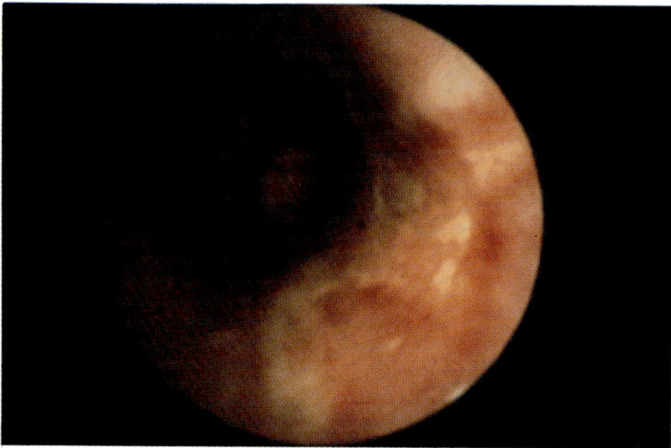

Plate XXXIII. Endoscopic appearance of CMV esophagitis, day 61. A shallow ulcer with serpiginous, reddened borders is seen in the distal esophagus. The ulcer base has a yellow, reticulated appearance.

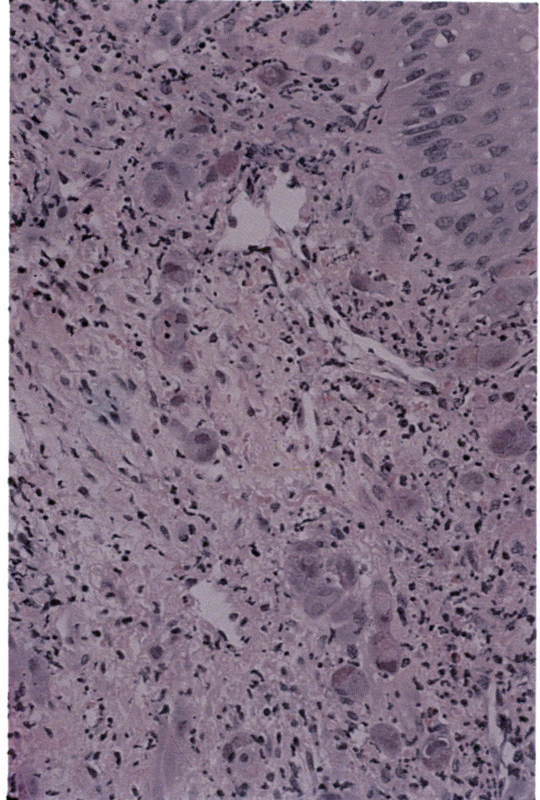

Plate XXXIV. Esophageal biopsy showing CMV infection, day 61. Large hyperchromatic cells containing both intranuclear and cytoplasmic inclusions are widely distributed in the subepithelial tissue. Immunohistochemical stains and in situ DNA hybridization would demonstrate additional infected cells which are neither large nor inclusion-bearing. The esophageal squamous epithelium (seen in the upper right) is never infected with CMV.

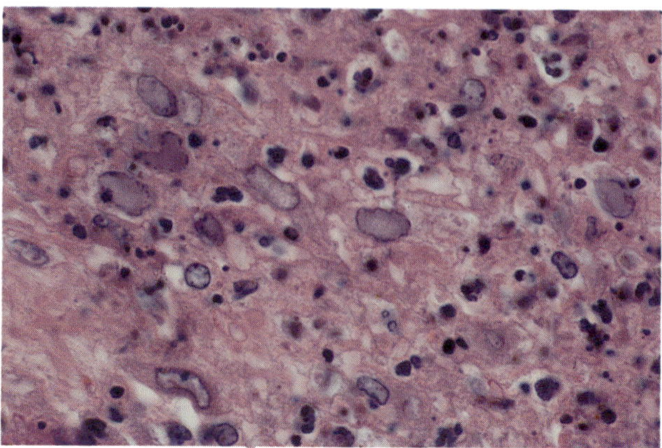

Plate XXXV. HSV infecting the lamina propria of the small intestine. Many cells display nuclear enlargement, chromatin margination and ground-glass nuclear inclusions. Heavy involvement of the lamina propria is unusual in HSV infection of the intestine.

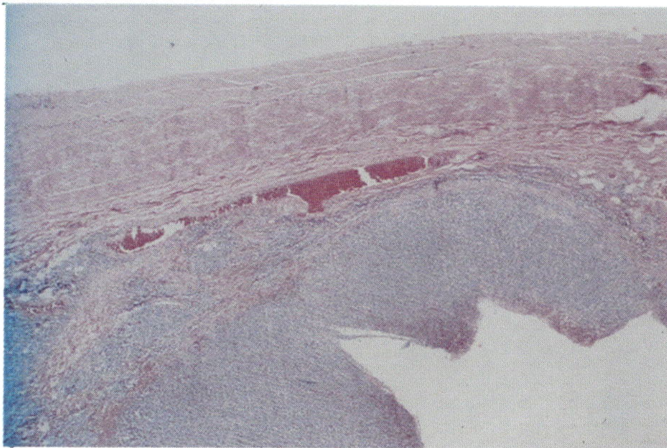

Plate XXXVI. EBV associated lymphoma infiltrating the intestinal mucosa in a boy treated for GVHD with CSP and a monoclonal antibody to T-lymphocytes. Although the GVHD improved, large, bizarre cells with atypical nucleoli characteristic of B-cell immunoblastic sarcoma rapidly formed tumor nodules in liver, spleen, lymph nodes and mesentery.

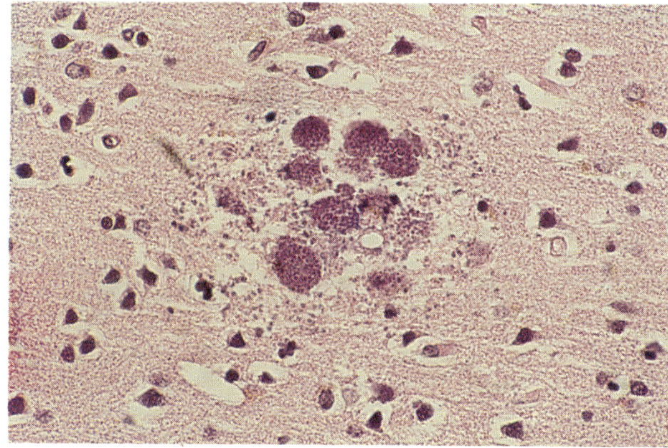

Plate XXXVII. Focal *Toxoplasma* encephalitis at autopsy, day 59. The large tissue cysts have released tachyzoites, which are proliferating and destroying cells. Toxoplasmosis following BMT usually results from reactivation in seropositive patients and is associated with GVHD.

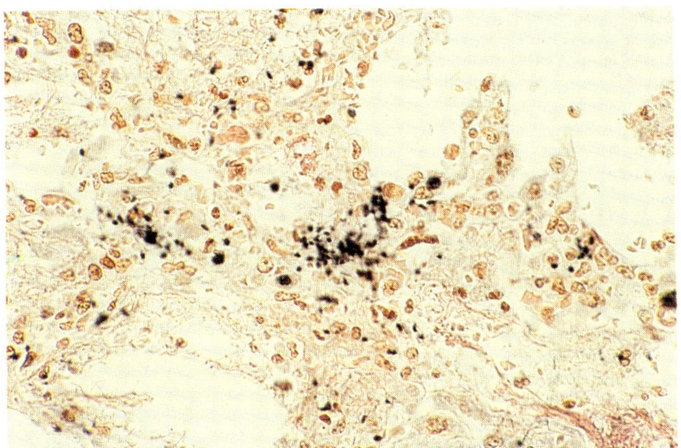

Plate XXXVIII. *Toxoplasma* pneumonia with immunocytochemical staining of tachyzoites, which appear as small, dark, circular and curved forms. Disseminated infection in the lungs and other organs is usually identified at autopsy, since immunocompromised marrow recipients produce a weak or negative serological response. Identification of parasites in a biopsy is diagnostic.

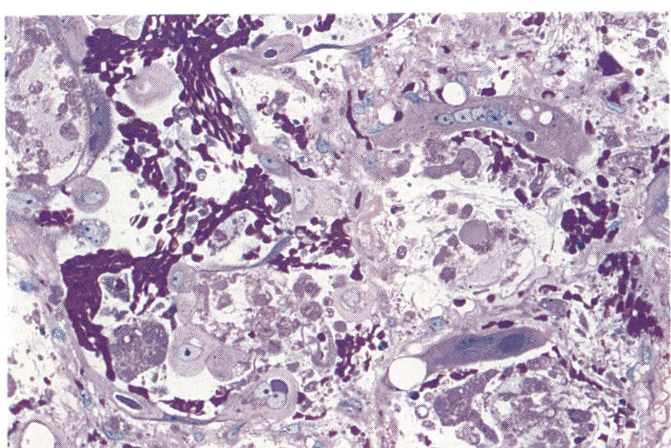

Plate XXXIX. Respiratory syncytial virus (RSV) pneumonia in a lung biopsy, day 48. The presence of dark purple cytoplasmic inclusions in multinucleated epithelial cells suggests the diagnosis but may be present with other viruses such as parainfluenza. During severe community outbreaks, infection may spread to hospitalized marrow recipients.

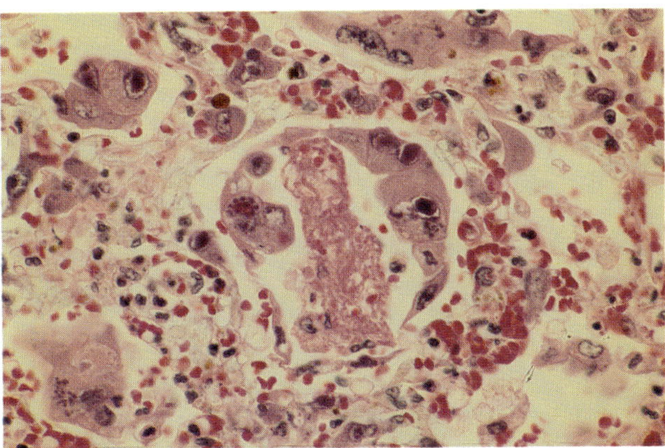

Plate XL. Severe CMV pneumonia at autopsy, day 81. Large oval nuclear inclusions as well as small clustered cytoplasmic inclusions are present.

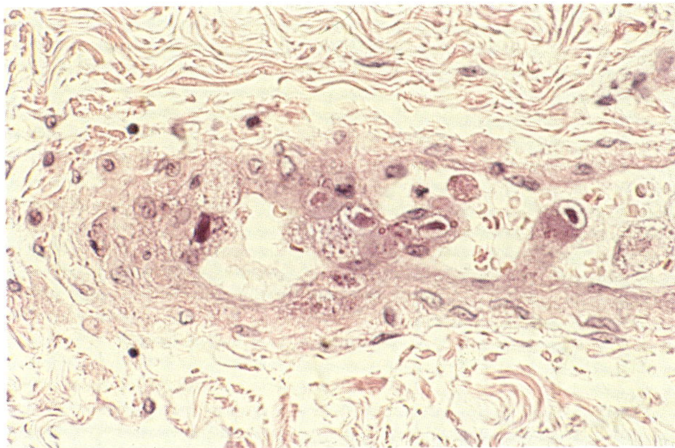

Plate XLI. Disseminated CMV with cutaneous vasculitis, day 71. Abdominal skin from autopsy shows a venule with microthrombosis and heavy CMV infection of the endothelium. Four days before death, the patient developed fever, jaundice, rising transaminases and shock. There was extensive CMV infection of lungs, liver, pancreas, adrenals and kidney glomeruli as well as hemorrhagic necrosis of subcutaneous fat. Despite the frequency of CMV dissemination after BMT, cutaneous involvement is rare.

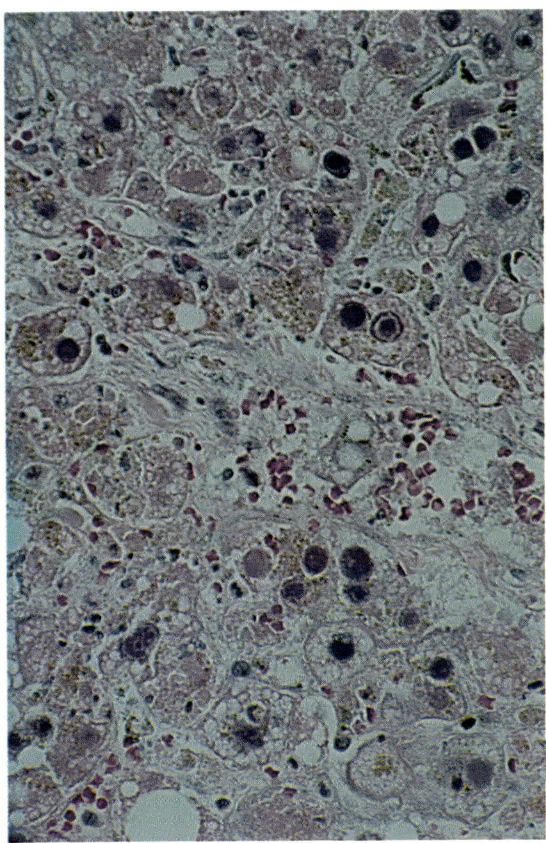

Plate XLII. Overwhelming adenovirus hepatitis at autopsy 92 days after allogeneic BMT for AML. Dark basophilic nuclear inclusions produce "smudge cells" with blurred nuclear margins. Occasional cells with a halo around the inclusion (right center) suggest a combined infection with CMV, which was confirmed by isolation of both viruses.

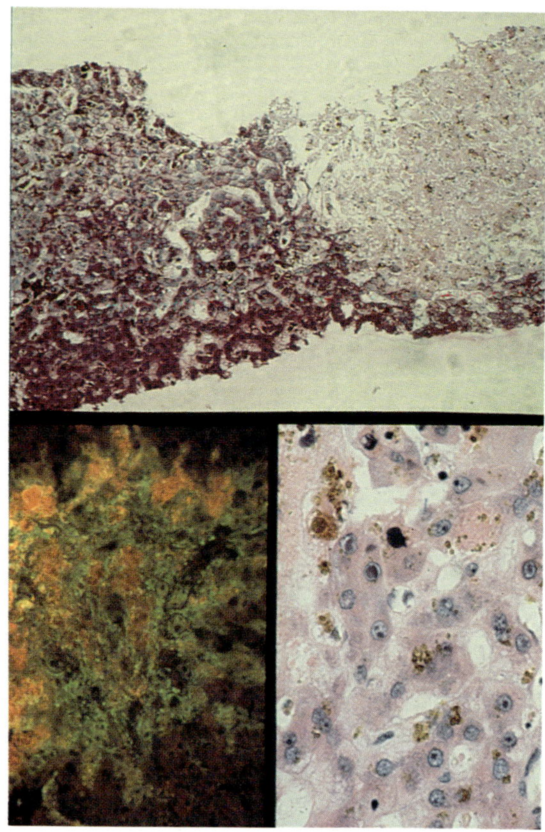

Plate XLIII. Varicella zoster virus (VZV) hepatitis in a percutaneous needle biopsy, day 79. At the top, a PAS stain demonstrates a pale necrotic area bordered by cells containing nuclear inclusions visible by H&E stain on the lower right. Immunofluorescence confirmed the presence of VZV (lower left) and intravenous acyclovir was begun within hours of the biopsy.

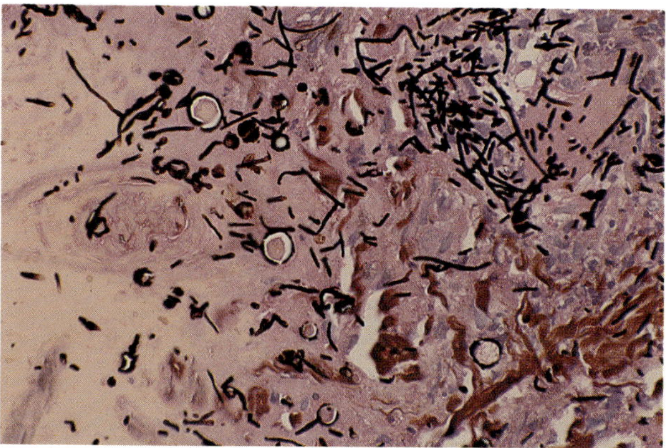

Plate XLIV. *Fusarium* hyphae invade the dermis in a pretransplant skin biopsy.

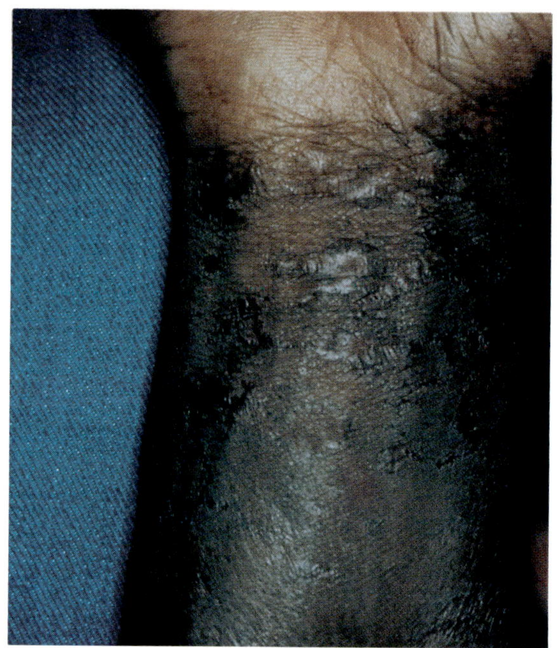

Plate XLV. Lichen planus-like chronic GVHD of the forearm of a 24-year-old black male 220 days after BMT of HLA-identical marrow.

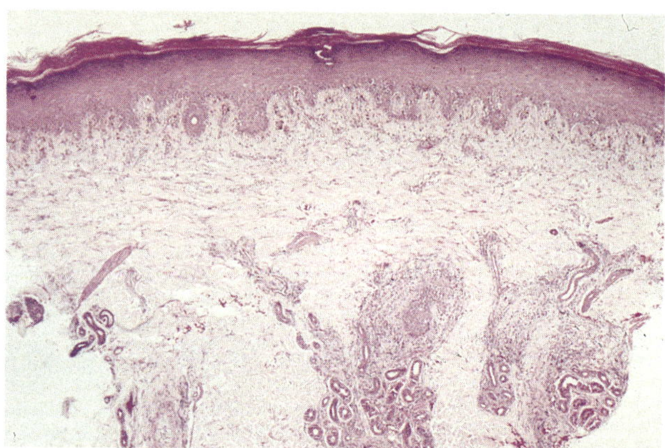

Plate XLVI. Lichen planus-like early chronic GVHD of skin, day 233. Biopsy of a papulosquamous lesion from the posterior neck demonstrates the characteristic features of the generalized or inflammatory type of chronic cutaneous GVHD. The thickened epidermis has hyper- and parakeratosis, hypergranulosis and acanthosis. The extensive destruction along the dermal-epidermal junction results in sawtooth-like changes of the rete ridges mimicking lichen planus. The papillary dermis has considerable perivascular inflammation. The lichenoid reaction also involves the hair follicles and eccrine glands seen deep in the reticular dermis. At this stage, treatment can prevent progression to fibrosis (see Plate LI).

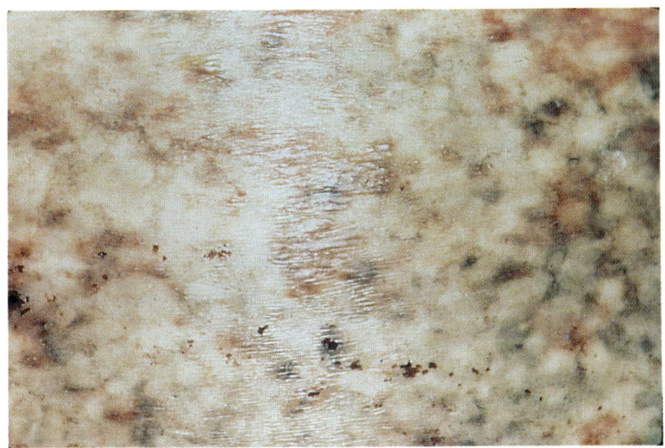

Plate XLVII. Poikiloderma in late chronic GVHD in a 2-year-old girl, day 450. Thinning of the epidermis and dermis are present along with telangiectasia and reticulated pigmentation.

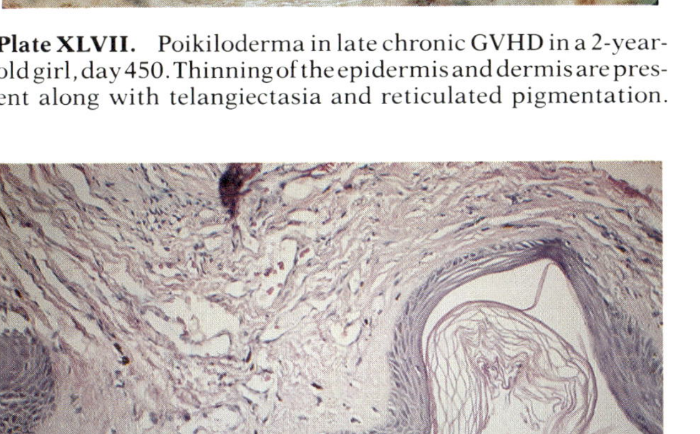

Plate XLVIII. Poikiloderma, day 719. The patient was treated vigorously for extensive chronic GVHD with corticosteroids plus several other immunosuppressive agents. Though he had extensive dyspigmentation, telangiectasia and atrophy of the skin, there were no contractures or scleroderma. Histologically, the epidermis is atrophic with loss of rete ridges. The fibrotic papillary dermis contains many telangiectatic vessels and there is intracellular melanin pigment. The deep dermal sweat glands remain despite earlier inflammatory involvement and the reticular dermal collagen is normal.

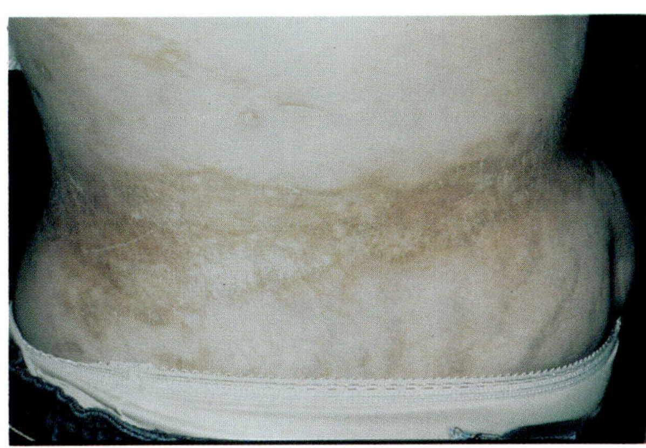

Plate XLIX. Localized late phase of chronic GVHD resembling morphea with atrophic plaque formation, induration and peripheral hyperpigmentation, day 684.

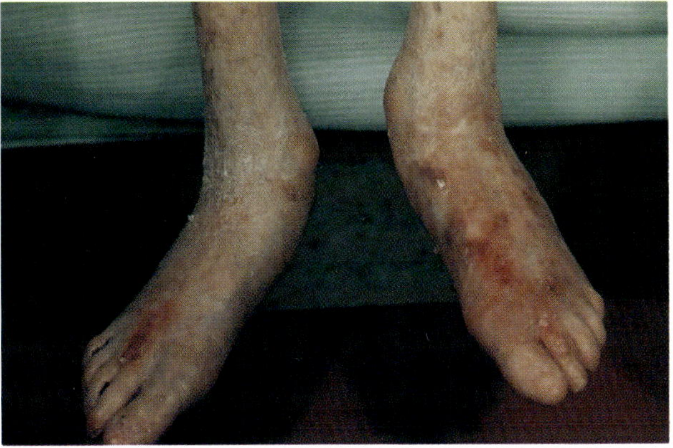

Plate L. Generalized scleroderma with atrophy, sclerodactyly and joint contracture, day 540 after HLA-identical BMT.

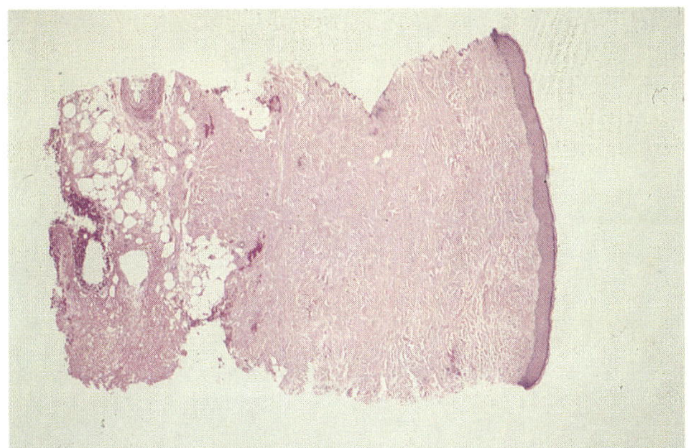

Plate LI. Late chronic GVHD of skin, day 959. As this patient's GVHD progressed, the epidermis became atrophic with straightening of the dermal-epidermal junction. All dermal appendages were destroyed. The reticular dermal collagen became increasingly sclerotic. A panniculitis seen at the base of the specimen resulted in fibrosis of the subcutaneous fat and large vessels. This histological picture corresponds to dense hidebound and sclerodermatous changes of late chronic GVHD.

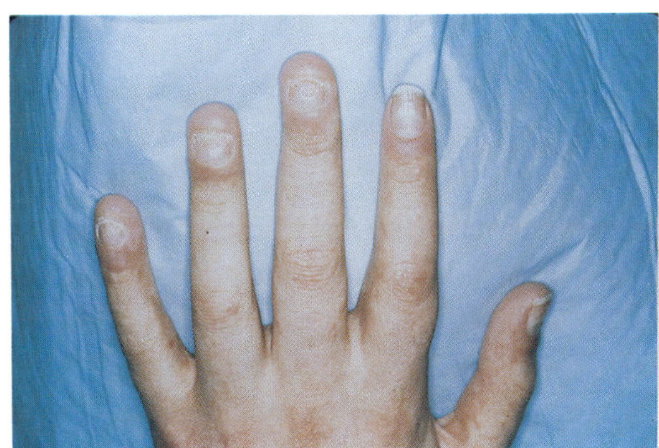

Plate LII. Periungal erythema and onychodystrophy 100 days after allogeneic BMT in a patient with ocular sicca and oral lesions of chronic GVHD.

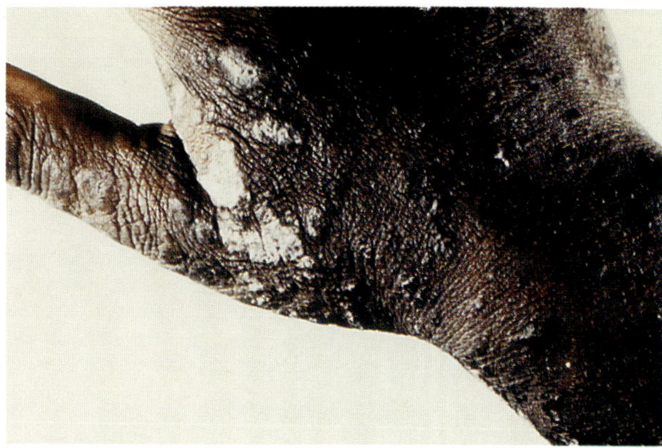

Plate LIII. Lichen planus-like chronic GVHD before treatment, day 220.

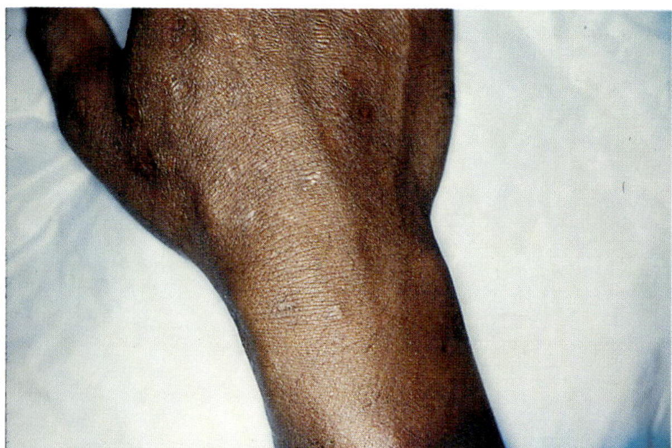

Plate LIV. Same patient shown in Plates XLV and LIII after treatment, day 770.

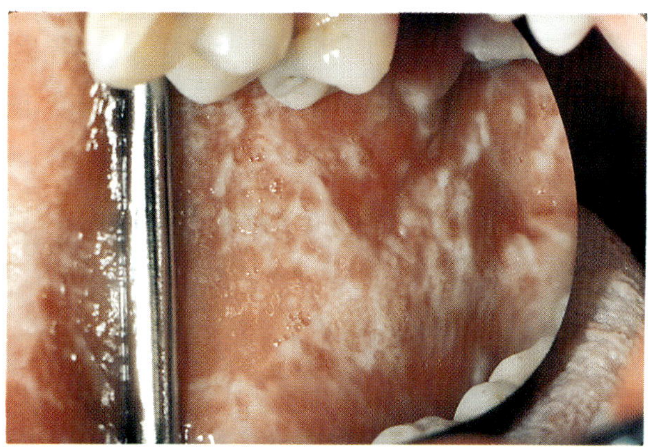

Plate LV. Lichenoid lesions of oral chronic GVHD showing erythema, white striae, plaque and ulcer formation, day 394.

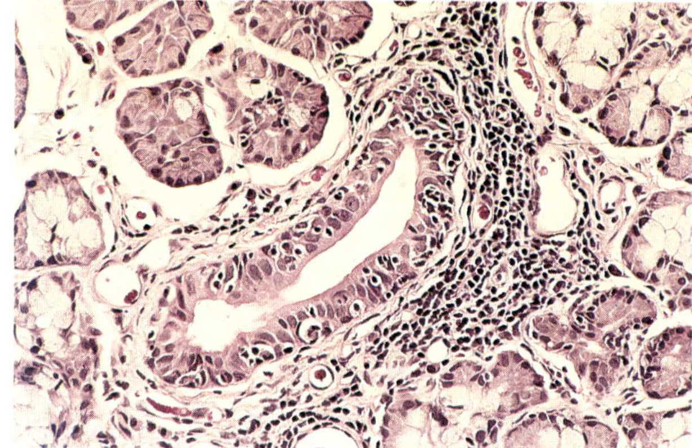

Plate LVI. Oral labial biopsy with early chronic GVHD, day 92. The minor salivary gland exhibits a periductal mononuclear inflammatory infiltrate which involves focally necrotic duct epithelium. There is inflammation of adjacent acini. This process leads to fibrosis with acinar atrophy in lobules drained by the affected ducts. The squamous surface epithelium (not present here) showed grade II lesions similar to those previously illustrated in skin (Plate XXI). The lip biopsy is valuable in the diagnosis and staging of chronic GVHD because it frequently mirrors destructive inflammatory changes in lacrimal, tracheal and esophageal glands as well as bile ducts.

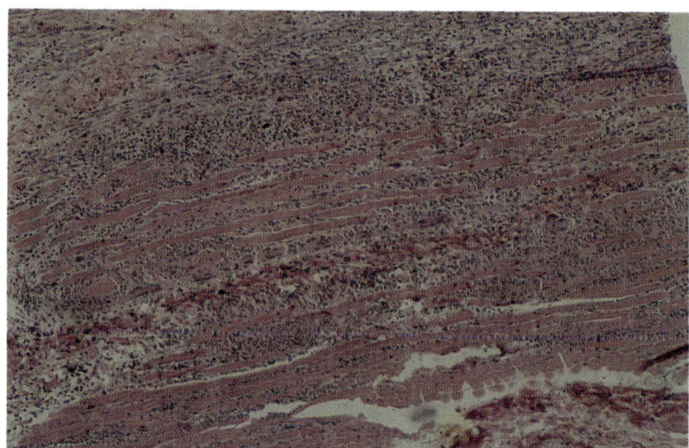

Plate LVII. Polymyositis in deltoid muscle biopsy associated with chronic GVHD, day 1129. There is extensive endomysial chronic inflammation associated with myocyte destruction. The condition responded to immunosuppressive therapy.

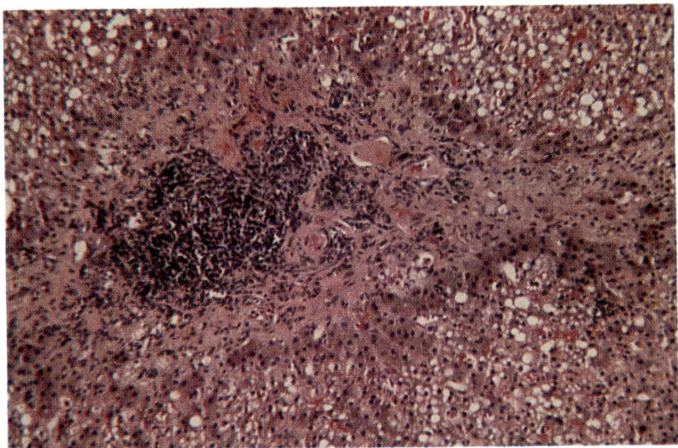

Plate LVIII. Chronic GVHD of liver, day 166. This biopsy shows a prominent plasmacytic infiltrate in the portal area and a paucity of interlobular bile ducts. The histological dichotomy between acute and chronic GVHD is less clear in liver than in skin. However, increased portal inflammation and loss of bile ducts are more common in chronic GVHD. Despite the frequency of chronic hepatic GVHD, cirrhosis and liver failure are rare and may reflect superinfection with hepatitis C virus.

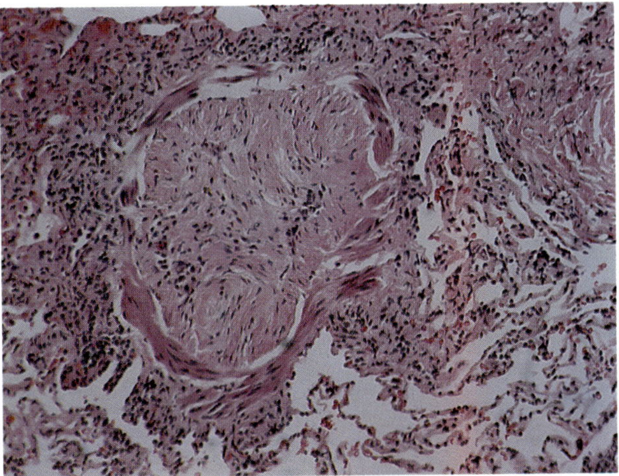

Plate LIX. Bronchiolitis obliterans in a lung biopsy, day 396. The patient had chronic GVHD with severe obstructive pulmonary disease. Similar small airway inflammation with fibrosis is seen in lung allograft rejection.

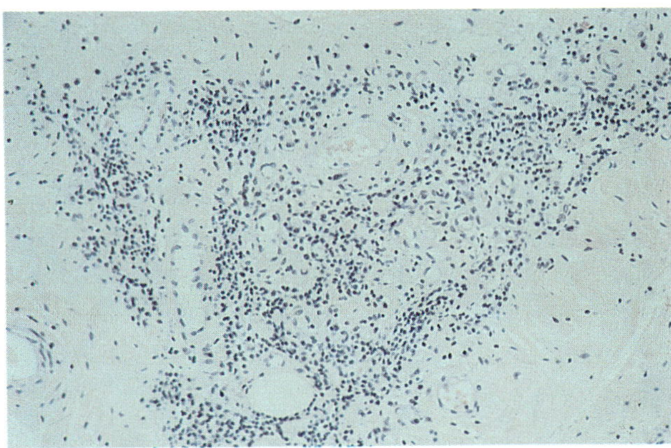

Plate LX. Atrophy and fibrosis of thymus associated with chronic GVHD in a 13-year-old, day 350. The patient had not received immunosuppressive drugs, so the destruction was presumably the result of chronic GVHD activity.

Acknowledgment

The editors gratefully acknowledge the contributions of the following investigators in providing these clinical and histologic color illustrations: Robert C. Hackman, MD, George E. Sale, MD, Keith M. Sullivan, MD, Mark Schubert, DDS, George B. McDonald, MD, Howard M. Shulman, MD.

Chapter 32
Other Viruses After Marrow Transplantation

Raleigh A. Bowden

Viral infections have been among the leading causes of morbidity and mortality following bone marrow transplantation (BMT). The most common virus infections after BMT include cytomegalovirus (CMV), herpes simplex virus (HSV), and varicella zoster virus (VZV) (1). In addition, Epstein-Barr virus (EBV) has been associated with a malignant lymphoproliferative complication seen in 0.6% of patients after BMT (2), although other clinical manifestations of EBV have not been described in the BMT setting. The herpesviruses are discussed in detail in other chapters in this book. The subject of this chapter is "other" viruses, which currently have received relatively less attention than the herpesvirus. This lack of attention is due, in part, to the necessity of coping with the more common viruses, which until only recently have not had effective treatment. The importance of the less common "other" viruses becomes evident as better control of herpesvirus infection in BMT recipients is achieved.

Included in this chapter is a discussion of: (1) "other" DNA viruses, which become latent and reactivate with immunosuppression (e.g., adenovirus and human herpesvirus type 6 [HHV6]); (2) respiratory viruses; and (3) less commonly reported but potentially problematic viruses in the BMT setting (e.g., parvovirus B19, the enteroviruses [Coxsackie virus and echovirus], rotavirus, measles, BK virus, and JC virus).

The goal of this chapter is to provide a review of virology, epidemiology, pathogenesis, immunity, and clinical manifestations of infection with each virus, with specific focus on experience in the BMT setting. Discussion includes a review of methods of diagnosis, prevention, and treatment. A summary of morbidity and mortality of each virus infection following BMT is also included.

Adenovirus

Virology and Epidemiology

Adenovirus is a nonenveloped DNA virus, measuring 70 nm in diameter. Adenovirus replication and assembly occurs in the nucleus, and virions are released when the cell is lysed. Adenovirus causes both lytic and latent infection. Infection may persist from days to years and may occur in host tissue (e.g., adenoidal) without causing apparent symptoms in immunocompetent hosts.

All adenovirus share a common group-specific complement-fixing antigen. There are at least 41 human adenovirus serotypes, although less than 40% of serotypes are implicated in human disease. Serotypes 1, 2, 5, and 6 are endemic to most areas, and types 4, 7, 14, and 21 are associated with epidemics in the general population. Primary infection is usually established early in life with either asymptomatic or symptomatic infection. By the age of 5, most people have been infected by one or more serotypes of adenovirus, resulting in latency with lifelong persistence of specific antibody.

Pathogenesis and Immunity

Transmission of adenovirus is either by respiratory droplet or the oral-fecal route. Adenovirus enters the mucosa and infects epithelial cells, resulting in inflammation and necrosis. Subsequent viremia may lead to infection of kidney, bladder, liver (Plate XLII), and lung, which are more common sites of invasive infection in BMT recipients than infection of the central nervous system seen in other settings. Because adenovirus becomes latent and chronic shedding in the absence of clinical disease can occur in the normal host, it is likely that many of the infections observed represent reactivation, although the exact proportion is unknown (3,4). Support for reactivation of adenovirus infection after BMT includes the nonseasonal pattern of virus isolation in this setting and the occurrence of virus shedding at a time similar to that of CMV infection (e.g., the median time of isolation of both CMV and adenovirus is 2–3 months after BMT).

There is no information available about reconstitution of specific immunity to adenovirus following BMT. It is likely, based on experience with the herpesviruses, that humoral immune responses will be unpredictable in the early post-transplant period, and cellular immunity has a primary role in the control of adenovirus infection.

Clinical Manifestations

In normal hosts, the most common presenting manifestations of adenovirus infection are respiratory and include pharyngitis, tracheitis, bronchitis, and pneumonitis (5). Adenovirus accounts for approximately 4 to 10% of viral pneumonia and bronchiolitis in children (adenovirus rarely causes disseminated infection with hepatitis, hemorrhagic cystitis, and enteritis in normal hosts outside the newborn period). These complications may be seen more commonly in immunocompromised patients (6). Severe disseminated adenovirus infection can occur in infants between the ages of 3 and 18 months. Serotypes 2, 3, 5, 7, and 21 are associated with illness in the general pediatric patient population. In addition, some fastidious serotypes, notably 40 and 41, are a significant cause of gastroenteritis in infants and young children (5–10%).

Most of the experience reported for adenovirus infection in immunocompromised hosts comes from descriptions following BMT (3,7,8) or following liver (9,10) or renal transplantation (11). Severity of infection appears to increase with increasing degrees of immunosuppression, as is common with other DNA viruses (1). In the largest published review of adenovirus infection in BMT recipients, Shields and colleagues (3) described adenovirus infection in 51 of 1,051 patients (5%) undergoing BMT from 1976 to 1982. The time from transplant to first viral isolation ranged from 13 to 199 days (mean, 44 days for those with serotypes 11, 34, or 35). An association of adenovirus infection with acute graft-versus-host disease (GVHD) was observed in this study.

A second retrospective study of adenovirus infection after BMT identified a similar incidence of adenovirus in 19 of 502 marrow transplants (4%) (7). Serotype 11 was the most common isolate in this study and was associated with hemorrhagic cystitis. Serotypes 1, 5, and 33 were also isolated. A virological survey of 96 pediatric marrow transplant recipients described adenovirus infection in 17 patients (18%), which was the second most common virus isolated after HSV (8). Type 12 was the most common isolate in this study. An association of adenovirus and GVHD in this study was also observed.

Table 32-1 summarizes the spectrum of adenovirus infection and disease in BMT recipients (3,7,8). It was not possible from the study by Shields and colleagues (3) to determine the incidence of asymptomatic infection in the patients reviewed, because a majority of patients had fever (N = 34), elevated liver enzyme levels (N = 43), elevated renal function studies (N = 13), and 31 were also infected with HSV or CMV, or both.

Invasive infection developed in 10 of the 51 infected patients from Shields and colleagues' (3) study. Seven of these 10 had infection identified in lung. Two of 5 patients with adenovirus in urine had clinical evidence of renal impairment, and 2 patients had virus in liver (Plate XLII), both with evidence of clinical hepatitis. Half the patients with disseminated infection died. No source of infection was identified but was presumed to be from reactivation of infection.

Table 32-1.
Manifestations of Adenovirus Infection After Marrow Transplant

	Shields et al. (3)	*Ambinder et al. (7)*	*Wasserman et al. (8)*
Total patients reviewed	1051	502	96
Total infections	51	19	17
Site cultured			
urine	22	10	9
stool	13	NR	11
throats	25	NR	3
hematuria	16	4	1
Tissue-documented (no. of patients)	10	NR	2
Pneumonia	7	NR	2
Renal	5	NR	1
Gut	2	NR	
Liver	2	NR	1
Spleen	2	NR	1
Adenovirus-associated mortality	5	2	1

An association noted between adenovirus serotype 11 in the urine and hemorrhagic cystitis in the study by Ambinder and co-workers (7) has been reported in at least three other studies (3,4,8). However, adenovirus was implicated as the cause of hemorrhagic cystitis in only 0.7% of patients in a center that reported a 20% incidence of hemorrhagic cystitis (7). Adenovirus type 5 has been reported as a cause of fulminant hepatitis after allogeneic transplantation (12).

Diagnostic Techniques

The diagnosis of adenovirus is made using routine tissue culture, immunofluorescence, or centrifugation culture techniques (13). By standard isolation in fibroblasts or heteroploid cells, the cytopathic effect of adenovirus is usually apparent within 5 to 7 days after inoculation. The diagnosis can also be made by demonstration of viral antigen in infected tissue. Serologies are presumably of limited value in the early post-BMT period because of variable ability of patients to mount an antibody response to infection and passive acquisition of antibody from blood products or intravenous immunoglobulin (IVIg).

Prevention and Treatment

There is no known form of prophylaxis of adenovirus infection for any clinical setting. There are also no known demonstrated antiviral agents effective for treatment, although both ganciclovir and phosphonacetic acid have shown in vitro activity against adenovirus. Alpha interferon (14), aerosolized ribavirin (15), and, more recently, intravenous ribavirin (16) have been used to treat either disseminated infection or hemorrhagic cystitis. In addition, treatment with human immune serum containing high titers of neutralizing antibody against adenovirus was associated with a successful outcome in a patient with combined immunodeficiency and disseminated infection (17).

Summary of Impact of Adenovirus Infection on Morbidity and Mortality After BMT

Adenovirus appears to infect approximately 5 to 18% of BMT recipients as a result of either primary respiratory or oral-fecal transmission or reactivation of latent virus. The proportion of each is not known. Adenovirus has similar epidemiology to CMV, and a majority of infections will be asymptomatic, usually becoming detectable during the second to third month after transplantation. When disseminated adenovirus infection occurs, it primarily affects the urinary tract, the liver, and the lungs, resulting in death in as many as 50% of patients. Serotype 11 is most commonly associated with hemorrhagic cystitis. GVHD is a risk factor for both development and severity of adenovirus infection. Current therapy consists of supportive care only because there are no proven means of prevention or treatment of adenovirus. Late infections can occur in the setting of chronic GVHD.

Respiratory Viruses

Virology and Epidemiology

Respiratory viruses are becoming increasingly appreciated as an important cause of morbidity and mortality after BMT. Such infections may occur in as many as 20% of patients during the winter months (18–20). Respiratory virus infection may be acquired before transplantation, with onset of clinical manifestations in the first few weeks after BMT. Alternatively, patients can acquire infection following BMT from either infected family members, health care workers, or other community exposures.

The most commonly identified respiratory viruses isolated following BMT, in order of frequency, are respiratory syncytial virus (RSV); parainfluenza types 1, 2, and 3; and influenza types A and B. For the purposes of this review, adenoviruses are described separately because they can be acquired by either respiratory or oral-fecal contact. Infection may also commonly result from reactivation in BMT recipients.

Table 32-2 shows a composite of 5 years of experience with respiratory virus isolates at Fred Hutchinson Cancer Research Center (FHCRC). This overview combined routine culturing data from all patients with upper or lower respiratory tract symptoms, beginning with a prospective study during the 1987 respiratory virus season (18). The data show a wide variation in the types and numbers of respiratory viruses recovered each year. Overall, RSV was most common, followed by parainfluenza types 1 and 3, then influenza type A. Review of the epidemiology in the general community virology laboratory (University of Washington Virology Laboratory) records for the 1991 to 1992 season showed the most common community isolate to be RSV, followed by influenza type A and parainfluenza type 1. The spectrum of respiratory viruses seen in the 1991 to 1992 season appeared to be an approximate reflection of the respiratory virus pattern isolated in the community.

Table 32-2.
Incidence and Type of Respiratory Viruses, FHCRC 1987–1992

	Influenza		*Parainfluenza*					
Season (ref)	*A*	*B*	*1*	*2*	*3*	*RSV*	*Rhinovirus*	*Total*
1987 (18)	1		9		2	1		13
1987–88	4	1	7	2	2	2		18
1988–89	2	1				3	21	27
1989–90 (14)						31	4	35
1990–91	2		1		3	5	2	13
1991–92	3		1	1	9	2	4	20
Total	12	2	18	3	16	44	31	126

The timing of infection in BMT recipients by month during the 1991 to 1992 season is shown in Figure 32-1. Isolation of respiratory viruses occurred from November to March; the highest number of isolates were identified in February. During this season, no single virus type predominated, in contrast to the predominance of RSV observed in 1989 to 1990.

Respiratory Syncytial Virus

RSV is classified as a pneumovirus in the paramyxovirus family. It contains single-stranded RNA, and there are at least two known antigenic

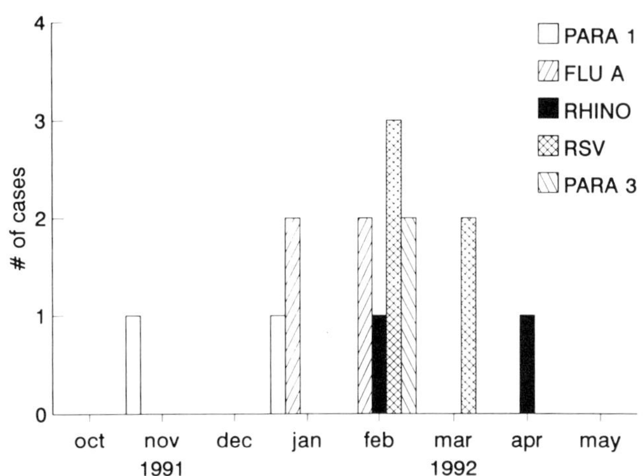

Figure 32-1. Type of respiratory virus isolated and number of cases by month during the 1991 to 1992 respiratory virus season at Fred Hutchinson Cancer Research Center. *Bars* on graph represent parainfluenza type 1 (PARA 1), parainfluenza type 3 (PARA 3), influenza type A (FLU A), rhinovirus (RHINO); and respiratory syncytial virus (RSV), as shown.

subgroups (A and B). The usual incubation period is 1 to 4 days. RSV is the major cause of pneumonia and bronchiolitis in otherwise healthy infants. It causes frequent reinfections, usually manifested as uncomplicated upper respiratory infection (URI) or febrile bronchitis in healthy adults. A high proportion of initial RSV infections are complicated by otitis media and lower respiratory tract involvement.

RSV is also the most commonly described respiratory virus in immunocompromised patients, including those with cancer (21), severe combined immunodeficiency (22), and following BMT (18,19,23,24) and solid organ transplantation (24–26).

Parainfluenza Virus

Parainfluenza, an enveloped paramyxovirus containing single-stranded RNA, is classified into four serotypes, of which the first three, types 1, 2, and 3, are the most common. Parainfluenza is antigenically more stable than influenza. The incubation period for parainfluenza is 1 to 4 days. The common presentation in normal children includes laryngotracheitis for parainfluenza type 1, croup or URI for type 2, and severe lower respiratory tract infection for type 3, although much clinical overlap occurs. Symptoms in normal adults may be manifested as nonspecific URI, sinusitis, or, less frequently, lower respiratory tract infection for all three common serotypes.

In the largest epidemiological review of parainfluenza infection after BMT, parainfluenza type 3 was most common (19 of 27 patients), followed in decreasing frequency by type 2 (4 patients), type 1 (3 patients), and type 4 (1 patient) (20).

Influenza

Influenza virus belong to the family of orthomyxoviruses and are enveloped, single-stranded, pleomorphic RNA viruses. Influenza is classified into three major types, of which type A is the most common, followed by type B. Influenza type C is uncommon, even in the normal population, has not been reported following BMT, and will not be discussed further.

The incubation period of influenza type A is short, (mean, 2 days). Transmission is by direct droplet spread or aerosolized respiratory secretions. Nearly all patients have upper respiratory symptoms with or without fever. Infection in BMT recipients may be associated with persistent high fever without the typical myalgias, headache, and shaking chills seen with typical influenza. Influenza type A can cause lower respiratory tract infection indistinguishable from other forms of interstitial pneumonia in BMT recipients and may be associated with high mortality.

Influenza type B is seen less commonly following BMT, presumably because it causes less frequent epidemics in the community, usually every 2 to 3 years. Influenza type B accounted for only 2 of 14 influenza isolates over 5 years at the FHCRC (see Table 32-2). Two BMT recipients have also been reported in an outbreak among 6 transplant recipients over a 3-week period at another institution (27).

Rhinovirus and Other Respiratory Viruses

Rhinovirus is classified as a picornavirus characterized by small, naked, single-stranded RNA. There are nearly 100 accepted serotypes, which usually cause mild URI symptoms in normal hosts. Rhinovirus is infrequently reported as a cause of upper respiratory tract infection after BMT. Two of 80 respiratory isolates in the 5-year experience from FHCRC were identified as rhinovirus (see Table 32-2), and one of 19 reported BMT pediatric respiratory isolates was identified as a rhinovirus (8). Lower respiratory infection with rhinovirus has been reported in infants and young children but not following BMT.

Coronavirus and measles are other causes of respiratory infections caused by RNA viruses. Infections by coronavirus has not been reported in BMT recipients. However, measles is a recognized cause of severe giant-cell pneumonia, developing with or without rash, and of severe central nervous system (CNS) disease in immunocompromised hosts (28).

Pathogenesis and Immunity

In general, respiratory viruses infect the epithelium of the respiratory tract. Viremia and disseminated infection are uncommon. Respiratory viruses replicate primarily in the ciliated epithelium, with resulting inflammation and necrosis. These viruses are also directly toxic to tissues. Both mechanical and cellular host responses can be impaired severely in normal hosts; presumably this impairment is even worse in the BMT setting, although it has not been specifically studied. It is not uncommon to see coinfection with agents such as CMV (19,20) or bacterial infection (20) in BMT recipients at the time of respiratory virus isolation.

Clinical Manifestations

Until recently, there has been little information about the incidence and severity of respiratory viral infections after BMT. Study of respiratory viruses is complicated by their relatively low frequency of detection, their diversity, and changing seasonal patterns from year to year. The pattern seen after BMT presumably reflects the viral epidemiology seen in the general community.

The morbidity associated with respiratory virus infections following BMT has been described in a number of published reviews (18–20). The first study reviewed all respiratory viruses isolated during a single season (18). This was a study of a cohort of 78 consecutive BMT recipients studied prospectively from January through April 1987, with cultures in all patients from the pretransplant evaluation and culturing of all symptomatic patients through the first 3 months after BMT. The goal was to determine incidence, severity, and outcome of respiratory virus infections. Fifteen of 78 patients (19%) had positive cultures for respiratory viruses, including adenovirus (see Table 32-2). Ten of 15 patients had virus recovered only prior to transplant, and 9 of 10 had upper respiratory symptoms (one was asymptomatic). Three patients had virus isolated only after BMT. Sinusitis and fever developed in one of these patients 80 days after transplantation, and the patient died with respiratory failure due to parainfluenza type 3 infection. Pneumonia developed in 2 patients 13 days (parainfluenza type 3) and 95 days (adenovirus) after BMT, respectively. The patient with parainfluenza type 3 infection recovered after aerosolized ribavirin treatment. The patient with adenovirus pneumonia died with hemorrhagic cystitis and disseminated infection.

Two patients had respiratory viruses isolated both before and after BMT. Parotitis and sinusitis developed on day 13 after BMT in one patient who had parainfluenza type 3 isolated 8 days prior to BMT; the patient recovered without antiviral treatment by day 31. The other had adenovirus in the throat, and gastrointestinal and lower respiratory tract symptoms developed after BMT. This patient survived. In summary, respiratory virus was isolated in 20% of patients during this single season. Most of the isolates were identified in the early post-transplant period, and the majority of patients had minimal morbidity. However, there were two respiratory virus–related deaths in 15 infected patients, one due to adenovirus and one due to RSV.

There are several reviews that focus on the morbidity and mortality of RSV after BMT. The largest reported outbreak occurred at FHCRC during 1989 to 1990 (19). This epidemic was observed 3 years after the initial report (18) and differed from the earlier report in that 31 of 33 recognized infections were caused by RSV (see Table 32-2) (19). In contrast to the previously reported season, the morbidity and mortality associated with the 1989 to 1990 epidemic was severe. Pneumonia developed in 18 of 31 patients (Figure 32-2, Plate XXXIX), 14 of whom died. Four different antigenic strains were identified in that epidemic, indicating that a common source was unlikely. RSV infection following BMT has also been reported in two smaller series. Eight patients were described by Hertz and associates (23); 6 had infection prior to marrow engraftment, and 4 of the 6 had fatal outcomes despite therapy with aerosolized ribavirin. In another study, infection developed in the first month after transplantation in 6 patients reported by Englund and colleagues (24). Three died despite therapy with aerosolized ribavirin.

The next largest respiratory virus experience following BMT was summarized in a report of parainfluenza viruses recovered over a 16-year period at the University of Minnesota (20). Twenty-seven of 1,253 patients (2%) had positive cultures for parainfluenza virus. Eight patients had upper respiratory involvement only; 19 of 27 (70%) had lower respiratory tract involvement with or without upper respiratory tract infection. Six of these 19 (32%) died with parainfluenza pneumonia. The most common type isolated was parainfluenza type 3, which accounted for 19 of the 27 isolates (70%). Sinusitis was commonly associated with all four serotypes. The median time of onset of infection was 23 days after BMT, with no obvious seasonal predilection.

Table 32-3 provides a broader perspective on severity of respiratory infection by describing the culture sites from which the different types of isolates were obtained from the FHCRC 5-year review of more than 2,400 transplantations. RSV, which was the major respiratory virus in this review, resulted in documented lower respiratory tract infection in approximately 50% of patients. The other major virus was parainfluenza type 3. Lower respiratory disease occurred in approximately 70% of patients from whom parainfluenza type 3 was isolated. A similar relative severity of parainfluenza type 3 compared with other parainfluenza serotypes in infants and young children has also been reported (15).

In the 1991 to 1992 season at FHCRC, there were 14 patients infected with respiratory viruses (excluding adenovirus). Eleven of 14 (79%) had virus isolated only from the upper respiratory tract (one rhinovirus, one parainfluenza type 1, 2 parainfluenza type 3, 3 influenza A viruses, and 4 RSV). Two patients with influenza type A had clinical sinusitis. No cultures were obtained from the sinuses. There were 3 patients

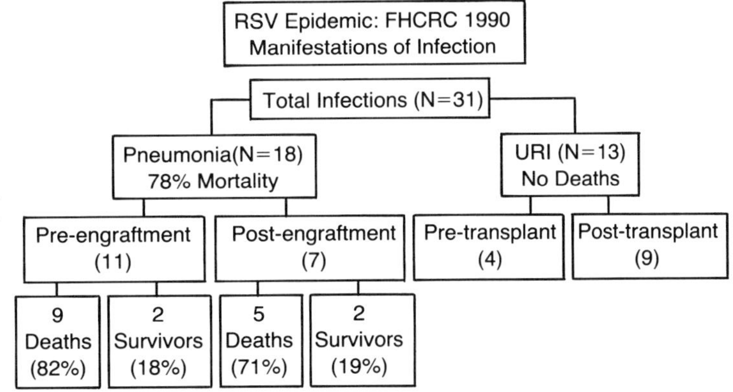

Figure 32-2. Mortality associated with respiratory syncytial virus (RSV) infection at Fred Hutchinson Cancer Research Center (FHCRC) during the 1989 to 1990 epidemic: Correlation with pneumonia or upper respiratory infection (URI) and engraftment status.

Table 32-3.
Site of Respiratory Virus Infection, FHCRC 1987–1992

		Culture Site—Respiratory*			
	Total Patients	*Upper (Throat or NP)*	*Sputum*	*Lower (BAL, ET or lung)*	*Unknown*
Influenza A	12	8		1	3
Influenza B	2	1		1	
Parainfluenza 1	18	6	8	4	
Parainfluenza 2	3	2		1	
Parainfluenza 3	16	12		4	
RSV	47	24		23	
Rhinovirus	29	28		1	
Total	127	81	8	35	3

First Positive Culture/Patient
*NP = nasopharyngeal; BAL = bronchoalveolar lavage; ET = endotracheal

with virologically documented pneumonia (one with parainfluenza type 1, one with influenza type A, and one with RSV). Clinical pneumonia without positive lower respiratory tract cultures developed in 2 additional patients, both with parainfluenza type 3 in their upper respiratory tract. All except one patient with parainfluenza type 3 died from pneumonia. Death was associated with isolation of virus prior to BMT in 3 patients and isolation pre-engraftment in 2.

Diagnosis of Respiratory Viruses

In general, respiratory viruses can be identified by several diagnostic methods utilizing secretions or tissue from the respiratory tract that contain respiratory epithelial cells. Although respiratory viruses can sometimes be recovered from throat cultures (e.g., adenovirus and influenza viruses), nasal swabs (29), washings/aspirates (30), or nasopharyngeal/throat swabs (31) are generally superior. Most articles comparing diagnostic techniques do so for diagnosis of RSV (29–31). Some argue that nasopharyngeal samples will miss cases of lower respiratory tract infection diagnosed by bronchoalveolar lavage (BAL) (31). There is debate about which source has the highest yield, and results may be affected by the age of the patient, the clinical setting, and the type of virus isolated. No studies have addressed which is the best type of specimen in the BMT setting, but it is likely that cultures from multiple sites will improve diagnostic yield.

Specimens can be examined by direct immunofluorescent staining of epithelial cells in respiratory secretions or lung tissue using various commercial enzyme immunoabsorbent assays or by inoculation of the specimen into cell culture. Serological diagnosis is unlikely to be useful in the transplant setting because of poor antibody responses to viruses (e.g., herpesviruses), the confounding effect of transient antibody acquired from blood products, or immunoglobulin administered in the early post-transplant period.

Prophylaxis of Respiratory Viruses

In general, the best form of prophylaxis is avoidance of exposure. Vaccines are available only for influenza types A and B. Their role for vaccination in the BMT setting is limited to annual vaccination of health care workers and family members in hopes of decreasing patient exposure. There are no studies evaluating the use of influenza vaccine in patients following BMT; however, this is unlikely to be a useful approach because infection often occurs when patients have little or no ability to mount an immune response early after BMT. Delaying BMT should be considered if feasible when a respiratory virus is identified prior to BMT, especially for viruses such as RSV or parainfluenza type 3, for which mortality is often high in the early post-transplant setting.

The use of amantadine prophylaxis after BMT has not been studied and, as with the vaccine strategy, may be more useful for health care workers, family members, and possibly patients before transplantation. Most published literature of prophylaxis deals with the use of amantadine for prevention of influenza, especially for prevention of transmission in hospital patients.

Treatment of Respiratory Viruses For Marrow Transplant Recipients

Supportive care and appreciation of potential complications, such as secondary bacterial infection in the lung, are the mainstays of treatment of respiratory virus infection. Ribavirin therapy, either aerosolized or intravenous, has not yet been shown to be of appreciable benefit for any of the respiratory viruses (19,23,24). Most of the treatment experience comes from the use of aerosolized ribavirin for the treatment of RSV (19,23,24), but there are also case reports about its use with other respiratory viruses, such as parainfluenza (20) or influenza type B (27). In the study of 27 patients with parainfluenza infections by Wendt and colleagues (20), 9 patients were treated with aerosolized ribavirin, 2 for upper respiratory tract infection and 7 for pneumonia. Seven of the 9 survived, compared with 14 of 18 patients not treated in that uncontrolled study.

Figure 32-3 depicts the 1989 to 1990 experience with RSV and outcome related to the use of aerosolized ribavirin in the first 100 days after transplantation (19). Because this was not a controlled study, it is not possible to draw conclusions about the efficacy of aerosolized ribavirin from this study. The mortality rate was high (78%) for patients in whom lower respiratory tract infection developed, regardless of whether the infection developed before or after engraftment. As mentioned previously in two smaller reports, there were 7 deaths in a total of 14 BMT recipients with RSV (23,24). All 7 died despite the use of aerosolized ribavirin. Intravenous ribavirin has recently become available for investigational use. It not clear which approach will be better because the aerosolized

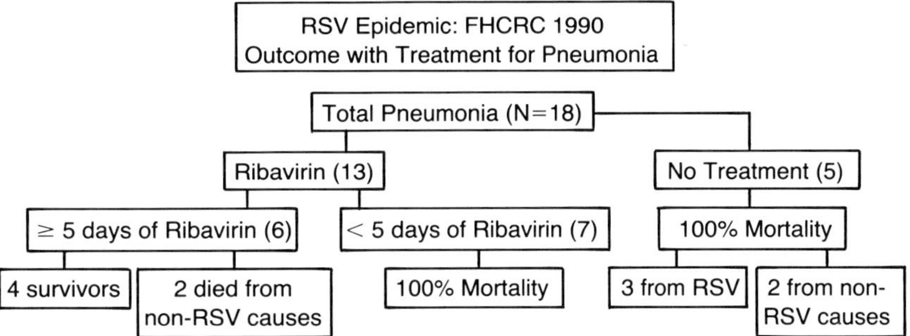

Figure 32-3. Mortality associated with respiratory syncytial virus (RSV) pneumonia at Fred Hutchinson Cancer Research Center (FHCRC) during the 1989 to 1990 epidemic: Relationship to the use of aerosolized ribavirin therapy and duration of treatment.

method may actually deliver more medication to the airway epithelium, which is the major site of infection. The use of oral ribavirin, which may be useful in patients with influenza type A, has not been reported in the BMT setting. Further studies are needed.

Immunoglobulin treatment using high titer RSV-specific globulin (RSVIg) in patients with lower respiratory tract infection has been investigated in infants with bronchiolitis and pneumonia (32,33). RSVIg appeared to shorten the duration of virus shedding and to improve oxygenation compared with control subjects (32). It is currently being studied for prophylaxis and therapy for RSV in young children at risk for severe disease. A Phase I study of patients with upper respiratory infection is also in progress at FHCRC in an effort to prevent progression to lower respiratory tract disease.

Summary of the Impact of Respiratory Virus Infection on Morbidity and Mortality after BMT

Respiratory viruses are being recognized as an increasingly important cause of viral infection after BMT, especially during the winter months. The epidemiology of respiratory infection varies each year and is dependent on the viruses present in the community. Because infection usually occurs in the first few weeks after BMT, it is presumed that many patients are infected prior to BMT. Although previously thought to be associated with minimal to moderate morbidity, recent larger epidemics have been associated with high mortality rates when infection progressed to pneumonia. RSV is the most commonly recognized respiratory virus, followed by parainfluenza and influenza viruses. There is no proven effective therapy for any of the respiratory viruses after BMT, although aerosolized ribavirin has been used. Specific IVIg and intravenous ribavirin are currently under investigation for RSV treatment.

Human Herpes Virus Type 6

Virology and Epidemiology

HHV6 is among the most ubiquitous virus in humans (34). HHV6 was first described in 1986 by Salahuddin and associates (35). Similar to other herpesviruses, it is enveloped and measures approximately 100 nm in diameter. HHV6 has been completely sequenced and most closely resembles CMV at the genomic level (36). HHV6 may contribute to the viral complications of BMT recipients for several reasons: (1) it is a herpesvirus and therefore has a latency state, (2) other herpesviruses cause significant morbidity and mortality after BMT, and (3) initial reports described isolation of the virus in immunosuppressed patients (34,35,37).

HHV6 was initially isolated from peripheral blood cells from patients with immune dysfunction, and has now been detected in the saliva of normal adults (38). It is a lymphotropic virus and grows preferentially in CD4 lymphocytes in vitro (39,40). Seroprevalence studies indicate that more than 90% of the healthy population is infected; most infections occur in early childhood. The only disease clearly associated with HHV6 is roseola infantum (38,41).

Clinical Manifestations and Diagnostic Techniques

Clinical manifestations of HHV6 in the BMT setting are not known. Asano and colleagues (42) first described recovery of HHV6 from peripheral blood mononuclear cell cocultivation from 3 pediatric BMT recipients with rash and fever. The largest study of HHV6 infection in the BMT population was done by Yoshikawa and associates (43). In this study, 25 patients were followed prospectively for isolation of HHV6 from blood and marrow and by serologies during the first 2 months after BMT. All patients and donors were seropositive for HHV6 prior to BMT, but no virus was cultured from any individual. HHV6 was isolated from 10 patients (40%) between days 14 and 22 after BMT. Two additional patients had significant increases in antibody titer. Four patients had a skin rash, and 3 of the 4 had concomitant febrile illnesses.

There have been additional reports ascribing both interstitial pneumonia (44) and marrow failure (45) to HHV6; however, further study is needed to determine whether HHV6 is a cofactor or a cause of these clinical syndromes.

HHV6 is a difficult virus to isolate in the laboratory. Isolation is best achieved by cocultivation of patient peripheral blood mononuclear cells (PBMC) with normal cord blood lymphocytes (46). The virus can be grown from saliva and has been isolated from kidney (47) as well as other tissues (34). Initial reports of serological testing used immunofluorescent techniques (35). More recently, anticomplement immunofluorescence has been shown to have increased sensitivity and specificity (46). However, as is the case with serological evaluation for other viruses, this approach is likely to be of limited value due to reasons already described.

Polymerase chain reaction (PCR) may be the best method for identification of HHV6 because of the difficulties in recovering the virus using standard culture techniques (34). Quantitative PCR techniques may be particularly useful in providing evidence for active replication of HHV6 in the absence of positive cultures.

The pathogenesis, immunology, prevention, and treatment, as well as the role of HHV6 in morbidity and mortality of BMT patients await further study and definition. HHV6 appears to be resistant to acyclovir in vitro at doses used in the clinical setting (48) but may be sensitive to other antivirals, such as phosphonoacetic acid (49). In summary, HHV6 is a relatively new member of the herpesvirus family, and its role as a cause of disease remains to be defined in the BMT setting. It is likely that reactivation infection will be common and may possibly be shown to be a cause of interstitial pneumonia and marrow suppression during the first few months after BMT.

Less Common Viruses

Parvovirus B19

Parvovirus are made of small, naked, single-stranded DNA, measuring 18 to 26 nm in diameter. Parvovirus infects a variety of animals, including cats and dogs. In 1975, a human parvovirus, B19, was isolated from asymptomatic blood donors. Seroepidemiological studies have shown evidence of past infection in approximately 60% of young adults. It is most likely spread by respiratory transmission or by blood. Viremia is readily detected by DNA probing. Parvovirus B19 has been grown from marrow cultures and has a predilection for the immature erythroid progenitor cell (50).

Parvovirus B19 commonly has been associated with aplastic crises in patients with hemolytic anemia. It is also the cause of erythema infectiosum, a self-limited disease of childhood characterized by fever, fatigue, myalgias, a lace-like rash, and a "slapped-cheek" appearance. Parvovirus B19 has also been associated with some cases of rheumatoid arthritis.

Little is known about the pathogenesis of parvovirus B19. Immunity is thought to be primarily humoral; neutralizing antibody to capsid protein has a major role in host defense (51). IgM antibody detection may be useful in the diagnosis of acute infection in normal persons. The reliability of serology in BMT recipients is questionable.

The first case of severe anemia caused by parvovirus B19 in a BMT recipient was reported by Weiland and colleagues (52). Inclusion cells were noted in the marrow with reticulocytopenia. Viremia was documented by electron microscopy, dot-blot hybridization, and PCR. Another BMT recipient has been reported with pure red-cell aplasia (53). Treatment is supportive.

Enteroviruses

Enteroviruses belong to the Picornavirus family. They include polioviruses, coxsackie viruses, echoviruses, and other serotypes simply referred to as enteroviruses. They measure 22 to 30 nm in diameter and are naked virons containing single-stranded RNA, which replicate in the cellular cytoplasm. Most of these viruses readily replicate in primate tissue culture, although many coxsackie A serotypes may require newborn mice for primary inoculation. Virus can be isolated from either throat or stool specimens. It may also be recovered from cerebrospinal or other body fluids.

Asymptomatic infection is common in normal hosts, and these viruses are most prevalent during the summer and fall months. Infection is usually by the fecal-oral route; shedding of virus from the oropharynx may persist for 1 to 4 weeks and from the lower gastrointestinal tract for up to 18 weeks. Viremic spread in the host is common, which can affect a variety of organs.

Infection by enteroviruses in BMT recipients has been reported (54,55). One outbreak of coxsackie A1–associated diarrhea affected patients in a 14-bed unit over a 3-week period, resulting in death in 6 of 7 infected patients (54). Diagnosis was made by the detection of coxsackie A1 antigen in stool or throat. Pathological examinations at autopsy revealed foamy vacuolated epithelium overlying the intestinal villi. Coxsackie virus was also identified in the stools of 4 of 78 patients with gastrointestinal infections in a large review of infectious gastroenteritis after BMT, making it the third most common infection after adenovirus and rotavirus (55). All 4 patients with coxsackie virus died; 2 had coinfections with adenovirus.

A case of fatal disseminated echovirus infection was reported by Biggs and associates (56) in a BMT recipient with pneumonitis and pericarditis. The pericardial fluid yielded echovirus type 11. The patient failed to respond to high doses of intravenous Ig or alpha-interferon. Treatment of all enterovirus is supportive.

Rotavirus

Rotavirus consist of double-stranded RNA measuring 60 to 70 nm in diameter and have a double-shelled capsid. They infect the duodenum and the jejunum, causing vomiting and diarrhea in normal hosts, occasionally accompanied by low-grade fever. Infection usually occurs in the winter, and transmission is by the oral-fecal route. Diagnosis is by electron microscopy or by enzyme-linked immunosorbent assay (ELISA).

Rotavirus was the second most frequent cause of diarrhea in one series of BMT recipients with gastroenteritis, resulting in death in 5 of 9 infected patients (55). There is no specific proven treatment.

Norwalk Virus

Norwalk virus are made of small, naked, DNA-containing virons that have been associated with outbreaks of diarrhea but have not been reported after BMT. Diagnosis is by electron microscopy. There is no known treatment short of supportive care.

BK Virus

BK virus is a polyomavirus that may cause mild respiratory infection in childhood, followed by latent infection in the kidney. It has been detected in the urine following BMT (57,58), renal transplants (59,60), and in pregnant women. BK virus can be detected by ELISA or DNA hybridization (57). Few clinical syndromes have been clearly associated with BK. Following BMT, it has been associated with transient hepatic dysfunction (57). Excretion was documented in 47% of 53 consecutive patients and was associated with late onset hemorrhagic cystitis (58,61). In that study, it was significantly more common following allogenic than autologous BMT. In another study, detectable levels of BK antigen developed in 11 of 25 patients (44%) 15 weeks after transplantation (62). Detection of both humoral and cellular immunity was documented and was higher in patients excreting BK than in those without BK antigenenuria. Treatment is supportive.

JC Virus

JC virus (JCV), another polyomavirus, is the cause of progressive multifocal leukoencephalopathy. It has been shown to reside in marrow mononuclear cells during latency; transmission to glial cells occurs via virus-infected lymphocytes (63). BMT recipients shed virus in the urine and can simultaneously be infected with more than one strain (64). There is no known treatment for JC virus.

Summary

More work is needed to define the epidemiology and impact of these less common viruses after BMT. Parvovirus may likely be identified as an important virus in this setting because infection appears to be frequent in the general population, because it may be transmitted by blood products, and because of its known infection of marrow progenitor cells. It is less clear what role the enteric viruses will have, although because diarrhea is a common post-transplant complication, more careful surveillance may result in increased appreciation for this group of viruses in patients with post-transplant diarrhea.

References

1. Bowden RA, Meyers JD. Infectious complications following marrow transplantation. In: Plasma therapy and transfusion technology, vol 6, no 2. 1985:285–302.
2. Zutter MM, Martin PJ, Sale GE, et al. Epstein-Barr virus lymphoproliferation after bone marrow transplantation. Blood 1988;72:520–529.
3. Shields AF, Hackman RC, Fife KH, Corey L, Meyers JD. Adenovirus infections in patients undergoing bone-marrow transplantation. N Engl J Med 1985;312:529–533.
4. Miyamura K, Minami S, Matsuyama T, et al. Adenovirus-induced late onset hemorrhagic cystitis following allogeneic bone marrow transplantation. Bone Marrow Transplant 1987;2:109–115.
5. Odio C, McCracken GH, Nelson JD. Disseminated adenovirus infection: a case report and review of the literature. Pediatr Infect Dis J 1984;3:46–49.
6. Zahradnik JM, Spencer MJ, Porter DD. Adenovirus infection in the immunocompromised patient. Am J Med 1980;68:725–732.
7. Ambinder RF, Burns W, Forman M, et al. Hemorrhagic cystitis associated with adenovirus infection in bone marrow transplantation. Arch Intern Med 1986;146: 1400–1401.
8. Wasserman R, August CS, Plotkin SA. Viral infections in pediatric bone marrow transplant patients. Pediatr Infect Dis J 1988;7:109–115.
9. Koneru B, Jaffe R, Esquivel CO, et al. Adenoviral infections in pediatric liver transplant recipients. JAMA 1987;258:489–492.
10. Michaels MG, Green M, Wald ER, Starzl TE. Adenovirus infection in pediatric liver transplant recipients. J Infect Dis 1992;165:170–174.
11. Myerowitz RL, Stalder H, Oxman MN, et al. Fatal disseminated adenovirus infection in a renal transplant recipient. Am J Med 1975;59:591–598.
12. Purtilo DT, White R, Filipovich A, Kersey J, Zelkowitz L. Fulminant liver failure induced by adenovirus after bone marrow transplantation (letter). N Engl J Med 1985;312:1707–1708.
13. Mahafzah AM, Landry ML. Evaluation of immunofluorescent reagents, centrifugation, and conventional cultures for the diagnosis of adenovirus infection. Diagn Microbiol Infect Dis 1989;12:407–411.
14. Meyers JD, Day LM, Lum LG, Sullivan KM. Recombinant leukocyte A interferon for the treatment of serious viral infections after marrow transplant: a phase I study. J Infect Dis 1983;148:551–556.
15. Ray CG. Respiratory viruses. In: Sherris JC, ed. Medical microbiology: an introduction to infectious diseases. New York: Elsevier, 1990:499–516.
16. Cassano WF. Intravenous ribavirin therapy for adenovirus cystitis after allogeneic bone marrow transplantation. Bone Marrow Transplant 1991;7:247–248.
17. Dagan R, Schwartz RH, Insel RA, Menegus MA. Severe diffuse adenovirus 7a pneumonia in a child with combined immunodeficiency: possible therapeutic effect of human immune serum globulin containing specific neutralizing antibody. Pediatr Infect Dis J 1984;3:246–251.
18. Ljungman P, Gleaves CA, Meyers JD. Respiratory virus infection in immunocompromised patients. Bone Marrow Transplant 1989;4:35–40.
19. Harrington RD, Hooton TM, Hackman R, et al. An outbreak of respiratory syncytial virus in a bone marrow transplant center. J Infect Dis 1992;165:987–993.

20. Wendt CH, Weisdorf DJ, Jordan MC, Balfour HH, Hertz MI. Parainfluenza virus respiratory infection after bone marrow transplantation. N Engl J Med 1992;326: 921–926.
21. Hall CB, Powell KR, MacDonald NE, et al. Respiratory syncytial viral infection in children with compromised immune function. N Engl J Med 1986;315:77–81.
22. Milner ME, de la Monte SM, Hutchins GM. Fatal respiratory syncytial virus infection in severe combined immunodeficiency syndrome. Am J Dis Child 1985;139:1111–1114.
23. Hertz MI, Englund JA, Snover D, Bitterman PB, McGlave PB. Respiratory syncytial virus-induced acute lung injury in adult patients with bone marrow transplants: a clinical approach and review of the literature. Medicine 1989;68:269–281.
24. Englund JA, Sullivan CJ, Jordan MC, Dehner LP, Vercellotti GM, Balfour HH Jr. Respiratory syncytial virus infection in immunocompromised adults. Ann Intern Med 1988;109:203–208.
25. Sinnott JT IV, Cullison JP, Sweeney MS, Hammond M, Holt DA. Respiratory syncytial virus pneumonia in a cardiac transplant patient. J Infect Dis 1988;158:650–651.
26. Pohl C, Green M, Wald ER, Ledesma-Medina J. Respiratory syncytial virus infections in pediatric liver transplant recipients. J Infect Dis 1992;165:166–169.
27. Aschan J, Ringden O, Ljungman P, Andersson J, Lewensohn-Fuchs I, Forsgren M. Influenza B in transplant patients. Scand J Infect Dis 1989;21:349–350.
28. Kaplan LJ, Daum RS, Smaron M, McCarthy CA. Severe measles in immunocompromised patients. JAMA 1992;267:1237–1241.
29. Wright AL, Taussig LM, Ray CG, Harrison HR, Holberg CJ. The Tucson childrens' respiratory study. II. Lower respiratory tract illnesses in the first year of life. Am J Epidemiol 1989;129:1232–1246.
30. Barnes SD, Leclair JM, Forman MS, Townsend TR, Laughlin GM, Charache P. Comparison of nasal brush and nasopharyngeal aspirate techniques in obtaining specimens for detection of respiratory syncytial viral antigen by immunofluorescence. Pediatr Infect Dis J 1989;8:598–600.
31. Derish MT, Kulhanjian JA, Frankel LR, Smith DW. Value of bronchoalveolar lavage in diagnosing severe respiratory syncytial virus infections in infants. J Pediatr 1992;119:761–763.
32. Hemming VG, Rodriguez W, Kim HW, et al. Intravenous immunoglobulin treatment of respiratory syncytial virus infections in infants and young children. Antimicrob Agents Chemother 1987;31:1882–1886.
33. Hemming VG, Prince GA, Rodriguez W, et al. Respiratory syncytial virus infections and intravenous gammaglobulins. Pediatr Infect Dis J 1988;7:S103-S106.
34. Cone R. Human herpesvirus 6: an update. In: de la Maza L, Peterson E, eds. Medical virology 10 (proceedings of the 1990 International Symposium on Medical Virology). New York: Plenum Press, 1991:141–164.
35. Salahuddin SZ, Ablashi DV, Markham PD, et al. Isolation of a new virus, HBLV, in patients with lymphoproliferative disorders. Science 1986;234:596–600.
36. Lawrence GL, Chee M, Craxton MA, Gompels UA, Honess RW, Barrell BG. Human herpesvirus 6 is closely related to human cytomegalovirus. J Virol 1990;64:287–299.
37. Becker WB, Engelbrecht S, Becker MLB, et al. Isolation of a new human herpesvirus producing a lytic infection of helper (CD4) T-lymphocytes in peripheral blood lymphocyte cultures—another cause of acquired immunodeficiency? S Afr Med J 1988;74:610–614.
38. Levy JA, Ferro F, Greenspan D, Lennette ET. Frequent isolation of HHV-6 from saliva and high seroprevalence of the virus in the population. Lancet 1990;1:1047–1050.
39. Takahashi K, Sonoda S, Higashi K, et al. Predominant CD4 T-lymphocyte tropism of human herpesvirus 6-related virus. J Virol 1989;63:3161–3163.
40. Agut H, Guetard D, Collandre H, et al. Concomitant infection by human herpesvirus 6, HTLV-1 and HIV-2. Lancet 1988;1:712.
41. Yoshiyama H, Suzuki E, Yoshida T, Kajii T, Yamamoto N. Role of human herpesvirus 6 infection in infants with exanthema subitum. Pediatr Infect Dis J 1990;9:71–74.
42. Asano Y, Yoshikawa T, Suga S, et al. Reactivation of herpesvirus type 6 in children receiving bone marrow transplants for leukemia. N Engl J Med 1991;324:634–635.
43. Yoshikawa T, Suga S, Asano Y, et al. Human herpesvirus-6 infection in bone marrow transplantation. Blood 1991;78:1381–1384.
44. Carrigan DR, Drobyski WR, Russler SK, Tapper MA, Knox KK, Ash RC. Interstitial pneumonitis associated with human herpesvirus-6 infection after marrow transplantation. Lancet 1991;2:147–149.
45. Knox K, Carrigan DR. In vitro suppression of bone marrow progenitor cell differentiation by human herpesvirus 6 infection. J Infect Dis 1992;165:925–929.
46. Lopez C, Pellett P, Stewart J, et al. Characteristics of human herpesvirus-6. J Infect Dis 1988;157:1271–1273.
47. Asano Y, Yoshikawa T, Suga S, et al. Human herpesvirus 6 harbouring in kidney. Lancet 1989;2:1391.
48. Burns WH, Sandford GR. Susceptibility of human herpesvirus 6 to antivirals in vitro. J Infect Dis 1990;162:634–637.
49. DiLuca D, Katsafanas G, Schirmer EC, Balachandran N, Frenkel N. The replication of viral and cellular DNA in human herpesvirus 6-infected cells. Virology 1990; 175:199–210.
50. Ozawa K, Kurtzman G, Young N. Productive infection by B19 parvovirus of human erythroid bone marrow cells in vitro. Blood 1987;70:384–391.
51. Kurtzman GJ, Cohen BJ, Field AM, Oseas R, Blaese RM, Young NS. Immune response to B19 parovirus and an antibody defect in persistent viral infection. J Clin Invest 1989;84:1114–1123.
52. Weiland HT, Salimans MM, Fibbe WE, Kluin PM, Cohen BJ. Prolonged parvovirus B19 infection with severe anaemia in a bone marrow transplant patient (letter). Br J Haematol 1989;71:300.
53. Niitsu H, Miura AB, Nobuo Y, Sugamura K. Pure red cell aplasia induced by B19 parvovirus during allogeneic bone marrow transplantation. Clin Transplant 1989;315.
54. Townsend TR, Bolyard EA, Yolken RH, et al. Outbreak of coxsackie A1 gastroenteritis: a complication of bone-marrow transplantation. Lancet 1982;1:820–823.
55. Yolken RH, Bishop CA, Townsend TR, et al. Infectious gastroenteritis in bone-marrow-transplant recipients. N Engl J Med 1982;306:1009–1012.
56. Biggs DD, Toorkey BC, Carrigan DR, Hanson GA, Ash RC. Disseminated echovirus infection complicating bone marrow transplantation. Am J Med 1990;88:421–424.
57. O'Reilly RJ, Lee FK, Grossbard E, et al. Papovavirus excretion following marrow transplantation: incidence

and association with hepatic dysfunction. Transplant Proc 1981;13:262–266.

58. Arthur RR, Shah KV, Baust SJ, Santos GW, Saral R. Association of BK viruria with hemorrhagic cystitis in recipients of bone marrow transplants. N Engl J Med 1986;315:230–234.

59. Coleman DV, Gardner SD, Field AM. Human polyomavirus infection in renal allograft recipients. Br Med J 1973;3:371–375.

60. Hogan TF, Borden EC, McBain JA, Padgett BL, Walker DL. Human polyomavirus infections with JC virus and BK virus in renal transplant patients. Ann Intern Med 1980;92:373–378.

61. Apperley JF, Rice SJ, Bishop JA, et al. Late-onset hemorrhagic cystitis associated with urinary excretion of polyomaviruses after bone marrow transplantation. Transplantation 1987;43:108–112.

62. Drummond JE, Shah KV, Saral R, Santos GW, Donnenberg AD. BK virus specific humoral and cell mediated immunity in allogeneic bone marrow transplant (BMT) recipients. J Med Virol 1987;23:331–344.

63. Houff SA, Major EO, Katz DA, et al. Involvement of JC virus-infected mononuclear cells from the bone marrow and spleen in the pathogenesis of progressive multifocal leukoencephalopathy. N Engl J Med 1988; 318:301–305.

64. Myers C, Frisque RJ, Arthur RR. Direct isolation and characterization of JC virus from urine samples of renal and bone marrow transplant patients. J Virol 1989;63:4445–4449.

Chapter 33
Gastrointestinal and Hepatic Complications

Margaret C. Shuhart and George B. McDonald

The incidence of intestinal and liver complications of bone marrow transplantation (BMT) has not changed much over the past 20 years, but the reason is not the lack of progress. In the 1970s, the major complications were intractable graft-versus-host disease (GVHD) of the intestine and liver and untreatable herpesvirus infections. The introduction of effective prophylaxis against GVHD has had a marked effect on the incidence of fatal GVHD. Antiviral agents have almost eliminated intestinal and hepatic infections caused by *herpes simplex virus* (HSV) and *cytomegalovirus* (CMV). These positive developments, however, have been counterbalanced by a higher incidence of fatal liver toxicity following cytoreductive therapy (veno-occlusive disease [VOD]) and by an increase in the number of transplants from unrelated donors that confer an increased risk of GVHD. In the 1990s, intestinal and liver diseases are still a cause of considerable morbidity in BMT recipients.

This chapter is organized by the problems that clinicians might encounter in caring for BMT recipients in the chronological order in which these problems are likely to appear.

Problems Before the Start of Cytoreductive Therapy

Several diseases of the intestine and the liver are relative contraindications to BMT because they may jeopardize post-transplant survival. Diagnosis and treatment of these diseases before transplantation can prevent some post-transplant complications.

Ulcers and Tumors in the Intestinal Tract

Mucosal ulcerations in the esophagus, stomach, and intestine may bleed profusely when platelet counts decrease after cytoreductive therapy. Symptoms of esophageal pain, heartburn, dysphagia, epigastric pain, nausea, and vomiting should be investigated with upper intestinal endoscopy before referral for BMT. In immunocompromised patients, "peptic" ulcers may have an infectious etiology (e.g., CMV, HSV, or fungal infection) (1,2). Rarely, peptic ulcers develop in patients with basophilic leukemia related to elevated serum histamine levels. In nontransplant recipients, gastric infection with *Helicobacter pylori* is often associated with idiopathic ulcers in the stomach and the duodenum (3). Treatment of *H. pylori*–associated gastroduodenal ulcers and peptic esophageal ulcers with medications that control acid secretion is usually successful, but large ulcers may not heal completely before several months. Treatment of *H. pylori* gastroduodenal infections with antibiotics has little immediate impact on ulcer healing but may lower the incidence of ulcer recurrence (4). There is no evidence that *H. pylori* gastric infection becomes disseminated in BMT recipients.

The goal of pre-BMT therapy in patients with inflammatory bowel diseases such as idiopathic ulcerative colitis or Crohn's disease is to minimize the extent of gross intestinal ulceration before cytoreductive therapy to lower the risk of bleeding after transplantation. Infection as the cause of colonic ulceration must also be ruled out. The most likely pathogens are CMV, *Entamoeba histolytica*, and *Clostridium difficile* (5). In 6 patients with Crohn's disease who underwent BMT, there was resolution of many of the manifestations of intestinal inflammation in the early post-BMT period, no serious bleeding, and no perforations. A similar experience has been reported in a patient with ulcerative colitis (6).

Patients who are to be transplanted for lymphoma, leukemia in relapse, or breast cancer may have intestinal involvement with malignant cells (7,8). Cytoreductive therapy results in necrosis of these cells (9). Both large intestinal ulcers and perforation due to tumor lysis have been seen, but the low frequency of this complication (estimated at one in 500 transplantations) does not warrant screening for intestinal involvement by tumor. Intra-abdominal abscesses and fistulae should be managed surgically before BMT.

Infections of the Intestine and Liver

Patients with chronic diarrhea should be investigated for organisms that are likely to disseminate during the period of immunosuppression following BMT. Intestinal parasites such as *E. histolytica* and *Strongyloides* can cause death in immunosuppressed hosts (10). *Giardia lamblia* and *Cryptosporidia* may lead to diarrhea after transplantation (11,12). Persistent eosinophilia in a patient from an area where parasites are endemic is an indication for screening for parasitic disease. Specific therapy is available for amoebiasis, strongyloidiasis, and giardiasis (2). Cryptosporidiosis has proven resistant to all therapy except withdrawal of immunosuppressive medication. Other treatable causes of diarrhea in patients with hematological malignancy include clostridial infections (*C. difficile*, *C. perfringens*, *C. septicum)* and overgrowth with *Candida albicans*. (2,13,14). Rarely, chronic *rotavirus* and *adenovirus* infections are present in suppressed hosts (2,15).

Pain in or near the anal canal in granulocytopenic patients is due to bacterial infection of perianal tissues until proved otherwise (16). These infections are usually polymicrobial, arising from either anal crypts or tears in the anal canal. Extensive supralevator and intersphincteric abscesses may be present without being apparent on external examination (17). Perianal infections must be dealt with before BMT, because extensive tissue necrosis and septicemia may result from uncontrolled infection (17). A recent National Institutes of Health study suggests that treatment consist of antibiotics to cover anaerobic as well as aerobic bacteria (16). Perianal HSV infection may also lead to painful ulcerations (18).

Tender hepatomegaly suggests either fungal infection or tumor, which may be differentiated by computed tomography (CT) or magnetic resonance imaging. The diagnosis of malignant cells in the liver is moot, because there is usually evidence of tumor elsewhere. The diagnostic focus is on whether viable fungi are present in the liver, an indication for systemic antifungal therapy before BMT (19). Differentiating active infection from fibrous remnants of previous fungal infection requires needle, laparoscopic, or surgical liver biopsy (20). *Candida* species are the most likely isolate. The same approach applies to asymptomatic patients whose abdominal imaging study shows intrahepatic lesions consistent with fungal infection.

Acute and Chronic Viral Hepatitis

Until 1990, the prevalence of viral hepatitis among candidates for BMT was 15 to 25%, largely due to prior exposure to blood products contaminated with hepatitis C virus (HCV) (21). Recent methods for screening blood products have resulted in a decrease in this percentage (22). The presence of hepatitis before transplantation carries three risks for BMT recipients: (1) an increased frequency of fatal liver toxicity (VOD) following cytoreductive therapy, (2) fulminant viral hepatitis after transplantation, and (3) progressive liver disease after recovery from BMT.

Liver Toxicity Following Cytoreductive Therapy

Four centers have identified pretransplant elevations of serum transaminase enzymes (AST) levels as an independent risk factor for liver toxicity following cytoreductive therapy (VOD) (21,23–25). A prospective study of 355 patients identified hepatitis as a risk factor for fatal liver toxicity, with a relative risk of 4.6 (25). Although even minor elevations of serum AST levels conferred risk, the incidence of fatal liver toxicity was higher with greater elevations of AST levels (8 of 10 patients with AST >164 IU/L died of VOD). We suggest deferring BMT during the acute phase of viral hepatitis. Decision making with regard to patients with chronic hepatitis or those with elevations of AST levels of unknown etiology is more difficult. Spontaneous resolution of chronic HCV over 6 to 12 months is not likely, but if drug-induced hepatitis is the cause of AST elevation, discontinuing the drug and deferring BMT is one option. Cirrhosis of the liver is a contraindication to high-dose cytoreductive therapy because the risk of fatal liver toxicity is very high.

Fulminant Viral Hepatitis

Fulminant hepatitis has been described in 3 BMT recipients who were carriers of the hepatitis B virus (HBV) (26–28) and in 2 patients who had chronic HCV (29). The pattern of clinical illness was similar: replication of virus during the period of immunosuppression after conditioning therapy, then development of hepatitis after reconstitution of the immune system after day 70. Similar fulminant hepatitis has been described in HBV-infected patients with hematological malignancy and in renal graft recipients following recovery of immune function (30,31). The presumed mechanism of hepatitis in these patients is immune-mediated hepatocyte injury rather than direct viral injury.

The risk of fulminant HBV after transplantation is probably less than 6 in 100, because more than 50 HBV-positive patients have been transplanted without fulminant hepatitis (28,32,33). There is some evidence that transplantation of HBV-immune donor marrow into an HBV-infected host facilitates elimination of HBV from the host (28,32–35). The risk of fulminant HCV is probably less than 1 in 100, given an estimated 15 to 25% prevalence of HCV-positive patients undergoing BMT over the last 2 decades and only 2 reported cases.

Chronic Hepatitis in Long-term Survivors

Patients undergoing BMT with chronic viral hepatitis may have an adverse long-term course. Progression of chronic hepatitis to cirrhosis has been noted in two studies of long-term BMT survivors (36,37). Both HBV and HCV also predispose patients to hepatocellular carcinoma. The frequency of these sequellae of chronic viral hepatitis in BMT recipients is not well defined.

Biliary Diseases

Patients may present for BMT with gallstones or sludge-like material in the gallbladder, the cystic duct, or the common bile duct. These conditions are asymptomatic in most patients, but may cause postprandial nausea and pain. Sepsis or a flu-like illness can result from bacterial cholangitis, without symptoms referable to the biliary tree. Symptomatic patients with gallstones in either the gallbladder or the biliary ducts should be considered for surgery before BMT because they may have infected bile and are at risk for uncontrolled sepsis after BMT. Endoscopic sphincterotomy and common duct stone removal is an alternative to surgery. Asymptomatic stones in the gallbladder (discovered with CT or ultrasound) can be left untreated.

Problems During the Early Posttransplant Period (From the Start of Cytoreductive Therapy to Day 100)

Nausea, Vomiting, and Anorexia

These symptoms are almost universal during and after conditioning therapy and are a common manifestation of acute GVHD. Infection with HSV and CMV was formerly a leading cause of these symptoms. Inability to eat is currently a major reason for prolonged hospitalization and parenteral nutrition.

Conditioning Therapy

Chemotherapy and total body irradiation (TBI) cause vomiting and anorexia by several mechanisms. One is related to the effects of chemotherapy on midbrain vomiting centers, causing symptoms during conditioning therapy (38). The intensity of vomiting tends to be worse with higher dose regimens, but antiemetic therapy dampens the severity of symptoms (Table 33-1) (39). Patients remain mildly nauseated and anorectic for 3 to 6 weeks (38). Elevated serum cytokine levels are one possible explanation for persistent anorexia in this early phase (40). Uncontrolled studies suggested that pentoxifylline may blunt these symptoms and allow earlier resumption of eating via its effects on release of tumor necrosis factor (41). Unfortunately, pentoxifylline itself may cause nausea at high doses. The third mechanism for nausea and anorexia is mucositis, which has its onset a few days before BMT and reaches a peak 10 to 14 days after BMT (38,42). Mucositis causes swelling, pain, and, in severe cases, sloughing of the oropharyngeal epithelium, and may be worsened by superinfection and methotrexate therapy (43,44). Mucosal involvement can extend into the hypopharynx and the esophagus, causing intense gagging, an inability to swallow, vomiting, and occasionally retrosternal pain. Opiate therapy for mucositis pain is effective (45) but can lead to gastric stasis, intestinal ileus, anorexia, and vomiting.

Acute GVHD

One of the earliest manifestations of acute GVHD involving the intestine is loss of appetite, followed by

Table 33-1.
Medication Schedules to Prevent Nausea and Vomiting During Cytoreductive Therapy[a]

Medications	*Dosing Schedule*	*Comments*
Schedule I		
Diphenhydramine	30 mg/m² intravenously 30 minutes before each metoclopramide dose × 6 doses for each chemotherapy infusion; continued every 4 hours × 6 doses after last dose of chemotherapy.	Antihistamine; not a potent antiemetic, but prevents extrapyramidal side effects of dopamine receptor antagonists and has sedative properties. Can be used alone in some infants and children at 0.5–1.0 mg/kg/dose every 4–6 hours.
Metoclopramide	40 mg/m² intravenously every 4 hours × 6 doses for each chemotherapy infusion.	Dopamine and serotonin receptor antagonist; extrapyramidal side effects; use cautiously in children.
Droperidol	3 mg/m² intravenously every 2 hours × 12 doses for each chemotherapy infusion.	Dopamine receptor antagonist; extrapyramidal side effects; use cautiously in children.
Schedule II		
Ondansetron by bolus dosing	0.15 mg/kg intravenously before chemotherapy, then at 4 and 8 hours after chemotherapy.	Serotonin receptor antagonist; doses may become less effective over time.
Lorazepam	0.25–2.0 mg intravenously every 4–6 hours.	Benzodiazepine; often a useful adjunct to ondansetron, especially for anticipatory vomiting, because of its sedative and anxiolytic effects.
Schedule III		
Ondansetron by bolus dosing	0.15 mg/kg intravenously before chemotherapy, then at 4 and 8 hours after chemotherapy.	Serotonin receptor antagonist; doses may become less effective over time.
Dexamethasone	10–20 mg intravenously 30–45 minutes before chemotherapy or with first dose of ondansetron.	Corticosteroid; useful as an adjunct to ondansetron for regimens that contain cis-platin. Side effects include hyperglycemia and mental status changes.

[a]The medications in schedules I and II are effective during cyclophosphamide and etoposide infusions. Nausea from busulfan is usually less problematic; preventive therapy with diphenhydramine and lorazepam may suffice. The medications in schedule III are effective for regimens that contain cis-platin.

nausea and vomiting. Before the introduction of cyclosporine (CSP)/methotrexate (MTX) prophylaxis for GVHD, these symptoms were often overlooked because diarrhea and abdominal pain dominated the clinical picture (46). A prospective study of 50 BMT recipients with unexplained vomiting that developed between days 20 and 100 found that 42% had unsuspected GVHD (47). In another study, 60% of patients with biopsy-proven GVHD affecting the stomach and the duodenum had nausea and vomiting as the primary symptom of acute GVHD (48). Immunosuppressive therapy using prednisone (1–2 mg/kg) is effective in treating these symptoms, particularly when they are the only manifestation of GVHD (48). Recent studies suggest that oral beclomethasone capsules are also effective. Some patients, however, progress to grade III to IV GVHD despite treatment. Anorexia and vomiting may also recur when immunosuppressive agents are tapered after successful treatment of GVHD, often as the only symptom. Endoscopic biopsy is often needed to confirm the diagnosis and to rule out intestinal infection (47,49) (Plates XXV and XXVI). If GVHD is confirmed on biopsy, reinstitution of prednisone therapy is usually effective.

Medications and Parenteral Nutrition

Oral nonabsorbable antibiotics (particularly nystatin), CSP, pentoxifylline, trimethoprim-sulfamethoxazole (TMP-SMX), and intravenous amphotericin are frequent causes of nausea and occasionally protracted vomiting. A temporal association between dosing and symptoms is often present, but not always, especially for TMP-SMX (50). Lipid infusions and high blood glucose and amino acid levels are also associated with nausea (51). Parenteral nutrition (TPN) may contribute to failure to resume eating by causing nausea and anorexia. Even after TPN has been stopped, appetite suppression may linger for 1 to 3 weeks (51,52).

Infections

CMV infection of the esophagus (Plates XXXIII and XXXIV) and the upper intestine was found in 38% of BMT recipients with unexplained vomiting in one prospective study during the pre-ganciclovir era (47). These infections were diagnosed a mean of 54 days after BMT. Although esophageal ulcers were present in almost all of these patients, esophageal symptoms were frequently absent. HSV esophagitis may present similarly (47,53). CMV and HSV esophagitis are now rare, owing to the use of prophylactic antiviral therapy. Currently, most cases of CMV enteritis represent infections that antedate BMT, primary (as opposed to reactivation) infections, or failure to continue prophylaxis due to toxicity from ganciclovir. Intravenous ganciclovir is highly effective in eliminating CMV from upper intestinal lesions, but symptoms and the endoscopic appearance are only minimally improved after 2 weeks of therapy (54). Factors contributing to persistence of nausea include the large size of CMV ulcers, acid-peptic reflux, and recurrence of CMV after ganciclovir is stopped. Current practice is to continue ganciclovir for an additional 2 weeks at a reduced dosage.

Fungal esophagitis can cause anorexia but not the incessant vomiting often seen with herpesvirus infections (55). Anorexia and vomiting may be manifestations of diseases of the central nervous system (e.g., subdural hematoma, intracerebral bleeding, or infections with *Aspergillus*, *Toxoplasma*, or viruses), but other neurological signs and symptoms usually dominate the clinical picture with these disorders. Systemic bacterial infection (bacteremia or focal abscesses), cholecystitis, acute pancreatitis, and acute viral hepatitis may also present with anorexia and vomiting.

Jaundice, Hepatomegaly, and Abnormal Liver Test Results

Jaundice in the first several weeks after BMT is most often secondary to liver toxicity following cytoreductive therapy (VOD), liver injury caused by other medications, and the cholestatic liver disease associated with sepsis (cholangitis lenta). Acute GVHD affecting the liver presents after day 15. Fungal infections of the liver are related to poor graft function and granulocytopenia. Viral hepatitis usually occurs after day 40. Two or more of these processes often coexist, presenting a diagnostic challenge.

Liver Toxicity Following Cytoreductive Therapy (VOD)

In the first few weeks after BMT, a clinical syndrome characterized by hepatomegaly, jaundice, and fluid retention develops in 10 to 60% of patients (21,23–25). This syndrome is due to damage to endothelial cells, sinusoids, and hepatocytes in zone 3 of the liver acinus (the area surrounding terminal hepatic venules) (56,57). The proximate cause of the damage is cytoreductive therapy. Histological changes in the liver include VOD of terminal hepatic venules, dilation and engorgement of sinusoids, and necrosis of hepatocytes (see Figure 16.3 and Plates V to X) (56–58). This syndrome, often called VOD of the liver, can vary in severity from mild, reversible disease to fatal disease associated with multiorgan failure (23,25,59).

Presenting Clinical Features and Differential Diagnosis

The diagnosis of VOD usually can be made on clinical grounds alone based on the triad of hepatomegaly, weight gain, and jaundice (Table 33-2) (21,23,59–61). Change in liver size and liver tenderness are usually the first signs of VOD, occurring 8 to 10 days after the start of cytoreductive therapy, or around day 1 after transplantation. Occasionally, liver pain is severe because the liver capsule is abruptly stretched. Renal sodium retention with resultant weight gain occurs at

Table 33-2.
Timing of the Onset of Signs of Liver Toxicity (Veno-occlusive Disease) Following Cytoreductive Therapy (190 Consecutive Patients)

Sign of Liver Toxicity	*Day of Onset (±SD) (Relative to Day 0, the Day of Transplantation)*
Hepatomegaly or liver tenderness	0.6±7.7
Weight gain >2% of baseline weight	0.7±4.3
Elevated serum bilirubin (>2 mg/dl or 34.2 μmol/L)	5.9±4.8

Reproduced by permission from McDonald GB, Hinds M, Fisher L, Schoch HG. Liver toxicity following cytoreductive therapy for marrow transplantation: risk factors, incidence and outcome. Hepatology 1991;14:162A.

about the same time (25,62,63) and is related to the development of intrasinusoidal hypertension due to obstruction to hepatic blood flow (64). In many patients, the early signs of VOD develop before marrow infusion and before therapy with CSP and MTX. Hyperbilirubinemia develops later, usually before day 12 (25,59). Peripheral edema develops in 60% and ascites in 20% of patients with VOD (25).

Liver biopsy is seldom needed to confirm the diagnosis of VOD before day 20, because clinical-histological correlations have shown that the clinical presentation described is highly correlated with damage to zone 3 of the liver acinus (21,23). Other less common liver diseases before day 20 include fungal infiltration, "hyperacute" GVHD, liver injury caused by other medications, and cholangitis lenta (46,61,62). Although jaundice is common to most of these conditions, fluid retention and weight gain are so characteristic of VOD as to be useful in the differential diagnosis. Passive liver congestion due to pericarditis or congestive heart failure may also present with hepatomegaly, weight gain, and jaundice, but other signs of cardiac disease are usually present. The difficulty in the differential diagnosis is not in separating VOD from other diseases, but in determining when several liver diseases (including VOD) are present simultaneously. When a firm diagnosis of VOD is needed, transvenous measurement of hepatic vein pressures and biopsy can be done, albeit with some risk because of thrombocytopenia. Experience from Barcelona (65) and Seattle (66) suggests that a hepatic venous pressure gradient (wedged minus free pressure) greater than 10 mm Hg is accurate in the diagnosis of VOD. Liver biopsy via the transvenous route can be done safely but faces a sampling problem (67), because the histological lesions of VOD can be patchy (see Chapter 16) (23,57). Imaging studies of the liver are useful to demonstrate hepatomegaly and ascites consistent with VOD and conversely the absence of infiltrative lesions. Ultrasound may demonstrate alterations in portal venous flow in advanced VOD but is not as useful in the early phases of the disease (68–70).

Clinical Course and Outcome

The incidence of BMT-related VOD and its severity varies widely, largely because of differences in conditioning regimens. We completed a year-long prospective study of VOD at our center. The overall incidence during 1987 to 1988 was 53%: 12% had mild disease, 26% had moderate disease, and 15% had severe disease (25). The outcome of VOD was usually apparent before day 20, because patients with severe VOD differed from those with nonsevere VOD in their degree of jaundice and amount of fluid retention (Table 33-3). A mathematical model that predicts severity of VOD based on the rate of increase of bilirubin levels and weight has been published (71). Platelet transfusion requirements were significantly higher in patients with severe VOD (see Table 33-3).

Published case fatality rates for BMT-related VOD range from 0 to 67% (23,24,59,63). These figures are dependent on how each center defines both VOD (exclusion of mild cases will inflate the fatality rate) and fatal VOD. It is often difficult to define the cause of death in BMT recipients and more difficult to state the role of liver dysfunction in causing death. Patients with VOD, as deeply jaundiced as they become, seldom die of liver failure, if liver failure is defined as development of hepatic coma and deranged liver synthetic function (72). Rather, the cause of death in patients who have persistent jaundice and fluid retention is multiorgan failure (25,62). Our data show that severe, irreversible VOD is significantly correlated with the development of renal and cardiopulmonary failure in the first 20 days after transplantation (Table 33-4). Organ failure before day 20 almost always follows development of VOD: Pulmonary infiltrates, pleural effusions, and cardiomegaly follow the onset of weight gain by approximately 1

Table 33-3.
Clinical Featuress of Patients with Veno-occlusive Disease of the Liver According to Severity of Disease

	Mild	*Moderate*	*Severe*
Weight gain (% increase)	7.0±3.5	10.1±5.3	15.5±9.2
Maximum serum bilirubin before day 20	4.7±2.9	7.9±6.6	26.0±15.2
Percent of patients with peripheral edema	23	70	85
Percent of patients with ascites	5	16	48
Platelet transfusion requirements to day 20	53.8±27.6	83.6±35.0	118.3±51.8
Day 100 mortality (all causes)(%)	3	20	98

Reproduced by permission from McDonald GB, Hinds M, Fisher L, Schoch HG. Liver toxicity following cytoreductive therapy for marrow transplantation: risk factors, incidence and outcome. Hepatology 1991;14:162A.

Table 33-4.
Relationship of Liver Toxicity (Veno-occlusive Disease [VOD]) to Multiorgan Failure Within 20 Days of Transplantation

	No VOD (n=86)(%)	*Mild or Moderate VOD (n=136)(%)*	*Severe VOD (n=54)(%)*
Renal failure	0	13(10)	29(54)
Cardiac failure	12(14)	35(26)	34(63)
Respiratory failure	1(1)	6(4)	23(43)

Reproduced by permission from McDonald GB, Hinds M, Fisher L, Schoch HG. Liver toxicity following cytoreductive therapy for marrow transplantation: risk factors, incidence and outcome. Hepatology 1991;14:162A.

week; renal insufficiency occurs at day 10, respiratory failure at day 12, and renal failure at day 15, on average (25,62).

Pathogenesis

Conditioning therapy is the proximate cause of VOD. Because endothelial cells are particularly sensitive to chemoradiotherapy, one hypothesis proposes that venular and sinusoidal endothelial injury during conditioning therapy results in local activation of the clotting cascade, first occluding sinusoidal pores that drain into venules, then causing postsinusoidal obstruction to venous blood flow (57,61,73). This hypothesis of endothelial injury and local coagulation is supported by the demonstration of denuded venular endothelium in animal models of early VOD (74) and the demonstration of clotting factors (fibrinogen and factor VIII) within VOD lesions in human autopsy specimens (73). Cytokine release during endothelial injury may contribute further to activation of coagulation (40,57). Tumor necrosis factor-alpha (TNF-α) mediates several procoagulant mechanisms, including the downregulation of anticoagulant factors and the upregulation of platelet activating factors and coagulant factors V and VIII (75–77). Several investigators have evaluated coagulation parameters in patients before, during, and after cytoreductive therapy (78–82). Levels of anticoagulation factors such as protein C, protein S, and antithrombin III are depressed during cytoreductive therapy and tend to remain depressed after BMT (78,80,82). Conversely, procoagulant factors (fibrinogen, vWF) are elevated (78,80,82). Mechanisms controlling the hepatic microcirculation may also have a role in the genesis of VOD (57). Endothelial injury may lead to release of endothelins, peptides with vasoconstrictive and platelet aggregating properties that may further promote venular narrowing (83).

Epidemiological studies have implicated many factors in the pathogenesis of VOD, the most important of which is the conditioning regimen itself (Table 33-5). The incidence of severe VOD is higher following conditioning with cyclophosphamide (CY)/TBI when the dose of TBI is greater than 10–12 Gy (25). The schedule of delivery (fractionated vs hyperfractionated) does not seem to influence the incidence of severe VOD, but some authors suggest that there is more VOD when TBI is delivered at higher dose rates (84) and conversely less VOD with lower dose rates (35,85). These studies, however, employed only 10 to 12 Gy TBI as a component of conditioning therapy.

Use of regimens that contain busulfan (BU) has been associated with a high incidence of VOD, particularly when BU doses exceed 16 mg/kg (86–88). However, blood levels following identical oral doses of BU vary widely from patient to patient, and toxicity is related to abnormally high blood levels (89,90). The pharmacokinetics of BU vary with age; children have lower steady-state concentrations and higher clearance rates than adults (91). Variability in BU pharmacokinetics is one explanation for the wide range in the incidence of VOD. One report has implicated the timing of BU administration in multiagent conditioning regimens; a higher incidence of VOD occurred when BU was administered first (87). The BCV conditioning regimen (carmustine [BCNU], CY and etoposide [VP-16]) has also been associated with a high incidence of severe VOD (25). Glutathione levels in hepatocytes and endothelial cells may be important in protecting these cells from high-dose cytoreductive therapy. Intracellular glutathione, which protects hepatocytes and endothelial cells from free oxygen radicals (92,93), is depleted by TBI, BU, and BCNU (57). In an animal model of VOD, glutathione depletion was needed to enhance the hepatic toxicity of cytotoxic drugs (94). Hepatocytes in zone 3 of the liver acinus are unique in that they are the predominant site of both glutathione S-transferases and the cytochrome P450 mixed-function oxidases, which bioactivate CY (95). The fact that VOD does not develop in all patients receiving the same doses of a given regimen and the variability in the reported incidence rates of VOD suggest that there is large individual variation in how the liver metabolizes cytotoxic agents and protects itself from damage.

Statistical analyses have identified additional independent risk factors for VOD (see Table 33-5) (21,23,24,35,56,63,78,79,84,85–89,95–106). The contradictory results of these analyses reflect variations in study design, definitions of VOD, patient population, and conditioning regimens, making comparison of the data difficult. Our analysis of risk factors took all putative risk factors into account and used severe VOD as an end point; we concluded that the factors in Table 33-6 were predictive of severe VOD (25). The most important of these additional risk factors are pretransplant hepatitis, fever, the inflammatory response during administration of cytoreductive therapy, and the infusion of mismatched donor marrow. Four large prospective studies reported an association between pretransplant hepatitis and VOD after BMT (21,23–25). In our analysis, hepatitis was a significant independent predictor of fatal VOD, with a relative risk of 4.6 (see Table 33-6). The mechanisms by which

Table 33-5.
Putative Risk Factors for Veno-occlusive Disease of the Liver after Marrow Transplantation

Risk Factors		*References*
Age	Increased risk age >10	106[a]
	Increased risk age >15	21[a]
	No effect	23[a],24[a],56,63,96,97
Sex	Increased risk with female sex	24[a],98[a]
	No effect	21[a],56,63,96,97,99
Diagnosis	Increased risk with malignancy other than ALL	21[a]
	Decreased risk with acute leukemia, first remission	23[a]
	Increased risk with leukemia (vs genetic disease)	96
	Increased risk with leukamia (vs aplastic anemia)	56
	No effect	24[a],63,99,106[a]
Relapse/remission status	Increased risk if in relapse	100
	No effect	21[a],23[a],24[a],63,96
Conditioning regimen	Increased risk if regimen included BU	56
	Decreased risk with fractionated BCNU (vs single dose)	99
	Increased risk with TBI >12 Gy	100
	Increased risk with BU >16 mg/kg, 3 (vs 2) alkylating agents, and order of BU administration	87
	Increased risk with BU >16 mg/kg	88
	Increased risk with increased blood levels of BU	89
	Increased risk with BU (vs CY/TBI)	86
	Increased risk with higher dose rate (Gy/min) TBI	84
	Decreased risk with lower dose rate (Gy/min) TBI	35,85
	No effect	21[a],23[a],63
Type of marrow graft	Decreased risk if autologous	100,101,
	No effect	21[a],23[a],96
Hepatitis at the time of transplant	Increased risk with elevated SGOT	21[a],23[a],24[a],56,101
	No effect	35,85,96,99,102,103,104
Previous liver disease	Increased risk with prior history of abnormal liver tests	97
	Increased risk with abnormal liver tests, hepatomegaly	56
	No effect	21[a],24[a],96
Liver tumor (in the past or at the time of transplant)	Increased risk with metastases at time of transplant	99
Antibiotic use	Increased risk with amphotericin use	98[a]
	Increased risk with ketoconazole	87
Methotrexate/cyclosporin	Increased risk with methotrexate for GVHD prophylaxis	98[a],105
T-cell depletion	Decreased risk with T-cell depletion for GVHD prophylaxis	104,106[a]
Deficiency of anticoagulant proteins (protein C, protein S, AT-III)	Increased risk with decreased protein C	78,79
CMV serology	Increased risk with positive serology	97

[a]These studies were analyzed by logistical regression (multivariate) models.
ALL = acute lymphoblastic leukemia; BU = busulfan; BCNU = carmustine; TBI = total body irradiation; Cy = cyclophosphamide; SGOT = serum glutamic oxaloacetic transaminase; CMV = cytomegalovirus; GVHD = graft-versus-host disease.

hepatitis confers increased risk are not known, but may relate to sensitized venular endothelium in patients with hepatitis or abnormal metabolism of cytotoxic drugs. Two prospective studies have implicated an intense inflammatory response as contributing to VOD (25,98), suggesting that release of cytokines such as TNF affects venular endothelium. Elevated TNF-α levels have been demonstrated in patients with VOD (40). There may also be a contribution of the type of donor marrow to VOD (see Table 33-6) (25). A recent study of T-lymphocyte–depleted BMT following CY/TBI conditioning reported a lower than expected incidence of VOD (104). In this report, the possible protective effect of T-cell depletion could not be separated from the lack of CSP or MTX prophylaxis, which may contribute to liver dysfunction after transplantation (105,107).

Prevention

Given that the pathogenesis of VOD is likely multifactorial, studies aimed at its prevention can approach the disease in several ways. Conditioning regimens can be altered to limit liver toxicity, whereas drugs that affect coagulation, venous patency, and cytokine release can be administered prophylactically.

Modification of Conditioning Regimens. Chemoradiotherapy doses have increased in the last 10 years in an attempt to decrease the relapse rate of malignancy after BMT. As a result, the incidence of VOD at our

Table 33-6.
Risk Factors for Severe Veno-occlusive Disease of the Liver Following Cytoreductive Therapy, Based on a Multivariate Analysis of Data from 355 Patients Transplanted During 1987 to 1988

Risk Factor	*Relative Risk*	*95% Confidence Interval*	*p* Value
Pretransplant acyclovir therapy	4.8	1.2–20.1	0.02
Pretransplant hepatitis	4.6	2.2–9.8	<0.00001
Vancomycin during cytoreductive therapy	2.9	1.4–6.0	0.003
Cytoreductive therapy with CY plus TBI (> 13 Gy), or BU/CY, or BCNU/CY/VP16	2.8	1.2–6.5	0.01
Mismatched or unrelated donor marrow	2.4	1.1–4.9	0.02
Past radiation therapy to the abdomen	2.2	1.0–4.9	0.04

Reproduced by permission from McDonald GB, Hinds M, Fisher L, Schoch HG. Liver toxicity following cytoreductive therapy for marrow transplantation: risk factors, incidence and outcome. Hepatology 1991;14:162A.
Cy = cyclophosphamide; TBI = total body irradiation; BU = busulfan; BCNU = carmustine; VP16 = etoposide.

institution has more than doubled (21,25). There is some evidence that conditioning regimens can be altered to diminish the risk of VOD. For example, fractionated doses rather than single-dose administration of BCNU were associated with a lower incidence of VOD (99). Similarly, administration of lower total doses of TBI (10 Gy) at 2 to 3 cGy/min may result in a low incidence of VOD (35,85); however, an increased risk of leukemic relapse will limit this approach. Because of the wide variation in pharmacokinetics of cytotoxic drugs, several centers have undertaken studies that measure levels of BU and CY metabolites after initial doses to adjust later doses. These studies will test the hypothesis that individualized dosing will limit liver toxicity while maintaining antitumor and immunosuppressive effects. Theoretically, shielding the liver during TBI might reduce regimen-related liver toxicity. Although this approach has not been studied formally, shielding has been used when VOD develops prior to completing TBI. No conclusion can be drawn regarding efficacy.

Heparin. Continuous infusion heparin has been given during conditioning therapy and through the first 2 weeks after BMT (108–111). Low doses of heparin (150 U/kg/day) can be tolerated by thrombocytopenic BMT recipients if the partial thromboplastin time is not prolonged (110). A randomized controlled study reported that a continuous infusion of heparin significantly reduced the incidence of VOD when compared with placebo (111). Two studies of prophylactic heparin in patients at high risk for fatal VOD did not suggest efficacy of heparin in preventing severe VOD (108,110).

Prostaglandin E_1. Prostaglandin E_1 (PGE_1) has vasodilatory and antithrombotic effects (112–114). In two trials in BMT recipients, PGE_1 was administered as a continuous infusion (97,115). One study encountered significant side effects (i.e., skin bullae, bone pain, hypotension) that may have been related to an effect of PGE_1 on CSP metabolism (115). Because many patients were withdrawn from the study, no conclusion could be made regarding efficacy. In a second study, patients prepared with low-dose CY/TBI were given PGE_1 and had a decreased incidence of VOD compared with a group of patients who did not receive PGE_1 (97).

Pentoxifylline. Pentoxifylline (PTX) is a xanthine derivative that has been demonstrated to down-regulate the production of TNF-α (41). Because TNF release is associated with regimen-related toxicity, it has been suggested that PTX may reduce the incidence and severity of VOD. In a Phase I-II trial, PTX was given to 30 BMT recipients from the start of conditioning therapy through hospital discharge (41). Treated patients appeared to have less severe liver and renal complications than historical control subjects, but a randomized trial of PTX showed no benefit over placebo (116).

Ursodeoxycholic Acid. Ursodeoxycholic acid is a nonhuman bile acid that increases bile flow (117) and causes less cell membrane damage than native human bile acids (118). A small pilot trial of ursodeoxycholic acid was reported to reduce the incidence of VOD compared with historical control subjects (119).

Treatment

The treatment of VOD is primarily supportive, with careful management of fluid overload and its attendant complications. Some pharmacological agents have been studied in an attempt to alter the natural history of established VOD. Rarely, surgical therapy (including liver transplantation) has been utilized in patients with severe disease or intractable ascites.

Supportive Therapy. Supportive treatment of VOD is based on the judicious management of sodium and water excess, with close attention to total body weight, urine output, and estimates of intravascular volume status. If patients become symptomatic due to excess extravascular volume, we attempt to achieve a sodium diuresis with spironolactone or furosemide, again paying close attention to intravascular volume status. Low-dose dopamine infusion has been abandoned, because studies in nonmarrow transplant recipients with the hepatorenal syndrome have shown a deleterious effect on sodium excretion (120). If ascites causes respiratory compromise, midline paracentesis is cautiously performed. Organ failure in patients with severe disease is managed with hemodialysis and mechanical ventilation, albeit with little impact on an already poor prognosis.

Tissue Plasminogen Activator. Given the evidence that coagulation factors are deposited in the subendothelial space of damaged venules in patients with VOD, thrombolysis has been proposed as therapy for established severe VOD. Uncontrolled studies show that therapy with tissue plasminogen activator (t-PA) and heparin may be effective (121,122). Six of 10 patients apparently responded to treatment with t-PA (20 mg) and heparin, with dramatic reductions in serum bilirubin and improvement in other signs and symptoms of VOD. Side effects of t-PA and heparin therapy included bleeding while on heparin, necessitating stopping the infusion. Fatal bleeding related to thrombolytic therapy has been reported in BMT recipients with VOD.

PGE_1. Results of a small uncontrolled study of PGE_1 infusion in established VOD have been reported (123). Nine patients were treated with continuous infusion PGE_1 within 1 to 10 days of diagnosis, with reduction in serum bilirubin levels, weight loss, and decrease in platelet transfusion requirements.

Surgical Approaches. In the past 15 years, we have treated 2 patients with peritoneovenous (Leveen) shunts for intractable ascites. Both patients died of complications related to shunt placement. Two patients with VOD have had successful portasystemic shunts for persistent ascites (124,125). To date, 3 patients have received liver transplants for their severe VOD and organ failure (126).

Acute GVHD

Acute GVHD usually occurs after day 15 as marrow engraftment appears (46,61,127,128), although a "hyperacute" form may develop earlier if CSP/MTX prophylaxis is not given (129). The syndrome of skin, gastrointestinal, and liver involvement develops in 30 to 70% of allogeneic BMT recipients (see Chapter 26). A maculopapular rash is usually the first manifestation of acute GVHD, with a characteristic distribution involving the palms, soles, and ears, and eventually spreading to the trunk, face, and extremities (Plates XVII, XIX, XX and XXIII). Gastrointestinal involvement, manifested by nausea, vomiting, and diarrhea, may be present (46). GVHD of the liver develops in approximately 70% of patients with acute GVHD, usually becoming apparent after cutaneous involvement is evident (61,128). Rarely, liver GVHD is noted as the initial manifestation of GVHD.

Liver test abnormalities usually consist of moderate to marked elevations in alkaline phosphatase and bilirubin levels, up to 20 times the upper limit of normal (41,61,130). Hepatocellular enzymes (AST, ALT) are also elevated, particularly in the early phases of GVHD, although seldom greater than 10 times their normal upper limit. Characteristic liver test abnormalities in the setting of typical skin and gastrointestinal GVHD are usually presumed to be secondary to liver GVHD. One must be cautious because of a high prevalence of other liver diseases in BMT recipients; diagnostic certainty can be difficult to achieve in a patient who has several liver diseases simultaneously. Liver disease that presents de novo in the absence of skin or intestinal GVHD or that persists despite immunosuppressive therapy usually requires a liver biopsy to evaluate for viral hepatitis, medication-induced liver injury, fungal infiltration, or persistent VOD. In the first 1 to 2 weeks of liver GVHD, however, a definitive histological diagnosis of GVHD may be difficult because a mild nonspecific lobular hepatitis (and not bile duct lesions) is seen early in GVHD (131,132). Characteristic findings of cholestasis and disrupted septal and interlobular bile duct epithelia are usually noted after 2 weeks of involvement (131–133) (see figures 16.6 and 16.7, Plates XXXI and XXXII). Intrahepatic peribiliary glands may also be involved (134). The combination of jaundice and elevated alkaline phosphatase levels typical of acute GVHD can also be seen with cholangitis lenta, liver injury caused by medications, fungal liver infection, and extrahepatic obstruction (46,61). Imaging studies (ultrasound, CT) can be useful in detecting biliary dilation and infiltrative lesions but cannot determine the presence or absence of GVHD.

Treatment of acute GVHD with immunosuppressive agents is covered in Chapter 26. A large retrospective study of GHVD treatment demonstrated that only 30% of patients with liver GVHD had resolution of liver abnormalities after initial treatment (135). Another 32% of these patients were not evaluable, because other liver diseases (VOD and infections involving the liver) obscured improvement due to immunosuppressive therapy. These patients with multifactorial liver disease had a worse response to immunosuppressive treatment. When jaundice is persistent despite treatment, it is difficult to know whether the GVHD is refractory to treatment or whether another liver disease is present. Liver imaging and measurement of hepatic venous pressure gradient (as a marker for persistent VOD) can provide objective evidence for the presence of other diseases and liver biopsy can indicate the degree of bile duct damage (as a marker for ongoing GVHD). Chronic GVHD of the liver will develop in more than half the patients with acute GVHD (136).

Cholangitis Lenta

Liver dysfunction can occur with fungemia, bacteremia, or localized abscess outside the liver (137–142), usually manifested as cholestasis with elevated bilirubin and serum alkaline phosphatase levels in patients who are persistently febrile. Liver histology reveals intrahepatic cholestasis with little or no evidence of hepatocellular necrosis (143,144). One pathogenic mechanism relates to circulating endotoxins and cytokines. Animal studies have shown that endotoxinemia causes a dose-dependent decrease in bile flow (145). Infections not usually associated with endotoxemia (e.g., staphylococcal sepsis) may also cause jaundice through the effect of cytokines and bacterial toxic products (141,142,146). Because infection usually occurs in the first days to weeks after transplantation, jaundice secondary to bacteremia may be confused with VOD, may contribute to the degree of hyperbilirubinemia in patients with VOD, or may mimic acute GVHD of the liver. There are no diagnostic tests for cholangitis lenta. Bacteremia is generally involved when persistent fever precedes cholestasis and cholestasis improves or resolves after treatment with antibiotics.

Infections of the Liver

Hepatic infections are not uncommon following BMT and may be difficult to diagnose because of a high prevalence of other liver diseases such as VOD and GVHD. Fungal infiltration most commonly develops in the first few weeks, whereas viral hepatitides usually have their onset after day 40 (46,61). Bacterial infections of the liver and the biliary tract are rare in the post-BMT setting.

Fungal Infection

Fungal liver disease develops when granulocytopenia is most profound, either soon after transplantation or later in patients with poor graft function. *Candida* species are most frequently involved, although other species, such as *Aspergillus*, *Trichosporon*, *Rhizopus*, and *Fusarium* are occasionally isolated (147–154). Fungal liver disease usually develops in patients with disseminated fungal disease; up to one third of all patients with disseminated visceral candidiasis have liver involvement (155). Rarely, infection isolated to the liver results from fungi gaining access to the portal vein by traversing intestinal mucosa (156). Most patients with proven fungal liver infection have had prior positive cultures for fungus, usually in surveillance cultures of stool, mouth, urine, and in blood cultures (153,154).

The clinical picture of fungal hepatitis is that of fever, tender hepatomegaly and increased serum alkaline phosphatase levels (19,155). In BMT recipients, this clinical triad may not be an accurate predictor of fungal liver infection. A case-control study of all autopsies done at the Hutchinson Center during 1980 to 1990 revealed almost identical clinical features during the last week of life in patients with and without fungal liver infection (154). A clinical diagnosis of fungal liver disease was never made in one third of patients who had fungal infection at autopsy, probably because imaging tests had a sensitivity of less than 25%. A definitive diagnosis of fungal liver disease requires visualization of liver-filling defects with CT, with guided fine-needle aspiration, or biopsy of the lesions (19,155,157). Rarely, yeast can invade vascular structures, resulting in hepatic infarcts or venous obstruction mimicking VOD (155). Massed fungi causing bile duct obstruction have also been reported (158,159). Patients with hepatic candidiasis are treated with intravenous amphotericin. Restoration of granulocyte function is the single most important factor in recovery from fungal liver infection. In those with discrete abscesses on CT, repeated imaging can be used to document regression of these lesions. However, regression of the size of lesions does not assure that the fungi have been eliminated; we have seen several patients whose signs and symptoms of fungal infection resolved, only to be reactivated months later following immunosuppressive drug treatment for chronic GVHD.

Viral Infection

Viral liver infections usually appear 6 to 10 weeks after BMT due to long incubation periods for primary infection and a lengthy period for viral activation from a latent phase. The presenting biochemical picture is usually that of mild to moderate increases in serum transaminase levels (AST, ALT), with variable degrees of hyperbilirubinemia. The clinical course may vary from asymptomatic or mild disease to fulminant hepatic necrosis and death.

Hepatitis C Virus. Infection with HCV is not uncommon among candidates for BMT (21,36). HCV is typically a chronic infection with fluctuating mild elevations in liver enzyme activity (160). Little is known about the natural history of HCV infection in the BMT population. In one series, 8 of 83 long-term survivors seroconverted 6 to 24 months after BMT, and all had continued abnormal transaminase levels on long-term follow-up (37). In another series, the prevalence of chronic hepatitis after BMT was high among patients who underwent transplantation with elevations of serum transaminase levels (36). Fatal reactivation of HCV infection has been reported in 2 BMT recipients following withdrawal of immunosuppressive therapy (29). Given the immune deficiency that occurs after transplantation, one cannot rely on antibody testing to confirm the diagnosis of HCV infection. Furthermore, patients receiving Ig therapy may passively acquire HCV antibody (161). We routinely measure serum HCV RNA by polymerase chain reaction in our patients with suspected HCV infection. There is no information about chronicity of HCV infection in BMT recipients, but by inference to HCV-infected solid organ transplant recipients, who may have a rapid progression to cirrhosis (162), the long-term course may be adverse. Results of treatment of HCV infection with interferon or ribavirin in BMT recipients have not been reported.

Hepatitis B Virus. The prevalence of acute HBV infection in BMT recipients is generally low if there is careful screening of blood products, but can be high in patients presenting from countries where HBV is endemic (28,32,33). During the immune-deficient period after BMT, patients with previous infection may have reactivation and replication of HBV (28). After immune reconstitution, the immune response to viremia may cause clinically apparent hepatitis and rarely has resulted in fulminant hepatic necrosis (26–28). There is evidence that grafting of HBV-immune marrow into an HBV-infected recipient may lead to elimination of the virus from the recipient (28,32–35).

CMV Hepatitis. Disseminated CMV infection has been reported to occur in 36 to 70% of allogeneic BMT recipients (163), particularly in those with GVHD, but its incidence has decreased markedly since the advent of prophylactic ganciclovir therapy. Liver involvement is usually seen only in patients with disseminated disease (163,164). CMV causes focal microabscesses in the liver lobule and occasionally involves bile duct epithelium (164–166). The clinical manifestations of CMV hepatitis are usually mild. Serum aminotransferase levels may be elevated to 10 times the normal upper limit, but these abnormalities are not specific. Massive hepatic necrosis from CMV hepatitis is rare (167). A definitive diagnosis requires immunohistochemical analysis and culture of tissue because typical CMV inclusion bodies may not be present (165,166). Ganciclovir is generally effective against CMV infection, although disseminated disease may be difficult to control (168). Foscarnet is used if marrow suppression secondary to ganciclovir is persistent or severe (169).

Adenovirus, Herpes Simplex Virus, and *Varicella Zoster Virus.* These viruses are important because they represent a common etiology for an uncommon condition, fulminant viral hepatitis (166,170–173). These viruses may also be treated effectively with antiviral drugs (173–175). The clinical presentation is that of a nonspecific viral prodrome accompanied by rapid increases in serum transaminase levels beyond 400 to 600 IU/L. The liver diseases that commonly cause transaminase elevations of more than 1,000 IU/L in BMT recipients are hepatitis caused by medications, liver ischemia, and these viruses. Prophylactic treatment with acyclovir has effectively eliminated infections with HSV and VZV, but acute *adenovirus* infections involving the lungs, intestine, and liver occur sporadically (170,171). Diagnoses of these viral infections can be made by liver biopsy using tissue immunohistochemical staining and viral culture methods (166,176) (Plates XLII and XLIII). Patients with HSV or VZV hepatitis should be treated with high-dose acyclovir (173,174,177). *Adenovirus* appears to be sensitive to high-dose ganciclovir and perhaps ribavirin (175), but clinical experience with these drugs for *adenovirus* infections is limited.

Epstein-Barr Virus. Infection with EBV usually presents as a mild clinical hepatitis, but can also lead to a malignant B-cell proliferative syndrome caused by EBV-transformed immunoblasts, which infiltrate the liver and the intestine (178,179). It is usually seen in immunosuppressed patients with GVHD or after monoclonal anti-T-cell antibody treatment and presents with jaundice, rapidly progressive painful hepatomegaly, and infiltration of other viscera (178,180) (Plate XXXVI). Histologically, there is portal infiltration with lymphocytes, demonstrated to be immunoblastic B cells (166,179).

Bacterial Infection

Bacterial liver abscesses and cholangitis are unusual in the BMT setting, likely due to infection prophylaxis during the period of granulocytopenia and the use of empiric antibiotics in patients with fever of undetermined source (181). Calculous and acalculous cholecystitis are a rare cause of abnormal liver test results in this patient population (166). Gall bladder infection is due primarily to gallbladder stasis in patients receiving TPN (182,183). More than 50% of patients have gallbladder sludge by day 20, presumably predisposing them to the development of cholecystitis (70,183). The effects of chemotherapy on mucus secretion and GVHD-induced cholestasis may also predispose to cholecystitis (70). In these immunodeficient patients, localized pain and tenderness are often absent until the gallbladder is gangrenous or perforation has occurred. Fortunately, cholecystitis is rare in these patients.

Latent mycobacterial infection may reactivate within the liver during prolonged immunosuppression after BMT (184,185). Although infections with atypical mycobacteria are seen commonly in patients with acquired immune deficiency syndrome (AIDS), we have seen only one patient with *Mycobacterium avium intracellulare* liver infection after BMT. Another case was caused by viable mycobacteria from earlier bacillus Calmette-Guerin (BCG) vaccination (184). Diagnosis of mycobacterial infection in the liver requires biopsy, cultures, and appropriate stains.

Liver Injury Caused by Medications

Many therapeutic agents used after transplantation are hepatotoxic. Biochemical abnormalities can be mild and nonspecific and may be overshadowed by concomitant VOD or acute GVHD. Rarely, toxicity can be severe and can result in fulminant hepatic failure.

TPN

TPN is the most uniformly administered "therapy." Liver abnormalities secondary to TPN consist of hepatic steatosis, hepatitis, and cholestasis (186–188). Biochemical indices include mild elevations in transaminase and alkaline phosphatase levels, which usually resolve after TPN is discontinued. Frank jaundice may develop in patients with TPN liver injury who are septic or receiving multiple transfusions (188–190). Prolonged TPN frequently results in gallbladder sludge formation, and jaundice may develop if thick inspissated sludge or stones impact in the common bile duct (191). Hepatic failure and fibrosis occur rarely in patients receiving long-term TPN (192).

Cyclosporine and Methotrexate

CSP is frequently used for GVHD prophylaxis and is usually begun just prior to allogeneic BMT. In a rat model, CSP caused abnormalities in bile flow at the canilicular level at doses in the therapeutic range (193). When serum bilirubin levels were compared in patients receiving low-dose intravenous CSP (1.5 mg/kg/day) versus standard-dose CSP (3 mg/kg/day), those receiving the lower dose had lower mean bilirubin levels during days 10 to 20 (107,194). Very high blood levels of CSP cause necrosis of hepatocytes in zone 3 of the liver acinus, with elevation of hepatocellular enzyme activity and bilirubin levels (166,195). Hepatotoxicity may develop with lesser doses in patients with coexisting liver disease (196,197). CSP may also potentiate chemoirradiation-induced hepatotoxicity (198). MTX alone or combined with CSP for GVHD prophylaxis is not usually hepatotoxic in the doses used, but several studies reported that peak serum bilirubin levels were higher in CSP/MTX-treated patients than in those who received CSP or MTX alone (199,200).

Antithymocyte Globulin and Anti-T-cell Monoclonal Antibodies

Antithymocyte globulin, used in the treatment of acute GVHD, may cause mild transient elevations in serum transaminase levels (201–203). A similar effect is seen in patients receiving anti-T-cell monoclonal antibodies (204,205). Serious liver toxicity has not been reported.

Antimicrobial Agents

TMP-SMX and ketoconazole are most commonly associated with hepatotoxicity. TMP-SMX, used for prophylaxis of bacterial infections and *Pneumocystis carinii* pneumonia, can cause cholestasis (206–209), microvesicular fat deposition (206), hepatitis (208), and, rarely, hepatocellular necrosis (210). Ketoconazole hepatotoxicity occurs in 5 to 10% of patients (211,212) and may cause fatal hepatic necrosis (213,214). Fluconazole has superceded ketoconazole and seems to be less hepatotoxic. Of the commonly used intravenous antibiotics, only mezlocillin is a common cause of hepatitis (215).

Idiopathic Hyperammonemia and Coma

A syndrome of hyperammonemia and coma has been described in patients who received high-dose chemotherapy, including conditioning for BMT (216). The earliest symptoms are progressive lethargy, confusion, weakness, and incoordination, which may initially be attributed to pain medications. Plasma ammonia levels increase to extreme levels and cause diffuse cerebral edema and elevated intracranial pressure. These patients usually have normal or mildly elevated liver test results, and the syndrome is not due to liver failure. The diagnosis is made by demonstrating high serum ammonia levels (usually > 500 μmol/L). The pathogenesis of this syndrome is unclear, but defects in hepatic enzymes that metabolize ammonium to urea have been reported in patients in whom postpartum hyperammonemia and coma developed (217). Primary treatment should be focused on decreasing the ammonia level with hemodialysis and ammonia-trapping therapy with sodium benzoate or sodium phenylacetate (216,218). The prognosis is generally poor; only 2 of 9 patients in one series survived (216).

Gastrointestinal Bleeding

Gross intestinal bleeding develops in 5 to 15% of BMT recipients (hematemesis, melena, or rectal bleeding) in the first 100 days, but many more have occult bleeding, particularly when platelet counts are low. Esophageal and small intestinal ulcers are the most common sites of severe bleeding.

Mucosal Trauma from Retching

Retching and vomiting during cytoreductive therapy are still common despite aggressive antiemetic therapy (37). Newer antiserotonin antagonist drugs combined with other antiemetics have reduced the incidence of vomiting in recent years (see Table 33-1) (38,39). Mucosal trauma to the midbody of the stomach is the most common cause of "coffee-ground" emesis (47). More severe bleeding results from Mallory-Weiss tears at the gastroesophageal junction and intramural esophageal hematomas, especially when platelet counts are less than 35,000/mm^3 (219,220). Persistent nausea and vomiting from day 20 to 90 are usually caused by acute GVHD, esophageal infection by HSV or CMV, and medications (e.g., TMP-SMX) (47,48,54). Endoscopic control of bleeding due to mucosal trauma is seldom needed, because bleeding usually ceases when platelet counts are brought to more than 60,000/mm^3. Intramural hematomas of the esophagus resolve in 10 to 14 days and do not require surgery (220).

Acid-peptic Ulcers

Ulcers present in the esophagus, the stomach, and the duodenum before BMT may bleed profusely when platelet counts decrease after conditioning therapy. Surgery may be necessary if bleeding persists because chronic ulcers are likely to expose submucosal arteries ("visible vessels"). After BMT, peptic esophagitis is a common endoscopic finding in patients who present with hematemesis (219). Bleeding from esophagitis is usually responsive to platelet infusions and control of peptic reflux. H_2-receptor antagonists should not be used in this setting because they depress granulocyte production (221–223). Omeprazole is very effective in blunting gastric acid production but may lead to colonization of the upper intestine with bacteria and fungi. We have also used intraesophageal antacid drips (3–5 mEq of neutralizing capacity/hour) to keep the esophagus alkaline.

Ulcers Caused by Infection

Bleeding ulcers caused by HSV, CMV, and *Candida* were common until recent years, but antiviral and antifungal prophylaxis has almost eliminated these lesions (168,224–226). HSV and fungal ulcers in the esophagus occurred throughout the post-BMT course, whereas most CMV ulcers developed after day 40. CMV was formerly the major cause of intestinal ulcers in BMT recipients, particularly in the esophagus, where large, shallow lesions were the site of blood loss (Plates XXXIII and XXXIV). Gastric and intestinal ulcers caused by CMV are deep and likely to cause severe bleeding. Isolated CMV ulcers have been resected successfully (227,228).

Other infections are less common causes of severe bleeding. HSV and fungal esophagitis may lead to persistent oozing of blood (55). *Candida* and *Aspergillus* infections in the intestine rarely may erode into submucosal blood vessels (1,229). Organisms that cause diffuse enteritis or colitis (*C. difficile, C. septicum, C. perfringens,* adenovirus, rotavirus) may lead to bleeding when platelet counts are low. EBV lymphoproliferative disease involving the stomach and the intestine can cause bleeding from ulcerated tumor nodules (178,179,230) (Plate XXXVI).

GVHD

A prospective study of severe intestinal bleeding identified acute GVHD as the cause in 60% of our patients (219), half of whom had a concomitant intestinal infection, usually CMV. Bleeding in acute GVHD is from extensive areas of mucosal ulceration in the distal small intestine and the cecum (230,231) (Plates XXVII and XXVIII). There may be hemorrhagic necrosis of the entire mucosa from stomach to rectum. The diagnosis of acute GVHD in patients with high-volume diarrhea and bleeding is usually obvious because of skin and liver involvement, but the exact site and nature of the bleeding lesions are often uncertain. Patients bleeding from GVHD tend to bleed steadily from large denuded areas rather than one discrete focus. When infection with CMV or fungus develops in intestinal mucosa already affected by GVHD, focal bleeding lesions may occur (230). Multiorgan failure and intestinal bleeding are frequent terminal events in patients with severe acute GVHD unresponsive to immunosuppressive therapy.

Management of bleeding in patients with acute GVHD is difficult. Correcting platelet and coagulation abnormalities may slow the bleeding. Immunosuppressive therapy (see Chapter 10) will limit the extent of mucosal necrosis, but re-epithelialization of the intestinal mucosa affected by GVHD is very slow. If bleeding persists, it is useful to rule out lesions other than GVHD (e.g., CMV ulcers, esophageal infections, peptic ulcers) and to determine whether the bleeding is coming from a single focus by using endoscopy and radionuclide blood pool scans. Focal lesions can be treated with endoscopic cautery, heater probe, or epinephrine intramucosal injection. These forms of therapy destroy tissue and lead to ulcers 0.5 to 2 cm in size within a few days. Unless the underlying disease process is eliminated, these endoscopic methods will not cure the bleeding problem. We have not been successful in resecting large segments of diffusely bleeding intestine involved with GVHD (230). Temporary control of bleeding has been achieved with angiographic embolization of mesenteric blood vessels and with octreotide (somatostatin analog) infusion intravenously.

Iatrogenic Causes of Bleeding

Endoscopic biopsy of intestinal mucosa is often needed to confirm diagnoses of GVHD and mucosal infections, but the incidence of significant bleeding at the site of biopsy is approximately 1 in 100 (47,232). Intramural duodenal hematomas also occurred after biopsy in 4 patients (47,220). To minimize this complication, platelet counts should be more than 60,000/mm^3 at the time of biopsy and maintained at that level for 10 to 14 days. Biopsy sites in mucosa involved with GVHD re-epithelialize slowly and may bleed days after the biopsy if platelet counts decrease. Bleeding from biopsy sites can often be controlled with endoscopic cautery or heater probe.

Dysphagia

Infections of the esophagus, formerly the most common cause of difficulty in swallowing, are now uncommon. Mucositis, acid-peptic esophagitis, and trauma are currently the leading causes.

Mucositis

Painful desquamation of the oral and the pharyngeal epithelium caused by conditioning therapy may lead to transfer dysphagia if the mucositis is severe (42,44,233) (Plates III and IV). Patients complain of pain on initiating a swallow and cannot move a bolus past the esophageal inlet. At endoscopy, there usually is extensive edema of tissues at and above the level of the cricopharyngeal muscle. Edema may also involve the airway and require intubation. Esophageal symptoms are unusual even with the most severe oral mucositis, but edema and necrosis of esophageal epithelium have been described (see Figure 16-2). HSV infections and MTX may also cause mucositis in the BMT setting (43).

Intramural Hematomas

The abrupt onset of severe retrosternal pain, hematemesis, and painful swallowing suggests development of an intramural hematoma in the wall of the esophagus (233,234). This condition occurs primarily in the first few weeks after BMT in patients whose platelet counts are less than 50,000/mm^3 (220). Symptoms may follow retching or may occur spontaneously. The diagnosis can be confirmed by an esophageal radiograph with swallowed contrast material (water-soluble contrast at first, then barium if there is no evidence of perforation into the mediastinum) and by a CT scan showing a thickened esophageal wall (220,235,236). Endoscopy is relatively contraindicated, as many intramural hematomas represent contained perforations that can be extended into complete perforations by insufflation of air (237). The hematoma may cause total esophageal obstruction. The course of intramural hematomas in BMT recipients is one of slow resolution over 1 to 3 weeks (220). Surgery is not necessary.

Esophageal Infections

Fungal infections of the esophagus are now unusual because of prophylaxis with antifungal drugs (55,225). Fungal esophagitis is due largely to *Candida albicans* and other *Candida* species, usually during the period of granulocytopenia following conditioning therapy (53). In granulocytopenic patients, the creamy adherent plaques typical of candidiasis are absent. Diagnosis depends on demonstrating branching hyphae or large numbers of yeast forms from brushings or biopsies of esophageal lesions. Cultures are not useful for diagnosis because they do not differentiate colonization from tissue infection. During periods of granulocytopenia, treatment with intravenous amphotericin is indicated. If granulocyte counts are greater than 1,000/mm^3 and there are no systemic symptoms of fungal infection, oral fluconazole (100–200 mg daily) is effective (55). Seemingly superficial *Candida* infections of the mouth and the esophagus should not be undertreated in BMT recipients, since swallowed yeast forms of *Candida* readily gain access to the portal venous circulation through the normal small intestine (156). Visceral *Candida* infections are usually preceded by evidence of superficial infection and positive blood cultures (149,153).

Bacterial esophagitis usually occurs as part of a mixed infection with fungi or viruses in patients with poor marrow function (53,238). The organisms are usually polymicrobial, derived from the oral flora. Diagnosis is made by finding large numbers of bacteria admixed with necrotic epithelial cells in biopsy specimens stained by tissue Gram stain.

The viruses that infect the esophagus are HSV, CMV, and, rarely, VZV (55). Nausea and vomiting are the most common presenting symptoms, but some patients have heartburn, painful swallowing and severe retrosternal pain (47,53,54). HSV causes small, 1- to 2-mm vesicles in the squamous epithelium of the mid and distal esophagus. The infected epithelial cells slough, leaving ulcers with reddened, raised borders (239,240). With extensive infection, ulcers may coalesce to form large areas of denuded epithelium. Because HSV infects only squamous epithelial cells in the esophagus, brushings and biopsy specimens must sample the edges and not the center of ulcers. HSV is identified by typical multinucleate cells with intranuclear inclusion bodies, by immunohistology showing specific staining of inclusion bodies using monoclonal antibodies to HSV antigens, and by viral culture (55,231). The diagnosis can be made by endoscopic brushings alone if low platelet counts preclude biopsy. If the epithelium of the entire esophagus has been sloughed because of HSV infection, diagnosis can be difficult, as no infected squamous cells remain except at the proximal margin of the ulcer and possibly in residual islands of squamous epithelium within the ulcer. Intravenous acyclovir is effective in eliminating virus, but large ulcers may heal slowly (241). HSV isolates resistant to acyclovir are usually responsive to foscarnet (242). VZV may produce a clinical and endoscopic picture identical to HSV esophagitis, but there is usually evidence of disseminated VZV infection in the skin and other viscera (55). Immunohistology of infected epithelial cells will differentiate HSV from VZV in the esophagus.

CMV esophagitis differs from HSV and VZV infection in several respects. CMV never infects squamous epithelium but involves endothelial cells and fibroblasts in the submucosal tissues of the esophagus (53,231,243) (Plate XXXIV). In most patients, the infection is systemic, not limited to the esophagus. The endoscopic appearance is of shallow, serpiginous ulcers with erythematous borders in the distal and midesophagus (240) (Plate XXXIII). Ulcers can be large, extending over 10 to 12 cm of the esophagus, but some normal-appearing epithelium is usually visible. Biopsy specimens must be obtained from the ulcer crater, a technique that requires platelet counts greater than 60,000/mm^3 to avoid bleeding. Diagosis of CMV is best made by placing biopsy material into veal infusion broth for transport to the virology laboratory. Shell-vial centrifugation culture methods provide a rapid (24 hr) result. Use of standard viral tissue culture for CMV is as accurate as centrifugation culture methods, but results are slower. CMV can be demonstrated by typical amphophilic intranuclear and intracytoplasmic inclusion bodies in large submucosal cells (Plate XXXIV). Immunohistology using early and intermediate CMV antigens and in situ DNA hybridization are more sensitive than routine staining because these methods identify infected cells that are neither megaloid nor inclusion-bearing (55). Viral culture methods are approximately twice as sensitive as immunohistological methods. Ganciclovir is effective in eliminating CMV from esophageal ulcers, but symptoms and ulcers respond slowly (54). Intravenous ganciclovir is given for 2 weeks at high dose and then for 2 or more weeks at a lower dose. Foscarnet is an alternative therapy that may be more effective than ganciclovir for CMV enteritis in patients with AIDS (244); experience with foscarnet for CMV enteritis in the BMT setting is limited.

Acid-peptic Esophagitis

Factors contributing to reflux esophagitis in BMT recipients include gastric stasis, the recumbent position, and poor salivary bicarbonate flow due to mucositis and acute GVHD. Patients with esophageal infection may complain of symptoms related to reflux, even when the infecting organism has been eliminated

(54). Treatment of gastroesophageal reflux with head-of-bed elevation and omeprazole (20 mg twice daily) is effective in relieving these symptoms. Development of peptic strictures in the weeks following BMT is rare.

Diarrhea

Diarrhea related to conditioning therapy is a common complication in the first few days after BMT. Acute GVHD, infectious enteritis, and medications cause most cases of diarrhea after day 20. Multiple etiologies may coexist.

Chemoradiotherapy Toxicity

Diarrhea in the first days after BMT is nearly always due to chemoradiotherapy toxicity to the intestine and is usually accompanied by anorexia. Histological findings after high-dose chemoradiotherapy include mucosal crypt aberrations, with nuclear atypia, epithelial flattening, and cell degeneration (232) (Plate XI). Surface epithelium and villous architecture are also distorted. This mucosal injury results in net fluid secretion by the intestine, peaking 1 to 2 weeks after the start of conditioning and returning to normal by day 12 to 15 (232,245) (Plate XII). Mucosal regeneration is complete by day 20 provided acute intestinal GVHD or enteric infection does not supervene.

Acute GVHD

More than 50% of patients with grade II to IV acute GVHD have gastrointestinal involvement, and diarrhea is the most common symptom (46,135,232). The onset of diarrhea can be sudden. A large-volume secretory diarrhea is characteristic (i.e., watery diarrhea persists even when there is no oral intake). The diarrheal fluid is watery, green in color, with ropy strands of mucoid material that reflect transmucosal protein loss (246). There is a rough correlation between the volume of diarrhea, the extent of intestinal involvement, and the severity of abdominal pain, nausea, and vomiting. In an allografted patient with skin and liver abnormalities typical of acute GVHD, the diarrheal syndrome described is almost diagnostic of intestinal GVHD. Supporting evidence for GVHD comes from a decreasing serum albumin level (from gut protein loss) and negative stool cultures for organisms that cause enteritis. CMV is about the only common cause of enteritis in BMT recipients which requires intestinal biopsy for diagnosis (247). If diarrhea develops in a CMV-seropositive patient who is not receiving prophylactic ganciclovir, an intestinal biopsy may be needed to differentiate GVHD from CMV enteritis. Otherwise, the predictive value of a negative stool culture for other viruses, bacteria, fungi, and parasites is high (247).

Occasionally, radiographs of the abdomen are useful, not so much to determine whether GVHD is present, but to ascertain the extent of involvement. Both plain radiographs and CT scans of the abdomen may reveal edema of the intestinal wall (248–250), but these findings are usually nonspecific and do not help to differentiate between infection and acute intestinal GVHD (249,250). Pneumatosis intestinalis may also be seen by plain radiograph or CT scan but is nonspecific (251). Findings on barium studies of the stomach and small bowel include bowel wall thickening, with effacement of mucosal folds, excess luminal fluid, and rapid transit (252,253). A definitive diagnosis of GVHD in problematic patients usually requires gastrointestinal biopsy. Although the yield from mucosal biopsy is higher with gastroduodenal than rectal biopsies (47,254), sigmoidoscopic rectal biopsy is easier, quicker, and less costly than upper endoscopic biopsy. When nausea and vomiting are present, we usually do gastroduodenal rather than rectal biopsies to rule out infection and other upper gastrointestinal pathology. In mild cases of intestinal GVHD, the gastroduodenal and rectosigmoid mucosa appear grossly normal, but moderately severe GVHD causes diffusely edematous and erythematous mucosa (Plate XXV). Severe, grade IV GVHD may lead to ulcerations and large areas of mucosal sloughing in the stomach, the small intestine, and the colon (230,231,255) (Plates XXVII and XXVIII). Even when the gross appearance is normal, gastrointestinal biopsies often reveal intestinal crypt cell necrosis and apoptotic bodies diagnostic of acute GVHD (49,231,232) (Plates XXVI, XXIX and XXX).

The pathogenesis of diarrhea in patients with GVHD involves several mechanisms. First, the areas of the intestine most involved with GVHD, the ileum and the cecum (46,231,252), are the segments most involved with retrieval of fluid from the intestinal lumen. A defect in fluid absorption in these areas leads to higher volumes of diarrhea than an absorption defect in the upper intestine or the distal colon. Second, the abrupt onset of diarrhea is associated more with mucosal edema than with crypt-cell necrosis. It is likely that abrupt protein-losing diarrhea and intestinal edema are caused by local release of cytokines such as TNF (40,256). In experimental situations in vivo and in vitro, cytokines cause increases in vascular permeability and increased flux of fluid across paracellular pores (257,258). Third, there is ongoing crypt-cell necrosis caused by alloimmune cytotoxic T lymphocytes in acute GVHD (259). Electron microscopy of rectal mucosa from patients with acute GVHD showed T cells extending pseudopods toward the nuclear membranes of epithelial cells (260). The target cells disintegrate in the process of apoptosis (231,232). In severe cases of GVHD, whole crypts are destroyed, then adjacent crypts, then whole segments of intestinal mucosa (231) (Plate XXX). Intestinal bleeding often accompanies diarrhea in patients with severe GVHD (219,230).

Successful treatment of acute GVHD with immunosuppressive therapy results in a dramatic reduction in stool volume, with resolution of accompanying symptoms of abdominal pain, nausea, and vomiting. In a retrospective study of acute GVHD treatment, 50% of patients with gastrointestinal GVHD responded to initial therapy with prednisone, CSP, or antithymocyte globulin (135). Patients with post-transplant gastrointestinal complications in addition to GVHD were less likely to respond to initial therapy. Octreotide, a somatostatin analogue, has been reported to reduce stool volume in patients with acute intestinal GVHD (261,262) by inhibiting gastrointestinal hormone and fluid secretion, enhancing sodium and chloride absorption, and decreasing intestinal motility (263). Our experience shows that octreotide infusions achieve a 30 to 50% reduction in diarrheal volume as long as the infusions are continued. Antidiarrheal medications such as opiates, lomotil, and loperamide must be used cautiously during the phase of acute GVHD characterized by intestinal edema, because these drugs may cause ileus and painful abdominal distention.

Enteric Infections

Enteric infections are now relatively uncommon after BMT, despite the use of nonabsorbable antibiotics that suppress normal microflora, allowing for overgrowth by aerobic and fungal organisms. Patients with acute GVHD are at risk for enteric infection, due to the immunological abnormalities associated with GVHD (264) and immunosuppressive therapy used to treat GVHD (135). In a recent prospective analysis of 150 consecutive patients with the onset of diarrhea after day 20, only 20 patients had documented enteric infection (247). Most of these were due to *C. difficile* astroviros and adenovirus.

Bacterial pathogens responsible for intestinal infections in normal hosts (*Salmonella, Shigella, Campylobacter*) almost never cause diarrhea in hospitalized BMT recipients. *C. difficile* is the most common bacterial cause of infectious diarrhea (247,265). Mean diarrheal volumes from *C. difficile* colitis in BMT recipients are lower than in those with acute GVHD; diagnosis depends on detection of *C. difficile* toxin in diarrheal fluid. Typical pseudomembranes involving the colonic mucosa are usually absent when patients are granulocytopenic; mucosal biopsy will identify GVHD when both *C. difficile* colitis and GVHD are present. Overgrowth of other clostridial species may cause typhlitis and focal necrotizing enteritis (13,266–268). Overgrowth of aerobic gram-negative organisms in the intestinal tract can cause a pseudomembranous enteropathy (264). Fungal overgrowth of the intestine is an overlooked cause of watery diarrhea in hospitalized nontransplant recipients (269–271) and may contribute to diarrhea after transplantation as well. Large numbers of *Candida* species were found in 21 of 150 patients with diarrhea, some of whom had no other explanation for diarrhea (247). Watery diarrhea secondary to small bowel involvement with both *Cryptosporidium* and *Giardia lamblia* was reported in a small number of patients (11,12). Treatment for cryptosporidiosis is unsatisfactory in non-BMT recipients; restoration of immune competence and therapy with spiramycin have been successfully used in some BMT recipients.

The incidence of viral gastrointestinal infection decreased in the past few years, likely due to antiviral prophylaxis in CMV- and HSV-seropositive patients and in patients with a CMV- or HSV-seropositive marrow donor. HSV infection is usually limited to the esophagus and only rarely causes intestinal disease (53,230) (Plate XXXV). Enteritis and colitis secondary to CMV may cause diarrhea with or without gastrointestinal bleeding (49,227,230, 231). Diffuse intestinal ulceration due to CMV with intestinal edema and protein loss identical to that of GVHD has been reported (253,272,273). Endoscopic examination with tissue biopsy for culture and immunohistochemistry is necessary for definitive diagnosis (231,274). The endoscopic appearance of discrete ulcerations is highly suggestive of viral involvement, and the diagnostic yield is highest if biopsy specimens are taken from the central portion of ulcerations. Treatment with ganciclovir eliminates CMV from tissue, but healing of ulcerations can be slow (54,275). Rotavirus, astrovirus adenovirus, and coxsackie viruses are sporadic causes of diarrhea (265,276). Severe necrotizing enteritis can result from adenovirus infection (170).

Medications

Oral nonabsorbable antibiotics used in gut decontamination are a frequent cause of diarrhea in patients who are eating. Magnesium salts (given during CSP therapy) and promotility agents, such as metaclopramide, may contribute to diarrhea.

Abdominal Pain

Abdominal pain is usually due to intestinal toxicity from chemoradiotherapy, hepatomegaly caused by VOD, and acute intestinal GVHD. Less common causes of abdominal pain, such as intestinal perforation and biliary colic, must be kept in mind.

Toxicity from Conditioning Therapy

Crampy abdominal pain in the immediate post-BMT period is commonly due to chemoradiotherapy-induced intestinal injury and is usually associated with diarrhea (46,232). Extensive mucosal necrosis, ulceration, and severe pain caused by conditioning therapy is unusual (230). Intestinal perforation may develop in the setting of lysis of a transmural lymphoma or metastatic carcinoma after conditioning therapy (7–9).

Patients with VOD often have right upper abdominal pain or tenderness secondary to hepatic enlargement (23,25,59). Although pain from VOD is usually only moderate and well localized, it can be severe and poorly localized, simulating a surgical abdomen (277). The diagnosis of VOD is strongly suggested by recent weight gain and hyperbilirubinemia, but abdominal imaging by plain radiography, ultrasound or CT scans may be needed to exclude other intra-abdominal pathology, such as a perforation, abscess, typhlitis, or hematoma.

Acute GVHD

Acute intestinal GVHD typically causes periumbilical crampy abdominal pain and diarrhea (46,128,246, 252,278). The presentation of these symptoms, along with nausea, vomiting, and a skin rash, make the diagnosis of acute GVHD likely. In some patients, the sudden onset of intestinal edema precedes skin rash and diarrhea and can cause a rigid, board-like abdomen with rebound tenderness (230,252); the diagnosis of acute GVHD may not be obvious. Intra-abdominal catastrophes may be ruled out by abdominal radiography (plain radiographs and CT). Surgical exploration should be performed only for clear indications, such as abscess or perforation, because little is to be gained from making the diagnosis of acute GVHD with laparotomy (230). Medical treatment of pain and diarrhea with opiates and anticholinergic medication may cause an ileus, with further exacerbation of pain. Intestinal decompression with a nasogastric or small intestinal sump tube may be needed until these medications can be cleared from the bloodstream.

Infection

Enteric infections are an uncommon cause of significant abdominal discomfort, with the exception of *C. difficile* colitis, which may cause colonic pain. Fungal abscesses of the liver and the spleen may cause abdominal pain, usually localized to the site of involvement (19). Acute pancreatitis is an infrequent cause of abdominal pain and may be due to viruses (particularly CMV) (279,280). Varicella zoster infection may present as abdominal pain, distention, and a clinical picture of intestinal pseudo-obstruction, before the appearance of typical zoster skin lesions.

Neutropenic enterocolitis (typhlitis) is a well-described complication in granulocytopenic hosts (13,266,267,281) and must be considered in any post-BMT recipient with the sudden onset of right-sided abdominal pain, fever, vomiting, and bloody diarrhea. The diagnosis is suggested by ultrasound or CT scan, typically revealing significant edema of the cecal wall (282,283). *Clostridium septicum* is most frequently implicated in typhlitis, but other clostridial species have been isolated (267,284,285). Patients often require surgical resection of the diseased bowel (281,286,287). Mortality is high despite aggressive medical and surgical therapy (281,286).

EBV-induced lymphoproliferative disorder has been described in BMT recipients given prolonged immunosuppressive therapy for acute GVHD (178–180). Infiltration of the liver, spleen, and intestinal wall with transformed B lymphocytes may cause severe pain due to organomegaly and ileus (178,230) (Plate XXXVI).

Hematomas

Spontaneous bleeding into the retroperitoneum, the abdominal wall, or the intra-abdominal viscera may develop in patients with low platelet counts, causing significant pain (288). Retroperitoneal hemorrhage may be asymptomatic but usually presents with lumbar or flank pain and less frequently abdominal discomfort. A CT scan is required for diagnosis. Rectus sheath hematomas often appear to have occurred spontaneously, but occasionally a history of minimal abdominal wall trauma can be elicited (289). Pain can be severe due to the rapid engorgement of a confined space. Occasionally, an abdominal wall mass can be palpated. The diagnosis is made by ultrasound or CT examination (288,290). Intramural hematomas of the small intestine can occur due to local ulceration from CMV or GVHD or at the site of duodenal biopsies (47,220). Patients usually present with abdominal pain and intestinal obstruction as the hematoma encroaches on the bowel lumen. The diagnosis is often suggested on a CT scan or contrast studies of the intestine.

Biliary and Pancreatic Pain

Gallbladder sludge develops in the majority of patients receiving prolonged TPN (70,182,183). When patients resume oral intake, gallbladder contraction forces this viscous, gel-like material through the cystic and common bile ducts and the ampulla of Vater. Nausea and epigastric abdominal pain are common symptoms. Pain usually resolves after patients have been eating for several days. Cholecystitis and gallbladder perforation are consequences of obstruction of the cystic duct by gallstones or sludge and infection of the gallbladder mucosa by enteric bacteria, fungi, and, rarely, CMV (291–293). The diagnosis of gallbladder disease, which requires surgery often must be made on clinical grounds, because the prevalence of gallbladder abnormalities at ultrasound (i.e., sludge and wall thickness) is high in BMT recipients without cholecystitis (70).

Biliary sludge can also obstruct the main pancreatic duct, causing acute pancreatitis (294). CMV infection may also cause pancreatitis (279,280), and pancreatic involvement with GVHD has been reported (295). However, acute pancreatitis is not common after transplantation.

Perforation

Intestinal perforation may occur rarely at the site of an ulceration (i.e., tumor, viral, fungal, or peptic) or diverticulum. The diagnosis is often delayed because immunodeficiency often masks the initial signs and symptoms. Perforation is rare with acute intestinal GVHD (230), which may present as an acute abdomen because of bowel wall edema.

Problems in Long-term Marrow Transplant Survivors (After Day 100)

Liver Disease

Liver disease after day 100 is usually due to chronic GVHD and chronic HCV infection. Liver injury caused by medications also causes abnormal liver chemistries and may be difficult to differentiate from liver involvement with GVHD and viruses.

Chronic GVHD

Chronic GVHD is a common cause of liver dysfunction after day 100 because 80% of patients with chronic GVHD have liver involvement (296,297). Typical biochemistry consists of elevated alkaline phosphatase (typically 5 to 15 times the normal upper limit) and transaminase levels, with variable elevation in total bilirubin levels (298,299). Patients may be asymptomatic or may experience pruritus, fatigue, and weight loss (see Chapter 26). The diagnosis of chronic GVHD of the liver is usually straightforward in patients with these typical liver test abnormalities and involvement of other systems (i.e., skin, mucous membranes, lacrimal glands) with chronic GVHD (300). A clinical diagnosis of isolated chronic GVHD of the liver is often difficult, however, because viral hepatitis and liver injury from medications may produce a similar biochemical picture (61). A liver biopsy is often needed to confirm the diagnosis prior to instituting immunosuppressive therapy. Characteristic histological findings include small bile duct injury with dropout, marked cholestasis, and a variable degree of portal inflammation (131,132,166) (see Figure 16-8, Plate LVIII). Bile duct abnormalities and portal inflammation are also seen in chronic HCV infection, making a definitive histological diagnosis difficult (132,301).

Patients with only liver and skin involvement have a limited form of the disease and tend to have a better prognosis than those with extensive multisystem disease (300). The major cause of death in patients with extensive chronic GVHD is infection. Immunosuppressive therapy usually controls liver disease activity, as measured by serum biochemical parameters (see Chapter 26). Several cases of progression to cirrhosis have been reported, but chronic viral hepatitis was not excluded in these patients (166,302–304). A trial of ursodeoxycholic acid in patients with chronic GVHD of the liver resulted in significant improvement in alkaline phosphatase, bilirubin, and transaminase levels during 6 weeks of therapy (299).

Chronic Viral Hepatitis

HCV infection is prevalent in patients presenting for BMT, but may also be acquired from an HCV-seropositive donor or from blood products that carry HCV despite negative serological screening by blood banks (21,36,305). The persistence of a chronic hepatitis is likely the most common manifestation of HCV infection in long-term BMT survivors (36,37,306) but may be unrecognized in patients with chronic GVHD of the liver. A false-positive anti-HCV serology can result from therapy with Ig (161). The diagnosis of chronic HCV infection can be certain in patients with fluctuating elevated transaminase levels and a positive polymerase chain reaction for HCV RNA in serum (305,307). Biopsy of the liver is not necessary to diagnose HCV infection but can be useful in gauging the severity of disease and progression to cirrhosis. The long-term prognosis of chronic HCV infections in recipients of solid organ transplants is an adverse one (162). There is no information regarding the prevalence of cirrhosis caused by HCV infection or the results of antiviral therapy in BMT survivors.

Liver Injury Caused by Medications

CSP, TMP-SMX, and azathioprine are medications most commonly implicated in causing liver injury after day 100 (61). CSP is an uncommon cause of liver injury if blood levels are kept in a therapeutic range. Renal transplant recipients on CSP therapy have a higher incidence of biliary and pancreatic disease than those receiving other immunosuppressive therapy (308). TMP-SMX has been associated with cholestasis, hepatitis, and microvesicular fat deposition (206–210). Azathioprine hepatotoxicty has been described primarily in renal allograft recipients and is believed to be due to an idiosyncratic reaction resulting in both cholestasis and hepatocellular injury (309). Prolonged use of azathioprine in non-BMT recipients has rarely been associated with peliosis hepatis, VOD, and nodular regenerative hyperplasia, all of which may cause portal hypertension and ascites (310–313).

Nodular Regenerative Hyperplasia

Nodular regenerative hyperplasia (NRH) is a histological diagnosis associated with noncirrhotic portal hypertension (314). It may be responsible for the development of ascites after day 100 in BMT recipients, as a late consequence of liver injury from cytoreductive therapy. The histological appearance is that of regenerative hepatocellular nodules without extensive fibrosis (315). Nodular regenerative hyperplasia represents an adaptation to heterogeneous blood flow distribution and is a sensitive indicator of intrahepatic vascular damage (314). The prevalence of NRH in autopsy liver tissue of BMT recipients ranges from 8 to 22%, but the histological diagnosis correlates poorly with clinical findings in these patients.

Chronic Fungal Liver Infection

Patients receiving immunosuppressive therapy for chronic GVHD are at risk for reactivating dormant fungi within the liver. These foci of infection represent fungal abscesses that developed after BMT but were incompletely treated. Clinical presentation includes fever and right upper abdominal tenderness or pain, but can present solely with abnormal liver test results, particularly an elevated alkaline phophatase level (19). *Candida* species are the most common isolate.

Esophageal Symptoms

Approximately 6% of patients with extensive chronic GVHD have esophageal involvement (296,300). Abnormalities include desquamation of the squamous epithelium, webs, submucosal fibrous rings, and long, narrow strictures in the upper and midesophagus (316,317). The most common symptom is dysphagia, but some patients present with insidious weight loss, retrosternal pain, and aspiration of gastric contents. The diagnosis is suggested by barium contrast radiographs and is confirmed by endoscopic inspection and biopsy of involved mucosa. Recurrent heartburn and pulmonary aspiration at night are probably due to a lack of effective esophageal peristalsis and poor salivary bicarbonate production, a result of salivary gland destruction. Although webs can be disrupted easily with dilators, dense strictures are difficult to dilate safely. An increased risk of esophageal perforation has been described (316). Advanced esophageal involvement can be prevented by prompt treatment of chronic GVHD in its early stages (300). Immunosuppressive drug treatment of patients with dense strictures will halt progression, but some of the damage is irreversible. Therapy with omeprazole or H_2-receptor antagonists should be considered if there is uncontrolled acid reflux.

Sporadic cases of fungal and, rarely, viral esophagitis occur in long-term BMT survivors, particularly those with chronic GVHD who receive immunosuppressive and antibiotic therapy.

Diarrhea and Weight Loss

The incidence of diarrhea decreases sharply after day 100, except in patients with ongoing acute GVHD refractory to treatment (230,252). There are sporadic cases of infectious enteritis among patients whose immune reconstitution is incomplete and among patients with chronic GVHD. The organisms most commonly found are *C. difficile* and rarely *Giardia lamblia* and *Cryptosporidia*. We have reported bacterial and fungal overgrowth in the jejunum of patients with chronic GVHD and diarrhea. Deficiency of secretory IgA is the likely explanation for overgrowth (stasis syndrome) (300,318). These patients respond to appropriate antibiotic or antifungal therapy.

Fifteen years ago we described a more severe malabsorption syndrome in patients with extensive untreated chronic GVHD (231,298). In these patients, the intestine was diffusely involved with submucosal and subserosal collagen deposition. This presentation disappeared after introduction of immunosupressive drug therapy for chronic GVHD.

Diarrhea secondary to pancreatic insufficiency has developed in some long-term BMT survivors. Its pathogenesis is unknown.

References

1. Eras P, Goldstein MJ, Sherlock P. Candida infection of the gastrointestinal tract. Medicine 1972;51:367–379.
2. McDonald GB, Rees GM. An approach to gastrointestinal problems in the immunocompromised patient. In: Yamada T, Alpers DH, Owyang C, Powell DW, Silverstein FE, eds. Textbook of gastroenterology. Philadelphia: JB Lippincott, 1991:900–927.
3. Peterson WL. *Helicobacter pylori* and peptic ulcer disease. N Engl J Med 1991; 324:1043–1048.
4. Graham DY, Lew GM, Klien PD, et al. Effect of treatment of *helicobacter pylori* infection on the long-term recurrence of gastric or duodenal ulcer. A randomized, controlled study. Ann Intern Med 1992;116:705–708.
5. Stenson WF, MacDermott RP. Inflammatory bowel disease. In: Yamada T, Alpers DH, Owyang C, Powell DW, Silverstein FE, eds. Textbook of gastroenterology. Philadelphia: JB Lippincott, 1991:1588–1645.
6. Yin JAL, Jowitt SN. Resolution of immune-mediated diseases following allogeneic bone marrow transplantation for leukaemia. Bone Marrow Transplant 1992;9: 31–33.
7. Herrmann R, Panahon AM, Barcos MP, Walsh D, Stutzman L. Gastrointestinal involvement in non-Hodgkin's lymphoma. Cancer 1980;46:215–222.
8. List AF, Greer JP, Cousar JC, et al. Non-Hodgkin's lymphoma of the gastrointestinal tract: an analysis of clinical and pathologic features affecting outcome. J Clin Oncol 1988;6:1125–1133.
9. Ferrara JJ, Martin EW Jr, Carey LC. Morbidity of emergency operations in patients with metastatic cancer receiving chemotherapy. Surgery 1982;92:605–609.
10. Walzer PD, Genta RM. Parasitic infections in the compromised host. New York: Marcel Dekker, 1989.
11. Collier AC, Miller RA, Meyers JD. Cryptosporidiosis after marrow transplantation: person-to-person transmission and treatment with spiramycin. Ann Intern Med 1984;101:205–206.
12. Bromiker R, Korman SH, Or R, et al. Severe giardiasis in two patients undergoing bone marrow transplantation. Bone Marrow Transplant 1989;4:701–703.
13. Kornbluth AA, Danzig JB, Bernstein LH. *Clostridium septicum* infection and associated malignancy. Report of 2 cases and review of the literature. Medicine 1989;68:30–37.
14. Myerowitz RL, Pazin GJ, Allen CM. Disseminated candidiasis. Changes in incidence, underlying diseases, and pathology. Am J Clin Pathol 1977;68:29–38.
15. Zahradnik JM, Spencer MJ, Porter DD. Adenovirus infection in the immunocompromised patient. Am J Med 1980;68:725–732.
16. Glenn J, Cotton D, Wesley R, Pizzo P. Anorectal infections in patients with malignant disease. Rev Infect Dis 1988;16:42–52.
17. Hiatt JR, Kuchenbecker SL, Winston DJ. Perineal gangrene in the patient with granulocytopenia: the importance of early diverting colostomy. Surgery 1986;100:912–915.
18. Kalb RE, Grossman ME. Chronic perianal herpes simplex in immunocompromised hosts. Am J Med 1986;80:486–490.

19. Thaler M, Pastakia B, Shawker TH, et al. Hepatic candidiasis in cancer patients: the evolving picture of the syndrome. Ann Intern Med 1988;108:88–100.
20. Gordon SC, Watts JC, Veneri RJ, Chandler FW. Focal hepatic candidiasis with perihepatic adhesions: laparoscopic and immunohistologic diagnosis. Gastroenterology 1990;98:214–217.
21. McDonald GB, Sharma P, Matthews DE, et al. Venocclusive disease of the liver after bone marrow transplantation: diagnosis, incidence, and predisposing factors. Hepatology 1984;4:116–122.
22. Aach RD, Stevens CE, Hollinger FB, et al. Hepatitis C virus infection in post-transfusion hepatitis. An analysis with first-and second-generation assays. N Engl J Med 1991;325:1325–1329.
23. Jones RJ, Lee KSK, Beschorner WE, et al. Venocclusive disease of the liver following bone marrow transplantation. Transplantation 1987;44:778–783.
24. Ganem G, Saint-Marc Girardin M-F, Kuentz M, et al. Venocclusive disease of the liver after allogeneic bone marrow transplantation in man. Int J Radiat Oncol Biol Phys 1988;14:879–884.
25. McDonald GB, Hinds M, Fisher L, Schoch HG, et al. Veno-occlusive disease of the liver and multiorgan failure after bone marrow transplantation: a cohort study of 355 patients. Ann Intern Med 1993;188:255–267.
26. Pariente EA, Goudeau A, Dubois F, et al. Fulminant hepatitis due to reactivation of chronic hepatitis B infection after allogeneic bone marrow transplantation. Dig Dis Sci 1988;33:1185–1191.
27. Webster A, Brenner MK, Prentice HG, Griffith PD. Fatal hepatitis B reactivation after autologous BMT. Bone Marrow Transplant 1989;4:207–208.
28. Chen PM, Fan S, Liu CJ, et al. Changing of hepatitis B virus markers in patients with BMT. Transplantation 1990;49:708–713.
29. Kanamori H, Fukawa H, Maruta A, et al. Case report: fulminant hepatitis C viral infection after allogeneic bone marrow transplantation. Am J Med Sci 1992;303: 109–111.
30. Hansen CA, Sutherland DE, Snover DC. Fulminant hepatic failure in an HBsAg carrier renal transplant patient following cessation of immunosuppressive therapy. Transplantation 1985;39:311–312.
31. Galbraith RM, Eddleston AL, Williams R, Zuckerman AJ. Fulminant hepatic failure in leukaemia and choriocarcinoma related to withdrawal of cytotoxic drug therapy. Lancet 1975;2:528–530.
32. Locasciulli A, Bacigalupo A, Van Lint MT, et al. Hepatitis B virus (HBV) infection and liver disease after allogeneic bone marrow transplantation: a report of 30 cases. Bone Marrow Transplant 1990;6:25–29.
33. Reed EC, Myerson D, Corey L, Meyers JD. Allogeneic marrow transplantation in patients positive for hepatitis B surface antigen. Blood 1991;77:195–200.
34. Ilan Y, Nagler A, Adler R, et al. Ablation of persistent hepatitis B by bone marrow transplantation from a hepatitis B-immune donor. Gastroenterology 1993;104: 1818–1821.
35. Lok ASF, Liang RHS, Chung H. Recovery from chronic hepatitis B (letter). Ann Intern Med 1992;116:957–958.
36. Locasciulli A, Bacigalupo A, Alberti A, et al. Predictability before transplant of hepatic complications following allogeneic bone marrow transplantation. Transplantation 1989;48:68–72.
37. Ljungman P, Duraj V, Magnius L, et al. Hepatitis C infection in allogeneic bone marrow transplant recipients. Clin Transplant 1991;5:283–286.
38. Chapko MK, Syrjala KL, Schilter I, Cummings C, Sullivan KM. Chemotherapy toxicity during bone marrow transplantation: time course and variation in pain and nausea. Bone Marrow Transplant 1989;4:181–186.
39. Viner CV, Selby PJ, Zelian GB, et al. Ondansetron—a new safe and effective antiemetic in patients receiving high-dose melphalan. Cancer Chemother Pharmacol 1990;25:449–453.
40. Holler E, Kolb HJ, Moller A, et al. Increased serum levels of tumor necrosis factor-α precede major complications of bone marrow transplantation. Blood 1990; 75:1011–1016.
41. Bianco JA, Appelbaum FR, Nemunaitas J, et al. Phase I–II trial of pentoxifylline for the prevention of transplant related toxicities following bone marrow transplantation. Blood 1991;78:1205–1211.
42. Schubert MM, Williams BE, Lloid ME, Donaldson G, Chapko M. Clinical assessement scale for the rating of oral mucosal changes following bone marrow transplantation. Cancer 1992;69:2469–2477.
43. Schubert MM, Peterson DE, Flournoy N, Meyers J, Truelove EL. Oral and pharyngeal herpes simplex virus infection following bone marrow transplantation: analysis of factors associated with infection. Oral Surg Oral Med Oral Pathol 1990;70:286–293.
44. Kolbinson DA, Schubert MM, Flournoy N, Truelove EL. Early oral changes following bone marrow transplantation. Oral Surg Oral Med Oral Pathol 1988;66:130–138.
45. Chapman CR, Hill HF. Patient-controlled analgesia in a bone marrow transplant setting. In: Foley KM, ed. Advances in pain research and therapy. New York: Raven, 1990:231–247.
46. McDonald GB, Shulman HM, Sullivan KM, Spencer GD. Intestinal and hepatic complications of human bone marrow transplantation. Gastroenterology 1986; 90:460–477, 770–784.
47. Spencer GD, Hackman RC, McDonald GB, et al. A prospective study of unexplained nausea and vomiting after marrow transplantation. Transplantation 1986; 42:602–607.
48. Weisdorf DJ, Snover DC, Haake R, et al. Acute upper gastrointestinal graft-versus-host disease: clinical significance and response to immunosuppressive therapy. Blood 1990;76:624–629.
49. Snover DC, Weisdorf SA, Vercellotti GM, Rank B, Hutton S, McGlave P. A histopathologic study of gastric and small intestine graft-versus-host disease following allogeneic bone marrow transplantation. Hum Pathol 1985;16:387–392.
50. Jaffe HS, Abrams DI, Ammann AJ, Lewis BJ, Golden JA. Complications of co-trimoxazole in treatment of AIDS-associated Pneumocystis carinii pneumonia in homosexual men. Lancet 1983;2:1109–1111.
51. Hansen BW, DeSomery DH, Hagedorn LW. Effects of enteral and parenteral nutrition on appetite in monkeys. J Parenter Ent Nutr 1977;1:83–88.
52. Martyn PA, Hansen BC, Jen K-LC. The effects of parenteral nutrition on food intake and gastric motility. Nurs Res 1984;33:336–342.
53. McDonald GB, Sharma P, Hackman RC, Meyers JD, Thomas ED. Esophageal infections in immunosuppressed patients after marrow transplantation. Gastroenterology 1985;88:1111–1117.
54. Reed EC, Wolford JL, Kopecky KJ, et al. Ganciclovir for the treatment of cytomegalovirus gastroenteritis in bone

marrow transplant patients. A randomized, placebo-controlled trial. Ann Intern Med 1990;112:505–510.
55. Baehr PH, McDonald GB. Infections of the esophagus. In: Surawicz CM, Owen RL, eds. Gastrointestinal and hepatic infections. Philadelphia: WB Saunders, 1993 (in press).
56. Shulman HM, McDonald GB, Matthews D, et al. An analysis of hepatic venocclusive disease and centrilobular hepatic degeneration following bone marrow transplantation. Gastroenterology 1980;79:1178–1191.
57. Shulman HM, Hinterberger W. Hepatic venocclusive disease—liver toxicity syndrome after bone marrow transplantation. Bone Marrow Transplant 1992;10:197–214.
58. Snover DC. Liver disease after bone marrow transplantation—pathology. In: Hoofnagle JH, Goodman Z, eds. Liver biopsy interpretation for the 1990's. Clinicopathologic correlations in liver disease. Thorofare: AASLD, 1991:239–254.
59. McDonald GB, Sharma P, Matthews DE, Shulman HM, Thomas ED. The clinical course of 53 patients with venocclusive desease of the liver after marrow transplantation. Transplantation 1985;36:603–608.
60. Rollins BJ. Hepatic veno-occlusive disease. Am J Med 1986;81:297–306.
61. McDonald GB, Shulman HM, Wolford HL, Spencer GD. Liver disease after bone marrow transplantation. Semin Liver Dis 1987;7:210–229.
62. McDonald GB. Liver disease after bone marrow transplantation. In: Hoofnagle JH, Goodman Z, eds. Liver biopsy interpretation for the 1990's. Clinicopathologic correlations in liver disease. Thorofare: AASLD, 1991: 841–853.
63. Brugieres L, Hartmann O, Benhamou E, et al. Veno-occlusive disease of the liver following high-dose chemotherapy and autologous bone marrow transplantation in children with solid tumors: incidence, clinical course and outcome. Bone Marrow Transplant 1988;3:53–58.
64. DiBona GF. Update on renal neurology: role of the renal nerves in formation of edema (editorial). Mayo Clin Proc 1989;64:469–472.
65. Carreras E, Granena A, Navasa M, et al. Transjugular liver biopsy in BMT. Bone Marrow Transplant, 1993;11:21–26.
66. Shulman HM, McDonald GB. Utility of transvenous liver biopsy and hepatic venous pressure measurements in Seattle marrow transplant recipients. Exp Hematol 1990;18:699.
67. McAfee JH, Keeffe E, Lee RG, Rosch J. Transjugular liver biopsy. Hepatology 1992;15:726–732.
68. Kriegshauser JS, Charboneau JW, Letendre L. Hepatic venocclusive disease after bone marrow transplantation: diagnosis with duplex sonography. Am J Roentgenol 1988;150:289–290.
69. Brown BP, Abu-Yousef M, Farner R, LaBrecque D, Gingrich R. Doppler sonography: a noninvasive method for evaluation of hepatic venocclusive disease. Am J Roentgenol 1990;154:721–724.
70. Hommeyer SC, Teefey SA, Jacobson AF, et al. Sonographic evaluation of patients with venocclusive disease of the liver: a prospective study. Radiology 1992;184:683–686.
71. Bearman SI, Anderson GL, Mori M, et al. Veno-occlusive disease of the liver: development of a model for predicting fatal outcome after marrow transplantation. J Clin Oncol (in press).
72. Shana CB, Gollan JL. Fulminant hepatic failure. In: Taylor MB, Gollan JL, Peppercorn MA, Steer ML, Wolfe MM, eds. Gastrointestinal emergencies. Baltimore: Williams & Wilkins, 1992:226–247.
73. Shulman HM, Gown AM, Nugent DJ. Hepatic veno-occlusive disease after bone marrow transplantation. Immunohistochemical identification of the material within occluded central venules. Am J Pathol 1987; 127:549–558.
74. Allen JR, Carstens LA, Katagiri GJ. Hepatic veins of monkeys with veno-occlusive disease. Arch Pathol 1969;87:279–289.
75. Jaattela M. Biology of disease. Biologic activities and mechanisms of action of tumor necrosis factor-alpha/cachectin. Lab Invest 1991;64:724–742.
76. Bevilacqua MP, Pober JS, Majeau GT, et al. Recombinant tumor necrosis factor induces procoagulant activity in cultured human vascular endothelium. Characterization and comparison with the actions of interleukin-1. Proc Natl Acad Sci USA 1986;83:533–537.
77. van der Poll T, Buller HR, ten Cate H, et al. Activation of coagulation after administration of tumor necrosis factor to normal subjects. N Engl J Med 1990;322:1622–1627.
78. Scrobohaci ML, Drouet L, Monem-Mansi A, et al. Liver veno-occlusive disease after bone marrow transplantation. Changes in coagulation parameters and endothelial markers. Thromb Res 1991;63:509–519.
79. Faioni EM, Krachmalnicoff A, Bearman SI, et al. Naturally occurring anticoagulants and bone marrow transplantation: plasma protein C predicts the development of veno-occlusive disease of the liver. Blood 1993;81:3458–3462.
80. Gordon B, Haire W, Kessinger A, Duggan M, Armitage J. High frequency of antithrombin 3 and protein C deficiency following autologous bone marrow transplantation for lymphoma. Bone Marrow Transplant 1991;8:497–502.
81. Harper PL, Jarvis J, Jennings I, Luddington R, Marcus RE. Changes in the natural anticoagulants following bone marrow transplantation. Bone Marrow Transplant 1990;5:39–42.
82. Collins P, Jones B, Uthayakumar, et al. Haemostatic changes in uncomplicated bone marrow transplants. Bone Marrow Transplant 1991;7(suppl 2):54.
83. Battistini B, D'Orleans-Juste P, Sirois P. Endothelins: circulating plasma levels and presence in other biologic fluids. Lab Invest 1993;68:600–628.
84. Vowels M, Lam-Po-Tang R, Zagars G, Ewing DP. Total body irradiation and Budd-Chiari syndrome. Abstracts of the annual meeting of the Royal College of Pathologists of Australia, 1979:306.
85. Sloane JP, Farthing MJG, Powles RL. Histopathological changes in the liver after allogeneic bone marrow transplantation. J Clin Pathol 1980;33:344–350.
86. Atkinson K, Biggs J, Noble G, Ashby M, Concannon A, Dodds A. Preparative regimens for marrow transplantation containing busulfan are associated with haemorrhagic cystitis and hepatic veno-occlusive disease but a short duration of leucopenia and little oro-pharyngeal mucositis. Bone Marrow Transplant 1987;2:385–394.
87. Meresse V, Hartmann O, Vassal G, et al. Risk factors of hepatic veno-occlusive disease after high-dose busulfan-containing regimens followed by autologous bone marrow transplantation: a study in 136 children. Bone Marrow Transplant 1992;10:135–141.
88. Vassal G, Deroussent A, Challine D, et al. Is 600 mg/

m² appropriate dosage of busulfan in children undergoing bone marrow transplantation? Blood 1992;79: 2475–2479.

89. Grochow LB, Jones RJ, Brundrett RB, et al. Pharmacokinetics of busulfan: correlation with veno-occlusive disease in patients undergoing bone marrow transplantation. Cancer Chemother Pharmacol 1989;25:55–61.

90. Hassan M, Oberg G, Ehrsson H, et al. Pharmacokinetics and metabolic studies of high-dose busulphan in adults. Eur J Clin Pharmacol 1989;36:525–530.

91. Grochow LB, Krivit W, Whitley CB, Blazar B. Busulfan disposition in children. Blood 1990;75:1723–1727.

92. Harlan JM, Levine JD, Callahan KS, Schwartz BR, Harker LA. Glutathione redox cycle protects cultured endothelial cells against lysis by extracellular generated hydrogen peroxide. J Clin Invest 1984;73:706–713.

93. Roberts DW, Bicci TJ, Benson RW, et al. Immunohistochemical localization and quantification of the 3-(cystein-S-yl)-acetominophen protein adduct in acetaminophen hepatotoxicicity. Am J Pathol 1991;95: 1130–1143.

94. Shulman HM, Luk K, Deeg HJ, Shuman WB, Storb R. Induction of hepatic veno-occlusive disease in dogs. Am J Pathol 1987;126:114–125.

95. Traber PG, Chianale J, Gumucio JJ. Physiologic significance and regulation of hepatocellular heterogeneity. Gastroenterology 1988;95:1130–1143.

96. Ozkaynak MF, Weinberg K, Kohn D, Sender L, Parkman R, Lenarsky C. Hepatic veno-occlusive disease post-bone marrow transplantation in children conditioned with busulfan and cyclophosphamide: incidence, risk factors, and clinical outcome. Bone Marrow Transplant 1991;7:467–474.

97. Gluckman E, Jolivet I, Scrobohaci ML. Use of prostaglandin E_1 for prevention of liver veno-occlusive disease in leukaemic patients treated by allogeneic bone marrow transplantation. Br J Haematol 1990; 74:277–281.

98. Nevill TJ, Barnett MJ, Klingemann H-G, Reece DE, Shepherd JD, Phillips GL. Regimen-related toxicity of a busulfan-cyclophosphamide conditioning regimen in 70 patients undergoing allogeneic bone marrow transplantation. J Clin Oncol 1991;9:1224–1232.

99. Ayash LJ, Hunt M, Antman K, et al. Hepatic veno-occlusive disease in autologous bone marrow transplantation of solid tumors and lymphomas. J Clin Oncol 1990;8:1699–1706.

100. Bearman SI, Appelbaum FR, Buckner CD, et al. Regimen-related toxicity in patients undergoing bone marrow transplantation. J Clin Oncol 1988;6:1562–1568.

101. Dulley FL, Kanfer EJ, Appelbaum FR, et al. Venocclusive disease of the liver after chemoradiotherapy and autologous bone marrow transplantation. Transplantation 1987;43:870–873.

102. Witherspoon RP, Storb R, Shulman HM, et al. Marrow transplantation in hepatitis-associated aplastic anemia. Am J Hematol 1984;17:269–278.

103. Lucarelli G, Galimbert M, Delfini C, et al. Marrow transplantation for thalassemia following busulphan and cyclophosphamide. Lancet 1985;1:1355–1357.

104. Soiffer RJ, Dear K, Rabinowe SN, et al. Hepatic dysfunction following T-cell-depleted allogeneic bone marrow transplantation. Transplantation 1991;52: 1014–1019.

105. Essell JH, Thompson JM, Harman GS, Johnson RA, Rubinsak JR. Marked increase in veno-occlusive disease of the liver associated with methotrexate use for graft-vs-host disease prophylaxis in patients receiving busulfan/cyclophosphamide. Blood 1993;79:2784–2788.

106. Radich JP, Sanders JE, Buckner CD, et al. Second allogeneic marrow transplantation for patients with recurrent leukemia after initial tranplant with TBI-containing regimens. J Clin Oncol 1993;11:304–313.

107. Stockschlaeder M, Storb R, Pepe M, et al. A pilot study of low-dose cyclosporin for graft-versus-host prophylaxis in marrow transplantation. Br J Haematol 1992;80:49–54.

108. Marsa-Vila L, Gorin NC, Laporte JP, et al. Prophylactic heparin does not prevent liver veno-occlusive disease following autologous bone marrow transplantation. Eur J Haematol 1991;47:346–354.

109. Rio B, Lamy T, Sittoun R. Preventive role of heparin for liver venocclusive disease (VOD). Bone Marrow Transplant 1988;3:266.

110. Bearman SI, Hinds MS, Wolford JL, et al. A pilot study of continuous infusion heparin for the prevention of hepatic veno-occlusive disease after bone marrow transplantation. Bone Marrow Transplant 1990;5:407–411.

111. Attal M, Huguet F, Rubie H, et al. Prevention of hepatic veno-occlusive disease after bone marrow transplantation by continuous infusion of low-dose heparin: a prospective randomized trial. Blood 1992; 79:2834–2840.

112. Oates JA, Fitzgerald GA, Branch RA, Jackson EK, Knapp HR, Roberts LJ. Clinical implications of prostaglandin and thromboxane A_2 formation. N Engl J Med 1988;319:689–698.

113. Simmet T, Peskar BA. Prostaglandin E_1 and arterial occlusive disease: pharmacologic considerations. Euro J Clin Invest 1988;18:549–554.

114. Vaughn DE, Plavin SR, Schafer AI, Loscalzo J. PGE_1 accelerated thrombolysis by tissue plasminogen acitvator. Blood 1989;73:1213–1217.

115. Bearman SI, Shen DD, Hinds M, et al. A phase I/II study of prostalandin E_1 for the prevention of hepatic toxicity after bone marrow transplantation. Brit J Haematol (in press).

116. Clift RA, Bianco JA, Appelbaum FR, et al. A randomized controlled trial of pentoxifylline for the prevention of regimen-related toxicities in patients undergoing allogeneic marrow transplantation. Blood (in press).

117. Batta AK, Salen G, Arora R, et al. Effect of ursodeoxycholic acid on bile acid metabolism in primary biliary cirrhosis. Hepatology 1989;10: 414–419.

118. Heuman DM, Mills AS, McCall J, Hylemon PB, Pandak WM, Vlahcevic ZR. Conjugates of ursodeoxycholate protect against cholestasis and hepatocellular necrosis caused by more hydrophobic bile salts. Gastroenterology 1991;100:203–211.

119. Essell JH, Thompson JM, Harman GS, et al. Pilot trial of prophylactic ursodiol to decrease the incidence of veno-occlusive disease of the liver in allogeneic bone marrow transplant patients. Bone Marrow Transplant 1992;10:367–372.

120. Hadengue A, Moreau R, Bacq Y, Gaudin C, Braillon A, Lebrec D. Selective dopamine DA_1 stimulation with fenoldopam in cirrhotic patients with ascites: a sys-

temic, splanchnic and renal hemodynamic study. Hepatology 1988;13:111–115.

121. Baglin TP, Harper P, Marcus RE. Veno-occlusive disease of the liver complicating ABMT successfully treated with recombinant tissue plasminogen activator (rt-PA). Bone Marrow Transplant 1990;5:439–441.

122. Bearman SI, Shuhart MC, Hinds MS, McDonald GB. Recombinant human tissue plasminogen activator for the treatment of established severe hepatic veno-occlusive disease of the liver after bone marrow transplantation. Blood 1993;80:2458–2462.

123. Ibrahim I, Pico JL, Maraninchi D, et al. Hepatic veno-occlusive disease following bone marrow transplantation treated by prostaglandin E_1. Bone Marrow Transplant 1991;7(suppl 2):53.

124. Murray JA, LaBrecque DR, Gingrich RD, Pringle KC, Mitros FA. Successful treatment of hepatic veno-occlusive disease in a bone marrow transplant patient with side-to-side portacaval shunt. Gastroenterology 1987;92:1073–1077.

125. Jacobson BK, Kalayoglu M. Effective early treatment of hepatic veno-occlusive disease with a central splenorenal shunt in an infant. J Pediatr Surg 1992;27:531–533.

126. Nimer SD, Milewicz AL, Champlin RE, Busuttil RW. Successful treatment of hepatic venoocclusive disease in a bone marrow transplant patient with orthotopic liver transplantation. Transplantation 1990;49:819–821.

127. Ferrara JLM, Deeg HJ. Graft-versus-host disease. N Engl J Med 1991;324:667–674.

128. Vogelsang GB, Hess AD, Santos GW. Acute graft-versus-host disease: clinical characteristics in the cyclosporine era. Medicine 1988;67:163–174.

129. Sullivan KM, Deeg HJ, Sanders J, et al. Hyperacute graft-versus-host disease in patients not given immunosuppression after allogeneic marrow transplantation. Blood 1986;67:1172–1175.

130. Yasmineh WG, Filipovich AH, Killeen AA. Serum 5′nucleotidase and alkaline phosphatase—highly predictive liver function tests for the diagnosis of graft-versus-host disease in bone marrow transplant recipients. Transplantation 1989;48:809–814.

131. Snover DC, Weisdorf SA, Ramsay AK, et al. Hepatic graft-versus-host disease: a study of the predictive value of liver biopsy in diagnosis. Hepatology 1984;4:123–130.

132. Shulman HM, Sharma P, Amos D, Fenster LF, McDonald GB. A coded histologic study of hepatic graft-versus-host disease after human bone marrow transplantation. Hepatology 1988;8:463–470.

133. Tanaka M, Umihara J, Chiba S, Ishikawa E. Intrahepatic bile duct injury following bone marrow transplantation. Analysis of pathological features based on three-dimensional and histochemical observation. Acta Pathol Jpn 1986;36:1793–1806.

134. Nakanuma Y. Graft-versus-host disease involves intrahepatic peribiliary glands. J Clin Gastroenterol 1988;10:233–234.

135. Martin PJ, Schoch G, Fisher L, et al. A retrospective analysis of therapy for acute graft-versus-host disease: initial treatment. Blood 1990;76:1464–1472.

136. Sullivan KM, Agura E, Appelbaum F, et al. Chronic graft-versus-host disease and other late complications of bone marrow transplantation. Semin Hematol 1991;28:249–258.

137. Zimmerman HJ, Fanf M, Utili R, Seeff LB, Hoofnagle J. Jaundice due to bacterial infection. Gastroenterology 1979;77:362–374.

138. Caruana JA, Montes M, Camara DS, Ummer A, Potmesil SH, Gage AA. Functional and histopathologic changes in the liver during sepsis. Surg Gynecol Obstet 1982;154:654–656.

139. Gimson AES. Hepatic dysfunction during bacterial sepsis. Intensive Care Med 1987;13:162–166.

140. Fang MH, Ginsberg AL, Dobbins WO. Marked elevation in serum alkaline phosphatase activity as a manifestation of systemic infection. Gastroenterology 1980;78:592–597.

141. Watanakunakorn C, Chan SJ, DeMarco DG, Palmer JA. *Staphylococcus aureus* bacteremia: significance of hyperbilirubinemia. Scand J Infect Dis 1987;19:195–203.

142. Quale JM, Mandel LJ, Bergasa NV, Straus EW. Clinical significance and pathogenesis of hyperbilirubinemia associated with *Staphylococcus aureus* septicemia . Am J Med 1988;85:615–618.

143. Lefkowitz JH. Cholestasis in the critically ill: pathology. In: Hoofnagle JH, Goodman Z, eds. Liver biopsy interpretation for the 1990's. Clinicopathologic correlations in liver disease. Thorofare: AASLD, 1991:66–75.

144. Banks JG, Foulis AK, Ledingham IM, MacSween RNM. Liver function in septic shock. J Clin Pathol 1982;35:1249–1252.

145. Fox ES, Briotman SA, Thomas P. Biology of disease. Bacterial endotoxins and the liver. Lab Invest 1990; 63:733–741.

146. Andrus T, Bauer J, Gerok W. Effects of cytokines on the liver. Hepatology 1991;13:364–375.

147. Meyers JD. Fungal infections in bone marrow transplant patients. Semin Oncol 1990;17:10–13.

148. Gardella S, Nomdedeu B, Bombi JA, et al. Fatal fungemia with arthritic involvement caused by Trichosporon beigelii in a bone marrow transplant recipient. J Infect Dis 1985;151:566–567.

149. Tollemar J, Ringden L, Bostrom L, Nilsson B, Sundberg B. Variables predicting deep fungal infections in bone marrow transplant recipients. Bone Marrow Transplant 1989;4:635–641.

150. Siegert W, Henze G, Wagner J, et al. Invasive *trichosporon cutaneum* (beigelii) infection in a patients with relapsed acute myeloid leukemia undergoing bone marrow transplantation. Transplantation 1988;46:151–153.

151. Liu KL, Herbrecht R, Bergerat JP, Koenig H, Waller J, Oberling F. Disseminated *trichosporon capitatum* infection in a patient with acute leukemia undergoing bone marrow transplantation. Bone Marrow Transplant 1990;6:219–221.

152. Minor RL Jr, Pfaller MA, Gingrich RD, Burns LJ. Disseminated *Fusarium* infections in patients following bone marrow transplantation. Bone Marrow Transplant 1989;4:653–658.

153. Goodrich JM, Reed EC, Mori M, et al. Clinical features and analysis of risk factors for invasive candidal infection after bone marrow transplantation. J Infect Dis 1991;164:731–740.

154. Rosetti F, Brawner D, Meyer W, Meyers JD, McDonald GB. Fungal liver disease in marrow transplant patients, 1980–1990: prevalence, risk factors and clinical features. Abstracts of the European Bone Marrow Transplant meeting, Stockholm, Sweden, 1992:111.

155. Lewis JH, Patel HR, Zimmerman HJ. The spectrum of hepatic candidiasis. Hepatology 1982;2:479–487.

156. Krause W, Matheis H, Wulf K. Fungaemia and

funguria after oral administration of *Candida albicans*. Lancet 1969;1:598–599.
157. Bondestam S, Jansson SE, Kivisaari L, et al. Liver and spleen candidiasis: imaging and verification by fine-needle aspiration biopsy. Br Med J 1981;282: 1514–1515.
158. Magnussen CR, Olson JP, Ona FV, Graziani AJ. Candida fungus balls in the common bile duct. Unusual manifestation of disseminated candidiasis. Arch Intern Med 1979;139:821–822.
159. Marucci RA, Whitely H, Armstrong D. Common bile duct obstruction secondary to infection with candida. J Clin Microbiol 1978;7:490–492.
160. Davis GL, Balart LA, Schiff ER, et al. Treatment of chronic hepatitis C with recombinant interferon alfa. N Engl J Med 1989;321:1501–1506.
161. Quinti I, Paganelli R, Scala E, et al. Hepatitis C virus antibodies in gamma globulin. Lancet 1990;336:1377.
162. Pereira BJG, Milford EL, Kirkman RL, Levey AS. Transmission of hepatitis C virus by organ transplantation. N Engl J Med 1991;325:454–460.
163. Meyers JD, Flourney N, Thomas ED. Risk factors for cytomegalovirus infection after bone marrow transplantation. J Infect Dis 1986;153:478–488.
164. Rees GM, Sarmiento JI, Myerson D, Coen D, Meyers JD, McDonald GB. Cytomegalovirus hepatitis in marrow transplant patients: clinical, histologic and histochemical analysis. Gastroenterology 1990;98:A470.
165. Snover DC, Hutton S, Balfour HH, et al. Cytomegalovirus infection of the liver in transplant recipients. J Clin Gastroenterol 1987;9:659–665.
166. Shulman HM, McDonald GB. Liver disease after bone marrow transplantation In: Sale GE, Shulman HM, eds. The pathology of bone marrow transplantation. New York: Masson, 1984:104–135.
167. Shusterman NH, Frauenenhoffer C, Kinsey D. Fatal massive hepatic necrosis in cytomegalovirus mononucleosis. Ann Intern Med 1978;88:810–812.
168. Meyers JD. Prevention and treatment of cytomegalovirus infections. Ann Rev Med 1991;42:179–187.
169. Jacobson MA, Drew WL, Feinberg J, et al. Foscarnet therapy for gancyclovir-resistant cytomegalovirus retinitis in patients with AIDS. J Infect Dis 1991;163: 1348–1351.
170. Shields AF, Hackman RC, Fife KH, et al. Adenovirus infections in patients undergoing bone marrow transplantation. N Engl J Med 1985;312:529–533.
171. Johnson PRE, Liu Yin JA, Morris DJ, Desai M, Cinkotai KI, McKeogh MM. Fulminant hepatic necrosis caused by adenovirus type 5 following bone marrow transplantation. Bone Marrow Transplant 1990;5:345–347.
172. Anuras S, Summers R. Fulminant herpes simplex hepatitis in an adult: report of a case in a renal transplant recipient. Gastroenterology 1976;70:425–428.
173. Johnson JR, Egans S, Gleaves CA, Hackman R, Bowden RA. Hepatitis due to herpes simplex virus in marrow-transplant recipients. Clin Infect Dis 1992;14:38–45.
174. Whitley RJ, Gnann JW Jr, Hinthorn D, et al. Disseminated herpes zoster in the immunocompromised host: a comparative trial of acyclovir and vidarabine. J Infect Dis 1992;165:450–455.
175. Taylor DL, Jeffries DJ, Taylor-Robinson D, Parkin JM, Tyms AS. The susceptibility of adenovirus infection to the anti-cytomegalovirus drug, ganciclovir (DHPG). FEMS Microbiol Lett 1988;49:337–341.
176. Marrie TJ, McDonald ATJ, Conern PE, Boadreau SJF. Herpes simplex hepatitis—use of immunoperoxidase to demonstrate the viral antigen in hepatocytes. Gastroenterology 1982;82:71–76.
177. Hayashi M, Takeyama K, Takayama J, Ohira M, Tobinai K, Shimoyama M. Severe herpes simplex virus hepatitis following autologous bone marrow transplantation: successful treatment with high dose intravenous acyclovir. Jpn J Clin Oncol 1991;21:372–376.
178. Martin PJ, Shulman HM, Schubach WH, et al. Fatal EBV-associated proliferation of donor B cells after treatment of acute graft-versus-host disease with a murine anti-T cell antibody. Ann Intern Med 1984; 101:310–315.
179. Zutter MM, Martin PJ, Sale GE, Shulman HM, et al. Epstein-barr virus lymphoproliferation after BMT. Blood 1988;72:520–529.
180. Hanto DW, Frizzera G, Gajl-Peczalska KJ, Simmons RL. Epstein-Barr virus, immunodeficiency, and B cell lymphoproliferation. Transplantation 1985;39:461–472.
181. Meyers JD. Infections in bone marrow transplant recipients. Am J Med 1986;81(suppl):27–38.
182. Messing B, Bories C, Kunstlinger F, Bernier J-J. Does total parenteral nutrition induce gallbladder sludge formation and lithiasis? Gastroenterology 1983;84: 1012–1019.
183. Frick MP, Snover DC, Feinberg SB, et al. Sonography of the gallbladder in bone marrow transplant patients. Am J Gastroenterol 1984;79:122–127.
184. Navari RM, Sullivan KM, Springmeyer SC, et al. Mycobacterial infections in marrow transplant patients. Transplantation 1983;36:509–513.
185. Peters M, Schurmann D, Mayr AC, Hetzer R, Pohle HD, Ruf B. Immunosuppression and mycobacteria other than *Mycobacterium tuberculosis*: results from patients with and without HIV infection. Epidemiol Infect 1989;103:293–300.
186. Baker AL, Rosenberg IH. Hepatic complications of total parenteral nutrition. Am J Med 1987;82:489–497.
187. Wagman LD, Burt ME, Brennan MF. The impact of total parenteral nutrition on liver function test in patients with cancer. Cancer 1982;49:1249–1257.
188. Balistreri WF, Bove KE. Hepatobiliary consequences of parenteral hyperalimentation. In: Popper H, Schaffner F, eds. Progress in liver diseases, vol 9. Philadephia: WB Saunders, 1990:567–602.
189. Robertson JF, Garden OJ, Shenkin A. Intravenous nutrition and hepatic dysfunction. JPEN 1986;10: 172–176.
190. Sittges-Serra A, Pallares R, Jaurrieta E, et al. Clinical and morphological studies of liver function in adult patients on total parenteral nutrition. In: Kleinberger G, Deutsch E, eds. New aspects of clinical nutrition. Basel: S. Karger, 1983:540–547.
191. Enzenauer RW, Montrey JS, Barcia PJ, Woods J. Total parenteral nutrition cholestasis: a cause of mechanical biliary obstruciton. Pediatrics 1985;76:905–908.
192. Stanko RT, Nathan G, Mendelow H, Adibi SA. Development of hepatic cholestasis and fibrosis in patients with massive loss of intestine supported by prolonged parenteral nutrition. Gastroenterology 1987;92:197–202.
193. Stone BG, Udani M, Sanghvi A, et al. Cyclosporin A-induced cholestasis. The mechanism in a rat model. Gastroenterology 1987;93:344–351.
194. Laupacis A, Keown PS, Ulan RA. Hyperbilirubinemia and cyclosporin A levels. Lancet 1981;2:1426–1427.

195. Tutschka PJ, Beschorner WE, Hess AD, Santos GW. Cyclosporin-A to prevent graft-versus-host diasease: a pilot study in 22 patients receiving allogeneic marrow transplants. Blood 1983;61:318–325.
196. Yee GC, Kennedy MS, Storb R, Thomas ED. Effects of hepatic dysfunction on oral cyclosporine pharmacokinetics in marrow transplant patients. Blood 1984; 64:1277–1279.
197. de Groen PC. Cyclosporine and the liver: how one affects the other. Transplant Proc 1990;22:1197–1202.
198. Deeg HJ, Shulman HM, Schmidt E, et al. Marrow graft rejection and venocclusive disease of the liver in patients with aplastic anemia conditioned with cyclophosphamide and cyclosporine. Transplantation 1986;42:497–501.
199. Storb R, Deeg HJ, Whitehead J, Appelbaum F, et al. Methotrexate and cyclosporine compared with cyclosporine alone for prophylaxis of acute graft-versus-host disease after bone marrow transplantation for leukemia. N Engl J Med 1986;314:729–735.
200. Storb R, Deeg HJ, Farewell V, Doney K, et al. Marrow transplantation for severe aplastic anemia: methotrexate alone compared with a combination of methotrexate and cyclosporine for prevention of acute graft-versus-host disease. Blood 1986;68:119–125.
201. Deeg HJ, Loughran TP, Storb R, et al. Treatment of human acute graft-versus-host disease with antithymocyte globulin and cyclosporine with or without methylprednisolone. Transplantation 1985;40:162–166.
202. Doney KC, Weiden PL, Buckner CD, et al. Treatment of severe aplastic anemia using antithymocyte globulin with or without an infusion of HLA haploidentical marrow. Exp Hematol 1981;9:829–834.
203. Storb R, Gluckman E, Thomas ED, et al. Treatment of established human graft-versus-host disease by antithymocyte globulin. Blood 1974;44:57–74.
204. Meeker TC, Lowder J, Maloney DG, et al. A clinical trial of anti-idiotype therapy for B cell malignancy. Blood 1985;65:1349–1363.
205. Dillman RO. Monoclonal antibodies in the treatment of cancer. CRC Crit Rev Oncol Hematol 1984;1:357–385.
206. Martinez-Hernandez A, Maddrey W. Intrahepatic cholestasis and phospholipidosis associated with the use of trimethoprim-sulfamethoxazole. Hepatology 1990;12:342–347.
207. Abi-Mansur P, Ardiaca MC, Allam C, Shamma'a M. Trimethoprim-sulfamethoxazole-induced cholestasis. Am J Gastroenterol 1981;76:356–359.
208. Steinbrecher UP, Mishkin S. Sulfamethoxazole-induced hepatic injury. Dig Dis Sci 1981;26:756–759.
209. Kowdley KV, Keefe EB, Fawaz KA. Prolonged cholestasis due to trimethoprim-sulfamethoxazole. Gastroenterology 1992;102:2148–2150.
210. Ransohoff DF, Jacobs G. Terminal hepatic failure following a small dose of sulfamethoxazole-trimethoprim. Gastroenterology 1981;80:816–819.
211. Lewis JH, Zimmerman HJ, Benson GD, Ishak KG. Hepatic injury associated with ketoconazole therapy. Analysis of 33 cases. Gastroenterology 1984;86:503–513.
212. Stricker BH, Blok AP, Bronkhorst FB, Van Parys GE, Desmet VJ. Ketoconazole-associated hepatic injury. A clinicopathological study of 55 cases. J Hepatology 1986;3:399–406.
213. Tilly H, Rueff B, Benhamou JP. Ketoconazole-induced fulminant hepatitis. Gut 1985;26:636–638.
214. Duarte PA, Chow CC, Simmons F, Ruskin J. Fatal hepatitis associated with ketoconazole therapy. Arch Intern Med 1984;144:1069–1070.
215. Parry MF, Neu HC. The safety and tolerance of mezlocillin. J Antimicrob Chemother 1982;9(suppl):273–280.
216. Mitchell RB, Wagner JE, Karp JE, et al. Syndrome of idiopathic hyperammonemia after high-dose chemotherapy: review of nine cases. Am J Med 1988;85:662–667.
217. Arn PH, Hauser ER, Thomas GH, Herman G, Hess D, Brusilow SW. Hyperammonemia in women with a mutation at the ornithine carbamoyltransferase locus. N Engl J Med 1990;322:1652–1655.
218. Batshaw ML, Brusilow S, Waber L, et al. Treatment of inborn errors of urea synthesis. Activation of alternative pathways of waste nitrogen synthesis and excretion. N Engl J Med 1982;306:1387–1392.
219. Wolford JL, McDonald GB. Gastrointestinal bleeding after marrow transplant: a prospective study of risk factors, etiology, and outcome. Gastroenterology 1987; 92:1697.
220. Wolford JL, McDonald GB. Intramural hematomas of esophagus, stomach and small intestine in marrow transplant patients. Gastroenterology 1988;94:A501.
221. Fitchen JH, Koeffler HP. Cimetidine and granulopoeisis: bone marrow culture studies in normal man and patients with cimetidine-associated neutropenia. Br J Haematol 1980;46:361–366.
222. Byron JW. Pharmacodynamic basis for the interaction of cimetidine with the bone marrow stem cells (CFU_s). Exp Hematol 1980;8:256–263.
223. Agura ED, Vila E, Petersen FB, Shields AF, Thomas ED. The use of ranitidine in bone marrow transplantation. Transplantation 1988;46:53–56.
224. Goodrich JM, Mori M, Gleaves CA, et al. Early treatment with ganciclovir to prevent cytomegalovirus disease after allogeneic bone marrow transplantation. N Engl J Med 1991;325:1601–1607.
225. Goodman JL, Winston DJ, Greenfield RA, et al. A controlled trial of fluconazole to prevent fungal infections in patients undergoing bone marrow transplantation. N Engl J Med 1992;326:845–851.
226. Perfect JR, Klotman ME, Gilbert CC, et al. Prophylactic intravenous amphotericin B in neutropenic autologous bone marrow transplant recipients. J Infect Dis 1992;165:891–897.
227. West JC, Armitage JO, Mitros FA, Klassen LW, Corry RJ, Ray T. Cytomegalovirus cecal erosion causing massive hemorrhage in a bone marrow transplant recipient. World J Surg 1982;6:251–255.
228. Sutherland DER, Chan FY, Foucar E, Simmons PL, Howard RJ, Najarian JS. The bleeding cecal ulcer in transplant patients. Surgery 1979;86:386–398.
229. Welsh RA, McClinton LT. Aspergillosis of lungs and duodenum with fatal intestinal hemorrhage. Arch Pathol 1954;57:379–382.
230. Spencer GD, Shulman HM, Myerson D, Thomas ED, McDonald GB. Diffuse intestinal ulceration after marrow transplantation: a clinical-pathological study of 13 patients. Hum Pathol 1986;17:621–633.
231. McDonald GB, Sale GE. The human gastrointestinal tract after allogeneic marrow transplantation. In: Sale GE, Shulman HM, eds. The pathology of bone marrow transplantation. New York: Masson, 1984:77–103.
232. Epstein RJ, McDonald GB, Sale GE, Shulman HM, Thomas ED. The diagnostic accuracy of the rectal biopsy in graft-versus-host disease: a prospective

study of thirteen patients. Gastroenterology 1980;78: 764–791.
233. Shay SS, Berendsen RS, Johnson LF. Esophageal hematoma. Four new cases, a review, and proposed etiology. Dig Dis Sci 1981;26:1019–1024.
234. Ackert JJ, Sherman A, Lustbader IJ, McCauley DI. Spontaneous intramural hematoma of the esophagus. Am J Gastroenterol 1989;84:1325–1328.
235. Demos TC, Okrent DM, Studlo JD, Flisak ME. Spontaneous esophageal hematoma diagnosed by computed tomography. J Comput Assist Tomogr 1986;10: 133–135.
236. Schweiger F, Depew WT. Spontaneous intramural esophageal hematoma. Diagnosis by CT scanning. J Clin Gastroenterol 1987;9:546–548.
237. Skillington PD, Matar KS, Gardner MA, et al. Intramural haematoma of the oesophagus complicated by perforation. Aust NZ J Surg 1989;59:430–432.
238. Walsh TJ, Belitsos NJ, Hamilton SR. Bacterial esophagitis in immuno-compromised patients. Arch Intern Med 1986;146:1345–1349.
239. McBane RD, Gross JB Jr. Herpes esophagitis: clinical syndrome, endoscopic appearance, and diagnosis in 23 patients. Gastrointest Endosc 1991;37:600–603.
240. Silverstein FE, Tytgat GNJ, eds. Atlas of gastrointestinal endoscopy, ed 2. Philadelphia: JB Lippincott, 1991.
241. Spruance SL, Stewart JC, Rowe NH, et al. Treatment of recurrent herpes labialis with oral acycovir. J Infect Dis 1990;161:185–190.
242. Safrin S, Assaykeen T, Follansbee S, et al. Foscarnet therapy for acyclovir-resistent mucocutaneous herpes simplex virus infection in 26 AIDS patients: preliminary data. J Infect Dis 1990;161:1078–1084.
243. Theise ND, Rotterdam H, Dieterich D. Cytomegalovirus esophagitis in AIDS: diagnosis by endoscopic biopsy. Am J Gastroenterol 1991;86:1123–1126.
244. Nelson MR, Connolly GM, Hawkins DA, et al. Foscarnet in the treatment of cytomegalovirus infection of the esophagus and colon in patients with the acquired immune deficiency syndrome. Am J Gastroenterol 1991;86:876–881.
245. Fegan C, Poynton CH, Whittaker JA. The gut mucosal barrier in bone marrow transplantation. Bone Marrow Transplant 1990;5:373–377.
246. Weisdorf SA, Salati LM, Longsdorf JA, et al. Graft-versus-host disease of the intestine: a protein-losing enteropathy characterized by fecal α_1-antitrypsin. Gastroenterology 1983;85:1076–1081.
247. Cox GJ, Hinds M, Tarr P, Ulness B, Meyers JD, McDonald GB. Etiology of acute diarrhea following marrow transplantation: a prospective study. Gastroenterology 1990;98:A443.
248. Maile CW, Frick MP, Crass JR, Snover DC, Weisdorf SA, Kersey JH. The plain radiograph in acute intestinal graft-versus-host disease. Am J Roentgenol 1985; 145:289–292.
249. Belli A-M, Williams MP. Graft versus host disease: findings on plain abdominal radiography. Clin Radiol 1988;39:262–264.
250. Jones B, Fishman EK, Kramer SS, et al. Computed tomography of gastrointestinal inflammation after marrow transplantation. Am J Roentgenol 1986;146: 691–696.
251. Navari RM, Sharma P, Deeg HJ, McDonald GB, Thomas ED. Pneumatosis cystoides intestinalis following allogeneic marrow transplantation. Transplant Proc 1983;25:1720–1724.
252. Fisk JD, Shulman HM, Greening RR, McDonald GB, Sale GE, Thomas ED. Gastrointestinal radiographic features of human graft-versus-host disease. Am J Roentgenol 1981;136:329–336.
253. Jones B, Kramer SS, Saral R, et al. Gastrointestinal inflammation after bone marrow transplantation: graft-versus-host disease or opportunistic infection? Am J Roentgenol 1988;150:277–281.
254. Roy J, Snover D, Weisdorf S, Mulvahill A, Filipovich A, Weisdorf D. Simultaneous upper and lower endoscopic biopsy in the diagnosis of intestinal graft-versus-host disease. Transplantation 1991;51:642–646.
255. Saito H, Oshimi K, Nagasako K, et al. Endoscopic appearance of the colon and small intestine of a patient with hemorrhagic enteric graft-vs.-host disease. Dis Colon Rectum 1990;33:695–697.
256. Piguet P-F, Grau GE, Allet B, Vassalli P. Tumor necrosis factor/cachectin is an effector of skin and gut lesions of the acute phase of graft-versus-host disease. J Exp Med 1987;166:1280–1289.
257. Remick DG, Kunkel RG, Larrick JW, Kunkel SL. Acute in vivo effects of human recombinant tumor necrosis factor. Lab Invest 1987;56:583–590.
258. Madara JL. Loosening tight junctions. Lessons from the intestine. J Clin Invest 1989;83:1089–1094.
259. Dilly SA, Sloane JP. Changes in rectal leukocytes after allogeneic bone marrow transplantation. Clin Exp Immunol 1987;67:951–958.
260. Gallucci BB, Sale GE, McDonald GB, Epstein R, Shulman HM, Thomas ED. The fine structure of human rectal epithelium in acute graft-versus-host disease. Am J Surg Pathol 1982;6:293–305.
261. Ely P, Dunitz J, Rogosheske J, Weisdorf D. Use of a somatostatin analogue, octreotide acetate, in the management of acute gastrointestinal graft-versus-host disease. Am J Med 1991;90:707–710.
262. Bianco JA, Higano C, Singer J, Appelbaum FR, McDonald GB. The somatostatin analog octreotide in the management of the secretory diarrhea of acute intestinal graft-versus-host disease in patients after bone marrow transplantation. Transplantation 1990; 49:1194–1195.
263. Dueno MI, Bai JC, Santangelo WC, Krejs GJ. Effect of somatostatin analogue on water and electrolyte transport and transit time in human small bowel. Dig Dis Sci 1987;32:1092–1096.
264. Beschorner WE, Yardley JH, Tutschka PJ, Santos G. Deficiency of intestinal immunity with graft-versus-host disease in humans. J Infect Dis 1981;144:38–46.
265. Yolken RH, Bishop CA, Townsend TR, et al. Infectious gastroenteritis in bone marrow transplant recipients. N Engl J Med 1982;306:1010–1012.
266. Nagler A, Pavel L, Naparstek E, Muggia-Sullam M, Slavin S. Typhlitis occurring in autologous bone marrow transplantation. Bone Marrow Transplant 1992;9:63–64.
267. Anonymous. Clostridium septicum infection and neutropenic enterocolitis (editorial). Lancet 1987;2:608.
268. Van Kessel LJP, Verbrugh HA, Stringer MF, Hoekstra JBL. Necrotizing enteritis associated with toxigenic type A *Clostridium perfringens*. J Infect Dis 1985;151: 974–975.
269. Kane JG, Chretien JH, Garagusi VF. Diarrhoea caused by *Candida*. Lancet 1976;1:335–336.
270. Gupta TP, Ehrinpreis MN. Candida-associated diarrhea in hospitalized patients. Gastroenterology 1990; 98:780–785.

271. Danna PL, Urban C, Bellin E, Rahal JJ. Role of candida in pathogenesis of antibiotic-associated diarrhoea in elderly patients. Lancet 1991;337:511–514.
272. Underwood JCE, Corbett CL. Persistent diarrhaea and hypoalbuminenia associated with cytomegalovirus enteritis. Br Med J 1978;1:1029–1030.
273. Tajima T. An autopsy case of primary cytomegalic inclusion enteritis with remarkable hypoproteinemia. Acta Pathol Jpn 1974;24:151–162.
274. Apperley JF, Goldman JM. Cytomegalovirus: biology, clinical features and methods for diagnosis. Bone Marrow Transplant 1988;3:253–264.
275. Reed EC, Shepp DH, Dandliker PS, Meyers JD. Gancyclovir treatment of cytomegalovirus infection of the gastrointestinal tract after marrow transplantation. Bone Marrow Transplant 1988;3:199–206.
276. Townsend TR, Bolyard EA, Yolken RH, et al. Outbreak of coxsackie A1 gastroenteritis: a complication of bone marrow transplantation. Lancet 1982;1:820–823.
277. Gottesman L, Turnbull AD, O'Reilly RJ. Surgical implications of hepatic venocclusive disease following bone marrow transplantation. J Surg Oncol 1988;37: 113–115.
278. Cox GJ, McDonald GB. Graft-versus-host disease of the intestine. Springer Semin Immunopathol 1990; 12:283–299.
279. Margreiter R, Schmid T, Dunser M, Tauscher T, Hengster P, Konigsrainer A. Cytomegalovirus (CMV) pancreatitis: a rare complication after pancreas transplantation. Transplant Proc 1991;23:1619–1622.
280. Parham DM. Post-transplantation pancreatitis associated with cytomegalovirus (report of a case). Hum Pathol 1981;12:663–665.
281. Mower WJ, Hawkins JA, Nelson EW. Neutropenic enterocolitis in adults with acute leukemia. Arch Surg 1986;121:571–574.
282. Frick MP, Maile CW, Crass JR, et al. Computed tomography of neutropenic colitis. Am J Roentgenol 1984;143:763–765.
283. Teefey SA, Montant MA, Goldfogel GA, Shuman WP. Sonographic diagnosis of neutropenic typhlitis. Am J Roentgenol 1987;149:731–733.
284. King A, Rampling A, Wight DGD, Warren RE. Neutropenic enterocolitis due to *Clostridium septicum* infection. J Clin Pathol 1984;37:335–343.
285. Hopkins DG, Kushner JP. Clostridial species in the pathogenesis of necrotizing enterocolitis in patients with neutropenia. Am J Hematol 1983;14:289–294.
286. Kunkel JM, Rosenthal D. Management of the ileocecal syndrome. Neutropenic enterocolitis. Dis Colon Rectum 1986;29:196–199.
287. Shamberger RC, Weinstein HJ, Delorey MJ, Levey RH. The medical and surgical management of typhlitis in children with acute nonlymphocytic (myelogenous) leukemia. Cancer 1986;57:603–609.
288. Scott WW, Fishman EK, Siegelman SS. Anticoagulants and abdominal pain. JAMA 1984;252:2053–2056.
289. Titone C, Lipsius M, Krakauer JS. "Spontaneous" hematoma of the rectus abdominis muscle: critical review of 50 cases with emphasis on early diagnosis and treatment. Surgery 1972;72:568–572.
290. Young JR, Cressman M, O'Hara PJ. Rectus sheath hematoma: diagnosis by computed tomography. Arch Intern Med 1981;141:820–822.
291. Warren GH, Marsh S. Granulomatous *Torulopsis glabrata* cholecystitis in a diabetic. Am J Clin Pathol 1982;78:405–410.
292. Valainis GT, Sachitano, Pankey GA. Cholecystitis due to *Torulopsis glabrata*. J Infect Dis 1987;156:244–245.
293. Ong EL, Ellis ME, Tweedle DE, Ferguson G, Haboubi NY, Knox WF. Cytomegalovirus cholecystitis and colitis associated with the acquired immunodeficiency syndrome. J Infect 1989;18:73–75.
294. Lee SP, Nicholls JF, Park HZ. Biliary sludge as a cause of acute pancreatitis. N Engl J Med 1992;326: 589–593.
295. Foulis AK, Farquharson MA, Sale GE. The pancreas in acute graft-versus-host disease in man. Histopathology 1989;14:1–9.
296. Sullivan KM, Shulman HM, Storb R, et al. Chronic graft-versus-host disease in 52 patients: adverse natural course and successful treatment with combination immunosuppression. Blood 1981;57:267–276.
297. Sullivan KM, Witherspoon RP, Storb R, et al. Prednisone and azathioprine compared with prednisone and placebo for treatment of graft-versus-host disease: prognostic influence of prolonged thrombocytopenia after allogeneic marrow transplantation. Blood 1988;72:546–554.
298. Shulman HM, Sullivan KM, Weiden PL, et al. Chronic graft-versus-host syndrome in man. A long-term clinicopathologic study of 29 Seattle patients. Am J Med 1980;69:204–217.
299. Fried RH, Murakami CS, Fisher LD, Willson RA, Sullivan KM, McDonald GB. Ursodeoxycholic acid treatment of refractory chronic graft-versus-host disease of the liver. Ann Intern Med 1992;116:624–629.
300. Sullivan KM, Agura E, Appelbaum, et al. Chronic graft-versus-host disease and other late complications of bone marrow transplantation. Semin Hematol 1991;28:249–258.
301. Scheuer PJ, Ashrafzahdeh P, Sherlock S, Brown D, Dusheiko GM. The pathology of hepatitis C. Hepatology 1992;15:567–571.
302. Knapp AB, Crawford JM, Rappeport JM, Gollan JL. Cirrhosis as a consequence of graft-versus-host disease. Gastroenterology 1987;92:513–519.
303. Yau JC, Zander AR, Srigley JR, et al. Chronic graft-versus-host disease complicated by micronodular cirrhosis and esophageal varices. Transplantation 1986; 41:129–130.
304. Stechschulte DJ, Fishback JL, Emami A, et al. Secondary biliary cirrhosis as a consequence of graft-versus-host disease. Gastroenterology 1990;98:223–225.
305. Sugitani M, Inchauspe G, Shindo M, Prince AM. Sensitivity of serological assays to identify blood donors with hepatitis C viraemia. Lancet 1992;339: 1018–1019.
306. Chen PM, Fan S, Hsieh RK, Tzeng CH, Chiou TJ, Liu JH. Liver disease in patients with liver dysfunction prior to bone marrow transplantation. Bone Marrow Transplant 1992;9:415–419.
307. Houghton M, Weiner A, Han J, Kuo G, Choo Q-L. Molecular biology of the hepatitis C viruses: implications for diagnosis, development and control of viral disease. Hepatology 1991;14:381–388.
308. Lorber MI, Van Buren CT, Flechner SM, et al. Hepatobiliary and pancreatic complications of cyclosporine therapy in 466 renal transplant recipients. Transplantation 1987;43:35–40.
309. DePinho R, Goldberg C, Leftkiowich J. Azathioprine and the liver. Evidence favoring idiosyncratic, mixed cholestasis-hepatocellular injury in humans. Gastroenterology 1984;86:162–165.

310. Read AE, Weisner RH, LaBrecque DR, et al. Hepatic venocclusive disease associated with renal transplantation and azathioprine therapy. Ann Intern Med 1986;104:651–655.
311. Adler M, Delhaye M, Deprez C, et al. Hepatic vascular disease after kidney transplantation: report of two cases and review of the literature. Nephrol Dial Transplant 1987;2:183–188.
312. Mion F, Napoleon B, Berger F, Chevallier M, Bonvoisin S, Descos L. Azathioprine induced liver disease: nodular regenerative hyperplasia of the liver and perivenous fibrosis in a patient treated for multiple sclerosis. Gut 1991;32:715–717.
313. Jones MC, Best PV, Catto GR. Is nodular regenerative hyperplasia of the liver associated with azathioprine therapy after renal transplantation? Nephrol Dial Transplant 1988;3:331–333.
314. Wanless IR. Micronodular transformation (nodular regenerative hyperplasia) of the liver: a report of 64 cases among 2500 autopsies and a new classification of benign hepatocellular nodules. Hepatology 1990; 11:787–797.
315. Snover DC, Weisdorf S, Bloomer J, McGlave P, Weisdorf D. Nodular regenerative hyperplasia of the liver following bone marrow transplantation. Hepatology 1989;9:443–448.
316. McDonald GB, Sullivan KM, Schuffler MD, Shulman HM, Thomas ED. Esophageal abnormalities in chronic graft-versus-host disease in humans. Gastroenterology 1981;80:914–921.
317. McDonald GB, Sullivan KM, Plumley TF. Radiographic features of esophageal involvement in chronic graft-versus-host disease. Am J Roentgenol 1984;142: 501–506.
318. Izutsu KT, Sullivan KM, Schubert MM, et al. Disordered salivary immunoglobulin secretion and sodium transport in human chronic graft-versus-host disease. Transplantation 1983;35:441–446.

Chapter 34
Neurological Complications of Bone Marrow Transplantation

Harry Openshaw and Neal E. Slatkin

Neurological Complications Affecting the Central Nervous System: Infectious, Vascular, and Metabolic

Neurological complications may occur at three stages of bone marrow transplantation (BMT): (1) from the conditioning agents used for marrow ablation, (2) during post-transplant pancytopenia; or (3) from immunosuppressive therapies and graft-versus-host disease (GVHD) (1–3). Figure 34-1 lists the neurological complications that may occur during these three stages and classifies the complications under the standard disease categories of infectious, cerebrovascular, metabolic, toxic, and immune-mediated disorders. A central nervous system (CNS) relapse of leukemia or lymphoma may masquerade as a late complication of BMT. Also, in patients undergoing transplantation for solid tumors, inheritable disorders, and experimentally for acquired immune deficiency syndrome (AIDS), clinicians must differentiate neurological manifestations of the original disease from complications of the transplant. Familiarity with BMT complications should permit ready recognition of most problems and early therapy or prevention to limit neurological morbidity.

CNS Infection

The neurological presentation of CNS infection in BMT recipients is usually an alteration in mental status, delirium or depression of sensorium, often without meningeal signs or obvious lateralizing neurological signs. A spinal fluid examination is indicated once a mass lesion has been excluded. For a suspected brain abscess, a stereotactic biopsy under appropriate platelet support may be diagnostic.

The blood-brain barrier restricts drug entry into the CNS except highly lipophilic compounds such as chloramphenicol, trimethoprim, and sulfonamides (4). Meningeal inflammation causes breakdown of the blood-brain barrier and allows entry of nonlipophilic drugs (e.g., β-lactam antibiotics). The status of the blood-brain barrier has not been specifically evaluated in BMT recipients, but clinically relevant changes may occur (e.g., breakdown in the blood-brain barrier from fractionated total body irradiation or maintenance of a closed barrier despite CNS infection due to pancytopenia and lack of meningeal inflammation).

Survival after BMT has improved over the last 10 years, in part as a consequence of advances in the management of infectious complications (5). Antimicrobial prophylaxis early in the transplant course is particularly effective for gram-negative organisms, and bacterial meningitis at this stage is now unusual. Also unusual, but still a risk, is bacterial meningitis in long-term survivors of BMT with chronic GVHD. Recently, meningitis due to penicillin-resistant *Streptococcus pneumoniae* was reported in 2 long-term survivors, both of whom were receiving chronic trimethoprim-sulfamethoxazole prophylaxis for *Pneumocystis carinii* infection (6).

In a clinical series of transplantations performed in the early 1970s, the incidence of CNS infection was 5%, and in two autopsy series from UCLA and Johns Hopkins, the incidence was 8% (2,7,8). *Aspergillus* accounted for 30 to 50% of CNS infections in all three series and is currently a major problem in BMT (Figure 34-2). The main risk occurs during the early granulocytopenic stage, and trials with antifungal prophylaxis have been disappointing (9). The other major fungal pathogen in BMT, *Candida albicans*, infects approximately 12% of BMT recipients, most in the first 35 days, and there is a high mortality (79%) (10). Unlike *Aspergillus*, however, CNS infection with *Candida* is relatively infrequent; it occurs in 3% of BMT recipients with systemic infection. Also, other chronic fungal meningitides (e.g., from *Cryptococcus neoformans*), which are frequent complications of immunosuppression in other disease processes, are rarely encountered in BMT recipients.

CNS infection with the protozoan *Toxoplasma gondii* is occasionally seen in BMT recipients, usually during the early post-transplant period after engraftment (11,12). Figure 34-3 shows magnetic resonance imaging (MRI) of a City of Hope patient in whom CNS toxoplasmosis developed after an autologous transplant and who had a good response to pyrimethamine and sulfadiazine.

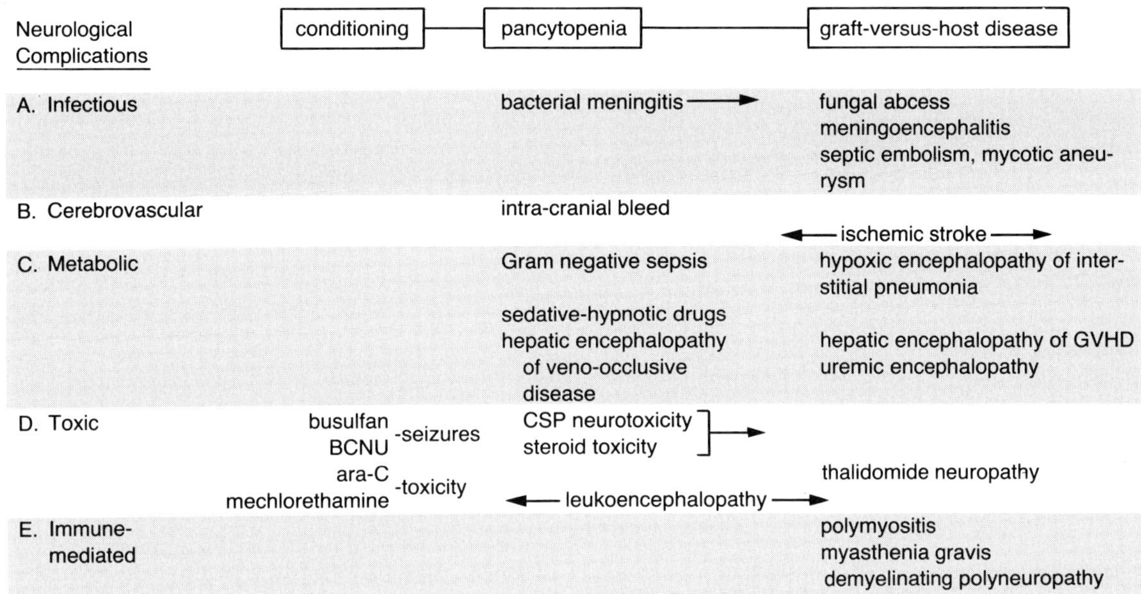

Figure 34-1. Neurological complications in allogeneic bone marrow transplantation organized by disease categories and the usual transplant stage of occurrence: bone marrow ablation, post-transplant pancytopenia, and graft-versus-host disease.

Recognized manifestations of cytomegalovirus (CMV) infection in BMT recipients include pulmonary, hepatic, and gastrointestinal involvement (see Chapter 28). For reasons that are uncertain, CMV chorioretinitis, a very common problem in patients with AIDS, is rarely diagnosed in BMT recipients (13). Similarly, CMV encephalitis is frequently recognized at least histopathologically in patients with AIDS but is rarely documented in BMT recipients (2,14). A neuropathological review of 28 BMT recipients who

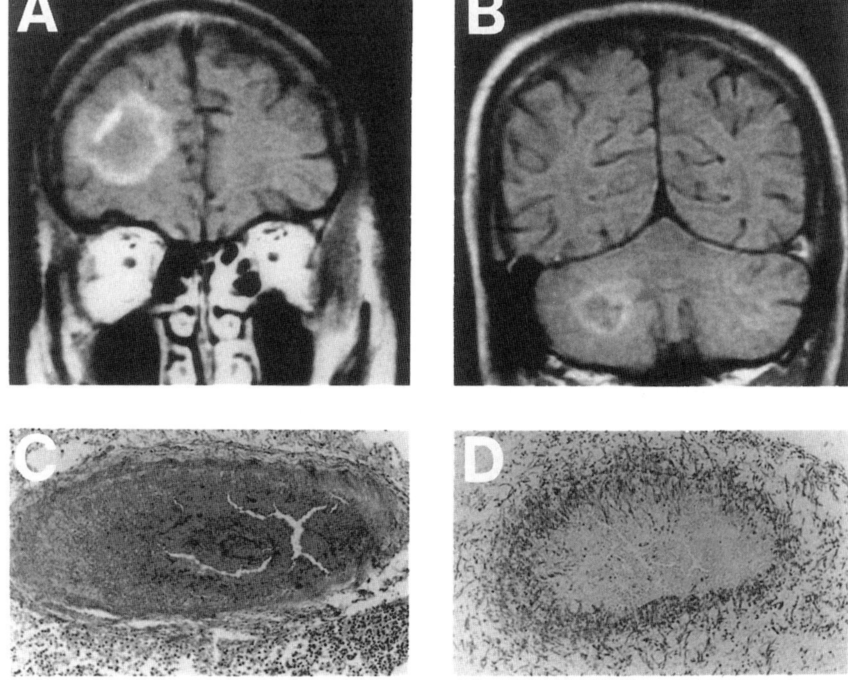

Figure 34-2. Magnetic resonance imaging (MRI) scan and histopathology of central nervous system (CNS) *Aspergillus* infection. Pulmonary aspergillosis developed in a 27 year-old man with Hodgkin's disease, as documented by bronchoscopy 5 months after autologous bone marrow transplantation (BMT). Gadolinium ring–enhanced lesions were documented on MRI scan in the right frontal lobe (A) and the right cerebellar hemisphere (B). CNS aspergillosis was confirmed at autopsy. (C, D) Postmortem histopathology of a 45-year-old woman in whom a locked-in syndrome developed, rapidly evolving to coma and death 2 months after allogeneic BMT for granulocytic sarcoma. A thrombosed branch of the basilar artery is shown in the subarchoid space with surrounding inflammatory cells (hematoxylin and eosin, ×100 magnification) as well as a mural invasion of the artery by septate, branching fungal hyphae (D. Gomori methanimine silver, ×100 magnification).

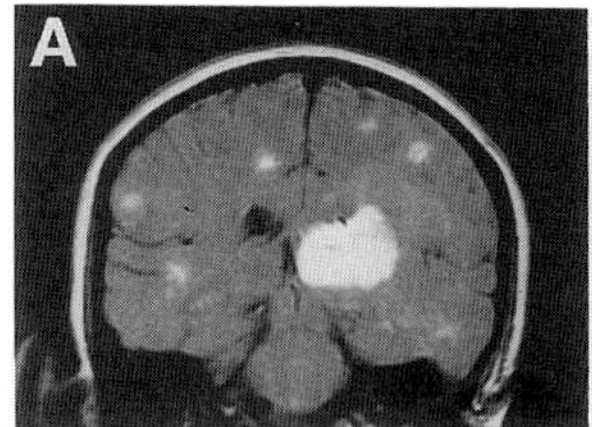

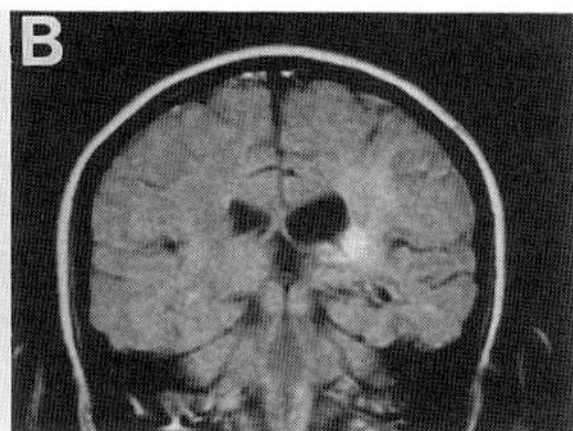

Figure 34-3. Magnetic resonance imaging (MRI) of central nervous system *Toxoplasma gondii* infection. At 3.5 months after autologous bone marrow transplantation for Hodgkin's disease, right-sided upper motor neuron clumsiness with sensory symptoms developed in a 21-year-old woman, and an MRI scan showed multiple gadolinium-enhancing lesions, the largest in the left parietotemporal area (A). Neurological recovery and almost complete resolution of the lesions on MRI scan occurred after 6 months of toxoplasmosis therapy with pyrimethamine and sulfadiazine (B).

died after systemic CMV infection noted microglial nodules compatible with CMV infection in 7, all of whom had a clinical course compatible with a nonfocal encephalitis (2). However, CMV cultures, detection of viral inclusion bodies, and immunocytochemical staining for CMV antigens were negative or not done in these patients. It remains to be established whether CMV encephalitis is a clinically important entity in BMT recipients.

Herpes simplex virus type 1 reactivates and is shed in the oral secretions in 80% of seropositive patients during the first few weeks after BMT (15). As described in Chapter 29, acyclovir prophylaxis prevents viral shedding (16) and is currently used routinely in many transplant centers. Despite the high incidence of viral reactivation, the clinical diagnosis of herpes simplex encephalitis is rarely made in transplant recipients. In immunocompetent individuals, herpes encephalitis usually occurs without any sign of mucocutaneous infection, and the infection is focal in the temporal lobes, most often presenting with seizures and psychiatric symptoms. Two fatal cases of herpes encephalitis were noted in patients treated at the transplantation unit at Johns Hopkins (2). Diagnosis in these patients was confirmed by viral culture and immunohistochemistry; unlike typical herpes encephalitis in otherwise normal individuals, however, the infection in these 2 patients was diffuse throughout the brain, and a subacute, mucocutaneous herpetic infection preceded the onset of CNS symptoms.

Active varicella zoster virus infection is present approximately half as often as herpes simplex and occurs later in the transplant course. The greatest incidence is during the fourth and fifth month after BMT (see Chapter 30). In a study from Seattle during the 1970s, clinical encephalitis developed in 4% of BMT recipients with active zoster or varicella (17). This study was done before the widespread use of antiviral drugs, and a follow-up study showed less morbidity in patients who received antiviral agents (18). Nevertheless, postherpetic neuralgia developed in 25% of the BMT recipients, and there were cases of facial nerve palsy and hearing loss associated with cranial zoster, as well as arm weakness with cervical zoster and neurogenic bladder with lumbosacral zoster. In nontransplant recipients with zoster, pleocytosis is present in most who have undergone spinal fluid examination, and it is likely that motor signs associated with zoster are caused by involvement of anterior horn cells in the spinal cord or motor nuclei in the brainstem (19). Hence, a mild meningoencephalitis with or without motor signs is probably more common in zoster than is usually acknowledged. The designation of varicella zoster encephalitis is usually reserved for the less common instances of diffuse encephalitis with a decrease in sensorium.

Adenovirus infection involving lung, liver, and kidney has been identified in BMT recipients, and there is a single report of fatal adenovirus meningoencephalitis in a patient with progressive GVHD 10 months after transplantation (20). Progressive multifocal leukoencephalopathy, the slow virus infection caused by polyomavirus JC has not yet been recognized in BMT recipients at the City of Hope and has been documented at Johns Hopkins in only 2 patients, one of whom had AIDS. This low incidence is surprising because the related polyomavirus BK is very often cultured from the urine in BMT recipients (15), and progressive multifocal leukoencephalopathy occurs in many of the hematological diagnoses that lead to transplantation, as well as in renal transplant recipients and in patients with AIDS.

Cerebrovascular Disease

In BMT recipients, intracranial hemorrhages are most frequently associated with thrombocytopenia and are usually fatal. The characteristic clinical course of a large intraparenchymal bleed is the abrupt onset of hemiparesis (or other neurological deficits localized to the cerebral hemispheres), followed by rapid depression of the sensorium and development of other brainstem signs from transtentorial herniation (Figure 34-4). A cerebellar bleed is more difficult to recognize because of the subtlety of the initial signs—abnormalities of gait and eye movement—which then progress to gaze paresis and coma. Spontaneous subdural hematomas can also be overlooked early in the course, particularly in BMT recipients who are sedated or encephalopathic for metabolic reasons, because subdural bleeds characteristically reduce the sensorium with no or mild lateralizing signs.

In one autopsy series of 105 transplant recipients, the number of hemorrhagic CNS lesions was very high: 13% had subarachnoid hemorrhages, 10% had subdural hematomas, and 5% had intraparenchymal hematomas (8). Computed tomography (CT) scans are preferable to MRI in evaluating patients suspected of

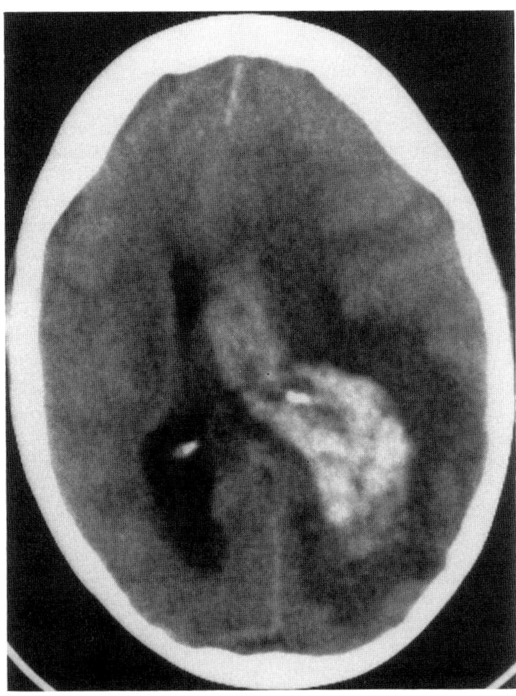

Figure 34-4. Computed tomography scan of intracranial hemorrhage. A 34-year-old woman with biphenotypic leukemia underwent allogeneic bone marrow transplantation; 1.5 months after transplant, a fatal massive left intraparenchymal hemorrhage developed, with rupture into the left lateral ventricle.

having acute intracranial bleeds because the hyperintense signal of blood is not seen on MRI until the formation of methemoglobin, 12 or more hours after the hemorrhage. Treatment of intracranial hemorrhages involves neurosurgical evacuation of the hematoma when feasible.

Ischemic strokes in BMT recipients may be embolic from endocarditis or thrombotic in association with the hypercoagulable state. Tumor embolization may, at least initially, be clinically indistinguishable from emboli of atheromatous disease or infectious endocarditis. An endarteritis associated with meningeal infection, particularly with *Aspergillus*, may occur and may be difficult to distinguish clinically from primary cerebrovascular disease (see Figure 34-2 C, D).

Levels of the circulating anticoagulant protein C, as well as levels of certain clotting factors, have been shown to be decreased in patients with breast cancer receiving chemotherapy and patients undergoing autologous BMT (21,22). There is one report of an ischemic stroke attributed to reduced protein C that occurred 11 months after allogeneic BMT (23). Prophylactic warfarin may be considered for patients with a hypercoagulable state and repeated episodes of transient cerebral ischemia; following a stroke, however, there is a danger of heparin converting a bland infarct to a hemorrhagic infarct, particularly within the first 72 hours of the stroke.

Nonbacterial thrombotic endocarditis occurs in BMT recipients as a consequence of a hypercoagulable state (24,25). Chemotherapy-induced endothelial damage and circulating immune complexes may also be contributing factors in nonbacterial thrombotic endocarditis. In an autopsy series of 91 allogeneic BMT recipients, there was a single case of bacterial endocarditis (group D *Streptococcus*) with stroke and 7 cases of nonbacterial thrombotic endocarditis; 2 of these patients suffered ischemic strokes. Neither septicemia nor GVHD were shown to be additional risk factors for nonbacterial thrombotic endocarditis (24). Because of the expectation of many more autologous transplantations for solid tumors and the association of high-dose chemotherapy with the hypercoagulable state—including high-dose cis-platinum, which is known to be associated with ischemic strokes (26)—it is likely that nonbacterial thrombotic endocarditis and ischemic stroke will become more frequent complications and will exceed in future clinical series the number of cases of hemorrhagic stroke after BMT.

Metabolic Encephalopathy

Metabolic encephalopathy in transplant recipients is most often associated with gram-negative sepsis or the use of sedative-hypnotic drugs. Hypoxic encephalopathy, which carries the risk of permanent neurological disability, may occur from interstitial pneumonia or from hypoxemia associated with red blood cell lysis in patients with the hemolytic uremic syndrome. Hepatic encephalopathy may occur from liver involvement in patients with GVHD or from fulminant hepatic failure in those with veno-occlusive disease. Renal failure with resultant uremic encephalopathy has been attributed to nephrotoxic drugs (including cyclosporine and tobramycin), the renal glomerulopathy that is rarely seen as a manifestation of GVHD, radiation nephritis, and the hemolytic uremic syndrome. Finally, electrolyte and acid-base imbalances occur frequently in very ill transplant recipients and are often associated with encephalopathy.

The characteristic clinical features of metabolic encephalopathy are delirium or depression of the sensorium, from lethargy to stupor or coma, usually, but not always, without lateralizing neurological signs. In hepatic coma, there may be abnormal neurological signs, including hemiplegia and brainstem signs with extensor or flexor posturing to noxious stimuli. Preservation of the pupillary light response and eye movements in the face of reflexive posturing argues for a metabolic rather than a structural etiology of coma. What can be misleading, especially in patients whose sensorium is clouded by sedative-hypnotic drugs, is unilateral pupillary dilation from a scopolamine patch (27) used sometimes in the first 2 weeks after BMT for mucositis-associated nausea. Recognition that the pupillary dilation in this instance is not from a structural lesion avoids the risk of breaking isolation to obtain a head scan.

Neurological Complications of Drug Treatment

As the use of autologous transplantation for solid tumors continues to expand, BMT recipients will be exposed increasingly to a variety of chemotherapeutic protocols with varying potentials for neurological toxicity. This chapter maintains a narrower focus, restricting discussion to allogeneic BMT treatment methods commonly used in conditioning regimens, as immunosuppressive therapy, or in the general supportive care of these patients. Emphasis is on neurological toxicities occurring the first year after transplantation. Brain tumors have rarely been reported as delayed secondary malignancies in BMT recipients, probably related to chemotherapy and radiation therapy of the primary hematological disease (28,29). Other long-term disabilities that may involve cognition and quality of life are discussed in Chapter 42.

Cyclosporine (CSP)

Neurological complications associated with cyclosporine (CSP) are common, generally reversible after temporary discontinuation of CSP, and diverse, ranging in severity from mild tremulousness to virtual coma. The initial suspicion that CSP neurotoxicity may be greater in bone marrow than in solid organ transplant recipients has not been substantiated, and there is no evidence that fractionated total body irradiation (FTBI) or intrathecal chemotherapy increases the risk of CSP toxicity (30–34).

Mechanism of CSP Neurotoxicity

The basis of CSP neurotoxicity is controversial. In animals, CSP at high doses has a direct neurotoxic effect, independent of alterations in blood pressure or renal function (35). Also compatible with a direct toxic effect is the reported association of hypocholesterolemia and CSP toxicity in liver transplant recipients (36). This association has been explained by an increase in serum free CSP levels, even though CSP entry into the CNS is normally restricted by the blood-brain barrier (37). Neurotoxicity has been seen when the trough serum level is above the therapeutic range; however, a strict predictable correlation between serum CSP levels and toxicity has not been found in individual patients monitored over time (38–40). Although CSP breakdown products are recognized as potential toxins, and abnormalities in CSP metabolism caused by the liver cytochrome P-450 enzymes have been postulated as a contributing factor in neurotoxicity, the precise role of CSP metabolites remains to be established (41,42). Speculatively, the increase of CSP neurotoxicity in patients receiving etoposide in the conditioning regimen may be the result of an effect on the liver, analogous to the described effect of erythromycin, ketoconazole, and calcium channel blockers in decreasing hepatic metabolism of CSP (38,43).

There are clinical and radiographic similarities between CSP toxicity and eclampsia, a condition of hypertensive encephalopathy in which vasospasm causes multifocal areas of brain ischemia and swelling (44,45). Headache and blurred vision are common to both diagnoses and are usually present prior to more severe neurological dysfunction, such as seizures. In a study of BMT recipients, a subacute blood pressure increase was the only factor that distinguished patients who had CSP seizures from other similarly treated patients (40). There is also evidence that CSP causes endothelial injury and the release of endothelins, vasoactive neuropeptides that have been implicated in cerebral vasospasm (46,47). Endothelin release may be triggered by or may cause microangiopathic hemolytic anemia, a condition found by multivariate analysis to have the highest correlation with CSP toxicity (43).

Radiographic Manifestations of CSP Neurotoxicity

CT and MRI abnormalities, primarily in the posterior temporal, parietal, and occipital lobe white matter, have been reported in some but not all patients with typical CSP encephalopathy (42,43,48–50). These lesions, thought to be focal areas of cerebral edema or ischemia, are radiolucent without contrast enhancement on CT and appear as fluffy areas of hyperintense signal on T2-weighted MRI (Figure 34-5). These areas of "leukoencephalopathy" usually resolve within 1 to 2 weeks as clinical improvement occurs, analogous to

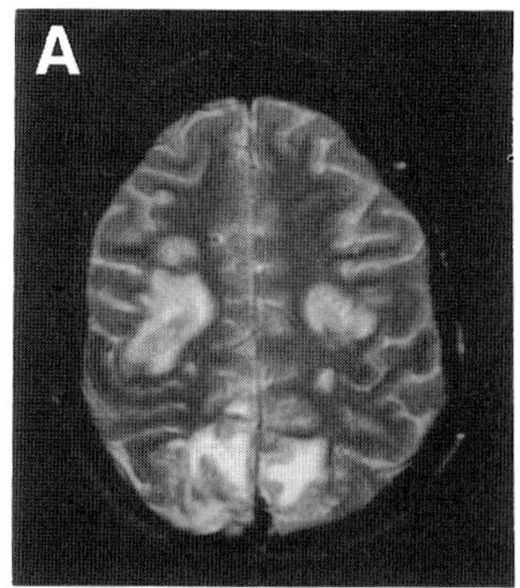

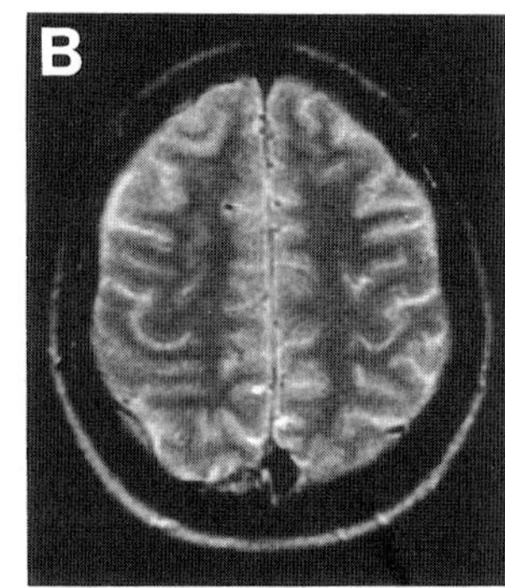

Figure 34-5. Magnetic resonance imaging (MRI) of cyclosporine (CSP) central nervous system toxicity. Abrupt onset of confusion with headache developed in this 20-year-old woman 5 weeks after allogeneic bone marrow transplantation for chronic myelogenous leukemia. Patches of bright signal on T_2-weighted images were present, especially in the parietal and occipital subcortical white matter (A). Later, a generalized seizure with encephalopathy occurred, and CSP was withheld for 4 days and then restarted at a lower dose. Repeat MRI scan showed resolution of the lesions (B).

the lesions described in hypertensive encephalopathy and eclampsia (51–53). Even on MRI, however, which is very sensitive in detecting cerebral edema, abnormalities when present only roughly correlate in number and extent with clinical severity, and it seems likely that cerebral ischemia and edema are not the only mechanisms of CSP encephalopathy.

Clinical Manifestations of CSP Neurotoxicity

Headache is a problem in approximately 20% of patients receiving CSP. These headaches, often unresponsive to narcotic analgesics, may be helped by propranolol, a drug used prophylactically for migraine (54). Also, in approximately 20% of patients receiving CSP, a fine sustension tremor is present. It seldom causes functional impairment and either decreases in severity as CSP is tapered or increases in amplitude when patients become encephalopathic (31,55). Except for the fairly characteristic clinical triad of prodromal headache, visual disturbance, and seizures, there is little to distinguish CSP encephalopathy from other metabolic or toxic encephalopathies. The earliest signs are usually disorientation, a mild confusion for names and faces, ideomotor apraxia, and impairment of concentration; memory deficits are common and dysphasia is less frequent. Lateralizing motor and sensory deficits are unusual and when present should prompt investigation with CT or MRI to exclude a structural lesion. As the encephalopathy deepens, agitation frequently occurs, and when sedative-hypnotic drugs are used, the clinical course is often characterized by alternating agitation and obtundation. If CSP is continued, myoclonic movements and eventually coma may occur (48,56). Even with discontinuation of CSP, encephalopathy usually persists for several days, or longer if large doses of sedative-hypnotic medications had been administered.

There are several reports of rapidly evolving pyramidal, cerebellar, and visual dysfunction in association with CSP. Cases of paraparesis and quadriparesis, with accompanying sensory levels and cerebellar syndromes with vestibular impairment, have been described, with good recovery even of severe deficits (30,57,58). Impaired vision to the point of cortical blindness may herald the onset of CSP-induced seizures, occur as a residual manifestation of ictal or postictal deficits, or occur as an isolated manifestation of CSP toxicity (59,60). Myalgia and muscle weakness infrequently occur with CSP use and remit with drug tapering, although a fatal case of rhabdomyolysis has been reported (61,62).

CSP Seizures

Multiple reports link CSP to seizures (57,58), more frequent in pediatric patients and especially early in the transplant course or during flares of GVHD when CSP and corticosteroid doses are increased (33,34, 63,64). Headache, visual disturbance, increased tremulousness, and mild confusion often occur prior to the seizure, which usually is single and generalized, but may be multiple and focal in onset. Partial seizures alone may occur occasionally with transient focal deficits such as cortical blindness and abnormal behavior (59,60,65,66). Hypomagnesemia and hypertension are often seen, relative to blood pressure levels for the several preceding days, and these conditions should be treated vigorously (67). CSP should be withheld for several days after the seizure, and then restarted at reduced dosage with careful attention to blood pressure. Anticonvulsant drugs are not of proved benefit in this setting, but their use is sanctioned by convention and certainly patients having more than one seizure should be treated. Single seizures lasting 3 or more minutes may be treated adequately with parenteral diazepam alone. As prophylaxis, phenytoin offers the advantage of a broad antiseizure spectrum, rapid intravenous loading, and perhaps reducing the half-life of CSP through increased hepatic metabolism (68). Phenytoin also enhances the metabolism of corticosteroids, which is an undesirable effect because corticosteroid serum levels are not readily available for dose adjustment. Therefore, valproic acid, an anticonvulsant free of these hepatic effects, may be preferred (69,70). There are no guidelines on how long to continue anticonvulsants, but the risk of additional seizures occurring once CSP is restarted appears to be very small, and anticonvulsants are generally used for only a few months at most.

Corticosteroids

A sense of well-being and even euphoria often accompany the initiation of corticosteroid treatment, and psychiatric symptoms occasionally occur with continued administration. Although described under the rubric of "steroid psychosis," vivid dreams and nonpsychotic mood disturbances are more frequent than frank psychotic depression, mania, or delirium (71). This toxicity is often dose-dependent, but when tapering of steroids is not feasible or is ineffective, neuroleptic and antianxiety medications may be valuable.

Proximal muscle weakness due to muscle protein catabolism is experienced by virtually all BMT recipients who receive the equivalent of 40 mg prednisone a day for more than 3 weeks (72,73). The typical symptoms of difficulty arising from a chair and difficulty washing hair are often mistakenly attributed in these patients to disuse atrophy alone. Muscle cramps and tenderness are less often reported in steroid myopathy and, when present, should prompt investigation to exclude an inflammatory myopathy (see section on polymyositis). Although corticosteroids do not affect the sensory and reflex examination, abnormalities in these systems due to prior chemotherapy may cloud the diagnostic picture, and a high index of clinical suspicion is often required for the diagnosis of steroid myopathy in BMT recipients. Serum creatinine phosphokinase levels are normal, the value of the 24-hour creatine/creatinine ratio remains to be determined, and electromyography often shows only slight abnormalities with myopathic motor units. Muscle biopsy may reveal type IIB fiber atrophy, but this finding is not specific to steroid myopathy. Treatment consists of switching from the more myotoxic fluorinated steroids (e.g., dexamethasone) to nonfluorinated agents (e.g., prednisone or methylprednisolone), tapering the steroids when feasible, and instituting daily physical therapy.

Thalidomide

Peripheral neuropathy, recognized in the 1960s soon after thalidomide was introduced as a sedative-hypnotic agent, can become symptomatic after 2 months of 100 mg/day, the starting dose used now experimentally for chronic GVHD (74). The problem begins with lower limb numbness and paresthesias, often accompanied by burning and hyperesthesia of the feet. With continued exposure, leg cramps and a stocking-glove pattern of sensory loss develops involving superficial sensation more than proprioception or vibration. In severe cases, upper motor neuron muscle weakness may occur, and deep tendon reflexes are paradoxically increased in association with the degree of sensory impairment, although distal wasting and depression of the ankle deep tendon reflexes also occur. There may be mild elevation of cerebrospinal fluid protein levels, and nerve conduction tests as well as morphological analysis indicate a large fiber, "dying-back" sensory neuropathy (i.e., initial degeneration in the distal region of the axon and progression of the degeneration proximal to the nerve cell body) (75). The extent of neurological recovery after discontinuation of thalidomide depends on the severity of symptoms and possibly patient age and duration of exposure. Motor signs revert more readily and completely than sensory symptoms, and distressing sensory complaints may be permanent in some patients (76).

Busulfan

Generalized seizures occur overall in approximately 10% of patients receiving high-dose busulfan (BU) (4 mg/kg/day for 4 days), probably more frequently in children, (77–80). BU readily crosses the blood-brain barrier, thus producing cerebrospinal-fluid-to-plasma-drug ratios of 1 or more, and it is presumed that seizures occur as a direct neurotoxic effect (81). Although myoclonic twitching may be seen shortly before or after the ictus, BU seizures usually are not focal and are seldom multiple or complicated. Prophylactic anticonvulsant treatment has been recommended when high-dose BU is used in BMT conditioning regimens (80,82). For such treatment to have value, a therapeutic drug level must be reached before the start of BU and maintained for 2 days after the last dose. An oral phenytoin loading dose of 18 mg/kg is generally adequate for this purpose, followed by a daily maintenance dose of 5 mg/kg.

Cytosine Arabinoside

Cytosine arabinoside (ara-C), a structural analogue of deoxycytidine, has been used for acute myeloid leukemia in conventional doses for 20 years (100–200 mg/m^2/day) and, to overcome cellular resistance, in high-dose form for 10 years (4–6 gm/m^2/day). Cerebellar toxicity, the principal neurological side effect of high-dose ara-C, has occurred in 10% of patients, and left permanent cerebellar disability in 3% (83). Much less often, seizures or transient encephalopathy have occurred with high-dose ara-C, and there have also been a few published cases of peripheral neuropathy, including two patients with clinical and electrophysiological features of acute demyelinating polyneuropathy consistent with the diagnosis of Guillain-Barré syndrome (see "Inflammatory Demyelinating Polyneuropathy" section). There is limited experience with high-dose ara-C used as a conditioning agent for BMT, and both cerebellar toxicity and a severe demyelinating neuropathy leading to the need for respiratory support have been reported (84,85).

Methotrexate

Low dose intravenous methotrexate (MTX) (10–15 mg/week), sometimes used for GVHD prophylaxis, has caused only occasional and minor neurotoxicity—headache, dizziness, and, rarely, seizures when given to patients with rheumatoid arthritis (86–88). High-dose MTX (5 gm/m^2/cycle), used mainly for osteogenic sarcomas, has been known to trigger transient leukoencephalopathy, similar in appearance but usually more extensive than the MRI abnormalities occasionally seen with CSP toxicity (89). The major progressive and permanent neurological disability from MTX in BMT recipients is delayed onset, chronic, and often fatal leukoencephalopathy resulting usually from the combination of intrathecal MTX and whole brain irradiation (90). The most common neurological signs include dysarthria, ataxia, dysphasia, spasticity and upper motor neuron weakness, seizures, confusion, and a decrease in sensorium. The incidence of leukoencephalopathy was 7% in a series of 415 BMT recipients in Seattle (91). All patients in whom leukoencephalopathy developed had received CNS therapy or prophylaxis with whole brain irradiation or intrathecal chemotherapy before BMT and all received intrathecal MTX after BMT. Onset of leukoencephalopathy was usually 4 to 5 months after BMT. An example from the City of Hope of post-transplant leukoencephalopathy is shown in Figure 34-6. Leukoencephalopathy with severe neurological sequelae and death has also been attributed to amphotericin B following FTBI in a BMT recipient (92). Unexpectedly, 5-fluorouracil and levamisole have recently been incriminated in leuko-

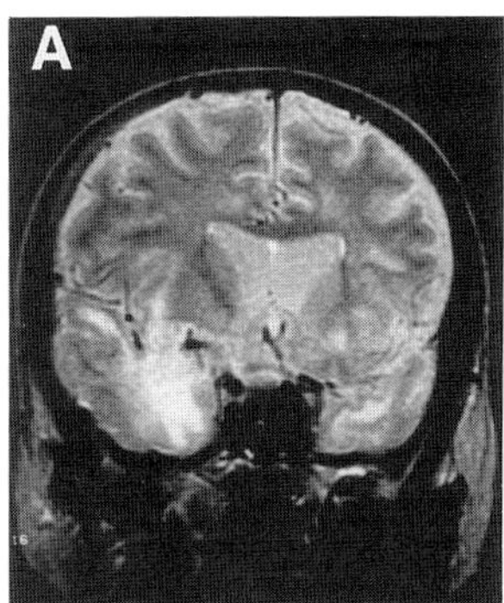

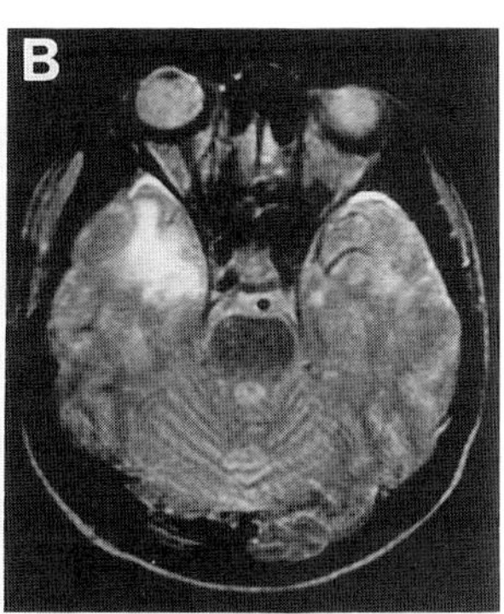

Figure 34-6. Magnetic resonance imaging of focal temporal lobe leukoencephalopathy. A 28-year-old man with acute lymphocytic leukemia underwent 2,400 cGy whole-brain irradiation in 1984, followed by 6 courses of 12 mg intrathecal methotrexate (MTX) prior to fractionated total body irradiation of 1,320 cGy over 5 days for an allogeneic bone marrow transplantation (BMT) in 1985. There was a relapse in the bone marrow in 1989 and in the central nervous system in 1991, and 11 additional courses of 12 mg intrathecal MTX was given before a second allogeneic BMT in 1991. Mild confusion developed during the conditioning with busulfan (BU) and etoposide, and there was a generalized seizure 4 days after BU was stopped and one day after cyclosporine was started. A profound memory disturbance then became manifest with a clear sensorium but a personality change, inappropriate behavior, and total lack of insight. Acyclovir was given for the possibility of herpes simplex encephalitis, but the severe neurological disability remained unchanged until his death from severe gastrointestinal and liver graft-versus-host disease 4 months after transplantation. Neuropathological examination of the brain was negative for viral inclusion bodies or other stigmata of encephalitis. Changes of a patchy leukoencephalopathy were present, most extensive in the temporal lobes.

encephalopathy in nontransplant recipients (93). As different chemotherapeutic protocols are introduced with FTBI and autologous BMT, there is the potential that other agents or combinations will provoke leukoencephalopathy.

Carmustine

High-dose carmustine (BCNU) (300–600 mg/m^2) is currently used in BMT conditioning regimens for patients with relapsed Hodgkin's disease. Intra-arterial BCNU for glioblastoma multiforme and for metastatic brain tumors has caused toxic encephalopathies with myoclonus and seizures (94,95). Because of these neurological toxicities, the dose of intra-arterial BCNU in a cooperative trial for glioblastoma multiforme was reduced from 200 to 100 mg/m^2 (96). In patients with relapsed Hodgkin's disease, seizures occurred in 2 of 61 who received intravenous BCNU (300 mg/m^2) with high-dose cyclophosphamide and etoposide as a conditioning regimen for autologous BMT (97). Similar toxicity with seizures has been anecdotally reported from other transplant centers, including the City of Hope, and prophylactic anticonvulsants are currently often used when BCNU is given at high doses, similar to the use of anticonvulsants for conditioning regimens with high-dose BU.

Mechlorethamine

Neurological toxicities have been encountered in patients receiving mechlorethamine in place of cyclophosphamide as a BMT conditioning regimen with FTBI. Otological and vestibular toxicity, as well as encephalopathy, were reported within days of administration of high-dose mechlorethamine (0.5–2.0 mg/kg); the incidence of toxicity varied directly in association with dose. In addition to the acute toxicity, chronic encephalopathic confusion and lethargy occurred in 50% of patients who survived at least 2 months after transplantation. All patients with chronic neurological toxicity had early acute mechlorethamine toxicity (98).

Antibiotics and Antiviral Drugs

Many of the antibiotics used after BMT have been associated with neurological toxicity: seizures from penicillin, pipracillin, metronidazole, and imipenem; encephalopathy from penicillin and metronidazole; hearing loss from aminoglycosides and vancomycin; peripheral neuropathy from metronidazole; and a myasthenic-like syndrome from aminoglycosides (99–102). Because toxicity is often enhanced by renal insufficiency, special caution applies to those BMT recipients taking CSP and at risk for CSP nephrotoxicity.

Much of the clinical experience with antiviral drugs comes from treating patients with AIDS, and it is often difficult to know whether a particular neurotoxicity is drug- or disease-related. Adenine arabinoside has been associated with tremors, hallucinations, and complex motor and behavioral disturbances (103,104), but this agent has been replaced largely by the less toxic acyclovir for herpetic infections. In BMT recipients, acyclovir (1,500–3,000 mg/m^2/day) has also caused tremulousness and agitation or lethargy, occasionally with epileptiform changes on electroencephalography (105). In the setting of renal failure, reversible stupor and coma and occasionally generalized seizures have followed both oral and intravenous administration of acyclovir (106–108). Delirium that improved after dose reduction was seen with ganciclovir (10 mg/kg/day) for CMV infection in a BMT recipient (109), and similar mental status changes have been noted in up to 5% of patients with AIDS receiving ganciclovir; seizures occur rarely and most often in patients also receiving imipenem (110). Foscarnit most often causes renal and electrolyte disturbances, and low calcium and magnesium levels caused by foscarnate have been associated with paresthesias, muscle cramps, and, rarely, seizures (111,112).

Immune-mediated Neurological Complications

It is still not known whether GVHD can affect the CNS. Allogeneic stimulation in an animal model has been shown to provoke major histocompatibility complex (MHC) class I and II antigen expression in the brain (113). Compatible with loss of the immunologically privileged status of the CNS associated with allogeneic stimulation, there have been recent reports of global neurological signs or chronic inflammatory cells in the brain of patients with systemic GVHD (114,115). Other etiologies, however, are possible in these patients, and published series of BMT recipients have failed to identify clinical cases that are definitively immune-mediated CNS disorders (2,3).

In contrast, it is well recognized that immune-mediated neurological complications of BMT affect the peripheral nervous system. These complications include myasthenia gravis, polymyositis, and inflammatory demyelinating polyneuropathy. The sine qua non of all three complications is lower motor neuron muscle weakness. Upper motor neuron muscle weakness is associated with a worse prognosis in BMT recipients because it is usually caused by a mass lesion in the brain or an epidural deposit with spinal cord compression. Signs that indicate an upper motor neuron lesion include spasticity, hyperactive deep tendon reflexes, extensor plantar responses, and clumsiness out of proportion to the degree of muscle weakness. Once these conditions have been excluded, the problem becomes one of determining the level of lower motor neuron involvement: anterior horn cell or motor root, peripheral nerve, neuromuscular junction, or muscle. Figure 34-7 shows an approach to this differential diagnosis of muscle weakness and the value of neurophysiological tests in this localization.

Weakness in a segmental distribution (i.e., in the distribution of a spinal nerve root) is inconsistent with a diagnosis of any of these conditions and suggests leptomeningeal disease or an epidural deposit at that particular spinal level. Much less commonly, herpes zoster infection produces weakness in a segmental distribution, as does subacute motor neuronopathy, which is rarely seen as a remote effect of lymphoma (19,116). Weakness of extraocular eye muscles is seen in virtually all patients with myasthenia gravis and tends to be a fluctuating weakness with characteristic fatigability and associated ptosis. Clinically, this weakness can be distinguished on repeat neurological examinations and differentiated from the fixed cranial nerve palsies associated with leptomeningeal disease or with intra-axial brainstem lesions. Ophthalmoplegia is only rarely seen in patients with acute inflammatory demyelinating polyneuropathy, the so called C. Miller Fisher variant of Guillain-Barré syndrome, and ophthalmoplegia has not been reported in patients with demyelinating polyneuropathy associated with BMT. Clinical features more consistent with polyneuropathy than myopathy include distal distribution of weakness, presence of sensory symptoms, and absence of deep tendon reflexes. Clearly, the last two features are often not

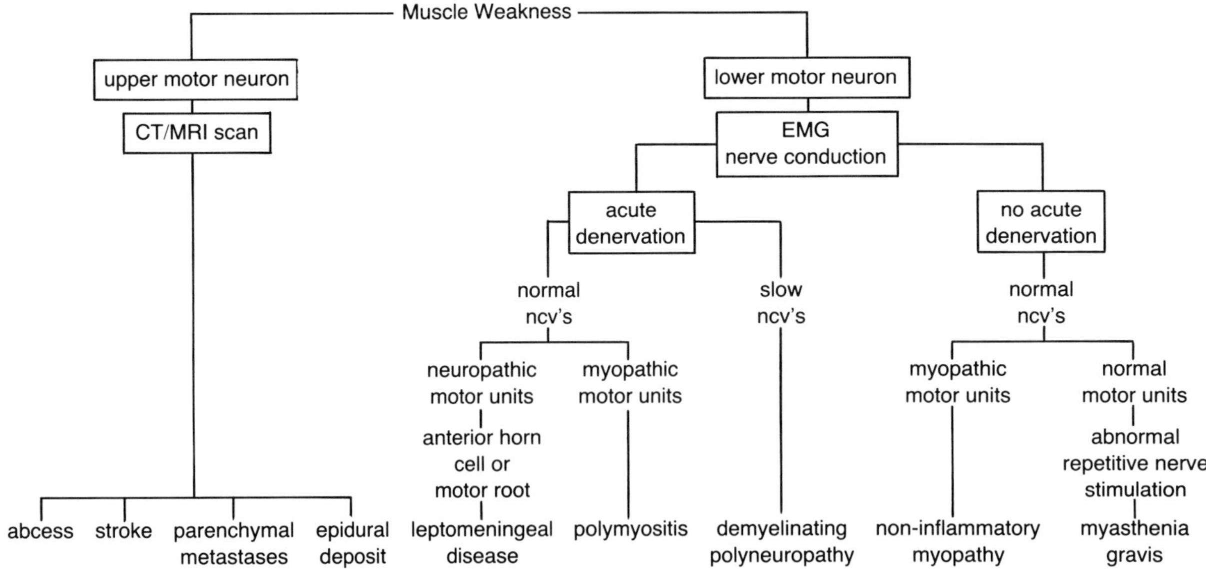

Figure 34-7. Diagnostic approach to bone marrow transplantation recipients with muscle weakness. A clinical distinction is first made regarding whether the weakness is upper or lower motor neuron in type, and a differential diagnosis is generated with the help of a head scan in the former and neurophysiological tests in the latter. EMG = electromyography; NCV = nerve conduction velocities.

helpful in many BMT recipients who have pre-existing neuropathy from vincristine, cis-platinum, or other causes. Muscle tenderness, subcutaneous swelling, and rash all favor an inflammatory myopathy over the usually milder myopathic weakness associated with disuse, corticosteroids, or other endocrine-metabolic myopathies, such as thyrotoxic myopathy.

Myasthenia Gravis

Myasthenia gravis is an immune-mediated disorder of the neuromuscular junction in which autoantibodies to the postsynaptic acetylcholine receptor produce a characteristic clinical syndrome of ptosis and extraocular muscle weakness, most often with proximal limb and facial muscle weakness. In early studies, detection of acetylcholine receptor antibodies appeared to be specific for myasthenia gravis, but more recently, autoantibodies without neuromuscular disease have been found in patients with certain hematological disorders, particularly acquired aplastic anemia, and in up to 40% of BMT recipients (117,118). Accordingly, it is somewhat surprising that so few cases of myasthenia gravis have been reported in BMT recipients (119–122). It may be that an unrecognized forme fruste of myasthenia gravis occurs commonly after BMT, and although partially treated by immunosuppression, it contributes to the weakness almost universally experienced after BMT. Diagnosis of myasthenia gravis is based on the distribution of muscle weakness, the clinical hallmarks of fatiguability and variability over time of clinical signs and symptoms, the therapeutic response to anticholinesterase drugs (the edrophonium test), and neurophysiological tests in which repetitive nerve stimulation produces a decremental response of the compound muscle action potential as a consequence of the loss of available acetylcholine receptors.

In 8 patients with myasthenia gravis after BMT from different transplantation centers, all patients had chronic GVHD, and, although most had detectable acetylcholine receptor antibody in the first few months after BMT, signs of myasthenia gravis were delayed until immunosuppressive drugs were tapered 2 to 4 years after BMT. For reasons that are difficult to explain, 5 of these 8 patients had undergone transplantation for aplastic anemia; 1 (with a seronegative donor) had acetylcholine receptor antibody both prior to transplantation (without neuromuscular disease) and (apparently donor-derived) after transplantation when symptoms of myasthenia gravis appeared. Thymoma, present in approximately 15% of patients with idiopathic myasthenia gravis, has not been identified in post-BMT myasthenia gravis.

Treatment of myasthenia gravis has improved greatly in the last 20 years because of better intensive care management of myasthenia crisis, the benefits of early thymectomy, prednisone and azathioprine, and the therapeutic effectiveness of plasmapheresis and immunoglobulin infusion. With recent advances also in the treatment of chronic GVHD and better survival after BMT, the number of cases of myasthenia gravis may very likely increase, making it more important to recognize early signs of myasthenia gravis and to avoid, or use with caution, drugs that affect neuromuscular transmission, including aminoglycoside antibiotics, certain cardiac antiarrhythmic agents, and parenteral magnesium.

Polymyositis

Polymyositis is a clinical syndrome characterized by proximal muscle weakness, often with muscle tenderness, dysphagia, and cardiac muscle involvement. There is elevation of creatinine phosphokinase and other muscle enzyme levels during disease activity, short duration (myopathic) motor units on electromyography with signs of acute denervation (fibrillation potentials and positive sharp waves), and necrotic myofibers with mononuclear inflammatory cells on muscle biopsy. Polymyositis may occur in patients with connective tissue disorders, systemic autoimmune diseases, and parasitic and viral infections—including toxoplasmosis, trichinosis, and cysticercosis, as well as human immunodeficiency virus and human T lymphotrophic virus type 1 infection (123).

There are several case reports of polymyositis associated with chronic GVHD after allogeneic BMT (124–127) (Plate LVII). Onset of weakness was from 100 days to 3 years after BMT, and treatment with steroids or azathioprine most often produced gratifying results. In 2 patients, myositis was thought to be the sole manifestation of GVHD (128,129), and there is a single case report of polymyositis after autologous BMT, with onset of muscle weakness 2 months after transplantation (130).

It is not difficult to differentiate polymyositis from myasthenia gravis and polyneuropathy. A potential problem arises when mild polymyositis goes unrecognized and accounts for a slower than usual functional recovery after BMT. Once recognized, it is important to exclude infectious causes of polymyositis and to exclude the occasional patient with drug-induced myositis (e.g., Xomazyme, a ricin-tagged antibody used experimentally for GVHD, has been implicated in cases of myopathy; and zidovudine (AZT), as well as the combination of lovastatin and CSP, can cause an inflammatory myopathy). Muscle weakness in patients with GVHD may also be caused by autoimmune hyperthyroidism (131) or, much more commonly, steroid myopathy; the dilemma in some patients is deciding whether steroids should be increased as therapy for polymyositis or decreased because of presumptive steroid myopathy. Further testing should help in this situation because, unlike polymyositis, patients with steroid or other endocrine myopathies have neither electromyography evidence of denervation nor inflammatory cells on muscle biopsy.

Inflammatory Demyelinating Polyneuropathy

Immune-mediated demyelinating polyneuropathy may occur acutely, often following viral infections, and lead rapidly to quadriplegia in the self-limited Guillain-Barré syndrome, or there may be a subacute onset and a progressive course in chronic inflammatory demyelinating polyneuropathy. The precise immune mechanism of Guillain-Barré syndrome and chronic inflammatory dysimmune polyneuropathy is uncertain, but plasmapheresis is often beneficial in both processes. Electrophysiological demonstration of nerve conduction slowing is necessary for the diagnosis of demyelinating neuropathy. In certain patients with immune-mediated demyelination, it may be helpful to document cerebrospinal fluid protein elevations and myelin breakdown with reactive macrophages on sural nerve biopsy (132).

Because of the known increased risk of Guillain-Barré syndrome in patients with Hodgkin's disease and other disorders with reduced cellular immunity (133), it is not surprising that Guillain-Barré–like cases have been anecdotally noted in BMT recipients. Compared with myasthenia gravis and polymyositis, there is greater clinical heterogeneity in these patients and less certainty as to the pathogenesis. Mention is made of mononeuritis multiplex in a transplant recipient whose neuropathy recovered after treatment of GVHD (1), and there are at least 5 other reports of a progressive demyelinating polyneuropathy in allogeneic BMT recipients, including 2 patients who were free of GVHD symptoms (134–137). Lymphocytes from a single patient studied showed a mitogenic response after stimulation with a crude peripheral nerve myelin extract, whereas lymphocytes from the donor and from the patient after neurological recovery were negative in this assay (137). No study of anti-GM_1 ganglioside antibody or other peripheral nerve antibody has been reported in BMT recipients, but treatment of demyelinating polyneuropathy in these patients has included plasmapheresis with variable success; prednisone, which is effective in nontransplant-associated chronic inflammatory demyelinating polyneuropathy; and intravenous gamma globulin, which has also been shown to be beneficial in some patients with immune-mediated polyneuropathy.

In contrast to these cases of polyneuropathy occurring 3 or more months after BMT and usually in the context of GVHD, there are some reports of demyelinating polyneuropathy with onset much earlier, within the first month after BMT. In 1 patient, a Guillain-Barré–like illness was attributed to high-dose ara-C (36 gm/m^2) used in the conditioning regimen (85), and rare similar cases with the same time course have been seen in nontransplant recipients who received high-dose ara-C (138). A demyelinating neuropathy also developed 20 days after an autologous BMT for non-Hodgkin's lymphoma, and the patient appeared to stabilize and improve after administration of corticosteroids (139). Finally, there have been 2 patients reported with quiescent chronic inflammatory demyelinating polyneuropathy who underwent BMT for hematological malignancies (allogeneic in 1, autologous in 1) and suffered severe exacerbations of the polyneuropathy at the time of conditioning or immediately after BMT, leading to quadriplegia and contributing to the patients' deaths (140). It is not clear what if any role immune-mediated demyelination has in early-onset polyneuropathy after BMT, but there is clearly need for caution in considering BMT for patients with a pre-existing inflammatory neuropathy.

Pretransplantation Neurological Screening

Pretransplant neurological screening may identify patients particularly prone for neurological complications and may lead to changes in treatment to minimize these complications. For example, anticonvulsant prophylaxis should be considered in BMT recipients with past seizures or a strong family history of epilepsy when these patients are on CSP or other drugs known to lower seizure threshold. Because of the cumulative toxicity of radiation therapy on the CNS, it may be prudent to use conditioning regimens without FTBI in brain-damaged patients and in patients with prior poliomyelitis at risk for postpoliomyelitis motor neuron disease. There is anecdotal evidence that regular exercise during corticosteroid treatment may reduce the muscle catabolic effect, and maintaining a conditioning program may be of particular value in patients who have been shown to be sensitive to the muscle toxicity of steroids but will require steroid prophylaxis because of the risk of GVHD. Caution is indicated when thalidomide is given long term to patients predisposed for other reasons to peripheral neuropathies (e.g., diabetics, alcoholics, individuals with high arches or other stigmata of congenital peripheral neuropathy, or patients who have had heavy exposure to vincristine or cis-platinum). Limited experience with inflammatory demyelinating polyneuropathy has suggested that this process may be exacerbated in association with BMT, and prospective BMT recipients with this diagnosis should at the least not be given conditioning regimens with high-dose ara-C, which has been shown to cause demyelinating neuropathy. Finally, careful medical evaluation of the bone marrow donor is justified not only to prevent transmissible infections but also to prevent the theoretically possible transmission of immune-mediated disease. When there is a marker for a particular disease process, such as acetylcholine receptor antibodies in myasthenia gravis, an argument can be made for the use of laboratory as well as clinical screening so the transplant team knows that a particular donor carries an increased risk.

References

1. Wiznitzer M, Packer RJ, August CS, Burkey ED. Neurological complications of bone marrow transplantation in childhood. Ann Neurol 1984;16:569–576.
2. Patchell RA, White CL, Clark AW, Beschorner WE, Santos GW. Neurologic complications of bone marrow transplantation. Neurology 1985;35:300–306.

3. Davis DG, Patchell RA. Neurological complications of bone marrow transplantation. Neurol Clin 1988;6: 377–387.
4. Schield WM. Drug delivery to the central nervous sysem: general principles and relevance to therapy for infections of the central nervous system. Rev Infect Dis 1989;7(suppl):S1669–S1690.
5. Wingard JR. Advances in the management of infectious complications after bone marrow transplantation. Bone Marrow Transplant 1990;6:371–383.
6. D'Antonio D, DiBartolomeo P, Iacone A, et al. Meningitis due to penicillin-resistant streptococcus pneumoniae in patients with chronic graft-versus-host disease. Bone Marrow Transplant 1992;9:299–300.
7. Winston DJ, Gale RP, Meyer DV, Young LS. Infectious complications of human bone marrow transplantation. Medicine 1979;58:1–31.
8. Mohrmann R, Mah V, Vinters HV. Neuropathologic findings after bone marrow transplantation: an autopsy study. Hum Path 1990;21:630–639.
9. Milliken ST, Powles RL. Antifungal prophylaxis in bone marrow transplantation. Rev Infect Dis 1990;12(suppl): S374–S379.
10. Verfaillie C, Weisdorf D, Haake R, Hostetter M, Ramsey NKC, McGlave P. Candida infections in bone marrow transplant recipients. Bone Marrow Transplant 1991; 8:177–184.
11. Lowenberg B, Van Gijn J, Prins E, Polderman AM. Fatal cerebral toxoplasmosis in a bone marrow transplant recipient with leukemia. Transplantation 1983;35:30–34.
12. Jehn U, Fink M, Gundlach P, et al. Lethal cardiac and cerebral toxoplasmosis in a patient with acute myeloid leukemia after successful allogeneic bone marrow transplantation. Transplantation 1984;38:430–433.
13. Palestine AG. Clinical aspects of cytomegalovirus retinitis. Rev Infect Dis 1988;10(suppl):S515–S521.
14. Cordonnier C, Feulihade F, Vernant JP, Marasult C, Rodet M, Rochant H. Cytomegalovirus encephalitis occurring after bone marrow transplantation. Scand J Haematol 1983;31:248–252.
15. Meyers JD. Infection in recipients of bone marrow transplants. Current clinical topics in infectious diseases. 1985;6:261–292.
16. Saral R, Burns WH, Laskin OL, et al. Acyclovir prophylaxis of herpes simplex virus infection. N Engl J Med 1981;305:63–67.
17. Atkinson K, Meyers JD, Storb R, Prentice RL, Thomas ED. Varicella zoster virus infection after marrow transplantation for aplastic anemia or leukemia. Transplantation 1980;29:47–50.
18. Locksley RM, Flournoy N, Sullivan KM, Meyers JD. Infection with varicella zoster virus infection after marrow transplantation. J Infect Dis 1985;152:1172–1181.
19. Thomas E, Howard FM. Segmental zoster paresis—a disease profile. Neurology 1971;173:843–845.
20. Davis D, Henglee PJ, Markesbery WR. Fatal adenovirus meningoencephalitis in a bone marrow transplant patient. Ann Neurol 1988;23:385–389.
21. Kaufman PT, Joneds RB, Greenberg CS, Peters WP. Autologous bone marrow transplantation and factor XII, factor VII, and protein C deficiencies. Cancer 1990;66:515–521.
22. Gordon B, Haire W, Kessinger A, Duggan M, Armitage J. High frequency of antithrombin 3 and protein C deficiency following autologous bone marrow transplantation and lymphoma. Bone Marrow Transplant 1991;8:497–502.
23. Gordon BG, Saving KL, McCallister JAM, et al. Cerebral infarction associated with protein C deficiency following allogeneic bone marrow transplantation. Bone Marrow Transplant 1991;8:323–325.
24. Patchell RA, White CL, Clark AW, Beschorner WE, Santos GW. Nonbacterial thrombotic endocarditis in bone marrow transplant patients. Cancer 1985;55:631–635.
25. Jerman MR, Fick RB. Nonbacterial thrombotic endocarditis associated with bone marrow transplantation. Chest 1986;90:919–922.
26. Doll DC, Ringenberg QS, Yarbro JW. Vascular toxicity associated with antineoplastic agents. Clin Oncol 1986;14:1405–1417.
27. Price BH. Anisocoria from scopalamine patches. JAMA 1985;254:1720–1721.
28. Witherspoon RP, Fisher LD, Schoch G, et al. Secondary cancers after bone marrow transplantation for leukemia or aplastic anemia. N Engl J Med 1989;321:784–789.
29. Kolb NJ, Bender-Gotze CH. Late complications after allogeneic bone marrow transplantation for leukemia. Bone Marrow Transplant 1990;6:61–72.
30. Atkinson K, Biggs J, Darveniza P, Boland J, Concannon A, Dodds A. Spinal cord and cerebellar-like syndromes associated with the use of cyclosporine in human recipients of allogeneic marrow transplants. Transplant Proc 1985;2:1673–1675.
31. Kahan BD, Flechner SM, Lorber MI, Golden D, Conley S, Van Buren CT. Complications of cyclosporine-prednisone immunosuppressive in 402 renal allograft recipients exclusively followed at a single center for from one to five years. Transplantation 1987;43:197–204.
32. Powell-Jackson PR, Carmichael FJL, Calne RY, Williams R. Adult respiratory distress syndrome and convulsions associated with administration of cyclosporine in liver transplant recipients. Transplantation 1984;38:341–343.
33. Grigg MM, Costanzo-Nordin MR, Celesia GG, et al. The etiology of seizures after cardiac transplantation. Transplant Proc 1988;3:937–944.
34. Ghany AM, Tutschka PJ, McGhee RB, et al. Cyclosporin-associated seizures in bone marrow transplant recipients given busulfan and cyclophosphamide preparative therapy. Transplantation 1991;52:310–315.
35. Famiglio L, Racusen L, Fivush B, Solez K, Fisher R. Central nervous system toxicity of cyclosporine in a rat model. Transplantation 1989;48:316–321.
36. De Groen PC, Aksamit AJ, Rakela J, Forbes GS, Krom RAF. Central nervous system toxicity after liver transplantation. The role of cyclosporine and cholesterol. N Engl J Med 1987;317:861–866.
37. Fazakerley JK, Webb HE. Cyclosporin, blood-brain barrier, and multiple sclerosis. Lancet 1985;2:889–890.
38. Kahan BD. Cyclosporine. N Engl J Med 1989;321:1725–1738.
39. Faynor SM, Moyer TP, Sterioff S, McDonald MW. Therapeutic drug monitoring of cyclosporine. Mayo Clin Proc 1984;59:571–572.
40. Slatkin NE, Eves CM, Stein AS, Forman SJ. Cyclosporin A associated seizures in bone marrow transplant recipients. Neurology 1990;40(suppl):248.
41. Lucey MR, Kolars JC, Merion RM, Campbell DA, Aldrich M, Watkins PB. Cyclosporin toxicity at therapeutic blood levels and cytochrome P-450 111A. Lancet 1990;335:11–15.

42. Kunzendorf U, Brockmoller J, Jochimsen F, Keller F, Walz G, Offermann G. Cyclosporin-metabolites and central nervous system toxicity. Lancet 1988;1:1223.
43. Reece DE, Frei-Lahr DA, Shepherd JD, et al. Neurologic complications in allogeneic bone marrow transplant patients receiving cyclosporin. Bone Marrow Transplant 1991;8:393–401.
44. Porapakkham S. An epidemiologic study of eclampsia. Obstet Gynecol 1979;54:26–30.
45. Crawford S, Varner MW, Digre KB, Servais G, Corbett JJ. Cranial magnetic resonance imaging in eclampsia. Obstet Gynecol 1987;70:474–477.
46. Zoja C, Furci L, Ghilardi F, et al. Cyclosporin-induced endothelial cell injury. Lab Invest 1986;55:455–462.
47. Lerman A, Hildebrand FL, Margulies KB, et al. Endothelin: a new cardiovascular regulatory peptide. Mayo Clin Proc 1990;65:1441–1445.
48. Lane RJM, Roche SW, Leung AAW, Greco A, Lange LS. Cyclosporin neurotoxicity in cardiac transplant recipients. J Neurol Neurosurg Psychiatry 1988;51:1434–1437.
49. Scheinman SJ, Reinitz ER, Petro G, Schwartz RA, Szmlac FS. Cyclosporine central neurotoxicity following renal transplantation. Transplantation 1990;49: 215–216.
50. Truwit CL, Denaro CP, Lake JR, DeMarco T. MR imaging of reversible cyclosporin A-induced toxicity. Am J Neuroradiol 1991;12:651–659.
51. Hauser RA, Lacey DM, Knight MR. Hypertensive encephalopathy. Magnetic resonance imaging demonstration of reversible cortical and white matter lesions. Arch Neurol 1988;45:1078–1083.
52. Jespersen CM, Rasmussen D, Hennild V. Focal intracerebral oedema in hypertensive encephalopathy visualized by computerized tomographic scan. J Intern Med 1989;225:349–350.
53. Beeson JH, Duda EE. Computed axial tomography scan demonstration of cerebral edema in eclampsia preceded by blindness. Obstet Gynecol 1982;60:529–532.
54. Gryn J, Goldberg J, Viner E. Propranolol for the treatment of cyclosporine-induced headaches. Bone Marrow Transplant 1992;9:211–212.
55. O'Sullivan DP. Convulsions associated with cyclosporin A. Bone Marrow J 1985;290:858.
56. Wilczek H, Ringden O, Tyden G. Cyclosporine-associated central nervous system toxicity after renal transplantation. Transplantation 1985;39:110.
57. Berden JHM, Hoitsma AJ, Merx JL, Keyser A. Severe central nervous system toxicity associated with cyclosporin. Lancet 1985;1:219–220.
58. Lind MJ, McWilliam L, Jip J, Scarfee JH, Morgenstern GR, Chang J. Cyclosporin associated demyelination following allogeneic bone marrow transplantation. Hematol Oncol 1989;7:49–52.
59. Ghalie R, Fitzsimmons WE, Bennett D, Kaizer H. Cortical blindness: a rare complication of cyclosporine therapy. Bone Marrow Transplant 1990;6:147–149.
60. Rubin AM, Kang H. Cerebral blindness and encephalopathy with cyclosporin A toxicity. Neurology 1987; 37:1072–1076.
61. Noppen M, Velkenifers B, Dierckx R, Bruyland M, Vanhalst L. Cyclosporine and myopathy. Ann Intern Med 1987;107:945–946.
62. Volin L, Jarventie G, Ruutu T. Fatal rhabdomyolysis as a complication of bone marrow transplantation. Bone Marrow Transplant 1990;6:59–60.
63. Joss DV, Barrett AJ, Kendra JR, Lucas CF, Desai S. Hypertension and convulsions in children receiving cyclosporin A. Lancet 1982;1:906.
64. Durrant S, Chipping PM, Palmer S, Gordon-Smith EC. Cyclosporin A, methylprednisone, and convulsions. Lancet 1982;2:829–830.
65. Noll RB, Roshni K. Complex visual hallucinations and cyclosporine. Arch Neurol 1984;41:329–330.
66. Appleton RE, Farrell K, Teal P, Hashimoto SA, Wong PKH. Complex partial status epilepticus associated with cyclosporin A therapy. J Neurol Neurosurg Psychiatry 1989;52:1068–1071.
67. Thompson CB, Sullivan KM, June CH, Thomas ED. Association between cyclosporin neurotoxicity and hypomagnesaemia. Lancet 1984;2:1116–1120.
68. Freeman DJ, Laupacis A, Keown PA, Stiller CR, Carruthers SG. Evaluations of cyclosporin-phenytoin interaction with observations on cyclosporin metabolites. Br J Clin Pharmacol 1984;18:887–893.
69. Fischman MA, Hull D, Bartus SA, Schweizer RT. Valproate for epilepsy in renal transplant recipients receiving cyclosporine. Transplantation 1989;48:542.
70. Hillebrand G, Castro LA, Van Scheidt W, Beukelmann D, Land W, Schmidt D. Valproate for epilepsy in renal transplant recipients receiving cyclosporine. Transplantation 1987;43:915–916.
71. Hall RCW, Popkin MK, Stickney SK, et al. Presentation of the steroid psychosis. J Nerv Ment Dis 1979;167:229–236.
72. Askari A, Vignos PJ, Moskowitz RW. Steroid myopathy in connective tissue disease. Am J Med 1976;61:485–492.
73. Khaleeli AA, Edwards RHT, Gohil K, et al. Corticosteroid myopathy: a clinical and pathological study. Clin Endocrinol 1983;18:155–166.
74. Fullerton PM, Kremer M. Neuropathy after intake of thalidomide (Distaval). Br Med J 1961;2:855–858.
75. Fullerton PM, O'Sullivan DJ. Thalidomide neuropathy: a clinical electrophysiological, and histological follow-up study. J Neurol Neurosurg Psychiatry 1968;31:543–551.
76. Clemmensen DJ, Olsen PZ, Andersen KE. Thalidomide neurotoxicity. Arch Dermatol 1984;120:338–341.
77. De La Camara R, Tomas JF, Figuera A, Berberana M, Fernandez-Ranada JM. High dose busulfan and seizures. Bone Marrow Transplant 1991;7:363–364.
78. Hartmann O, Banhamou E, Beaujean F, et al. High-dose busulfan and cyclophosphamide with autologous bone marrow transplantation support in advanced malignancies in children: a phase II study. J Clin Oncol 1986;12:1804–1810.
79. Marcus RE, Goldman JM. Convulsions due to high-dose busulphan. Lancet 1984;2:8417–8418.
80. Vassal G, Deroussent A, Hartmann O, et al. Dose-dependent neurotoxicity of high-dose busulfan in children: a clinical and pharmacological study. Cancer Res 1990;50:6203–6207.
81. Hassan M, Ehrsson H, Smedmyr B, et al. Cerebrospinal fluid and plasma concentrations of busulfan during high-dose therapy. Bone Marrow Transplant 1989;4: 113–114.
82. Grigg AP, Shepherd JD, Phillips GL. Busulphan and phenytoin. Ann Intern Med 1989;111:1049–1050.
83. Baker WJ, Royer GL, Weiss RB. Cytarabine and neurological toxicity. J. Clin Oncol 1991;9:679–693.
84. Vogler WR, Winton EF, Heffner LT, et al. Ophthalmological and other toxicities related to cytosine arabinoside and total body irradiation as preparatory regimen for

bone marrow transplantation. Bone Marrow Transplant 1990;6:405–409.

85. Johnson NT, Crawford SW, Sargur M. Acute acquired demyelinating polyneuropathy with respiratory failure following high-dose systemic cytosine arabinoside and marrow transplantation. Bone Marrow Transplant 1987;2:203–207.
86. Weinblatt ME. Toxicity of low dose methotrexate in rheumatoid arthritis. J Rheumatol 1985;12(suppl):35–39.
87. McKendry RJR, Cyr M. Toxicity of methotrexate compared with azathioprine in the treatment of rheumatoid arthritis. Arch Intern Med 1989;149:685–689.
88. Wernick R, Smith DL. Central nervous system toxicity associated with weekly low-dose methotrexate treatment. Arthritis Rheum 1989;32:770–775.
89. Ebner F, Ranner G, Slavc I, et al. MR findings in methotrexate-induced CNS abnormalities. Am J Neuroradiol 1989;110:959–964.
90. Bleyer WA. Neurological sequelae of methotrexate and ionizing radiation: a new classification. Cancer Treat Rep 1981;65(suppl):89–98.
91. Thompson CB, Sanders JE, Fournoy N, Buckner CD, Thomas ED. The risks of central nervous system relapse and leukoencephalopathy in patients receiving marrow transplants for acute leukemia. Blood 1986;67:195–199.
92. Devinsky O, Lemann W, Evans AC, Moeller JR, Rottenberg DA. Akinetic mutism in a bone marrow transplant recipient following total body irradiation and amphotericin B chemoprophylaxis. Arch Neurol 1987;44:414–417.
93. Hook CC, Kimmel DW, Kvols LK. Multifocal inflammatory leukoencephalopathy with 5-fluorouracil and levamisole. Ann Neurol 1992;31:262–267.
94. Hochberg FH, Pruitt AA, Beck DO, DeBrun G, Davis K. The rationale and methodology for intra-arterial chemotherapy with BCNU as treatment for glioblastoma. J Neurosurg 1985;63:876–880.
95. Madajewicz S, West CR, Hyung CP, et al. Phase II study—intra-arterial BCNU therapy for metastatic brain tumors. Cancer 1981;47:653–657.
96. Shapiro WR, Green SB. Re-evaluating the efficacy of intra-arterial BCNU. J Neurosurg 1987;66:313–314.
97. Jagannath S, Armitage JO, Dicke KA, et al. Prognostic factors for response and survival after high-dose cyclophosphamide, carmustine, and etoposide with autologous bone marrow transplantation for relapsed Hodgkin's disease. J Clin Oncol 1989;7:179–185.
98. Sullivan KM, Storb R, Shulman HM. Immediate and delayed neurotoxicity after mechlorethamine preparation bone marrow transplantation. Ann Intern Med 1982;97:182–189.
99. Snavely SR, Hodges GR. The neurotoxicity of antibacterial agents. Ann Intern Med 1984;101:92–104.
100. Frytak S, Moertel CG, Childs DS. Neurologic toxicity associated with high-dose metronidazole therapy. Ann Intern Med 1978;88:361–362.
101. Eng RHK, Munsif AN, Yangco BG, Smith SM, Chmel H. Seizure propensity with Imipenem. Arch Intern Med 1989;149:1881–1883.
102. Kusumi RK, Plouffe JF, Wyatt RH, Fass RJ. Central nervous system toxicity associated with metronidazole therapy. Ann Intern Med 1980;93:59–60.
103. Burge DR, Chow AW, Sacks SL. Neurotoxic effects during vidarabine therapy for herpes zoster. Can Med Assoc J 1985;132:392–395.
104. Feldman S, Robertson PK, Lott L, Thornton D. Neurotoxicity due to adenine arabinoside therapy during varicella-zoster virus infections in immunocompromised children. J Infect Dis 1986;154:889–893.
105. Wade JC, Meyers JD. Neurologic symptoms associated with parenteral acyclovir treatment after marrow transplantation. Ann Intern Med 1983;98:921–925.
106. Spiegal DM, Lau K. Acute renal failure and coma secondary to acyclovir therapy. JAMA 1986;255:1882–1883.
107. Cohen SMZ, Minkove JA, Zebley JW, Mulholland JH. Severe but reversible neurotoxicity from acyclovir. Ann Intern Med 1984;100:920.
108. Swan SK, Bennett WM. Oral acyclovir and neurotoxicity. Ann Intern Med 1989;111:188.
109. Davis CL, Springmeyer S, Gmerek BJ. Central nervous system side effects of ganciclovir. N Engl J Med 1990;322:933–934.
110. De Armand B. Safety considerations in the use of ganciclovir in immunocompromised patients. Transplant Proc 1991;23:26–29.
111. Jacobsen MA, O'Donnell JJ. Approaches to the treatment of cytomegalovirus retinitis: ganciclovir and foscarnet. J Acquired Immune Deficiency Syndrome 1991;4(suppl):S11–S15.
112. Chrisp P, Clissold SP. Foscarnet: a review of its antiviral activity, pharmacokinetic properties and therapeutic use in immunocompromised patients with cytomegalovirus retinitis. Drugs 1991;41:104–129.
113. Hickey WF, Kimura H. Graft-vs.-host disease elicits expression of class I and class II histocompatibility antigens and the presence of scattered T lymphocytes in rat central nervous system. Proc Natl Acad Sci USA 1987;84:2082–2086.
114. Rouah E, Gruber R, Shearer W, Armstrong D, Hawkins EP. Graft-versus-host disease in the central nervous system: a real entity? Am J Clin Pathol 1988;89:543–546.
115. Marosi C, Budka H, Grimm G, et al. Fatal encephalitis in a patient with chronic graft-versus-host disease. Bone Marrow Transplant 1990;6:53–57.
116. Schold SC, Cho ES, Somasundaram M, et al. Subacute motor neuronopathy: a remote effect of lymphoma. Ann Neurol 1979;5:271–287.
117. Lefvert AK, Bjorkholm M. Antibodies against the acetylcholine receptor in hematological disorders: implication for the development of myasthenia gravis after bone marrow grafting. N Engl J Med 1987; 317:170.
118. Lefvert AK, Bolme P, Hammarstrom L, et al. Bone marrow grafting selectively induces the production of acetylcholine receptor antibodies, immunoglobulins bearing related idiotypes, and anti-idiotypic antibodies. Ann NY Acad Sci 1987;505:825–827.
119. Bolger GB, Sullivan KM, Spence AM, et al. Myasthenia gravis after allogeneic bone marrow transplantation: relationship to chronic graft-versus-host disease. Neurology 1986;36:1087–1091.
120. Grav JM, Casademont J, Monforte R, et al. Myasthenia gravis after allogeneic bone marrow transplantation: report of a new case and pathogenetic considerations. Bone Marrow Transplant 1990;5:435–437.
121. Seely E, Drachman D, Smith BR, et al. Post bone marrow transplantation (BMT) myasthenia gravis: evidence for acetylcholine receptor (AChR) abnormality. Blood 1984;64(suppl):221a.
122. Smith CI, Aarli JA, Biberfeld P, et al. Myasthenia

gravis after bone marrow transplantation: evidence for a donor origin. N Engl J Med 1983;309:1565–1568.
123. Dalakas MC. Polymyositis, dermatomyositis, and inclusion-body myositis. N Engl J Med 1991;325: 1487–1498.
124. Sullivan KM, Shulman HM, Storb R, et al. Chronic graft-versus-host disease in 52 patients: adverse natural course and successful treatment with combination immunosuppression. Blood 1981;57:267–276.
125. Anderson BA, Young PV, Kean WF, et al. Polymyositis in chronic graft-versus-host disease. Arch Neurol 1982;39:188–190.
126. Reyes MG, Noronha P, Thomas W, et al. Myositis of chronic graft versus host disease. Neurology 1983; 33:1222–1224.
127. Urbano-Marquez A, Estruch R, Grav JM, et al. Inflammatory myopathy associated with chronic graft-versus host disease. Neurology 1986;36:1091–1093.
128. Pier N, Dubowitz V. Chronic graft versus host disease presenting with polymyositis. Bone Marrow J 1983; 286:2024.
129. Slatkin NE, Sheibani K, Forman SJ, et al. Myositis as the major manifestation of chronic graft versus host disease (GVHD). Neurology 1987;37(suppl):205.
130. Schmidley JW, Galloway P. Polymyositis following autologous bone marrow transplantation in Hodgkins disease. Neurology 1990;40:1003–1004.
131. Mulligan SP, Joshua DE, Joasoo A, et al. Autoimmune hyperthyroidism associated with chronic graft-versus-host disease. Transplantation 1987;44:463–464.
132. Asbury AK, Bolis L, Gibbs CJ. Autoimmune neuropathies: Guillain-Barre syndrome. Ann Neurol 1990; 27(suppl):1–79.
133. Lisak RP, Mithell M, Zweiman B, et al. Guillain-Barre syndrome and Hodgkin's disease: three cases with immunological studies. Ann Neurol 1977;1:72–78.
134. Granena A, Grau JM, Carreras E, et al. Subacute sensorimotor polyneuropathy in a recipient of an allogeneic bone marrow graft. Exp Hematol 1983: 11(suppl 113):10–12.
135. Maguire H, August C, Sladky J. Chronic inflammatory demyelinating polyneuropathy: a previously unreported complication of bone marrow transplantation. Neurology 1989;39(suppl):410.
136. Greenspan A, Deeg HJ, Cottler-Fox M, Sirdofski M, Spitzer TR, Kattah J. Incapacitating peripheral neuropathy as a manifestation of chronic graft-versus-host disease. Bone Marrow Transplant 1990;5: 349–352.
137. Eliashiv S, Brenner T, Abramsky O, et al. Acute inflammatory polyneuropathy following bone marrow transplantation. Bone Marrow Transplant 1991;8:315–317.
138. Paul M, Joshua D, Rahme N, et al. Fatal peripheral neuropathy associated with axonal degeneration after high-dose cystosine arabinoside in acute leukemia. Br J Haematol 1991;79:521–523.
139. Bierman P, Bashir R, Openshaw H, Slatkin N. Inflammatory polyradiculoneuropathy in autologous bone marrow transplantation (BMT). Neurology 1991;41 (suppl):199–200.
140. Openshaw H, Hinton DR, Slatkin NE, Bierman PJ, Hoffman FM, Snyder DS. Exacerbation of inflammatory demyelinating polyneuropathy after bone marrow transplantation. Bone Marrow Transplant 1991; 7:411–414.

Chapter 35

Management of ABO Incompatibility in Allogeneic Bone Marrow Transplantation

Irena Sniecinski

ABO incompatibility between donor and recipient is encountered in 20 to 30% of all allogeneic bone marrow transplantations (BMTs). The incompatibility may be major, which occurs when the recipient plasma contains isohemagglutinins directed against donor red blood cell (RBC) antigens (e.g., group O recipient and group A donor). Alternatively, there could be a minor incompatibility, in which the donor plasma contains isohemagglutinins directed against the recipient RBC antigens (e.g., group A recipient and group O donor). In some instances, there could be a bidirectional ABO incompatibility (i.e., when the recipient is group A and the donor is group B).

Donor-recipient ABO incompatibility is not considered to be a contraindication to successful BMT. Previous studies showed no significant effect of major or minor ABO mismatch on the incidence of graft rejection, the incidence of graft-versus-host disease (GVHD), and survival (1–6). Nevertheless, patients undergoing ABO incompatible BMT are at risk for development of several immunohematological complications (Table 35-1). Major ABO incompatibility between marrow donor and recipient has the potential risk of severe hemolytic reaction caused by infusion of a large red cell mass with the marrow cells (7). Continuing production of isohemagglutinins by the recipient under this stimulus in the post-transplant period may then result in delayed erythropoiesis, persistent hemolysis, or both (1,8–21). Potential adverse outcomes of minor ABO incompatibility include rapid immune hemolysis at the time of infusion of donor marrow as a result of passive transfer of isohemagglutinins in the marrow plasma, or delayed immune hemolysis caused by red cell isohemagglutinins produced transiently by the donor marrow lymphocytes (2, 22–27).

Table 35-1.
Immunohematological Complications of ABO incompatible Bone Marrow Transplantation

Major ABO Incompatibility
Immediate hemolysis of the RBC infused with the donor marrow
Delayed hemolysis of the RBCs produced by engrafted marrow
Delayed onset of erythropoiesis
Minor ABO Incompatibility
Immediate hemolysis of the recipient RBCs by the isohemagglutinins infused with the marrow
Delayed hemolysis of recipient RBCs due to persistent production of isohemagglutinins by the marrow lymphocytes
Major and Minor ABO Incompatibility
Immediate hemolysis caused by the recipient or donor isohemagglutinins
Delayed hemolysis caused by the recipient or donor isohemagglutinins

RBC = red blood cell.

A number of methods are available for prevention of hemolysis in the setting of ABO incompatible BMT. This chapter reviews the various approaches for preventing both immediate and delayed immunohematological problems and discusses current recommendations regarding optimal management.

Major ABO Incompatibility

The marrow aspirate usually contains approximately the same concentration of RBCs as one unit of whole blood; thus, a severe hemolytic transfusion reaction at the time of BMT might occur due to interaction of donor-type RBCs with pre-existing host-derived isohemagglutinins. Hemolysis occurring by this mechanism can be eliminated using the following methods of preparation for a major ABO incompatible BMT: (1) in vitro removal of the incompatible RBCs from the marrow aspirate prior to its infusion, and (2) in vivo removal of circulating isohemagglutinins from the recipient.

Early attempts to prevent hemolysis at the time of marrow infusion involved the removal of the anti-A or anti-B isohemagglutinins from the recipient before BMT by plasmapheresis or immunoadsorption (28–35). Subsequently, several techniques of RBC depletion from marrow grafts have been developed and successfully used in ABO-mismatched transplants (8–15, 36–48).

Because the technique is simple and poses no risk

to the recipient, the current practice is to deplete RBCs from all marrows involving major ABO incompatibility and to lower recipient isohemagglutinins only when they are present in high titers, which may result in delayed erythropoiesis and hemolysis after BMT (14,49). Some transplant centers restrict the use of RBC depletion to ABO incompatible human leukocyte antigen (HLA)–matched sibling BMT and recommend isohemagglutinin depletion for management of matched-unrelated donors (MUD), partially mismatched family donors, and transplants for aplastic anemia (50).

Red Cell Removal from Donor Marrow

The main objective of RBC removal from donor marrow is to remove the majority of RBCs while preserving the hematopoietic progenitors to ensure timely engraftment. Several manual and automated techniques have been developed to remove the RBCs selectively from the marrow. Some techniques isolate the mononuclear cell–rich preparation where the cells necessary for engraftment are found, whereas others utilize the entire buffy coat, containing both mononuclear and polymorphonuclear cells.

Buffy coat can be prepared by gravity sedimentation or differential centrifugation. Sedimentation under gravity is a simple technique that requires no special equipment (8,9,36–38). The marrow aspirate is placed in a standard blood transfusion bag and mixed with 6% hydroxyethyl starch at a ratio of 8:1. The bag is hung in an inverted position, and the marrow cells are allowed to separate at room temperature for 30 to 60 minutes under visual monitoring. The sedimented RBCs are removed through a port in the lower end of the inverted bag, and the supernatant plasma and buffy coat layer are resuspended before infusion. With this single-step technique, a median of 75% nucleated cells and 55% colony forming units can be recovered. The hematocrit of the buffy coat after sedimentation is 1 to 4%, with a volume of residual RBCs ranging from 0.4 to 21.8 mL. The red cell–rich sediment may be treated again with hydroxyethyl starch to increase the recovery of nucleated cells to 86.2% and the recovery of colony forming units to 98.2%, while removing 97.8% of RBCs (36).

Other sedimenting agents, including Plasmagel, Dextran, and Ficoll-Hypaque, have been evaluated and found to be less effective in this procedure (37,38).

An alternative method of buffy coat preparation from marrow is differential centrifugation using a COBE-2991 cell processor or discontinuous flow cell separators (H-30 or V-50 models; Haemonetics, Inc, Braintree, MA). Centrifugation of the marrow using these instruments yields a buffy coat concentrate containing 75% of the original nucleated cells and 57 to 83% of the colony forming units (10, 39, 40). The average volume of the RBCs remaining in the concentrate varies from 8 to 38 mL (10,40). This method is less time-consuming and tedious than the gravity sedimentation technique. In addition, it provides a better closed processing system and a more objective and reproducible separation.

Overall, sedimentation and centrifugation methods of preparation of buffy coat from marrow leave a considerable volume of RBCs in the final concentrate and do not entirely eliminate the risk of acute hemolysis associated with infusion of the ABO-incompatible marrow. Several cases of adverse reactions associated with transfusion of buffy coat concentrate from ABO-incompatible donors have been reported (8,10,36). Most of these reactions represented transient episodes of hemoglobinuria, chills, fever, or hypertension, although in 1 patient, acute shortness of breath, wheezing, and back pain developed (10).

A mononuclear cell–rich concentrate can be prepared by processing the marrow in a cell separator, either with or without density gradient. In the former technique, the buffy coat is prepared, then layered over a density gradient, and subsequently centrifuged to yield an enriched fraction of mononuclear cells (14, 41–44). Density gradient separation of the mononuclear cell concentrate assures 60% recovery of granulocyte-macrophage colony forming units and removal of 99% of RBCs.

Automated nondensity gradient methods for preparing mononuclear cell concentrates require the availability of one of the following continuous flow cell separators: Fenwal CS-3000 Plus (Baxter Healthcare, Deerfield, IL) or Spectra (COBE BCT, Lakewood, CO). Both cell separators are capable of preparing the marrow concentrate preferentially enriched with mononuclear cells (45–48). Recovery of the hematopoietic stem cells was found to be superior to the sedimentation methods. Results of marrow processing with these instruments are presented in Table 35-2 (48).

Removal of Isohemagglutinins from Recipient

The alternate approach to prevention of acute hemolysis is removal of isohemagglutinins from the plasma of BMT recipients (28–35). The goal of this approach is to decrease the titer of the potentially offending isohemagglutinins prior to marrow infusion. Depletion of isohemagglutinins may be achieved through the use of plasma exchange, plasma immunoadsorption, or whole blood immunoadsorption, usually carried out daily over 3 to 4 days prior to marrow infusion, with the goal of reducing the isohemagglutinin titers to 1:16 or lower (29). Some investigators have supplemented these techniques with pre-BMT transfusion of donor-type blood or purified A or B substance to absorb completely the recipient's isohemagglutinins (29–31). Others utilize in vivo absorption of isohemagglutinins by administering small volumes of donor-type incompatible RBCs without plasma exchange or immunoadsorption (34). The incompatible RBCs are infused 12 to 24 hours prior to BMT. This method has been used safely even in recipients with isohemagglutinin titers as high as 1:256.

Table 35-2.
ABO-incompatible Bone Marrow Processing

		Spectra (n = 14)			*CS-3000 Plus (N = 10)*	
Volume (ml)	Initial		1072 ± 288	Initial		1124 ± 262
	Final		151 ± 33	Final		204 ± 9.0
% Recovery		15 ± 3			19 ± 5	
RBC (ml)	Initial		318 ± 68	Initial		338 ± 68
	Final		5.0 ± 1.5	Final		6.6 ± 4.9
% Recovery		1.6 ± 0.5			1.9 ± 1.1	
MNC ($\times 10^9$)	Initial		5.3 ± 1.7	Initial		5.8 ± 2.2
	Final		4.5 ± 1.5	Final		3.5 ± 0.8
% Recovery		84 ± 11			63 ± 21	
PMN ($\times 10^9$)	Initial		9.7 ± 2.5	Initial		9.4 ± 3.3
	Final		1.3 ± 0.7	Final		1.3 ± 0.6
% Recovery		15 ± 11			15 ± 9	

RBC = red blood cell; MNC = mononuclear leukocyte; PMN = polymorphonuclear leukocyte.

Drawbacks and Limitations of Red Cell and Isohemagglutinin Depletion Methods

The major risks of RBC depletion from marrow include stem-cell loss during processing and the hazard of infusing small amounts of incompatible RBCs. Stem-cell loss appears to be acceptable for matched sibling grafts because there have been no reports of delayed engraftment caused by insufficient number of stem cells retained in the marrow after processing with any method of RBC depletion. However, there is some concern that this stem-cell loss might carry an increased risk of graft failure in patients with aplastic anemia and recipients of MUD transplants (50). The risk for development of a serious hemolytic reaction to the small volume of the residual RBCs in the processed marrow is insignificant.

Isohemagglutinin depletion techniques have several drawbacks, including citrate toxicity, thrombocytopenia, and the risk of disease transmission. Moreover, plasma exchange and immunoadsorption are sometimes followed by rebound of antibody in the post-transplant period, leading to severe delayed hemolysis in some patients (1,11,29,35).

Although both methods are very effective in preventing the immediate hemolysis in the setting of major ABO-mismatched BMT, neither is 100% successful in preventing clinically significant delayed hemolysis. This risk has been estimated to be approximately 10% and appears to be increased in patients with high pretransplant isohemagglutinin titers and in patients receiving cyclosporine (CSP)/prednisone (PSE) for GVHD prophylaxis (12).

Delayed hemolysis usually begins several weeks after BMT as donor-derived RBCs produced by engrafted marrow start to appear in the circulation (Figure 35-1). Hemolysis is caused by the continuing synthesis of isohemagglutinins by residual host lymphocytes and plasma cells. Common laboratory findings include a positive direct antiglobulin test result and the presence of isohemagglutinins directed against donor-type RBCs in recipient plasma or eluate. The persistence of functional host-derived lymphocytes and plasma cells that have survived the BMT conditioning regimen can also result in delayed erythroid engraftment and increased RBC transfusion requirement (2,12,16,29). The mechanism appears to involve the interaction of host-derived anti-donor isohemagglutinins with ABO antigens present on donor-derived erythroid progenitors (12,17,19). Studies utilizing marrow cultures have demonstrated that A and B antigens are expressed on early and late erythroid progenitors,

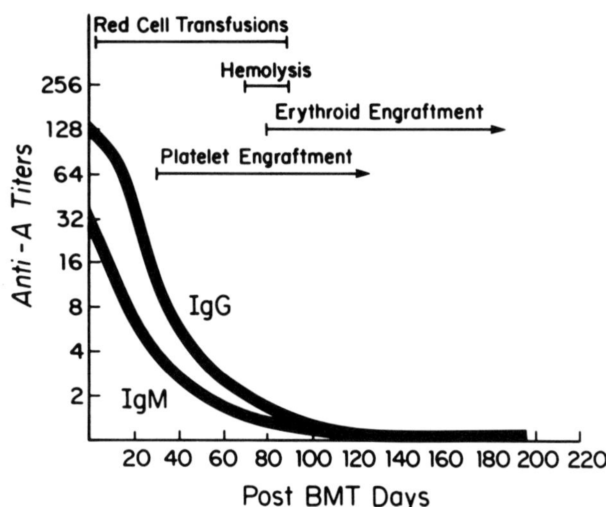

Figure 35-1. Post-transplant course in a patient with no red cell production and high isohemagglutinin titers. Hemolysis occurred when titers were low. Resolution coincided with undetectable isohemagglutinins. Findings of hemolysis were present even though donor marrow-derived red cells were undetectable, suggesting intramedullary hemolysis. *Upper curve* represents immunoglobulin G (IgG) isohemagglutinins, and *lower curve* represents IgM isohemagglutinins.

and isohemagglutinin-containing autologous sera have been shown to suppress the growth of these colonies (17,19,51,52).

Persistence of isohemagglutinins has been observed in 18% of recipients of major ABO-incompatible marrow receiving CSP/PSE for GVHD prophylaxis (12). In most of these patients, erythroid engraftment occurred spontaneously within 6 months when antibody titers decreased. However, in some patients, isohemagglutinin-induced RBC aplasia persisted for many months; in 1 patient, RBC production was suppressed for more than 5 years. To decrease the frequency of this complication, some investigators recommend removal of isohemagglutinins from CSP/PSE-immunosuppressed recipients prior to infusion of RBC-depleted marrow (14,49).

Management of Major ABO Incompatibility

Prior to BMT, immunoglobulin M (IgM) and IgG isohemagglutinin titers should be measured in all patients having major ABO incompatibility with their marrow donors. Patients with IgG isohemagglutinin titers of 256 or less should receive RBC-depleted marrow. Removal of RBCs from marrow concentrates should be carried out using a technique that maximizes mononuclear and clonogenic cell recovery, providing a dose of at least 0.5×10^8 mononuclear cells/kg of recipient body weight. The residual RBCs in the processed marrow should not exceed 10 mL. Patients with IgG isohemagglutinin titers above 256 should be considered for plasma exchange or immunoadsorption in addition to receiving RBC-depleted marrow. The exchange should decrease the titer of isohemagglutinin to 16 or below. Transfusion of incompatible RBCs for in vivo absorption of isohemagglutinins not removed by these procedures is not recommended because of the risk of delayed hemolysis caused by antibody rebound in the post-transplant period.

Following BMT, all patients should be monitored by immunohematological testing for the appearance of donor-derived RBCs and changes in recipient isohemagglutinin titers. Group O RBCs should be used for transfusions until the recipient changes to donor ABO type (Table 35-3). If donor-type platelets are not readily available, the volume of the incompatible plasma administered with platelets should be minimized before transfusion. To prevent the occurrence of transfusion-associated GVHD, all cellular blood products should be irradiated with 1,500 to 3,000 cGy before transfusion.

Patients who demonstrate high isohemagglutinin titers before BMT have a very high probability of antibody return after BMT and should be followed with weekly testing of isohemagglutinins titers. An increasing titer usually heralds delayed onset of erythropoiesis, hemolysis, or both. Patients demonstrating these complications should be considered for removal of antibody by plasma exchange or immunoadsorption when the titer of returning antibody during the post-transplant period is greater than 1:16.

Minor ABO Incompatibility

Minor ABO mismatch is present in 15 to 20% of HLA-matched donor-recipient pairs. Patients receiving marrow from a minor ABO-incompatible donor are at risk for development of immediate immune hemolysis caused by isohemagglutinins infused with the marrow or delayed immune hemolysis caused by isohemagglutinins produced by the marrow lymphocytes or plasma cells.

Immediate hemolysis in the setting of minor ABO incompatible BMT has not been life-threatening (2). Nevertheless, prophylaxis against this complication is recommended when the donor isohemagglutinin titer is 128 or higher.

A more serious consequence of minor ABO incompatible BMT is the occurrence of delayed hemolysis due to isohemagglutinins produced by lymphocytes transfused with the marrow (22–27). Hemolysis is usually abrupt in onset, appearing 9 to 16 days after BMT (Figure 35-2). The direct antiglobulin test result is usually positive, and antibody of donor specificity can be eluted from the recipient's RBCs. The frequency of clinically significant hemolysis varies from 15 to 71%

Table 35-3.
Recommended Blood Groups for Red Blood Cells and Platelet/Plasma Components in ABO-incompatible Bone Marrow Transplantations

Major ABO Incompatibility	*Minor ABO Incompatibility*	*Major and Minor ABO Incompatibility*
1. Give recipient-type RBCs 2. Give donor-type platelets and plasma concentrates Example Patient O; donor A Group O RBCs Group A or AB platelets and plasma concentrates	1. Give group O RBCs 2. Give recipient-type plasma and platelet concentrates Example Patient B; donor O Group O RBCs Group B or AB platelets and plasma concentrates	1. Give group O RBCs 2. Give group AB platelets and plasma concentrates Example Patient A; donor B Group O RBCs Group AB platelets and plasma concentrates

RBC = red blood cell.

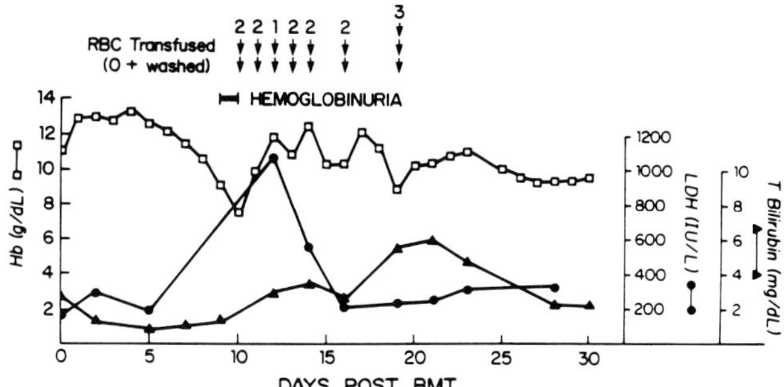

Figure 35-2. ABO minor mismatched bone marrow transplantation (BMT) (donor O+, recipient B+). Flow chart shows hematological and biochemical evidence for hemolysis. Fourteen units of packed O+ red cells were required to maintain the hemoglobin concentration between day 10 and day 19 after BMT. Note that mutant hemoglobin (Hb), lactic dehydrogenase (LDH), and total bilirubin levels were normal for the first 5 days after BMT. During the hemolytic episode, no incompatible isohemagglutinins were infused; red blood cells (RBCs) transfused were washed group O; platelets were group O washed and resuspended in fresh AB plasma.

(23,26–27). Although the hemolysis is self-limiting and without significant morbidity in most patients, in 10 to 15% it has been associated with serious complications, including renal failure and delayed engraftment (22,25).

The risk for development of clinically significant hemolysis appears to be increased in patients undergoing T-cell–depleted BMT (24,26,27). In one study (27), a strongly reactive donor-derived anti-A antibody was identified in 8 of 9 recipients following minor ABO-incompatible, T-cell–depleted BMT. Also, patients receiving non-T-cell–depleted marrow and CSP/PSE for GVHD prophylaxis without methotrexate (MTX) were at increased risk for delayed hemolysis after BMT (23,53). In patients with minor ABO-incompatible, unrelated donors, hemolysis also affected the bystander transfused group O RBCs (53).

In this setting, the operative mechanism for antibody production is an unimpeded, donor-derived B-lymphocyte response to recipient RBC-mismatched antigens. The production of antibody by donor memory B lymphocytes is enhanced by ex vivo removal of T lymphocytes or suppression of T-lymphocyte function by CSP. Both appear to have similar enhancing effects on the function of transplanted B lymphocytes. The "bystander" hemolysis most likely results from complement activation by the immune reaction between donor-derived antibody and recipient-derived A or B antigens, with subsequent complement binding to antigen-negative RBC (51). Unlike the situation in major ABO-mismatched BMTs, pretransplant isohemagglutinin titers do not appear to predict the incidence or severity of hemolysis following minor ABO-mismatched transplantations (23,24). Post-transplant immunosuppression with MTX may prevent the development of hemolysis, even in patients receiving CSP (53).

There are two approaches to minimize the risk of immediate and delayed RBC hemolysis in minor ABO incompatible BMT recipients: (1) removal of plasma from the donor marrow, and (2) pre-BMT dilution of recipient RBCs with group O RBCs. To prevent the risk of immediate hemolysis, plasma is removed from the marrow if the donor has an isohemagglutinin titer of 128 or more. This removal can be done by centrifuging the marrow and removing the supernatant plasma from the marrow concentrate (2). No substantial loss of stem cells is associated with this procedure.

Dilution of patient RBCs with group O cells might be accomplished by prophylactic transfusion or by RBC exchange. The second approach has been found to be more successful in preventing or decreasing the severity of delayed immune hemolysis after BMT (53,54).

Management of Minor ABO-mismatched BMT

Before BMT, IgM and IgG isohemagglutinin titers should be measured in all marrow donors who are minor ABO-incompatible with their prospective recipients. Presence of an isohemagglutinin titer of 128 or more is an indication for removal of plasma from the marrow before BMT. To prevent the occurrence of severe delayed hemolysis in the post-transplant period, prophylactic RBC exchange of the marrow recipient should be performed in all patients receiving post-transplant immunosuppression with CSP without concurrent MTX. RBC exchange should be carried out regardless of the donor's isohemagglutinin titer and until 80% of the patient's RBC mass is replaced with group O RBC. All RBC transfusions required in the pretransplant period should also be from group O donors.

Following BMT, recipients should be monitored for development of immune hemolysis using direct antiglobulin and antibody screening tests. These tests should be performed every 2 days during the first 3 post-transplant weeks. Group O packed or washed RBCs should be used for transfusion. To prevent transfusion of significant volumes of ABO-incompatible plasma, platelet concentrates should be either of the recipient type or volume-depleted if of donor type. All cellular blood products should be irradiated with 1,500 to 3,000 cGy before transfusion to avoid transfusion-associated GVHD.

Management of Bidirectional ABO Mismatch

Patients receiving bidirectional ABO-mismatched marrow are at a potential risk for complications related to both major and minor ABO incompatibilities. To reduce the potential for severe acute and delayed hemolysis, the following guidelines for management of these patients are recommended:

1. Appropriate titers should be performed on marrow donor and recipient.
2. RBC and plasma depletion of the marrow before infusion.
3. RBC exchange of the recipient prior to BMT.
4. Plasma exchange of the recipient when the recipient's isohemagglutinin IgG titer is above 256.
5. Group O red cell products and group AB plasma products should be used for the pretransplant and post-transplant transfusion support.

Summary

ABO incompatible BMT creates the risk of immunohematological problems resulting from both donor-versus-host and host-versus-donor antibody production. Various approaches have been developed to prevent and treat those immunohematological complications. Some methods prevent the occurrence of clinically significant problems and others only reduce the severity of the clinical manifestations of adverse interaction between the incompatible immune systems of donor and recipient. Immunohematological problems should always be anticipated, and close monitoring and appropriate measures are necessary when a major or minor ABO blood group mismatch exists between the donor and the recipient.

References

1. Buckner CD, Clift RA, Sanders JE, Gray W, Storb R, Thomas ED. ABO-incompatible marrow transplants. Transplantation 1978;26:233–238.
2. Lasky LC, Warkentin PI, Kersey JH, Ramsay NKC, McGlave PB, McCullough J. Hemotherapy in patients undergoing blood group incompatible bone marrow transplantation. Transfusion 1983;23:277–285.
3. Gale RP, Feig S, Ho W, et al. ABO blood group system and bone marrow transplantation. Blood 1977;50:185–194.
4. Marmont AM, Damasio EE, Bacigalupo A, et al. A to O bone marrow transplantation in severe aplastic anaemia: dynamics of blood group conversion and demonstration of early dyserythropoiesis in the engrafted marrow. Br J Haematol 1977;36:511–518.
5. Bleyer WA, Blaese RM, Bujack JS, et al. Long-term remission from acute myelogenous leukemia after bone marrow transplantation and recovery from acute graft-versus-host reaction and prolonged immunoincompetence. Blood 1975;45:171.
6. Biggs JC, Concannon AJ, Dodds AJ, et al. Allogenic bone marrow transplantation across the ABO barrier. Med J Aust 1979;2:173–175.
7. Goldfinger D. Acute hemolytic transfusion reaction—a fresh look at pathogenesis and considerations regarding therapy. Transfusion 1977;17:85–98.
8. Dinsmore RE, Reich LM, Kapoor N, et al. ABH incompatible bone marrow transplantation: removal of erythrocytes by starch sedimentation. Br J Haematol 1983;54:441–449.
9. Ho WG, Champlin RE, Feig SA, Gale RP. Transplantation of ABH incompatible bone marrow: gravity sedimentation of donor marrow. Br J Haematol 1984;57: 155–162.
10. Braine HG, Sensenbrener LL, Wright SK, Tutschka PJ, Saral R, Santos GW. Bone marrow transplantation with major ABO blood group incompatibility using erythrocyte depletion of marrow prior to infusion. Blood 1982;60:420–425.
11. Warkentin PI, Yomtovian R, Hurd D, et al. Severe delayed hemolytic transfusion reaction complicating an ABO-incompatible bone marrow transplantation. Vox Sang 1983;45:40–47.
12. Sniecinski IJ, Oien L, Petz LD, Blume KG. Immunohematologic consequences of major ABO-mismatched bone marrow transplantation. Transplantation 1988; 45:530–534.
13. Sniecinski IJ, Petz LD, Oien L, Blume KG. Immunohematologic problems arising from ABO incompatible bone marrow transplantation. Transplant Proc 1987;19: 4609–4611.
14. Blacklock HA, Prentice HG, Evans JPM, et al. ABO-incompatible bone marrow transplantation: removal of red blood cells from donor marrow avoiding recipient antibody depletion. Lancet 1982,2:1061–1064.
15. Jin NR, Hill R, Segal G, et al. Preparation of red-blood-cell-depleted marrow for ABO-incompatible marrow transplantation by density-gradient separation using the IBM 2991 blood cell processor. Exp Hematol 1987;15:93–98.
16. Gmür JP, Burger J, Schaffner A, et al. Pure red cell aplasia of long duration complicating major ABO-incompatible bone marrow transplantation. Blood 1990;75:290–295.
17. Barge AJ, Johnson G, Witherspoon R, Torok-Storb B. Antibody-mediated marrow failure after allogeneic bone marrow transplantation. Blood 1989;74:1477–1480.
18. Cockerill KJ, Lyding J, Rander AR. Red cell aplasia due to host type isohemagglutinins with exuberant red cell progenitor production of donor type in an ABO mismatched allogeneic bone marrow transplant recipient. Eur J Haematol 1989;43:195–200.
19. Marmont AM, Frassoni F, van Lint MT, et al. Isohemagglutinin induced pure red cell aplasia following ABO incompatible marrow transplant for severe aplastic anemia. Resolution after plasma exchange. Exp Hematol 1983;11 (suppl 11):51.
20. Heyll A, Aul C, Runde V, Arning M, Schneider W, Wernet P. Treatment of pure red cell aplasia after major ABO incompatible bone marrow transplantation with recombinant erythropoietin (letter). Blood 1991;77:907.
21. Hows J, Chipping PM, Palmer S, Gordon-Smith. Regeneration of peripheral blood cells following ABO incompatible allogeneic bone marrow transplantation for severe aplastic anemia. Br J Haematol 1983;53:145–151.
22. Branch DR, Sniecinski I, Spruce W, Krance R, Petz LD, St. Jean J. Delayed immune hemolytic anemia following ABO minor mismatched bone marrow transplantation. Blood 1984;64:216.
23. Hows J, Beddow K, Gordon-Smith E, et al. Donor derived RBC antibodies and immune hemolysis after allogeneic BMT. Blood 1986;67:177–181.
24. Haas RJ, Rieber P, Helmig M, Strobel E, Belohradsky BH, Heim MU. Acquired immune haemolysis by anti-A 1 antibody following bone marrow transplantation. Blut 1986;53:401–404.
25. Rowley S, Braine H. Probable hemolysis following minor ABO incompatible marrow transplantation (IMT) (abstract). Blood 1982;60(suppl 1):171a.

26. Robertson VM, Henslee PJ, Jennings CD, Hill MG, Thompson JT, Dickson LG. Early appearance of anti-A isohemagglutinin after allogeneic, ABO minor incompatible, T cell depleted bone marrow transplant. Transplant Proc 1987;19:4612–4617.
27. Hazelhurst GR, Brenner MK, Wimperis JZ, et al. Hemolysis after T-cell depleted bone marrow transplantation involving minor ABO incompatibility. Scand J Haematol 1986;37:1–3.
28. Hershko C, Gale RP, Ho W, Fitchen J. ABH antigens and bone marrow transplantation. Br J Haematol 1980;44:65–73.
29. Bensinger WI, Buckner CD, Thomas ED, Clift RA. ABO-incompatible marrow transplants. Transplantation 1982;33:427–429.
30. Curtis JE, Messner HA. Bone marrow transplantation for leukemia and aplastic anemia: management of ABO incompatibility. CMA 1982;126:649–655.
31. Berkman EM, Caplan S, Kim CS. ABO-incompatible bone marrow transplantation: preparation by plasma exchange and in vivo antibody absorption. Transfusion 1978;18:504–508.
32. Bensinger WI, Baker DA, Buckner CD, Clift RA, Thomas ED. Immunoadsorption for removal of A and B blood-group antibodies. N Engl J Med 1981;304:160–162.
33. Osterwalder B, Gratwohl A, Nissen C, Speck B. Immunoadsorption for removal of anti-A and anti-B blood group antibodies in ABO-incompatible bone marrow transplantation. Blut 1986;53:379–390.
34. Tichelli A, Gratwohl A, Wenger R, et al. ABO incompatible bone marrow transplantation: in vivo adsorption, an old forgotten method. Transplant Proc 1987; 19:4632–4637.
35. Bensinger WI, Buckner CD, Clift RA, Williams BM, Banaji M, Thomas ED. Comparison of techniques for dealing with major ABO-incompatible marrow transplants. Transplant Proc 1987;19:4600–4608.
36. Warkentin PI, Hilden JM, Kersey JH, Ramsay NKC, McCullough J. Transplantation of major ABO-incompatible bone marrow depleted of red cells by hydroxyethyl starch. Vox Sang 1985;48:89–104.
37. Ma DDF, Biggs JC. Comparison of two methods for concentrating stem cells for cryopreservation and transplantation. Transfusion 1982;22:217–219.
38. Wells JR, Sullivan A, Cline MJ. A technique for the separation and cryopreservation of myeloid stem cells from human bone marrow. Cryobiology 1979;16:201–210.
39. Gilmore MJ, Prentice HG, Corringham RE, et al. A technique for the concentration of nucleated marrow cells for in vitro manipulation and cryopreservation using the IBM-2991. Vox Sang 1983;45:294–302.
40. Anderson NA, Cornish JM, Godwin V, Gunstone MJ, Oakhill A, Pamphilon DH. Bone marrow processing on the Haemonetics V50 cell separator. Transfusion Sci 1990;11:201–204.
41. English D, Lamberson R, Graves V, et al. Semi-automated processing of bone marrow grafts for transplantation. Transfusion 1989;29:12–16.
42. Gilmore MJ, Prentice HG, Blacklock MA, et al. A technique for rapid isolation of bone marrow mononuclear cells using Ficoll-Metrizoate and the IBM 2991 blood cell processor. Br J Haematol 1982;50:619–621.
43. Humblet Y, Lefebvre P, Jacques JL, et al. Concentration of bone marrow progenitor cells by separation on a Percoll gradient using the Haemonetics model 30. Bone Marrow Transplant 1988;3:63–67.
44. Smith JW, Halpern LN, Johnson KA, et al. Mononuclear cell purification by continuous density gradient separation in the Haemonetics V-50. Bone Marrow Transplant 1987;2:74.
45. Areman EM, Cullis H, Spitzer T, Sacher RA. Automated processing of human bone marrow can result in a population of mononuclear cells capable of achieving engraftment following transplantation. Transfusion 1991;31:724–730.
46. Dragani A, Angelini A, Iacone A, D'Antonio D, Torlontano G. Comparison of five methods for concentrating progenitor cells in human marrow transplantation. Blut 1990;60:278–281.
47. Lyding J, Zander A, Rachell M, et al. Bone marrow concentration using COBE Spectra. J Clin Apheresis 1990;5:156.
48. Sniecinski I, Park HS, Nowicki B, Moreland M. Bone marrow processing for transplantation: comparison of two automated techniques. Transfusion 1992;32(suppl): 605.
49. Sniecinski I, Salvage G. Oien L. Optimal management of ABO incompatible marrow transplants by hemapheresis (abstract). J Clin Apheresis 1990;5:176–177.
50. Bensinger WI, Deeg JH. Transfusion support and donor considerations in marrow transplantation. In: Sacher RA, Au Buchon JP, eds. Marrow transplantation: practical and technical aspects of stem cell reconstitution. American Association of Blood Banks, 1992.
51. Blacklock HA, Katz F, Michalevicz R, et al. A and B blood group antigen expression on mixed colony cells and erythroid precursors: relevance for human allogeneic bone marrow transplantation. Br J Hematol 1984;58:267–276.
52. Sieff C, Bicknell D, Caine G, Robinson J, Lam G, Greaves MF. Changes in cell surface antigen expression during hemopoietic differentiation. Blood 1982;60:703–713.
53. Gajewski J, Petz LD, Calhoun L, et al. Hemolysis of transfused group O red blood cells in minor ABO-incompatible unrelated-donor bone marrow transplants in patients receiving cyclosporine without post-transplant methotrexate. Blood 1992;79:3076–3085.
54. Sniecinski I, Salvage G, Oien L. Management of minor ABO incompatible marrow transplants. Proceedings of the Joint Congress of the International Society of Blood Transfusion and American Association of Blood Banks, 1990:54.

Chapter 36

Immunological Reconstitution Following Bone Marrow Transplantation

Robertson Parkman

Reconstitution of the immune system following bone marrow transplantation (BMT) is characterized by (1) a lack of sustained transfer of clinically significant donor derived T- and B-lymphocyte immunity, (2) a recapitulation of normal lymphoid ontogeny, and (3) the effects of acute and chronic graft-versus-host disease (GVHD) and their therapies. Other factors that can influence immunological reconstitution include the donor-recipient relationship (autologous, syngeneic, allogeneic [histocompatible or matched unrelated donor]), intervening infections, and recipient age, among others.

Transfer of Donor Immunity

When adequate pretransplant chemoradiotherapy is given, all normal recipient hematopoiesis, T-lymphocyte immunity, and the majority of B-lymphocyte immunity are eliminated. When unmanipulated marrow is transplanted, either autologous or allogeneic, the possibility exists that the donor-derived antigen-specific T and B lymphocytes contained within the marrow may contribute to the recipient's immunocompetence following transplantation.

T-lymphocyte Immunity

Antigen-specific T-lymphocyte immunity is necessary for clinical control of DNA and RNA viral, protozoan, and fungal infections. Through their control of specific antibody production by B lymphocytes, T lymphocytes are also necessary for control of infections with encapsulated respiratory bacteria. Assessments of the transfer of donor T-lymphocyte immunity have failed to demonstrate clinically significant transfer (1–7). Following BMT, recipients are at high risk for infections with DNA viruses to which the recipients had pretransplant immunity. In vitro evaluation for the presence of antigen-specific T-lymphocyte proliferation early after BMT fails to detect antigen-specific T-lymphocyte immunity to DNA viral antigens, which is usually not detected until viral reactivation (either clinical or subclinical) occurs, resulting in the production of new antigen-specific T lymphocytes.

The lack of transfer of significant antigen-specific T-lymphocyte immunity may be caused by several factors. First, long-lived antigen-specific T lymphocytes may reside in the fixed lymphoid tissues of the donor rather than in the peripheral circulation. Second, the drugs, especially methotrexate (MTX), used as prophylaxis for GVHD may result in the selective destruction of antigen-specific T lymphocytes that are stimulated in vivo by the presence in the recipient of viral antigens. Thus, GVHD prophylaxis may result in the depletion of donor-derived antigen-specific T lymphocytes.

B-lymphocyte Immunity

Whereas it is clear that clinically significant donor-derived T-lymphocyte immunity is not transferred following BMT, donor-derived antibody production can be detected early following BMT (8–14). Investigators have studied the production of antibodies to a variety of antigens (e.g., tetanus toxoid, diphtheria toxoid, polio virus, hepatitis virus) following BMT. Increased antibody production has been shown when either the donor or the recipient were immunized prior to BMT. The maximal antibody response was obtained when both the donor and the recipient were immunized (12). If the patients were not immunized, antibody production was not maintained, and in most patients clinically significant antibody levels were no longer detectable one year following BMT. Evaluation of the transfer of B-lymphocyte immunity is confounded by the fact that studies to detect antibody production following BMT have not used immunoglobulin (Ig) isotyping to determine the source of the antibodies (i.e., donor or recipient B lymphocytes) (14). Because nondividing antibody-producing B lymphocytes and plasma cells are resistant to the cytoablative effects of many of the chemoradiotherapeutic agents used as preparation for BMT, increased antibody production by host cells might be expected when patients are immunized immediately following transplantation. Both the transferred donor and the residual recipient nondividing antibody-producing B lymphocytes can persist for their normal life span, at the end of which defects in antibody production would be detected. Increased post-transplant antibody production following donor and recipient immunization can be due to the transfer of (1) immune donor B lymphocytes, (2) antigen-primed donor antigen-presenting cells, or (3) immune donor T lymphocytes that cooperate with either donor or recipient antigen-specific B lymphocytes.

Routine administration of intravenous immunoglobulin (IVIg) to BMT recipients negates the need for antibody production early following BMT (15). BMT recipients are incapable of normal antibody production to the capsular polysaccharide antigens of encapsulated respiratory bacteria for a prolonged period following BMT (16–19). When Ig replacement therapy ceases, recurrent pyogenic infections can develop if patients do not receive prophylactic antibiotics. Definable defects in antibody production can be detected in all BMT recipients.

Normal Lymphoid Ontogeny

Lymphoid ontogeny can be characterized in terms of both cellular and molecular differentiation. The progeny of the pluripotent hematopoietic stem cells that are destined for T-lymphocyte differentiation express CD7 as their first distinctive surface antigen (20). $CD34^+$, $CD7^+$ cells are present in both the fetal yolk sac and the fetal liver. In fetal life, $CD34^+$, $CD7^+$ cells are present in the fetal thymus after 7 to 8 weeks of gestation. Cytoplasmic $CD3^+$ cells can be detected at 8 to 9 weeks of fetal life, followed by the surface expression of CD2 (Figure 36-1). With the expression of CD2, the surface expression of rearranged T-cell receptor (TCR) genes can be detected, with both TCR-$\alpha\beta$ and TCR-$\gamma\delta$ present (21–26). At the early stages of thymic diffferentiation, the TCR-$\alpha\beta^+$ cells express low levels of surface TCR and CD3 but no CD4 or CD8 (double-negative stage of thymic differentiation). The double-negative thymocytes then quickly traverse a stage of $CD8^{low}$ expression to become $CD3^{low}$, $CD4^+$, $CD8^+$ (double positive) thymocytes.

Positive and negative selection occurs at the double-positive thymocyte stage (27–29). Positive selection is

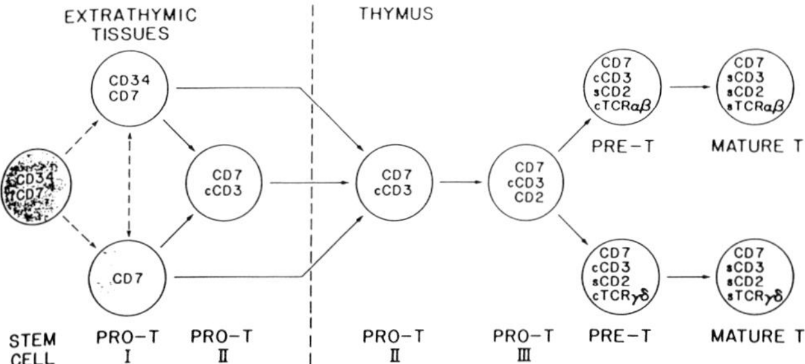

Figure 36-1. T-lymphocyte differentiation (Reproduced by permission from Haynes BF, Denning SM, Singer KH, Kurtzberg J. Ontogeny of T-cell precursors: a model for the initial stages of human T-cell development. Immunol Today 1989;10:87–91.)

a result of interactions between the TCR-$\alpha\beta$ receptor and the thymic epithelium, resulting in proliferation and clonal expansion of T lymphocytes, whose specificity is for exogenous (nonself) antigens. Following their positive selection, the double-positive thymocytes differentiate into $CD3^+$, $CD4^+$, TCR-$\alpha\beta$ or $CD3^+$, $CD8^+$, TCR-$\alpha\beta$ single-positive thymocytes that are exported to the peripheral circulation as single-positive mature peripheral blood T lymphocytes. Negative selection also occurs at the double-positive thymocyte stage. The interaction of double-positive TCR-$\alpha\beta$ thymocytes with self antigens expressed on marrow-derived dendritic cells present in the thymus results in an apoptotic signal, death of the cell, and clonal deletion of cells with specificity for self antigens.

In early fetal life, the frequency of TCR-$\gamma\delta$ thymocytes is equal to that of TCR-$\alpha\beta$ cells; nevertheless, our understanding of the differentiation of TCR-$\gamma\delta$ thymocytes is less complete than of TCR-$\alpha\beta$ cells (21). Development of TCR-$\gamma\delta$ cells is characterized by rearrangements of the δ variable and joining regions. Different joining regions are used in fetal as opposed to adult differentiation. TCR-$\gamma\delta$ thymocytes do not express significant surface CD4 and CD8. Following their export from the thymus, TCR-$\gamma\delta$ T lymphocytes selectively migrate to epithelial organs, including skin, uterus, and gut. The mechanisms involved in positive and negative selection of TCR-$\gamma\delta$ thymocytes are imperfectly understood.

In addition to the surface and molecular changes that occur during T-lymphocyte differentiation, a series of functional changes occur that can be measured by proliferation following stimulation with nonspecific stimuli such as mitogen (e.g., phytohemagglutinin [PHA]) or calcium ionophore and phorbol ester (30). The first proliferative responses that can be demonstrated in thymocytes following PHA stimulation requires the presence of exogenous growth factors, either interleukin-7 (IL-7) or IL-2 (22). The requirement for exogenous growth factors demonstrates that cells capable of expressing cytokine receptors following stimulation are present earlier in ontogeny than thymocytes capable of cytokine production. In normal lymphoid ontogeny, PHA-responsive, IL-2–dependent cells are followed by the appearance of PHA-responsive, IL-2–producing cells. Later in ontogeny, thymocytes capable of responding to allogeneic lymphocytes can be identified. Following their export to the peripheral circulation, T lymphocytes can be sensitized following exposure to specific antigen. Antigen-specific in vitro proliferation is first detected only in the presence of exogenous IL-2, followed by normal proliferation without exogenous IL-2, demonstrating that antigen-specific, IL-2–dependent T lymphocytes develop before antigen-specific IL-2–producing T lymphocytes (Figure 36-2).

Phenotypic Analysis of BMT Recipients

The T lymphocytes present following BMT can be derived from either the mature T lymphocytes in the

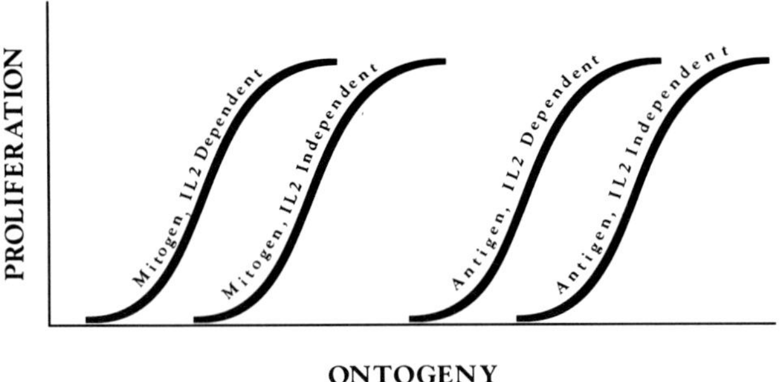

Figure 36-2. Ontogeny of T-lymphocyte proliferation.

marrow inoculum or the transplanted pluripotent hematopoietic stem cells. The most accurate assessment of lymphoid ontogeny following BMT will be observed in the recipients of T-cell–depleted (TCD) marrow in whom there is no significant contribution by the mature donor-derived T lymphocytes.

Recipients of unmanipulated autologous marrow achieve an absolute lymphocyte count of 500/μL more rapidly than do recipients of untreated histocompatible bone marrow (15 vs 27–30 days) (31,32). The delay in normalization of the absolute lymphocyte count in allogeneic recipients may be due in part to the routine administration of post-transplant MTX as prophylaxis against acute GVHD. Recipients of TCD allogeneic marrow have a mean day of absolute lymphocyte count recovery of 25, compared with 31 for recipients of unmanipulated histocompatible marrow, possibly due to the lack of post-transplant MTX therapy (33). Recipients of autologous marrow purged with 4-hydroperoxycyclophosphamide (4-HC) display variable and prolonged lymphopenia. Normalization of the absolute number of $CD3^+$ T lymphocytes is delayed in a pattern that parallels the delay in the absolute lymphocyte count. Autologous recipients recover their $CD3^+$ T-lymphocyte count 6 to 8 weeks after BMT, whereas allogeneic recipients normalize their $CD3^+$ T-lymphocyte counts 12 weeks after BMT. Acute GVHD has no effect on the recovery of $CD3^+$ T lymphocytes.

Normalization of the percentage and absolute number of $CD8^+$ T lymphocytes is more rapid than that of $CD4^+$ T lymphocytes (31,33–36). $CD8^+$ T lymphocytes reach normal values 4 months after BMT, whereas significant decreases in $CD4^+$ T lymphocytes exist for the first 6 months after BMT. More rapid normalization of $CD8^+$ T-lymphocyte levels in conjunction with reduced $CD4^+$ levels results in an inversion of the normal CD4/CD8 ratio, which does not normalize until 6 to 9 months after BMT. Natural killer cells ($CD16^+$, $CD8^{dim}$) reappear early after BMT and during the first month represent the major lymphoid population (37). The presence of natural killer cells in addition to the $CD8^+$, $CD3^+$ T lymphocytes further increases the total number of $CD8^+$ lymphocytes and contributes to the inversion of the CD4/CD8 ratio.

In addition to the presence of mature $CD3^+$ single-positive T lymphocytes, phenotypic T lymphocytes, which are normally found in the peripheral circulation only during fetal life or in the adult thymus during postnatal life, can be detected (38). $CD3^{dim}$ double-negative and $CD3^+$ double-positive T lymphocytes can be detected. In addition, T lymphocytes expressing CD1, normally found only on thymocytes, are present in the peripheral circulation (39). Some patients have the sustained presence of increased numbers of TCR-γδ T lymphocytes. These findings are consistent with the recapitulation of lymphoid ontogeny that occurs following BMT.

The number of B lymphocytes, as determined by either the presence of surface immunoglobulin or CD20 expression, returns to normal levels 1 to 2 months after BMT and is unaffected by TCD (37,40). B lymphocytes expressing CD5 occur at increased frequency following transplantation, suggesting that post-transplant B lymphocytes are predisposed to anti-antibody production or are activated. Defects in mucosal IgA production exist for up to 1 year after BMT. Without replacement of IVIg, transplant recipients have reduced levels of IgG, IgA, and IgM during the first 6 months after BMT (40). Patients without chronic GVHD normalize their IgG levels in 8 to 9 months, their IgM levels in 9 to 12 months, and their IgA levels in 2 to 3 years. Patients with chronic GVHD may have elevated levels of IgM and IgG starting 6 to 9 months after BMT (Figure 36-3).

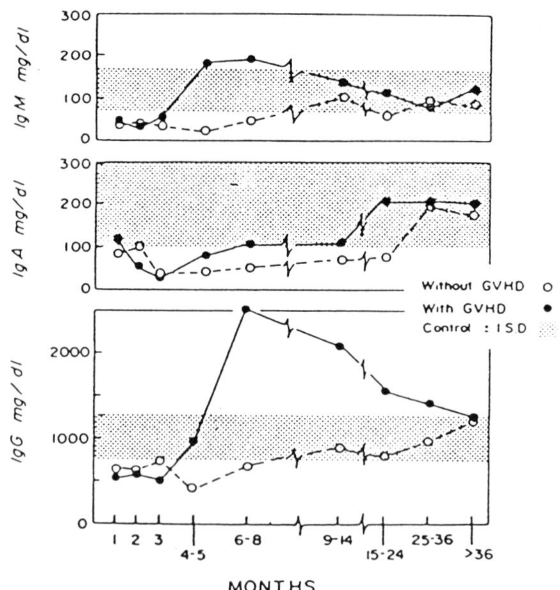

Figure 36-3. Median values of serum immunoglobulin G (IgG), IgA, and IgM in patients after bone marrow transplantation. *Shaded area* represents values of marrow donors. (Reproduced by permission from Noel DR, Witherspoon RP, Storb R, et al. Does graft-versus-host disease influence the tempo of immunologic recovery after allogeneic human marrow transplantation? An observation on long-term survivors. Blood 1978;51:1087–1105.)

Functional Analysis of T-lymphocyte Reconstitution

The recovery of T-lymphocyte function following BMT can be assayed in terms of the response to either nonspecific stimuli (e.g., PHA, anti-CD3 antibody) or specific antigenic stimulation (e.g., tetanus toxoid, herpes virus antigens). Recipients of non-TCD marrow show decreased proliferation to stimulation with PHA or anti-CD3 antibody for the first 1 to 2 months after BMT (33). By the third month, addition of exogenous IL-2 can normalize the proliferation response to PHA stimulation when the proliferation is corrected for the percentage of $CD3^+$ T lymphocytes (41,42). By 4 to 6 months, proliferation responses to mitogenic stimulation normalize without the addition of exogenous IL-2, suggesting that normal IL-2 production is present. The addition of exogenous IL-1 rarely improves the proliferation response to mitogenic stimulation, demonstrating that normal IL-1 production by monocytes and other antigen-presenting cells is present following BMT.

Direct measurement of IL-2 following BMT demonstrates decreased IL-2 production. Regardless of the type of BMT and whether acute GVHD is present or absent, recipients of histocompatible marrow have decreased IL-2 production early after BMT, as do long-term survivors with chronic GVHD (43,44). Long-term survivors (>12 mo) without chronic GVHD have IL-2 production that is similar to that of their donors. When $CD4^+$ T lymphocytes were isolated early after BMT, their IL-2 production was relatively normal on a per cell basis, suggesting that the defects in IL-2 production are due in part to the quantitative decrease in the number of $CD4^+$ T lymphocytes, in addition to the recapitulation of lymphoid ontogeny.

Recipients of TCD allogenic marrow have prolonged defects in their proliferation response to PHA as compared with recipients of non-TCD marrow. Patients who receive haploidentical T-cell–depleted marrow for severe combined immunodeficiency have no phenotypic T lymphocytes for 1 to 2 months after BMT, at which time $CD3^{dim}$ T lymphocytes first appear. Three months after BMT, a proliferation response to PHA stimulation in the presence of exogenous IL-2 is first detected (45). The proliferative response to PHA in the absence of exogenous IL-2 normalizes 4 to 6 months after BMT if no immunosuppression (e.g., cyclosporine [CSP]/steroids) is administered. The time course of responsiveness to mitogenic stimulation and the need for exogenous IL-2 parallels the time course of normal lymphoid ontogeny (see Figure 36-2). Analogous results can be seen in adult recipients of TCD marrow, in whom the proliferative response to PHA without exogenous IL-2 was not normalized until 6 months after BMT (33).

T-lymphocyte immunity is characterized by the capacity for development of antigen-specific responses. Patients' immunological response to specific antigens can be determined after either herpes virus reactivation/infection or specific immunization (e.g., phage $\phi\chi174$, tetanus toxoid). Protection against infection with opportunistic organisms does not correlate with normal mitogen-induced proliferation but with reconstitution of antigen-specific T-lymphocyte function, which includes cytotoxic T lymphocytes (CTLs), cytokine production (IL-2, IL-4, γ-interferon), and cooperation with B lymphocytes in specific antibody production.

Herpes viruses that are latent in BMT recipients are a source of infection following BMT. Acquisition of antigen-specific T-lymphocyte reactivity to herpes virus antigens following BMT is common and can be used to assess the reconstitution of post-BMT antigen-specific T-lymphocyte function. T-lymphocyte proliferation responses to herpes simplex (HSV), varicella zoster (VZV), and cytomegalovirus (CMV) are rarely detected during the first month after allogeneic BMT regardless of the donor immune status. By 40 days post-BMT, a T-lymphocyte proliferation response to HSV can be detected, followed by acquisition of responses to VZV and CMV (6,7). The sequential acquisition of immunological responsiveness parallels the time course of viral reactivation (HSV <VZV <CMV). Routine administration of acyclovir delays the appearance of antigen-specific proliferation to HSV and VZV by inhibiting viral reactivation (6). Acquisition of antigen-specific T-lymphocyte proliferation, however, does not mean that normal T-lymphocyte function is present. Assessment of cytokine production has demonstrated decreased γ-interferon production following herpes virus antigen stimulation in the presence of normal proliferation. When CTL function was assessed against VZV- and CMV-infected autologous fibroblasts, an absence of a CTL response was noted in some patients when normal proliferation was present, suggesting that reconstitution of CTL activity lags behind acquisition of antigen-specific proliferation (46).

Assessment of the antigen-specific T-lymphocyte proliferation to herpes virus antigens of recipients of unpurged autologous marrow demonstrates that some patients acquire antigen-specific proliferation by 1 month following BMT (7). More rapid acquisition of T-lymphocyte responsiveness in recipients of autologous as compared with allogeneic marrow may be due to the lack of administration of immunosuppressive drugs (e.g., MTX, CSP, steroids), which interfere with normal lymphoid ontogeny or eliminate antigen-specific T lymphocytes transferred at the time of BMT.

Immunization of BMT recipients during the first 3 months after BMT with tetanus or diphtheria toxoids does not result in the development of antigen-specific T-lymphocyte function, as measured by in vitro antigen-induced proliferation. Antigen-specific T-lymphocyte function routinely develops in patients without chronic GVHD who are immunized more than 100 days after BMT; however, immunization of patients with chronic GVHD does not result in detectable antigen-specific T-lymphocyte function in the majority of patients. It is not clear whether the lack of antigen-specific T-lymphocyte function is due to the immunosuppression that patients with chronic GVHD received or an absence of antigen-specific T-lymphocyte precursors.

Functional Analysis of B-lymphocyte Reconstitution

Specific antibody production requires the interaction of antigen-specific T and B lymphocytes. Therefore, defective antibody production can be due to defects in either T or B lymphocytes. B-lymphocyte function can be determined following either nonspecific stimulation, which does not require antigen-specific T lymphocytes; or antigen-specific stimulation, which does require immunocompetent T lymphocytes. The proliferative response of B lymphocytes to mitogenic stimulation, *Staphylococcus aureus* Cowan strain A, or crosslinked anti-IgM antibodies (anti-Mμ) returns to normal 2 months after BMT regardless of the type of transplant and parallels the recovery of phenotypic B lymphocytes (33). Thus, the functional capacity of B lymphocytes to respond to mitogenic stimulation normalizes early following BMT.

Because specific antibody production requires T- and B-lymphocyte interaction, in vitro Ig production following polyclonal T-lymphocyte stimulation is a more accurate assessment of B-lymphocyte immunocompetence than mitogenic stimulation. In vitro stimulation of T and B lymphocytes with pokeweed mitogen and nonmitogenic doses of *Staphylococcus aureus* Cowan strain A has revealed markedly reduced IgM and IgG production for the first 3 months after BMT (47–49). Histocompatible recipients of both TCD and unmodified marrow have normal IgM production after 4 to 6 months. Recipients of unmodified marrow have normal IgG production by 7 to 9 months, whereas recipients of TCD marrow do not normalize their IgG production until one year after BMT. Normal production of IgM without IgG production 4 to 6 months after BMT represents defective Ig switching (IgM to IgG), which is secondary to defects in T-lymphocyte function (34).

Specific antibody production in vivo can best be assessed by evaluation of antibody-positive recipients, who receive marrow from antibody-negative donors; and of antibody-negative recipients, who are transplanted from antibody-positive donors. In the absence of immunization or viral reactivation, sustained (<1 yr) antibody production is not observed (13). Recipients who have antibody to tetanus or diphtheria toxoids and hepatitis virus prior to BMT have detectable antibody early after BMT, but sustained antibody production is not present one year after BMT (50). Antibody-negative recipients, who receive marrow from antibody-positive donors, have detectable antibody after BMT, but antibody production is not sustained. Thus, without antigenic stimulation, sustained antibody production does not occur following BMT. When antibody-positive patients are immunized immediately (0–14 days) following BMT, a transient increase in antibody titer can be observed (12). Immunization later in the post-BMT period does not result in specific antibody production unless antigen-specific T lymphocytes are generated. Once the pre-existing antigen-specific donor or recipient B lymphocytes die, specific antibody production is no longer possible. Specific antibody production is possible only when new antigen-specific T and B lymphocytes develop.

Immunization with new antigens, such as keyhole limpet hemocyanin (KLH) or phage $\phi\chi174$, to which neither the donor nor the recipient has been immunized, provides the most accurate assessment of the recipient's capacity to produce specific antibody (16,34). Primary immunization during the first 2 to 3 months following BMT of either allogeneic or syngeneic recipients results in absent or minimal IgM antibody production. Primary immunization more than 3 months after BMT produces a heterogeneous response; patients without chronic GVHD have a normal primary IgM response, whereas patients with chronic GVHD have a markedly reduced primary response. Repeat immunization to determine the recipient's secondary antibody response and the capacity of the recipient to switch from IgM to IgG antibody production varies with the chronic GVHD status of the recipient. Patients without chronic GVHD have a normal secondary response and normal Ig switching, whereas patients with chronic GVHD have a reduced secondary antibody response that remains primarily IgM (Figure 36-4). Thus, patients with chronic GVHD have a reduced capacity to make specific antibodies to new antigens and an inability to switch from IgM to IgG antibody production.

Immunization with pneumococcal polysaccharide vaccine results in a lack of antibody production during the first 3 months after allogeneic BMT. Reconstitution

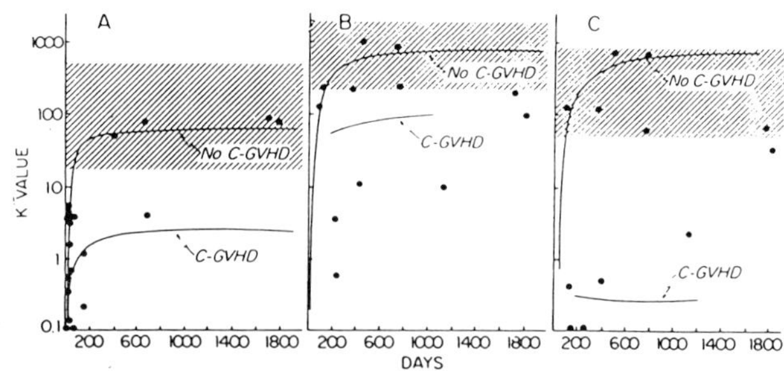

Figure 36-4. Maximum antibody activity following primary (A) and secondary (B) $\phi\chi174$ phage injection in normal subjects and allogeneic and syngeneic bone marrow transplant recipients. (C) IgG antibody activity of the secondary response. *Hatched area* represents the 5th to 95th percentile response for normal subjects. The *curves* represent the estimated means for data from allogeneic recipients with or without chronic graft-versus-host disease (GVHD). The *dots* represent individual data points from syngeneic transplant recipients. (Reproduced by permission from Witherspoon RP, Kopecky K, Storb RF, et al. Immunological recovery in 48 patients following syngeneic marrow transplantation for hematological malignancy. Transplantation 1982;33:143–149.)

of the capacity to produce antibody to polysaccharide antigens is delayed in allogeneic recipients without chronic GVHD, as compared with their capacity to respond to protein antigens (34). Transplant recipients are similar to normal newborns, who can respond to protein antigens but not to polysaccharide antigens (51,52). Thus, reconstitution of B-lymphocyte function following BMT, like that of T lymphocytes, recapitulates normal lymphoid ontogeny.

Antibodies to the capsular polysaccharide of *Hemophilus influenze*, polyribosylphosphate (PRP), develop in normal individuals because of antigenic cross-reactivity between PRP and the capsular polysaccharide of the K stains of *Escherichia coli* that naturally occurs in the gastrointestinal tract (53). Measurement of anti-PRP antibodies therefore assesses the capacity of BMT recipients to produce antibody to a naturally occurring bacterial polysaccharide. In the absence of the capacity to make antipolysaccharide antibodies, patients should receive prophylactic antibiotics or IVIg.

Effect of GVHD on Immunological Reconstitution

Acute GVHD following histocompatible BMT has little effect on the tempo of lymphoid reconstitution as measured by absolute lymphocyte count or the absolute number of $CD3^+$ T lymphocytes. Transient depression of the absolute lymphocyte count and $CD3^+$ T-lymphocyte counts occurs following administration of anti-T-lymphocyte immunosuppression, especially antithymocyte globulin (ATG) and anti-T-lymphocyte monoclonal antibodies. In the absence of specific immunosuppression, the tempo of T- and B-lymphocyte recovery is unaffected by acute GVHD. The presence of acute GVHD or its treatment with ATG is associated with a decreased primary antibody response to KLH, even if chronic GVHD does not develop (16). Thus, acute GVHD in humans, as in mice, may result in a sustained immunodeficiency in the absence of chronic GVHD, presumably due to thymic damage (54,55).

Transient elevation of IgE levels and production of specific IgE antibodies have been demonstrated early following BMT (14–28 days) and correlate with the presence of acute GVHD (56,57). IgE production is normally stimulated by IL-4 and suppressed by γ-interferon, suggesting that imbalances in these cytokines occur early following BMT (58).

The most apparent abnormalities due to GVHD are seen in chronic GVHD. Patients with chronic GVHD have a decreased capacity to develop an antigen-specific T-lymphocyte response and to produce specific antibodies, particularly to polysaccharide antigens, while having an increased incidence of autoantibodies (e.g., anti-DNA, erythrocyte, thyroid) (59). Immunization of patients with chronic GVHD with recall antigens, such as tetanus and diphtheria toxoids, or new antigens, such as KLH, has revealed sustained defects in antibody production, including decreased primary primary antibody production, decreased Ig switching, and decreased secondary antibody production (see Figure 36-4) (40,60). In particular, patients with chronic GVHD have a prolonged inability to produce antibodies to polysaccharide antigens, which are the primary antigenic determinants of the encapsulated respiratory bacteria. Analysis of the infectious complications of chronic GVHD before routine administration of prophylactic antibiotics and IVIg showed an increased incidence of infections with encapsulated respiratory bacteria, including sepsis, pneumonitis, and sinusitis (61). Routine administration of prophylactic antibiotics and IVIg has markedly reduced infection complications; however, the inability of patients with chronic GVHD to produce protective antibodies to bacterial polysaccharide antigens remains. Vaccines composed of polysaccharide antigens coupled to an immunogenic carrier protein can immunize normal infants at 2 to 6 months of age, a time when they are unable to respond to nonconjugated polysaccharide vaccines, suggesting that conjugated polysaccharide vaccines may have a future role in the immunization of patients with chronic GVHD (62).

In vitro analysis of the cellular basis of the immunodeficiency present in patients with chronic GVHD has demonstrated a variety of cellular defects. Decreases in the number and function of $CD4^+$ helper T lymphocytes have been described, in addition to the presence of activated (DR expressing) $CD4^+$ and $CD8^+$ suppressor T lymphocytes (63–66). Limiting dilution analysis has identified a decrease in the frequency of helper T-lymphocyte precursors early after BMT in all patients and a sustained decrease in the frequency of CTL and helper T-lymphocyte precursors in patients with chronic GVHD (67). Intrinsic B-lymphocyte defects that result in a lack of normal responsiveness to T-lymphocyte stimulation have been identified (68). Thus, no single primary defect can explain the immunodeficiency associated with chronic GVHD.

Murine experiments have demonstrated defects in thymic epithelium function following acute GVHD (54,55). Administration of CSP can inhibit the differentiation of double-positive thymocytes into $CD3^+$ single-positive thymocytes (69). The combined effects of thymic damage and CSP may result in defects in both positive and negative thymic selection. Defective positive thymic selection would result in a reduction in the frequency of mature T lymphocytes with specificity for exogenous antigens, whereas reduced negative selection would result in an increased frequency of autoreactive T lymphocytes.

Transfer of Immunologically Mediated Diseases Following BMT

The chemoradiotherapy that BMT recipients receive ablates all their T-lymphocyte immunity and the majority of their B-lymphocyte immunity. Transplantation of a donor immune system with a genetically determined predilection to produce autoimmune or IgE antibodies will result in recipients with autoimmune or allergic diseases. When nonallergic recipients were transplanted with marrow from skin test–positive donors who had clinical allergies, skin test reactivity was detected in 8 of 11 long-term survivors; clinical allergic rhinitis developed in 7 and clinical asthma developed in 2 without a prior history of asthma (70). Thus, the clinical transfer of IgE-mediated hypersensitivity can occur following BMT.

Thrombocytopenia developed in one recipient transplanted with marrow from a donor who produced an antiplatelet antibody; the thrombocytopenia ultimately resolved but with persistent autoantibody production (71). The transfer of anti-acetylcholine receptor antibody production from a donor with myasthenia gravis has resulted in clinical myasthenia gravis in the recipient (72).

Immunization

Immunization with protein antigens in the immediate post-BMT period can result in short-lived increases in antibody titer. However, sustained antibody production following immunization with protein antigens can occur only when adequate T-lymphocyte immunocompetence recovers. The onset of antigen-specific T-lymphocyte function in patients without chronic GVHD occurs 3 to 6 months following BMT. Antigen-specific T-lymphocyte proliferation and in vivo production of specific antibody routinely develop in patients reimmunized with tetanus and diphtheria toxoids during this period (Table 36-1). Immunization with unconjugated polysaccharide vaccines during the same period rarely results in the production of protective antibody. No studies have been published on the potential use of conjugated polysaccharide vaccines in post-transplant recipients. Protective T- or B-lymphocyte immunity rarely develop in patients with chronic GVHD, even after repeated immunizations. Routine administration of IVIg to patients with chronic GVHD abrogates the need for routine immunization with protein or polysaccharide antigens.

Because of delays in the production of antibodies to viral vaccines, the use of inactivated polio virus vaccine is preferable to the use of live oral polio vaccine for initial vaccination of BMT recipients. Transplant recipients without chronic GVHD can be immunized with the inactivated polio vaccine 6 to 12 months after BMT. Because of the risks associated with administration of live attenuated viral vaccines, immunization with the measles-mumps-rubella vaccine is not advocated in patients without chronic GVHD until 1 to 2 years following BMT unless the social environment demands early immunization (73–75). Patients with chronic GVHD who are receiving IVIg are not at risk of infection, and vaccination with a live viral vaccine in the presence of IVIg replacement therapy is ineffective. The efficacy of immunization can be confirmed by the measurement of specific antibody levels.

Table 36-1.
Immunization Following Bone Marrow Transplantation

Vaccine	*Patients Without Chronic GVHD*	*Patients with Chronic GVHD*
Diphtheria-tetanus toxoid	3–6 mo	3–6 mo
Oral polio virus (Sabin)	Not recommended	Not recommended
Inactivated polio virus (Salk)	6–12 mo	Not indicated if on IVIg
Measles-mumps-rubella	1–2 yr	Not recommended

GVHD = graft-versus-host disease; IVIg = intravenous immunoglobulin.

References

1. Meyers JD, Flournoy N, Thomas ED. Cytomegalovirus infection and specific cell-mediated immunity after marrow transplant. J Infect Dis 1980;142:816–824.
2. Meyers JD, Flournoy N, Thomas ED. Cell-mediated immunity to varicella-zoster virus after allogeneic marrow transplant. J Infect Dis 1980;141:479–487.
3. Meyers JD, Flournoy N, Thomas ED. Infection with herpes simplex virus and cell-mediated immunity after marrow transplant. J Infect Dis 1980;142:338–346.
4. Wade JC, Day LM, Crowley JJ, Meyers JD. Recurrent infection with herpes simplex virus after marrow transplantation: role of the specific immune response and acyclovir treatment. J Infect Dis 1980;149:750–756.
5. Quinnan GV, Kirmani N, Rook AH, et al. Cytotoxic T cells in cytomegalovirus infection: HLA-restricted T-lymphocyte and non-T-lymphocyte cytotoxic responses correlate with recovery from cytomegalovirus infection in bone marrow transplant recipients. N Engl J Med 1982;307:7–13.
6. Ljungman P, Wilczek H, Gahrton G, et al. Long-term acyclovir prophylaxis in bone marrow transplant recipients and lymphocyte proliferation responses to herpes virus antigens in vitro. Bone Marrow Transplant 1986;1:185–192.
7. Gratama JW, Verdonck LF, Van Der Linden JA, et al. Cellular immunity to vaccinations and herpes-virus infections after bone marrow transplantation. Transplantation 1986;41:719–724.
8. Lum LG, Seigneuret MC, Storb R. The transfer of antigen-specific humoral immunity from marrow donors to marrow recipients. J Clin Immunol 1986;6:389–396.
9. Shiobara S, Lum LG, Witherspoon RP, Storb R. Antigen-specific antibody responses of lymphocytes to tetanus toxoid after human marrow transplantation. Transplantation 1985;41:587–592.
10. Lum LG, Munn NA, Schanfield MS, Storb R. The detection of specific antibody formation to recall antigens after human bone marrow transplantation. Blood 1986;67:582–587.
11. Lum LG. A review: the kinetics of immune reconstitution after human marrow transplantation. Blood 1987;69:369–380.
12. Wimperis JZ, Brenner MK, Prentice HG, et al. Transfer of a functioning humoral immune system in transplantation of T-lymphocyte-depleted bone marrow. Lancet 1986;339–343.

13. Wahren B, Gahrton G, Linde A, et al. Transfer and persistence of viral antibody-producing cells in bone marrow transplantation. J Infect Dis 1984;150:358–365.
14. Witherspoon RP, Schanfield MS, Strob R, Thomas ED, Giblett ER. Immunoglobulin production of donor origin after marrow transplantation for acute leukemia or aplastic anemia. Transplantation 1978;26:407–408.
15. Sullivan KM, Kopecky KJ, Jocom J, et al. Immunomodulatory and antimicrobial efficacy of intravenous immunoglobulin in bone marrow transplantation. N Engl J Med 1990;323:705–712.
16. Witherspoon RP, Strob R, Ochs HD, et al. Recovery of antibody production in human allogeneic marrow graft recipients: influence of time posttransplantation, the presence or absence of chronic graft-versus-host disease, and antithymocyte globulin treatment. Blood 1981;58:360–368.
17. Winston DJ, Gale RP, Meyer DV, Young LS, the UCLA Bone Marrow Transplantation Group. Infectious complications of human bone marrow transplantation. Medicine 1979;58:1–31.
18. Winston DJ, Ho WG, Schiffman G, et al. Pneumococcal vaccination of recipients of bone marrow transplant. Arch Intern Med 1983;143:1735–1737.
19. Ambrosino DM. Impaired polysaccharide responses in immunodeficient patients: relevance to bone marrow transplant patients. Bone Marrow Transplant 1992; 7(suppl 3);48–51.
20. Haynes BF, Denning SM, Singer KH, Kurtzberg J. Ontogeny of T-cell precursors: a model for the initial stages of human T-cell development. Immunol Today 1989;10:87–91.
21. Ferrick DA, Ohashi PS, Wallace V, Schilham M, Mak TW. Thymic ontogeny and selection of $\alpha\beta$ and $\gamma\delta$ T cells. Immunol Today 1989;10:403–407.
22. Toribio ML, Alonso JM, Barcena A, et al. Human T-cell precursors: involvement of the IL-2 pathway in the generation of mature T cells. Immunol Rev 1988;104: 55–79.
23. Haynes BF, Martin ME, Kay HH, Kurtzberg J. Early events in human T cell ontogeny. J Exp Med 1988;168: 1061–1080.
24. Campana D, Janossy G, Coustan-Smith E, et al. The expression of T cell receptor-associated proteins during T cell ontogeny in man. J Immunol 1989;142:57–66.
25. Haynes BF, Singer KH, Dennings SM, Martin ME. Analysis of expression of CD2, CD3 and T cell antigen receptor molecules during early human fetal thymic development. J Immunol 1988;141:3776–3784.
26. Lobach DF, Haynes BE. Ontogeny of the human thymus during fetal development. J Clin Immunol 1987;7:81–97.
27. Marrack P, Lo D, Brinster R, et al. The effect of thymus environment on T cell development and tolerance. Cell 1988;53:627–634.
28. Russell, Lo DY. Positive and negative selection of an antigen receptor on T cells in transgenic mice. Nature (London) 1988;336:73–76.
29. Zuniga-Pflucker JC, Longo DL, Kruisbeek AM. Positive selection of CD4-8$^+$ T cells in the thymus of normal mice. Nature (London) 1989;338–376.
30. Parkman R, Merler E. Discontinuous density gradient analysis of the developing human thymus. Cell Immunol 1973;8:382–331.
31. Atkinson K. Reconstruction of the haemopoietic and immune systems after marrow transplantation. Bone Marrow Transplant 1990;5:209–226.
32. Linch DC, Knott LJ, Thomas RM, et al. T cell regeneration after allogeneic and autologous bone marrow transplantation. Br J Haematol 1983;53:451–458.
33. Keever CA, Small TN, Flomenberg N, et al. Immune reconstitution following bone marrow transplantation: comparison of recipients of T-cell depleted marrow with recipients of conventional marrow grafts. Blood 1989;73:1340–1350.
34. Friedrich W, O'Reilly RJ, Koziner B, Gebhard DR, Good RA, Evans RL. T lymphocyte reconstitution in recipients of bone marrow transplants with and without GVHD: imbalances of T cell subpopulations having unique regulatory and cognitive functions. Blood 1982; 59:696–701.
35. Forman SJ, Nocker P, Gallagher M, et al. Pattern of T cell reconstitution following allogeneic bone marrow transplantation for acute hematological malignancy. Transplantation 1982;34:96–98.
36. Atkinson K. T cell sub-populations defined by monoclonal antibodies after HLA-identical sibling marrow transplantation. II. Activated and functional subsets of the helper-inducer and the cytotoxic-suppressor subpopulations defined by two colour fluorescence flow cytometry. Bone Marrow Transplant 1986;1:121–132.
37. Ault KE, Antin JH, Ginsburg D, et al. Phenotype of recovering lymphoid cell populations after marrow transplantation. J Exp Med 1985;161:1483–1502.
38. Gratama JW, Fibbe WE, Visser JW, Kliunnelemans HC, Ginsel LA, Bolhuis RL. CD3$^+$, 4$^+$ and/or 8$^+$ T cells and CD3$^+$, 4$^-$, 8$^-$ T cells repopulate at different rates after allogeneic bone marrow transplantation. Bone Marrow Transplant 1989;4:291–296.
39. Rappeport JM, Dunn MJ, Parkman R. Immature T lymphocytes in the peripheral blood of bone marrow transplant recipients. Transplantation 1983;36:674–680.
40. Noel DR, Witherspoon RP, Storb R, et al. Does graft-versus-host disease influence the tempo of immunologic recovery after allogeneic human marrow transplantation? An observation on long-term survivors. Blood 1978;51:1087–1105.
41. Roosnek EE, Brouwer MC, Vossen JM, et al. The role of interleukin-2 in proliferative responses in vitro of T cells from patients after bone marrow transplantation. Transplantation 1987;43:855–860.
42. Welte K, Liobanu N, Moore MAS, Gulati S, O'Reilly RJ, Mertelsmann R. Defective interleukin-2 production in patients after bone marrow transplantation and in vitro restoration of defective T-lymphocyte proliferation by highly purified interleukin 2. Blood 1984;64:380–385.
43. Brkic S, Tsoi M-S, Mori T, et al. Cellular interactions in marrow-grafted patients. Transplantation 1985;39: 30–35.
44. Cooley MA, McLachlan K, Atkinson K. Cytokine activity after human bone marrow transplantation. Br J Haematol 1989;73:341–347.
45. O'Reilly RJ, Keever CA, Small TN, Brochstein J. The use of HLA-non-identical T-cell-depleted marrow transplants for correction of severe combined immunodeficiency disease. Immunodeficiency Rev 1989;1:273–309.
46. Reusser P, Riddell SR, Meyers JD, Greenberg PD. Cytotoxic T-lymphocyte response to cytomegalovirus after human allogeneic bone marrow transplantation: pattern of recovery and correlation with cytomegalovirus infection and disease. Blood 1991;78:1373–1380.
47. Witherspoon RP, Lum LG, Storb R, Thomas ED. In vitro regulation of immunoglobulin synthesis after human

marrow transplantation. II. Deficient T and non-T-lymphocyte function within 3–4 months of allogeneic, syngeneic or autologous marrow grafting for hematologic malignancy. Blood 1982;59:844–850.
48. Ringden O, Witherspoon R, Storb R, Ekelund E, Thomas ED. B cell function in human marrow transplantation recipients assessed by direct and indirect haemolysis-in-gel. J Immunol 1979;123:2729–2734.
49. Witherspoon RP, Goehle S, Kretschmer M, Storb R. Regulation of immunoglobulin production after human marrow grafting: the role of helper and suppressor T cells in acute graft-versus-host disease. Transplantation 1986;41:328–335.
50. Lum LG. The kinetics of immune reconstitution after human marrow transplantation. Blood 1987;69:369–380.
51. Peltola H, Kayhta H, Sivonen A, Makela PH. Haemophilus influenzae type B capsular polysaccharide vaccine in children. A double-blind field study of 100,000 vaccinees 3 months to 5 years of age in Finland. Pediatrics 1977;60:730–733.
52. Wilkens J, Wehrle PF. Further characterization of responses of infants and children to meningococcal polysaccharide vaccine. J Pediatr 1979;94:828–832.
53. Schneerson R, Robbins JB. Induction of serum Haemophilus influenzae type b capsular antibodies in adult volunteers fed cross-reacting Escherichia coli 075: K100:H5. N Engl J Med 1975;292:1093–1096.
54. Seddik M, Seemayer TA, Lapp WS. T cell functional defect associated with thymic epithelial cell injury induced by a graft-versus-host reaction. Transplantation 1980;29:61–66.
55. Seddik M, Seemayer TA, Lapp WS. The graft-versus-host reaction and immune function. Transplantation 1984;37:281–286.
56. Saryan JA, Rappeport J, Leung DY, Parkman R, Geha RS. Regulation of human immunoglobulin E synthesis in acute graft-versus-host disease. J Clin Invest 1983; 71:556–564.
57. Ringden O, Persson U, Johansson SG, et al. Markedly elevated serum IgE levels following allogeneic and syngeneic bone marrow transplantation. Blood 1983; 61:1190–1195.
58. Findleman FD, Holmes J. Lymphokine control of in vitro immunoglobulin isotype selection. Annu Rev Immunol 1990;8:303–333.
59. Graze PR, Gale RP. Chronic graft versus host disease: a syndrome of disordered immunity. Am J Med 1979;66: 611–620.
60. Witherspoon RP, Kopecky K. Storb RF, et al. Immunological recovery in 48 patients following syngeneic marrow transplantation for hematological malignancy. Transplantation 1982;33:143–149.
61. Atkinson K, Storb R, Prentice RL, et al. Analysis of late infections in 89 long-term survivors of bone marrow transplantation. Blood 1979;53:720–731.
62. Anderson PW, Pichichero ME, Insel RA, Betts R, Eby R, Smith DH. Vaccines consisting of periodate-cleaved oligosaccharides from the capsule of Haemophilus influenzae type b coupled to a protein carrier: structural and temporal requirements for priming the human infant. J Immunol 1986;137:1181–1186.
63. Reinherz EL, Parkman R, Rappeport J, Rosen FS, Schlossman SF. Aberrations of suppressor T cells in human graft-versus-host disease. N Engl J Med 1979; 300:1061–1068.
64. Lum LG, Seigneuret MC, Storb RF, Witherspoon RP, Thomas ED. In vitro regulation of immunoglobulin synthesis after marrow transplantation. I. T-cell and B-cell deficiencies in patients with and without chronic graft-versus-host disease. Blood 1981;58:431–439.
65. Hansen JA, Atkinson K, Martin PJ, Storb R, Longton G, Thomas ED. Human T lymphocyte phenotypes after bone marrow transplantation: T cells expressing "Ia like" antigen. Transplantation 1983;36:277–281.
66. Lum LG, Seigneuret MC, Oreutt-Thordarson N, et al. The regulation of immunoglobulin synthesis after HLA-identical bone marrow transplantation. VI. Differential rates of maturation of distinct functional groups within lymphoid subpopulations in patients after human marrow grafting. Blood 1985;65:1422–1433.
67. Rozans MK, Smith BR, Burakoff SJ, Miller RA. Long-lasting deficit of functional T cell precursors in human bone marrow transplant recipients revealed by limiting dilution methods. J Immunol 1986;136:4040–4048.
68. Storek J, Saxon A. Reconstitution of B cell immunity following bone marrow transplantation. Bone Marrow Transplant 1992;9:395–408.
69. Jenkins MK, Schwartz RH, Pardoll DM. Effects of cyclosporine A on T cell development and clonal deletion. Science 1988;241:1655–1658.
70. Agosti JM, Sprenger JD, Lum LG, et al. Transfer of allergen-specific IgE-mediated hypersensitivity with allogeneic bone marrow transplantation. N Engl J Med 1988;319:1623–1628.
71. Minchinton RM, Waters AH, Kendra J, Barrett AJ. Autoimmune thrombocytopenia acquired from an allogeneic bone-marrow graft. Lancet 1982:627–629.
72. Smith CIE, Aarli JA, Biberfeld P, et al. Myasthenia gravis after bone-marrow transplantation. N Engl J Med 1983;309:1565–1568.
73. Ljungman P, Duraj V, Magnius L. Response to immunization against polio after allogeneic marrow transplantation. Bone Marrow Transplant 1991;7:89–93.
74. Engelhard D, Handsher R, Naparstek E, et al. Immune response to polio vaccination in bone marrow transplant recipients. Bone Marrow Transplant 1991;8:295–300.
75. Ljungman P, Fridell E, Lonnqvist B, et al. Efficacy and safety of vaccination of marrow transplant recipients with a live attenuated measles, mumps, and rubella vaccine. J Infect Dis 1989;159:610–615.

Chapter 37
Critical Care and Respiratory Failure

Stephen W. Crawford

Critical illness requiring intensive care occurs in 24 to 40% of bone marrow transplant (BMT) recipients because of the need for cardiac monitoring, mechanical ventilation, hemodialysis, or other forms of intensive care (1,2). The incidence of these complications increases with the age of the patient, the intensity of the cytoreductive regimen, transplantation for malignant disease, and allogeneic, autologous, or syngeneic BMT. With careful selection of candidates, transplant units may experience a lower proportion of critically ill patients.

Many of the complications of BMT are similar to those of other recipients of intensive chemoradiotherapy. Thus, the principles and approaches to critical care of BMT recipients are similar to those for other immunosuppressed patients. The primary features that distinguish BMT recipients from other immunosuppressed patients are the prevalence of graft rejection, graft-versus-host disease (GVHD), and chemoradiotherapy regimen–related toxicities (RRTs). In some regards, BMT recipients may present a less confusing clinical diagnostic picture than other immunosuppressed patients because specific complications tend to occur within well-defined periods. These intervals are determined by the timing and intensity of cytoreductive therapies and the pattern of immune reconstitution that follows.

A standard approach for critical care of BMT recipients is to transfer critically ill marrow recipients to a centralized intensive care unit. Some centers provide intensive care within the BMT unit. Such localized units are specialized to care for immunosuppressed patients, in contrast to a general medical or surgical intensive care unit. The range and severity of complications associated with BMT require involvement of medical specialists, such as intensivists, pulmonologists, nephrologists, and gastroenterologists who are experienced with immunosuppressed patients. Intensivists or a critical care team may provide primary care responsibility, or the intensivists and other medical subspecialists may serve as consultants to the transplant team. The involvement of surgeons familiar with the complications of BMT and experience in treating immunosuppressed and pancytopenic patients may be critical. Surgical specialists most likely to be involved in the urgent care of BMT recipients are thoracic surgeons, general surgeons, otolaryngologists, and, occasionally, neurosurgeons.

Appropriate nursing expertise is crucial to efficient care of critically ill BMT recipients. Regardless of intensive care unit setting, critically ill BMT recipients should be treated by nurses skilled and experienced in oncology practices.

Critical Care Complications After BMT

BMT recipients experience many of the same complications as oncology patients receiving intensive antineoplastic therapies. Bacteremia or serious bacterial infections are noted in up to 50% of marrow recipients (3). Central venous access catheters, neutropenia, and immunosuppression to prevent GVHD pose risks for bacterial and fungal infections. Increasingly, *Aspergillus* and *Candida* species colonization and infection are emerging as frequent problems (4). RRT commonly cause desquamation of the oropharyngeal and gastrointestinal mucosa (mucositis) within the first 3 weeks after transplantation (5). The mucositis and opiate analgesics administered to temper the pain increase the risk of pulmonary aspiration and mandate intravenous alimentation (6).

Congestive cardiomyopathy syndromes and pleuropericarditis associated with radiotherapy, cyclophosphamide (CY), and anthracycline-containing preparative regimens may occur in up to 5% of BMT recipients. Pericardial tamponade often necessitates surgical removal of pericardial fluid. Atrial tachyarrhythmias are seen frequently in association with pleuropericarditis, and central nervous system complications may occur with specific drug treatments. Both Guillian-Barré syndrome and peripheral neuropathies have been described after cytosine arabinoside administration. Toxicity due to cyclosporine (CSP) may cause altered sensorium, seizures, and coma.

BMT-related complications have been reviewed elsewhere (7). Complications that predispose to or are associated with critical illness are listed in Table 37-1. Several complications that may result in critical illness are specific to BMT and are covered extensively in other chapters in this text. Most notable among these complications are relapse, rejection, GVHD, and hepatic venoocclusive disease (VOD).

Table 37-1.
Complications of Bone Marrow Transplantation with Critical Care Implications

Graft failure
Relapse of malignancy
Secondary malignancy
Reactions to marrow infusion
Bronchospasm
Anaphylaxis
Hypotension
Pulmonary fat emboli
Graft-versus-host disease
Acute
Chronic
Gastrointestinal disease
Oral mucositis
Esophagitis/gastritis
Hemorrhage
Diarrheal syndromes
Hepatic insufficiency
VOD
Drug toxicity
Infection
Cardiac disease
Tachyarrhythmias
Myocarditis
Pericarditis
Pericardial effusion
Renal insufficiency
Hepatorenal syndrome
Nephrotoxicity
Respiratory disease
Pneumonia
Aspiration
Infection
Idiopathic
ARDS
Interstitial
Chronic fibrosis
Airflow obstruction
Bronchiolitis
Pleural effusion
Diaphragmatic paralysis
Neuromuscular
Metabolic encephalopathy
Leukoencephalopathy
Seizures
Polyneuropathy
Infection
Bacterial
Viral
Herpes group
Varicella zoster
Respiratory viruses
RSV
Adenovirus
Influenza
Parainfluenza
Fungal
Candida species
Filamentous fungi
Pneumocystis carinii
Protozoal

VOD = veno-occlusive disease; ARDS = adult respiratory distress syndrome; RSV = respiratory syncytial virus.

Incidence and Significance of Pulmonary Complications

Overall, pulmonary disease develops in 40 to 60% of patients at some time after BMT, and up to 40% require intensive care (2,8). Incidence depends on transplant characteristics, such as degree of human leukocyte antigen (HLA) disparity and donor source (allogeneic, syngeneic, or autograft), specific conditioning regimen agents and doses, underlying disease, and age of the patient (9,10). Thus, the incidence of pulmonary complications among patients transplanted for hematological malignancy and who receive total body irradiation (TBI) for conditioning is higher than that of patients transplanted for aplastic anemia who receive only CY. Pneumonia is the leading infectious cause of death, and, until recently, cytomegalovirus (CMV) was the most common cause of fatal pulmonary infection (4). The incidence of some pulmonary infections, such as *Pneumocystis carinii* and perhaps bacterial pneumonia, has decreased due to the routine use of prophylactic antimicrobial agents. However, diffuse "idiopathic" pulmonary injury continues, with an incidence of 10 to 15% and a mortality rate exceeding 60%. Many of these idiopathic pneumonias are attributed to toxicity from intensive cytoreductive chemotherapy and irradiation.

Significant pulmonary dysfunction is found in some long-term survivors months and even years after successful BMT (11,12). Airflow obstructive defects occur in at least 10% of patients with chronic GVHD and have been seen rarely in recipients of autologous marrow (13). The obstruction is most often demonstrated to be obliterative bronchiolitis and may progress to profound respiratory insufficiency and death.

Temporal Sequence of Complications

Specific complications tend to occur within well-defined periods that correspond to the state of immune reconstitution following BMT (4,14). Knowledge of these periods makes diagnostic decisions in marrow recipients easier than in many other immunosuppressed patients.

Specific complications may be grouped according to the time of presentation relative to the day of BMT (15). The groupings are based in part on the fact that chronic GVHD occurs approximately at or beyond day 100, delimiting a "late" from an "early" period. The early period can be subdivided further into the period of profound neutropenia that exists for a variable period before BMT and usually for maximum of 3 weeks after BMT, and the period of acute GVHD, which begins 2 to 3 weeks after BMT. A list of complications and their approximate timing and incidence after allogeneic BMT is shown in Table 37-2.

Complications within the first 30 days are dominated by RRT. Pancytopenia is the rule. Pulmonary edema syndromes due to excess fluid administration have been reported in up to half of BMT recipients (16). Also, congestive heart failure due to cardiotoxic

Table 37-2.

	Approximate Incidence
Early complications (<100 days)	
Pulmonary edema syndromes	0–50%
Infectious pneumonia	30–40%
Bacterial	2–30%
Fungal	10–20%
Viral	20–30%
Protozoal	<5%
Idiopathic pneumonia	10–20%
Oral mucositis	50–70%
Pulmonary VOD	Rare
Late complications (>100 days)	
Bronchopneumonia	20–30%
Idiopathic pneumonia	10–20%
Viral pneumonia	0–10%
Obstructive airflow	10–20%
Pulmonary vascular changes	50%

VOD = veno-occlusive disease.

chemotherapy, adult respiratory distress syndrome (ARDS) due to chemoradiotherapy injury or sepsis, and pulmonary hemorrhage in the presence of thrombocytopenia contribute to diffuse infiltrates. These patients frequently suffer from multiorgan disease with RRT or, among allogeneic marrow recipients, grade II to IV (moderate to severe) acute GVHD. Severe oral mucositis is common and may result in recurrent aspiration of oral secretions. Secondary infection of the denuded oral mucosa with herpes simplex virus (HSV) or gram-negative bacilli may delay healing and increase the risk of pneumonia. Thus, pancytopenia, hepatic and renal failure, desquamative skin lesions, and mucositis complicate both evaluation and management. During this period, diffuse pulmonary infiltrates rarely are infectious, and opportunistic infections are not prevalent (17).

Days 30 to 100 to 150 are dominated by viral pneumonias, especially CMV, as causes for diffuse pulmonary infiltrates (9,17). Onset varies from insidious to rapid progression of tachypnea, hypoxia, and respiratory failure. Unfortunately, there is little clinically to distinguish the similar presentations of pneumonias of other etiologies. During this period, granulocyte number and function usually have returned to normal, but defects in humoral and cell-mediated immunity persist. Opportunistic and idiopathic pneumonias are also common during this period.

Three to 5 months after BMT, the immune function of marrow recipients usually returns toward normal except in those with chronic GVHD (18). Thus, late pneumonias predominate among allogeneic marrow recipients with chronic GVHD, because the major risk for pneumonia appears to be prolonged impairment in immunity (19,20). Viral pneumonias are seen but become less common after day 100. Pneumocystis infection occasionally presents in patients with chronic GVHD and inadequate prophylaxis. Idiopathic pneumonias, possibly due to radiation or cytotoxic agents, are clinically identical in presentation to other diffuse pneumonias. Late after BMT, diffuse pulmonary disease is often insidious in onset.

Progressive airflow obstruction consistent with obliterative bronchiolitis develops in approximately 10% of allogeneic marrow recipients with chronic GVHD (12). This pattern is frequently recognized late after BMT, although it may occur at any time. Also, diffuse idiopathic pneumonia develops in 10 to 20% of marrow recipients. Little is known about the pathogenesis and predisposing factors for these late processes.

Pretransplant Evaluation

The evaluation before BMT should include a thorough physical examination, chest radiographs, pulmonary function studies, and electrocardiograms. The primary concern is for diagnosing pre-existing infection, pulmonary limitation, and cardiac disease. Clinical experience suggests that transplant recipients with invasive fungal infection, especially *Aspergillus*, have a high rate of mortality. For this reason, it is crucial that unexplained focal lung, renal, and hepatic lesions be evaluated fully before BMT. Biopsy or resection of focal lesions often is advisable for diagnosis and potential cure of a suspected infection.

Pulmonary function abnormalities in total lung volume, diffusing capacity, or oxygenation before BMT have been shown to increase the risk of mortality among patients with malignancy, whereas airflow obstruction does not (21). Abnormal pulmonary function studies likely modify the risks associated with age, relapse, and GVHD, and in the absence of other factors rarely represent sufficient risk to contraindicate BMT.

Left ventricular failure may be evaluated by echocardiography or radionuclide ventriculography. However, routine measurement of left ventricular ejection fraction is not warranted because a prospective study did not document a significantly increased risk of cardiac toxicity among patients with a history of unresponsiveness to anthracycline administration or with an ejection fraction below 50% (22). It is prudent to obtain a complete cardiac evaluation, including stress testing, if there is a history of angina, although data regarding the risk associated with coronary vascular disease are not available.

Diagnostic Procedures

Radiographic Techniques

Routine posterior-anterior and lateral view chest radiographs are advisable on a weekly basis during the early period after marrow infusion due to the high frequency of pulmonary complications. In many cases, chest radiographs are the first clinical indication of pulmonary disease. Among patients with abnormalities, the pattern of infiltration is key to the diagnostic approach. The distinction between diffuse and localized pulmonary disease is useful in generating a differential diagnosis and in formulating a diagnostic approach (Figure 37-1) (14,23).

The most common presentation of pulmonary disease after BMT is diffuse pulmonary infiltrates, which may be seen in patients with CMV pneumonia, idiopathic pneumonia, pulmonary edema, and bacterial or fungal pneumonia. Air bronchograms are suggestive of bacterial infection (24). Pulmonary edema syndromes typically present with enlarged pericardial silhouette and pleural effusions, and interstitial septal lines may be present. Both viral-associated and idiopathic pneumonias may be very similar in appearance, with reticular and alveolar infiltrates. Pleural effusions suggest pulmonary edema because they are rare with these pneumonias.

Similar to the situation in acute leukemia, localized parenchymal disease at any time after BMT is due to infection in the majority of patients (17,25). Computerized tomography (CT) is useful both for diagnosis in localized pulmonary disease and for defining the extent of involvement. Central consolidation with a surrounding zone of attenuation ("halo" sign) is reportedly typical for invasive pulmonary aspergillosis (26). Also, CT may reveal the presence of additional lesions in the contralateral thoracic cavity or mediastinum, which would mitigate against surgical resection and may lead to other diagnostic biopsies. CT of the head and abdomen should be performed prior to any attempted biopsies of focal lung lesions to exclude metastatic lesions in view of the high prevalence of disseminated fungal disease.

Pulmonary and Systemic Artery Catheters

Placement of a flow-directed pulmonary artery (PA) catheter (Swan-Ganz catheter) is frequently indicated in the management of critically ill marrow recipients. At the Fred Hutchinson Cancer Research Center, 12% of marrow recipients are monitored with these catheters at some time after BMT. Sepsis syndrome or the combination of hepatic VOD, diffuse pulmonary infiltrates, and hypotension or renal insufficiency pose dilemmas in fluid management. Assessment of left ventricular function, filling pressures, and vascular resistance are useful in preventing congestive pulmonary edema and maximizing cardiac performance. PA catheters may be placed safely via a percutaneous route using the Seldinger technique in most patients. Thrombocytopenia, although a concern, does not appear to be a contraindication provided the procedure is performed by an experienced operator. It is prudent to provide platelet transfusion prior to placement in patients with counts less than 50,000/mm^3 when possible. Internal jugular and femoral veins provide readily compressible and accessible sites in most patients. Fluoroscopy rarely may be necessary to guide the pulmonary artery catheter past a tunnelled right atrial (Hickman or Groshong) catheter.

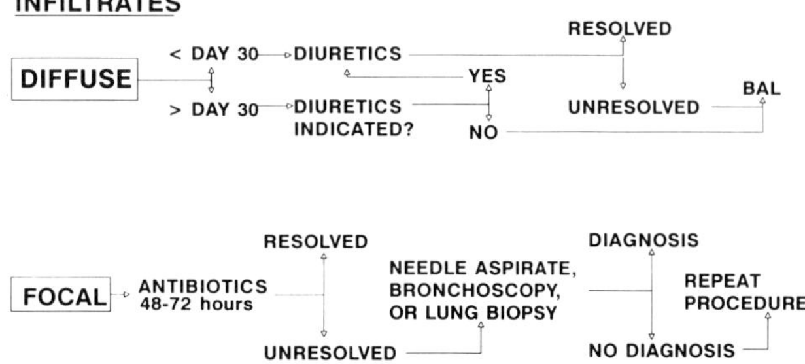

Figure 37-1. Diagnostic approach to pulmonary infiltrates after marrow transplantation.

Percutaneous placement of arterial catheters in radial, dorsalis pedis, or femoral arteries also appears to be safe in BMT recipients with thrombocytopenia. Placement is indicated for arterial pressure monitoring in patients with prolonged hypotension, those requiring infusions of multiple vasoactive drugs, as well as those requiring frequent arterial blood gas analysis for respiratory failure.

Fiberoptic Bronchoscopy

Fiberoptic bronchoscopy with bronchoalveolar lavage (BAL) is the procedure of choice to evaluate diffuse infiltrates (27,28). There is a high prevalence of viral infection, notably CMV, and a low prevalence of other opportunistic infections. Advancements in rapid virological and microbiological testing applied to BAL specimens permit sensitive and specific detection of viral as well as bacterial and *Pneumocystis carinii* infections (27,29–32). Rapid centrifugation (shell vial) culture appears to be the most sensitive method of detecting viral infection. Fluorescent antibody staining with monoclonals has increased sensitivity over cytology alone (33). BAL is a safe diagnostic procedure for the evaluation of pulmonary infiltrates in BMT recipients and may be performed in profoundly thrombocytopenic patients with little risk of bleeding or infection (34–38). Although BAL can document the presence of viral and bacterial infection, negative results do not exclude the presence of fungal infection and do not confirm the diagnosis of idiopathic pneumonia. Use of additional invasive procedures must be individualized on the basis of the likelihood of undiagnosed treatable infection.

Other bronchoscopic techniques may be of less benefit than BAL. Transbronchial lung biopsy does not appear to improve the diagnostic yield in marrow recipients with diffuse infiltrates, is not specific for idiopathic processes, and may be unsafe in thrombocytopenic patients (39–41). It is unclear whether protected specimen brushings add to the diagnostic yield of BAL, although they may improve the recovery of fungal elements.

Fine-needle Aspiration

Transthoracic aspiration by thin (18–22 gauge) needles is useful for sampling peripheral lung lesions that may not be approached easily by fiberoptic bronchoscopy (42–44). The diagnostic yield of fungal infection with transthoracic thin-needle aspiration is probably highest from mass-like lesions and lower from diffuse or infiltrative ones. The diagnosis is usually made on the basis of histological staining of the specimen rather than culture.

Depending on operator experience and location of the lesion, the complication rate may be as low as 15% in patients with platelet counts of at least 30,000/mm^3 (17). Transthoracic thin-needle aspiration may be the procedure of choice for lesions in which filamentous fungi are highly suspected. The procedure yields a diagnosis of fungal infection in approximately two thirds of patients with focal lung lesions that persist or develop after administration of broad-spectrum antibiotics. Of the one third of transthoracic thin-needle aspirations with no specific diagnosis, the negative predictive value for fungal infection is only 50% (17). A negative test result does not exclude the most common infectious cause for the lesion. Transthoracic thin-needle aspiration is not necessary if lung resection is planned.

Thoracotomy

The role and yield of open lung biopsy for the diagnosis and management of diffuse pulmonary infiltrates in immunocompromised hosts have received much attention (45–54). Most reports note that thoracotomy may be undertaken with acceptable morbidity and mortality, even in severely immunosuppressed patients, as long as the platelet count is adequate (usually >50,000/mm^3). Open lung biopsy has the highest probability of rendering a specific diagnosis of the procedures available and had been the mainstay of diagnosis for diffuse pulmonary infiltrates prior to the advent of rapid and sensitive virological diagnostic techniques. Open biopsy is currently reserved for marrow recipients with nondiagnostic BAL results. This situation frequently occurs late after BMT, when viral infections are less frequent and the possibility of opportunistic infections is increased. The morbidity of open lung biopsy may be diminished in the hands of a surgeon who is skilled in the use of a thoracoscope. Thorascopically directed biopsy permits diagnostic tissue to be obtained without a formal thoracotomy incision.

Lung biopsy also has a role in diagnosis and management of focal lung lesions. Surgical resection of a focal fungal lesion may be diagnostic and also curative (17). Caution must be exercised, however, in discounting fungal disease on the basis of a negative open lung biopsy sample. Despite the relatively large tissue specimen that can be sampled, the diagnoses may not be evident in the pathological examination. Invasive filamentous fungi, because of their focal nature and accompanying large degree of tissue infarction and hemorrhage, may not be seen in as many as 20% of patients in whom they are present (50,55). Therefore, it is difficult to withdraw or withhold empirical antifungal therapy in neutropenic patients despite "negative" results. Also, open lung biopsy may be a useful diagnostic tool to detect *Legionella* infections in marrow recipients with nondiagnostic transthoracic thin-needle aspiration results.

Critical Care and Pulmonary Diseases

Sepsis

Evaluation and treatment of sepsis in BMT recipients pose several distinct problems. Bacteremia is very common and documented in at least 50% of marrow recipients. However, although gram-negative enteric organisms are common, gram-positive cocci and yeast are being seen with increasing regularity. The prevalence of coagulase-negative staphylococci and *Candida* species influences antibiotic choices and prompts the empirical addition of antistaphylococcal agents and amphotericin more frequently.

Systemic viral infections are seen more often after BMT than after conventional chemotherapy. CMV viremia has been associated with high cardiac output and low systemic vascular resistance, suggestive of sepsis due to bacterial or fungal causes. However, the elevated pulmonary vascular resistance typical of bacterial sepsis is usually absent when associated with CMV. It is unclear whether this apparent sepsis response is due to viremia or concomitant processes often associated with CMV infection, such as GVHD.

The syndrome of clinical sepsis after allogeneic BMT presents the problem of differentiation between bacterial or fungal sepsis and acute GVHD. The cardiovascular responses in patients with acute GVHD may be indistinguishable from those of endotoxemia. Acute GVHD may be associated with high levels of circulating tumor necrosis factor (TNF) and other vasoactive cytokines. Markedly decreased systemic vascular resistance, tachycardia, increased stroke volume and cardiac output, and relative hypotension similar to a bacterial sepsis response may be seen with the acute onset of GVHD. These patients have fever, diffuse cutaneous hyperemia, and bounding peripheral and precordial pulses. ARDS, azotemia, and altered sensorium may follow.

The frequent finding of relative intravascular volume expansion due to excessive administration of crystalloid fluids early after BMT further confuses evaluation and treatment of clinical sepsis in marrow recipients (16). In addition to exogenous fluid administration, intravascular volume may be increased due to fluid and sodium retention from hepatic VOD. However, blood loss, often from occult gastrointestinal sources, may complicate the assessment of intravascular volume in marrow recipients with sepsis.

Given the potential complexities of diagnosis and management, central hemodynamic monitoring with a flow-directed pulmonary artery catheter is useful. Such monitoring allows support of arterial pressure to at least a mean of 60 mm Hg with vasoactive drugs such as dopamine or norepinephrine while avoiding excessive volume administration. Pulmonary artery wedge pressures above 18 mm Hg should be avoided, especially in patients with diffuse pulmonary infiltrates suggesting ARDS. Positive inotropic support with dobutamine or amrinone is given to those patients with a low stroke volume index (or low left ventricular stroke work index) despite "normal" pulmonary artery occlusion pressures. Such patients have diminished myocardial function, although there is adequate left ventricular diastolic filling pressures (or preload).

Pleural Disease

Although pleural effusions are common in the first weeks after BMT, they are rarely related to an identifiable infectious source. Pleural effusions may be associated with fluid retention of any cause, especially with ascites secondary to hepatic VOD. Bilateral pleural effusions in the presence of weight gain can be approached conservatively without diagnostic thoracentesis (14). Cautious diuresis often produces satisfactory results.

Bacterial empyema has been very rare after BMT, probably because of the frequent administration of broad-spectrum antibiotics during the neutropenic period. However, a large unilateral or rapidly accumulating effusion in the presence of fever or ipsilateral chest pain should be evaluated promptly by thoracentesis. Pleural involvement of invasive *Aspergillus* species infection is frequently seen in these settings and is difficult to confirm by culture or cytological examination. Unusual causes of pleural effusion include chylothorax, *Candida* empyema, and *Legionella feelii* empyema.

Diffuse Infiltrates

Idiopathic (Interstitial) Pneumonia Syndrome

BMT recipients with diffuse pulmonary infiltrates are usually evaluated with diagnostic procedures such as BAL or lung biopsy. If no infectious etiology is found after cytological, histological, microbiological, and virological studies, the process is referred to as "idiopathic pneumonia syndrome" (56). Previously, the term *interstitial pneumonia* was used to describe the syndrome of diffuse pulmonary inflammation with fever and tachypnea that was not due to bacterial or fungal infection (57). However, the term *interstitial pneumonia* is ambiguous because it implies that parenchymal rather than airspace inflammation is predominant. The pathological processes associated with the clinical syndrome frequently are not primarily "interstitial." It is preferable to refer to these pneumonias as "diffuse," on the basis of the radiographic and clinical presentation, and to use the term *idiopathic pneumonia syndrome* to describe those cases without an identifiable pathogen.

The term *idiopathic pneumonia syndrome* does not suggest a specific etiological and pathogenetic process. Factors associated with this diffuse pulmonary injury syndrome include a multitude of drugs, radiation, and systemic infections leading to ARDS (58,59). Although pulmonary injury associated with these factors appears similar in radiographic and clinical presentations, the pathological patterns may vary widely. Few of the pathologies are pathognomonic, and most are only suggestive of the possible etiology of the injury. The histopathology of these pneumonias usually displays either diffuse alveolar damage consistent with ARDS or mononuclear interstitial infiltrates (usually referred to as idiopathic interstitial pneumonia) (60). Processes also included in the idiopathic pneumonia syndrome are pulmonary hemorrhage and edema. Less common are thromboemboli and leukemic infiltrate (9).

It is estimated that idiopathic pneumonia develops in 10 to 20% of allogeneic marrow recipients, and recipients of syngeneic BMT have a similar incidence (11%) (61). The incidence of idiopathic pneumonia appears lower among autologous marrow recipients, although this may be due to differences in conditioning regimens (62). The incidence of diffuse idiopathic pneumonia syndrome is highest during the second week after BMT and then is relatively constant throughout the next 12 weeks (9).

Risk factors for idiopathic pneumonia syndrome appear to be related largely to the type of conditioning therapy before BMT. Both increased dose and dose rate of TBI are risks (63). Also, patients with lymphoma with prior chest radiotherapy appear to be at greater risk after BMT that includes TBI, whereas patients with aplastic anemia who do not receive TBI are at lower risk (64). Fractionated irradiation schedules reduce the incidence compared with single exposure (9). Reports of the effects of recipient age and presence of acute GVHD have been conflicting (9,65). Recent data from Seattle suggest that acute GVHD is a risk for idiopathic pneumonia among marrow recipients with severe aplastic anemia (Unpublished observations).

There are several possible causes for the lung injury designated as the diffuse idiopathic pneumonia syndrome. It appears clear that RRT is a major contributor. Irradiation and chemotherapeutic agents used in pre-BMT conditioning regimens may cause pulmonary injury through metabolic toxicity or hypersensitivity reactions (63,66,67). Other causes are pulmonary responses to sepsis. Sepsis is common after BMT and sepsis-related pulmonary toxicity may account for a proportion of cases of diffuse idiopathic pneumonia syndrome with a histology consistent with ARDS. Also, administration of large volumes of blood products during the BMT procedure may lead to pulmonary vascular injury through leukoagglutination reactions (68).

Several unusual causes of diffuse idiopathic pneumonia after BMT include leukemic infiltration due to relapse of primary malignancy, injection of malignant cells with reinfused autologous marrow, and fat embolization due to marrow infusion (25,69–71).

The syndrome is one of fever, nonproductive cough, tachypnea, hypoxemia, and diffuse intra-alveolar or interstitial infiltrates on chest radiography. However, this presentation is nonspecific and cannot be differentiated readily from pulmonary edema syndromes or viral pneumonia. Some cases of idiopathic pneumonia present with few symptoms and are detected by changes noted on routine radiography or pulmonary function testing. It is unknown whether such a cryptogenic presentation alters the prognosis.

Restrictive respiratory defects are not common during the first several weeks after BMT among marrow recipients in whom diffuse pneumonia does not develop (72). Four studies of long-term lung function after BMT report a decline in diffusing capacity over time, and only two document a decline in lung volumes of approximately 10% (73–76). Factors that appear to be associated with decline in lung function include pneumonia after BMT, TBI, and GVHD. There are no demonstrated differences in restrictive lung defects or declines in diffusion between autologous and allogeneic marrow recipients (76). Obstructive airflow defects were seen only in patients with GVHD after BMT.

The mortality rate associated with diffuse idiopathic pneumonia syndrome after BMT is 50 to 70% (9,77). Rapid deterioration with oxygenation failure is typical, and assisted mechanical ventilation and positive end-expiratory pressure are frequently required. Although 20% of marrow recipients ventilated for respiratory failure survive the episode, the subsequent mortality rate is high and the survival rate plateaus at 3% (78,79). Recurrent respiratory failure, complications of GVHD, and relapse of malignancy are common causes of death. Long-term survivors seem to have near normal lung function. Unfortunately, clinical factors present at the time of respiratory failure do not appear to predict survival.

No proven efficacious treatment exists for idiopathic pneumonia syndrome after BMT. There are no prospective studies to indicate that treatment for idiopathic pneumonias with various histologies respond differently. For most patients, there is no reason to obtain tissue to define the histology of a pneumonia documented by bronchoscopy to be noninfectious. Treatment approaches remain similar regardless of specific histology. Fever in marrow recipients should be presumed to represent bacterial infection, and empirical antibiotics should be begun after appropriate cultures are obtained.

Supportive management, including assisted mechanical ventilation, is appropriate, at least for a limited period to determine the likely course of disease. Treatment of ARDS-like conditions after BMT with corticosteroids has not been evaluated in clinical trials and carries the risk of increasing the incidence of infection. However, success with this approach among autologous marrow recipients has been reported (80).

Studies of suppression of inflammatory mediators, such as TNF, are of potential importance. Administration of intravenous or oral pentoxifylline, a phosphodiesterase inhibitor with anti-TNF properties, to patients with idiopathic pneumonia after BMT appears effective in decreasing elevated TNF levels. Prospective studies of mortality and resolution of pneumonia are still required.

Pulmonary Edema Syndromes

Reductions in the total amount of sodium and fluids administered have resulted in a decrease in the radiographic evidence of pulmonary edema after BMT, which had occurred in up to 50% of patients at some centers (16). However, in addition to iatrogenic causes, RRT likely contributes to edema syndromes. Sloane and colleagues (81) described a syndrome of severe pulmonary edema associated with pulmonary hemorrhage. In their report of 32 autopsies of patients transplanted for leukemia, 10 died with lesions characterized histologically by intra-alveolar and, to some degree, interstitial edema with fibrin and erythrocytes. Cellular infiltrates, fibrosis, and hyaline membranes were notably absent.

Pulmonary edema may also be due to cardiac dysfunction. Anthracyclines in excess of 500 mg/m^2, and high-dose Cy have been associated with cardiac decompensation (82–86). Cardiac and pericardial toxicity have been associated with TBI and Cy, often in the setting of prior anthracycline administration (85,87). Fortunately, the incidence of cardiac decompensation appears low (88).

Hepatic VOD is frequently associated with pulmonary edema. A syndrome of weight gain, hyperbilirubinemia, and ascites may develop in as many as 60% of adults transplanted for hematological malignancies (89). The syndrome is often associated with interstitial pulmonary edema, pleural effusions, and renal failure. Pulmonary edema also develops in association with acute GVHD and may be due in part to diffuse alveolar damage and capillary leak.

A radiographic appearance of diffuse interstitial markings with an increase in the cardiothoracic ratio in the absence of overt clinical symptoms is common. This state usually occurs within the first 2 weeks after BMT. The abnormalities of pulmonary edema may be identical to and readily confused with idiopathic pneumonia. Distinctions between pulmonary edema and pneumonia often cannot be made with certainty without pulmonary artery catheterization. However, recent increase in total body weight should prompt a trial of diuretic therapy prior to consideration of invasive diagnostic procedures. Noninvasive assessment of cardiac function with ultrasonographic or radionuclide techniques is often warranted to guide treatment.

Pulmonary Hemorrhage

Diffuse alveolar hemorrhage among both autologous and allogeneic marrow recipients is more common in the first weeks after marrow infusion (55,90). After autologous BMT, a syndrome of "diffuse alveolar hemorrhage" was reported in 21% of recipients. The syndrome was characterized histologically by diffuse alveolar damage with alveolar erythrocytes and clinically by diffuse infiltrates, hypoxemia, and progressively bloody return from BAL. This syndrome was associated with older patient age, malignancy, fever, severe oral-pharyngeal mucositis, renal failure, and a high mortality (90).

Many cases of alveolar hemorrhage after BMT are probably due to diffuse lung injury in the presence of thrombocytopenia. The majority of marrow recipients have normal clotting parameters at the time of hemorrhage. Local anticoagulant activity within the lungs of marrow recipients may account for some cases, similar to the local perturbations of coagulation involved in the pathogenesis of ARDS in the non-BMT setting.

Pulmonary hemorrhage presents radiographically as either focal or diffuse alveolar opacification. Rapid onset of radiographic pulmonary densities in the absence of overt clinical change in thrombocytopenic marrow recipients suggests alveolar hemorrhage. Such presentations are common, especially in the presence of ecchymosis in other soft tissues (such as sclerae), but it is often difficult clinically to confirm alveolar hemorrhage. Hemoptysis is rare. BAL demonstration of grossly bloody alveolar fluid and hemosiderin-laden macrophages without evidence of airway bleeding may support the clinical suspicion but is not diagnostic. Diagnostic procedures should be undertaken primarily to evaluate for potential infectious etiologies. Therapy should be directed at correcting thrombocytopenia; clotting deficits, if any; and azotemia. BMT recipients rarely die because of the bleeding itself but rather as a result of the process causing the underlying lung injury.

Clinical Approach to Diffuse Infiltrates

In general, a trial of diuretics or pulmonary artery catheterization may help differentiate the presentation of diffuse infiltrates due to idiopathic pneumonia syndrome from pulmonary edema due to volume excess or left ventricular failure. Pulmonary infection is confirmed by histological or cytological demonstration of infection or culture from BAL or open lung biopsy.

Marrow recipients with diffuse pulmonary infiltrates within 30 days after BMT usually do not require invasive diagnostic evaluation because of the low prevalence of infectious causes (see Figure 37-1) (55). A thorough clinical evaluation and empiric treatment with broad-spectrum antibiotics are recommended. Empirical diuresis and sodium restriction should be instituted. Occasionally, pulmonary artery wedge measurement (or cardiac echocardiography) to exclude pulmonary edema and to guide therapy is recommended if renal insufficiency or respiratory compromise exist. Bleeding disorders should be corrected and adequate platelet support provided to prevent further pulmonary hemorrhage. Outbreaks of viral pneumonias due to respiratory syncytial virus and *Parainfluenza* virus have recently been recognized in BMT units (91–93). Thus, if clinical deterioration ensues, fiberoptic bronchoscopy with BAL, as well as nasopharyngeal and throat swabs for virological studies, should be performed to exclude treatable pulmonary infection, especially during fall and winter months.

Marrow recipients with diffuse infiltrates after 30 days generally should undergo fiberoptic bronchoscopy with BAL. In addition to bacterial, fungal, and cytological stains, a quantitative bacterial culture should be performed. These specimens should be processed with rapid detection techniques for viral pathogens. Direct fluorescent monoclonal antibody stains and centrifugation culture (shell vial) are indicated if the patient or donor are seropositive for CMV (27,94).

Focal Infiltrates

Focal, multifocal, or patchy infiltrates in the first 30 days after BMT frequently represent bacterial or fungal infection during this period of granulocytopenia. Bacteria are an unusual cause for diffuse infiltrates. The proportion of focal infiltrates that resolve spontaneously or with empirical antibacterial therapy is unknown. Focal radiographic lesions with a mass-like appearance that develop or persist despite antibiotics at any time after BMT are pulmonary fungal infections in the majority of patients. Occasionally, *Legionella, Pseudomonas,* and, rarely, *Nocardia* species are identified within localized lesions.

Noninfectious causes of focal lung lesions after BMT include resolving (sterile) abscess, lymphoma or Hodgkin's disease, and organizing pneumonia with bronchiolitis obliterans. Clinical history of recent bacteremia, previous solid tumor, or clinical acute pneumonia that is resolving are important to the differential diagnosis. Unfortunately, absence of fever and clinical symptoms does not exclude the diagnosis of filamentous fungal infection.

Clinical Approach to Focal Lesions

Unlike the case for diffuse infiltrates, the clinical approach to localized lesions does not change significantly as time after BMT passes. BMT recipients with focal pulmonary lesions should be evaluated aggressively because there is a high probability of infection. CT scanning of the chest should be included in the diagnostic evaluation. Fungal infection often reveals a mass-like appearance of the lesion, with a zone of attenuation highly suggestive of tissue invasion. Additional lesions, not appreciated on plain chest radiography, may also be seen.

The diagnostic approach to localized lesions is dictated by radiographic appearance and location. Areas of bronchopneumonia are approached with fiberoptic bronchoscopy and BAL, whereas peripheral, consolidated lesions are amenable to percutaneous needle aspiration for diagnosis. A nondiagnostic evaluation by any technique should be repeated or alternative measures for diagnosis attempted. If bronchoscopy or needle aspiration are nondiagnostic, the most definitive study is biopsy at thoracotomy. Surgical resection should be considered when the pulmonary lesions can be removed completely because this procedure may be both diagnostic and curative in patients with localized fungal infection.

The presentation of basilar infiltrates without mass-like consolidation within the first several weeks after marrow infusion in the setting of oral mucositis should prompt evaluation for recurrent aspiration. A history of recurrent cough induced by attempts at swallowing or nocturnal paroxysms of cough in the setting of severe mucositis is common. The appropriate approach to such patients is conservative: moderating administration of sedatives, encouraging pulmonary toilet, and avoidance of mucosal bleeding by adequate platelet support. Most patients receive broad-spectrum antibiotics. Rarely, tracheal intubation is required to avoid massive aspiration in profoundly obtunded patients or acute airway obstruction in the presence of severe upper airway bleeding.

Respiratory Failure Without Infiltrates

Airflow Obstruction and Bronchiolitis

Several centers report that chronic airflow obstruction develops in 6 to 10% of allogeneic marrow recipients (12,95). Most of these cases are among long-term survivors with chronic GVHD. The most common histology found in the lungs of these patients is an obliterative bronchiolitis pattern (11). A similar pattern has been reported in 2 patients after autologous BMT (13). In addition, the obliterative bronchiolitis lesions in the lungs of BMT recipients are occasionally but not invariably accompanied by interstitial infiltrates of mononuclear cells (11,96,97).

The onset of airflow obstruction more than 100 days after BMT is strongly related to the development of chronic GVHD (11,12). Factors associated with the increased risk of GVHD, such as increasing age and HLA-nonidentical marrow grafts, are not independent risk factors for the development of obliterative bronchiolitis. However, administration of methotrexate (MTX) after BMT for the prophylaxis of GVHD is associated with airflow obstruction. Also, there is a higher incidence of decreased levels of immunoglobulin G (IgG) among patients with obliterative bronchiolitis than in other marrow recipients (95). This hypogammaglobulinemia may be a manifestation of the immunological lesion responsible for the airway disease or merely may be related to the presence of chronic GVHD (18,98).

The etiology of obliterative bronchiolitis after BMT is unknown. Those causes recognized in otherwise normal hosts, such as recurrent aspiration, viral infection with influenza, adenovirus or measles, and bacterial or *Mycoplasma* infection, have not been found consistently in marrow recipients with obliterative bronchiolitis. The strong association between chronic GVHD and the development of obliterative bronchiolitis suggests an immunological mechanism inducing bronchial epithelial injury (11,12). The lung epithelium may be the target of immune-mediated injury in patients with chronic GVHD through the expression of Ia antigens and subsequent activation of donor cytotoxic T cells. The association with the administration of MTX also raises the possibility of direct drug-related injury to the pulmonary bronchial epithelium.

Airflow obstruction is occasionally seen within 100 days after BMT. Histology is available for few of these cases, and the defect is possibly related to infection. This early presentation is often associated with acute GVHD.

Typical manifestations of airflow obstruction due to obliterative bronchiolitis after BMT are insidious progression of tachypnea; dyspnea on exertion; and dry, nonproductive cough. Fever is not common (99). There may be few physical findings. Chest auscultation may reveal scattered expiratory wheezing and occasionally diffuse inspiratory crackles but is sometimes normal. Rarely, acute and profound wheezing is noted. Chest radiographs are commonly normal. The diagnosis of airflow obstruction is made among asymptomatic BMT recipients by routine pulmonary function testing. When the presentation is more than 150 days after BMT, evidence of chronic GVHD is usually present, although the condition may occur at any time after BMT.

The syndrome is often progressive and results in death due to respiratory failure. A more rapid onset and faster rate of progression are associated with a worse outcome (99). Control of chronic GVHD with increased immunosuppression may achieve stabilization of the airway disease (11,99,100). Patients with gradual declines in airflow tend to have more benign courses. Marrow recipients with the onset of airflow obstruction beyond 150 days after BMT tend to have a more gradual decline in lung function. Airflow may stabilize in 50% of these patients. Reversal of the obstruction is uncommon.

There are no prospective studies of the treatment of obliterative bronchiolitis after BMT. Obstructive airflow in the presence of chronic GVHD is managed primarily by controlling the GVHD with increased immunosuppression. Experience with obliterative bronchiolitis among the recipients of heart-lung transplantations suggests that the addition of azathioprine (1.0–1.5 mg/kg/day) to CSP may be effective in arresting the decline in airflow in these patients (101). In addition, aerosolized bronchodilator treatment for symptomatic patients is appropriate. Early and aggressive antibiotic treatment for any potential lower respiratory infection should be initiated. Prophylactic trimethaprim-sulfamethoxazole (or other forms of anti-*Pneumocystis* prevention) should be continued for the duration of immune suppression. Routine intravenous replacement of immunoglobulin for those with low class or subclass levels is usual (102).

Similar immunosuppressive management is recommended for airflow obstruction that develops early in the BMT course in the absence of chronic GVHD. Evaluation for possible airway infection by respiratory viruses or fungus should be undertaken in rapidly developing obstruction, especially in the presence of acute GVHD.

Early recognition and treatment may improve outcome. Therefore, routine spirometry after BMT among patients with chronic GVHD is encouraged to detect the insidious onset of this process.

Pulmonary VOD

Pulmonary VOD is a rare complication after BMT (103,104). Three cases of pulmonary VOD were reported in children with acute lymphocytic leukemia, 2 of which were associated with carmustine (BCNU). BCNU was also associated with the development of pulmonary VOD in 2 non-BMT recipients after treatment for glioma (105). Pulmonary VOD has been a very rare complication after cytoreductive conditioning for BMT with CY and TBI but has been reported in a child with acute lymphocytic leukemia who previously received multiagent chemotherapies (57,104).

Pulmonary VOD presents with insidious dyspnea on exertion, hypoxemia, and resting tachypnea within 3 to 4 months after BMT. Chest radiography has been reported to be normal. Clinical examination, electrocardiography, and ultrasound studies are consistent with pulmonary hypertension. Perfusion-ventilation radionuclide scans have been normal, excluding the diagnosis of pulmonary embolism that may present similarly. Pulmonary function studies have failed to demonstrate airflow obstruction consistent with bronchiolitis. The diagnostic procedure of choice is right-sided heart catheterization with a pulmonary angiogram. Right-sided heart catheterization reveals elevated pulmonary artery pressure, with normal pulmonary artery wedge pressures. Angiography excludes the presence of thrombi as a cause for the pulmonary hypertension.

Pulmonary VOD has been recognized most often at autopsy after conventional chemotherapy treatment for malignancy. These patients had an insidious course, with progressive hypoxemia and dyspnea on exertion due to pulmonary hypertension. Prompt recognition and diagnosis appear important because response to high-dose corticosteroid therapy (methylprednisolone, 2.0 mg/kg/day) occurred in 2 of 3 patients reported (103).

Pulmonary Vascular Changes

Pulmonary endothelial-cell swelling and localized thrombosis in small vessels have been reported in up to 50% of autopsies after BMT (81). However, venous thromboembolism has rarely been reported perhaps because of the profound thrombocytopenia that develops after cytoreductive conditioning (106). Right atrial catheters serve as a nidus for thrombosis, and fibrinolytic agents are frequently used to dissolve the clots that occlude these catheters (107,108). Although these clots rarely cause clinically significant pulmonary compromise, small recanalized thromboemboli of various age occasionally are seen histologically at autopsy.

Bone fragment embolization that was apparently without sequelae has been reported after marrow infusion (109). In addition, pulmonary ossification may occur rarely in canine models of BMT (110). Areas of intravascular calcification may represent organization and dystrophic calcification of pulmonary thromboemboli and not necessarily embolic bone spicules from the marrow infusion.

Clinical Approach to Respiratory Failure Without Pulmonary Infiltrates

Patients who present with marked tachypnea or hypoxemia after BMT in the absence of radiographic infiltrates should be evaluated for the presence of obstructive airways disease, pulmonary VOD, and pulmonary vascular disease. Diagnostic evaluation should include full pulmonary function testing and arterial blood gas analysis. The absence of airflow obstruction rules out bronchiolitis. If restrictive ventilatory defects are noted, CT of the chest should be performed to look for subtle interstitial disease suggestive of idiopathic pneumonia not otherwise noted on routine radiography. Evaluation would then proceed as for diffuse infiltrates. Patients with hypoxemia but no obstructive or restrictive lung defects should proceed to echocardiography to look for right ventricular failure and pulmonary arterial hypertension typical of pulmonary VOD. If these signs are present, right-sided heart catheterization should be performed to confirm the diagnosis of pulmonary VOD. In the rare patient with dyspnea despite normal pulmonary function testing and echocardiography, exercise pulmonary function testing is indicated to detect pulmonary vascular disease or myocardial limitations.

Ethical Considerations in Critical Care

The mortality rate among BMT recipients in intensive care units is high (1,78,79,111,112), probably due to underlying immune suppression, multiple organ injuries from RRT, and a high proportion of patients with underlying fatal malignancies.

The difficulties in dealing with critical complications of BMT are exemplified by respiratory failure. Long-term survival (>6 mo) after assisted mechanical ventilation for respiratory failure occurs in only 3% of patients, but clinical characteristics present at the time of onset of respiratory failure cannot be used to predict outcome (78,79). A therapeutic trial of respiratory support may be useful because survival after ventilation for 9 or more days appears uncommon.

Given the poor prognosis associated with respiratory failure, it is important to establish in advance patients' wishes regarding advanced life support (113). Patients at increased risk can be identified before BMT. The risk factors are 20 years of age or older, receipt of an HLA-nonidentical graft, and malignancy in relapse at time of BMT. More than half of patients with all 3 risk factors receive assisted mechanical ventilation (78).

In the absence of the known wishes of a BMT recipient regarding institution of life support and an inability to predict outcome accurately, it is reasonable to apply life support on a limited-time basis. A trial of support for a prestated time period can allow time to establish a firm prognosis. Continued decline in respiratory function over several days or development of progressive multiple organ failure is an indication of futile intervention (112). Similarly, clinical experience suggests that respiratory failure associated with pulmonary infection may represent a situation from which survival is exceedingly unlikely. In such patients, it may be appropriate to withhold or withdraw life support after informing patients (or surrogates) of the prognosis (114).

Clinical experience shows that cardiopulmonary resuscitation (CPR) in the event of sudden cardiac arrest after BMT carries the same dismal prognosis as it does in the setting of malignancy. Survival to hospital discharge is rarely achieved. It is appropriate to explain these facts to patients at risk and to withhold CPR. In addition, BMT centers ethically may adopt a policy of withholding CPR from all BMT candidates (115). Although CPR may not alter the outcome in the event of sudden cardiac arrest, there may be medical indications for otherwise providing life support. Consultation with an institutional ethics committee may help not only with decisions regarding individual cases, but also in developing institutional policies regarding withholding and withdrawing life support.

References

1. Afessa B, Tefferi A, Hoagland HC, Letendre L, Peters SG. Outcome of recipients of bone marrow transplants who require intensive-care unit support. Mayo Clin Proc 1992;67:117–122.
2. O'Quin T, Moravec C. The critically ill bone marrow transplant patient. Semin Oncol Nursing 1988;4:25–30.
3. Petersen FB, Buckner CD, Clift RA, et al. Laminar air flow isolation and decontamination: a prospective randomized study of the effects of prophylactic systemic antibiotics in bone marrow transplant patients. Infection 1986;14:115–121.
4. Meyers JD. Infection in bone marrow transplant recipients. Am J Med 1986;81(suppl 1A):27–38.
5. Atkinson K, Biggs JC, Ting A, Concannon AJ, Dodds AJ, Pun A. Cyclosporin A is associated with faster engraftment and less mucositis than methotrexate after allogeneic bone marrow transplantation. Br J Haematol 1983;53:265–270.
6. Kolbinson DA, Schubert MM, Flournoy N, Truelove EL. Early oral changes following bone marrow transplantation. Oral Surg Oral Med Oral Pathol 1988;66:130–138.
7. Press OW, Schaller RT, Thomas ED. Bone marrow transplant complications. In: Toledo-Pereyra LH, ed. Complications of organ transplantation. New York: Marcel Dekker, 1987:399–424.
8. Krowka MJ, Rosenow EC, Hoagland HC. Pulmonary complications of bone marrow transplantation. Chest 1985;87:237–246.
9. Meyers JD, Flournoy N, Thomas ED. Nonbacterial pneumonia after allogeneic marrow transplantation: a review of ten years' experience. Rev Infect Dis 1982;4:1119–1132.
10. Weiner RS, Bortin MM, Gale RP, et al. Interstitial pneumonitis after bone marrow transplantation: assessment of risk factors. Ann Intern Med 1986;104:168–175.
11. Chan CK, Hyland RH, Hutcheon MA, et al. Small-airways disease in recipients of allogeneic bone marrow transplants. Medicine 1987;66:327–340.
12. Clark JC, Schwartz DA, Flournoy N, Sullivan KM, Crawford SW, Thomas ED. Risk factors for airflow obstruction in recipients of bone marrow transplants. Ann Intern Med 1987;107:648–656.
13. Paz HL, Crilley P, Patchefsky A, Schiffman RL, Brodsky I. Bronchiolitis obliterans after autologous bone marrow transplantation. Chest 1992;101:775–778.
14. Clark JG, Crawford SW. Diagnostic approaches to pulmonary complications of marrow transplantation. Chest 1987;91:477–479.
15. van der Meer JWM, Guiot HFL, van den Broek PJ, van Furth R. Infections in bone marrow transplant recipients. Semin Hematol 1984;21:123–140.
16. Dickout WJ, Chan CK, Hyland RH, et al. Prevention of acute pulmonary edema after bone marrow transplantation. Chest 1987;92:303–309.
17. Crawford SW, Hackman RC, Clark JG. Biopsy diagnosis and clinical outcome of focal pulmonary lesions after marrow transplantation. Transplantation 1989;48:266–271.
18. Witherspoon RP, Matthews D, Storb R, et al. Recovery of in vivo cellular immunity after human marrow grafting: influence of time postgrafting and acute graft-versus-host disease. Transplantation 1984;37:145–150.
19. Wingard JR, Santos GW, Saral R. Late-onset interstitial pneumonia following allogeneic bone marrow transplantation. Transplantation 1985;39:21–23.
20. Sullivan KM, Meyers JD, Flournoy N, Storb R, Thomas ED. Early and late interstitial pneumonia following human bone marrow transplantation. Int J Cell Cloning 1986;4:107–121.
21. Crawford SW, Fisher L. Predictive value of pulmonary function tests before marrow transplantation. Chest 1992;101:1257–1264.
22. Bearman SI, Petersen FB, Schor RA, et al. Radionuclide ejection fraction in the evaluation of patients being considered for bone marrow transplantation: risk for cardiac toxicity. Bone Marrow Transplant 1990;5:173–177.
23. Crawford SW, Meyers JD. Respiratory disease in the marrow transplant patient. In: Shelhamer J, Pizzo PA, Parrillo JE, Masur H, eds. Respiratory disease in the immunosuppressed host. New York: J.B. Lippincott, 1991:595–623.
24. Pagani JJ, Kangarloo H. Chest radiography in pediatric allogeneic bone marrow transplantation. Cancer 1980; 46:1741–1745.
25. Tenholder MF, Hooper RG. Pulmonary infiltrates in leukemia. Chest 1980;78:468–473.

26. Kuhlman JE, Fishman EK, Burch PA, Karp JE, Zerhouni EA, Siegelman SS. Invasive pulmonary aspergillosis in acute leukemia. The contribution of CT to early diagnosis and aggressive management. Chest 1987;92:95–99.
27. Crawford SW, Bowden RA, Hackman RC, Gleaves CA, Meyers JD, Clark JG. Rapid detection of cytomegalovirus pulmonary infection by bronchoalveolar lavage and centrifugation culture. Ann Intern Med 1988;108:180–185.
28. Williams D, Yungbluth M, Adams G, Glassroth J. The role of fiberoptic bronchoscopy in the evaluation of immunocompromised hosts with diffuse pulmonary infiltrates. Am Rev Respir Dis 1985;131:880–885.
29. Gleaves CA, Smith TF, Shuster EA, Pearson GR. Comparison of standard tube and shell vial cell culture techniques for the detection of cytomegalovirus in clinical specimens. J Clin Microbiol 1985;21:217–221.
30. Linder J, Vaughan WP, Armitage JO, et al. Cytopathology of opportunistic infection in bronchoalveolar lavage. Am J Clin Pathol 1987;88:421–428.
31. Kahn FW, Jones JM. Diagnosing bacterial respiratory infection by bronchoalveolar lavage. J Infect Dis 1987;155:862–869.
32. Thorpe JE, Baughman RP, Frame PT, Wesseler TA, Staneck JL. Bronchoalveolar lavage for diagnosing acute bacterial pneumonia. J Infect Dis 1987;155:855–861.
33. Emanuel D, Peppard J, Stover D, Gold J, Armstrong D, Hammerling U. Rapid immunodiagnosis of cytomegalovirus pneumonia by bronchoalveolar lavage using human and murine monoclonal antibodies. Ann Intern Med 1986;104:476–481.
34. Weiss SW, Hert RC, Gianola FG, Clark JC, Crawford SW. Complications of fiberoptic bronchoscopy in thrombocytopenic patients. Am Rev Respir Dis 1992;145:A244.
35. Stover DE, Zaman MB, Hajdu SI, et al. Bronchoalveolar lavage in the diagnosis of diffuse pulmonary infiltrates in the immunosuppressed host. Ann Intern Med 1984;101:1–7.
36. Williams D, Yungbluth M, Adams G, Glassroth J. The role of fiberoptic bronchoscopy in the evaluation of immunocompromised hosts with diffuse pulmonary infiltrates. Am Rev Respir Dis 1985;131:880–885.
37. Broaddus C, Dake MD, Stulbarg MS, et al. Bronchoalveolar lavage and transbronchial biopsy for the diagnosis of pulmonary infections in the acquired immunodeficiency syndrome. Ann Intern Med 1985;102:747–752.
38. Martin WJ II, Smith TF, Sanderson DR, Brutinel WM, Cockerill FR III, Douglas WW. Role of bronchoalveolar lavage in the assessment of opportunistic pulmonary infections: utility and complications. Mayo Clin Proc 1987;62:549–557.
39. Springmeyer SC, Silvestri RC, Sale GE, et al. The role of transbronchial biopsy for the diagnosis of diffuse pneumonias in immunocompromised marrow transplant recipients. Am Rev Respir Dis 1982;126:763–765.
40. Nishio JN, Lynch JP. Fiberoptic bronchoscopy in the immunocompromised host: the significance of a "nonspecific" transbronchial biopsy. Am Rev Respir Dis 1980;121:307–312.
41. Haponik EF, Summer WR, Terry PB, Wang KP. Clinical decision making with transbronchial lung biopsies: the value of nonspecific histologic examination. Am Rev Respir Dis 1982;125:524–529.
42. Castellino RA, Blank N. Etiologic diagnosis of focal pulmonary infection in immunocompromised patients by fluoroscopically guided needle aspiration. Radiology 1979;132:563–567.
43. Berquist TH, Bailey PB, Cortese DA, Miller WE. Transthoracic needle biopsy: accuracy and complications in relation to location and type of lesion. Mayo Clin Proc 1980;55:475–481.
44. Khouri NF, Stitik FP, Erozan YS, et al. Transthoracic needle aspiration biopsy of benign and malignant lung lesions. Am J Radiol 1985;144:218–288.
45. Greenman RL, Goodall PT, King AB. Lung biopsy in immunocompromised hosts. Am J Med 1975;59:488–496.
46. Rossiter SJ, Miller DC, Churg AM, et al. Open lung biopsy in the immunosuppressed patient: is it really beneficial? J Thorac Cardiovasc Surg 1979;77:338–343.
47. Burt ME, Flye MW, Webber BL, et al. Prospective evaluation of aspiration needle, cutting needle, transbronchial, and open lung biopsy in patients with pulmonary infiltrates. Ann Thorac Surg 1981;32:146–153.
48. Jaffe JP, Maki DG. Lung biopsy in immunocompromised patients: one institution's experience and an approach to management of pulmonary disease in the compromised host. Cancer 1981;48:1144–1153.
49. Prober CG, Whyte H, Smith CR. Open lung biopsy in immunocompromised children with pulmonary infiltrates. Am J Dis Child 1984;138:60–63.
50. McCabe RE, Brooks RG, Mark JBD, Remington JS. Open lung biopsy in patients with acute leukemia. Am J Med 1985;78:609–616.
51. Cockerill FR, Wilson WR, Carpenter HA, et al. Open lung biopsy in immunocompromised patients. Arch Intern Med 1985;145:1398–1404.
52. Cheson BD, Samlowski WE, Tang TT, et al. Value of open lung biopsy in 87 immunocompromised patients with pulmonary infiltrates. Cancer 1985;55:453–459.
53. Fitzgerald W, Bevelaqua FA, Garay SM, et al. The role of open lung biopsy in patients with the acquired immunodeficiency syndrome. Chest 1987;91:659–661.
54. Stulbarg MS, Golden JA. Open lung biopsy in the acquired immunodeficiency syndrome (AIDS). Chest 1987;91:639–640.
55. Crawford SW, Hackman RC, Clark JG. Open lung biopsy diagnosis of diffuse pulmonary infiltrates after marrow transplantation. Chest 1988;94:949–953.
56. Clark JG, Hansen JA, Hertz MI, Parkman R, Jensen L, Peavy H. NHLBI workshop summary: idiopathic pneumonia syndrome following bone marrow transplantation. Am Rev Respir Dis 1993; (in press).
57. Hackman RC. Lower respiratory tract. In: Sale GE, Shulman HM, eds. The pathology of bone marrow transplantation. New York: Masson, 1984:156–170.
58. Grossman J, Kahn F. Noninfectious pulmonary disease in the immunocompromised host. Semin Respir Med 1989;10:78–88.
59. Ognibene FP, Martin SE, Parker MM, et al. Adult respiratory distress syndrome in patients with severe neutropenia. N Engl J Med 1986;315:547–551.
60. Crawford SW, Hackman RC. Clinical presentation, pathology and outcome of idiopathic pneumonia after marrow transplantation. Am Rev Respir Dis 1990; 141:A48.
61. Appelbaum FR, Meyers JD, Flournoy N. Nonbacterial nonfungal pneumonia following marrow transplantation in 100 identical twins. Transplantation 1982; 33:265–268.
62. Wingard JR, Sostrin MB, Vriesendorp HM, et al.

Interstitial pneumonitis following autologous bone marrow transplantation. Transplantation 1988;46:61–65.
63. Keane TJ, van Dyk J, Rider WD. Idiopathic interstitial pneumonia following marrow transplantation: the relationship with total body irradiation. Int J Radiat Oncol Biol Phys 1981;7:1365–1370.
64. Appelbaum FR, Sullivan KM, Buckner CD, et al. Treatment of malignant lymphoma in 100 patients with chemotherapy, total body irradiation, and marrow transplantation. J Clin Oncol 1987;5:1340–1347.
65. Weiner RS, Bortin MM, Gale RP, et al. Interstitial pneumonitis after bone marrow transplantation: assessment of risk factors. Ann Intern Med 1986;104:168–175.
66. Gross NJ. The pathogenesis of radiation-induced lung damage. Lung 1981;159:115–125.
67. Ginsberg SJ, Comis RL. The pulmonary toxicity of antineoplastic agents. Semin Oncol 1982;9:34–51.
68. Popovsky MA, Abel MD, Moore SB. Transfusion-related acute lung injury associated with passive transfer of anti-leukocyte antibodies. Am Rev Respir Dis 1983; 128:185–189.
69. Glorieux P, Bouffet E, Philip I, et al. Metastatic interstitial pneumonitis after autologous bone marrow transplantation: a consequence of reinjection of malignant cells? Cancer 1986;58:2136–2139.
70. Lipton JH, Russell JA, Burgess KR, et al. Fat embolization and pulmonary infiltrates after bone marrow transplantation. Med Pediatr Oncol 1987;15:24–27.
71. Paradinas FJ, Sloane JP, Depledge MH, et al. Pulmonary fat embolisation after bone marrow transplantation. Lancet 1983;1:715–716.
72. Springmeyer SC, Silvestri RC, Flournoy N, et al. Pulmonary function of marrow transplant patients: I. Effects of marrow infusion, acute graft-versus-host-disease, and interstitial pneumonitis. Exp Hematol 1984;12:805–810.
73. Springmeyer SC, Flournoy N, Sullivan KM, Storb R, Thomas ED. Pulmonary function changes in long-term survivors of allogeneic marrow transplantation. In: Recent advances in bone marrow transplantation. New York: Alan R. Liss, 1983:343–353.
74. Sutedja TG, Apperley JF, Hughes JMB, et al. Pulmonary function after bone marrow transplantation for chronic myeloid leukaemia. Thorax 1988;43:163–169.
75. Prince DS, Wingard JR, Saral R, Santos GW, Wise RA. Longitudinal changes in pulmonary function following bone marrow transplantation. Chest 1989;96:301–306.
76. Tait RC, Burnett AK, Robertson AG, et al. Subclinical pulmonary function defects following autologous and allogeneic bone marrow transplantation: relationship to total body irradiation and graft-versus-host disease. Int J Radiat Oncol Biol Phys 1991;20:1219–1227.
77. Weiner RS, Dicke KA (for the Advisory Committee of the International Bone Marrow Transplant Registry). Risk factors for interstitial pneumonitis following bone marrow transplantation for severe aplastic anemia: a preliminary report. Transplant Proc 1987;19:2639–2642.
78. Crawford SW, Schwartz DA, Petersen FB, Clark JG. Mechanical ventilation after marrow transplantation: risk factors and clinical outcome. Am Rev Respir Dis 1988;137:682–687.
79. Crawford SW, Petersen FB. Long-term survival from respiratory failure after marrow transplantation. Am Rev Respir Dis 1992;145:510–514.
80. Chao NJ, Duncan SR, Long GD, Horning SJ, Blume KG. Corticosteroid therapy for diffuse alveolar hemorrhage in autologous bone marrow transplant recipients. Ann Intern Med 1991;114:145–146.
81. Sloane JP, Depledge MH, Powles RL, Morgenstern GR, Trickey BS, Dady PJ. Histopathology of the lung after bone marrow transplantation. J Clin Pathol 1983; 36:546–554.
82. Alexander J, Dainiak N, Berger HJ, et al. Serial assessment of doxorubicin cardiotoxicity with quantitative radionuclide angiocardiography. N Engl J Med 1979; 300:278–283.
83. Henderson IC, Frei E. Adriamycin and the heart. N Engl J Med 1979;300:310–311.
84. Gottdiener JS, Mathisen DJ, Borer JS, et al. Doxorubicin cardiotoxicity: assessment of late left ventricular dysfunction by radionuclide cineangiography. Ann Intern Med 1981;94:430–435.
85. Appelbaum FR, Strauchen JA, Graw RG. Acute lethal carditis caused by high-dose combination therapy. Lancet 1976;7950:58–62.
86. Gottdiener JS, Appelbaum FR, Ferrans VJ, et al. Cardiotoxicity associated with high-dose cyclophosphamide therapy. Arch Intern Med 1981;141:758–763.
87. Trigg ME, Finlay JL, Bozdech M, Gilbert E. Fatal cardiac toxicity in bone marrow transplant patients receiving cytosine arabinoside, cyclophosphamide, and total body irradiation. Cancer 1987;59:38–42.
88. Baello EB, Ensberg ME, Ferguson DW, et al. Effect of high-dose cyclophosphamide and total-body irradiation on left ventricular function in adult patients with leukemia undergoing allogeneic bone marrow transplantation. Cancer Treat Rep 1986;70:1187–1193.
89. McDonald GB, Sharma P, Matthews DE, Shulman HM, Thomas ED. Venocclusive disease of the liver after bone marrow transplantation: diagnosis, incidence, and predisposing factors. Hepatology 1984;4:116–122.
90. Robbins RA, Linder J, Stahl MG, et al. Diffuse alveolar hemorrhage in autologous bone marrow transplant recipients. Am J Med 1989;87:511–518.
91. Hertz MI, Englund JA, Snover D, Bitterman PB, McGlave PB. Respiratory syncytial virus-induced acute lung injury in adult patients with bone marrow transplants: a clinical approach and review of the literature. Medicine 1989;68:269–281.
92. Ljungman P, Gleaves CA, Meyers JD. Respiratory virus infections in immunocompromised patients. Bone Marrow Transplant 1989;4:35–40.
93. Wendt CH, Weisdorf DJ, Jordan MC, Balfour HH, Hertz MI. Parainfluenza virus respiratory infection after bone marrow transplantation. N Engl J Med 1992;326:921–926.
94. Emanuel D, Peppard J, Stover D, Gold J, Armstrong D, Hammerling U. Rapid immunodiagnosis of cytomegalovirus pneumonia by bronchoalveolar lavage using human and murine monoclonal antibodies. Ann Intern Med 1986;104:476–481.
95. Holland HK, Wingard JR, Beschorner WE, Saral R, Santos GW. Bronchiolitis obliterans in bone marrow transplantation and its relationship to chronic graft-v-host disease and low serum IgG. Blood 1988;72:621–627.
96. Ralph DD, Springmeyer SC, Sullivan KM, et al. Rapidly progressive airflow obstruction in marrow transplant recipients. Am Rev Respir Dis 1984;129:641–644.
97. Kurzrock R, Sanders A, Kanojia M, et al. Obstructive lung disease after allogeneic marrow transplantation. Transplantation 1984;37:156–169.
98. Witherspoon RP, Storb R, Ochs HD, et al. Recovery of

antibody production in human allogeneic marrow graft recipients: influence of time post-transplantation, presence or absence of chronic graft-versus-host disease, and antithymocyte globulin treatment. Blood 1981; 58:360–368.

99. Clark JG, Crawford SW, Madtes DK, Sullivan KM. Obstructive lung disease after allogeneic marrow transplantation: clinical presentation and course. Ann Intern Med 1989;111:368–376.

100. Urbanski SJ, Kossakowska AE, Curtis J, et al. Idiopathic small airways pathology in patients with graft-versus-host disease following allogeneic bone marrow transplantation. Am J Surg Pathol 1987;11:965–971.

101. Glanville AR, Baldwin JC, Burke CM, et al. Obliterative bronchiolitis after heart-lung transplantation: apparent arrest by augmented immunosuppression. Ann Intern Med 1987;107:300–304.

102. Sullivan KM, Kopecky KJ, Jocom J, et al. Immunomodulatory and antimicrobial efficacy of intravenous immunoglobulin in bone marrow transplantation. N Engl J Med 1990;323:705–712.

103. Hackman RC, Madtes DK, Petersen FB, Clark JG. Pulmonary veno-occlusive disease following bone marrow transplantation. Transplantation 1989;47:989–992.

104. Troussard X, Bernaudin JF, Cordonnier C, et al. Pulmonary veno-occlusive disease after bone marrow transplantation. Thorax 1984;39:956–957.

105. Lombard CM, Churg A, Winokur S. Pulmonary veno-occlusive disease following therapy for malignant neoplasms. Chest 1987;92:871–876.

106. Allen BT, Day DL, Dehner LP. CT demonstration of asymptomatic pulmonary emboli after bone marrow transplantation: case report. Pediatr Radiol 1987; 17:65–67.

107. Sanders JE, Hickman RO, Aker S, Hersman J, Buckner CD, Thomas ED. Experience with double lumen right atrial catheters. J Parenter Enter Nutr 1982;6:95–99.

108. Petersen FB, Clift RA, Hickman RO, et al. Hickman catheter complications in marrow transplant recipients. J Parenter Enter Nutr 1986;10:58–62.

109. Abrahams C, Catchatourian R. Bone fragment emboli in the lungs of patients undergoing bone marrow transplantation. Am J Clin Pathol 1983;79:360–363.

110. Sale GE, Storb R. Bilateral diffuse pulmonary ectopic ossification after marrow allograft in a dog: evidence for allotransplantation of hemopoietic and mesenchymal stem cells. Exp Hematol 1983;11:961–966.

111. Denardo SJ, Oye RK, Bellamy PE. Efficacy of intensive care for bone marrow transplant patients with respiratory failure. Crit Care Med 1989;17:4–6.

112. Torrecilla C, Cortes JL, Chamorro C, Rubio JJ, Dominquez de Villota E. Prognostic assessment of the acute complications of bone marrow transplantation requiring intensive therapy. Intensive Care Med 1988;14:393–398.

113. Schneiderman LJ, Arras JD. Counseling patients to counsel physicians on future care in the event of patient incompetence. Ann Intern Med 1985;102:693–698.

114. Schneiderman LJ, Jecker NS, Jonsen AR. Medical futility: its meaning and clinical implications. Ann Intern Med 1990;112:949–954.

115. American Thoracic Society Bioethics Task Force. Withholding and withdrawing life-sustaining therapy. Am Rev Respir Dis 1991;144:726–731.

Chapter 38
Growth and Development After Bone Marrow Transplantation

Jean E. Sanders

Use of marrow ablative doses of chemotherapy or chemoradiotherapy followed by marrow infusion for an ever-increasing number of children and young adults with malignant and nonmalignant disorders has resulted in an increasing number of long-term disease-free survivors. An understanding of the late effects resulting from the agents used in bone marrow transplantation (BMT) preparative regimens and the treatment received prior to BMT is important to appreciate and anticipate the effects on growth and development after BMT. The agents used in preparatory regimens for BMT are designed to suppress the patient's immune system and to eradicate abnormal cells. Consequently, the doses given are not limited by marrow toxicity. The most common regimens utilize high-dose cyclophosphamide (CY) given alone or in combination with other agents, such as busulfan (BU) or total body irradiation (TBI). Other chemotherapy agents that have been used in preparative regimens include high dose carmustine (BCNU), melphalan, etoposide (VP16), and thiotepa, and other irradiation regimens include thoracoabdominal irradiation (TAI) or total lymphoid irradiation (TLI).

Both chemotherapy and irradiation are known to affect the function of the neuroendocrine system and, therefore, growth and development (1). Endocrine gland secretions act as catalysts to promote normal growth, and normal growth and development require balanced endocrine gland function. Growth- and maturation-promoting hormones include growth hormone (GH), thyroid hormones, androgens, and estrogens. The adrenal glucocorticoids are antagonistic to growth.

This chapter reviews the effects of the agents used in BMT preparative regimens on the endocrine system and the subsequent effects on growth and development.

Thyroid Function

Conventional chemotherapy does not impair thyroid function, but irradiation to the thyroid gland has been associated with development of compensated hypothyroidism, overt hypothyroidism, thyroiditis, and thyroid neoplasms (2). After irradiation, the onset of thyroid dysfunction begins as asymptomatic compensated hypothyroidism within the first year in 30 to 55% of children and progresses to overt hypothyroidism over the next several decades. The presence of hypothyroidism contributes to diminished linear growth in young children. Among 1,677 patients treated with 7.5 to 44 Gy mantle radiotherapy for Hodgkin's disease, the actuarial risk for development of thyroid disease at 20 years was 52%; incidence was 67% 26 years after irradiation exposure (3). The risk for development of thyroid malignancies was 1.7% beyond 19 years, which was significantly greater than the expected risk of 0.07% in normal age-matched control subjects (3).

Chemotherapy Preparative Regimens

Following BMT, thyroid function has most frequently been evaluated by determination of thyroid-stimulating hormone (TSH) and thyroxine (T4) plasma levels. Other studies less often performed include free T4, T3, resin T3 uptake (RT_3U), and TSH response to thyrotropin-stimulating hormone. Results of reported studies, (Table 38-1) show that chemotherapy regimens including CY, BU plus CY, and other chemotherapy agents plus CY have not resulted in the development of thyroid function abnormalities (4–7). Idiopathic thyroiditis developed at age 14 (10 years after BMT) in one child of 50 transplanted for severe aplastic anemia after a preparative regimen with CY (200 mg/kg) (4). None of the thyroid function studies demonstrated an etiology for the thyroiditis. Because the incidence of idiopathic thyroiditis in normal school age children is approximately 1%, it is probable that this patient's thyroiditis was a random event.

Irradiation Preparative Regimens

Compensated hypothyroidism and overt hypothyroidism often occur following any irradiation-containing preparative regimen (TLI or TBI) (4,7–9). Among 143 children given 7.5 Gy single-exposure TLI or 7.8 to 10.0 Gy single-exposure TBI, compensated hypothyroidism

Table 38-1.
Thyroid Function after Bone Marrow Transplantation

	TSH[a] *(% abnormal)*	T_4 *(% abnormal)*	*Median Follow-up (Yr)*	*Reference*
Chemotherapy preparative regimens				
CY	1/50 (2%)	1/50 (2%)	9	4
BU + CY	0/39	0/30	2	5, 6, 7
Other[4] + CY	0/5	0/5	2	6
Total lymphoid irradiation				
CY + 7.5 Gy (single exposure)	11/27 (41%)	0/27	5	8
Total body irradiation				
CY + 7.8–8.8 Gy (single exposure)	9/26 (35%)	0/26	5	8
CY + 10.0 Gy (single exposure)	10/23 (56%)	2/23 (9%)	3	9
CY + 9.5–10.0 Gy (single exposure)	19/67 (28%)	9/67 (13%)	8	4, 7
CY + 12.0–15.75 Gy Fractionated	13/113 (12%)	3/113 (3%)	4	4, 7
CY + 13.75 Gy Fractionated	0/18	0/18	3	8

[a]Number of patients with abnormal values/total number studies.
[b]Other includes carmustine, cytarabine, 6-TG, and melphalan.
TSH = thyroid stimulating hormone; T_4 = thyroxine; CY = cyclophosphamide; BU = busulfan.

developed in 28 to 56%, and overt hypothyroidism developed in 9 to 13% (see Table 38-1). These findings are in contrast to the 10 to 14% incidence of compensated hypothyroidism and less than 5% overt hypothyroidism observed among 131 children after 12.0 to 15.75 Gy fractionated TBI. In these longitudinal studies, patients receiving single-exposure TBI have usually been followed more than 5 years after irradiation exposure, whereas those given fractionated exposure TBI have usually been followed less than a median of 4 years after irradiation. Although fractionated TBI appears to result in less development of thyroid function abnormalities, data from nontransplant irradiation studies indicate a risk for development of thyroid dysfunction over many years (3). The development of abnormal thyroid function was not associated with sex, age at transplant, or occurrence of acute or chronic graft-versus-host disease (GVHD). More detailed evaluation of the hypothalamic-pituitary-thyroid neuroendocrine axis with free thyroxine, RT_3U, thyrotropin-stimulating hormone, and microsomal and thyroglobulin antibody has demonstrated that the major effect of irradiation is at the level of the end organ (thyroid gland) and not at the level of the hypothalamus or the pituitary gland (7). Autoimmune thyroiditis developed 4 years after BMT in one patient transplanted after CY and 3.0 Gy TBI for severe aplastic anemia (10). It was discovered that the patient's marrow donor had compensated autoimmune thyroiditis. Studies of patient and donor T and B cells led to the speculation that this autoimmune disorder was transferred from the donor to the recipient. This problem developed in no other patient following BMT, including those with chronic GVHD.

Treatment

All patients in whom overt hypothyroidism develops should receive treatment with thyroxine, but the benefit of thyroid replacement in patients with compensated hypothyroidism is unclear. Although the carcinogenic potential of thyroid irradiation has been well documented, the ability of thyroid replacement to reduce the incidence of radiation-associated thyroid carcinoma is unproven (2,3). Recommendations from pediatric endocrinologists vary with respect to treatment of compensated hypothyroidism after irradiation therapy. Among patients in whom benign thyroid nodules developed after conventional irradiation therapy, treatment with thyroxine decreases the risk of recurrence of these nodules but does not decrease the risk of thyroid carcinoma (11). Thyroid masses (4 papillary carcinoma, one toxic goiter, and one adenoma) developed in at least 6 children with untreated abnormal thyroid function between 4 and 14 years after single 10.0 Gy exposure TBI in 5 patients and 7 years after 15.75 Gy fractionated exposure TBI. The adenoma was found at autopsy, but the other 5 patients have been treated successfully with thyroidectomy for 4 and radioactive iodine thyroid ablation for one. All 5 are receiving replacement therapy with thyroid hormone. All patients should be evaluated annually with physical examinations and tests of thyroid function.

Growth

Height growth is a continuous and finely regulated phenomenon that in infancy is determined largely by nutrition, in childhood by GH, and in puberty by the synergistic action of GH and sex steroids (1). Thus, GH has a major role in the growth process. Conventional chemotherapy may result in subnormal growth due to an effect on the GH-somatomedin-chondrocyte axis, but GH studies have not been performed consistently. Data are conflicting as to whether intensive chemotherapy regimens with or without the use of prophylactic cranial irradiation are associated with persistant growth impairment because often only growth rates are reported (12–16). Diminished bone formation and reduced osteoblast function has been observed in animal models after administration of chemotherapeutic agents (17).

Because GH secretion is episodic, determination of GH levels usually involves a stimulus to enhance pituitary GH secretion, followed by multiple venous blood samplings. Commonly used stimuli include exercise; sleep; or pharmacological agents such as clonidine, levodopa, arginine, and insulin. Failure to attain a normal circulating GH level after two stimuli defines classic GH deficiency. Children who have received cranial irradiation have had variable responses to the provocative stimuli used, which may be due to the use of different pharmacological agents, variations in the interval between irradiation and testing, or neurosecretory defects (18–20). Although the 24-hour spontaneous pulsatile GH secretion test is considered to be the most physiological assessment of GH secretion, it is impractical due to the large volumes of blood required (5 mL every 20 min for 24 hr) (21,22). The 12-hour overnight sampling schedule has been shown to be well tolerated, reliable, and reproducible (23).

Chemotherapy Preparative Regimens

Normal growth rates have been reported in long-term studies of children who received BMT preparative regimen with CY only (24). When tested, these children always had normal GH levels. Some children with chronic GVHD requiring treatment with corticosteroids did have decreased growth velocity during the time of disease activity. However, once chronic GVHD was controlled, growth rates returned to normal and "catch up" growth was observed.

BU, an alkylating agent frequently combined with CY in BMT preparative regimens, is an agent that effects dividing as well as nondividing cells and is known to cross the blood-brain barrier (25,26). Data on the effect of BU on growth velocity as well as GH secretion are just now becoming available. Among 35 girls and 45 boys transplanted for thalassemia major following a preparative regimen of 14 mg/kg BU plus 200 mg/kg CY, those 9 years of age or less at BMT had normal growth velocity, whereas those 10 to 12 years of age at BMT demonstrated decreased growth velocity with no pubescent growth spurt (5). Follow-up of a total of 35 children during the first 3 years after administration of 16 mg/kg BU plus 200 mg/kg CY and BMT for leukemia demonstrated decreasing growth velocity (7,27). All had progressive decrease in standardized height growth with increasing years after BMT (Table 38-2). GH deficiency was present in 6 of 11 patients in one series but in none of 7 in another series of patients transplanted for leukemia. Methods of GH testing differed between these two studies, and not all patients had GH testing in one. These early results show that recipients of BU-containing preparative regimens will require careful follow-up, with special attention to growth and occurrence of GH deficiency. Additional patients with longer follow-up are needed for definitive determination of the effect of BU on GH deficiency and growth velocity.

Table 38-2.
Standardized Height Growth

	Preparative Regimen			
	N	*BU + CY*[a,b]	*N*	*CY + TBI*[a,c]
Before transplantation	35	−0.2	88	−0.4
Year + 1	35	−0.6	88	−0.6
Year + 2	26	−0.90	50	−0.90
Year + 3	1	−1.4	20	−1.6
Year + 4	...	...	13	−1.8
Year + 5	...	...	10	−2.0
Year + 6	...	...	6	−2.3
Year + 8	...	...	4	−3.2

[a]Values expressed as standard deviation Z scores.
[b]Data from references 7 and 27.
[c]Data from references 7, 27, 29, and 30.
BU = busulfan; CY = cyclophosphamide; TBI = total body irradiation.

Central Nervous System Irradiation

Central nervous system (CNS) irradiation has been associated with the development of GH deficiency, which appears to be related to the child's age at time of irradiation, the radiation dose received, and the length of time after irradiation (18). Many children referred for BMT have received 18 to 24 Gy CNS irradiation prior to BMT. When TBI is included in the preparative regimen, the total CNS irradiation dose will usually exceed 30 Gy, the estimated threshold for development of GH deficiency (28). GH deficiency may be expected to develop in the majority of patients who receive this total dose of CNS irradiation 2 to 3 years after irradiation, whereas GH deficiency may not develop in patients who receive lower doses of CNS irradiation for 5 to 10 years after irradiation. Thus, it may be expected that nearly all children who have received CNS irradiation in addition to TBI are likely to experience development of GH deficiency, but GH deficiency may not develop in those who receive only TBI until just prior to or after their growth period, depending on their age at TBI.

Irradiation Preparative Regimens

Growth hormone levels after TBI-containing preparative regimens and BMT have been determined for more than 200 children following stimulation with insulin, arginine, levodopa, glucagon, or clonidine, or by sleep (12-hour overnight spontaneous secretion) (4,7,24,27,29–31). Studies were usually performed from 1 to 8 years (median, 2 yr) after TBI and BMT. Overall, more than half were reported to have subnormal GH levels. Less than half who had not received prior cranial irradiation demonstrated GH deficiency.

In addition, during the first 2 years after BMT, those without chronic GVHD grew significantly better than those with chronic GVHD (31). This finding may be due to chronic GVHD itself or to the therapy with corticosteroids. None of these patients demonstrated "catch-up" growth after treatment was stopped and chronic GVHD was no longer active. Whereas one explanation may be related to the growth-suppressive effects of glucocorticoids, failure to achieve "catch-up" growth after completion of treatment suggests that other factors, such as GH deficiency and irradiation to the long bones, may also contribute to poor growth.

Height velocity with respect to time after BMT has been determined utilizing standard deviation (SD) Z scores calculated for height (height minus mean height for age and sex) divided by the SD of height for age and sex for a total of 98 TBI recipients and 35 BU-CY recipients (see Table 38-2) (7,27,29,30). Combined results of each of these separate studies demonstrate that with each additional year after TBI, the height Z score (standardized height growth) progressively decreases. By 5 years after TBI, all patients were more than 2 SD below the mean, and at 8 years more than 3 to 4 SD below the mean. It appears as though patients receiving BU-CY may have the same pattern of a progressive decrease in standardized height growth during the first 2 to 3 years after BMT, which does not differ substantially from that observed for TBI patients (7,27).

Evaluation of growth velocity in centimeters growth in height per year plotted according to chronological age on standardized growth velocity curves has consistently demonstrated progressive decrease in velocity with increasing patient age (Figure 38-1) (7). Among 112 girls, 30 had received 10.0 Gy single-exposure TBI and 82 had received 12.0 to 15.75 Gy fractionated TBI; of 154 boys, 48 received 10.0 Gy TBI and 106 received fractionated TBI. Growth velocity was similar for both groups of patients and did not differ with respect to whether cranial irradiation had or had not been given. Also, the type of TBI administered (single or fractionated exposure) had no major effect on growth velocity (see Figure 38-1). Growth rates were at or below the 3rd percentile at most ages, and no pubescent growth spurt was observed. Among 56 children less than 11 years of age at BMT, final median adult height is less than the 10th percentile for both boys and girls (Table 38-3). Among 87 patients 11 to 16 years of age at BMT, median final height achieved for 21 girls and 46 boys is near the 50th percentile for sex.

Treatment

GH can stimulate growth of epiphyseal cartilage and subsequent bone growth directly via the action of insulin-like growth factor-I (IGF-I). When insufficient GH is secreted, growth velocity and bone maturation are retarded, and the divergence of the growth rate from normal increases with age unless replacement therapy is initiated. Studies of children with hypopituitarism have shown that the final height achieved is related to height at the start of treatment (32). The total height gained from GH therapy has been shown to be inversely related to patient age at the start of treatment and positively related to duration of therapy. Treatment started before the child's height drops below the 3rd percentile results in the greatest final height in response to GH treatment. Because growth before puberty has been demonstrated to be the major determinant of final height, treatment with GH during this period should be optimized. After cranial irradiation, GH deficiency may develop in children with previously normal GH secretion at the time of puberty due to an inability to produce an increased amount of GH to promote the growth spurt (33,34). In addition, BMT patients also have the problem of impaired gonadal function (7,24,31). At the time of puberty, use of low-dose sex hormone treatment along with GH may result in improved height velocity and final height (35).

Despite documentation of GH deficiency and decreased growth rates, relatively few children have

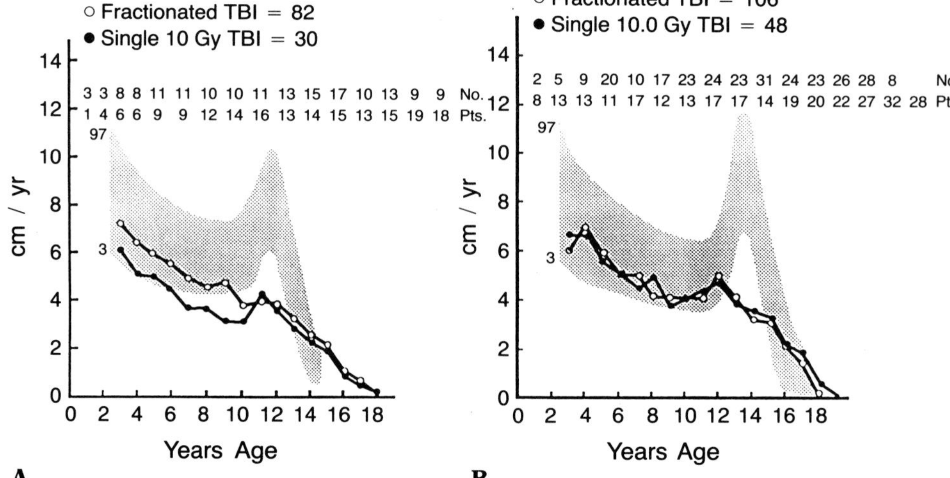

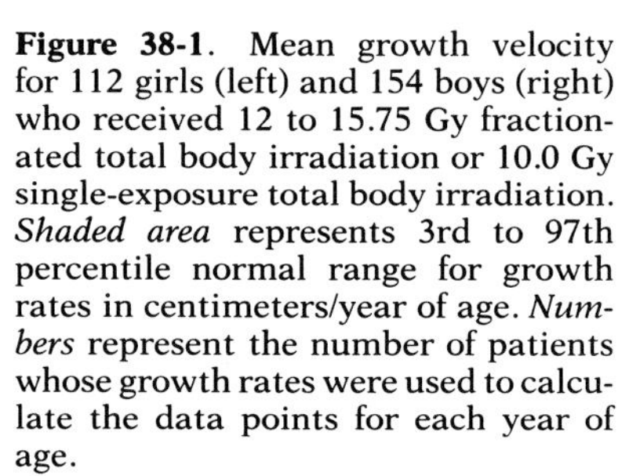

Figure 38-1. Mean growth velocity for 112 girls (left) and 154 boys (right) who received 12 to 15.75 Gy fractionated total body irradiation or 10.0 Gy single-exposure total body irradiation. *Shaded area* represents 3rd to 97th percentile normal range for growth rates in centimeters/year of age. *Numbers* represent the number of patients whose growth rates were used to calculate the data points for each year of age.

Table 38-3.
Final Adult Height

	N	*Girls*	*N*	*Boys*
United States standards				
Height percentile				
Centimeters: 10th–90th (50th)		156.3–169.4 (162.5)		166.3–182.4 (174.5)
Inches: 10th–90th (50th)		61.5–66.7 (64.0)		65.5–71.8 (68.7)
TBI recipients				
Age at TBI ≤10 years	27		29	
Centimeters: range (median)		129.5–162.6 (152.4)		129.5–167.6 (147.5)
Inches: range (median)		51–64 (60)		51–66 (62)
Age at TBI 11–17 years	21		46	
Centimeters: range (median)		129.5–167.5 (162.5)		152.4–182.9 (167.6)
Inches: range (median)		51–66 (64)		60–72 (66)

TBI = total body irradiation.

received therapy with GH supplementation after BMT (7,36). Those children treated with GH have not demonstrated the "catch-up" growth response that has been observed among nonirradiated GH-deficient patients. However, therapy did appear to improve height velocity SD score from -0.13 to +2.2 in one series of 13 children treated for 2 years (35). In this group, the height SD score did not change, indicating that although "catch-up" growth was not observed, further negative deviation from normal did not occur. The median age at start of treatment was 12.2 years, which may account for the relatively blunted response. Studies of early GH treatment during the pretransplant period have not been reported. When studied, IGF-I levels have usually been low or low-normal in most of the patients with GH deficiency, although this level has not correlated well with growth rates during the first 2 years after BMT (7,37).

Initially, treatment with human GH was limited due to the limited supply of the drug. However, with the availability of recombinant GH, this is no longer a problem. Reports of leukemia occurring in patients treated with human GH raised concern that there might be a causal relationship between GH therapy and development of leukemia (38–40). The Lawson Wilkins Pediatric Endocrine Society and the Human Growth Foundation of the United States convened a workshop in 1988 to review known leukemia cases in 22,000 GH-treated patients in Europe, North America, Japan, and Australia since 1959 (41). Of 15 cases of leukemia, 4 occurred after a brief period of GH therapy or there were compelling reasons to suspect another cause for the leukemia. The 11 suspect cases developed during 150,000 patient-years of risk, including the periods of treatment and follow-up, so that the incidence of leukemia was aproximately 1 per 21,000 patient-years of risk. The expected annual leukemia incidence among hypopituitary patients treated was estimated to be 1 per 42,000 patient-years. After review of all available data, workshop participants concluded that there may be a small increase in leukemia incidence associated with GH treatment of GH-deficient patients; however, it was not clear that this incidence was directly related to GH therapy. In absolute terms, a current estimate of individual risk, assuming a 10-year GH treatment course, would be 1 per 2,400 (0.042%), which is not different from the SEER estimate of new cases of leukemia reported in the United States (1 per 2,400/year). Thus, treatment of GH-deficient children after BMT should not contribute significantly to an increased risk of leukemia.

Oral-facial Growth

Irradiation to bone produces epiphyseal, metaphyseal, and diaphyseal injury which affects subsequent bone growth (42). The effect is related to patient age at the time of irradiation as well as the site irradiated, the dose schedule, and the total dose of irradiation (43). Irradiation to the head and neck of growing children, especially those less than 6 years of age, results in altered growth of the facial skeleton (44). Cephalometric measurements of facial bones have been used to study facial growth before and after TBI and BMT. When results obtained from the TBI patients were compared with measurements obtained from healthy age-matched nontransplant children, the TBI recipients showed significantly reduced length of both the maxilla and the mandible, which was most pronounced in mandibular growth (45). There was also a significant reduction in vertical growth of the upper face, which was particularly evident in the posterior area, especially in patients less than 6 years of age. Development of secondary teeth was often affected, with delayed or arrested tooth formation, shortening and blunting of tooth roots, incomplete calcification, premature closure of apices, and dental caries (46,47). Five children who were GH-deficient and who received treatment with GH were studied at time of initiation of GH therapy and after 1 to 2 years of therapy (48). GH therapy appeared to have a stimulating influence on mandibular growth, with increases in mandibular length that exceeded corresponding values of those not given GH by 150%. There was also improved vertical growth of the condyles, suggesting that condylar cartilage is the most likely site of mandibular growth activity. GH promotes longitudinal bone growth by stimulating differentiation of epiphyseal plate precursor cells and increases responsiveness to IGF-I. Treatment with GH, however, did not improve the disturbed root development of the teeth. Thus, the stimulating effect of dental development on the growth of the alveolar processes was absent.

Puberty

Puberty is accompanied by significant changes in hormonal activity, secondary sexual characteristics, and growth velocity. The normal pubertal growth rate is 1.5 to 2.0 times greater than the prepubertal growth rate (49). In the absence of pubertal sex hormone secretion, the increased growth velocity associated with the pubertal growth spurt does not occur, and development of secondary sexual characteristics is delayed or absent. Gonadal hormone production and germ-cell viability are affected by high doses of alkylating agents and irradiation, with variables related to patient age, sex, and type and dose of therapy (50). Azoospermia develops in prepubertal boys who have received a cumulative dose of greater than 350 mg/kg CY, whereas doses of 200 mg/kg or less result in minimal alteration of spermatogenesis. The effects of high-dose BU on the prepubertal testes have not been reported. Irradiation to the prepubertal testes results in damage to the germinal epithelium that does not become apparent until after puberty (51). Boys who received more than 24 Gy testicular irradiation have had delayed or arrested development of secondary sexual characteristics, with elevated gonadotropin and low testosterone values. Primary ovarian failure usually occurs following total cumulative doses of more than 500 mg/kg CY to prepubertal girls (50). No data are available regarding delayed effects of high-dose BU or irradiation on the prepubertal ovary.

Sex hormones indirectly stimulate linear growth by increasing endogenous GH secretion (52). This stimulation leads to increasing circulating and tissue levels of IGF-I, which activates growth at the level of bone and cartilage. Treatment with low-to-moderate doses of sex hormones promotes increased linear growth, but high doses of sex hormones result in a greater influence on skeletal maturation with resultant compromise in final adult height via the mechanism of premature epiphyseal closure. Children with idiopathic GH deficiency usually have a late but normal pubertal growth spurt. Children with hypogonadotropic hypogonadism have an absence of sex hormone production, delayed puberty, delayed pubertal growth spurt, and an increase in final adult height (35). Thus, interruption in either production of pubertal GH or sex hormone production is likely to result in both delayed pubescence and decreased linear height.

Chemotherapy Preparative Regimens

Following high-dose CY and BMT for aplastic anemia, 20 of 23 girls and 17 of 21 boys who were prepubertal at time of administration of CY and have now been followed long enough to be more than 12 years of age have nearly all demonstrated normal development of secondary sexual characteristics (Tables 38-4, 38-5) (24,53). Among these 20 girls, menarche occurred between 11 to 16 (median, 13) years of age for 19, and one had delayed puberty, with menarche occurring at approximately 18 years of age. All have normal gonadotropin levels. Ovarian function is normal; 10 women have given birth to 14 normal children (see Table 38-4). Among the 17 boys, development was delayed for 2. Leydig cell function was normal for all, but 2 had evidence of Sertoli cell damage with elevated follicle-stimulating hormone (FSH). Semen analysis demonstrated normal sperm counts in 5 and azoospermia in 2. Seven of these men have fathered 10 normal children (see Table 38-5).

Gonadal function after 14 mg/kg BU plus 200 mg/kg CY and allogeneic BMT for thalassemia has been reported for 30 prepubertal patients (15 girls, 15 boys) who ranged in age from 9.3 to 17.2 years (54). Thirteen girls had evidence of primary ovarian failure, with increased gonadotropin levels (see Table 38-4), and 2 patients had hypogonadotropic hypogonadism. All girls had low estradiol levels both before and after transplantation. Among the 15 boys, post-transplant luteinizing hormone (LH) and FSH concentrations were within the normal range. However, after gonadotropin-releasing hormone stimulation, 3 had

Table 38-4.
Pubertal Development—Girls

	Preparative Regimen		
	CY[a]	*BU CY*[b]	*CY + TBI*[c]
Prepuberty at transplant	23	15	58
Current age			
< 12 years	3	...	16
≥ 12 years	20	15	42
Development			
Normal	19	ND	12
Delayed	1	ND	30
LH: prepubertal	...	2	
Normal	20	...	12
Elevated	...	13	30
FSH: prepubertal	...	2	...
Normal	20	0	12
Elevated	...	13	30
Estradiol			
Normal	20	...	12
Low	...	15	30
Pregnancies			
Number Girls	10	...	...
Number Live Births	14	...	...
Hormone supplement	0	ND	9

[a]Data from references 24 and 53.
[b]Data from reference 54.
[c]Data from references 7 and 53.
CY = cyclophosphamide; BU = busulfan; TBI = total body irradiation; ND = no data; LH = luteinizing hormone; FSH = follicle stimulating hormone.

Table 38-5.
Pubertal Development—Boys

	Preparative Regimen		
	CY[a]	*BU-CY*[b]	*CY + TBI*[c]
Prepuberty at transplant	21	15	93
Current Age			
≤ 12 years	4	...	28
> 12 years	17	15	65
Development			
Normal	14	ND	14
Delayed	2	ND	51
LH: prepubertal		10	...
Normal	17	3	52
Elevated	0	2	13
FSH: prepubertal		10	
Normal	15	3	35
Elevated	2	2	30
Testosterone			
Normal	17		5
Low	0	15	60
Children fathered			
Number men	7	...	...
Number children	10	...	...
Hormone supplement	...	ND	17

[a]Data from references 24 and 53.
[b]Data from reference 54.
[c]Data from references 7 and 53.
CY = cyclophosphamide; BU = busulfan; TBI = total body irradiation; ND = no data; LH = luteinizing hormone; FSH = follicle stimulating hormone.

normal responses, 2 had elevated FSH responses, and 10 had lower LH or FSH responses than the prepubertal control subjects with normal gonadal function. Responses to stimulation with gonadotropin-releasing hormone were reduced for 12 of the 15 boys. These gonadal function results must be interpreted with caution, however, because patients with thalassemia major treated with chelation and transfusion frequently show delayed or absent puberty.

TBI Preparative Regimens

Following TBI, delayed development of secondary sexual characteristics has been observed in 30 of 42 girls and in 51 of 65 boys currently 12 years of age or older (see Tables 38-4, 38-5) (7,53). Those with delayed puberty all had elevated gonadotropin levels and subnormal sex hormone levels, indicating primary gonadal failure. Among the boys, all 18 with testicular irradiation in addition to TBI had testicular failure requiring hormone supplementation for development of secondary sexual characteristics. The 14 boys in whom secondary sexual characteristics developed at an appropriate age had received fractionated TBI rather than single-dose TBI. Among the 12 girls in whom secondary sexual characteristics developed within an appropriate age range, 6 had received 10.0 Gy single-exposure TBI and 6 had received 12.0 Gy fractionated TBI. None of the girls have become pregnant, and none of the young men have fathered children.

It is recommended that the development of secondary sexual characteristics be monitored carefully after patients reach 11 years of age and that Tanner Developmental Scores be determined annually. Because normal production of sex hormones is necessary for promotion of the pubertal growth spurt in addition to promoting sexual maturation, children with evidence of gonadal failure and delayed development of secondary sexual characteristics may benefit from supplementation with sex hormones. This supplementation should be achieved with gradually increasing sex hormone doses to prevent premature advancement of bone age. These patients also should have growth rates carefully followed and should have GH determinations performed.

Gonadal Function After Puberty

Alkylating agent therapy administered to adult women may impair reproductive function (55). Ovarian atrophy has been observed following treatment with BU (56). After CY, ovarian biopsies have demonstrated loss of ova, which suggests that CY acts directly on the oocyte (57). The reversibility of this loss of ova is related to patient age and the total dose of CY received. Because CY acts by first-order kinetics and the number of oocytes normally decreases steadily with increasing age, equivalent drug doses in older patients whose ova are more depleted than those of younger patients may explain why the likelihood of infertility is increased in older women. For example, a cumulative total dose of 5.2 gm CY given to a 40-year-old woman will result in ovarian failure, whereas a cumulative total dose of 20 gm given to a woman 25 years of age is needed to produce ovarian failure (57).

The predominant gonadal lesion after alkylating agent therapy in adult men is localized to the germinal epithelium (58). Testicular biopsies from men treated with CY have demonstrated Sertoli cell damage, with germinal aplasia and absent spermatogonia and spermatozoa (59,60). This level of damage is usually reflected in an elevated FSH level and azoospermia. Leydig cell function is spared, as evidenced by normal LH and testosterone levels. The degree of testicular function compromise is related to total dose of CY, but age does not appear to be a factor. Azoospermia develops in patients who receive more than a cumulative total dose of 18 gm CY, but oligospermia develops in those who receive less than 250 mg/kg CY given as low doses of CY for short periods; this condition is often reversible. Recovery of spermatogenesis may occur after a period of a year or more.

Chemotherapy Preparative Regimens

Women

Ovarian function has been evaluated in 65 women between 13 and 38 years of age at time of receiving 200 mg/kg CY and BMT for aplastic anemia (53,61–64). All women had normal menstrual periods prior to CY administration and therefore were considered as having normal ovarian function. Follow-up studies with measurement of FSH, LH, and estradiol as well as histories of menstruation, constitutional symptoms related to menopause, and hormone replacement therapy administered were obtained 1 to 13 (median, 3 yr) years after BMT (Table 38-6) (53,61–64). All women less than 26 years of age at time of CY administration had evidence of ovarian function recovery; gonadotropin levels returned to normal and menstruation returned between 0.25 and 3 (median, 0.75 yr) years after BMT. Seven of 19 women 26 to 38 years of age never demonstrated evidence of ovarian recovery but had primary ovarian failure, with elevated LH and FSH levels as well as low estradiol levels. These women received estrogen/progesterone cyclic hormone supplementation. Chronic GVHD was not a factor associated with ovarian recovery or fertility. Twenty-four pregnancies for 17 women resulted in 19 live births and 5 abortions.

After a BMT preparative regimen with BU plus CY, 50 women were evaluated for return of ovarian function (see Table 38-6). None of these women evaluated 1 to 2 years after BMT demonstrated return of normal ovarian function. All have LH and FSH levels elevated in the menopausal range and all have low estradiol levels, indicating primary ovarian failure. These women have symptoms of ovarian failure, which have been controlled with cyclic hormone supplementation.

Table 38-6.
Ovarian Function in Postpubertal Women

	Preparative Regimen			
	CY[a]	*BU + CY*	*CY + TAI/TLI*[b]	*CY + TBI*[c]
Number women	65	50	3	380
Age at transplant (yr)	13–38	15–45	15–22	13–50
Years follow-up	1–13	1–4	1–5	1–12
LH-FSH levels				
Normal Elevated	58	0	1	8
Elevated	7	50	2	372
Estradiol levels				
Normal	58	0	1	8
Low	7	50	2	372
Menstruation				
Absent	7	50	1	372
Time to recovery (yr)	0.25–3.0 (0.75)	...	3	3–7 (5)
Pregnancies				
Number women	17	...	1	7
Number live births	19	...	1	4
Number abortions	5	...	...	5

[a]Data from references 53, 61, 62, 63, and 64.
[b]Data from references 63 and 65.
[c]Data from reference 53, 61, 63, and 66.
CY = cyclophosphamide; BU = busulfan; TAI = thoracoabdominal irradiation; TLI = total lymphoid irradiation; TBI = total body irradiation; LH = luteinizing hormone; FSH = follicle stimulating hormone.

Table 38-7.
Testicular Function in Postpubertal Men

	Preparative Regimen		
	CY	*BU + CY*	*CY + TBI*
Number Men	82	34	417
Age at transplant (yr)	14–41 (22)	13–39 (28)	13–57 (30)
Years follow-up	1–15 (4)	1–3 (1)	1–17 (4)
LH levels			
Normal	79	32	334
Elevated	3	2	83
FSH levels			
Normal	72	2	41
Elevated	10	32	376
Testosterone levels			
Normal	81	ND	ND
Low	1	ND	ND
Semen analysis			
Normal	28	1	5
Azoospermia	3	4	318
Not done	34	29	94
Children fathered			
Number men	18	1	5
Number children	27	1	9

[a]Data from references 53 and 63.
CY = cyclophosphamide; BU = busulfan; TBI = total body irradiation; LH = luteinizing hormone; FSH = follicle stimulating hormone; ND = no data.

Men

Testicular function has been evaluated in 82 men between 1 to 15 (median, 4 yr) years after 200 mg/kg CY and BMT (Table 38-7) (53). Follow-up studies demonstrated that Leydig cell function was normal in more than 95% with normal LH and normal testosterone values. Sertoli cell function was normal in most; FSH levels were normal in 87%. Eighteen of these men have fathered 27 children, all of whom are reported normal.

Following a preparative regimen of BU (16 mg/kg) and CY (120 or 200 mg/kg), 34 men had testicular function studied between 1 and 3 years after BMT (53). LH levels were normal for the majority, but FSH levels were elevated for 32 of 34 men. Semen analysis demonstrated that one of 5 men who submitted specimens for analysis had return of spermatogenesis; this man has fathered a child 2 years after transplantation.

Thoracoabdominal Irradiation Preparative Regimens

Women

Three women ages 15 to 22 at time of BMT have been evaluated after BMT preparative regimens containing TAI (63,65). All 3 had evidence for primary ovarian failure for the first 3 years after TAI, with elevated LH and FSH and low estradiol levels. The one patient followed for more than 3 years recovered ovarian function approximately 4 years after BMT, became pregnant, and delivered a normal child.

Total Body Irradiation Preparative Regimens

Women

From 1 to 12 years after a BMT preparative regimen containing TBI, 380 women have been evaluated for return of ovarian function (53,61,63,66). These patients were 13 to 45 years of age at BMT and all were menstruating prior to initiation of the preparative regimen. After BMT, ovarian failure developed in all women for at least 3 to 6 years as determined by elevated LH, and FSH levels, low estradiol levels, and amenorrhea. Between 3 to 7 (median, 5 yr) years after BMT, 10 women demonstrated ovarian recovery, with return of LH, FSH, and estradiol levels to normal. All women with ovarian recovery were less than 26 years of age at time of BMT. The majority of women who recovered received 12.0 Gy fractionated TBI, although 3 women received 10.0 Gy single-exposure TBI. A total of 9 pregnancies occurred among 6 women, resulting in the birth of 4 normal infants and 5 abortions. Information regarding the fetal products of conception are not available. It may be reasonable to expect an increased risk of fetal malformations or abortion, but precise data are not available. Chronic GVHD did not influence recovery of ovarian function. More than half the women with primary ovarian failure experienced symptoms of menopause, with vasomotor instability, insomnia, osteoporosis, vaginitis, and vaginal atrophy (61,67). In addition, women with chronic GVHD are at increased risk for development of vaginal strictures and web formation secondary to vaginal mucosal involvement with chronic GVHD. Vaginal dilation and systemic control of chronic GVHD are necessary, in addition to systemic cyclic estrogen/progestrones, to control symptoms. Because it is not possible to predict which women will recover ovarian function, it is recommended that all receive cyclic hormone therapy beginning approximately 3 months after TBI.

Men

After BMT with TBI-containing preparative regimens, a total of 417 men have been evaluated for return of testicular function between 1 to 12 years after BMT (53). In general, Leydig cell function was preserved, with normal LH and testosterone levels, but Sertoli cell function was damaged, as evidenced by elevated FSH levels in the majority of men studied (see Table 38-7). Of the 323 men who submitted semen for analysis, only 5 demonstrated return of spermatogenesis. These 5 men have fathered 9 normal children. All received 10.0 Gy single-exposure TBI. None of those receiving fractionated TBI demonstrated recovery of spermatogenesis. One study describes a high incidence of sexual dysfunction following TBI for malignant diseases in 51 men, more than half of whom had chronic GVHD (68). The areas of dysfunction included erectile failure, ejaculation problems, and decreased libido.

Summary

These evaluations of endocrine function following BMT demonstrate that the occurrence of abnormalities that may influence subsequent growth and development of children usually do not occur after a preparative regimen of CY. In general, children have normal thyroid function, normal growth rates, and normal pubertal maturation. Among postpubertal women, return of ovarian function depends on the woman's age at the time CY is administered. All women less than 26 years of age experience ovarian function recovery approximately 9 months after CY, whereas older women usually enter early menopause. Patient age does not affect testicular function; most men demonstrate normal gonadal function with normal gonadotropin levels 1 or more years after CY. A total of 70 children have been born to these patients.

Multiple endocrine function abnormalities, which affect normal growth and development of children, frequently occur after BMT regimens that include BU or TBI. Patients are at risk for development of thyroid function abnormalities for many years after TBI, and these patients are also at risk for development of thyroid malignancy. After BU or TBI, growth rates are usually less than normal. GH deficiency develops in many of these patients, but treatment with GH has been infrequent. The final adult height of patients less than 10 years of age when TBI was administered is less than the 10th percentile. Gonadal function damage by BU or TBI results in the majority of patients having delayed onset of puberty. Among postpubertal patients, most women and men have permanent damage to the gonad, with primary ovarian failure or azoospermia. A few patients have experienced ovarian or testicular recovery 3 to 7 years after TBI. Those who recover gonadal function may be fertile. A total of 21 pregnancies have resulted in the birth of 15 normal children.

All patients who receive BMT must have continued long-term follow-up evaluations to detect the occurrence of endocrine gland dysfunction. Initiation of appropriate hormone therapy when abnormal endocrine function is detected may improve the growth and development of children and prevent late effects associated with ovarian failure.

References

1. Lowrey GJ. Growth and development of children. Chicago: Year Book Medical, 1986:
2. Fleming ID, Black TL, Thompson EI, Pratt C, Rao B, Hustu O. Thyroid dysfunction and neoplasia in children receiving neck irradiation for cancer. Cancer 1985; 55:1190–1194.

3. Hancock SL, Cox RS, McDougall R. Thyroid diseases after treatment of Hodgkin's disease. N Engl J Med 1991;325:599–606.
4. Sanders JE, Buckner CD, Sullivan KM, et al. Growth and development after bone marrow transplantation. In: Buckner CD, Gale RP, Lucarelli G, eds. Advances and controversies in thalassemia therapy: bone marrow transplantation and other approaches. New York: Alan R. Liss, 1989:375–382.
5. Manenti F, Galimberti M, Lucarelli G, et al. Growth and endocrine function after bone marrow transplantation for thalassemia. In: Buckner CD, Gale RP, Lucarelli G, eds. Advances and controversies in thalassemia therapy: bone marrow transplantation and other approaches. New York: Alan R. Liss, 1989:273–280.
6. Urban C, Schwingshandl J, Slavc I, et al. Endocrine function after bone marrow transplantation without the use of preparative total body irradiation. Bone Marrow Transplant 1988;3:291–296.
7. Sanders JE. Endocrine problems in children after bone marrow transplant for hematologic malignancies. Bone Marrow Transplant 1991;8:2–4.
8. Katsanis E, Shapiro RS, Robison LL, Haake RJ, Kim T, Pescovitz OH. Thyroid dysfunction following bone marrow transplantation: long-term follow-up of 80 pediatric patients. Bone Marrow Transplant 1990; 5:335–340.
9. Sklar CA, Kim TH, Ramsay NKC. Thyroid dysfunction among long-term survivors of bone marrow transplantation. Am J Med 1982;73:688–694.
10. Wyatt DT, Lum LG, Casper J, Hunter J, Camitta B. Autoimmune thyroiditis after bone marrow transplantation. Bone Marrow Transplant 1990;5:357–361.
11. Fogelfeld L, Wiviott MBT, Shore-Freedman E, et al. Recurrence of thyroid nodules after surgical removal in patients irradiated in childhood for benign conditions. N Engl J Med 1989;320:835–840.
12. Robinson LL, Nesbit ME Jr, Sather HN, Meadows AT, Ortega JA, Hammond GD. Height of children successfully treated for acute lymphoblastic leukemia: a report from the late effects study committee of Children's Cancer Study Group. Med Pediatr Oncol 1985;13:14–21.
13. Berry DH, Elders MJ, Crist WM, et al. Growth in children with acute lymphocytic leukemia: a pediatric oncology group study. Med Pediatr Oncol 1983;11:39–45.
14. Kirk JA, Raghupathy P, Stevens MM, et al. Growth failure and growth-hormone deficiency after treatment for acute lymphoblastic leukaemia. Lancet 1987;1:190–193.
15. Wells RJ, Foster MB, D'Ercole AJ, McMillan CW. The impact of cranial irradiation on the growth of children with acute lymphocytic leukemia. Am J Dis Child 1983;137:37–39.
16. Starceski PJ, Lee PA, Blatt J, Finegold D, Brown D. Comparable effects of 1800- and 2400-rad (18- and 24-Gy) cranial irradiation on height and weight in children treated for acute lymphocytic leukemia. Am J Dis Child 1987;141:550–552.
17. Friedlaender GE, Tross RB, Dogannis AC, Kirkwood JM. Effects of chemotherapeutic agents on bone. J Bone Joint Surg 1984;66:602–606.
18. Shalet SM. Irradiation-induced growth failure. Clin Endocrinol Metab 1986;15:591–606.
19. Romshe CA, Zipf WB, Miser A, Miser J, Sotos JF, Newton WA. Evaluation of growth hormone release and human growth hormone treatment in children with cranial irradiation-associated short stature. J Pediatr 1984;104:177–181.
20. Bercu BB, Damond FB Jr. Growth hormone neurosecretory dysfunction. Clin Endocrinol Metab 1986; 15:537–590.
21. Albertsson-Wikland K, Rosberg S. Analyses of 24-hour growth hormone profiles in children: relation to growth. J Clin Endocrinol Metab 1988;67:493–500.
22. Saggese G, Cesaretti G, Cinquanta L, et al. Evaluation of 24-hour growth hormone spontaneous secretion: comparison with a nocturnal and diurnal 12-hour study. Horm Res 1991;35:25–29.
23. Richards GE, Cavallo A, Meyer WJ III. Diagnostic validity of 12-hour integrated concentration of growth hormone. Am J Dis Child 1987;141:553–555.
24. Sanders JE, Buckner CD, Sullivan KM, et al. Growth and development in children after bone marrow transplantation. Horm Res 1988;30:92–97.
25. Hassan M, Oberg G, Ehrsson H. Pharmacokinetic and metabolic studies of high-dose busulphan in adults. Eur J Clin Pharmacol 1989;36:525–530.
26. Hassan M, Ehrsson H, Smedmyr B, et al. Cerebrospinal fluid and plasma concentrations of busulfan during high-dose therapy. Bone Marrow Transplant 1989; 4:113–114.
27. Wingard JR, Plotnick LP, Freemer CS, et al. Growth in children after bone marrow transplantation: Busulfan plus cyclophosphamide versus cyclophosphamide plus total body irradiation. Blood 1992;79:1068–1073.
28. Shalet SM, Clayton PE, Price DA. Growth and pituitary function in children treated for brain tumors or acute lymphoblastic leukaemia. Horm Res 1988;30:53–61.
29. Leiper AD, Stanhope R, Lau T, et al. The effect of total body irradiation and bone marrow transplantation during childhood and adolescence on growth and endocrine function. Br J Haematol 1987;67:419–426.
30. Hovi L, Rajantie J, Perkkiö M, Sainio K, Sipilä I, Siimes MA. Growth failure and growth hormone deficiency in children after bone marrow transplantation for leukemia. Bone Marrow Transplant 1990;5:183–186.
31. Sanders JE, Pritchard S, Mahoney P, et al. Growth and development following marrow transplantation for leukemia. Blood 1986;68:1129–1135.
32. Joss E, Zuppinger K, Schwartz HP, Roten H. Final height of patients with pituitary growth failure and changes in growth variables after long-term hormonal therapy. Pediatr Res 1983;17:676–679.
33. Mauras N, Blizzard RM, Link K, Johnson ML, Rogol AD, Veldhuis JD. Augmentation of growth hormone secretion during puberty: evidence for a pulse amplitude-modulated phenomenon. J Clin Endocrinol Metab 1987;64:596–601.
34. Moëll C. Disturbed pubertal growth in girls after acute leukaemia: a relative growth hormone insufficiency with late presentation. Acta Paediatr Scand [Suppl] 1988;343:162–166.
35. Bourguignon J-P. Linear growth as a function of age at onset of puberty and sex steroid dosage: therapeutic implications. Endocr Rev 1988;9:467–488.
36. Papadimitriou A, Uruena M, Hamill G, Stanhope R, Leiper AD. Growth hormone treatment of growth failure secondary to total body irradiation and bone marrow transplantation. Arch Dis Child 1991;66:689–692.
37. Dopfer R, Ranke M, Blum W, Ehninger G, Niethammer D. Influence of allogeneic bone marrow transplantation

on the endocrine system in children. Transplant Proc 1989;21:3070–3073.

38. Endo M, Kaneko Y, Shikano T, Minami H, Chino J. Possible association of human growth hormone treatment with an occurrence of acute myeloblastic leukaemia with an inversion of chromosome 3 in a child with pituitary dwarfism. Med Pediatr Oncol 1988;16:45–47.
39. Sasaki U, Hara M, Watanabe S. Occurrence of acute lymphoblastic leukemia in a boy treated with growth hormone for growth retardation after irradiation to the brain tumor. J Clin Oncol 1988;18:81–84.
40. Delemarre-Van De Waal HA, Odink RJH, De Grauw TJ, De Waal FC. Leukaemia in patients treated with growth hormone (letter). Lancet 1988;1:1159.
41. Fisher DA, Job J-C, Preece M, Underwood LE. Leukaemia in patients treated with growth hormone. Lancet. 1988;1:1159–1160.
42. Parker RG, Berry HC. Late effects of therapeutic irradiation on the skeleton and bone marrow. Cancer 1976;37:1162–1171.
43. Probert JC, Parker BR. The effects of radiation therapy on bone growth. Radiology 1975;114:155–162.
44. Rosenberg SW, Kolodney H, Wong GY, Murphy ML. Altered dental root development in long-term survivors of pediatric acute lymphoblastic leukemia. Cancer 1987;59:1640–1648.
45. Dahllöf G, Forsberg C-M, Ringdén O, et al. Facial growth and morphology in long-term survivors after bone marrow transplantation. Eur J Orthod 1989;11:1–9.
46. Dahllöf G, Barr M, Bolme P, et al. Disturbances in dental development after total body irradiation in bone marrow transplant recipients. Oral Surg Oral Med Oral Pathol 1988;65:41–44.
47. Dahllöf G, Heimdahl A, Bolme P, Lönnqvist B, Ringdén O. Oral condition in children treated with bone marrow transplantation. Bone Marrow Transplant 1988;3:43–51.
48. Dahllöf G, Forsberg C-M, Näsman M, et al. Craniofacial growth in bone marrow transplant recipients treated with growth hormone after total body irradiation. Scand J Dent Res 1991;99:44–47.
49. Cutter GB, Cassosta FG, Ross JR. Pubertal growth: physiology and pathophysiology. Recent Prog Horm Res 1986;42:443–470.
50. Ray H, Mattison D. How radiation and chemotherapy affect gonadal function. Contemp Obstet Gynecol 1985;109:106–115.
51. Shalet SM, Beardwell CG, Jacobs HS, Pearson D. Testicular function following irradiation of the human prepubertal testes. Clin Endocrinol 1978;9:483–490.
52. Pescovitz OH. The endocrinology of the pubertal growth spurt. Acta Paediatr Scand [Suppl] 1990;367:119–125.
53. Sanders JE, the Seattle Marrow Transplant Team. The impact of marrow transplant preparative regimens on subsequent growth and development. Semin Hematol 1991;28:244–249.
54. De Sanctis V, Galimberti M, Lucarelli G, Polchi P, Ruggiero L, Vullo C. Gonadal function after allogeneic bone marrow transplantation for thalassaemia. Arch Dis Child 1991;66:517–520.
55. Uldall PR, Kerr DNS, Tacchi D. Amenorrhea and sterility. Lancet 1972;1:693–694.
56. Belohorsky B, Siracky J, Sandor L, Klauber E. Comments on the development of amenorrhea caused by Myleran in cases of chronic myelosis. Neoplasia 1960;4:397–402.
57. Warne GL, Fairley KF, Hobbs JB, Martin FIR. Cyclophosphamide-induced ovarian failure. N Engl J Med 1973;289:1159–1162.
58. Shalet SM. Effects of cancer chemotherapy on gonadal function of patients. Cancer Treat Rev 1980;7:131–152.
59. Etteldorf JN, West CD, Pitcock JA, Williams DL. Gonadal function, testicular histology, and meiosis following cyclophosphamide therapy in patients with nephrotic syndrome. J Pediatr 1976;88:206–212.
60. Fairley KF, Barrie JU, Johnson W. Sterility and testicular atrophy related to cyclophosphamide therapy. Lancet 1972;1:568–569.
61. Sanders JE, Buckner CD, Amos D, et al. Ovarian function following marrow transplantation for aplastic anemia or leukemia. J Clin Oncol 1988;6:813–818.
62. Jacobs P, Dubovsky DW. Bone marrow transplantation followed by normal pregnancy. Am J Hematol 1981; 11:209–212.
63. Hinterberger-Fischer M, Kier P, Kalhs P, et al. Fertility, pregnancies and offspring complications after bone marrow transplantation. Bone Marrow Transplant 1991;7:5–9.
64. Schmidt H, Ehninger G, Dopfer R, Waller HD. Pregnancy after bone marrow transplantation for severe aplastic anemia. Bone Marrow Transplant 1987;2:329–332.
65. Calmard-Oriol P, Dauriac C, Vu Van H, Lacroze M, Landriot B, Guyotat D. Successful pregnancy following allogeneic bone marrow transplantation after conditioning by thoraco-abdominal irradiation. Bone Marrow Transplant 1991;8:229–230.
66. Russell JA, Hanley DA. Full-term pregnancy after allogeneic transplantation for leukemia in a patient with oligomenorrhea. Bone Marrow Transplant 1989; 4:579–580.
67. Schubert MA, Sullivan KM, Schubert MM, et al. Gynecological abnormalities following allogeneic bone marrow transplantation. Bone Marrow Transplant 1990;5:425–430.
68. Baruch J, Benjamin S, Treleaven J, Wilcox AH, Barron JL, Powles R. Male sexual function following bone marrow transplantation. Bone Marrow Transplant 1991;7(suppl. 2):52.

Chapter 39

Delayed Complications After Bone Marrow Transplantation

H. Joachim Deeg

Currently more than 6,000 patients a year undergo allogeneic bone marrow transplantation (BMT), and at least 4,000 to 5,000 are transplanted annually with autologous marrow. With some diagnoses, the success rate has continued to improve, and a growing number of patients have been followed for many years, some more than 2 decades after BMT. Most of these patients lead a normal and productive life, whereas chronic or delayed complications have developed in some (1).

Etiology of Delayed Complications

Some delayed complications (e.g., chronic graft-versus-host disease [GVHD] and immunodeficiency) are directly transplant-related; others (e.g., infertility or cataracts) are due to the intensity of the preparative regimen. Others are related to the underlying diagnosis (e.g., disease recurrence), and many are of multifactorial etiology (e.g., chronic pulmonary disease or secondary malignancies) (Figure 39-1). Problems may arise because of direct, therapy-related trauma (e.g., destruction of skeletal growth plates), because of damage related to graft-host interactions (e.g., lymphoproliferative disorders), or because of repair processes that result in scar formation (e.g., bladder dysfunction or respiratory impairment). Chronic GVHD, disease recurrence, infections, neurological complications, impairment of growth and development, and infertility are discussed elsewhere in this volume. Table 39-1 lists delayed complications discussed herein.

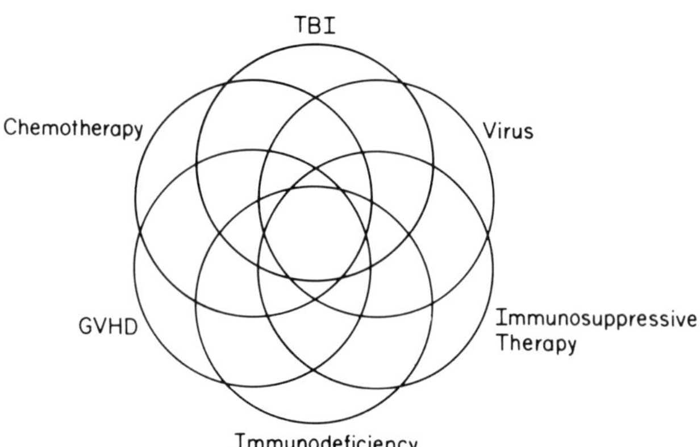

Figure 39-1. Multifactorial etiology of delayed post-transplant complications. TBI = total body irradiation; GVHD = graft-versus-host disease.

Table 39-1.
Delayed Complications of Bone Marrow Transplantation

Airway and pulmonary disease
Autoimmune dysfunction
Neuroendocrine dysfunction
Ophthalmological problems
Avascular necrosis of the bone
Dental problems
Genitourinary dysfunction
Secondary malignancies
Psychosocial effects and rehabilitation

Airway and Pulmonary Disease

Pulmonary tissue is sensitive to various cytotoxic agents and irradiation. The reponses to injury are particularly prominent in the interstitium. As a consequence, the repair process may result in scar formation in the interstitial space, which in turn interferes with effective gas exchange and respiratory kinetics. In addition, lungs and airways are prominent targets for viral, bacterial, and fungal infections that, if protracted or associated with incomplete parenchymal repair, further impair pulmonary function. Finally, the bronchial tree can serve as a target of a graft-versus-host reaction, which may result in severe structural and functional damage. As a result, delayed or chronic pulmonary complications are frequent, affecting approximately 10 to 15% of patients after BMT. Delayed interstitial pneumonitis, restrictive lung disease, obstructive lung disease, and bronchiolitis obliterans have all been reported.

Late Onset Interstitial Pneumonitis

Late interstitial pneumonitis has been observed almost exclusively in patients with chronic GVHD (see Chapter 26). Some reported patients showed marked interstitial fibrosis. However, these patients improved on immunosuppressive therapy and failed to respond to bronchodilators (2). These observations suggest an immune mechanism, although this hypothesis is currently considered controversial.

Lymphocytic bronchitis is often associated with a nonproductive cough, dyspnea, wheezing, and occasionally with bronchospasm. Histologically, lymphocytes infiltrate the proximal bronchial mucosa, the submucosa, and the muscularis, and there is an associated loss of ciliae (3). Mucosal and submucosal gland necrosis contribute to the loss of mucous ciliary clearance. Most of these patients also have other typical clinical and pathological findings of chronic GVHD.

Restrictive Disease

Restrictive defects of ventilatory function are common in BMT recipients. In one study, even among otherwise healthy long-term survivors, approximately 20% showed a mean loss in total lung capacity of 0.81 liters, a decrease in vital capacity of 0.54 liters, and an impairment of diffusing capacity of 4.4 mL/min/mm Hg one year after BMT (4). Lung function improved over the subsequent 3 to 4 years. The restrictive pulmonary changes were not correlated with any particular conditioning regimen or chronic GVHD. Patients with interstitial pneumonitis early after BMT tend to experience development of more severe restrictive changes subsequently. Generally, these changes do not produce severe symptoms and do not require therapeutic intervention.

A more recent study comparing results after autologous and allogeneic BMT found marked defects of diffusing capacity, as well as static and dynamic lung volumes, particularly in patients with GVHD (5). There were no significant differences between patients given autologous BMT and allogeneic BMT recipients without evidence of GVHD.

Obstructive Disease

The pathogenesis of obstructive pulmonary disease after BMT is largely unknown (6). Obstructive changes might represent sequelae to extensive restrictive changes in the small airways, or, as in obstructive bronchiolitis, may be due to small airway destruction. Repeated aspirations triggered, for example, by esophageal abnormalities or by purulent sinus secretions may contribute to airway inflammation and obstructive lung disease.

Obstructive defects are present in 10 to 15% of patients with chronic GVHD. These patients may present with cough, dyspnea, and wheezing, on the average 1 to 1.5 years after transplantation. The one minute forced expiratory volume is often markedly reduced; in addition, immunoglobulin G (IgG) and IgA levels in serum are usually low. There is no response to bronchodilator treatment, and only 30 to 40% of patients improve with immunosuppressive therapy (6).

Bronchiolitis Obliterans

Progressive bronchiolitis obliterans affects approximately 10% of all patients with active chronic GVHD. The clinical and pathological findings of bronchiolitis obliterans after BMT are similar to those seen after lung or heart-lung transplants. It is thought that the histological changes (Plate LIX) are due to a graft-versus-host reaction, possibly aggravated by infections that are prominent clinically (7). Pulmonary infections develop in more than 20% of allogeneic BMT recipients without GVHD and in more than 60% of those with chronic GVHD (8).

The clinical course of bronchiolitis can vary from mild, with slow deterioration, to diffuse necrotizing fatal bronchiolitis of the small airways. Bronchiolitis obliterans has been observed as early as 3 months and generally within 2 years of marrow grafting. Chest radiographs may show hyperinflation of the lungs and flattening of the diaphragm. Recurrent pneumothoraces have been reported. Pulmonary function tests show a marked reduction in forced midexpiratory flow to 10 or 20% of predicted values and moderate to severe reduction in forced vital capacity. The diffusion capacity is usually normal. Pulmonary ventilation scans show decreased activity patterns corresponding to areas of obliteration of bronchiolar walls along with atelectatic areas. Significant morbidity among patients with bronchiolitis obliterans is due to recurrent respiratory tract infections, often caused by *Pseudomonas aeruginosa*.

Characteristically, this disease does not respond well to conventional therapy of chronic GVHD, although immunosuppression with glucocorticoids is helpful in some patients.

Autoimmune Dysfunction

Any immune reactivity of transplanted allogeneic cells against the host, by definition, would be termed *alloreactivity*. However, because the donor-derived immune system replaces the patients' autochthonous immunity, donor-derived cells need to be "instructed" to accept the new (host) environment as self, and any reactivity against those determinants would become autoreactivity. The process of instruction is not always successful, in part because of thymic damage, and host-reactive cells are not eliminated. Thus, in addition to alloaggression there would be autoimmunity. These problems are discussed in detail elsewhere (see Chapter 17).

One manifestation of autoimmunity is the presence

of autoantibodies, which are observed frequently after BMT. Most commonly detected are rheumatoid factor, antinuclear, anti-smooth muscle, and antimitochondrial antibodies (9). Most patients are asymptomatic, and the significance of circulating autoantibodies in the context of GVHD is unclear. In some instances, however, such as in myasthenia gravis, autoantibodies cause severe clinical problems (10). The antiacetylcholine receptor antibodies mediating this problem are of donor allotype. Generally, the disease occurs in patients with chronic GVHD and manifests itself more than 1 or 2 years after BMT. It is also possible that patterns of abnormal immune reactivity of the donor are transferred with the marrow from the donor to the patient. This has been shown convincingly, for example, with atopic asthma.

Several hematological problems can also be mediated by autoantibodies, including immune thrombocytopenia, anemia, and neutropenia. Incidence is low, but manifestations can persist for years after BMT. To what extent these problems are related to GVHD remains to be determined.

Neuroendocrine Dysfunction

Problems related to hormone deficiencies are discussed elsewhere in this volume (see Chapter 38).

Ophthalmological Problems

As described elsewhere, the eyes are targets of acute and chronic GVHD. In addition, the eyes may show changes related to the conditioning regimen (in particular, total body irradiation [TBI], and, occasionally chemotherapeutic agents), the treatment of GVHD (glucocorticoids), and infections.

Irradiation is known to cause cataracts (11). Not surprisingly, posterior capsular cataracts develop in patients conditioned with TBI beginning approximately 1 year after BMT. For patients given single-dose TBI (usually 920–1,000 cGy), the incidence at 5 to 6 years is 80%. Among patients given fractionated TBI, the incidence of cataracts is lower; approximately 50% at doses greater than 1,200 cGy, and 30 to 35% at doses 1,200 cGy or less. Among chemotherapy-conditioned patients, the incidence is 20%. The incidence of cataracts is higher in patients who also received cranial irradiation before BMT and in patients treated with glucocorticoids. Approaches to cataract prevention are experimental. Treatment may require implantation of an artificial lens.

Other ocular complications, in particular infections, have generally been related to chronic GVHD. GVHD and infections may also lead to scar formation (e.g., synechiae, ectropion) and even corneal perforation. Long-term antibiotic coverage and artificial tears can prevent some infections and scarring. Obstruction of the nasolacrimal duct, related to GVHD or conditioning-induced fibrosis, has been observed in some patients (12).

Aseptic Necrosis of the Bone

Aseptic (avascular) necrosis, particularly of the humerus or femur heads, has long been recognized as a side effect of glucocorticoid therapy. Because many patients receive glucocorticoid therapy before and after transplantation, it is not surprising that this complication is common in this patient population. Necrosis may occur with great delay even after short courses of high-dose therapy, as for treatment of acute GVHD. The exact incidence of this complication has not been determined. Some patients show improvement when glucocorticoids are discontinued, but others have required treatment in the form of hip or knee joint replacement.

Dental Problems

The oral mucosa is a prime target of chronic GVHD (see Chapter 26). Frequently there is also an oral sicca syndrome, which may result in poor oral hygiene, recurrent infection, and dental decay. However, severe dental decay also occurs in nontransplant recipients given head or neck irradiation. It is not surprising, therefore, that an oral sicca syndrome, periodontal disease, and cavities can occur in patients without GVHD. The problem is most prevalent in children conditioned with TBI. Many of these problems can be prevented by diligent hygiene, fluoride treatment, and other supportive measures.

In addition, irradiation may interfere with the development of teeth and facial bones in children (13). There may be poor calcification, micrognathia, mandibular hypoplasia, root blunting, and apical closure. The changes are most severe in children less than 7 years of age at the time of BMT. Only omission of irradiation from conditioning regimens can prevent these problems.

Genitourinary Tract Dysfunction

Hemorrahagic cystitis develops in 5 to 10% of patients and is usually an acute problem. In most instances, it is caused by the effect of the cyclophosphamide (CY) metabolite acrolein on the bladder mucosa. However, severe hemorrhagic cystitis may also follow busulfan (BU) administration (14). Most patients recover quickly, and hematuria ceases. Infrequently, patients will have protracted hematuria, and scarring of the bladder wall with volume loss may present a chronic problem manifested by urinary frequency. CY-induced cystitis can usually be prevented by administration of the acrolein inhibitor Mesna. Viruria, for example, with adenovirus or polyomavirus, has also been implicated in hematuria.

Radiation nephritis may develop after high-dose irradiation. Doses of TBI used in preparation for BMT are generally thought to be insufficient to induce clinically relevant radiation nephritis. However, in patients who have received aggressive antitumor therapy (e.g., with platinum compounds) before BMT may be at risk of suffering renal damage. Chronic renal failure has indeed been observed in children with acute lymphoblastic leukemia or neuroblastoma following autologous or allogeneic BMT (15).

Case reports have documented the development of a hemolytic uremic syndrome or microangiopathic hemolytic anemia associated with renal failure, particularly in cyclosporine (CSP)-treated patients, either during therapy or following discontinuation (16). The mechanism is not clear. Presumably, the intensity of the conditioning regimen itself or chemoradiotherapy given prior to BMT and resulting in endothelial damage sets the stage. CSP may further alter the pathways of prostaglandin synthesis, which, in conjunction with endothelial damage, might interfere with coagulation homeostasis.

Finally, there are some case reports describing a delayed-onset nephrotic syndrome as a possible manifestation of chronic GVHD.

Secondary Malignancies

Conditions under which malignancies occur at a significantly higher frequency than in the population at large include congenital conditions of chromosomal instability, such as ataxia telangiectasia or Fanconi anemia; immunosuppression or chronic antigenic stimulation, both resulting in disruption of normal regulatory mechanisms; and infection with viruses, such as Epstein-Barr virus (EBV), known from laboratory investigations to immortalize cell lines.

Extensive studies in survivors of the atomic bomb explosions in Hiroshima and Nagasaki have shown clearly the effects of various radiation doses (gamma rays or neutrons) on the development of malignancies. Most striking is the increased incidence of diseases of the blood and blood-forming organs, especially leukemia. Similar observations have been made in both children or adults irradiated for medical indications (e.g., acne or ankylosing spondylitis). Finally, secondary cancers develop in patients treated with chemotherapy, radiation, or both, for Hodgkin's disease, non-Hodgkin's lymphoma, leukemia, and solid tumors. An increased incidence of malignant tumors has also been reported in patients receiving immunosuppressive therapy after renal transplantation.

In the 1960s and 1970s, several investigators reported the development of lymphomas in mice transplanted with marrow from an allogeneic donor. It appeared that a graft-versus-host reaction transformed from an immunological into a neoplastic disorder. Others provided evidence that these lymphomas were virus-induced. Subsequent studies in large animals focused on the conditioning regimen, especially TBI, as a risk factor for post-transplant development of secondary malignancies.

Rhesus Monkeys

In 1981, Broerse and colleagues (17) reported their observations on tumor development in rhesus monkeys observed since 1964. Monkeys were exposed either to x-ray irradiation (300–860 cGy; 30 cGy/min) or to fission neutrons (230–440 cGy; ^{235}U; 8 cGy/min) and were rescued with autologous marrow cells.

Among 20 x-ray–irradiated monkeys, malignant tumors developed in eight 7.5 to 15 (median, 11.5 yr) years after TBI. Among 9 monkeys irradiated with fission neutrons, malignant tumors developed in six 4 to 15 (median, 8 yr) years after TBI. Among 21 control animals followed for 15 to 20 years, malignant tumor developed in none. Thus, the tumor incidence for 100 observation years was 4.1 for x-ray–irradiated, 7.6 for fission neutron–treated, and zero for control monkeys. The tumors included predominantly carcinomas and sarcomas. The authors concluded that both qualities of irradiation carried a significant risk of inducing tumors and that the latency interval was longer with x-ray irradiation than with fission neutrons.

Dogs

The Seattle group reported similar results in a canine model; they observed a six-fold increased risk in TBI-treated dogs (see Chapter 1) (18).

Clinical Studies

In the 1970s, several case reports described the post-transplant occurrence of leukemia in donor-derived cells. One study suggested that approximately 5% of leukemic recurrences after BMT were in donor-derived cells (19).

Because the number of long-term surviving patients has continued to increase, it has become possible to carry out more detailed analyses. Results in 2,246 patients transplanted between May 1970 and February 1987 have been presented (20). Of these patients, 1,926 were transplanted for a hematological malignancy and 320 for severe aplastic anemia; 1,980 patients received allogeneic marrow grafts from an human leukocyte antigen (HLA)-identical or partially matched family member, 152 from a monozygotic twin donor, and 13 from an unrelated HLA-phenotypically matched donor. In addition, 101 patients were infused with autologous marrow. Patients with a hematological malignancy were conditioned with CY (120 mg/kg), plus 920 to 1,575 cGy TBI (single dose or in multiple fractions from dual opposing cobalt sources), or chemotherapy only, usually BU and CY. Patients with severe aplastic anemia, 287 of whom had an HLA-matched sibling donor, were generally conditioned with CY (200 mg/kg) only. The remaining patients were given 120 to 200 mg/kg CY or another alkylating agent along with 920 or 1,200 cGy TBI.

Of 2,246 patients at risk at the beginning of treatment, 347 were at risk after year 5 and 85 after year 10. Secondary malignancies were observed in 35 patients. Among 16 non-Hodgkin's lymphomas, 11 were associated with EBV, 2 were of T-cell type, and 3 were not otherwise classifiable. A new leukemia developed in 6 patients; in 2 patients, leukemia occurred in host cells, but had a phenotype different from the original disease. In 4 patients, leukemia was in donor cells. Thirteen malignancies were solid tumors, including 3 glioblastomas multiforme, 3 squamous-cell carcinomas (2 of the oral cavity and one of the vulva), 3 malignant melanomas, one basal-cell carcinoma, and 3 adenocarcinomas (one each of lung, liver, and rectum). Thirty of the patients died of the secondary cancers, whereas 5 survived with successful treatment.

The risk for development of any type of secondary malignancy was highest during year one (1.2 cases/100 observation years) and declined subsequently (20). The risk was significantly associated with the use of antithymocyte globulin (ATG) or antibody 64.1 (anti-CD3) used for the treatment of acute GVHD after BMT with use of TBI as part of the conditioning regimen (Table 39-2). The development of a lymphoproliferative disorder was also associated with T-cell depletion of the marrow and BMT from an HLA-nonidentical donor (see Table 39-2). The risk for a solid tumor was associated with the use of ATG.

A recent update including 4,294 patients shows secondary malignancies in 82 patients (Witherspoon RP, Deeg HJ. Unpublished observations). The spectrum of malignancies is comparable to that reported previously (Table 39-3). Seven malignancies occurred in patients conditioned without the use of irradiation, 5 in patients with aplastic anemia, and 2 in patients with a malignant disorder. The remaining malignancies developed in 75 patients conditioned with a TBI-containing regimen. Therefore, the probability for development of a secondary malignancy at 15 years is approximately 6% for patients prepared without irradiation and 20% in patients conditioned with TBI.

Table 39-2.
Significant Risk Factors for the Development of a Post-transplant Second Malignancy[a]

Variable	*Multivariate p Value*	*Relative Risk (95% CI)*
All secondary malignancies		
Treatment of GVHD with		
ATG	0.0003	4.2 (2.1–8.7)
64.1	0.0090	13.6 (3.8–48.0)
TBI	0.0021	3.9 (1.2–12.8)
Lymphoproliferative disorders		
Treatment of GVHD with		
64.1	0.0018	15.6 (4.0–61.8)
ATG	0.0054	4.9 (1.6–14.5)
T-cell depletion of marrow	0.0149	12.4 (2.6–59.9)
HLA-nonidentity	0.0252	3.8 (1.2–11.8)
Solid tumors		
Treatment of GVHD with ATG	0.0308	4.3 (1.3–14.2)

[a]According to the Multivariate Stepwise Proportional-Hazards model.
CI = confidence interval; GVHD = graft-versus-host disease; ATG = antithymocyte globulin; TBI = total body irradiation; 64.1 = an anti-CD3 monoclonal antibody.

Table 39-3.
Post-transplant Malignancies[a]

Type of Malignancy	*No. Patients*
Lymphoproliferative disorder	21
Basal-cell carcinoma	15
Squamous-cell carcinoma	10
Acute lymphoblastic leukemia	6
Adenocarcinoma	6
Papillary carcinoma of the thyroid	3
Carcinomas, other	4
Glioblastome multiforme	4
Myelodysplastic syndrome	3
Malignant melanoma	3
Sarcoma	2
Acute myeloid leukemia	2
Miscellaneous	5
Total	82

[a]Observed among 4,294 patients transplanted for malignant or nonmalignant disease after conditioning with chemotherapy alone or combined with total body irradiation.

Preliminary data from the International Bone Marrow Transplant Registry (Horowitz MM. Personal communication) show 109 secondary malignancies among 9,732 patients, for an approximate incidence of 0.6/100 person years, a figure similar to that observed in the Seattle population. The group at Hôpital Saint Louis in Paris recently reported results in patients with severe aplastic anemia conditioned with a combination of thoracoabdominal irradiation and CY (21). Analysis of 147 patients followed for up to 10 years shows a projected incidence of secondary malignancies of 25%, as compared with approximately 6% among Seattle patients prepared with CY only (22). These data suggest that it is the conditioning regimen (i.e., the use of irradiation) that represents the highest risk for tumor development in these patients, rather than a genetic predisposition.

Most secondary malignancies after BMT have been fatal. However, a recent report suggests that patients with a polyclonal B-cell lymphoproliferative disorder respond to anti-CD21 or CD24 monoclonal antibodies; patients with monoclonal tumors fail to do so (23). EBV-related disease is discussed in detail in Chapter 31.

Central and Peripheral Nervous System

Peripheral and central nervous systems are both frequently affected by complications after BMT. Most of these complications occur in the acute post-transplant period, but some are delayed (see Chapter 34). In addition to infections, hemorrhage, and structural abnormalities, there may also be hypothalamic-pituitary dysfunction, impaired memory, shortened attention span, and defects of verbal fluency. Children may score lower than control subjects in visual-motor and processing tasks and various I.Q. tests (24).

Psychosocial Effects and Rehabilitation

Research on issues of survivorship in cancer patients in general and BMT patients in particular has begun only recently (25,26). It is clear, however, that long-term adjustments and rehabilitation depend strongly on events along the way. Not only acute complications, related, for example, to poor engraftment, but also chronic and delayed problems have a major impact (27).

Changes in body image due to skin disfigurement, weight loss, and weakness, in addition to medications, especially glucocorticoids or CSP, and their side effects, may be the most significant factors. Along with the fear of disease recurrence, these factors may lead to severe depression, changes in partner relationships, and family roles. Patients may change their life priorities and perspectives, which in turn affects their families.

As the interval from BMT extends, adjusting to the day-to-day environment becomes more important. Whereas patients without chronic problems move toward normal activities within one or 2 years after BMT, patients with chronic GVHD or pulmonary disease may be crippled for years. Major adjustments in lifestyle and occupation may be necessary in patients in whom joint contractures or muscle wasting develop. Problems with sexuality arise sooner or later after BMT, both in adolescents and in adults. Healthy partners may put inappropriate demands on BMT recipients, which further contributes to intramarital stress, and in addition to social and financial demands, may result in marital dysfunction and divorce.

Problems with employment and insurance may occur because many insurance companies are reluctant to provide health or life protection. Open communication is extremely helpful. However, the possibility of late sequelae (e.g., secondary malignancy) also needs to be considered.

Effects of conditioning and transplantation on growth and development of pediatric patients are discussed elsewhere (see Chapter 38). Early detection of potential problems and health maintenance are important, possibly for several decades. The desire to be equal to their peers may cause problems with compliance in this age group. A multidisciplinary approach involving adolescent medicine physicians and endocrinologists along with group therapy appears most promising. Rehabilitation must begin at the time of diagnosis and should involve a long-term treatment plan (25).

References

1. Deeg HJ. Delayed complications and long-term effects after bone marrow transplantation. Hematol Oncol Clin North Am 1991;4:641–657.
2. Raschko JW, Cottler-Fox M, Abbondanzo SL, Torrisi JR, Spitzer TR, Deeg HJ. Pulmonary fibrosis after bone marrow transplantation responsive to treatment with prednisone and cyclosporine. Bone Marrow Transplant 1989;4:201–205.
3. Beschorner WE, Saral R, Hutchins GM, Tutschka PJ, Santos GW. Lymphocytic bronchitis associated with graft-versus-host disease in recipients of bone-marrow transplants. N Engl J Med 1978;299:1030–1036.
4. Springmeyer SC, Flournoy N, Sullivan KM, Storb R, Thomas ED. Pulmonary function changes in long-term survivors of allogeneic marrow transplantation. In: Gale RP, ed. Recent advances in bone marrow transplantation. New York: Alan R. Liss, 1983:343–353.
5. Tait RC, Burnett AK, Robertson AG, et al. Subclinical pulmonary function defects following autologous and allogeneic bone marrow transplantation: relationship to total body irradiation and graft-versus-host disease. Int J Radiat Oncol Biol Phys 1991;20:1219–1227.
6. Clark JG, Schwartz DA, Flournoy N, Sullivan KM, Crawford SW, Thomas ED. Risk factors for airflow obstruction in recipients of bone marrow transplants. Ann Intern Med 1987;107:648–656.
7. Holland HK, Wingard JR, Beschorner WE, Saral R, Santos GW. Bronchiolitis obliterans in bone marrow transplantation and its relationship to chronic graft-v-host disease and low serum IgG. Blood 1988;72:621–627.
8. Sullivan KM, Mori M, Sanders J, et al. Late complications of allogeneic and autologous marrow transplantation. Bone Marrow Transplant 1992;10:127–134.
9. Rouquette-Gally AM, Boyeldieu D, Prost AC, et al. Autoimmunity after allogeneic bone marrow transplantation. Transplantation 1988;46:238–240.
10. Smith CI, Aarli JA, Biberfeld P, et al. Myasthenia gravis after bone marrow transplantation: evidence for a donor origin. N Engl J Med 1983;309:1565–1568.
11. Deeg HJ, Flournoy N, Sullivan KM, et al. Cataracts after total body irradiation and marrow transplantation: a sparing effect of dose fractionation. Int J Radiat Oncol Biol Phys 1984;10:957–964.
12. Hanada R, Ueoka Y. Obstruction of nasolacrimal ducts closely related to graft-versus-host disease after bone marrow transplantation. Bone Marrow Transplant 1989;4:125–126.
13. Dahllöf G, Barr M, Bolme P, et al. Disturbances in dental development after total body irradiation in bone marrow transplant recipients. Oral Surg Oral Med Oral Pathol 1988;65:41–44.
14. Atkinson K, Biggs J, Noble G, et al. Preparative regimens for marrow transplantation containing busulphan are associated with haemorrhagic cystitis and hepatic veno-occlusive disease but a short duration of leucopenia and little oro-pharyngeal mucositis. Bone Marrow Transplant 1987;2:385–394.
15. Tarbell NJ, Guinan EC, Niemeyer C, Mauch P, Sallan SE, Weinstein HJ. Late onset of renal dysfunction in survivors of bone marrow transplantation. Int J Radiat Oncol Biol Phys 1988;15:99–104.
16. Juckett M, Perry EH, Daniels BS, Weisdorf DJ. Hemolytic uremic syndrome following bone marrow transplantation. Bone Marrow Transplant 1991;7:405–409.
17. Broerse JJ, Hollander CF, Van Zwieten MJ. Tumor induction in Rhesus monkeys after total body irradiation with X-rays and fission neutrons. Int J Radiat Biol 1981;40:671–676.
18. Deeg HJ, Prentice R, Fritz TE, et al. Increased incidence of malignant tumors in dogs after total body irradiation and marrow transplantation. Int J Radiat Oncol Biol Phys 1983;9:1505–1511.

19. Boyd CN, Ramberg RE, Thomas ED. The incidence of recurrence of leukemia in donor cells after allogeneic bone marrow transplantation. Leuk Res 1982;6:833–837.
20. Witherspoon RP, Fisher LD, Schoch G, et al. Secondary cancers after bone marrow transplantation for leukemia or aplastic anemia. N Engl J Med 1989;321:784–789.
21. Socié G, Henry-Amar M, Cosset JM, Devergie A, Girinsky T, Gluckman E. Increased incidence of solid malignant tumors after bone marrow transplant for severe aplastic anemia. Blood 1991;78:277–279.
22. Witherspoon RP, Storb R, Pepe M, Longton G, Sullivan KM. Cumulative incidence of secondary solid malignant tumors in aplastic anemia patients given marrow grafts after conditioning with chemotherapy alone (letter). Blood 1992;79:289–290.
23. Fischer A, Blanche S, Le Bidois J, et al. Anti-B-cell monoclonal antibodies in the treatment of severe B-cell lymphoproliferative syndrome following bone marrow and organ transplantation. N Engl J Med 1991;324: 1451–1456.
24. McGuire T, Sanders JE, Hill D, Buckner CD, Sullivan K. Neuropsychological function in children given total body irradiation for marrow transplantation (abstract). Exp Hematol 1991;19:578.
25. Nims JW. Survivorship and rehabilitation. In: Whedon MB, ed. Bone marrow transplantation, principles, practice and nursing insights. Boston: Jones & Bartlett, 1991:334–345.
26. Wingard JR, Curbow B, Baker F, Piantadosi S. Health, functional status, and employment of adult survivors of bone marrow transplantation. Ann Intern Med 1991;114:113–118.
27. Andrykowski MA, Altmaier EM, Barnett RL, Otis ML, Gingrich R, Henslee-Downey PJ. The quality of life in adult survivors of allogeneic bone marrow transplantation: correlates and comparison with matched renal transplant recipients. Transplantation 1990;50:399.

Chapter 40
Management of Relapse After Bone Marrow Transplantation

David S. Snyder

Cure of leukemia is the goal of therapy with bone marrow transplantation (BMT). Unfortunately, relapse of the original disease remains a problem of varying degree depending on a number of factors, including stage of the disease at the time of BMT, source of bone marrow, T-cell depletion, details of the preparatory regimen, graft-versus-host disease (GVHD) prophylaxis, and the subsequent incidence of GVHD.

With the aid of highly sensitive molecular biological techniques, it is becoming clear that minimal residual disease may persist or recur and yet not necessarily lead to cytogenetic or clinical relapse, especially in chronic myeloid leukemia (CML). Rarely, leukemia may recur or arise in donor cells. Secondary malignancies such as B-cell lymphoproliferative diseases may develop as a complication of the conditioning regimen, viral reactivation, or immunosuppression and must be distinguished from relapse of the primary disease.

Prophylaxis with cytokines such as interferon may be effective in preventing relapse in high-risk patients who have undergone BMT, in particular for CML. Leukemia that relapses after intensive, myeloablative BMT conditioning regimens is generally considered to be incurable. However, reinduction therapy is sometimes effective in achieving a subsequent remission, which may be long-lasting in some patients. Options for post-BMT therapy of relapsed leukemia include additional chemotherapy, differentiation-inducing agents (e.g., all-trans retinoic acid for acute promyelocytic leukemia), immunotherapy with various cytokines to induce graft-versus-leukemia (GVL) effects, and, finally, a second BMT for selected patients. Success rates for second BMTs are low, whereas fatal complication rates, including regimen-related toxicities of veno-occlusive disease (VOD) and interstitial pneumonitis (IP), and GVHD are high.

The decision regarding whether to treat a patient aggressively when leukemia relapses after BMT is difficult. Quality-of-life issues must be weighed carefully in balancing the risks and benefits of attempting a second BMT versus those of choosing alternative therapies or supportive care only.

Incidence of Relapse of Leukemia After BMT

BMT is the only proven modality capable of curing patients with CML. Long-term disease-free survival (DFS) rates of 50 to 75% (1–3) have been reported for patients transplanted while in chronic phase (CP). For patients transplanted for more advanced stages of CML, the DFS rates are lower, ranging from 15 to 30% (3–5); higher relapse rates account for most of the increased rates of failure. For patients with acute myeloid leukemia (AML) and acute lymphoblastic leukemia (ALL), BMT can often lead to prolonged DFS, with reported rates of 40 to 65% for patients transplanted with early stage disease, and 10 to 40% for patients with more advanced disease (2,6–9).

In this first section, the risk factors associated with relapse of leukemia, in particular, the inverse relation between the incidence of GVHD and relapse, are reviewed. There is a complex interrelation between GVHD and relapse, such that any intervention designed to minimize the incidence of GVHD is usually associated with a higher relapse rate.

Risk Factors for Relapse of Leukemia After BMT

The stage of disease at the time of BMT is a significant risk factor for relapse. For patients with CML, clinical relapse rates for patients transplanted in CP are generally less than 20%, whereas for patients transplanted in accelerated phase (AP) or blast crisis (BC), the relapse rates are as high as 40 to 80% (1–5) (Figure 40-1). Cytogenetic or molecular relapse rates may be considerably higher, and are discussed in more detail later. Relapse rates for patients with AML or ALL transplanted while in first complete remission are reported to be 5 to 30%, compared with 40 to 80% for patients who were at more advanced stages of disease (2,6–15).

The presence of various chromosomal abnormalities in patients before BMT may be important risk factors for relapse (3–5,16,17). The specific components of the conditioning regimen may influence

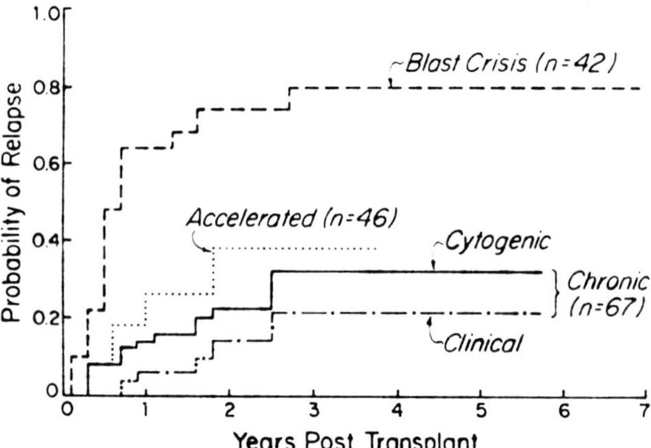

Figure 40-1. Kaplan-Meier product limit estimates for probability or relapse after a allogeneic bone marrow transplantation. (Reproduced by permission from Thomas ED, Clift RA, Fefer A, et al. Marrow transplantation for the treatment of chronic myelogenous leukemia. Ann Intern Med 1986;104:155–163.)

relapse rates. The traditional preparative regimen in general use for BMT is the combination of total body irradiation (TBI) and cyclophosphamide (CY). However, there are a number of alternative regimens available, including radiation-containing regimens (e.g., fractionated TBI [FTBI]/etoposide [15,18]) and nonradiation regimens (e.g., busulfan/CY [14,19] or busulfan/CY/etoposide [13]). The relative superiority of any one of these regimens over another can only be determined in randomized control Phase III studies. Differences in the total dose and fractionation scheme of TBI may be associated with differences in relapse rates, although overall survival may not be different (11,20–22).

Perhaps most significant is the inverse relation between GVHD and relapse; absence of GVHD is associated with higher relapse rates (1,7–9,23,24). Maneuvers designed to reduce the risk of relapse, such as T-lymphocyte depletion of donor marrow, are clearly associated with higher relapse rates, perhaps most strikingly for patients with CML in CP (1,25).

The concept of a GVL effect has been invoked as one explanation for this relation between GVHD and relapse. It has been postulated that alloreactive T lymphocytes that mediate GVHD reactions may recognize antigenic differences expressed on residual leukemic cells as well as on normal host tissues. There is some evidence from animal models and from clinical experience suggesting that GVL and GVHD effects may actually be independent phenomena (26).

In some cases of relapse of leukemia after BMT, the transformed cells are actually of donor origin (27–32). Whether such events represent a new malignancy arising in donor cells or some type of genetic transformation of donor cells by host leukemic cells is difficult to determine.

For patients with CML, it may be important to distinguish hematological relapse from cytogenetic or molecular relapse. It has been apparent for some time that as many as 50% of patients with Philadelphia chromosome (Ph)-positive CML have persistence or reappearance of the Ph chromosome after BMT. In most of these patients, the chromosomal marker disappears during the course of the first year after BMT with no clinical sequelae. However, some of these patients do progress to hematological relapse, especially if they were transplanted beyond CP, received T-cell–depleted marrow, or have progressively increasing percentages of Ph cells in post-BMT karyotypes (33–37).

Molecular relapse or persistence of disease is defined by the detection of bcr-abl mRNA or rearranged DNA in post-BMT marrow samples. The incidence of this finding may be as high as 50 to 80%, at least transiently (38–42). It is unclear how often molecular relapse progresses to clinical relapse; therefore, it is unclear how these data should be used in making clinical decisions about the need for further therapy. Molecular techniques were helpful in documenting the development of a new lymphoproliferative disease, as opposed to relapse of CML, in a patient transplanted in lymphoid blast crisis (43). This concept of molecular relapse or persistence of disease is applicable to acute leukemias as well if specific markers analogous to the bcr-abl fusion gene are available (e.g., t(15;17) in acute promyelocytic leukemia, and rearranged T-cell receptor or immunoglobulin genes in T- and B-cell ALL).

It is important to distinguish relapse of the original leukemia from other neoplastic processes that may develop after BMT. B-cell lymphoproliferative disorders may arise after BMT, often as a consequence of immunosuppression, T-cell depletion, or activation of latent Epstein-Barr viral infection (44–46). Such patients may benefit from reduction of immunosuppression, antiviral therapy, or standard chemotherapy. Other secondary malignancies, including solid tumors and leukemia, may develop in patients treated with BMT for leukemia or aplastic anemia (47). There may be significant prognostic and therapeutic implications depending on whether a patient has relapsed after BMT or has developed a new malignancy.

Treatment Options for Leukemia Relapsing After BMT

Prophylaxis Against CNS Relapse

The most effective way to deal with the problem of relapse of leukemia after BMT may be to identify those patients at greatest risk for relapse and to intervene prophylactically with either chemotherapy or immunotherapy. The Seattle group studied the specific issue of isolated central nervous system (CNS) relapse in patients transplanted for AML or ALL (48). They evaluated the relative risks and benefits of post-transplant intrathecal methotrexate (IT-MTX) in these patients. The probability of CNS relapse was reduced from 38 to 7% in patients with ALL who received IT-MTX, compared with those who did not. In contrast, there was no such protection demonstrated for patients with AML, in part because the incidence of CNS relapse was much lower in this group (2% compared with 13% in patients with ALL). There was a 7% risk for development of leukoencephalopathy in patients who received radiation and/or IT chemotherapy before transplant and post-transplant IT-MTX. The authors concluded that for patients with ALL, but not for patients with AML, the benefit of IT-MTX in reducing post-transplant CNS relapse outweighed the risk for development of leukoencephalopathy.

Immunotherapy as Prophylaxis Against Relapse After BMT

There is considerable evidence that immunological mechanisms (i.e. GVL effects), account for at least some of the therapeutic benefits of BMT. Several groups have studied the feasibility of using cytokines to manipulate the donor or host immune response against residual leukemia cells to augment or create GVL effects after either allogeneic or autologous BMT. This topic has been reviewed recently by Klingemann and Phillips (49). One approach would be to identify patients at higher risk for relapse after BMT based on a number of established risk factors and to treat them with interleukin 2 (IL-2) or α-interferon (α-IFN) early after BMT to augment natural killer (NK) cell and/or other killer cell activity to reduce the risk of relapse.

The Vancouver BMT group reported the results of a Phase I trial to establish the maximum tolerated dose of daily recombinant α-2b-IFN administered subcutaneously to a group of patients undergoing BMT for hematological malignancies considered to be at high risk for relapse (50). Myelosuppression was the limiting toxicity, with a maximum tolerated dose of 1.0×10^6 IU/m^2. These authors did not demonstrate any change in either NK or IL-2-activated NK activity as a result of the IFN therapy. They raised cautions about potentially increased risks of GVHD and neurotoxicity from the IFN.

The Dana-Farber transplant group, as well as other investigators (51–53), studied the impact of prolonged infusion of low-dose recombinant IL-2 (rIL-2) after autologous and T-cell depleted allogeneic BMT (54). Thirteen marrow recipients received rIL-2 at a dose of 2×10^5 U/m^2/day by continuous intravenous infusion for 90 days, beginning a median of 85 days after BMT. Toxicity was minimal. All patients demonstrated a marked increase in NK cell number and activity. The impact of this approach on relapse rates and infectious complications needs to be established in prospective studies.

Immunotherapy as Treatment of Relapsed CML After BMT

Leukemia that relapses after BMT is generally considered to be incurable. However, it may be possible at least to achieve a subsequent remission and possibly long-term DFS in a small percentage of such patients using one of a variety of therapeutic approaches. In this section, the experience with immunotherapy for relapsed CML is discussed. In following sections, results from reinduction chemotherapy, differentiation-inducing agents, and second BMTs are reviewed.

α-IFN has been proven to be an active agent for patients with CML in CP, with hematological response rates up to 75% and major cytogenetic response rates of approximately 25% (55). Several investigators have extrapolated from this experience to treat CML patients who relapse after BMT with α-IFN. Arcese and colleagues (56) treated 18 patients with CML with hematological [4] or cytogenetic [14] relapse after T-cell depleted allogeneic BMT with α-2b-IFN. The 4 patients with hematological relapse achieved long-lasting hematological remission, although there was no reduction in Ph-positive bone marrow cells. Six of the 14 patients with cytogenetic relapse progressed to hematological relapse, whereas 8 of 14 remain in hematological remission; 2 of these 8 have achieved complete cytogenetic and molecular remission.

Investigators from Munich treated 3 patients with hematological relapse after BMT for CML in CP with α-IFN in combination with transfusion of donor buffy coat cells to induce a GVL effect (57). All 3 patients had complete hematological and cytogenetic remission, persisting for 32 to 91 weeks after treatment. GVHD developed in 2 patients, requiring immunosuppressive therapy.

The Hammersmith group described their experience using donor buffy coat cells alone to treat 2 patients who relapsed cytogenetically after allogeneic BMT for CML (58). Both patients received T-cell–depleted marrow, one from a matched unrelated donor and the other from her HLA-identical brother. Significant GVHD developed in both patients after BMT that responded to immunosuppressive therapy. Both patients received buffy coat cells from their original donor after they relapsed cytogenetically. Extensive GVHD developed in one patient after the infusion, and the other patient had only minimal GVHD. Both patients achieved hematological, cytogenetic, and molecular remissions, as documented by the absence of bcr-abl transcripts by polymerase chain reaction (PCR) assay, 23 and 65 months after BMT, respectively.

The Seattle group reported their results of treating 18 patients with relapsed CML after BMT with α-IFN (59). Relapse was defined as more than 90% Ph-positive metaphases and hematological parameters consistent with CP of CML. Only one of the 18 patients received T-cell–depleted marrow. The doses of α-IFN ranged from 3 to 6×10^6 U/m^2/day. Six of the 18 patients had complete disappearance of the Ph chromosome, and 2 patients had a partial response ($<$ 35% Ph-positive metaphases). Nine patients had no significant response. Two patients had significant worsening of GVHD, and almost all patients had chronic systemic side effects, mainly fatigue.

The group from Hadassah University in Jerusalem reported on their experience using concomitant IL-2 and α-IFN to treat 10 patients with CML at various stages of the disease, including one patient who relapsed after BMT (60). Eight of the 10 patients had hematological responses, and one patient had elimination of the Ph marker, even by PCR. These investigators found the side effects to be tolerable, and they speculated on the potential benefit of this combined cytokine treatment in patients with evidence of minimal residual disease after BMT.

Chemotherapy for Relapsed Leukemia After BMT

Patients who relapse after BMT for leukemia may not necessarily be refractory to additional reinduction chemotherapy. There are a few reports in the literature describing attempts to reinduce remissions using standard combination chemotherapy. A significant percentage of these patients may achieve a CR, although it is unclear whether any of them are actually cured.

The Westminster group (61) described their experience with 63 children and adolescents with ALL who relapsed between 75 and 1,126 days after allogeneic BMT. Nineteen of these patients were reinduced with standard combination chemotherapy; 7 achieved CR, of whom 5 were alive in CR 88 to 1,240 days after relapse. For 3 of these 5 patients, the duration of remission was already longer than the time interval between their BMT and relapse. This phenomenon of a longer remission after chemotherapy compared with that after first BMT is referred to as "inversion." The other 2 patients died during a second BMT. Actuarial survival was 26%. Favorable outcome after reinduction chemotherapy was predicted by the pace of the disease. The 5 long-term survivors had "slow" disease, as defined by an interval of more than 2 years between diagnosis and first relapse (either before or after BMT). The other predictive factor was that patients who relapsed more than 500 days after BMT were more likely to respond and survive compared with patients who relapsed less than 500 days after BMT.

The University of Minnesota transplant group reported on 65 patients with ALL who had relapsed after either allogeneic, autologous, or syngeneic BMT (62). Twelve of these patients elected not to receive additional therapy, and their median survival from the time of relapse was only 36 days (range, 13–167 days). For the 53 patients who did receive additional chemotherapy, the median survival was 168 days (range, 18 days to 4.7 yr). Fifty-two of these 53 patients were treated with multidrug induction regimens; 29 of 52 (56%) achieved CR. Six patients were alive 1 to 5 years after relapse; 2 were off therapy in CR, 2 were in CR still on therapy, one was in relapse on therapy, and one was on therapy after a second relapse after BMT. Actuarial survival was 8%. Independent predictors of prolonged survival for these 52 patients were longer time interval from BMT to relapse (i.e., > 100 days compared with < 100 days), younger age at diagnosis, and the use of a preparative regimen that contained fractionated TBI. Factors that were not significant included type of BMT (i.e., autologous vs other), GVHD, and the number of induction attempts before BMT.

The European Group for Bone Marrow Transplantation (EBMT) reported their experience with 117 patients with relapsed leukemia (41 with AML; 76 with ALL) after BMT (63). Relapses occurred between 3 and 30 months after BMT and were found in recipient cells in all patients analyzed. In 10 patients, there were new cytogenetic abnormalities. Of the 117 patients, 74 received further chemotherapy; 21 of 50 patients with ALL and 11 of 24 patients with AML achieved a CR. The median survival for these patients was 12 months, compared with 4 months for untreated patients or treated patients who did not achieve CR. Predictive factors for successful remission induction were long interval between BMT and relapse in ALL (but not in AML) patients and isolated extramedullary relapse. Factors not predictive of success included presenting blast count, karyotype, and remission status at time of BMT.

The Seattle group described their results of treating patients who relapsed with acute leukemia after matched or mismatched allogeneic or syngneic BMT (64). Ninety-five of 455 (21%) patients with AML relapsed a median of 6.5 months after BMT. Sites of relapse were as follows: 83 of 95 were in bone marrow (76 marrow only, 7 marrow plus additional site); 12 of 95 were isolated extramedullary relapses in testis, CNS, bone, among others. Of these 95 patients with relapse, 62 received further therapy; 55 of 62 received chemotherapy, 6 of 62 received radiation alone to isolated extramedullary sites of relapse, and one of 62 received a second BMT. Twenty of the 62 achieved a CR. Patients who relapsed more than 100 days after BMT did better than patients who relapsed less than 100 days after BMT (15 of 23 CR compared with one of 14). The use of ara-C as reinduction chemotherapy was also predictive of a favorable response. The median disease-free survival for all treated patients was 6 months (range, 0.4–53+ mo).

For patients with ALL, 130 of 366 (36%) relapsed (86 in marrow only; 14 in marrow plus additional site; and 30 isolated extramedullary relapse with 18 testis, 12 CNS, plus other sites). Ninety-four patients received additional therapy, and 52 achieved a CR. The majority of these 94 patients were treated with chemotherapy alone (63 of 94); 12 received radiation alone; 14 received radiation followed by chemotherapy; 4 received IT-MTX alone; and one underwent a second BMT as initial therapy for the relapse. Remissions were more likely in late relapse patients (> 1 yr from BMT) compared with early relapse patients (< 100 days after BMT) (65 vs 7%). The median survival for treated patients was 10.5 months (range, 5–109+ mo). Eighteen patients with either AML or ALL underwent a second BMT at some point after their relapse, and the results are discussed later.

In a recent case report (65), the Vancouver group described the course of a 35-year-old woman with CML in CP who relapsed with lymphoid BC after receiving an allogeneic BMT from her histocompatible brother. The patient had been conditioned with busulfan/CY and had received CSP and MTX for GVHD prophylaxis. She had cytogenetic evidence of complete donor engraftment by 25 days after BMT. However, by day 100, there were 50% Ph-positive metaphases detected in her bone marrow, and by day 126, she had hematological evidence of lymphoid BC of her CML with additional chromosomal abnormalities other than the Ph chromosome. She was treated with daunorubicin, vincristine, and prednisone for 4 weeks, and by day 273, she was in CR and 100% of bone marrow metaphases were male. CSP had been discontinued at day 120. She remained in hematological and cytogenetic CR 19 months after BMT (15 mo after the onset of BC), although a bcr-abl rearrangement was detectable in her bone marrow by PCR assay at that time. This patient demonstrates that sustained donor hematopoiesis is achievable after chemotherapy for BC relapse after BMT for CML. The authors speculated that stopping the CSP may have allowed a GVL effect to emerge, which possibly contributed to the maintenance of remission.

Differentiating Agent as Treatment of Relapsed Acute Promyelocytic Leukemia

There has been considerable progress in understanding the molecular basis of the translocation t(15;17), which is uniquely associated with acute promyelocytic leukemia (PML) (66–69). It is now known that the PML (or myl) gene is translocated from chromosome 15q22 to a region of chromosome 17q21 that contains the retinoic acid receptor-alpha (RAR-α) gene. How this newly created fusion gene causes the development of acute PML is currently unclear. However, it has been shown both experimentally and clinically that all-trans retinoic acid can induce remissions in patients with acute PML, probably via an interaction with the altered RAR-α that induces differentiation of the malignant promyelocytes (70–72). Success has been achieved using all-trans retinoic acid in patients with acute PML ocurring de novo, relapsing after chemotherapy, or with refractory disease. This approach has recently been applied to the setting of acute PML relapsing after BMT.

The Victoria, Australia group reported their experience treating one man with acute PML who relapsed after undergoing allogeneic BMT from an HLA-matched sister while in a first CR induced by standard induction chemotherapy (73). The patient relapsed cytogenetically at day 213 and hematologically by day 252 after BMT. The patient had 44% blasts and 32% abnormal promyelocytes in the bone marrow, laboratory features of disseminated intravascular coagulation (DIC), and 100% of metaphases showed 46XY, t(15;17). He was treated with all-trans retinoic acid for 108 days. The DIC cleared after 7 days of therapy. Bone marrow examination on day 34 revealed a hypocellular marrow, with fibrosis and marrow necrosis. The patient achieved a CR hematologically and cytogenetically by day 47, with 100% normal female metaphases in his bone marrow. He then relapsed hematologically on day 108; the all-trans retinoic acid was stopped and chemotherapy was begun, but he died 12 days later. Toxicity of the all-trans retinoic acid included hyperleukocytosis requiring leukaphereses and hydroxyurea, bone pain, and dry skin. The authors concluded that this experience supports the concept that remission after all-trans retinoic acid is due to elimination of the malignant clone via terminal differentiation and death of malignant cells. In this patient, hematopoiesis was then re-established, at least transiently, by residual donor stem cells. It remains to be determined how useful this agent will ultimately be in treating relapsed acute PML after BMT.

Second BMTs for Relapsed Leukemia After BMT

It is generally assumed that if leukemia recurs after BMT, then the malignant cells must be resistant to almost any other form of therapy, and the patient is therefore incurable. This assumption may not be correct. In previous sections of this chapter, the results of immunotherapy and reinduction chemotherapy for relapsed leukemia after BMT are reviewed. A significant percentage of patients may achieve CR with these approaches, although it is uncertain whether any of the patients are actually cured.

A second BMT represents another option for treating these patients. As is reviewed chronologically in the following section, certain carefully selected patients may benefit with prolonged DFS. The availability of effective, alternative conditioning regimens is the key to the success of this approach. The problems of refractory leukemia and life-threatening toxicity from a second BMT remain major obstacles.

The UCLA transplant group reported on 4 patients with acute leukemia who had relapsed 10 to 17 months after allogeneic BMT from HLA-matched siblings while in remission and then underwent a second BMT using the original donors (74). For the first BMT, patients were conditioned with CY for 2 days followed by TBI, given either as a single dose or in 6 fractions. All patients received standard course MTX for GVHD prophylaxis. The patients were treated with conventional chemotherapy after they relapsed following the BMT; 3 of 4 achieved a CR. They then proceeded to a second BMT using one of two conditioning regimens: busulfan followed by CY in 2 patients, or high-dose ara-C followed by fractionated TBI in 2 patients. MTX was used again for GVHD prophylaxis. Two patients remained in continuous CR 11 and 23 months after the second BMT, compared with remission durations of 10 and 17 months, respectively, after the first BMT. (i.e., inversions). Toxicity was considerable; one patient died from VOD and *Candida* infection 2 weeks after BMT, gastrointestinal toxicity occurred in all 3 surviving patients, and chronic respiratory compromise occurred in one patient who received TBI before both the first and the second BMT.

Previously, the Westminster group (61) treated 19 patients with ALL who relapsed after BMT with chemotherapy. Two of the 7 patients who achieved a remission were then treated with a second BMT. Both patients died, one from infection and gastrointestinal toxicity from ara-C just before the BMT and the other in CR from severe acute gastrointestinal and liver GVHD on day 27 after BMT.

The Sydney, Australia group (75) reported their results of second BMTs in 9 patients relapsing 3 to 32 months after first BMT. The patients had a variety of hematological malignancies, including CML, ALL, AML at various stages, and one patient with acute myelofibrosis. All patients were conditioned initially with CY and fractionated TBI and received grafts from HLA-identical siblings. All patients were then reconditioned while in relapse with high-dose melphalan (plus CY in one patient; ara-C/adriamycin in another) and received marrow from their original donors. CSP was used for GVHD prophylaxis both times. Three of the 9 patients died from relapse, whereas 3 of 9 were alive without disease 81, 36, and 33 months, respectively, after the second BMT. The rate of marrow engraftment, the incidence of acute GVHD, and IP were similar after both first and second BMTs, but nephrotoxicity and oropharyngeal mucositis from melphalan were significant complications after the second BMTs.

City of Hope reviewed their results of second BMTs in 5 patients who relapsed with hematological malignancies 7 months to 8 years after first BMT (76). All 5 patients had been conditioned with TBI-containing regimens before the first BMT. A novel, nonradiation regimen consisting of busulfan/etoposide was used before the second BMT, and the same sibling donors were used as for the first BMT. All 5 patients engrafted and entered CR. Two patients were alive in CR 2 and 10 months after second BMT. One of these 2 patients is currently alive and well more than 6 years following second BMT. Two other patients relapsed again 8 and 17 months after second BMT; one patient died with acute respiratory failure. Thus, remissions could be induced with the two drugs in this new regimen, although the durability of response and the immunosuppressive potential of the regimen were unclear.

The Seattle group reported on 26 patients with recurrent leukemia who relapsed 1.5 to 78 months (median, 26 mo) after first BMT who were then treated with a second BMT (77). All patients had received CY/TBI as the conditioning regimen before the first BMT. For the second preparative regimen, 20 patients received busulfan or dimethylbusulfan plus CY, one patient received dimethylbusulfan alone, and 5 patients received multiagent chemotherapy with TBI. Fourteen patients died from toxicities, including VOD and IP; 5 patients died from relapse. Seven patients (27%) were alive after 12 to 38 months (median, 26 mo); 5 of 7 (19%) were disease-free and 2 had recurrent leukemia (Figure 40-2). Chronic GVHD developed in 2 of the 5 disease-free survivors. All the survivors had been conditioned with nonradiation regimens before the second BMT, and 6 of 7 survivors relapsed more than 2 years after the first BMT.

The Seattle group expanded on their experience with second BMTs in a recent abstract (78), in which they reported the results of second BMTs for 77 patients with relapsed AML [30], refractory anemia with excess blasts [2], CML [28], ALL [15], and lymphoma [2]. All patients had received a TBI-containing regimen for their first BMT and a nonradiation regimen for the second (busulfan/CY for 69 patients, and BCNU/etoposide/CY for 8). The probability of DFS was 15% at a median follow-up of 32 months. Relapse occurred in 65% and severe VOD in 26%. Thirty percent of patients died before day 50, mainly from VOD. By multivariate analysis, the significant determinants of DFS were severe VOD (relative risk of death, 9.0) and GVHD of grade II or higher (relative risk of death, 0.5).

The EBMT reported that 32 of 74 patients who had relapsed with ALL or AML after BMT and were then treated with reinduction chemotherapy achieved a CR (63). Of these 32 patients, 9 underwent a second BMT while in CR: 4 with AML and 5 with ALL. The interval from first BMT to relapse ranged from 7 to 31 months (median, 12 mo). They were conditioned for the second BMT with a variety of regimens, including CY/TBI (5), high-dose ara-C (2), melphalan (1), and busulphan (1). Five of these patients died early from graft-related complications (GVHD [3], VOD [1], congestive heart failure [1]). Three patients died after relapsing 6, 9, and 12 months after the second BMT. Only one patient with ALL was alive and disease-free 15 months after the second BMT.

In the study from Seattle (64) cited earlier, in which

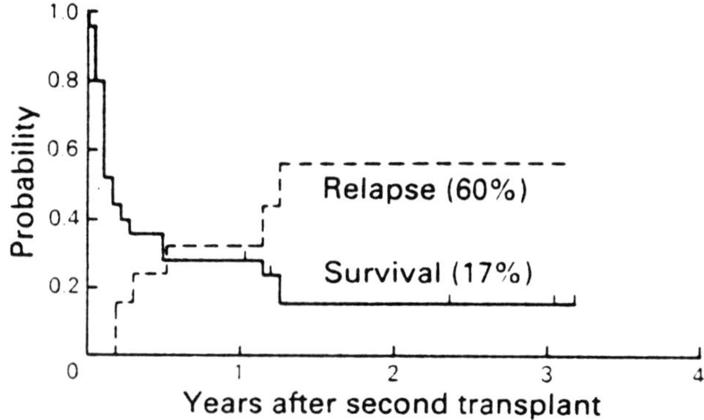

Figure 40-2. Kaplan-Meier product limit estimates of disease-free survival (*broken line*) and relapse (*dotted line*) for 26 patients measured from the time of second bone marrow transplantation. Surviving patients are represented by *tic* marks. (Reproduced by permission from Sanders JE, Buckner CD, Clift RA, et al. Second marrow transplants in patients with leukemia who relapse after allogeneic marrow transplantation. Bone Marrow Transplant 1988;3:11.

62 of 95 patients with AML and 94 of 130 patients with ALL who had relapsed after BMT were then treated with additional therapy, 18 of these patients underwent a second BMT. Of these 18 patients, 13 had AML and 5 had ALL. Seven had undergone syngeneic and 11 allogeneic BMT. Eleven patients were retransplanted while in relapse, and 7 patients (5 with AML, 2 with ALL) were in CR. Of these 7 patients, only one with AML remained alive and disease-free more than 3 years after the second BMT. One of the 11 patients retransplanted in relapse was alive in continued remission 46 months after the second BMT. The remaining 16 patients died from relapse [7], sepsis [2], fungemia [2], IP [2], VOD [1], and other causes [2].

The Johns Hopkins BMT Unit originally described 11 leukemia patients who underwent a second BMT after relapsing following a first BMT (79) and then updated the results for these 11 patients plus an additional 12 patients (80). The group of 23 patients included 12 with CML, 7 with AML, and 4 with ALL. Generally, patients who had received fractionated TBI before their first BMT received busulfan/CY for the second BMT (with or without etoposide), and vice versa. The marrow donors were the same for both transplants for all patients. All 23 patients engrafted a median of 21 days after the second BMT. Acute GVHD occurred in 8 patients, and chronic GVHD occurred in 8 of 12 allogeneic patients who had survived more than 100 days. With a median follow-up of 24 months after the second BMT, the probabilities of event-free survival and relapse were 38 and 24%, respectively. Fourteen patients died, 4 from relapse and 10 from BMT-related toxicity. Patients with CML appeared to do better than patients with AML or ALL (7 of 12 patients alive, disease-free with CML, compared with 2 of 11 patients with AML or ALL).

The London transplant group with the Royal Postgraduate Medical School published their results of second BMTs for 16 patients who relapsed with CML after undergoing a first BMT with T-cell–depleted bone marrow (81). The median number of days from first BMT to cytogenetic and hematological relapse was 494 and 557 days, respectively; median number of days from first to second BMT was 1,211 days. Marrow for second BMTs came from the same HLA-identical siblings used for the first BMT, but the marrows were unmanipulated for the second BMT. Eleven patients were in second CP at the time of second BMT, and 5 patients were in AP or third CP. All 16 patients had received TBI-containing regimens for their first BMT. For conditioning before the second BMT, 4 patients received mitoxantrone/etoposide/total lymphoid irradiation; the other 12 patients received busulfan either alone (8), or in combination with CY (3) or melphalan (1). All patients were given CSP either alone or with MTX or methylprednisolone as prophylaxis against GVHD. The actuarial DFS was 49% at 4 years. Eight patients were alive at 4 years in hematological and cytogenetic CR. Five of these patients were analyzed serially by PCR for detection of bcr-abl transcripts, and 4 of 5 were negative at the time of their most recent study. One patient has been persistently positive 6, 8, and 18 months after second BMT. Five of the 8 patients conditioned wtih busulfan alone are alive in CR. Eight patients died, from IP [2], GVHD [2], BC [2], and infection [2]. Time to relapse after first BMT of less than one year was a high risk factor for poor outcome after second BMT. The authors speculated that GVL mechanisms in this patient population may have been responsible for much of the anti-leukemic effect; therefore, less intensive reconditioning regimens, such as busulfan alone, may lead to better outcomes overall by minimizing transplant-related toxicity.

Investigators at the M.D. Anderson Cancer Center recently reported their experience with second BMTs in 17 patients who had relapsed a median of 9 months after first BMT for ALL [8], AML [5], CML [3], or lymphoma [1] (82). The median interval between transplants was 14 months. Fourteen were allogeneic from HLA-identical siblings, and 3 were syngeneic. The same donor was used for both transplants in all patients except one, for whom a second matched sibling was used. Fourteen patients had been conditioned with TBI-containing regimens for their first BMT and were then conditioned with a variety of nonradiation regimens for their second BMT. Of the 3 patients who were conditioned with chemotherapy alone for their first BMT, 2 received TBI-containing regimens for their second BMT, and one was conditioned with the same chemotherapy regimen used for the first BMT. Most of the allogeneic recipients received CSP alone or with other immunosuppressive agents for GVHD prophylaxis during the second BMT. Only one of the 17 patients received T-cell–depleted marrow for the second BMT; 4 other patients had received T-cell–depleted marrows for their first BMT. Eight patients were in CR before the second BMT, and 9 had active disease. Median survival overall was 9 months. Six of the 9 patients transplanted with active disease achieved a CR; one patient in BC of CML entered a second CP; and 2 patients died of relapse. Median DFS was 4 months, with a probability of 3-year DFS of 12%. Two patients remained alive in continuous CR at 37 and 55 months. A third patient survived in CR after receiving further chemotherapy for a relapse 17 months after the second BMT. Four patients died before day 100: 2 with IP; one with GVHD; and one with persistent AML, aspergillosis, and IP. Of the 10 patients who died after day 100, 8 died from relapse; one from GVHD and one from IP, both in remission. No significant risk factors emerged from this study, including interval between transplants. Five patients had inversions (i.e., the duration of CR after second BMT was longer than that after first BMT). The authors concluded that second transplants should be done in selected patients, that toxicities are significant, and that novel conditioning regimens such as CY/BCNU/etoposide merit further study.

Table 40-1 summarizes the international experience with second BMT.

Table 40-1.
Experience With Second Bone Marrow Transplantation

Group, Ref	*No. Patients*	*Interval from BMT1 to BMT2 (mo) (range)*	*No. Patients (interval <1 yr)*	*Inversions*[a]	*Patients with CCR (> 1yr)*	*Patients Who Died (< 100 days)*
Seattle(77)	26	16 (1–76)	6	2	5	15
MDACC(82)	17	14 (6–24)	6	5	2	4
Hopkins(79)	11	16 (4–62)	3	3	4	4
EBMTG(63)	9	14 (8–44)	1	0	1	4
Sidney(75)	9	14 (4–33)	4	2	1	4
Duarte(76)	5	17 (7–96)	1	1	1	1
UCLA(74)	4	11 (10–17)	2	2	1	1
Total (%)	81 (100)		23 (28)	15 (19)	15 (19)	33 (41)

[a]Inversions = remission after BMT2 longer than after BMT1.
BMT = bone marrow transplantation; CCR = continuous complete remission; UCLA = University of California at Los Angeles; MDACC = M.D. Anderson Cancer Center; EBMTG = European Bone Marrow Transplant Group.
(Reproduced by permission from Spinolo JA, Yau JC, Dickie KA, et al. Second bone marrow transplants for relapsed leukemia. Cancer 1992;69:405–409.)

Summary

The questions of who should receive additional therapy for relapse after first BMT, and in particular, who should undergo a second transplantation are difficult to answer. Atkinson (83) recently discussed this issue after reviewing the international experience with second transplants and made the following observations. In general, long-term leukemia-free survival (LFS) rates are strikingly different for patients relapsing early (< 6 mo? < 12 mo?) after first BMT, compared with later relapse. For patients relapsing within 6 months after first BMT, LFS after second BMT is less than 10%, compared with more than 30% for those relapsing later than 6 months after first BMT. Transplant-related mortality (e.g., VOD and IP) is more common after second than first BMT. It is probably of benefit to maximize GVL effects by using less intense GVHD prophylaxis and by using unmanipulated marrows for second transplantations. Other good risk factors for a favorable outcome after second BMT include good risk leukemia (CML in CP, acute leukemia in CR) and a high Karnofsky performance score before second BMT.

The challenges of overcoming resistant disease that relapses or persists after a first BMT and of limiting cumulative toxicity from a second BMT are difficult. Patients who were conditioned with TBI-containing regimens should be reconditioned with nonradiation regimens to minimize the risk of IP and other toxicities. The availability of effective, alternative conditioning regimens, as mentioned, is one key to the potential success of second transplantations. Several alternatives to the traditional CY/TBI regimen have been developed and include FTBI/etoposide (15,18), busulfan/CY (14,19), busulfan/etoposide (76), BCNU/etoposide/CY (84), and busulfan/CY/etoposide (13). More experience with these regimens will need to be acquired to define their toxicities, antileukemic and immunosuppressive activities, especially in heavily pretreated patients, such as potential candidates for second BMT.

The goals and expected outcomes of a second BMT or additional chemotherapy must be clearly defined for patients who relapse after first BMT. The potential for cure is obviously much less after a second compared with a first BMT. The risk/benefit ratios are tipped heavily toward risk in considering a second BMT. Alternatives to second BMT, such as additional standard chemotherapy or immunotherapy to augment GVL, may be more attractive for patients who have only a very small chance of cure of their leukemia. For many patients, the approach of supportive care only, geared toward palliation of symptoms and maximizing quality and quantity of time out of hospital, may be the best alternative.

References

1. Goldman JM, Gale RP, Horowitz MM, et al. Bone marrow transplantation for chronic myelogenous leukemia in chronic phase. Ann Intern Med 1988;108: 806–814.
2. Snyder D, Blume K, Chao N, et al. Fractionated total body irradiation (FTBI) and etoposide (VP-16): an effective preparative regimen for allogeneic bone marrow transplantation (BMT) for patients with leukemia in first complete remission (CR) (abstract). Proc ASCO 1991;10:220.
3. Thomas ED, Clift RA, Fefer A, et al. Marrow transplantation for the treatment of chronic myelogenous leukemia. Ann Intern Med 1986;104:155–163.
4. McGlave P, Arthur D, Haake R, et al. Therapy of chronic myelogenous leukemia with allogenic bone marrow transplantation. J Clin Oncol 1987;5:1033–1040.
5. Thomas ED, Clift RA. Indications for marrow transplantation in chronic myelogenous leukemia. Blood 1989; 73:861–864.
6. Forman SJ, Krance RA, O'Donnell MR, et al. Bone marrow transplantation for acute nonlymphoblastic leukemia during first complete remission. Transplantation 1987;43:650–653.

7. Barrett AJ, Horowitz MM, Gale RP, et al. Marrow transplantation for acute lymphoblastic leukemia: Factors affecting relapse and survival. Blood 1989;74:862–871.
8. Doney K, Fisher LD, Appelbaum FR, et al. Treatment of adult acute lymphoblastic leukemia with allogeneic bone marrow transplantation. Multivariate analysis of factors affecting acute graft-versus-host disease, relapse, and relapse-free survival. Bone Marrow Transplant 1991;7:453–459.
9. Weisdorf DJ, Nesbit ME, Ramsay NKC, et al. Allogeneic bone marrow transplantation for acute lymphoblastic leukemia in remission: Prolonged survival associated with acute graft-versus-host disease. J Clin Oncol 1987;5:1348–1355.
10. Chao NJ, Forman SJ, Schmidt GM, et al. Allogeneic bone marrow transplantation for high-risk acute lymphoblastic leukemia during first complete remission. Blood 1991;78:1923–1927.
11. Clift RA, Buckner CD, Appelbaum FR, et al. Allogeneic marrow transplantation in patients with acute myeloid leukemia in first remission: a randomized trial of two irradiation regimens. Blood 1990;76:1867–1871.
12. Dopfer R, Henze G, Bender-Götze C, et al. Allogeneic bone marrow transplantation for childhood acute lymphoblastic leukemia in second remission after intensive primary and relapse therapy according to the BFM- and CoALL-protocols: results of the German Cooperative Study. Blood 1991;78:2780–2784.
13. Vaughan WP, Dennison JD, Reed EC, et al. Improved results of allogeneic bone marrow transplantation for advanced hematologic malignancy using busulfan, cyclophosphamide and etoposide as cytoreductive and immunosuppressive therapy. Bone Marrow Transplant 1991;8:489–495.
14. Tutschka PJ, Copelan EA, Klein JP. Bone marrow transplantation for leukemia following a new busulfan and cyclophosphamide regimen. Blood 1987;70:1382–1388.
15. Blume KG, Forman SJ, O'Donnell MR, et al. Total body irradiation and high-dose etoposide: a new preparatory regimen for bone marrow transplantation in patients with advanced hematologic malignancies. Blood 1987; 69:1015–1020.
16. Schouten HC, van Putten WLJ, Hagemeijer A, et al. The prognostic significance of chromosomal findings in patients with acute myeloid leukemia in a study comparing the efficacy of autologous and allogeneic bone marrow transplantation. Bone Marrow Transplant 1991;8:377–381.
17. Forman SJ, O'Donnell MR, Nademanee AP, et al. Bone marrow transplantation for patients with Philadelphia chromosome-positive acute lymphoblastic leukemia. Blood 1987;70:587–588.
18. Schmitz N, Gassmann W, Rister M, et al. Fractionated total body irradiation and high-dose VP-16-213 followed by allogeneic bone marrow transplantation in advanced leukemias. Blood 1988;72:1567–1573.
19. Copelan EA, Biggs JC, Avalos BR, et al. Radiation-free preparation for allogeneic bone marrow transplantation in adults with acute lymphoblastic leukemia. J Clin Oncol 1992;10:237–242.
20. Frassoni F, Bacigalupo A, Marmont A, Scarpati D, Corvò R, Vitale V. Total body irradiation dose and relapse risk after marrow transplantation for leukemia. Blood 1991;77:2543–2544.
21. Clift RA, Buckner CD, Appelbaum FR, et al. Allogeneic marrow transplantation in patients with chronic myeloid leukemia in the chronic phase: a randomized trial of two irradiation regimens. Blood 1991;77:1660–1665.
22. Socie G, Devergie A, Girinsky T, et al, for the advisory committee of GEGMO. Influence of the fractionation of total body irradiation on complications and relapse rate for chronic myelogenous leukemia. Int J Radiat Oncol Biol Phys 1991;20:397–404.
23. Sullivan KM, Weiden PL, Storb R, et al. Influence of acute and chronic graft-versus-host disease on relapse and survival after bone marrow transplantation from HLA-identical siblings as treatment of acute and chronic leukemia Blood 1989;73:1720–1728.
24. Sullivan KM, Storb R, Buckner CD, et al. Graft-versus-host disease as adoptive immunotherapy in patients with advanced hematologic neoplasms. N Engl J Med 1989;320:828–834.
25. Marmont AM, Horowitz MM, Gale RP, et al. T-cell depletion of HLA-identical transplants in leukemia. Blood 1991;78:2120–2130
26. Slavin S, Ackerstein A, Naparstek E, Or R, Weiss L. Hypothesis: the graft-versus-leukemia (GVL) phenomenon: is GVL separable from GVHD? Bone Marrow Transplant 1990;6:155–161.
27. Boyd CN, Ramberg RC, Thomas ED. The incidence of recurrence of leukemia in donor cells after allogeneic bone marrow transplantation. Leuk Res 1982;6:833–837.
28. Marmont A, Frassoni F, Bacigalupo A, et al. Recurrence of Ph-positive leukemia in donor cells after marrow transplantation for chronic granulocytic leukemia. N Engl J Med 1984;310:903–905.
29. Browne PV, Lawler M, Humphries P, McCann SR. Donor-cell leukemia after bone marrow transplantation for severe aplastic anemia. N Engl J Med 1991;325:710–713.
30. Witherspoon RP, Schubach W, Neiman P, Martin P, Thomas ED. Donor cell leukemia developing six years after marrow grafting for acute leukemia. Blood 1985; 65:1172–1174.
31. Stein J, Zimmerman PA, Kochera M, et al. Origin of leukemic relapse after bone marrow transplantation: comparison of cytogenetic and molecular analyses. Blood 1989;73:2033–2040.
32. Fialkow PJ, Thomas ED, Bryant JI, Neiman PE. Leukemic transformation of engrafted human marrow cells in vivo. Lancet 1971;1:251–255.
33. Sessarego M, Frassoni F, Defferrari R, et al. Karyotype evolution of Ph positive chronic myelogenous leukemia patients relapsed in advanced phases of the disease after allogeneic bone marrow transplantation. Cancer Genet Cytogenet 1991;57:69–78.
34. Calabrese G, Di Bartolomeo P, Stuppia L, et al. Cytogenetics in patients with chronic myelogenous leukemia treated with bone marrow transplantation. Cancer Genet Cytogenet 1989;41:49–59.
35. Sessarego M, Frassoni F, Defferrari R, et al. Cytogenetic follow-up after bone marrow transplantation for Philadelphia-positive chronic myeloid leukemia. Cancer Genet Cytogenet 1989;42:253–261.
36. Arthur CK, Apperley JF, Guo AP, Rassool F, Gao LM, Goldman JM. Cytogenetic events after bone marrow transplantation for chronic myeloid leukemia in chronic phase. Blood 1988;71:1179–1186.
37. Cooperative Study Group on Chromosomes in Transplanted Patients. Cytogenetic follow-up of 100 patients submitted to bone marrow transplantation for Philadel-

phia chromosome-positive chronic myeloid leukemia. Eur J Haematol 1988;40:50–57.
38. Lange W, Snyder DS, Castro R, Rossi JJ, Blume K. Detection by enzymatic amplification of bcr-abl mRNA in peripheral blood and bone marrow cells of patients with chronic myelogenous leukemia. Blood 1989; 73:1735–1741.
39. Roth MS, Antin JH, Ash R, et al. Prognostic significance of Philadelphia chromosome-positive cells detected by the polymerase chain reaction after allogeneic bone marrow transplant for chronic myelogenous leukemia. Blood 1992;79:276–282.
40. DeLage R, Soiffer RJ, Dear K, Ritz J. Clinical significance of bcr-abl gene rearrangement detected by polymerase chain reaction after allogeneic bone marrow transplantation in chronic myelogenous leukemia. Blood 1991;78:2759–2767.
41. Snyder DS, Rossi JJ, Wang J-L, et al. Persistence of bcr-abl gene expression following bone marrow transplantation for chronic myelogenous leukemia in chronic phase. Transplantation 1991;51:1033–1040.
42. Ganesan TS, Min GL, Goldman JM, Young BD. Molecular analysis of relapse in chronic myeloid leukemia after allogeneic bone marrow transplantation. Blood 1987;70:873–876.
43. Miller WJ, Shapiro RS, Gonzalez-Sarmiento R, Kersey JH. Molecular genetic rearrangements distinguish pre- and post-bone marrow transplantation lymphoproliferative processes. Blood 1987;70:882–885.
44. Shapiro RS, McClain K, Frizzera G, et al. Epstein-Barr virus associated B cell lymphoproliferative disorders following bone marrow transplantation. Blood 1988; 71:1234–1243.
45. Schubach WH, Miller G, Thomas ED. Epstein-Barr virus genomes are restricted to secondary neoplastic cells following bone marrow transplantation. Blood 1985;65:535–538.
46. Fischer A, Blanche S, Le Bidois J, et al. Anti-B-cell monoclonal antibodies in the treatment of severe B-cell lymphoproliferative syndrome following bone marrow and organ transplantation. N Engl J Med 1991; 324:1451–1456.
47. Witherspoon RP, Fisher LD, Schoch G, et al. Secondary cancers after bone marrow transplantation for leukemia or aplastic anemia. N Engl J Med 1989;321:784–789.
48. Thompson CB, Sanders JE, Flournoy N, Buckner CD, Thomas ED. The risks of central nervous system relapse and leukoencephalopathy in patients receiving marrow transplants for acute leukemia. Blood 1986;67:195–199.
49. Klingemann H-G, Phillips GL. Immunotherapy after bone marrow transplantation. Bone Marrow Transplant 1991;8:73–81.
50. Klingemann H-G, Grigg AP, Wilkie-Boyd K, et al. Treatment with recombinant interferon (α-2β) early after bone marrow transplantation in patients at high risk for relapse. Blood 1991;78:3306–3311.
51. Higuchi CM, Thompson JA, Petersen FB, Buckner CD, Fefer A. Toxicity and immunomodulatory effects of interleukin-2 after autologous bone marrow transplantation for hematologic malignancies. Blood 1991; 77:2561–2568.
52. Gottlieb DJ, Brenner MK, Heslop HE, et al. A phase I clinical trial of recombinant interleukin-2 following high dose chemo-radiotherapy for haematological malignancy: applicability to the elimination of minimal residual disease. Br J Cancer 1989;60:610.
53. Blaise D, Olive D, Stoppa AM, et al. Hematologic and immunologic effects of the systemic administration of recombinant interleukin-2 after autologous bone marrow transplantation. Blood 1990;76:1092–1097.
54. Soiffer RJ, Murray C, Cochran K, et al. Clinical and immunologic effects of prolonged infusion of low-dose recombinant interleukin-2 after autologous and T-cell-depleted allogeneic bone marrow transplantation. Blood 1992;79:517–526.
55. Talpaz M, Kantarjian H, Kurzrock R, Trujillo JM, Gutterman JU. Interferon-alpha produces sustained cytogenetic responses in chronic myelogenous leukemia. Ann Intern Med 1991;114:532–538.
56. Arcese W, Mauro FR, Alimena G, et al. Interferon therapy for Ph1 positive CML patients relapsing after T cell-depleted allogeneic bone marrow transplantation. Bone Marrow Transplant 1990;5:309–315.
57. Kolb HJ, Mittermuller J, Clemm C, et al. Donor leukocyte transfusions for treatment of recurrent chronic myelogenous leukemia in marrow transplant patients. Blood 1990;76:2462–2465.
58. Cullis JO, Jiang YZ, Schwarer AP, Hughes TP, Barrett AJ, Goldman JM. Donor leukocyte infusions for chronic myeloid leukemia in relapse after allogeneic bone marrow transplantation. Blood 1992;79:1379–1381.
59. Higano CS, Raskind WH, Singer JW. Use of alpha interferon for the treatment of chronic myelogenous leukemia in chronic phase after allogeneic bone marrow transplantation. Blood 1992;80:1437.
60. Nagler A, Ackerstein A, Naparstek E, Ben-Neriah S, Barak V, Slavin S. Concomitant treatment of chronic myelogenous leukemia (CML) with recombinant human interleukin-2 (IL2) (abstract). Blood 1991;78(suppl 1):238a.
61. Barrett AJ, Joshi R, Tew C. How should acute lymphoblastic leukaemia relapsing after bone-marrow transplantation be treated? Lancet 1985;1:1188–1191.
62. Bostrom B, Woods WG, Nesbit ME, et al. Successful reinduction of patients with acute lymphoblastic leukemia who relapse following bone marrow transplantation. J Clin Oncol 1987;5:376–381.
63. Frassoni F, Barrett AJ, Granena A, et al. Relapse after allogeneic bone marrow transplantation for acute leukaemia: a survey by the E.B.M.T. of 117 cases. Br J Haematol 1988;70:317–320.
64. Mortimer J, Blinder MA, Schulman S, et al. Relapse of acute leukemia after marrow transplantation: natural history and results of subsequent therapy. J Clin Oncol 1989;7:50–57.
65. Nevill TJ, Barnett MJ, Robinson KS, Greer W, Phillips GL. Return to durable donor haematopoiesis after blast phase relapse of chronic myeloid leukaemia following marrow transplantation. Br J Haematol 1992;80:256–258.
66. Chen S-J, Zhu Y-J, Tong J-H, et al. Rearrangements in the second intron of the RARA gene are present in a large majority of patients with acute promyelocytic leukemia and are used as molecular marker for retinoic acid-induced leukemic cell differentiation. Blood 1991; 78:2696–2701.
67. Chang K-S, Stass SA, Chu D-T, Deaven LL, Trujillo JM, Freireich EJ. Characterization of a fusion cDNA (RARA/myl) transcribed from the t(15;17) translocation breakpoint in acute promyelocytic leukemia. Mol Cell Biol 1992;12:800–810.
68. Chang K-S, Lu J, Wang G, et al. The t(15;17) breakpoint in acute promyelocytic leukemia cluster within two different sites of the myl gene: targets for the detection

of minimal residual disease by the polymerase chain reaction. Blood 1992;79:554–558.

69. Kastner P, Perez A, Lutz Y, et al. Structure, localization and transcriptional properties of two classes of retinoic acid receptor α fusion proteins in acute promyelocytic leukemia (APL): structural similarities with a new family of oncoproteins. EMBO J 1992;11:629–642.
70. Fenaux P, Degos L. Treatment of acute promyelocytic leukemia with all-trans retinoic acid. Leuk Res 1991; 15:655–657.
71. Chen Z-X, Xue Y-Q, Zhang R, et al. A clinical and experimental study on all-trans retinoic acid-treated acute promyelocytic leukemia patients. Blood 1991; 78:1413–1419.
72. Chomienne C, Balitrand N, Ballerini P, Castaigne S, De Thé H, Degos L. All-trans retinoic acid modulates the retinoic acid receptor-α in promyelocytic cells. J Clin Invest 1991;88:2150–2154.
73. Bashford J, Szer J, Wiley JS, Buckley M, Garson OM, Van der Weyden MB. Treatment of acute promyelocytic leukaemia relapsing after allogeneic bone marrow transplantation with all-trans-retinoic acid: suppression of the leukaemic clone. Br J Haematol 1991;79: 331–334.
74. Champlin RE, Ho WG, Lenarsky C, et al. Successful second bone marrow transplants for treatment of acute myelogenous leukemia or acute lymphoblastic leukemia. Transplant Proc 1985;17:496–499.
75. Atkinson K, Biggs J, Concannon A, Dodds A, Dale B, Norman J. Second marrow transplants for recurrence of haematological malignancy. Bone Marrow Transplant 1986;1:159–166.
76. Blume KG, Forman SJ. High dose busulfan/etoposide as a preparatory regimen for second bone marrow transplants in hematologic malignancies. Blut 1987;55:49–53.
77. Sanders JE, Buckner CD, Clift RA, et al. Second marrow transplants in patients with leukemia who relapse after allogeneic marrow transplantation. Bone Marrow Transplant 1988;3:11–19.
78. Radich J, Sanders J, Buckner CD, Martin P, Petersen FB. Second allogeneic bone marrow transplants for patients relapsing after initial transplant with TBI-containing regimens (abstract). Blood 1991;78(suppl 1):241a.
79. Wagner JE, Santos GW, Burns WH, Saral R. Second bone marrow transplantation after leukemia relapse in 11 patients. Bone Marrow Transplant 1989;4:115–118.
80. Wagner JE, Vogelsang GB, Zehnbauer BA, Griffin CA, Shah N, Santos GW. Relapse of leukemia after bone marrow transplantation: effect of second myeoloablative therapy. Bone Marrow Transplant 1992;9: 205–209.
81. Cullis JO, Schwarer AP, Hughes TP, et al. Second transplants for patients with chronic myeloid leukaemia in relapse after original transplant with T-depleted donor marrow: feasibility of using busulphan alone for re-conditioning. Br J Haematol 1992;80:33–39.
82. Spinolo JA, Yau JC, Dicke KA, et al. Second bone marrow transplants for relapsed leukemia. Cancer 1992;69:405–409.
83. Atkinson K. Who should get second transplants? (Abstract). J Cell Biochem [A] 1992;16(suppl):179.
84. Radich J, Sanders J, Buckner CD, Martin P, Petersen FB. Second marrow transplants utilizing a preparative regimen of cyclophosphamide, etoposide and carmustine (abstract). Blood 1990;76(suppl 1):560a.

Chapter 41
Psychological Issues in Bone Marrow Transplantation

David K. Wellisch and Deane L. Wolcott

Hope is the earliest and the most indispensable of virtues. If life is to be sustained, hope must remain, even where confidence is wounded, trust impaired.

Erik Erikson

This chapter is oriented toward three basic goals. The first and foremost is to provide a deeper level of understanding of patients undergoing bone marrow transplantation (BMT) and their families. The second is to delineate interventions that facilitate psychological management of patients and their families. With these two goals in mind, it is expected that the third major goal of the chapter can be achieved: improved adaptation to and coping with the rigors of the BMT process.

This chapter has three basic sections. The first section is primarily oriented toward BMT patients in terms of delineation of psychological reactions to BMT and to interventions for those reactions. These are subdivided into "usual" and "unusual" reactions, with attendant interventions. The second section is oriented toward families of BMT patients. A key theme in this section is that BMT is a biomedical experience for patients but a psychological experience for the entire family unit. The family of a BMT recipient includes several relationships: (1) the donor-recipient dyad; (2) the patient and spouse/significant other; (3) the patient and their children; and (4) the patient and their parents. All these relationships are discussed in terms of expected reactions and possible interventions. The third section is oriented toward the staff that cares for BMT recipients. They form a complex psychological matrix that often is ignored. A key theme in this section is the idea that psychological coping, adapting, and integrity of the medical and nursing staff have direct implications for the capacity of patients and their families to cope with BMT. In this section, the notion of the BMT unit as a "psychological system" is a key feature.

BMT Patients

Selection for BMT

The psychological processes involved in BMT start with selection for BMT. A key question at this point is, are there psychiatric contraindications for BMT? The psychological literature on BMT offers few answers to this question, having focused substantially more on outcome and follow-up than on pretransplant evaluation. Some data can be obtained from studies of transplantation of other organs, such as liver, kidney, and heart. Surman (1), in a review of psychiatric aspects of organ transplantation, delineates several areas to focus on as key risk factors. Two of the most frequent and crucial include recent alcohol or drug abuse (2,3) and a pattern of obvious medical noncompliance (4). Surman (1) comes to two basic conclusions on this issue, both of which apply to potential transplant patients. (1) Most patients with psychiatric contraindications to organ transplantation are capable of successful intraoperative and postoperative outcomes, and (2) rather than deny transplantation on psychiatric grounds, the question becomes, what psychiatric services are necessary to bring this patient through the transplant process? If these services are not available, where can this be achieved?

The psychiatric consultation group at UCLA has been interested in the issue of prediction of psychological adaptation to and coping with BMT through systematic assessment of patients. We have developed a system of assigning BMT recipients a "level" of perceived psychosocial adjustment ranging from level I (good adjustment) to level III (poor adjustment) (5). Table 41-1 depicts a set of 7 psychosocial characteristics and how they manifest themselves within three levels of BMT recipients. This system has enabled us to do several things, including predict or adjust workload in psychiatric management of the BMT recipient population in the hospital at any one time; predict staff stress, especially for nurses on the unit; talk in "shorthand" about patient/family problems; and develop more fine-tuned orientation toward interventions that "fit" each of the three patient levels. As can be observed from Table 41-1, level III patients virtually always present with pre-existing psychiatric diagnoses, which can involve both DSM-III-R Axis I (e.g., anxiety disorder, major depression) or Axis II (e.g., character disorders, substance abuse) (6). This group has been able to undergo transplantation at

Table 41-1.
Psychosocial Levels of Adjustment of BMT Recipients

Psychosocial Characteristics	*Level 1*	*Level 2*	*Level 3*
Prior psychiatric history	None	Some history of depression, anxiety, or trauma; personality disorder features; some history of significant loss.	Significant history. May involve chemical dependency, multiple or significant loses, serious personality disorder, severe anxiety disorder, or phobias; major depression.
Quality of family/social support	Good to excellent: social/family members present and available; willing to focus on patient's needs	Good to fair: some separation difficulties; some conflict and dependency problems.	Dysfunctional: enmeshed or disengaged boundaries; extremely conflictual; focused on individual needs at expense to patient.
Prior history of coping	Good to excellent: adapts to problems and changes flexibly. Has extensive repertoire of coping behaviors.	Good to Fair: some flexibility in coping repertoire and some variations in coping responses, with general limitations. Some negativistic patterns of responding when under stress.	Fair to poor: decompensation under stress; negativistic patterns; rigid style; history of self-destructive behaviors; limited repertoire of coping behavior; impulsive or aggressive responses.
Coping with disease and treatment	Resolution of feelings about diagnosis. Considers treatment options with realistic balance of hope and concern for future.	Denial; lack of clarity; ambivalence over treatment choice.	Extreme denial; confusion over disease course; severe ambivalence about treatment.
Quality of affect	Appropriate fears; some anxiety; appropriate sadness.	Moderate fears and anxiety; moderate depression.	Generalized anxiety; moderate to severe depression; extreme fears and anger.
Mental status (past and present)	No cognitive impairment or disorder of attention; normal sleep-wake cycle; normal activity level and responsiveness.	Some history or current impairment in cognitive function, attention, sleep-wake cycle, activity level, or responsiveness.	Global disorder of cognitive functions (perception, thinking, memory, orientation); attention (awareness and consciousness; difficulties with mobilizing, shifting, sustaining, and directing attention; hyperalert or hypoalert); severe disruption of normal sleep-wake cycles; reduced or heightened activity level and responsiveness (movements, speech).
Proneness to anticipatory anxiety	Not prone to anticipatory anxiety.	Moderate to high: anticipatory anxiety beginning with actual day of chemotherapy/radiation.	Severe anticipatory anxiety, nausea, vomiting beginning prior to day of chemotherapy/radiation.

UCLA despite these manifest or latent disorders with intensive involvement and planning with the psychiatry service.

Of the 7 psychosocial characteristics present in Table 41-1, the most important in anticipating problems are (1) prior psychiatric history, (2) quality of family/social support, and (3) prior history of coping (in that order) in prediction of adjustment to BMT (5). These three issues, therefore, become critical in our evaluation of how difficult BMT will be for patients.

Psychosocial "Stages" of BMT

Usual and Expected Problems

In a now classic article on psychological evaluation of BMT, Brown and Kelly (7) described 8 characteristic psychological stages of BMT: (1) decision to accept BMT, (2) initial admission evaluation and case planning, (3) entry into isolation/conditioning regime, (4) actual transplant, (5) graft rejection versus take, (6) potential graft-versus-host disease (GVHD), (7) preparation for discharge, and (8) adaptation out of hospital. Table 41-2 depicts these stages, associated psychological reactions and symptoms, and characteristic psychiatric interventions. As Table 41-2 shows, the psychological reactions to BMT unfold along with the medical events associated with BMT. Table 41-2 reflects a typical course of behavioral response during allogenic BMT transplantation for acute lymphoblastic leukemia (ALL) or chronic myeloid leukemia (CML). If autologous BMT is done without total body irradiation (TBI), then the responses tend to be somewhat milder. These stages and possible psychological reactions must be evaluated in the context of Table 41-1 in terms of the levels of psychological adaptation of patients. Level II and especially level III patients bring to BMT a history of poorer psychological integration; more significant

Table 41-2.
Stages of BMT-associated Psychological Reactions/Interventions

Stage of BMT	*Possible Psychological Reactions*	*Intervention Possibilities*
1. Decision-making	1. Ambivalence—anxiety (mild to severe) 2. Denial (of potential problems with BMT) 3. Refusal (rare)	1. Education (best) 2. Formation of oncologist/patient treatment alliance 3. Referral for psychological evaluation or counseling
2. Initial admission evaluation and care planning	1. Denial persists 2. Anxiety (mild to severe) 3. Affect blunted (2^0 to denial, "numbness")	1. Solidification of treatment alliance 2. Introduction of psychological services 3. Evaluation of patient's personality/coping 4. Psychopharmacology if needed
3. Conditioning regimen; entry into reverse isolation	1. Patient personality characteristics accentuate 2. Anxiety heightens—dependency needs escalate 3. Concerns about dying, aloneness, possible claustrophobia appear 4. Neuropsychiatric complications of steroids, other medications, and infections begin to appear	1. Relaxation techniques 2. Psychotherapy 3. Psychopharmacology 4. Begin evaluation of impact of medications on brain/central nervous system (CNS)
4. Actual BMT	1. Let down—"is this all there is to it?" 2. Mounting sense of bond/gratitude to donor	Continue as per last phase
5. Graft rejection vs take (medical "nadir")	1. Anxiety reaches peak—regression evident 2. Depression symptoms (2^0 to medical nadir) 3. Regret—"If I knew I would be this sick I would not have done this" (not infrequent) 4. Anger at staff—Increased dependency on staff 5. Neuropsychiatric disregulation (per previous phases) 6. Frustration, especially for action-oriented patients	1. Increase psychological support 2. Increase psychopharmacological agents, as needed 3. Seriously evaluate impact/necessity of all medications on brain/CNS 4. Continuity of structure critical
6. If graft takes, possible development of GVHD	1. Depression and } Two dominant 2. Anger } reactions 3. Underlying grief forming—"I thought I'd get through this without permanent changes"	1. Maintain high level of psychological support 2. Facilitate ventilation 3. Intervene vigorously if depression escalates
7. Preparation for discharge	1. Mixture of relief/anxiety 2. Separation anxiety possible from unit 3. Denial frequently about return to life tasks (overestimation) 4. Grief to depression (?) about body image changes (i.e., GVHD) now viewed as possibly permanent	1. Discharge educational counseling critical 2. Creation of interim structure/schedule of medical visits 3. Referral for psychological counseling (infrequent) 4. Referral to post-BMT support group
8. Adaptation out of hospital	1. Neuropsychological (cognitive) deficits 2. Body image changes 3. Slower (than anticipated) energy return 4. Sexual problems 5. Slower (than anticipated) return to work/school Nos. 1 through 5 all fuel mild to severe grief reactions that can become depression.	1. Post-BMT support group 2. General cancer support group 3. Individual psychological counseling 4. Family counseling 5. Psychopharmacological agents, especially antidepressants

CNS = central nervous system; GVHD = graft-versus-host disease.
Adapted from Brown NH, Kelly MJ. Stages of bone marrow transplantation: a psychiatric perspective. Psychosom Med 1976;38:439–446.

losses and trauma; a more dysfunctional or primitive set of defenses and coping responses to the stresses of BMT; and a greater capacity to regress to pathological levels of behavior under the impact of conditioning, isolation, pain, and metabolic- or drug-induced delirium during transplantation.

As Table 41-2 shows, stages III and V contain the most severe psychological responses for patients. In stage III, during conditioning, several factors are set in motion simultaneously that have major impact. Overall, this is the point where "the train has left the station" and there is no going back after the onset of conditioning. This fact is coupled with placement in reverse isolation, which can generate substantial feelings of aloneness and claustrophobia, which in turn may produce a sense of feeling "trapped," escalating anxiety. This reaction was personified in a 25-year-old Filipino-American man transplanted for ALL at UCLA. At this stage of his BMT, he revealed frightening memories, previously repressed, of being in an underground bunker while under enemy attack in Vietnam. This post-traumatic stress disorder was revived by the entry into reverse isolation and required extensive staff education, psychotherapy, and psychopharmacological (anxiolytic) intervention. On the medical side, the introduction of radiation to the brain and the central nervous system (CNS), as well as the introduction of steroid and narcotics for pain, all disorient the patient, compounding the sense of loss of control psychologically at this stage (8).

In stage V, patients are again confronted with a series of intense psychological issues, some for the first time during BMT. The key psychological issue is the breakdown of denial, which involves previously held denial that engraftment might not take place at all. Although initially well educated during the informed consent conducted before BMT, studies show retention of such information by patients is severely limited (9,10). The second crisis involves the realization that substantial trauma, pain, and debility have been induced by conditioning, which is more than the patient was able to grasp during informed consent sessions. Third is the realization that all of this debility might not rapidly (or ever) go away even if survival is achieved. Disillusionment may be projected onto both the family and the physicians at this point. For level I patients, this can take the form of a question ("why did no one tell me I would feel like this?"), whereas for level III patients, it can take the form of a raging, paranoid attack ("you all lied to me and tricked me into this; I would never have done this if I had not been lied to about what I would feel.") This represents a potential crisis for the working alliance of the patient/family/staff. For level I patients, fewer of the possible interventions are necessary at these two stages (III and V) than for level II or III patients, who may need the entire spectrum of possible interventions.

"Usual" BMT Recipient Psychological Reactions

Five psychological/neurological reactions are ubiquitous in BMT recipients regardless of procedure (i.e., allogeneic, autologous with/without TBI) and should be regarded as normal responses. These include (1) anxiety, (2) grief, (3) regression, (4) ambivalence, and (5) neuropsychiatric disregulation of the brain or the CNS.

Anxiety in BMT recipients is an emotional and physiological response to actual external threats and to the pressure of internal emotional states that may be unacceptable. The question becomes the proportion of the anxiety to the threat. A second question becomes, does the focus of the anxiety become displaced from its original source to another source, procedure, or person? Mild to moderate anxiety is to be expected consistently throughout BMT, probably reaching its height during the medical nadir during the engraftment phase. The conscious dangers of fear of death and loss of denial produce the highest level of anxiety. When anxiety becomes severe, it overflows the psyche and becomes more physiological (11). This produces gross motor restlessness, otherwise known as agitation. Agitation in BMT recipients is a symptom that calls for intervention.

Grief in BMT recipients is a response to losses and is a normal and expected development. It is often confused with depression; it mimics the signs and symptoms of depression, but it is not a maladjustment but a functional adjustment (11). Grief in BMT recipients takes shape during engraftment and can be expected to be present in all stages thereafter, especially in the post-hospitalization phase as losses and decreased abilities to function as previously are fully realized. Grief waxes and wanes, whereas depression remains fixed and grows in intensity. Grief leads to self preoccupation and withdrawal, processes accentuated by reverse isolation and drug-induced delirium and disorientation. Grief in BMT recipients rarely embodies suicidal thoughts or feelings of personal worthlessness. BMT patients can be expected to say, "I intensely dislike what I am going through but I still feel like a worthwhile person." The same patient who has crossed the line between normal grief and clinical depression might say, "I have been destroyed by what I am going through, feel worthless, no longer human, and wish I would die." Such feelings or thought patterns clearly call for intervention.

Regression is an anxiety-binding defense mechanism in which the personality may experience loss of mature emotional development and revert to a lower level of integration, adjustment, and expression. The individual in regression seeks to regain both control over anxieties and to regain gratifications of an earlier period of life (11). All patients regress in the face of the psychological and medical impacts of BMT, especially during the conditioning phase, when these factors are most intense. For level I and usually level II patients, regression characteristically stops during the engraftment phase. For level III patients, regression may become a free-fall leading to infantile behaviors and inducing disgust and rejection in the staff. This condition obscures underlying feelings of panic about caring for such a primitive, passive, and needy patient. When normal regression becomes a free-fall and an infantile personality core is exposed, it may produce life-threatening noncompliance in BMT patients. A clinical example of this was a 16-year-old boy who was not able to be transplanted for aplastic anemia but was given a course of antithymocyte globulin. His parents were so infantile and needy that they were unable to be supportive and they stopped coming to the hospital midcourse in his treatment. The patient regressed to the point of nearly autistic withdrawal and refused to be touched and examined medically. Psychological intervention was minimally successful; the patient was ultimately discharged home to die. Such regression always calls for intensive psychological interventions.

Ambivalence represents contradictory feelings and attitudes toward the same person or situation (11). One of the two feeling components of ambivalence may remain repressed and unconscious, thus giving rise to anxiety and feelings of guilt. The repressed feeling may be one of hostility and may be felt toward one to whom a person is indebted, such as a physician or a nurse. Such a feeling is often not tolerable consciously. BMT recipients are very likely to have ambivalence toward the health care team members who care for them. Conscious feelings of gratitude and dependency are almost certain to be countered by far less tolerable feelings of hostility about the trauma, pain, and suffering induced by BMT, especially for patients who earlier had fewer physical effects of their disease. Sudden emergence of such hostile feelings, especially when the patient is regressed, are not be to understood as a collapse of the doctor-patient relationship, but rather the normal expression of a previously repressed but expected realm of feeling toward the treating physician.

Neuropsychiatric disregulation is to be expected along a continuum in all BMT recipients. Wolcott and Stuber (8) reported delirium to be clinically common during and immediately after conditioning. High-dose cyclophosphamide (CY) has been associated with transient water intoxication, euphoria, and feelings of unreality (8,12,13). Immediate and delayed neurotoxicity has been reported secondary to mechlorethamine (nitrogen mustard) administration during conditioning. This neurotoxicity can take the form of delirium; diffuse electroencephalographic slowing occurs in the acute phase. Delayed neuropsychological problems have included communicating hydrocephalus occurring 2 to 8 months after transplantation (8,14). Patchell and colleagues (15) reported on the incidence and etiology of CNS complications in 77 children and adults who died after BMT. Problems developed in 62% (48 of 77), whereas altered mental states due to metabolic and/or hypoxia developed in 56%. GVHD calls for use of steroid and cyclosporine, which both have well-known and documented psychiatric side effects, including organic affective syndromes and encephalopathy (16,17). A crucial issue at this point is the pretransplant integrity of the patient's brain and CNS, which may be very different for level III BMT recipients, who may have abused alcohol or drugs earlier in life, had head trauma, and had poorer prenatal care. In a very provocative report on outcome of liver transplantation in alcoholics, each carefully matched with a nonalcoholic liver transplant recipient, the alcoholic transplant recipients had longer lengths of stay, more mortality, more serious medical complications, and more episodes of delirium and prolonged encephalopathy after transplantation than the other group (18). These findings suggest that neuropsychiatric disregulation may follow the same gradient of intensity as all other psychological adaptational difficulties from level I to level III patients.

"Unusual" Psychological Reactions

Five unusual psychological reactions are harbingers of significant danger in BMT recipients and always call for rapid and definitive psychological or medical intervention. These reactions include (1) persistent suicidal ideation or frank suicidality, (2) depression that clearly departs from the normal grief reaction, (3) disruptive anxiety, (4) pathological regression up to and including frank psychiatric decompensation, and (5) organic delirium.

Suicidal ideation for cancer patients in general is probably not a rare phenomenon. There seems to be a consensus in the literature that actual suicide in cancer patients is a relatively rare phenomenon, including BMT recipients (19–21). This incidence, however, may not relate to the actual incidence of suicide in cancer patients because it is far more likely to occur at home (versus hospital), with family reluctance to report it (22). Breitbart (23), in a combined review of the literature and assessment of 1,080 psychiatric consultations at Memorial Sloan-Kettering Cancer Center involving suicidal ideation, developed a set of 8 key variables to predict cancer patients at increased suicide risk: (1) advanced illness/poor prognosis; (2) depression and hopelessness; (3) pain (uncontrolled); (4) delirium; (5) loss of control/sense of hopelessness; (6) preexisting psychopathology; (7) prior suicide history, personal or in family; and (8) exhaustion and fatigue. In surveying this list, it is readily apparent that several of these factors such as advanced illness/poor (or guarded) prognosis, delirium, pain, loss of control, and exhaustion/fatigue are frequent co-factors in BMT. Two cases of suicidal behavior after BMT were described by Jenkins and Roberts (24). The two patients were both young adults (early 20s); one was a man, and the other was a woman with two young children. The man achieved a completed suicide; the woman suffered a serious overdose with antidepressant medication and survived only to die of septicemia and deterioration several weeks later. Two key factors are shared by these two patients: Both had persistent GVHD that became chronic, visible, and disfiguring; and both were given repeated courses of steroids. Thus, the emotional dynamics of hopelessness, loss of control, and depression, which were possibly partially biologically induced by steroids, seemed to form a lethal combination in these two patients. A key issue is early intervention before these factors build to a lethal level.

Depression in cancer patients can be very difficult to differentiate from sadness and grief, especially in the advanced stages of illness. However, identification and timely intervention for depression can be crucial in the survival of BMT recipients. The frequency of depression in cancer patients varies widely over studies based on types of ratings (e.g., clinician reports vs predefined criteria). In a review of studies of cancer patients that varied by stage and site, the highest frequency of depression was present in patients who (1) had advanced disease, (2) were in the hospital (as opposed to outpatient status), and (3) had Karnofsky scores of 40 or less (25). This profile essentially includes all BMT recipients in the midst of transplantation after conditioning. However, even though BMT is a "depressogenic" procedure, not all patients become clinically depressed during BMT. Massie (25) describes 3 key areas in the vulnerability to depression: (1) family history (has there been previous depression or suicide?); (2) personal history (has there been previous psychiatric illness such as depression, affective disorder, or alcoholism/drug abuse?); and (3) are there contributing illness/treatment factors such as steroids, suspect chemotherapeutic agents (i.e., interferon), valium, or phenobarbital, or other metabolic or neurological problems creating mild to moderate delirium that have gone unrecognized? Many signs and symptoms can be present in BMT recipients that may be depression or may be treatment-induced. Somatic symptomatology has less value in diagnosing depression in BMT recipients. The most central symptoms include severity of dysphoric mood; degree of feelings of hopelessness, guilt, and worthlessness; and presence of suicidal ideation (25). Although symptoms of grief ebb and flow, these symptoms of depression remain fixed and steadily escalate over time if left untreated.

Anxiety in BMT recipients is another ubiquitous emotional reaction that is expected but can escalate to disruptive and disorganizing levels. Allowing anxiety to rise to a disruptive level fragments coping in patients and reverberates within family and staff, with subsequent declines in their coping and abilities to support the patient. Four basic types of anxiety can be seen in BMT recipients: (1) situational/reactive anxiety related to crises; (2) anxiety related to medical influences, which can involve poorly controlled pain and abnormal metabolic states, such as hypoxia, sepsis, delirium, or pulmonary embolism. Anxiety can also be drug-induced. Steroids such as dexamethasone and prednisone can produce anxiety at high dosages or during rapid taper. These steroids are commonly administered to BMT recipients. Neuroleptics given for emesis control can often produce akathesias, which induce agitation and motor restlessness and mimic anxiety. (3) Anxiety relating to a preexisting anxiety disorder, which can be expected in level III patients (see Table 41-1); and (4) special anxiety-provoking medical situations, such as isolation following the conditioning regimen or bone marrow biopsies during BMT (26).

Pathological regression can take many forms in BMT recipients. Such patients tend to group into three clusters (6). (1) an anxious/fearful cluster; (2) a dramatic, emotional, or erratic cluster; or (3) an "odd" or eccentric cluster (27). Under the stresses of BMT, each of these three clusters may regress to dysfunctional levels that interfere in compliance with medical regimes and frustrate efforts of staff to care for them.

The anxious/fearful cluster includes patients who are obsessive-compulsive, avoidant, dependent, or passive-aggressive. They can become "collapsed" under extreme stress and become infantile in their dependency needs. The staff response in such a circumstance can be to feel overwhelmed by their infantile neediness. The dramatic, emotional, or erratic cluster includes patients who are histrionic, narcissistic, antisocial, or borderline in personality maladjustment. Such patients can become hostile, act-out, confrontational, and demanding in histrionic ways under stress. The staff response is to feel irritated, threatened, or demeaned by such patients. The staff can feel like such patients have "bitten the hand that feeds them" and withdraw from contact with them down to a minimal level. The odd/eccentric cluster includes patients who are paranoid, schizoid, or schizotypal. These patients start from a socially isolated, suspicious, and hypersensitive interpersonal stance. They often bring unusual "private" perceptions and ways of thinking to the BMT context. Their response to extreme pressure in BMT can be alarming withdrawal, frank paranoia, and primitive reactions that reflect a sense of losing sight of the BMT procedures being directed toward helping them. Instead they feel attacked and withdraw further into eccentric self-defensive postures. The staff feels alarmed by such reactions, which are often sensed by the patient, leading to further staff-patient alienation. Approximately 10% of the general population has such personality disorders, almost exactly the percentage of level III BMT recipients found in the UCLA matrix (5). The key is to stem such dangerous regressions or accentuations of dysfunctional personality styles by organizing psychiatric intervention early; checking carefully for contributing organic factors (especially drugs or metabolic delirium); and facilitating a clear, organized set of rules, expectations, and consistent figures with whom these more unusual and dysfunctional patients deal.

Delirium in BMT Recipients

Delirium, or acute organic mental disorder, is clinically quite common in adult BMT recipients (BMTRs) during the late BMT conditioning regimen (BMTCR) and early post-BMT periods. Multiple factors appear to contribute to delirium during this critical phase of BMT. Delirium may be associated with grossly inappropriate and potentially dangerous behavior. The onset of delirium in BMTRs should always result in careful medical and psychiatric evaluation and institution of aggressive measures to diagnose and reverse any correctible medical contributing factors. Active behavioral control measures and psychiatric interventions to reverse the psychiatric symptoms of delirium are also essential.

The cardinal symptoms of delirium are altered level of consciousness (e.g., fluctuating alertness, agitation, lethargy), altered sensory/perceptual function (e.g., illusions, hallucinations), impaired concentration and memory (e.g., registration of new information, immediate recall, short-term memory), impaired higher cognitive functions (e.g., reasoning, abstract thinking), delusions (often paranoid), impaired social judgment, impulsiveness, and an abnormal sleep-wake cycle. These symptoms often have their onset over a few hours, may have a very clear waxing and waning course (often worse at night), and typically resolve over 2 to 4 days without neurological or psychiatric sequelae.

The keys to early diagnosis of delirium are having a high index of suspicion in BMTRs during the high

Table 41-3.
Potential Pathophysiological Mechanisms of Delirium in Bone Marrow Transplantation Recipients

Common Pathophysiological Mechanisms	*Example*
Inadequate cerebral energy metabolism	Generalized cerebral hypoxia
Metabolic imbalance	Hyponatremia; hypoglycemia
Infection	Sepsis, CNS, other
Medication toxicity	CNS anticholinergic medications; analgesics/opiates; antineoplastic agents
Direct CNS Insult	Trauma; CNS radiation (part of TBI); CNS mass lesion; CNS neoplastic process
Intoxication/withdrawal states	Benzodiazepine intoxication; alcohol withdrawal
Circadian rhythm disruption	Sleep-wake cycle disruption
Specific psychological/ environmental factors	Prolonged immobilization; severe social isolation; very limited sensory stimulation
Hormonal imbalance	Addison's (myxedema madness); hypercalcemia

Specific common contributing factors to delirium
1. Metabolic imbalance: acute GVHD with diarrhea, liver dysfunction
2. Anti-nausea medication toxicity: benzodiazepine/ odansetron, thorozine, metaclopiamine
3. Analgesic/opiate medication toxicity
4. Infection/sepsis
5. Sleep deprivation
6. High fevers, relative social isolation, lack of orienting cues
7. Respiratory insufficiency: interstitial pneumonia (hopefully declining frequency with effective anti-cytomegalovirus treatment)
8. Possible role of CNS toxicity of conditioning regimen
9. High degree of stress/distress, with anxiety and fear

CNS = central nervous system; GVHD = graft-versus-host disease.

delirium incidence phases of BMT (especially stage III; see Table 41-2); careful mental status examination whenever the patient's mental status or social behavior are acutely altered; training of BMT nursing staff to perform screening mental status examinations; and easy access to psychiatric consultation to confirm the psychiatric diagnosis and to institute the psychiatric component of the delirium treatment plan.

Although attempted or completed suicide is relatively rare in hospitals and in BMTRs, clinically, the vast majority of medical in-patients who attempt or complete suicide are delirious at the time of the suicidal crisis. There are anecdotal reports of completed suicide in delirious BMTRs. Inadequately supervised delirious patients often will act in ways that compromise their medical care (e.g., pulling out intravenous/central catheters), and not infrequently will attempt (often ineffectively and impulsively) to assault staff members. Because the onset of delirium is often a prodrome of a potentially serious underlying medical problem (e.g., early sepsis, respiratory insufficiency), the onset of delirium should always be regarded as a serious medical event and inspire a very thorough medical re-evaluation.

The common general pathophysiological mechanisms of delirium are outlined in Table 41-3. Delirium is usually multifactorial in origin. Frequently it is impossible to determine which of the several factors present that could plausibly have contributed to the delirium are most clinically important. Delirium treatment interventions must often be directed toward reversing each of the potential contributing factors. Delirium rarely occurs before or very early in the course of the BMT conditioning regimen. Delirium at this treatment phase is commonly associated with a primary CNS disease process, serious infection, or psychoactive substance intoxication or withdrawal state. The onset of delirium later during the BMT hospitalization course is often associated with infection; interstitial pneumonia with respiratory compromise; GVHD with metabolic imbalance or liver or renal dysfunction; or the neuropsychiatric toxicity of immunosuppressant medications, such as cyclosporine. The general principles of management of delirium are outlined in Table 41-4.

Table 41-4.
Key Principles of Assessment and Management of Delirium in BMT Recipients

1. Early diagnosis. Based on high index of suspicion, routine nursing staff screening, mental status examination, early or routine psychiatric consultation.
2. Comprehensive medical re-evaluation based on the diagnosis of delirium. Correct all correctible medical factors potentially contributing to delirium.
3. Psychiatric consultation. Confirm diagnosis; treat psychotic symptoms with low-dose high-potency neuroleptics; minimize medications with known deliriogenic potential; evaluate risk for dangerous behavior; and institute needed patient observation measures, physical restraints, and chemical restraints. Treat secondary anxiety/agitation.
4. Restore normal patient sleep-wake cycle as rapidly as possible.
5. Educate patients and their family concerning the causes of delirium, its frequency in the BMT setting, the principles of its management as they relate to family member interactions with the delirious patient, its generally favorable prognosis, and its differentiation from the functional psychoses.
6. Provide an environment that seems safe to the patient, with regular brief patient contacts with staff members, regular provision of orienting cues, and much contact with family members/close friends and familiar objects.
7. Frequent psychiatric reassessment until delirium clears.
8. Psychopharmacological interventions. Use of low-dose high-potency neuroleptics (e.g., Haldol), with frequent reassessment of symptomatic response and dosage modification.

BMT = bone marrow transplantation.

Psychological/Psychobiological Interventions

General Principles

Five key guiding principles of psychological intervention for BMT recipients pave the way for effective management.

1. Tailor the interventions to the person. All too often the reverse is attempted; patients are fitted into rigid psychological interventions. To be effective, one should consider both the level of adjustment of the patient as well as the stage of BMT. We have learned, for example, that level II patients seem to benefit from one type of psychotherapy (supportive, clarifying), whereas this approach is contraindicated for level III patients, who require a more limit-setting and confrontational type of psychotherapy. It has also been our experience that level I and often level II patients can learn and utilize relaxation training interventions in the absence of the therapist. Level III patients require the presence of the therapist to benefit from such an intervention (28).
2. The goal of psychological interventions for BMT recipients is increasing their sense of control. If the patient can be taught a skill, given an insight, or a medicine that increases a sense of control, then negative symptoms can be expected to dissipate. If for some reason the psychological intervention reduces the patient's sense of control, then it is an iatrogenic intervention, which could involve pushing level III patients into an uncovering psychotherapy that makes them face previously repressed feelings or memories, or overmedicating a patient, which increases subclinical delirium.
3. Build a treatment plan for psychological care versus intervention when psychological symptoms become crises. Mental health consultants are best utilized as resources to help staff build an ongoing, clearly understood care plan, which is mainly administered by the staff with help from the mental health consultants.
4. Environmental stability is intrinsic to BMT recipients' coping and adaptation. This stability involves continuity of care by the same health providers as much as possible. Information about tests, treatments, and results should be given by the same person whenever possible. The more the structure remains stable and predictable, the better it is a "container" for patient anxieties or conflicts.
5. The combination of human intervention (therapy) plus psychopharmacological medications is usually better than drugs alone. Derogatis and Wise (29) continually reflect this point of view in their management program for anxiety and depression in medically ill patients.

Psychotherapy

Psychotherapy is a procedure that deals with underlying feelings, defenses, and memories so that they become conscious, organized, understood, and ultimately more bearable for patients. Returning to the concept of levels of psychological adaptability for BMT recipients, psychotherapy has seemed appropriate for two of three levels of BMT recipients (5,28). Level I patients do not seem to require psychotherapy. They come to the BMT context with a well-organized, functional set of defense mechanisms with which to cope. They come without the traumas and losses so characteristic of level II and III patients. The most they seem to need from a mental health consultant is occasional supportive visits. They do benefit from learning relaxation techniques, which is discussed later.

Level II patients seem to require and benefit most from psychotherapy. We have found that level II patients have often had significant losses or separation difficulties that have gone previously unacknowledged and unmourned. Emotional reactions to these do arise during BMT, and psychotherapy of a supportive, clarifying kind is indicated and helpful. The key is not to uncover material that moves beyond the patient's conscious awareness, but to attend to the issues that dominate the patient's consciousness. A good example of such a level II patient was a 34-year-old man undergoing conditioning for BMT who suddenly began acutely grieving his parents' divorce when he was a child and his own divorce three years prior. We supported him in expressing these grief states, clarified with him why these feelings would come up at this time, and carefully organized staff and family support to reduce his unstated but underlying fears of abandonment in the face of his growing dependency needs and feelings of vulnerability. We learned that he had dealt with previous losses through incessant activity, thus keeping his mind deflected and preoccupied from feelings of grief. The enforced inactivity, regressive push, and dependency state of BMT accentuated this emotional crisis for him.

Level III patients often require a different kind of psychotherapy. They have the same or even more traumatic losses than level II patients but different responses. Their response to the pressure of BMT combined with the emerging presence of chaotic or traumatic feelings and emotional states that were previously buried is to decompensate or to act-out in disruptive or challenging ways to the staff. This action can take forms such as life-threatening noncompliance, denigration, or endless needy behaviors like pressing the bell every 2 to 5 minutes for the nurse. For supportive therapy to be useful, such patients first require confrontational, limit-setting, and organizing psychotherapeutic interventions. An example of this profile was a patient in his early 20s who during his BMT became extremely volatile, denigrating, and sarcastic to staff and began a pattern of pitting staff against staff ("The night nurse told me to call her as often as I needed. How come you can't be warm like her?"). The staff felt a mixture of intimidation, anger, and shame at their own feelings about him. They began to reduce contact with him to a minimum which increased his sarcasm and hostility. Psychotherapy with him involved several steps. First, the staff and mental health consultants met to assess the situation and to draw up a meticulous intervention/care plan that reduced his ability to split the staff. Second, in psychotherapy, he was confronted about the effects of his behavior or his ability to get his needs met. Such confrontation in the management of the patient with a serious character disorder or borderline personality disorder is an essential part of the process (30). This process led to the beginning of a therapeutic relationship in which he was able to reveal a life history of abuse at the hands of parents and grandparents that he was re-enacting in the hospital. Such level III patients are prone to lack the ability to discriminate between the staff on whom they depend from earlier abusive dependency figures, and therefore attack out of defensive needs (31). This is extremely confusing and demoralizing to the staff, who have no idea why such a negative cycle of interaction has developed (32). Often, use of medications plus psychotherapy combined can be helpful for level III patients, less so for level II patients, and rarely if ever for level I patients. Psychotherapy, as reflected in Table 41-2, can be most useful in stages 3 through 5, when feelings of loss of control, loss of body integrity, and escalation of negative somatopsychic feelings are highest. It can be a primary intervention for feeling states involving grief, loss, and earlier stages of depression.

Behavioral Techniques

Three types of behavioral techniques have been useful in the BMT setting: (1) relaxation training, (2) systematic desensitization, and (3) contingency management. Relaxation training, otherwise known as progressive relaxation, progressive muscle relaxation, or Jacobson's modified progressive relaxation technique, is a form of self-regulation based on the proposition by Jacobson (33) that relaxation and anxiety are mutually exclusive states. In such training, patients are instructed to close their eyes and concentrate on sequentially relaxing one muscle group at a time from head to toes. Clinical evidence supports this technique in aiding control of psychological distress, mainly anxiety, and for physiological relaxation of muscles and decreased skin resistance (34–36). We have often used this procedure with patients undergoing BMT in a two-step procedure. During step one, the therapist teaches the patient the technique and practices with them to an acceptable level of competency. During step two, the therapist makes an audiotape of his/her instructions to the patient, which guides them through the steps (muscle groups) involved in the procedure. The patient is then instructed to repeat and practice this technique at least twice each day in addition to when anxiety increases to an uncomfortable level. In our experience, level I through III patients can all easily learn this procedure and benefit from its use. However, level I and II patients can and will make use of the tape in the absence of the therapist, whereas level III patients rarely are able to do so. This may reflect the trend toward noncompliance but also the dependency on the person-to-person interaction in level III patients.

In a review of the subject, Mastrovito (37) relates criteria for good and poor patient candidates for such procedures. Good candidates include (1) patients who have anxiety, pain, or a conditioned response to chemotherapy that is not controlled by usual methods; (2) patients who have a great need for self-control and who are hesitant to use medication to control pain or distress; and (3) patients who have heard of the benefits and know that such intervention is available and ask for it. Poor candidates include (1) patients who have a CNS complication of cancer (delirium or dementia); (2) patients who have a history of serious mental illness and in whom cooperation would be marginal; and (3) patients who are not motivated to try and who are disinterested and unenthusiastic after initial exposure to the technique. In applying this technique to BMT recipients, Mastrovito's point about a patient's need for self-control is very evident. This is a nonpharmacologic intervention that enhances sense of control and is totally under the patient's own management in terms of frequency and timing.

Systematic desensitization has its basic utility as a counter-conditioning procedure for phobias and related anxiety disorders. The basic procedure is to induce a deeply relaxed individual to confront, first in imagination, then in reality, a series of increasingly anxiety-provoking stimuli. The goal is to eliminate the conditioned association between those stimuli and anxiety and to substitute (condition) an associated relaxation response to that same set of stimuli (38). The most common procedure used to achieve this aim is progressive muscle relaxation or another form of relaxation, such as regulated deep breathing. In a well-designed, randomized therapy outcome study, systematic desensitization showed superior effects over supportive counseling and no treatment in dealing with conditioned anticipatory nausea and vomiting (39). The applications of this counter-conditioning procedure to the BMT situation are potentially multiple. They include high anxiety, potentially phobic situations, such as bone marrow aspirations; needles in general; and claustrophobic situations, such as reverse isolation during total body irradiation.

Contingency management involves work with the staff that treats patients and formation of a care plan for the entire unit to follow, based on behavioral and learning theory principles. Two of these principles that are particularly crucial are positive and negative reinforcement. A positive reinforcer is a stimulus that increases the probability of evocation of the behavior it follows. A negative reinforcer is a stimulus that increases, when removed, the probability of evocation of the behavior it follows (40). When a behavior that is viewed as dysfunctional, noxious, or even dangerous is positively reinforced, it becomes conditioned and will increase in frequency. This is often the case in the BMT context prior to proper formation of a coordinated, goal-oriented care plan. For example, a regressed patient becomes noncompliant with necessary health maintenance behaviors, such as oral care to reduce infection, after conditioning. The staff can unwittingly reinforce such noncompliance with over-attention to the noncompliance. Another example might be the patient who leans on the bell and rings every few minutes for staff—soon driving them to desperation. A noteworthy example, as described previously, was a 16-year-old patient in our Center being treated for aplastic anemia with ATG because no HLA match was found. During hospitalization several things happened, including abandonment by his dysfunctional parents, which led to profound regression and noncompliance. He became so noncompliant that he refused self-care and also refused to be examined by the unit physicians. The staff became increasingly desperate about his condition and their relationship with him. A behavioral program using nursing staff attention as a positive reinforcer and withdrawal of that attention as a negative reinforcer was developed. The staff decided that compliance with mouth care secondary to a serious dental infection or surgery and with physical examinations were two key target behaviors. The staff was ambivalent about the behavioral program, feeling it was possibly unethical or cruel. Many pharmacological interventions were tried, with no positive results. Only when the staff organized around the behavioral program did the patient begin to settle down and comply with the necessities of treatment (41). Obviously, such an intervention program has to be considered and constructed for only the most severely regressed or noncompliant patients; only with such organization can these situations be brought back under control. Such a program does have ethical considerations and these should be carefully considered and balanced with the dangers that nonimplementation presents.

Psychopharmacological Therapy for BMT Recipients

In general, psychopharmacological treatment of psychiatric disorders in adult BMT recipients should be conceptualized as one component of overall medical and psychiatric care of the psychiatric disorder. Many psychiatric disorders at all phases after BMT are at least partially caused by ongoing medical symptoms or organ system dysfunction. Many of the medications commonly used after BMT, especially those with immunosuppressant properties, may contribute to psychiatric disorders. Most psychiatric disorders have a better prognosis if psychotherapeutic (including behavioral and stress management) treatment is administered in concert with any psychopharmacological interventions.

All psychopharmacological agents carry risks for acute medical and psychiatric toxicity, and chronic use is associated with substantial risks for some classes of agents. Thus, initiation of treatment with psychopharmacological agents is a significant medical decision that carries a responsibility to ensure comprehensive treatment of the psychiatric disorder, including appropriately close follow-up of treatment response.

In the early post-BMT phase, acute reactive anxiety symptoms/disorders and acute organic mental disorders are quite common. Anxiety disorders may be coincidentally pharmacologically treated by the antinausea (e.g., lorazepam) and analgesic regimens commonly used for medical symptom control early after BMT. However, sedative-hypnotics and analgesics may also precipitate or exacerbate delirium, another very common psychiatric disorder early after BMT. In the first few months after BMT, hospitalization discharge anxiety disorders, including those with many characteristics of post-traumatic stress disorder, and depressive disorders are common. Major depressive episodes and manic depressive episodes do occur and should always receive careful psychiatric assessment and treatment. During later post-transplant phases, each of these disorders may still occur, and significant marital/family problems also occur.

Table 41-5 provides guidelines for the use of psychopharmacological agents in adult BMT recipients. Rational psychopharmacological treatment of BMT recipients requires ensuring the following.

1. Accuracy of the psychiatric diagnosis, the certainty and strength of the indication for psychopharmacological treatment, and that the patient receives the appropriate combination of psychotherapeutic and psychopharmacological care.
2. That the patient's medical status has been fully and appropriately evaluated, to reasonably rule out organically based psychiatric disorders, or that the syndrome is a psychiatric presentation of a medical disorder (e.g., hypothyroidism). All medical disorders that are potentially contributing to the patient's psychiatric disorder should receive optimal treatment.
3. That the psychopharmacological agent and dose regimen have been selected after thoughtful consideration of the patient's medical and psychiatric history and current status. Coexisting medical disease states, as they relate to the choice of psychopharmacological agent and to the dosing regimen, must be considered in the treatment plan.
4. The patient's psychiatric status and response to treatment must be monitored closely and frequently, so that appropriate changes to the psychopharmacological regimen are made in a timely way.

Optimally, the decision to initiate psychopharmacological care in adult BMTRs should be made after consultation with a psychiatrist knowledgeable about psychiatric disorders in this population and of the many nuances of psychopharmacological and psychotherapeutic treatment of psychiatric disorders after BMT. The authors recommend that psychiatric consultation should always be sought when psy-

Table 41-5.
Guidelines for Commonly Used Psychopharmacological Agents in Adult BMT Recipients

Class/Agent	*Indications*	*Usual Total 24-hr Dose Range[a] (mg/day)*	*Half-life*
Benzodiazepines[b]			
Oxazepam (Serax)	Anxiety, insomnia	30–120	Medium
Lorazepam (Ativan)	Insomnia	2–6	Medium
Flurazepam (Dalmane)	Insomnia	15–30	Long
Triazolam (Halcion)	Insomnia	0.125–0.5	Short
Diazepam (Valium)	Anxiety, insomnia	10–30	Long
Neuroleptics[c]	**All:** delirium, severe acute prepsychotic anxiety, dementia with agitation/lability, brief reactive psychosis, severe acute emotional or behavioral lability, hypomanic/manic state		
Haloperidol (Haldol)		1–10	Long
Droperidol (Inapsone)		1–10	Short
Perphenazine (Trilafon)		4–16	Long
Fluphenazine (Prolixin)		2–10	Long
Lithium carbonate[d]	Prophylaxis of bipolar affective disorder, manic episode	600–1,200	Related to renal function
Antidepressants[e]	**All:** Major depressive episode, severe organic depressive syndrome. **Some:** panic attacks, adjuvant for chronic pain (e.g., peripheral neuropathy), insomnia		
Amitriptyline (Elavil)		75–150	Long
Imipramine (Tofranil)		75–150	Long
Trazodone (Desyrel)		200–400	Long
Fluxoxetine (Prozac)		20–40	Very long
Doxepin (Sinequan)		75–150	Long
Nortriptyline (Pamelor)		40–100	Long
Protriptriptyline (Vivactil)		10–60	

[a]Benzodiazepines, neuroleptics, and lithium carbonate usually given in 2–4 divided doses/day. Antidepressants given 1–3 doses/day. All dose ranges are for otherwise healthy adults less than 65 years of age and are for the specified indications. Higher doses may be used after psychiatric consultation. Variable interval between treatment onset and initial clinical effects.
[b]Regular, higher dose, or chronic use beyond a few weeks can be associated with risk for dependence and development of a withdrawal syndrome with sudden discontinuation. Do not stop suddenly, especially early after transplantation.
[c]Psychiatric consultation recommended when indications for neuroleptics exist. Behavioral and psychotherapeutic interventions often combined with neuroleptics. Acute extrapyramidal syndromes may develop, including neuroleptics malignant syndrome.
[d]Psychiatric consultation *essential* for management of patients with major affective disorder or in whom manic psychosis develops. Lithium carbonate should be very cautiously used in patients with impaired renal function. Lithium dosage is guided by serum levels. Narrow toxic-therapeutic ratio.
[e]Psychiatric consultation strongly recommended for patients with severe depression or those being treated with antidepressants after transplantation. Many depressed chronic dialysis patients do not require antidepressants.

chopharmacological treatment is contemplated in the following clinical situations.

1. Patients with severe or worsening depression, in whom suicidal risk may be present.
2. When antidepressants have been used in appropriate doses for appropriate periods with minimal or no clinical benefit.
3. Patients with psychotic symptoms or those with evidence of a significant organic mental disorder.
4. Whenever lithium carbonate or neuroleptics are contemplated for treatment of a psychiatric disorder.
5. For patients with severe recurrent acute or chronic anxiety symptoms, especially for those with panic attacks, significant phobias, or symptoms of post-traumatic stress disorder.
6. For patients who have been on a schedule of multiple daily doses of sedative-hypnotic medications (e.g., all benzodiazepines) for more than 2 to 3 months.
7. For patients with a history of significant substance abuse disorder.

Families of BMT Recipients

Four basic subsystems of the BMT patients' family are important to consider in the context of the BMT experience: (1) The donor-recipient dyad; (2) the patient/spouse or patient/significant other dyad; (3) the patient and his/her children; and (4) the patient and his/her parents.

The Donor-Recipient Dyad

The donor-recipient dyad comes with more than a genetic-biological HLA match. It comes with a history of sibling rivalry that is centered around competition for parental attention and affection (28). This dyad comes to BMT with a spectrum of adjustment and adaptation to this universal psychodynamic factor. In the majority of cases, we have seen a mature and functional sibling bond; however, a minority have presented a life history of dysfunctional resolution of such conflicts. In previous research, we found the donor to often feel like their "brother's keeper" and to have a sense of personal failure if the recipient dies or has problems (28). Thus, for the donor, it is not "the process failed," but rather, "I failed." In a study on donors' psychological adjustment, approximately 20% evidenced psychological problems directly related to the BMT experience (42). These findings are strikingly similar to a study of kidney donation (relative-to-relative) where at one year follow-up, 24% of the donors had worse scores on depression (43).

The issue of the donor's interpersonal role in the family is important to consider. The "black sheep" kidney donor has been found to end up with significantly more negative feelings about the experience at one year post-transplant (44). Our experience has revealed some interesting and troubling family interactions with "black sheep" donors—in some of the interactions, the donor appeared to hold the family/recipient hostage around the BMT; in others, the donor fantasized restoration of self-esteem and family-esteem around donation. Several studies of donors in the earlier renal transplant literature found unconscious resentment and impulsiveness in decision-making (45–47), which led to concerns that a "volunteer might not be a volunteer." It also led to recommendations that "it is important to screen out those (donors) whose relationships with the recipient contain an excess of negative feelings" (47). Because this screening is often not possible in the context of allogeneic BMT, attention to the possible underlying conflicts of the donor-recipient relationship becomes even more important. In practical terms, this means obtaining some history of this relationship and intervening as early as possible if that history involves unresolved hostility or conflict. Second, educating the donors about possible psychological sequelae of the donation can also be important.

The Patient/Spouse or Patient/Significant Other Dyad

The key figures in the emotional support of BMT recipients are usually the spouse or the partner. Given the mean age of the majority of BMT recipients, these spouses are likely to be young adults less than 45 years of age, with maximal job and parental responsibilities. They typically take a leave of absence from work or child care responsibilities to accompany the patient through BMT. The greater a sense of fragmentation a spouse feels between these various roles and responsibilities, the less quality support they can offer for the patient.

We have found that spouses accompany patients through the "phases" of BMT described in Table 41-2. Often the spouse has pushed the patient to consent to BMT, hoping for "the answer" out of a chronic, recurrent illness situation. When conditioning is performed and the patient becomes dramatically more ill and dependent, the spouse often feels trapped and overwhelmed. We have seen a range of spouse accommodation; some become overgiving, martyr-like, and self-sacrificing. They have trouble leaving the hospital. A midrange group are able to separate, freely allow others to provide care for patients, and use their support systems for emotional help. Another group of spouses are disconnected, visit infrequently, and may or may not be dysfunctional. Some are avoidant, others cannot detach from outside responsibilities.

We provide a separate group for spouses and family members that patients do not attend. We try to apply social work interventions to facilitate a reduced sense of fragmentation in the lives of the spouses. Individual psychological consultation and therapy are frequently necessary for spouses. Key issues for the patient-spouse interactions arise during preparation for discharge and posthospitalization phases. As is evident in the data on follow-up, sexual reconnection can be laden with anxiety and problems (48–50). Counseling around these issues is particularly crucial to reduce fears of infection secondary to sexual contact and to restore normal interaction after the profound dependencies created during BMT. Lack of attention to this factor can maintain extreme dysfunction in the relationship after BMT. Maintenance of the coping skills and mental health of the spouse is key to supporting the patient. Dysfunction in the spouse can be a serious harbinger of reduction of coping in the patient.

Patient/Child Relationships

This young adult population will very frequently have children who are preadolescents or sometimes adolescents. These children are reactive to many things, but none more fundamental than the enforced separation from the parents that BMT requires. The children of these patients are frequently the "hidden" members of the families who never visit or are never seen by the staff. Preadolescent children of BMT recipients may be less verbal than adolescent children. They may have fantasies that the parental illness is their fault due to normal but conflictual ambivalent feelings about parents. Such children may need assurance that this is not true, as well as help in cognitively integrating BMT and how it is expected to help their parent.

Adolescents may have different issues with parental BMT. For them, the procedure may mean role shifts and increased responsibilities at home, which promote resentment and possibly defiance or acting-out. Although older children may be able to talk about such issues, younger children may need help in acting them out in play or through drawings. We advocate that children visit during BMT, if at all possible, to reduce separation trauma. However, preparation for what the parent presents is absolutely essential. Unprepared children can be traumatized, especially after conditioning.

A very common question about such children centers around when they may need referral for psychological help. Table 41-6 subdivides preadolescents and

Table 41-6.
Behaviors of Children of BMT Recipients Indicating Need for Psychological Intervention

Developmental Phase	*Behavior of Concern*
Preadolescence	
	Potential need for referral
	Sudden learning problems
	Distractibility
	Episodes of sadness
	Sleep problems
	Appetite problems
	Some withdrawal from peers/playing
	Absolute need for referral
	Cruelty to animals
	Fire setting
	Stealing
	Loss of toilet training (if previously established)
	Refusal to go to school
	Chronic sleep problems
	Chronic eating disorders (anorexia, obesity)
	Sudden aggression toward peers
	Serious withdrawal
	Somatic identification with ill parent
	Suicidality
Adolescence	
	Potential need for referral
	Same as preadolescents
	Absolute need for referral
	Stealing
	Drug abuse
	Promiscuity
	Running away episodes
	Somatic identification with ill parent
	Suicidality
	Chronic sleep, eating, grooming problems
	Rage reactions

adolescents and details general criteria that reflect potential and absolute need for psychological help. The key is to refer prior to the behavior becoming serious enough to interfere with or fragment the patient-child bond. Of the many behaviors listed in Table 41-6, somatic identification with the ill parent is a harbinger of long-term or lifetime psychosomatic disability. This identification will be present in children who are in grief but cannot articulate to or gain support from the family to talk about their feelings. Such a pattern forms the basis for the unresolved grief reaction and the adult somatatizing personality (51). When death is impending, children should be informed in terms that are comprehensible (52). The parent will frequently require staff help to achieve this difficult but necessary step. If the child is given no advanced preparation, the capacity to trust the surviving parent can be undermined. Children can cope with this information if they are provided proper support and attention. Frequently, adult anxieties about children are projected onto them and they are then excluded in a pseudo-"protective" stance by the adults. Childhood grief responses may be different from those of adulthood. Grief may provoke confusion in adults, whereas their children carry on their usual interests and play activities.

BMT Recipients and Their Parents

The young adulthood developmental status of BMT patients has important implications for the relationship with parents during and after BMT. In a classic study of the developmental phases of young adulthood (ages 18–40), Levinson (53) articulated the shifts in the young adult from dependent child to "becoming one's own man/woman" and the need to be seen as an equal and "not as a kid." These shifts create three major challenges for the BMT recipient's parents: (1) the dilemma of nurturing and supporting their ill child while attempting to respect and maintain the child's autonomy, which, for BMT recipients in their 20s is an autonomy recently structuralized; (2) the dilemma of not feeling rejected by their ill child's sometimes extreme behavior in the service of their autonomy; and (3) the dilemma of both wishing to control the child's medical care and suffering the anxiety of sharing or relinquishing such control.

Intervention with such parents can take place in several spheres. It has been shown that staff will perceive themselves to be in conflict with approximately 20% of the families on a BMT unit (54). This conflict may frequently occur between parents of a BMT recipient and the staff and is often displaced away from the parent-patient interaction. Instead of the parents struggling with the patient or the patient's spouse for control, they struggle with the staff. This can take the form of questioning or second-guessing the staff, which debilitates the staff and can quickly create a schism in patient-staff and parent-staff alliances. The staff can easily lose empathy for the parents, fail to see the desperation underlying these behaviors, and withdraw support for them entirely. Such parents can be seen by mental health consultants individually, as a couple, or in a family group, depending on their level of distress or dysfunction. A key issue is to facilitate the maintenance of empathy in staff and parents. It is important that the parents be viewed as having a special and profound grief: that of having a child with a life-threatening illness in the prime of life. However, it is equally important that limits be set for the parents so they do not undermine the relationship and care of the BMT recipient secondary to conflict with staff.

Psychological Issues of Staff Who Care for BMT Recipients

The relationship of staff, patients, and families on the BMT unit form a triangle that is a "psychological system." Conflict or dysfunction between any parts of this system effect all others. In a classic study of systematic functioning of the psychiatric hospital, it was discovered that on wards where staff was depressed or distressed, patient recovery was dramatically less successful than on wards where staff was psychological intact (55). This same observation may easily be related to the BMT unit.

We have observed two key emotional dynamics present in staff on BMT units that are central to their emotional functioning: guilt and grief in relation to the patients. The dynamic of guilt was unconsciously expressed in a staff group by a nurse who related a fragment of a recent dream.

I dreamed Paul McCartney finally noticed me. . . . I have always loved him. As he was walking toward me closer and closer, I saw that he had a GVHD and scleroderma type skin.

This dream seemed to reflect several important things for this young BMT nurse. The dream revealed the sense that anyone who she cares about and gets close to will have signs of fatal illness, possibly induced by closeness to her. At a more conscious level, staff often has expressed guilt about being the agents of treatments that create so much suffering, symptomatology, and dysfunction in this youthful patient group. They often lose the perspective that the illness is the real culprit and feel a powerful sense of personal guilt. A secondary question is, "are we normal to want to work on a BMT unit at all?" This question leads to the issue of grief secondary to the repetitive close attachments and breaking of those attachments by death that such a staff has to endure. Attending to the task of mourning such losses is a primary reason why the creation of support groups for BMT staff, especially nursing staff, is a sine qua non of staff integrity and function.

Lack of attention to these issues leads to staff "burn-out" and ultimately to staff turnover. Burn-out is a syndrome of physical and emotional exhaustion involving the development of negative self-concept, negative job attitudes, and loss of ability to be concerned or feel for patients (56). Some key strategies for combating burn-out appear in Table 41-7. Many of these skills and perceptions can be focused on and developed in a regularly programmed staff support group. Emotional danger signs for BMT staff can include (1) depression that is characterized by lack of energy, excessive irritability, and sleep disorders; (2) dreams laden with conflictual material symbolizing conscious defenses being overwhelmed by cancer-generated feelings; (3) inability to detach oneself from the job, characterized by inability to stop calling in or thinking about patients during off time; (4) repetitive accidents; or (5) guilt over taking time off from work. These signs can warrant psychological consultation and possible brief or longer term psychotherapy to alleviate such symptomatic patterns. This consultation should never be undertaken with a mental health consultant to the BMT unit. Rather, the consultant can act as referral and triage resources for the staff member.

A final issue is the struggle on the BMT unit to strike a balance between patient care and research. This struggle can sometimes lead to fragmentation between physicians and nurses on a BMT unit. Extreme positions and perceptions of the other's professional group can be assumed, especially during intense periods of stress when patients are dying. Nurses can take the position that physicians choose inappropriate BMT candidates and select patients for research goals, ignoring quality-of-life issues. Physicians can take the position that nurses lack the vision and proper scientific perspective necessary to advance the field (28). This is an instance where the psychological system of the BMT unit is fraying, with patient care usually reduced as a result. Mental health consultation can sometimes reinstitute functional communication at this juncture and heal painful splits between the staff subgroups (28).

Table 41-7.
Key Strategies for Combating BMT Staff Burn-out

Training in interpersonal coping skills
Availability of a support system
Recognition and analysis of personal feelings (i.e, anger, guilt)
Use of humor
Creation of effective boundary between work and personal life
Strategies to maintain physical health

Adapted from Maslach C. The burnout syndrome and patient care. In: Garfield C, ed. Stress and Survival. St. Louis: C.V. Mosby, 1979.

References

1. Surman OS. Psychiatric aspects of organ transplantation. Am J Psychiatry 1989;146:972–982.
2. Frierson RL, Lippmann SB. Heart transplantation patients rejected on psychiatric considerations. Psychosomatics 1987;28:347–355.
3. Mai FM, McKenzie FN, Kostuk WJ. Psychiatric aspects of heart transplantation: preoperative evaluation and postoperative sequelae. Br Med J 1986;292:311–313.
4. Schroeder JS, Hunt S. Cardiac transplantation update 1987. JAMA 1987;258:3142–3145.
5. Futterman AD, Wellisch DK, Bond G, Carr CR. The psychosocial levels system: a new rating scale to identify and assess emotional difficulties during bone marrow transplantation. Psychosomatics 1991;32:177–186.
6. American Psychiatric Association. Diagnostic and statistical manual of mental Disorders (third edition-revised). Washington DC: American Psychiatric Association, 1987.
7. Brown HN, Kelly MJ. Stages of bone marrow transplantation: a psychiatric perspective. Psychosom Med 1976;38:439–446.
8. Wolcott DL, Stuber ML. Psychiatric aspects of bone marrow transplantation. In: Craven J, Rodin G, eds. Psychiatric aspects of organ transplantation. New York: Oxford University Press, 1992:1–31.
9. Penman DT, Holland JC, Bahna GF, et al. Informed consent for investigational chemotherapy: patients' and physicians' perceptions. J Clin Oncol 1984;2:849–855.

10. Morrow GR. How readable are subject consent forms? JAMA 1980;244:56–58.
11. Noyes AP, Kolb LC. Modern clinical psychiatry. Philadelphia: WB Saunders, 1963.
12. DeFronzo RA, Broine H, Colvin OM. Water intoxication in man after cyclophosphamide therapy. Ann Intern Med 1973;78:861–869.
13. Lesko L. Bone marrow transplantation. In: Holland JC, Rowland JH, eds. Handbook of psychooncology. New York: Oxford University Press, 1989:163–173.
14. Sullivan KM, Storb R, Shulman HM, et al. Immediate and delayed neurotoxicity after mechlorethamine preparation for bone marrow transplantation. Ann Intern Med 1982;97:182–189.
15. Patchell RA, White CL, Clark AW, et al. Central nervous system complications of bone marrow transplantation: a clinical and pathological study. Ann Neurol 1982; 12:80.
16. De Groen PC, Aksamit AJ, Rokela J, et al. Central nervous system toxicity after liver transplantation: the role of cyclosporine and cholesterol. N Engl J Med 1987;317:861–866.
17. Ling MHM, Perry P, Tsuang MT. Side effects of corticosteroid therapy: psychiatric aspects. Arch Gen Psychiatry 1981;38:471–477.
18. Gastfriend DR, Surman OS, Gaffey G, et al. Outcome of liver transplantation in alcoholics. Presented at the American Psychiatric Association 143rd Annual Meeting, New York, NY, May 12–17, 1990.
19. Forman B. Cancer and suicide. Gen Hosp Psychiatry 1979;1:108–114.
20. Bolund C. Suicide and cancer: I. Demographics and social characteristics of cancer patients who committed suicide in Sweden 1973–1976. J Psychosoc Oncol 1985;3:17–30.
21. Bolund C. Suicide and cancer: II. Medical and care factors in suicides by cancer patients in Sweden 1973–1976. J Psychosoc Oncol 1985;3:31–52.
22. Holland JC. Psychological aspects of cancer. In: Holland JC, Frei G, eds. Cancer medicine, ed 2. Philadelphia: Lea & Febiger, 1978.
23. Breitbart W. Suicide. In: Holland JC, Rowland JH, eds. Handbook of psychooncology. New York: Oxford University Press, 1989:291–299.
24. Jenkins PL, Roberts DJ. Suicidal behavior after bone marrow transplantation. Bone Marrow Transplant 1991;7:159–161.
25. Massie MJ. Depression. In: Holland JC, Rowland JH, eds. Handbook of psychooncology. New York: Oxford University Press, 1989:283–290.
26. Massie MJ. Anxiety, panic and phobias. In: Holland JC, Rowland JH, eds. Handbook of psychooncology. New York: Oxford University Press, 1989:300–310.
27. Massie MJ. Personality disorders. In: Holland JC, Rowland JH, eds. Handbook of psychooncology. New York: Oxford University Press, 1989:310–319.
28. Futterman AD, Wellisch DK. Psychodynamic themes of bone marrow transplantation. Hematol Oncol Clin North Am 1990;4:699–709.
29. Derogatis LR, Wise TN. Anxiety and depressive disorders in the medical patient. Washington, D.C.: American Psychiatric Press, 1989.
30. Buie DH, Adler G. The uses of confrontation with borderline patients. Int J Psychoanal Psychother 1972; 1:90–108.
31. Adler G, Buie DH. Aloneness and borderline psychopathology: the possible relevance of child development issues. Int J Psychoanal 1979;60:83–96.
32. Adler G. Helplessness in the helpers. Br J Med Psychol 1972;45:315–326.
33. Jacobson E. Progressive muscle relaxation. Chicago: University of Chicago Press, 1938.
34. Goldfried MR. Reduction of generalized anxiety through a variant of systematic desensitization. In: Goldfried MR, Mersbaum M. eds. Behavior change through self-control. New York: Holt, Rinehart & Winston, 1973.
35. Goldfried MR, Trier CS. Effectiveness of relaxation on an active coping skill. J Abnorm Psychol 1974;83:348–355.
36. Paul GL. Physiological effects of relaxation training and hypnotic suggestion. J Abnorm Psychol 1969;74:425–437.
37. Mastrovito R. Behavioral techniques: progressive relaxaton and self-regulatory therapies. In: Holland JC, Rowland JH, eds. Handbook of psychooncology. New York: Oxford University Press, 1989:492–501.
38. Redd W. Management of anticipatory nausea and vomiting. In: Holland JC, Rowland JH, eds. Handbook of psychooncology. New York: Oxford University Press, 1989:421–433.
39. Morrow GR, Morrell BS. Behavioral treatment for the anticipatory nausea and vomiting induced by cancer chemotherapy. N Engl J Med 1982;307:1476–1480.
40. Yates AJ. Behavior therapy. New York: John Wiley & Sons, 1970:24–43.
41. Namir S, Wellisch DK. The hated adolescent: reactions of family and hospital staff to an aplastic anemia patient. Family Systems Med 1985;3:313–325.
42. Wolcott DL, Wellisch DK, Fawzy FI, et al. Psychological adjustment of adult bone marrow transplant donors whose recipient survives. Transplantation 1986;41:484–488.
43. Simmons R. Psychological reaction to giving a kidney. In: Levy, NB, ed. Psychonephrology, vol 1. New York: Plenum Publishing, 1981:227–245.
44. Kemph JP. Renal failure, artificial kidney and kidney transplant. Am J Psychiatry 1966;122:1270–1275.
45. Cramond WA, Knight PR, Lawrence JR. The psychiatric contribution to a renal unit undertaking chronic hemodialysis and renal homotransplantation. Br J Psychiatry 1967;113:1201–1212.
46. Fellner CH, Marshall JR. Twelve kidney donors. JAMA 1968;206:2703–2707.
47. Cramond WA. Medical, moral and legal aspects of organ transplantation and long-term resuscitative measures. Psychological, social and community aspects. Med J Aust 1968;2:622–627.
48. Hengeveld MH, Houtman RB, Zwaan FE. Psychological aspects of bone marrow transplantation: a retrospective study of 17 long-term survivors. Bone Marrow Transplant 1988;3:69–75.
49. Altmaier EM, Gingrich RD, Fyfe MA. Two-year adjustment of bone marrow transplant survivors. Bone Marrow Transplant 1991;7:311–316.
50. Baruch J, Benjamin S, Treleaven J, et al. Male sexual function following bone marrow transplantation. Presented at the Annual Conference of the British Psycho-Oncology Society, St. Bartholomews Hospital, London, England, Dec 9, 1991.
51. Bowlby J. Childhood mourning and its implications for psychiatry. Am J Psychiatry 1961;118:481–495.
52. Hollingsworth C. Children's reaction to illness or death

of parent. In: Pasnau RO, ed. Psychosocial aspects of medical practice: children and adolescents. Menlo Park, CA: Addison-Wesley Publishing, 1982:48–60.
53. Levinson DJ. The seasons of a man's life. New York: Ballantine Books, 1978.
54. Zabora J, Fetting J, Shanley V, et al. Predicting conflict with staff among families of cancer patients during prolonged hospitalizations. J Psychosoc Oncol 1989;7: 103–111.
55. Stanton A, Schwartz MS. The mental hospital. New York: Basic Books, 1954.
56. Maslach C. The burnout syndrome and patient care. In: Garfield C, ed. Stress and survival. St. Louis: C.V. Mosby, 1979.

Chapter 42
Assessment of Quality of Life Following Bone Marrow Transplantation

Gerhard M. Schmidt

Survival of patients with malignant disease represents a major medical achievement, but full recovery to a prediagnosis level of "health" is more elusive. The World Health Organization defines health as "complete physical, mental and social well-being and not merely the absence of disease and infirmity" (1). In circumstances where medical intervention with toxic drugs does not have a readily apparent impact on quantity of survival, quality of survival becomes a pertinent end point. The Karnofsky Index applied by medical caregivers for evaluation of the functional aspect of quality of life was developed in 1948 for patients with cancer (2). However, function alone may be too narrow a focus to evaluate an individual's perception of well-being. During the past three decades, the concept of quality of life (QOL) has expanded. The evolution of clinical and behavioral sciences methodology has resulted in the inclusion of patient perspective of physical, mental, and social health (3), which has resulted in a surge of activity in QOL research. *QOL* first appeared in medical literature as an index term in 1977, with 28 citations, and has since risen to 167 in 1989 (4). There are numerous "generic" or general clinical measures that assess functional status alone, and several have been specifically designed for the field of clinical oncology (5–9). Most instruments, however, utilize patient-derived data, with the expectation of providing personal QOL aspects, whereas caregiver-rated instruments are useful in describing functional status (10,11). Generic instruments typically fail to address disease and treatment-specific issues (12–14). They have been used in the setting of chronic disease primarily to aid health policy decisions in resource allocation. In contrast, disease-specific QOL instruments can be more responsive in detecting an improvement within the setting of a randomized placebo-controlled trial (15). Disease-specific instruments have been developed either as investigator-designed instruments or with patient-derived attributes (16–18). A comprehensive review of QOL measures commonly used in oncology was recently summarized (19). In this comparison, the 136-question Sickness Impact Profile with a "yes or no" format emerged as the "gold standard" among general QOL measures, although disease- and site-specific questions are lacking.

There are several reasons to measure QOL in bone marrow transplantation (BMT) survivors: (1) to assess whether problems are transient and whether they are related to the underlying disease or a consequence of the treatment (20); (2) to identify groups who would benefit from early intervention in either physical rehabilitation or psychological support to prevent psychosocial decompensation; (3) to evaluate possible differences in perceived outcome based on treatment, socioeconomic and educational status, and ethnic or cultural background; and (4) to help identify and provide alternative treatment options. Most reports of BMT outcomes do not address the issue of QOL despite a considerable potential for acute, delayed, and chronic toxicity (21–24). This deficit may be explained by problems in measurement, which include difficulties in both definition and instrumentation (3,20,25–27).

QOL is a complex concept with diverse dimensions and often with variance among authors as to which exact dimensions to include (28). The need of intervention across all phases of the BMT process has been recognized by several investigators in an attempt to minimize complications, to promote rehabilitation, and to assist in successful coping with illness (29). In addition, psychological and social support given as an adjunct to appropriate medical care may enhance both quality and quantity of life of cancer patients (30–33). A recent study examined the cost-effectiveness of BMT and found that "cost per additional year of life" was lower for BMT when compared with liver, heart, pancreas, and kidney transplantation (34). However, others have suggested that it is important to also focus on quality in addition to quantity by including measurements of QOL into similar research in the future (35).

Quality of Life Assessments in BMT Recipients

Studies, methodologies, and results examining QOL in BMT survivors are summarized in Table 42-1. One

Table 42-1.
Summary of Quality of Life Studies in Bone Marrow Transplantation

Center, Year, Ref	*Sample Size (Response Rate)*	*Methodology*	*Study Goal*	*Results*
UCLA, 1986 (36,37)	26 (72%)	IDQ, POMS, Simmons Scale (39), SAS-SR	Adaptation post-BMT for both recipients and donors	75% were doing well; 10–20% may benefit from psychological support
Leiden, 1988 (41)	17 (89%)	IDQ, SCL-90, BDI, KPS	Psychosocial aspects of BMT	Close link of physical condition and psychological state; some felt to be inadequately prepared
Kentucky, 1989 (42)	23 (96%)	FLIC, POMS	Documentation of function and psychosocial aspects	Older age was the only variable associated with poorer physical outcome
Kentucky, 1989 (43)	16 (70%)	FLIC, POMS, SIP	Function and psychosocial aspects over time	Results showed little change in functional status over time
Kentucky/Iowa, 1990 (45)	29 (88%)	FLIC, POMS, SIP, SEAS, PAIS, SER, PHQ	Comparison with renal transplant recipients	Both groups perceived their health as poorer than a typical person their age
Seattle, 1990 (48)	100 (N/A)	SIP, BDI, BES	Function and psychosocial aspects	Functioning returned to normal at one year except in the domains of work, recreation, and stamina
Johns Hopkins University, 1991 (49)	135 (86%)	MOS, KPS	Health, function, and employment as measures of rehabilitation	Rehabilitation was achieved comparable to survivors given less intensive treatment for cancer
Iowa, 1991 (51)	12 (80%)	IDQ	Comparison to chemotherapy	Objectively, BMT recipients are doing worse, but, subjectively, survivors rate their health as positively as chemotherapy patients
City of Hope, 1992 (52)	212 (90%)	IDQ, KPS	Value of telephone interview in allogeneic BMT recipients	90% participation; 69% returned to full-time work, younger patients do better
Stanford, 1992 (53)	58 (98%)	IDQ	Quality of life in recipients of autologous BMT	No long-term morbidity in surviving adult patients
City of Hope, 1992 (17,18)	119 (N/A) 195 (N/A)	QOL-BMT	Definition of QOL by BMT survivors; development of BMT-specific QOL instrument	The meaning of QOL was defined by allogeneic BMT survivors, and a tentative BMT-specific QOL instrument was proposed

IDQ = Investigator Designed Questionnaire; POMS (38) = Profile of Moods Status; SAS-SR (40) = Social Adjustment Scale-Self Report; FLIC (5) = Functional Living Index; SIP (44) = Sickness Impact Profile; BDI (56) = Beck Depression Inventory; BES (48) = BMT Events Scale; SLC-90 (57) = Symptom Checklist-90; MOS (50) = Medical Outcome Study (short form general health survey); KPS (2) = Karnofsky Performance Status; PAIS (46) = Psychological Adjustment to Illness Scale; SEAS (47) = Sleep, Energy, and Appetite Scale; SER (47) = Symptom Experience Report; PHQ (47) = Perceived Health Questionnaire; BMT-QOL (17,18) = Quality of Life—Bone Marrow Transplant Instrument; BMT = bone marrow transplantation.

of the first studies addressing health status and psychosocial functioning as perceived by adult survivors of allogeneic marrow transplantation was done by Wolcott and colleagues (36) at the University of California Los Angeles. The variables studied included (1) demographics, (2) health status, (3) general health perception, (4) social adjustment, (5) mood state, (6) self-esteem, (7) recipient-donor relationship, and (8) recipient attitude about BMT. A parallel study examined the same variables except for health status and social adjustment in bone marrow donors (37). This strategy allowed comparison of BMT recipients' and donors' psychological and social adjustment after BMT. Twenty-six of 36 (72%) adult recipients, at least one year after BMT, completed a demographic questionnaire, a current medical status form, and a 63-item investigator-constructed questionnaire inquiring about systemic symptoms specifically related to BMT, as well as global self-perceived current health to assess physical limitations. Psychological interactions were assessed using (1) the Profile of Moods States (POMS) (38) to measure mood disturbances—the POMS is a 65-question self-report checklist with 6 subscales, including tension/anxiety, depression, anger, fatigue, vigor, and confusion/bewilderment; (2) the Simmons Scale (39) to document improvement of self-esteem; and (3) the Social Adjustment Scale-Self Report (SAS-SR) (40) to measure various role-function areas. They found that approximately 25% reported chronic physical symptoms, high rates of infections, and high medical care utilization. In contrast, approximately 75% of BMT long-term survivors were doing well psychosocially and medically, whereas 15 to 20% experienced increased emotional stress, low self-esteem, and suboptimal life satisfaction. Deterioration of the marrow recipient's health status showed a greater adverse impact on the donor's psychosocial status than on other members of the family. This study suggested that psychological support might be beneficial and necessary to both donors and recipients in the 10 to 20% of transplantations that lead to chronic physical dysfunction.

A retrospective study from the University of Leiden examined the psychological adaptation of 17 survivors one to five years after BMT (41). Most patients showed excellent emotional tolerance and effective adjustment, but several felt inadequately prepared for the emotional and sexual problems after discharge from the hospital.

A QOL study performed at the University of Kentucky was designed to assess current physical and psychosocial functioning as a function of age and time after BMT in adult survivors of allogeneic BMT (42). Twenty-three of 24 (96%) consecutive adult subjects completed the POMS and the Functional Living Index (FLIC) at least 2 months after BMT (5). Slight modifications in wording were made to adapt the latter questionnaire for BMT recipients. Finally, the patients were asked (1) whether they would still decide to receive a transplant, and (2) the extent to which their course of transplantation corresponded to their expectations. The data presented in this study suggested greater mood disturbances but similar overall functioning in BMT survivors when compared with patients with other cancers. The study confirmed that younger age was associated with better post-BMT functioning, but did not find that time since BMT was a determinant of better physical or psychological functioning. More than one third of patients reported that their course of transplantation and its sequelae were worse than expected, but only one patient indicated that he would not make the same choice again.

A follow-up study at Kentucky incorporated a second and a third assessment at approximately one-year intervals to learn if the perceptions of physical and emotional health changed longitudinally with time after transplantation in the same patients (43). In addition to the FLIC and POMS questionnaires, patients completed a shortened version of the Sickness Impact Profile (SIP) (44). This study confirmed the previous findings of much greater illness-related dysfunction among BMT survivors than among a sample of renal transplant recipients, particularly in the Alertness Behavior subscale of the SIP. The data also indicated that there was very little change in psychosocial functioning with passage of time.

A third study from Kentucky attempted to identify pretransplant and post-transplant variables that might correlate with outcomes using renal transplant survivors as a comparison group (45). In addition to the POMS, FLIC, and SIP questionnaires, this study utilized the Psychological Adjustment to Illness Scale (PAIS) (46); the Sleep, Energy, and Appetite Scale (SEAS); the Symptom Experience Report (SER); and the Perceived Health Questionnaire (PHQ), using a 10-step, health-ladder technique (47) to examine differences in the study group. As shown in Table 42-2, the BMT and renal transplant (RT) groups did not differ regarding perceptions of their current physical health, health of a typical person of their age, or their expected health 6 months in the future (all $P < 0.05$). Patient analyses indicated that both groups perceived their current physical health as poorer than that of a typical person their age, and both groups expected their health to continue to be rated poorer. This study showed that 55% of the BMT patients and 31% of the RT patients were employed outside their home. Furthermore, 38% of BMT recipients and 45% of RT recipients were either not employed or retired for health-related reasons ($X^2 = 6.29$, not significant). Multivariate analysis confirmed that age at BMT, education, and dose of radiation were significant predictors of post-BMT QOL. Sex differences, initial disease, time since BMT, and chronic graft-versus-host disease were found to be unrelated. The study also revealed that it was far more difficult to explain interpatient variability with regard to affective status than it was to account for variability in functional or physical health status. It was concluded that prediction of post-BMT affective status also requires consideration of personality, coping style, social support, or expectations for post-BMT QOL.

In a QOL study from the Seattle group, 100 adult BMT survivors were assessed with self-report measures prior to BMT and followed one year later using the SIP, BMT Events Scale (BES), and coping scale (48). It was discovered that 3 of 12 areas of functioning on the SIP were impaired for more than 25% of the patients. These three impaired areas were work (41%), recreation, and pastimes (37%). Overall physical impairment on the SIP was best predicted by SIP pretransplant, sex, and use of social support as a

Table 42-2.
Current Employment Status for Bone Marrow and Renal Transplantation Groups

	BMT		*RT*	
Employment status	*n*	*%*	*n*	*%*
Employed outside home	16	55	9	31
Retired, health-related	4	14	2	7
Not working, health-related	7	24	11	38
Not working, not health-related	2	7	7	24

n = 29 BMT recipients and 29 RT recipients.
BMT = bone marrow transplantation; RT = renal transplantation.
(Reproduced by permission from Andrykowski MA, Altmaier EM, Barnett RL, Otis ML, Gingrich R, Henslee-Downey PJ. The quality of life in adult survivors of allogeneic bone marrow transplantation: correlates and comparison with matched renal transplant recipients. Transplantation 1990;50:399–406.)

coping style. Physical impairment at one year was not predicted by diagnosis, bone marrow status, conditioning regimen, or age. Twenty-two percent reported mild to severe depression at one year. The most common concern of survivors included uncertainty about the future (86%), worry about relapse (83%), fatigue (81%), having to slow down the pace of life (79%), thoughts about dying (78%), and worry about their families (77%). They concluded that although most survivors return to normal functioning one year after BMT, distress related to consequences of the disease and the transplantation procedure lingered.

The question of whether control of the underlying disease and the presence of complications or other illness would be major determinants of an individual's health and functional ability after allogeneic BMT was addressed at the Johns Hopkins University (49). Furthermore, the investigators hypothesized that post-BMT vocational status would not only be influenced by health and functional ability, but also by age, education, and previous history of employment. The previously validated Medical Outcome Study (MOS) short form (50) was used to assess health perception, physical and social functioning, pain, and significant illness. The Karnofsky score was either physician-rated or self-reported. Employment and job discrimination were examined in multiple-choice questions. One hundred and thirty-five of 157 (86%) completed the mailed survey. Most patients (93%) reported they could do normal activities with no or only minor physical problems (Karnofsky scores ≥ 80). Global health was described as good to excellent by 67% of patients. Perceived health, physical function, and social functioning were reported to be good or excellent for most patients with modal scores near the top of the range (Table 42-3). Most patients perceived that social activities (80%) or physical functional abilities (67%) were unimpaired or only slightly affected. Sixty-five percent had returned to full- or part-time employment, and one third were not employed or attending school. Job discrimination and problems in obtaining insurance were reported by 23 and 39%, respectively. A minority of patients had limitations of physical functioning, judged their overall health as poor and their social function as limited by health, and experienced pain. Moderate or severe pain was uncommon (13%). Demographic, health, and functional variables were tested for their association with employment or school attendance (or loss thereof). A multivariate logistical regression analysis revealed that loss of employment was associated with lower social functioning, chronic graft-versus-host disease, greater job discrimination, and female gender (Table 42-4). The study concluded that despite the intensity of BMT, high rates of eventual rehabilitation were achieved, comparable to outcomes in survivors given less intensive treatment for cancer.

A study from the University of Iowa sought to extend these findings by directly comparing BMT survivors to a matched sample of maintenance chemotherapy patients (51). BMT recipients surviving 2 or more years were eligible. Twelve previous patients (80%) also participated, and a sample of patients matched with regard to age, sex, and diagnosis agreed to participate as well. The investigator-designed interview was constructed to obtain information in the areas of physical, personal, psychological, and social functioning, and the 30-minute interview was conducted over the telephone by a psychologist or a physician's assistant. BMT survivors demonstrated more symptoms and side effects, required more help with self-care, and experienced more disruption of their sexual functioning and vocational status than maintenance chemotherapy patients. However, subjectively, BMT survivors rated their health as positively as chemotherapy patients.

Table 42-3.
Measures of Health and Functional Status in 135 survivors of Bone Marrow Transplantation

Measures	*Number of Survivors with Scores (%)*	*Range of Possible Scores*	*Mean Score*	*Median Score*	*Mode*	*Standard Error*
Self-reported measures						
Karnofsky performance status	116 (86)[a]	40 to 100	89.7	90.0	90.0	0.96
Health perception scale	133 (99)	4 to 20	14.1	16.0	17.0	0.41
Function						
Physical	133 (99)	6 to 36	30.4	33.0	36.0	0.61
Social	133 (99)	1 to 6	5.2	6.0	6.0	0.09
Pain[b]	134 (99)	1 to 5	4.0	4.0	5.0	0.10
Global health statement	132 (99)	1 to 5	3.5	4.0	4.0	0.09
Physician-rated measures						
Karnofsky performance status[c]	79 (59)	40 to 100	92.8	100	100	1.40
Clinically significant illness	135 (100)	0 to 1	...	0	0	...

[a]There were no significant differences between the 116 subjects who completed this item and the 19 who did not.
[b]The higher the score, the less the experience of pain.
[c]There were no significant differences between those with and those without physician-scored performance ratings. Seventy of these 79 patients had both self-reports and physician ratings.
(Reproduced by permission from Wingard JR, Curbow B, Baker F, Piantadosi S. Health, functional status, and employment of adult survivors of bone marrow transplantation. Ann Intern Med 1991;114:113–117.)

Table 42-4.
Factors Associated with Employment for Patients Who Had Been Employed before Transplantation

Factor	*Odds Ratio (95% CI)*	*p* Value
Currently employed		
Social function	7.42 (2.51–21.92)	<0.001
Physician-rated illness	0.19 (0.07–0.53)	0.002
Currently attending school	0.16 (0.04–0.55)	0.004
Perceived job discrimination	0.48 (0.26–0.89)	0.02
Global health	2.92 (1.06–8.05)	0.04
Currently employed or attending school		
Social function	20.98 (4.52–97.31)	<0.001
Married	0.09 (0.02–0.37)	<0.001
Chronic graft-versus-host disease	0.07 (0.02–0.35)	0.001
Perceived job discrimination	0.28 (0.12–0.61)	0.002
Highest grade of education	1.39 (1.05–1.83)	0.02
Male gender	3.50 (1.02–11.98)	0.05
Loss of employment among subjects who had been employed before transplantation		
Chronic graft-versus-host disease	12.73 (2.99–54.24)	<0.001
Social function	0.08 (0.02–0.33)	<0.001
Perceived job discrimination	3.22 (1.56–6.66)	0.002
Male gender	0.24 (0.07–0.86)	0.03

[a]As analyzed by multivariate logistical regression.
Reproduced by permission from Wingard JR, Curbow B, Baker F, Piantadosi S. Health, functional status, and employment of adult survivors of bone marrow transplantation. Ann Intern Med 1991;114:113–117.

In view of the relatively small samples in these studies, the goals at City of Hope National Medical Center and Stanford University were to conduct brief and simple interviews with the greatest number of individuals possible (52). The investigator-designed instrument included three domains of quality of life: (1) productive activity and functioning, (2) health status and treatment-related physical symptoms, and (3) qualitative aspects of daily life. Patients graded the overall quality of life on a scale of 1 to 10, 1 representing the worst and 10 representing the best possible. Most interviews took place by telephone (95%), with the minority in person. Interviews were conducted with a parent for children less than 14 years of age at the time of the survey. Two hundred thirty-five allogeneic marrow recipients were contacted at least one year after BMT to obtain information on their quality of life; 212 (90%) participated. In this study, most patients were 3 years or longer after BMT and rated their quality of life at 8 or higher, and all of the pediatric survivors had a Karnofsky score of 90 or 100%.

Table 42-5 also shows the changes in productive activities (i.e., school enrollment and employment) and marital status after BMT for women and men from prediagnosis to the time of the QOL survey. Although slightly different patterns are apparent for women and men, subgrouping of patients results in groups too small for statistical analysis. Most of the adults (134 or 89%) were either employed or in school full-time prior to their diagnosis leading to BMT. At the time of the survey, 92 (69%) of these patients had returned to full-time activity, whereas another 7 (5%) patients had resumed work or school part-time. Twenty-six percent (35 patients) had not returned to their former activities at all one to 13 years (median, 3 yr) after BMT. Three patients had been active part-time prior to diagnosis; one continued part-time and 2 had gone on to full-time activity when surveyed. Fourteen patients were not active outside of the home before diagnosis; 21% of those patients had begun full- or part-time activity at the time of survey, whereas most (79%) remained at home.

Changes in school enrollment following BMT for pediatric patients are also summarized. The majority (90%) of the 40 pediatric transplant recipients attending school full-time prior to diagnosis had returned to full-time attendance or employment. Only 2 patients

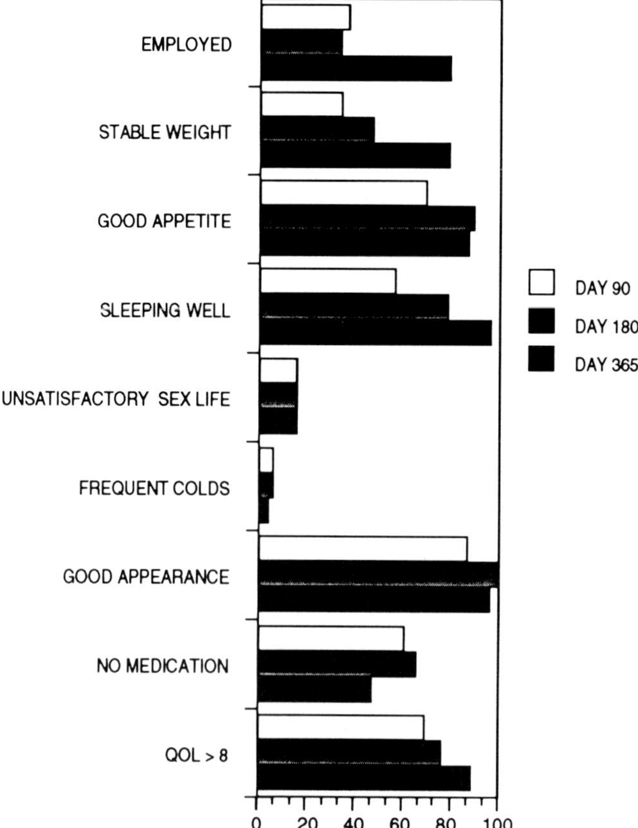

Figure 42-1. Quality of life (QOL) issues after autologous bone marrow transplantation. Note the progressive involvement in overall QOL between days 90 and 365. (Reproduced by permission from Chao NJ, Tierny DK, Bloom JR, et al. Dynamic assessment of quality of life following autologous bone marrow transplantation. Blood 1992;80:825–830.)

Table 42-5.
Changes in Productive Activity and Marital Status at Time of Survey

	Patients ≥ 18 Years at Transplant		*Patients ≤ 18 Years at Transplant*	
Status at Post-BMT Survey	*Female (n = 67)*	*Male (n = 95)*	*Female (n = 22)*	*Male (n = 28)*
Work, school activity				
Number (%) that:				
Returned to full time	30/48 (63%)	62/86 (72%)	16/17 (94%)	20/23 (87%)
Reduced to part time	4/48 (8%)	3/86 (4%)	0/17	2/23 (9%)
Stopped work or school	14/48 (29%)[a]	21/86 (24%)[b]	1/17 (6%)[c]	1/23 (4%)[c]
Increased part to full time	1/2 (50%)	1/1 (100%)	...	0/1
Returned to part time	1/2 (50%)	0/1	...	1/1 (100%)
Started up full time	2/11 (18%)	0/3	4/4 (100%)[d]	4/4 (100%)[e]
Started up part time	1/11 (9%)	0/3	0/4	0/4
Remained inactive	8/11 (73%)	3/3 (100%)	0/4	0/4
Marital status				
Remained married	40/48 (83%)[f]	42/26 (91%)[g]	Not applicable	
Became separated	1/48 (2%)[h]	1/46 (2%)[i]		
Became divorced	7/48 (15%)[j]	3/46 (7%)[k]		
Remained single	11/17 (65%)	36/49 (73%)		
Became married	6/17 (35%)	13/49 (27%)[m]		

[a]Median time post-BMT for the 14 patients was 4 years (1–13).
[b]Median time post-BMT for the 21 patients was 3 years (1–10).
[c]School-aged at transplant and young adult at survey.
[d]Ages at transplant were 1, 1, 1, and 5 years.
[e]Ages at transplant were 3, 5, 5, and 6 years.
[f]Including committed live-in relationships: one live-in remained so; another married after BMT.
[g]Including two patients involved in committed live-in relationships who remained so involved after BMT.
[h]Separated at 13.0 years post-BMT.
[i]Separated at 3.5 years post-BMT.
[j]Couples with female BMT patients divorced between 3.9 and 9.4 years post-BMT.
[k]Couples with male BMT patients divorced between 2.5 and 10.6 years post-BMT.
[l]Includes one female BMT patient who entered into a live-in relationship.
[m]Includes one male BMT patient who entered into a live-in relationship.
(Reproduced by permission from Schmidt GM, Niland JC, Fonbuena PP, et al. Extended follow up in 212 long-term allogeneic bone marrow transplant survivors: addressing issues of quality of life. Transplantation 1993;55:551.)

had not returned to school or work at all, 2.7 and 9.5 years after BMT, respectively. Eight children had not been enrolled in school before diagnosis (4 preschoolers); all were enrolled in school or employed full-time when surveyed 1.6 years to 11 years after BMT (median, 7.2 yr).

The presence of physical symptoms and perception of general sense of well-being was also analyzed in this study. Older transplant recipients were observed to have significantly higher incidence of chronic graft-versus-host disease, frequency of common colds, and skin changes when compared with pediatric transplant recipients ($p < 0.01$). Older patients were also more likely to require regular medications. Younger survivors were rated with a higher Karnofsky performance status and global-subjective score. Thus, this study, which also included a large number of pediatric BMT survivors, extended the previous observation that younger patients may overcome procedure-related toxicity more completely than older persons. There were no significant differences between patients receiving total body irradiation as part of the conditioning regimen and those who did not, with the exception of increased cataract development in pediatric patients receiving total body irradiation.

A similar perception of QOL and return to functionality were demonstrated at Stanford University. In autologous BMT survivors (age, 18 or older), 58 (98%) patients completed the interview, and a progressive improvement in overall QOL between day 90 and 365 was demonstrated (Figure 42-1) (53). Seventy-eight percent of the patients were employed; 88% reported a subjective above average to excellent QOL one year following autologous BMT; 14% reported sexual difficulties; and 5% experienced problems with sleeping or frequent colds. Whereas early QOL studies concentrated on investigator-focused areas, such as the relationship between clinical problems such as graft-versus-host disease and functionality, more recent studies have attempted to address more subjective areas, such as patient family interactions. Recent investigations at the City of Hope led to the proposal of a new BMT-specific instrument to examine the impact of this procedure on the lives of the survivors based on insights collected from patients on their definitions of QOL (17,18,54).

Perspective and Future Recommendations

The integration of behavioral sciences and technological advances have only recently been recognized as enhancing medical care delivery. QOL studies in BMT are one facet in which long term consequences of a technically "successful" procedure can be assessed for both quality and duration of survival. The salient features in the studies cited are that most survivors of BMT are doing functionally well and are able to return to what they themselves consider a normal life. However, chronic physical symptoms occur in approximately 25% of BMT survivors. Similar to the association of the radiation dose with poorer post-BMT physical status (55), it may be important to identify other possible causal relationships between diminished QOL and disease- or transplant-related factors. This information could maximize the likelihood that patients will be able to resume a normal, productive life (42). Although function appears to be easier to measure, interpatient variability in affective status is far more difficult to assess (45).

Evidence is emerging that global overall or aggregated measures ("I feel fine!") of QOL do not provide adequate measures of adjustment. Multidimensional QOL analysis provides more of an opportunity to study cause and effect and to intervene appropriately when necessary. Examples include survivors with profound functional limitations due to severe chronic GVHD who would benefit from rehabilitation or new treatments but are appreciative for every moment alive. Another illustration is the case of an introverted adolescent who has problems adapting to treatment-induced changes of appearance and has suicidal ideation. In both cases, global responses of a high or low subjective QOL rating do not provide the necessary details for treatment alteration or psychosocial intervention.

Symptoms or problems in adaptation are often mediated by a patient's own perspective of their situation. The factors of gratitude and philosophical outlook on life changes are more elusive to assess, demonstrating limitations in methodology. Also, a prospective comparison with norms for the general population is lacking, and it remains unclear what constitutes an appropriate comparison group. Similarly, information on events between diagnosis and BMT and the previous perceptions of the treatment experience is missing in most QOL studies. This may represent an opportunity to compare BMT with other treatment modalities. Questions of whether routine screening reliably identifies distressed survivors and whether appropriate intervention is effective need to be examined. Neurobehavioral assessment tools should be included in future QOL studies to identify any defects associated with certain treatments. These issues, and relatively small sample sizes, make conclusions from QOL research in the field of BMT tentative. Future prospective, longitudinal QOL investigation is needed.

Although there is an array of available tools with previously validated psychometric characteristics, there is a need for refining methodology. This refinement is justified by innovations in conceptual hypotheses, by identification of more cogent variables for a target population, and by practicality of the instrument itself. There is currently no single ideal QOL tool. In grouping existing instruments or in designing a new survey, several factors should be taken into account: (1) it should be couched in language appealing to patients, with a patient-derived (rather than investigator-derived) format; (2) the questionnaire must be varied enough to elicit information on the many facets of QOL without being so cumbersome that patients fatigue or lose interest; and (3) it must be scientifically reliable and easy to administer. Lengthy and complex questionnaires may be rejected by those who may have the most unfavorable long-term BMT outcomes, and any conclusion from studies with less than perfect compliance remains speculative. QOL instruments should not cause emotional distress or impose a cost burden to subjects. Finally, the cost of QOL research must be limited.

Studies involving deeply personal and perceptional issues are limited due to subjects' possible lack of candor. Plausible examples include reluctance to reveal negative feelings about treatment or its outcome for fear of appearing ungrateful to the medical staff, and reluctance to be truthful about sexual dysfunction, a problem compounded by differences in cultural taboos in the diverse population surveyed.

QOL issues after intensive medical care will become more prominent in a society with increasing medical sophistication and limited resources. The outcome of such care will be monitored closely by patients, their families, health maintenance providers, and the public, as well as the scientific or medical community. Health care professionals will have to demonstrate increasing communicative skills and vigorous mechanisms of quality documentation at all levels. Behavioral and psychosocial research has been somewhat detached from clinical medicine; the current challenge is to find a way to ask the relevant question, to pick the right measurement tool, and to strive toward resolution in a rational and scientific method.

References

1. World Health Organization. WHO Chron 1943;1:29.
2. Karnofsky DA, Burchenal JH. The clinical evaluation of chemotherapeutic agents in cancer. In: MacLeod CM, ed. Evaluation of chemotherapeutic agents. New York: Columbia University Press, 1949:199–205.
3. Deyo RA. The quality of life, research, and care. Ann Intern Med 1991;114:695–697.
4. Grant MM, Padilla GV, Ferrell BR, Rhiner M. Assessment of quality of life with a single instrument. Semin Oncol Nurs 1990;4:260–270.
5. Schipper H, Clinch J, McMurray A, Levitt M. Measuring the quality of life of cancer patients: the functional living index-cancer. J Clin Oncol 1984;2:472–483.
6. Padilla GV, Presant GV, Grant MM. Quality of life

index for patients with cancer. Res Nurs Health 1983;6:117–126.
7. Selby PJ, Chapman JA, Etazadi-Amoli J. The development of a method of assessing the quality of life for cancer patients. Br J Cancer 1984;20:849–859.
8. Aaronson NK, Bullinger M, Ahmedzai S. A modular approach to quality of life assessment in cancer clinical trials. Recent Results Cancer Res 1988;111:231–249.
9. Jones DR, Fayers PM, Simons J. Measuring and analyzing quality of life in cancer clinical trials: a review. In: Aaronson NK, Beckman J, eds. The quality of life of cancer patients. New York: Raven, 1987:41–62.
10. Kaplan G, Meier P. Non-parametric estimations from incomplete observations. J Am Stat Assoc 1958; 53:457–481.
11. Spitzer WO, Dobson AJ, Hall J, et al. Measuring the quality of life in cancer patients. J Chronic Dis 1981; 34:585–597.
12. Bergner M, Bobbitt RA, Carter WB, Gilson BS. The sickness impact profile: development and final revision of a health status measure. Med Care 1981;19:787–805.
13. Hunt SM, McKenna SP, McEwen J. The Nottingham Health Profile: subjective status and medical consultations. Soc Sci Med 1981;15:221–229.
14. Anderson JP, Bush JW, Berry CC. Classifying function for health outcome and quality of life evaluation: self versus individual models. Med Care 1986;24:454–469.
15. Gelber RD, Gelman R, Goldhirsch A. A quality-of-life-oriented endpoint for comparing therapies. Biometrics 1989;45:781–795.
16. Padilla GV, Ferrell BR, Grant MM, Rhiner M. Defining the content domain of quality of life for cancer patients with pain. Cancer Nurs 1990;13:108–115.
17. Ferrell BR, Grant MM, Schmidt GM, et al. The meaning of quality of life for bone marrow transplant survivors: part I. The impact of bone marrow transplant on quality of life. Cancer Nurs 1992;15:153–160.
18. Ferrell BR, Grant MM, Schmidt GM, et al. The meaning of quality of life for bone marrow transplant survivors: part II. Improving quality of life for bone marrow transplant survivors. Cancer Nurs 1992;15:247–253.
19. Cella DF, Tulsky DS. Measuring quality of life today: methodological aspects. Oncology 1990;4:29–38.
20. Bloom JR. Quality of life after cancer: a policy perspective. Cancer 1991;67 (suppl):855–859.
21. Deeg HJ, Flournoy N, Sullivan KM, et al. Cataracts after total body irradiation and marrow transplantation: a sparing effect of dose fractionation. Int J Radiat Oncol Biol Phys 1984;10:957–964.
22. Deeg HJ, Sanders J, Martin P, et al. Secondary malignancies after marrow transplantation. Exp Hematol 1984; 12:660–666.
23. Deeg HJ, Storb R, Thomas ED. Bone marrow transplantation: a review of delayed complications. Br J Haematol 1984;57:185–208.
24. Wolcott DL, Fawzy FI, Wellisch DK. Psychiatric aspects of bone marrow transplantation: a review of current issues. Psychiatric Med 1987;4:299–317.
25. Feinstein AR. An additional basic science for clinical medicine: III The challenges of comparison and measurement. Ann Intern Med 1983;99:705–712.
26. Aaronson NK, Meyerowitz BE, Bard M, et al. Quality of life research in oncology: past achievements and future priorities. Cancer 1991;67(suppl):839–843.
27. Aaronson NK. Methodologic issues in assessing the quality of life of cancer patients. Cancer 1991; 67(suppl):844–850.
28. Ferrell BR, Wisdom C, Wenzl C. Quality of life as an outcome variable in the management of cancer pain. Cancer 1989;63(suppl):2321–2327.
29. Brown HN, Kelly MJ. Stages of bone marrow transplantation: a psychiatric perspective. Psychosom Med 1976; 6:439–446.
30. Spiegel D, Kraemer HC, Bloom JR, Gottheil E. Effect of psychosocial treatment of survival of patients with metastatic breast cancer. Lancet 1989;334:888–891.
31. House JS, Landis KR, Umberson D. Social relationships and health. Science 1988;241:540.
32. Forester B, Kornfeld DS, Fleiss JL. Psychotherapy during radiotherapy: effects on emotional and physical distress. Am J Psychiatry 1985;142:22.
33. Morgenstern H, Gellert GA, Walter SD, Ostfeld AM, Siegel BS. The impact of a psychosocial support program on survival with breast cancer: the importance of selection bias in program evaluation. J Chronic Dis 1984;37:273.
34. Welch HG, Larson EB. Cost effectiveness of bone marrow transplantation in acute nonlymphocytic leukemia. N Engl J Med. 1989;321:807–812.
35. Andrykowsky MA. Cost effectiveness of BMT (letter). N Engl J Med 1990;322:703.
36. Wolcott DL, Wellisch DK, Fawzy FI, Landsverk J. Adaptation of adult bone marrow transplant recipient long-term survivors. Transplantation 1986;41:478–484.
37. Wolcott DL, Wellisch DK, Fawzy FI, Landsverk J. Psychological adjustment of adult bone marrow transplant donors whose recipient survives. Transplantation 1986;41:484–488.
38. McNair DM, Lorr M, Droppleman LF. Manual for the profile of mood states. San Diego: Education and Industrial Testing Service, 1981.
39. Simmons RG, Klein SD, Simmons RL. Gift of life: the social and psychological impact of organ transplantation. In: New York: John Wiley and Sons, 1977.
40. Weissman MM, Sholomskas D, John K. The assessment of social adjustment: an update. Arch Gen Psychiatry 1981;38:1250.
41. Hengeveld MW, Houtman RB, Zwaan FE. Psychological aspects of bone marrow transplantation: a retrospective study of 17 longterm survivors. Bone Marrow Transplant 1988;3:69.
42. Andrykowski MA, Henslee PJ, Farrall MG. Physical and psychosocial functioning of adult survivors of allogeneic bone marrow transplantation. Bone Marrow Transplant 1989;4:75–81.
43. Andrykowski MA, Henslee PJ, Barnett RL. Longitudinal assessment of psychosocial functioning of adult survivors of allogeneic bone marrow transplantation. Bone Marrow Transplant 1989;4:505–509.
44. Bergner M, Bobbitt RA, Carter WB, Gilson B. The sickness impact profile: development and final revision of a health status measure. Med Care 1981;19:787–805.
45. Andrykowski MA, Altmaier EM, Barnett RL, Otis ML, Gingrich R, Henslee-Downey PJ. The quality of life in adult survivors of allogeneic bone marrow transplantation: correlates and comparison with matched renal transplant recipients. Transplantation 1990;50:399–406.
46. Derogatis LR. The psychosocial adjustment to illness scale (PAIS). J Psychosom Res 1986;30:77.
47. Cantril H. The patterns of human concern. New Brunswick, NJ: Rutgers University Press, 1965.
48. Syrjala KL, Georgiadou F, Hazlewood L, Donaldson G, Hutchinson F. Recovery from marrow transplantation

(MT): physical and psychological functioning at one year post-transplant (abstract). Exp Hematol 1990; 18:660.

49. Wingard JR, Curbow B, Baker F, Piantadosi S. Health, functional status, and employment of adult survivors of bone marrow transplantation. Ann Intern Med 1991; 114:113–117.
50. Stewart AL, Hays RD, Ware JE. The MOS short-form general health survey: reliability and validity in a patient population. Med Care 1988;26:724–732.
51. Altmaier EM, Gingrich RD, Fyfe MA. Two-year adjustment of bone marrow transplant survivors. Bone Marrow Transplant 1991;7:311–316.
52. Schmidt GM, Niland JC, Fonbuena PP, et al. Extended follow up in 212 long-term allogeneic bone marrow transplant survivors: addressing issues of quality of life. Transplantation 1993;5:551–557.
53. Chao NJ, Tierny DK, Bloom JR, et al. Dynamic assessment of quality of life following autologous bone marrow transplantation. Blood 1992;80:825–830.
54. Schmidt GM, Fonbuena PP, Niland JC, et al. Development of a visual analog tool to measure quality of life in long-term survivors of allogeneic marrow transplantation (abstract). Blood 1991;78:291.
55. Andrykowski MA, Altmaier EM, Barnett RL, et al. Cognitive dysfunction in adult survivors of allogeneic marrow transplantation: relationship to dose of total body irradiation. Bone Marrow Transplant1990;6:269–276.

Part IV
Allogeneic Marrow Transplantation for Acquired Diseases

Chapter 43
Bone Marrow Transplantation for Aplastic Anemia

Rainer Storb

Aplastic anemia is a disease that is characterized by pancytopenia and hypocellular marrow (1). It has been associated with hepatitis, chloramphenicol, phenylbutazone, benzene, insecticides, gold, and other agents, but in the majority of patients no etiological factor for the disease can be found. Fanconi anemia is a congenital form of aplastic anemia. Finally, there seems to be a relationship between aplastic anemia and acquired paroxysmal nocturnal hemoglobinuria. Patients with the following findings appear to have a particularly unfavorable prognosis: granulocytes of less than 0.5×10^9/L, platelet counts of less than 20×10^9/L, reticulocyte values less than 1% in the face of anemia, and hypoplastic marrow with more than 70% lymphoid cells. Mortality in such severe cases of aplastic anemia is 80 to 90%; most patients die within the first 6 months of diagnosis. Possible pathophysiological mechanisms of disease include deficiencies of hematopoietic stem cells, a defective microenvironment, impairment of cellular interactions needed to sustain hematopoiesis, and immunological suppression of marrow function. An appreciation of these various pathophysiological mechanisms has led to application of treatment strategies, including immunosuppressive therapy and bone marrow transplantation (BMT).

Important progress was made with the clinical observation that acquired aplastic anemia can be corrected by intravenous infusion of syngeneic marrow (1–5). The recovery of marrow function seen in some of the patients treated with syngeneic marrow stimulated interest in broader application of BMT for treatment of aplastic anemia. In 1972, a publication described the results of the first 4 transplants of marrow from human leukocyte antigen (HLA)–identical sibling donors (6). The report showed that allogeneic BMT could cure the disease; 2 patients are alive now, 20 years later. It also described two of the three major transplant-related problems—graft rejection and acute graft-versus-host disease (GVHD)—findings that were amplified in a subsequent publication describing a larger series of patients (7). A report appearing in 1976 drew attention to the third problem: chronic GVHD (8). The impact of each of the three problems on the outcome of marrow grafting has changed over the last 21 years. The risks of graft rejection and of acute GVHD have lessened, whereas the problem of chronic GVHD has persisted. Also, new problems related to BMT have appeared (e.g., secondary malignancies) (9). Overall survival after BMT has improved significantly. New challenges have appeared in the form of HLA-nonidentical and unrelated marrow grafts.

This chapter reviews the changes that have occurred in BMT for aplastic anemia over the past 21 years.

Syngeneic Bone Marrow Grafts

Data on 26 patients with aplastic anemia of various etiologies treated by syngeneic grafts have been reported in the literature. The first 12 patients listed in Table 43-1 were transplanted in Seattle (2,5), and the remaining 14 patients have been transplanted elsewhere (2–4). One of the 26 patients was unevaluable for response. Eleven showed prompt and sustained increases of their peripheral blood cell counts along with marrow recovery, and they are surviving between 0.5 and 29 years after BMT. In 4 patients, repeated marrow grafts without preceding immunosuppression were carried out. Either no or only transient responses were seen. However, the patients have survived for 2 to 18 years. In 10 patients, a second marrow infusion after treatment with cyclophosphamide (CY) (50 mg/kg/day on 4 consecutive days) led to prompt and complete recovery in 9; the tenth patient required a third marrow infusion following CY and total body irradiation (TBI). After initial marrow recovery, pure red-cell aplasia developed in this patient. Despite therapy with antithymocyte globulin (ATG), the problem persisted and the patient died from liver failure due to iron overload 9 years after the initial BMT. One other patient died 7 years after BMT from complications of diabetes, a problem that preceded his aplastic anemia. Overall, the results with syngeneic transplants suggest that some cases of aplastic anemia are caused by a defect in hematopoietic stem cells, which can be corrected by simple intravenous infusion of syngeneic marrow. There are, however, other cases in which the infused twin marrow transplant either fails to engraft or fails following a period of transient recovery of hematopoietic function. These cases may represent an immune etiology or be the result of unknown factors

Table 43-1.
Bone Marrow Grafts from Monozygous Twins

Patient No.	*Age (yr)*	*Etiology*	*Conditioning Regimen*			*Outcome*	*Years after Marrow Graft*
			First	*Second*[a]	*Third*[b]		
1	9	Idiopathic	None	...	...	Complete remission	>29
2	18	Chloramphenicol	None	...	...	Complete remission	>28
3	35	600 cGy TBI	None	...	...	Complete remission	>22
4	18	PNH	None	...	...	Complete remission	>18
5	19	Idiopathic	None	...	...	Complete remission	>16
6	44	Pure red-cell aplasia	None	CY, 50 × 4	CY + TBI	Death from complications of iron overload	†9
7	53	Idiopathic	None	CY, 50 × 4	...	Cure of aplastic anemia; death from complications of diabetes	†7
8	23	Idiopathic	None	CY, 50 × 4	...	Complete remission	>10
9	64	Idiopathic	None	CY, 50 × 4	...	Complete remission	>8
10	10	Idiopathic	None	CY, 50 × 4	...	Complete remission	>2
11	11	Idiopathic	None	CY, 50 × 4	...	Complete remission	>0.5
12	12	Idiopathic	None	...	...	Complete remission	>0.5
13	3	Drug	None	None	...	No response	>18
14	7	Drug	None	...	...	Complete remission	>16
15	66	Drug	None	...	...	Complete remission	1[c]
16	54	Pure red-cell aplasia	None	...	...	Not evaluable	1[c]
17	9	Idiopathic	None	...	...	Complete remission	>14
18	32	Idiopathic	None	None	None	Transient response	>14
19	15	Hepatitis	None	CY, 50 × 4	...	Complete remission	>1.5
20	18	Idiopathic	None	None	...	Transient response	>8
21	10	Idiopathic	None	None	...	Transient response	>2
22	15	Idiopathic	None	CY, 50 × 4	...	Complete remission	>2.5
23	13	Idiopathic	None	CY, 50 × 4	...	Complete remission	>1
24	24	PNH	None	CY, 50 × 4	...	Complete remission	>1
25	25	Drug	None	...	...	Complete remission	>16
26	15	Idiopathic	Yes	...	...	Complete remission	>1

[a]CY, 50 × 4 = cyclophosphamide, 50 mg/kg on each of 4 days.
[b]CY + TBI = cyclophosphamide, 60 mg/kg on each of 2 days, plus 6 × 200 cGy of total body irradiation.
[c]Reportedly lost for follow-up.
†Patient died.
PNH = paroxysmal nocturnal hemoglobinuria.
Data from (2–5).

whereby the dysfunction of marrow can be overcome by conditioning with CY and another BMT.

HLA-Identical Related Bone Marrow Transplants

Most transplantations have used marrow from HLA-identical family members. In preparation for an allogeneic HLA-identical BMT, recipients are treated by intensive immunosuppressive therapy to prevent graft rejection mediated by residual host immune function. Immunosuppressive agents used have included CY, given either alone at a dose of 50 mg/kg/day intravenously on 4 successive days or at a reduced dose in combination with TBI or limited-field radiation, such as total lymphoid irradiation (TLI) or thoracoabdominal irradiation (TAI) (Table 43-2). This approach at immunosuppression is utilized regardless of etiology of the severe aplastic anemia, with the exception of those patients whose aplasia is due to Fanconi anemia. Patients with Fanconi anemia are known to be particularly susceptible to the toxicity from alkylating agents and irradiation. They have therefore been treated with reduced doses of immunosuppression, either lower doses of CY or TAI.

All patients with the diagnosis of aplastic anemia who are candidates for BMT should have cytogenetic studies performed to rule out a diagnosis of myelodysplasia, as manifested by clonal cytogenetic abnormalities. Myelodysplastic patients are at high risk for development of leukemia after BMT if given CY alone. To eradicate the premalignant clone, they require more intensive conditioning, such as the addition of TBI or busulfan (BU) (10). For further discussion on myelodysplasia, see Chapter 47.

Graft Rejection

In the early 1970s, graft rejection was the major cause of failure of marrow transplants following CY (7,8,11–16) (Figure 43-1). Rejection is likely to be due to sensitization of the recipient to blood cells from the marrow donor, an assumption that is strongly supported by animal studies (17). Avoiding transfusions prior to BMT

Table 43-2.
HLA-identical Bone Marrow Grafts for Severe Aplastic Anemia: Worldwide Results in the 1980s and 1990s.

Transplant Team, Ref	*Year of Report*	*Year of Transplantation*	*Number of Patients*	*Age Range in Years (Median)*	*Transfused*	*Conditioning Program*	*Prevention of GVHD*	*Rejection (%)*	*GVHD (%) Acute*	*GVHD (%) Chronic*	*Living (%)*	*Range of Follow-up (Median)*
UCLA (55)	1983	1977–1981	46	2–44 (19)	Yes	CY + 300 cGy TBI	MTX	2	70	. . .	63	9 mo–4.5 yr (2 yr)
Boston (31)	1985	1977–1984	40	2–35 (17)	Yes	PAPAPA-CY	MTX	10	53	>35	61	<10 mo–11 yr (5 yr)
Seattle (54)	1986	1971–1981	81	2–17 (13)	Yes	CY	MTX	18	30	30	71	10–20 yr
Seattle (18,19)	1986	1972–1984	50	3–32 (17)	No	CY	MTX	10	23	37	82	1–12 yr (7 yr)
Minneapolis (32)	1987	1977–1986	58	2–45 (18)	Yes	CY + 750 cGy TLI	MTX/ATG + Pred	5	38	12–54	70	<6 mo–8 yr
EBMT (43)	1988	1981–1988	218	1–50	Yes	CY ± TLI, TAI, or TBI	MTX or CSP	. . .	. . .	. . .	63	<1–6 yr
Seattle (26,27)	1988	1976–1981	42	1–49 (20)	Yes	CY	MTX	14	36	60	67	7–11 yr
London (37)	1989	1979–1985	49	3–47 (22)	Yes	CY	CSP	17	50	37	69	1.8–7.8 yr (5.8 yr)
IBMTR (29)	1989	1978–1986	625	. . .	Yes	CY		20				
						CY + TLI or TAI	MTX or CSP	9	. . .	. . .	. . .	. . .
						CY + TBI		5				
UCLA (34)	1990	1984–1988	29	0.7–41 (19)	Yes	CY + 300 cGy TLI	MTX/CSP	23	22	. . .	78	7 mo–5 yr (2 yr)
EBMT (56)	1990	1970–1988	171	1–15	Yes	CY ± TLI, TAI, or TBI	MTX or CSP	. . .	. . .	. . .	63	1 mo–15 yr (4.5 yr)
Seattle (5,48)	1991–1992	1981–1990	35	1–18 (10)	Yes	CY	MTX/CSP	24	15	30	94	1–10.5 yr (5 yr)
Paris (33)	1991	1980–1989	107	5–46 (19)	Yes	CY + 600 cGy TAI	MTX, CSP, or MTX/CSP	3	32	55	62	1–10 yr (3¾ yr)
IBMTR (30)	1992	1980–1987	595	1–<40	Yes	CY + TLI, TAI, or TBI	MTX, CSP, or MTX/CSP	10	40	45	63	>2–>7 yr
Seattle (5)	1992	1988–1991	29	2–46 (24)	Yes	CY/ATG	MTX/CSP	3	15	30	93	6 mo–3.5 yr (2 yr)

GVHD = graft-versus-host disease; CY = cyclophosphamide; TBI = total body irradiation; PAPAPA = alternating procarbazine and antithymocyte globulin; TLI = total lymphoid irradiation; TAI = thoracoabdominal irradiation; ATG = antithymocyte globulin; MTX = methotrexate; CSP = cyclosporine; Pred = prednisone.

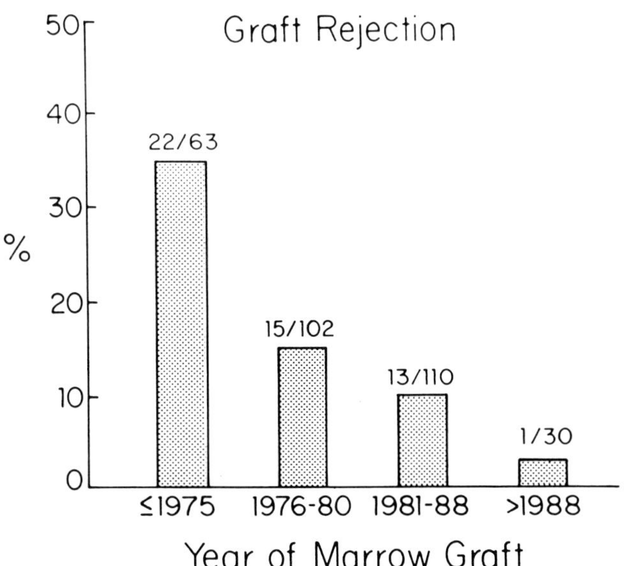

Figure 43-1. The incidence of graft rejection versus year of marrow graft from human leukocyte antigen–identical family members following cyclophosphamide (5). Number of rejections/number of patients transplanted.

has lessened the incidence of rejection and has improved survival (18,19) (Figure 43-2). Factors significantly associated with rejection among multiply-transfused patients given CY were a low marrow cell dose (less than 3×10^8 marrow cells/kg body weight) and positive in vitro tests of cell-mediated immunity of recipient against donor cells, consistent with the concept of transfusion-induced sensitization (20–23). Mortality among rejecting patients was 80%, compared with 25% among patients with sustained first graft. As a consequence of the high incidence of rejection, survival of patients transplanted in the 1970s was only 40 to 45% (6–8,11–16) (see Figure 43-2).

Two forms of graft rejection may occur. Patients may experience either primary rejection without any sign of hematological function of the graft or, more frequently, late rejection after initial recovery of hematopoiesis. Late rejection may be seen weeks or months after BMT. The outlook is poor for patients with primary graft rejection, although some patients have been successfully retransplanted. Patients with late graft rejection can often be rescued by a second BMT. Regimens to condition patients for a second BMT include CY combined with TBI or limited-field irradiation (8,24), or a combination of CY and ATG, which resulted in successful engraftment in 15 of 19 patients and 50% survival (25).

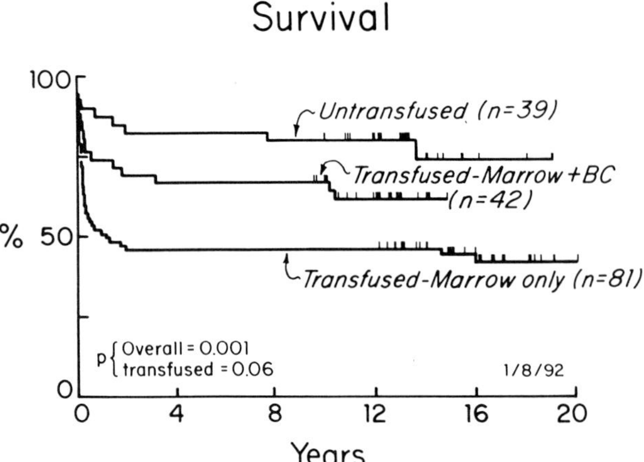

Figure 43-2. Bone marrow transplants from human leukocyte antigen–identical family members after cyclophosphamide (5). Survival of untransfused versus transfused patients given marrow only versus transfused patients given marrow and buffy coat cell infusions (BC). All were administered long-term methotrexate after transplantation. Deaths at 10.5 and 15.5 years are from cancer. *Tick marks* indicate surviving patients.

During the late 1970s and the 1980s, various approaches were developed to reduce the risk of graft rejection. Table 43-2 summarizes the results obtained with these approaches over the last decade. In Seattle, patients continue to be conditioned with CY, with as many marrow cells as possible being infused. Between the mid-1970s and the mid-1980s, multiply transfused patients have been given, in addition to the marrow, unirradiated buffy-coat cells from the marrow donor (26,27) to increase the number of stem cells, as well as to provide donor lymphoid cells, which may be beneficial in enhancing hematopoietic engraftment. This approach resulted in a decrease in the incidence of rejection, at the price, however, of a higher incidence of de novo chronic GVHD (28). Survival improved compared with that of patients not given buffy-coat infusions (see Figure 43-2), a finding that was not confirmed by retrospective analyses carried out through the International Bone Marrow Transplant Registry (IBMTR) (29,30). Other transplant teams increased the intensity of the pretransplant immunosuppression by combining CY with TBI, limited-field irradiation, or other agents. Smith and colleagues (31) used procarbazine and ATG on alternating days combined with CY and found a reduction in the incidence of rejection, although a previous prospective randomized study failed to support their findings (8). Some investigators combined CY with 750 cGy TLI (32), whereas others combined CY with 600 cGy TAI (33). A decrease in the incidence of graft rejection was seen with both approaches. Such decreases were not seen when the TLI dose was only 300 cGy (34). Overall, the irradiation-based regimens reduce the risk of graft rejection. However, the addition of the irradiation may adversely affect other transplant outcomes (15,33,35), and patients may be at increased risk for development of secondary malignancy.

Among CY-treated patients, it was noted that buffy-coat cell transfusions were not the only reason for a decrease in the incidence of rejection, and the year BMT was performed emerged as an independent significant factor during the 1980s (22) (see Figure 43-1). It was hypothesized that this variation could be due to the introduction of cyclosporine (CSP) in lieu of methotrexate (MTX) for GVHD prevention, as was suggested by Hows and associates (36,37), and also by retrospective IBMTR analyses (29). The Seattle team found no differences in the incidence of rejection in patients transplanted concurrently and treated with either of the two GVHD prevention protocols (5,38). Thus, other factors may explain the reduced rejection incidence, including the use of modified blood products such as buffy-coat–poor red blood cells and platelets before BMT, as well as the use of single donor platelets, which is known to reduce the risk of rejection in experimental animals (17). Recent results in a canine BMT model have shown that the risk of sensitization to minor (but not to major) histocompatibility antigens by blood transfusions can be minimized when the transfusion product is exposed to gamma irradiation (2,000 cGy), thereby all but eliminating the risk of DLA-identical marrow graft rejection (39). These experimental data strongly suggest that transfusion products for human BMT candidates should be irradiated before transfusion, both before and after BMT.

A regimen combining alternating CY and ATG was found to be effective in conditioning patients for a second BMT after failure of the first (25). Because of its impressive immunosuppressive qualities, this regimen is now being explored for first marrow grafts, and buffy-coat cell transfusions are omitted, which should reduce the risk of chronic GVHD. The CY/ATG regimen has been used to condition 29 mostly multiply transfused patients. The preliminary results are encouraging; only one patient rejected the graft, and 27 of the 29 patients are surviving (5).

Acute GVHD

Grade II to IV acute GVHD has a strong adverse influence on survival in patients transplanted for severe aplastic anemia. Seattle data show an actuarial probability of survival at 11 years of 45% for patients with preceding grade II to IV acute GVHD, compared with greater than 80% among patients with grade 0 and I acute GVHD (40). IBMTR data show a 31% 5-year actuarial probability of survival for patients with grades II to IV acute GVHD, compared with 80% among patients with no or mild acute GVHD. During the 1970s, MTX was the most commonly used agent given after BMT to prevent acute GVHD. Nevertheless, grade II to IV acute GVHD developed in approximately 40 to 50% of patients so treated (40).

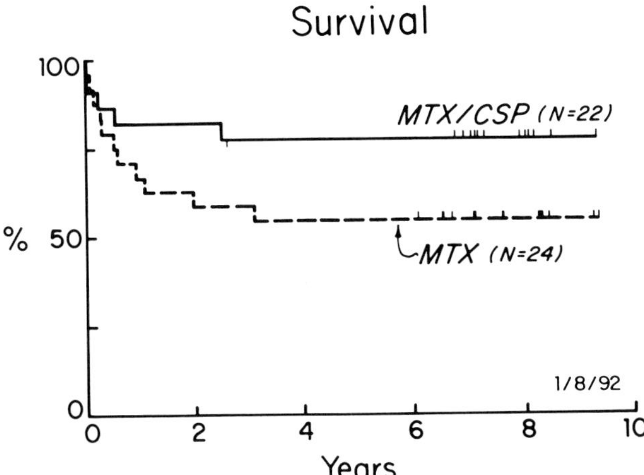

Figure 43-3. Human leukocyte antigen–identical marrow grafts following cyclophosphamide (38). Survival of adult patients randomized to either receive methotrexate (MTX) or a combination of MTX/cyclosporine (CSP) for graft-versus-host disease prophylaxis. *Tick marks* indicate surviving patients. One patient died at 2.5 years from an accident.

Increasing patient age and previous pregnancy of the marrow donor are important risk factors for the development of acute GVHD (41,42). Laminar airflow isolation is of some benefit in reducing the incidence of acute GVHD in MTX-treated patients (40).

Because of the high mortality associated with acute GVHD, a number of studies were carried out in the 1980s to investigate whether the incidence of this complication could be reduced and survival improved. CSP has been studied as a single agent to prevent acute GVHD. A retrospective study reported by Hows and colleagues (36,37) concluded that survival was increased in patients given CSP compared with historical control subjects receiving MTX; however, the incidence of acute GVHD was unchanged. Retrospective analyses by the EBMT group also showed that CSP favorably influenced survival compared with results in historical control patients given MTX (43–45). However, results of several controlled prospective trials showed no significant differences in incidence of acute GVHD or in survival among patients given CSP compared with those given MTX (46).

Data in experimental animals led to the clinical introduction of a combination of a short course of MTX combined with CSP. Two randomized trials showed significant reductions in incidence and severity of acute GVHD in patients given this combination versus those receiving either MTX or CSP alone (38,47). Importantly, no grade IV acute GVHD was seen in patients given the combination. The reduction in acute GVHD resulted in improved survival (Figure 43-3); particularly gratifying results were seen among pediatric patients (Figure 43-4) (48). Maintenance of adequate CSP levels may be helpful to prevent acute GVHD, although recent data suggest that optimal doses of both MTX and CSP are important in controlling acute GVHD (49).

Combined CSP and prednisone may also be effective in reducing the incidence of acute GVHD, although no randomized controlled studies have been reported to assess the contribution of prednisone in GVHD prevention. Triple therapy with MTX/CSP and prednisone did not result in improvement compared with CSP and MTX alone in one study (50), whereas another study (51) suggested some improvement with a three-drug combination compared with CSP and prednisone alone.

Most recent data show only approximately 15 to 18% incidence of acute grade II to III GVHD in patients with aplastic anemia given MTX/CSP, and there has been no mortality associated with this complication (5).

Chronic GVHD

With the decreased incidence of rejection and acute GVHD, chronic GVHD has emerged as the major

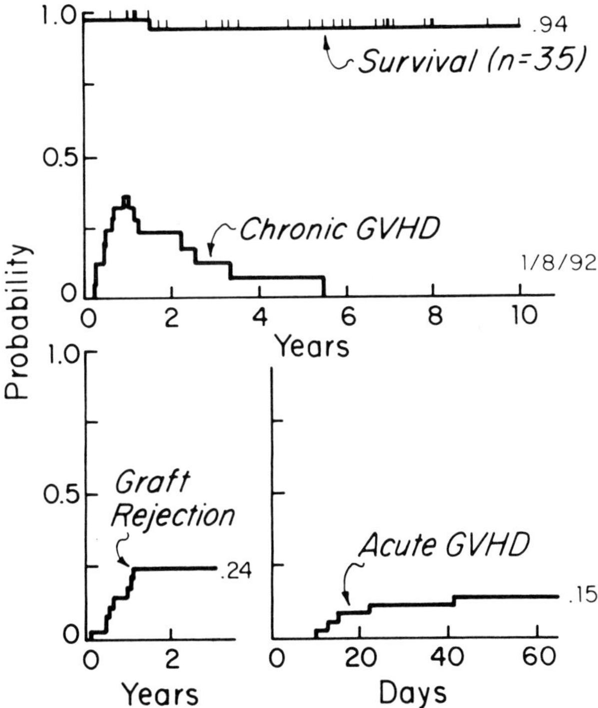

Figure 43-4. Marrow grafts from human leukocyte antigen–identical family members in 35 children, 18 years and younger, prepared with cyclophosphamide and given post-grafting immunosuppression with methotrexate/cyclosporine (MTX/CSP) (5,48). Shown is the probability of survival (*upper panel*), prevalence of chronic graft-versus-host disease (GVHD) (*upper panel*), cumulative incidence of graft rejection (*lower left*), and cumulative incidence of acute GVHD, grades II to III (*lower right*). *Tick marks* indicate surviving patients.

complication of BMT for aplastic anemia despite the progressive reduction in the incidence of acute GVHD. Chronic GVHD incidence has remained unchanged over the past 21 years, 25–55% (28,52) (see Table 43-2). Multivariate analyses have identified three risk factors for the development of chronic GVHD: (1) preceding acute GVHD, (2) increasing patient age, and (3) use of buffy-coat cells in addition to the marrow to prevent rejection (28). Because of their adverse influence on chronic GVHD, buffy-coat cell infusions are no longer used. Gluckman and associates (33) suggest that radiation-based conditioning programs might also lead to an increase in chronic GVHD.

Chronic GVHD is associated with significant morbidity and requires prolonged immunosuppressive therapy, although ultimately immunosuppression can be discontinued in many patients as chronic GVHD resolves (52). One third of affected patients may die, usually from gram-positive infections. The worst survival is seen in patients with progressive chronic GVHD, which develops from acute GVHD, whereas survival is slightly better in patients with quiescent chronic GVHD, which may develop after a transient episode of acute GVHD, and in those with de novo chronic GVHD, which develops without preceding acute GVHD.

A number of treatments, including prednisone, azathioprine, CY, procarbazine, CSP, and thalidomide, have been given either alone or in combination for the treatment of chronic GVHD beginning in a systematic manner in 1976 (52). Has the survival of patients affected by chronic GVHD been changed since the introduction of therapy? Results in Figure 43-5 suggest improvements in survival over time, but these trends are as yet not statistically significant. This finding then focuses attention on measures to prevent the development of chronic GVHD. Most cases of chronic GVHD are diagnosed during the time when CSP is tapered until shortly after the drug is discontinued 6 months after BMT. Perhaps continuing CSP at "therapeutic levels" for longer periods after the marrow graft would benefit those patients deemed at highest risk for development of chronic GVHD (e.g., those with preceding acute GVHD and older patients).

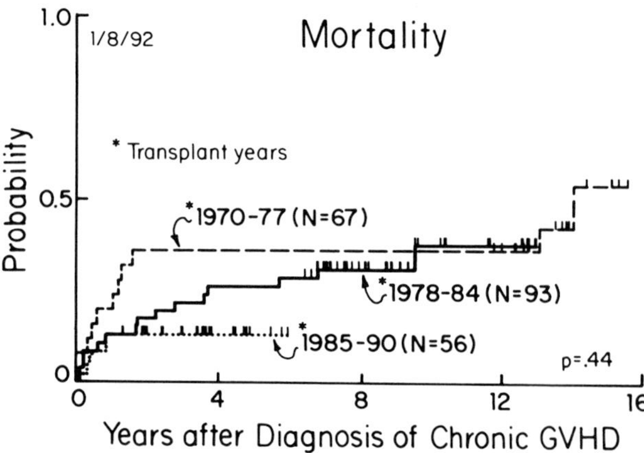

Figure 43-5. Marrow grafts from human leukocyte antigen–identical family members after cyclophosphamide (5). Mortality among patients diagnosed to have chronic graft-versus-host disease (GVHD) by transplant year.

Interstitial Pneumonia

In 1989, Weiner and co-workers (53) reviewed IBMTR data from 547 patients with aplastic anemia receiving HLA-identical marrow grafts for the risk of interstitial pneumonia. They found an incidence of interstitial pneumonia of 17%; 37% of cases were associated with cytomegalovirus (CMV) infection, 22% with other organisms, and in 41% of cases no organisms were identified. The mortality due to interstitial pneumonia was 11%. They found that four factors predicted the development of interstitial pneumonia: (1) the use of MTX rather than CSP after BMT; (2) moderate to severe acute GVHD; (3) TBI compared to CY in the preparative regimen; and (4) increased patient age.

Seattle data in part agree with the IBMTR findings (5). An analysis of the interstitial pneumonia incidence among 329 patients showed an overall incidence of 16% over a 21-year period, of which 44% were due to CMV, 37% due to a variety of other infectious organisms, and 19% of unknown etiology. The cumulative mortality was 7%. TBI was a significant risk factor for the development of interstitial pneumonia, as was the presence of acute GVHD. However, the analysis failed to show adverse influences of patient age or MTX prophylaxis on the development of interstitial pneumonia, consistent with findings made in prospective randomized trials comparing MTX to CSP for GVHD prophylaxis (46). The reasons for the differences between the Seattle and the IBMTR data may be related to the fact that the IBMTR compares results in recent CSP-treated patients to those in earlier MTX-treated individuals rather than comparing concurrent trials.

Survival

Although 40 to 45% survival was the rule during the 1970s, survival has markedly improved during the 1980s (see Table 43-2). This improvement is due to reductions in the incidence of graft rejection and acute GVHD. Two principal approaches have been pursued with regard to containing the problem of rejection. CY remained the principal immunosuppressant used to condition patients for BMT. In some centers, CY was combined with biological approaches (e.g., ATG or viable buffy-coat cell infusions from the marrow donor) or with other immunosuppressive drugs (e.g., procarbazine before or CSP after BMT). In most centers, CY was combined with some form of irradiation, either TBI or limited-field irradiation. With regard to GVHD prevention, MTX was the principal drug in the 1970s and early 1980s; it was replaced later by CSP in some centers or used in combination with CSP by other investigators. Seattle patients have all been conditioned with CY. Multiply transfused patients given MTX after BMT showed an overall survival of 67%, with observations ranging from 7 to 11 years (18,19); survival for similarly treated untransfused patients was 82% at 1 to 12 years (26,27); and pediatric patients given postgrafting MTX and observed for 10 to 20 years had a survival of 71% (54).

Since the mid-1980s, all patients, children and adults, have been given a combination of MTX and CSP as GVHD prophylaxis. Approximately 94% of pediatric patients 19 years and younger survive with observation ranging from 2 to 10 years (48), whereas survival for both pediatric and adult patients conditioned with CY/ATG is now at 93% (5). In the latter group, the observation period is still very short; the lead patient is at only 3.5 years. Figure 43-6 illustrates the improvement in survival seen over the past 21 years in Seattle. Smith and colleagues (31) in Boston reported a survival of 61% between less than 10 months to 11 years in patients given the combination of procarbazine, ATG, and CY; rejection was 10%. Hows and associates (37) in London also avoided irradiation and used CY alone followed by CSP after BMT. They reported that rejection was 17%, acute GVHD 50%, and survival 69%, with observation ranging from 1.8 to 7.8 years.

The use of TBI combined with CY began in the latter half of the 1970s, and the addition of limited-field irradiation was initiated by Ramsay and colleagues (55) in Minneapolis in the early 1980s. Feig and coworkers (56) at UCLA conditioned patients with CY and 300 cGy TBI, a regimen that virtually eliminated the problem of rejection but led to an increase in acute GVHD and interstitial pneumonia; survival was 63% with observation ranging from 9 months to 4.5 years. McGlave and associates (32) in Minneapolis conditioned patients with CY along with 750 cGy TLI. Patients were given MTX, ATG, and prednisone for GVHD prevention. The rejection rate was 5%, the incidence of acute GVHD was 38%, and survival was 70%, with observation ranging from less than 6 months to 8 years (32). The EBMT group reviewed results in patients given CY either alone or in combination with limited-field irradiation or TBI and postgrafting MTX or CSP (43). They reported an overall survival of 63%, with observation ranging from less than 1 to 6 years. They noted that in this retrospective analysis, CSP-treated patients survived better than earlier patients given MTX. A subsequent report by the EBMT summarized results in pediatric patients less than 15 years of age (57). Survival was reported to be 63%, with observation ranging from 1 month to 15 years. Champlin and associates (34) at UCLA described conditioning with CY and 300 cGy TLI followed by MTX/CSP after grafting. Rejection in this small group of patients was 23%, acute GVHD 22%, and survival 78%, with observation ranging from 7 months to 5 years. The authors concluded that 300 cGy TLI was not sufficient to suppress rejection, a finding that is in contrast to that reported by McGlave and colleagues (32) from Minnesota with a combination of CY and 750 cGy TLI. Gluckman and associates (33) in Paris conditioned patients with CY and 600 cGy TAI along with postgrafting immunosuppression with MTX, CSP, or MTX/CSP. Their report showed rejection to occur in 3%, acute GVHD in 32%, chronic GVHD in 55%, and survival in 62%, with observation ranging from 1 to 10 years. Two retrospective analyses by the IBMTR, one in 1989 (29) and one in 1992 (30), showed that the incidence of graft rejection is higher in patients given CY alone compared with those given CY combined with some form of irradiation. Acute GVHD incidence was 40% with a variety of postgrafting immunosuppressive regimens. The incidence of chronic GVHD was 45%, and survival was 63% between 2 years to more than 7 years after BMT.

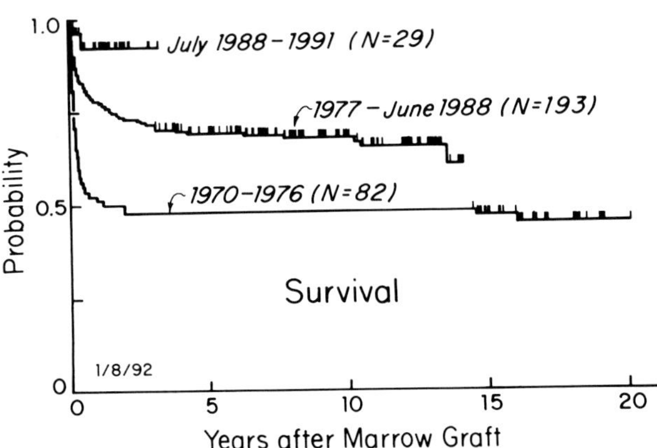

Figure 43-6. Marrow grafts from human leukocyte antigen–identical family members after cyclophosphamide (5). Survival by transplant year. *Tick marks* indicate surviving patients. Three late deaths were from cancer.

This overview shows that survival of patients transplanted for aplastic anemia has improved during the 1980s (from 40–45% to 60–90% or more). In part, improvement is due to a decrease in the incidence of graft rejection, which results from more intensified conditioning programs and from changes in transfusion practice before BMT. Improved survival also results in part from a decline in the incidence of and mortality from acute GVHD following the introduction of the MTX/CSP combination. Serious problems still exist with chronic GVHD.

Current results with the CY/ATG conditioning regimen match those with limited-field irradiation–based programs with regard to rejection, and they seem superior with regard to survival and avoidance of long-term sequelae (5).

Influence of Etiology of Aplastic Anemia on Outcome of the Marrow Graft

It is now well established that BMT can cure aplastic anemia resulting from causes other than an idiopathic etiology. Cure has been achieved in patients with paroxysmal nocturnal hemoglobinuria, pregnancy-associated aplastic anemia, Blackfan-Diamond anemia, Fanconi anemia, and hepatitis-associated aplastic anemia. With regard to hepatitis-associated aplastic anemia, there was concern that liver damage due to hepatitis might either lead to increased liver damage from CY or that the damaged liver might not be able to activate CY. Neither of these concerns proved valid (58). Marrow grafts were successful even when CY was administered at times of highly abnormal liver function test results, and there were no problems with veno-occlusive disease of the liver. Also, there were no long-term sequelae related to the procedure in these patients.

Patients with Fanconi anemia, an autosomal recessive disease, have spontaneous chromosomal aberrations, in particular multiple breakages, gaps, fragments, and exchange figures in all body cells. These patients have an unusual sensitivity to toxicity from alkylating agents. As a result, various transplant teams have reduced exposure to these agents. Hows and colleagues (59) used low-dose CY (5 mg/kg/day × 4), followed by TBI (200 cGy × 3 fractions). Six of 10 recipients with HLA-identical sibling grafts are surviving, with a median follow-up of 3.2 years. Gluckman and associates (60) utilized CY (5 mg/kg/day × 4), followed by a single dose of TAI (500 cGy). Thirteen of their 19 patients are alive, with a median follow-up of 6 years. Flowers and co-workers (61) reported the use of CY alone, initially at a dose of 200 mg/kg over 4 days. More recently, these investigators dropped the dose of CY progressively to 140 mg/kg over 4 days. Seven of 12 patients are alive, with the longest survivor at 18 years. One of the 12 died at 10.5 years from a head and neck carcinoma, whereas one, having received a marrow graft from a sibling with latent Fanconi syndrome, died at 1.5 years with poor marrow graft function. Whichever the approach, survival in these patients is projected to be approximately 60%. The lowest dose of CY that will still permit sustained engraftment in these patients not treated with an irradiation-based regimen is unknown.

Late Effects

As more and more patients become long-term survivors, several late effects after BMT have become apparent.

Growth and Development

A recent survey compared the neuroendocrine function in patients with aplastic anemia given a CY conditioning regimen to that of patients with leukemia given a CY/TBI–based regimen (62); (see Chapter 38). No thyroid function abnormalities were noted in children given CY, whereas significant abnormalities were noted in those given CY/TBI. Similarly, children transplanted following CY had normal growth velocity and growth hormone levels, results that are at variance with the decreased growth velocity noted among children given CY/TBI.

Fertility

Findings similar to those on growth and development have been made with regard to gonadal function during and after puberty (62); (see Chapter 38). However, there was some evidence that high-dose CY in women older than 40 years may result in amenorrhea. Fifty-nine children have been born to patients conditioned with CY, whereas childbirth was an exceptional event in patients given CY/TBI.

Secondary Malignant Tumors

Data on 330 patients with aplastic anemia who were conditioned with CY and followed for up to 20 years after BMT have been analyzed by Witherspoon and colleagues (63). The cumulative cancer incidence was 3.8% at 15 years. Specifically, squamous-cell carcinomas of tongue, maxillary sinus, buccal mucosa, extremity, or vulva developed in 5 of the patients. Three of the 5 died from their cancer, whereas 2 were cured by surgery. All 5 had chronic GVHD and all were treated with prolonged courses of prednisone and azathioprine. One of the 5 had a history of smoking and alcoholism, and one had Fanconi anemia, a disease in which cancer is more common than in the general population. Figure 43-7 contrasts the data in patients conditioned by CY alone (63) with those reported by Socié and associates (64), who used a conditioning regimen consisting of CY and TAI. CY/TAI–conditioned patients had a cumulative cancer incidence of 22% at 8 years, compared with 3.8% at 15 years in CY-conditioned patients. These data show

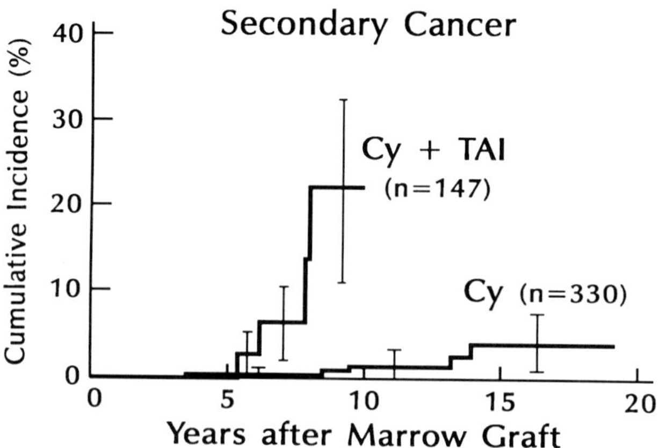

Figure 43-7. Human leukocyte antigen–identical marrow grafts for aplastic anemia. Shown is the incidence of secondary malignant tumors in 147 patients reported from Paris (64) who were conditioned with a combination of cyclophosphamide and thoracoabdominal irradiation (CY + TAI) versus 330 patients conditioned with CY reported from Seattle (63).

that radiation-based regimens should be avoided in HLA-identical BMT recipients because of the associated risk of late cancer.

Grafts from Alternative Bone Marrow Donors

Generally, the results of marrow grafts from alternative donors have been much less encouraging than those of grafts from genotypically HLA-identical siblings. In part, this difference is related to the fact that recipients of marrow grafts from alternative donors have all first been treated with extended courses of immunosuppressive therapy (usually ATG; in some instances CSP, or both) and they are considered BMT candidates only after failure to respond to immunosuppression. By the time a marrow graft is considered, patients are often infected and refractory to platelet transfusions, complications that may adversely influence the outcome of BMT. In part, the results of marrow grafts from alternative donors are worse because of increased risks of both graft rejection and GVHD due to the greater genetic disparity between donor and recipient.

HLA-nonidentical Related Grafts

Patients who are HLA-haploidentical with their marrow donors and who are phenotypically identical for the HLA antigens on the nonshared haplotype generally do well following BMT. Initially, CY was used as a single agent to condition such patients. Nine patients were so treated; all engrafted and 8 are living (one died from an accident after more than 3 years with sustained engraftment) (5,65). EBMT surveys from 1987 and 1988 reported 45% survival for phenotypically HLA-identical marrow grafts (45,65).

For patients who were less well matched, initial reports described the use of CY alone (5,65). Most of these patients rejected their grafts. Only 2 of 7 one-HLA-locus–mismatched patients are surviving (more than 6 years), and there are no survivors among two HLA-loci–mismatched recipients. More recently, CY (60 mg/kg on each of 2 days) was combined with TBI (200 cGy on each of 6 days) (5). Early infections, GVHD, and graft failure continue to be problems; currently, 5 of 11 one- or two-HLA-loci–mismatched patients are living. EBMT surveys showed 25% projected survival for one-HLA-locus–mismatched and 11% for two or more HLA-loci–mismatched recipients (45,66). Similar results were reported by Camitta and associates (67).

Unrelated Bone Marrow Grafts

Even less information is available on unrelated BMTs. One report described 15 such transplants following CY and 6 X 200 cGy TBI; only 4 survived between 1.2 and 4.2 years after grafting (5). Most deaths were due to early infections present at the time of BMT, graft failure, or complications associated with acute and chronic GVHD. Reports by Gajewski and colleagues (68) and Hows and associates (69) summarized the worldwide data. For phenotypically HLA-identical unrelated recipients, they reported survival of 9 of 29 patients, compared with 6 of 17 patients with partially mismatched unrelated grafts.

These results show that transplants of marrow from alternative donors are possible, but early infections, graft rejection, and GVHD still pose formidable barriers to success. Until better ways of controlling these complications are found, marrow grafts from alternative donors will remain a treatment of last resort, when all other therapies have been exhausted. The only exceptions to this recommendation are patients who have a phenotypically HLA-matched family member. In these patients, BMT is the therapy of choice.

Alternatives to Bone Marrow Grafting

Since 1970, when Mathé in Paris (70) described the use of ATG for treating patients with aplastic anemia, immunosuppressive therapy has been used in patients for whom no marrow donor could be identified. No prospective studies have been carried out in which BMT was compared with immunosuppressive therapy. However, since 1978, the Seattle team has treated a number of patients with ATG along with oxymetholone at the same center where marrow grafts are carried out. In many patients, methylprednisolone was administered along with ATG (71). Figure 43-8 shows the survival of 172 patients under age 51 years given ATG, compared with that of a concurrent group of 181 patients of comparable age given either phenotypically or genotypically HLA-identical marrow grafts from family members after CY. Marrow grafting offers significantly improved survival regardless of patient age.

The data from the EBMT registry (43) differed somewhat from the Seattle data. Although there was a

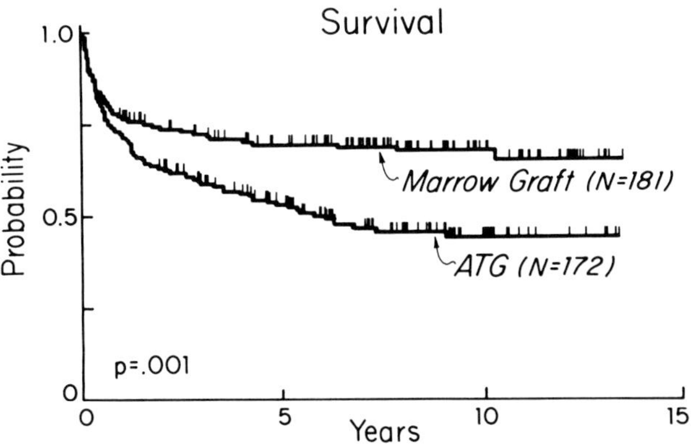

Figure 43-8. Survival of patients with aplastic anemia less than 51 years of age given either a bone marrow transplantation after conditioning with cyclophosphamide or treated with immunosuppressive therapy with antithymocyte globulin (5,70). *Tick marks* indicate surviving patients as of December 1991.

significant advantage overall for patients undergoing BMT, this advantage appeared to be restricted mainly to pediatric patients, whereas in older patients, survival after ATG and marrow grafting was identical. It is not clear why the data obtained at multiple centers differ from those obtained at a single center. In any event, the survival curves of ATG-treated patients continually change because of development of late leukemia, paroxysmal nocturnal hemoglobinuria, and recurrence of aplastic anemia, whereas survival curves are more stable for patients who were treated with BMT. In general, patients who have an HLA-identical family member donor should be offered a marrow graft as first choice, whereas in all other patients, therapy with ATG may be attempted first. Only after failure of ATG should BMT from an alternative donor be considered.

Conclusions

The improved survival of patients with aplastic anemia treated with HLA-identical BMT is due in part to the decreased incidence of graft rejection. The decline in rejection, in turn, results from the more judicious use of transfusions before BMT, the removal of sensitizing white blood cells from transfusion products, and improvements in the immunosuppressive qualities of the conditioning programs used to prepare patients for BMT. With regard to the latter, irradiation-based programs have been effective, although the CY/ATG program looks impressive (only 1 rejection among 29 patients transplanted). With regard to transfusions before BMT, in vitro irradiation of all blood products may further reduce the risk of sensitization to minor histocompatibility antigens. The incidence and severity of acute GVHD have declined with the introduction of the MTX/CSP regimen, and this decline has also contributed to improved survival. Chronic GVHD is difficult to treat and emphasis should be on prevention rather than on treatment. Whether an extended course of CSP beyond 6 months after BMT will further reduce the risk of chronic GVHD is currently under study.

As more and more patients become long-term survivors, the problem of long-term sequelae from the initial conditioning programs and from postgrafting immunosuppression must be considered, in particular, secondary cancer. Perhaps less toxic conditioning programs can be designed. Radiation-based regimens should not be used in HLA-identical recipients because of the higher likelihood of inducing secondary cancer, the potential deleterious effects on growth and development in pediatric patients, and the problem of sterility.

References

1. Camitta BM, Storb R, Thomas ED. Aplastic anemia. Pathogenesis, diagnosis, treatment, and prognosis. N Engl J Med 1982;306:645–652, 712–718.
2. Appelbaum FR, Fefer A, Cheever MA, et al. Treatment of aplastic anemia by bone marrow transplantation in identical twins. Blood 1980;55:1033–1039.
3. Lu DP. Syngeneic bone marrow transplantation for treatment of aplastic anaemia: report of a case and review of the literature. Exp Hematol 1981;9:257–263.
4. Champlin RE, Feig SA, Sparkes RS, Gale RP. Bone marrow transplantation from identical twins in the treatment of aplastic anaemia: implication for the pathogeneis of the disease. Br J Haematol 1984;56:455–463.
5. Storb R, Longton G, Anasetti C, et al. Changing trends in marrow transplantation for aplastic anemia. Bone Marrow Transplantation 1992;10:45–52.
6. Thomas ED, Buckner CD, Storb R, et al. Aplastic anaemia treated by marrow transplantation. Lancet 1972;1:284–289.
7. Storb R, Thomas ED, Buckner CD, et al. Allogeneic marrow grafting for treatment of aplastic anemia. Blood 1974;43:157–180.
8. Storb R, Thomas ED, Weiden PL, et al. Aplastic anemia treated by allogeneic bone marrow transplantation: a report on 49 new cases from Seattle. Blood 1976;48 817–841.
9. Witherspoon RP, Fisher LD, Schoch G, et al. Secondary cancers after bone marrow transplantation for leukemia or aplastic anemia. N Engl J Med 1989;321:784–789.
10. Appelbaum FR, Storb R, Ramberg RE, et al. Allogeneic marrow transplantation in the treatment of preleukemia. Ann Intern Med 1984;100:689–693.
11. Gale RP, Cline MJ, Fahey JL, et al. Bone-marrow transplantation in severe aplastic anaemia. Lancet 1976;2:921–923.
12. van Bekkum DW, Bach FH, Bergan JJ, et al. Marrow transplants from histocompatible, allogeneic donors for aplastic anemia. A report from the ACS/NIH bone marrow transplant registry. JAMA 1976;236:1131–1135.
13. Gluckman E, Barrett AJ, Arcese W, Devergie A, Degoulet P. Bone marrow transplantation in severe aplastic anemia: a survey of the European Group for Bone Marrow Transplantation (E.G.B.M.T.). Br J Haematol 1981;49:165–173.
14. Elfenbein G, Kallman C, Braine H, et al. Analysis of factors related to bone marrow graft rejection in aplastic anemia: usefulness of measures of broad alloimmunity as predictors. Transplant Proc 1981;8: 1539–1543.
15. Bortin MM, Gale RP, Rimm AA, for the Advisory Committee of the International Bone Marrow Registry. Allogeneic bone marrow transplantation for 144 patients with severe aplastic anemia. JAMA 1981;245: 1132–1139.
16. Bacigalupo A, Giorgio FD, Congiu M, et al. Treatment of severe aplastic anemia in Europe 1970–1983. A report of the EBMT SAA working party. Exp Hematol 1985;13(suppl 17):56–57.
17. Storb R, Deeg HJ. Failure of allogeneic canine marrow grafts after total body irradiation: allogeneic "resistance" vs transfusion induced sensitization. Transplantation 1986;42: 571–580.
18. Storb R, Thomas ED, Buckner CD, et al. Marrow transplantation in thirty "untransfused" patients with severe aplastic anemia. Ann Intern Med 1980;92:30–36.
19. Anasetti C, Doney KC, Storb R, et al. Marrow transplantation for severe aplastic anemia: long term outcome in fifty "untransfused" patients. Ann Intern Med 1986;104: 461–466.

20. Storb R, Prentice RL, Thomas ED. Marrow transplantation for treatment of aplastic anemia. An analysis of factors associated with graft rejection. N Engl J Med 1977;296:61–66.
21. Storb R, Prentice RL, Thomas ED, et al. Factors associated with graft rejection after HLA-identical marrow transplantation for aplastic anaemia. Br J Haematol 1983;55:573–585.
22. Deeg HJ, Self S, Storb R, et al. Decreased incidence of marrow graft rejection in patients with severe aplastic anemia: Changing impact of risk factors. Blood 1986;68:1363–1368.
23. Niederwieser D, Pepe M, Storb R, Loughran TP Jr, Longton G, for the Seattle Marrow Transplant Team. Improvement in rejection, engraftment rate and survival without increase in graft-versus-host disease by high marrow cell dose in patients transplanted for aplastic anemia. Br J Haematol 1988;69:23–28.
24. Champlin RE, Feig SA, Gale RP. Case problems in bone marrow transplantation. I. Graft failure in aplastic anemia: its biology and treatment. Exp Hematol 1984;12:728–733.
25. Storb R, Weiden PL, Sullivan KM, et al. Second marrow transplants in patients with aplastic anemia rejecting the first graft: use of a conditioning regimen including cyclophosphamide and antithymocyte globulin. Blood 1987;70:116–121.
26. Storb R, Doney KC, Thomas ED, et al. Marrow transplantation with or without donor buffy coat cells for 65 transfused aplastic anemia patients. Blood 1982;59:236–246.
27. Anasetti C, Storb R, Longton G, et al. Donor buffy coat cell infusion after marrow transplantation for aplastic anemia (letter). Blood 1988;72:1099–1100.
28. Storb R, Prentice RL, Sullivan KM, et al. Predictive factors in chronic graft-versus-host disease in patients with aplastic anemia treated by marrow transplantation from HLA-identical siblings. Ann Intern Med 1983;98:461–466.
29. Champlin RE, Horowitz MM, van Bekkum DW, et al. Graft failure following bone marrow transplantation for severe aplastic anemia: risk factors and treatment results. Blood 1989;73: 606–613.
30. Gluckman E, Horowitz MM, Champlin RE, et al. Bone marrow transplantation for severe aplastic anemia: influence of conditioning and graft-versus-host disease prophylaxis regimens on outcome. Blood 1992;79:269–275.
31. Smith BR, Guinan EC, Parkman R, et al. Efficacy of a cyclophosphamide-procarbazine-antithymocyte serum regimen for prevention of graft rejection following bone marrow transplantation for transfused patients with aplastic anemia. Transplantation 1985,39:671–673.
32. McGlave PB, Haake R, Miller W, Kim T, Kersey J, Ramsay NKC. Therapy of severe aplastic anemia in young adults and children with allogeneic bone marrow transplantation. Blood 1987;70:1325–1330.
33. Gluckman E, Socie G, Devergie A, Bourdeau-Esperou H, Traineau R, Cosset JM. Bone marrow transplantation in 107 patients with severe aplastic anemia using cyclophosphamide and thoraco-abdominal irradiation for conditioning: long-term follow-up. Blood 1991;78: 2451–2455.
34. Champlin RE, Ho WG, Nimer SD, et al. Bone marrow transplantation for severe aplastic anemia. Transplantation 1990; 49:720–724.
35. Graze PR, Feig S, Tesler A, et al. (The UCLA Bone Marrow Transplantation Team). Bone marrow transplantation for aplastic anemia: conditioning with cyclophosphamide plus low-dose total-body irradiation. In: Baum SJ, Ledney GD, eds. Experimental hematology today. New York: Springer-Verlag, 1979: 185–191.
36. Hows J, Palmer S, Gordon-Smith EC. Cyclosporine and graft failure following bone marrow transplantation for severe aplastic anemia. Br J Haematol 1985;60:611–617.
37. Hows JM, Marsh JCW, Yin JL, et al. Bone marrow transplantation for severe aplastic anaemia using cyclosporin: long-term follow-up. Bone Marrow Transplant 1989;4:11–16.
38. Storb R, Deeg HJ, Farewell V, et al. Marrow transplantation for severe aplastic anemia: methotrexate alone compared with a combination of methotrexate and cyclosporine for prevention of acute graft-versus-host disease. Blood 1986;68: 119–125.
39. Bean MA, Storb R, Graham T, et al. Prevention of transfusion-induced sensitization to minor histocompatibility antigens on DLA-identical canine marrow grafts by gamma irradiation of marrow donor blood. Transplantation 1991;52:956–960.
40. Storb R, Prentice RL, Buckner CD, et al. Graft-versus-host disease and survival in patients with aplastic anemia treated by marrow grafts from HLA-identical siblings. Beneficial effect of a protective environment. N Engl J Med 1983;308:302–307.
41. Gale RP, Bortin MM, van Bekkum DW, et al. Risk factors for acute graft-versus-host disease. Br J Haematol 1987;67:397–406.
42. Flowers MED, Pepe MS, Longton G, et al. Previous donor pregnancy as a risk factor for acute graft-versus-host disease in patients with aplastic anemia treated by allogeneic marrow transplantation. Br J Haematol 1990;74:492–496.
43. Bacigalupo A, Van Lint MT, Congiu M, Marmont AM. Bone marrow transplantation (BMT) for severe aplastic anaemia (SAA) in Europe: a report of the EBMT-SAA Working Party. Bone Marrow Transplant 1988;3:44–45.
44. Bacigalupo A, Hows J, Gluckman E, et al. Bone marrow transplantation (BMT) versus immunosuppression for the treatment of severe aplastic anaemia (SAA): a report of the EBMT SAA Working Party. Br J Haematol 1988;70:177–182.
45. Gordon-Smith EC, Hows J, Bacigalupo A, et al. Bone marrow transplantation for severe aplastic anaemia (SAA) from donors other than HLA identical siblings: a report of the EBMT working party. Bone Marrow Transplant 1987;2:100.
46. Storb R, Deeg HJ, Fisher LD, et al. Cyclosporine v methotrexate for graft-v-host disease prevention in patients given marrow grafts for leukemia: long-term follow-up of three controlled trials. Blood 1988;71:293–298.
47. Storb R, Deeg HJ, Whitehead J, et al. Methotrexate and cyclosporine compared with cyclosporine alone for prophylaxis of acute graft versus host disease after marrow transplantation for leukemia. N Engl J Med 1986;314:729–735.
48. Storb R, Sanders JE, Pepe M, et al. Graft-versus-host disease prophylaxis with methotrexate/cyclosporine in children with severe aplastic anemia treated with cyclophosphamide and HLA-identical marrow grafts. Blood 1991;78:1144–1149.
49. Nash RA, Pepe MS, Storb R, et al. Acute graft-versus-

host disease: analysis of risk factors after allogeneic marrow transplantation and prophylaxis with cyclosporine and methotrexate. Blood 1992;80:1838–1845.
50. Storb R, Pepe M, Anasetti C, et al. What role for prednisone in prevention of acute graft-versus-host disease in patients undergoing marrow transplants? Blood 1990;76:1037–1045.
51. Schmidt GM, Chao NJ, Snyder DS, et al. Cyclosporin A/prednisone/methotrexate (CSA/PSE/MTX) versus CSA/PSE for the prevention of acute graft versus host disease (GVHD): a prospective randomized study for patients in complete remission (abstract). Blood 1989; 74(suppl 1):244a.
52. Sullivan KM, Agura E, Anasetti C, et al. Chronic graft-versus-host disease and other late complications of bone marrow transplantation. Semin Hematol 1991;28: 250–259.
53. Weiner RS, Horowitz MM, Gale RP, et al. Risk factors for interstitial pneumonia following bone marrow transplantation for severe aplastic anemia. Br J Haematol 1989;71:535–543.
54. Sanders JE, Whitehead J, Storb R, et al. Bone marrow transplantation experience for children with aplastic anemia. Pediatrics 1986;77:179–186.
55. Ramsay NK, Kim TH, McGlave P, et al. Total lymphoid irradiation and cyclophosphamide conditioning prior to bone marrow transplantation for patients with severe aplastic anemia. Blood 1983;62:622–626.
56. Feig SA, Champlin R, Arenson E, et al. Improved survival following bone marrow transplantation for aplastic anaemia. Br J Haematol 1983;54:509–517.
57. Locasciulli A, van't Veer L, Bacigalupo A, et al. Treatment with marrow transplantation or immunosuppression of childhood acquired severe aplastic anemia: a report from the EBMT SAA Working Party. Bone Marrow Transplant 1990;6:211–217.
58. Witherspoon RP, Storb R, Shulman H, et al. Marrow transplantation in hepatitis-associated aplastic anemia. Am J Hematol 1984;17:269–278.
59. Hows J, Durrant S, Swirsky D, Yin J, Worsley A, Gordon-Smith E. Fanconi's anemia treated by allogeneic marrow transplantation (abstract). Exp Hematol 1987;15:566.
60. Gluckman E, Devergie A, Dutreix J. Bone marrow transplantation for Fanconi anemia. In: Schroeder-Kurth TM, Auerbach AD, Obe G, eds. Fanconi anemia, clinical, cytogenetic and experimental aspects. Berlin Heidelberg: Springer-Verlag, 1989: 60–67.
61. Flowers ME, Doney KC, Storb R, et al. Marrow transplantation for Fanconi anemia with or without leukemic transformation: an update of the Seattle experience. Bone Marrow Transplant 1992;9:167–173.
62. Sanders JE, the Seattle Marrow Transplant Team. The impact of marrow transplant preparative regimens on subsequent growth and development. Semin Hematol 1991;28:244–249.
63. Witherspoon RP, Storb R, Pepe M, Longton G, Sullivan KM. Cumulative incidence of secondary solid malignant tumors in aplastic anemia patients given marrow grafts after conditioning with chemotherapy alone (letter). Blood 1992;79:289–290.
64. Socie G, Henry-Amar M, Cosset JM, Devergie A, Girinsky T, Gluckman E. Increased incidence of solid malignant tumors after bone marrow transplantation for severe aplastic anemia. Blood 1991; 78:277–279.
65. Beatty PG, Di Bartolomeo P, Storb R, et al. Treatment of aplastic anemia with marrow grafts from related donors other than HLA genotypically-matched siblings. Clin Transplant 1987; 1:117–124.
66. Bacigalupo A, Hows J, Gordon-Smith EC, et al. Bone marrow transplantation for severe aplastic anemia from donors other than HLA identical siblings: a report of the BMT Working Party. Bone Marrow Transplant 1988;3:531–535.
67. Camitta B, Ash R, Menitove J, et al. Bone marrow transplantation for children with severe aplastic anemia: use of donors other than HLA-identical siblings. Blood 1989;74:1852–1857.
68. Gajewski JL, Chattopadhyay A. Treatment of aplastic anemia with bone marrow transplants from closely matched unrelated donors. In: Champlin RE, Gale RP, eds. New strategies in bone marrow transplantation. New York: Wiley-Liss, 1991:101–108.
69. Hows JM, on behalf of the Severe Aplastic Anaemia Working Party of the EBMTG, and the IMUST Study Group. Unrelated donor transplants for severe acquired aplastic anemia (SAA) Abstract. J Cell Biochem 1992;(suppl 16A):177.
70. Mathé G, Amiel JL, Schwarzenberg L, et al. Bone marrow graft in man after conditioning by autilymphocytic serum. Br Med J 1970;2:131–136.
71. Doney K, Kopecky K, Storb R, et al. Long-term comparison of immunosuppressive therapy with anti-thymocyte globulin to bone marrow transplantation in aplastic anemia. In: Shahidi NT, ed. Aplastic anemia and other bone marrow failure syndromes. New York: Springer-Verlag, 1990:104–114.

Chapter 44

Allogeneic Bone Marrow Transplantation for Chronic Myeloid Leukemia

Richard Champlin and Philip McGlave

Chronic myeloid leukemia (CML) is a hematological malignancy characterized by excessive clonal proliferation of myeloid cells and their progenitors (1). The disease arises from the malignant transformation of a pluripotential hematopoietic stem cell (2,3). CML is characterized by panmyelosis and the presence of the Philadelphia chromosome (Ph) (4), a reciprocal translocation between chromosomes 9 and 22 t(9;22)(q34;q11) (5). Patients typically present with symptoms related to leukocytosis, thrombocytosis, or splenomegaly (6,7). Frequently, leukocytosis is discovered in asymptomatic patients presenting for screening physical and laboratory examinations.

Clinically, the disease can be divided into several phases (1,6,7). An initial *chronic phase* is present in most patients, during which cells mature normally to granulocytes, erythrocytes, and platelets. After a variable period, the disease inevitably undergoes transformation to an *acute phase* (blastic crisis) characterized by maturation arrest at the level of the myeloblast or the lymphoblast (1,7,8). A transient *accelerated phase* can be identified in some patients prior to development of overt blast crisis, whereas others present in an accelerated phase or blast crisis with no antecedent history of a chronic phase.

Although CML may have a prolonged course, it is a universally fatal disease with conventional therapy. During the chronic phase, leukocytosis, splenomegaly, and systemic symptoms can be controlled with intermittent or continuous treatment with hydroxyurea or busulfan (BU) (1), but available chemotherapeutic agents have no selectivity for the malignant cells and are incapable of eradicating the disease or delaying transformation (9). The median duration of the chronic phase is approximately 3 years (9–14). Treatment with single agent or combination chemotherapy, splenectomy, or splenic irradiation may control clinical signs and symptoms of disease, but none of these therapies significantly delay transformation to the accelerated phase or blast crisis.

The accelerated phase is defined by a number of clinical parameters, including rapid doubling of white blood cells, 10% or more blasts in peripheral blood or marrow, 20% or more circulating basophils plus eosinophils, increasing splenomegaly, development of lymphadenopathy or chloromas, development of cytopenias, and resistance to chemotherapy treatment (15–17). These clinical or hematological signs usually signal a markedly shortened survival or an imminent transformation to blast crisis. Development of additional nonrandom chromosome abnormalities—clonal evolution—often precedes or accompanies these clinical features of transformation (18). Blast crisis is characterized by maturation arrest in the leukemic clone, resulting in accumulation of myeloid or lymphoid blasts. Available chemotherapy is of limited benefit (19,20). Combination chemotherapy for blast crisis can induce a second chronic phase in some patients, but this treatment only slightly prolongs survival. Treatment of lymphoid blast crisis with vincristine and prednisone–based therapy may induce a transient remission. Myeloid blast crisis is generally treated with chemotherapy regimens successful in patients with acute myeloblastic leukemia (AML), although this therapy is usually ineffective for CML blast crisis. Median duration of survival for patients in blast crisis ranges from 2 to 5 months in most studies. The natural course of CML has not been substantially modified by conventional chemotherapeutic agents or by aggressive combination therapy (21,22).

The annual rate of death for patients with chronic phase CML is 5 to 10% for the first 1 to 2 years after diagnosis, and increases to 25% per year thereafter, corresponding to the incidence of transformation. Median survival from diagnosis is approximately 4 years (9–14). Patients sometimes survive for many years in chronic phase. In one series, approximately 10% of patients were alive at 7 years using only conventional chemotherapy (11). In the absence of bone marrow transplantation (BMT), no therapy has altered the natural history of the disease. Intensive chemotherapy may produce cytogenetic remissions, but these have been transient. Recently, however, initial treatment with alpha-interferon has been reported to control leukocytosis in approximately 80% of patients (23). Unlike other chemotherapeutic agents that have been commonly used for treatment of CML, alpha-interferon can suppress the growth of Ph-positive cells and allow re-establishment of diploid hematopoiesis in some patients (23). In one study, 73% of newly diagnosed patients achieved hematological remission, and 19% had complete cytogenetic remission, with no detectable Ph-positive cells on at least one cytogenetic evaluation. An analysis of these patients showed that the probability of relapse-free survival was better in patients with hematological remission associated with major cytogenetic responses, suggesting that interferon may have a role in altering the natural history of the disorder in some patients who are sensitive to this agent. Patients failing to achieve a cytogenetic remission appear to have similar survival as with conventional chemotherapy. Other studies, however, have not seen a survival advantage related to cytogenetic response to interferon (24). Randomized controlled trials involving larger numbers of patients are ongoing to determine if alpha-interferon prolongs the duration of chronic phase or improves overall survival (25).

It is impossible to predict when an individual patient will transform from a stable chronic phase to an accelerated phase or blast crisis. Prognostic factors at diagnosis predicting earlier transformation include marked splenomegaly, a higher percentage of blasts, peripheral blood or marrow basophilia, age, race, and additional cytogenetic abnormalities (9–14). On the basis of these parameters, patients may be categorized into high, intermediate, and low-risk groups, with median survivals of approximately 2, 3, and 5 years, respectively.

Genetic Basis of CML

CML is a clonal malignancy of a pluripotential hematopoietic stem cell. The Ph chromosome can be identified in more than 95% of patients with CML (5). The Ph translocation results in transposition of the cellular abl (c-abl) gene from its usual position on chromosome 9 to chromosome 22 (26–30). The normal proto-oncogene c-abl contains more than 230 kb and 12 exons that encode for a p145 protein with tyrosine kinase activity. The breakpoint on chromosome 9 occurs within a large 200-kb region at the 5′ end of the c-abl gene that leaves exons 2 through 11 as integral parts of the fusion gene. The breakpoint on chromosome 22 occurs within a limited 5.8-kb DNA segment termed the *breakpoint cluster region* or *bcr,* which resides on a gene composed of 140 kb and 23 exons, now designated the BCR gene. The bcr consists of 6 exons, which correspond to exons XIII through XVIII of the BCR gene. The function of the normal BCR gene is not known, although a p160 bcr protein has been characterized as a serine/threonine kinase (31). The site of the breakpoint in the bcr varies. Transposition of c-abl into the BCR gene results in the creation of an abnormal fusion gene termed *bcr-abl,* which occurs either between bcr exons 3 and 4 or between bcr exons 2 and 3 and abl exon 2. The messenger RNA (mRNA) transcript that results from the fusion gene is 8.5 kb and is translated into a p210 protein with augmented tyrosine kinase activity (32). Conflicting data have been reported regarding the prognostic significance of the location of the breakpoint within BCR (33–35).

bcr-abl rearrangement can be found in virtually all patients with CML, even those with a variant translocation not apparently involving chromosome 9 or with no gross cytogenetic evidence of the Ph chromosome (36,37). The p210 tyrosine kinase gene product may represent a cancer-specific marker and likely has a central role in the development of this malignancy. The p210 protein has been shown to transform hematopoietic cells in vitro, suggesting that it may have a causal role in the development of CML (38). Expression of this protein in a mouse model using a retroviral vector can result in development of CML or acute lymphoblastic leukemia (ALL)–like disease (39).

The Ph chromosome is also found in 10% of children and 25 to 35% of adults with ALL, as well as 2% of patients with AML. In half of patients, a novel bcr-abl fusion gene is created that results from the splicing of abl exon 2 to a site within the first intron of the BCR gene (40–42). This "ALL" bcr-abl gene is transcribed as a 7-kb mRNA, which is translated into a p190 protein that also has tyrosine kinase activity. The reason that CML develops in some patients with the "CML" bcr-abl recombination and ALL develops in others is unknown. Presumably other factors are involved, such as the nature of the target cell in which the transforming event occurs, or possibly the coexpression of other oncogenes that determine the specific phenotype of the leukemia.

Activation or suppression of other oncogenes is likely involved in the transformation process from a stable chronic phase. Altered expression of the p53 gene located on chromosome 17 is found in a significant percentage of patients with CML in advanced stages (43,44). This gene product appears to act as a suppressor oncogene that may allow for accelerated cell proliferation if it is inactivated. Other evidence suggests activation of c-myc or c-myb may be involved (45,46).

BMT from Related Donors

Allogeneic or syngeneic BMT is an effective treatment for CML, capable of producing long-term disease-free survival (47–49). The objective is cure of CML by eradication of the leukemic clone with marrow ablative chemoradiotherapy and restoration of hematopoiesis by transplantation of normal donor-derived stem cells. In addition, the donor-derived allogeneic marrow cells confer an important graft-versus-leukemia (GVL) effect, which acts to prevent recurrence of the disease. Approximately 20% of syngeneic transplant recipients transplanted in blast crisis have survived free of disease more than 5 years, demonstrating that the intensive marrow ablative therapy can eradicate even far advanced disease in some patients (50). Better results have been reported for patients receiving syngeneic BMT while in chronic phase; the actuarial continuous remission rate and survival are each approximately 65% at more than 5 years.

More than 4,000 patients with CML have received allogeneic BMT from an human leukocyte antigen (HLA)–identical sibling donor (47–49,51–54). Although most patients achieve a complete hematological and cytogenetic remission from the marrow ablative preparatory regimen, overall results are dependent on the stage of the disease at the time of transplantation. For patients undergoing BMT during blast crisis, approximately 10 to 20% become long-term survivors and remain in continuous complete remission. Patients who are in accelerated phase have approximately a 35 to 40% chance of 5-year disease-free survival, whereas patients undergoing transplantation in chronic phase have had a 50 to 60% chance of long-term disease-free survival (Figure 44-1). The major cause of treatment failure for patients with advanced CML is leukemia relapse. Patients transplanted in blast crisis have a 60% relapse rate, compared with 20% for patients in chronic phase (Figure 44-2).

Most patients have received high-dose cyclophosphamide (CY) and total body irradiation (TBI) as the antileukemic preparative regimen prior to BMT. The combination of BU and CY without radiotherapy appears equally effective (55–57). It has not been possible to improve the antileukemic efficacy of the preparative regimen with additional systemic chemotherapy or radiation without a concomitant increase in toxicity (58).

In a recent Phase III trial from Seattle, 134 patients with CML in chronic phase up to age 55 received a transplant from an HLA- identical sibling and were randomized to receive either a regimen of CY (60 mg/kg IV on each of the successive 2 days) followed by 6 days of 2.0 Gy TBI (median age, 38) or a regimen consisting of BU (4 mg/kg on each of 4 successive days) followed by CY (60 mg/kg on each of 2 successive days). With a median follow-up of 2 years, approximately 80% of patients in both arms are alive, with a relapse rate of approximately 10% (Figure 44-3). To date, there are no statistically significant differences in the long-term control of the

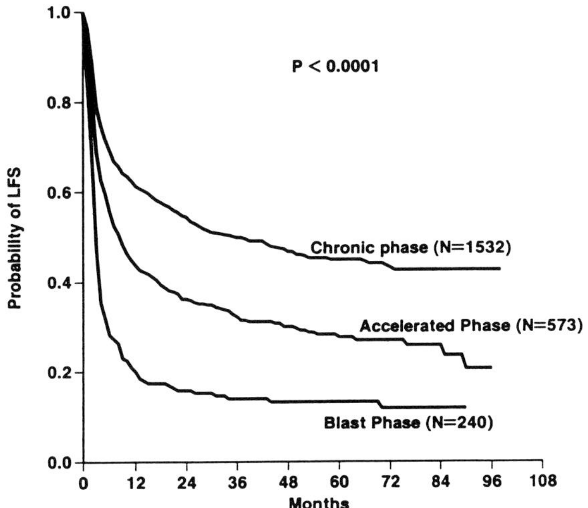

Figure 44-1. Leukemia-free survival after bone marrow transplantation from an human leukocyte antigen–identical sibling depending on stage. (Data from the International Bone Marrow Transplant Registry.)

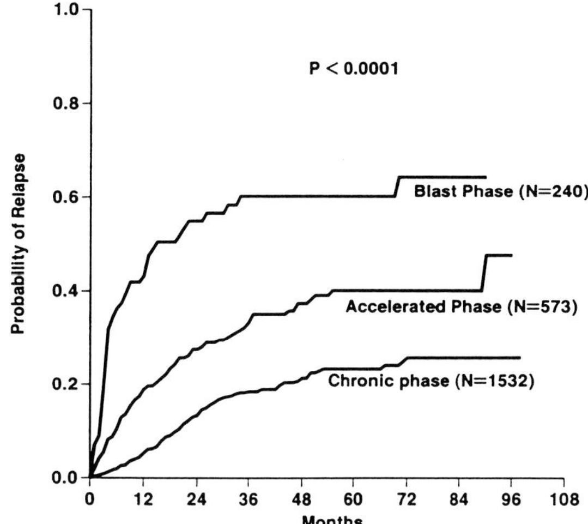

Figure 44-2. Probability of relapse after bone marrow transplantation from an human leukocyte antigen–identical sibling depending on stage. (Data from the International Bone Marrow Transplant Registry.)

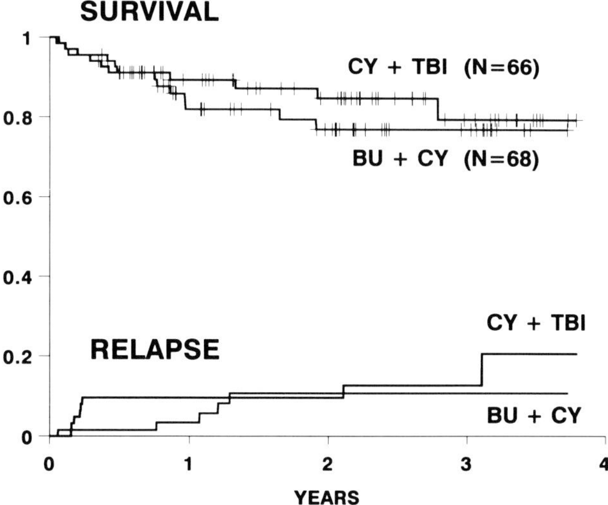

Figure 44-3. Relapse and survival after bone marrow transplantation from an human leukocyte antigen–identical sibling using cyclophosphamide/total body irradiation (CY/TBI) or busulfan/CY as the preparative regimen for chronic phase chronic myelogenous leukemia. (Data from the Seattle program [59].)

disease for patients receiving either of these two preparatory regimens (59).

A study was conducted at the City of Hope and Stanford examining the effectiveness of a regimen of hyperfractionated TBI (13.2 Gy in 11 fractions over 4 days) combined with etoposide (VP16; 60 mg/kg given as a single infusion over 4 hours on day -3) followed by BMT from an HLA-identical sibling donor. Sixty-eight patients received this regimen and 79% are alive and in continued complete remission, with a median follow-up of 30 months (Figure 44-4) (60).

The major limitation of allogeneic BMT is the risk of transplant-related complications. The high-dose chemotherapy and radiation preparative regimens are sufficiently immunosuppressive that graft rejection is rare with transplantation of unmodified HLA-matched marrow. Acute graft-versus-host disease (GVHD) is a major problem, however; it occurs in 20 to 35% of patients receiving combination post-transplant immunosuppressive therapy (61). Life-threatening regimen-related toxicity and infectious complications may occur, which are discussed elsewhere in this volume. In all, 20 to 30% of patients have died from treatment-related complications within 6 months of the procedure (47–60).

The major prognostic factors predicting transplant outcome are stage of disease, age, and interval from diagnosis to BMT (51–54) (Figure 44-5). Patients transplanted in the first two decades of life have better long-term, disease-free survival than patients transplanted in the fifth decade. Nevertheless, allogeneic BMT offers the only potential for long-term control of the disease, which makes it a reasonable treatment option for patients even in their fifth and sixth decade of life (48,50,55). Patients in chronic phase who are transplanted within one year of diagnosis also have improved survival (47,51,54). Thomas and colleagues (51) reported that survival of patients transplanted within one year of diagnosis

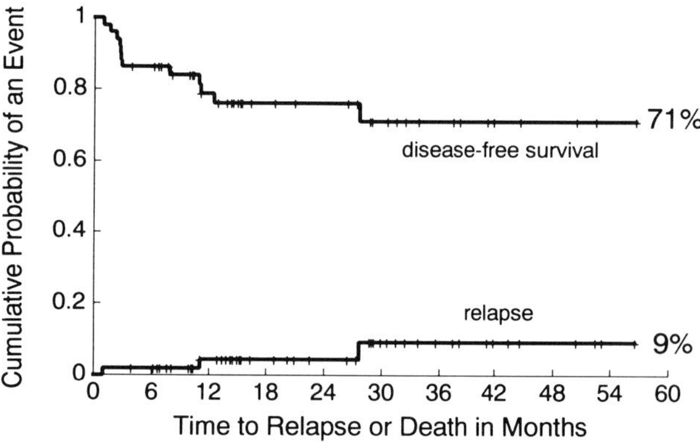

Figure 44-4. Relapse and disease-free survival in patients receiving hyperfractionated total body irradiation and etoposide as the preparative regimen for chronic phase chronic myelogenous leukemia. (Data from Stanford and City of Hope [60].)

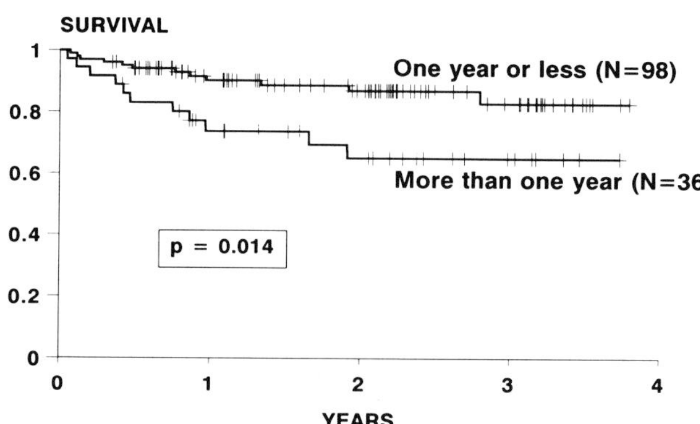

Figure 44-5. Survival after bone marrow transplantation for chronic phase chronic myelogenous leukemia depending on interval from diagnosis to transplant. (Data from the Seattle program [51].)

was approximately 80% at 2 years, compared with 44% in patients in chronic phase at 1 to 3 years. In a recent analysis by the International Bone Marrow Transplant Registry, the advantage in actuarial survival for patients transplanted during the first year is approximately 10% (62). This effect of interval from diagnosis to BMT was due to a lower risk of treatment-related mortality and also a lower relapse rate. Prior therapy with BU was also associated with a greater risk of transplant-related mortality than use of hydroxyurea.

Clonal evolution, the development of additional chromosome abnormalities, in patients with chronic phase CML often precedes the development of clinical features of transformation (18). Presence of an additional Ph chromosome or trisomy 8 in BMT recipients has been associated with an increased risk of relapse in one report (63), but in other studies, clonal evolution as an isolated finding has not had prognostic implications (60,64).

Splenomegaly is a characteristic feature in CML and a major site of disease involvement. Presence of marked splenomegaly at diagnosis is reported to be an adverse prognostic factor after BMT, and some investigators have recommended pretransplant splenectomy or splenic radiation to eliminate a potential site of residual disease (65). However, the presence of splenomegaly at the time of BMT has not been associated with a greater risk of relapse (66). Marked splenomegaly at the time of transplantation can impair the response to platelet transfusions and delay the time to hematological recovery (67). Prior splenectomy is associated with a shorter interval to engraftment, but possibly a higher risk of GVHD (68). Routine use of splenectomy is recommended only for patients with marked splenomegaly or hypersplenism.

The development of myelofibrosis is a feature of accelerated CML and is a poor prognostic feature in patients receiving standard chemotherapy. This myelofibrosis can be reversed by allogeneic BMT (60,69). The presence of myelofibrosis prolongs the interval to hematological recovery and increases the risk of graft failure (70).

Timing of Transplantation

The best results of allogeneic BMT have been achieved in patients during chronic phase. In addition, superior survival is reported for patients transplanted within one year of diagnosis (51,62). If a transplantation is to be performed, delaying the procedure in a clinically stable patient can only increase the risk of treatment failure. The risks and potential benefits of early BMT must be balanced against the risk of delaying the treatment (i.e., transformation to blast crisis). Given the risk of transplant-related complications, some patients have opted to delay transplantation. There are, however, no reliable tests to detect imminent transformation of the leukemia, and results are clearly inferior if transplantation is performed after development of accelerated phase or blast crisis. For patients who are clinically stable, there is a relatively constant risk of transformation, approximately 25% per year (11).

Preliminary data using alpha-interferon in patients with early chronic phase CML have prompted some centers to delay the use of BMT in adults for approximately one year to allow for a trial of interferon (23). Those failing to have hematological control and those without a complete cytogenetic remission within this interval could then be referred for allogeneic BMT. This approach would delay incurring the risks associated with BMT, and a small fraction of patients achieve remissions exceeding 5 years with interferon treatment alone. The concerns with this approach is progression of the CML while on interferon therapy, which would compromise the success of subsequent BMT or if interferon therapy may increase treatment complications after subsequent marrow transplantation. In a preliminary analysis at the M.D. Anderson Cancer Center, prior interferon therapy did not lead to a greater risk of graft failure, GVHD, or other transplant complications (71). Because the time to BMT is an important prognostic factor, this approach could adversely affect the rate of long-term survival.

Minimal Residual Disease After BMT

Considerable recent data indicate that high-dose preparative regimens do not completely eliminate all malignant cells in patients with CML. Up to 50% of patients have had small numbers of Ph chromosome–positive cells identified by cytogenetic analysis (72,73). These cytogenetic relapses do not necessarily lead to clinical recurrence. Many patients receiving unmodified transplants have remained in hematological remission, and the Ph-positive cells may spontaneously disappear in later analyses. In recipients of T-cell–depleted marrow, however, more than 90% of patients with cytogenetic relapse progress to a clinical hematological relapse (73), indicating that these residual malignant cells are capable of proliferating and re-establishing the disease. These data support the concept of an active GVL effect mediated at least in part by alloreactive T cells to prevent leukemic relapse after transplantation.

A more sensitive technique to detect minimal residual disease utilizes the polymerase chain reaction (PCR) to detect bcr-abl transcripts (74–80). Several recent studies have documented detection of Ph-positive cells with this technique in the majority of patients following BMT. The prognostic significance of this finding is uncertain, but patients with consistently positive results or increasing numbers of Ph-positive cells have a high rate of relapse (77–80). In patients remaining in remission, the rate of positive assays decreases over time. Fluorescence in situ hybridization (FISH) is also being applied for assessment of minimal residual disease as another means to quantify subclinical residual disease (81).

Graft-versus-leukemia

An additional GVL effect, largely mediated by alloreactive T cells, is important to prevent leukemic relapse following BMT. This GVL effect appears to be particularly important in patients transplanted for CML. GVL has been closely associated with the presence of GVHD (82–85). This antileukemic effect correlates best with the presence of chronic GVHD. The impact of acute GVHD is uncertain, but the lowest rate of relapse occurs in patients with both acute and chronic GVHD.

GVHD does not develop in patients receiving transplants from identical twin donors. These patients have at least twice the risk of relapse of CML, compared with transplant recipients from HLA-identical siblings (Figure 44-6) (85). T-cell depletion of donor

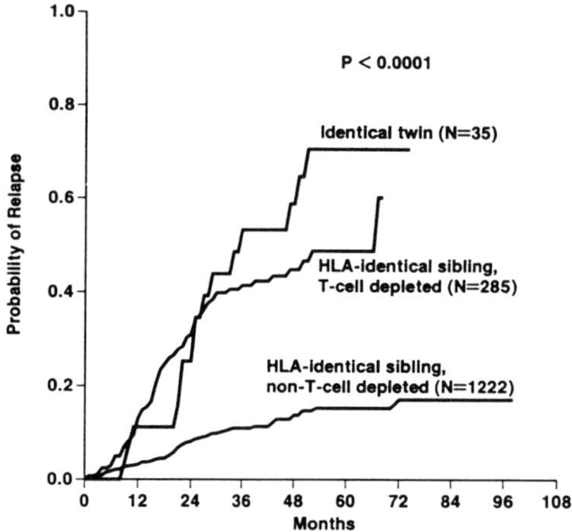

Figure 44-6. Probability of relapse for patients receiving bone marrow transplantation for chronic phase chronic myelogenous leukemia using T-cell–depleted or non-T-cell–depleted marrow from an human leukocyte antigen–identical sibling or using syngeneic non-T-cell–depleted marrow. (Data from the International Bone Marrow Transplant Registry.)

marrow is the most effective means of preventing acute and chronic GVHD, but this benefit has been offset by the substantial increase in the risk of leukemic relapse (86,87). The net effect has been worsening of disease-free survival in most studies. The increase in leukemic relapse is more striking for patients with CML than other forms of leukemia (87). In a study of the International Bone Marrow Transplant Registry, 12% of patients with CML in chronic phase receiving unmodified HLA-identical BMTs relapsed at 5 years, compared with a relapse rate of more than 50% in T-cell–depleted transplant recipients (62). Even recipients of T-cell–depleted marrow in whom GVHD develops have an increased relapse rate compared with patients receiving unmodified allografts without GVHD (87), suggesting an effect of T lymphocytes independent of GVHD. The high relapse rate with T-cell–depleted BMT indicates that viable leukemic cells survive the preparative regimen, which are capable of reestablishing the disease in most patients. Consistent with these data is the observation that Ph-positive metaphases can be detected intermittently for many months in many patients receiving unmodified marrow, even though many never experience a hematological relapse. In contrast, patients with detectable Ph-positive cells following T-cell–depleted transplantation generally progress to overt hematological relapse (73). The GVL effect presumably must be operative over an extended period.

The recognition and effector mechanisms that mediate GVL and the cell populations involved are incompletely understood (88–92). CD4- and CD8-positive T-cell clones reactive with leukemic cells have been described, and cytotoxic T lymphocytes are likely to be the primary effector cells (88,89). Lymphokine activated killer (LAK) and natural killer (NK) cells may also be important in this process (90,91). The joining region of the p210 bcr-abl fusion protein could conceivably serve as a target for a leukemia- specific immune response (93).

It is uncertain whether GVL can be distinguished from GVHD in humans or whether the same or different cell populations mediate each process. Following allogeneic BMT, stable chimerism with donor-derived hematopoiesis is the rule, although mixed chimerism occurs in some patients. The GVL effect may result from reactivity directed against host hematopoietic tissue. Such an effect would prevent competitive repopulation by both normal and leukemic host-derived hematopoietic cells, and this potential mechanism would not require recognition of leukemia specific antigens.

It is conceivable that different cellular subsets are responsible for GVHD and GVL. CD4-positive T cells recognize antigens presented with class II major histocompatibility complex (MHC) antigens. CD8-positive lymphocytes recognize antigens presented in the context of class I loci. CD4-positive cells mediate acute GVHD in MHC class II disparate recipients, whereas CD8-positive cells are primarily responsible in class I disparate transplants in mice (94). Depletion of the CD8-positive cytotoxic/suppressor subset of T lymphocytes is sufficient to reduce or prevent GVHD in most donor-recipient murine strain combinations that are MHC-compatible but mismatched for minor histocompatibility loci. Champlin and associates (95) recently reported that selective depletion of CD8-positive cells in combination with post- transplant cyclosporine (CSP) resulted in a significantly reduced rate of acute GVHD, without an increase in the rate of leukemic relapse. Improved methods to selectively enhance the GVL effect may be possible.

GVHD Prophylaxis

Recommendations for prevention and control of acute GVHD are complex in patients with CML, given the interaction of T cells, GVHD, and leukemic relapse. With transplantation of unmodified marrow, administration of multiagent post-transplant immunosuppressive therapy using CSP with methotrexate (MTX) or CSP and corticosteroids results in a significantly lower incidence of acute GVHD than single-agent immunosuppressive therapy (61,96). In patients with AML, the CSP/MTX combination was associated with a higher rate of leukemic relapse than CSP alone, thus abrogating any improvement in leukemia-free survival. However, in patients with CML, the relapse rate was not affected by the CSP/MTX combination, and overall results were improved (61).

Although T-cell depletion is the most effective means to prevent acute and chronic GVHD, the marked increase in leukemic relapse associated with this procedure offsets this benefit. Several centers are examining modifications of this approach to reduce the risk of relapse. Innovative approaches include further intensification of the preparative regimen to increase antileukemic cytotoxicity, subtotal T-cell depletion, selective depletion of T-cell subsets that primarily induce GVHD, or administration of interferon-alpha or other cytokines to suppress minimal residual leukemia after transplantation (97). It is unclear if any of these innovations will improve treatment outcome, and T-cell depletion should not be used routinely to prevent GVHD in patients with CML except in the context of a controlled clinical trial.

Treatment of Relapsed CML After BMT

A number of treatment options may be considered for patients with recurrent CML after allogeneic BMT. Second transplants are one option, particularly for patients who had a remission greater than one year (98–100). Patients initially prepared with a TBI-containing preparative regimen cannot tolerate further TBI, but may receive a BU/CY regimen. Patients relapsing after a T-cell–depleted BMT may achieve a prolonged remission with an unmodified (non-T-cell–depleted) second transplant.

The risks of a second BMT are substantial, and other alternatives may be considered. Patients who recur into chronic phase may respond to interferon (101).

Reinduction of hematological and cytogenetic remission has been achieved by infusion of donor buffy-coat cells, which frequently also induce transient GVHD (102,103). These intriguing reports suggest that the post-transplant chimeric state may be manipulated to induce an enhanced GVL effect.

Transplants from Unrelated Donors

Transplantation using marrow obtained from suitably HLA-matched related donors is the only proven curative therapy for CML (47,104). Unfortunately, fewer than 40% of otherwise eligible patients will have an HLA-identical sibling donor or a suitable, partially HLA-mismatched related donor (105,106). Investigators considered CML an ideal disease to test the efficacy of unrelated donor BMT. The natural history of CML includes a prolonged chronic phase (11), which may allow time to locate a suitably matched unrelated donor.

Several clinical studies have demonstrated that therapy for CML with unrelated donor BMT results in sustained donor engraftment, disappearance of the Ph chromosome, and clinical remissions in some patients. These reports also defined particular risks associated with this approach, including early mortality, graft failure, a high incidence of moderate or severe acute and extensive chronic GVHD, prolonged convalescence, and the development of Epstein-Barr virus (EBV)–associated lymphoma (107–111). In some patients, successful transplants were achieved using unrelated donors with nonidentity detected by serological testing at the HLA A, B, or DR locus rather than HLA-identical unrelated donors.

Engraftment After Unrelated Donor Transplantation

Failure to establish hematological engraftment (primary graft failure) and loss of an established graft (late graft failure) are problems encountered in unrelated donor BMT therapy for CML. In one recent analysis, 22 of 196 patients experienced primary graft failure, and an additional 10 patients experienced late graft failure (112). The incidence of graft failure far exceeded that observed in matched sibling BMT therapy for leukemia, but was similar to that observed in phenotypically one-HLA–mismatched related donor transplantation (106). Recent observations suggest that some cases of graft failure after unrelated donor BMT may occur because of HLA structural polymorphisms not recognized by current serological HLA typing methods (113).

The high incidence of graft failure compels investigators to develop contingency plans for CML unrelated donor BMT candidates because prolonged hospitalization, transfusion dependency, and death from pancytopenia can be anticipated when graft failure occurs. One approach to the problem of graft failure is the storage of autologous peripheral blood or marrow stem cells prior to transplantation. These "back-up cells" can be expected to re-establish autologous hematopoiesis after failure of unrelated donor marrow to engraft. An alternative approach is performance of a second unrelated donor transplantation. Unrelated donors may not be available for a second donation in a timely fashion. Moreover, the National Marrow Donor Program (NMDP) and other organizations have implemented policies governing the approach of unrelated donors for repeat donation to protect these individuals from coercion and potentially harmful effects of second donation (114). These considerations suggest that groups performing unrelated donor BMT for CML should have a prearranged plan for graft failure that can be implemented early in the transplant course. Unrelated donor transplant candidates should be educated to understand the risks of graft failure and its sequelae.

GVHD and Prophylaxis After Unrelated Donor Transplant

The probability for development of grade III to IV acute GVHD after unrelated donor BMT for CML is approximately 55%, and the probability for development of extensive chronic GVHD is similar (112). These are higher incidences than expected in a comparable group of CML recipients receiving matched sibling donor BMT, but similar to those observed in patients who receive one or two HLA-mismatched related donor marrow BMTs (105,106). This high incidence of acute GVHD is observed not only in recipients of one-HLA–mismatched unrelated donor bone marrow, but also in recipients of HLA-matched marrow, suggesting that standard serological testing of HLA may not identify important structural MHC polymorphisms that provoke GVHD reactions after unrelated donor BMT for CML.

In one recent study, the use of unrelated donor marrow depleted of T lymphocytes resulted in a 20% incidence of grade III to IV acute GVHD, which was signficantly lower than the 60% incidence observed in recipients of non-T-cell–depleted marrow. Similarly, the 22% incidence of extensive chronic GVHD observed in recipients of T-cell–depleted marrow was significantly lower than the 59% incidence observed in recipients of non-T-cell–depleted marrow (112). The widespread use of T-cell depletion in this setting, however, must be viewed with great caution. Long-term follow-up of patients with CML receiving T-cell–depleted, related donor marrow transplants has revealed extraordinarily high relapse rates not seen in comparable patients receiving non-T-cell–depleted marrow (53,104,115). T-lymphocyte depletion may also increase the risk of graft failure and EBV lymphoma, problems that have been encountered in unrelated donor BMTs for CML (108,112,116). The long-term effects of T-cell depletion on relapse and on disease-free survival cannot be appreciated fully without prolonged, careful assessment of patients with CML receiving unrelated donor marrow.

Outcome of Unrelated Donor Transplant

Conclusions concerning the efficacy of unrelated donor BMT for CML must still be considered preliminary. Follow-up of CML unrelated donor recipients has been relatively short, and the groups studied have heterogeneous characteristics that may affect long-term outcome. Analysis of the largest group studied to date shows several transplant characteristics that independently predict a poorer outcome (112) (Table 44-1). Use of unrelated donor marrow mismatched at the A, B, or DR locus rather than serologically HLA-matched marrow is associated with poorer disease-free survival. These data indicate that, if possible, a fully matched donor should be chosen. Long-term disease-free survival, however, has been documented on many occasions in which marrow obtained from unrelated donors mismatched at one HLA A, B, or DR locus was used. It has not yet been determined if certain parameters of HLA donor/recipient nonidentity measured by serological testing of HLA (e.g. non identity within an HLA noncrossreactive group rather than an HLA crossreactive group) will have an adverse effect on outcome, as has been seen in the related donor setting (105,106). Similarly, it is not known if newly developed molecular methods for determining HLA nonidentity (described in Chapter 51) will predict donor/recipient combinations that can be associated with poor outcome.

Transplantation in patients with advanced disease rather than in the chronic phase also has an independent, adverse effect on disease-free survival. In one analysis, 45% of chronic phase patients transplanted within one year of diagnosis (n = 30) were surviving disease-free at a median of 1.5 years. In this study, disease-free survival of 85 chronic phase patients transplanted greater than one year after diagnosis (36%), as well as 51 patients transplanted in accelerated phase (27%), 16 in second chronic phase (22%), or 14 in blast crisis (0%), was less favorable (Figure 44-7) (112). These data suggest a role for unrelated donor BMT therapy for patients with CML in chronic phase, preferably early in the disease course.

An independent beneficial effect of younger recipient age on outcome has also been identified. The incidence of disease-free survival is significantly better for patients with CML who are less than 20 years of

Table 44-1.
Factors Associated with Leukemia-free Survival Following Unrelated Donor Marrow Transplant (Proportional Hazards Analysis)

Characteristic	*p* Value	*Favorable*
Level of donor-recipient disparity	0.01	Serological HLA A, B, DR match
Recipient age (per decade)	0.02	Younger age
Disease status at transplantation	0.04	First chronic phase

HLA = human leukocyte antigen.

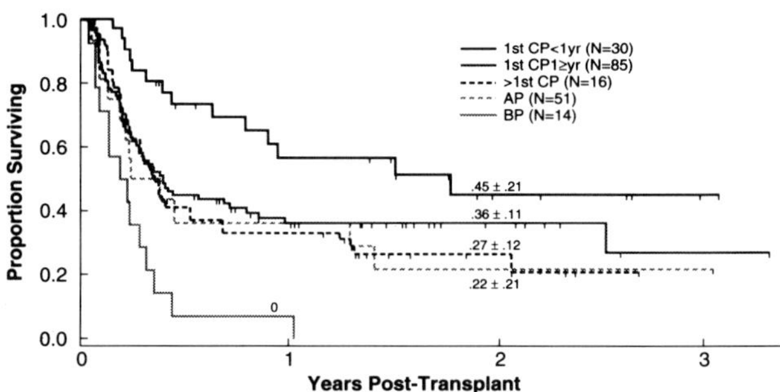

Figure 44-7. Disease-free survival after bone marrow transplantation from an unrelated donor according to disease stage and interval from diagnosis to transplant. (Data from the National Marrow Donor Program.)

age than for older recipients of unrelated donor transplantation. The incidence of disease-free survival is similar in patients with CML receiving unrelated donor transplantations in their third, fourth, or fifth decades. These data suggest no *a priori* reason for setting an arbitrary upper age limit of less than 55 years for adults undergoing unrelated donor BMT for CML. This is of particular importance because CML is a disease of middle age.

The adverse impact of risk factors may be additive. For example, older recipients with advanced CML receiving unrelated donor marrow mismatched at one HLA locus have poorer disease-free survival than recipients with only one of these risk features. Patients who do not survive unrelated donor BMT for CML usually die within the first 6 months following transplantation of complications commonly associated with related donor transplantation. Most common primary or contributing causes of death include infection, acute and chronic GVHD, and pneumonia (112). Relapse is uncommon; it occurred in less than 10% of chronic phase patients transplanted to date. Valid estimates of relapse will not be available, however, without much longer patient follow-up. It has not yet been determined if the use of unrelated donors bestows a GVL effect that will supersede the effect attributed to matched sibling donor transplant therapy for CML (85).

Convalescence Following Unrelated Donor Transplantation

Prolonged convalescence can be anticipated in some patients following unrelated donor BMT. In one recent analysis, only 51% of survivors assessed at one year had normal Karnofsky activity levels. Forty percent of patients had mild or moderate impairment of activity, whereas 9% had profound impairment of activity (112). No association between impaired activity levels at one year and use of mismatched rather than matched marrow or of transplant at older rather than younger age (Table 44-2) could be identified. These observations

Table 44-2.
Karnofsky Activity Assessment of Younger (<30 years) and Older (≥30 years) Patients with Chronic Myelogenous Leukemia at One Year Following Unrelated Donor Marrow Transplant

	AGE		
Score	*<30 (%)*	*≥30 (%)*	*Total (%)*
100	18 (55)	20 (48)	38 (51)
90–80	12 (36)	18 (42)	30 (40)
70–30	3 (9)	4 (10)	7 (9)

suggest that the issues of early mortality and prolonged convalescence should be raised in patients undergoing counseling prior to unrelated donor BMT for CML.

Summary

CML is a a disease of the hematopoietic stem cell. Until the advent of BMT, the course of CML, although sometimes prolonged, led inexorably to death. Marrow transplant from an HLA- matched sibling donor can cure some patients with CML. Best results are observed in chronic phase recipients; however, prolonged disease-free survival has been observed in patients undergoing transplant with more advanced disease. Although alpha-interferon therapy has efficacy in patients with CML, it is not curative. The advantages of delaying BMT for a trial of alpha-interferon are questionable in the context of an overall strategy to cure patients with an available, suitably matched related donor.

Experience with related donor marrow transplant therapy has taught several important lessons concerning the biology of CML. Patients receiving marrow inocula depleted of T lymphocytes experience a reduced incidence of GVHD; however, the incidence of hematological relapse increases markedly. These observations emphasize the existence of dormant, malignant clones surviving even after ablative therapy, and evoke hypotheses concerning an ongoing antileukemia effect provided by lymphocyte subsets in the allogeneic graft. The presence of very small numbers of bcr/abl-positive cells in the recipient can be detected by sensitive molecular genetic techniques and does not always predict hematological relapse. This observation underscores the complex and not yet fully understood interactions between donor and residual host hematological and immunological cells.

Preliminary studies suggest that the donor pool can be expanded to include HLA phenotypically matched and, in selected patients, one-HLA–mismatched or unrelated donors. These alternative donor transplants are associated with a higher incidence of acute and chronic GVHD, as well as graft failure. Younger patients transplanted early in the disease course fare best. Development of the NMDP in the United States and donor registries in other countries, as well as recent innovations in HLA typing methodology (see Chapter 51) may increase the efficacy of the unrelated donor search.

References

1. Champlin RE, Golde DW. Chronic myelogenous leukemia: recent advances. Blood 1985;65:1039–1047.
2. Fialkow PJ, Jacobson RJ, Papayannopoulou TH. Chronic myelocytic leukemia: clonal origin in a stem cell common to the granulocyte, erythrocyte, platelet and monocyte/macrophage. Am J Med 1977;63:125–130.
3. Fialkow PJ, Martin PJ, Najfeld V, et al. Evidence for a multistep pathogenesis of chronic myelogenous leukemia. Blood 1981;58:158–163.
4. Nowell PC, Hungerford DA. Chromosome studies on normal and leukemic human leukocytes. J Nat Cancer Institute 1959;25:85–109.
5. Rowley JD. The Philadelphia chromosome translocation: A paradigm for understanding leukemia. Cancer 1990;65:2178–2184.
6. Spiers ASD. The clinical features of chronic granulocytic leukemia. Clin Hematol 1977;6:77–95.
7. Canellos GP. Clinical characteristics of the blast phase of chronic granulocytic leukemia. Hematol Oncol Clin North Am 1990;4:359–368.
8. Bakhshi A, Minowada J, Arnold A, et al. Lymphoid blast crises of chronic myelogenous leukemia represent stages in the development of B-cell precursors. N Engl J Med 1983;309:826–831.
9. Sokal JE. Evaluation of survival data for chronic myelocytic leukemia. Am J Hematol 1976;1:493–500.
10. Kantarjian HM, Smith TL, McCredie KB, et al. Chronic myelogenous leukemia: a multivariate analysis of the associations of patient characteristics and therapy with survival. Blood 1985;66:1326–1335.
11. Sokal JE, Baccarani M, Tura S, et al. Prognostic discrimination among younger patients with chronic granulocytic leukemia: relevance to bone marrow transplantation. Blood 1985;66:1352–1357.
12. Tura S, Baccarani M, Corbelli G, et al. Staging of chronic myeloid leukemia. B J Hematol 1981 47:105–109.
13. Kantarjian HM, Keating MJ, Smith TL, Talpaz M, McCredie KB. Proposal for a simple synthesis prognostic staging system in chronic myelogenous leukemia. Am J Med 1990;88:1–8.
14. Italian Coop Study Group on CML. Confirmation and improvement of Sokal's prognostic classification of Ph+ chronic myeloid leukemia: the value of early evaluation of the course of the disease. Ann Hematol 1991;63:307–314.
15. Karanas A, Silver RT. Characteristics of the terminal phase of chronic granulocytic leukemia. Blood 1968;32: 445–459.
16. Theologides A. Unfavorable signs in patients with chronic myelocytic leukemia. Ann Intern Med 1972;76: 95–99.
17. Kantarjian H, Talpaz M. Definition of the accelerated phase of CML. J Clin Oncol 1988;6:180–181.
18. Spiers AS, Baikie AG. Cytogeneitic evolution and clonal proliferation in acute transformation of chronic granulocytic leukemia. Br J Cancer 1968;22:192–204.
19. Coleman M, Silver R, Pajak T, et al. Combination chemotherapy for terminal phase chronic myelocytic leukemia. Blood 1980;55:29–36.
20. Marks SM, Baltimore D, McCaffrey R. Terminal trans-

ferase as a predictor of initial responsiveness to vincristine and prednisone in blastic chronic myelogenous leukemia: a co- operative study. N Engl J Med 1978;298:812–814.
21. Clarkson B. Chronic myelogenous leukemia: is aggressive treatment indicated? J Clin Oncol 1985;3:135.
22. Gale RP, Butturini A. Can intensive chemotherapy cure chronic myelogenous leukemia. Leukemia 1992;6:863–865.
23. Talpaz M, Kantarjian H, Kurzrock R, Trujillo JM, Gutterman JU. Interferon-alpha produces sustained cytogenetic responses in chronic myelogenous leukemia. Philadelphia chromosome- positive patients. Ann Intern Med 1991;114:532–538.
24. Ozer H, George S, Pettenati M, et al. Subcutaneous a-interferon in untreated chronic phase Philadelphia chromosome positive chronic myelogenous leukemia: no evidence for significant improvement in response duration or survival. Blood 1992;80 (suppl 1):358a.
25. Italian Group on Chronic Myeloid Leukemia . A prospective comparison of a-IFN and conventional chemotherapy in Ph+ chronic myeloid leukemia. Clinical and cytogenetic results at 2 years in 322 patients. Haematologica 1992;77:204–214.
26. Bartram CR, deKlein A, Hagemeijer A, et al. Translocation of the c-abl oncogene adjacent to a translocation break point in chronic myelocytic leukemia. Nature 1983;306:277–280.
27. Heisterkamp N, Stephenson JR, Groffen J, et al. Localization of the c-abl oncogene adjacent to a translocation break point in chronic myelocytic leukemia. Nature 1983;306:239–242.
28. Groffen J, Stephenson JR, Heisterkamp N, et al. Philadelphia chromosomal breakpoints are clustered within a limited region, bcr, on chromosome 22. Cell 1985;36: 93–99.
29. Heisterkamp N, Stam K, Groffen J, et al. Structural organization of the bcr gene and its role in the Ph1 translocation. Nature 1985;315:758–761.
30. Clark SS, Crist WM, Witte ON. Molecular pathogenesis of Ph- positive leukemias. Annu Rev Med 1989;40:113–122.
31. Maru Y, Witte ON. The *BCR* gene encodes a novel serine/threonine kinase activity within a single exon. Cell 1991;67:459–468.
32. Lugo TG, Pendergast A-M, Muller AJ, Witte ON. Tyrosine kinase activity and transformation potency of *bcr-abl* oncogene products. Science 1990;247:1079–1082.
33. Shtalrid M, Talpaz M, Kurzrock R, et al. Analysis of breakpoints within the *bcr* gene and their correlation with the clinical course of Philadelphia-positive chronic myelogenous leukemia. Blood 1988;72:485–490.
34. Dreazen O, Berman M, Gale RP. Molecular abnormalities of bcr and c-abl in chronic myelogenous leukemia associated with a long chronic phase. Blood 1988;71: 797–799.
35. Mills KI, Benn P, Birnie GD. Does the breakpoint within the major breakpoint cluster region (M-bcr) influence the duration of the chronic phase in chronic myeloid leukemia? An analytical comparison of current literature. Blood 1991;78:1155–1161.
36. Morris CM, Heisterkamp N, Kennedy MA, Fitzgerald PH, Groffen J. Ph-negative chronic myeloid leukemia: molecular analysis of ABL insertion into M-BCR on chromosome 22. Blood 1990;76:1812–1818.
37. Kurzrock R, Gutterman JA, Talpaz M. The molecular genetics of Philadelphia chromosome-positive leukemias. N Engl J Med 1988;319:990–998.
38. Gishizky ML, Witte ON. Initiation of dysregulated growth of multipotent progenitor cells by bcr-abl in vitro. Science 1992;256:836–839.
39. Daley GQ, Van Etten RA, Baltimore D. Induction of chronic myelogenous leukemia in mice by the P210$^{bcr/abl}$ gene of the Philadelphia chromosome. Science 1990; 247:824–830.
40. Kawasaki ES, Coyne MY, McCormick FF, et al. Diagnosis of CML and ALL by detection of leukemia specific sequences amplified in vitro. Proc Natl Acad Sci USA 1988;85:5698–5702.
41. Heisterkamp N, Jenkins R, Thibodeau S, Testa JR, Weinberg K, Groffen J. The *bcr* gene in Philadelphia chromosome positive acute lymphoblastic leukemia. Blood 1989;73:1307–1311.
42. Witte ON. Closely related BCR/ABL oncogenes are associated with the distinctive clinical biologies of Philadelphia chromosome positive chronic myelogenous and acute lymphocytic leukemia. Curr Topics Microbiol Immunol 1988;141:42–49.
43. Ahuja H, Bar-Eli M, Advani SH, Benchimol S, Cline MJ. Alterations in the p53 gene and the clonal evolution of the blast crisis of chronic myelocytic leukemia. Proc Natl Acad Sci USA 1989;86:6783–6787.
44. Mashal R, Shtalrid M, Talpaz M, et al. Rearrangement and expression of *p53* in the chronic phase and blast crisis of chronic myelogenous leukemia. Blood 1990;75: 180–189.
45. Ratajczak MZ, Hijiya N, Catani L, et al. Acute- and chronic- phase chronic myelogenous leukemia colony-forming units are highly sensitive to the growth inhibitory effects of c-*myb* antisense oligodeoxynucleotides. Blood 1992;79:1956–1961.
46. Sawyers CL, Callahan W, Witte ON. Dominant negative MYC blocks transformation by *ABL* oncogenes. Cell 1992;70:901–910.
47. Thomas ED, Clift RA. Indications for marrow transplantation in chronic myelogenous leukemia. Blood 1989; 73:861–864.
48. Champlin RE, Goldman JM, Gale RP. Bone marrow transplantation in chronic myelogenous leukemia. Semin Hematol 1988;25:74–80.
49. Snyder DS, McGlave PB. Treatment of chronic myelogenous leukemia with bone marrow transplantation. Hematol/Oncol Clin North Am 1990;4:535–557.
50. Fefer A, Cheever MA, Greenberg PD, et al. Treatment of chronic granulocytic leukemia with chemoradiotherapy and transplantation of marrow from identical twins. N Engl J Med 1982;306:63–68.
51. Thomas ED, Clift RA, Fefer A, et al. Marrow transplantation for the treatment of chronic myelogenous leukemia. Ann Intern Med 1986;104:155–163.
52. Speck B, Bortin MM, Champlin R, et al. Allogeneic bone marrow transplantation for chronic myelogenous leukemia. Lancet 1984;1:665–668.
53. Goldman JM, Gale RP, Bortin MM, et al. Bone marrow transplantation for chronic myelogenous leukemia in chronic phase: increased risk of relapse associated with T-cell depletion. Ann Intern Med 1988;108:806–814.
54. Martin PJ, Clift RA, Fisher LD, et al. HLA-identical marrow transplantation during accelerated-phase chronic myelogenous leukemia: analysis of survival and remisssion duration. Blood 1988;72:1978–1984.
55. Wagner JE, Zahurak M, Piantodosi S, et al. Bone marrow transplantation of chronic myelogenous leuke-

mia in chronic phase: evaluation of risks and benefits. J Clin Oncol 1992;10:779–789.
56. Copelan EA, Grever MR, Kapoor N, Tutschka PJ. Marrow transplantation following busulfan and cyclophosphamide for chronic myelogenous leukaemia in accelerated or blastic phase. Br J Haematol 1989;71: 487–491.
57. Biggs JC, Szer J, Crilley P, et al. Treatment of chronic myeloid leukemia with allogeneic bone marrow transplantation after preparation with BuCy2. Blood 1992; 80:1352–1357.
58. Clift RA, Buckner CD, Appelbaum FR, et al. Allogeneic marrow transplantation in patients with chronic myeloid leukemia in the chronic phase: a randomized trial of two irradiation regimens. Blood 1991;77:1660–1665.
59. Buckner CD, Clift RA, Appelbaum FR, Thomas ED. A randomized study comparing two transplant regimens for CML in chronic phase. Blood 1992;80(suppl 1):72a.
60. Blume K, Forman S. High dose etoposide (VP-16)-containing preparatory regimens in allogeneic and autologous bone marrow transplantation for hematologic malignancies. Semin Oncol 1992;19(suppl 13): 63–66.
61. Storb R, Deeg HJ, Pepe M, et al. Methotrexate and cyclosporine versus cyclosporine alone for prophylaxis of graft-versus-host disease in patients given HLA-identical marrow grafts for leukemia: long-term follow-up of a controlled trial. Blood 1989;73:1729–1734.
62. Goldman J, McGlave P, Szydlo R, Gale RP, Horowitz MM. Impact of disease duration and prior treatment on outcome of bone marrow transplantation for chronic myelogenous leukemia. Exp Hematol 1992;62:830.
63. Przepiorka D, Thomas ED. Prognostic significance of cytogenetic abnormalities in patients with chronic myelogenous leukemia. Bone Marrow Transplant 1988; 3:113–119.
64. Goldman JM, Apperly JF, Jones L, et al. Bone marrow transplantation for patients with chronic myelogenous leukemia. N Engl J Med 1986;314:202–207.
65. Gluckman E, Devergia A, Bernheim A, et al. Splenectomy and bone marrow transplantation in chronic granulocytic leukemia. Lancet 1983;1:1392–1393.
66. Gratwohl A, Hermans J, Biezen AV, et al. No advantage for patients who receive splenic irradiation before bone marrow transplantation for chronic myeloid leukaemia: results of a prospective randomized study. Bone Marrow Transplant 1992;10:147–152.
67. Banaji M, Bearman SI, Buckner CD, et al. The effects of splenectomy on engraftment and platelet transfusion requirements in patients with chronic myelogenous leukemia undergoing marrow transplantation. Am J Hematol 1986;22:275–283.
68. Baughan ASJ, Worsley AM, McCarthy DM, et al. Haematological reconstitution and severity of graft-versus-host disease after bone marrow transplantation for chronic granulocytic leukaemia: the influence of previous splenectomy. Br J Haematol 1984;56:445–454.
69. McGlave PB, Brunning RD, Hurd DD, et al. Reversal of severe myelofibrosis and osteosclerosis following allogeneic bone marrow transplantation for chronic myelogenous leukemia. Br J Hematol 1982;52:189–194.
70. Rajantie J, Sale GE, Deeg HJ, et al. Adverse effect of severe marrow fibrosis on hematological recovery after chemoradiotherapy and allogeneic bone marrow transplantation. Blood 1986;67:1693–1697.
71. Giralt S, Kantarjian H, Giglio A, et al. Interferon treatment does not adversely affect the outcome of allogeneic bone marrow transplant for CML. J Clin Oncol 1993;11:1055–1061.
72. Arthur CK, Apperley JF, Guo AP, et al. Cytogenetic events after bone marrow transplantation for chronic myeloid leukemia in chronic phase. Blood 1988;71: 1179–1186.
73. Offit K, Burns JP, Cunningham I, et al. Cytogenetic analysis of chimerism and leukemia relapse in chronic myelogenous leukemia patients after T cell-depleted bone marrow transplantation. Blood 1990;75:1346–1355.
74. Lee MS, Chang KS, Freireich E, et al. Detection of minimal residual bcr-abl transcripts by a modified polymerase chain reaction. Blood 1988;72:893–897.
75. Sawyers CL, Timson L, Kawasaki ES, Clark SS, Witte ON, Champlin R. Molecular relapse in chronic myelogenous leukemia patients after bone marrow transplantation detected by polymerase chain reaction. Proc Natl Acad Sci USA 1990;87:563–567.
76. Snyder DS, Rossi JJ, Wang J-L, et al. Persistence of bcr-abl gene expression following bone marrow transplantation for chronic myelogenous leukemia in chronic phase. Transplantation 1991;51:1033–1040.
77. DeLage R, Soiffer RJ, Dear K, Ritz J. Clinical significance of *bcr-abl* gene rearrangement detected by polymerase chain reaction after allogeneic bone marrow transplantation in chronic myelogenous leukemia. Blood 1991;78:2759–2767.
78. Thompson JD, Brodsky I, Yunis JJ. Molecular quantification of residual disease in chronic myelogenous leukemia after bone marrow transplantation. Blood 1992;79:1629–1635.
79. Hughes TP, Morgan GJ, Martiat P, Goldman JM. Detection of residual leukemia after bone marrow transplant for chronic myeloid leukemia: role of polymerase chain reaction in predicting relapse. Blood 1991;77:874–878.
80. Roth MS, Antin JH, Ash R, et al. Prognostic significance of Philadelphia chromosome-positive cells detected by the polymerase chain reaction after allogeneic bone marrow transplant for chronic myelogenous leukemia. Blood 1992;79:276–282.
81. Tkachuk DC, Westbrook CA, Andreeff M, et al. Detection of bcr-abl fusion in chronic myelogenous leukemia by in situ hybridization. Science 1990;250:559–562.
82. Weiden PL, Sullivan KM, Flournoy N, Storb R, Thomas ED. Antileukemic effect of chronic graft-versus-host disease: contribution to improved survival after allogeneic marrow transplantation. N Engl J Med 1981;304: 1529–1532.
83. Sullivan KM, Weiden PL, Storb R, et al. Influence of acute and chronic graft-versus-host disease on relapse and survival after bone marrow transplantation from HLA-identical siblings as treatment of acute and chronic leukemia. Blood 1989;73:1720–1728.
84. Sullivan KM, Storb R, Buckner CD, et al. Graft-versus-host disease as adoptive immunotherapy in patients with advanced hematologic neoplasms. N Engl J Med 1989;320:828–834.
85. Horowitz MM, Gale RP, Sondel PM, et al. Graft-versus-leukemia reactions after bone marrow transplantation. Blood 1990;75:555–562.
86. Champlin R. T-cell depletion to prevent graft-versus-host disease after bone marrow transplantation. Hematol Oncol Clin North Am 1990;4:687–698.
87. Marmont AM, Horowitz MM, Gale RP, et al. T-cell depletion of HLA-identical transplants in leukemia. Blood 1991;78:2120- 2130.

88. Sosman JA, Oettel KR, Smith SD, Hank JA, Fisch P, Sondel PM. Specific recognition of human leukemic cells by allogeneic T-cells: II. Evidence for HLA-D restricted determinants on leukemic cells that are crossreactive with determinants present on unrelated nonleukemic cells. Blood 1990;75:2005–2016.
89. Truitt RL, Atasoylu AA. Contribution of CD4+ and CD8+ T cells to graft-versus-host disease and graft-versus-leukemia reactivity after transplantation of MHC-compatible bone marrow. Bone Marrow Transplant 1991;8:51–58.
90. Delmon L, Ythier A, Moingeon P, et al. Characterization of antileukemia cells' cytotoxic effector function. Implications for monitoring natural killer responses following allogeneic bone marrow transplantation. Transplantation 1986;42:252–256.
91. Hauch M, Gazzola MV, Small T, et al. Anti-leukemia potential of interleukin-2 activated natural killer cells after bone marrow transplantation for chronic myelogenous leukemia. Blood 1990;75:2250–2262.
92. Barrett A, Jiang YZ. Immune responses to chronic myeloid leukaemia. Bone Marrow Transplant 1992;9: 305–311.
93. Chen W, Peace DJ, Rovira DK, You S, Cheever MA. T-cell immunity to the joining region of $p210^{BCR\text{-}ABL}$ protein. Proc Natl Acad Sci USA 1992;89:1468–1472.
94. Korngold R, Sprent J. T cell subsets and graft-versus-host disease. Transplantation 1987;44:335–339.
95. Champlin R, Ho W, Gajewski J, et al. Selective depletion of $CD8^{+}$ T-lymphocytes for prevention of graft-versus-host disease after allogeneic bone marrow transplantation. Blood 1990;76:418–423.
96. Forman SJ, Blume KG, Krance RA et al. A prospective randomized study of acute graft-versus-host disease in 107 patients with leukemia: methotrexate/prednisone versus cyclosporine/prednisone. Transplant Proc 1987; 21:2605–2607.
97. Klingemann H-G, Grigg AP, Wilkie-Boyd K, et al. Treatment with recombinant interferon (a-2β) early after bone marrow transplantation in patients at high risk for relapse. Blood 1991;78:3306–3311.
98. Mrsic M, Horowitz MM, Atkinson K, et al. Second HLA-identical sibling transplants for leukemia recurrence. Bone Marrow Transplant 1992;9:269–275.
99. Cullis JO, Schwarer AP, Hughes TP, et al. Second transplants for patients with chronic myeloid leukaemia in relapse after original transplant with T-depleted donor marrow: feasibility of using busulphan alone for re-conditioning. Br J Haematol 1992;80:33–39.
100. Sanders JE, Buckner CD, Clift RA, et al. Second marrow transplants in patients with leukemia who relapse after allogeneic marrow transplants. Bone Marrow Transplant 1988;3:11–19.
101. Higano CS, Raskind WH, Singer JW. Use of a interferon for the treatment of relapse of chronic myelogenous leukemia in chronic phase after allogeneic bone marrow transplantation. Blood 1992;80:1437–1442.
102. Kolb HJ, Mittermüller J, Clemm C, et al. Donor leukocyte transfusions for treatment of recurrent chronic myelogenous leukemia in marrow transplant patients. Blood 1990;76:2462–2465.
103. Cullis JO, Jiang YZ, Schwarer AP, Hughes TP, Barrett AJ, Goldman JM. Donor leukocyte infusions for chronic myeloid leukemia in relapse after allogeneic bone marrow transplantation. Blood 1992;79:1379–1381.
104. McGlave P. Bone marrow transplants in chronic myelogenous leukemia: an overview of determinants of survival. Semin Hematol 1990;27:23–30.
105. Beatty PG, Clift RA, Mickelson EM, et al. Marrow transplantation from related donors other than HLA-identical siblings. N Engl J Med 1985;313:765–771.
106. Anasetti C, Amos D, Beatty PG, et al. Effect of HLA compatibility on engraftment of bone marrow transplants in patients with leukemia or lymphoma. N Engl J Med 1989;320:197–204.
107. Hows JM, Yin JL, Marsh J, et al. Histocompatible unrelated volunteer donors compared with HLA nonidentical family donors in marrow transplantation for aplastic anemia and leukemia. Blood 1986;68: 1322–1328.
108. McGlave P, Scott E, Ramsay N, et al. Unrelated donor bone marrow transplantation therapy for chronic myelogenous leukemia. Blood 1987;70:877–881.
109. Beatty PG, Ash R, Hows JM, McGlave PB. The use of unrelated bone marrow donors in the treatment of patients with chronic myelogenous leukemia: experience of four marrow transplant centers. Bone Marrow Transplant 1989;4:287–290.
110. Ash RC, Caper JT, Chitambar CR, et al. Successful allogeneic transplantation of T-cell depleted bone marrow from closely HLA-matched unrelated donors. N Engl J Med 1990;322:485–494.
111. McGlave PB, Beatty P, Ash R, Hows JM. Therapy for chronic myelogenous leukemia with unrelated donor bone marrow transplantation: results in 102 cases. Blood 1990;75:1728–1732.
112. McGlave PB, Bartsch G, Anasetti C, et al. Unrelated donor bone marrow transplantation therapy for chronic myelogenous leukemia: initial experience of the National Marrow Donor Program (NMDP). Blood 1993;81:543–550.
113. Fleischhauer K, Kernan NA, O'Reilly RJ, Dupont B, Yang SY. Bone marrow allograft rejection by host-derived allocytotoxic T lymphocytes recognizes a single amino acid at position 156 of the HLA-B44 class I antigen. N Engl J Med 1990;323:1818–1822.
114. Stroncek DF, McGlave P, Ramsay N, McCullough J. Effects on donors of second bone marrow collections. Transfusion 1991;31:819–822.
115. Apperley JF, Mauro FR, Goldman JM, et al. Bone marrow transplantation for chronic myeloid leukaemia in first chronic phase: importance of a graft-versus-leukaemia effect. Br J Haematol 1988;69:239–245.
116. Shapiro RS, McClain K, Frizzera G, et al. Epstein-Barr virus associated B cell lymphoproliferative disorders following bone marrow transplantation. Blood 1988; 71:1234–1243.

Chapter 45

Allogeneic Bone Marrow Transplantation for Acute Myeloid Leukemia

Gwynn D. Long and Karl G. Blume

Allogeneic bone marrow transplantation (BMT) for acute myeloid leukemia (AML) has evolved over the past 2 decades from salvage therapy administered only to patients with end-stage leukemia to an accepted form of postremission therapy administered early in the course of the disease (1,2). Initial attempts at human marrow transplantation were generally unsuccessful but demonstrated at least transient engraftment in some patients and provided a framework for future studies (3–5). Subsequent advances in supportive care (including transfusional and nutritional support and antibiotics) and tissue typing have helped to usher in the modern era of human BMT.

In 1974, the Seattle group reported the treatment outcome of 16 patients with refractory hematological malignancies (7 with AML) employing myeloablation with high-dose cyclophosphamide (CY) and 1,000 cGy total body irradiation (TBI) followed by marrow grafting from identical twins (6). All patients engrafted, and complete remissions were achieved in 86%. Two patients failed to achieve remission, one patient died of viral hepatitis, and 5 patients relapsed between 3 and 7 months after BMT. An updated report in 1977 indicated that 6 patients (3 with AML) remained alive and disease-free 4 to 6 years later (7). In 1981, the same group of investigators reported on 34 patients with refractory leukemia (11 of whom were included in the original report) who received marrow transplants from identical twins (8). Twenty-four patients (70%) achieved complete remission and 8 (24%) were alive and disease-free at a median follow-up of 80 months after BMT. The primary cause of failure was recurrent leukemia in 14 patients. These studies demonstrated that infusions of identical twin marrow can restore hematopoiesis following myeloablative doses of chemoradiotherapy and that a significant portion of patients with refractory leukemia can apparently be cured with this procedure.

Allogeneic BMT for Patients with Relapsed AML

Thomas and colleagues (9) reported the results of 100 patients with end-stage acute leukemia grafted with marrow from human leukocyte antigen (HLA)–identical siblings in 1977. Fifty-four patients had AML, all of whom were prepared with 1,000 cGy single-dose TBI plus several different high-dose chemotherapy regimens. At the time of the report, 7 patients with AML were alive and in continuous complete remission between 11 months and 4.5 years after transplantation. Early deaths were due to graft-versus-host disease (GVHD), bacterial or fungal infections, and interstitial pneumonitis (primarily due to cytomegalovirus). Figure 45-1, from an update of this trial, reveals that 6 patients remained in continuous complete remission between 11 and 14 years after

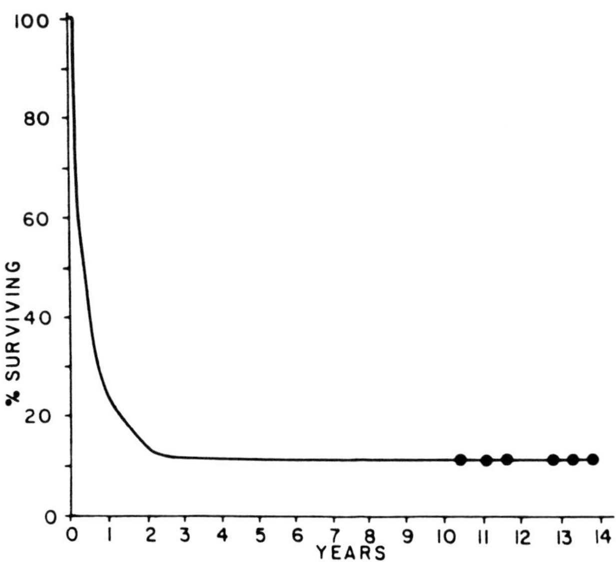

Figure 45-1. Kaplan-Meier estimate of the disease-free survival of 54 patients with relapsed acute myeloid leukemia who underwent allogeneic bone marrow transplantation from human leukocyte antigen–identical sibiling donors. (Reproduced by permission from Fefer A, Thomas ED. Marrow transplantation in the treatment of acute leukemia. In: Henderson ES, Lister TA, eds. Leukemia. Philadelphia: WB Saunders, 1990:431–441.)

BMT and were cured of their disease (10). As of 1992, the patients are between 17 and 20 years post-BMT, except for one patient who had hepatitis before transplantation and died of a hepatoma 16 years later (Thomas ED. Personal communication). Other early studies also demonstrated that a minority of patients with refractory disease could become long-term survivors after BMT (11,12).

The early encouraging results with allogeneic BMT in refractory acute leukemia led to the use of the procedure earlier in the course of the disease when patients were in better clinical condition. The justification for such an approach was based on the fact that the prognosis for patients with relapsed AML treated with standard chemotherapy remains uniformly poor (13). An initial report in 1983 suggested that the outcome of patients undergoing BMT in early relapse was similar to patients transplanted in second remission (14). Figure 45-2 shows the probability of leukemia-free survival in patients with various stages of AML transplanted in Seattle between 1973 and 1985 (15). The estimated 5-year disease-free survival for patients in untreated first relapse chemotherapy-resistant first relapse or second remission was 30, 21, and 28%, respectively. The probability of relapse, after BMT was 36% for patients in untreated first relapse, 56% in resistant first relapse, and 37% in second remission. Patients transplanted at time of first relapse are spared the considerable morbidity and mortality associated with attempts at remission reinduction and are likely to be in reasonably good clinical condition at the time of BMT. The currently available data support the concept that BMT in early relapse is equivalent to BMT in second remission and that evaluation for BMT should be initiated as soon as possible for patients with histocompatible donors following the detection of recurrent disease (see Figure 45-2).

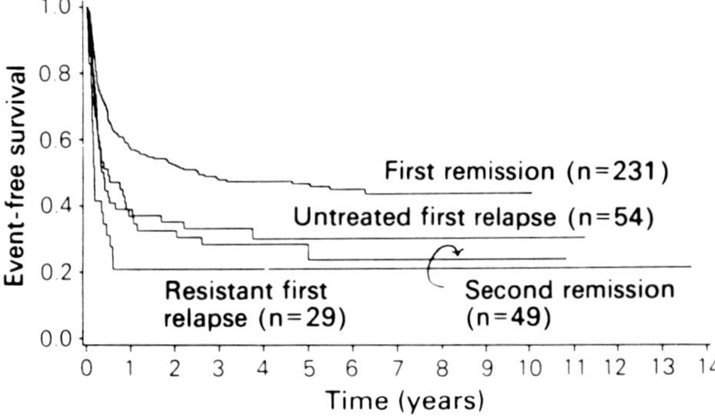

Figure 45-2. Effect of remission status on the probability of disease-free survival after allogeneic bone marrow transplantation for patients with acute myeloid leukemia. (Reproduced by permission from Clift RA, Buckner CD, Thomas ED, et al. The treatment of acute non-lymphoblastic leukemia by allogeneic marrow transplantation. Bone Marrow Transplant 1987;2:243–258.)

A study reported in 1985 suggested that even patients who fail to achieve a first remission after induction chemotherapy should be considered for allogeneic BMT. Three of 9 patients with AML refractory to induction therapy were alive and well between 3 and 60 months after BMT (16). A more recent study described 16 patients with AML who had failed at least 2 cycles of induction therapy and were prepared with high-dose therapy and allografted from HLA-identical sibling donors (17). At the time of the report, 8 patients were alive and disease-free between 18 months and 11 years after BMT. These observations indicate that patients with AML refractory to induction therapy can be salvaged with BMT and that newly diagnosed patients should be HLA-typed so that potential donors can be identified more quickly if the patient fails to enter remission with initial treatment. Patients with appropriate donors should not be treated with more than 2 induction attempts before proceeding to BMT to avoid additional toxicity with little chance of achieving remission.

Allogeneic BMT for Patients with AML in First Remission

The majority of patients with AML in first remission will relapse if treated with conventional chemotherapy only (18). Patients in first remission are theoretically ideal candidates for BMT because their leukemic burden is minimal, the residual leukemic population is less likely to have become resistant to therapy, and patients are generally in good clinical condition. Several studies in both children and adults from multiple institutions demonstrated that patients undergoing BMT in first remission have a superior outcome (12,15,19–28). Five-year disease-free survival figures range from 45 to 65% in studies with sufficient follow-up; relapse rates were between 10 and 25% (see Figure 45-2). The incidence of relapse in these patients is lower than in patients with more advanced disease. The primary causes of failure are transplant-related complications, including GVHD, interstitial pneumonitis, and infection.

Several reports have been published that have attempted to identify prognostic factors for patients undergoing BMT for AML in first remission. The Seattle group reported that patients under age 20 at time of BMT had a better outcome than older patients, but no significant difference was noted in the prognosis of patients between 20 and 50 years of age (15). At least 2 other groups failed to demonstrate a significant impact of age on disease-free survival following BMT (28–30). Figure 45-3 shows that relapse rates and disease-free survival were not significantly different in patients under age 18, compared with patients between 18 and 45 years of age (28). Other reports demonstrated that BMT is a reasonable treatment option for patients between ages 30 and 50 (31–33), whereas patients over age 50 suffer significantly higher rates of transplant-related complications, and allogeneic BMT should probably not be considered as

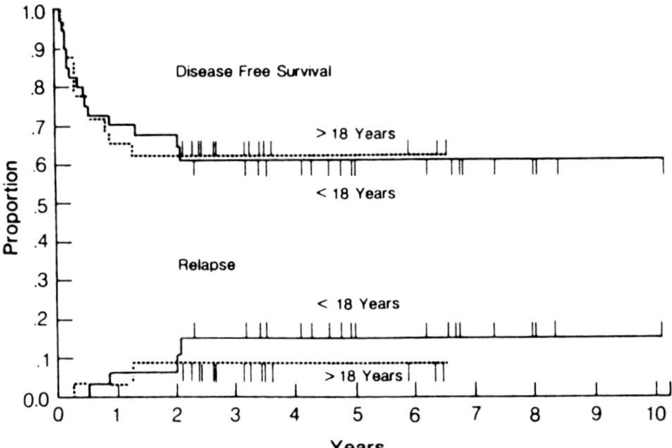

Figure 45-3. Effect of age on the probabilities of disease-free survival and relapse in 73 patients undergoing allogeneic bone marrow transplantation for acute myeloid leukemia in first complete remission. (Reproduced by permission from McGlave PB, Haake RJ, Bodstrom BC, et al. Allogeneic bone marrow transplantation for acute nonlymphocytic leukemia in first remission. Blood 1988;72:1512–1517.)

first-line therapy in such patients (31). In the pediatric patient population, no difference was observed in the outcome of patients under age 6 in a collaborative study from the Children's Cancer Study Group (27), and another report suggested that even patients with AML in first remission less than 2 years of age could expect a good outcome following BMT (34). These data indicate that patients under age 50 with HLA-identical sibling donors should be offered allogeneic BMT as a treatment option during first remission of AML.

Some studies have suggested that patients with a high white blood cell count at presentation or with French American British (FAB) classification M4 or M5 subtypes of AML have an unfavorable prognosis even with BMT (28,30,35), although others have failed to confirm the importance of these pretransplant characteristics (27,29). Other factors that have not proved to be prognostically significant include time from diagnosis to complete remission and time from achieving remission to BMT (28,29). Although certain chromosomal translocations have proved to be highly predictive of early relapse in some chemotherapy trials, such data are not yet available in studies of BMT for AML.

Preparative Regimens for Patients with AML

The purpose of the preparative regimen in allogeneic BMT is two-fold: (1) to eradicate the leukemic clone, and (2) to immunosuppress recipients to allow permanent and functional marrow engraftment. Early studies at Seattle in patients with advanced disease utilized TBI (920–1,000 cGy) administered as a single fraction after infusion of high-dose CY. When patients were grafted in remission, the relapse rate was significantly decreased, but the incidence of transplant-related complications was not (19). In an attempt to decrease regimen-related toxicity, the Seattle group compared high dose CY plus either 1,000 cGy single-fraction TBI or 200 cGy TBI per day for 6 days. A randomized trial in patients with AML in first remission demonstrated a survival advantage for the cohort treated with fractionated radiotherapy (36). The relapse rate was similar in the two groups, but the overall frequency of nonrelapse deaths was lower in the fractionated TBI group, resulting in an overall survival advantage that has persisted even after 10 years of follow-up (37).

In 1983, investigators from Memorial Sloan-Kettering Cancer Center described a regimen utilizing hyperfractionated TBI (38). A total dose of 1,320 cGy TBI was administered in 11 fractions over 4 days, with CY given after rather than prior to radiotherapy as in previous studies. Partial lung shielding with lead blocks was utilized, with supplemental electron beam therapy to the chest wall and testicular boost radiation. Overall relapse-free survival was significantly improved in patients with AML treated with the hyperfractionated TBI compared with historical control subjects prepared with CY followed by single-fraction TBI. The incidence of interstitial pneumonitis was also significantly decreased in the hyperfractionated TBI group. Although this study utilized historical control subjects, the hyperfractionated TBI with lung shielding appeared to decrease both the relapse rate and the regimen-related toxicity compared with single-fraction TBI. A more recent study from the University of Minnesota did not reveal an advantage for hyperfractionated TBI, again compared with historical control subjects who received single-fraction TBI (35). In this report, CY was administered before the hyperfractionated TBI and lung shielding was not utilized, perhaps explaining the lack of a difference in the incidence of interstitial pneumonitis between the two groups. A trend toward improved survival and lower relapse was seen in the hyperfractionated TBI group, but the difference was not statistically significant.

Studies in Seattle established 1,575 cGy administered in 225 cGy daily fractions as the maximum tolerated radiotherapy dose if combined with high-dose CY and allografting in patients with advanced leukemia (39). A recent randomized trial compared 1,200 cGy fractionated TBI with 1,575 cGy fractionated TBI in patients with AML in first remission (40). All patients received uniform GVHD prophylaxis with methotrexate (MTX) and cyclosporine (CSP). A significant increase in acute GVHD was observed in the higher dose TBI group, presumably because the toxicity of the higher dose radiation prevented administration of scheduled doses of MTX and CSP. The relapse rate was significantly decreased in the group receiving 1,575 cGy, but transplant-related toxicity was increased, resulting in no difference in overall relapse-free survival (Figure 45-4).

These results suggest an advantage for fractionated

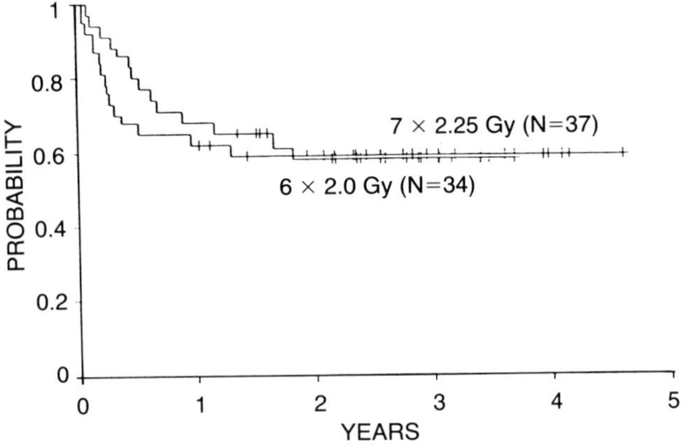

Figure 45-4. Probability of relapse-free survival after allogeneic bone marrow transplantation for acute myeloid leukemia in first remission with two irradiation regimens. (Reproduced by permission from Clift RA, Buckner CD, Appelbaum FR, et al. Allogeneic marrow transplantation in patients with acute myeloid leukemia in first remission: a randomized trial of two irradiation regimens. Blood 1990; 76:1867–1871.)

radiotherapy over single-fraction TBI, with decreased toxicity and no increase in relapse rates. No particular radiotherapy regimen, however, can be recommended as clearly superior to all others. The clinical situation may dictate which regimen is preferable. For example, a higher radiation dose might be indicated for patients with more advanced disease, in whom the risk of relapse may outweigh the risks of regimen-related toxicity. Better understanding of the pathogenesis and prevention of such complications as interstitial pneumonitis and veno-occlusive disease (VOD) of the liver may allow for safer administration of higher dose radiotherapy.

The combination of high-dose CY and TBI as developed in Seattle has been the most commonly used preparative regimen for allogeneic BMT for AML over the past 20 years. This regimen is associated with a relapse rate of approximately 25% in patients transplanted during first remission of AML (15). Relapse rates are correspondingly higher in patients with more advanced disease. Several groups of investigators have attempted to modify the CY and TBI regimen by adding additional agents or substituting other drugs for CY in an attempt to improve the antileukemic effect and thus decrease relapse rates. Investigators from the City of Hope National Medical Center reported a Phase I/II study in 1987 utilizing high-dose etoposide (VP16) and hyperfractionated TBI in patients with advanced leukemia (41). Patients were treated with 1,320 cGy TBI in 11 fractions over 4 days, followed by a single dose of VP16 and allografting. The study established 60 mg/kg as the maximum tolerated dose of VP16 in combination with TBI. Hepatic toxicity precluded further dose escalation. At the time of the report, the actuarial disease-free survival of patients with acute leukemia was 42%, with a relapse rate of 32%. Investigators in Germany reported similar results, with a 3-year disease-free survival rate of 56% and a relapse rate of 12% in patients with advanced acute leukemia (42). A Phase II trial was subsequently carried out in patients with acute leukemia in first remission and chronic myelogenous leukemia in first chronic phase at the City of Hope and Stanford University. Forty-one patients with AML in first remission were transplanted, with an actuarial disease-free survival of 67% and a relapse rate of only 7 % (Figure 45-5) (43). These data indicate that the combination of high-dose VP16 and fractionated TBI is an effective preparatory regimen for AML. Prospective randomized trials, however, will be required to determine the ultimate efficacy of the regimen in comparison with the standard regimen, CY and TBI.

The substitution of high-dose melphalan for CY in combination with TBI in a prospective randomized trial in patients with AML in first remission resulted in equivalent disease-free survival with the 2 preparative regimens (44). The combination of high-dose cytarabine and TBI with and without CY also demonstrated similar results to CY and TBI in comparable patient groups (45,46). Recently, a Phase I study combining busulfan (BU) with CY and fractionated TBI was reported (47). Thirty-six patients with advanced hematological malignancies were treated. The maximum tolerated doses were 6.9 mg/kg BU and 47 mg/kg CY when combined with 1,200 cGy fractionated TBI. Dose-limiting toxicity was hepatic and pulmonary. The actuarial probability of survival for patients treated on this dose level was 67% at 18 months, and no severe regimen-related toxicity was observed. The actuarial probability of relapse was 17% for patients with advanced myeloid malignancies, with a significantly higher relapse rate for patients with lymphoid malignancies.

Preparative regimens that do not contain TBI have also been developed. In 1983, Santos and colleagues

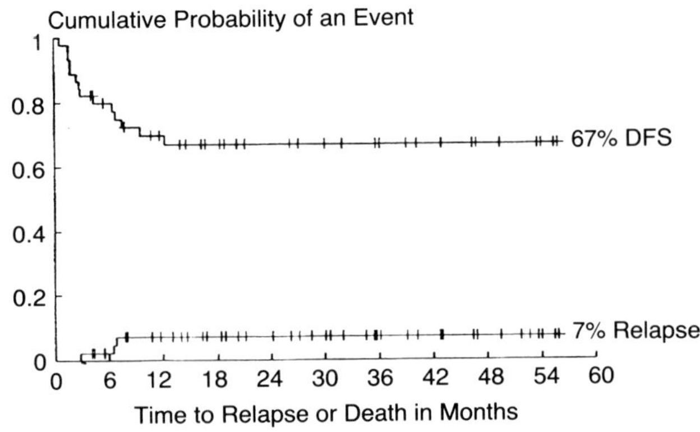

Figure 45-5. Probabilities of disease-free survival (DFS) and relapse for 41 patients with acute myeloid leukemia in first remission following preparation for allogeneic bone marrow transplantation with fractionated total body irradiation and etoposide.

from Johns Hopkins, described the treatment of patients with AML with high-dose BU and CY without radiotherapy followed by allogeneic BMT (48). BU was administered orally over a 4-day period, with a total dose of 16 mg/kg, and CY was administered intravenously at 50 mg/kg on 4 successive days, for a total dose of 200 mg/kg. Primary causes of death were GVHD, with infection and interstitial pneumonitis primarily due to cytomegalovirus. At the time of the report, the disease-free survival was 44% in patients with AML in first remission, with no relapses in a group of 18 patients. In 1989, these same investigators reported an update of results utilizing this regimen in 99 patients with AML (49). All patients engrafted. Disease-free survival at 3 years for 49 patients in first remission was 45%; 4 patients relapsed. A subgroup of the patients who had received intravenous CSP for GVHD prophylaxis had a relapse-free survival of 64%. Fifty patients were transplanted in second or third remission or early relapse, with a disease-free survival of 31%; only 9 patients relapsed. The incidence of transplant-related toxicities such as interstitial pneumonitis and hepatic VOD was similar to that reported for TBI-containing regimens.

In an attempt to reduce regimen-related toxicity, other investigators have decreased the dose of CY to 120 mg/kg in combination with the same dose of BU (50). This initial study demonstrated that this modified regimen was well tolerated and was sufficiently immunosuppressive to allow engraftment in 48 of 49 evaluable patients. A multicenter trial utilizing this regimen in 127 patients with AML was reported in 1991 (51). The 3-year leukemia-free survival for patients in first complete remission was 63%, with an actuarial relapse rate of 14%. The disease-free survival for patients in second remission or initial relapse was 33%, with a relapse rate of 41%. Fatal VOD of the liver and cardiomyopathy occurred in 5% of patients. These studies suggest that the combination of BU and CY may be a viable alternative to CY and TBI.

The results of a recent French collaborative trial, however, indicate that BU/CY may not be as effective as the TBI-containing regimen (52). One hundred and one patients with AML in first complete remission were prospectively randomized to CY (120 mg/kg) plus BU (16 mg/kg) or to CY (120 mg/kg) plus TBI (1,000 cGy single fraction in 7 patients, and a median dose of 1,200 cGy fractionated in 43 patients) followed by allogeneic BMT from HLA-identical sibling donors. The two groups of patients were well matched in terms of pretransplant characteristics, such as age, sex, FAB classification, white blood cell count at diagnosis, and time from diagnosis to complete remission and to BMT. GVHD prophylaxis was identical for the two groups, with no difference in the incidence of acute or chronic GVHD. The patients prepared with CY and TBI had a significantly better actuarial 2-year disease-free survival than the patients prepared with BU and CY (72 vs 47%) and a significantly lower relapse rate (14 vs 34%). The nonrelapse regimen–related mortality was also lower in the TBI group (8 vs 27%), although this difference was not statistically significant. The relapse rate in the BU group was higher in this study than in previous reports (51), perhaps because the time from achieving complete remission to BMT was shorter in this randomized trial, and patients remaining in remission for long periods are less likely to relapse regardless of the treatment used. The authors also suggested that the decreased toxicity from the TBI regimen might be explained by use of lung shielding in all patients, and the higher relapse rate in the BU group was due at least in part to variability in absorption and bioavailability. This study underscores the importance of prospectively randomized trials as opposed to the use of historical control subjects to evaluate the impact of new preparative regimens for BMT.

Chemotherapy Versus BMT for First Remission AML

Modern chemotherapy regimens utilizing cytarabine and an anthracycline result in complete remissions in approximately 70% of patients under 60 years of age with newly diagnosed AML (18). Once remission is achieved, the vast majority of patients will relapse during the next one to 2 years. A retrospective review of 760 patients who achieved complete remission between 1974 and 1979 on three different Cancer and Leukemia Group B protocols followed by maintenance chemotherapy demonstrated a median duration of remission of 1.1 years and a 16.4% disease-free survival at 8 years, with a minimum follow-up of all patients of 6 years (53). The use of consolidation and intensification chemotherapy in place of maintenance chemotherapy resulted in 10 to 25% of such patients being alive and well at 2 years (18,54). As reported more recently, intensive postremission chemotherapy with high-dose cytarabine and daunorubicin can achieve a 5-year disease-free survival of approximately 30 to 50% (55–57).

Controversy still exists regarding whether patients with AML in first remission who have HLA-matched sibling donors should proceed to marrow transplantation during remission or at the time of first relapse. Several studies have compared the outcome of BMT and chemotherapy for patients with AML in first remission (Table 45-1). A retrospective study from the Royal Marsden Hospital, initially reported in 1980 and updated in 1982, demonstrated a significant improvement in relapse-free survival in patients undergoing BMT, compared with conventional chemotherapy (21,58). Three more recent studies demonstrated a statistically significant advantage for BMT over chemotherapy. Relapse-free survival in these studies ranged from 48 to 66% with BMT, compared with 13 to 21% after chemotherapy (59–62). The Seattle investigators reported a prospective comparison in 1984 (59). Patients had been followed between 2 and 6 years, and the estimated 5-year disease-free survival was 49% for the transplanted group and 20% for the chemotherapy group. In a follow-up analysis published in 1988, all patients had been observed for a minimum of 5 years,

Table 45-1.
Bone Marrow Transplantation Versus Chemotherapy for AML in First Remission

Study Group, Years, Ref	*Treatment*	*No. Patients*	*DFS (%)*	*p Value*
Royal Marsden, 1980–1982 (21,58)	BMT	53	54	<0.05
	CT	51	21	
UCLA, 1985 (65)	BMT	23	40	>0.4
	CT	44	27	
Genova, 1985 (60)	BMT	19	64	<0.05
	CT	18	13	
Seattle, 1984–1988 (59,61)	BMT	33	48	<0.05
	CT	43	21	
M. D. Anderson, 1988 (68)	BMT	11	36	0.24
	CT	27	15	
Spain, 1988 (69)	BMT	14	70	<0.10
	CT	13	17	
France, 1989 (62)	BMT	20	66	<0.002
	CT	20	16	
Sweden, 1989 (64)	BMT	11	100	<0.001
	CT	15	7	
St. Jude/Seattle, 1990 (70)	BMT	19	43	0.33
	CT	42	31	
UCLA, 1992 (66)	BMT	28	45	NS
	CT	54	38	
ECOG, 1992 (67)	BMT	54	42	NS
	CT	29	30	

AML = acute myeloid leukemia; DFS = disease-free survival; BMT = bone marrow transplantation; CT = chemotherapy; NS = not significant.

with an actual 5-year disease-free survival of 48% for the BMT group, 21% for the chemotherapy group, and 10% for a group of patients with suitable donors who did not undergo BMT (Figure 45-6) (61). A French collaborative study was also designed and performed as a prospective comparison. All patients received uniform remission induction and consolidation chemotherapy before going on to BMT or to additional chemotherapy (62). An update of that study utilizing high-dose cytarabine and daunorubicin as "superconsolidation" in the chemotherapy group still demonstrated a significant disease-free survival advantage for the patients undergoing BMT (63). In a pediatric study from Sweden, all 11 patients with AML in first complete remission who underwent allogeneic BMT were alive and well for more than 2 years after transplantation, compared with only one of 15 children who were treated with chemotherapy alone after remission (64). The other studies listed in Table 45-1 all demonstrate a trend toward improved disease-free survival in the BMT group, although this trend is not statistically significant.

To date, no study has demonstrated an advantage for patients treated with chemotherapy compared with BMT. In a UCLA study from 1985, the relapse rate was significantly lower in the BMT group, but overall survival was not improved due to nonrelapse-related deaths in the transplanted patients (65). There was a trend toward better survival in the BMT group, but because of the small number of patients, statistical significance could not be expected. A more recent trial from the same group employed consolidation chemotherapy with high-dose cytarabine and daunorubicin (66). As in the previous report, the decreased relapse rate in the BMT group was offset by increased procedure-related complications, resulting in no significant difference in overall disease-free survival between the 2 groups. A prospective multicenter trial was recently reported by investigators from the Eastern Cooperative Oncology Group (67). All patients were induced with one or 2 cycles of daunorubicin, cytarabine, and thioguanine, with a complete remission rate of 68%. Patients under age 41 with HLA-matched sibling donors were assigned to undergo allogeneic BMT; all other patients were randomized to receive maintenance chemotherapy with thioguanine and cytarabine for 2 years or a single cycle of consolidation chemotherapy with high-dose cytarabine and amsacrine. In the subset of patients less than 41 years of age, the 4-year disease-free survival was 14% in the group treated with maintenance chemotherapy, 30% in the group treated with consolidation therapy, and 42% in the group of patients assigned to BMT. All patients were evaluated by intent to treat; 9 of 54 patients in the BMT group relapsed before transplantation, so that only 45 patients were transplanted in first remission. The relapse rate in the BMT group was only 13%, whereas relapse largely accounted for the failures in the chemotherapy groups. Similar results were obtained in the studies from M.D. Anderson (68) and Spain (69), as well as in a pediatric group study (70), which included only patients less than 20 years of age.

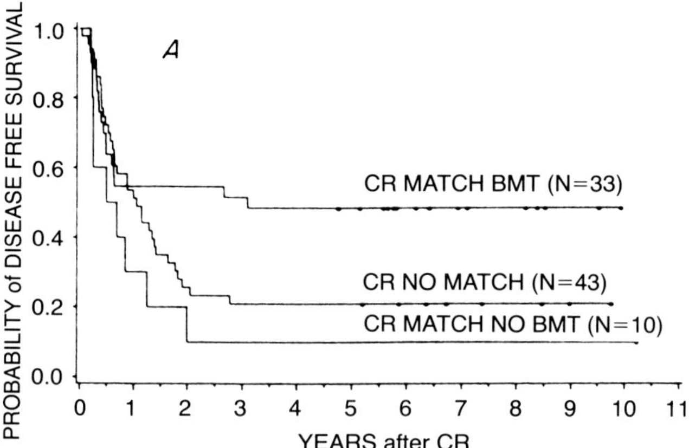

Figure 45-6. Kaplan-Meier estimates of the probability of disease-free survival of patients with acute myeloid leukemia in first remission who (1) had no matched family donor, (2) had a matched donor but were not transplanted, or (3) had a matched family donor and underwent allogeneic bone marrow transplantation (BMT). (Reproduced by permission from Appelbaum FR, Fisher LD, Thomas ED, et al. Chemotherapy versus marrow transplantation for adults with acute nonlymphocytic leukemia: a five-year follow-up. Blood 1988;72:179–184.)

Graft-versus-Leukemia Effect in Patients with AML

The principal role of allogeneic BMT is to re-establish hematopoietic and immunological function in recipients after myeloablative chemoradiotherapy. Some evidence suggests that the marrow graft may also exert an antileukemic effect (graft-versus-leukemia). Relapse rates are decreased in patients in whom significant acute or chronic GVHD develops compared with patients with no or mild GVHD (71). Several studies demonstrated that the relapse rate for patients with AML in first remission is higher in recipients of syngeneic marrow grafts (in whom GVHD does not develop), compared with recipients of allogeneic marrow grafts. Data compiled from 6 different centers revealed a relapse rate of 18% with allogeneic BMT, compared with 59% with syngeneic BMT (72). A more recent retrospective multicenter study confirmed the relationship between syngeneic grafts and an increased risk of relapse (73). This study also confirmed the antileukemic effect of acute and chronic GVHD, but noted that GVHD is not beneficial in terms of overall leukemia-free survival due to the significant mortality associated with this immunological complication. Patients with more advanced disease also appear to have a lower relapse rate after allogeneic versus syngeneic BMT (74). Studies are ongoing at multiple centers in an effort to define the graft-versus-leukemia effect and to develop methods to potentiate that effect while controlling GVHD (see Chapter 19).

Alternative Donors

Although allogeneic BMT is effective therapy for patients with early and advanced leukemia, only approximately 25 to 35% of otherwise eligible patients have HLA-matched sibling donors (see Chapter 51). Other potential donors include partially matched family members or matched unrelated volunteer donors. In 1985, investigators in Seattle reported a study involving 105 patients with hematological malignancies who underwent BMT from related donors who were fully or partially phenotypically HLA-identical (75). HLA incompatibility was associated with delayed engraftment, an increased risk of graft rejection, and an increased incidence of and earlier onset of acute GVHD, compared with a group of historical control subjects with HLA-identical sibling donors. The probability of survival for patients with acute leukemia in remission with one-HLA-locus–incompatible marrow donors was not significantly different from the control subjects despite the increased incidence of complications. A more recent report from the same group substantiates the relationship between HLA incompatibility and graft rejection and suggests that one-locus mismatches are the limit of incompatibility for allogeneic BMT with currently available immunosuppressive therapies (76). Approximately 40% of the patients and control subjects in this study had AML, and no difference in the incidence of graft failure was observed based on diagnosis.

Only approximately 10% of patients have appropriate partially matched non-sibling related donors for BMT; therefore, more than 50% of otherwise eligible patients do not have suitable family member donors. Several centers have explored the use of phenotypically HLA-matched unrelated volunteer donors for allogeneic BMT. Investigators from the Medical College of Wisconsin described their results in 55 patients (13 with AML) prepared with intensive chemoradiotherapy and grafted with T-cell–depleted marrow from closely HLA-matched unrelated donors (77). The incidence of acute GVHD was 53% in recipients of partially matched marrow and only 17% in recipients of phenotypically identical marrow. Actuarial disease-free survival was 48% in patients with acute leukemia in first remission and 32% in patients with more advanced disease.

The Seattle group compared the outcome of 52 patients with phenotypically matched unrelated donors with 104 age- and disease-matched control subjects transplanted from HLA-identical sibling donors (78). The majority of the patients in the study had chronic myelogenous leukemia (56%), and all patients with AML were in relapse or second or greater remission. All patients received uniform GVHD prophylaxis, and the incidence of moderate to severe acute GVHD was 79% in the unrelated donor group, compared with 36% in the related donor group. The probability of disease-free survival, however, was similar in the two groups (41 vs 46%).

The National Marrow Donor Program (NMDP) is a national volunteer bone marrow donor registry that facilitated marrow donations from unrelated donors for 459 patients through November 1990 (79). BMT was performed at 29 different centers. Ninety-four percent of evaluable patients engrafted, and moderate to severe acute GVHD developed in 64% of patients. The actuarial probability of disease-free survival at 2 years was 40% in patients with acute leukemia in first or second remission or chronic myelogenous leukemia in first chronic phase.

These studies suggest that the outcome of BMT utilizing closely matched related or unrelated donors for patients with AML may be comparable to the outcome of patients with HLA-identical sibling donors (see Chapter 51).

Second Transplants for Relapsed AML after Allogeneic BMT

Leukemic relapse remains a significant problem following BMT for AML, especially for patients with advanced disease at the time of transplantation. The majority of relapses occur within 2 years after marrow grafting, although late relapses have been reported up to 7 years after BMT (80). In rare cases, these relapses occurred in cells of donor origin, suggesting that a new variant of leukemia had developed. The prognosis for patients with recurrent leukemia is extremely poor. Few patients can tolerate additional chemotherapy, and the vast majority die within months of relapse.

Second BMTs have been attempted in some patients with relapsed leukemia (see Chapter 40). Two of 4 patients who received second BMTs for recurrent acute leukemia at UCLA were alive and disease-free 11 and 23 months after the second BMT (81). A larger series of patients was reported by investigators at Seattle in 1988 (82). Twenty-six patients with recurrent leukemia received a second BMT between 1.5 and 78 months after the initial BMT. Regimen-related toxicity was significant; fatal VOD of the liver developed in 23% of patients, and fatal pneumonitis (infectious and idiopathic) developed in 34%. Overall disease-free survival was 19%, with a median follow-up of 32 months and a relapse rate of 60%. No patient who underwent second BMT within one year of the first survived more than 100 days, and only 1 of 15 patients grafted within 2 years of the initial BMT was alive with recurrent disease. In contrast, 5 of 11 patients whose second BMT was more than 2 years after the first were alive and free of disease at the time of the report.

Similar results were recently reported from Johns Hopkins University (83). The projected actuarial disease-free survival of 23 patients after second BMT was 29% at 4 years, with a probability of relapse of 42%. The principal causes of failure were therapy-related toxicities in the first 11 patients treated. Subsequently, patients who experienced serious transplant-related toxicities during their first BMT were excluded from consideration for second BMT, and 6 of 12 more recently retransplanted patients are alive and free of leukemia between 4 and 39 months after their second myeloablative procedure.

These studies suggest that a second BMT might be efficacious in selected patients. Candidates for second BMT should have had at least a one-year disease-free interval after the initial BMT and should not have experienced any significant regimen-related toxicities, such as VOD, pneumonitis, or severe GVHD, during the first marrow grafting procedure.

Summary and Future Directions

Allogeneic BMT has evolved into a widely accepted and effective form of therapy for patients with AML. Patients under age 50 with relapsed AML who have a matched sibling donor should undergo BMT because approximately 25 to 30% of such patients will become long-term survivors, whereas chemotherapy alone offers no chance for control of their disease. Available data suggest that the outcome for patients transplanted in early relapse is equivalent to BMT in second remission; therefore, patients with available donors should proceed to transplantation as soon as possible after detection of relapse. Transplantation is also an effective therapy for patients with AML who fail initial induction therapy.

The role of BMT for patients in first complete remission remains somewhat controversial. Although all comparative studies demonstrate decreased relapse rates in BMT recipients, some studies do not reveal a significant improvement in disease-free survival because of transplant-related complications such as GVHD, interstitial pneumonitis, infections, and VOD. All studies demonstrate improved disease-free survival with BMT, although not always significant by log-rank analysis. Marrow transplantation from matched sibling donors is appropriate for patients in first remission under the age of 50 years. As new strategies are developed to control GVHD and to prevent such complications as VOD of the liver and interstitial pneumonitis, the transplant-related failure rate should decrease so that the lower relapse rates achieved with BMT will translate into improved survival.

Prospective randomized trials to compare BMT and chemotherapy for patients in first remission are ongoing and are likely to continue for the foreseeable future until adequate patient numbers and follow-up periods are achieved to answer the question of superior therapy with certainty. Perhaps subgroups of patients will be identified who benefit significantly from one approach or the other. These clinical trials rely on "biological randomization"— patients with matched sibling donors are offered BMT and patients without donors are treated with chemotherapy. Another approach would be to randomize patients with matched donors to BMT during first remission or at the time of first relapse. Theoretically, if 25% of patients treated with chemotherapy become long-term disease-free survivors and if 25 to 30% of patients who relapse can be salvaged with BMT, then the outcome for patients managed with this strategy might approach the 50% disease-free survival generally observed in patients transplanted in first remission. One risk of such an approach is that complications will develop in some patients during consolidation and intensification chemotherapy or at the time of relapse, which would make them ineligible for BMT despite having a suitable donor. The development of better preparatory regimens and advances in the prevention of transplantation-related toxicities will also undoubtedly impact on the issue of chemotherapy versus BMT.

Several preparatory regimens have been developed for patients with AML. To date, no single regimen has proved to be ideal in terms of antileukemic effect or toxicity. New combinations of agents are being explored, as well as better methods of delivery of old agents, such as using the first dose pharmacokinetics of BU to determine subsequent dose adjustments (Buckner CD. Personal communication). Novel approaches to bone marrow ablation, such as antibody-radionuclide conjugates (84), are also being explored.

The scope of allogeneic BMT has been expanded to patients who do not have HLA-identical sibling donors through the utilization of partially matched family donors or unrelated volunteer donors. Marrow transplantation from phenotypically matched or one-

HLA-locus–mismatched family donors should be considered for all patients with AML. Marrow grafting from unrelated donors, however, should currently be offered only to patients with AML beyond first remission due to the increased incidence of severe acute GVHD.

Impressive progress has been made in the past 2 decades, both in basic immunology and clinical transplantation, so that currently more than one-half of newly diagnosed patients with AML who achieve remission and have available donors can expect to be cured of their disease.

References

1. Thomas ED, Storb R, Clift RA, et al. Bone marrow transplantation. N Engl J Med 1975;292:832–843, 895–902.
2. Thomas ED. Marrow transplantation for malignant diseases. J Clin Oncol 1983;1:517–531.
3. Thomas ED, Lochte HL, Lu WC, Ferrebee JW. Intravenous infusion of bone marrow in patients receiving radiation and chemotherapy. N Engl J Med 1957;257: 491–496.
4. Thomas ED, Lochte HL, Ferrebee JW. Irradiation of the entire body and marrow transplantation: some observations and comments. Blood 1959;14:1–23.
5. Thomas ED, Lochte HL, Cannon JH, Sahler OD, Ferrebee JW. Supralethal whole body irradiation and isologous marrow transplantation in man. J Clin Invest 1959;38:1709–1716.
6. Fefer A, Einstein AB, Thomas ED, et al. Bone-marrow transplantation for hematologic neoplasia in 16 patients with identical twins. N Engl J Med 1974;290: 1389–1393.
7. Fefer A, Buckner CD, Thomas ED, et al. Cure of hematologic neoplasia with transplantation of marrow from identical twins. N Engl J Med 1977;297:146–148.
8. Fefer A, Cheever MA, Thomas ED, et al. Bone marrow transplantation for refractory leukemia in 34 patients with identical twins. Blood 1981;57:421–430.
9. Thomas ED, Buckner CD, Banaji M, et al. One hundred patients with acute leukemia treated by chemotherapy, total body irradiation, and allogeneic marrow transplantation. Blood 1977;49:511–533.
10. Fefer A, Thomas ED. Marrow transplantation in the treatment of acute leukemia. In: Henderson ES, Lister TA, eds. Leukemia. Philadelphia: WB Saunders, 1990: 431–441.
11. Santos GW, Sensenbrenner LL, Anderson PN, et al. HL-A-identical marrow transplants in aplastic anemia, acute leukemia, and lymphosarcoma employing cyclophosphamide. Transplant Proc 1976;8:607–610.
12. Blume KG, Beutler E, Bross KJ, et al. Bone marrow ablation and allogeneic marrow transplantation in acute leukemia. N Engl J Med 1980;302:1041–1046.
13. Grever MR. Treatment of patients with acute nonlymphocytic leukemia not in remission. Semin Oncol 1987;14:416–424.
14. Appelbaum FR, Clift RA, Buckner CD, et al. Allogeneic marrow transplantation for acute nonlymphoblastic leukemia after first relapse. Blood 1983;61:949–953.
15. Clift RA, Buckner CD, Thomas ED, et al. The treatment of acute non-lymphoblastic leukemia by allogeneic marrow transplantation. Bone Marrow Transplant 1987;2:243–258.
16. Zander AR, Dicke KA, Keating M, et al. Allogeneic bone marrow transplantation for acute leukemia refractory to induction chemotherapy. Cancer 1985;56: 1374–1379.
17. Forman SJ, Schmidt GM, Nademanee AP, et al. Allogeneic bone marrow transplantation as therapy for primary induction failure for patients with acute leukemia. J Clin Oncol 1991;9:1570–1574.
18. Mayer RJ. Current chemotherapeutic treatment approaches to the management of previously untreated adults with de novo acute myelogenous leukemia. Semin Oncol 1987;14:384–396.
19. Thomas ED, Buckner CD, Clift RA, et al. Marrow transplantation for acute nonlymphoblastic leukemia in first remission. N Engl J Med 1979;301:597–599.
20. Mannoni P, Vernant JP, Rodet M, et al. Marrow transplantation for acute nonlymphoblastic leukemia in first remission. Blut 1980;41:220–225.
21. Powles RL, Clink HM, Bandini G, et al. The place of bone-marrow transplantation in acute myelogenous leukaemia. Lancet 1980;1:1047–1050.
22. Forman SJ, Spruce WE, Farbstein MJ, et al. Bone marrow ablation followed by allogeneic marrow grafting during first complete remission of acute nonlymphocytic leukemia. Blood 1983;61:439–442.
23. Dinsmore R, Kirkpatrick D, Flomenberg N, et al. Allogeneic bone marrow transplantation for patients with acute nonlymphocytic leukemia. Blood 1984;63: 649–656.
24. Zwaan FE, Hermans J, Barrett AJ, Speck B. Bone marrow transplantation for acute nonlymphoblastic leukaemia: a survey of the European Group for Bone Marrow Transplantation (E.G.B.M.T.). Br J Haematol 1984;56:645–653.
25. Bacigalupo A, Frassoni F, Van Lint MT, et al. Bone marrow transplantation (BMT) for acute nonlymphoid leukemia (ANLL) in first remission. Acta Haematol 1985;74:23–26.
26. Sanders JE, Thomas ED, Buckner CD, et al. Marrow transplantation for children in first remission of acute nonlymphoblastic leukemia: an update. Blood 1985;66: 460–462.
27. Feig SA, Nesbit ME, Buckley J, et al. Bone marrow transplantation for acute non-lymphocytic leukemia: a report from the Childrens Cancer Study Group of sixty-seven children transplanted in first remission. Bone Marrow Transplant 1987;2:365–374.
28. McGlave PB, Haake RJ, Bostrom BC, et al. Allogeneic bone marrow transplantation for acute nonlymphocytic leukemia in first remission. Blood 1988;72:1512–1517.
29. Forman SJ, Krance RA, O'Donnell MR, et al. Bone marrow transplantation for acute nonlymphoblastic leukemia during first complete remission. Transplantation 1987;43:650–653.
30. Weisdorf DJ, McGlave PB, Ramsay NK, et al. Allogeneic bone marrow transplantation for acute leukaemia: comparative outcomes for adults and children. Br J Haematol 1988;69:351–358.
31. Klingemann HG, Storb R, Fefer A, et al. Bone marrow transplantation in patients aged 45 years and older. Blood 1986;67:770–776.
32. Blume KG, Forman SJ, Nademanee AP, et al. Bone marrow transplantation for hematologic malignancies in patients aged 30 years or older. J Clin Oncol 1986;4:1489–1492.
33. Aschan J, Ringden O, Tollemar J, et al. Improved survival in marrow recipients above 30 years of age

with better prevention of graft-versus-host disease. Transplant Proc 1990;22:195–197.
34. Johnson FL, Sanders JE, Ruggiero M, Chard RL, Thomas ED. Bone marrow transplantation for the treatment of acute nonlymphoblastic leukemia in children aged less than 2 years. Blood 1988;71:1277–1280.
35. Kim TH, McGlave PB, Ramsay N, et al. Comparison of two total body irradiation regimens in allogeneic bone marrow transplantation for acute non-lymphoblastic leukemia in first remission. Int J Radiat Oncol Biol Phys 1990;19:889–897.
36. Thomas ED, Clift RA, Hersman J, et al. Marrow transplantation for acute nonlymphoblastic leukemia in first remission using fractionated or single-dose irradiation. Int J Radiat Oncol Biol Phys 1982;8:817–821.
37. Thomas ED. Total body irradiation regimens for marrow grafting. Int J Radiat Oncol Biol Phys 1990;19: 1285–1288.
38. Shank B, Chu F, Dinsmore R, et al. Hyperfractionated total body irradiation for bone marrow transplantation. Results in seventy leukemia patients with allogeneic transplants. Int J Radiat Oncol Biol Phys 1983;9: 1607–1611.
39. Clift RA, Buckner CD, Thomas ED, et al. Allogeneic marrow transplantation using fractionated total body irradiation in patients with acute lymphoblastic leukemia in relapse. Leuk Res 1982;6:401–407.
40. Clift RA, Buckner CD, Appelbaum FR, et al. Allogeneic marrow transplantation in patients with acute myeloid leukemia in first remission: a randomized trial of two irradiation regimens. Blood 1990;76:1867–1871.
41. Blume KG, Forman SJ, O'Donnell MR, et al. Total body irradiation and high-dose etoposide: a new preparatory regimen for bone marrow transplantation in patients with advanced hematologic malignancies. Blood 1987; 69:1015–1020.
42. Schmitz N, Gassmann W, Rister M, et al. Fractionated total body irradiation and high-dose VP 16-213 followed by allogeneic bone marrow transplantation in advanced leukemias. Blood 1988;72:1567–1573.
43. Snyder D, Blume K, Chao N, et al. Fractionated total body irradiation and etoposide: an effective preparative regimen for allogeneic bone marrow transplantation for patients with leukemia in first complete remission (abstract). Proc Am Soc Clin Oncol 1991;10:220.
44. Helenglass G, Powles RL, McElwain TJ, et al. Melphalan and total body irradiation (TBI) versus cyclophosphamide and TBI as conditioning for allogeneic matched sibling bone marrow transplants for acute myeloblastic leukaemia in first remission. Bone Marrow Transplant 1988;3:21–29.
45. Riddell S, Appelbaum FR, Buckner CD, et al. High-dose cytarabine and total body irradiation with or without cyclophosphamide as a preparative regimen for marrow transplantation for acute leukemia. J Clin Oncol 1988;6:576–582.
46. Messner HA, Curtis JE, Minden MM. The combined use of cytosine arabinoside, cyclophosphamide, and total body irradiation as preparative regimen for bone marrow transplantation in patients with AML and CML. Semin Oncol 1985;12(suppl 3):187–189.
47. Petersen FB, Buckner CD, Appelbaum FR, et al. Busulfan, cyclophosphamide and fractionated total body irradiation as a preparatory regimen for marrow transplantation in patients with advanced hematological malignancies: a phase I study. Bone Marrow Transplant 1989;4:617–623.
48. Santos GW, Tutschka PJ, Brookmeyer R, et al. Marrow transplantation for acute nonlymphocytic leukemia after treatment with busulfan and cyclophosphamide. N Engl J Med 1983;309:1347–1353.
49. Geller RB, Saral R, Piantadosi S, et al. Allogeneic bone marrow transplantation after high-dose busulfan and cyclophosphamide in patients with acute nonlymphocytic leukemia. Blood 1989;73:2209–2218.
50. Tutschka PJ, Copelan EA, Klein JP. Bone marrow transplantation for leukemia following a new busulfan and cyclophosphamide regimen. Blood 1987;70:1382–1388.
51. Copelan EA, Biggs JC, Thompson JM, et al. Treatment for acute myelocytic leukemia with allogeneic bone marrow transplantation following preparation with BuCy2. Blood 1991;78:838–843.
52. Blaise D, Maraninchi D, Archimbaud E, et al. Allogeneic bone marrow transplantation for acute myeloid leukemia in first remission: a randomized trial of busulfan-cytoxan versus cytoxan-total body irradiation as a preparative regimen: a report from the Groupe d'Etudes de la Greffe de Moelle Osseuse. Blood 1992;79:2578–2582.
53. Preisler HD, Anderson K, Rai K, et al. The frequency of long-term remission in patients with acute myelogenous leukemia treated with conventional maintenance chemotherapy: a study of 760 patients with a minimal follow-up time of 6 years. Br J Haematol 1989;71:189–194.
54. Champlin R, Gale RP. Acute myelogenous leukemia: recent advances in therapy. Blood 1987;69:1551–1562.
55. Wolff SN, Herzig RH, Fay JW, et al. High-dose cytarabine and daunorubicin as consolidation therapy for acute myeloid leukemia in first remission: long-term follow-up and results. J Clin Oncol 1989;7:1260–1267.
56. Champlin R, Gajewski J, Nimer S, et al. Postremission chemotherapy for adults with acute myelogenous leukemia: improved survival with high-dose cytarabine and daunorubicin consolidation treatment. J Clin Oncol 1990;8:1199–1206.
57. Phillips GL, Reece DE, Shepherd JD, et al. High-dose cytarabine and daunorubicin induction and post-remission chemotherapy for the treatment of acute myelogenous leukemia in adults. Blood 1991;77:1429–1435.
58. Powles RL, Watson JG, Morgenstern GR, Kay HE. Bone marrow transplantation in leukaemia remission (letter). Lancet 1982;1:336–337.
59. Appelbaum FR, Dahlberg S, Thomas ED, et al. Bone marrow transplantation or chemotherapy after remission induction for adults with acute nonlymphoblastic leukemia. Ann Intern Med 1984;101:581–588.
60. Marmont A, Bacigalupo A, Van Lint MT, Frassoni F, Carella A. Bone marrow transplantation versus chemotherapy alone for acute nonlymphoblastic leukemia. Exp Hematol 1985;13(suppl 17):40.
61. Appelbaum FR, Fisher LD, Thomas ED, et al. Chemotherapy versus marrow transplantation for adults with acute nonlymphocytic leukemia: a five-year follow-up. Blood 1988;72:179–184.
62. Reiffers J, Gaspard MH, Maraninchi D, et al. Comparison of allogeneic or autologous bone marrow transplantation and chemotherapy in patients with acute myeloid leukaemia in first remission: a prospective controlled trial. Br J Haematol 1989;72:57–63.
63. Reiffers J, Stoppa AM, Rigal-Huguet F, et al. Allogeneic versus autologous bone marrow transplantation versus chemotherapy for treatment of acute myeloid leukemia

in first complete remission. Bone Marrow Transplant 1991;7(suppl 2):36.
64. Ringden O, Bolme P, Lonnqvist B, Gustafsson G, Kreuger A. Allogeneic bone marrow transplantation versus chemotherapy in children with acute leukemia in Sweden. Pediatr Hematol Oncol 1989;6:137–144.
65. Champlin RE, Ho WG, Gale RP, et al. Treatment of acute myelogenous leukemia: a prospective controlled trial of bone marrow transplantation versus consolidation chemotherapy. Ann Intern Med 1985;102:285–291.
66. Schiller GJ, Nimer SD, Territo MC, Ho WG, Champlin RE, Gajewski JL. Bone marrow transplantation versus high-dose cytarabine-based consolidation chemotherapy for acute myelogenous leukemia in first remission. J Clin Oncol 1992;10:41–46.
67. Cassileth PA, Lynch E, Hines JD, et al. Varying intensity of postremission therapy in acute myeloid leukemia. Blood 1992;79:1924–1930.
68. Zander AR, Keating M, Dicke K, et al. A comparison of marrow transplantation with chemotherapy for adults with acute leukemia of poor prognosis in first complete remission. J Clin Oncol 1988;6:1548–1557.
69. Conde E, Iriondo A, Rayon C, et al. Allogeneic bone marrow transplantation versus intensification chemotherapy for acute myelogenous leukaemia in first remission: a prospective controlled trial. Br J Haematol 1988;68:219–226.
70. Dahl GV, Kalwinsky DK, Mirro J, et al. Allogeneic bone marrow transplantation in a program of intensive sequential chemotherapy for children and young adults with acute nonlymphocytic leukemia in first remission. J Clin Oncol 1990;8:295–303.
71. Weiden PL, Sullivan KM, Flournoy N, et al. Antileukemic effect of chronic graft-versus-host disease: contribution to improved survival after allogeneic marrow transplantation. N Engl J Med 1981;304:1529–1533.
72. Gale RP, Champlin RE. How does bone-marrow transplantation cure leukaemia? Lancet 1984;2:28–30.
73. Ringden O, Horowitz MM. Graft-versus-leukemia reactions in humans. Transplant Proc 1989;21:2989–2992.
74. Fefer A, Sullivan KM, Weiden P, et al. Graft versus leukemia effect in man: the relapse rate of acute leukemia is lower after allogeneic than after syngeneic marrow transplantation. Prog Clin Biol Res 1987; 244:401–408.
75. Beatty PG, Clift RA, Mickelson EM, et al. Marrow transplantation from related donors other than HLA-identical siblings. N Engl J Med 1985;313:765–771.
76. Anasetti C, Amos D, Beatty PG, et al. Effect of HLA compatibility on engraftment of bone marrow transplants in patients with leukemia or lymphoma. N Engl J Med 1989;320:197–204.
77. Ash RC, Casper JT, Chitambar CR, et al. Successful allogeneic transplantation of T-cell-depleted bone marrow from closely HLA-matched unrelated donors. N Engl J Med 1990;322:485–494.
78. Beatty PG, Hansen JA, Longton GM, et al. Marrow transplantation from HLA-matched unrelated donors for treatment of hematologic malignancies. Transplantation 1991;51:443–447.
79. Kernan NA, Bartsch G, Ash RC, et al. Analysis of 462 transplantations from unrelated donors facilitated by the National Marrow Donor Program. N Engl J Med 1993;328:593–602.
80. Witherspoon R, Flournoy N, Thomas ED, Ramberg R, Buckner CD, Storb R. Recurrence of acute leukemia more than two years after allogeneic marrow grafting. Exp Hematol 1986;14:178–181.
81. Champlin RE, Ho WG, Lenarsky C, et al. Successful second bone marrow transplants for treatment of acute myelogenous leukemia or acute lymphoblastic leukemia. Transplant Proc 1985;17:496–499.
82. Sanders JE, Buckner CD, Clift RA, et al. Second marrow transplants in patients with leukemia who relapse after allogeneic marrow transplantation. Bone Marrow Transplant 1988;3:11–19.
83. Wagner JE, Vogelsang GB, Zehnbauer BA, Griffin CA, Shah N, Santos GW. Relapse of leukemia after bone marrow transplantation: effect of second myeloablative therapy. Bone Marrow Transplant 1992;9:205–209.
84. Appelbaum FR, Brown P, Sandmaier B, et al. Antibody-radionuclide conjugates as part of a myeloablative preparative regimen for marrow transplantation. Blood 1989;73:2202–2208.

Chapter 46
Allogeneic Bone Marrow Transplantation for Acute Lymphoblastic Leukemia

Nelson J. Chao and Stephen J. Forman

Acute lymphoblastic leukemia (ALL) is a hematological malignancy characterized by rapid proliferation and subsequent accumulation of immature lymphocytes and their progenitor cells. Although this type of leukemia is most common in children, approximately 20% of adult patients present with this variant of acute leukemia. Over the past 2 decades, there has been substantial improvement in the initial management of both adults and children with ALL. Several large studies have resulted in complete remission rates between 80 and 90%, even in the adult population. In addition, studies to date in the pediatric patient population indicate that approximately 50 to 75% of children with ALL, particularly those with good risk features, can be cured. In general, long-term survival for adults with ALL has not been as good as that achieved in children. Remission rates were lower and disease-free survival clearly inferior. This chapter reviews the progress that has been made using bone marrow transplantation (BMT) to achieve long-term disease-free survival for both adults and children with ALL.

Diagnosis and Classification

ALL comprises a heterogeneous group of disorders based on morphological, immunological, and cytogenetic characteristics. Various features have emerged as important prognostic indicators and therefore are highly relevant to the decision-making process concerning the timing of BMT. Utilizing the French American British (FAB) morphological classification, three types of lymphoblasts, termed *L1*, *L2*, and *L3*, have been described (1,2). This classification is based on the spectrum of cell properties, including the size of the nucleus relative to the cytoplasm, the number and size of nucleoli, and the degree of cytoplasmic basophilia. In childhood ALL, 85% of patients have L1 morphology, whereas adult patients with ALL tend to have predominantly L2 characteristics.

In addition, ALL cells can be characterized immunologically based on the presence of lymphocyte antigens related to T-cell or B-cell ontogeny (3,4). In general, immunological identification is based on characterization of cell surface antigens, including the expression of common ALL antigen (CD10), T-cell antigens, or immunoglobulin molecules. Recent studies indicate that most cases of common ALL are committed to B-lymphocyte lineage (but are not mature B cells), based on the detection of intracytoplasmic immunoglobulin and immunoglobulin gene rearrangements (5–7). In children, approximately 75% of cases are of the common ALL phenotype; the remainder are T-cell or null phenotype. In adults, only 50% of the cases demonstrate the common ALL phenotype, and T-cell ALL accounts for more than 20%. B-cell ALL is rare in both children and adults.

With improvement in both morphological and immunological characterization of cells, investigators have noted leukemic cells in patients expressing both lymphoid and myeloid features (8–10). Cases of myeloid leukemia have been described in which blasts reacted with antibodies against T-cell markers (CD2 and CD7) in addition to having T-cell receptor β-chain gene rearrangements (11). Several series also described patients whose leukemias had lymphoid appearance but with serologically defined myeloid antigens. Patients with biphenotypic acute leukemias appear to have an inferior long-term disease-free survival compared with patients with ALL who have only lymphoid characteristics.

Cytogenetic analysis has emerged as a very important part of the clinical evaluation and therapeutic decision-making for patients with ALL. Several types of chromosomal abnormalities have been noted. Most children with L1 morphology demonstrate high hyperdiploidy, with trisomies involving some or all of chromosomes 4, 6, 8, 10, 12, 13, 18, and 21 (12). There are 3 nonrandom structural abnormalities found frequently in patients with ALL, the most common of which is the Philadelphia (Ph) chromosome, t(9;22)(q34;q11) (13). This chromosome is found in approximately 20% of adults with ALL, but in less than 10% of children with the disease. Although the Ph chromosome is formed by a translocation between chromosomes 9 and 22, and morphologically appears the same as in chronic myeloid leukemia (CML), molecular studies suggest that the break point on chromosome 22 is different in most cases of the 2 disorders. The product of the translocation may have a different size from that found in CML. Molecular analysis may be needed to distinguish patients with Ph-positive ALL from patients presenting in lymphoid blast crisis of CML (14). The second most common translocation is between chromosome 4 and 11, t(4;11)(q21;q23) (15,16). Most of the patients with this abnormality have L2 morphology. This type of ALL is often associated with a high white blood cell count (WBC) and occurs more frequently in children under the age of one. The third and most recently discovered specific translocation of ALL is the t(1;19)(q23;q13) found in pre-B ALL (12). In addition, patients with the L3 morphology typical of Burkitt's leukemia/lymphoma have a specific cytogenetic abnormality: t(8;14)(9q24;q32) (17,18).

Prognostic Features

Many studies of ALL have examined prognostic factors present at diagnosis to determine the intensity and type of therapy, including BMT, that should be administered. Utilizing morphological criteria, most studies have found no difference in remission rate in the L1 versus L2 morphologies (19). However, data on the L3 subtypes suggest that these patients have lower remission rates, shorter durations of remission, and a higher incidence of central nervous system (CNS) involvement, similar to Burkitt's lymphoma (20). Immunologically, data from studies in childhood ALL indicate that patients with the common ALL phenotype have a better prognosis than those with T-cell or null-cell phenotype (4,21). Children with B-cell ALL have the worst prognosis. Recent studies in the adult patient population, using combination chemotherapy, suggest that T-cell ALL, which formerly had a poor outcome in children and adults, is now the most favorable subtype in adults (22,23). Similar to ALL in children, adult B-cell ALL has a low rate of remission with poor long-term survival. In 7 studies of 43 patients, the complete remission rate was only 35% with most patients relapsing rapidly (24). The current available data suggest that adults with T-cell ALL treated with chemotherapy have the best chance for long-term disease-free survival and cure, whereas those with common ALL have an intermediate prognosis. Those with null-cell ALL have an inferior prognosis. Patients with biphenotypic morphology or B-cell ALL also appear to have an unfavorable outcome.

Age has also emerged as an important prognostic factor (23–27). It has already been mentioned that there is a difference in outcome between children and adults and that children under the age of one with ALL do poorly. In 2 large studies of adult patients, the best limits that predicted poor prognosis were age greater than or equal to 25 years in one study and 35 years in the second study. Increasing age beyond the "cut-off" age was associated with shorter remissions and decreased survival (23,24,26,28).

Although a high WBC at presentation may influence the remission rate, it also has an adverse effect on remission duration. Few long-term survivors were observed in patients who had markedly elevated WBC at diagnosis. Recent studies suggest a "cut-off" of a high WBC of 25,000/μL in one study and 35,000/μL in a second study (23–25,28).

The success of the initial induction therapy also influences the duration of remission. Several studies have indicated that patients achieving remission within 4 weeks have a significantly better outcome than those who achieve it later (25,26).

Cytogenetic analysis has emerged as an important predictor for survival in patients with ALL and influences not only the rate of remission but also the duration (19). More than 80% of adults with a normal karyotype achieve a remission, whereas only half of those patients with chromosome abnormalities do (27,29). Those with a particularly poor prognosis include those with the following chromosomal translocations: t(9;22), t(4;11), and t(8;14). An abnormal karyotype is an adverse risk factor independent of age, immune phenotype, or the initial WBC (12). Some investigators have hypothesized that the poor outcome of common ALL in adults is explained by the higher frequency of the t(9;22) translocation.

BMT for Patients with ALL

Early BMT studies of patients with refractory leukemia demonstrated that it was possible to achieve short-term control of the disease in most patients, with a few becoming long-term disease-free survivors. In an original series of 16 patients receiving marrow grafts from identical twins during the refractory stage of hematological neoplasia, 6 patients achieved an unmaintained remission that is now longer than 15 years (30). This series was followed by a report from Seattle in 1977 of 100 patients (46 with ALL) with refractory acute leukemia treated with chemotherapy and total body irradiation (TBI) followed by BMT (31). Seven patients with ALL were free of recurrent leukemia from one to 4.5 years following BMT, with a Kaplan-Meier curve demonstrating a plateau of surviving patients living beyond 2 years. Since publication of this report, one patient with ALL died of pneumonia at 9 years and one patient died of chronic active hepatitis at 17 years, whereas 4 are alive and well 17 to 19 years following BMT (Thomas ED. Personal communication). These studies provided the basis for examination of the role of allogeneic BMT in other circumstances, including in patients with relapsed disease and ultimately in patients with poor prognostic features at diagnosis.

In 1979, investigators from Seattle reported 22 patients with ALL who underwent transplantation in second or subsequent remission and were compared with a concurrent group of 26 patients receiving transplants in relapse using identical conditioning regimens. Patients in remission had a lower incidence of recurrent leukemia, a lower death rate from nonleukemic causes, and improved survival. More than half the patients receiving transplants while in remission were alive and well one to 3 years after marrow grafting (32).

BMT for Adult Patients with ALL Not in First Remission

Although remarkable strides have been achieved in the primary therapy of newly diagnosed patients with ALL, several subgroups of patients with ALL continue to suffer relapses following the induction of remission (25,33–35). As described earlier, patients with ALL have been identified whose prognosis is poor based on pretreatment characteristics. Some of the identified risk factors for relapse include age over 30 years; a WBC at presentation in excess of 25,000/μL; extramedullary disease; the chromosomal translocation t(9;22), t(4;11), or t(8;14); null-cell phenotype; and the requirement for induction chemotherapy beyond 4 weeks to attain a complete remission (CR) (25,36,37). If a patient presents without any of these adverse factors, the probability of continued remission at 5 years (equivalent to cure) is 37 to 72% (25,35–39). However, any of the listed poor prognostic variables places the patient in an unfavorable or "high-risk" group, with an overall probability of continued remission at 5 years of only 18 to 28% (25,36–38).

The principle cause of failure from primary chemotherapy is recurrence of leukemia. Relapses can occur in the marrow or in extramedullary sites, such as the testes or the central nervous system. Patients with an isolated extramedullary relapse, both adults and children, are at high risk for subsequent marrow relapse. Treatment of relapsed adult patients with standard doses of chemotherapy can be successful in achieving a second remission. However, second remissions frequently last less than 6 months, and nearly all patients eventually succumb to their disease or to the toxicities associated with reinduction therapy attempts. BMT from a fully histocompatible sibling donor offers a disease-free survival advantage for adult patients.

The experience with allogeneic BMT for patients in second or subsequent remission or in relapse is summarized in Table 46-1 (39–44,56–71). In most of these studies, the data for adults are not reported separately from those attained in children. BMT for ALL patients with advanced disease (i.e. past the stage of second CR) results in a disease-free survival of approximately 20% and is superior to any other form of therapy. The main cause for failure in this group is leukemic recurrence. Data from the City of Hope and Stanford for patients transplanted in CR2 or CR3 demonstrate a disease-free survival of 41%, compared with 19% for patients transplanted while in relapse. BMT for patients in CR2 is associated with a significantly better outcome due to a lower relapse rate. Overall, disease-free survival is 40 to 50%, with a range of 10 to 65%. The relapse rate after BMT ranges from 12 to 65%, with an average of approximately 30 to 40%. The differences in the disease-free survival and relapse rates may be related to patient selection criteria, inclusion of pediatric patients, and the preparatory regimen.

BMT for Children with ALL

The prognosis of children who suffer a relapse depends on the site of relapse and the duration of the first remission. Children who relapse after a remission

Table 46-1.
BMT for Patients with ALL Not in First Complete Remission (CR)

Institutions, Ref	*No. Patients (Children)*[a]	*Preparative Regimens*	*Follow-up in Years (Median)*	*Disease-free Survival (%)*	*Relapse (%)*
Patients in CR2					
Leiden, Westminster, Basel (56)	96 (NS)	CY/TBI	3 (1)	34	34
Seattle (43)	48 (0)	CY/TBI	9 (2)	10	65
Johns Hopkins (40)	36 (NS)	CY/TBI	8.9 (4.9)	43	26
City of Hope (71)	30 (NS)	AraC/CY/TBI, FTBI/CY	5 (2.7)	46	30
Memorial Sloan-Kettering (39)	28 (NS)	TBI/CY	2.4 (1.2)	65	NS
Genova (41)	25 (NS)	CY/TBI	2 (NS)	32	NS
Kiel, Ulm. Leiden (44) (note: CR2->CR2)	18 (NS)	FTBI/VP16	2.9 (0.6)	63	12
Westminster (42)	11 (5)	CY/TBI (VP)	2.6 (1)	10	NS
Patients in CR3 or Relapse					
Seattle (43)	103 (0)	CY/TBI	17 (5)	10	NS
Leiden, Westminter, Basel (56)	39 (NS)	CY/TBI	2.5 (1)	33	73
City of Hope (71)	21 (NS)	AraC/CY/TBI, FTBI/CY	7 (2.7)	20	43
Johns Hopkins (40)	20 (NS)	CY/TBI	8.8 (6)	25	48
Memorial Sloan-Kettering (39)	16 (NS)	TBI/CY	2 (0.9)	19	NS

[a]Number in parentheses represents the subgroup of children from the total number of patients.
ALL = acute lymphoblastic leukemia; NS = not specified; CY/TBI = cyclophosphamide plus total body irradiation; araC = cytosine arabinoside; FTBI = fractionated TBI; VP16 = etoposide.

Table 46-2.
BMT for Children with ALL

Institutions, Ref	*No. Patients*	*Remission*	*Preparative Regimens*	*Follow-up in Years (Median)*	*Disease-free Survival (%)*	*Relapse (%)*
Seattle (51)	57	CR2	CY/TBI	10.4 (NS)	40	42
Tubingen, Berlin, Munchen, Ulm, Wien, Hanover, Kiel, Essen (49)	51	CR2	CY/TBI; TBI/VP16	NS	52	NS
Nancy, Creteil, Lyon, Paris, Poitiers, Lille, Pessac (47)	32	CR1	CY/TBI	6.8 (2.5)	84	3.50
Genova (72)	31	CR2	CY/TBI	2.5 (NS)	47	NS
Memorial Sloan-Kettering (48)	31	CR2	FTBI/CY	6.9 (4.8–5.1)	64	13
	12	CR3			42	25
	16	CR4/relapse			23	64
Case Western Reserve (50)	20	CR2	AraC/FTBI	6.6 (2.8)	58	17
Cordoba, Sevilla, Jurez, Huelva (52)	16	CR2	TBI/CY	5.9 (4.1)	58	NS
Minnesota (53)	15	CR2=; >CR2	CY/TBI	4 (NS)	43	NS

BMT = bone marrow transplantation; ALL = acute lymphoblastic leukemia; CR = complete remission; NS = not specified; CY/TBI = cyclophosphamide plus total body irradiation; araC = cytosine arabinoside; FTBI = fractionated TBI; VP16 = etoposide.

of 3 or more years have a high likelihood of achieving a second CR (45). Some investigators suggest that BMT not be utilized in patients who achieve a second CR until a second relapse occurs (45,46). Children, especially those who relapse several years after completion of therapy, occasionally become long-term disease-free survivors with second-line standard conventional therapy. In contrast, children who suffer a relapse within 18 months of attaining a CR, and especially those who relapse on therapy, have a dismal outlook; less than 5% become long-term disease-free survivors, even with the use of modern chemotherapy. Such patients should be considered for BMT. The increased intensity of initial remission induction and maintenance therapy programs also limits the success of reinduction attempts, because the cells causing relapse are often highly drug-resistant because of prior chemotherapy.

The BMT data for children are presented in Table 46-2 (47–53,72). The largest study was performed by the Seattle Bone Marrow Transplant Group (51). Fifty-seven children between the ages of 3 and 17 received an allogeneic BMT during second CR of ALL. The actuarial disease-free survival was 40%, with a "plateau" extending from 2.5 to 10.4 years (Figure 46-1). There was no significant prognostic factor associated with the probability of relapse following BMT. The BMT group at Memorial Sloan-Kettering Cancer Center reported even more encouraging data (48). In their study of children with ALL who received BMT while in second CR, the duration of the initial remission had no effect on the probability of relapse following BMT. The only pretransplant factor associated with improved outcome was the disease status at the time of BMT; thus, the earlier the transplant, the more favorable the outcome (Figure 46-2). Overall, the disease-free survival for children transplanted in second CR is 40 to 62%, with a relapse rate of 13 to 40%.

Allogeneic BMT has been compared with chemotherapy by the group in Cordoba, Spain (52). In that study, 76 patients aged 2 to 17 years with recurrent ALL achieved a second remission. Twenty-one patients had a histocompatible sibling donor and underwent allogeneic BMT. The remaining 55 patients received continued intensive chemotherapy. Eleven patients were alive in the BMT group, compared with 7 in the chemotherapy group (Figure 46-3). The probability of remaining in CR in the BMT group was 58.5%, compared with 10.9% in the chemotherapy group ($p < 0.005$). Although there might have been a selection bias in patients undergoing BMT, these encouraging results suggest that allogeneic BMT is associated with excellent disease-free survival and should be offered to such patients who have a fully histocompatible sibling.

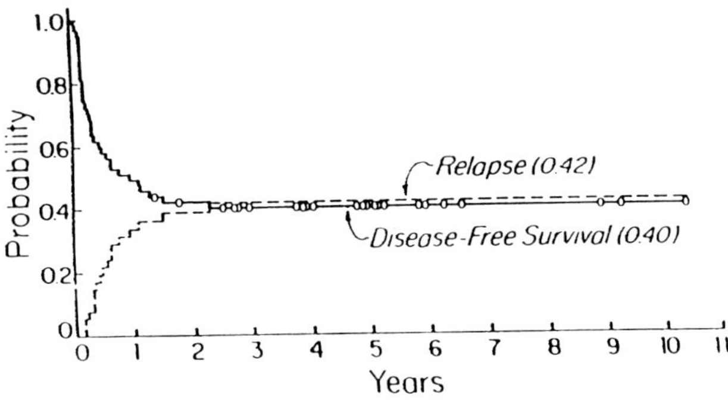

Figure 46-1. Kaplan-Meier product limit estimates for probability of disease-free survival and relapse for 57 children with acute lymphoblastic leukemia transplanted in complete remission. *Open circles* indicate living patients. (Reproduced by permission from Sanders JE, Thomas ED, Buckner CD, Doney K. Marrow transplantation for children with acute lymphoblastic leukemia in second remission. Blood 1987;70:324.)

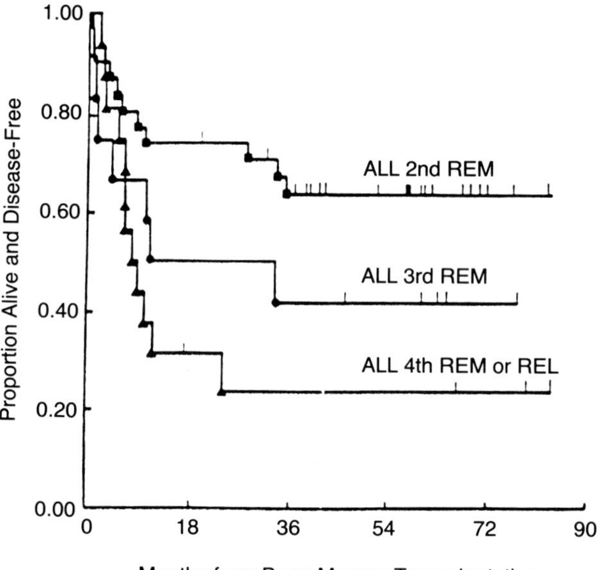

Figure 46-2. Disease-free survival among 59 children receiving transplants for acute lymphoblastic leukemia (ALL), stratified to their disease status at the time of bone marrow transplantation. Thirty-one patients received transplants in second remission (REM), 12 in third remission, and 16 in fourth remission or relapse (REL). *Tick marks* indicate living patients. (Reproduced by permission of the New England Journal of Medicine, from Brochstein JA, Kernan NA, Groshen S, et al. Allogeneic bone marrow transplantation after hyperfractionated total-body irradiation and cyclophosphamide in children with acute leukemia. N Engl J Med 1987;317:1618.)

BMT for Patients with ALL in First CR

Analyses of the clinical and biological characteristics of patients with ALL have identified patients who will be unlikely to achieve a cure of their disease with chemotherapy only. Although a proportion will become long-term disease-free survivors, most will still relapse. Patients who have "high risk" or unfavorable ALL may therefore benefit from high-dose radiochemotherapy followed by allogeneic BMT if they are treated early in the course of their disease, prior to first relapse. Several studies have investigated this approach in patients with "high risk" ALL who were treated with myeloablative therapy followed by allogeneic BMT while in first CR. In one series of 53 patients (median age, 24 yr; range, infancy to 50 yr), the selection criteria for BMT included WBC ≥ 25,000/μL or more; the chromosomal translocations t(9;22), t(4;11), or t(8;14); age 30 years or older; extramedullary leukemia; and time to achieve CR (>4 weeks) (54). Although no doubt exists about the contribution of these risk factors to poor prognosis of ALL, their individual potency as high-risk predictors remains uncertain. Approximately two-thirds of the patients had at least one risk factor, and the remaining patients had 2 or more high-risk features at presentation. Although the time to achieve CR may be related to the intensity of the induction regimen (and therefore more applicable to current intensive induction therapies), all but 5 patients received anthracyclines as part of the induction therapy. The majority of the patients (89%) were transplanted within the first 4 months after achieving CR. BMT in first CR led to prolonged disease-free survival in this patient population, who would otherwise be expected to do poorly. An update of this study with 63 high-risk patients who had a median follow-up of 71 months (range, 2 mo to 12.4 yr) demonstrates an actuarial disease-free survival of 62% and a relapse rate of 11% (Figure 46-4).

This approach has also been utilized in the treatment of a pediatric population of patients who were believed to be at risk for early relapse. Thirty-two children with high-risk ALL in first CR were treated with cyclophosphamide (CY) and TBI, followed by an allogeneic BMT (47). The main reasons for pursuing BMT in this group of patients were a WBC greater than 100,000/μL, structural chromosomal abnormalities, and resistance to initial induction chemotherapy. With a median follow-up of 30 months (range, 7–82 mo), the projected probability of surviving without disease at 5 years was 84.4%. The estimated chance of relapse in 5 years after BMT was only 3.5%.

The data for allogeneic BMT for adult patients with ALL in first CR are presented in Table 46-3 (40,41, 43,54–56,73,74). Disease-free survival ranged from 42 to 71%, with a relatively low relapse rate ranging from 6 to 50%. This wide range of disease-free survival and relapse rates may be related to differ-

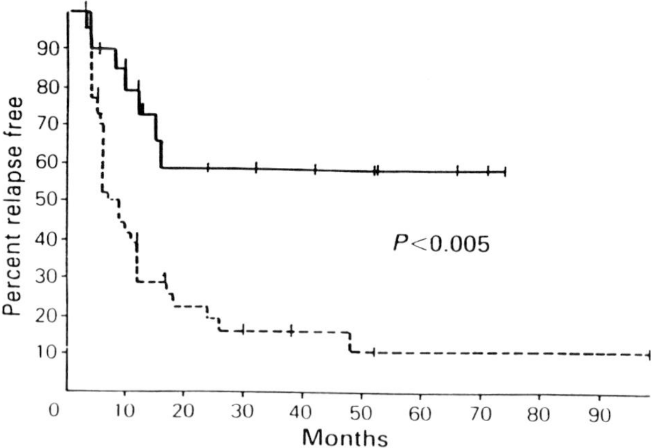

Figure 46-3. Probability of remaining in complete remission. The *solid line* represents the bone marrow transplantation group (n=21; 58.5±12.4% disease-free survival [DFS], 95% confidence limits). The *broken line* represents the chemotherapy group (n=40; 10.9 ±6.1% relapse-free survival, 95% confidence limits). *Tick marks* indicate living patients. (Reproduced by permission from Torres A, Martinez F, Gomez P, et al. Allogeneic bone marrow transplantation versus chemotherapy in the treatment of childhood acute lymphoblastic leukemia in second complete remission. Bone Marrow Transplant 1989;4:609–611.)

Table 46-3.
BMT for Patients in CR1

Institutions, Ref	*No. Patients (Children)*[a]	*Preparative Regimens*	*Follow-up in Years (Median)*	*Disease-free Survival (%)*	*Relapse (%)*
Leiden, Westminter, Basel (56)	57 (NS)	CY/TBI	3 (1)	58	6
Stanford/City of Hope (54)	53 (2)	AraC/CY/TBI, FTBI/CY, FTBI/VP16	10.2 (4.8)	61	10
Seattle (43)	41 (0)	CY/TBI	10 (2)	22	50
Westminster (73)	32 (9)	VIPER, VVRAPID, VVRAPID-X	9 (4.2)	50	31
Bordeaux, Creteil, Lyon, Marseille (74)	27 (8)	CY/TBI	12 (4.7)	59	14
Marseille (55)	25 (3)	FTBI/CY, FTBI/MEL	5 (3.3)	71	9
Johns Hopkins (40)	18 (NS)	CY/TBI	6 (4.8)	42	20
Genova (41)	7 (NS)	CY/TBI	2 (NS)	57	NS

[a]Number in parentheses represents the subgroup of children from the total number of patients.
BMT = bone marrow transplantation; CR = complete remission; NS = not specified; CY/TBI = cyclophosphamide plus total body irradiation; araC = cytosine arabinoside; FTBI = fractionated TBI; VP16 = etoposide; VIPER = vincristine, prednisolone, CY, TBI; VVRAPID = vincristine, araC, VM26, prednisolone, daunorubicin, TBI; VVRAPID-X = vincristine, araC, VM26, prednisolone, daunorubicin, TBI × 2; MEL = melphalan.

ences in patient selection and to the preparatory regimen used for BMT.

Timing of BMT

The optimum timing of BMT for patients with ALL remains an important question (57). The studies presented in Table 46-3 suggest that BMT should be considered during first CR for the majority of patients under the age of 50 years with high-risk ALL who have a histocompatible sibling donor. Patients presenting with high-risk characteristics have a poor outcome when treated with modern intensive chemotherapy, with disease-free survival of only 18 to 28% (36–38). For them, BMT offers an excellent chance of disease-free survival and cure. Moreover, the results with BMT are likely to improve further as some causes for transplant-related morbidity and mortality (i.e., graft-versus-host disease [GVHD] and cytomegalovirus [CMV]-associated interstitial pneumonia) are now more effectively prevented or treated.

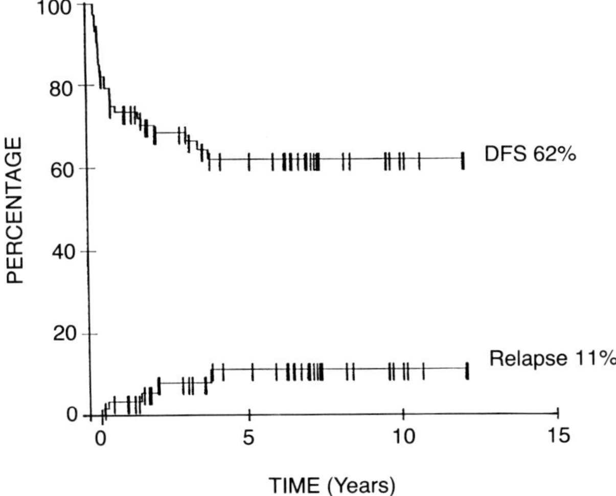

Figure 46-4. Actuarial disease-free survival and relapse for 63 patients transplanted with high-risk acute lymphoblastic leukemia in first complete remission. *Tick marks* indicate living patients. Updated results from (54).

One may consider to reserve BMT for patients with high-risk ALL after recurrence of their disease and attainment of a second remission. However, this approach requires that patients who relapse enter a second CR, retain or regain a good performance status, and are immediately accepted at a BMT center. Unfortunately, many patients who relapse will die of their illness (resistant or progressive disease) or from chemotherapy-associated complications. Such complications from reinduction chemotherapy, if they do not result in death, are still likely to affect biological reserves and can impact unfavorably on the final outcome. For these various serious complications, a sizable fraction of these patients will never be transplanted.

Studies evaluating the outcome of BMT in patients with acute myeloid leukemia who have relapsed based on whether they underwent immediate BMT, as opposed to an attempt at achieving a second CR, suggest nearly equivalent results (58). Such data do not exist for patients with ALL. The decision concerning whether to reinduce patients who have a histocompatible sibling is a judgment that is based on the condition of the patient, the duration of the preceding CR, and the prognostic features associated with the leukemia. Patients with a long first CR without cytogenetic abnormalities may benefit from an attempt to achieve a second CR because attainment of a second CR occurs in the range of 50 to 87% and is dependent on the patient's age. However, this range may be lowered with the use of more intensive primary chemotherapy (57). In contrast, patients with leukemia who relapse within one year and who may have cytogenetic abnormalities should proceed directly to treatment with BMT. The ultimate role of BMT as a treatment modality in first CR of ALL remains to be determined and will require a trial in which the outcome of BMT performed in first CR is compared prospectively with that of "best" chemotherapy.

Improvements in BMT for ALL

Sequential studies from multiple BMT centers have led to improvements in the area of transplant-related complications, including GVHD and CMV-associated interstitial pneumonia. Although this progress should translate into improved disease-free survival, leukemic relapse is still a significant problem, particularly for those patients with advanced or poor-risk disease. Therefore, there is a need for more effective antileukemic regimens. Although a clinically significant graft-versus-leukemia effect has been demonstrated in many series, it cannot be solely relied on to prevent leukemic relapse.

Several different preparatory regimens have been designed, each based on substituting a different chemotherapeutic agent for CY or substituting chemotherapy for TBI. Definitive results require Phase III trials comparing fractionated TBI and CY with any new regimen.

High-dose fractionated TBI in combination with high-dose cytosine arabinoside (ara-C) has been employed by several centers (50,59–61). Three groups, including investigators at Case Western Reserve, the Pediatric Oncology Group (POG), and UCLA, have utilized this regimen. The best result thus far was reported from Case Western Reserve, where 20 pediatric patients with ALL in second remission were transplanted, 58% of whom were alive and in continued CR, with a relapse rate under 20% (50). However, studies performed by the POG and UCLA groups have not shown a significant improvement in relapse-free survival with this regimen and investigators have observed considerable toxicity.

Investigators at Johns Hopkins University and Ohio State University attempted to approach this problem by substituting busulfan (BU) for TBI (62,63). The rationale for the substitution was the desire to minimize the long-term side effects of TBI, with the goal of determining the efficacy of high-dose combined alkylator therapy in eliminating the leukemic cells. These regimens include either high-dose BU (16 mg/kg) and CY (200 mg/kg), as utilized at Johns Hopkins University, or BU (16 mg/kg) and CY (120 mg/kg), as utilized at Ohio State University. At Ohio State University, 13 patients with ALL not in first remission received BMT after preparation with BU and CY, and 7 have remained free of disease. These nonradiation-dependent regimens have shown activity in the treatment of patients with advanced ALL, suggesting that TBI or fractionated TBI is not an absolute requirement for successful treatment of ALL with BMT.

In 1987, the City of Hope group studied the substitution of etoposide (VP16) for CY in allogeneic BMT (64). A Phase I/II study indicated that a VP16 dose of 60 mg/kg was the maximum tolerated dose when combined with fractionated TBI (1,320 cGy in 11 fractions). In this study, 36 patients with ALL were treated, 28 of whom were in relapse. The actuarial disease-free survival was 57%, with a 32% relapse rate, suggesting that the regimen had significant activity in patients with refractory ALL. Studies from the Universities of Kiel, Ulm, and Leiden utilized the same regimen in a group of 17 patients with ALL (44). Ten of the 17 patients were in relapse at the time of BMT, and 64% of the group survive in remission, with a median follow-up of 18 months (range, 6–35 mo). This regimen has also been utilized in high-risk patients undergoing BMT during their first CR. Twenty-six patients have been transplanted, 81% of whom are alive, with a median follow-up of 21 months after BMT. One patient relapsed 25 months after BMT.

BMT for Patients with Ph-positive ALL

As discussed earlier, Ph-positive ALL is a variant of ALL that carriers an exceptionally poor prognosis. Although patients can achieve a CR, the median remission duration is less than one year. Occasional patients become long-term disease-free survivors with intensive current chemotherapy. Two studies suggest that BMT can be effective therapy for these patients and that long-term disease-free survival can be attained using this approach (65,66).

At the City of Hope and Stanford, 27 patients with Ph-positive ALL received allogeneic BMT. Six of 10 patients transplanted in first CR are alive after BMT, with a median follow-up of 2.4 years. Two patients died from GVHD and sepsis, one from cardiomyopathy, and one from relapse. Analysis of the first CR patients demonstrates an actuarial disease-free survival of 44%, with a relapse rate of 20%. Four of 17 patients transplanted with more advanced disease (not in first CR) are alive and well, with a median follow-up of 5.2 years. The major cause of death was relapse (6 patients) and GVHD or infection (7 patients).

The International Bone Marrow Transplant Registry has recently reported the data from 21 BMT teams on 32 HLA-identical siblings who underwent BMT for Ph-positive ALL in first CR. There were 14 deaths from transplant-related complications and 7 relapses, with 11 patients alive and free of leukemia. The 3-year actuarial probability of disease-free survival was 36 ± 17%, with the probability of relapse 38 ± 22%. Considering the poor prognosis for patients with this variant of ALL, BMT performed early during the course of this disease is currently the treatment of choice if a suitable donor is available. The poor prognosis of patients with Ph-positive ALL also suggests that in the absence of a matched sibling donor, an unrelated donor should be sought.

BMT for Patients with Remission-induction Failure

Despite improved remission rates for patients with ALL, a small proportion of patients will not achieve a CR, even with the best available therapy. Often, these patients have one or more defined poor prognostic factors at presentation. After failing to enter a remission with first-line chemotherapy, these patients are usually treated again with second or third-line regimens, but these attempts are most often unsuccessful. Even when such therapy is finally successful in achieving a remission, very few of these patients will go on to become long-term disease-free survivors. Allogeneic BMT has been utilized as an approach for patients who fail induction therapy in an attempt to achieve both a remission and a cure (61). In a study from the City of Hope and Stanford of 22 patients with primary induction failure (5 of whom had ALL), all patients were treated with high-dose preparatory regimens followed by allogeneic BMT from a histocompatible donor (61). Despite the poor prognosis of this patient population and their poor physical condition after receiving aggressive induction therapy, 38% of the whole group became long-term disease-free survivors. All patients achieved a remission following BMT.

The results of this study suggest that allogeneic BMT should be considered as a therapeutic approach for all patients who fail to enter a remission after 2 courses of standard chemotherapy. The preparatory regimen can be used in these circumstances to attain a remission and to potentially cure the patient. It seems unlikely that the use of a third induction attempt would be useful in the ultimate control of the leukemia in such patients. BMT should be considered early in the course of their therapy. Any further attempts with remission induction therapy are more likely to result in toxicity that will preclude the option of BMT and are unlikely to achieve a remission.

Management of the Central Nervous System

In general, development of a CNS relapse in patients with ALL portends a poor prognosis, both for the effect it has on the CNS and because it is a harbinger of systemic relapse. Most patients with ALL have had some form of CNS prophylaxis with radiation or chemotherapy prior to the first systemic relapse. Patients who relapse in the CNS require additional therapy to control the disease prior to BMT. Previous prophylactic intrathecal therapy and CNS radiation does not necessarily preclude the use of TBI in the preparation for BMT. However, some caution needs to be exercised for patients who will be undergoing BMT after suffering a CNS relapse. Usually, it is unnecessary to reirradiate the patients' brain or to irradiate the spinal cord prior to BMT because this approach usually leads to more toxicity. In general, these patients can be managed with either intrathecal methotrexate or the combination of methotrexate, ara-C, and hydrocortisone until there is clearing of the leukemic cells from the spinal fluid. Following BMT, these patients receive 5 intrathecal methotrexate injections during the first 100 days followed by one monthly methotrexate injection for 18 months. This approach, designed in Seattle, can result in control of the leukemia without substantially increasing the risk of leukoencephalopathy. The risk of CNS damage caused by cranial radiation, intrathecal chemotherapy, and high-dose chemotherapy has been documented and is related to the amount of intrathecal chemotherapy following the BMT procedure (67). Currently, our approach for patients undergoing their first induction without any evidence of CNS disease is to administer intrathecal methotrexate as prophylaxis for a total of 5 times prior to the BMT procedure. Cranial radiation is not necessary if patients receive a preparatory regimen containing fractionated TBI.

Biological Therapy Following BMT

As described, despite the use of allogeneic BMT in patients with advanced disease to attain a cure, many patients still relapse. In general, methods to improve the results of this therapy in such patients have focused primarily on changes in the preparatory regimen and modification of GVHD prophylaxis. Some investigators have noted the potential use of biological therapy following BMT either to enhance an already present graft-versus-leukemia effect or to exploit the direct antileukemic activity of the biological agent. Two studies have examined the possibility of administering interferon after BMT (68,69). A study from Seattle indicated that the relapse rate for patients receiving interferon appears to be decreased, without a concomitant increase in GVHD (69). A prospective randomized trial utilizing interferon in the post-transplant setting addressing the issue of leukemia relapse is underway.

The only interleukin so far to receive consideration for use as a immunomodulator following BMT is interleukin-2. When used in autologous patients, there does not appear to be a negative effect on engraftment (70); however, exacerbation of GVHD remains a serious concern.

Conclusions

As we enter the third decade of clinical BMT for ALL, remarkable strides have been made in understanding the biology and characteristic features of the disease. This understanding allows for more informed decision-making for the patient who suffers from this disease. Concurrently, significant improvements have occurred with clinical care of patients. BMT now provides a curative potential for a large number of patients in various stages of this disease. Continued basic research will result in enhanced knowledge of the underlying disease and the physiology of the host tolerance toward BMT. With this knowledge, more specific and less toxic therapies will be available for these patients. This third decade will demonstrate how effective and how much more improvement can be achieved in the care of patients with ALL.

References

1. Bennett JM, Catousky D, Daniel MT. Proposals for the classification of acute leukemias. Br J Haematol 1976;33:451–457.

2. Brearley RL, Johnson S, Lister TA. Acute lymphoblastic leukemia in adults: clincopathological correlations with the French-American-British (FAB) cooperative group classification. Eur J Cancer 1979;15:909–914.
3. Foon KA, TR. Immunologic classification of leukemia and lymphoma. Blood 1986;68:1–31.
4. Greaves MF, Lister TA. Prognostic importance of immunologic markers in adult acute lymphoblastic leukemia. N Engl J Med 1981;304:119–120.
5. Korsmeyer SJ, Hilter P, Ravetch JV, et al. Developmental hierarchy of immunoglobulin gene rearrangements in human leukemia pre-B cells. Proc Natl Acad Sci USA 1981;78:7096–7100.
6. Korsmeyer SJ, Arnold A, Bakhshi A, et al. Immunoglobulin gene rearrangement and cell surface antigen expression in acute lymphocytic leukemias of T cell and B cell precursor origins. J Clin Invest 1983;71:301–313.
7. Vogler LB, Crist W, Bockman DE, et al. Pre-B-cell leukemia. A new phenotype of childhood lymphoblastic leukemia. N Engl J Med 1978;298:872–878.
8. Mirro J, Zipf T, Pui CH. Acute mixed lineage leukemia: clinicopathologic correlations and prognostic significance. Blood 1985;66:1115–1123.
9. Sobol RE, Mick R, Royston I, et al. Clinical importance of myeloid antigen expression in adult acute lymphoblastic leukemia. N Engl J Med 1987;316:1111–1117.
10. Schiffer C. Hybrid leukemias. In: Gale RP, Hoelzer D, eds. Acute lymphoblastic leukemia. New York: Wiley-Liss, 1990:129–142.
11. Norton JD, Campana D, Hoffbrand AV, et al. Rearrangement of immunoglobulin and T cell antigen receptor genes in acute myeloid leukemia with lymphoid-associated markers. Leukemia 1987;1:757–761.
12. Michael PM, Levin MD, Garson OM. Translocation 1;19—a new cytogenetic abnormality in acute lymphocytic leukemia. Cancer Genet Cytogenet 1984;12: 333–341.
13. Bloomfield CD, Lindquist L, Brunning RD, et al. The Philadelphia chromosome in acute leukemia. Virchows Arch [B] 1978;29:81–91.
14. Rodenhuis S, Slater RM, Behrendt H, Veerman AJP. Distinguishing the Philadelphia chromosome of acute lymphoblastic leukemia from its counterpart in chronic myelogenous leukemia (letter). N Engl J Med 1985; 313:51.
15. Arthur DC, Bloomfield CD, Lindquist LL, Nesbit ME. Translocation 4;11 in acute lymphoblastic leukemia: clinical characteristics and prognostic significance. Blood 1982;59:96–99.
16. Levin MD, Michael PM, Garson OM, et al. Clinicpathological characteristics of acute lymphoblastic leukemia with the 4;11 chromosome translocation. Pathology 1984;16:63–66.
17. Mitelman F, Andersson-Anvret M, Brandt L, et al. Reciprocal 8;14 translocation in EBV-negative B-cell acute lymphocytic leukemia with Burkitt-type cells. Int J Cancer 1979;24:27–33.
18. Berger R, Bernheim A. Cytogenetic studies in Burkitt's lymphoma-leukemia. Cancer Genet Cytogenet 1982;7: 231–244.
19. Michael PM, Garcon OM, Ekert H, et al. A prospective study of childhood acute lymphocytic leukemia: hematologic, immunologic, and cytogenetic correlations. Med Pediatr Oncol 1988;14:153–161.
20. Magrath IT, Ziegler JL. Bone marrow involvement in Burkitt's lymphoma and its relationship to acute B-cell leukemia. Leuk Res 1979;4:33–59.
21. Greaves MF, Janossy G, Peto J, et al. Immunologically defined subclasses of acute lymphoblastic leukemia in children. Their relationship to presentation features and prognosis. Br J Haematol 1981;48:179–195.
22. Bitran JD. Prognostic value of immunologic markers in adults with acute lymphoblastic leukemia (letter). N Engl J Med 1978;299:1317.
23. Clarkson B, Ellis S, Little C, et al. Acute lymphoblastic leukemia in adults. Semin Oncol 1985;12:160–179.
24. Hoelzer D, Gale RP. Acute lymphoblastic leukemia in adults: recent progress, future directions. Semin Hematol 1987;24:27–39.
25. Hoelzer D, Thiel E, Loffler H, et al. Prognostic factors in a multicenter study for treatment of acute lymphoblastic leukemia in adults. Blood 1988;71:123–131.
26. Hoelzer D, Thiel E, Loffler H, et al. Intensified therapy in acute lymphoblastic and acute undifferentiated leukemia in adults. Blood 1984;64:38–47.
27. Reaman G, Zeltzer P, Bleyer WA, et al. Acute lymphoblastic leukemia in infants less than one year of age: a cumulative experience of the Children's Cancer Study Group. J Clin Oncol 1985;3:1513–1521.
28. Marcus RE, Catovsky D, Johnson SA, et al. Adult acute lymphoblastic leukemia: a study of prognostic features and response to treatment over a ten year period. Br J Cancer 1986;53:175–180.
29. Bloomfield CD, Goldman AL, Alimena G, et al. Chromosomal abnormalities identify high-risk and low-risk patients with acute lymphoblastic leukemia. Blood 1986;67:415–420.
30. Fefer A, Einstein AB, Thomas ED, et al. Bone marrow transplantation for hematologic neoplasia in 16 patients with identical twins. N Engl J Med 1974;290: 1389–1393.
31. Thomas ED, Buchner CD, Banaji M, et al. One hundred patients with acute leukemia treated by chemotherapy, total body irradiation, and allogeneic marrow transplantation. Blood 1977;49:511–533.
32. Thomas ED, Sanders JE, Flournoy N, et al. Marrow transplantation for patients with acute lymphoblastic leukemia in remission. Blood 1979;54:468–476.
33. Baccarani M, Corbelli G, Amadori S, al. Adolescent and adult acute lymphoblastic leukemia: prognostic features and outcome of therapy. A study of 293 patients. Blood 1982;60:677–684.
34. Barnett MJ, Greaves ML, Amess JAL, et al. Treatment of acute lymphoblastic leukemia in adults. Br J Haematol 1986;64:455–468.
35. Gottlieb AJ, Weinberg V, Ellison RR, et al. Efficacy of daunorubicin in the therapy of adult acute lymphoblastic leukemia. A prospective randomized trial by Cancer and Leukemia Group B. Blood 1984;64:267–274.
36. Gaynor J, Chapman D, Little C, et al. A cause-specific hazard rate analysis of prognostic factors among 199 adults with acute lymphoblastic leukemia: the Memorial Hospital experience since 1969. J Clin Oncol 1988;6:1014–1030.
37. Hussein KK, Dahlberg S, Head D, et al. (Southwest Oncology Group). Treatment of acute lymphoblastic leukemia in adults with intensive induction consolidation and maintenance chemotherapy. Blood 1989;73: 57–63.
38. Kantarjian HM, Walters RS, Keating MJ, et al. Results of the vincristine, doxorubicin, and dexamethasone regimen in adults with standard- and high-risk acute lymphocytic leukemia. J Clin Oncol 1990;8:994–1004.
39. Dinsmore R, Kirkpatrick D, Flomenberg N, Gulati S,

Shank B, O'Reilly RJ. Allogeneic marrow transplantation for acute lymphoblastic leukemia in remission: the importance of early transplantation. Transplant Proc 1983;15:1397–1400.

40. Wingard JR, Piantadosi S, Santos GW, et al. Allogeneic bone marrow transplantation for patients with high-risk acute lymphoblastic leukemia. J Clin Oncol 1990;8:820–830.
41. Van Lint M, Bacigalupo A, Frassoni F, et al. Bone marrow transplantation (BMT) for acute lymphoblastic leukemia (ALL) in remission. Haematology 1986;71: 135–138.
42. Barrett A, Dendra JR, Lucas CF, et al. Bone marrow transplantation for acute lymphoblastic leukemia. Br J Hematol 1982;52:181–188.
43. Doney K, Fisher LD, Appelbaum FR, et al. Treatment of adult acute lymphoblastic leukemia with allogeneic bone marrow transplantation. Multivariate analysis of factors affecting acute graft-versus-host disease, relapse, and relapse-free survival. Bone Marrow Transplant 1991;7:453–459.
44. Schmitz N, Gassman W, Rister M, et al. Fractionated total body irradiation and high dose VP16–213 followed by allogeneic bone marrow transplantation in advanced leukemias. Blood 1988;72:1567–1573.
45. Rivera GK. Therapeutic options for children with acute lymphocytic leukemia who fail on contemporary protocols. In: Gale RP, Champlin RE, eds. Bone marrow transplantation. Current controversies. New York: Alan R. Liss, 1989:31–45.
46. Chessells JM, Rodgers DM, Leiper AD, et al. Bone marrow transplantation has a limited role in prolonging second marrow remission in childhood lymphoblastic leukemia. Lancet 1986;1:1239–1241.
47. Bordigoni P, Vernant J, Souillet G, et al. Allogeneic bone marrow transplantation for children with acute lymphoblastic leukemia in first remission: a cooperative study of the groupe d'etude de la greffe de moelle osseuse. J Clin Oncol 1989;7:747–753.
48. Brochstein JA, Kernan NA, Groshen S, et al. Allogeneic bone marrow transplantation after hyperfractionated total-body irradiation and cyclophosphamide in children with acute leukemia. N Engl J Med 1987;317: 1618–1624.
49. Dopfer R, Henze G, Bender-Goetze C, et al. Allogeneic bone marrow transplantation for childhood acute lymphoblastic leukemia in second remission after intensive primary and relapse therapy according to the BFM- and CoALL-protocols: results of the German Cooperative Study. Blood 1991;78:2780–2784.
50. Coccia PF, Strandjord SE, Warkentin PI, et al. High-dose cytosine arabinoside and fractionated total-body irradiation: an improved preparative regimen for bone marrow transplantation of children with acute lymphoblastic leukemia in remission. Blood 1988;71:888–893.
51. Sanders JE, Thomas ED, Buckner CD, Doney K. Marrow transplantation for children with acute lymphoblastic leukemia in second remission. Blood 1987; 70:324–326.
52. Torres A, Martinez F, Gomez P, et al. Allogeneic bone marrow transplantation versus chemotherapy in the treatment of childhood acute lymphoblastic leukemia in second complete remission. Bone Marrow Transplant 1989;4:609–612.
53. Woods W, Nesbit ME, Ramsay NK, et al. Intensive therapy followed by bone marrow transplantation for patients with acute lymphocytic leukemia in second or subsequent remission: determination of prognostic factors (a report from the University of Minnesota Bone Marrow Transplantation Team). Blood 1983;61: 1182–1189.
54. Chao NJ, Forman SJ, Schmidt GM, et al. Allogeneic bone marrow transplantation for high-risk acute lymphoblastic leukemia during first complete remission. Blood 1991;78:1923–1927.
55. Blaise D, Gaspard AM, Stoppa AM, et al. Allogeneic or autologous bone marrow transplantation for acute lymphoblastic leukemia in first complete remission. Bone Marrow Transplant 1990;5:7–12.
56. Zwaan FE, Hermans J, Barrett AJ, Speck B. Bone marrow transplantation for acute lymphoblastic leukaemia: a survey of the European Group for Bone Marrow Transplantation (E.G.B.M.T.). Br J Haematol 1984;58: 33–42.
57. Ramsay NKC, Kersey JH. Indications for marrow transplantation in acute lymphoblastic leukemia. Blood 1990;75:815–818.
58. Appelbaum FR, Clift RA, Buckner CD, et al. Allogeneic marrow transplantation for acute nonlymphoblastic leukemia after first relapse. Blood 1983;61:949–953.
59. Blume KG. Marrow transplantation for acute lymphoblastic leukemia: new preparatory regimens. In: Gale RP, Champlin RE, eds. Bone marrow transplantation. Current controversies. New York: Alan R. Liss, 1989: 47–56.
60. Champlin R, Jacobs A, Gale RP, et al. High-dose cytarabine in consolidation chemotherapy or with bone marrow transplantation for patients with acute leukemia: preliminary results. Semin Oncol 1985;12: 190–195.
61. Forman SJ. Allogeneic marrow transplantation for acute lymphoblastic leukemia. In: Champlin RE, Gale RP, eds. New strategies in bone marrow transplantation. New York: Wiley-Liss, 1991:119–130.
62. Tutschka PJ, Copelan EA, Klein JP. Bone marrow transplantation for leukemia following a new busulfan and cyclophosphamide regimen. Blood 1987;70:1382–1388.
63. Santos GW, Tutschka PJ, Brookmeyer R, et al. Marrow transplantation for acute nonlymphocytic leukemia after treatment with busulfan and cyclophosphamide. N Engl J Med 1983;309:1347–1353.
64. Blume KG, Forman SJ, O'Donnell MR, et al. Total body irradiation and high-dose etoposide: a new preparatory regimen for bone marrow transplantation in patients with advanced hematologic malignancies. Blood 1987; 69:1015–1020.
65. Barrett AJ, Horowitz MM, Ash RC, et al. Bone marrow transplantation for Philadelphia chromosome positive acute lymphoblastic leukemia. Blood 1992;79:3067–3070.
66. Forman SJ, O'Donnell M, Nademanee AP, et al. Bone marrow transplantation for patients with Philadelphia chromosome-positive acute lymphoblastic leukemia versus intensification chemotherapy for acute myelogenous leukaemia in first remission: a prospective controlled trial. Br J Haematol 1988;68:219–226.
67. Thompson CB, Sanders JE, Flournoy N, Buckner CD, Thomas ED. The risks of central nervous system relapse and leukoencephalopathy in patients receiving marrow transplants for acute leukemia. Blood 1986;67:195–199.
68. Klingemann H-G, Grigg AP, Wilkie-Boyd, K, et al. Treatment with recombinant interferon (a-2b) early after bone marrow transplantation in patients at high risk for relapse. Blood 1991;78:3306–3311.

69. Meyers JD, Flournoy N, Sanders JE, et al. Prophylactic use of human leukocyte interferon after allogeneic marrow transplantation. Ann Intern Med 1987;107:809–816.
70. Blaise D, Olive D, Stoppa AM, et al. Hematologic and immunologic effects of the systemic administration of recombinant interleukin-2 after autologous bone marrow transplantation. Blood 1990;76:1092–1097.
71. Blume KG, Forman SJ, Krance RA, Henke M, Findley DO, Hill LR. Bone marrow transplantation for acute leukemia. Hematology and Blood Transfusion 1985;29:39–41.
72. Frassoni F, Bacigalupo A, Van Lint MT, et al. Bone marrow transplantation versus chemotherapy for patients under 15 years of age in 2nd remission acute lymphoblastic leukemia (ALL). Exp Hematol 1985;13 (suppl 17):41–42.
73. McCarthy DM, Barett AJ, MacDonald D, et al. Bone marrow transplantation for adults and children with poor risk acute lymphoblastic leukemia in first complete remission. Bone Marrow Transplant 1988;3:315–322.
74. Vernant JP, Marit G, Maraninchi D, et al. Allogeneic bone marrow transplantation in adults with acute lymphoblastic leukemia in first complete remission. J Clin Oncol 1988;6:227–231.

Chapter 47

Allogeneic Bone Marrow Transplantation for Myelodysplastic and Myeloproliferative Disorders

Frederick R. Appelbaum

The myelodysplastic and myeloproliferative disorders include a wide spectrum of clonal hematopoietic diseases. The major distinction between the myelodysplastic and myeloproliferative diseases is that in myelodysplasia, clonal proliferation is generally ineffective, resulting in the development of progressive pancytopenias, whereas in the myeloproliferative disorders, increased peripheral counts are the rule, at least until the disease enters its terminal phase. Recently, as our understanding of normal hematopoiesis has increased, so too has our understanding of this group of disorders. One important insight came with the demonstration that these disorders all arise from neoplastic transformation at a level of differentiation close to, if not identical with, the hematopoietic stem cell, so that myeloid cells, platelets, red cells, B and even T lymphocytes often derive from the same altered clone (1–3). This observation may explain why these disorders are incurable with conventional therapies. Only with complete eradication of the marrow and replacement using marrow from a normal donor have cures been achieved. However, the recent gains in knowledge of hematopoiesis have also led to a number of nontransplant treatment strategies, including the use of low-dose chemotherapy, differentiating agents, and hematopoietic growth factors, which, although not curative, have proven to be of benefit for some patients. Given this increased number of treatment options, optimal management of any patient, and particularly the appropriate use of bone marrow transplantation (BMT) in these disorders, requires an understanding of the natural history of these specific syndromes, as well as up-to-date knowledge of the results obtainable with each intervention. In this chapter, these points are discussed from the particular point of view of BMT. For a more complete discussion of the pathophysiology of each of these disorders, readers are referred to a number of excellent reviews (4–8) or to any of the standard textbooks of hematology.

Myelodysplasia

Disease Definition

The myelodysplastic syndrome (MDS) includes a group of clonal hematopoietic disorders characterized by impaired maturation of hematopoietic cells and development of progressive peripheral cytopenias. The French American British (FAB) Cooperative Group recognizes 5 distinct forms of pathology in MDS: (1) refractory anemia (RA), (2) refractory anemia with ringed sideroblasts (RARS), (3) refractory anemia with excess blasts (RAEB), (4) refractory anemia with excess blasts in transformation (RAEB-t), and (5) chronic myelomonocytic leukemia (CMMoL) (Table 47-1) (9–11). This classification system is used widely and has been of considerable benefit in making sense of these closely related disorders, but it can be criticized on 2 counts. First, it ignores the syndrome of hypoplastic myelodysplasia, which should

Table 47-1.
Classification of Myelodysplastic Syndrome by the FAB Cooperative Group

Classification	*% Marrow Blasts*	*% Peripheral Blood Blasts*	*Ringed Sideroblasts > 15% of Bone Marrow*	*Monocytes > 1,000/μL*
Refractory anemia	< 5	≤ 1	−	−
Refractory anemia with ringed sideroblasts	< 5	≤ 1	+	−
Refractory anemia with excess blasts	5–20	< 5	−/+	−
Refractory anemia with excess blasts in transition	20–30	> 5	−/+	−/+
Chronic myelomonocytic leukemia	≤ 20	< 5	−/+	+

FAB = French American British Classification.
+= always present; − = always absent; −/+ = variable.

be included; and second, it includes the syndrome of CMMoL which some have argued might be placed more appropriately in the myeloproliferative group of diseases.

RA, RARS, RAEB, and RAEB-t have common features, and it is not unusual for a patient's disease to progress from one category to the next. Common to all subtypes are dysplastic features of the marrow, including dyserythropoiesis often with ringed sideroblasts, dysgranulopoiesis with hypogranulation, and dysmegakaryocytopoiesis with micromegakaryocytes. Even experienced pathologists often will not agree on the exact subtype of MDS in a given patient.

Clinical and Laboratory Features

In the past, MDS has been considered to be a relatively rare disease, with a reported incidence of approximately 1 per 100,000 per year. However, recent studies suggest a much higher incidence, particularly if mild forms of the disease are included; in one screening study of elderly patients, an incidence of 1 per 1,000 in persons over age 55 was found (12). The disease is much more common in the elderly, with a median onset above age 60. Although uncommon in the young, MDS can occur in children. Most cases arise de novo, but MDS occurring 4 to 5 years after prior chemotherapy for Hodgkin's disease or other cancers is a well-recognized phenomenon. Patients often have no symptoms referable to MDS, whereas others present with fatigue and weakness. Splenomegaly is found in less than 20% of patients, and other findings on physical examination are usually absent.

The laboratory findings dictate the subcategory of MDS. In RA, anemia is invariably seen, and the reticulocyte count is usually low. Peripheral blood granulocytes and platelets may be normal or diminished. Leukemic blasts are rarely seen in the periphery and make up less than 5% of marrow cells. RARS has features essentially identical to RA, except that ringed sideroblasts make up 15% or more of the marrow cellularity. In RAEB, blasts make up from 5 to 20% of the marrow cells and can comprise up to 5% of the peripheral white blood cell count (WBC). Thrombocytopenia is common. RAEB-t is similar to RAEB, but the blast count is more than 5% in the peripheral blood or above 20% but less than 30% in the marrow. If greater than 30% blasts are seen in the marrow, the diagnosis of acute myelogenous leukemia (AML) is made. CMMoL shows features similar to RAEB, but the circulating monocyte count must be greater than 1,000/μL.

A clonal chromosomal abnormality is seen in 40 to 60% of patients. The most common abnormalities are loss of part or all of chromosome 7, trisomy 8, isochromosome 17, 5q-, and 20q-. These abnormalities are also seen in some patients with AML and in that setting are associated with a poor prognosis. Of interest, some chromosomal abnormalities seen in patients with AML, such as t(8:21), t(15:17), and inv(16), are almost never seen in patients with MDS, and in patients with AML are associated with a relatively favorable prognosis.

Natural History

If the major form of therapy is supportive care, the prognosis for patients with MDS is extremely variable. Some patients will survive for very long periods, whereas others will die within the first year from diagnosis. The FAB classification schema has prognostic significance in that patients with RA or RARS survive longer than patients with RAEB or RAEB-t. Several recent studies examining prognostic factors in large numbers of patients identified the most important clinical variables for predicting survival to be percent of blasts in marrow, extent of neutropenia, and degree of thrombocytopenia (13–15). Thus, although some patients enjoy prolonged survival after diagnosis, the median survival for patients with MDS is less than one year if there are more than 10% blasts in the marrow, platelets are less than 40,000/μL, or granulocytes are less than 1,000/μL. The Bournemouth scoring system is a simple system that gives one point for each of the following: hemoglobin below 10 gm/dL, granulocytes below 2,500/μL, platelets below 100,000/μL, and bone marrow blast count above 5% (16). As shown in Figure 47-1, the median survival for patients with a score of 0 or one is almost 5 years, but it is less than 2 years for patients with a score of 2 or 3 and less than one year for patients with a score of 4. Although it is still uncertain whether patients with primary MDS behave differently than patients with MDS secondary to previous exposure to chemotherapy, most experience suggests that patients with secondary MDS have a modestly worse prognosis, stage for stage (17).

Death in patients with MDS is usually due either to disease progression to AML or to the complications of pancytopenia. Patients with RAEB and RAEB-t have a much higher likelihood of progressing to AML with an incidence of 35 to 65% within 2 years of diagnosis, compared with an incidence of 5 to 10% for patients with RA. Infection and hemorrhage associated with low peripheral blood counts are the most common

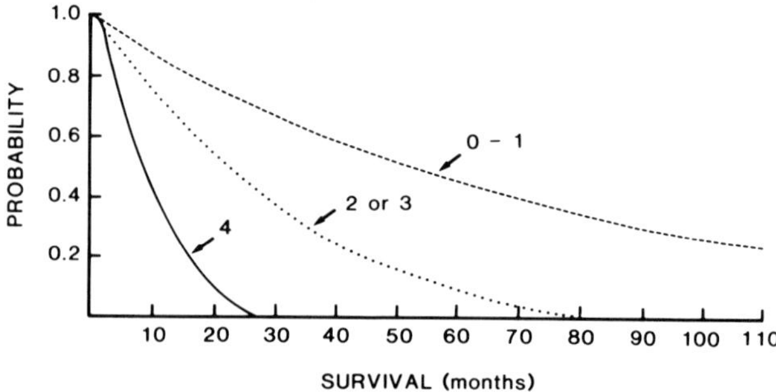

Figure 47-1. Survival of patients with myelodysplastic syndrome categorized using the Bournemouth scoring system (16).

causes of death in MDS, accounting for 35 to 50% of all deaths. Because this is a disease of the elderly, nonhematological deaths are also seen and account for 10 to 20% of deaths.

Nontransplant Therapies

Hormonal Therapy

An occasional patient with MDS will respond to treatment with corticosteroids, and, in one study, these responses correlated with increased colony growth in vitro with the addition of steroids to patients' cultures (18). However, responses to glucocorticoids are uncommon, and given the increased risk of infection with these agents, glucocorticoids should not be used routinely in the treatment of MDS. Androgens have also been studied, but in a randomized trial were shown to be of no benefit (19). Danazol, a synthetic androgen with activity in immune thrombocytopenia, has been reported to improve platelet counts in approximately 25% of patients with MDS, moderate thrombocytopenia, and fewer than 20% marrow blasts (20). Although the mechanism of danazol's activity is uncertain, a decrease in monocyte Fc-receptor numbers was seen, suggesting that danazol may reverse accelerated platelet clearance.

Differentiating Agents

The demonstration that various compounds can induce myeloid differentiation in vitro led to testing similar agents in patients with MDS. Among this group, 13-cis retinoic acid is the most extensively studied. Results from clinical Phase I to II trials indicate apparent responses in approximately 20% of patients and also noted hepatic and dermatological toxicity that limited patient compliance. Two prospective randomized trials of 13-cis retinoic acid in patients with MDS have been reported (21,22). Complete hematological responses were seen in neither study, and there was no improvement in either progression-free or overall survival. Recent studies in acute promyelocytic leukemia suggest that all trans-retinoic acid may be a more effective differentiating agent than cis retinoic acid, although reasons for this possible difference are not apparent. All transretinoic acid has not been widely studied in MDS, but trials are now in progress.

Trials of other differentiating agents have been negative or are too preliminary to allow conclusions. Although there is substantial experience with low-dose cytarabine, this agent almost certainly works as a cytotoxic agent and is not a differentiating agent.

Hematopoietic Growth Factors

Hematopoietic growth factors have been studied extensively in patients with MDS. This activity has been fueled by the hope that hematopoietic growth factors might increase normal counts in pancytopenic patients, both by stimulating normal cell growth and by inducing abnormal progenitors to differentiate more normally. Both of these activities have been documented in patients with MDS, but the extent and duration of such responses have been limited. The two most studied agents have been granulocyte-macrophage colony stimulating factor (GM-CSF) and, to a lesser extent, granulocyte colony stimulating factor (G-CSF). A summary of 5 Phase I to II studies suggests that when given to patients with MDS, GM-CSF results in an increase in granulocyte counts in approximately 75% of patients (23–27). Improvements in other cell lineages are less common, but 15% of patients will show an increase in platelet counts and decreased red-cell transfusion requirement. Hematological responses are usually limited in their duration to less than 6 months. A multi-institutional randomized trial of GM-CSF has been completed and reported in preliminary form and appears to confirm the results of the Phase I to II trials (Seigel R. Personal communication). Although not as extensively studied, G-CSF appears to provide responses in patients with MDS with a frequency and duration very similar to that of GM-CSF (28,29). As with GM-CSF, G-CSF does not provide a consistent platelet response. Two small studies of interleukin-3 (IL-3) have been reported, which suggest that IL-3 also can result in granulocyte elevations, has at best an inconsistent effect on platelets, and has considerable toxicity (30,31). None of these myeloid growth factors delay the progression to AML, and, in fact, a concern with their use is the possible stimulation of malignant progenitors. In some individuals, the percentage of marrow blasts has increased with the use of GM-CSF or G-CSF. This effect has been seen more commonly in patients with more than 15% blasts and has usually, but not always, been reversible with discontinuation of the growth factor.

Erythropoietin (EPO) has been studied in patients with low-risk MDS, usually RA or RARS, whose major problem is anemia. Most of these patients had high endogenous EPO levels, but with high doses of exogenous EPO, 20% either became red-cell transfusion–independent or had a decreased need for transfusions (32).

Chemotherapy

Chemotherapeutic approaches to MDS have ranged from low-dose single-agent therapy to the aggressive multiagent regimens used in the treatment of AML. The original rationale for the use of low-dose cytarabine was that it induces differentiation of human leukemic cell lines in culture. Over the past decade, a number of mostly anecdotal reports of the use of cytarabine administered for 7 to 21 days at 20 mg/m^2, either subcutaneously or by continuous infusion, have been published (33,34). These reports have been summarized recently by Cheson and associates (35). The complete response rate was 16% and another 20% of patients had minor responses. Moderate to severe myelosuppression developed in virtually all patients following the use of cytarabine, demonstrating that if low-dose cytarabine works, it does so by a cytotoxic and not a differentiating effect. Furthermore, 10% of patients died from treatment-related causes, demonstrating the substantial risk with this therapy. Recently, a trial was completed in which patients were randomized to low-dose cytarabine or supportive care only (36). Similar to the previously published trials, only 8% of treated patients achieved a complete response, and there was no discernible difference in survival between the treated and control groups. When examined by FAB classification, responses were least common in patients with RA or RARS; in these patients, low-dose cytarabine probably negatively influenced survival. In patients with RAEB or RAEB-t, responses were more common and there was at least a trend toward improved survival.

Intensive AML-like combination chemotherapies for patients with MDS using cytarabine plus anthracyclines have been the subject of a number of studies (37). Complete response (CR) rates in these studies have averaged approximately 40% and have ranged from as low as 13% to as high as 52%. In general, the highest CR rates were seen in younger patients with primary MDS who had not received previous therapy. The average duration of complete response in these studies was consistently less than 12 months. When compared with results in patients with de novo AML, intensive chemotherapy of MDS results in a lower CR rate and shorter remission duration. Treatment-related deaths are more frequent, in part because there is a significantly longer interval between chemotherapy and granulocyte recovery and a higher frequency of regenerative failure. Furthermore, there is a higher incidence of drug resistance, in some cases associated with increased expression of the multidrug resistance phenotype.

Bone Marrow Transplantation

Allogeneic BMT was initially attempted in the treatment of patients with MDS based on the incurability of the disease with conventional measures and the observation that BMT could cure patients with other forms of incurable hematological malignancies. As shown in Table 47-2, there are now at least 7 publications detailing the outcome of allogeneic BMT in the treatment of patients with MDS (38–44). In addition, an eighth publication summarizes registry data but may include many of the patients reported in the other 7 primary articles (45). The 3-year event-free survival in these 7 studies ranges from 40 to 67%; many patients are alive without evidence of disease for longer than 5 years after transplant and some as far from transplant as 15 years. Results from Seattle are representative of most studies and are shown in Figure 47-2. The long-term disease-free survival in these studies offers strong evidence that MDS is curable with BMT.

Table 47-2.
Primary Reports of Bone Marrow Transplantation for Myelodysplastic Syndrome

Authors, Ref	*No. Patients*	*Preparative Regimen*	*% Transplant-related Mortality*	*Event-free Survival (%)*
Appelbaum (38)	59	CY/TBI	39	45
Longmore (39)	23	Ara-C/CY/TBI BCV	35	43
O'Donnell (40)	20	Ara-C/CY/TBI BU/CY VP16/TBI	45	40
Bélanger (41)	8	CY/TBI BU/CY	25	50
Kolb (42)	7	CY/TBI	38	50
Bunin (43)	6	BU/CY/Ara-C/TBI	33	50
Tricot (44)	7	Ara-C/CY/TBI	29	67

CY/TBI = cyclophosphamide plus total body irradiation; ara-C = cytosine arabinoside; BCV = carmustine, CY, etoposide; BU/CY = bulsufan plus CY; VP16/TBI = etoposide plus TBI.

Treatment failure after BMT is due mainly to transplant-related complications, including interstitial pneumonia and graft-versus-host disease (GVHD), as well as disease recurrence. In the 7 studies cited, death from transplant-related complications occurred in 25 to 45% of patients. This incidence is somewhat higher than reported in other transplant settings and may reflect the older age and the prior therapy of these patients. In most of the reports, younger age and shorter time from diagnosis to transplant were two prognostic factors impacting on nonmalignant deaths but not on relapse rates.

Relapse has been another important reason for treatment failure. The likelihood of relapse after transplantation is dependent on the FAB classification. None of 23 patients reported by the Seattle group and none of the 9 patients summarized by the European Transplant Registry who were transplanted for RA or RARS have relapsed after transplantation (38,45). In contrast, relapse rates for patients transplanted for RAEB or RAEB-t have ranged from 25 to 44% in the larger studies.

Although available results demonstrate that MDS is curable with BMT, a substantial number of questions remain, including the choice of preparative regimen, the possibility of extending the source of donor marrow, and the overall place of BMT in the management of patients with MDS. As noted in Table 47-2, a variety of preparative regimens has been employed in the treatment of MDS, and although few firm conclusions can be drawn, several principles seem evident. First, preparative regimens that include cyclophosphamide (CY) alone, such as used in the treatment of aplastic anemia, seem inadequate to eradicate the malignant clone (46). The largest experience has been with CY plus 12 Gy total body irradiation (TBI). This

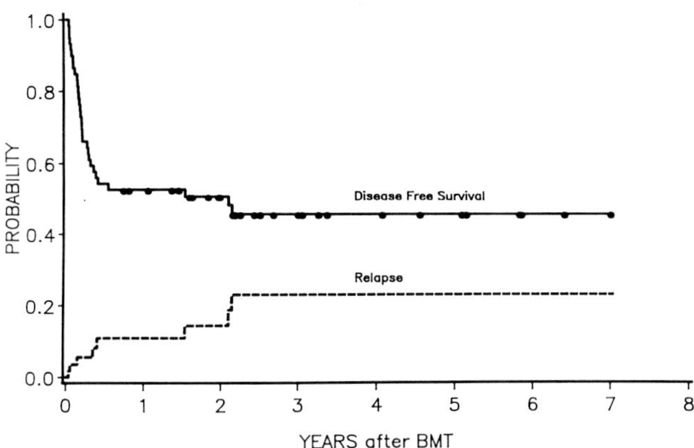

Figure 47-2. Probability of disease-free survival and relapse among 59 patients transplanted in Seattle for myelodysplasia. *Solid circles* represent patients alive in complete remission (39).

regimen appears to be an excellent choice for patients with RA or RARS. For patients with RAEB or RAEB-t, relapse is common with CY plus 12 Gy TBI; therefore, more aggressive regimens using, for example, higher doses of TBI or additional chemotherapy might be considered. A combination of busulfan (BU) (16 mg/kg) and CY (120 mg/kg), similar to that used in the treatment of AML, has also been studied in MDS. Whether this regimen is as good as or better than CY plus 12 Gy TBI for patients with less advanced MDS (i.e., RA, RARS) is unknown. For some patients, such as those who have already received dose-limiting radiotherapy for a prior malignancy, BU/CY would seem to be a very reasonable alternative to CY/TBI. For patients with more aggressive forms of MDS (i.e., RAEB, RAEB-t), there is no evidence to suggest that BU/CY can lower relapse rates.

Because only approximately one-third of patients will have human leukoycte antigen (HLA)–identical family members to serve as marrow donors, alternative sources of marrow must be considered if BMT is to have a wider impact in MDS. As noted in Chapter 51, for most hematological malignancies, use of family member donors mismatched for a single antigen results in survival very similar to that seen using completely matched donors, whereas survival following BMT from family donors mismatched for two or more antigens is considerably worse (47). Although experience in the use of unrelated matched donors is still limited, it appears that survival will not be as good as with matched family member donors, owing to an increased incidence of GVHD and infection. There is only a very limited published experience with the use of partially matched or unrelated donors in the treatment of patients with MDS. This limited experience has been consistent with expectations based on results in other hematological malignancies; 3 of 6 patients transplanted for MDS with partially matched or unrelated donors survived in one study, and 6 of 14 survived in our study (38,43). There is almost no experience with autologous BMT in patients with MDS. Whether one could possibly isolate a pure population of normal hematopoietic progenitors from a frankly dysplastic marrow is unknown. Some patients with MDS treated with intensive chemotherapy enter a clinical complete remission, and some of these patients have undergone autologous BMT, but results are as yet quite preliminary.

Role of BMT in MDS

The appropriate place of BMT in the treatment of any individual patient with MDS requires consideration of the patient's disease status, age, and the source of marrow, at a minimum. As noted earlier, the natural history of MDS is extremely variable, but groups of patients can be identified with a median survival of less than one year, including those with more than 10% blasts in the marrow, less than 40,000 platelets/μL, or less than 1,000 granulocytes/μL. Given the otherwise incurable nature of MDS, BMT is certainly warranted for any such patient who is age 55 or less and for whom a suitable donor can be identified (i.e., an HLA-matched or single-antigen mismatched family member or matched unrelated donor). Extending the use of BMT for patients with less advanced myelodysplasia (i.e., those with a Bournemouth score of 2 or 3 who have a median survival without transplant of less than 2 years) is reasonable, particularly if patients are younger and have well-matched donors. For patients with RA or RARS who have no significant cytopenias other than anemia, it is difficult to justify the use of BMT until the patient shows evidence of disease progression to a more aggressive state. However, these patients require careful observation so that the opportunity to intervene with BMT when it becomes appropriate is not lost. The use of two or three antigen-mismatched donors for patients with MDS and the use of BMT in patients above age 55 are areas of active investigation appropriate for patients with high-risk disease.

Myeloproliferative Disorders

Disease Definition

The myeloproliferative disorders are a group of diseases that include chronic myeloid leukemia (CML), juvenile chronic myeloid leukemia (JCML), polycythemia vera (PV), essential thrombocytosis (ET), and agnogenic myeloid metaplasia with myelofibrosis (AMM). All these diseases are characterized by the slow but relentless progressive expansion of a clone of hematopoietic cells generally limited to a single myeloid lineage, and all these disorders frequently eventuate in a myeloid blast crisis similar to AML. Like the myelodysplastic syndromes, all of the myeloproliferative disorders appear to result from neoplastic transformation at the level of a multipotent or possibly pluripotent hematopoietic stem cell. One of the myeloproliferative disorders, CML, is dealt with in Chapters 44 and 56 and will not be discussed herein.

Polycythemia Vera

Clinical and Laboratory Features

PV is characterized by expansion of the total red-cell mass and is often accompanied by an increase in myelopoiesis, thrombopoiesis, and splenomegaly. The median age at onset is 60 years, but the disease can occur in patients as young as age 20. Patients usually present with symptoms related to an increase in blood volume and viscosity, most often with headache, weakness, pruritus, or dizziness. Circulatory disturbances of the central nervous system ranging from transient ischemia to stroke are the most dangerous presenting symptoms. Physical findings include facial rubor, conjunctival erythema, and splenomegaly, which is seen in 90% of patients. The hematocrit is elevated in virtually all patients unless bleeding or iron deficiency complicate the picture. Moderate leukocytosis (10,000–20,000 cells/μL) and thrombocytosis (400,000–800,000/μL) are common. Marrow hyperplasia, including not only erythroid hyperplasia but myeloid hyperplasia, is the rule. No specific chromosomal abnormality is associated with PV. In vitro cultures of marrow from patients with PV typically show autonomous growth of erythroid colonies. The distinction between PV and either secondary polycythemia or other myeloproliferative disorders is sometimes difficult; therefore, the National Polycythemia Vera Study Group has established criteria for the diagnosis of PV (Table 47-3).

Natural History and Nontransplant Therapies

Treatment of PV is palliative. In most patients, the initial objective of therapy is to reduce the hematocrit to normal levels using phlebotomies every other day or so. Phlebotomy alone does not control thrombocytosis and thrombotic complications; therefore some form of myelosuppressive therapy is advisable in most patients. In the past, BU was often used, but is no longer recommended because of the unpredictable severe marrow suppression sometimes seen, nonhematopoietic toxicities, and secondary AML. In the early 1980s, the PV Study Group conducted a large Phase III study comparing phlebotomy alone or combined with either chlorambucil or ^{32}P therapy (48). The phlebotomy alone arm proved the best, with a median survival of 12.7 years, compared with 8.8 years in the chlorambucil arm and 11.8 years in the ^{32}P arm. The reasons for excess deaths in the arms using myelosuppressive agents were mostly due to an excess incidence of AML. More recently, hydroxyurea at a dose of 15 mg/kg/day (individually adjusted) appears to yield excellent results.

No matter which initial therapy is chosen, patients will eventually fail treatment. Sometimes the disease progresses to a more aggressive myeloproliferative disorder, including AML, but more often a postpolycythemia myeloid metaplasia with progressive pancytopenia and splenic enlargement develop. In other patients, life-threatening thrombotic complications are the reason for treatment failure.

BMT

The role of BMT in PV is more hypothetical than realized. Given that PV is a disease of the hematopoietic stem cell, it should be curable with BMT, but given an average survival with conventional therapy of 10 years and the average age of onset of the disease of close to 60, BMT has been virtually untested as a treatment for PV. As shown in Table 47-4, we are aware of 3 patients who have undergone BMT, all of whom had eradication of their malignant clone and one of whom is reported to be surviving. Given the utility of BMT in other hematopoietic disorders, it appears reasonable to consider this approach in younger patients with appropriate donors who have failed first-line therapy with phlebotomy and hydroxyurea.

Table 47-3.
Clinical Characteristics of the Myeloproliferative Diseases

	Disease				
Characteristic	*CML*	*Polycythemia Vera*	*Essential Thrombocytosis*	*Myeloid Metaplasia with Myelofibrosis*	*JCML*
Hematocrit	Decreased	Increased	+/−	Decreased	Decreased
White cell count	Usually > 50,000	<25,000	<25,000	<25,000	>50,000
Differential	All stages, from promyelocytes to PMNs	WNL	WNL	Leukoerythroblastic smear	As in CML
Platelets	Normal or increased	Normal or increased	Dramatically increased	Normal increase or decrease	Decreased
Bone marrow	Myeloid hyperplasia	Myeloid and erythroid hyperplasia	Increased megakaryocytes	Fibrosis	See CML
Special studies	Ph chromosome	Increased RBC mass	...	...	Increased fetal Hgb

CML = chronic myelogenous leukemia; JCML = juvenile CML; PMNs = polymorphonuclear leukocytes; WNL = within normal limits; RBC = red blood cell; Hgb = hemoglobin.

Table 47-4.
Available Data on Bone Marrow Transplantation for Myeloproliferative Diseases[a]

Disease	*No. Patients*	*No. CR*	*No. Alive*	*Source*
Polycythemia vera	3	3	1	IBMTR-2, FHCRC-1
Essential thrombocythemia	3	3	0	IBMTR-2, FHCRC-1
AMM	10	7	4	IBMTR-2, FHCRC-6, other-2
JCML	14	14	6	FHCRC-14

[a]Data were obtained by conducting literature searches using MEDLINE and CANCERLIT, by review of the Fred Hutchinson Cancer Research Center (FHCRC) database, and with the generous assistance of D'Yetta Kosar and Mary Horowitz of the International Bone Marrow Transplant Registry (IBMTR) statistical center. The analysis has not been reviewed or approved by the Advisory Committee of the IBMTR.
AMM = agnogenic myeloid metaplasia; JCML = juvenile chronic myelogenous leukemia.

Essential Thrombocythemia

Clinical and Laboratory Features

Essential (or primary) thrombocythemia (ET) is the least common of the myeloproliferative disorders and is characterized by the isolated expansion of the megakaryocytic lineage. Although seen in all age groups, the average age at diagnosis is in the 50s. The most common presenting symptoms involved thromboembolic events both of the microcirculation and of large vessels. Other cases are diagnosed serendipitously during evaluation of other diseases. Physical examination is relatively unremarkable, but in 40 to 50% of patients, splenomegaly is detected, and in 20%, hepatomegaly is found. The hallmark of the disease is an increased platelet count, usually above 600,000/μL. The increased platelet count is accompanied by hyperplasia of marrow megakaryocytes, absence of the Ph chromosome, increased red-cell mass, or increased marrow fibrosis. In virtually all patients, thrombocythemic platelets function abnormally. They are relatively resistant to the aggregating effects of epinephrine and they are also relatively unresponsive to the inhibitory effects of prostaglandin D. Thus, it is not surprising that both excessive thrombosis and increased bleeding can be found in association with ET. Curiously, reduction of platelet counts to normal in the thrombocythemic patients can reverse both problems.

Natural History and Nontransplant Therapies

Previous studies have estimated that 65 to 75% of patients with ET will survive 10 years from diagnosis. Most deaths were due to thrombotic complications, many of which were sudden and unpredictable. Transformation to AML is seen in 10 to 15% of patients. The blasts in these patients may be of either myeloid or megakaryocytic morphology. Therapy of patients with ET and life-threatening hemorrhagic or thrombotic episodes requires rapid reduction of platelet levels with plateletpheresis, in combination with initiation of myelosuppressive therapy. The best drug to use to lower platelet counts is controversial. Hydroxyurea is probably preferred over other alkylating agents, although BU, melphalan, and a variety of others have been used with success. Alpha-interferon was reported to be successful in lowering platelet counts in 60% of patients but is accompanied by more systemic side effects than most low-dose alkylators (49). Recently, anagrelide, a drug that appears to inhibit megakaryocytic maturation and platelet release, has been shown to be remarkably effective in reducing platelet counts for prolonged periods in patients with ET (50).

BMT

As is the situation with PV, BMT for ET remains mostly a theoretical issue. We are aware of only 3 patients with ET who have undergone BMT, and although all 3 successfully engrafted and achieved complete remission, none of the 3 is a long-term survivor. Given the long natural history of this disorder, further trials of BMT should be limited to younger patients in whom uncontrollable thrombocytosis with recurrent bleeding or thrombotic episodes develop or who show signs of leukemic transformation.

Agnogenic Myeloid Metaplasia

Agnogenic myeloid metaplasia (AMM), also sometimes called idiopathic myelofibrosis, is a myeloproliferative disorder characterized by marrow fibrosis, splenomegaly, anemia, and a leukoerythroblastic blood picture in the periphery. The majority of patients with AMM are in their mid-50s, but occasional patients in the pediatric age group are seen. Most patients present with chief complaints due to anemia, but fever, night sweats, anorexia, and weight loss are not uncommon. Splenomegaly is present in 90% of patients and hepatomegaly in 70%. The diagnosis is established by examination of the peripheral blood and marrow. The peripheral smear invariably demonstrates a leukoerythroblastic pattern, with teardrop poikilocytosis, nucleated red cells, and immature myeloid elements. Bone marrows are usually not aspirable, and on bone marrow biopsy, bone marrow fibrosis and osteosclerosis are the rule. Large numbers of blast cells are usually not seen and, if present, suggest that the diagnosis might instead be M7 AML, a disease which in the past had been called acute myelofibrosis or acute myelosclerosis. Most patients with AMM are anemic, but WBC and platelet counts are more variable; both increased and decreased counts are seen. AMM is a clonal disorder of a multipotent hematopoietic stem cell. Genetic analyses have demonstrated the multipotent nature of the malignant cell but have also shown that the increased connective tissue in the marrow in this disorder is of nonclonal origin and therefore a secondary phenomenon (51). Although no single cytogenetic abnormality is associated with AMM, approximately 40% of patients will have a clonal chromosomal abnormality, frequently of chromosomes 1, 5, 7, 9, 11, or 13. A new, or second, abnormality often heralds the conversion to an acute leukemic–like picture.

Natural History and Nontransplant Therapies

Survival after diagnosis of AMM is quite varied, ranging from 1 to 30 years but averages approximately 5 years. Not surprisingly, a poor prognosis is associated with the presence of anemia, thrombocytopenia, hepatomegaly, and B symptoms at diagnosis. Some investigators view the disease as comprised of two groups: one with a fulminate course and a median survival of less than 2 years and a separate group accounting for approximately half the patients, with a median survival of approximately 10 years (52). Nontransplant therapy in patients with AMM is aimed at treating the anemia, the thrombocytopenia, and the problems associated with an enlarged spleen, including pain, portal hypertension, and hypersplenism. Anemia is usually treated with transfusion therapy, and in one third of patients androgens appear to decrease transfusion requirements. Corticosteroids are used in patients with a hemolytic component of their disease. Platelet transfusions are used in patients with active bleeding, but long-term effective replacement is usually not possible due to poor transfusion increments, in part because of hypersplenism as well as development of alloimmunization. Treatment of splenic enlargement is a controversial issue, and splenectomy, splenic irradiation, BU, and alpha-interferon have all been used. Splenectomy is effective in alleviating splenic pain and portal hypertension in most patients, but only approximately 50% of patients will show improvements in either red-cell requirements or platelet counts. The procedure is associated with a 10% mortality and is frequently complicated by bleeding and infection. BU or local irradiation to the spleen can control splenic pain temporarily but can also lead to a decrease in peripheral blood counts.

BMT

BMT is the only therapy currently available that offers any hope of cure for patients with AMM. However, as in all of the other myeloproliferative syndromes, except CML, there is little experience with BMT in AMM. Reasons for this likely include uncertainty about whether the fibrotic component of the disease process is reversible with BMT and reluctance to submit older patients with a chronic disease to the dangers of BMT. In CML, marrow fibrosis accompanies the disease in as many as 20% of patients. The observation that BMT was possible in such patients and led to rapid reversal of the fibrosis provided initial evidence that BMT might have a role in the treatment of myelofibrosis. In 1986, experience concerning the effects of marrow fibrosis on engraftment of allogeneic marrow in 47 patients was reported (53). Thirty-two patients had either mild or moderate fibrosis (grade 1 or 2) and 15 had severe fibrosis (grade 3 or 4). In most patients, the fibrosis was secondary to CML, but in 4 the diagnosis of AMM or a closely related variant was made. Whereas prompt and complete engraftment is the rule in patients without fibrosis, 2 of 32 (6%) patients with mild or moderate fibrosis and 5 of 15 (33%) with severe fibrosis failed to engraft. Furthermore, even in those patients who did engraft, the rate of myeloid and platelet recovery was slower in patients with severe fibrosis than in those without. Reversal of fibrosis was observed in 12 of 15 patients with severe and 24 of 29 patients with mild fibrosis. Fibrosis reappeared in 6 of the former and in one of the latter group and occurred concomitantly with either graft rejection or leukemic relapse. These data suggest that marrow fibrosis should not be viewed as a contraindication to transplantation, but severe fibrosis does pose an additional risk.

In addition to the 4 patients with AMM mentioned, there are published reports of 2 additional patients transplanted successfully for AMM (54), and we are aware of 4 other patients treated similarly, for a total of 10 patients transplanted for AMM, of whom 4 are known to be alive and well. These results argue for the continued investigation of the use of BMT for younger patients with AMM.

Juvenile Chronic Myeloid Leukemia

Clinical and Laboratory Features

JCML is a myeloproliferative disorder characterized by hepatosplenomegaly, leukocytosis, thrombocytopenia, and increased fetal hemoglobin. Most patients are less than 2 years of age at diagnosis, and 95% are less than age 4. Patients characteristically present with malaise, bleeding, and fever. Pallor, hepatosplenomegaly, lymphadenopathy, and an eczematous facial rash are commonly found on physical examination. Laboratory findings include an elevated WBC, often over 100,000/μL with occasional blasts, anemia, and thrombocytopenia; bone marrow examination shows myeloid and erythroid hyperplasia. The Ph chromosome is not present in patients with JCML, but in 40% of patients a clonal chromosomal abnormality is found. Recent laboratory studies suggest that the elevated counts seen in patients with JCML are due, at least in part, to an abnormally exuberant response to endogenously produced GM-CSF by the cells of the malignant clone (55).

Natural History and Nontransplant Therapy

JCML usually follows an aggressive downhill course. Death from bone marrow failure occurs an average of

9 months after diagnosis. Therapies normally useful in adult CML, such as BU or hydroxyurea, are rarely of use in JCML. Intensive induction chemotherapy similar to that used in AML results in complete remission in a minority of patients. Recently, the use of 13-cis retinoic acid was found to result in favorable responses in 4 of 8 patients (56).

BMT

In Seattle, 14 children between the ages of 2 and 5 years with JCML were treated with CY, TBI, and allogeneic BMT (57). Six patients received marrow from an HLA-identical sibling and 8 received marrow from family members matched for one haplotype and mismatched on the other for between one and 3 antigens. Five of the patients died of transplant-related complications and 3 of recurrence of their disease. The other 6 survived in continuous remission for between 6 months and 11.5 years, including 3 of 6 recipients of HLA-identical marrow transplants and 3 of the 8 recipients of partially matched marrow. Given the extremely aggressive nature of this myeloproliferative disease and the absence of any other curative approach, marrow transplantation is clearly warranted. In the past, because of the pace of this disease and the time required to find an unrelated matched donor, most marrow donors have had to come from within the family even if partially histoincompatible. Given the recent demonstration of the activity of 13-cis retinoic acid and the growth of the National Marrow Donor Program, consideration of the use of unrelated matched donors for patients with JCML should be given.

Summary

The results presented herein demonstrate that high-dose chemotherapy followed by allogeneic BMT can eradicate the malignant clone and allow prolonged disease-free survival in patients with myelodysplastic and myeloproliferative syndromes. Because the natural history of these disorders varies so widely, the correct time to proceed to transplantation remains a difficult issue. For patients less than age 55 with MDS who are neutropenic, thrombocytopenic, or who have increasing numbers of blasts, and who have HLA-identical donors, BMT should be considered the treatment of choice. Although the indications for BMT are less easily defined in the myeloproliferative syndromes, BMT should be considered for patients with JCML at any stage of disease and for patients with ET, PV, or AMM with either life-threatening cytopenias or with disease that shows signs of leukemic transformation.

References

1. Prchal JT, Throckmorton DW, Carroll AJ, Fuson EW, Gams RA, Prchal JF. A common progenitor for human myeloid and lymphoid cells. Nature 1978;274:590–591.
2. Janssen JWG, Buschle M, Layton M, et al. Clonal analysis of myelodysplastic syndromes: evidence of multipotent stem cell origin. Blood 1989;73:248–254.
3. Tefferi A, Thibodeau SN, Solbert LA. Clonal studies in a myelodysplastic syndrome using X-linked restriction fragment length polymorphisms. Blood 1990;75:1770–1773.
4. Doll DC, List AF. Myelodysplastic syndromes. Semin Oncol 1992;19:1–3.
5. Cheson BD. The myelodysplastic syndromes: current approaches to therapy. Ann Intern Med 1990;112:932–941.
6. List AF, Garewal HS, Sandberg AA. The myelodysplastic syndromes: biology and implications for management. J Clin Oncol 1990;8:1424–1441.
7. Heyman MR. Recent advances in biology and treatment of myelodysplasia. Current Opinion Oncol 1991;3:44–53.
8. Greenberg PL. Treatment of myelodysplasic syndromes. Blood Rev 1991;5:42–50.
9. Bennett JM, Catovsky D, Daniel MT, et al. Proposals for the classification of the acute leukaemias. French-American-British (FAB) co-operative group. Br J Haematol 1976;33:451–458.
10. Bennett JM, Catovsky D, Daniel MT, et al. Proposals for the classification of the myelodysplastic syndromes. Br J Haematol 1982;51:189–199.
11. Bennett JM, Catovsky D, Daniel MT, et al. Proposed revised criteria for the classification of acute myeloid leukemia. A report of the French-American-British Cooperative Group. Ann Intern Med 1985;103:620–625.
12. Hamblin TJ, Oschier DG. The myelodysplastic syndrome—a practical guide. Hematol Oncol 1987;5:19–34.
13. Tricot G, Vlietinck R, Boogaerts MA, et al. Prognostic factors in the myelodysplastic syndromes: importance of initial data on peripheral blood counts, bone marrow cytology, trephine biopsy and chromosomal analysis. Br J Haematol 1985;60:19–32.
14. Coiffier B, Adeleine P, Gentihomme O, Felman P, Treille-Ritouet D, Bryon PA. Myelodysplastic syndromes. A multiparametric study of prognostic factors in 336 patients. Cancer 1987;60:3029–3032.
15. Sanz GF, Sanz MA, Vallespì T, et al. Two regression models and a scoring system for predicting survival and planning treatment in myelodysplastic syndromes: a multivariate analysis of prognostic factors in 370 patients. Blood 1989;74:395–408.
16. Mufti GJ, Stevens JR, Oscier DG, Hamblin TJ, Machin D. Myelodysplastic syndromes: a scoring system with prognostic significance. Br J Haematol 1985;59:425–433.
17. Kantarjian HM, Keating MJ. Therapy-related leukemia and myelodysplastic syndrome. Semin Oncol 1987;4:435–443.
18. Bagby GC Jr, Gabourel JD, Linman JW. Glucorticoid therapy in the preleukemia syndrome (hemopoietic dysplasia). Identification of responsive patients using in-vitro techniques. Ann Intern Med 1980;92:55–58.
19. Najean Y, Pecking A. Refractory anemia with excess of blast cells: prognostic factors and effect of treatment with androgens or cytosine arabinoside. Results of a prospective trial in 58 patients. Cancer 1979;44:1976–1982.
20. Cines DB, Cassileth PA, Kiss JE. Danazol therapy in myelodysplasia. Ann Intern Med 1985;103:58–60.
21. Koeffler HP, Heitjan D, Mertelsmann R, et al. Random-

ized study of 13-cis retinoic acid v placebo in the myelodysplastic disorders. Blood 1988;71:703–708.
22. Clark RE, Ismail SA, Jacobs A, Payne H, Smith SA. A randomized trial of 13-cis retinoic acid with or without cytosine arabinoside in patients with the myelodysplastic syndrome. Br J Haematol 1987;66:77–83.
23. Vadhan-Raj S, Keating M, LeMaistre A, et al. Effects of recombinant human granulocyte macrophage colony stimulating factor in patients with myelodysplastic syndromes. N Engl J Med 1987;317:1545–1552.
24. Antin JH, Smith BR, Holmes W, Rosenthal DS. Phase I/II study of recombinant human granulocyte-macrophage colony-stimulating factor in aplastic anemia and myelodysplastic syndrome. Blood 1988;72:705–713.
25. Ganser A, Völkers B, Greher J, et al. Recombinant human granulocyte-macrophage colony-stimulating factor in patients with myelodysplastic syndromes-A phase I/II trial. Blood 1989;73:31–37.
26. Herrmann F, Lindemann A, Klein H, et al. Effect of recombinant granulocyte-macrophage colony-stimulating factor in patients with myelodysplastic syndrome with excess blasts. Leukemia 1989;3:335–338.
27. Thompson JA, Lee DJ, Kidd P, et al. Subcutaneous granulocyte-macrophage colony-stimulating factor in patients with myelodysplastic syndrome: toxicity, pharmacokinetics, and hematological effects. J Clin Oncol 1989;7:629–637.
28. Negrin RS, Haeuber DH, Nagler A, et al. Treatment of myelodysplastic syndromes with recombinant human granulocyte colony-stimulating factor. A phase I-II trial. Ann Intern Med 1989;110:976–984.
29. Negrin RS, Haeuber DH, Nagler A, et al. Maintenance treatment of patients with myelodysplastic syndromes using recombinant human granulocyte colony-stimulating factor. Blood 1990;76:36–43.
30. Ganser A, Seipelt G, Lindemann A, et al. Effects of recombinant human interleukin-3 in patients with myelodysplastic syndromes. Blood 1990;76:455–462.
31. Kurzrock R, Talpaz M, Estrov Z, Rosenblum MG, Gutterman JU. Phase I study of recombinant human interleukin-3 in patients with bone marrow failure. J Clin Oncol 1991;9:1241–1250.
32. Stein R, Abels R, Krantz S. Pharmacologic doses of recombinant human erythropoietin in the treatment of myelodysplastic syndromes. Blood 1991;78:1658–1665.
33. Wisch JS, Griffin JD, Kufe DW. Response of preleukemic syndromes to continuous infusion of low-dose cytarabine. N Engl J Med 1983;309:1599–1602.
34. Griffin JD, Spriggs D, Wisch JS, Kufe DW. Treatment of preleukemic syndromes with continuous intravenous infusion of low-dose cytosine arabinoside. J Clin Oncol 1985;3:982–991.
35. Cheson BD, Jasperse DM, Simon R, Friedman MA. A critical appraisal of low-dose cytosine arabinoside in patients with acute nonlymphocytic leukemia and myelodysplastic syndromes. J Clin Oncol 1986;4:1857–1864.
36. Miller KB, Kim K, Morrison FS, et al. Evaluation of low dose ara-C versus supportive care in the treatment of myelodysplastic syndromes: an intergroup study by the Eastern Cooperative Oncology Group and the Southwest Oncology Group (abstract 771). Blood 1988;72 (suppl 1):72:215a.
37. Cheson BD. Chemotherapy and bone marrow transplantation for myelodysplastic syndromes. Semin Oncol 1992;19:85–94.
38. Appelbaum FA, Barrall J, Storb R, et al. Bone marrow transplantation for patients with myelodysplasia. Ann Intern Med 1990;112:590–597.
39. Longmore G, Guinan EC, Weinstein HJ, Gelber RD, Rappeport JM, Antin JH. Bone marrow transplantation for myelodysplasia and secondary acute nonlymphoblastic leukemia. J Clin Oncol 1990;8:1707–1714.
40. O'Donnell MR, Nademanee AP, Snyder DS, et al. Bone marrow transplantation for myelodysplastic and myeloproliferative syndromes. J Clin Oncol 1987;5:1822–1826.
41. Bélanger R, Gyger M, Perreault C, Bonny Y, St-Louis J. Bone marrow transplantation for myelodysplastic syndromes. Br J Haematol 1988;69:29–33.
42. Kolb HJ, Holler E, Bender-Götze C, et al. Myeloablative conditioning for marrow transplantation in myelodysplastic syndromes and paroxysmal nocturnal haemoglobinuria. Bone Marrow Transplant 1989;4:29–34.
43. Bunin NJ, Casper JT, Chitambar C, et al. Partially matched bone marrow transplantation in patients with myelodysplastic syndromes. J Clin Oncol 1988;6:1851–1855.
44. Tricot G, Boogaerts MA, Verwilghen RL. Treatment of patients with myelodysplastic syndromes: a review. Scand J Haematol 1986;36(suppl 45):121–127.
45. DeWitte T, Zwaan F, Hermans J, et al. Allogeneic bone marrow transplantation for secondary leukaemia and myelodysplastic syndrome: a survey by the Leukaemia Working Party of the European Bone Marrow Transplantation Group (EBMTG). Br J Haematol 1990;74:151–155.
46. Appelbaum FR, Storb R, Ramberg RE, et al. Allogeneic marrow transplantation in the treatment of preleukemia. Ann Intern Med 1984;100:689–693.
47. Anasetti C, Amos D, Beatty PG, et al. Effect of HLA compatibility on engraftment of bone marrow transplants in patients with leukemia or lymphoma. N Engl J Med 1989;320:197–204.
48. Berk PD, Goldbert JD, Donovan PB, Fruchtman SM, Berlin NI, Wasserman LR. Therapeutic recommendations in polycythemia vera based on Polycythemia Vera Study Group protocols. Semin Hematol 1986;23:132–143.
49. Talpaz M, Kurzrock R, Kantarjian H, O'Brien S, Gutterman JU. Recombinant interferon-alpha therapy of Philadelphia chromosome-negative marrow proliferative disorders with thrombocytosis. Am J Med 1989;86:554–558.
50. Silverstein MN, Petitt RM, Solberg LA Jr, Fleming JS, Knight RC, Schacter LP. Anagrelide: a new drug for treating thrombocytosis. N Engl J Med 1988;318:1292–1294.
51. Greenberg BR, Woo L, Veomett IC, Payne CM, Ahmann FR. Cytogenetics of bone marrow fibroblastic cells in idiopathic chronic myelofibrosis. Br J Haematol 1987;66:487–490.
52. Manoharan A. Myelofibrosis: prognostic factors and treatment. Br J Haematol 1988;69:295–298.
53. Rajantie J, Sale GE, Deeg HJ, et al. Adverse effect of severe marrow fibrosis on hematologic recovery after chemoradiotherapy and allogeneic bone marrow transplantation. Blood 1986;67:1693–1697.
54. Dokal I, Jones L, Deenmamode M, Lewis SM, Goldman JM. Allogeneic bone marrow transplantation for primary myelofibrosis. Br J Haematol 1989;71:158–160.
55. Evans PM, Czepulkowski B, Gibbons B, Swanbury GJ, Chessells JM. Childhood monosomy 7 revisited. Br J Haematol 1988:69:41–45.

56. Castleberry RP, Emanuel P, Gualtieri R, et al. Preliminary experience with 13-cis retinoic acid in the treatment of juvenile chronic myelogenous leukemia (abstract 670). Blood 1991;78(suppl 1):170a.

57. Sanders JE, Buckner CD, Thomas ED, et al. Allogeneic marrow transplantation for children with juvenile chronic myelogenous leukemia. Blood 1988;71:1144–1146.

Chapter 48

Allogeneic and Syngeneic Bone Marrow Transplantation for Multiple Myeloma

Gösta Gahrton

Multiple myeloma is a fatal disease, with a median survival of approximately 3 years. Conventional chemotherapy usually consists of a combination of melphalan plus prednisone based on the original trial by Alexanian and colleagues (1). Their patients received either melphalan alone or a combination of melphalan and prednisone. The patients were treated for 4 days every 6 weeks. Melphalan alone produced a 32% response rate, whereas the addition of prednisone increased the response to approximately 60%. Because of the higher response rate and ease of management, the combination is currently favored.

Many attempts have been made to improve the response rate and survival in patients with multiple myeloma by adding other drugs or using new combinations. Only one study has demonstrated results superior to the melphalan and prednisone combination (2). In this study, intermittent melphalan plus prednisone was compared with alternating treatment every 21 days with VMCP (vincristine, melphalan, carmustine [BCNU], and prednisone) and VBAP (vincristine, BCNU, adriamycin, and prednisone). The median survival with these combinations was 42 months, as compared with 23 months for melphalan and prednisone. A subsequent analysis of this study indicated that the increased survival was due mainly to a higher response rate in poor-risk stage II patients (3). More recent attempts to improve the results by adding interferon either to melphalan plus prednisone for initial treatment or for maintenance of remission have resulted in an improved response rate (4–6); however, the effect on survival was only marginal.

In the early 1980s, attempts were made to use marrow ablative treatment with subsequent bone marrow transplantation (BMT). Fefer and associates (7) and Highby and colleagues (8) used marrow from identical twin donors and the Royal Marsden group (9,10) used autologous marrow. These studies demonstrated that intensive treatment with marrow rescue could induce complete remissions of long duration in some patients and provided the basis for increased attempts to cure myeloma by intensive chemoradiotherapy and BMT.

Preparative Regimens for BMT in Patients with Multiple Myeloma

The myeloma cell is highly sensitive to irradiation and several cytotoxic drugs. Both melphalan and cyclophosphamide (CY) have been cornerstones in the conventional cytotoxic drug treatment of multiple myeloma. Total body irradiation (TBI) in combination with one of these drugs has been the most common preparative regimen for patients with multiple myeloma. In the European Group for Bone Marrow Transplantation (EBMT) study (11), 33 of 90 patients received variants of the Seattle protocol (12) combining TBI and CY. Forty-three patients received TBI and CY combined with other drugs, usually melphalan. Five patients received TBI and melphalan alone; 9 patients received cytotoxic drugs only, without TBI. In 6 of these patients, busulfan (BU) was used in combination with CY, a combination originally used by Tutschka and associates (13) for conditioning of patients with leukemia. Although the BUCY regimen seemed promising, there was no significant difference between results with BU or other combinations in the EBMT study, neither with respect to response to treatment nor with respect to survival. However, patients conditioned with BU-containing combinations were followed for a shorter time than those conditioned with TBI and other drugs. Thus, it is too early to draw conclusions about the relative merits of the regimens. In the EBMT study, there was no indication that combining TBI with several drugs gave better results than TBI and CY alone.

The BUCY combination was used in 20 of the patients with myeloma who received an allogeneic BMT and in one who received a syngeneic BMT in the series by the Seattle group (14,15). The results seemed to be at least as successful in inducing response and prolonging survival as TBI with CY.

Syngeneic BMT

Fefer and co-workers (7) and Osserman and colleagues (16) published the first reports of syngeneic BMT in patients with multiple myeloma. These Seattle patients were prepared with CY and TBI. The patients were transplanted in partial response after being treated with melphalan and prednisone. Both relapsed but survived for 24 and 32 months. Buckner and associates (15) reported 6 additional transplants from syngeneic donors. At the time of transplantation, 7 of the recipients were in a progressive stage after chemotherapy. Three of these patients were alive and well 726 to 3,560 days after BMT. Two died of interstitial pneumonia. Four died with multiple myeloma, 2 of whom survived for 1,596 and 1,759 days.

In the EBMT study, 6 patients received marrow from syngeneic donors; 3 were receiving second- or third-line treatment (17). Five were stage III patients. Two patients had not responded to previous treatment, whereas 3 were in partial remission and one was in complete remission. The results were amazingly good. One patient died at day 483, but 5 were alive 177, 693, 709, 1,045, and 1,128 days after BMT. However, all but one patient survived with signs of multiple myeloma. It is too early to predict the outcome for these patients. The presence of abnormal immunoglobulin in plasma or urine and myeloma cells in the marrow indicates that the disease probably will progress.

Immediate transplant-related mortality for recipients of syngeneic marrow appears to be lower than for those receiving allogeneic marrow. The one patient in the Seattle study reported to have a small persistent serum monoclonal spike at 9.5 years is now living and well 13 years after transplantation, and the monocolonal spike has disappeared (Fefer A., Personal communication). Thus, the results of syngeneic transplants indicate that prolonged survival may be obtained, but most patients probably will relapse if transplanted with advanced disease. Patients with identical twins are candidates for BMT early in the course of the disease.

Allogeneic BMT

The first promising case reports of allogeneic transplants were published in the mid 1980s (18–20). Of 3 patients reported from the Huddinge group (19), one was resistant to melphalan and prednisone but went into a complete remission following BMT. She was without signs of multiple myeloma for 4 years but then relapsed. Among the patients reported by the Bologna group, one was well and in complete remission 67 months following transplantation (21). Following these promising reports, allogeneic BMT was performed throughout Europe. In 1983, the EBMT started a registry of allogeneic marrow grafts for myeloma at Huddinge Hospital. At the last update, 26 centers had reported their results to the registry (11).

Number of Allogeneic BMTs Performed

The exact number of allogeneic BMTs performed for multiple myeloma is not known. Ninety BMTs using human leukocyte antigen (HLA)–matched sibling donors had been reported to the EBMT registry at the end of 1989 (11). The annual number reported to the registry was approximately 20 for the years 1987 to 1989, a number presumably increasing since that time. Six patients who received grafts from donors other than siblings were reported from 1983 until the end of 1989. In the International Bone Marrow Transplant Registry (IBMTR), there were 77 reports of BMTs until the end of 1989 (17). However, European transplants are usually reported both to the EBMT and the IBMTR. Thus, only approximately 23 patients transplanted in the United States or elsewhere outside Europe can be added to those reported to the EBMT registry. The Seattle group (15) performed 14 marrow transplants with matched allografts and 3 with partially matched allografts as reported in 1989. These patients are not reported in the IBMTR registry. Additional patients have probably been transplanted during 1990 and 1991. Thus, an estimated 200 patients worldwide have received an allogeneic BMT for multiple myeloma by the end of 1991. The great majority of the marrow donors have been HLA-matched siblings. Only a small fraction of transplants has utilized other donors, such as matched or partially matched relatives or matched unrelated donors.

Because most of the European case reports of allogeneic BMT (19–24) are reported to the EBMT registry and because most of the European data are also reported to the IBMTR, this review is mainly based on the studies by Gahrton and colleagues (11) and the Seattle group (14,15).

Response to BMT

The response rate to BMT using matched sibling donors is seen in Tables 48-1 to 48-3. Complete remission was defined as the disappearance of the monoclonal immunoglobulin determined by conventional electrophoresis or immunofixation and no myeloma cells in the marrow. Because 18 patients

Table 48-1.
Complete Remission (CR) Following BMT by Line of Treatment Before BMT

Number Lines of Treatment Before BMT	*Total No. Patients*	*No. Evaluable following BMT*	*Following BMT*		
			No. CR	*% of Total*[a]	*% of Evaluable*[a]
One	33	25	20	61	80
Two	31	24	11	35	45
Three or more	26	18	8	31	44
Total	90	67	39	43	58

[a]There was a significant ($p = 0.01$) trend toward higher frequency of remission with lower number of treatment lines (Chi-square test). Patients who had received only one line of treatment before BMT had a significantly ($p = 0.006$) higher fraction in CR after BMT than those who had received two or more lines of treatment (Fisher's exact test). Data from the EBMT study (1991) (11).
BMT = bone marrow transplantation.

Table 48-2.
Complete Remission (CR) Following BMT by Status at Conditioning for BMT

Status at Conditioning	Total No. Patients Before BMT	No. Evaluable Following BMT	Following BMT No. CR	% of Total[a]	% of Evaluable[a]
CR	7	6	6	67	100
Partial remission	34	26	15	44	58
No response	22	18	10	45	56
Progression	27	17	8	30	47
Total	90	67	39	43	58

[a]There were significantly ($p = 0.039$) higher fraction of patients in CR following BMT in the group who was in CR before BMT than in the other groups (Fisher's exact test). Data from the EBMT study (1991) (11).
BMT = bone marrow transplantation.

died before engraftment and 5 were not evaluable at the time of analysis, remission status could be evaluated in only 67 of the 90 patients. Thirty-nine (58%) of these patients had no signs of myeloma, whereas 28 (42%) had either persistent plasma cells in the marrow or light chains or abnormal immunoglobulin detectable in the urine or serum.

The pretransplant characteristics of patients in the EBMT study were highly heterogenous. An attempt was made to correlate the response following grafting to pretreatment factors (i.e., the number of treatment attempts before BMT, the response to treatment, and the stage at diagnosis and at the time of BMT). As expected, patients who had received only one course of treatment before BMT were more likely to enter a complete remission after BMT than patients who had received 2 or more courses of treatment (see Table 48-1). Also, a complete remission before BMT was associated with a better prognosis compared with having progressive disease or disease that did not respond to treatment (see Table 48-2). Stage I at

Table 48-3.
Complete Remission (CR) Following BMT by Stage at Diagnosis

Stage at diagnosis	Total No. Patients at Diagnosis	No. Evaluable Following BMT	Response to BMT No. CR		% of Total[a]	% of Evaluable[a]
IA	13	11	10	11	79	91
IB	1	1	1			
IIA	14	6	4	5	33	71
IIB	1	1	1			
IIIA	52	40	17	23	38	48
IIIB	9	8	6			
Total	90	67	39		43	58

[a]There was a significantly ($p = 0.01$) higher frequency of CR in stage I (A + B) versus stages II + III (A + B) (Fisher's exact test). Data from the EBMT study (1991) (11).
BMT = bone marrow transplantation.

diagnosis or at transplantation was associated with a higher chance of entering a complete remission following BMT than being in stage II or stage III (see Table 48-3).

Radiographic bone lesions were disregarded in the definition of response. In fact, radiographic bone lesions usually did not change significantly following BMT. The lesions in the bone were rated as major lytic lesions, minor lytic lesions, osteoporosis, or none. Only 7 patients showed improvement (i.e. major lytic lesions changed to minor lesions in 3, and minor lesions disappeared in 4). However, new bone lesions appeared in 3 patients, and in 2 there was progression of the lesions.

In the Seattle study (14), there were 12 complete remissions in both marrow and monoclonal immunoglobulin among 20 patients who received allografts after preparation with BUCY. Eight patients died within the first 100 days after grafting. Four died later of graft-versus-host disease (GVHD) or myeloma. Eight are living in complete remission 6 to 42 months after BMT.

Graft-versus-Host Disease

GVHD does not appear to be more common following allogeneic BMT for multiple myeloma than for other hematological malignancies. GVHD prevention reported in the EBMT study, as well as in the Seattle study, consisted in most patients of methotrexate (MTX) and cyclosporine (CSP). However, many other preventive methods have been used, such as CSP alone, CSP with prednisolone, pretreatment of the marrow with monoclonal antibodies against T cells, and combinations of all these agents. In the EBMT study, there was no clear difference in the incidence of GVHD between patients who had been given the MTX-CSP combination or other types of GVHD prevention. Forty-six percent of the patients who could be evaluated had no signs of GVHD, and only 10% had grade III or IV GVHD (Table 48-4). It appears that until other methods of preventing GVHD have proved to be superior to MTX-CSP, this regimen is preferable. Relapse is one of the most important causes of failure to cure patients with multiple myeloma. The MTX component may have some advantage in preventing relapse.

Table 48-4.
Graft-versus-host Disease (GVHD)[a]

Acute GVHD	No. Patients (%)
Grade 0	37 (46)
Grade I	22 (28)
Grade II	13 (16)
Grade III	4 (5)
Grade IV	4 (5)
Total	80 (100)

[a]Data from the EBMT Study (1991) (11).

Survival and Relapse-free Survival Following Transplants from HLA-matched Sibling Donors

The EBMT study consisted mainly of patients in stage III who had received more than one line of treatment and who were either not responding or in partial remission. Nevertheless, the median survival was 26 months from BMT, and the actuarial survival was 40%, with a maximum follow-up of 78 months (Figure 48-1). Twelve of the patients were still alive 36 to 78 months after BMT. There was no single pretreatment factor that predicted for duration of survival. Thus, within the age group 23 to 55 years, survival in patients above and below 40 years of age was similar. Stage I patients tended to do better than stage II and III patients, but this difference was not significant (Figure 48-2). Also, there was a trend toward better survival among patients who were in complete remission at the time of BMT, but this trend was not statistically significant (Figure 48-3). Patients who received only first-line treatment before BMT had a tendency toward better survival than the other groups (Figure 48-4). Also, patients who were treated within 12 months of diagnosis tended to have a longer survival than those who were transplanted later in the course of the disease.

Sixty-seven of the patients in the EBMT study could be evaluated for survival following engraftment. Complete remission following BMT significantly predicted for a prolonged survival (Figure 48-5). Another post-BMT factor that predicted for survival was acute GVHD (Figure 48-6). Those who had grade I GVHD had the best survival, whereas those who had grades III or IV GVHD experienced a significantly poorer treatment outcome.

Among the 39 patients who were in complete remission following BMT, the median relapse-free survival following engraftment was 48 months (Figure 48-7). Of these patients, 11 were still in complete remission 24 to 68 months after BMT.

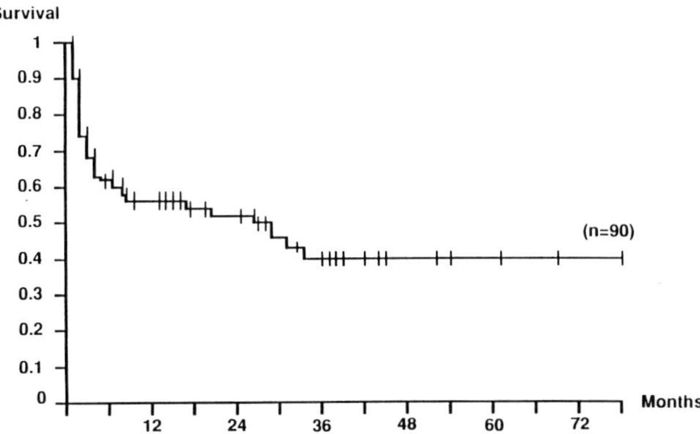

Figure 48-1. Kaplan-Meier curve for actuarial survival after bone marrow transplantation. Data from the EBMT study (1991) (11).

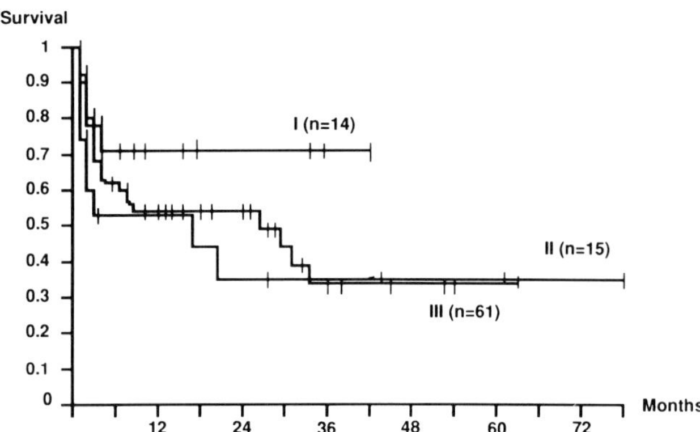

Figure 48-2. Actuarial survival after bone marrow transplantation according to stage of the disease at diagnosis. The Kaplan-Meier curves show a slight trend toward better survival among patients with stage I disease at diagnosis than among patients with stage II or III disease, but the difference was not significant. Data from the EBMT study (1991) (11).

It is too early to speculate that these patients are cured. However, it is obvious that it is possible to obtain a sustained complete remission without further treatment following BMT. It is particularly interesting to note that 7 of the patients that were in continuous complete remission more than 24 months after BMT were either not responding to treatment before BMT or were in a progressive stage of the disease.

Myeloma cells in the marrow, monoclonal light chains in urine, or abnormal immunoglobulin in serum usually disappeared within 1 to 6 months. However, the disappearance rate of immunoglobulin following BMT varied considerably. The median time

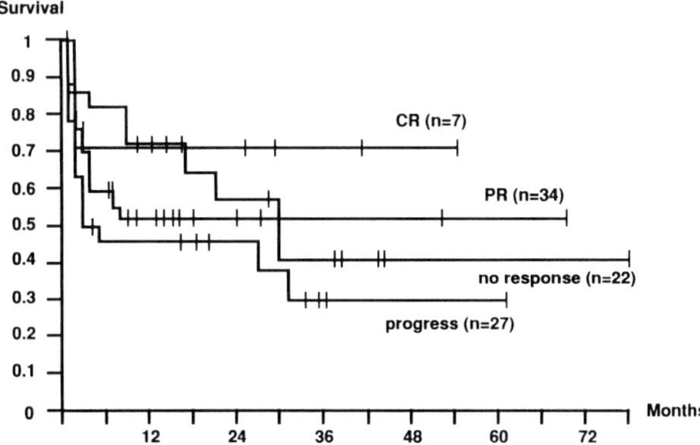

Figure 48-3. Actuarial survival after bone marrow transplantation (BMT) according to the response status before conditioning. The Kaplan-Meier curves show a tendency toward improved survival among patients with a better response before BMT, but the difference was not significant. CR = complete remission; PR = partial remission. Data from the EBMT study (1991) (11).

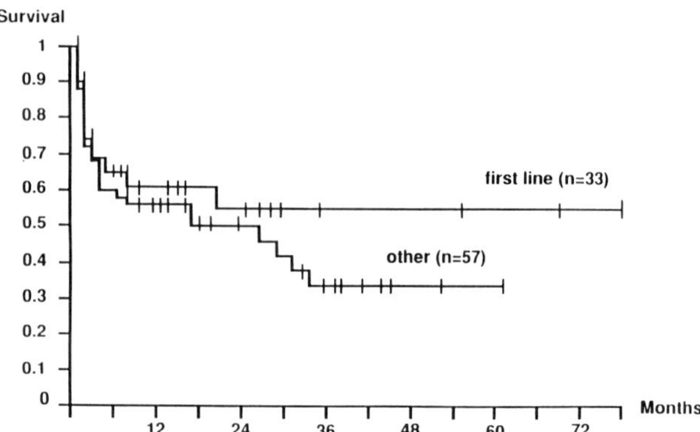

Figure 48-4. Actuarial survival after bone marrow transplantation (BMT) according to the number of lines of treatment regimens used before BMT. The Kaplan-Meier curves show a slight but not significant trend toward improved survival in patients who received only first-line treatment, as compared with those who received two or more lines of treatment. Data from the EBMT study (1991) (11).

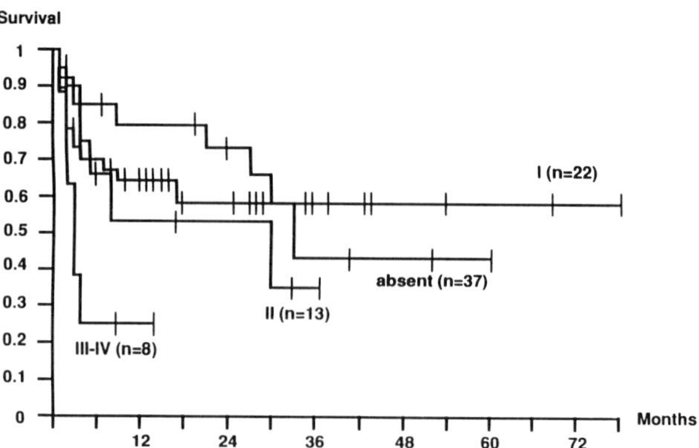

Figure 48-6. Actuarial survival after bone marrow transplantation according to the degree of graft-versus-host disease (GVHD). The Kaplan-Meier curves show that patients with grade I GVHD had significantly better survival than those with Grade III or IV, whereas those who had no GVHD or grade II GVHD were in a middle position. Data from the EBMT study (1991) (11).

was approximately 4 months, but in isolated patients, disappearance occurred as long as 2 years following BMT without any additional treatment.

The 20 patients in Seattle prepared with BU/CY and given an allogeneic graft showed an actuarial disease-free survival of 32% at three years.

Causes of Death

The causes of death following allogeneic BMT in patients with multiple myeloma are mainly the same as those following BMT for other hematological malignancies. At an average follow-up of 78 months from the start of BMT, 47 patients were alive and 43 patients died in the EBMT study. In the Seattle study, 8 were alive and 12 died. The causes of death were mainly the same in both studies (Table 48-5). Interstitial pneumonitis was an important cause of death, as were fungal and bacterial infections. Although recurrence was usually not the main immediate cause of death, most patients who died because of infections, hemorrhage, or organ failure also had signs of myeloma at death.

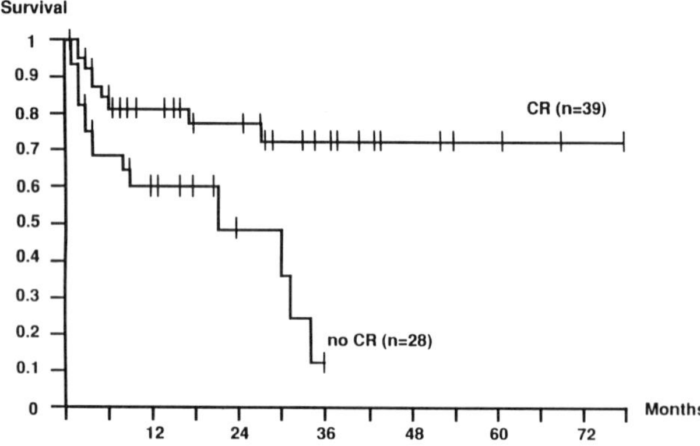

Figure 48-5. Actuarial survival after bone marrow transplantation according to whether patients were in complete remission (CR) after engraftment. The Kaplan-Meier curves show significantly ($p = 0.0001$, two-sided log rank test) better survival among patients who entered CR after engraftment than among those who did not. Data from the EBMT study (1991) (11).

BMT Using Non-sibling Donors

The experience with the use of marrow from non-sibling donors is very limited in patients with multiple myeloma. In the EBMT study, 6 patients received marrow from non-sibling donors, 3 of whom were unrelated. The patients were usually in poor condition at the time of BMT, and the transplant-related death

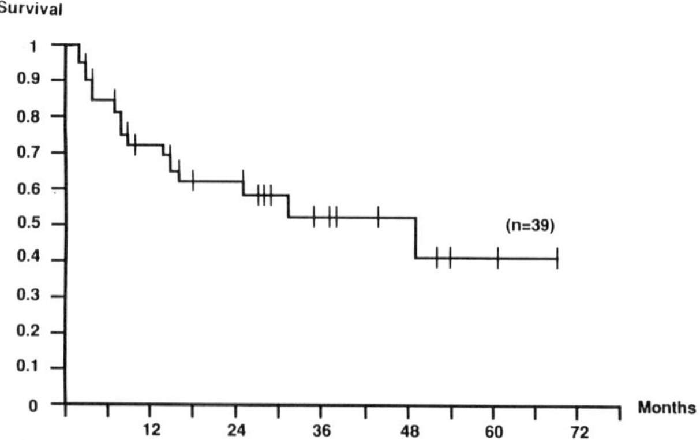

Figure 48-7. Actuarial relapse-free survival after bone marrow transplantation (BMT) among patients who entered complete remission after BMT. Data from the EBMT study (1991) (11).

Table 48-5.
Causes of Death after Allogeneic BMT for Multiple Myeloma

	EBMT Study (11) (n = 90)	*Seattle Study (15) (n = 17)*
Interstitial pneumonitis	9	3
Recurrence of myeloma	8	2[a]
GVHD	6	3
Bacterial or fungal infection	6	2
Hemorrhage	5	0
Organ failure	4	2
Other causes	5	0
Total	43	12

[a]Seven patients had signs of multiple myeloma, but it was not the main cause of death.
BMT = bone marrow transplantation; GVHD = graft-versus-host disease.

rate was high. Five of the 6 patients died within 75 days, and only one patient, who received the graft from an HLA-identical related donor, was alive 200 days after BMT. This patient still had signs of disease at the time of the report.

It is too early to predict the outcome of non-sibling donor BMT. To date, only patients with a poor prognosis have been selected for this type of BMT. Most probably the results will not be inferior to those seen in chronic myeloid leukemia if patients with less poor prognostic parameters are selected for BMT earlier in the course of the disease (25).

Prospects for the Future

Allogeneic BMT appears to be an option for younger patients with multiple myeloma. The disease is less common in the age group under 55 (i.e., in patients generally considered to be candidates for allogeneic BMT). In the Swedish population, the incidence of multiple myeloma was 545 per year, and only 38 of these patients are under 55 years of age (26). The relative rarity of patients suitable for BMT should in no way diminish the effort to cure them.

Multiple myeloma is a disease that is never cured with conventional treatment; it has a median survival of slightly less than 3 years. This grim outlook provides the basis for undertaking aggressive chemoradiotherapy with BMT. However, some patients with stage I disease may survive much longer, which makes it difficult to judge which patients should be selected for BMT. The data from the 2 main studies (11,14) indicate that patients who are in an early stage of the disease, who have not received several lines of treatment, and who are still responsive have a greater chance to be long-term survivors following BMT. The balance between the risk of transplant-related death and the chance for long-term survival must be weighed in selecting the right patients for BMT. There are no absolute guidelines. In young patients with disease that has required cytotoxic drug treatment and who have had a good response, the chance of obtaining long-term survival after BMT is good. Thus, this patient group should be considered as candidates for BMT. However, because of the risk of transplant-related mortality, it is also reasonable to wait until the patient no longer responds to first-line treatment but is still responsive to second-line treatment. This stage appears to be a clear indication for BMT. However, it is also possible to perform BMT in patients resistant to chemotherapy. The data from both the EBMT study and the Seattle group indicate that patients who are resistant and probably have no chance for long-term survival with any conventional treatment may sometimes benefit from BMT, with complete remission and long-term survival. In summary, except for those with stage I disease, patients with multiple myeloma who have an HLA-matched donor should be considered for allogeneic BMT at any stage of disease, the sooner the better.

The role of allogeneic BMT as compared with autologous BMT is not yet defined. Further studies must be done to clarify which approach is preferable. Transplant-related mortality is somewhat less with autologous BMT, and patients could probably be transplanted up to 60 or even 65 years of age (see Chapter 57). However, as has been shown for other hematological malignancies, the relapse rate may well be higher after autologous BMT, not only because of the lack of a graft-versus-myeloma effect that might be present following allogeneic BMT, but also because of contamination of the marrow inoculum with malignant clonogenic cells. The decision between an allogeneic or an autologous graft is often determined by the age of the patient and the availability of an HLA-matched donor.

Because of the seemingly high relapse rate or even lack of complete remission following BMT, post-BMT treatment may be an option. Interferon added to melphalan-prednisone has been tried, both for induction of response (4) and for maintenance of response (5,11). It appears that interferon treatment in these settings may be of value. Thus, trials of interferon for post-BMT treatment should be explored (27). Interferon or other forms of postgrafting treatment, such as other biological response modifiers, may prove to eradicate minimal residual disease following BMT. Chromosomal rearrangements that have been identified in patients with multiple myeloma (28–32) could be used for detection of minimal residual disease by sensitive molecular techniques, such as the polymerase chain reaction (32,33). Although new preparative regimens are being studied, none have proved superior to CY and TBI. The combination of BU with CY shows promise. Other preparative regimens are being explored by several marrow transplant teams and improvements may yet be found.

Improvement of the general technology of BMT is occurring as a result of research projects in many transplant centers. Some examples are use of ganciclovir for prevention of cytomegalovirus pneumonia, use of hematopoietic growth factors made available through recombinant technology, and use of agents that down-regulate tumor necrosis factor-alpha, thus reducing regimen-related toxicity. Progress in all these areas should lead to a cure for an increasing number of patients with multiple myeloma.

References

1. Alexanian R, Haut A, Khan A, et al. Treatment for multiple myeloma: combination chemotherapy with different melphalan dose regimens. JAMA 1969;208: 1680–1685.
2. Salmon SE, Haut A, Bonnet J, et al. Alternating combination chemotherapy and levamisole improves survival in multiple myeloma. A Southwest Oncology Group Study. J Clin Oncol 1983;1:453–461.
3. Salmon SE, Cassady JR. Plasma cell neoplasm. In: De Vita VT Jr, ed. Cancer: principles and practice of oncology. New York: J.B. Lippincott, 1989:1853.
4. Mellstedt H, Österborg A, Björkholm M, et al. Treatment of multiple myeloma with interferon alpha: the Scandinavian experience. Br J Haematol 1991; 79:21–25.
5. Mandelli F, Avvisati G, Amadori S, et al. Maintenance treatment with recombinant interferon alfa-2b in patients with multiple myeloma responding to conventional induction chemotherapy. N Engl J Med 1990; 322:1430–1434.
6. Westin J, Cortelezzi A, Hjort M, et al. Interferon therapy during the plateau phase of multiple myeloma: an update of a Swedish multicenter study. In: Pileri A, Boccadoro M, eds. III International Workshop On Multiple Myeloma: from biology to therapy. Torino: 1991:134–135.
7. Fefer A, Greenberg PD, Cheever MA, et al. Treatment of multiple myeloma with chemoradiotherapy and identical twin bone marrow transplantation (abstract). Proc Am Soc Clin Oncol 1982;1:C731.
8. Highby DJ, Brass C, Fitzpatrick J, Henderson ES. Bone marrow transplantation in multiple myeloma: a case report with protein studies (abstract). Proc Am Soc Clin Oncol 1982:C747.
9. McElwain TJ, Powles RL. High-dose intravenous melphalan for plasma cell leukaemia and myeloma. Lancet 1983;1:822–824.
10. Selby P, McElwain TJ, Nandi AC, et al. Multiple myeloma treated with high dose intravenous melphalan. Br J Haematol 1987;66:55–62.
11. Gahrton G, Tura S, Ljungman P, et al. Allogeneic bone marrow transplantation in multiple myeloma. N Engl J Med 1991;325:1267–1273.
12. Thomas ED, Storb R, Clift RA, et al. Bone marrow transplantation. N Engl J Med 1975;292:832–843,895–902.
13. Tutschka PJ, Copelan EA, Klein JP. Bone marrow transplantation for leukemia following a new busulfan and cyclophosphamide regimen. Blood 1987;70:1382–1388.
14. Bensinger WI, Buckner CD, Clift RA, et al. A phase I study of busulfan and cyclophosphamide in preparation for allogeneic marrow transplant for patients with multiple myeloma. J Clin Oncol 1992;10:1492–1497.
15. Buckner CD, Fefer A, Bensinger WI, et al. Marrow transplantation for malignant plasma cell disorders: summary of the Seattle Experience. Eur J Haematol 1989;43:186–190.
16. Osserman EF, Dire LB, Dire J, Sherman WH, Hersman JA, Storb R. Identical twin marrow transplantation in multiple myeloma. Acta Haematol 1982;68:215–223.
17. Gahrton G, Ljungman P, Tura S, et al. Allogeneic bone marrow transplantation in multiple myeloma. In: Champlin RE, Gale RP, eds. New strategies in bone marrow transplantation. UCLA Symposia on molecular and cellular biology, new series. New York: Wiley-Liss, 1991:395–404.
18. Ozer H, Han T, Nussbaum-Blumenson A, Henderson ES, Fitzpatrick J, Highby DJ. Allogeneic BMT and idiotypic monitoring in multiple myeloma. AACR Abst 1984;84:161.
19. Gahrton G, Ringdén O, Lönnqvist B, Lindquist R, Ljungman P. Bone marrow transplantation in three patients with multiple myeloma. Acta Med Scand 1986;219:523–527.
20. Tura S, Cavo M, Baccarani M, Ricci P, Gobbi M. Bone marrow transplantation in multiple myeloma. Scand J Haematol 1986;36:176–179.
21. Tura S, Cavo M, Rosti G, et al. Allogeneic bone marrow transplantation for multiple myeloma. Bone Marrow Transplant 1989;4:106–108.
22. Gallamini A, Buffa F, Bacigalupo A, et al. Allogeneic bone marrow transplantation in multiple myeloma. Acta Haematol 1987;77:111–114.
23. Nikoskelainen J, Kokela K, Katka K, et al. Allogeneic bone marrow transplantation in multiple myeloma: a report of four cases. Bone Marrow Transplant 1988; 3:495–500.
24. Samson D, Kanfer E, Taylor J, et al. Allogeneic BMT for multiple myeloma: the Riverside experience (abstract). Br J Haematol 1990;74(suppl 1):53.
25. McGlave PB, Beatty P, Ash R, Hows JM. Therapy for chronic myelogenous leukemia with unrelated donor bone marrow transplantation: results in 102 cases. Blood 1990;75:1728–1732.
26. National Board of Health and Welfare. The Cancer Registry. Cancer Incidence in Sweden 1988. Stockholm, Sweden, 1991.
27. Attal M, Huguet F, Schlaifer D, et al. Maintenance treatment with recombinant alpha interferon after autologous bone marrow transplantation for aggressive myeloma in first remission after conventional induction chemotherapy. Bone Marrow Transplant 1991;8: 125–128.
28. Gahrton G, Zech L, Nilsson K, Lönnqvist B, Carlström A. Two translocations, t(11;14) and t(1;6), in a patient with plasma cell leukemia and 2 populations of plasma cells. Scand J Haematol 1980;24:42–46.
29. Philip P. Chromosomes of monoclonal gammopathies. Cancer Genet Cytogenet 1980;2:79.
30. Barlogie B, Alexanian R. Biology and therapy of multiple myeloma. Acta Haematol 1978;78:171–174.
31. Lisse IM, Drivsholm A, Christoffersen P. Occurrence and type of chromosomal abnormalities in consecutive malignant monoclonal gammopathies: correlation with survival. Cancer Genet Cytogenet 1988;35:27–36.
32. Kokkinou S, Juliusson G, Ohrling M, Gahrton G. Chromosome analysis in B-cell mitogen-stimulated cells from myeloma patients: high incidence of clonal abnormalities in Bence-Jones and non-secretory subtypes. Blood 1990;76:357a.
33. Deane M, Samson D. Detection of minimal residual myeloma after bone marrow transplantation. Br J Haematol 1991;79:134–135.

Chapter 49
Allogeneic Bone Marrow Transplantation for Lymphomas

Richard J. Jones

The term *lymphoma* refers to a heterogeneous group of malignancies of the lymphoreticular system, ranging from some of the slowest-growing to some of the fastest-growing cancers in humans, and from incurable to curable with standard therapy. Although the lymphomas encompass more than 10 distinct diseases with markedly different biologies, it now appears that all lymphomas can be functionally divided into two groups based on their clinical behavior: indolent and aggressive lymphomas (Table 49-1). With few exceptions, lymphomas within each group share similar clinical presentations and prognoses that facilitate common approaches to treatment.

Indolent lymphomas share characteristics of slow growth, long median survivals (ranging from 7–11 yr) even untreated, and responsiveness to gentler forms of therapy, such as oral chemotherapy. In contrast to patients with aggressive lymphomas, patients with indolent lymphomas rarely have sustained remissions and are probably incurable with conventional-dose therapy. Indolent lymphomas are unheard of in childhood and are rare in young adults, gradually increasing in incidence with age. Indolent lymphomas include all non-Hodgkin's lymphomas (NHLs) classified as low-grade by the Working Formulation; 2 NHLs classified as intermediate-grade in the Working Formulation (follicular large-cell and diffuse small cleaved cell) that most evidence now suggests behave indolently; and a relatively newly described lymphoma, diffuse intermediate differentiated lymphocytic NHL (also called mantle zone lymphoma) that was not included in the Working Formulation (see Table 49-1). Chronic lymphocytic leukemia (CLL) is the leukemic manifestation of small (or well differentiated) lymphocytic lymphomas, with a natural history that parallels that expected for small lymphocytic lymphomas. Both diseases can be viewed as a single entity with a full spectrum of presentation between adenopathy alone and a strictly leukemic form.

Aggressive lymphomas comprise more than 50% of the new cases of lymphomas. They are characterized by fast explosive growth, frequent constitutional symptoms (fever, night sweats, or weight loss), rapid progression when unresponsive, and the requirement for aggressive forms of therapy. Virtually all lymphomas that arise in children are aggressive lymphomas. Aggressive lymphomas include all NHLs classified as high grade in the Working Formulation and 2 NHLs classified as intermediate-grade in the Working Formulation (diffuse large cell and diffuse mixed lymphoma) that clearly behave aggressively (see Table 49-1). All types of Hodgkin's disease can also be approached as aggressive lymphomas, with similar clinical behaviors to aggressive NHLs. In contrast to indolent lymphomas, approximately half the patients with aggressive lymphomas are curable with aggressive first-line therapy. However, very few patients with aggressive lymphomas who progress during initial treatment with combination chemotherapy or relapse afterward will experience a prolonged survival with conventional-dose salvage therapy (1–3). This finding is in contrast to patients with relapsed indolent lymphomas, who can have a prolonged survival after conventional-dose salvage therapy, although cure is similarly unlikely.

Over the past 20 years, high-dose cytotoxic therapy followed by bone marrow transplantation (BMT) has become effective salvage therapy, and probably the treatment of choice, for patients who have failed

Table 49-1.
Functional Classification of Lymphomas

Indolent lymphomas
Follicular small-cleaved
Follicular mixed small-cleaved and large cell
Small lymphocytic/chronic lymphocytic leukemia
Diffuse intermediate-differentiated lymphocytic (mantle zone)
Follicular large cell
Diffuse small-cleaved cell
Aggressive lymphomas
Diffuse mixed small-cleaved and large cell
Diffuse large cell
Diffuse large cell (immunoblastic)
Diffuse small noncleaved cell (Burkitt's lymphoma)
Lymphoblastic lymphoma
Hodgkin's disease

first-line chemotherapy for aggressive lymphomas. The role of BMT for patients with indolent lymphomas is much less clear. Many fewer patients have undergone BMT for indolent lymphomas and the follow-up is much shorter than for aggressive lymphomas, probably because of the relatively long survival and the older age of patients with indolent lymphomas.

Clinical Trials

Background

Historically, there have been differences with regard to the type of transplant (allogeneic or autologous) primarily employed for the various hematological malignancies. Because of the clear presence of a clinically significant graft-versus-leukemia effect (4–9) and concern regarding bone marrow contamination with leukemia, allogeneic BMT has generally been preferred over autologous BMT for patients with acute leukemia. Conversely, autologous BMT has been predominantly used in patients with NHL and Hodgkin's disease, probably because bone marrow involvement has been perceived to be a lesser problem in the lymphomas. Moreover, initial studies were unable to establish a graft-versus-lymphoma effect associated with allogeneic BMT (10,11).

Recent data indicate that there is little reason to favor a different type of transplant for patients with acute leukemia than for those with aggressive lymphomas. Although the pattern of relapse after autologous BMT suggests that failure to eradicate lymphoma remaining in the patient is a more important cause of disease progression than infusion of lymphoma cells with the autologous graft, several studies now suggest that relapse following autologous BMT can be the result of infusing viable lymphoma cells with the autologous marrow grafts (12,13). This finding is not surprising because morphological involvement of bone marrow by NHL and Hodgkin's disease is common, and occult involvement may be universal. Approximately 10% of patients at initial diagnosis and 25 to 50% of patients at relapse have morphological involvement of bone marrow by Hodgkin's disease (14,15); morphological bone marrow involvement is approximately twice as common in patients with aggressive NHL (16,17). Even more importantly, recent studies now clearly demonstrate the existence of a clinically significant graft-versus-lymphoma effect associated with allogeneic BMT for patients with aggressive NHL and Hodgkin's disease (18). Because at least 50% of patients with lymphoma relapse after autologous BMT, allogeneic BMT should be considered for these patients because of its superior antitumor activity. Allogeneic BMT should be particularly attractive in this group of patients because of their relatively young age. In fact, the average age of the lymphoma population (< 30 years for Hodgkin's disease and approximately 45 years for NHL) is less than the average age of patients with acute myeloid leukemia (19).

Aggressive Lymphomas

There have been few reported trials of allogeneic BMT in patients with NHL (10,18,20,21) or Hodgkin's disease (10,11,18,21,22), and most of these reports have involved small numbers of patients (Table 49-2). The largest series was from Seattle and included 60 patients who underwent allogeneic BMT for refractory lymphoma (10). The majority of the patients were in resistant relapse (i.e., no longer sensitive to conventional-dose salvage therapy) at the time of BMT. All patients were treated with cyclophosphamide plus total body irradiation (Cy/TBI) and received methotrexate after transplantation as graft-versus-host disease (GVHD) prophylaxis. The overall event-free survival in this relatively poor risk group of patients was approximately 20% in both allogeneic and autologous BMT recipients, and in patients with both Hodgkin's disease and NHL. However, the relapse rate after allogeneic BMT was nearly 20% lower

Table 49-2.
Bone Marrow Transplantation for Lymphoma

No. Patients	*Preparative Regimen*	*Types of Lymphoma*	*% Patients with Sensitive Relapse*	*Continuous Complete Remission (% of Total)*	*Transplant-related Mortality (%)*	*Median Follow-up (Mo)*	*Ref*
60	CY/TBI (10–15.75 Gy)	NHL(A)-49/HD-11	18	23	36	24	(10)
19	CY/TBI (12 Gy) or BUCY	NHL(A)-9/HD-10	100	47	47	44	(18)
17	CYaraCTBI (14 Gy)	NHL(A)-10/HD-7	47	47	23	27	(21)
20	CY/TBI (12–14.4 Gy) or BUCY	HD	45	15	40	26	(11)
8	CBV	HD	0	12.5	50	29	(22)
8	BUCY	NHL(A)	75	50	12.5	26	(20)
6	TBI (13.2 Gy)	NHL(A)	100	67	17	18	(23)
4	CyaraCTBI	NHL(I)	0	75	25	19	(21)
17	CyTBI (8–14 Gy)	CLL	?	53	35	29	(37)

CY = cyclophosphamide; TBI = total body irradiation; araC = cytosine arabinoside; BU = busulfan; NHL(A) = aggressive non-Hodgkin's lymphoma; NHL(I) = indolent non-Hodgkin's lymphoma; HD = Hodgkin's disease; CLL = chronic lymphocytic leukemia; CBV = cyclophosphamide, BCNU, VP = 16.

than the relapse rate after autologous BMT, although differences did not reach statistical significance.

Likewise, a Johns Hopkins University study of BMT in 50 patients with relapsed Hodgkin's disease found that the actuarial relapse rate of 17% in allogeneic patients in sensitive relapse (i.e., still responsive to conventional-dose salvage therapy) was substantially lower than the 34% relapse rate in similar autologous BMT recipients (11). This difference also did not reach statistical significance. There was no difference in the actuarial event-free survival between the allogeneic (56% of patients in sensitive relapse) and autologous (51%) BMT recipients. The most important prognostic factor for outcome following BMT was the status of the lymphoma at the time of BMT (i.e., sensitive relapse versus resistant relapse). The type of preparative regimen, Cy/TBI versus busulfan-cyclophosphamide (BUCY), did not influence the outcome. The majority of the transplant-related deaths in this study were a result of interstitial pneumonitis; inadequate pulmonary function in the setting of prior chest irradiation predicted death from interstitial pneumonitis. Other smaller studies of allogeneic BMT in patients with aggressive lymphomas have shown similar results (see Table 49-2). A study of allogeneic BMT in patients with Hodgkin's disease in resistant relapse revealed a poor event-free survival (22). Conversely, three studies found only approximately a 30% relapse rate after allogeneic BMT for Hodgkin's disease and aggressive NHL in patients who were primarily in sensitive relapse (20,21,23). Again, both Cy/TBI and BUCY appeared to produce similar results. There did not appear to be any difference between the incidence of or complications from acute and chronic GVHD in any of the studies of allogeneic BMT in patients with lymphomas and that seen in age-matched patients with acute leukemia undergoing allogeneic BMT.

Allogeneic Graft-versus-lymphoma Effect

The existence of an immunological antitumor effect associated with allogeneic BMT was established in animal models more than 20 years ago (24–26). Multiple studies have now established a clinically significant antitumor effect, independent of the cytotoxic preparative regimen, against acute leukemias and chronic myeloid leukemia (4–9). The mechanisms responsible for this graft-versus-leukemia effect are not completely understood. Although GVHD, especially chronic GVHD, accounts for much of this graft-versus-tumor activity (4–9), allogeneic BMT appears to generate an immunological antileukemia effect independent of clinically significant GVHD (8,9).

As already mentioned, initial reports were unable to prove the existence of a similar graft-versus-tumor effect, associated with allogeneic BMT against lymphomas (10,11). However, the inability to document a graft-versus-lymphoma effect was likely the result of the limited statistical power of small sample sizes rather than biological differences between lymphomas and leukemias. There was a trend toward improved lymphoma control with allogeneic BMT in both studies. Moreover, it is unlikely that biological differences would be responsible, because lymphomas and acute lymphocytic leukemia are similar immunologically (27).

The results of BMT for relapsed Hodgkin's disease or aggressive NHL were analyzed in 118 consecutive patients at Johns Hopkins University to determine what characteristics, including type of graft, influenced outcome (18). The 38 patients, who were less than 50 years of age and had a human leukocyte antigen (HLA)–matched related donor underwent allogeneic BMT and the other 80 patients underwent purged autologous BMT. As previously shown (11,28), patient response to conventional salvage therapy before BMT was the only factor that influenced the event-free survival after BMT in a multivariate analysis. Patients in sensitive relapse had a significantly improved probability of event-free survival compared with those in resistant relapse ($p < 0.001$). Having sensitive disease also had a favorable influence on the probability of relapse after BMT.

Although the type of graft was not a significant prognostic factor for event-free survival after BMT, it was an independent prognostic factor for the probability of relapse after BMT in multivariate analysis (18). The actuarial event-free survival of patients in sensitive relapse was 41% for autologous BMT recipients and 47% for allogeneic BMT recipients (Figure 49-1*A*; $p = 0.8$). However, the allogeneic BMT recipients had a significantly lower relapse rate than the autologous BMT recipients. The actuarial probability of relapse after BMT was 46% for patients with sensitive disease undergoing autologous BMT, compared with only 18% for allogeneic graft recipients in sensitive relapse (Figure 49-1*B*; $p = 0.02$). The difference in relapse rates between allogeneic and autologous BMT recipients was similar for patients with Hodgkin's disease (24% difference) and NHL (29% difference). There were too few relapses (only 2 patients) in the patients who received allogeneic grafts for sensitive lymphomas to determine if the development of GVHD was associated with a decrease in relapse rate, as has been previously reported in patients undergoing allogeneic BMT for leukemia (5–7).

All the autologous marrows were morphologically free of lymphoma at the time of BMT and were purged in an attempt to eradicate any occult lymphoma cells that may have been present in the infused marrow. Nonetheless, it is possible that some of the difference in relapse rates between autologous and allogeneic BMT recipients was the result of infusing viable lymphoma cells with the autologous marrow. However, relapse rates and patterns of relapse in studies of patients with lymphomas undergoing purged autologous BMT (18,29,30) are similar to studies that did not use purging (28,31,32). Thus, failure to eradicate lymphoma in these patients appears to be a more important cause of disease progression than infusion

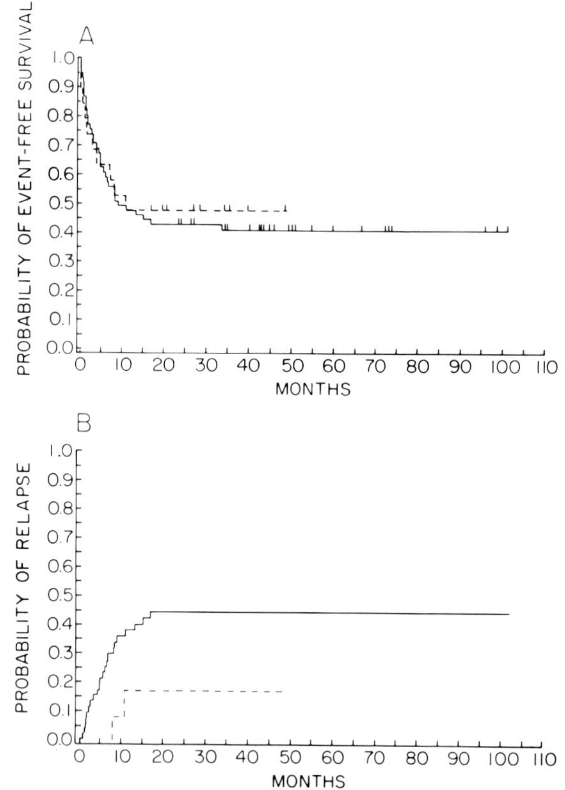

Figure 49-1. Actuarial probability of event-free survival (A) and relapse (B) in 61 patients who underwent autologous bone marrow transplantation (BMT) (*solid lines*) and 19 patients who underwent allogeneic BMT (*broken lines*) for aggressive lymphomas in sensitive relapse.

of occult lymphoma cells with the autologous marrow. The decreased relapse rate after allogeneic BMT likely results primarily from an immunological graft-versus-lymphoma effect.

As seen in patients with acute leukemia (4), the improved control of lymphoma with allogeneic BMT did not lead to an improvement in event-free survival (18). The beneficial graft-versus-lymphoma effect with allogeneic BMT was offset by increased peritransplant mortality, largely resulting from GVHD. Whereas 18 of 38 allogeneic BMT recipients (47%) died of causes directly related to BMT, 17 of 80 autologous BMT recipients (21%) died of transplant-related causes ($p = 0.007$). Acute GVHD developed in 24 of the 38 allogeneic BMT recipients (63%), and chronic GVHD developed in 8 of 25 allogeneic BMT recipients (32%) who survived at least 100 days. The majority of the deaths (11 of 18) resulting from allogeneic BMT were related to GVHD.

Indolent Lymphomas

There have been very few studies of allogeneic BMT in patients with indolent lymphomas. Indolent lymphomas affect an older group of patients (median age, > 55 yr) (33,34), and these patients can expect long-term survival (median, 7–11 yr) (33,34). Older patients undergoing allogeneic BMT have a high transplant-related mortality, largely resulting from the complications of GVHD; the long natural history makes it difficult to determine the role of BMT in these diseases because of the long follow-up needed after BMT to show an improvement in survival. A total of 7 patients who underwent allogeneic BMT for low-grade NHL have been reported (20,21,35). The largest series contained 4 patients (see Table 49-2) (21); 3 of the 4 are alive without disease. However, these 4 patients are very young for this disease (median age, 32 yr; range, 26–38 yr), and the follow-up was very short (median, 19 mo; range, 10 to 32 mo).

The largest experience with allogeneic BMT in patients with indolent lymphoid malignancies is in CLL; 26 patients are reported in the literature (36,37). The largest series was a collection of 17 patients from the European Bone Marrow Transplant Group (see Table 49-2) (37). Most of the patients had advanced-stage disease, although 5 had early stage CLL. The median age of the 17 patients was 40 (range, 32 to 49 yr), and the follow-up was short (median, 29 mo; range, 7 to 48 mo). The preparative regimen was Cy/TBI; 6 patients received additional chemotherapy with etoposide, chlorambucil, or melphalan. GVHD prophylaxis involved methotrexate alone in one patient, cyclosporine (CSP) alone in 2 patients, CSP and methotrexate in 11 patients, and CSP and T-cell depletion in 3 patients. Acute GVHD developed in all patients; 2 patients died directly as a result of GVHD. An additional 3 patients died of transplant-related causes, 3 relapsed, and 9 are alive and free of disease.

Autologous GVHD

A syndrome similar to GVHD develops spontaneously in 5 to 10% of patients undergoing autologous or syngeneic BMT (38–40). This syndrome clinically resembles GVHD, but it is a mild, self-limited disease that generally involves only the skin. Histological changes of this "autologous GVHD" are also identical to those of allogeneic GVHD. Autologous GVHD was controversial until the development of animal models for the syndrome (41–43). In these models, a syndrome similar to GVHD developed in rats or mice treated with CSP after syngeneic BMT. CSP-induced GVHD after syngeneic BMT in rats appears to be mediated by autoreactive T lymphocytes directed against class II histocompatibility (HLA-DR or Ia) antigens (44). Thus, autologous/syngeneic GVHD is an autoimmune syndrome, mediated by T lymphocytes that recognize Ia antigen, that develops after BMT. CSP appears to augment the development of autoreactive lymphocytes after BMT by blocking mechanisms that delete autoreactive T cells in the thymus (45).

GVHD after syngeneic BMT in animals exhibits antitumor activity similar to allogeneic GVHD against tumors that express Ia antigen (46,47). Because most lymphomas (including Reed-Sternberg cells of Hodgkin's disease) express Ia antigens (27), autologous GVHD could potentially produce a clinical immunological antilymphoma effect without increasing post-transplant toxicity. Autologous GVHD can be induced with CSP at a dose of 1 mg/kg/day beginning on the day of BMT and continuing for 28 days in the majority of patients undergoing autologous BMT for lymphomas (48). As in animals with syngeneic GVHD, autoreactive lymphocytes recognizing a public epitope of the Ia antigen appear to mediate clinical autologous GVHD. Other groups have now confirmed these clinical results by inducing autologous GVHD, including finding Ia-restricted autoreactive lymphocytes in patients with autologous GVHD (49,50). Preliminary results in patients with aggressive NHLs in sensitive relapse suggest that there may be a clinically significant antitumor effect, similar to that seen in the animal models, associated with autologous GVHD (51).

Conclusions

Allogeneic BMT for Aggressive Lymphomas

Although there have been very few patients with lymphomas who have undergone allogeneic BMT, a number of conclusions can still be reached. Allogeneic BMT for lymphomas presents no special procedural considerations compared with age-matched allogeneic BMT for other diseases. The incidence of transplant related complications, especially GVHD, can be expected to be similar to that seen with age-matched allogeneic BMT for other diseases. Although most studies of allogeneic BMT in patients with lymphomas have used Cy/TBI-based preparative therapy, there is no evidence that any preparative regimen produces superior results. Most importantly, allogeneic BMT generates immunological antitumor activity against lymphomas that appears to decrease the relapse rate in patients by approximately 25 to 30% compared with autologous BMT. The magnitude of this graft-versus-lymphoma effect is similar to the better recognized graft-versus-leukemia effect associated with allogeneic BMT. However, this immunological graft-versus-tumor effect has not translated into an improvement in event-free survival for allogeneic BMT recipients. The beneficial graft-versus-lymphoma effect associated with allogeneic BMT is offset by increased transplant-related mortality, largely resulting from GVHD.

Nevertheless, its superior antitumor activity makes allogeneic BMT an important approach for continued study in patients with lymphomas. In fact, allogeneic and autologous BMT have the same advantages and disadvantages and produce similar results in patients with aggressive lymphomas as in patients with acute leukemia. Hence, the same approach should be used in deciding which type of transplant (autologous versus allogeneic) is best for patients with aggressive lymphomas as for patients with acute leukemia.

Therefore, allogeneic BMT from HLA-matched siblings may be preferred over autologous BMT for patients with relapsed Hodgkin's disease or aggressive NHL at low risk for the complications of GVHD. This approach would particularly pertain to patients with Hodgkin's disease or Burkitt's and lymphoblastic lymphomas, whose median ages are less than 30. The immunological antilymphoma activity of allogeneic BMT may outweigh the toxicity of GVHD in these patients. Only approximately one third of the patients who are likely to benefit from allogeneic BMT for lymphoma will have an HLA-identical sibling. Because of the increased toxicity of GVHD with partially matched related or matched unrelated transplants, and because of the superb overall results with autologous BMT in these diseases, autologous BMT should probably be chosen over allogeneic BMT when an HLA-identical sibling donor is not available.

Allogeneic BMT for Indolent Lymphomas

The number of patients with indolent lymphoid malignancies (CLL and indolent lymphomas) is too small and the follow-up is too short to draw any conclusions about the effectiveness of allogeneic BMT in these diseases. Moreover, patients with indolent lymphoid malignancies are at high risk for the complications of allogeneic BMT because of their older median age. The long survival associated with these diseases, regardless of stage, also makes the high transplant-related mortality associated with allogeneic BMT unattractive. Although allogeneic BMT could be considered in the small number of patients (approximately 10%) who are less than 60 years of age, the prognosis of these younger patients is even better than the general population with indolent lymphomas (52). Furthermore, there is currently no definitive evidence that BMT can be curative in patients with indolent lymphomas. For these reasons, autologous BMT should probably be preferred over allogeneic BMT in patients with indolent lymphomas because of its relatively lower transplant-related mortality.

CLL has been separated from the other lymphoid malignancies in reports of allogeneic BMT, probably because of the bone marrow involvement in this disease. However, CLL is biologically the same disease as small lymphocytic lymphoma, with the same natural history. Moreover, bone marrow involvement is present at diagnosis in the majority of patients with indolent lymphomas without affecting prognosis (16,53), and a frank leukemic presentation occurs in approximately 25% of patients with indolent lymphoma. Therefore, when considering BMT, CLL is probably best approached similarly to the other indolent lymphomas.

Allogeneic BMT as a Model for Improving Autologous BMT

Improvements in the outcome of allogeneic BMT will require decreasing the toxicity of GVHD without eradicating the immunological antitumor activity associated with allogeneic BMT. Substantial improvement in the outcome of autologous BMT for lymphomas requires enhancing the antitumor activity of the procedure. It is unlikely that major advances can be made in improving the antitumor activity of cytotoxic preparative regimens. Current preparative regimens are at or near nonhematological dose-limiting toxicity, hindering further increases in the intensity of, or the addition of new cytotoxic agents to, these preparative regimens. Immunological approaches that mimic the immunological antitumor activity of allogeneic BMT (i.e., autologous GVHD or post-transplant interleukin-2) probably offer the best chance for increasing tumor control with autologous BMT.

References

1. Longo DL, Duffey PL, Young RC, et al. Conventional-dose salvage combination chemotherapy in patients relapsing with Hodgkin's disease after combination chemotherapy: the low probability for cure. J Clin Oncol 1992;10:210–218.
2. Santoro A, Bonfante V, Bonadonna G. Salvage chemotherapy with ABVD in MOPP-resistant Hodgkin's disease. Ann Intern Med 1982;96:139–143.
3. Santos GW, Yeager AM, Jones RJ. Autologous bone marrow transplantation. Ann Rev Med 1989;40:99–112.
4. Kersey JH, Weisdorf D, Nesbit ME, et al. Comparison of autologous and allogeneic bone marrow transplantation for treatment of high-risk refractory acute lymphoblastic leukemia. N Engl J Med 1987;317:461–467.
5. Weiden PL, Flournoy N, Thomas ED, et al. Antileukemic effect of graft-versus-host disease in human recipients of allogeneic-marrow grafts. N Engl J Med 1979;300:1068–1073.
6. Weiden PL, Sullivan KM, Flournoy N, Storb R, Thomas ED. Antileukemic effect of chronic graft-versus-host disease. N Engl J Med 1981;304:1529–1533.
7. Sullivan KM, Storb R, Buckner CD, et al. Graft-versus-host disease as adoptive immunotherapy in patients with advanced hematologic neoplasms. N Engl J Med 1989;320:828–834.
8. Butturini A, Bortin MM, Gale RP. Graft-versus-leukemia following bone marrow transplantation. Bone Marrow Transplant 1987;2:233–242.
9. Horowitz MM, Gale RP, Sondel PM, et al. Graft-versus-leukemia reactions after bone marrow transplantation. Blood 1990;75:555–562.
10. Appelbaum FR, Sullivan KM, Buckner CD, et al. Treatment of malignant lymphoma in 100 patients with chemotherapy, total body irradiation, and marrow transplantation. J Clin Oncol 1987;5:1340–1347.
11. Jones RJ, Piantadosi S, Mann RB, et al. High-dose cytotoxic therapy and bone marrow transplantation for relapsed Hodgkin's disease. J Clin Oncol 1990;8:527–537.
12. Gribben JG, Freedman AS, Neuberg D, et al. Immunologic purging of marrow assessed by PCR before autologous bone marrow transplantation for B-cell lymphoma. N Engl J Med 1991;325:1525–1533.
13. Vaughan WP, Weisenburger DD, Sanger W, Gale RP, Armitage JO. Early leukemic recurrence of non-Hodgkin lymphoma after high-dose anti-neoplastic therapy with autologous marrow rescue. Bone Marrow Transplant 1987;1:373–378.
14. Bartl R, Frisch B, Burkhardt R, Huhn D, Papenberger R. Assessment of bone marrow histology in Hodgkin's disease: correlation with clinical factors. Br J Haematol 1982;51:345–360.
15. Rosenberg SA. Hodgkin's disease of the bone marrow. Cancer Res 1971;31:1733–1736.
16. Bennett JM, Cain KC, Glick JH, Johnson GJ, Ezdinli E, O'Connell MJ. The significance of bone marrow involvement in non-Hodgkin's lymphoma: the Eastern Cooperative Oncology Group Experience. J Clin Oncol 1986;4:1462–1469.
17. Conlan MG, Bast M, Armitage JO, Weisenburger DD. Bone marrow involvement by non-Hodgkin's lymphoma: the clinical significance of morphologic discordance between the lymph node and bone marrow. J Clin Oncol 1990;8:1163–1172.
18. Jones RJ, Ambinder RF, Piantadosi S, Santos GW. Evidence of a graft-versus-lymphoma effect associated with allogeneic bone marrow transplantation. Blood 1991;77:649–653.
19. DeVita VT, Jaffe ES, Mauch P, Longo DL. Lymphocytic lymphomas. In: DeVita VT, Hellman S, Rosenberg SA, eds. Cancer, principal and practice of oncology. Philadelphia: J.B. Lippincott, 1989:1741–1798.
20. Copelan EA, Kapoor N, Gibbins B, Tutschka PJ. Allogeneic marrow transplantation in non-Hodgkin's lymphoma. Bone Marrow Transplant 1990;5:47–50.
21. Lundberg JH, Hansen RM, Chitambar CR, et al. Allogeneic bone marrow transplantation for relapsed and refractory lymphoma using genotypically HLA-identical and alternative donors. J Clin Oncol 1991;9:1848–1859.
22. Phillips GL, Reece DE, Barnett MJ, et al. Allogeneic marrow transplantation for refractory Hodgkin's disease. J Clin Oncol 1989;7:1039–1045.
23. Nademanee AP, Forman SH, Schmidt GM, et al. Allogeneic bone marrow transplantation for high risk non-Hodgkin's lymphoma during first complete remission. Blut 1987;55:11–18.
24. Owens AH Jr, Santos GW. The effect of cyclophosphamide and allogeneic and parental spleen cells on the course of L1210 leukemia. Exp Hematol 1965;8:15–17.
25. Bortin MM, Rimm AA, Saltzstein EC. Graft versus leukemia: quantification of adoptive immunotherapy in murine leukemia. Science 1973;179:811–813.
26. Bortin MM, Rimm AA, Saltzstein EC, Rodey GE. Graft versus leukemia. Transplantation 1973;16:182–188.
27. Foon KA, Todd RF, III. Immunologic classification of leukemia and lymphoma. Blood 1986;68:1–31.
28. Philip T, Armitage JO, Spitzer G, et al. High-dose therapy and autologous bone marrow transplantation after failure of conventional chemotherapy in adults with intermediate-grade or high-grade non-Hodgkin's lymphoma. N Engl J Med 1987;316:1493–1498.
29. Takvorian T, Canellos GP, Ritz J, et al. Prolonged disease-free survival after autologous bone marrow transplantation in patients with non-Hodgkin's lymphoma with a poor prognosis. N Engl J Med 1987; 316:1499–1505.
30. Gulati SC, Shank B, Black P, et al. Autologous bone marrow transplantation for patients with poor-prognosis lymphoma. J Clin Oncol 1988;6:1303–1313.
31. Carella AM, Congiu AM, Gaozza E, et al. High-dose chemotherapy with autologous bone marrow transplantation in 50 advanced resistant Hodgkin's disease patients: an Italian study group report. J Clin Oncol 1988;6:1411–1416.

32. Jagannath S, Armitage JO, Dicke KA, et al. Prognostic factors for response and survival after high-dose cyclophosphamide, carmustine, and etoposide with autologous bone marrow transplantation for relapsed Hodgkin's disease. J Clin Oncol 1989;7:179–185.
33. Horning SJ, Rosenberg SA. The natural history of initially untreated low-grade non-Hodgkin's lymphomas. N Engl J Med 1984;311:1471–1475.
34. Rosenberg SA. The low-grade non-Hodgkin's lymphomas: challenges and opportunities. J Clin Oncol 1985;3:299–310.
35. Appelbaum FR, Thomas ED, Buckner CD, et al. Treatment of non-Hodgkin's lymphoma with chemoradiotherapy and allogenic marrow transplantation. Hematol Oncol 1983;1:149–157.
36. Bandini G, Michallet M, Rosti G, Tura S. Bone marrow transplantation for chronic lymphocytic leukemia. Bone Marrow Transplant 1991;7:251–253.
37. Michallet M, Corront B, Hollard D, et al. Allogeneic bone marrow transplantation in chronic lymphocytic leukemia: 17 cases. Report from the EBMTG. Bone Marrow Transplant 1991;7:275–279.
38. Rappeport J, Mihm M, Reinherz E, Lopansri S, Parkman R. Acute graft-versus-host disease in recipients of bone-marrow transplants from identical twin donors. Lancet 1979;2:717–720.
39. Hood AF, Vogelsang GB, Black LP, Farmer ER, Santos GW. Acute graft-vs-host disease. Development following autologous and syngeneic bone marrow transplantation. Arch Dermatol 1987;123:745–750.
40. Einsele H, Ehnigner G, Schneider EM, et al. High frequency of graft-versus-host like syndromes following syngeneic bone marrow transplantation. Transplantation 1988;45:579–585.
41. Glazier A, Tutschka PJ, Farmer ER, Santos GW. Graft-versus-host disease in cyclosporin A-treated rats after syngeneic and autologous bone marrow reconstitution. J Exp Med 1983;158:1–8.
42. Cheney RT, Sprent J. Capacity of cyclosporine to induce auto-graft-versus-host disease and impair intrathymic T cell differentiation. Transplant Proc 1985;17:528–530.
43. Bryson JS, Jennings CD, Caywood BE, Kaplan AM. Induction of a syngeneic graft-versus-host disease like syndrome in DBA/2 mice. Transplantation 1989;48:1042–1047.
44. Hess AD, Horwitz L, Beschorner WE, Santos GW. Development of graft-vs-host disease like syndrome in cyclosporine-treated rats after syngeneic bone marrow transplantation. J Exp Med 1985;161:718–730.
45. Jenkins MK, Schwartz RH, Pardoll DM. Effects of cyclosporine A on T cell development and clonal deletion. Science 1988;241:1655–1658.
46. Geller RB, Esa AH, Beschorner WE, Frondoza CG, Santos GW, Hess AD. Successful in vitro graft-versus-tumor effect against an Ia-bearing tumor using cyclosporine-induced syngeneic graft-versus-host disease in the rat. Blood 1989;74:1165–1171.
47. Hess AD, Noga SJ. Syngeneic graft versus host disease (SGVHD): an autoimmune therapeutic approach for residual leukemia (abstract). Blood 1991;78:188a.
48. Jones RJ, Vogelsang GB, Hess AD, et al. Induction of graft-versus-host disease following autologous bone marrow transplantation. Lancet 1989;2:754–757.
49. Dale BM, Atkinson K, Kotasek D, Biggs JC, Sage RE. Cyclosporine-induced graft vs host disease in two patients receiving syngeneic bone marrow transplants. Transplant Proc 1989;21:3816–3817.
50. Carella AM, Gaozza E, Congiu A, et al. Cyclosporine-induced graft-versus-host disease after autologous bone marrow transplantation in hematological malignancies. Ann Hematol 1991;62:156–159.
51. Jones RJ, Vogelsang GB, Ambinder RF, Santos GW, Hess AD. Autologous marrow transplantation (ABMT) with cyclosporine (CSA)-induced autologous graft-versus-host disease (GVHD) for relapsed aggressive non-Hodgkin's lymphoma (NHL), (abstract). Blood 1991;78:287a.
52. Lee JS, Dixon DO, Kantarjian HM, Keating MJ, Talpaz M. Prognosis of chronic lymphocytic leukemia: a multivariate regression analysis of 325 untreated patients. Blood 1987;69:929–936.
53. Gallagher CJ, Gregory WM, Jones AE, et al. Follicular lymphoma: prognostic factors for response and survival. J Clin Oncol 1986;4:1470–1480.

Chapter 50

Bone Marrow Transplantation for the Acquired Immune Deficiency Syndrome

Rein Saral and H. Kent Holland

In 1981, a series of articles appeared in the medical literature documenting the occurrence of opportunistic infections in homosexual men (1–3). This was the first clinical recognition of infection by the human immunodeficiency virus (HIV) causing the acquired immune deficiency syndrome (AIDS). In the past decade, the enormous public health implications of HIV disease have begun to be understood. An unprecedented research effort has defined the causative agent (HIV) and determined the molecular structure of the virus (4–10). The multiple clinical problems confronted by patients with HIV have been described and continue to present challenges both diagnostically and therapeutically for physicians involved in the care of these patients (11). The immunological consequences of infection with HIV have also been described, and efforts continue to define further the mechanisms responsible for the immunodeficiency that results from infection (12,13).

Malignancy and Immunodeficiency

The increased frequency of cancer in patients with impaired immune functions has been recognized for at least 2 decades (14). Studies in patients with genetically determined immunodeficiency have demonstrated an increased incidence of malignancy. Patients with ataxia telangiectasia, an autosomal recessive disease, have disorders of both cellular and humoral immunity, with a 60- to 180-fold excess risk for development of cancer (15). Non-Hodgkin's lymphomas (NHLs) and leukemia are common malignancies seen in this patient population, although solid tumors are also observed. The Wiskott-Aldrich syndrome, a sex-linked disease, is associated with a high risk of malignancy. Patients with this disorder have defects in their immunoglobulin (Ig) production, T-cell and platelet (PLT) dysfunction, and a 100-fold increased risk of NHL (16). These B-cell lymphomas are high grade, with a propensity for extranodal presentation and a high likelihood of brain involvement. Patients with severe combined immunodeficiency, combined variable immunodeficiency, and infantile sex-linked hypogammaglobulinemia are at increased risk for malignancy (14).

Until the outbreak of AIDS, the most common form of acquired immunodeficiency was that associated with solid organ transplantation and bone marrow transplantation (BMT). Use of immunosuppressive drugs to prevent graft rejection has improved survival and allowed a marked increase in the use of organ transplantation as a therapeutic modality. However, there is a significant increase in the incidence of cancer in organ and bone marrow transplant recipients who receive post-transplant immunosuppression (17,18). There is a marked increase in lymphoid malignancies in transplant recipients, similar to that observed in selected populations with genetically determined immunodeficiency.

Malignancy and HIV Infection

Shortly after the recognition and description of AIDS, an association was made between certain malignancies and AIDS. Kaposi's sarcoma was first recognized in young homosexual men at the same time opportunistic infections were reported in a similar patient population (19). In 1982, an outbreak of Burkitt's-like lymphoma was reported in homosexual men, and in 1984, NHL in 90 homosexual men was described by Ziegler and colleagues (20,21). Other studies emphasized the emergence of lymphomas in HIV-positive patients (22–26). The striking findings in these reports were the young age of the patients, the high-grade nature of the lymphoma, the extranodal involvement, and the primary involvement of the brain. In a recent analysis of nearly 100,000 patients with AIDS, approximately 3% had NHLs (27). On the basis of this analysis, the risk of NHL is estimated to be at least 60 times greater for patients with AIDS than for the general population. Of 2,824 NHLs in HIV-positive patients, 1,695 (60%) occurred in patients under the age of 40, and 2,701 (96%) occurred in patients under the age of 60. The majority of lymphomas diagnosed in patients with AIDS are high-grade B-cell types, although T-cell lymphomas have been reported (28). Large-cell immunoblastic and small uncleaved (Burkitt's) lymphomas account for approximately two-thirds of the AIDS-related NHLs diagnosed. The remaining lymphomas are intermediate-grade diffuse large-cell lymphomas. The high frequency of Burkitt's lymphomas is notable because it accounts for only 5% of all cases of NHL reported in the United States. Stage IV disease is seen in a large number of patients with marrow involvement, especially those with Burkitt's lymphomas. Primary central nervous system (CNS) disease is common; it occurs in approximately 20 to 25% of those who present with NHL. CNS involvement by lymphomas generally presents as mass lesions, but diffuse leptomeningeal disease may also be seen (29).

Antiretroviral therapies (e.g., zidovudine), prophylaxis, and treatment of herpesvirus, bacterial and fungal infections, and *Pneumocystis carinii* have led to prolonged survival of patients with AIDS (30,31). However, this prolonged survival results in increases in the prevalence of NHL. In a study of 55 symptomatic patients with AIDS who received zidovudine-containing regimens, NHLs developed in 8, at a median of 24 months after initiating therapy (23). Using Kaplan-Meier methodology, the estimated probability for development of lymphoma was 29% after 30 months of therapy and 46% after 36 months. Patients in whom lymphomas developed had less than 100 CD4 cells/mm^3 for a median of 18 months and less than 50 CD4 cells/mm^3 for a median of 15 months. NHLs may occur independently of CD4 cell count in patients with AIDS but appear to be increased if the CD4 cell count decreases below 50 mm^3. Current studies suggest that between 2,900 and 9,800 cases of AIDS-associated lymphomas per year will occur in the early 1990s (32). When one considers that there are approximately 38,000 cases of NHL per year in the United States, the significant impact of AIDS on this disease is apparent.

Mechanisms of Malignancy

The potential mechanisms by which lymphoid malignancies develop in HIV-infected and other immunocompromised patients continue to be the object of many studies. Advances in molecular immunology and molecular biology will provide tools to elucidate specific pathways that lead to malignant transformation.

Chromosomal translocations have been described in these B-cell malignancies, emphasizing their potential role in malignant transformation. In Burkitt's lymphoma, oncogene activation occurs when the *c-myc* gene located at chromosome 8 is translocated to the Ig gene heavy-chain region on chromosome 14 (33). Translocation of the *bcl-1* gene from chromosome 11 to chromosome 14 has been observed in leukemia, lymphoma, and multiple myeloma, and translocation of the *bcl-2* gene from chromosome 18 to chromosome 14 in lymphoma (34,35). Other translocations have been observed and correlated with disease characteristics (36).

The association between Epstein-Barr virus (EBV) and B-cell lymphomas has been observed and recognized for nearly 30 years (37). Two forms of Burkitt's lymphoma have been classified. The endemic/high incidence form of the disease is restricted to areas of Africa and New Guinea, and the Epstein-Barr genome is consistently detected in the tumor (38). The low incidence/sporadic form is seen globally, but Epstein-Barr viral genome is detected in only 15 to 20% of patients. In both diseases, chromosome translocations involving the *c-myc* oncogene are observed; however, there are differences at the molecular level in the breakpoint locations on the chromosome (39). Burkitt's lymphoma in patients with AIDS more closely resembles the sporadic form in both the translocation breakpoint and the presence of EBV in the lymphoma (40,41).

EBV has been associated with non-Burkitt's B-cell lymphomas, especially in patients with chronic immunosuppression (42–44). Large cell immunoblastic B-cell lymphomas that occur in this setting may contain EBV, which may reflect viral-induced B-cell activation in the absence of normal T-cell surveillance, resulting in genetic events that lead to malignant transformation. Studies of the primary CNS lymphoma in patients with AIDS suggest that EBV is present consistently, a finding similar to those in CNS lymphomas that occur in allograft recipients (45,46). Many of the systemic immunoblastic lymphomas in patients with AIDS contain EBV, but absence of the virus in similar lymphomas in some patients with AIDS suggests the importance of other mechanisms in the process of malignant transformations.

The importance of tumor suppressor genes in the pathogenesis of all forms of cancer has been recognized by many investigators (47). Losses of or mutations in specific tumor suppressor genes appear to be important in the process of malignant transformation (48–50). In addition, the binding of viral proteins to suppressor gene proteins, or inactivation of these proteins, may be important mechanisms that enhance the process of transformation (51,52).

Cytokines are a group of proteins that are important in the proliferation and differentiation of lymphohematopoietic cells. Although cytokines are important under normal conditions, they may also be important in enhancing malignant transformation. Interleukin-6 (IL-6) is an example of a cytokine that may have a role in the development of non-Hodgkin's B-cell lymphoma in HIV-infected patients. This cytokine is a B-cell growth and differentiation factor (53). HIV infection can lead to increased IL-6 production. HIV-infected monocytes producing IL-6 promote the proliferation of activated B cells, which could enhance the process of malignant transformation (54,55).

It is obvious that multiple factors are responsible for the increased prevalence of lymphoma in patients with AIDS. It is also clear that further investigation will establish the cascade of events that leads to malignant transformation and the development of lymphoma. This knowledge is of fundamental importance in understanding the molecular basis of neoplasia and will allow scientists to develop better therapeutic and prophylactic strategies to treat or prevent these malignancies.

Treatment of Non-Hodgkin's Lymphoma in Patients with AIDS

Treatment of lymphoma in patients with AIDS presents a therapeutic challenge. A number of effective chemotherapeutic regimens have been developed for the treatment of high-grade lymphomas in patients in whom the disease develops de novo without an apparent risk factor (e.g., organ transplantation, HIV infection). Complete response rates of 60 to 80% with long-term disease-free survival have been observed using a variety of chemotherapeutic regimens (e.g., CHOP [cyclosphosphamide, adriamycin, vincristine and prednisone]; ProMACE-MOPP [prednisone, methotrexate, adriamycin, cyclophosphamide (CY), etoposide-mechlorethamine, vincristine, procarbazine, prednisone]). Use of similar regimens to treat HIV-infected patients with lymphomas has not yielded similar results. Although remissions are achieved with chemotherapy, the ultimate fate of this group of patients is death. The reasons for failure include refractory disease or relapse, or relentless progression of the underlying immunodeficiency with the development of opportunistic infections (22,56–58).

Rationale for BMT for AIDS

The rationale for considering BMT as a therapy for patients with HIV infection is presented in Table 50-1. The major reservoir of cells containing HIV is lymphocytes (primarily $CD4^{+}$), macrophages, myeloid cells, Lagerhan-dendritic cells, B lymphocytes transformed by EBV, and microglial cells (59–67). These are precisely the cells that are destroyed by preparative regimens used prior to BMT. These cells are reconstituted from donor-derived progenitor cells after BMT. Studies demonstrate that patients who receive high-dose chemotherapy with or without total body irradation (TBI) followed by allogeneic BMT reconstitute their lymphohematopoietic systems with donor-derived cells (68,69). This complete chimerism has been proved using cytogenetic and molecular (e.g., restriction fragment length polymorphism [RFLP]) techniques in the majority of patients (70,71). Thus, lymphoid and hematopoietic cells are of donor origin following allogeneic BMT, including monocyte/macrophage populations such as Kupffer's cells in the liver, alveolar macrophages in the lung, and microglial cells in the CNS (72–74). Investigators have demonstrated that EBV may be of donor origin following allogeneic BMT because recipient B cells have been eradicated and replaced by donor B cells (75).

Table 50-1.
Rationale for Bone Marrow Transplantation in HIV-positive Patients

1. Ablate HIV-containing cells resident in the hematopoietic-lymphoid reservoir
2. Reconstitute host with uninfected donor hematopoietic-lymphoid precursors
3. Prevent infection of donor-derived cells by HIV

HIV = human immunodeficiency virus.

If the preparative regimen effectively destroys the lymphohematopoietic reservoir of HIV, the next important consideration is protecting donor cells from infection by HIV because these donor cells are susceptible to infection by residual host HIV. If the reservoir of virus is destroyed and donor cells are free of HIV, then immune reconstitution should occur in a similar time frame as described in other patient populations following BMT (76). A testable hypothesis is the use of BMT preceded by a marrow lethal preparative regimen to eradicate the reservoir of HIV and to reconstitute the patient with donor cells utilizing therapies to prevent donor cells from being infected by HIV.

As is discussed later in this chapter, there are a number of theoretical approaches to preventing HIV infection of donor cells following allogeneic BMT or conferring resistance to the virus in autologous lymphohematopoietic progenitor cells. The initial approach was based on preclinical studies and clinical trials, which suggested that antiretroviral chemotherapy might be capable of limiting or preventing the infection of permissive cells by HIV. Zidovudine, a reverse transcriptase inhibitor, has demonstrated efficacy in treating patients with HIV infection (77–79). Early preclinical studies suggested that this compound, at concentrations achievable in humans, was capable of inhibiting infectivity and cytopathic effects of HIV in CD4 lymphocyte cell lines and human peripheral mononuclear cells (80). In vivo studies demonstrated that zidovudine inhibited murine and feline retroviral infection and disease when the drug was administered at the time of initial viral exposure (81–83). These studies suggested that zidovudine could be used as prophylaxis against HIV infection. A major concern in using zidovudine in patients undergoing BMT was its effects on marrow function. Because zidovudine suppressed hematopoiesis in patients with AIDS, it was felt that its use as prophylaxis for pre-BMT and immediate postallogeneic BMT recipients could cause the marrow engraftment to be jeopardized. In unpublished studies, it was determined that zidovudine did suppress but did not prevent growth of hematopoietic colonies in vitro at concentrations used in therapy. In addition, use of zidovudine in a rat allogeneic BMT model did not prevent or delay engraftment (84).

On the basis of these observations, it appeared reasonable to consider a clinical trial of allogeneic BMT in patients with HIV infection. Patients would receive marrow ablative therapy with high-dose chemotherapy and TBI to destroy the reservoir of cells containing HIV. Marrow from an HLA-identical sibling would be administered to reconstitute a new lymphohematopoietic system, and antiretroviral therapy would be given prior to and following BMT as prophylaxis to prevent or retard HIV infection of donor cells.

Because patients with HIV infection had a high likelihood for developing of malignant disease, they were obviously a group to consider for BMT. Currently, the Emory group considers BMT for HIV-positive patients with NHL in first or subsequent remission after initial chemotherapy or for those patients who continue to have disease but who respond to chemotherapy (chemosensitive disease) and who have an human leukocyte antigen (HLA)–matched family member donor who is HIV-negative. Patients are excluded if they have active opportunistic infection or significant organ dysfunction. We also consider BMT for HIV-positive patients who have a malignant disease for which BMT is the treatment of choice, including patients with acute or chronic leukemia and other lymphohematopoietic malignant diseases, such as Hodgkin's disease.

Experience with BMT and HIV

The experience with BMT in HIV-positive patients is limited. Initial studies by the National Institutes of Health (NIH) group and others did not employ a preparative regimen to reduce the viral burden. Patients with HIV were given marrow and peripheral blood with antiretroviral therapy in varying combinations (85–88). Donors were HIV seronegative identical twins. The investigators reasoned that infusion of immune competent cells in conjunction with antiviral therapy would restart a functioning immune system and exert an antiviral effect. These studies did not demonstrate a significant effect on the virus, although transient improvements in immune responses were observed. Several HIV positive patients received BMTs utilizing a preparative regimen without the use of antiretroviral therapy to inhibit viral replication and infection of donor cells. The results were poor with no evidence that HIV viral burden was effected (80,89–91).

The Hopkins and Emory group have performed 8 BMTs in patients with HIV infections. Five of the 8 patients received allogeneic BMTs, and 3 received syngeneic BMTs. Seven of the 8 patients received a preparative regimen of CY (50 mg/kg daily for 4 days) and TBI (3 Gy daily for 4 days with lung shielding on the third day), and one patient received busulfan (Bu; 4 mg/kg daily for 4 days) and CY (50 mg/kg daily for 4 days). All patients received intravenous zidovudine starting 2 weeks prior to BMT and continuing indefinitely, with a switch to oral administration at the time of discharge from the hospital.

Only one of 8 patients died less than 30 days following BMT. Complications occurring during this period were not different from those experienced by non-HIV–positive BMT recipients. A major concern was the effect of zidovudine on engraftment. All patients who survived for longer than 30 days engrafted. Complete chimerism (using cytogenetic or RFLP analysis) was demonstrated in patients who received an allogeneic BMT. Although myeloid engraftment and recovery were noted in all patients surviving more than 30 days, prolonged thrombocytopenia requiring transfusion was observed in several patients. All patients had slow recovery of erythroid function and required red-cell transfusion support.

Six of 8 patients have been studied to determine the effect of the preparative regimen and zidovudine on HIV. Three allogeneic and 3 syngeneic BMT recipients were evaluated with quantitative cultures for the virus and polymerase chain reaction (PCR) for viral sequences (RNA and DNA) in blood, marrow, and tissues (if available). Two of the 3 allogeneic recipients had evidence of viral eradication by culture or by PCR analysis following transplantation. The first patient died of recurrent lymphoma 47 days following BMT. Extensive studies of organs (including brain) at autopsy failed to reveal HIV in any organ (84). The second patient with lymphoma had disappearance of HIV by quantitative culture and by PCR analysis following BMT. Cultures remained negative from 40 days until 120 days after BMT when HIV was detected. The patient subsequently died of complications from graft-versus-host disease (GVHD). Both patients received a preparative regimen containing CY followed by TBI. Neither of these patients received zidovudine therapy prior to BMT (e.g., virus was zidovudine-naive). The third allogeneic recipient received zidovudine for months prior to consideration for BMT and was given a preparative regimen of BU followed by CY because he had received significant radiation treatment prior to BMT. This patient remained culture-positive after BMT.

All 3 syngeneic transplant recipients had advanced HIV disease. Their CD4 lymphocyte counts ranged from 10 to 100 mm^3 prior to BMT, and all had received zidovudine for more than 6 months prior to transplantation. Pretransplant HIV was obtained from all 3 patients, and these isolates were tested for sensitivity to zidovudine. Two of the 3 patients had highly resistant virus (>10μmol/L zidovudine required for inhibition), and the third had virus inhibited by 2μmol/L zidovudine. This finding is in contrast to the one allogeneic recipient who had disappearance of virus after BMT and had pre-BMT isolate that was inhibited by 0.02μmol/L zidovudine. None of the 3 syngeneic recipients showed clearance of virus, although their CY/TBI conditioning regimen was identical to that of allogeneic recipients. All 3 remained culture-positive from some site (blood or marrow) in the post-BMT period, although a decrease in virus titer was detected in all patients.

The importance of viral sensitivity to zidovudine is demonstrated in Figure 50-1. Allogeneic BMT recipients with zidovudine-sensitive virus had complete disappearance of HIV by quantitative culture by 6 weeks following BMT with a multi-log reduction in virus. In contrast, a patient with virus resistant to zidovudine had a less dramatic effect on viral load. However, in the 2 patients with highly resistant virus,

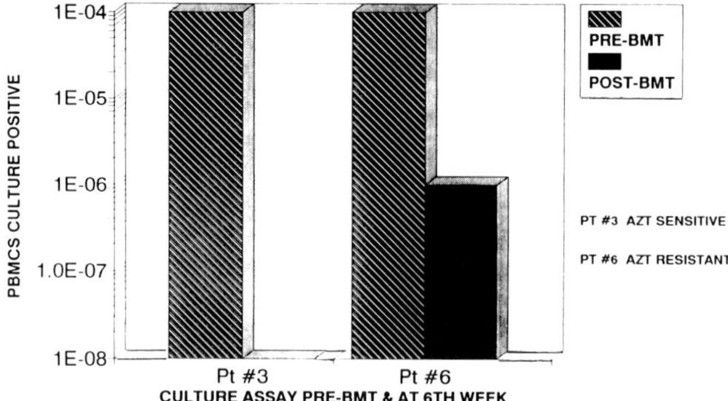

Figure 50-1. Representative human immunodeficiency virus type 1 (HIV-1) cultures performed on 2 patients who underwent bone marrow transplantation (BMT). Quantitative cultures of peripheral blood mononuclear cells (PBMCs) were assayed at 10^3, 10^4, 10^5, 10^6, and 10^7 PBMCS to detect the presence of HIV-1 infection. Patient 3 underwent allogeneic BMT for lymphoma, and the pre-BMT HIV-1 isolate was noted to be zidovudine (AZT)–sensitive, as defined by an IC_{50} of <0.1 μmol in vitro. Quantitative HIV-1 cultures before BMT were positive at a cell dose of 10^4; post-BMT quantitative HIV-1 cultures were negative up to a dose concentration of 10^7. Patient 6 underwent a syngeneic BMT, and the pre-BMT HIV-1 isolate was noted to be AZT-resistant, as defined by an IC_{50} of >10 μmol in vitro. Despite the presence of resistant HIV-1, quantitative culture performed at the 6th week demonstrated a 2-log reduction, from 10^4 pre-BMT to 10^6 PBMCs cultured positive.

quantitative cultures demonstrated a 1- to 2-log reduction in virus in blood or bone marrow, suggesting that the preparative regimen was effective in cytoreducing cells that are reservoirs of the virus. The results also suggest the importance of utilizing effective therapy to prevent infection of donor cells by HIV.

An important consideration in using BMT as a therapeutic approach to HIV-positive patients is the ability to reconstitute immune function in the post-BMT period. Preliminary studies suggest that immune reconstitution is possible (84).

In an attempt to transfer immune responses adoptively from donor to patient, the donor was immunized with a common recall antigen (e.g., tetanus toxoid) and the recipient was immunized shortly after infusion of marrow. Patients who were unable to mount a proliferative response to the antigens prior to BMT were able to do so following immunization, suggesting that immune reconstitution is possible following transplantation in this patient population. Clearly, sustained immune function is dependent on preventing infection of donor cells by HIV and is theoretically and practically possible.

These preliminary studies evaluating BMT in HIV-positive patients are similar to the early studies evaluating BMT in the treatment of refractory hematopoietic malignancy (92). Complete responses have been observed, and patients who failed to achieve complete responses had significant reduction in the number of HIV-infected cells.

BMT and AIDS: Future Directions

What is necessary to improve the therapeutic potential of BMT in HIV-positive patients? Table 50-2 outlines a multitherapeutic approach to evaluate new strategies to control HIV disease by BMT.

Preparative regimens used in HIV-positive patients are directed not only at destroying those cells containing virus, but also against the underlying tumor for which BMT is undertaken. In fact, the reservoir of HIV-containing cells may require preparative regimens that differ from those used to treat and ablate malignant cells. Use of antibodies coupled with radioisotopes to target malignant cells has been an area of research directed at developing more effective and less toxic alternatives to TBI (93). A similar strategy could be used to target HIV-containing cells to provide a more effective way of eradicating this cell population. Other efforts to eradicate this reservoir are discussed later in this chapter, but the optimal preparative regimen for HIV has not yet been developed.

Current studies evaluating BMT have been performed utilizing HLA-identical family member donors or identical twins, but, as a result of increasing experience with unrelated HLA-identical volunteer donors, it may be possible to expand the donor pool (94).

An intriguing possibility is the application of autologous BMT to HIV-positive patients. Extensive research has been devoted to identifying the pluripotent progenitor cells that reconstitute the lymphohe-

Table 50-2.
Bone Marrow Transplantation for HIV-1–infected Host—Multitherapeutic Approach

I. Ablate latent proviral HIV-1–infected hematopoietic-lymphoid cellular reservoir with marrow-lethal therapy (e.g., cyclophosphamide and total body irradiation)
II. Reconstitute host with uninfected hematopoietic-lymphoid progenitor stem cells from:
  1. Marrow from HLA–identical sibling donor
  2. Autologous CD34+ positively selected progenitor stem cells
III. Inhibition of HIV-1 infection of reconstituting donor/autologous CD34+ hematopoietic stem cells
  1. Pharmacological: AZT, DDI
  2. Gene vector therapy: insertion of gene vectors into hematopoietic stem cells designed to inhibit HIV-1 (e.g., decoy TAT gene, hammerhead ribozymes)
IV. Augmentation of host cytotoxic T-lymphocyte (CTL) response to residual latent HIV-1–infected cells
  1. Adoptive immune transfer of donor-to-host immunity by vaccinating donor against HIV-1 antigens
  2. Ex-vivo augmentation of donor CTL cells against HIV-1 antigen with reinfusion of CTL cellular clones after transplantation
  3. Lymphokine gene therapy

HIV = human immunodeficiency virus; HLA = human leukocyte antigen; AZT = zidovudine; DDI = dideoxyinosine.

matopoietic system following marrow lethal therapy. These studies have identified putative stem cells in preclinical models and in humans (95–99). Early progenitor cells in humans express antigens that allow isolation of these cells using different techniques. Although the exact characteristics that define the true stem cell remain controversial, CD34 is an antigen that appears to be present on early progenitor cells (100–103). Studies have been performed isolating CD34 cells from patients with HIV infection. Using PCR technology, these cells do not appear to contain HIV gene sequences (104,105), which raises the possibility that virus-negative progenitor cells may be obtained from HIV-infected patients. Assuming that these cells can be purified from marrow or peripheral blood, autologous BMT becomes a feasible option for HIV-positive patients. Positive selection of CD34 cells from marrow and peripheral blood is currently being investigated as a means to reconstitute non-HIV–positive patients with malignancy undergoing autologous BMT (106). These studies demonstrated that 50 to 70% of the cells selected by positive selection techniques are CD34-positive. A more effective way of purification will be necessary before these positive selection techniques will suffice in HIV-positive patients. An alternative approach would be the development of "purging" techniques to destroy HIV-positive cells in a manner analogous to that in use to remove malignant cells in patients undergoing autologous BMT. A combination of positive selection and "purging" may be necessary to obtain an HIV-negative progenitor cell population for autologous BMT as a therapeutic approach in HIV-positive patients.

A major requirement for successful eradication of HIV is the ability to inhibit HIV infection of reconstituting lymphohematopoietic cells, whether their source is allogeneic, syngeneic, or autologous. This inhibition may be accomplished if effective antiviral therapy is available. Zidovudine has been used as prophylaxis against infection of repopulating hematopoietic-lymphoid cells following BMT. Clinical studies demonstrate that resistance develops in a significant number of HIV-positive patients receiving zidovudine as a single-agent therapy (107). In addition, studies demonstrate that zidovudine may not be as effective prophylactically as suggested in earlier reports. Extensive research has defined a number of antiviral compounds that have activity against HIV (31). The compounds currently in clinical use are reverse-transcriptase inhibitors, which inhibit the rate of HIV DNA synthesis. Didanosine and dideoxycytosine, both reverse transcriptase-inhibitors, have been studied as single agents in HIV-infected patients (108–110). Didanosine may be active against HIV isolates resistant to zidovudine (111). Studies suggest that combination therapy with didanosine and zidovudine given either simultaneously or in an alternating regimen may be more effective in treating HIV-positive patients than single-agent therapy (112). Whether the efficacy is due to lower occurrence of viral resistance is unclear. However, studies are in progress evaluating the combination as prophylaxis against HIV infection of hematopoietic-lymphoid cells following BMT. Other compounds that inhibit the viral regulatory protein TAT gene expression or inhibit the HIV protease are being developed and will enter clinical trials in the future (113,114). These agents have mechanisms of action quite different from the reverse-transcriptase inhibitors and may prove valuable as single agents or in combination with reverse-transcriptase inhibitors. Studies have also demonstrated synergistic antiviral (HIV) activity in vitro with the combination of zidovudine and alpha-interferon, but this combination has shown toxicity in clinical studies (115). Although the concept of complete pharmacological prophylaxis against HIV infection remains unproven, it remains a goal that may yet be achieved.

The concept of providing a resistance gene to infection with HIV in permissive cells has become feasible with new developments in molecular biology and gene transfer. The ability to define and purify a pluripotent progenitor cell that can repopulate a human hematopoietic lymphoid system represents a major step in implementing such a strategy. If a resistance gene or genes can be introduced into these cells and stable expression of these genes can be achieved, it would provide a very effective method of prophylaxis against HIV. For this approach to be practical, vector systems are needed to introduce a resistance gene with a high degree of efficiency and stable expression of the gene into hematopoietic progenitor stem cells and their progeny. Extensive research has defined retroviral vectors that may be used to transduce cells with a specified gene or genes. Although the technology currently does not exist to introduce genes into human pluripotent progenitor cells, efforts are preceding in several laboratories investigating retroviral vectors and other viral vector systems, as well as direct gene transfer into cells. In vitro studies suggest that introduction of specific genetic sequences into cells may render them incapable of supporting HIV replication. Production of high levels of RNA transcripts encoding the HIV (transactivation response [TAR] element) in cells is capable of inhibiting HIV replication in cells (116). This approach has been evaluated in peripheral blood CD4-positive cells as a prelude to Phase I studies in humans (117). The concept of intracellular immunization, a genetic alteration of cells mediated by gene transfer to inhibit viral replication, has generated other strategies to inhibit viral gene function, including the use of antisense RNA and ribozymes (118). Use of ribozymes has great appeal theoretically because these catalytic RNAs recognize and cleave specific nucleotide sequences. The genetic variability encountered in naturally occurring HIV isolates may be overcome using a multivariate ribozyme to target multiple cleavage sites in the HIV genome (119).

Use of immune therapy to facilitate destruction of HIV-containing cells before or after BMT may augment the effect of the preparative regimen. Investigators are currently evaluating several candidate vaccines against HIV. Although research to date has not produced an effective vaccine, the concept of adoptively transferring immune responses from donor to recipient has been well described in the BMT population (120). Recent studies by Riddell and colleagues (121) in Seattle using antigen-specific T-cell clones to restore viral immunity provide a novel strategy to exert a therapeutic antiviral effect against HIV. They were able to generate $CD3^+$, $CD8^+$, and $CD4^-$ cytomegalovirus (CMV)-specific cytotoxic T-cell clones from CMV-seropositive donors, which were propagated in vitro for 1 to 3 months prior to adoptive transfer. Infusion of these cells provided persistent reconstitution of cytotoxic T-cell responses against CMV. Because cytotoxic lymphocytes (CD8+) against HIV can be demonstrated in patients with HIV infection, these cells may be isolated and expanded in vitro. For this strategy to work, the cells cloned from the patient must be free of latent HIV. By using CD8+ lymphocytes, the major reservoir of the virus will be avoided, but all T-cell clones will need to be examined carefully to exclude virus-positive cells.

Another approach to reducing the reservoir of HIV-containing cells is based on efforts to augment cytotoxic T-lymphocyte responses in vivo against HIV-containing cells using HIV-positive cells transduced with lymphokine genes. This approach is based on studies which demonstrate that insertion of cytokine genes (e.g., IL-2, IL-4) into tumor cells enhances their recognition by major histocompatibility complex (MHC) class I–restricted $CD8^+$ cytotoxic T cells. In preclinical studies, cytokine transfection of murine tumor cells with IL-2 or IL-4 enhanced recognition of these tumor cells in vivo with the generation of a T-cell–dependent immune response that in one study resulted in the cure of animals with established tumor (122,123). A similar approach to HIV infection is possible in humans and is testable using the simian immunodeficiency virus (SIV) model system, which is analogous to human disease.

All of the therapeutic approaches outlined to facilitate destruction of HIV-containing cells and the approaches to preventing donor cells from infection with the virus are testable with currently available technology. A systematic approach to introducing new therapies when technology has evolved from the preclinical to the clinical arena will help determine the success or lack of success of each component of therapy. In all likelihood, a multitherapeutic approach utilizing several strategies will be necessary to alter permanently the reservoir of HIV to create a virus-free state.

The rising incidence of neoplastic disease in HIV-positive patients presents therapeutic challenges. Use of potentially curative therapies such as BMT should not be denied to this patient population. Efforts at eradicating the cause of the immunodeficiency as well as its manifestations (e.g., lymphoma) are essential when contemplating therapeutic maneuvers in HIV-positive patients. We believe BMT may be applied as therapy for patients who are HIV-positive and have a malignancy for which BMT is treatment of choice. Therapy in these patients will allow us to refine the procedure so that its use may be applied to other HIV-positive patients in the future. We believe that this approach may define principles for using BMT to eradicate nonmalignant cells transformed by exogenous agents, such as viruses, so that the disease caused by these agents may be eradicated.

References

1. Gottlieb MS, Schroff R, Schanker HM, et al. Pneumoncystis carinii pneumonia and mucosal candidiasis in previously healthy homosexual men: evidence of a new acquired cellular immunodeficiency. N Engl J Med 1981;305:1425–1431.
2. Masur H, Michelis MA, Greene JB, et al. An outbreak of community-acquired Pneumoncystis carinii pneumonia: initial manifestation of cellular immune dysfunction. N Engl J Med 1981;305:1431–1438.
3. Siegal FP, Lopez C, Hammer GS, et al. Severe acquired immunodeficiency in male homosexuals, manifested by chronic perianal ulcerative herpes simplex lesions. N Engl J Med 1981;305:1439–1444.
4. Barre-Sinoussi F, Chermann JC, Rey F, et al. Isolation of a T-lymphotropic retrovirus from a patient at risk for acquired immunodeficiency syndrome (AIDS). Science 1983;220:868–871.
5. Gallo RC, Salahuddin SZ, Popovic M, et al. Frequent detection and isolation of cytopathic retroviruses (HTLV-III) from patients with AIDS and at risk for AIDS. Science 1984;224:500–503.
6. Popovic M, Sarngadharan MG, Read E, et al. Detection, isolation, and continuous production of cytopathic retroviruses (HTLV-III) from patients with AIDS and pre-AIDS. Science 1984;224:500–504.
7. Clavel F, Guetard F, Brun-Vezinet F, et al. Isolation of a new human retrovirus from West African patients with AIDS. Science 1986;233:343–346.
8. Ratner L, Haseltine W, Patarca R, et al. Complete nucleotide sequence of the AIDS virus, HTLV-III. Nature 1985;313:277–284.
9. Wain-Hobson S, Songio P, Danos O, et al. Nucleotide sequence of the AIDS virus, LAV. Cell 1985;40:9–17.
10. Alizon M, Wain-Hobson S, Montagnier L, et al. Genetic variability of the AIDS virus: nucleotide sequence analysis of two isolates from African patients. Cell 1986;46:63–74.
11. Chaisson RE, Volberding PA. Clinical manifestations of HIV infection. In: Mandell GL, Douglas RG, Bennett JE, eds. Principles and practice of infectious diseases, vol I. New York: Churchill Livingstone, 1990:1059–1092.
12. Fauci AS. The human immunodeficiency virus: infectivity and mechanisms of pathogenesis. Science 1988;239:617–622.
13. Fauci AS, Schnittman SM, Poli G, Koenig S, Pantaleo G. NIH Conference. Immunopathogenic mechanism in human immunodeficiency virus (HIV) infection. Ann Intern Med 1991;114:678–693.
14. Groopman JE, Broder S. Cancer in AIDS and other immunodeficiency states. In: DeVita VT Jr, Hellman S, Rosenberg SA, eds. Cancer: principles and practice of oncology, ed 3. Philadelphia: J.B. Lippincott, 1989:1953–1970.
15. Morrell D, Cromarie E, Swift M. Mortality and cancer incidence in 263 patients with ataxia telangiectasia. J Natl Cancer Inst 1986;77:89–92.

16. Cotelingham JD, Witebsky FG, Hsu SM, Blaese RM, Jaffe ES. Malignant lymphoma in patients with the Wiskott-Aldrich syndrome. Cancer Invest 1985;3:515–522.
17. Pearson J. Lymphomas complicating organ transplantation. Transplant Proc 1983;15:2790–2797.
18. Witherspoon RP, Fisher MD, Schoch G, et al. Secondary cancers after bone marrow transplantation for leukemia or aplastic anemia. N Engl J Med 1989;321:784–789.
19. Hymes KB, Cheung T, Greene JB, et al. Kaposi's sarcoma in homosexual men—a report of eight cases. Lancet 1981;2:598–600.
20. Ziegler JL, Drew WL, Miner, et al. Outbreak of Burkitt's-like lymphoma in homosexual men. Lancet 1982;2:631–633.
21. Ziegler JL, Beckstead JA, Volberding PA, et al. Non-Hodgkin's lymphoma in 90 homosexual men. Relation to generalized lymphadenopathy and the acquired immunodeficiency syndrome (AIDS). N Engl J Med 1984;311:565–570.
22. Knowles DM, Chamulak GA, Subar M, et al. Lymphoid neoplasia associated with the acquired immunodeficiency syndrome (AIDS). Ann Intern Med 1988;108:744–753.
23. Pluda JM, Yarchoan R, Jeffe ES, et al. Development of non-Hodgkin's lymphoma in a cohort of patients with severe human immunodeficiency virus (HIV) infection on long-term antiretroviral therapy. Ann Int Med 1990;113:276–282.
24. Kaplan LD, Abrams DI, Feigal E, et al. AIDS-associated non-Hodgkin's lymphoma in San Francisco. JAMA 1989;261:719–724.
25. Opportunistic non-Hodgkin's lymphomas among severely immunocompromised HIV-infected patients surviving for prolonged periods on antiretroviral therapy-United States. Morb Mortal Wkly Rep 1991;40:591, 597–600.
26. Rabkin CS, Hilgartner MW, Hedberg KW, et al. Incidence of lymphomas and other cancers in HIV-infected and HIV-uninfected patients with hemophilia. JAMA 1992;267:1090–1094.
27. Beral V, Peterman T, Berkelmam R, Jaffe H. AIDS-associated non-Hodgkin's lymphoma. Lancet 1991;337:805–809.
28. Herndier BG, Shiramizu BT, Jewett NE, Aldape KD, Reyes GR, McGrath MS. Acquired immunodeficiency syndrome-associated T-cell lymphoma: evidence for human immunodeficiency virus type 1-associated T-cell transformation. Blood 1992;79:1768–1774.
29. Gill PS, Levine AM, Meyer PR, et al. Primary central nervous system lymphoma in homosexual men. Clinical, immunologic and pathologic features. Am J Med 1985;78:742–748.
30. Broder S, Mitsuya H, Yarchoan R, Pavlalies GN. Antiretroviral therapy in AIDS. Ann Intern Med 1990;113:604–618.
31. Yarchoan R, Pluda JM, Perno CF, Mitsuya H, Broder S. Antiretroviral therapy of human immunodeficiency virus infection: current strategies and challenges for the future. Blood 1991;78:859–884.
32. Gail MH, Pluda JM, Rabkin CS, et al. Projections of the incidence of non-Hodgkin's lymphoma related to acquired immunodeficiency syndrome. J Natl Cancer Inst 1991;83:695–701.
33. Dalla-Favera R, Bregni M, Erikson J, Patterson D, Gallo RC, Croce CM. Human c-myc oncogene is located on the region of chromosome 8 that is translocated in Burkitt lymphoma cells. Proc Natl Acad Sci USA 1982;79:7824–7827.
34. Tsujimoto Y, Yunis J, Onotoro-Showe L, Erikson L, Nowell PC, Croce CM. Molecular cloning of the chromosonal breakpoint of B-cell lymphomas and leukemias with the T (11;14) chromosome translocation. Science 1984;224:1403–1406.
35. Tsujimoto Y, Cossman J, Jaffe E, Croce CM. Involvement of the bcl-2 gene in human follicular lymphoma. Science 1985;228:1440–1443.
36. Schouten HC, Sanger WG, Weisenburger DD, Anderson J, Armitage JO. Chromosomal abnormalities in untreated patients with non-Hodgkin's lymphoma: associations with histology, clinical characteristics, and treatment outcome. Blood 1990;75:1841–1847.
37. Epstein MA, Achong BG, Barr YM. Virus particles in cultured lymphoblasts from Burkitt's lymphoma. Lancet 1964;1:702–703.
38. Magrath I. The pathogenesis of Burkitt's lymphoma. Adv Cancer Res 1990;55:133–270.
39. Pellici P-G, Knowles DM, Magrath I, Dalla-Favera R. Chromosomal breakpoints and structural alterations of the c-myc locus differ in endemic and sporadic forms of Burkitt's lymphoma. Proc Natl Acad Sci USA 1986;83:2984–2988.
40. Negri A, Barriga F, Knowles DM, Magrath IT, Dalla-Favera R. Different regions of the immunoglobulin heavy chain locus are involved in chromosomal translocations in distinct pathogenetic forms of Burkitt's lymphoma. Proc Natl Acad Sci USA 1988;85:2748–2752.
41. Subar M, Neil A, Inghirami G, Knowles DM, Dalla-Favera R. Frequent c-myc oncogene activation and infrequent presence of Epstein-Barr virus genome in AIDS-associated lymphoma. Blood 1988;72:667–671.
42. Hanto DW, Frizzera G, Gajl-Peczalska KJ, et al. Epstein-Barr virus-induced B-cell lymphoma after renal transplantation. Acyclovir therapy and transition from polyclonal to monoclonal B-cell proliferation. N Engl J Med 1982;306:913–918.
43. Shearer WT, Ritz J, Finegold MJ, et al. Epstein-Barr virus-associated B-cell proliferations of diverse clonal origins after bone marrow transplantation in a 12-year-old patient with severe combined immunodeficiency. N Engl J Med 1985;312:1151–1159.
44. Hochberg FH, Miller G, Schooley RT, Hirsch MS, Feorino P, Henle W. Central nervous system lymphoma related to Epstein-Barr virus. N Engl J Med 1983;309:745–748.
45. Hamilton-Dutoit SJ, Karkov J, Franzmann MB, Pallesen G. AIDS-related central nervous system lymphoma. In: Haase AT, Gluckman JC, Racz P, eds. Modern pathology of AIDS and other retroviral infections. Basel: Karger, 1990:110–129.
46. Nakleh KE, Manivel JC, Copenhaver CM, Sung JH, Strickler JG. In situ hybridization for detection of Epstein-Barr virus in central nervous system lymphomas. Cancer 1991;67:444–448.
47. Stanbridge EJ, Nowell PC. Origins of human cancer revisited. Cell 1990;63:867–874.
48. Chen Y-C, Chen P-J, Yeh S-H, et al. Deletion of the human retinoblastoma gene in primary leukemias. Blood 1990;76:2060–2064.
49. Sugimoto K, Toyoshima H, Sakai R, et al. Mutations of the p53 gene in lymphoid leukemia. Blood 1991;77:1153–1156.
50. Mashal R, Shtalrid M, Talpaz M, et al. Rearrangement and expression of p53 in the chronic phase and blast

crisis of chronic myelogenous leukemia. Blood 1990; 75:180–189.
51. Hollingsworth RE, Lee WH. Tumor suppressor genes: new propects for cancer research. J Natl Cancer Inst 1991;83:91–96.
52. DeCaprio JA, Ludlow JW, Lynch D, et al. The product of the retinoblastoma susceptibility gene has properties of a cell cycle regulatory element. Cell 1989;58: 1085–1095.
53. Kishimoto T. The biology of interleukin-6. Blood 1989;74:1–10.
54. Birx DL, Redfield RR, Tencer K, Fowler A, Burke DS, Tosato G. Induction of interleukin-6 during human immunodeficiency virus infection. Blood 1990;76:2303–2310.
55. Scala G, Quinto I, Ruocco MR, et al. Expression of an exogenous interleukin-6 gene in human Epstein-Barr virus B-cells confers growth advantage and in vitro tumorigenicity. J Exp Med 1990;172:61–68.
56. Levine AM, Wernz JC, Kaplan L, et al. Low-dose chemotherapy with central nervous system prophylaxis and zidovudine maintenance in AIDS-related lymphoma: a prospective multi-institutional trial. JAMA 1991;266:84–88.
57. Pluda JM, Yarchoan R, Broder S. The occurrence of opportunistic non-Hodgkin's lymphomas in the setting of infection with the human immunodeficiency virus. Ann Oncol 1991;2:191–200.
58. Gill PS, Levine AM, Krailo M, et al. AIDS-related malignant lymphoma: results of prospective treatment trials. J Clin Oncol 1987;5:1322–1328.
59. Ammann AJ, Abrams D, Conant M, et al. Acquired immune dysfunction in homosexual men: immunologic profiles. Clin Immunol Immunopathol 1983;27:315–325.
60. Klatzmann D, Barre-Sinoussi F, Nugeyre MT, et al. Selective tropism of lymphadenopathy associated virus (LAV) for helper-inducer T lymphocytes. Science 1984;225:59–63.
61. Dalgleish AG, Beverly PC, Clapham PR, Crawford DH, Greaves MF, Weiss RA. The CD4 (T4) antigen is an essential component of the receptor for the AIDS retrovirus. Nature 1984;312:763–767.
62. Klatzmann DE, Champagne E, Chamaret S, et al. T-lymphocyte T4 molecule behaves as the receptor for human retrovirus LAV (letter). Nature 1984;312:767–768.
63. Ho DD, Rota TR, Hirsch MS. Infection of monocyte/macrophages by human T lymphotropic virus type III. J Clin Invest 1986;77:1712–1715.
64. Gartner S, Markovits P, Markovitz DM, Kaplan MH, Gallo RC, Popovic M. The role of monoclear phagocytes in HTLV III/LAV infection. Science 1986;233:215–219.
65. Maddon PJ, Dalgleish AG, McDougal JS, Clapham PR, Weiss RA, Axel R. The T4 gene encodes the AIDS virus receptor and is expressed in the immune system and the brain. Cell 1986;47:333–348.
66. Montagnier L, Gruest J, Chamaret S, et al. Adaptation of lymphadenopathy associated virus (LAV) to replication in EBV-transformed B lymphoblastoid cell lines. Science 1986;225:63–66.
67. Salahuddin SZ, Ablashi DV, Hunter EA, et al. HTLV-III infection of EBV-genome-positive B lymphoid cells with or without detectable T4 antigens. Int J Cancer 1987;39:198–202.
68. Borgaonkar DS, Bias WB, Sroka BM, Hutchinson JR, Santos GW. Identification of graft versus host cells in bone marrow transplants by the quinacrine banding technique of chromosome identification. Acta Cytol 1974;18:263–267.
69. Thomas ED, Buckner CD, Banaji M. One hundred patients with acute leukemia treated by chemotherapy, total body irradiation, and allogeneic marrow transplantation. Blood 1977;49:511–533.
70. Blazar BR, Om HT, Arthur DC, Kersey JH, Filipovich AH. Restriction fragment length polymorphisms as markers of engraftment in allogeneic marrow transplantation. Blood 1985;6:1436–1444.
71. Ginsburg D, Antin JH, Smith BR, Orkin SH, Rappeport JM. Origins of cell populations after bone marrow transplantation. J Clin Invest 1985;75:596–603.
72. Thomas ED, Ramberg RE, Sale GE, Sparkes RS, Golde DW. Direct evidence for a bone marrow origin of the alveolar macrophage in man. Science 1976;192:1016–1017.
73. Gale RP, Sparkes RS, Golde DW. Bone marrow origin of hepatic macrophages (Kuppfer cells) in humans. Science 1978;201:937–938.
74. Hicky WF, Kimura H. Perivascular microglial cells of the CNS are bone-marrow derived and present antigen in vivo. Science 1988;239:290–292.
75. Gratama JW, Oosterveer MA, Zwaan FE, Lepoutre J, Klein G, Ernberg I. Eradication of Epstein-Barr virus for sites of viral latency. Proc Natl Acad Sci USA 1985;85:8693–8696.
76. Lum LG. A review: the kinetics of immune reconstitution after human marrow transplantation. Blood 1987;69:369–380.
77. Fischl MA, Richman DD, Grieco HH, et al. The efficacy of azidothymudine (AZT) in the treatment of patients with AIDS and AIDS-related complex: a double-blind placebo-controlled trial. N Engl J Med 1987;317:185–191.
78. Fischl M, Parker C, Pettinelli C, et al. A randomized controlled trial of a reduced daily dose of zidovudine in patients with the acquired immunodeficiency syndrome. N Engl J Med 1990;323:1009–1014.
79. Volberding PA, Lagakos SW, Koch MA, et al. Zidovudine in asymptomatic human immunodeficiency virus infection. A controlled trial in persons with fewer than 500 CD-4 positive cells per cubic millimeter. N Engl J Med 1990;322:941–949.
80. Mitsuyasu R, Volberding P, Groopman J, Champlin R. Bone marrow transplantation for identical twins in the treatment of acquired immunodeficiency syndrome and Kaposi's sarcoma. J Cell Biochem 1984;8A(suppl):19.
81. Tavares L, Roneker C, Johnston K, Lehrman SN, de Noronha F. 3′-Azido-3′-deoxythymidine in feline leukemia virus-infected cats: a model for therapy and prophylaxis of AIDS. Cancer Res 1987;47:3190–3194.
82. Ruprecht RM, O'Brien LG, Rossoni LD, Nusinoff-Lehrman S. Supression of mouse viraemia and retroviral disease by 3′-Azido-3′-deoxythymidine. Nature 1986;323:467–469.
83. Sharpe AH, Jaenisch R, Ruprecht RM. Retroviruses and mouse embryos: a rapid model for neurovirulence and transplacental antiviral therapy. Science 1987;236: 1671–1674.
84. Holland HK, Saral R, Rossi JJ, et al. Allogeneic bone marrow transplantation, zidovudine, and human immunodeficiency virus type 1 (HIV-1) infection: studies in a patient with non-Hodgkin's lymphoma. Ann Intern Med 1989;111:973–981.
85. Davis KC, Hayward A, Ozturk G, Kohler PF. Lympho-

cyte transfusion in case of acquired immunodeficiency syndrome (letter). Lancet 1983;1:599–600.
86. Lane HC, Masur H, Longo DL, et al. Partial immune reconstitution in a patient with the acquired immunodeficiency syndrome. N Engl J Med 1984;311:1099–1103.
87. Vilmer E, Rhodes-Feuilette A, Rabian C, et al. Clinical and immunological restoration in patients with AIDS after marrow transplantation using lymphocyte transfusions from the marrow donor. Transplantation 1987; 44:25–29.
88. Lane HC, Zunich KM, Wilson W, et al. Syngeneic bone marrow transplantation and adoptive transfer of peripheral blood lymphocytes combined with zidovudine in human immunodeficiency virus (HIV) infection. Ann Intern Med 1990;113:512–519.
89. Hassett JM, Zaroulis CG, Greenberg ML, Siegal FP. Bone marrow transplantation in AIDS (letter). N Engl J Med 1983;309:665.
90. Vilmer E, Rouzioux C, Barre F, et al. Screening for lymphadenopathy/AIDS virus in bone marrow-transplant recipients (Letter). N Engl J Med 1986;314:1252.
91. Verdonk LF, de Gast GC, Lange JM, Schuurman HJ, Dekker AW, Bast BJ. Syngeneic leukocytes together with suramin failed to improve immunodeficiency in a case of transfusion-associated AIDS after syngeneic bone marrow transplantation. Blood 1988;71:666–671.
92. Thomas ED, Buckner CD, Rudolph RH. Allogeneic marrow grafting for hematologic malignancy using HLA-matched donor-recipient sibling pairs. Blood 1971;38:267–287.
93. Bianco JA, Sandmaier B, Brown PA, et al. Specific marrow localization of an 131I-labeled anti-myeloid antibody in normal dogs: effects of a "cold" antibody pretreatment dose on marrow localization. Exp Hematol 1989;17:929–934.
94. Beatty PG, Hansen JA, Longton GM, et al. Marrow transplantation from HLA-matched unrelated donors for treatment of hematologic malignancies. Transplantation 1991;51:443–447.
95. Spangrude GJ, Heimfeld S, Weissman IL. Purification and characterization of mouse hematopoietic stem cells. Science 1988;241:58–62.
96. Spangrude GJ, Smith LG, Uchida N, et al. A perspective on mouse hematopoietic stem cells. Blood 1991; 78:1395–1402.
97. Smith LG, Weissman IL, Heimfeld S. Clonal analysis of hematopoietic stem-cell differentiation in vivo. Proc Natl Acad Sci USA 1991;88:2788–2792.
98. Baum CM, Weissman IL, Tsukamoto AS, Buckle AM, Peault B. Isolation of a candidate human hematopoietic stem-cell population. Proc Natl Acad Sci USA 1992;89:2804–2808.
99. Sutherland HJ, Lansdorp PM, Henkelman DH, Eaves AC, Eaves CJ. Functional characterization of individual human hematopoietic stem cells cultured at limiting dilution on supportive marrow stromal layers. Proc Natl Acad Sci USA 1990;87:3584–3588.
100. Civin CI, Strauss LC, Brovall C, Fackler MJ, Schwartz JF, Sharper JH. Antigenic analysis of hematopoiesis. III. A hematopoietic progenitor cell surface antigen defined by a monoclonal antibody raised against KG-1a cells. J Immunol 1984;1331:157–165.
101. Civin CI, Banquerigo ML, Strauss LC, Loken MR. Antigenic analysis of hematopoiesis. VI. Flow cytometric characterization of My-10-positive progenitor cells in normal human bone marrow. Exp Hematol 1987; 15:10–17.
102. Andrews RG, Singer JW, Bernstein ID. Monoclonal antibody 12-8 recognizes a 115-kd molecule present on both unipotent and multipotent hematopoietic colony-forming cells and their precursors. Blood 1986;67:842–845.
103. Andrews RG, Singer JW, Bernstein ID. Human hematopoietic precursors in long-term culture: single CD34+ cells that lack detectable T cell, B cell, and myeloid cell antigens produce multiple colony-forming cells when cultured with marrow stromal cells. J Exp Med 1990;172:355–358.
104. Davis BR, Schwartz DH, Marx JC, et al. Absent or rare human immunodeficiency virus infection of bone marrow stem/progenitor cells in vivo. J Virol 1991; 65:1985–1990.
105. von-Laer D, Hufert FT, Fenner TE, et al. CD34+ hematopoietic progenitor cells are not a major reservoir of the human immunodeficiency virus. Blood 1990;76:1281–1286.
106. Berenson RJ, Bensinger WI, Hill R, et al. Stem cell selection-clinical experience. Prog Clin Biol Res 1991;333:403–413.
107. Larder BA, Darby G, Richman DD. HIV with reduced sensitivity to zidovudine (AZT) isolated during prolonged therapy. Science 1989;243:1731–1734.
108. Merigan TC, Skowion G, Bozzette SA, et al. Circulating p24 antigen levels and responses to dideoxycytidine in human immunodeficiency (HIV) infection. Ann Intern Med 1989;110:189–194.
109. Cooley TP, Kunches LM, Saunders CA, et al. Once-daily administration of 2′,3′-dideoxyinosine (ddI) in patients with the acquired immunodeficiency syndrome or AIDS-related complex: results of a Phase I trial. N Engl J Med 1990;322:1340–1345.
110. Lambert JS, Seidlin M, Reichmann RC, et al. 2′,3′-dideoxyinosine (ddI) in patients with the acquired immunodeficiency syndrome or AIDS-related complex: a phase I trial. N Engl J Med 1990;322:1333–1340.
111. Richmann DD. Susceptibility to nucleoside analogue of zidovudine-resistant isolates of human immunodeficiency virus. Am J Med 1990;88(suppl 5B):85–105.
112. Kahn JO, Lagakos SW, Richman DD, et al. A controlled trial comparing continued zidovudine with didanosine in human immunodeficiency virus infection. New Engl J Med 1992;327:581–587.
113. Mitsuya H, Yarchoan R, Broder S. Molecular targets for AIDS therapy. Science 1990;249:1533–1544.
114. DeClerq E. Perspectives for the chemotherapy of AIDS. Anticancer Res 1987;7:1023–1038.
115. Hartshorn KL, Vogt MW, Chou TC, et al. Synergistic inhibition of human immunodeficiency virus in vitro by azidothymidine and recombinant alpha A interferon. Antimicrob Agents Chemother 1987;31:268–272.
116. Sullenger BA, Gallardo HF, Ungers GE, Gilboa E. Overexpression of TAR sequences renders cells resistant to human immunodeficiency virus replication. Cell 1990;63:601–608.
117. Smith CA, Gallardo HF, Sullenger BA, Ungers GE, Terry L, Gilboa E. Decreased susceptibility to HIV replication in peripheral blood CD4+lymphocytes genetically altered with retroviral vectors expressing TAR decoy RNA. Blood 1991;78:284a.
118. Baltimore D. Intracellular immunization. Nature 1988;335:395–396.
119. Sarver N, Cantin EM, Chang PS, et al. Ribozymes as

potential anti-HIV-1 therapeutic agents. Science 1990; 247:1222–1225.

120. Donnenberg AD, Hess AD, Duff SC, et al. Regeneration of genetically restricted immune functions after human bone marrow transplantation: influence of four different strategies for graft-versus-host disease prophylaxis. Transplant Proc 1987;19:144–152.

121. Riddell SR, Watanabe KS, Goodrich JM, Cheng RL, Agha ME, Greenberg PD. Restoration of viral immunity in immunodeficient humans by the adoptive transfer of T cell clones. Science 1992;257:238–241.

122. Fearon ER, Pardoll DM, Itaya T, et al. Interleukin-2 production by tumor cells bypasses T helper function in the generation of an antitumor response. Cell 1990;60:397–403.

123. Golumbek PT, Lazenby AJ, Levitsky HI, et al. Treatment of established renal cancer by tumor cells engineered to secrete interleukin-4. Science 1991;254:713–716.

Chapter 51

Bone Marrow Transplantation from HLA-Partially Matched Related Donors and Unrelated Volunteer Donors

Claudio Anasetti and John Hansen

Patients who might benefit from the bone marrow transplantation (BMT) of normal hematopoietic stem cells need access to a suitably matched donor. Usually, this has been an human leukocyte antigen (HLA) genotypically identical sibling. However, less than 30% of patients in North America have such a matched sibling. Until recently, there have been limited options for the remaining patients. A few have found partially HLA-matched relatives, and increasing numbers are being transplanted with marrow from HLA-matched, unrelated volunteer marrow donors.

Histocompatibility

Polymorphism and HLA Typing

The HLA system is described in detail in Chapter 4. Briefly, HLA genes are highly polymorphic and encode 2 classes of histocompatibility molecules, the class I HLA-A, B, and C antigens; and the class II HLA-DR, DQ, and DP antigens (Table 51-1) (1). HLA antigens were originally defined serologically by typing with alloantisera. Individual HLA antigens characteristically express multiple serological specifications, many of which crossreact with other antigens. Certain well-defined crossreactive specificities, such as the determinants that define A9, Bw22, and DRw6, are referred to as public specificities because they are associated with 2 or more distinct antigens. Antigens that share a public specificity are said to belong to the same crossreactive group (CREG) (Table 51-2). Serological specificities that define a single antigen are referred to as private antigens and, in the past, private antigens were assumed to represent unique molecules. Although HLA-A2 is defined as a private specificity by serology, HLA-A2 molecules are not all the same. Analysis by isoelectrical focusing (IEF) gel electrophoresis has shown that HLA-A2 represents a family of related but distinct structural variants (2). Protein and gene sequencing experiments have shown that these variants have unique primary structures, but they all react with anti-A2 antisera and monoclonal antibodies (Table 51-3; 4-2) (1). Similarly, at least 7 different alleles encode molecules of the B27 antigen family (3,4). Each of the A2 and B27 variants appear to be functionally relevant because each can be distinguished by cytotoxic T-cell clones (CTLs) (4–5). More than 93 IEF-defined variants can be identified among 55 HLA-A and B private antigens (2). Because serology alone does not identify all known structural variants, complete phenotyping for HLA-A, B, and C requires a 2-step process. Level 1 typing involves serological identification of private antigens, and level 2 typing involves use of IEF to identify structural variants not recognized by serology. However, IEF does not identify all structural variants. There are at least 2 distinct B27 alleles (B*2701 and B*2707) that encode molecules which cannot be distinguished by IEF. Nevertheless B27HS and B27LH can be distinguished by CTL, and they differ in primary sequence by 5 amino acids (see Table 51-3) (4). Definitive typing for HLA-A, B, and C will require the use of molecular methods capable of identifying individual alleles. This technology will hopefully be available in the clinical laboratory within the next few years.

Serological analysis with alloantisera has also provided the ground work for elucidation of the class II HLA-DR and DQ antigens, and in vitro assays for measuring T-cell recognition of HLA-D determinants have greatly facilitated study of the functional polymorphism of these genes. Compatibility for the HLA-D region can be determined directly by incubating cells from patient and donor in reciprocal one-way mixed lymphocyte cultures (MLC) (*patient* + $donor_x$ and *donor* + $patient_x$; where $donor_x$ or $patient_x$ represent the irradiated stimulator cell) (6). HLA-D compatibility also can be determined indirectly by typing with a panel of HLA-D-homozygous typing cells (HTC) in a modified MLC assay (6). A series of HLA-D specificities has been defined by HTC, and characteristically each "Dw" specificity is included completely within a well-defined DR specificity (Tables 51-4; 4-3). In some

Table 51-1.
HLA alloantigens Recognized by the World Health Organization (WHO) HLA Nomenclature Committee, 1991[a]

A	*B*	*B*	*C*	*D*	*DR*	*DQ*
A1	(B5)	**B52(5)**	**Cw1**	**Dw1**	**DR1**	(DQ1)
A2	**B7**	**B53**	**Cw2**	(Dw2)	**DR103**	**DQ2**
A203	**B703**	**B54(22)**	(Cw3)	**Dw3**	(DR2)	(DQ3)
A210	**B8**	**B55(22)**	**Cw4**	**Dw4**	(DR3)	**DQ4**
A3	(B12)	**B56(22)**	**Cw5**	(Dw5)	**DR4**	**DQ5(1)**
(A9)	**B13**	**B57(17)**	**Cw6**	(Dw6)	(DR5)	**DQ6(1)**
(A10)	(B14)	**B58(17)**	**Cw7**	(Dw7)	(DR6)	**DQ7(3)**
A11	(B15)	**B59**	**Cw8**	(Dw8)	**DR7**	**DQ8(3)**
(A19)	(B16)	**B60(40)**	**Cw9(w3)**	**Dw9**	**DR8**	**DQ9(3)**
A23(9)	(B17)	**B61(40)**	**Cw10(w3)**	**Dw10**	**DR9**	
A24(9)	**B18**	**B62(15)**		Dw11(w7)	**DR10**	
A2403	(B21)	**B63(15)**		**(Dw12)**	**DR11(5)**	
A25(10)	(B22)	**B64(14)**		(Dw13)	**DR12(5)**	
A26(10)	**B27**	**B65(14)**		(Dw14)	**DR13(6)**	
(A28)	**B35**	**B67**		**Dw15**	**DR14(6)**	
A29(19)	**B37**	(B70)		**Dw16**	**DR1403**	
A30(19)	**B38(16)**	**B71(70)**		**Dw17(w6)**	**DR1404**	
A31(19)	**B39(16)**	**B72(70)**		**Dw18(w6)**	**DR15(2)**	
A32(19)	**B3901**	**B73**		**Dw19(w7)**	**DR16(2)**	
A33(19)	**B3902**	**B75(15)**		**Dw20**	**DR17(3)**	
A34(10)	(B40)	**B76(15)**		**Dw21**	**DR18(3)**	
A36	**B4005**	**B77(15)**		**Dw22**		
A43	**B41**	**B7801**		(Dw23)		
A66(10)	**B42**					
A68(28)	**B44(12)**	(Bw4)		Dw24(52)	(DR52)	
A69(28)	**B45(12)**	(Bw6)		Dw25(52)		
A74(19)	**B46**			Dw26(52)	**DR53**	
	B47					
	B48					
	B49(21)					
	B50(21)					
	B51(5)					
	B5102					
	B5103					

[a]**Bold type** indicates private specificity; parentheses indicate a public specificity.
HLA = human leukocyte antigen.
Reproduced by permission from Bodmer JG, Marsh SGE, Albert ED, et al. Nomenclature for factors of the HLA system, 1991. Tissue Antigens 1992;39:161–173.

Table 51-2.
HLA-A and B Crossreactive Groups[a]

A locus													
1.	A1	A3	A11	A36									
2.	A9	A23	A24										
3.	A10	A25	A26	A34	A66	A43							
4.	A19	A29	A30	A31	A32	A33	A74						
5.	A2	A28	A68	A69									
B locus													
1.	B5	B18	B35	B51	B52	B53	B70	B71	B72				
2.	B12	B21	B44	B45	B49	B50							
3.	B14	B64	B65										
4.	B8	B59											
5.	B15	B17	B46	B57	B58	B62	B63	B70	B71	B72	B75	B76	B77
6.	B16	B38	B39	B67									
7.	B37												
8.	B7	B27	B42	B73									
9.	B7	B22	B54	B55	B56	B67							
10.	B7	B40	B41	B48	B60	B61							
11.	B13	B47											

[a]As defined by the National Marrow Donor Program, Histocompatibility Committee.
HLA = human leukocyte antigen.

Table 51-3.
Isoelectrical Focusing–defined HLA-A and B Variants and Alleles

Private Specificity	*IEF Variant*	*Allele*[a]
HLA-A1	NK	A*0101
HLA-A2	A2.1	A*0201
	A2.2F	A*0202
	A2.3	A*0203
	ND	A*0204
	A2.2y	A*0205
	A2.4a	A*0206
	A2.4b	A*0207
	A2.4c	A*0208
	A2-OZB	A*0209
	A2-LEE	A*0210
	A2.5	A*0211
	ND	A*0212
HLA-B8	NK	B*0801
HLA-B27[b]	B27f-LH/B27f-HS	B*2701 (LH); B*2707(HS)
	B27.2/B27e	B*2702
	B27d	B*2703
	B27.3/B27b	B*2704
	B27.1/B27a	B*2705
	B27.4	B*2706

[a]Alleles defined by sequencing.
[b]B27f-LH and B27f-HS cannot be distinguished by isoelectrical focusing (IEF), but they react differently with cytotoxic T lymphocytes, and sequencing has revealed a substantial difference in their primary sequence. B*2707 differs with B*2701 by substitution of 5 amino acids (4).
HLA = human leukocyte antigen; NK = none known; ND = not defined.
From the World Health Organization WHO HLA Nomeclature Committee, 1991.

cases, for example, HLA-DR4, which is well defined by serology, HLA-D typing can distinguish a series of unique specificities that all share DR4 (Dw4, Dw10, Dw13, Dw14, and Dw15).

However, additional alleles encoding DR4 products have been identified for which no HTC specificities are known. There are at least 12 alleles that encode distinct members of the DR4 family (DRB1*0401 to *0412). HLA-D typing combined with DR and DQ serology has been an important part of donor matching. However, both methods essentially have been replaced by direct molecular typing for DRB, DQA, and DQB alleles. The molecular method most commonly used involves hybridization of sequence-specific oligonucleotide probes (SSOP) to polymerase chain reaction (PCR)–amplified DNA (7,8). The standard DR phenotypes (DR1–DRw18, 52, and 53) as well as the HTC-defined HLA-D specificities (Dw1–Dw25) can be predicted by knowing which alleles are expressed at the DRB1, DRB3, DRB4, and DRB5 loci (Table 51-4; 4-3). Thus, by selecting the appropriate primers and hybridization probes, SSOP/PCR–based typing can be used to recapitulate both DR serology and HLA-D typing, and, more importantly, the individual alleles that encode the DR, DQ, and DP antigens can be identified.

Crossmatching for Anti-HLA Antibodies

Donor selection for BMT requires not only matching for the relevant HLA antigens or alleles, but also crossmatch testing to determine if the recipient has been sensitized to antigens of the donor. Patients may be alloimmunized by pregnancy or blood transfusions, and if sensitization to donor alloantigens occurs, it may result in a significant increase in the risk of marrow graft failure. Donor-specific immunity can be demonstrated by testing the patient's blood for antibodies or T cells reactive with donor cells. Standard procedures for crossmatching the patient's serum with donor lymphocytes include the National Institutes of Health two-stage complement-dependent microcytotoxicity (CDC) assay, modified Amos or antiglobulin method using T cells as target cells for identifying anti-HLA class I antibodies, and the B-cell CDC crossmatch for identifying anti-HLA class II antibodies (9).

HLA Haplotypes and Segregation in Families

The HLA antigens inherited together from one parent are referred to as an HLA haplotype (Figure 51-1). Two haplotypes, one from each parent, comprise the genotype of each individual. Assuming that the parents are unrelated and monogamous, the number of HLA antigens occurring within a family is limited to those expressed by the 4 available parental haplotypes. Parental haplotypes can segregate among the offspring in 4 different combinations, and the chance that any one sibling is HLA-identical with another is 25%. Nevertheless, it is possible to occasionally find family members who are partially matched for HLA even though they have not inherited the same 2

Table 51-4.
HLA-DR and D (HTC-defined) Antigens and Alleles[a]

DR Antigen	*HLA-D*	*DRB*	*Allele*
DR4	Dw4	DRB1	*0401
DR4	Dw10	DRB1	*0402
DR4	Dw13(13.1)	DRB1	*0403
DR4	Dw14(14.1)	DRB1	*0404
DR4	Dw15	DRB1	*0405
DR4	Dw13(13.2)	DRB1	*0407
DR4	Dw14(14.2)	DRB1	*0408
DR4	Dw "blank"[b]	DRB1	*0409
DR4	Dw "blank"[b]	DRB1	*0410
DR4	Dw "blank"[b]	DRB1	*0411
DR4	Dw "blank"[b]	DRB1	*0412

[a]DR antigens are serologically defined and HLA-D antigens are defined by T cells in a modified-mixed lymphocyte culture assay using HLA-homozygous typing cells (HTC). HLA-DR and D antigens are encoded by the DRB1 locus.
[b]indicates Dw "blank" (i.e., undefined DR-associated Dw specificity). Although the sequence of the peptide can be predicted from the known sequence of the gene, serological reagents and HTC do not exist that can distinguish these Dw "blanks" from one another.
HLA = human leukocyte antigen.

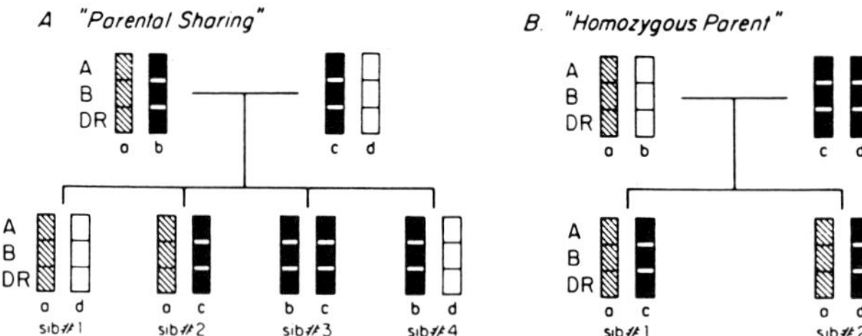

Figure 51-1. Segregation of human leukocyte antigen (HLA) haplotypes and partial sharing of HLA antigens within a family. (A) Two parents share 2 phenotypically similar haplotypes (haplotypes "b" and "c"). (B) One parent is HLA-homozygous, and 2 distinct but phenotypically similar haplotypes (haplotypes "c" and "d") segregate within the family.

haplotypes. There are 2 reasons for this fortuitous matching. First, the frequency of HLA antigens is highly variable; some are common, whereas others occur rarely. Second, certain HLA haplotypes show a feature referred to as positive linkage disequilibrium. The antigens expressed by these haplotypes, also known as extended haplotypes, are found together more often than predicted by the frequency of their genes in the general population. The reason for this preferential association of antigens on certain haplotypes is unknown, but presumably it has occurred because of genetic selection.

When a family study is performed in search of an HLA-identical sibling donor, all members of the immediate family should be typed for HLA-A, B, and DR, and each of the 4 parental haplotypes identified. If an HLA-identical sibling is not found, the parental haplotypes should be reviewed for homozygosity or sharing of antigens. The parents, siblings, children, and sometimes an uncle, aunt, cousin, or even a grandparent who share a haplotype with the patient may have a second haplotype that is partially matched with the patient. Figure 51-1A illustrates a family in which the parents share 2 similar haplotypes, "b" and "c." The patient (sib #2, "a/c") has a unique genotype, and none of the siblings are HLA-identical with the patient. However, the patient and the father ("a/b") share the paternal "a" haplotype and may be matched phenotypically for the HLA-A, B, and DR antigens of their nonshared haplotypes ("b" and "c"). Figure 51-1B illustrates a family in which the mother ("c/d") appears to be HLA-homozygous. Although the patient (sib #1, "a/c") has a unique genotype, the patient and sib #2 ("a/d") share the paternal "a" haplotype; each has inherited one of the two maternal haplotypes ("c" and "d"); and, depending on the degree of similarity for the "c" and "d" haplotypes, they may be matched for the maternal HLA-A, B, and DR loci.

Donor and Recipient Matching

As improvements in HLA typing have increased the sensitivity of histocompatibility testing, the definition of "a match" has become more difficult to standardize. Before molecular methods were available for identifying specific HLA genes, typing was limited to definition of phenotype. Using SSOP/PCR, it is now possible routinely to define genotypes for the DR, DQ, and DP loci. A molecular analysis also can be done for HLA-A, B, and C, but not on a routine basis. Clinical typing for class I antigens continues to be based on serology augmented by IEF as needed to identify variants that cannot be recognized by serology. IEF, however, will not identify all molecular variants (see Table 51-3). Class I typing will remain limited to phenotyping, and definitive matching for HLA-A, B, and C will not be possible until molecular typing for class I alleles can also be performed routinely.

To accommodate the transition from classic to molecular typing and to classify systematically different degrees of donor and recipient disparity, we developed a matching scheme that utilizes 4 match grades: (1) identity (phenotypic or genotypic); (2) micromismatch; (3) minor mismatch; and (4) major mismatch (Table 51-5). According to this system, a patient and donor are classified as HLA-A and B phenotypically identical if they cannot be distinguished by serology and IEF. A micromismatch is assigned if the antigens are identical by serology but differ by IEF. A minor mismatch is assigned if the antigens belong to the same CREG, and a major mismatch is assigned if the antigens are distinct and noncrossreactive (see Tables 51-1, 51-2). A patient and donor are classified as genotypically identical for DR if the same DRB alleles are identified by SSOP/PCR typing. Assignment of phenotypic identity for DRB is based on HLA-D (HTC) typing. A micromismatch is assigned if the patient and donor HLA-D specificities are identical by HLA-D typing but differ by SSOP/PCR (e.g., Dw14.1 and Dw14.2 are encoded by distinct alleles but cannot be distinguished by HLA-D typing). Class II minor mismatches are specificities that can be distinguished by HLA-D typing but not by serology (e.g., Dw4 and Dw10, which both type as DR4 by serology). Class II major mismatches are DR antigens distinguishable by serology (e.g., DR1 and DR4).

Ideally, every BMT donor and recipient should be HLA genotypically identical, whether they are related or unrelated. However, this is not possible in the majority of patients; therefore, some degree of HLA disparity must be accommodated if these transplants are to be undertaken. The minimal requirements for matching may vary in different clinical situations. As described later in this chapter, a one-HLA-locus major mismatch in haploidentical transplants and a one-locus minor mismatch in unrelated donor transplants can be tolerated with reasonable success, although these limited mismatches are associated with significant increases in the incidence and severity of graft-versus-host disease (GVHD).

In addition to classifying matching according to the degree of overall disparity for each locus (see Table 51-5), matching should also be described in terms of the vector of incompatibility (Table 51-6). Incompatibility

Table 51-5.
Classification of Donor and Recipient Matching for HLA-A, B, and D According to Degree of Genetic Disparity at Each Locus

HLA Antigen	*Match*[a]	*Method*[b]	*Example*
Class I, HLA-A, B	Genotypic identity	SSOP	B*2701 vs B*2701
	Phenotypic identity	Serology	B7 vs B7
		IEF	B27.1 vs B27.1
	Micromismatch	IEF	B27.1 vs B27.2
		SSOP	B*2701 vs B*2702
	Minor mismatch	Serology	B7 vs B27 (CREG)
	Major mismatch	Serology	B7 vs B8 (non-CREG)
Class II, HLA-DRB	Genotypic identity	SSOP	DRB1*0401 (Dw4) vs DRB1*0401 (Dw4)
	Phenotypic identity	HLA-D or SSOP	Dw4 vs Dw4
	Micromismatch	SSOP	DRB1*0404 (Dw14.1) vs DRB1*0408 (Dw14.2)
	Minor mismatch	HLA-D or SSOP	Dw4 (DR4) vs Dw10 (DR4)
	Major mismatch	Serology or SSOP	DR1 vs DR4

[a]"Genotypic identity" is defined as matching for individual genes. "Phenotypic identity" is defined as matching for individual gene products or antigens as identified by serology, IEF, or HLA-D typing.
[b]Serology represents level 1 typing; IEF for class I and HLA-D (HTC-defined) for class II represent level 2 typing. SSOP typing of the DRB loci can recapitulate the classic specificities defined by serology and HLA-D typing, as well as identify individual alleles.
HLA = human leukocyte antigen; SSOP = sequence-specific oligonucleotide prove; IEF = isoelectrical focusing; CREG = crossreactive group.

Table 51-6.
Matching for HLA-A, B, and D According to the Vector of Genetic Disparity[a]

		Vector and Number of Incompatible Loci[b]		
Recipient	*Donor*	*Rejection*	*GVHD*	*Overall*
Haploidentical Related Donor				
[A1,B8,Dw3] / **A2,B44,Dw7**	[A1,B8,Dw3] / **A3,B7,Dw2**	3	3	3
[A1,B8,Dw3] / **A1**,B35.1,Dw1	[A1,B8,Dw3] / **A3**,B35.1,Dw1	1 major	0	1 major
[A1,B8,Dw3] / **A2,B44**,Dw4	[A1,B8,Dw3] / **A1,B8**,Dw4	0	2	2
Unrelated Donor				
A1,B8,Dw3 / A3.1,B7,Dw2	A1,3.1 B7,8 Dw2,w3	0	0	0
A1,B8,Dw3 / A2.1,**B44**,Dw2	A1,2.1 B8 Dw2,w3	0	1 major	1 major
A1,B8,Dw3 / **A3**,B7,Dw2	A1,**11** B7,8 Dw2,w3	1 minor	1 minor	1 minor
A1,B8,Dw3 / **A2.1**,B8,Dw3	**A1,2.2 B8**,44 Dw3,**w7**[c]	>3	1 micro	>3

[a]Related donors share one haplotype with the patient (indicated by [ ]). Haplotypes of unrelated donors ("URD") are usually not known. Incompatible antigens are identified by bold type.
[b]Numbers indicate the number of mismatches for the HLA-A,B, and DRB loci. One locus mismatches are further defined as major, minor or micro.
[c]The donor is incompatible for A1, A2.2, B8 and Dw3, and the patient is incompatible for one micro mismatch (A2.1 vs A2.2).

in the donor defines the genetic risk of rejection ("rejection vector"). Incompatibility in the recipient defines the genetic risk of GVHD ("GVHD vector"), and combining the two defines the "overall" incompatibility. The distinction between "overall" and donor or recipient incompatibility becomes relevant when the patient or donor is homozygous for one or more HLA loci. Examples of matching by vector are illustrated for both haploidentical related and unrelated donors in Table 51-6. The maximum disparity for HLA-A, B, and D in a haploidentical BMT is a "3-antigen mismatch," and the maximum disparity for an unrelated donor BMT where donor and recipient are both heterozygous is a "6-antigen mismatch." If the maximum disparity is a "one-locus" mismatch, the degree of disparity is further defined as micro, minor, or major (see Table 51-5).

Transplants from HLA-Partially Matched Related Donors

Graft Failure

The first indication of donor engraftment is an increase of peripheral granulocyte counts. More than 95% of the patients who engraft achieve a count of at least 100 cells/mm^3 by day 21 after BMT, and graft failure is likely to occur if severe granulocytopenia persists beyond 21 days (10). To demonstrate donor engraftment in sex-mismatched transplants, peripheral blood lymphocytes and marrow cells can be tested by in situ DNA hybridization with a Y-body–specific probe (11). If donor and recipient are sex-matched, chimerism can be determined by restriction fragment length polymorphism (RFLP) or PCR/SSOP using probes specific for polymorphic or variable tandem repeated sequences (12). Graft failure may also occur after an initial take. In this circumstance, studies of chimerism are essential to confirm the gradual disappearance of donor cells and the reappearance of host cells and to exclude nonalloimmune mechanisms of marrow suppression, such as drug toxicity or viral infections. Following graft failure, functional studies may demonstrate that residual host lymphocytes have specific cytolytic T-lymphocyte (CTL) activity against donor alloantigens, or the patient's serum may be active in antibody-dependent cell-mediated cytotoxicity (ADCC) of donor cells (13,14). These findings have been interpreted to indicate alloimmune-mediated rejection as the mechanism for graft failure. Primary graft failure occurs most commonly in sensitized patients with a positive pretransplant antidonor crossmatch, whereas late graft failure occurs most commonly after transplantation of T-cell–depleted donor marrow (10,15). Graft failure of either type is usually associated with persistent aplasia. In certain patients, recovery of autologous myeloid cells can occur, especially if the conditioning regimen did not include total body irradiation (TBI) but consisted of chemotherapy only or if the patient is treated with hemopoietic growth factors, GM-CSF or G-CSF (16). If there is no recovery of myeloid function despite growth factor therapy, a second BMT from the same or different donor can be attempted, but the success of second transplants has been limited (10,17).

Relevance of the Pretransplant Conditioning Regimen

Marrow transplants from HLA-partially matched relatives have been performed for patients with severe aplastic anemia, myelodysplastic syndrome, leukemia, lymphomas, and myelomas. Pretransplant immunosuppression with cyclophosphamide (CY) alone (200 mg/kg over 4 days) was sufficient to allow sustained engraftment in 9 patients with severe aplastic anemia transplanted from an HLA-A, B, and D phenotypically identical donor (18). In contrast, only 4 of 11 patients transplanted from haploidentical relatives incompatible for one HLA-A, B, or D locus, and 0 of 3 patients transplanted from a 2-locus–incompatible donor had sustained engraftment with the same preparative regimen. Conditioning with busulfan (BU) (13–16 mg/kg over 4 days), in addition to CY (120–200 mg/kg over 2–4 days) was used for 11 patients with myelodysplastic syndrome, lymphomas, or myelomas. Nine patients transplanted from a one-locus–incompatible donor and one of 2 transplanted from 2-locus–incompatible donor engrafted. These data suggest combining BU and CY provides more immunosuppression than CY alone. Pretransplant conditioning with CY (120 mg/kg over 2 days) and TBI (920–1,575 cGy) allowed engraftment in 98% of 930 patients with hematological malignancy transplanted from a genotypically HLA-identical sibling, compared with 88% of 276 patients transplanted from an HLA-haploidentical partially matched donor ($p < 0.0001$) (10). Among the latter, the rate of graft failure was 17% in patients conditioned with 1,200 cGy TBI (over 6 days), 12% in patients conditioned with 1,575 cGy (over 7 days), 9% in patients conditioned with 1,320 to 1,440 cGy (120 cGy t.i.d. for 11–12 doses), and 5% in patients given 1,000 cGy in a single dose. Thus, donor incompatibility for HLA represents a significant barrier to achieving sustained engraftment, but host resistance and alloimmune-mediated rejection can be overcome by increasing the intensity of the pretransplant conditioning regimen. Further escalation of the dose of TBI and addition of other immunosuppressive chemotherapeutic agents, however, may not be possible because of significant toxicity already encountered with higher doses of TBI (1,575 cGy over 7 days and 1,000 cGy on one day) and with the BU and CY regimen. New immunosuppressive agents that can increase the immunosuppressive activity of these established regimens without additional toxicity are needed.

Significance of Prior Alloimmunization

Prior alloimmunization to donor histocompatibility antigens has a profound effect on the probability of achieving sustained engraftment. In a recent update of the results of haploidentical BMT in 522 patients surviving at least 21 days after the marrow infusion at the Fred Hutchinson Cancer Research Center (FHCRC), the rate of graft failure was 62% in patients with a positive pretransplant crossmatch, compared with 7% in patients with a negative crossmatch (p = 7.82E-10) (Table 51-7). The antiglobulin crossmatch and the B-cell crossmatch at 22 or 37°C correlated best with graft failure (19). Autoreactive antibodies were observed in 4 patients, but all were successfully engrafted. Alloimmunized patients who tested positive for anti-HLA antibodies by screening against a random cell panel but were crossmatch negative with the donor did not demonstrate an increased risk of graft failure.

Graft failure in a crossmatch-positive patient is most likely the result of alloimmune rejection mediated by sensitized radioresistant host T cells, although a role for the antibody cannot be excluded. Removal of antidonor antibody through plasma exchange followed by CY (120 mg/kg) and TBI (1,200–1,575 cGy); the addition of total lymphoid irradiation (600 cGy in 4 fractions over 2 days) prior to CY (120 mg/kg) and TBI (1,575 cGy); or the addition of antithymocyte globulin (ATG) (10 mg/kg/day, day −2 to day +3) to the standard regimen of CY (120 mg/kg) and TBI (1,575 cGy) has not resulted consistently in sustained marrow engraftment.

Table 51-7.
Risk Factors for Graft Failure in Haploidentical Transplants: Positive Crossmatch and HLA Mismatching[a]

	Proportion of Patients With Graft Failure[b]	
	Crossmatch-positive (%)	*Crossmatch-negative (%)*
Vector of HLA disparity		
None or GVH only[c]	0/0 (0)	2/75 (3)
Rejection ≤ GVH[d]	10/17 (59)	22/350 (6)
Rejection > GVH[e]	3/4 (75)	11/76 (15)
Total	13/21 (62)	35/501 (7)

[a]Primary and secondary graft failure in patients with malignancy surviving more than 20 days after transplantation from an HLA-haploidentical donor.
[b]Data represents incidence of graft failure in patients with a positive and negative antidonor crossmatch.
[c]Transplants in which there was no donor HLA incompatibility (rejection vector): the donor was either HLA-identical or homozygous at the mismatched HLA locus.
[d]Transplants in which the degree of donor HLA incompatibility (rejection vector) was equal to or less than the degree of recipient incompatibility (GVH vector). Donor and recipient were HLA-mismatched; the donor was either heterozygous or homozygous at the mismatched locus, and the patient was heterozygous at the mismatched locus.
[e]Transplants in which the degree of donor HLA incompatibility was greater than the degree of recipient incompatibility. Donor and recipient were HLA-mismatched; the donor was HLA heterozygous, and the patient was homozygous at the mismatched locus.
HLA = human leukocyte antigen; GVH = graft-versus-host.

Despite a negative CDC crossmatch, marrow graft failure occurred in 7% of HLA-haploidentical graft recipients conditioned with CY and TBI. It is possible that some of these patients were alloimmunized even though anti-donor HLA antibodies were not detectable in the standard CDC assays. The binding of antibodies to human lymphocytes can be detected by immunofluorescence analysis using flow cytometry. Several laboratories have standardized conditions for use of a crossmatch assay by flow microfluorimetry (FMF) (19). Simultaneous 2-color immunofluorescence using fluoresceinisothyocianate-conjugated antihuman immunoglobulin (Ig) and a phycoerhytrin-conjugated B-cell–specific antibody allows discrimination of anti-class II HLA-DR and DQ antibodies reactive only against B cells from anti-class I HLA-A, B, and C antibodies reactive against all lymphocytes. In controlled sensitivity assays, the microfluorimetry crossmatch demonstrated at least 10-fold greater sensitivity than any of the CDC crossmatch assays. However, a direct comparison of the predictive value of these assays has not been performed.

HLA-mismatching and Graft Failure

Donor HLA incompatibility is associated with increased graft failure. In patients with a negative crossmatch, the graft failure rate was 3% if there was no donor incompatibility for HLA-A, B, or D. However, the graft failure rate was 8% if the donor was incompatible for one or more loci. The vector of HLA mismatch affects both the risk of GVHD and the risk of graft failure. Recipients homozygous at the mismatched locus have a significantly lower rate of GVHD (p = 0.03; Figure 51-2) but a higher rate of graft failure than heterozygous recipients (p = 0.0054; see Table 51-7).

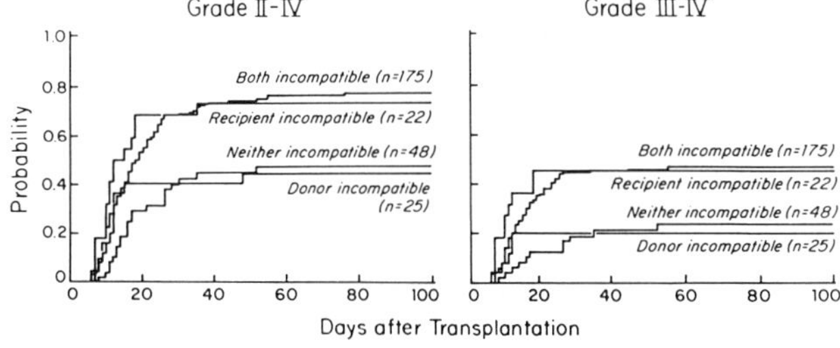

Figure 51-2. Probability of acute graft-versus-host disease (GVHD) (grades II–IV, left; grades III–IV, right) in patients transplanted for hematological neoplasms. Patients and donors shared one human leukocyte antigen (HLA) haplotype and differed for one HLA locus on their nonshared haplotypes. The probability of acute GVHD is shown for recipients homozygous for the mismatched locus (donor is incompatible for one HLA locus in the direction of host-versus-graft only); for heterozygous recipients transplanted from homozygous donors (recipient is incompatible for one HLA locus in the direction of graft-versus-host only); and for heterozygous recipients transplanted from heterozygous donors (both are incompatible for one HLA locus in both directions).

Effect of Marrow Cell Dose, Hematopoietic Growth Factors, T-cell Depletion, and Post-transplant Immunosuppression

In haploidentical transplants, higher doses of nucleated donor marrow cells correlated with a more rapid increase in the peripheral blood neutrophils after BMT, but within the range of nucleated donor marrow cells administered to these patients (1.0–5.0 × 10^8/kg) there was no suggestion that a higher marrow dose could prevent either primary or secondary graft failure (10). Efficacy of granulocyte-macrophage colony stimulating factor (GM-CSF) in facilitating engraftment of marrow from HLA-incompatible donors remains to be established. However, pilot studies of GM-CSF administered from day 0 to 27 in patients transplanted from an HLA-identical sibling or unrelated donor have begun and suggest that this growth factor does not increase the incidence or severity of acute GVHD (20,21). Studies from Memorial Sloan-Kettering and the International Bone Marrow Transplant Registry (IBMTR) have reported that T-cell depletion of donor marrow is associated with an increased rate of graft failure that is proportional to the degree of donor HLA incompatibility (see also Chapter 11) (13,22). In contrast, more powerful post-transplant immunosuppression can decrease the incidence of graft failure. At FHCRC, crossmatch-negative patients had a graft failure rate of 5% when treated with cyclosporine (CSP) plus methotrexate (MTX), but 9% when treated with MTX alone ($p = 0.03$).

Graft-versus-Host Disease

Recipient HLA incompatibility, but not donor incompatibility, determines the risk of acute GVHD (23). One-HLA-locus–incompatible but homozygous recipients who are matched with their donor in the direction of GVH have a lower incidence of acute GVHD than one-locus–incompatible heterozygous recipients ($p = 0.03$) (see Figure 51-2). HLA homozygosity in the donor does not decrease the incidence of GVHD. The incidence of acute GVHD in one-locus–incompatible transplants in homozygous recipients is similar to that seen in phenotypically HLA-matched BMT.

The incidence and severity of acute GVHD correlate with the degree of recipient HLA incompatibility (Figure 51-3) but is also significantly affected by the type of therapy used for GVHD prophylaxis. MTX given on days 1, 3, 6, and 11 and weekly thereafter until day 102 was the standard therapy for GVHD prophylaxis until 1985. In patients receiving MTX as the only immunosuppressive agent, the probability of grades II to IV GVHD was 35% for recipients of HLA phenotypically identical BMT, 73% for recipients of one-locus–incompatible BMT, 76% for recipients of 2-locus–incompatible BMT, and 84% for recipients of 3-locus–incompatible BMT (24). When it became apparent that the combination of cyclosporine (CSP) and MTX was superior to either agent alone in HLA-identical sibling BMT, the same regimen was adopted

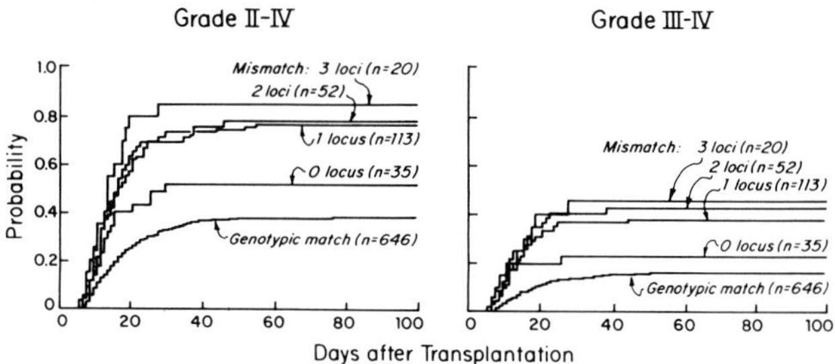

Figure 51-3. Probability of acute graft-versus-host disease (GVHD) (grades II–IV, left; grades III–IV, right) in 396 haploidentical bone marrow transplantations classified according to the degree of recipient incompatibility ("GVHD" vector) for 0, 1, 2, or 3 HLA-A, B, and D loci compared with probability of acute GVHD in HLA-genotypically identical sibling transplantations. All patients received cyclosporine plus methotrexate as GVHD prophylaxis.

for HLA-partially matched BMT. In a multivariate analysis of 474 patients who received CSP + MTX who achieved sustained engraftment, HLA incompatibility was a significant risk factor for acute GVHD (relative risk = 1.95 per HLA locus; $p < 0.0001$) (see Figure 51-3) (23). The risk of severe acute GVHD was significantly less, and time of onset was delayed in the CSP + MTX group (relative risk = 0.35; $p < 0.0001$). Incidence of severe acute GVHD was decreased from 53 to 28% in one-locus–incompatible recipients and from 63 to 47% in 2-locus–incompatible recipients. A third independent factor associated with a lower risk of severe GVHD was younger age of the patient (relative risk = 1.23 per decade; $p = 0.0094$). Diagnosis and stage of disease at the time of the BMT, patient and donor sex, donor age, donor relationship, and marrow cell dose were not significant risk factors for acute GVHD. BMT from HLA-haploidentical family members was associated with a higher probability for development of chronic GVHD (49 vs 33%) and an earlier median day of chronic GVHD onset (159 vs 201 days) compared with BMT from HLA-identical siblings (25).

One-HLA-A- or B-locus–incompatible recipients had a significantly lower incidence of acute GVHD when receiving CSP + MTX rather than MTX alone, but there was no apparent benefit from CSP + MTX in patients incompatible for one HLA-D locus. There was no significant difference in the incidence of acute GVHD for one-locus mismatches at HLA-A, B, or D. In one-HLA-A-locus–incompatible transplants, mismatching for antigens belonging to the same cross-reactive group (minor mismatch) results in less acute GVHD than mismatching for noncrossreacting A locus antigens (major mismatch). The difference between minor and major mismatches is seen in patients receiving either CSP + MTX or MTX alone (Figure 51-4).

A major mismatch for the serologically defined HLA-DR antigens was associated with an increased rate of acute GVHD (Figure 51-5). However, in the case

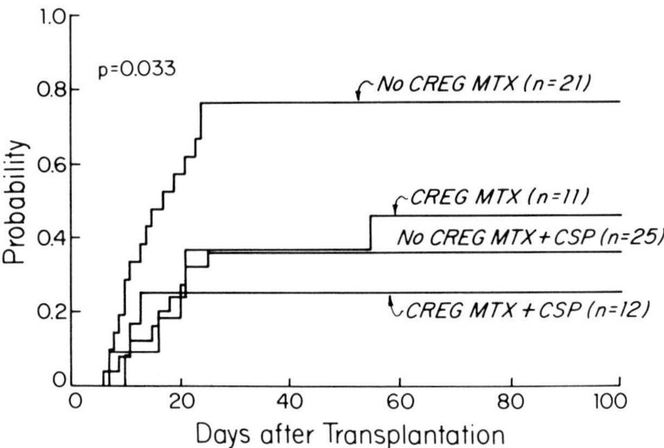

Figure 51-4. Probability of grade III to IV acute graft-versus-host disease (GVHD) in 69 haploidentical bone marrow transplantations in which the donor was incompatible for one class I human leukocyte antigen A (HLA-A) locus ("GVHD" vector). *Curves* represent minor (crossreactive group ["CREG"]) and major ("no-CREG") mismatches stratified according to the type of GVHD prophylaxis (methotrexate [MTX] only or MTX and cyclosporine [CSP]).

of a minor mismatch, where patient and donor are matched for HLA-DR by serological typing but mismatched for an HLA-D specificity defined by HTC or mismatched for a DRB1 allele defined by PCR/SSOP, there was also an increased risk of GVHD. A DR minor mismatch such as Dw4 (DR4) versus Dw14 (DR4) appears to have the same GVHD risk as a DR major mismatch such as DR4 vs DR5.

To assess the value of the MLC assay for predicting GVHD, donor versus recipient MLC responses for HLA-A, B, and D phenotypically identical or one-DR-locus–mismatched transplants were classified as "compatible" (relative response [RR] $< 10\%$), weakly reactive (RR $= 10–35\%$), or strongly reactive (RR $> 35\%$). There was a trend for a higher RR to be associated with increased GVHD, but the difference was not significant ($p = 0.4$) (see Figure 51-5, right panel). These data suggest that the MLC does not contribute to donor selection. Compatibility for HLA-DRB1 alleles and avoidance of DR major and minor mismatches as defined by SSOP typing appear to be the most important factors to minimize the risk of acute GVHD.

Depletion of mature T cells from the donor marrow is effective in decreasing both acute and chronic GVHD and associated morbidity (see also Chapter 11). Prevention of GVHD requires depletion of more than 99% (2 logs) of clonable T cells (15), and removal of fewer donor T cells requires administration of post-transplant immunosuppression for effective prevention of GVHD (26). Except in patients with congenital severe combined immunodeficiency disease (SCID), T-cell depletion has been complicated by an increased rate of marrow graft failure, worse with higher degrees of donor HLA mismatch (22,27). In patients with chronic myelogenous leukemia (CML), T-cell–depleted transplants have also been associated with an increased probability of post-BMT relapse (15). Attempts to compensate for graft failure and relapse by intensifying the conditioning regimen have resulted in more treatment-related toxicity and death. T-cell depletion by various methods has not improved disease-free survival in either HLA-matched, HLA-haploidentical, or unrelated donor transplants except for those patients with SCID (15,22,27).

Immune Reconstitution

T lymphocytes recognize foreign peptides presented by self-HLA but not necessarily by allogeneic HLA molecules, a phenomenon defined as HLA restriction. Therefore, mature T cells transplanted to an HLA-disparate recipient may not recognize antigen presented by host antigen-presenting cells (APC), thereby failing to help immune reconstitution. However, new T cells derived from hematopoietic stem cells must differentiate within the host thymus and as a result of positive and negative selection will also recognize antigen presented by host APC (as well as donor-derived APC). This process has been confirmed by studies in children with SCID receiving T-cell–depleted HLA-haploincompatible transplants (28). These recipients most often become split chimerae: T cells originate from the donor, whereas B cells and antigen-presenting cells originate from the recipient. Studies of these patients have demonstrated that the repertoire of T cell antigen receptors eventually expressed by donor-derived T cells is determined by the HLA restriction elements of the recipient.

The high-dose chemotherapy and radiation administrated to patients with hematological malignancy may

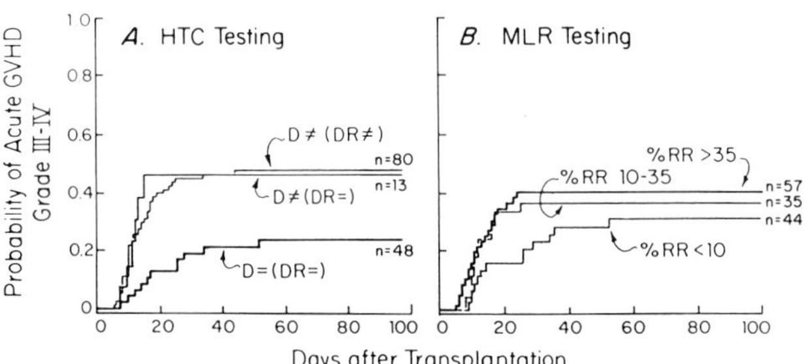

Figure 51-5. Relevance of homozygous typing cell (HTC) or mixed leukocyte reaction (MLR) testing of donors and recipients to occurence of acute graft-versus-host disease (GVHD). *Figures* represent the probability of grades III to IV acute GVHD in haploidentical HLA-A, B-identical transplants variably matched for HLA-D. (A) Probability of GVHD for donors and recipients matched for HLA-D (HTC-defined) or mismatched for HLA-D and DR (serologically defined), or mismatched for D but matched for DR. (B) Probability of GVHD for donors and recipients matched according to the strength of the donor antirecipient MLC response as measured by percent relative response (%RR). The donor MLC responses were classified as "compatible" (RR<10%), "weakly reactive" (RR=10–35%), and "strongly reactive" (RR>35%).

impair thymic function, thereby causing further delay in immune reconstitution. GVHD and the immunosuppressive therapy administered for prevention or treatment of GVHD may also contribute to a prolonged state of immunodeficiency. Serum Ig levels are significantly lower in recipients of HLA-haploidentical or unrelated donor grafts 3 to 4 months after BMT, compared with recipients of HLA-matched sibling grafts. These observations may explain in part the increased infections that occur in these patients and provide a rationale for replacement Ig therapy, although the clinical benefit of replacement therapy has not yet been proved. Successful prevention of GVHD should allow faster reconstitution of both T-cell and B-cell immunity.

Relapse

Relapse of leukemia after HLA-identical sibling BMT is less frequent in recipients in whom clinically significant GVHD develops than in syngeneic BMT or allogeneic BMT recipients without GVHD (see Chapter 19). Patients with acute lymphoblastic leukemia (ALL) in whom GVHD develops after BMT from haploidentical donors also had a lower risk of relapse than patients without GVHD (23). The probability of leukemic relapse in patients without clinically significant GVHD was the same whether the marrow donor was an HLA-genotypically identical sibling or haploidentical relative. These data suggest that HLA disparity in absence of acute GVHD has no antileukemic effect. In one analysis, chronic but not acute GVHD was associated with a lower relapse rate in patients with acute myeloid leukemia (AML) or CML (23). Because recipients of one-HLA-locus–incompatible transplants have a higher incidence of acute GVHD than recipients of HLA-identical sibling transplants, we would expect to see a lower incidence of leukemic relapse. After BMT for ALL or AML in remission or CML in chronic phase, the probability of relapse was 22% in 61 recipients of one-HLA-antigen–incompatible grafts, compared with 37% in 561 recipients of HLA-identical sibling grafts ($p = 0.09$). There was also a trend for a lower probability of relapse in unrelated donor transplants compared with HLA-identical sibling transplants. In a study of 52 HLA-matched unrelated donor and 104 HLA-identical sibling transplants, the incidence of relapse was 16 and 25%, respectively ($p = 0.34$) (29). Among unrelated donor transplants, there was also a trend for a lower probability of relapse in 42 one-HLA-locus minor mismatches, compared with 70 HLA matches (12 vs 23%; $p = 0.19$) (30).

Survival

Immunodeficiency Disorders

Most children with SCID (57 to 77% in different series) have become long-term survivors after BMT of T-cell–depleted marrow from a haploidentical parent incompatible for 2 or 3 HLA antigens (see also Chapter 64). If these children have residual natural killer cells or T-cell function, T-cell–depleted haploidentical grafts may be rejected in absence of conditioning therapy. Sustained engraftment can be achieved by conditioning with CY and BU. Although the post-transplant course should not be complicated by acute GVHD, significant morbidity and mortality may occur from opportunistic infections before full immune reconstitution is achieved.

Aplastic Anemia

Patients with moderate or severe aplastic anemia who lack an HLA-identical sibling donor are usually treated first with immunosuppressive therapy involving ATG or CSP because of the complications associated with HLA-mismatched BMT, especially graft failure. Patients who fail to show significant improvement in hematopoietic function within 100 days can be classified as nonresponders and at that time be considered for BMT from an HLA-partially matched related or a matched unrelated donor. Higher rates of engraftment can be achieved by adding TBI to CY, but infections, usually acquired before transplantation, and GVHD continue to impair the success of treatment. Three of 6 one-locus–mismatched and 2 of 5 2-locus–mismatched recipients are alive between 1 or 6 years after BMT in Seattle (31). In a report on 60 patients from the IBMTR, 27% of aplastic patients transplanted from a haploidentical donor were alive at 2 years (22).

Leukemia

The probability of survival following HLA-haploidentical BMT correlates best with the overall degree of HLA compatibility (23,24). Recipients of HLA-A, B, or D phenotypically identical or one-locus–incompatible BMT for AML in first remission (Figure 51-6, right upper panel), ALL in first or second remission (see Figure 51-6, left upper panel), or CML in chronic phase (see Figure 51-6, left lower panel) had a probability of survival indistinguishable from recipients of HLA-genotypically identical BMT. Too few "good risk" patients were transplanted from a 2- or 3-locus–incompatible donor to allow a significant analysis of the results. "Poor risk" patients receiving 2- or 3-locus–incompatible BMT for acute leukemia in relapse (see Figure 51-6; right lower panel represents data for patients with AML) had a lower survival rate than HLA-matched "poor risk" patients due to mortality from GVHD and infection. GVHD prophylaxis with CSP + MTX did not significantly improve survival.

Transplants from Unrelated Donors

Background

The first unrelated donor BMT achieving sustained engraftment was performed in 1972 in a patient with

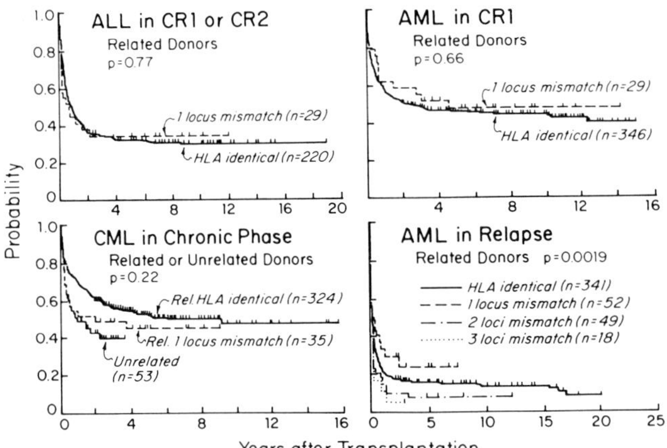

Figure 51-6. Probability of disease-free survival for patients with leukemia in remission transplanted from a human leukocyte antigen (HLA)–genotypically identical sibling or a haploidentical family member mismatched for one HLA locus (*top*). (Bottom left) Disease-free survival for patients with chronic myelogenous leukemia (CML) in chronic phase transplanted from HLA-A, B, or D identical unrelated donors, an HLA-identical sibling, or a haploidentical family member mismatched for one HLA locus. (Bottom right) Disease-free survival for patients with leukemia in relapse transplanted from an HLA-genotypically identical sibling or a haploidentical family member mismatched for 1, 2, or 3 HLA loci.

SCID (32). In 1979, the first successful unrelated donor BMT was performed for a patient with leukemia, a 10-year-old girl with ALL in second remission (33). The patient had a remarkably benign post-BMT course, with no evidence of acute or chronic GVHD. Unfortunately, she relapsed and died 23 months later from refractory leukemia. The publication of additional case reports between 1973 and 1983 (34–39) clearly established the feasibility of unrelated donor marrow BMT and provided an increasing impetus for the recruitment of larger numbers of HLA-typed unrelated volunteers.

Establishment of a National Network of Unrelated Donors

The first local marrow donor programs were developed during the early 1980s (40–45). However, unrelated donor searches were very difficult, time-consuming, and usually nonproductive. Public interest in unrelated BMT came to the attention of the United States Congress, and a special appropriation was enacted for the establishment of a National Donor Registry through the Office of Naval Research. The goals of the contract were to recruit a large number of HLA-typed volunteers who gave informed consent; establish a National Coordinating Center to facilitate the donor search process and communication between donor and transplant centers; and improve the safety and efficacy of unrelated donor transplants. In July 1986, a contract was awarded to establish a National Marrow Donor Registry, and this Registry became known as the National Marrow Donor Program (NMDP) (46). After an initial start-up phase, the NMDP became operational in September 1987. In December 1987, the program provided its first HLA-matched unrelated donor marrow for BMT. In May 1989, primary responsibility for the Federal contract was transferred from the Navy to the National Heart, Lung and Blood Institute (NHLBI), Department of Health and Human Services (DHHS). During the first 4 years, the American Red Cross was the recipient of the Federal contract, but in October 1990, NMDP was incorporated as an independent nonprofit organization. As of May 1992, NMDP has recruited more than 600,000 HLA-A, and B–typed volunteer donors, processed formal donor searches for more than 5,475 patients, and provided HLA-matched unrelated donor marrow for more than 1,125 transplants. The NMDP network includes 106 donor centers and 57 transplant centers. Currently, the program grows by 15,000 to 20,000 new donors and facilitates more than 40 transplants each month. Requests for donor searches are submitted to NMDP by member transplant centers, the centralized donor file is searched, and, if a potential match is found, requests for additional HLA typing or marrow donation are forwarded to the appropriate donor center.

Probability of Finding a Donor

The number of private antigens encoded by the HLA-A, B, and DRB1 loci exceeds 87 (see Table 51-1). By calculating all possible combinations of these antigens present in any individual, the number of unique HLA-A, B, and DR phenotypes present in the population is estimated to be more than 47 million. If these phenotypes were randomly distributed in the population, the chance of finding an HLA match would be very small for all patients. HLA alleles, however, are not randomly distributed, and certain antigens and haplotypes occur much more frequently than others (see Chapter 4). For patients with the most common haplotypes, it was possible to find HLA-identical unrelated donors when the National Registry contained only 20,000 donors (47). Now that the Registry contains more than 600,000 donors, the chance of finding matches has improved significantly. The Seattle team has performed more than 400 unrelated donor transplants since 1979. A total of 14 transplants were done through 1986, but subsequently the annual number has increased to 13, 52, 70, 90, and 114 from 1987 through 1991, respectively (Table 51-8). Although the number of preliminary searches has remained relatively constant since 1989, the percent of patients transplanted has increased steadily from 18% in 1989 to 36% in 1992.

GVHD in Unrelated Donor Transplants

The incidence and severity of acute GVHD in 151 patients transplanted from an HLA-A, B, and D

Table 51-8.
Unrelated Donor Searches Initiated and Transplants Performed at the Fred Hutchinson Cancer Research Center

Year	*Preliminary Searches*	*URD Transplants (%)*
1988	243	52 (21)
1989	397	70 (18)
1990	401	90 (22)
1991	313	114 (36)
1992	351	127 (36)

URD = unrelated donor.

phenotypically identical donor for treatment of hematological malignancy was evaluated. Donor selection was based on serological and HTC typing (48), and matching for HLA-DRB1, DRB3, DRB5, and DQB1 alleles was confirmed by PCR/SSOP. Despite matching for HLA-A, B, DRB, and DQB, DPB1 compatibility was observed in only 22% of recipients; 55% of recipients were incompatible for one DPB1 locus, and 23% were incompatible for 2 DPB1 loci. The incidence of grades II to IV and grades III–IV acute GVHD was 75 and 37%, respectively. Recipient incompatibility for DPB1 did not influence significantly the risk of acute GVHD or survival. HLA-A and B matching in this study was assessed only by serological typing, identity for HLA-C was not evaluated, and the contribution of mismatching for the IEF-defined HLA-A or B microvariants remains to be determined. Thus, the increased GVHD seen in these patients may be due to undetected or undefined HLA disparity. However, it is also possible that the increased GVHD observed in unrelated donor transplant recipients may be caused by a greater degree of mismatching for non-HLA–linked minor histocompatibility antigens among unrelated individuals (49).

The effect of mismatching for HLA-A, B, or D in unrelated donor transplants has been evaluated in 112 consecutive patients less than 36 years of age who received CSP + MTX as GVHD prophylaxis (30). The patient and unrelated donor were HLA-A, B, and D phenotypically identical in 70 cases, there was a class I minor mismatch in 21 cases, and a class II minor mismatch in 21 cases. The probability of grades II to IV acute GVHD was 78% for the identical group and 94% for the minor mismatch group ($p < 0.001$). The probability of grades III to IV acute GVHD was 36% for the identical and 51% for the minor mismatch group ($p = 0.05$). When analyzed separately, HLA class I or II minor mismatches were associated with similar acute GVHD rates. At day 100 post-transplant, 66% of the identical and 64% of the minor mismatch group were alive in remission with sustained donor grafts. The cumulative incidence of clinically extensive chronic GVHD was 60% for the phenotypically identical unrelated donor group, and 74% for the minor mismatch unrelated donor group, and there was no significant difference in survival at 2 to 3 years (33% for each).

Survival

Nonmalignant Disorders

An initial report from NMDP described results of unrelated donor BMT in 41 patients with a variety of congenital diseases, including immunodeficiency syndromes. The probability of survival was 52% at 2 years (27). Fifteen patients with severe aplastic anemia have been transplanted in Seattle from unrelated volunteer donors. Eleven transplants were HLA-identical and 4 were incompatible for one HLA-A, B, or D minor mismatch. All patients were conditioned with a regimen containing CY and TBI (1,200 cGy). Eleven patients died: 3 in the early post-BMT period from infection most likely acquired before BMT, 2 with graft failure, 3 with acute GVHD and infection or hemorrhage, 2 with chronic GVHD and infection or hemorrhage, and one with a secondary lymphoma. Four patients (25%) survive at 1.7 to 5 years after BMT. A joint report of 40 unrelated transplants for patients with nonmalignant disorders from 5 BMT centers, which included 15 patients from FHCRC, reported a 28% survival rate (50). This preliminary experience does not differ from that observed in similar late-stage patients transplanted from HLA-matched sibling donors in the early 1970s and emphasizes the need to transplant patients early in the course of the disease before they become infected or sensitized to HLAs by multiple blood transfusions.

Acute Leukemia

Initial reports on small series of patients have indicated that unrelated donor BMT can be successful in patients with acute leukemia (51,52). A search for an HLA-matched unrelated donor was initiated at the FHCRC for 345 patients with acute leukemia referred from June 1979 through December 1989, and an unrelated donor BMT was performed in 64 patients (19%). BMT was offered only to patients at or beyond first relapse. The median time from initiation of the search to BMT was 165 days. In 36 cases, the patient and donor were HLA-A, B, and D identical, in 27 there was a minor mismatch at one locus, and in one there was a minor mismatch at 2 loci. Median patient age at BMT was 20 years (range, 1–49 yr); 34 patients had ALL and 30 had AML; 3 patients were in first complete marrow remission after an extramedullary relapse, 14 were in second remission, 8 in third remission, 11 in first relapse, and 28 in second, subsequent, or refractory relapse. Sixty-one patients were prepared with CY + TBI and 3 with chemotherapy only. All patients received unmodified marrow. GVHD prophylaxis was CSP + MTX for 60 patients, MTX alone for 2, and prednisone + CSP for 2. Ten of 25 patients transplanted while in remission survive at 2 to 6 years (Kaplan-Meier [KM] estimate, 39%), and 8 of 39 patients transplanted in relapse survive at 2 to 3 years (KM estimate, 16%). Patients less than 20 years of age had better survival than older patients. Survival of patients

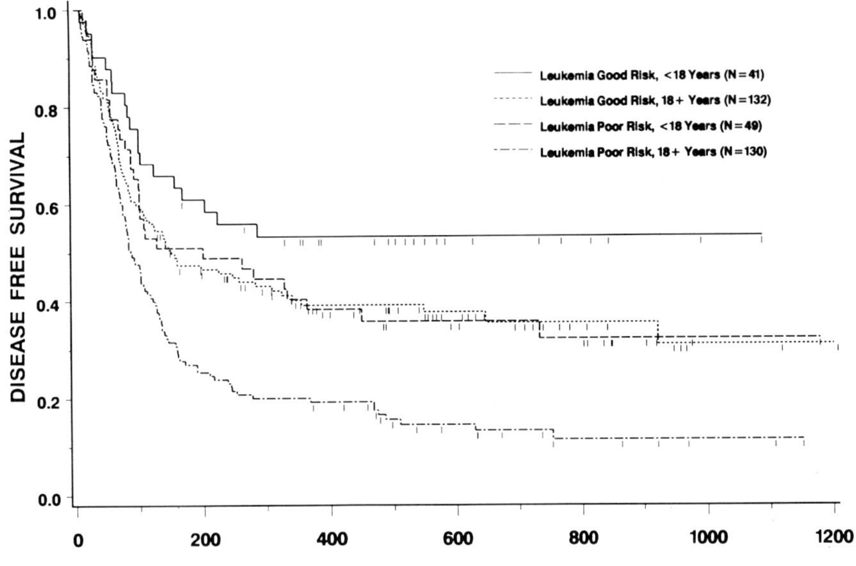

Figure 51-7. Probability of disease-free survival shown as a function of time after bone marrow transplantation with patients stratified by leukemia risk and age. Events are recorded at time of relapse or death. *Tick marks* represent patients alive in remission. Good risk was defined as patients with acute leukemia in first or second remission or chronic myelogenous leukemia in primary chronic phase. Poor risk was defined as patients with more advanced disease.

who did not proceed to an unrelated donor BMT correlated with the disease stage at the time of the initial donor search. The probability of survival at 3 to 5 years was 17% for patients in first relapse or second remission and 0% for patients at or beyond second relapse. A Cox model using time-dependent treatment covariates evaluated the effect of unrelated BMT on survival from initiation of the donor search. The estimated death rate among patients receiving unrelated donor BMT was increased by a factor of 6.3 ($p = 0.0001$) in the period immediately following BMT, as compared with alternative therapies (i.e., chemotherapy or autologous marrow BMT). This hazard ratio subsequently declined by approximately 5/1,000 per day ($p = 0.0001$) indicating that, by approximately one year after BMT, surviving unrelated graft recipients are at lower risk of death than surviving patients treated with alternative therapies. This initial study (Anasetti C, Anderson G. Unpublished observations) indicated that BMT from an unrelated donor is feasible in approximately 20% of the patients with relapsed acute leukemia. Although associated with an increased early mortality, unrelated donor transplant recipients have a better probability of long-term survival than those receiving current alternative therapies.

NMDP reported on the outcome of unrelated donor BMT in patients with acute leukemia. The probability of disease-free survival at 1.5 years was 45% for 58 patients transplanted in first or second remission and 19% for 98 patients with more advanced disease (27). Younger age of the patient is associated with better survival. The probability of disease-free survival in patients with either acute or chronic leukemia whose transplant was facilitated by NMDP is shown in Figure 51-7. These results indicate that BMT from an unrelated donor can be effective treatment for patients with acute leukemia. Outcome depends on the stage of disease at the time of BMT, with best results achieved at first or second remission.

Chronic Myeloid Leukemia

Reports from 4 different centers and a combined study from the NMDP have shown that CML is curable by unrelated donor BMT (27,53,54). CML has become the most frequent indication for unrelated donor BMT (27). Ninety-eight patients with CML received an unrelated donor BMT at the FHCRC. Fifty-three were in chronic phase, 24 in accelerated phase, 10 in a second chronic phase, and 11 in blast crisis. Median patient age was 33 years (range, 5–51 yr). In 73, the patient and donor were HLA-A, B, and DR–identical by serological testing and identical for DRB1 alleles by SSOP/PCR. Patients less than 36 years were eligible for a one-locus minor mismatched transplant: 11 transplants were mismatched for one HLA-A or B crossreactive antigen, and 14 were incompatible for one HLA-DR minor. Patients were conditioned with CY and TBI and transplanted with unmodified marrow with CSP + MTX used for GVHD prophylaxis. In patients with CML in chronic phase, the probability for development of acute GVHD grades II to IV was 75% for HLA-A, B, and D–identical transplant and 93% for a one-locus minor mismatch ($p < 0.01$). The Kaplan-Meier estimate of survival for patients transplanted in chronic phase was 40±5%, with no deaths observed after 647 days (see Figure 51-6). No patient in this group has had clinical relapse. The median follow-up of surviving patients is 725 days (range, 365–1,139 days). Age of the patient and HLA mismatch of the donor did not significantly affect survival. Results were compared with a cohort of patients similar for age and interval to

BMT who were transplanted from an HLA-identical sibling at FHCRC. Disease-free survival for the control subjects was 56±5% at 3 years (p = 0.04). After an unrelated BMT, 9 of 24 (37%) patients transplanted in accelerated phase are alive, disease-free from 693 to 1,840 days (median, 784 days); 4 of 10 patients transplanted in second chronic phase are alive and disease-free from 1,161 to 2,472 days (median, 1,646 days); and one of 11 patients transplanted in blast crisis survives at 599 days.

Conclusions

HLA incompatibility between recipient and marrow donor represents a risk factor for graft failure and GVHD that has been only partially overcome by improving immunosuppressive regimens. Increasing knowledge of the structure of HLA and development of powerful new typing technology have made possible precise and definitive HLA matching of patients and unrelated donors. Large registries of volunteer donors have provided a match to a growing proportion of patients in need of BMT and allowed long-term disease-free survival for patients with a variety of diseases. Unrelated donor transplants, however, are associated with an increased incidence of graft failure and GVHD compared with HLA-matched sibling transplants. Such increase may be due to disparities for undetected HLA determinants or to non-HLA–linked histocompatibility genes. Because of the complexity of the HLA system and its extreme polymorphism, HLA-identical marrow donors will not be found for most patients. The clinical reality is that a certain degree of donor-recipient genetic disparity is inevitable, and the degree and type of mismatching between unrelated donors and recipients will be variable. Therefore, it is still necessary to improve methods for BMT that can result in survival despite some amount of HLA disparity. Future research in this field will be aimed at decreasing the toxicities associated with the preparative regimens, improving hematopoietic recovery by administration of recombinant growth factors, and exploring novel immunosuppressive agents and new modalities for prevention and treatment of graft rejection and GVHD.

References

1. Bodmer JG, Marsh SGE, Albert ED, et al. Nomenclature for factors of the HLA system, 1991. Tissue Antigens 1992;39:161–173.
2. Yang SY. Nomenclature for HLA-A and HLA-B alleles detected by ID-IEF gel electrophoresis. In: Dupont B, ed. Histocompatibility testing 1987. New York: Springer-Verlag, 1989:54–57.
3. Choo SY, Antonelli P, Nisperos B, Nepom GT, Hansen JA. Six variants of HLA-B27 identified by isoelectric focusing. Immunogenetics 1986;23:24–29.
4. Choo SY, Fan L, Hansen JA. A novel HLA-B27 allele maps B27 allospecificity to the region around position 70 in the $\alpha 1$ domain. J Immunol 1991;147:174–180.
5. Ezquerra T, Domenech N, van der Poel J, Strominger JL, Vega MA, Lopez de Castro JA. Molecular analysis of an HLA-A2 functional variant CLA defined by cytotoxic T lymphocytes. J Immunol 1986;137:1642–1649.
6. Dupont B, Braun DW, Yunis EF, Carpenter CB. HLA-D by cellular typing. In: Terasaki PI, ed. Histocompatibility testing 1980. Los Angeles, UCLA Press, 1980:229–267.
7. Angelini G, Preval C, Gorski J, Mach B. High-resolution analysis of the human HLA-DR polymorphism by hybridization with sequence specific oligonucleotide probes. Proc Natl Acad Sci USA 1986;83:4489–4493.
8. Petersdorf EW, Smith AG, Mickelson EM, Martin PJ, Hansen JA. Ten HLA-DR4 alleles defined by sequences polymorphisms within the DRB1 first domain. Immunogenetics 1991;33:267–275.
9. NIH lymphocyte microcytotoxicity technique. In: NIAID manual of tissue typing techniques. (DHEW publication No. [NIH] 80–545.) Atlanta: National Institute of Allergy and Infectious Disease. 1979;39.
10. Anasetti C, Amos D, Beatty PG, et al. Effect of HLA compatibility on engraftment of bone marrow transplants in patients with leukemia or lymphoma. N Engl J Med 1989;320:197–204.
11. Durnam DM, Anders KR, Fisher L, O'Quigley JO, Bryant EM, Thomas ED. Analysis of the origin of marrow cells in bone marrow transplant recipients using a Y-chromosome-specific in situ hybridization assay. Blood 1989;74:2220–2226.
12. Blazar BR, Orr HT, Arthur CD, Kersey JH, Filipovich AH. Restriction fragment length polymorphisms as markers of engraftment in allogeneic marrow transplantation. Blood 1985;66:1436–1444.
13. Kernan NA, Flomenberg N, Dupont B, O'Reilly RJ. Graft rejection in recipients of T-cell-depleted HLA-nonidentical marrow transplants for leukemia. Transplantation 1987;43:842–847.
14. Barge AJ, Johnson G, Witherspoon R, Torok-Storb B. Antibody-mediated marrow failure after allogeneic bone marrow transplantation. Blood 1989;74:1477–1480.
15. Martin PJ, Kernan NA. T-cell depletion for the prevention of graft-vs.-host disease. In: Burakoff SJ, Deeg HJ, Ferrara J, Atkinson K, eds. Graft versus host disease: immunology, pathophysiology, and treatment. New York: Marcel Dekker, 1990:371–387.
16. Nemunaitis J, Singer JW, Buckner CD, et al. The use of recombinant human granulocyte-macrophage colony-stimulating factor in graft failure after bone marrow transplantation. Blood 1990;76:245–253.
17. Kernan NA, Bordignon C, Heller G, et al. Graft failure after T-cell-depleted human leukocyte antigen identical marrow transplants for leukemia: I. Analysis of risk factors and results of secondary transplants. Blood 1989;74:2227–2236.
18. Beatty PG, Di Bartolomeo P, Storb R, et al. Treatment of aplastic anemia with marrow grafts from related donors other than HLA genotypically-matched siblings. Clin Transplant 1987;1:117–124.
19. Anasetti C. The role of the immunogenetics laboratory in marrow transplantation. Arch Pathol Lab Med 1991;115:288–292.
20. Nemunaitis J, Buckner CD, Appelbaum FR, et al. Phase I/II trial of recombinant human granulocyte-macrophage colony-stimulating factor following allogeneic bone marrow transplantation. Blood 1991;77:2065–2071.
21. Nemunaitis J, Anasetti C, Storb R, et al. Phase II trial of recombinant human granulocyte-macrophage colony-stimulating factor (rhGM-CSF) in patients undergoing

allogeneic bone marrow transplantation from unrelated donors. Blood 1992;79:2572–2577.

22. Ash RC, Horowitz MM, Gale RP, et al. Bone marrow transplantation from related donors other than HLA-identical siblings: effect of T-cell depletion. Bone Marrow Transplant 1991;7:443–452.
23. Anasetti C, Beatty PG, Storb R, et al. Effect of HLA incompatibility on graft-versus-host disease, relapse, and survival after marrow transplantation for patients with leukemia or lymphoma. Hum Immunol 1990; 29:79–91.
24. Beatty PG, Clift RA, Mickelson EM, et al. Marrow transplantation from related donors other than HLA-identical siblings. N Engl J Med 1985;313:765–771.
25. Sullivan KM, Agura E, Anasetti C, et al. Chronic graft-versus-host disease and other late complications of bone marrow transplantation. Semin Hematol 1991;28:250–259.
26. Ash RC, Casper JT, Chitambar CR, et al. Successful allogeneic transplantation of T-cell-depleted bone marrow from closely HLA-matched unrelated donors. N Engl J Med 1990;322:485–494.
27. Kernan NA, Bartsch G, Ash RC, et al. Retrospective analysis of 462 unrelated marrow transplants facilitated by the National Marrow Donor Program (NMDP) for treatment of acquired and congenital disorders of the lymphohematopoietic system and congenital metabolic disorders. N Engl J Med 1993;328:593–602.
28. Robert JL, Volkman DJ, Buckley RH. Modified MHC restriction of donor-origin T-cells in humans with severe combined immunodeficiency transplanted with haploidentical bone marrow stem cells. J Immunol 1989;143:1575–1579.
29. Beatty PG, Hansen JA, Thomas ED, et al. Marrow transplantation from HLA-matched unrelated donors for treatment of hematologic malignancies. Transplantation 1991;2:443–446.
30. Beatty PG, Anasetti C, Hansen JA, et al. Marrow transplantation from unrelated donors for treatment of hematologic malignancies: effect of mismatching for one HLA locus. Blood 1993;81:249–253.
31. Storb R, Longton G, Anasetti C, et al. Changing trends in marrow transplantation for aplastic anemia. Bone Marrow Transplant 1992;10:45–52.
32. O'Reilly RJ, Dupont B, Pahwa S, et al. Reconstitution in severe combined immunodeficiency by transplantation of marrow from an unrelated donor. N Engl J Med 1977;297:1311–1318.
33. Hansen JA, Clift RA, Thomas ED, Buckner CD, Storb R, Giblett ER. Transplantation of marrow from an unrelated donor to a patient with acute leukemia. N Engl J Med 1980;303:565–567.
34. Speck B, Zwaan FE, van Rood JJ, Ernisse JG. Allogeneic bone marrow transplantation in a patient with aplastic anemia using a phenotypically HLA-A identical unrelated donor. Transplantation 1973;16:24–28.
35. Horowitz SD, Bach FH, Groshong T, Hong R. Treatment of severe combined immunodeficiency with bone marrow from an unrelated, mixed-leucocyte-culture-nonreactive donor. Lancet 1975;2:431–433.
36. Lohrmann HP, Dietrich M, Goldmann SF, et al. Bone marrow transplants for aplastic anemia from a HLA and MLC-identical unrelated donor. Blut 1975;31:347–354.
37. Foroozonfar N, Hobbs JR, Hugh-Jones K, et al. Bone marrow transplant from an unrelated donor for chronic granulomatous disease. Lancet 1977;1:210–213.
38. Gordon-Smith ED, Fairhead SM, Chipping PM, et al. Bone marrow transplantation for severe aplastic anemia using histocompatible unrelated volunteer donors. Br Med J 1982;225:835–837.
39. Duquesnoy RJ, Zeevi A, Marrari M, Hackbart S, Camitta B. Bone marrow transplantation for severe aplastic anemia using a phenotypically HLA-identical, SB-compatible unrelated donor. Transplantation 1983;35:566–571.
40. McCullough J, Bach FH, Coccia P, et al. Bone marrow transplantation from unrelated volunteer donors: summary of conference on scientific, ethical, legal, financial, and other practical issues. Transfusion 1982;22:78–81.
41. James DCO. Organization of a hospital bone marrow panel. In: Smit Sibinga CTh, Das PC, Opelz G eds. Transplantation and blood transfusion. Boston: Martinus Nijoff, 1984:131–139.
42. McElligott MC, Menitove JE, Aster RJ. Recruitment of unrelated persons as bone marrow donors. Transfusion 1986;26:309–314.
43. McCullough J, Roger G, Dahl R, et al. Development and operation of a program to obtain volunteer bone marrow donors unrelated to the patient. Transfusion 1986;26:315–323.
44. Beatty PG, Atcher C, Hess E, Meyer DM, Slichter SJ. Recruiting blood donors into a local bone marrow donor registry. Transfusion 1989;29:778–782.
45. McCullough J, Scott EP, Halagan N. Effectiveness of a regional bone marrow donor program. JAMA 1988; 259:3286–3289.
46. McCullough J, Hansen J, Perkins H, Stroncek D, Bartsch G. The National Marrow Donor Program: how it works, accomplishments to date. Oncology 1989;3:63–72.
47. Beatty PG, Dahlberg S, Mickelson EM, et al. Probability of finding HLA-matched unrelated marrow donors. Transplantation 1988;45:714–718.
48. Petersdorf EW, Smith AJ, Mickelson E, et al. The role of HLA-DPB1 disparity in the development of acute graft-versus-host disease following unrelated donor marrow transplantation. Blood 1993;81:1923–1932.
49. Martin PJ. Increased disparity for minor histocompatibility antigens as potential cause of increased GVHD risk in marrow transplantation from unrelated donors compared with related donors. Bone Marrow Transplant 1991;8:217–223.
50. Hows JM, Szydlo R, Anasetti C, Camitta B, Gajewsky J, Gluckman E. Unrelated donor marrow transplants for severe acquired aplastic anemia. Bone Marrow Transplant 1992;10(suppl 1):102–106.
51. Hows J, Yin JL, Marsh J, et al. Histocompatible unrelated volunteer donors compared with HLA nonidentical family donors in marrow transplantation for aplastic anemia and leukemia. Blood 1986;68:1322–1328.
52. Gingrich RD, Ginder GD, Goeken NE, et al. Allogeneic marrow grafting with partially mismatched, unrelated marrow donors. Blood 1988;71:1375.
53. McGlave P, Scott E, Ramsay N, McCullough J, Kersey J. Unrelated donor bone marrow transplantation therapy for chronic myelogenous leukemia. Blood 1987;70:877–881.
54. Beatty PG, Ash R, Hows JM, McGlave PG. The use of unrelated bone marrow donors in the treatment of patients with chronic myelogenous leukemia: experience of four marrow transplant centers. Bone Marrow Transplant 1989;4:287–290.

Part V
Autologous Marrow Transplantation for Acquired Diseases

Chapter 52
Autologous Bone Marrow Transplantation for Non-Hodgkin's Lymphoma

Philip J. Bierman and James O. Armitage

Very high-dose chemotherapy or radiation therapy supported by autologous bone marrow transplantation (BMT) has been shown to cure some patients with sensitive malignancies who have failed to be cured with standard therapies. Thus, resistance of the tumor cells in some patients is "relative" rather than "absolute." Because non-Hodgkin's lymphomas are highly chemotherapy-sensitive and sometimes cured by chemotherapy at standard doses, one might expect that high-dose therapy and BMT would make a major contribution to their treatment. Currently, non-Hodgkin's lymphomas are the diseases most frequently treated with autologous BMT (1,2).

Non-Hodgkin's Lymphomas

Non-Hodgkin's lymphomas represent malignancies of lymphocytes and display a tremendous variation in clinical aggressiveness. They vary from some of the most indolent neoplasms (e.g., follicular small-cleaved cell non-Hodgkin's lymphomas) to the most rapidly growing and most aggressive (e.g., Burkitt's or small noncleaved cell lymphomas). Non-Hodgkin's lymphomas are being diagnosed with increasing frequency. Their incidence has increased 60% between 1973 and 1989 (3). Approximately 41,000 new cases will be diagnosed in the United States in 1992, and these will account for nearly 20,000 deaths (3). Because some aggressive non-Hodgkin's lymphomas are associated with infection by the human immunodeficiency virus (HIV), there is an increase in their frequency based solely on the large numbers of patients with the acquired immune deficiency syndrome (AIDS). It has been estimated that as many as 8 to 27% of new non-Hodgkin's lymphomas in 1992 in the United States will be associated with HIV infection (4). However, the disease is also becoming more frequent in patients not affected by HIV. When comparing the period 1973 to 1975 with the period 1987 to 1989, the largest increase in incidence was seen in the oldest age groups (3). The explanation for this latter increase is not known.

Classification

One of the difficulties in any discussion of non-Hodgkin's lymphomas relates to the classification of these varied disorders. Numerous classification schemes have been popular over the past few decades. Although the previously used methods of classification seemed to have little in common, they all were able to predict clinical outcome. However, translation between the various systems was difficult and hindered communication between physicians and interpretation of the literature. In an attempt to resolve this dilemma, the Working Formulation (5) for the classification of non-Hodgkin's lymphomas was developed as a method of translating nomenclature between the various classification systems in use at the time (Table 52-1). The Working Formulation has since become the most widely used classification system for non-Hodgkin's lymphomas. This system divides patients into low-grade, intermediate-grade, and high-grade lymphomas and has great utility in predicting clinical outcome. The majority of non-Hodgkin's lymphomas seen in the United States are tumors of B lymphocytes, although lymphoblastic lymphomas are usually tumors of T lymphocytes, as are approximately half of the diffuse mixed-cell lymphomas. The

Table 52-1.
Working Formulation of Non-Hodgkin's Lymphomas

Low grade	
A.	Small lymphocytic
B.	Follicular small cleaved
C.	Follicular mixed
Intermediate grade	
D.	Follicular large
E.	Diffuse small cleaved
F.	Diffuse mixed
G.	Diffuse large
High grade	
H.	Immunoblastic
I.	Lymphoblastic
J.	Small noncleaved

major criticism of the Working Formulation has been the failure to separate lymphomas into T-cell and B-cell phenotypes.

Small lymphocytic lymphomas are a malignancy of small "well-differentiated lymphocytes" that are morphologically and immunologically similar to the cells of chronic lymphocytic leukemia (CLL). Small lymphocytic lymphomas are often considered to represent the solid tissue counterpart of CLL. These lymphomas accounted for 4% of the lymphomas studied by the Working Formulation. Small lymphocytic lymphomas are usually composed of B lymphocytes and are sometimes associated with the t(11;14) chromosomal abnormality, as well as trisomy 12, which may be associated with a poorer prognosis (6). These lymphomas are generally disseminated at the time of diagnosis. Eighty-one percent of patients studied by the Working Formulation presented with stage IV disease. Patients with small lymphocytic lymphomas occasionally have disease in extranodal sites, such as the stomach and the orbit. When patients with small lymphocytic lymphomas secrete immunoglobulin M (IgM) they have a disease that is indistinguishable from macroglobulinemia of Waldenstrom. Small lymphocytic lymphomas are not rapidly fatal in most patients, and survival beyond 5 years is frequent, even for patients who are managed without specific therapy (7,8). These lymphomas, however, are usually not curable with chemotherapy despite initial responses to a wide variety of agents. Prolonged failure-free survival may sometimes be observed following radiation therapy for patients who present with localized disease (8). Diffuse intermediate lymphoma is a newly recognized category of lymphoma that is not included in the Working Formulation (9,10). This subtype is being diagnosed with increasing frequency and clinically occupies an intermediate site between small lymphocytic lymphomas and diffuse small-cleaved cell lymphomas. Diffuse intermediate lymphomas, like small lymphocytic lymphomas, are B-cell neoplasms that are frequently associated with the t(11;14) chromosomal translocation.

The follicular lymphomas accounted for approximately one third of the cases studied by the Working Formulation. They include follicular small-cleaved cell, follicular mixed, and follicular large-cell subtypes. These are tumors of B lymphocytes and are frequently associated with the t(14;18)(q32;q21) chromosomal translocation (6,11). These tumors tend to be widely disseminated at diagnosis. Although highly responsive to chemotherapy and radiation, they are rarely cured with these modalities. Because patients with low-grade follicular lymphomas are often asymptomatic, they are sometimes managed initially with observation alone. Median survival for patients with low-grade follicular lymphomas may be 8 to 10 years (12–14). Inclusion of the follicular large-cell lymphomas in the intermediate-grade category of the Working Formulation would suggest that it has a more aggressive course and might be curable with conventional chemotherapy. Although this is a controversial issue, there is evidence to suggest that this is the case, particularly for patients with less advanced disease (15,16).

Diffuse small-cleaved cell lymphomas are unusual in the United States (17); they account for 7% of the lymphomas studied by the Working Formulation. Some of these cases undoubtedly represent the diffuse counterpart of the follicular small-cleaved cell lymphoma because they often display similar biological characteristics, such as the t(14;18) translocation, and may also have a similar, indolent course. Like those with follicular low-grade lymphomas, patients with diffuse small-cleaved lymphomas often have stage IV disease at diagnosis. However, other tumors that fit into this category can have a more aggressive course. These lymphomas may be associated with a T-cell immunophenotype rather than the B-cell immunophenotype seen in follicular lymphomas, and they may have a high expression of the Ki-67 antigen (17).

Diffuse mixed, diffuse large-cell, and immunoblastic lymphomas can be considered one entity clinically. Inclusion of immunoblastic lymphomas in the high-grade category of the Working Formulation is unfortunate in this regard. These lymphomas comprise approximately one third of those studied by the Working Formulation and represent the most common types of non-Hodgkin's lymphomas seen in adults. These lymphomas can begin in lymph nodes or in extranodal sites and may present in a localized or disseminated manner. These tumors are chemotherapy-responsive and are curable in a significant proportion of patients.

Both lymphoblastic lymphomas and small noncleaved cell lymphomas are extremely rapidly growing neoplasms and occur frequently in children (18,19). They comprise 9% of the cases studied by the Working Formulation. Lymphoblastic lymphomas are closely related to T-cell acute lymphoblastic leukemia, whereas small noncleaved lymphomas represent the solid tumor counterpart of L3 or Burkitt cell acute lymphoblastic leukemia. These tumors have a propensity to spread to the central nervous system (CNS) and the blood, and rapid staging and prompt institution of therapy is important. Both are frequently chemotherapy-curable when they occur in children but have a poorer prognosis in adults.

Staging

Staging of cancer usually involves collection of data before the onset of therapy and assists in determining prognosis. The choice of therapy for non-Hodgkin's lymphomas is dictated by the extent of disease determined by the staging evaluation. The most popular staging system utilized for non-Hodgkin's lymphomas has been the Ann Arbor system (20) (Table 52-2). This staging system collects data about sites of involvement and the presence or absence of systemic symptoms. This system was originally developed for Hodgkin's disease and works better for this disease than for non-Hodgkin's lymphomas, because the latter

Table 52-2.
Ann Arbor Staging System For Lymphomas

Stage I: Involvement of a single lymph node region (I) or of a single extralymphatic organ or site (I_E).
Stage II: Involvement of 2 or more lymph node regions on the same side of the diaphragm (II), or localized involvement of extralymphatic organ or site and of 1 or more lymph node regions on the same side of the diaphragm (II_E).
Stage III: Involvement of lymph node regions on both sides of the diaphragm (III), which may also be accompanied by localized involvement of extralymphatic organ or site (III_E) or by involvement of the spleen (III_S), or both (III_{SE}).
Stage IV: Diffuse or disseminated involvement of one or more extralymphatic organs or tissues with or without associated lymph node enlargement.
Symptom Status A: Asymptomatic.
Symptom Status B:
1. Unexplained weight loss of more than 10% of body weight in 6 months prior to admission; or
2. Unexplained fever, with temperatures above 38°C; or
3. Night sweats.

have a much higher frequency of extranodal involvement and are more often widely disseminated at diagnosis. A variety of other staging systems has been developed to take into account other prognostic factors, such as serum lactic dehydrogenase (LDH) levels, serum beta-2 microglobulin levels, diameter of the largest mass, and number of extranodal sites. Although these systems are quite different from the Ann Arbor system, they can also predict clinical course and treatment outcome accurately. In an attempt to standardize staging for patients with diffuse mixed, diffuse large-cell, and immunoblastic lymphoma, a large study was undertaken to find a compromise system. This led to the development of the International Prognostic Index (21) (Table 52-3). Patients classified as low risk with this system had a 5-year survival of 73%, compared with 26% for patients with high-risk disease. This system is likely to be utilized widely for patients with the common aggressive non-Hodgkin's lymphomas.

The actual staging of patients with non-Hodgkin's lymphomas begins with a careful history and physical examination. Routine laboratory tests, including a complete blood count with differential, platelet count, and a chemistry screening panel are performed. The staging evaluation should also include a serum LDH level and might include a serum beta$_2$-microglobulin level. Computerized tomography scans of the chest, the abdomen, and the pelvis are performed routinely. A gallium scan with single-photon emission computed tomography (SPECT) imaging is also often useful in patients with aggressive non-Hodgkin's lymphomas. SPECT imaging can be particularly useful, if shown to be positive before therapy, in determining the presence of viable tumor cells in residual masses following therapy. Other imaging studies should be done when appropriate for a particular patient's circumstances.

Table 52-3.
International Prognostic Factors Index For Non-Hodgkin's Lymphomas

Risk Category	*Number of Risk Factors*
Low	0, 1
Low-intermediate	2
High-intermediate	3
High	4, 5
Risk factors	
Age > 60	
Ann Arbor Stage III or IV	
> 1 extranodal site	
Performance status 2, 3, or 4	
Lactic dehydrogenase levels > normal	

In addition to the initial diagnostic biopsy, a marrow aspirate and biopsy should also be performed.

Primary Therapy

The initial treatment of patients with low-grade non-Hodgkin's lymphomas is highly controversial. If patients have low bulk disease and are asymptomatic, many physicians would suggest no initial therapy and treatment only when symptoms develop. This is an approach based on the long natural history of the disease and the failure to demonstrate survival differences among patients treated aggressively and those managed with single-agent chemotherapy or observation alone (12,22,23). This "watch and wait" option is frequently chosen for elderly patients. Patients with localized low-grade lymphomas can be cured with radiation therapy, or a combination of radiation therapy and chemotherapy (24,25). In patients with bulky or symptomatic disease, or those who are not comfortable without initial therapy, treatment options include single-agent chemotherapy; combination chemotherapy; multimodality therapy, including both chemotherapy and radiation; and low-dose total body radiotherapy. Each of these treatment choices has been shown to yield a high proportion of complete remissions and a prolonged disease-free survival. Unfortunately, it cannot be shown whether overall survival is increased or whether these treatments have curative potential for patients with disseminated disease at the time of diagnosis. Because the treatment outcome is ultimately poor for these patients, studies have been initiated utilizing high-dose therapy and autologous BMT as part of the primary therapy for patients with low-grade lymphomas. The results of these studies are too early to report.

It has been less than 20 years since the first demonstrations that patients with aggressive non-Hodgkin's lymphomas could be cured with chemotherapy (26). Since then, a large number of chemotherapy regimens with curative potential have been developed (27). Patients with the more common intermediate-grade lymphomas should always be treated initially with a combination chemotherapy regimen. For patients with localized disease (Ann Arbor stage I or minimal Ann Arbor stage II), the duration of chemotherapy can be reduced (e.g., from 6 to 3 courses) and local radiotherapy administered to the sites of known disease (28–30). With either a full course of chemotherapy or a combination of chemotherapy and radiotherapy, the results are excellent, with disease-free survival seen in 75% or more of patients. The curability of advanced stage non-Hodgkin's lymphomas represents one of the major successes of modern oncology. Utilizing effective combination chemotherapy regimens, the majority of patients achieve a complete remission, and between 30 to 50% of patients achieve long-term, disease-free survival (27,31). However, 50% or more of these patients eventually die of disease, and autologous BMT has been considered as part of the primary therapy for high-risk, younger patients with aggressive non-Hodgkin's lymphomas. A number of completed pilot studies suggest that the treatment results might be improved with this approach (32–37); however, no definitive trial has been completed.

For patients with lymphoblastic and small noncleaved cell lymphomas, initial treatment results are age-dependent. The majority of children with these lymphomas appear to be cured with combination chemotherapy regimens that usually include prophylactic treatment to the CNS (18,19). For adults, treatment with similar regimens yields poorer results. Patients who have minimal disease have a high cure rate, but patients with bulky disease, high LDH, and CNS or marrow involvement have a very poor outcome (38,39). It has been suggested that these latter patients may be candidates for high-dose therapy and autologous BMT as part of their primary therapy. A pilot study from The Netherlands suggests that the results can be improved with this approach (40). Nine adult patients with poor-risk lymphoblastic lymphomas underwent autologous BMT in first remission. There was no transplant-related mortality, and disease-free survival was estimated to be 67%. These results are encouraging; however, no comparative trial has been completed.

Salvage Therapy

If patients with non-Hodgkin's lymphomas relapse following initial therapy or fail to achieve an initial complete remission they have a poor ultimate outcome. Patients with low-grade lymphomas can achieve a second complete remission with a variety of salvage therapies and still have prolonged survival. However, all of these patients will eventually die of lymphoma unless they die of some other condition first. For younger patients, this poor ultimate outlook is often considered to be unacceptable despite the fact that 5 to 10 years of survival might be achieved with repeated salvage treatments. In these patients, high-dose therapy and autologous BMT are being used with increasing frequency.

Despite the substantial progress in treatment of the common aggressive non-Hodgkin's lymphomas such as diffuse large-cell lymphomas, at least 50% of patients will relapse from complete remission or fail to achieve an initial complete remission. A variety of salvage chemotherapy regimens have been developed for this population (41,42). Most of these regimens have employed combinations of cisplatin, etoposide, and ifosfamide. Complete remission rates as high as 35 to 40% have been reported, but overall it appears that less than 10% of patients with relapsed intermediate-grade non-Hodgkin's lymphomas can be cured with conventional salvage chemotherapy. These patients have made up the largest group of patients treated with high-dose therapy and autologous BMT. Autologous BMT has also been utilized for patients with high-grade lymphomas following failure of primary chemotherapy. BMT has been used less often in these patients due to the relatively low frequency of these histological subtypes and concerns about occult contamination of the marrow with malignant cells.

Results of High Dose Therapy and Autologous BMT in Patients with Non-Hodgkin's Lymphomas

More than 30 years ago the first attempts at using stored autologous marrow to treat chemotherapy- and radiation-induced myelosuppression were reported (43,44). However, this technique came into wide use following the first reports from the National Cancer Institute, in which high dose BACT chemotherapy (carmustine, cytarabine, cyclophosphamide, and 6-thioguanine) followed by autologous BMT was used in a group of patients with non-Hodgkin's lymphomas (45,46). The BACT chemotherapy used in these early trials was not permanently marrow-ablative, since some patients were treated with the identical BACT regimen without BMT. Patients treated with BMT did, however, have significantly faster bone marrow recovery, and these studies established the fact that high-dose chemotherapy could cure some patients who were previously considered incurable. Since then, autologous BMT has been used with increasing frequency for a wide variety of malignancies, as well as for non-Hodgkin's lymphomas (1,2). The International Bone Marrow Transplant Registry estimates that more than 2,000 transplants are being performed each year for non-Hodgkin's lymphomas.

The use of high-dose therapy and autologous BMT is based on the assumption that some patients have lymphomas that are resistant to the doses of drugs that can be administered safely in standard chemotherapy regimens but might be sensitive if the doses of drugs or radiation could be significantly escalated (47). This concept is illustrated by the 3 columns in Figure 52-1. As the intensity of therapy is increased, treatment-related toxicity also increases. Because most of the agents used to treat cancer suppress the marrow, at some point an unacceptable mortality related to myelosuppression is reached. If myelosuppression could be ignored as a factor in selecting

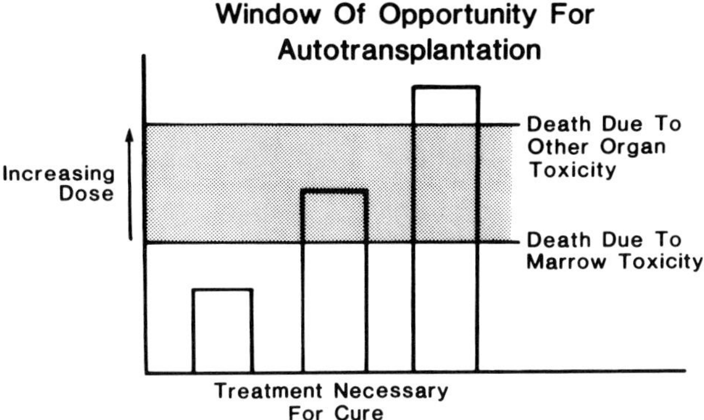

Figure 52-1. Patients represented by the middle column are the best candidates for autologous bone marrow transplantation because this technique allows administration of chemotherapy or radiation in doses that would otherwise be intolerable due to severe myelosuppression.

therapy, the intensity of treatment could be increased significantly until toxicity from damage to other organs supervened. Certain agents, such as the alkylating agents and radiotherapy, follow this pattern, and it is no accident that these are the agents usually utilized in high-dose therapy and autologous BMT. Some agents, such as vincristine and doxorubicin, have important early toxicity in organs other than marrow and are not suitable for dose escalation in transplantation. Utilization of autologous BMT to treat patients with lymphomas depends on identifying subgroups of patients who fit into the "window" illustrated in Figure 52-1. This window illustrates that cure can be accomplished at a dose of therapy above that which causes unacceptable deaths from myelotoxicity without marrow support and below that which causes an unacceptable frequency of deaths from damage to other organs.

Perhaps the most important issue in selecting patients with lymphomas for autologous BMT is one of timing. Patients with a high probability of cure using conventional treatments should not be subjected to the rigors of autologous BMT. Similarly, one would not want to withhold BMT until treatment resistance increased to the point where dose escalation could no longer cure the patient or preceding treatments had so weakened the patient that surviving a transplant would not be expected.

The decision to recommend BMT is easiest for patients with end-stage, refractory lymphomas in whom no alternative therapy is likely to produce a satisfactory outcome. Unfortunately, results suggest that these patients are unlikely to benefit from BMT. Currently, the most popular setting in which to perform an autologous BMT for patients with lymphomas is at the first sign of treatment failure when patients are still well and the tumor is still sensitive to chemotherapy administered at usual doses. In this setting, a significant proportion of patients can be cured with autologous BMT. This observation was demonstrated in one of the largest reports of patients undergoing BMT for lymphoma. Patients with chemotherapy-sensitive relapsed non-Hodgkin's lymphomas could be cured 35 to 40% of the time with this technique (48).

It is possible that the most effective time to perform autologous BMT would be as part of primary therapy for patients with lymphomas. This process would require the ability to identify patients in whom the cure rate with standard therapy was low, that the mortality of BMT was also very low, and that the increase in dose intensity available with BMT would overcome the patient's resistance to standard chemotherapy. Studies are now underway to test the hypothesis that autologous BMT should be performed very early in patients with poor prognosis lymphomas. Investigators from City of Hope have reported results of autologous BMT in 20 first remission patients (37). Patients in this report were believed to have a poor prognosis with conventional chemotherapy alone, based on elevated LDH levels, bulky disease, extranodal disease, or advanced stage. Results of BMT in these patients are displayed in Figure 52-2 and demonstrate a disease-free survival estimated to be 84%. Results of additional pilot studies performed to date (Table 52-4) suggest that very high cure rates can be achieved in patients with aggressive non-Hodgkin's lymphomas when autologous BMT is performed as part of the primary therapy. It must be noted, however, that some of the patients in these trials would have been cured without the risk and expense associated with autologous BMT. It is unclear from these studies whether all high-risk patients were transplanted, or whether only selected patients

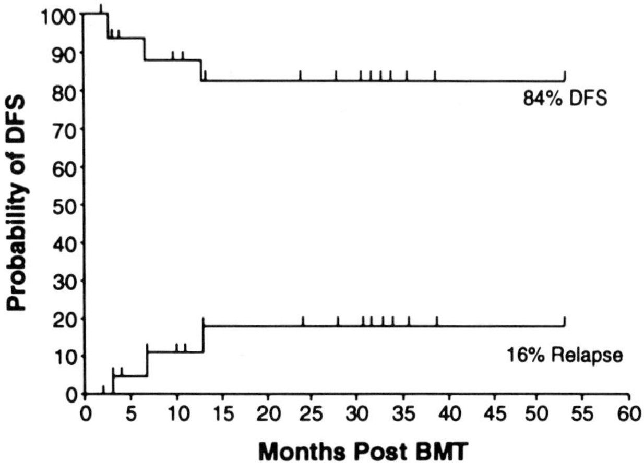

Figure 52-2. Probability of disease-free survival and relapse in patients with poor prognosis lymphoma following autologous bone marrow transplantation in first complete remission. (Reproduced by permission from Nademanee A, Schmidt GM, O'Donnell MR, et al. High-dose chemoradiotherapy followed by autologous bone marrow transplantation as consolidation therapy during first complete remission in adult patients with poor-risk aggressive lymphoma: a pilot study. Blood 1992;80:1130–1134.)

Table 52-4.
Use of Early Autologous Bone Marrow Transplantation for High-risk Non-Hodgkin's Lymphomas

Reference	*No. of Patients*	*Disease Status at Time of Transplant*	*Outcome*	*Comments*
(32)	17	1st PR	13 CCR (8–75 mo); 75% actuarial survival	
(33)	14	1st CR (6) 1st PR (8)	11 CCR (35–73 mo); 79% actuarial survival	Survival significantly better than similar high-risk patients who did not undergo early transplantation
(34)	15	1st PR	6 CCR (19–61 mo)	
(35)	21	1st CR	14 CCR (5–72 mo); 66% actuarial DFS	
(36)	12	1st CR	8 CCR (8–52 mo); 66% actuarial DFS	Outcome superior to historical patients with similar prognostic factors treated with chemotherapy alone
(37)	20	1st CR	17 CCR (2–54 mo); 84% actuarial DFS	

PR = partial remission; CR = complete remission; CCR = continuous complete remission; DFS = disease-free survival.

received BMT. In addition, some of these high-risk patients might be salvaged with BMT after relapse, rather than receiving BMT up front. Although these reports clearly demonstrate that BMT can be safely performed for high-risk patients in first remission, a randomized clinical trial should be carried out to document the efficacy of this approach. Pilot studies often incorporate subtle and invisible selection factors that limit comparisons to historical control subjects.

Low-grade Lymphomas

Patients with disseminated low-grade lymphomas are rarely cured with standard therapies, but have a median survival that may exceed 10 years. Experience with BMT in these patients is limited compared with that of more aggressive histological subtypes. The prolonged natural history of these lymphomas mandates long follow-up to determine whether this treatment is truly curative. Most patients with low-grade lymphomas have been treated with autologous BMT after relapse from complete remission or after failure to achieve a complete remission. Because of the high frequency of marrow involvement in these lymphomas, most studies have utilized some method of treating the marrow **in vitro** in an attempt to eliminate the risk of infusing contaminating tumor cells. Some investigators have utilized hematopoietic progenitor cells derived from the peripheral blood (by repetitive apheresis procedures) in the hopes that the frequency of circulating tumor cells would be lower than that found in the marrow. In both situations, the treatment regimen utilized has generally been high-dose chemotherapy and total body irradiation (TBI). The very high level of radiosensitivity seen in follicular lymphomas treated with low doses of TBI as part of their primary therapy makes the inclusion of TBI seem a particularly logical treatment in this group of patients.

At least 3 large series have been reported in which patients with follicular, low-grade lymphomas have been treated with high-dose therapy and autologous BMT (Table 52-5). Patients transplanted at Dana-Farber Cancer Institute and St. Bartholomew's Hospital were generally in second or third remission at the time of BMT and had minimal disease status, defined as less than 10 to 20% marrow involvement and lymph nodes no greater than two cm in diameter (49,50). Marrow was purged in these studies with anti-B-cell monoclonal antibodies and complement. In Nebraska, most patients were transplanted with autologous peripheral stem cells, although a small group received unpurged marrow (51). Disease-free survival in this series was similar to that observed

Table 52-5.
Autologous Bone Marrow Transplantation For Low-Grade Non-Hodgkin's Lymphomas

Reference	*No. Patients*	*Transplant Regimen*	*Rescue Source*	*Early Deaths (%)*	*Outcome*
(49)	51	CY, TBI	Purged marrow	1 (2)	32 CCR; 47% projected DFS
(50)	38	CY, TBI	Purged marrow	2 (5)	22 CCR (2 mo to 5 yr)
(51)	33	CY, TBI, or BEAC	Unpurged marrow or PSCs	3 (9)	16 CCR (median follow-up, 21 mo); 42% projected DFS

CY = cyclophosphamide; TBI = total body irradiation; CCR = continuous complete remission; DFS = disease-free survival; BEAC = carmustine, etoposide, cytarabine, cyclophosphamide; PSC = peripheral stem cells.

following BMT with purged marrow. No difference in overall survival or disease-free survival was observed between the small number of patients receiving unpurged marrow and those transplanted with peripheral stem cells. Among patients receiving peripheral stem cells, there was no difference in outcome among patients with histological evidence of marrow involvement and those without marrow involvement. A high proportion of patients in these reports achieved complete remission following BMT, although many of the patients were transplanted while in second or third remission. Treatment-related mortality was low, and a significant percentage of patients in each series remain free of disease, although follow-up is relatively short. It will take a prolonged period of observation to be certain that patients with low-grade lymphomas are indeed cured with BMT.

Intermediate-grade and Immunoblastic Lymphomas

Early trials of autologous BMT in patients with relapsed large-cell lymphomas showed that a small number of patients could be cured with this approach, even when treated late in the course of their disease (52–54). In 1984, a study was published in which BMT outcome was shown to be dependent on an individual's sensitivity to conventional chemotherapy administered prior to transplantation (55). This concept was subsequently validated in a larger multi-institutional report of 100 patients who received autologous BMT for non-Hodgkin's lymphomas (48). Results of this study are displayed in Table 52-6 and Figure 52-3. Patients who had never achieved a complete remission with standard chemotherapy (primary refractory) had an extremely poor outlook, with no long-term disease-free survivors. Patients who had been in complete remission and subsequently relapsed and were resistant to standard doses of chemotherapy at the time of BMT (resistant relapse) were occasionally cured. The 3-year disease-free survival was estimated to be 14% for this group. The best results were seen in patients who had relapsed from complete remission but had achieved at least a partial remission with standard chemotherapy salvage regimens (sensitive relapse). These patients had a long-term, disease-free survival rate estimated to be 36% at 3 years. Selected

Table 52-6.
Autologous Bone Marrow Transplantation for non-Hodgkin's Lymphomas: Results According to Chemotherapy Sensitivity

	Primary Refractory (%)	*Resistant Relapse (%)*	*Sensitive Relapse (%)*
Partial Remission	47	14	9
Complete Remission	28	45	86
Actuarial 3-year disease-free survival	0	14	36

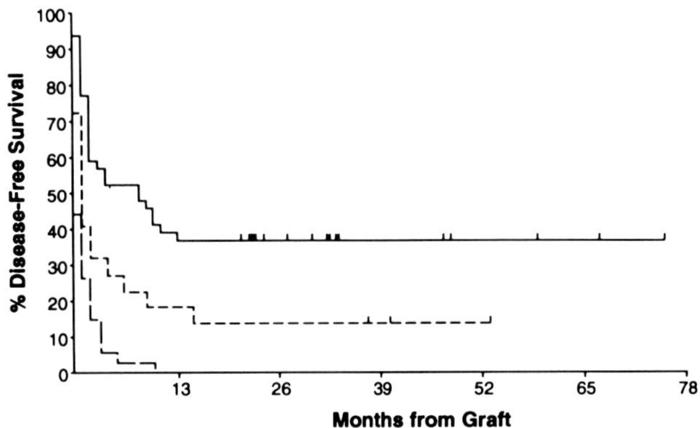

Figure 52-3. Actuarial 3-year disease-free survival following autologous bone marrow transplantation for non-Hodgkin's lymphoma for patients in sensitive relapse (*solid line*), resistant relapse (*dashed line*); and those without prior complete remission (*broken line*). (Reproduced by permission from Philip T, Armitage JO, Spitzer G, et al. High-dose therapy and autologous bone marrow transplantation after failure of conventional chemotherapy in adults with intermediate-grade or high-grade non-Hodgkin's lymphoma. N Engl J Med 1987;316:1493–1498.)

results of selected series of autologous BMT for intermediate- and high-grade lymphomas are listed in Table 52-7 (34,48,56–61). Although long-term disease-free survival exceeding 50% has been reported, it appears that only 20 to 25% of patients will be cured. The different treatment outcomes can be explained by differences in pretreatment prognostic factors, as well as differences in BMT regimens and selection criteria between institutions.

The improved outcome for patients with chemotherapy-sensitive disease at the time of BMT has been consistently demonstrated in reports of BMT for intermediate-grade non-Hodgkin's lymphomas. The Seattle group has been able to separate patients into those with "advanced lymphoma" (i.e., resistant first relapse, second or subsequent relapse, or third remission) and "less advanced lymphoma" (i.e., first or second remission, untreated relapse, or sensitive relapse) (58). The 5-year actuarial survival was 16% for the former group and 42% for the latter. The influence of performance status at the time of BMT has also been noted. In the Seattle experience, patients with advanced disease and a performance status less than 80% had a 7% actuarial survival, compared with 21% for patients with advanced disease with a performance status greater than 80% (58). A superior outcome associated with higher performance status in patients following BMT for lymphoma has been noted by other investigators (59,62,63). The presence of bulky disease has had an adverse effect on BMT outcome in some series (62,63), whereas others have found this variable to be unimportant (34). High-grade histology in comparison with intermediate-grade histology has been associated with higher relapse rates or inferior survival in some reports (57,58), whereas other investigators

Table 52-7.
Autologous Bone Marrow Transplantation for Intermediate-grade and High-grade non-Hodgkin's Lymphomas

Reference	*No. Patients*	*ED (%)*	*Outcome*	*Comments*
(48)	100	21	19% actuarial DFS	—
(34)	50	18	14% CCR (19–78 mo)	Some patients received 2 transplants
(56)	25	24	40% actuarial DFS	—
(57)	46	7	60% actuarial DFS	7 patients had low-grade lymphomas
(58)	101	21	11% EFS	27 patients had low-grade lymphomas or other lymphoproliferative disorders
(59)	66	21	16% DFS	2 patients had mycosis fungoides or malignant histiocytosis
(60)	70	13	16 CCR (12–78 mo)	15 patients had low-grade lymphomas
(61)	44	34	57% actuarial DFS	9 patients had low-grade lymphomas

ED = early death; DFS = disease-free survival; CCR = continuous complete remission; EFS = event-free survival.

have not found that BMT outcome is significantly influenced by histology (60,61). Patients with transformed lymphomas have had inferior outcomes in some reports (56,64), and others have reported good results following BMT in patients with transformed lymphomas (49). Patients with T-cell lymphomas have results equivalent to those with B-cell lymphomas (60,63). These results as well as others demonstrate superior results for patients who were transplanted earlier in the course of their disease, at a time of chemotherapy sensitivity, with less bulky disease, and a higher performance status.

All patients with intermediate-grade non-Hodgkin's lymphomas should be evaluated for BMT following relapse from a front-line chemotherapy regimen. Trials utilizing high-dose therapy and autologous BMT as part of the primary therapy of patients with poor prognosis, aggressive non-Hodgkin's lymphomas are now being reported (see Table 52-4). It is hoped that the use of early BMT might provide a significant improvement over the results attainable with standard therapy. Such trials, however, need to be approached cautiously. Treatment-related deaths in excess of 10% in patients who are receiving BMT as consolidative therapy in first complete remission are unacceptable because some of these patients might otherwise have been cured. For a patient to accept such a risk, it is necessary to demonstrate conclusively that the cure rate with early BMT is superior to standard therapy. It is not necessarily true that transplants performed during first complete remission will be superior to the combination of best primary therapy followed by BMT at the first signs of relapse. Prospective randomized trials will be necessary to answer these questions. These trials would require large numbers of patients and are unlikely to be completed without the cooperation of multiple institutions. Variations in histology and other pretransplant patient characteristics, as well as differences in transplant preparative regimens, will make such studies even more difficult to perform.

High-grade Lymphomas

Lymphoblastic lymphomas and small noncleaved cell (Burkitt's) lymphomas are highly aggressive malignancies. In children, standard therapy has improved to the point that at least 50% of all subgroups can be cured (18,19). However, adult patients can be divided into those with a cure rate in excess of 50% and those with a low probability of cure. Patients in the latter category include those with initial CNS or marrow involvement and high LDH levels. These high-risk patients have also been considered for high-dose therapy followed by autologous BMT in initial remission (35,40). Studies to date suggest that the previously poor treatment outcome can be improved by early BMT. Unfortunately, no prospective, randomized trials have been completed to document the apparent increase in efficacy. Because of the rarity of these tumors, it would be difficult to carry out such trials.

When patients with small noncleaved cell lymphomas undergo BMT after relapse, there is concern about transfusing tumor cells with the marrow. Reports of early disseminated relapse following autologous transplantation suggest that this may be a real possibility (65). At least one group of investigators suggested that patients at risk to relapse can be identified by a marrow culture method (66). A number of investigators would not feel comfortable performing autologous BMT in relapsed patients with small noncleaved cell lymphomas with unpurged marrow because of these concerns.

Treatment Regimens

Treatments that can be utilized for dose escalation and autologous BMT for patients with lymphomas are limited. A perfect treatment regimen would have only myelotoxicity and no significant extramedullary toxicity. Unfortunately, there are no such regimens available. Most high-dose preparative regimens utilized in patients with lymphomas include one or more alkylating agents, etoposide, occasionally other drugs such as cytarabine, and sometimes TBI. Examples of some of the most frequently used regimens are listed in Table 52-8.

There have been no prospective studies comparing transplant regimens for non-Hodgkin's lymphomas. Investigators from Memorial Sloan-Kettering have suggested that the use of an etoposide, cyclophospha-

Table 52-8.
Popular Preparative Regimens for Autologous Bone Marrow Transplantation for Non-Hodgkin's Lymphomas

Regimen	*Total Dose Administered*
CBV	Cyclophosphamide, 4.8–7.2 gm/M^2
	Carmustine, 300–600 mg/M^2
	Etoposide, 750–2,400 mg/M^2
BEAC	Carmustine, 300 mg/M^2
	Etoposide, 600–800 mg/M^2
	Cytarabine, 800 mg/M^2
	Cyclophosphamide, 140 mg/kg or 6 gm/M^2
BEAM	Carmustine, 300 mg/M^2
	Etoposide, 400–800 mg/M^2
	Cytarabine, 800–1,600 mg/M^2
	Melphalan, 140 mg/M^2
CY-TBI	Cyclophosphamide, 120–200 mg/kg
	Total body irradiation, 800–1,320 cGy
VP16, CY, TBI	Etoposide, 60 mg/kg or 750 mg/M^2
	Cyclophosphamide, 100–120 mg/kg
	Total body irradiation, 1,200–1,375 cGy

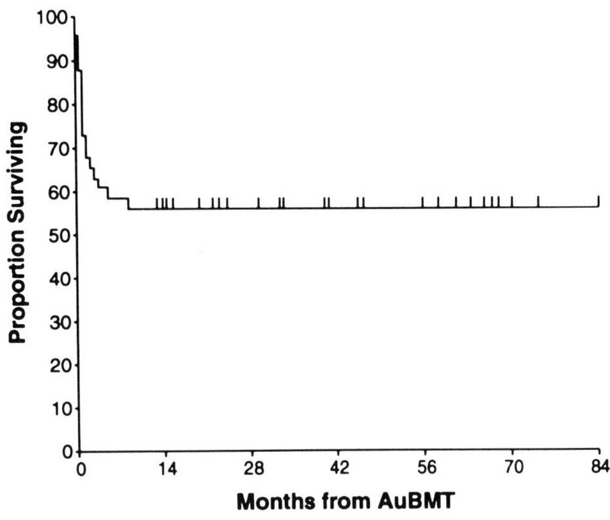

Figure 52-4. Disease-free survival following autologous bone marrow transplantation in patients conditioned with total body irradiation, etoposide, and cyclophosphamide. (Reproduced by permission from Gulati S, Yahalom J, Acaba L, et al. Treatment of patients with relapsed and resistant non-Hodgkin's lymphoma using total body irradiation, etoposide, and cyclophosphamide and autologous bone marrow transplantation. J Clin Oncol 1992;10:936–941.)

mide, TBI regimen has yielded results superior to cyclophosphamide and TBI alone (Figure 52-4) (61). The patients listed in Table 52-7 were conditioned with a wide variety of regimens, and differences in pretransplant variables make any comparisons difficult. The optimal dose of any particular agent within a transplant regimen is unknown. For example, the CBV (cyclophosphamide, carmustine, and etoposide) regimen is widely used for autologous BMT for patients with both non-Hodgkin's lymphomas and Hodgkin's disease. However, the doses of CBV used by different investigators vary widely. It is currently unclear if patients who receive the highest doses of drugs in this regimen have a superior treatment outcome compared with those receiving lower doses. Regimens that contain the highest doses may be associated with increased risk of toxicity (67). It will be difficult to resolve these issues without comparative trials.

The role of radiotherapy in autologous BMT for lymphomas is equally unclear. TBI is widely utilized for BMT in patients with low-grade and lymphoblastic lymphomas; however, the majority of patients undergoing BMT for intermediate-grade lymphomas and small non-cleaved cell lymphomas probably do not receive TBI. Unfortunately, there are no prospective trials comparing the relative efficacy of regimens containing radiotherapy and those that contain only drugs. Most reports have shown no clear survival benefit in patients who have received TBI as compared with chemotherapy (48,56,58,68). Radiation does appear to be associated with increased toxicity, primarily pulmonary complications (48,58), especially in patients who have had previous radiation therapy. Localized radiation may also be delivered to areas of bulky disease in patients undergoing autologous BMT. Some investigators favor the use of this approach immediately prior to BMT in an effort to reduce the extent of bulky disease in a manner similar to the way conventional chemotherapy is administered prior to BMT. It has been difficult to show a survival advantage with this approach, although a trend toward improved survival has been noted in some patients receiving involved-field radiation prior to BMT (57). Other investigators have chosen to administer radiation as "consolidation therapy" following BMT. Again, a survival advantage is difficult to demonstrate with this approach. The use of post-BMT radiotherapy may, however, improve survival in patients who only achieve a partial remission following BMT (68). A number of ongoing studies are testing the hypothesis that radiotherapy can be delivered directly to the tumor in an attempt to avoid much of the toxicity associated with its use (69). In these situations, patients receive antibodies labeled with radioactive molecules that deliver the radiotherapy directly to the tumor. A number of early trials suggested that this approach might allow the use of radiotherapy in BMT for lymphomas at a very high dose with reduction in toxicity.

Marrow Purging

One of the most controversial areas regarding the use of high dose therapy and autologous BMT to treat patients with lymphomas deals with the necessity of treating the marrow in vitro to eliminate the possibility of infusing any contaminating tumor cells. A wide variety of methods have been developed to accomplish this goal, including the use of chemotherapeutic agents, immunological maneuvers, and mechanical maneuvers aimed at eliminating tumor cells (see

Chapters 13 and 14). In addition, other investigators have attempted specifically to select the cells that lead to myeloid engraftment rather than attempt to eliminate malignant cells (e.g., reverse purging, positive selection).

Although it is quite clear that these approaches can reduce or eliminate tumor cells in in vitro systems (see Chapter 15), it is unclear whether they have any definite impact on the results of BMT. Most relapses following autologous BMT for lymphoma occur at sites of previous disease, rather than at new locations. This finding suggests that relapse following BMT results from inadequacies of the preparative regimen rather than from reinfusion of contaminated marrow. Furthermore, it is unclear whether transplanted lymphoma cells are clonogenic and capable of contributing to relapse. Several reports have failed to demonstrate a benefit from purging (57,58,60,61,68).

At least 3 indirect lines of evidence, however, suggest a possible rationale for purging in BMT for non-Hodgkin's lymphomas. The first line of evidence relates to reports of early leukemic relapses in patients following unpurged BMT (65). Most of these patients had high-grade lymphoma, which suggests the possibility that viable marrow cells may be infused at the time of BMT. Another report studied the role of purging in a group of patients undergoing BMT for B-cell non-Hodgkin's lymphomas (70). All patients were shown by PCR to have evidence of the t(14;18) translocation in their marrow at the time of harvest and were purged using a monoclonal antibody. Following BMT, disease-free survival was significantly better in the patients without detectable lymphoma cells in their marrow after purging compared with those who still had cells detectable by PCR. Actuarial disease-free survival in these patients is displayed in Figure 52-5. Another piece of evidence supporting a possible role for purging deals with a group of patients with intermediate-grade lymphomas who had their marrows studied in vitro utilizing a cell culture method designed to detect the presence of tumor cells (71). Those patients in whom tumor cells could be detected by this system had a much poorer survival than patients who received marrow in which tumor cells could not be cultured (Figure 52-6). These studies could be interpreted as demonstrating the need for purging the marrow in at least some patients undergoing autologous BMT. However, an alternate hypothesis would be that both studies demonstrated a method to identify patients with highly aggressive lymphomas that are likely to resist the action of chemotherapy and thus are likely to relapse. It would seem to be reasonable to avoid infusion of tumor cells whenever possible. To this end, patients in whom tumor cell contamination of the marrow seems likely are usually transplanted with marrow that has been treated in vitro or with peripheral blood stem cells in hopes of infusing a minimal number of lymphoma cells.

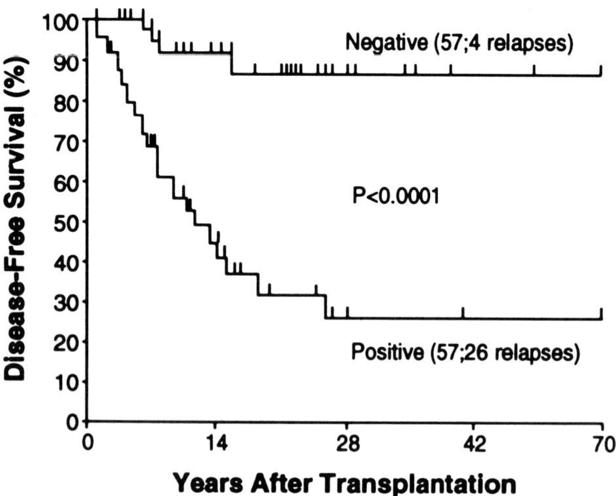

Figure 52-5. Actuarial probability of disease-free survival after autologous bone marrow transplantation. "Negative" denotes patients without detectable lymphoma cells following purging, and "positive" denotes patients in whom residual lymphoma cells were detected. (Reproduced by permission from Gribben JG, Freedman AS, Neuberg D, et al. Immunologic purging of marrow assessed by PCR before autologous bone marrow transplantation for B-cell lymphoma. N Engl J Med 1991;325:1525–1533.)

Future Considerations

Autologous BMT is a treatment that is being used with increasing frequency for patients with non-Hodgkin's lymphomas. Although results appear to be superior to those achieved with standard-dose salvage regimens, it is important to note that no comparative trials have

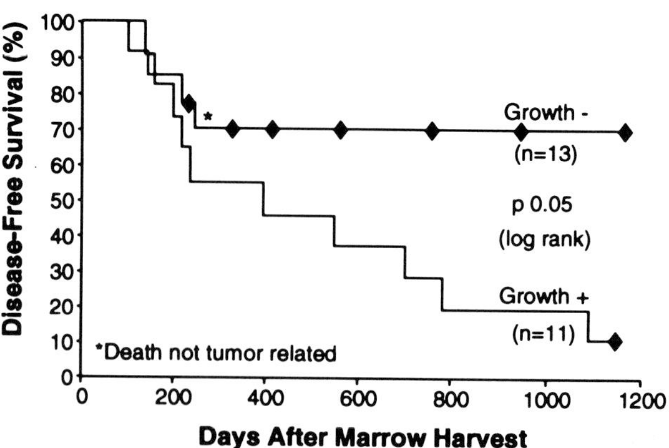

Figure 52-6. Actuarial survival of patients with non-Hodgkin's lymphoma who achieved complete remission after autologous bone marrow transplantation segregated on the basis of culture evidence of lymphoma in their marrow. (Reproduced by permission from Sharp JG, Joshi SS, Armitage JO, et al. Significance of detection of occult non-Hodgkin's lymphoma in histologically uninvolved bone marrow by a culture technique. Blood 1992;79:1074–1080.)

been completed. Only 50% of patients referred to transplant centers are ever transplanted, and selection bias may account for the observed difference in results (72,73). Patients with a poor performance status and those with comorbid illness may be excluded from protocols, and only the "best" patients may ever undergo BMT (73). In addition, patients with rapidly progressive disease may also be excluded from BMT protocols because they may not be able to travel to transplant centers and undergo pretransplant evaluation and marrow harvesting. No prospective trials comparing autologous BMT with conventional salvage chemotherapy have been performed. A retrospective review of 34 patients with relapsed non-Hodgkin's lymphomas referred to the University of Nebraska between 1983 and 1987, however, revealed an actuarial 5-year disease-free survival of 40% for patients who received autologous BMT, compared with 0% for patients treated with conventional cisplatin-based salvage chemotherapy (56). Another study retrospectively compared the results of autologous BMT and conventional salvage chemotherapy among patients with non-Hodgkin's lymphomas who had failed an initial intensive chemotherapy regimen (74). Median survival and freedom from progression were significantly longer in patients treated with BMT than those treated only with conventional salvage chemotherapy regimens. These results suggest that BMT is the preferred approach for patients after failure of initial chemotherapy, but no prospective trial has been completed. An international prospective trial is currently underway in which patients with relapsed intermediate- or high-grade non-Hodgkin's lymphomas receive 2 cycles of DHAP (dexamethasone, cytarabine, and cisplatin) salvage chemotherapy. Patients who respond to DHAP are subsequently randomized to 4 more cycles of DHAP or autologous BMT (75). Final results of this study are not available, but the interim analysis has shown no difference in survival between the 2 groups.

Numerous questions remain regarding the use of autologous BMT for patients with non-Hodgkin's lymphomas. Some of these questions deal with issues such as timing, preparative regimen, and purging. However, many fundamental questions remain regarding the value of autologous BMT in comparison with conventional salvage chemotherapy, as well as questions regarding the optimal source of marrow rescue. Allogeneic BMT has been used less frequently for patients with non-Hodgkin's lymphomas, compared with autologous BMT (see Chapter 49). Allogeneic BMT eliminates the possibility of infusing malignant cells with marrow. In addition, there is evidence to suggest that a graft-versus-lymphoma effect exists that is similar to the graft-versus-leukemia effect seen following allogeneic BMT for leukemia (see Chapter 19) (76,77). The end results of allogeneic BMT are no better than autologous BMT due to the increased mortality associated with allogeneic BMT. However, these results suggest that autologous BMT results can be improved. Currently, various techniques are being evaluated to experimentally induce a graft-versus-lymphoma effect following autologous BMT (78). The use of peripheral stem-cell transplantation is also increasing. This technique allows the use of high-dose therapy regimens in patients whose marrow cannot be harvested due to tumor involvement or radiation therapy. Results of peripheral stem-cell transplantation for non-Hodgkin's lymphomas are at least as good as the results seen following autologous BMT (79).

Many more patients could be treated with BMT. The treatment-related mortality of autologous BMT for lymphomas continues to decrease, and if the results of studies to test the utilization of early treatment in the course of the disease are positive, utilization of BMT for non-Hodgkin's lymphomas will increase dramatically. Currently, autologous BMT should be considered a "standard" therapy for patients with chemotherapy-sensitive, relapsed non-Hodgkin's lymphomas.

The different criteria for patient selection, as well as variations in preparative regimens and purging, all without controlled clinical trials, show that autologous BMT studies for lymphoma still require further scientific proof. Controlled trials must now be done before autologous BMT can be widely applied in hospitals not participating in such studies.

References

1. Advisory Committee of the International Autologous Bone Marrow Transplant Registry (ABMTR). Autologous bone marrow transplants: different indications in Europe and North America. Lancet 1989;2:317–318.
2. Gratwohl A. Bone marrow tranplantation activity in Europe 1990. Bone Marrow Transplant 1991;8:197–201.
3. Gloeckler Ries, LA. Non-Hodgkin's lymphoma. Cancer Statistics Review 1973–1989. NIH publication No. 92-2789. Bethesda, MD: National Institutes of Health,
4. Gail MH, Pluda JM, Rabkin CS, et al. Projection of the incidence of non-Hodgkin's lymphoma related to acquired immunodeficiency syndrome. J Natl Cancer Inst 1991;83:695–701.
5. Non-Hodgkin's Lymphoma Pathologic Classification Project. National Cancer Institute sponsored study of classifications of non-Hodgkin's lymphomas. Cancer 1982;49:2112–2135.
6. Levine EG, Arthur DC, Frizzera G, et al. There are differences in cytogenetic abnormalitites among histologic subtypes of the non-Hodgkin's lymphomas. Blood 1985;66:1414–1422.
7. Simon R, Durrleman S, Hoppe RT, et al. The non-Hodgkin lymphoma pathologic classification project. Ann Intern Med 1988;109:939–945.
8. Morrison WH, Hoppe RT, Weiss LM, et al. Small lymphoyctic lymphoma. J Clin Oncol 1989;7:598–606.
9. Weisenburger DD, Nathwani BN, Diamond LW, et al. Malignant lymphoma, intermediate lymphocytic type: a clinicopathologic study of 42 cases. Cancer 1981; 48:1415–1425.
10. Perry DA, Bast MA, Armitage JO, et al. Diffuse intermediate lymphocytic lymphoma. A clinicopathologic study and comparision with small lymphocytic lymphoma and diffuse small cleaved cell lymphoma. Cancer 1990;66:1995–2000.
11. Offit K, Wong G, Filippa D, et al. Cytogenetic analysis

of 434 consecutively ascertained specimens of non-Hodgkin's lymphoma: clinical correlations. Blood 1991;77:1508–1515.
12. Horning SJ, Rosenberg SA. The natural history of initally untreated low-grade non-Hodgkin's lymphomas. N Engl J Med 1984;311:1471–1475.
13. Gallagher CJ, Gregory WM, Jones AE, et al. Follicular lymphoma: prognostic factors for response and survival. J Clin Oncol 1986;4:1470–1480.
14. Bastion Y, Berger F, Bryon P-A, et al. Follicular lymphomas: assessment of prognostic factors in 127 patients followed for 10 years. Ann Oncol 1991;2(suppl 2):123–129.
15. Anderson JR, Vose JM, Bierman PJ, et al. Clinical features and prognosis of follicular large cell lymphoma (FLCL): a report from the Nebraska lymphoma study group (NLSG). Proc Am Soc Clin Oncol 1992;11:330.
16. Kantarjian HM, McLaughlin P, Fuller LM, et al. Follicular large cell lymphoma: analysis and prognostic factors in 62 patients. J Clin Oncol 1984;2:811–819.
17. Leith CP, Spier CM, Grogan TM, et al. Diffuse small cleaved-cell lymphoma: a heterogeneous disease with distinct immunobiologic subsets. J Clin Oncol 1992; 10:1259–1265.
18. Murphy SB, Fairclough DL, Hutchison RE, et al. Non-Hodgkin's lymphomas of childhood: an analysis of the histology, staging, and response to treatment of 338 cases at a single institution. J Clin Oncol 1989;7:186–193.
19. Picozzi VJ, Coleman CN. Lymphoblastic lymphoma. Semin Oncol 1990;17:96–103.
20. Carbone PP, Kaplan HS, Musshoff K, et al. Report of the Committee on Hodgkin's Disease Staging Classification. Cancer Res 1971;31:1860–1861.
21. Shipp M, Harrington D, Anderson J, et al. Development of a predictive model for aggressive lymphoma: the international NHL prognostic factors project. Proc Am Soc Clin Oncol 1992;11:319.
22. Ezdinli EZ, Anderson JR, Melvin F, et al. Moderate versus aggressive chemotherapy of nodular lymphocytic poorly differentiated lymphoma. J Clin Oncol 1985;3:769–775.
23. Young RC, Longo DL, Glatstein E, et al. The treatment of indolent lymphomas: watchful waiting v aggressive combined modality treatment. Semin Hematol 1988; 25(suppl 2):11–16.
24. Paryani SB, Hoppe RT, Cox RS, et al. Analysis of non-Hodgkin's lymphomas with nodular and favorable histologies, stages I and II. Cancer 1983;52:2300–2307.
25. McLaughlin P, Fuller LM, Velasquez WS, et al. Stage I-II follicular lymphoma. Cancer 1986;58:1596–1602.
26. DeVita VT, Canellos GP, Chabner B, et al. Advanced diffuse histiocytic lymphoma, a potentially curable disease. Lancet 1975;1:248–250.
27. DeVita VT, Hubbard SM, Young RC, et al. The role of chemotherapy in diffuse aggressive lymphomas. Semin Hematol 1988;25(suppl 2):2–10.
28. Mauch P, Leonard R, Skarin A, et al. Improved survival following combined radiation therapy and chemotherapy for unfavorable prognosis stage I-II non-Hodgkin's lymphomas. J Clin Oncol 1985;3:1301–1308.
29. Connors JM, Klimo P, Fairey RN, et al. Brief chemotherapy and involved field radiation therapy for limited-stage, histologically aggressive lymphoma. Ann Intern Med 1987;107:25–30.
30. Longo DL, Glatstein E, Duffey P, et al. Treatment of localized aggressive lymphomas with combination chemotherapy followed by involved-field radiation therapy. J Clin Oncol 1989;7:1295–1302.
31. Fisher RI, Gaynor E, Dahlberg S, et al. A phase III comparison of CHOP vs. m-BACOD vs. proMACE-cytaBOM vs. MACOP-B in patients with intermediate or high-grade non-Hodgkin's lymphoma: preliminary results of SWOG-8516 (intergroup 0067), the national high priority lymphoma study. Proc Am Soc Clin Oncol 1992;11:315.
32. Philip T, Hartmann O, Biron P, et al. High-dose therapy and autologous bone marrow transplantation in partial remission after first-line induction therapy for diffuse non-Hodgkin's lymphoma. J Clin Oncol 1988;6:1118–1124.
33. Gulati SC, Shank B, Black P, et al. Autologous bone marrow transplantation for patients with poor-prognosis lymphoma. J Clin Oncol 1988;6:1303–1313.
34. Gribben JG, Goldstone AH, Linch DC, et al. Effectiveness of high-dose combination chemotherapy and autologous bone marrow transplantation for patients with non-Hodgkin's lymphomas who are still responsive to conventional-dose therapy. J Clin Oncol 1989;7:1621–1629.
35. Santini G, Congiu AM, Coser P, et al. Autologous bone marrow transplantation for adult advanced stage lymphomblastic lymphoma in first CR. A study of the NHLCSG. Leukemia 1991;5(suppl 1):42–45.
36. Baro J, Richard C, Calavia J, et al. Autologous bone marrow transplantation as consolidation therapy for non-Hodgkin's lymphoma patients with poor prognostic features. Bone Marrow Transplant 1991;8:283–289.
37. Nademanee A, Schmidt GM, O'Donnell MR, et al. High-dose chemoradiotherapy followed by autologous bone marrow transplantation as consolidation therapy during first complete remission in adult patients with poor-risk aggressive lymphoma: a pilot study. Blood 1992;80:1130–1134.
38. Coleman CN, Picozzi VJ, Cox RS, et al. Treatment of lymphoblastic lymphoma in adults. J Clin Oncol 1986;4:1628–1637.
39. Coiffier B, Bryon P-A, Ffrench M, et al. Intensive chemotherapy in aggressive lymphomas: updated results of LNH-80 protocol and prognostic factors affect ing response and survival. Blood 1987;70:1394–1399.
40. Verdonck LF, Dekker AW, de Gast GC, et al. Autologous bone marrow transplantation for adult poor-risk lymphoblastic lymphoma in first remission. J Clin Oncol 1992;10:644–646.
41. Bierman P, Armitage JO. Salvage therapy for patients with relapsed or refractory aggressive non-Hodgkin's lymphoma. Oncology 1987;1:11–20.
42. Cabanillas F. Ifosfamide combinations in lymphoma. Semin Oncol 1990;17(suppl 4):58–62.
43. Kurnick NB, Montano A, Gerdes JC, Feder BH. Preliminary observations on the treatment of postirradiation hematopoietic depression in man by the infusion of stored autogenous bone marrow. Ann Intern Med 1958;49:973–986.
44. Clifford P, Clift RA, Duff JK. Nitrogen-mustard therapy combined with autologous marrow infusion. Lancet 1961;1:687–690.
45. Appelbaum FR, Herzig GP, Ziegler JL, et al. Successful engraftment of cryopreserved autologous bone marrow in patient with malignant lymphoma. Blood 1978; 52:85–95.
46. Applebaum FR, Deisseroth AB, Graw RG, et al. Prolonged complete remission following high dose chemotherapy of Burkitt's lymphoma in relapse. Cancer 1978;41:1059–1063.
47. Frei E, Canellos GP. Dose: a critical factor in cancer chemotherapy. Am J Med 1980;69:585–594.

48. Philip T, Armitage JO, Spitzer G, et al. High-dose therapy and autologous bone marrow transplantation after failure of conventional chemotherapy in adults with intermediate-grade or high-grade non-Hodgkin's lymphoma. N Engl J Med 1987;316:1493–1498.
49. Freedman AS, Ritz J, Neuberg D, et al. Autologous bone marrow transplantation in 69 patients with a history of low-grade B-cell non-Hodgkin's lymphoma. Blood 1991;77:2524–2529.
50. Rohatiner AZS, Price CGA, Arnott S, et al. Myeloablative therapy with autologous bone marrow transplantation as consolidation of remission in patients with follicular lymphoma. Ann Oncol 1991;2(suppl 2):147–150.
51. Bierman P, Vose A, Armitage J, Kessinger A. High-dose therapy followed by autologous hematopoietic rescue for follicular low grade non-Hodgkin's lymphoma. Proc Am Soc Clin Oncol 1992;11:317.
52. Gorin NC, David R, Stachowiak J, et al. High dose chemotherapy and autologous bone marrow transplantation in acute leukemias, malignant lymphomas and solid tumors. Eur J Cancer 1981;17:557–568.
53. Tanner NM, Spitzer G, Zander AR, et al. High-dose chemoradiotherapy and bone marrow transplantation in patients with refractory lymphoma. Eur J Cancer Clin Oncol 1983;19:1091–1096.
54. Philip T, Biron P, Herve P, et al. Massive BACT chemotherpy with autologous bone marrow transplantation in 17 cases of non-Hodgkin's malignant lymphoma with a very bad prognosis. Eur J Cancer Clin Oncol 1983;19:1371–1379.
55. Philip T, Biron P, Maraninchi D, et al. Role of massive chemotherapy and autologous bone-marrow transplantation in non-Hodgkin's malignant lymphoma. Lancet 1984;2:391.
56. Vose JM, Armitage JO, Bierman PJ, et al. Salvage therapy for relapsed or refractory non-Hodgkin's lymphoma utilizing autologous bone marrow transplantation. Am J Med 1989;87:285–288.
57. Colombat P, Gorin N-C, Lemonnier M-P, et al. The role of autologous bone marrow transplantation in 46 adult patients with non-Hodgkin's lymphomas. J Clin Oncol 1990;8:630–637.
58. Petersen FB, Appelbaum FR, Hill R, et al. Autologous marrow transplantation for malignant lymphoma: a report of 101 cases from Seattle. J Clin Oncol 1990;8:638–647.
59. Phillips GL, Fay JW, Herzig RH, et al. The treatment of progressive non-Hodgkin's lymphoma with intensive chemoradiotherapy and autologous marrow transplantation. Blood 1990;75:831–838.
60. Weisdorf DJ, Haake R, Miller WJ, et al. Autologous bone marrow transplantation for progressive non-Hodgkin's lymphoma: clinical impact of immunophenotype and in vitro purging. Bone Marrow Transplant 1991;8:135–142.
61. Gulati S, Yahalom J, Acaba L, et al. Treatment of patients with relapsed and resistant non-Hodgkin's lymphoma using total body irradiation, etoposide, and cyclophosphamide and autologous bone marrow transplantation. J Clin Oncol 1992;10:936–941.
62. Armitage JO, Jagannath S, Spitzer G, et al. High dose therapy and autologous marrow transplantation as salvage treatment for patients with diffuse large cell lymphoma. Eur J Cancer Clin Oncol 1986;22: 871–877.
63. Vose JM, Peterson C, Bierman PJ, et al. Comparison of high-dose therapy and autologous bone marrow transplantation for T-cell and B-cell non-Hodgkin's lymphomas. Blood 1990;76:424–431.
64. Schouten HC, Bierman PJ, Vaughan WP, et al. Autologous bone marrow transplantation in follicular non-Hodgkin's lymphoma before and after histologic transformation. Blood 1989;74:2579–2584.
65. Vaughan WP, Weisenburger DD, Sanger WG, et al. Early leukemic recurrence of non-Hodgkin lymphoma after high-dose anti-neoplastic therapy with autologous marrow rescue. Bone Marrow Transplant 1987;1:373–378.
66. Philip T, Biron P, Philip I, et al. Massive therapy and autologous bone marrow transplantation in pediatric and young adults Burkitt's lymphoma (30 courses on 28 patients: a 5-year experience). Eur J Cancer Clin Oncol 1986;22:1015–1027.
67. Wheeler C, Antin JH, Churchill WH, et al. Cyclophosphamide, carmustine, and etoposide with autologous bone marrow transplantation in refractory Hodgkin's disease and non-Hodgkin's lymphoma: a dose finding study. J Clin Oncol 1990;8:648–656.
68. Goldstone AH, Singer CRJ, Gribben JG, et al. Fifth report of EBMTG experience of ABMT in malignant lymphoma. Bone Marrow Transplant 1988;3(suppl 1):33–36.
69. Appelbaum, FR. Radiolabeled monoclonal antibodies in the treatment of non-Hodgkin's lymphoma. Hematol Oncol Clin North Am 1991;5:1013–1025.
70. Gribben JG, Freedman AS, Neuberg D, et al. Immunologic purging of marrow assessed by PCR before autologous bone marrow transplantation for B-cell lymphoma. N Engl J Med 1991;325:1525–1533.
71. Sharp JG, Joshi SS, Armitage JO, et al. Significance of detection of occult non-Hodgkin's lymphoma in histologically uninvolved bone marrow by a culture technique. Blood 1992;79:1074–1080.
72. Brandwein JM, Smith AM, Langley GR, et al. Outcome of patients with relapsed or refractory non-Hodgkin's lymphoma referred for autologous bone marrow transplantation. Blood 1990;76:530a.
73. Surbone A, Armitage JO, Gale RP. Autotransplantations in lymphoma: better therapy or healthier patients? Ann Intern Med 1991;114:1059–1060.
74. Bosly A, Coiffier B, Gisselbrecht, et al. Bone marrow transplantation prolongs survival after relapse in aggressive-lymphoma patients treated with the LNH-84 regimen. J Clin Oncol 1992;10:1615–1623.
75. Philip T, Chauvin F, Armitage J, et al. Parma international protocol: pilot study of DHAP followed by involved-field radiotherapy and BEAC with autologous bone marrow transplantation. Blood 1991;77:1587–1592.
76. Jones RJ, Ambinder RF, Piantadosi S, et al. Evidence of a graft-versus-lymphoma effect associated with allogeneic bone marrow transplantation. Blood 1991;77:649–653.
77. Chopra R, Goldstone AH, Pearce R, et al. Autologous versus allogeneic bone marrow transplantation for non-Hodgkin's lymphoma: a case-controlled analysis of the European bone marrow transplant group registry data. J Clin Oncol 1992;10:1690–1695.
78. Klingemann H-G, Phillips GL. Immunotherapy after bone marrow transplantation. Bone Marrow Transplant 1991;8:73–81.
79. Vose JM, Bierman PJ, Anderson JR, et al. High-dose chemotherapy with hematopoietic stem cell rescue for non-Hodgkin's lymphoma (NHL): evaluation of event-free survival based on histologic subtype and rescue product. Proc Am Soc Clin Oncol 1992;11:318.

Chapter 53
Transplantation for Hodgkin's Disease

Gordon L. Phillips

Hodgkin's disease is a relatively uncommon malignant disease of unknown and perhaps variable etiology. Histologically, the tumor mass is comprised mainly of reactive cells; the characteristic malignant Reed-Sternberg cells (and variants) are of uncertain derivation and are seen with differing frequencies in the recognized subtypes (lymphocyte predominance, nodular sclerosis, mixed cellularity, and lymphocyte depletion).

Hodgkin's disease arises in lymph nodes and usually spreads in a stepwise manner to contiguous nodes. Accordingly, although precise staging is very important, a discussion of staging is beyond the scope of this chapter; standard source materials should be consulted regarding the Ann Arbor system (which has recently been revised as the Cotswolds classification). Radiotherapy remains the mainstay of treatment for limited-stage Hodgkin's disease, whereas chemotherapy with multiagent drug regimens is indicated for more disseminated disease. Combined modality therapy (i.e., chemotherapy plus radiotherapy) is highly efficient in producing tumor eradication but is more toxic than either modality alone. In any case, optimal use of these modalities will cure approximately 75% of patients with Hodgkin's disease (1). These general points, and certain others, are summarized in Table 53.1.

Table 53-1. Salient Features of Hodgkin's Disease

Incidence	2.5/100,000; 800 new cases per year in Canada, 8,000 in United States
Age distribution	Biphasic, with age peaks at 25 to 30 and 60+ years
Etiology	Unknown; may vary with different histologies (e.g., nodular sclerosis, mixed cellularity, lymphocyte predominance, lymphocyte depletion)
Relevant cell	Reed-Sternberg cell or variants; precursor unknown
Manner of spread	Usually contiguous in a nodal pattern
Natural history	Variable; usually chronically progressive and ultimately fatal if not controlled
Therapy	
Limited stage	Primarily radiotherapy
Advanced stage	Primarily chemotherapy
Outcome	Curability estimated to be approximately 75% with optimal treatment; secondary malignancy a major late complication of therapy

Despite the successes noted with standard radiotherapy and chemotherapy regimens, some patients with Hodgkin's disease remain incurable. Because strong evidence exists supporting the utility of dose-intensive cytotoxic therapy (2–4), dose escalation of these agents to levels requiring rescue with marrow reconstituting ("stem") cells might be postulated to be effective in producing cure in some of these patients. Accordingly, during the past decade, myeloablative therapy and marrow transplantation, especially (but not exclusively) using the patient's own (autologous) marrow, has been employed increasingly for the treatment of certain patients with Hodgkin's disease (5).

Role of Bone Marrow Transplantation

To understand the role of bone marrow transplantation (BMT) in the therapy of Hodgkin's disease, it is important to be aware of the results achieved with current conventional primary chemotherapy regimens such as MOPP/ABVD (mechlorethamine, vincristine [Oncovin], procarbazine, prednisone/doxorubicin [Adriamycin], bleomycin, vinblastine, dacarbazine) (6) or MOPP/ABV "Hybrid" (7) in the treatment of patients with advanced Hodgkin's disease. For example, the results in 165 such patients aged 16 to 65 who were treated with MOPP/ABV Hybrid at a single center between 1980 and 1989 have recently been analyzed and reported. One hundred fifty eight (93%) achieved an initial complete remission, and the actuarial failure-free survival was 72% at 8 years. There were 3 toxic deaths (1.8%). Only the presence of "B" symptoms at diagnosis was identified as a negative prognostic feature for failure-free survival—even these patients had a failure-free survival of 62% (8).

However, patients whose disease is not cured by regimens such as MOPP/ABV Hybrid are only occasionally curable with alternative therapies containing putatively non-crossresistant agents (9). In contrast with these results, and as discussed more fully later, are those of numerous series using myeloablative therapy and autologous BMT (5,10), which consistently suggest a durable remission rate of 30 to 50% in similar patients. Despite this apparent improvement, it is difficult to exclude the possibility that patient selection is, at least to a degree, responsible for these results, because it is likely that some patients otherwise eligible for BMT were not transplanted for a variety of reasons (e.g., rapid progression, co-morbid disease, marrow involvement, refusal). Prospective randomized trials designed to address this issue have not been performed, due not only to the difficulty in performing such trials in general, but also to the absence of accepted standard conventional therapy as well as autologous BMT regimens, and finally to the potentially large number of patients that would be required to convincingly demonstrate a difference (11).

Timing Considerations and Patient Selection

For this discussion, we assume that current optimal primary chemotherapy consists of regimens such as MOPP/ABV(D) (12–14). If other, less effective primary therapies are used, salvage chemotherapy in standard dose may be more effective (15), and the following discussion of optimal timing of BMT may be less applicable (16). Similar considerations may also be pertinent in patients with recurrent disease who receive conventional salvage therapy; whether the precise regimen (or other details of therapy, such as the duration between the time given and entry onto a conditioning regimen) are important is unknown but at least arguable. Unfortunately, these details are not provided in most published reports.

The issue of timing is discussed primarily in terms of disease status, which is not only an estimate of the extent and various biological features of the tumor (especially the degree of chemoresistance), but also a rough measure of cumulative organ toxicity due to prior therapy. Using this approach, BMT may be undertaken (1) as primary treatment; (2) during an initial complete remission induced by conventional chemotherapy; (3) after conventional chemotherapy has failed to produce complete remission (i.e., "primary induction failure"); (4) after relapse, in place of conventional salvage therapy; and (5) after relapse, following the use of conventional salvage therapy (Table 53-2).

Although transplant regimens could be used as primary treatment in patients with Hodgkin's disease, it is not clear whether a single course of currently used myeloablative regimens requiring hematological support would be more efficacious than conventional therapy such as MOPP/ABV(D); the transplant regimen would certainly be more toxic and more expensive. In addition, given the effectiveness of primary chemotherapy regimens such as MOPP/ABV(D), a randomized trial of several hundred patients would be needed to test the relative effectiveness of chemotherapy versus BMT as primary treatment. For these reasons, it is most unlikely that BMT regimens will be used as the sole systemic therapy in patients with Hodgkin's disease.

The use of BMT as consolidation therapy for patients in an initial complete remission is a frequent strategy for many other hematological malignancies, especially in patients in whom reliable signs portending relapse can be identified. Although use of these augmented-dose marrow transplant regimens is likely to decrease relapse rates if used in this manner, the

Table 53-2. Evaluation of Autologous Bone Marrow Transplantation by Disease Status in Hodgkin's Disease

Disease Status[a]	*Considerations*	*Indication for Routine Transplantation*	*Comments*
Primary treatment	More toxic and expensive than conventional chemotherapy; may or may not be as effective and would be difficult to prove	No	Unlikely to be tested in a clinical trial
Initial complete remission	More toxic and expensive than conventional chemotherapy; unless precisely selected, many patients may be overtreated	No	Currently, applies to few (if any) patients; precise patient selection is critical for clinical trials
Primary induction failure	High degree of tumor resistance to chemotherapy	Strong	Favorable situation regarding cumulative toxicity from primary therapy
Untreated first relapse	Probably optimal timing for most patients	Strong	Exposes few patients potentially curable with nontransplant modalities to risks of transplantation
Sensitive relapse or later complete remission	Probably less favorable than untreated first relapse, but cumulative toxicity may be increased	Strong	Not used as extensively as in non-Hodgkin's lymphomas
Resistant relapse	High degree of tumor cell chemotherapy resistance and cumulative toxicity	Marginal	Relatively few patients will be cured

[a]Following regimens such as MOPP/ABV(D) (mechlorethamine, vincristine, procarbazine, prednisone/doxorubicin, bleomycin, vinblastine, dacarbazine).

attendant toxicity may minimize potential gains. Conversely, toxicity may be more modest in this setting due to the relatively low cumulative doses of prior therapy.

To date, only a limited experience of BMT as consolidation therapy has been published. Carella and associates (17) transplanted patients selected as having a poor prognosis despite being in an initial complete remission induced with MOPP/ABVD, using an intensive combination chemotherapy regimen and unmanipulated autologous marrow. At the time of this report, 13 of these 15 patients were well, whereas one relapsed and another died of treatment-related causes. Although these results are interesting, a convincing demonstration of the utility of this approach will be difficult, undoubtedly requiring a randomized clinical trial with clearly defined high-risk patients (who are relatively uncommon) and many years of follow-up. Even if instituted, such a trial could be complicated in its interpretation by the fact that relapses in the conventional therapy arm could be salvaged successfully with transplant regimens. Therefore, it is unlikely that BMT regimens will soon become routine management for patients in first remission. However, the precise definition of a poor-prognosis group would provide an impetus to study this strategy further.

Of course, some patients will fail to obtain an initial complete remission with MOPP/ABV(D) induction, and such "primary induction failure" patients have a poor prognosis with conventional salvage therapy. Intensive therapy and BMT is strongly indicated for these patients, and, likely depending on the extent of tumor resistance, durable complete remission can be produced in a surprising number of patients (18). Of course, one would expect those patients with some degree of chemosensitivity (i.e., those in partial remission) to have better results than those with lesser degrees of tumor response. However, this expectation may be difficult to assess, because some patients with persistent radiological masses will not have residual viable tumor in those masses. This possibility should be evaluated carefully before a transplant is considered in this situation.

In the majority of patients, it is likely that the optimal time to employ a marrow transplant is at the first sign of recurrence after exposure to primary conventional therapy with MOPP/ABV(D) (11,16), so called untreated (or untested) relapse; almost all of these patients are incurable with conventional chemotherapy, yet retain an element of chemosensitivity and are usually not heavily pretreated. Results in 53 patients so treated in Vancouver are depicted in Figure 53-1: an event-free survival of 62% (95% confidence interval [CI] 41 to 78%) is noted; 2 patients died of nonrelapse causes.

Despite these results, this postulate remains arguable (16); these findings have never been addressed in a randomized clinical trial. In any case, it should be appreciated that these patients, although homogenous with regard to disease status, are undoubtedly heterogeneous with regard to certain features of tumor biology (e.g., tumor burden and aggressiveness), and

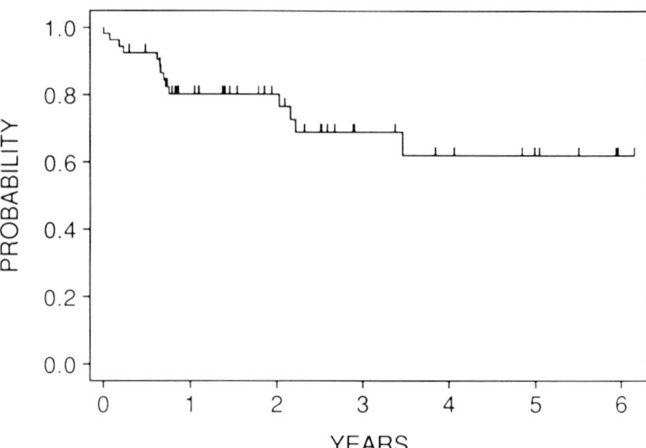

Figure 53-1. Event-free survival in 53 patients with Hodgkin's disease in first untested relapse given autologous bone marrow transplantation.

certain clinical correlates of tumor biology (e.g., duration of previous response) may override that of disease status alone (19). If follows that subgroups *within* the group of patients in untreated relapse might be able to be identified and appropriate therapy applied (19). In cases of relatively good prognosis, this could conceivably involve conventional therapy, although BMT regimens would be expected to be even more effective in this situation. For those patients anticipated to do poorly with current transplant regimens, more experimental transplant approaches may be used.

Also, the presence of marrow involvement with tumor, assessed histologically, may be relatively unusual at the time of first recurrence (18). Even if demonstrated, marrow involvement may not be an absolute contraindication to the use of peripheral blood—or even marrow—autotransplants, if remission can first be reinduced with conventional therapy. Obviously, the feasibility of allogeneic BMT would not be affected in this case.

Alternatively, conventional-dose salvage chemotherapy can be used to document residual chemosensitivity and, if successful, to produce a state of minimal residual disease (also called "sensitive relapse"). This is a frequent tactic in the treatment of non-Hodgkin's lymphomas before autologous BMT (5), although there are no convincing data to suggest the superiority of this approach. The main negative feature of "chemotherapy testing" is the potential increase in post-transplant toxicity due to the cumulative effects of conventional salvage-therapy. Such toxicity could preclude or complicate subsequent BMT; for this reason, first untreated relapse remains the preferred indication over sensitive relapse.

Finally, although some patients with end-stage Hodgkin's disease can be cured with BMT, this timing is not recommended because it maximizes the probability of both the emergence of resistant tumor cells and the acquisition of cumulative hematological and nonhematological toxicity due to the use of conventional-dose salvage therapy. Also, if one postpones consideration of BMT until the presence of more advanced disease status after unsuccessful salvage therapy (16), it is inevitable that some patients will be lost before the transplant can be undertaken and that transplanted patients will suffer a high early mortality due to toxicity and a high relapse rate. Therefore, if such patients are selected for transplantation, they should be chosen very carefully.

Preparative Regimens

General Considerations

The effectiveness of conditioning regimens is critical with regard to outcome, because autotransplants depend on them entirely—and allotransplants at least partially—for antitumor effects. Conditioning regimens must be considered in the context of disease status; unfortunately, it is unrealistic to expect current myeloablative regimens reliably to rescue patients completely unreponsive to conventional chemotherapy. It is much more likely that such regimens will be most successful in patients having at least some degree of responsiveness to conventional-dose therapy. Assessment of the efficacy of any therapy—including conditioning regimens—may be difficult in Hodgkin's disease and the non-Hodgkin's lymphomas due to persistence of radiographic masses in relatively inaccessible sites that may represent either residual tumor or nonmalignant tissue. Therefore, some "partial responses" may actually represent complete tumor eradication, a fact that should be borne in mind when assessing the activity of a regimen based on initial response alone.

There are a number of considerations regarding the construction of conditioning regimens. First, the agents employed should be active against Hodgkin's disease in conventional doses, and even more effective in escalated doses (3), although the degree of dose escalation permitted by marrow transplantation is usually less than anticipated (20). Second, drugs should be selected to avoid severe overlapping nonhematological toxicity, a more serious problem with escalated- than with conventional-dose therapy. Third, agents should be selected to minimize the presence of extreme tumor resistance, usually by selecting multiple drugs to which the patient is unlikely to have been exposed, or which have specific pharmacological or especially synergistic considerations. Very few conditioning regimens are composed entirely of multiple myelosuppressive agents in conventional doses. However, the use of agents in conventional dose added to augmented-dose agents is relatively common (10). Finally, as implied, patients with end-stage Hodgkin's disease must be considered to represent a paradoxical relationship between the disease status and transplant-related toxicity, in that patients with advanced disease are precisely those who require more potent cytoreduction but are less likely to be able to tolerate the resultant complications (21). Consequently, if an untested regimen is assessed in very heavily pretreated patients, excessive toxicity may produce a high treatment-related death rate and give an overestimate of the regimen's toxicity—and an underestimate of its usefulness—compared with treatment of a less heavily pretreated population.

The alkylating agents (as a class) are best suited for use in conditioning regimens, although agents of other classes are active in Hodgkin's disease and should also be considered. As noted in Table 53-3, the agents most frequently included in conditioning regimens for Hodgkin's disease are the chloroethylnitrosoureas (especially carmustine [BCNU], melphalan, cyclophosphamide (CY), and etoposide [VP16-213]). In general, these agents fulfill the criteria noted.

Myeloablative Therapy

Although the combination of CY and total body irradiation (TBI) is frequently used as pretransplant conditioning for many hematological malignancies (25), this regimen has been used relatively infrequently in patients with Hodgkin's disease (10), in part due to the increased incidence of severe or fatal pulmonary toxicity noted in patients previously exposed to thoracic radiotherapy who receive conditioning with TBI (26). However, regimens including TBI may be both safe and effective in patients who have not had prior mediastinal radiotherapy (27–30).

Many more patients have received conditioning regimens consisting of intensive combination chemotherapy alone, most of which are derivations of the "BACT" regimen BCNU, arabinosyl cytosine [cytarabine], cyclophosphamide, and thioguanine) developed at the National Cancer Institute several decades ago (31). As indicated in Table 53-3 in a simplified

Table 53-3.
Representative Conditioning Regimens

Author, Year, Ref	*Cytarabine* (*mg/m*^{2})	*Carmustine (BCNU)* (*mg/m*^{2})	*Cyclophosphamide* (*mg/m*^{2})	*Melphalan* (*mg/m*^{2})	*Etoposide (VP16-213)* (*mg/m*^{2})
Jagannath, 1989 (22)	. . .	300	6,000	. . .	600–900[b]
Gribben, 1989 (23)	800–1,600	300	. . .	140	400–800
Wheeler, 1990 (24)[a]	. . .	450	7,200	. . .	2,000
Reece, 1991 (18)	. . .	600	7,200	. . .	2,400[b]

[a]Maximum tolerated doses in Phase I study.
[b]VP16-213 given as twice daily infusion × 3 days.

fashion, the most popular combination of drugs—CY, BCNU, and etoposide (VP16-213) (CBV)—has been used in varying doses and schedules; only a few representative regimens are detailed. Wheeler and colleagues (24) performed a Phase I study of this combination and suggested that the maximal cumulative doses of CY, BCNU, and VP16-213 are likely in the range of 7,200,450, and 2,000 mg/m^2, respectively.

With currently available data, it is most difficult to assess accurately the relative superiority of the various CBV regimens. That said, the various CBV regimens can be divided roughly into 2 groups, those using "lower" (e.g., Jagannath and colleagues [22] versus "higher" (e.g., Reece and associates [18]) doses of (especially) VP16-213 and BCNU; relatively little variation in CY doses are noted. As expected, the antilymphoma effects appear to be greater with the higher-dose regimens, but toxicity is also increased (32). It is unclear whether the former consideration outweighs the latter; a randomized trial would be required to answer this question definitively. In any case, high-dose regimens should be used primarily in those patients likely to survive and benefit from their use (i.e., heavily pretreated patients).

The other BACT variant used widely is BCNU, VP16-213, cytarabine, and melphalan (BEAM) (23). Melphalan is an attractive agent to include in conditioning regimens because it is not a component of primary therapy and has been shown to produce durable complete remission as a single agent in the autotransplant setting (33). Conversely, cytarabine in conventional doses is not usually considered an active agent in Hodgkin's disease.

Whether the CBV and BEAM regimens could be improved by further manipulation of the dose or schedule of these agents or by addition or substitution of other cytotoxic agents in unknown. Modifications should be evaluated, however, because all these regimens fail to cure a substantial proportion of patients with relapsed or progressive Hodgkin's disease. In addition, other "standard" conditioning regimens should be considered for additional clinical testing. For example, Jones and colleagues (24) reported that the combination of busulfan (BU) and CY originally developed to treat acute myeloid leukemia (34) (with cumulative doses of 16 and 200 mg/kg, respectively) is active in transplant regimens for Hodgkin's disease as well. This finding is somewhat surprising, as the activity of BU for Hodgkin's disease has not been evaluated extensively (35) (likely due to its excessive myelotoxicity), and it is unlikely that CY alone, even at this dose, would produce satisfactory results. Of course, evaluation of such regimens implies an eventual comparison with an accepted standard; although the CBV regimen may be accepted as such, there is no single schedule of CBV that is widely accepted as standardized, thus complicating such a trial.

Regimens such as CBV may also increase lung toxicity in patients who have previously had mediastinal radiotherapy, although likely to a lesser degree than TBI (18). Also, certain CBV regimens can produce satisfactory immunosuppression for a successful allogeneic BMT (using a histocompatible sibling), at least for patients with Hodgkin's disease (36), a disease characterized by a degree of intrinsic immunosuppression.

Sequential use of 2 conditioning regimens and autotransplants has also been evaluated. This approach potentially allows the use of a greater number of cytotoxic agents, in augmented doses and in greater cumulative doses, and has been employed by Ahmed and colleagues (37), who used a "CBV-like" regimen followed by a second regimen of vinblastine, cytarabine (or thio-TEPA), mitoxantrone, and carboplatin. This approach requires further evaluation, but many patients failed to receive the second course for a variety of reasons, and this general approach must be considered potentially quite toxic unless cumulative toxicity is minimized, a feature that may require substantial dose reductions.

A related approach has been reported by Gianni and associates (38), who used a sequential regimen of high-dose CY and growth factor support to optimize blood stem-cell collection followed by cycle-active therapy (vincristine, methotrexate with leukovorin rescue, and cisplatin or etoposide) and finally by the conditioning regimen of TBI (1,250 cGY) and melphalan (160 mg/m^2) and blood stem-cell reinfusion. Local radiotherapy was given on recovery if needed. In a group of 25 heavily pretreated patients with progressive Hodgkin's disease, an event-free survival of 49% was produced, with no toxic deaths. In addition to the lack of fatal toxicity, the sequential nature of this therapy is attractive in an antitumor sense, and more information regarding this approach is awaited.

An alternative and arguably complementary approach to improving antitumor responses with conditioning regimen modification is that of immune targeting with isotopes or toxins. Although such an approach has been tested in other diseases, the development of appropriate monoclonal antibodies is hampered in Hodgkin's disease by the confusion regarding the identity (and therefore the antigenic characteristics) of the relevant "stem cell." On the basis of observations that antiferritin monoclonal antibodies tend to accumulate in Hodgkin's disease sites, attempts have been made to use ferritin as a vehicle for directed therapy. However, results using anti-ferritin labeled radioconjugates have been less than encouraging (39) and have not led to an obvious place in standard treatment or in the transplant setting.

Peritransplant Radiotherapy

Although the value of conventional local radiotherapy given in the peritransplant period is unproven, it is nonetheless a commonly used tactic, especially in patients with bulky disease. Such an approach is justified in theory, because patients tend to relapse in sites of bulky disease, and local radiotherapy is effective given as conventional therapy (2). Also,

requires the presence of graft-versus-host disease, the simplest approach for its exploitation is the more widespread use of allogeneic BMT.

An alternative approach toward producing a state of "autologous graft-versus-host disease" has been suggested by Jones and associates (59), and Phase II clinical trials are underway in non-Hodgkin's lymphomas; such could also be applicable for Hodgkin's disease. The use of α-interferon, interleukin-2 (IL-2), or other cytokines, could also be useful as immunomodulators.

It is likely that the combination of basic improvements in the management of allogeneic BMT-related problems and the more widespread availability of alternative donors will produce an increase in the use of allogeneic BMT in Hodgkin's disease over the next few years. This prediction is even more likely if marrow not predisposed to leukemogenesis is deemed very desirable for transplantation.

Results

Autologous Marrow and Blood Cell Transplants

As indicated in Table 53-5, an increasing number of studies have been reported in peer-reviewed journals that include more than 15 patients and in which patients with Hodgkin's disease receiving autologous marrow or blood cell transplants can be clearly discerned; series including patients with non-Hodgkin's lymphomas in which patients with Hodgkin's disease could not easily be separated are not listed (56). As expected, these patients were heterogeneous in terms of patient-, disease-, and treatment-related factors. However, virtually all had progressed following multiagent primary chemotherapy. Although this format invites comparison, the heterogeneity of these studies must be emphasized—such comparisons should be undertaken with caution.

Most patients responded; the complete response rate was at least 50%. Also, and as indicated, an apparent "partial response" may in fact represent a full complete response. Nonrelapse mortality occurred in slightly more than 10% of patients and varied greatly among the studies; as expected, those treating patients with more advanced disease and those using more intensive doses of therapy generally had more toxicity. Although not always described in detail, at least some of these deaths were due to sepsis and (at least in theory) could have been reduced by the use of hematopoietic growth factors. Many of these other deaths were due to pulmonary toxicity, at least arguably related to the use of high doses of BCNU (18,29).

Although patients who did not remit obviously had poorer outcomes, relapse from documented complete remission was relatively uncommon. Accordingly, disease-free survivals of 30 to 40% are common; occasional series reported up to 50% (18). Although unproven, most investigators believe these differences are due mostly to disease- rather than treatment-related factors.

Prognostic factors for durable remission are not consistent, an observation that may be related to small numbers of patients. As expected, however, features of advanced, chemoresistant disease portend a poor outcome.

Allogeneic Marrow Transplants

As noted previously, fewer reports have dealt with allogeneic BMT for Hodgkin's disease, regardless of series size (61). Again, heterogeneity prevents a simple analysis, although some patients who could not undergo autotransplantation were cured with allotransplants (Tables 53-6,53-7).

Hematopoietic Growth Factors

As detailed, there are clearly circumstances in which delayed blood count recovery is noted following BMT for Hodgkin's disease (62). Although death due to pancytopenic complications alone in patients who are not heavily pretreated is uncommon (18), more rapid recovery would be useful in all patients.

A number of Phase II studies, including several specifically in Hodgkin's disease (63,64), have reported the use of available hematopoietic growth factors—currently either granulocyte-macrophage colony stimulating factor (GM-CSF) or granulocyte colony-stimulating factor (G-CSF)—in enhancing neutrophil recovery, but generally without hastening of platelet recovery, as compared with historical series. Complications from these growth factors have generally been minor, and their effects on morbidity and hospitalization (and therefore cost) have been variable although often favorable.

Two Phase III studies have been reported. Nemunaitis and co-workers (65) noted favorable effects of yeast GM-CSF at a dose of 250 μg/day for 14 to 21 days on the kinetics of neutrophil recovery in a heterogeneous group of patients with lymphoid malignancy, but no benefit was shown in the subgroup of patients with Hodgkin's disease, perhaps indicating the presence of extensively damaged marrow. In contrast, Gulati and colleagues (66) found benefit for both neutrophils and platelet recovery (as well as diminished hospitalization costs) in the group of patients with Hodgkin's disease treated with GM-CSF following autologous BMT. Newer hematopoietic growth factors (especially in combination) that act on less-mature cells than G-CSF and GM-CSF may further hasten post-transplant marrow recovery.

Economic Considerations

Although not directly related to the issue of increasing the cure rate in patients with Hodgkin's disease who require an autotransplant, the changing climate of medical economics is such that this issue bears discussion. Relatively little on this topic had been published (67), probably due to the disparity between the cure rates with conventional chemotherapy versus

Table 53-5.
Representative Published Results in Autologous Bone Marrow Transplantation Studies for Hodgkin's Disease

Author, Year, Ref	*No. Patients*	*Disease Status*						*Conditioning Regimen*	*Stem-cell Source*	*CR/PR*	*Non-relapse Deaths*	*Alive Without Progression*	*Event-free Survival*	*Adverse Prognostic Factors*
		PIF	*CR*	*UR*	*SR*	*RR*	*NSR*							
Philip et al. 1986 (10)	17	11	...	...	3	3	...	Various; usually BACT (+ TBI in 4)	Marrow	9/0	9	3	NS	NS
Carella et al. 1988 (17)	50	18	...	7	13	12	...	CBV	Marrow	24/16	2	12	>40% at 3 yr	NS
Jagannath et al. 1989 (22)	61	...	...	17	12	32	...	CBV (+ LRT in selected patients)	Marrow	29/18	4	23	38% at 2 yr	>2 prior regimens, poor performance status
Gribben et al. 1989 (23)	44	22	NS	NS	NS	NS	...	BEAM (+ LRT in selected patients)	Marrow	22/16	2	20	NS	Large tumor mass at time of transplant
Phillips et al. 1989 (28)	26	5	...	8	...	13	...	CY+TBI (+ LRT in selected patients)	Marrow	18/3	6	7	38% at 4.5 yr[a]	Lower performance status and longer diagnosis to transplant
Hurd et al. 1990 (60)	33	NS	NS	NS	NS	NS	NS	CBV (+ LRT in selected patients)	Marrow: 23 Blood: 8 Both: 2	25/NS	0	12	32% at 28 mo	Marrow involvement at the time of blood cell harvest
Jones et al. 1990 (27)	28	...	...	...	20	8	...	CY + TBI or BUCY (4)	Purged marrow	NS	6	10	Approximately 50% at 20 mo	Resistant relapse status
Kessinger et al. 1991 (50)	56	3	NS	NS	NS	NS	NS	CBV (+ LRT in selected patients)	Blood	29/18	4	28	37% at 3 yr	Marrow involvement at transplant
Gianni et al. 1991 (38)	25	16	...	9	...	...	...	CY → VCR + MTX/LV + CDDP or VP16-213 + MEL + LRT	Blood	18/NS	0	12	49% at 3 yr	Failure to achieve remission with primary therapy
Reece et al. 1991 (18)	56	12	...	32	1	6	..	CBV +/− MVPP and LRT	Marrow	44/2	12[b]	30	47% at 5 yr	Low performance status
Total	396										45	157		

[a]Overall, not EFS.
[b]Progressed from CR/PR.
PIF = primary induction failure; CR = complete remission; UR = untested relapse; SR = sensitive relapse; RR = resistant relapse; NSR = nonspecified relapse; PR = partial remission; BACT = carmustine (BCNU) + arabinosyl cytosine + cyclophosphamide (CY) + thioguanine; TBI = total body irradiation; NS = not specified; CBV = CY + BCNU + etoposide (VP16-213); LRT = local radiotherapy; BEAM = BCNU + VP-16 + cytosine arabinoside + melphalan (MEL); BUCY = busulfan + CY; VCR = vincristine; MTX = methotrexate; LV = levcouorin; CDDP = cisplatin; MVVP = mustargen + vinblastine + prednisone + procarbazide.

Table 53-6.
Representative Published Results in Allogeneic and Syngeneic Bone Marrow Transplantation Studies for Hodgkin's Disease

Author, Year, Ref	*No. Patients*	*Disease Status*						*Conditioning Regimen*	*Marrow Source*	*Non-relapse Deaths*	*Alive without Progression*	*Event-free Survival*	*Adverse Prognostic Factors*
		PIF	*CR*	*UR*	*SR*	*RR*	*NSR*						
Appelbaum, 1985 (55)	8	...	...	...	...	...	8	TBI[a](1) CY ± BCNU ± TBI[a] (3) CY + TBI[b] (1) CY + TBI[c] (3)	HLA-identical sibs (8)	5	2		Very heavily pretreated. Prior chest irradiation in 4; 3 died of NRM, 1 of relapse
Phillips, 1986 (54)	3	3	...	...	...	...	...	CY + TBI[b] (3)	HLA-identical sibs (3)	1	2		Very heavily pretreated. Prior chest irradiation in 1; this patient alive and well
Phillips, 1989 (36)	8	4	...	...	...	4	...	CY + BCNU + VP16-213 (8)	HLA-identical sibs (8)	4	1		Very heavily pretreated. Prior chest radiotherapy in 5; all are dead, including 1 relapse
Lundberg, 1990 (57)	7	3	...	1	3	...	...	CBV + LRT (1) CY + CA + TBI[d] + LRT (3) BUCY (3) + LRT (1)	HLA-matched sibs (6) Unrelated donor (1)	2	3		Four had received prior mediastinal radiation; all received non-TBI conditioning; all are dead, including 2 relapses
Jones, 1990 (27)	22	...	...	...	9	12	1	CY + TBI[b] (number NR) CY + TBI[d] (number NR) BUCY (number NR)	HLA-identical sibs (21) Syngeneic (1)	11	5		Almost all patients were "tested" with conventional chemotherapy; disease status was strongest predictor of EFS; no survivors except those in SR

[a]1,000 cGy.
[b]1,200 cGy.
[c]1,400 cGy.
[d]1,440 cGy.
PIF = primary induction failure; CR = complete remission; UR = untested relapse; SR = sensitive relapse; RR = resistant relapse; NSR = nonspecified relapse; TBI = total body irradiation; CY = cyclophosphamide; BCNU = carmustine; VP16-213 = etoposide; LRT = local radiotherapy; CA = cytosine arabinoside; BUCY = busulfan + CY; HLA = human leukocyte antigen; NR = not reported; NRM = nonrelapse mortality; EFS = event-free survival.

Table 53-7.
Representative Published Results in Allogeneic and Syngeneic Bone Marrow Transplantation Studies for Lymphoma; Hodgkin's Disease patients not Discernable

Author, Year, Ref	*No. Patients*	*Disease Status*						*Conditioning Regimen*	*Marrow Source*	*Non-relapse Deaths*	*Alive Without Progression*	*Event-free Survival*	*Adverse Prognostic Factors*
		PIF	*CR*	*UR*	*SR*	*RR*	*NSR*						
Appelbaum, 1987 (56)	73	2	12	7	...	52	...	CY + TBI[a] (19) CY + TBI[b] (35) CY + TBI[c] (5) CY + TBI[d] (14)	Syngeneic (13) HLA-identical sibs (NR) HLA-mismatched relatives (NR)	NR	14		Disease status and prior chest radiotherapy only predictors of LFS
Gribben, 1987 (61)	42	NR	27	NR	NR	NR	NR	CY + TBI[e] (42)	NR	...	18		Disease status did, but marrow source did not, influence relapse rate or survival
Jones, 1991 (46)	38	...	...	...	19	19	...	CY + FTBI[b] (number NR) BUCY (4) (number NR)	HLA-identical sibs (NR) HLA-mismatched relatives (NR)	NR	9		

[a]1,000 cGy.
[b]1,200 cGy.
[c]1,440 cGy.
[d]1,575 cGy.
[e]dose NR.
PIF = primary induction failure; CR = complete remission; UR = untested relapse; SR = sensitive relapse; RR = resistant relapse; NSR = nonspecified relapse; TBI = total body irradiation; CY = cyclophosphamide; HLA = human leukocyte antigen; FTBI = fractionated TBI; NR = not reported; LFS = lymphoma-free survival; BUCY = busulfan + CY.

those with autotransplant regimens in patients with relapsed Hodgkin's disease, and the assumption that saving lives is ultimately "cost-effective," especially when long-term survivors are relatively asymptomatic (68).

Nevertheless, in an attempt to apply this therapy more widely, it would clearly be desirable to decrease the "unit cost" of autologous BMT. This reduction can be achieved most simply by optimal patient selection (especially by avoiding patients with end-stage diseases, who are unlikely to be cured and are most likely to suffer toxicity that adds to expense) and the use of various measures to ameliorate hematological toxicity (primarily utilizing hematopoietic growth factors) and perhaps nonhematological toxicity as well.

Summary

The increasing use of BMT regimens in providing curative therapy for some patients with Hodgkin's disease not considered curable by other means has several implications for routine management of these patients. First, and probably most importantly, oncologists who manage the primary care of patients with Hodgkin's disease should be aware that the vast majority of such patients who fail conventional chemotherapy need to be evaluated *promptly* for BMT, with the understanding that most patients should be transplanted soon after relapse; delayed referral will result in fewer cures (69). Second, eradication of in vivo tumors needs to be improved; however, it is not clear how this is to be done, because severe nonhematological toxicity may preclude further dose escalation unless suitable cytoprotectants are found. Third, the role of autologous blood stem cell and allogeneic BMT should be evaluated more fully. Conceivably, blood or allogeneic marrow may replace autologous marrow not only in situations of marrow contamination, but perhaps in other cases as well. It is likely that hematopoietic growth factors will be increasingly useful, both in reducing toxicity and in increasing the patient population eligible for transplantation.

Certain of these questions have been, and others should now be, addressed in clinical (especially Phase III) trials. However, an important but less obvious goal is to make marrow transplant regimens available to all patients with Hodgkin's disease who require them. This process will require examination of the reasons why suitable patients with Hodgkin's disease do not undergo BMT, as has been done for acute myeloid leukemia and allogeneic BMT (70). It is currently unclear exactly how many patients with Hodgkin's disease are being transplanted; however, the European Bone Marrow Transplant Group and the North American Autologous Marrow Transplant Group are collecting data to answer this question.

References

1. Urba WJ, Longo DL. Hodgkin's disease. N Engl J Med 1992;326:678–687.
2. Kaplan HS. Evidence for a tumoricidal dose level in the radiotherapy of Hodgkin's disease. Cancer Res 1966; 26:1221–1224.
3. Frei III E, Canellos GP. Dose: a critical factor in cancer chemotherapy. Am J Med 1980;69:585–594.

4. Carde P, MacKintosh FR, Rosenberg SA. A dose and time response analysis of the treatment of Hodgkin's disease with MOPP chemotherapy. J Clin Oncol 1983; 1:146–153.
5. Armitage JO. Bone marrow transplantation in the treatment of patients with lymphoma. Blood 1989; 73:1749–1758:
6. Bonadonna G, Valagussa P, Santoro A. Alternating non-cross-resistant combination chemotherapy or MOPP in stage IV Hodgkin's disease. Ann Intern Med 1986; 104:739–746.
7. Klimo P, Connors JM. MOPP/ABV hybrid program: combination chemotherapy based on early introduction of seven effective drugs for advanced Hodgkin's disease. J Clin Oncol 1985;3:1174–1182.
8. Hoskins P, Klimo P, Fairey R, O'Reilly SE, Voss N, Connors JM. MOPP/ABV hybrid chemotherapy for advanced Hodgkin's disease (HD). 7 year experience at a single centre (abstract). Presented at the Fourth International Conference on Malignant Lymphoma, Lugano, Switzerland, June 6–9, 1990.
9. Buzaid AC, Lippman SM, Miller TP. Salvage therapy of advanced Hodgkin's disease. Critical appraisal of curative potential. Am J Med 1987;83:523–532.
10. Phillips GL, Reece DE. Clinical studies of autologous bone marrow transplantation in Hodgkin's disease. Clin Haematol 1986;15:151–166.
11. Phillips GL, Reece DE, Connors JM. Bone marrow transplantation in Hodgkin's disease. Bone Marrow Transplant 1992;10(suppl 1):64–66.
12. Canellos GP, Propert K, Cooper R, et al. MOPP vs. ABVD vs. MOPP alternating with ABVD in advanced Hodgkin's disease: a prospective randomized CALGB trial (abstract). Proc Am Soc Clin Oncol 1988;7:230.
13. Glick J, Tsiatis A, Chen M, Rassiga A, Mann R, O'Connell M. Improved survival with MOPP/ABVD compared to BCVPP ± radiotherapy (RT) for advanced Hodgkin's disease: 6-year ECOG results (abstract). Blood 1990;76(suppl 1):350a.
14. Glick J, Tsiatis A, Schilsky R, et al. A randomized Phase III trial of MOPP/ABVD Hybrid vs sequential MOPP/ABVD in advanced Hodgkin's disease: preliminary results of the intergroup trial. ECOG, CALGB, and SWOG, Philadelphia, PA, Boston, MA, Chicago, IL (abstract). Proc Am Soc Clin Oncol 1991;10:271.
15. Santoro A, Bonfante V, Bonadonna G. Salvage chemotherapy with ABVD in MOPP-resistant Hodgkin's disease. Ann Intern Med 1982;96:139–143.
16. Desch CE, Lasala MR, Smith TJ, Hillner BE. The optimal timing of autologous bone marrow transplantation in Hodgkin's disease patients after a chemotherapy relapse. J Clin Oncol 1992;10:200–209.
17. Carella AM, Congiu AM, Gaozza E, et al. High-dose chemotherapy with autologous bone marrow transplantation in 50 advanced resistant Hodgkin's disease patients: an Italian Study Group report. J Clin Oncol 1988;6:1411–1416.
18. Reece DE, Barnett MJ, Connors JM, et al. Intensive chemotherapy with cyclophosphamide, carmustine, and etoposide followed by autologous bone marrow transplantation for relapsed Hodgkin's disease. J Clin Oncol 1991;9:1871–1879.
19. Lohri A, Barnett M, Fairey RN, et al. Outcome of treatment of first relapse of Hodgkin's disease after primary chemotherapy: identification of risk factors from the British Columbia experience 1970 to 1988. Blood 1991;77:2292–2298.
20. Herzig GP. Autologous marrow transplantation in cancer therapy. Prog Hematol 1981;12:1–23.
21. Bearman SI, Appelbaum FR, Back A, et al. Regimen-related toxicity and early posttransplant survival in patients undergoing marrow transplantation for lymphoma. J Clin Oncol 1989;7:1288–1294.
22. Jagannath S, Armitage JO, Dicke KA, et al. Prognostic factors for response and survival after high-dose cyclophosphamide, carmustine, and etoposide with autologous bone marrow transplantation for relapsed Hodgkin's disease. J Clin Oncol 1989;7:179–185.
23. Gribben JG, Linch DC, Singer CRJ, McMillan AK, Jarrett M, Goldstone AH. Successful treatment of refractory Hodgkin's disease by high-dose combination chemotherapy and autologous bone marrow transplantation. Blood 1989;73:340–344.
24. Wheeler C, Antin JH, Churchill WH, et al. Cyclophosphamide, carmustine, and etoposide with autologous bone marrow transplantation in refractory Hodgkin's disease and non-Hodgkin's lymphoma: a dose-finding study. J Clin Oncol 1990;8:648–656.
25. Thomas ED. The use and potential of bone marrow allograft and whole-body irradiation in the treatment of leukemia. Cancer 1982;50:1449–1454.
26. Pecego R, Hill R, Appelbaum FR, et al. Interstitial pneumonitis following autologous bone marrow transplantation. Transplantation 1986;42:515–517.
27. Jones RJ, Piantadosi S, Mann RB, et al. High-dose cytotoxic therapy and bone marrow transplantation for relapsed Hodgkin's disease. J Clin Oncol 1990;8: 527–537.
28. Phillips GL, Wolff SN, Herzig RH, et al. Treatment of progressive Hodgkin's disease with intensive chemoradiotherapy and autologous bone marrow transplantation. Blood 1989;73:2086–2092.
29. Horning SJ, Chao NJ, Negrin RS, et al. The Stanford experience with high-dose etoposide cytoreductive regimens and autologous bone marrow transplantation in Hodgkin's disease and non-Hodgkin's lymphoma: Preliminary data. Ann Oncol 1991;2(suppl 1):47–50.
30. Philip T, Dumont J, Teillet F, et al. High dose chemotherapy and autologous bone marrow transplantation in refractory Hodgkin's disease. Br J Cancer 1986;53:737–742.
31. Graw Jr RG, Lohrmann H-P, Bull MI, et al. Bone-marrow transplantation following combination chemotherapy immunosuppression (B.A.C.T.) in patients with acute leukemia. Transplant Proc 1974;6:349–354.
32. Phillips GL, Reece DE. High-dose chemotherapy with cyclophosphamide, BCNU and VP16-213 (CBV) and bone marrow transplantation for advanced Hodgkin's disease. In: Zander A, Barlogie B, eds. Autologous bone marrow transplantation in lymphoma, Hodgkin's disease and multiple myeloma. Heidelberg: Springer-Verlag, 1993 (in press).
33. Russell JA, Selby PJ, Ruether BA, et al. Treatment of advanced Hodgkin's disease with high dose melphalan and autologous bone marrow transplantation. Bone Marrow Transplant 1989;4:425–429.
34. Santos GW, Tutschka PJ, Brookmeyer R, et al. Marrow transplantation for acute nonlymphocytic leukemia after treatment with busulfan and cyclophosphamide. N Engl J Med 1983;309:1347–1353.
35. Kaplan HS. Chemotherapy. In: Hodgkin's disease, ed 2. Cambridge, MA: Harvard University Press, 1980:442–477.
36. Phillips GL, Reece DE, Barnett MJ, et al. Allogeneic marrow transplantation for refractory Hodgkin's disease. J Clin Oncol 1989;7:1039–1045.
37. Ahmed T, Feldman E, Ciavarella D, et al. Sequential autologous bone marrow transplantation (BMT) for high risk Hodgkin's disease (HD) (abstract). Proc Am Soc Clin Oncol 1991;10:223.

38. Gianni AM, Siena S, Bregni M, et al. Prolonged disease-free survival after high-dose sequential chemo-radiotherapy and haemopoietic autologous transplantation in poor prognosis Hodgkin's disease. Ann Oncol 1991; 2:645–653.
39. Vriesendorp HM, Blum JE, Herpst JM, et al. Refractory Hodgkin's disease: treatment with polyclonal yttrium labeled antiferritin (abstract). Proc Am Soc Clin Oncol 1990;9:256.
40. Jagannath S, Dicke KA, Armitage JO, et al. High-dose cyclophosphamide, carmustine, and etoposide and autologous bone marrow transplantation for relapsed Hodgkin's disease. Ann Intern Med 1986;104:163–168.
41. Yahalom J, Gulati S, Shank B, Clarkson B, Fuks Z. Total lymphoid irradiation, high-dose chemotherapy and autologous bone marrow transplantation for chemotherapy-resistant Hodgkin's disease. Int J Radiat Oncol Biol Phys 1989;17:915–922.
42. Fouillard L, Gorin NC, Laporte JP, Douay L, Isnard F, Najman A. Recombinant human granulocyte-macrophage colony-stimulating factor plus the BEAM regimen instead of autologous bone marrow transplantation (letter). Lancet 1989;1:1460.
43. Neidhart J, Mangalik A, Kohler W, et al. Granulocyte colony-stimulating factor stimulates recovery of granulocytes in patients receiving dose-intensive chemotherapy without bone marrow transplantation. J Clin Oncol 1989;7:1685–1692.
44. Brandwein JM, Callum J, Sutcliffe SB, Scott JG, Keating A. Analysis of factors affecting hematopoietic recovery after autologous bone marrow transplantation for lymphoma. Bone Marrow Transplant 1990;6:291–294.
45. Chao NJ, Nademanee AP, Long GD, et al. Importance of bone marrow cytogenetic evaluation before autologous bone marrow transplantation for Hodgkin's disease. J Clin Oncol 1991;9:1575–1579.
46. Jones RJ, Ambinder RF, Piantadosi S, Santos GW. Evidence of a graft-versus-lymphoma effect associated with allogeneic bone marrow transplantation. Blood 1991;77:649–653.
47. Rosenberg SA. Hodgkin's disease of the bone marrow. Cancer Res 1971;31:1733–1736.
48. Bartl R, Frisch B, Burkhardt R, Huhn D, Pappenberger R. Assessment of bone marrow histology in Hodgkin's disease: correlation with clinical factors. Br J Haematol 1982;51:345–360.
49. Joshi SS, Novak DJ, Messbarger L, Maitreyan V, Weisenburger DD, Sharp JG. Levels of detection of tumor cells in human bone marrow with or without prior culture. Bone Marrow Transplant 1990;6:179–183.
50. Kessinger A, Bierman PJ, Vose JM, Armitage JO. High-dose cyclophosphamide, carmustine, and etoposide followed by autologous peripheral stem cell transplantation for patients with relapsed Hodgkin's disease. Blood 1991;77:2322–2325.
51. Körbling M, Holle R, Haas R, et al. Autologous blood stem-cell transplantation in patients with advanced Hodgkin's disease and prior radiation to the pelvic site. J Clin Oncol 1990;8:978–985.
52. Beatty PG, Clift RA, Mickelson EM, et al. Marrow transplantation from related donors other than HLA-identical siblings. N Engl J Med 1985;313:765–771.
53. Nitzberg MC, Newburger PE, Raymond J. Marrow donors and international cooperation. Lancet 1988; 1:117–118.
54. Phillips GL, Herzig RH, Lazarus HM, Fay JW, Griffith R, Herzig GP. High-dose chemotherapy, fractionated total-body irradiation, and allogeneic marrow transplantation for malignant lymphoma. J Clin Oncol 1986;4:480–488.
55. Appelbaum FR, Sullivan KM, Thomas ED, et al. Allogeneic marrow transplantation in the treatment of MOPP-resistant Hodgkin's disease. J Clin Oncol 1985; 3:1490–1494.
56. Appelbaum FR, Sullivan KM, Buckner CD, et al. Treatment of malignant lymphoma in 100 patients with chemotherapy, total body irradiation, and marrow transplantation. J Clin Oncol 1987;5:1340–1347.
57. Lundberg JH, Hansen RM, Chitambar CR, et al. Allogeneic bone marrow transplantation for relapsed and refractory lymphoma using genotypically HLA-identical and alternative donors. J Clin Oncol 1991; 9:1848–1859.
58. Horowitz MM, Gale RP, Sondel PM, et al. Graft-versus-leukemia reactions after bone marrow transplantation. Blood 1990;75:555–562.
59. Jones RJ, Vogelsang GB, Hess AD, et al. Induction of graft-versus-host disease after autologous bone marrow transplantation. Lancet 1989;1:754–757.
60. Hurd DD, Haake RJ, Lasky LC, et al. Treatment of refractory and relapsed Hodgkin's disease: intensive chemotherapy and autologous bone marrow or peripheral blood stem cell support. Med Pediatr Oncol 1990;18:447–453.
61. Gribben J, Goldstone AH, Ernst P, et al. Bone marrow transplantation for non-Hodgkin's lymphoma in remission—allogeneic versus autologous (abstract). Bone Marrow Transplant 1987;2(suppl 1):204.
62. Hill RS, Mazza P, Amos D, et al. Engraftment in 86 patients with lymphoid malignancy after autologous marrow transplantation. Bone Marrow Transplant 1989;4:69–74.
63. Devereaux S, Linch DC, Gribben JG, McMillan A, Patterson K, Goldstone AH. GM-CSF accelerates neutrophil recovery after autologous bone marrow transplantation for Hodgkin's disease. Bone Marrow Transplant 1989;4:49–54.
64. Taylor KM, Jagannath S, Spitzer G, et al. Recombinant human granulocyte colony-stimulating factor hastens granulocyte recovery after high-dose chemotherapy and autologous bone marrow transplantation in Hodgkin's disease. J Clin Oncol 1989;7:1791–1799.
65. Nemunaitis J, Rabinowe SN, Singer JW, et al. Recombinant granulocyte-macrophage colony-stimulating factor after autologous bone marrow transplantation for lymphoid cancer. N Engl J Med 1991;324:1773–1778.
66. Gulati SC, Bennett CL. Granulocyte-macrophage colonystimulating factor (GM-CSF) as adjunct therapy in relapsed Hodgkin disease. Ann Intern Med 1992; 116:177–182.
67. McMillan A, Goldstone A. What is the value of autologous bone marrow transplantation in the treatment of relapsed or resistant Hodgkin's disease? Leuk Res 1991;15:237–243.
68. Vose JM, Kennedy BC, Bierman PJ, Kessinger A, Armitage JO. Long-term sequelae of autologous bone marrow or peripheral stem cell transplantation for lymphoid malignancies. Cancer 1992;69:784–789.
69. Armitage JO, Bierman PJ, Vose JM, et al. Autologous bone marrow transplantation for patients with relapsed Hodgkin's disease. Am J Med 1991;91:605–611.
70. Berman E, Little C, Gee T, O'Reilly R, Clarkson B. Reasons that patients with acute myelogenous leukemia do not undergo allogeneic bone marrow transplantation. N Engl J Med 1992;326:156–160.

Chapter 54

Autologous Bone Marrow Transplantation for Acute Myeloid Leukemia

Andrew M. Yeager

Historical Perspective

Autologous marrow, previously collected and cryopreserved, was first used to reconstitute normal hematopoiesis after intensive antitumor therapy (chemotherapy with or without irradiation) in patients with refractory lymphomas, carcinomas, and chronic myeloid leukemia (CML) (1–5). In patients with end-stage refractory acute myeloid leukemia (AML), the long-term relapse-free survival observed in some after marrow-lethal chemoradiotherapy and syngeneic bone marrow transplantation (BMT) (6) suggested that similar antileukemic effects might be obtained with autologous marrow, collected in hematological remission, as the source of hematopoietic stem cells. The development of cryobiological methods for the reproducible and safe preservation and storage of marrow cell suspensions (see Chapter 23) provided a technological foundation for the more widespread clinical application of autologous BMT in AML.

The first successful autologous BMT in a patient with first relapse of AML (chloromas) was reported by Gorin and colleagues in 1977 (7,8). The marrow, collected in first remission and stored in liquid nitrogen without additional treatment, was infused after a pretransplant chemotherapeutic conditioning regimen (TACC: thioguanine, cytosine arabinoside, cyclophosphamide [CY], and lomustine). By today's standards, the cell dose was low (0.5×10^8 nucleated marrow cells/kg), but hematological reconstitution was prompt. Thirty days after transplantation, the chloromas had resolved; the patient was in complete clinical and hematological remission for 83 days after autologous BMT, then developed testicular and central nervous system relapses (but remained in hematological remission). This case demonstrated the feasibility of autologous marrow collection and storage, the responsiveness of the leukemia to high-dose chemotherapy and stem-cell rescue, and the rapidity of hematological reconstitution after intensive polychemotherapy and autologous BMT in AML.

Since the mid-1970s, the interest in application of autologous BMT for AML has increased substantially in both Europe and North America. The patterns of and indications for autologous BMT for AML differ somewhat between Europe and North America (9). Initially, more trials of autologous BMT for AML were carried out in Europe, especially in first remission and often without ex vivo marrow treatment. In contrast, autologous BMTs in second or subsequent remission with immunologically or pharmacologically treated ("purged") marrow were predominantly conducted in American centers.

Although there are numerous published reports of autologous BMT for AML, these studies are confounded by many factors, including age range of the patient population, types and intensity of previous AML chemotherapy regimens, durations of remission at the time of autologous BMT, whether the autologous marrow has been purged ex vivo (and by which method), and whether the graft is cryopreserved in liquid nitrogen or maintained at 4°C. Interpretation of results of many studies is further compromised by the small number of patients studied and the relatively low statistical power.

General Considerations

The effectiveness of autologous BMT in patients with acute leukemia depends on at least 3 factors: (1) whether the collected and cryopreserved marrow suspension contains adequate numbers of stem cells for hematological reconstitution; (2) whether viable AML cells in the infused marrow suspension are capable of causing post-transplant relapse; and (3) whether the pretransplant conditioning regimen effectively eradicates residual leukemia in the patient. In autologous BMT for acute leukemia, the origin of leukemic relapse—whether from residual disease in vivo, infused viable tumor cells in the autologous marrow, or both—is an unresolved but critical issue. A strategy to address this question by molecular genetics techniques is discussed.

Comparing the outcome of autologous BMT for AML with the results of allogeneic BMT in similar groups of patients may not be appropriate, because allogeneic graft-versus-host disease (GVHD) and graft-versus-leukemia (GVL) effects, absent in the autologous BMT setting, may affect leukemic relapse rate and disease-free survival (10–12). Although it has been suggested that the outcome of autologous BMT for acute leukemia may also be compared with that of allogeneic BMT in which no clinical GVHD is observed (13,14), this view must be countered by the strong possibility, supported by preclinical studies, that allogeneic GVL effects can occur without manifestations of GVHD (11,12).

In contrast, comparison of autologous BMT with syngeneic BMT, in which the infused marrow is free of tumor cell contamination and the risk for development of substantial GVHD is negligible, is valid. The total number of syngeneic BMTs for AML is small, and use of historical control subjects or registry data on syngeneic BMT is further compromised by the heterogeneity of both the AML chemotherapy and the pretransplant conditioning regimens, which may differ in their antitumor effectiveness.

In addition to determination of relapse rate and event-free survival, the antileukemic effectiveness of autologous BMT for AML in second or subsequent remission may be estimated by comparing durations of previous and post-transplant remissions. In general, the durations of chemotherapy-induced subsequent remissions of AML are shorter than first remission; post-transplant remissions that exceed preceding remissions (so called remission inversions) would strongly suggest that the intensive antineoplastic therapy and stem-cell rescue provide substantially more antileukemic effects than expected with conventional chemotherapy alone (15). In addition, an attractive aspect of using remission inversions to measure antileukemic effectiveness of autologous BMT is the fact that each patient serves as his or her own control. Only approximately one half of patients who relapse with AML will successfully attain a subsequent remission, which introduces an unavoidable selection bias in autologous BMT for AML in other than first remission.

Critical analysis of studies of autologous BMT for first-remission AML merits some additional considerations. In these patients, determination of remission inversions cannot be made. As with studies of autologous BMT in second and later remission, patient selection has a role: Those who never attain a first remission or whose remissions are so tenuous that autologous marrow collection cannot be carried out are excluded from analysis. Most clinical studies of autologous BMT for first-remission AML do not have a complementary chemotherapy arm, so it is difficult to discern whether the observed relapse-free survival after BMT is substantially different from that in the chemotherapy cohort. To address this issue, several large-scale multicenter randomized prospective trials are being conducted in both adults and children to compare outcome of autologous BMT with conventional chemotherapy and with allogeneic BMT (16,17).

Time-censoring, or time-selection bias, is perhaps one of the most important variables in critical analysis and interpretation of the autologous BMT studies

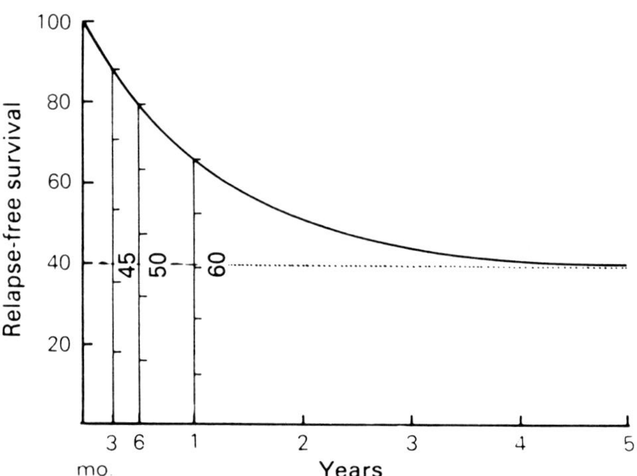

Figure 54-1. The time-censoring effect may explain better outcome (lower relapse rate and higher relapse-free survival) when autologous bone marrow transplantation for acute myeloid leukemia is carried out in patients with longer remission durations. In this hypothetical example, the plateau for disease-free survival with conventional chemotherapy is 40% at 5 years. With time from attaining remission, relapsed patients are excluded from analysis, and the probability of relapse-free survival among the remaining cohort increases proportionately. For example, if the cohort of surviving patients is followed from 3, 6, or 12 months after attaining remission (rather than at "zero time" after attaining remission), the corresponding relapse-free survival would be 45, 50, or 60%, respectively. (Reprinted by permission from Gale RP, Armitage JO, Butturini A. Is there a role for autotransplants in acute leukemia? Bone Marrow Transplant 1989;4:217–219.)

for AML in first remission. As illustrated in Figure 54-1, the apparently low relapse rates and high relapse-free survival observed after autologous BMT late in first remission (e.g., after 6–12 mo or longer) may attribute the antileukemic effect to the transplant, when in fact the beneficial effects are due primarily to effective conventional chemotherapy alone. Selection for autologous BMT of patients with longer first remission durations obviously excludes those who have already relapsed and selects a subgroup of patients who, by virtue of not relapsing earlier, are much more likely to have been cured of AML with conventional chemotherapy (14,18–21).

On the Need for Marrow Purging

One of the most controversial and unresolved areas of autologous BMT for AML is the need for and choice of ex vivo marrow treatment, or "purging." Early in the clinical application of autologous BMT for AML, there was a high level of interest among many centers in the use of methods to eliminate occult clonogenic tumor cells from the autologous marrow cell suspension, because residual tumor in the autologous marrow might be responsible for post-transplant relapse; other centers have consistently used untreated marrow for trials of autologous BMT for AML. Encouraging relapse-free survival has been reported after autologous BMT with either untreated or treated marrow in these patients, and arguments for and against purging have been presented. Most trials of autologous BMT with unpurged marrow for AML in first remission, where there is a chance for cure with conventional chemotherapy alone, have been undertaken in a nonprospective fashion. In contrast, until recently, the only substantive trials of autologous BMT for AML in second or subsequent remission have been conducted with purged marrow. These patients have a negligible chance for cure with conventional chemotherapy.

As evidence against marrow purging, mathematical modeling (22) and preclinical studies in rodent AML (23–25) have suggested that the contribution of autologous BMT to the leukemic burden is small and that the major contribution to relapse is residual leukemia in vivo not eradicated by the preparative regimen. It has also been suggested that cryopreservation may reduce or eliminate leukemic cells from the graft (26). Others have suggested that more in vivo chemotherapy (e.g., consolidation or maintenance) is responsible for better outcome of autologous BMT; this view has been argued in unpurged autologous BMT, especially for first-remission AML. Unfortunately, many of the studies that support this argument were those in which patients were transplanted late in remission, again introducing the time-censoring bias.

Some would argue empirically that the marrow purging process, the cost of which is not negligible, adds little risk and may be beneficial. More objective studies that support the value of ex vivo marrow treatment include correlations of relapse-free survival after autologous BMT with the sensitivity to chemopurging agents of occult AML cells cultured from remission marrows (27) and correlation of antileukemic effectiveness with the intensity of the chemopurging effect against normal committed hematopoietic progenitors (28). Multicenter retrospective analyses of European Bone Marrow Transplant Registry data suggest that the relapse rate is significantly lower after autologous BMT in patients transplanted with purged versus unpurged marrow when the remission duration is less than 6 months and the time to attain first remission exceeds 40 days (29,30). These observations are consistent with more effective eradication of aggressive AML that is incompletely eradicated by in vivo chemotherapy and is present in the autologous marrow graft. In addition, the plateau in relapse-free survival was attained earlier in recipients of chemically purged marrow, suggesting a more effective elimination of AML cells capable of causing later relapses (30).

Randomized prospective studies that compare the outcome of purged and unpurged autologous BMT in AML, with a third arm consisting of a chemotherapy cohort, would probably be the best method to address this question, but the logistics of such a trial are daunting, and large numbers of patients would need to be enrolled. Other novel and potentially highly instructive studies are being developed to identify the sources of relapse of AML after autologous BMT and to determine the kinetics of autologous hematopoietic and lymphoid reconstitution after autologous BMT. For example, techniques for safe retroviral vector–mediated introduction of marker genes into normal and leukemic marrow cells have been developed; these cells or their progeny can be identified by appropriate molecular biological techniques such as polymerase chain reaction (31). Clinical trials of autologous BMT with gene-marked unpurged marrow are currently being introduced in patients with AML (32). Identification of the marker gene in at least some of the leukemic cells at relapse after autologous BMT would indicate that the tumor cells in the autologous marrow graft were at least in part responsible for the recurrence of leukemia. The efficiency of ex vivo manipulation to reduce or eradicate leukemic cells in the marrow suspension could also be assessed in this system.

Selection of Patients and Timing of Autologous BMT

The likelihood of long-term relapse-free survival is negligible with conventional chemotherapy in patients with AML in second or subsequent remission, and allogeneic BMT from related histocompatible donors is associated with a substantial chance for cure in these patients. In patients with second- or subsequent-remission AML who lack a related donor, or who are older than acceptable age limits for allogeneic BMT, autologous BMT with chemically or immunologically purged marrow can lead to long-term relapse-free survival (33–36). The risk of transplant-related complications, such as hepatic veno-occlusive disease, is higher in third- than in second-remission patients, and argument can therefore be made for proceeding with autologous BMT in an earlier remission (33). The experiences with unpurged autologous BMT in patients with AML in remission other than first is extremely limited (37,38), but these preliminary single-institution results are nevertheless encouraging.

The selection of patients for autologous BMT during the first remission of AML is somewhat more problematic; undoubtedly a proportion of these patients will be cured after receiving aggressive conventional chemotherapy regimens. Furthermore, the optimal methods for ex vivo marrow treatment (if any) and for in vivo pretransplant chemoradiotherapeutic conditioning regimens are not universally established. Good results with both unpurged and purged autologous BMT have been reported for AML in first remission, although the time-selection bias must be taken into account. In the absence of a suitable related allogeneic donor, the data with autologous BMT in first-remission AML are at least as good as, and may be somewhat better than, any reported chemotherapy regimens. One multicenter report suggests that the disease-free survival after allogeneic and autologous BMT is comparable (16). The role of autologous BMT for AML in first remission may be defined by ongoing prospective trials that compare autologous BMT with conventional chemotherapy.

Clinicians may therefore consider several factors in selection of patients for autologous BMT for first remission AML. For example, would this patient most likely be referred for syngeneic or related allogeneic BMT if an appropriate suitable donor were identified? Patients at especially high risk for recurrence of AML by virtue of prognostic factors at diagnosis (e.g., karyotypic abnormalities, high leukocyte count, presence of extramedullary leukemia) or lack of response to remission-induction chemotherapy might benefit from autologous BMT, as they might from allogeneic BMT. At least one study did not demonstrate any adverse influence of karyotypic abnormalities on relapse-free survival after autologous BMT (39), and a multivariate analysis did not show any of these prognostic factors to be significant for poorer outcome (i.e., lower survival or higher risk of relapse) (40). Although a retrospective analysis of data from multiple European transplant centers has suggested that the outcome after autologous BMT for secondary AML (e.g., after treatment for Hodgkin's disease or other neoplasm) is worse than for de novo AML (30), others have reported encouraging long-term relapse-free survival after autologous BMT with chemically purged marrow in patients transplanted in first remission for AML after treatment for Hodgkin's disease (41).

Autologous Transplantation of Unpurged Marrow

In Relapse

Initial studies of autologous BMT with untreated remission marrow for patients with fully relapsed AML demonstrated high response rates (remissions in 55% to more than 90% of patients) (42–50), similar to that described in recipients of syngeneic BMT for end-stage leukemia (6) (Table 54-1). Unlike the syngeneic BMT experience, however, there was no apparent plateau in disease-free survival after autologous BMT for relapsed AML. Nevertheless, these studies showed substantial antileukemic effects of intensive polychemotherapy or chemotherapy plus total body irradiation (TBI) regimens and the hematopoietic repopulating ability of autologous remission marrows stored in liquid nitrogen for several months or longer.

Despite these less-than-promising studies, there has been renewed interest by some centers in the application of autologous BMT for AML in first relapse, using marrow obtained in first remission and including single or double autologous BMT. Using a busulfan (BU)/CY preparative regimen and a single transplant, Chopra and associates (38) showed a 70% relapse rate (6 of 9 patients) and a 33% relapse-free survival, all with remission inversions, after autologous BMT for AML in first relapse, not significantly different from the 48% disease-free survival in the 25 patients transplanted in second remission with the same regimen. The double autologous BMT procedure relies on successive intensive in vivo tumor purges, and has obvious limitations. The Rome group further suggested that different preparative regimens be used for each autologous BMT (51), an approach that has theoretical advantages and may reduce the risk of tumor cross-resistance to drugs. The prolonged relapse-free survival, with remission inversions, in 2 of 3 patients transplanted for first relapse AML with a BAVC regimen (BCNU, amsacrine, VP-16 [etoposide], and cytosine arabinoside) first and then a CY/TBI regimen is encouraging (51), but larger series are needed to confirm the usefulness of this procedure. Unresolved issues in single- or double-autologous BMT for AML in relapse include the optimal time to proceed with autologous BMT ("early" versus later relapse) and the rapidity with which the diagnosis of early relapse of AML can be made and the patient referred for prompt autologous BMT.

In Second or Later Remission

Transplantation of untreated autologous remission marrow for AML in second or subsequent remission has had, for the most part, limited success (see Table 54-1). A single-center trial in 15 adults with second or later remission of AML given autologous BMT after a "CVB" (CY, BCNU, and VP16) preparative regimen showed an actuarial relapse rate exceeding 80% (11 of 15 patients) and only 2 long-term relapse-free survivors with remission inversions (52). The European Cooperative Bone Marrow Transplantation Group reported a 23% survival and 59% actuarial relapse rate among 18 adults given autologous BMT for second-remission AML (53).

Two important studies readdressed the question of autologous BMT with unpurged marrow in second-remission AML (37,38); in these studies, there was no apparent time-selection bias, because patients were transplanted at a median of 2 months after attaining second remission. Meloni and colleagues (37) showed low regimen-related mortality and long-term relapse-free survival in 10 of 17 patients transplanted with unpurged second-remission marrow after a BAVC preparative regimen. The actuarial relapse rate was 45%, and the disease-free survival was 59%, with remission inversions observed in all 10 patients (compared with 1 inversion among the 6 patients who relapsed). Chopra and associates (38) reported on 25 patients in second remission given unpurged autologous BMT after conditioning with BU and CY. Four patients died with transplant-related complications, 9 relapsed at a median of 6 months (range, 3–13 mo) after autologous BMT (actuarial relapse rate, 43%), and 12 were in unmaintained second remission (10 with remission inversions) at a median of 26+ months (range, 15+ to 60+) after transplantation (disease-free survival, 48%).

Questions remain about the possible selection biases in these 2 trials, the intensity (or lack thereof) of

Table 54-1.
Autologous Transplants with Unpurged Marrow for Acute Myeloid Leukemia in Second or Subsequent Remission or in First Relapse

Preparative Regimen[a]	*No. Patients*	*Median Age (yr) (Range)*	*Remission Status at BMT (No. Patients)*	*No. BMT-related Deaths*	*No. Relapses*	*Median Time to Relapse (mo) (Range)*	*Actuarial Relapse Rate (%)*	*No. Relapse-free Surivors*	*Median Duration of Relapse-free Survival (mo) (Range)*	*Actuarial Relapse-free Survival (%)*	*No. Inversions*	*Author, Year, Ref*
COATA or BAVC	13	28 (6–41)	ER1	4	5	5 (4–10)	NR	4	4+ (0.5+ to 28+)	NR	. . .	Meloni et al. 1985 (47)
BAVC → CY/TBI[b]	3	28 (9–36)	ER1	1	0	. . .	. . .	2	46+, 53+	NR	2/2	Meloni et al. 1989 (51)
BAVC	17	24 (1–47)	CR2	1	6	4.5 (2–18)	45	10	39+ (24+ to 63+)	59	10/10	Meloni et al. 1990 (37)
BUCY 120 or 200	34	40 (21–60)	CR2 (25)	4	9	6 (3–13)	43	12	26+ (15+ to 60+)	48	10/12	Chopra et al. 1991 (38)
			ER1 (9)	0	6	4.5 (1–24)	70	3	16+, 38+, 38+	33		
CY/BCNU/VP16	15	32 (21–55)	CR2 (10) CR3 (4) CR4 (1)	2	11	5.2 (1.9–13)	NR	2	57+, 81+	14	2/2	Spinolo et al. 1990 (52)

[a]For descriptions of preparative regimens, see text and original references.
[b]Double autografts.
ER1 = first (early) relapse; CR = complete remission; NR = not reported.

regimens used to induce first and subsequent remissions, and the potentially different antileukemic effects of the pretransplant conditioning regimens used. Nevertheless, if other centers can demonstrate relapse-free survival in patients given autologous BMT with unpurged second-remission marrow similar to that shown in these provocative reports, then the need for purging of autologous marrow in patients with second-remission AML may be questioned.

In First Remission

Several centers have shown encouraging results with autologous BMT with untreated marrow for first-remission AML, usually without simultaneous comparative chemotherapy arms or any indication that the patients transplanted were at especially high risk for relapse after conventional chemotherapy regimens (48–50,54–61) (Table 54-2). CY/TBI was most often used as the preparative regimen, but high-dose melphalan (48,49), "BACCT" (BCNU, adriamycin, CY, cytosine arabinoside, and thioguanine) (50), and BU/CY (61) have also been employed. In these relatively small series, none of these regimens appeared to have unusually severe nonhematological toxicity or superior antileukemic effects. These initial reports demonstrated relapse-free survival rates of approximately 50 to 60% and relapse rates of 30 to 40% after autologous BMT with unpurged marrow, but factors such as time-selection bias (as discussed) may have influenced at least some of these early reports. In one study from Glasgow, for example, the range of durations of first remission at time of BMT was substantial (16–90 weeks), and 4 of the 5 relapses observed in this trial were in patients with remission durations below the median (i.e., <26 wk) (54,55). An alternative explanation to time-selection bias is that the lower frequency of relapses after autologous BMT late in first remission correlates with more cycles of consolidation and maintenance chemotherapy, suggesting that these successive courses of chemotherapy provide a more effective in vivo elimination of residual leukemia from the marrow. A retrospective analysis for the European Bone Marrow Transplant Group (53) showed a 33% relapse rate and 45% survival among 60 patients transplanted for AML in first remission, mostly with untreated marrows. These relapse and survival rates were superior to those for patients undergoing autologous BMT in second remission with untreated or purged marrow.

As these trials of autologous BMT with unpurged marrow for first-remission AML have matured and accrued more patients, the relapse-free survival is somewhat lower (approximately 35–50%) and the relapse rates higher (approximately 40–50%) than initially reported (56,59,62,63). In part, this finding may reflect BMT earlier in first remission, thus decreasing the time-selection bias for which the initial studies were criticized (54–56). In some of these series, a number of patients who relapsed after BMT have successfully attained durable second remissions with conventional chemotherapy; this has seldom been the case in other studies of autologous BMT for AML, where post-transplant relapses are often refractory to salvage therapy.

Not all reports of autologous BMT with unpurged marrow for first-remission AML have been positive, however. One study from Seattle (64), in which 13 patients who received untreated autologous BMT after CY/TBI at a median first-remission duration of 3 months (range, 1 to 13 mo), showed a high relapse rate (8 of 13; actuarial relapse rate, 67%). The 2-year relapse-free survival was 22%, not substantially different from the relapse-free survival expected at that time for recipients of conventional chemotherapy for AML. The durations of first remission before transplantation were shorter (2–4 mo) in the 3 long-term survivors and longer (5–13 mo) in the 8 patients who relapsed; there was no favorable effect of time-selection in this small series.

A novel approach to unpurged autologous BMT for first-remission AML involves double autologous BMT in an attempt to decrease minimal residual disease, to increase the effectiveness of the in vivo marrow purging, and thus decrease the leukemic relapse rate (50,65). Marrow collected soon after hematological recovery following the first BMT may contain fewer occult tumor cells and may be used for the second autologous BMT. The London group compared the outcome in 76 patients (50 given single autologous BMT, 26 given double autologous BMT) after the BACCT regimen and following the same remission-induction and consolidation AML therapy. The 5-year relapse-free survival was 50%, and the relapse rate was 47% for the entire group; for the double-transplant group, the 3-year disease-free survival and actuarial relapse rate were 67 and 30%, respectively. The antileukemic effect of the double autologous BMT was suggested by the timing of relapses: Most of the relapses after double autologous BMT occurred more than one year after transplant, whereas virtually all relapses in the single-transplant group occurred within one year of the procedure. Practical limitations to the applicability of the double autologous BMT technique may be substantial; more than 50% of otherwise eligible patients in the London series could not undergo a second autologous BMT because of relapse, persistent marrow hypoplasia (especially thrombocytopenia), unacceptable nonhematological organ dysfunction, or patient refusal (65). Larger series will be required to determine the feasibility of the double autologous BMT approach for AML in remission.

Autologous Transplantation with Marrow Treated (Purged) Ex Vivo

The concern that high relapse rates observed in some early trials of autologous BMT with untreated marrow were caused at least in part by contamination of the autologous marrow graft by viable occult leukemic

Table 54-2.
Autologous Transplantation with Unpurged Marrow for Acute Myeloid Leukemia in First Remission

Preparative Regimen[a]	No. Patients	Median Age (yr) (Range)	Median Duration of CR1 at BMT (Mo) (Range)	No. BMT-related Deaths	No. Relapses	Median Time to Relapse (mo) (Range)	Actuarial Relapse Rate (%)	No. Relapse-free Survivors	Median Duration of Relapse-free Survival (mo) (Range)	Actuarial Relapse-free Survival (%)	Comments	Author, Year, Ref
CY/TBI	54	36 (15–54)	5+ (2+ to 17+)	6	19	7 (2–27)	44	29	26+ (3+ to 102+)	51	. . .	Burnett et al. 1990 (56)
	32	40 (16–58)	3.8+	3	17	NR	60	12	NR	35	Prospective trial compared with allogeneic BMT	Löwenberg et al. 1990 (115)
	13	18 (13–38)	3+ (1+ to 13+)	2	8	11 (2–12)	67	3	2+, 46+, 50+	22	. . .	Stewart et al. 1985 (64)
	12	43 (15–57)	7+ (3+ to 12+)	1	5	9 (3–14)	NR	7	10+ (7+ to 72+)	NR	. . .	Löwenberg et al. 1987 (59)
	45	37 (12–62)	5+ (2+ to 10+)	7	11	NR	36	23	26+ (2+ to 67+)	51	. . .	Carella et al. 1990 (63)
BUCY120	20	40 (16–53)	6+ (2.5 to 13.5)	2	7	8 (2–11)	38±11	11	20+ (11+ to 36+)	55±11	. . .	Beelen et al. 1989 (61)
BUCY200	9	9 (0.5–17)	6+	0	0	. . .	NR	9	18+ (5+ to 36+)	NR	. . .	Solh et al. 1991 (163)
BACCT	76 (26 double autografts)	40 (16–57)	6+ (0.5+ to 12+)	5 (1)	30 (7)	8 (0–26) (14 [7–21])	47 (30)	39 (18)	38+ (7+ to 125+) (46+ [8+ to 125+])	50 (67)	26/76 had double autografts	McMillan et al. 1989 (65)
AraC/CY/TBI	33	37 (1–54)	4+	9	9	NR	48	14	18+	31	Prospective trial compared with allogeneic BMT	Ferrant et al. 1990 (40)
CY/VP16/AraC	7	43 (25–62)	(2+ to 4+)	0	1	8	NR	6	5+ (1+ to 17+)	NR	. . .	Koeppler et al. 1990 (142)
L-PAM	7	16 (10–52)	5+ (2+ to 6+)	0	0	. . .	. . .	7	5+ (3+ to 20+)	NR	Double autograft	Maraninchi et al. 1984 (48,49)
	11	10 (1–16)	4+ (2+ to 16+)	0	4	15 (12–20)	NR	7	29+ (15+ to 56+)	NR	Double autograft	Michel et al. 1988 (60)

[a]For descriptions of preparative regimens, see text and original references.
ER1 = first (early) relapse; CR = complete remission; NR = not reported.

Table 54-3.
Autologous Transplantation with Marrow Treated Ex Vivo for Acute Myeloid Leukemia in Second or Subsequent Remission or Early Relapse

Preparative Regimen[a]	*No. Patients*	*Median Age (yr) (Range)*	*Remission Status at BMT (No. Patients)*	*Marrow Purging*	*Median Duration of CR at BMT (mo) (Range)*	*No. BMT-related Deaths*	*No Relapses*
PIP/TBI	12	28 (18–48)	REL1	Albumin density gradient	. . .	0	4+ 5 no responses
CY/TBI	7		CR≥1	Mafosfamide	5.5+ (2+ to 23+)	2	4
	30	35 (17–53)	CR≥2	Mafosfamide	3+ (1+ to 8+)	2	14
BUCY200	98	30 (1–56)	CR2 (82)	4HC	2.5+ (0.5+ to 7.0+)	15	38
			CR3 (16)			6	5
	13	5 (1–21)	CR2	4HC	1+ (1+ to 12+)	0	5
BUCY200 ± AraC or CY/TBI	24	33 (10–61)	CR2 (7)	4HC	1.5+ (1+ to 5+)	3	2
			CR3 (8)			2	5
			CR4 (1)			0	1
			ER (8)			1	6
CY/VP16/TBI	10	38 (20–48)	CR2 or 3	4HC + VP16	2+ (1+ to 9+)	2	5
CY/TBI or BU/CY or BU/VP16	48	37 (11–57)	CR2 (36)	MoAbs αCD-14 andαCD-15	2+ (0 to 15+)	15	15
			CR3 (7)			1	1
			ER1 (5)				
CY/TBI, CY/AraC, or BU/CY	12	40 (25–49)	CR1 (2)	MoAb αCD33	2+(1+ to 6+)	0	7
			CR2 (10)				

[a]For descriptions of preparative regimens, see text and original references.
ER1 = first (early) relapse; CR = complete remission; NR = not reported; 4HC = 4-hydroperoxycyclophosphamide; MoAb = monoclonal antibody.

cells led to the focus by several groups on ex vivo treatment or "purging" of autologous marrow to remove these tumor cells (46,66). Many techniques to accomplish this challenging task have been evaluated in in vitro models, preclinical animal tumor systems, and some clinical trials (67) and are discussed elsewhere in this volume (See Chapters 13, 14, and 15). Some of the major approaches to ex vivo marrow treatment in which clinical trials have been conducted are summarized below and in Tables 54-3 and 54-4.

Physical Separation Methods

Physical methods to remove leukemic cells from autologous marrow cell suspensions are based on the suggestion that leukemic blasts are consistently different (i.e., larger and less dense) from normal hematopoietic progenitors (43,68). There was no evidence that marrow separation by albumin density-gradient centrifugation improved relapse-free survival (43), and this technique has virtually been abandoned in clinical autologous BMT. Preclinical studies suggested that counterflow centrifugal elutriation, which separates heterogeneous cell populations on the basis of size and buoyant density, might effectively separate neoplastic cells from marrow suspensions (68). This may be the case for solid tumor contamination of the marrow, but leukemic and lymphoma cells are sufficiently heterogeneous and are elutriated along with a similar distribution to normal marrow populations (68). For this reason, counterflow centrifugal elutriation has not been evaluated in clinical trials of autologous BMT for AML. However, recent data from the use of counterflow centrifugal elutriation to select pluripotential hematopoietic stem cells in rodents (69) and to deplete allogeneic marrow grafts of lymphocytes before clinical BMT (70,71) suggest that physical separation techniques may be applied in conjunction with other methods for ex vivo treatment of the fractionated marrow cell suspension.

Pharmacological Purging

Most clinical trials of autologous BMT with treated marrow have used pharmacological methods to reduce or eliminate tumor cells from the cell suspension. The rationale for incubation with antineoplastic agents is in large part based on the concept of differential sensitivity of neoplastic versus normal hematopoietic progenitors to these compounds (72). Advantages to this approach include the ability to expose cells to concentrations of drugs that substantially exceed peak plasma levels attained in vivo after administration of maximally tolerated doses (73). Nevertheless, tumor cell heterogeneity and de novo or acquired drug resistance may limit the effective removal of leukemic cells by antineoplastic agents.

The largest preclinical and clinical experiences with pharmacological marrow treatment have been

Median Time to Relapse (mo) (Range)	Actuarial Relapse Rate (%)	No. Relapse-free Survivors	Median Duration of Relapse-free Survival (mo) (Range)	Actuarial Relapse-free Survival (%)	No. Inversions	Author, Year, Ref
3.5 (2–7)	NR	3	3+, 3+, 5+	NR	NR	Zander et al. 1979 (43)
3 (0–4.5)	. . .	1	9+	. . .	. . .	Gorin et al. 1986 (77)
5 (0.4–30)	65	14	19+	34	11/14	Körbling et al. 1989 (84)
(2–23)	58	29	46+ (0.5–106+)	30	26/34	This publication
. . .	55	5	. . .	27	. . .	
5 (2–6)	39	8	24+ (16+ to 33+)	61	6/8	Lenarsky et al. 1990 (164)
6, 9	73	2	19+, 37+	19	NR	Rosenfeld et al. 1989 (36)
5 (3.5–10)	. . .	1	14+	. . .	. . .	
4	. . .	0	. . .	. . .	. . .	
3 (0–9)	. . .	1	21+	. . .	. . .	
NR	NR	3	28+ (14+ to 45+)	NR	3/3	Gulati et al. 1989 (89)
				51		Ball et al. 1992 (35)
11 (3–39)	39	15	30+ (7+ to 87+)	30	11/15	
11	NR	3	4+, 20+, 29+	NR	. . .	
8 (3–17)	58	5	12+ (1+ to 33+)	29	NR	Robertson et al. 1992 (94)

with two congeners of CY: mafosfamide (4-sulfoethylthiocyclophosphamide, Asta Z 7557) and 4-hydroperoxycyclophosphamide (4HC) (73). Both compounds hydrolyze in aqueous solution to form 4-hydroxycyclophosphamide, the primary product of CY activation, which is then metabolized intracellularly to the active alkylating agent phosphoramide mustard. Studies in a rodent model of AML showed that incubation of mixtures of leukemic and normal marrow cells with graded concentrations of 4HC eliminated tumor cells yet spared normal hematopoietic stem cells and suggested the feasibility of this method in clinical autologous BMT (74).

Of practical importance is the fact that the enzyme aldehyde dehydrogenase inactivates CY metabolism by converting the intermediate aldophosphamide to the inactive compound carboxyphosphamide rather than to phosphoramide mustard. Erythrocytes have substantial levels of aldehyde dehydrogenase, and contamination of the marrow cell suspension by excess erythrocytes may interfere with the effectiveness of 4HC or mafosfamide treatment (75). Standardization of the red-cell content of the marrow graft or separation of marrow mononuclear cells to provide an erythrocyte-free cell suspension are important considerations in the consistent processing of autologous marrow cells in clinical trials (see Chapter 14).

Most clinical trials of autologous BMT with chemically purged marrow in the United States used 4HC, whereas those in Europe used mafosfamide. Several European studies with mafosfamide used individualized drug incubation concentrations, designed to spare approximately 5% of normal committed hematopoietic progenitors (CFC-GM) based on a preincubation dose-response sensitivity of each patient's marrow CFC-GM to the mafosfamide (76,77). Dose adjustment of the mafosfamide concentration with which autologous marrow suspensions are treated may be associated with a significantly lower risk of relapse in patients transplanted for first-remission AML (29,78), although effects on disease-free survival have not been clearly evident. In the case of 4HC, there has been a more consistent usage of the same drug incubation concentration for each patient, despite the known interpatient differences in the 4HC sensitivity of committed progenitor cell populations (79), and individualized 4HC incubation regimens have not been evaluated.

In Relapse

As with unpurged autologous BMT, the initial experiences with chemically purged autologous BMT for fully relapsed AML showed a high likelihood of tumor clearance but no sustained relapse-free survival (77,80,81); nevertheless, these studies demonstrated that hematological reconstitution could occur after infusion of remission marrow treated ex vivo with mafosfamide (see Table 54-3). Unlike allogeneic BMT for AML in early first relapse (i.e., less than 30% blasts in the marrow), which may provide relapse-free survival comparable to BMT in second remission, autologous BMT for AML in early relapse with cryopreserved 4HC-treated remission marrow has not

Table 54-4.
Autologous Transplantation with Marrow Treated Ex Vivo for Acute Myeloid Leukemia in First Remission

Preparative Regimen[a]	*No. Patients*	*Median Age (yr) (Range)*	*Median Duration of CR at BMT (mo) (Range)*	*Marrow Purging*	*No. BMT-related Deaths*	*No. Relapses*	*Median Time to Relapse (mo) (Range)*	*Actuarial Relapse Rate (%)*	*No. Relapse-free Survivors*	*Median Duration of Relapse-free Survival (mo) (Range)*	*Actuarial Relapse-free Survival (%)*	*Author, Year, Ref*
TACC	18	23.7 (3–44)	NR	Mafosfamide	5	5	8 (4–18.5)	NR	8	Approximately 8+ (2.5+ to 60+)	NR	Cahn et al. 1986 (85)
CY/TBI	9	39 (30–44)	5+ (2+ to 23+)	Mafosfamide	3	1	3	NR	5	26+ (8+ to 27+)	NR	Gorin et al. 1986 (77)
	22	35 (17–50)	4+ (2+ to 6+)	Mafosfamide	1	7	3.5 (0–9)	36	14	31+	61	Körbling et al. 1989 (84)
BUCY200	48	25 (4–56)	2.5+ (1.5+ to 15+)	4HC	6	19	6 (3–18)	49	23	18+ (1+ to 132+)	41	This publication
CY/VP16/TBI	4	32 (22–45)	2+ (1+ to 3+)	4HC + VP16	0	2	NR	NR	2	14+, 33+	NR	Gulati et al. 1989 (89)
CY/TBI	7	43 (34–46)	10+ (6+ to 14+)	MoAbs αCD14 αCD15	0	3	10, 16, 22	49	4	24+ (12+ to 50+)	51	Ball et al. 1992 (35)
BAVC	6	19 (5–37)	3+ (2+ to 7+)	MoAb αCD15	1	2	8, 9	NR	3	35+, 35+, 47+	NR	deFabritiis et al. 1989 (92)

[a]For descriptions of preparative regimens, see text and original references.
ER1 = first (early) relapse; CR = complete remission; NR = not reported; 4HC = 4-hydroperoxycyclophosphamide; MoAb = monoclonal antibody.

been encouraging; some patients did not attain remission, and the relapse rate was high (36). Other approaches to increase the antitumor effectiveness and decrease post-transplant relapses, such as more intensive pretransplant conditioning regimens, combination ex vivo purging techniques, or post-transplant immunotherapy, may be useful in this group of high-risk AML patients.

In Second or Subsequent Remission

Some early reports of autologous BMT with mafosfamide-purged marrow for AML in second or later remission were not encouraging (77,80,81), leading at least one group to conclude that autologous BMT with chemically purged marrow was of little value in patients with poor-risk leukemias (see Table 54-3). However, a report from The Johns Hopkins Oncology Center in 1986 suggested that long-term relapse-free survival could be achieved in patients with second or third remission AML given autologous BMT with 4HC-treated marrow after BU/CY conditioning (33). The incubation concentration of 4HC (100 μg/mL) was based on phase I dose escalation trials from that institution (82). An update of this series shows long-term relapse-free survival in 9 patients (all with remission inversions), for an actuarial relapse-free survival of 32% and an actuarial relapse rate of 50% (83). Similar results have subsequently been reported in 30 patients with AML in second or subsequent remission who received mafosfamide-purged autologous BMT and a CY/TBI preparative regimen (84). In this series, the actuarial relapse rate was 65%, and the relapse-free survival was 34%, with remission inversions in 11 of 14 patients.

Current results of autologous BMT with 4HC-treated marrow at The Johns Hopkins Oncology Center include 98 patients with AML (82 in second and 16 in third remission). Twenty-one patients (15 in second and 6 in third remission) died with transplant-related complications, mostly sepsis during aplasia or hepatic veno-occlusive disease. Forty-three patients (38 second and 5 third remission) relapsed at a median of 6 months (range, 2–23 mo) after BMT; the actuarial relapse rate was 58% for second and 55% for third remission (Figure 54-2A). Thirty-four patients (29 in second and 5 in third remission) were alive without relapse at a median of 46+ months (range, 0.5+ to 106+ mo) after autologous BMT; the disease-free survival was 30% for second and 27% for third remission (Figure 54-2B). Twenty-six of these patients have had remission inversions, compared with only 2 of the 43 who relapsed. Unlike allogeneic BMT, for which the risk of leukemic relapse increases with later remission numbers, the actuarial relapse rates in The Johns Hopkins Oncology Center series were not significantly different for patients given autologous BMT with 4HC-treated marrow in first versus later remissions.

In First Remission

Although the therapeutic role of autologous BMT with purged marrow for AML in second or subsequent remission appears to be more firmly established by the studies described, its application in first remission is less well defined (see Table 54-4). Some pilot studies of autologous BMT with chemically purged marrow included patients with first-remission AML, but with a few exceptions (77) there was no evidence that these patients were selected for BMT in first remission because of being at an especially high risk for relapse. Trials with mafosfamide purging and either a CY/TBI or a TACC chemotherapy regimen showed relapse rates of 30 to 50% and relapse-free survivals of 45 to 60% (77, 84,85). In at least one of these series, the relapse rate after autologous BMT in first remission was not

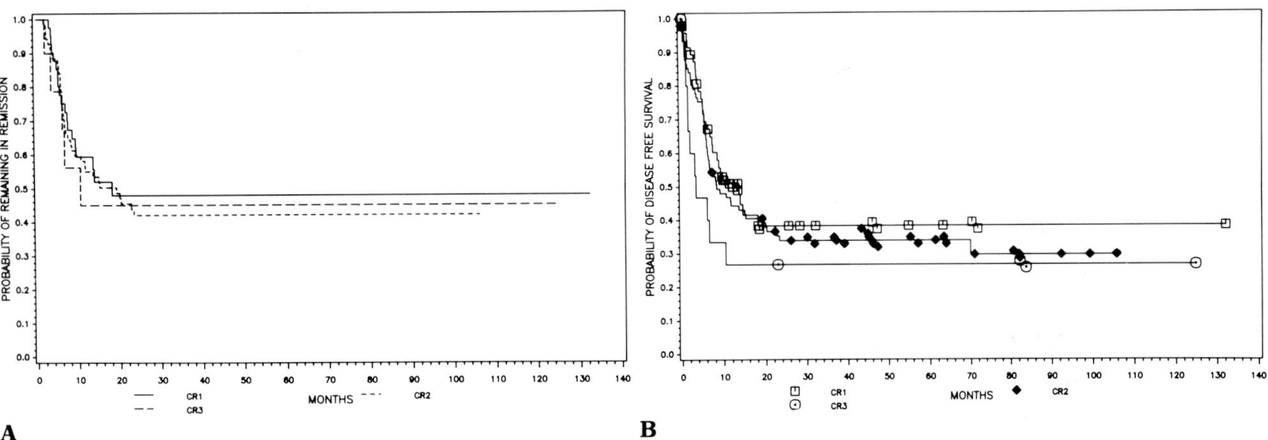

Figure 54-2. Probability of remaining in remission (A) and disease-free survival (B) for 146 patients with acute myeloid leukemia in first remission (48 patients; *open squares*), second remission (82 patients; *solid diamonds*), or third remission (16 patients; *open circles*) transplanted with 4-hydroperoxycyclophosphamide–purged marrow and a busulfan/cyclophosphamide preparative regimen. Individual living patients are indicated by the symbols.

significantly different from that observed in patients transplanted with mafosfamide-treated marrow for second or later remission (84). As with autologous BMT using unpurged marrow, interpretation of the results of autologous BMT with mafosfamide-purged marrow for first-remission AML is problematic; there were no discernible pretransplant factors to identify whether any of these first-remission patients were at especially high risk for relapse with conventional antileukemic chemotherapy alone.

Investigators at The Johns Hopkins Oncology Center carried out autologous BMT with a BU/CY preparative regimen and 4HC-treated marrow in 48 patients with first-remission AML, virtually all of whom had poor prognostic features (e.g., high leukocyte count at diagnosis, failure to attain remission with first-line induction chemotherapy, presence of extramedullary leukemia at diagnosis) and who were transplanted early in first remission (median, 2.5+ mo; range, 1.5+ to 15+ mo). Six patients died with transplant-related complications. Nineteen patients relapsed at a median of 6 months (range, 3–18 mo) after autologous BMT, for an actuarial relapse rate of 49% (see Figure 54-2A). Twenty-three patients remained in remission at a median of 18+ months (range, 1+ to 132+ mo) after BMT, for an actuarial relapse-free survival of 41% (Figure 54-2B). These data suggest that autologous BMT with chemically purged marrow can produce sustained relapse-free survival in relatively poor prognosis first-remission AML.

Retrospective analysis of data from the European Bone Marrow Transplant Group in 671 unpurged and mafosfamide-treated autologous BMT for first-remission AML (29,30) shows better disease-free survival (63 vs 34%) and significantly lower probability of relapse (23 vs 55%) in the recipients of chemically purged marrow who received preparative regimens that included TBI. These studies supported the advantage of marrow purging with mafosfamide in a group of relatively high-risk first-remission patients, (i.e., those whose time from diagnosis to first remission exceeded 40 days [indicative of potentially less sensitivity of leukemia to remission-induction chemotherapy] (30). Because time-censoring bias has been a concern in some reports of autologous BMT for AML, it is of note that this analysis also showed the advantage for purging to be most evident in patients transplanted within 6 months of remission (if anything, indicative of less in vivo tumor purging as a result of fewer cycles of chemotherapy). The plateau for continued remission occurred sooner in recipients of purged versus unpurged marrow, potentially incriminating the graft as a source of a few tumor cells that lead to disease recurrence despite an effective in vivo tumor purge by the intensive pretransplant chemoradiotherapy (30). This retrospective analysis did not explore fully the role of non-TBI regimens on relapse rate and disease-free survival, because a substantial number of the patients studied received one of several polychemotherapeutic pretransplant conditioning regimens.

Prolonged hematological recovery, especially of platelets, occurs in patients with AML given either mafosfamide- or 4HC-treated autologous BMT. The time to attain neutrophils in excess of 0.5×10^9/L and platelets exceeding 50×10^9/L are significantly longer in recipients of chemically purged autologous BMT for AML than observed after allogeneic or syngeneic BMT in similar groups of patients. However, similar delays in recovery of peripheral blood counts have been reported after autologous BMT with unpurged marrow for first-remission AML (54–56). In contrast, the kinetics of hematological reconstitution are more rapid in recipients of mafosfamide- or 4HC-treated autologous BMT for acute lymphoblastic leukemia (ALL) than for AML (86). These findings suggest that the prolonged marrow aplasia and hypoplasia after autologous BMT for AML may reflect damage to the marrow stem-cell compartment by the specific antileukemic chemotherapy and possibly an increased fragility of the stem-cell pool to cryopreservation in AML (86,87). Because there is a fairly close correlation between the residual CFC-GM content of the chemically purged marrow and the rate of hematological reconstitution, especially of neutrophils, (79,88), clinicians may anticipate the expected duration of aplasia and requirements for broad-spectrum antibiotics and transfusion support.

Combination Pharmacological Purging

In vitro studies have suggested that incubation of marrow with chemotherapeutic agents in addition to 4HC or mafosfamide may enhance cytotoxicity against neoplastic cells without substantially increased toxicity against hematopoietic progenitors (see Chapter 14), and post-transplant relapses have been correlated with relative resistance of occult leukemic cells to 4HC (27). One clinical trial examined autologous BMT with marrow treated ex vivo with 4HC plus VP16 (89); the concentration of 4HC (100 μmol/L) was approximately 35% of that used in the trial reported from The Johns Hopkins Oncology Center, and one of 2 VP16 concentrations (4.25 or 8.5 μmol/L) was used. The pretransplant conditioning regimen also included both CY and VP16, in addition to TBI. Hematological reconstitution was not substantially different from that seen after autologous BMT with 4HC- or mafosfamide-treated marrow. Two of 4 patients transplanted in first remission and 5 of 10 patients transplanted in second or third remission relapsed; there were 2 transplant-related deaths. Three patients in second or third remission and 2 in first remission were alive without relapse at a median of 28+ months (range, 14+ to 45+ mo) after autologous BMT. Although these results are encouraging in second- and third-remission patients, the relapse-free survival in this study, which uses a lower incubation concentration of 4HC, was not clearly superior to that observed in patients in similar remission given marrow treated with 4HC alone. Furthermore, complementary evaluation of marrows for leukemic colony growth and sensitivity to 4HC and

VP16 might have provided potentially instructive comparisons with sensitivity of normal progenitors and correlations with outcome.

Immunological Purging

Immunological purging of autologous marrow in AML has received attention as appropriate AML-specific monoclonal antibodies, which react with the CD14, CD15, and CD33 myeloid antigens commonly expressed on leukemic colony-forming cells but to a much lesser degree on primitive normal hematopoietic cells, have been developed (90) (see Table 54-3, 54-4). Most techniques relied on coincubation of marrow cells with monoclonal antibodies and complement. Other measures, such as pretreatment of cells with neuraminidase, may increase reactivity of leukemic blasts with some monoclonal antibodies, as shown with anti-CD15 (91). The initial trial of autologous BMT with marrows treated ex vivo with both anti-CD15 (PM-81) and anti-CD14 (AML-2-23) monoclonal antibodies and complement showed relapse-free survival in high-risk patients conditioned with a CY/TBI regimen (34). Prolonged thrombocytopenia was common but similar to that reported with both chemically purged and unpurged autologous BMT for AML. Another study reported treatment of autologous marrow with one anti-CD15 murine monoclonal antibody (S4-7) and complement and a BAVC preparative regimen. Six of 7 patients showed reasonably prompt hematological reconstitution, but there was one death during aplasia. Three patients remained in unmaintained first remission at 35, 35, and 47 months after BMT (92). Of interest was the finding that a substantial proportion of leukemic cells from 2 of the 3 patients who relapsed after BMT did not react against the anti-CD15 monoclonal antibody; although possibly indicative of an ineffective ex vivo purge of the autologous marrow, this finding could also be compatible with failure of eradication of residual (although heterogeneous with regard to antigen density and expression) leukemia in vivo by the pretransplant regimen. These clinical observations are consistent with in vitro studies demonstrating relative resistance to immunological purging of leukemic cells with low antigen density (93).

A multicenter report of autologous BMT with doubly immunopurged marrow (both anti-CD15 and anti-CD14 monoclonal antibodies) included 55 patients (7 in first remission, 36 in second remission, 7 in third remission, and 5 in first relapse); most were treated with CY/TBI or BU/CY (35). The relapse-free survival and actuarial relapse rate were 51 ± 10 and 49 ± 20%, respectively, in first-remission patients. For patients transplanted in second or third remission, the relapse-free survival and actuarial relapse rate were 30 ± 9 and 39 ± 8%, respectively; 11 of the 15 patients alive and in remission after BMT for second- or third-remission AML have shown inversions of remission duration, compared with only 1 of the 15 second/third-remission patients who relapsed. However, the first-remission transplants were carried out relatively late in remission (median duration of first remission, 10 mo; range, 6–14 mo), suggesting potential time-selection bias. Of interest is the observation, albeit in a small series, of attainment of second remission and sustained relapse-free survival in 3 of 5 patients transplanted in first relapse; other series of autologous BMT with purged or unpurged marrow have not reported sustained relapse-free survival in these groups of patients.

A third study by investigators at The Dana Farber Cancer Institute recently carried out autologous BMT with anti-CD33 (anti-My9) purging of marrow in 12 patients with AML (10 in second remission); this monoclonal antibody reacts with malignant cells from most patients with AML, as well as some committed (e.g., BFU-E, CFC-GM) and pluripotential (CFU-GEMM) normal hematopoietic progenitors. Seven patients relapsed at a median of 8 months (range, 3–17 mo) after BMT, and 5 patients were in unmaintained remissions at a median of 12+ months (range, 1+ to 33+ mo), for a disease-free survival of 29%, similar to that seen after autologous BMT with two-antibody–treated or chemically purged marrow (94).

These studies demonstrate that autologous BMT with immunologically purged marrow can provide relapse-free survival that is comparable but not superior to, that observed after chemically purged marrow in second- and perhaps later-remission AML. However, the data are too limited at this time to support routinely autologous BMT with immunologically purged marrow for first-remission AML.

Immunotoxins are produced by linking a monoclonal antibody to a cytotoxin, such as ricin A, and may be used to provide targeted toxin delivery to cells reacting with the monoclonal antibody. Immunotoxins have been developed in which ricin has been linked to the anti-CD13 monoclonal antibodies AML-2-23 and MCS-2 (95). Preclinical evaluation indicates that these immunotoxins are highly active against myeloblasts from patients with AML, and these agents may be clinically useful for ex vivo marrow treatment and possibly for in vivo treatment to decrease minimal residual leukemia. As yet, however, there are no clinical trials of autologous BMT with immunotoxin-purged marrow in AML.

Autologous Transplantation with Long-term Cultured Marrow

Long-term cultures of leukemic marrow cells on marrow-derived stromal layers allow proliferation of pluripotential hematopoietic stem cells and suppress the growth of neoplastic cells (96,97). Normal stem cells derived from long-term leukemic marrow cultures in murine lymphoblastic leukemia have established normal hematopoiesis without leukemic recurrence in lethally irradiated allogeneic or syngeneic recipients (96). The first application of this technique in 1986 was associated with an 8-month remission in a patient with first relapse of AML (98).

Autologous BMT with long-term cultured marrow in patients with relapsed leukemia or myelodysplasia has shown disappointingly high relapse rates (99). The best results of rescue with long-term cultured cells has been observed in patients transplanted for AML in first remission; of 15 patients thus treated, the relapse rate was low (one patient), and 12 patients were alive and free of relapse at a median of approximately 12+ months (range, 2+ to 60+ mo) after BMT, for a disease-free survival of approximately 75% (99,100). Hematopoietic recovery was substantially slower than observed after autologous BMT with unpurged or chemically purged marrow.

In contrast to its potential utility for autologous BMT with positively selected stem cells in CML (101,102), long-term marrow cultures for autologous stem-cell transplantation appear to be of little (if any) value in relapsed or recurrent AML, and its use in first-remission patients is not clear. Whereas autologous BMT with long-term cultured marrow has been carried out in first remission AML, there has been no evidence of any factors indicating this to be a population at high risk for relapse with conventional chemotherapy. The technique itself is labor- and equipment-intensive; the large-scale marrow culture system for the first patient treated required 60 800-mL culture flasks incubated for 10 days. The long durations of marrow hypoplasia and relatively high incidence of graft failure in these single-institution trials raise additional questions about the applicability of this technique.

Autologous Transplantation with Peripheral Blood Stem Cells

Under steady-state conditions, hematopoietic stem cells and primitive progenitors are found with relatively low frequency in the peripheral circulation (103); various methods may be used to increase the percentage of these primitive peripheral blood stem cells and then collect these cells by several aphereses. Peripheral blood stem cells have successfully reconstituted hematopoiesis after intensive myeloablative therapy in patients with lymphomas and other solid tumors. A theoretical advantage to this procedure over autologous marrow collection may be the collection of fewer contaminating leukemic blasts (if carried out in remission); clearly, apheresis procedures do not expose patients to the risks, albeit small, of anaesthesia required for marrow collection. As reviewed by Körbling (104), the possibility that peripheral blood cell collections have fewer contaminating tumor cells for autologous transplantation may be balanced or outweighed by the possible mobilization of tumor cells by the techniques used (e.g., chemotherapy, cytokines) to mobilize marrow-derived stem cells. Initial studies have shown the feasibility of collection and infusion of autologous peripheral blood stem cells in patients with AML (105–107).

Transplantation of autologous peripheral blood stem cells for first-remission AML has shown prompt hematological reconstitution (within 2 to 4 weeks), shorter hospitalizations, and relapse-free survival of 20 to 40% (104,108–110). A retrospective analysis of data from the European Bone Marrow Transplant Group suggested similar relapse rates and disease-free survival between recipients of peripheral blood stem cells or autologous BMT (purged or unpurged) for first-remission AML (111), similar to results of a single-center nonrandomized comparison of autologous BMT with mafosfamide-purged marrow versus untreated peripheral blood stem cells (104). Although the 2-year relapse-free survival was not significantly different between the 2 groups (51% in the BMT group vs 35% in the peripheral blood cell group), there was a trend in favor of the BMT group, with evidence of a plateau in relapse-free survival (104).

Additional prospective studies of transplantation of autologous peripheral blood stem cells for AML in first remission are justified and may also be worthy of study in later remissions. The issue of mobilization of leukemic cells along with stem cells during the apheresis procedures, the minimal and optimal numbers of peripheral blood stem cells to be collected, and the number of aphereses needed to collect the requisite number of cells are unanswered questions at this time. Whether addition of peripheral blood stem cells to autologous BMT will enhance the rate of hematopoietic recovery without jeopardizing antileukemic effect is also unknown; a prospective randomized study in recipients of autologous BMT for solid tumors has shown that this approach does not hasten hematological reconstitution (112). Finally, it is not clear whether methods for purging with immunological or pharmacological agents to eradicate occult leukemic cells, as is currently used for bone marrow, will be applicable, safe, or useful in treatment of autologous peripheral blood stem cells.

Comparative Trials of Autologous BMT

Retrospective analyses of patients in the first remission of AML receiving chemotherapy, allogeneic, or autologous BMT have suggested that BMT patients fare better, especially after allogeneic BMT, than recipients of conventional treatment only (113,114). Retrospective reviews are confounded by a multiplicity of preparative regimens and, quite probably, selection and time-censoring biases. Appreciation and clarification of the role of autologous BMT for first-remission AML may best be made through prospective (ideally, randomized) trials that compare the effectiveness of autologous BMT with chemotherapy. The comparison between autologous and allogeneic BMT may be of interest, especially with regard to disease-free survival, because the higher relapse rate seen after autologous BMT may balance the higher risk of mortality from allogeneic BMT (e.g., GVHD, interstitial pneumonitis). However, as discussed, comparison of relapse rates after autologous and allogeneic BMT may be problematic; the allogeneic GVL effect may influence this measure of antileukemic effectiveness.

Obviously, allogeneic BMT arms in comparative trials are not truly randomly assigned but have the "biological randomization" of having a histocompatible-related donor.

Several European prospective trials have compared autologous BMT with unpurged marrow versus allogeneic BMT, and a few have included a third conventional chemotherapy arm. Substantial losses of patients between the remission induction and BMT steps have been observed (40,114,115); at least 2 prospective trials lost 40 to 50% of potentially eligible autologous BMT patients because of inadequate marrow collection, relapse before BMT, refusal to participate, or medical co-morbidity (40,115). These studies have shown lower relapse-free survival and higher relapse rates among the autologous BMT recipients than after allogeneic BMT, although these differences were not consistently statistically significant. One study suggested that either autologous or allogeneic BMT was superior to conventional chemotherapy alone, in which the relapse-free survival was less than 10%; however, this study did not include formal randomization to the chemotherapy arm (115). Furthermore, analysis of data on an intention-to-treat basis showed significant differences in disease-free survival in favor of allogeneic BMT, largely related to a higher procedure-related mortality in the autologous BMT group and to the fact that a number of patients randomized to autologous BMT relapsed before transplantation was carried out (40).

Two prospective studies, one in adults and one in children, are worthy of consideration. The Bordeaux-Grenoble-Marseilles-Toulouse (BGMT) group compared the outcome in adults with AML treated with conventional chemotherapy, allogeneic BMT, or unpurged double autologous BMT with high-dose melphalan in a prospective controlled trial (114,116). The best outcome (relapse rate, 18%; disease-free survival, 66%) was among the allograft recipients, with an intermediate relapse rate and disease-free survival (50 and 41%, respectively) in the autologous BMT patients, and with the highest relapse rate (83%) and lowest disease-free survival (16%) in the chemotherapy recipients (114,116). Interpretation of this study is somewhat clouded because additional conventional-dose antileukemic chemotherapy was given between the 2 autologous BMTs. A cooperative Italian prospective study compared outcome in 98 children with AML who attained remission with the same induction-consolidation regimens and then received allogeneic BMT from HLA-compatible donors after CY/TBI (18 patients) or randomization to autologous BMT with unpurged marrow after BAVC regimen (32 patients) or conventional chemotherapy (32 patients). The 2-year disease-free survival after allogeneic BMT (76%) was superior to that of autologous BMT recipients (31%) or chemotherapy alone (12%). Sixteen patients (17%) were not evaluable because of protocol or randomization violations, and an intention-to-treat analysis was not presented (117).

Although techniques for and clinical trials of autologous BMT with unpurged or chemically purged marrow have been developed, the application of more intensive combination chemotherapy regimens, sometimes with newer agents or higher doses of more commonly used drugs, have shown impressive effects on relapse rate and relapse-free survival in newly diagnosed patients with AML (118,119). Several prospective trials have suggested an advantage for allogeneic BMT over conventional chemotherapy only (120–122), but the role of autologous BMT for first-remission AML is still controversial. To determine whether autologous BMT with chemically purged marrow for first-remission AML is superior to the results of chemotherapy alone, prospective multicenter North American trials are being conducted in both adults and children. Preliminary analyses of these trials suggest that autologous BMT is clearly no worse, and may be somewhat better, than chemotherapy alone in providing long-term relapse-free survival in patients with AML (17), and in adults may provide relapse-free survival comparable to that seen after allogeneic BMT from a histocompatible-related donor (16).

Future Directions

Post-transplant relapse remains the major therapeutic challenge in autologous BMT for AML. That relapse may be due to tumor cells in the marrow graft, residual AML in vivo, or both, dictates several possible approaches to reduce postautograft recurrence of AML.

Ex Vivo Autograft Treatment

More intensive ex vivo treatment of marrow to eliminate occult tumor cells from the cell suspension is supported by the observed correlations between in vitro sensitivity to 4HC of leukemic cell colonies and lower relapse rates and better disease-free survival in recipients of 4HC-treated marrow (27); this topic is discussed in detail elsewhere (see Chapter 14). For example, the addition of vincristine and methylprednisolone to ex vivo purging with 4HC substantially increases cytotoxicity against leukemic cells without much additional toxicity to committed hematopoietic progenitors in vitro (123,124). This triple-drug combination has had limited but encouraging use in patients autografted for AML in early relapse and appears to allow satisfactory hematopoietic reconstitution (124); application of this combination-agent purging in remission AML has as not yet been studied.

Preclinical studies have shown that combined treatment with monoclonal antibodies or immunotoxins and one (e.g., mafosfamide or 4HC) (125–128) or 2 (e.g., 4HC and VP16; VP16 and cytosine arabinoside) chemotherapeutic agents (129,130) provides at least additive antileukemic effects without undue toxicity to normal hematopoietic cells. These represent yet other avenues for investigation in optimizing antileukemic effects and sparing of stem cells in clinical purging of autologous marrow grafts. Especially in relapsed leukemia, the issue of multidrug resistance must be considered. An intriguing study has shown that multidrug-resistant neoplastic cell lines and leukemic blasts can be lysed with complement and a monoclonal antibody directed against P-glycoprotein, the cell-surface product of the multiple drug resistance (MDR) gene; incubation with VP16 led to further decreases in tumor cells (131). Although there was no appreciable toxicity of the monoclonal antibody toward committed hematopoietic progenitors (i.e., CFC-GM, CFU-GEMM, BFU-E), the combination of VP16 and monoclonal antibody led to approximately a 2-log reduction. It is not known whether processing of autografts by these combined immunopharmacological methods to remove drug-resistant cells will adversely affect engraftment by eradication of more primitive hematopoietic precursors; the finding of MDR gene expression in primitive human hematopoietic cells (including long-term culture-initiating cells) (132) supports this concern.

Stem-cell Selection

An alternative to ex vivo marrow treatment, which is designed to eliminate occult tumor cells by a process of "negative selection," the purification of primitive hematopoietic repopulating cells (stem cells) from the marrow graft ("positive selection") may be considered (133). The CD34 antigen identifies a population of primitive hemopoietic cells that are present with very low frequency in the marrow and peripheral blood but may increase after stem-cell mobilization techniques such as chemotherapy and cytokines. The feasibility of hematological reconstitution by transplantation of CD34-positive cells after intensive myelosuppressive therapy has been demonstrated in preclinical studies (134) and in limited clinical trials in patients with solid tumors (113). Identification of cells bearing CD34 but not HLA-DR antigens may therefore define a population of very primitive stem cells that provides hematopoietic reconstitution after transplantation into autologous recipients; this approach has been suggested in autologous BMT for CML (111,135). The CD34-positive selection methods may have limited application in autologous BMT for AML, because CD34 is expressed on malignant cells from at least some patients with AML (136).

Pretransplant Conditioning Regimens

Development of more effective in vivo cytoreductive preparative regimens to eradicate residual leukemia in the patient is another approach to decreasing relapse rates after autologous BMT. Readers are directed to Chapters 8 and 9 for a more detailed discussion of principles, choices, and toxicities of pretransplant conditioning regimens.

Most autologous BMT in the leukemias have been carried out with the same regimens (e.g., CY/TBI, BU/CY) that were developed and found to be effective in allowing engraftment and relapse-free survival in allogeneic BMT recipients. Regimens such as VP16 and TBI (137); cytosine arabinoside and TBI (138); and addition of VP16 (139), melphalan (140), or TBI (141) to BU and CY are effective for allogeneic BMT and may be useful in autologous BMT for AML. Limited preliminary studies of high-dose CY, cytosine arabinoside, and VP16 before autologous BMT for first-remission AML are encouraging (142).

Allogeneic BMT conditioning regimens include intensive immunosuppression to prevent graft rejection by host immune mechanisms, but regimens for autologous BMT do not require immunosuppressive properties. For example, the BAVC, BACCT, and TACC regimens are all less immunosuppressive than BU/CY or CY/TBI; at least one small nonrandomized study found similar disease-free survival in patients with first-remission AML given unpurged autologous BMT after either CY/TBI or BAVC (143). Newer and probably minimally immunosuppressive regimens for autologous BMT in AML include VP16 and BU (144). The challenge is to increase the in vivo antileukemic "purge" without unacceptable extramedullary toxicity.

Immunotherapeutic Approaches After Autologous BMT

Immune-mediated elimination of residual leukemic cells is demonstrated by the GVL effect in allogeneic BMT settings, but GVL is not operative in conventional syngeneic or autologous BMT. Humoral modulation of antileukemic effect is supported by preclinical studies in which post-transplant administration of a monoclonal antibody specific for AML antigens prevents leukemic relapses in a rodent model of minimal residual AML without adversely affecting kinetics of engraftment by normal cells (145). Post-transplant passive immunotherapy may therefore be a relatively simple method to reduce relapses after autologous BMT, but no clinical trials have been conducted. Selection of appropriate monoclonal antibodies for such trials, as well as the purification, timing, and dosage of administration of monoclonal antibody after transplant, are all controversial aspects of this therapeutic approach.

Administration of interleukin-2 (IL-2) and lymphokine-activated killer (LAK) cells has been associated with tumor regressions in patients with refractory malignancies, and preclinical studies have shown that transplantation of IL-2–activated syngeneic marrow is curative in rodent models of AML (146,147). Infusion of IL-2 at tolerable dosage levels is associated with increased LAK cells (148,149), interferon-γ, and tumor necrosis factor, and may actually enhance the rate of hematopoietic recovery (150). A preliminary report in 8 patients with AML in remission or relapse treated with a 21-day course of IL-2 after hematological reconstitution following autologous BMT suggests that this approach may be associated with decreased relapse rates (149). A longer course (90 days) of lower-dose IL-2 appears to be tolerated in patients receiving T-cell–depleted allografts and autografts for lymphoid malignancies (151) but has not been evaluated in patients receiving autologous BMT for AML. Interferon α-2B (IF-α2B), which has some immunomodulatory effects in allogeneic BMT (152), is also myelosuppressive; no large-scale trials have studied IF-α2B after autologous BMT for AML, and the possible inhibitory effects on normal hematopoiesis may limit its usefulness.

The antineoplastic effects of host cellular immunity are supported by the observations of lower relapse rates in patients in whom clinically apparent GVHD develops after allogeneic BMT for AML (12,153,154). Immunological GVL effects may be operative against neoplastic cells that bear Ia (class II) antigens on the cell surface (155–157). The recent description of mild, generally self-limited cutaneous GVH-like reactions in patients given short-course cyclosporine (CSP) after autologous BMT with unpurged or chemically purged marrow for the treatment of AML (158,159) suggests that this technique may be used to induce an immunological GVL effect in recipients of autologous BMT (and, perhaps, syngeneic BMT as well). Rodent studies and limited clinical observations indicate that autologous GVH reactions are associated with the development of anti-Ia cytotoxic T lymphocytes (160,161) and have an antitumor effect against Ia-positive myeloma in a rodent model (155). Whether the disrupted immunoregulation observed in patients in whom autologous GVHD develops after CSP is associated with an autograft-versus-tumor effect as well is unknown at this time. Cellular expression of Ia antigen may be increased by administration of agents such as interferon (155,162) to enhance the antitumor effects of CSP-induced autologous GVHD.

References

1. Kurnick NB, Montano A, Gerdes JC, Feder BH. Preliminary observations on the treatment of postirradiation hematopoietic depression in man by the infusion of stored autogenous bone marrow. Ann Intern Med 1958;49:973–986.
2. McFarland W, Granville NB, Dameshek W. Autologous bone marrow infusion as an adjunct in therapy of malignant disease. Blood 1959;14:503–521.
3. Clifford P, Clift RA, Duff JK. Nitrogen-mustard therapy combined with autologous marrow infusion. Lancet 1961;1:687–690.
4. Buckner CD, Rudolph RH, Fefer A, et al. High-dose cyclophosphamide therapy for malignant disease. Cancer 1972;29:357–365.
5. Buckner CD, Clift RA, Fefer A, Neiman PE, Storb R, Thomas ED. Treatment of blastic transformation of chronic granulocytic leukemia by high dose cyclophosphamide, total body irradiation and infusion of cryopreserved autologous marrow. Exp Hematol 1974;2:138–146.
6. Fefer A, Cheever MA, Thomas ED, et al. Bone marrow transplantation for refractory acute leukemia in 34 patients with identical twins. Blood 1981;57:421–430.
7. Gorin NC, Stachowiak J, Hirsch-Marie F, et al. Greffe de moelle autologue après aplasie thérapeutique définitive entraînant une rémission complète dans un cas de leucémie aiguë myéloblastique chimiorésistante. Nouv Presse Med 1977;6:2741–2745.
8. Gorin NC, Najman A, Duhamel G. Autologous bone marrow transplantation in acute myelocytic leukaemia. Lancet 1977;1:1050.
9. Gorin NC, Gale RP, Armitage JO. Autologous bone marrow transplants: different indications in Europe and North America. Lancet 1989;2:317–318.
10. Powles R, Treleaven J, Millar J, et al. How do allogeneic bone marrow transplants cure leukaemia? The role of graft versus host disease. Bone Marrow Transplant 1991;7(suppl 2):9–10.
11. Slavin S, Ackerstein A, Naparstek E, Or R, Weiss L. The graft-versus-leukemia (GVL) phenomenon: is GVL separable from GVHD? Bone Marrow Transplant 1990; 6:155–161.
12. Brenner MK, Heslop HE. Graft-versus-leukaemia effects after marrow transplantation in man. Bailliere's Clin Haematol 1991;4:727–749.
13. Kersey JH, Weisdorf D, Nesbit ME, et al. Comparison of autologous and allogeneic bone marrow transplantation for treatment of high-risk refractory acute lymphoblastic leukemia. N Engl J Med 1987;317:461–467.
14. Gale RP, Butturini A. Autotransplants in leukemia. Lancet 1989;2:315–317.
15. Linch DC, Burnett AK. Clinical studies of ABMT in acute myeloid leukemia. Clin Haematol 1986;15:167–186.
16. Cassileth PA, Anderson J, Lazarus HM, et al. An ECOG trial of autologous bone marrow transplantation (AUTOBMT) in first remission (CR) of acute myeloid leukemia (AML) (abstract no. 2117). Blood 1990; 76(suppl 1):532a.
17. Ravindranath Y, Yeager A, Krischer J, et al. Intensive consolidation chemotherapy (ICC) vs. purged autologous bone marrow transplantation (ABMT) early in remission for treatment of childhood acute myeloid leukemia (AML): preliminary results of Pediatric Oncology Group (POG) Study 8821 (abstract). Proc ASCO 1992;11:283.
18. Gale RP, Armitage JO, Butturini A. Is there a role for autotransplants in acute leukemia? Bone Marrow Transplant 1989;4:217–219.
19. Gale RP, Horowitz MM, Butturini A. Autotransplants in acute leukemia. Br J Haematol 1991;78:135–137.
20. Keating A. Is marrow purging necessary or clinically useful? Bone Marrow Transplant 1991;7(suppl 1):61–65.
21. Gray R, Wheatley K. How to avoid bias when comparing bone marrow transplantation with chemotherapy. Bone Marrow Transplant 1991;7(suppl 3):9–12.
22. Schultz FW, Martens ACM, Hagenbeek A. The contribution of residual leukemic cells in the graft to leukemia relapse after autologous bone marrow transplantation: mathematical considerations. Leukemia 1989;3:530–534.
23. Hagenbeek A, Martens ACM. Toxocity of ASTA Z 7557 (INN mafosfamide) to normal and leukemic stem cells: implications for autologous bone marrow transplantation. Invest New Drugs 1984;2:237–243.
24. Hagenbeek A, Martens ACM. Reinfusion of leukemic cells with the autologous marrow graft: preclinical studies on lodging and regrowth of leukemia. Leuk Res 1985;9:1389–1395.

25. Hagenbeek A, Martens ACM. On the fate of leukemic cells infused with the autologous marrow graft. Haematol Bluttransfus 1987;30:553–559.
26. Hagenbeek A, Martens ACM. Cryopreservation of autologous marrow grafts in acute leukemia: survival of in vivo clonogenic leukemic cells and normal hemopoietic stem cells. Leukemia 1989;3:535–537.
27. Miller CB, Zehnbauer BA, Piantadosi S, Rowley SD, Jones RJ. Correlation of occult clonogenic leukemia drug sensitivity with relapse after autologous bone marrow transplantation. Blood 1991;78:1125–1131.
28. Rowley SD, Jones RJ, Piantadosi S, et al. Efficacy of ex vivo purging for autologous bone marrow transplantation in the treatment of acute nonlymphoblastic leukemia. Blood 1989;74:501–506.
29. Gorin NC, Aegerter P, Auvert B, et al. Autologous bone marrow transplantation for acute myelocytic leukemia in first remission: a European survey of the role of marrow purging. Blood 1990;75:1606–1614.
30. Gorin NC, Labopin M., Meloni G, et al. Autologous bone marrow transplantation for acute myeloblastic leukemia in Europe: further evidence of the role of marrow purging by mafosfamide. Leukemia 1991;5:896–904.
31. Cornetta K, Moen RC, Culver K, et al. Amphotropic murine leukemia retrovirus is not an acute pathogen for primates. Hum Gene Ther 1990;1:15–30.
32. Brenner M, Mirro J Jr, Hurwitz C, et al. Autologous bone marrow transplant for children with AML in first complete remission: use of marker genes to investigate the biology of marrow reconstitution and the mechanism of relapse. Hum Gene Ther 1991;2:137–159.
33. Yeager AM, Kaizer H, Santos GW, et al. Autologous bone marrow transplantation in patients with acute nonlymphocytic leukemia, using ex vivo marrow treatment with 4-hydroperoxycyclophosphamide. N Engl J Med 1986;315:141–147.
34. Ball ED, Mills LE, Coughlin CT, Beck JR, Cornwell GG III. Autologous bone marrow transplantation in acute myelogenous leukemia: in vitro treatment with myeloid cell-specific monoclonal antibodies. Blood 1986;68: 1311–1315.
35. Ball ED, Mills L, Hurd D, McMillan R, Gingrich R. Autologous bone marrow transplantation for acute myeloid leukemia using monoclonal antibody-purged bone marrow. Prog Clin Biol Res 1992;377:97–111.
36. Rosenfeld C, Shadduck RK, Przepiorka D, Mangan KF, Colvin M. Autologous bone marrow transplantation with 4-hydroperoxycyclophosphamide purged marrows for acute nonlymphocytic leukemia in late remission or early relapse. Blood 1989;74:1159–1164.
37. Meloni G, de Fabritiis P, Petti MC, Mandelli F. BAVC regimen and autologous bone marrow transplantation in patients with acute myelogenous leukemia in second remission. Blood 1990;75:2282–2285.
38. Chopra R, Goldstone AH, McMillan AK, et al. Successful treatment of acute myeloid leukemia beyond first remission with autologous bone marrow transplantation using busulfan/cyclophosphamide and unpurged marrow: the British Autograft Group experience. J Clin Oncol 1991;9:1840–1847.
39. Schouten HC, van Putten WLJ, Hagemeijer A, et al. The prognostic significance of chromosomal findings in patients with acute myeloid leukemia in a study comparing the efficacy of autologous and allogeneic bone marrow transplantation. Bone Marrow Transplant 1991;8:377–381.
40. Ferrant A, Doyen C, Delannoy A, et al. Allogeneic or autologous bone marrow transplantation for acute nonlymphocytic leukemia in first remission. Bone Marrow Transplant 1991;7:303–309.
41. Geller RB, Vogelsang GB, Wingard JR, et al. Successful marrow transplantation for acute myelocytic leukemia following therapy for Hodgkin's disease. J Clin Oncol 1988;6:1558–1561.
42. Dicke KA, Zander AR, Spitzer G, et al. Autologous bone marrow transplantation in relapsed adult acute leukemia. Exp Hematol 1979;7(suppl 5):170–187.
43. Zander AR, Verma DS, Spitzer G, et al. Autologous bone marrow transplantation in acute leukemia. Int J Radiat Oncol Biol Phys 1979;5:1709–1710.
44. Gorin NC. Autologous bone marrow transplantation for acute leukemia in Europe. Exp Hematol 1984;12(suppl 15):123–125.
45. Hervé P, Rozenbaum A, Plouvier E, et al. Autologous bone marrow transplantation in acute myeloid leukemia in relapse or in complete remission. Cancer Treat Rep 1982;66:1983–1985.
46. Gorin NC. Autologous bone marrow transplantation in acute non-lymphocytic leukemia. Blood Transfus Immunohematol 1985;28:463–475.
47. Meloni G, de Fabritiis P, Papa G, et al. Cryopreserved autologous bone marrow infusion following high dose chemotherapy in patients with acute myeloblastic leukemia in first relapse. Leuk Res 1985;9:407–412.
48. Maraninchi D, Mascret B, Gastaut JE, et al. Bone marrow transplantation strategies in acute leukaemia. Lancet 1984;2:1401.
49. Maraninchi D, Gastaut JA, Hervé P, et al. High dose melphalan and autologous marrow transplantation in acute leukemias in relapse or remission. Exp Hematol 1984;12(suppl 15):130–131.
50. Goldstone AH, Anderson CC, Linch DC, et al. Autologous bone marrow transplantation following high dose chemotherapy for the treatment of adult patients with acute myeloid leukaemia. Br J Haematol 1986;64:529–537.
51. Meloni G, de Fabritiis P, Pulsoni A, Sandrelli A, Simone F, Mandelli F. Acute myelogenous leukemia in first relapse treated with two consecutive autologous bone marrow transplantations: a pilot study. Eur J Haematol 1989;42:441–444.
52. Spinolo JA, Dicke KA, Horwitz LJ, et al. High dose chemotherapy and unpurged autologous bone marrow transplantation for acute leukaemia in second or subsequent remission. Cancer 1990;66:619–626.
53. Gorin NC, Hervé P, Aegerter P, et al. Autologous bone marrow transplantation for acute leukaemia in remission. Br J Haematol 1986;64:385–395.
54. Burnett AK, Tansey P, Watkins R, et al. Transplantation of unpurged autologous bone marrow in acute myeloid leukaemia in first remission. Lancet 1984;2:1068–1070.
55. Burnett AK, Tansey P, Alcorn M, Maharaj D, McDonald GA, Robertson AG. Autologous bone marrow transplantation in first remission of acute myeloid leukaemia. Exp Hematol 1984;12(suppl 15):126–127.
56. Burnett AK, Pendry K, Rawlinson PS, et al. Autograft to eliminate minimal residual disease in AML in first remission—update on the Glasgow experience. Bone Marrow Transplant 1990;6(suppl 1):59–60.
57. Löwenberg B, Hagenbeek A, Sizoo W, de Gast GC, Verdonck LF. Bone marrow transplantation strategies in acute leukaemia. Lancet 1984;2:1400–1401.
58. Löwenberg B, Abels J, van Bekkum DW, et al. Transplantation of non-purified autologous bone marrow in patients with AML in first remission. Cancer 1984;54: 2840–2843.

59. Löwenberg B, Abels J, van Bekkum DW, et al. Treatment of patients with acute myeloid leukemia in first remission with marrow ablative therapy and autologous bone marrow transplantation. Haematol Bluttransfus 1987;10:233–236.
60. Michel G, Maraninchi D, Demeocq F, et al. Repeated courses of high dose melphalan and unpurged autologous bone marrow transplantation in children with acute nonlymphoblastic leukemia in first complete remission. Bone Marrow Transplant 1988;3:105–111.
61. Beelen DW, Quabeck K, Graeven U, Sayer HG, Mahmoud HK, Schaefer UW. Acute toxicity and first clinical results of intensive postinduction therapy using a modified busulfan and cyclophosphamide regimen with autologous bone marrow rescue in first remission of acute myeloid leukemia. Blood 1989;74:1507–1516.
62. de Gast GC, Zwaan FE, Hagenbeek T, Verdonck LF, Löwenberg B. Autologous bone marrow transplantation in first remission AML—its relative value. Bone Marrow Transplant 1991;6(suppl 1):52–54.
63. Carella AM, Piatti G, Gaozza E. Autologous BMT in patients with acute non lymphoblastic leukemia (ANLL) in first complete remission (CR-1) (abstract no. 602). Exp Hematol 1990;18:708.
64. Stewart P, Buckner CD, Bensinger W, et al. Autologous marrow transplantation in patients with acute nonlymphocytic leukemia in first remission. Exp Hematol 1985;13:267–272.
65. McMillan AK, Goldstone AH, Linch DC, et al. High-dose chemotherapy and autologous bone marrow transplantation in acute myeloid leukemia. Blood 1990;76:480–488.
66. Santos GW, Kaizer H. Bone marrow transplantation in acute leukemia. Semin Hematol 1982;19:227–239.
67. Trickett AE. Tumour cell purging for autologous bone marrow transplantation. Med Lab Sci 1990;47:120–131.
68. Keng PC, Rubin P, Constine LS, Frantz C, Nakissa N, Gregory P. Characterization of the biophysical properties of human tumor and bone marrow cells as a preliminary step to the use of centrifugal elutriation in autologous bone marrow transplantation. Int J Radiat Oncol Biol Phys 1984;10:1913–1922.
69. Jones RJ, Wagner JE, Celano P, et al. Separation of pluripotent hematopoietic stem cells from spleen colony-forming cells. Nature 1990;347:188–189.
70. Noga SJ, Donnenberg AD, Schwartz CL, et al. Development of a simplified counterflow centrifugal elutriation procedure for depletion of lymphocytes from human bone marrow. Transplantation 1986;41:220–229.
71. Wagner JE, Donnenberg AD, Noga SJ, et al. Bone marrow graft engineering by counterflow centrifugal elutriation: results of a phase I-II clinical trial. Blood 1990;75:1370–1377.
72. Bruce WR, Meeker BE, Valeriote FA. Comparison of the sensitivity of normal hematopoietic and transplanted lymphoma colony forming cells to chemotherapeutic agents administered in vivo. J Natl Cancer Inst 1966;37:233–243.
73. Santos GW, Colvin OM. Pharmacological purging of bone marrow with reference to autografting. Clin Haematol 1986;15:67–83.
74. Sharkis SJ, Santos GW, Colvin M. Elimination of acute myelogenous leukemic cells from marrow and tumor suspensions in the rat with 4-hydroperoxycyclophosphamide. Blood 1980;55:521–523.
75. Jones RJ, Zuehlsdorf M, Rowley SD, et al. Variability in 4-hydroperoxycyclophosphamide activity during clinical purging for autologous bone marrow transplantation. Blood 1987;70:1490–1494.
76. Douay L, Gorin NC, Laporte JP, Lopez M, Najman A, Duhamel G. ASTA Z 7557 (INN mafosfamide) for the in vitro treatment of human leukemic bone marrows. Invest New Drugs 1984;2:187–190.
77. Gorin NC, Douay L, Laporte JP, et al. Autologous bone marrow transplantation using marrow incubated with Asta Z 7557 in adult acute leukemia. Blood 1986;67:1367–1376.
78. Rizzoli V, Mangoni L, Carlo-Stella C, et al. Autologous marrow transplantation in first remission acute myeloid leukemia using marrow purged with mafosfamide. Bone Marrow Transplant 1991;7(suppl 2):37.
79. Rowley SD, Zuehlsdorf M, Braine HG, et al. CFU-GM content of bone marrow graft correlates with time to hematologic reconstitution following autologous bone marrow transplantation with 4-hydroperoxycyclophosphamide-purged bone marrow. Blood 1987;70:271–275.
80. Hervé P, Cahn JY, Plouvier E, et al. Autologous bone marrow transplantation for acute leukemia using transplant chemopurified with metabolite of oxazaphosphorines (ASTA Z 7557, INN mafosfamide). Invest New Drugs 1984;2:245–252.
81. Hervé P, Cahn JY, Plouvier E, et al. Autologous bone marrow transplantation in acute leukemia using marrow cells chemopurified with a cyclophosphamide derivative (ASTA Z 7557). Exp Hematol 1984;12(suppl 15):133–134.
82. Kaizer H, Stuart RK, Brookmeyer R, et al. Autologous bone marrow transplantation in acute leukemia: a phase I study of in vitro treatment of marrow with 4-hydroperoxycyclophosphamide to purge tumor cells. Blood 1985;65:1504–1510.
83. Yeager AM. Autologous bone marrow transplantation in patients with acute nonlymphocytic leukemia, using ex vivo marrow treatment with 4-hydroperoxycyclophosphamide: an update: In: Powles RL, Gordon-Smith EC, eds. Clinical papers in bone marrow transplantation: an anthology. 1993 (in press).
84. Körbling M, Hunstein W, Fliedner TM, et al. Disease-free survival after autologous bone marrow transplantation in patients with acute myelogenous leukemia. Blood 1989;74:1898–1904.
85. Cahn JY, Hervé P, Flesch M, et al. Autologous bone marrow transplantation (ABMT) for acute leukemia in complete remission: a pilot study of 33 cases. Br J Haematol 1986;63:457–470.
86. Douay L, Laporte JP, Mary J-Y, et al. Difference in kinetics of hematopoietic reconstitution between ALL and ANLL after autologous bone marrow transplantation with marrow treated in vitro with mafosfamide (ASTA Z 7557). Bone Marrow Transplant 1987;2:33–43.
87. Köppler H, Pflüger KH, Havemann K. Hematopoietic reconstitution after high-dose chemotherapy and autologous nonfrozen bone marrow rescue. Ann Hematol 1991;63:253–258.
88. Rowley SD, Davis JM, Piantadosi S, Jones RJ, Yeager AM, Santos GW. Density-gradient separation of autologous bone marrow grafts before ex vivo purging with 4-hydroperoxycyclophosphamide. Bone Marrow Transplant 1990;6:321–327.
89. Gulati SC, Shank B, Sarris A, et al. Autologous bone marrow transplant using 4-HC, VP-16 purged bone marrow for acute non-lymphoblastic leukemia. Bone Marrow Transplant 1989;4(suppl 1):116–118.
90. Ball ED. In vitro purging of bone marrow for autologous marrow transplantation in acute myelogenous

leukemia using myeloid-specific monoclonal antibodies. Bone Marrow Transplant 1988;3:387–392.
91. Ball ED, Vredenburgh JJ, Mills LE, et al. Autologous bone marrow transplantation for acute myeloid leukemia following in vitro treatment with neuraminidase and monoclonal antibodies. Bone Marrow Transplant 1990;6:277–280.
92. De Fabritiis P, Ferrero D, Sandrelli A, et al. Monoclonal antibody purging and autologous bone marrow transplantation in acute myelogenous leukemia in complete remission. Bone Marrow Transplant 1989;4:669–674.
93. Janssen WE, Lee C, Gross S, Gee AP. Low antigen density leukemia cells: selection and comparative resistance to antibody-mediated marrow purging. Exp Hematol 1989;17:252–257.
94. Robertson MJ, Griffin J, Soiffer R, et al. Human bone marrow depleted of CD33 positive cells mediates delayed but durable reconstitution of hematopoiesis. Blood 1992;79:2229–2236.
95. Myers DE, Uckun FM, Ball ED, Vallera DA. Immunotoxins for ex vivo marrow purging in autologous bone marrow transplantation for acute nonlymphocytic leukemia. Transplantation 1988;46:240–245.
96. Hays EF, Hale L. Growth of normal hemopoietic cells in cultures of bone marrow from leukemic mice. Eur J Cancer Clin Oncol 1982;18:413–418.
97. Coulombel L, Kalousek DK, Eaves CJ, Gupta CM, Eaves AC. Long-term marrow culture reveals chromosomally normal hematopoietic progenitor cells in patients with Philadelphia-chromosome-positive myelogenous leukemia. N Engl J Med 1983;308:1493–1498.
98. Chang J, Coutinho L, Morgenstern G, et al. Reconstitution of haemopoietic system with autologous marrow taken during relapse of acute myeloblastic leukaemia and grown in long-term culture. Lancet 1986;1:294–295.
99. Chang J, Morgenstern GR, Coutinho LH, et al. The use of bone marrow cells grown in long-term culture for autologous bone marrow transplantation in acute myeloid leukaemia: an update. Bone Marrow Transplant 1989;4:5–9.
100. Chang J. The use of bone marrow cells grown in long-term culture for autologous bone marrow transplantation in acute myeloid leukaemia: an update. In: Powles RL, Gordon-Smith EC, eds. Critical papers in bone marrow transplantation: an anthology. 1993 (in press).
101. Verfaillie C, Blakolmer K, McGlave P. Purified primitive human hematopoietic progenitor cells with long-term in vitro repopulating capacity adhere selectively to irradiated bone marrow stroma. J Exp Med 1990;172:509–520.
102. Barnett MJ, Eaves CJ, Phillips GL, et al. Autografting with curative intent in chronic myeloid leukemia (CML) (abstract no. 590). Exp Hematol 1990;18:705.
103. Bensinger WI, Berenson RJ. Peripheral blood and positive selection of marrow as a source of stem cells for transplantation. Prog Clin Biol Res 1990;337:93–98.
104. Körbling M, Fliedner TM, Holle R, et al. Autologous blood stem cell (ABSCT) versus purged bone marrow transplantation (pABMT) in standard risk AML: influence of source and cell composition of the autograft on hemopoietic reconstitution and disease-free survival. Bone Marrow Transplant 1991;7:343–349.
105. Reiffers J, Bernard P, David B, et al. Successful autologous transplantation with peripheral blood hemopoietic cells in a patient with acute leukemia. Exp Hematol 1986;14:312–315.
106. Tilly H, Bastit D, Lucet J-C, Esperou H, Monconduit M, Piguet H. Haemopoietic reconstitution after autologous peripheral blood stem cell transplantation in acute leukaemia. Lancet 1986;2:154–155.
107. To LB, Dyson PG, Branford AL, et al. Peripheral blood stem cells collected in very early remission produce rapid and sustained autologous haemopoietic reconstitution in acute non-lymphoblastic leukaemia. Bone Marrow Transplant 1987;2:103–108.
108. Reiffers J, Marit G, Rice A, et al. Peripheral blood stem cell transplantation in patients with acute myeloid leukemia. In: Dicke KA, ed. Autologous bone marrow transplantation: proceedings of the Fifth International Symposium. Omaha: University of Nebraska Press, 1990:873–827.
109. Juttner CA, To LB, Haylock DN, et al. Approaches to blood stem cell mobilization. Initial Australian clinical results. Bone Marrow Transplant 1988;3(suppl 1):22–24.
110. Sanz GF, de la Rubia J, Martín G et al. Busulfan (BU) and cyclophosphamide (CY) followed by autologous peripheral stem cell transplantation (PSCT) for patients with AML in first remission (abstract no. 2017). Blood 1991:78(suppl 1):507a.
111. Reiffers J, Körbling M, Labopin M, Gorin NC. Autologous blood stem cell transplantation versus autologous bone marrow transplantation for acute myeloid leukemia in first complete remission. Bone Marrow Transplant 1991;7(suppl 2):144.
112. Lobo F, Kessinger A, Landmark JD, et al. Addition of peripheral blood stem cells collected without mobilization techniques to transplanted autologous bone marrow did not hasten marrow recovery following myeloablative therapy. Bone Marrow Transplant 1991;8:389–392.
113. Hermans J, Suciu S, Stijnen T, et al. Treatment of acute myelogenous leukemia. An EBMT-EORTC retrospective analysis of chemotherapy versus allogeneic or autologous bone marrow transplantation. Eur J Cancer Clin Oncol 1989;25:545–550.
114. Reiffers J, Gaspard MH, Maraninchi D, et al. Comparison of allogeneic or autologous bone marrow transplantation and chemotherapy in patients with acute myeloid leukaemia in first remission: a prospective controlled trial. Br J Haematol 1989;72:57–63.
115. Löwenberg B, Verdonck LJ, Dekker AW, et al. Autologous bone marrow transplantation in acute myeloid leukemia in first remission: results of a Dutch prospective study. J Clin Oncol 1990;8:287–294.
116. Reiffers J, Stoppa AM, Attal M, et al. Superiority of allogeneic bone marrow transplantation as treatment for acute myeloid leukemia (AML) in first remission (abstract no. 759). Blood 1991;78(suppl 1):192a.
117. Arcese W, Amadori S, Testi AM, et al. Allogeneic vs autologous BMT vs intensive chemotherapy in childhood ANLL during first complete remission: AIEOP experience. Bone Marrow Transplant 1991;7(suppl 3):71–74.
118. Mayer RJ. Acute leukemias in adults: an overview of recent strategies. J Cancer Res Clin Oncol 1990; 116:94–96.
119. Wolff SN, Herzig RH, Fay JW, et al. High-dose cytarabine and daunorubicin as consolidation therapy for acute myeloid leukemia in first remission: long-term follow-up and results. J Clin Oncol 1989;7:1260–1267.
120. Appelbaum FR, Dahlberg S, Thomas ED, et al. Bone

marrow transplantation or chemotherapy after remission induction for adults with acute nonlymphoblastic leukemia. A prospective comparison. Ann Intern Med 1984;101:581–588.

121. Champlin RE, Ho WG, Gale RP, et al. Treatment of acute myelogenous leukemia. A prospective controlled trial of bone marrow transplantation versus consolidation chemotherapy. Ann Intern Med 1985;102:285–291.

122. Elmongy MB, Barnett MJ, Bow E, et al. Allogeneic bone marrow transplantation (BMT) vs. high dose cytarabine (HIDAC)-based chemotherapy (CTX) regimens in first remission acute myeloid leukemia (abstract no. 769). Proc ASCO 1991;10:227.

123. Zuehlsdorf M, Rowley SD, Braine HG, et al. Increased ratio of cytotoxicity for K562 and human CFU-GM by sequential incubations of 4-hydroperoxycyclophosphamide (4-HC) and methylprednisolone (MP) compared to 4-HC alone (abstract). Blood 1986;68(suppl 1):294a.

124. Rowley SD, Miller CB, Piantadosi S, Davis JM, Santos GW, Jones RJ. Phase I study of combination drug purging for autologous bone marrow transplantation. J Clin Oncol 1991;9:2210–2218.

125. Hervé P, Wijdenes J, Racadot E. Perspectives of monoclonal antibodies in the acute leukemias. Bone Marrow Transplant 1989;4(suppl 1):198–201.

126. De Fabritiis P, Bregni M, Lipton J, et al. Elimination of clonogenic Burkitt's lymphoma cells from human bone marrow using 4-hydroperoxycyclophosphamide in combination with monoclonal antibodies and complement. Blood 1985;65:1064–1070.

127. Uckun FM, Gajl-Peczalska K, Myers DE, et al. Marrow purging in autologous bone marrow transplantation for T-lineage acute lymphoblastic leukemia: efficacy of ex vivo treatment with immunotoxins and 4-HC against fresh leukemic marrow progenitor cells. Blood 1987;69:361–366.

128. LeBien TW, Anderson JM, Vallera DA, et al. Increased efficacy in selective elimination of leukemic cell line clonogenic cells by a combination of monoclonal antibodies BA-1, BA-2, BA-3 plus complement and mafosfamide (Asta-Z-7557). Leuk Res 1986;10:139–143.

129. Stiff PJ, Schultz WC, Bishop M, Marks L. Anti-CD33 monoclonal antibody and etoposide/cytosine arabinoside combinations for the ex vivo purification of bone marrow in acute nonlymphocytic leukemia. Blood 1991;77:355–362.

130. Lemoli RM, Gasparetto C, Scheinberg DA, Moore MAS, Clarkson BD, Gulati SC. Autologous bone marrow transplantation in acute myelogenous leukemia: in vitro treatment with myeloid-specific monoclonal antibodies and drugs in combination. Blood 1991; 77:1829–1836.

131. Aihara M, Aihara Y, Schmidt-Wolf G, et al. A combined approach for purging multidrug-resistant leukemic cells lines in bone marrow using a monoclonal antibody and chemotherapy. Blood 1991;77:2079–2084.

132. Chaudhary PM, Roninson IB. Expression and activity of P-glycoprotein, a multidrug efflux pump, in human hematopoietic stem cells. Cell 1991;66:85–94.

133. Civin CI, Strauss LC, Fackler MJ, Trischmann TM, Wiley JM, Loken MR. Positive stem cell selection—basic science. Prog Clin Biol Res 1990;333:387–401.

134. Berenson RJ, Andrews RG, Bensinger WI, et al. Antigen CD34+ marrow cells engraft lethally irradiated baboons. J Clin Invest 1988;81:951–955.

135. Verfaillie CM, Miller WJ, Boylan K, McGlave PB. Selection of benign primitive hematopoietic progenitors in chronic myelogenous leukemia on the basis of HLA-DR antigen expression. Blood 1992;79:1003–1010.

136. Geller RB, Zahurak M, Hurwitz CA, et al. Prognostic importance of immunophenotyping in adults with acute myelocytic leukaemia: the significance of the stem-cell glycoprotein CD34 (My10). Br J Haematol 1990;76:340–347.

137. Blume KG, Forman SJ, O'Donnell MR, et al. Total body irradiation and high-dose etoposide: a new preparatory regimen for bone marrow transplantation in patients with advanced hematologic malignancies. Blood 1987;69:1015–1020.

138. Coccia PF, Strandjord SE, Warkentin PI, et al. High-dose cytosine arabinoside and fractionated total-body irradiation: an improved preparative regimen for bone marrow transplantation of children with acute lymphoblastic leukemia in remission. Blood 1988;71:888–893.

139. Jones RJ, Santos GW. New conditioning regimens for high risk marrow transplants. Bone Marrow Transplant 1989;4(suppl 4):15–17.

140. Phillips GL, Shepherd JD, Barnett MJ, et al. Busulfan, cyclophosphamide, and melphalan conditioning for autologous bone marrow transplantation in hematologic malignancy. J Clin Oncol 1991;9:1880–1888.

141. Petersen FB, Buckner CD, Appelbaum FR, et al. Busulfan, cyclophosphamide and fractionated total body irradiation as a preparatory regimen for marrow transplantation in patients with advanced hematological malignancies: a phase I study. Bone Marrow Transplant 1989;4:617–623.

142. Koeppler H, Pflueger KH, Wolf M, Weide R, Havemann K. High-dose chemotherapy with noncryopreserved autologous bone marrow transplantation for acute myeloid leukemia in first complete remission. Haematol Bluttransfus 1990;33:699–701.

143. Meloni G, de Fabritiis P, Carella AM, et al. Autologous bone marrow transplantation in patients with AML in first complete remission. Results of two different conditioning regimens after the same induction and consolidation therapy. Bone Marrow Transplant 1990; 5:29–32.

144. Linker CA, Damon LE, Ries CA, Rugo HS. Busulfan/etoposide preparative regimen for autologous purged bone marrow transplantation for treatment of ANLL (abstract no. 1154). Blood 1991;78(suppl 1):291a.

145. Wagner JE, Johnson RJ, Santos GW, Kim BK, Shin HS. Systemic monoclonal antibody therapy for eliminating minimal residual leukemia in a rat bone marrow transplant model. Blood 1989;73:614–618.

146. Long GS, Hiserodt JC, Harnaha JB, Cramer DV. Lymphokine-activated killer cell purging of leukemia cells from bone marrow prior to syngeneic transplantation. Transplantation 1988;46:433–438.

147. Charak BS, Brynes RK, Groshen S, Chen S-C, Mazumder A. Bone marrow transplantation with interleukin-2-activated bone marrow followed by interleukin-2 therapy for acute myeloid leukemia in mice. Blood 1990;76:2187–2190.

148. Heslop HE, Gottlieb DJ, Bianchi ACM, et al. In vivo induction of gamma interferon and tumor necrosis factor by interleukin-2 infusion following intensive chemotherapy or autologous marrow transplantation. Blood 1989;74:1374–1380.

149. Higuchi CM, Thompson JA, Petersen FB, Buckner CD,

Fefer A. Toxicity and immunomodulatory effects of interleukin-2 after autologous bone marrow transplantation for hematologic malignancies. Blood 1991; 77:2561–2568.

150. Heslop HE, Duncombe AS, Reittie JE, et al. Interleukin-2 infusion after autologous bone marrow transplantation enhances hemopoietic regeneration. Transplant Proc 1991;23:1704–1705.

151. Soiffer RJ, Murray C, Cochran K, et al. Clinical and immunologic effects of prolonged infusion of low-dose recombinant interleukin-2 after autologous and T-cell-depleted allogeneic bone marrow transplantation. Blood 1992;79:517–526.

152. Klingemann H-G, Grigg AP, Wilkie-Boyd K, et al.Treatment with recombinant interferon (α-2β) early after bone marrow transplantation in patients at high risk for relapse. Blood 1991;78:3306–3311.

153. Weiden PL, Sullivan KM, Flournoy N, Storb R, Thomas ED. Antileukemic effect of graft-versus-host disease in human recipients of allogeneic-marrow grafts. N Engl J Med 1979;300:1068–1073.

154. Weiden PL, Sullivan KM, Flournoy N, Storb R, Thomas ED. Antileukemic effect of chronic graft-versus-host disease. Contribution to improved survival after allogeneic marrow transplantation. N Engl J Med 1980;304:1529–1533.

155. Geller RB, Esa AH, Beschorner WE, Frondoza CG, Santos GW, Hess AD. Successful in vitro graft-versus-tumor effect against an Ia-bearing tumor using cyclosporine-induced syngeneic graft-versus-host disease in the rat. Blood 1989;74:1165–1171.

156. Schlossman SF, Chess L, Humphreys RE, Strohminger JL. Distribution of Ia-like molecules on the surface of normal and leukemic human cells. Proc Natl Acad Sci USA 1976;73:1288–1292.

157. Griffin JD, Mayer RJ, Weinstein HJ, et al. Surface marker analyses of acute myeloblastic leukemia: identification of differentiation-associated phenotypes. Blood 1983;62:557–563.

158. Talbot DC, Powles RL, Sloane JP, et al. Cyclosporine-induced graft-versus-host disease following autologous bone marrow transplantation in acute myeloid leukaemia. Bone Marrow Transplant 1990;6:17–20.

159. Yeager AM, Vogelsang GB, Jones RJ, Farmer ER, Altomonte V, Santos GW. Induction of cutaneous graft-versus-host disease by administration of cyclosporine to patients undergoing autologous bone marrow transplantation for acute myeloid leukemia. Blood 1992; 79:3031–3035.

160. Hess AD, Horwitz L, Beschorner WE, Santos GW. Development of graft-versus-host disease like syndrome in cyclosporine-treated rats after syngeneic bone marrow transplantation. I. Development of cytotoxic T lymphocytes with apparent polyclonal anti-Ia specificity, including autoreactivity. J Exp Med 1985;161:718–730.

161. Jones RJ, Vogelsang GB, Hess AD, et al. Induction of graft-versus-host disease after autologous bone marrow transplantation. Lancet 1989;1:754–757.

162. Noga SJ, Hess AD. The anti-tumor effect of cyclosporine A (CSA) induced autoimmune graft-vs-host disease (AIGVHD) is potentiated by gamma interferon (IFN) (abstract no. 465). Exp Hematol 1991;19:580.

163. Solh H, Saunders EF, Freedman M. Autologous bone marrow transplantation (ABMT) following high-dose busulfan (Bu) and cyclophosphamide (Cy) using unpurged marrow in children with acute nonlymphoblastic leukemia (ANL) (abstract no. 2019). Blood 1991;78(suppl 1):507a.

164. Lenarsky C, Weinberg K, Petersen J, et al. Autologous bone marrow transplantation with 4-hydroperoxycyclophosphamide purged marrows for children with acute nonlymphoblastic leukemia in second remission. Bone Marrow Transplant 1990;6:425–429.

Chapter 55
Autologous Bone Marrow Transplantation for Acute Lymphoblastic Leukemia

Jerome Ritz, Norma K. Ramsay, and John H. Kersey

Autologous bone marrow transplantation (BMT) for relapsed acute lymphoblastic leukemia (ALL) was undertaken more than 3 decades ago (1). The demonstration that this approach could provide effective treatment for children with ALL who had relapsed after initial therapy was accomplished early in the 1980s (2,3). As discussed in other chapters, autologous BMT has now been used successfully in combination with high-dose chemoradiotherapy for treatment of a variety of other hematological malignancies, including non-Hodgkin's lymphomas and acute myeloid leukemia (AML), as well as solid tumors. Autologous BMT offers a therapeutic alternative for patients with ALL at high risk for relapse who do not have human leukocyte antigen (HLA)–compatible donors and are therefore not candidates for allogeneic BMT.

The results of autologous BMT for ALL vary considerably depending on the stage of disease at the time of BMT as well as other factors, such as age and duration of response to previous conventional dose therapy. The best clinical results have been achieved in high-risk patients transplanted in first remission and in pediatric patients who relapse after a long (>2 yr) initial remission. These patients appear to have excellent long-term leukemia-free survival (>50%) following this approach, but high relapse rates continue to represent a significant limitation in other patient groups, suggesting that further improvements in therapy are necessary. New approaches to improve the effectiveness of autologous BMT and to prevent relapse, such as the development of better preparative regimens and better methods for in vitro purging of autologous marrow, as well as the use of post-transplant immunotherapy, are currently being tested.

Prognostic Factors in ALL

ALL is characterized by uncontrolled proliferation of malignant lymphoblasts in the marrow, which spread to other organs including blood, lymph nodes, central nervous system, gonads, and other extramedullary sites. The various subtypes of ALL are defined by clinical features, response to therapy, cellular immunophenotypes, cytogenetics, and, more recently, molecular genetics (4). Clinical features that have been found to be particularly important in defining groups of patients at high risk for treatment failure include age and white blood cell (WBC) count at diagnosis. Infants, older adults, and individuals with high WBC counts have a particularly poor outcome with conventional therapy. Cell marker (immunophenotype) analysis has demonstrated that most cases (approximately 85%) of ALL originate from B-lymphocyte precursors; only rare cases have characteristics of mature (surface immunoglobulin $[Ig]^{+}$) B lymphocytes (5). Approximately 15% of cases of ALL originate in T lymphocytes and their precursors. Initial immunophenotypic studies suggested that distinct phenotypic subsets of ALL with different degrees of responsiveness to chemotherapy could be identified (6). However, as chemotherapeutic regimens have improved, immunophenotype has not continued to be important as an independent predictor of outcome in most patients. An exception is a rare leukemia in which some of the cells have T-lymphocyte characteristics and other cells have a myeloid immunophenotype (7). In cases where ALL immunophenotype does not have prognostic significance, analysis of cell-surface markers remains important for determining eligibility for autologous BMT and for selecting appropriate methods for purging marrow of residual ALL cells.

Specific molecular genetic abnormalities also define types of ALL with a poor prognosis following conventional intensive chemotherapy regimens (8,9). A well-characterized subtype of ALL is the result of the fusion of the *bcr* and *abl* genes resulting in a 185-kd protein product; this form of ALL is identified by the t(9;22) translocation (Philadelphia chromosome). *Bcr-abl*–positive ALL represents approximately 4% of childhood ALL and approximately 20% of adult ALL and is seldom cured with standard chemotherapy. Other molecular genetic rearrangements of B-lineage cells result in very specific translocations and subtypes of leukemia. Several have been defined both cytogenetically and at the molecular genetic level and include Burkitt translocations involving the *myc* oncogene and one of the immunoglobulin genes, t(4;11) and t(1;19). Specific abnormalities in T-lineage

ALL include a rearrangement between TCRα/δ and TAL/SCL (SCL represents a helix-loop-helix transcriptional activating protein) (10,11). Additional molecular genetic rearrangements including T-cell receptor loci have been described involving the rhombitin gene, resulting in a t(11;14) translocation.

Of the molecular genetic rearrangements noted, t(9;22), t(4;11) and the Burkitt translocations generally have a very poor prognosis. In addition, hypodiploidy (less than 44 chromosomes) has been associated with a high rate of treatment failure. Although the incidence of these abnormalities in pediatric patients with ALL is low, conventional therapy is not highly effective in patients with these characteristics, and more aggressive therapy should be considered early in the course of treatment.

General Indications for Autologous BMT in ALL

As a result of steady improvements in chemotherapy over the past 20 years, more than 60% of children with ALL are now cured with intensive induction regimens followed by 2 years of maintenance therapy (12). On the basis of clinical criteria such as age and WBC count at the time of presentation, it is possible to identify distinct subsets of patients with even more favorable prognosis. Thus, for most children, BMT is only considered following relapse. Nevertheless, certain factors at diagnosis portend a very poor prognosis and can be used to identify subsets of pediatric patients in whom more aggressive therapy is indicated. For example, the presence of the Philadelphia chromosome and other structural chromosomal abnormalities described indicate an extremely poor prognosis in children and adults, and in such patients, first remission BMT is warranted. In general, any patient with high-risk ALL, which has often been defined as a predicted event-free survival of less than 30 to 40% with chemotherapy, should be a candidate for BMT (13). Adults have a lower likelihood of long-term survival, and only approximately 30 to 35% are alive 5 years after initial diagnosis (14–16). Thus, in many centers, adults with ALL are considered for BMT in first remission. Following relapse, second remissions can often be achieved both in pediatric and adult patients with intensive reinduction chemotherapy regimens, but ultimate survival following second remission is usually poor despite initial responsiveness to conventional-dose chemotherapy (17). More aggressive therapy using BMT is therefore considered for almost all patients who fail conventional dose therapy.

As with other hematological malignancies, the initial demonstration that BMT could provide effective therapy for ALL occurred in the setting of allogeneic BMT using marrow from HLA-compatible sibling donors. In ALL, the results of allogeneic BMT continue to be the standard to which results of autologous BMT are compared (18–20). Moreover, autologous BMT is generally reserved for patients who do not have HLA-compatible allogeneic donors. However, less than 30% of patients have a matched sibling donor, and the majority of patients are therefore not eligible for allogeneic BMT. In recent years, use of alternative sources of donor marrow has received intensive investigation, and increasing numbers of patients with ALL have been transplanted using matched unrelated donors or less than fully matched family donors (see Chapter 51). Nevertheless, the ability to find appropriate allogeneic donors remains limited for the majority of patients with ALL, and unrelated donor BMTs continue to be associated with relatively high rates of severe graft-versus-host disease (GVHD), graft failure, and BMT-related mortality (21). Although improvements in unrelated allogeneic donor BMTs are continually being made, autologous BMT often remains the best alternative for patients who lack a matched sibling donor.

Timing of Autologous BMT in ALL

As noted, one important issue in the timing of autologous BMT is the stage of the disease during which BMT should be considered. Early BMT has advantages in that it is provided at a time when the disease has not become refractory to chemoradiotherapy. When harvested in first remission, autologous marrow has received less chemotherapy than marrow obtained in later remissions and is therefore more likely to engraft promptly and completely after BMT. In addition, contamination of marrow with residual leukemia is likely to be less in first remission. Nevertheless, peritransplant morbidity and mortality remain sufficiently high so that patients who are likely to have an excellent chance of cure with chemotherapy alone are not considered for BMT unless they fail chemotherapy. Experience with autologous transplantation in first remission has therefore been limited. For example, although adults and children with *bcr-abl*/t(9;22) leukemia have a very poor prognosis with chemotherapy, insufficient data have been reported to demonstrate whether autologous BMT in first remission is preferred over chemotherapy. Nevertheless, some high-risk patients have become long-term survivors with BMT, and preliminary results from some centers are encouraging (22,23). The use of autologous BMT for selected high-risk patient groups should be considered an important issue for careful study.

Children and adults who relapse after receiving combination chemotherapy can often be induced into a second remission, although they ultimately have a very poor prognosis. Patients who fail to achieve complete remission with their initial induction regimen also have a poor prognosis. Because of the inability of conventional-dose chemotherapy to maintain long-term remissions in these patients, they should be considered as candidates for autologous (or allogeneic) BMT. One possible exception is children who relapse after a first remission of more than 18 to 24 months or

Table 55-1.
Eligibility for Bone Marrow Transplantation in Acute Lymphoblastic Leukemia

	First Remission	*Second or Later Remission*	*Chemotherapy Failure*
Pediatric patients (age <18 years)	No	Yes	Yes
Specific high-risk features t(9;22) t(4;11) Burkitt translocation Hypodiploid (< 44 chromosomes) Certain uncommon phenotypes (e.g., T lymphocyte/myeloid)	Yes	Yes	Yes
Adult patients (age ≥ 18 years)	Yes	Yes	Yes

who relapse after discontinuation of primary chemotherapy; some patients in these categories have become long-term survivors with chemotherapy alone (17,24).

Autologous BMT should be considered for all patients with ALL who have failed chemotherapy or who are in second or subsequent remission, with the possible exceptions described. Patients who have undergone multiple relapses should also be considered as candidates for BMT because some of these patients have become long-term survivors following autologous or allogeneic BMT. However, unlike allogeneic BMT, autologous BMT can be performed only if "remission" marrow is available for transplant. This requirement thus generally restricts autologous BMT to those patients who can achieve complete hematological remission and excludes patients with ALL that is refractory to conventional-dose chemotherapy. Groups of patients with ALL currently eligible for autologous BMT are summarized in Table 55-1.

Choice of Donors for BMT

In patients with ALL, a variety of marrow sources, including HLA-identical siblings, partially HLA-mismatched related donors, HLA-matched unrelated donors, partially HLA-mismatched unrelated donors, and autologous marrow, have been used to support patients following myeloablative therapy. To begin the process of considering these various options, HLA typing should be performed soon after a patient has been identified as a potential candidate for BMT. Because the largest BMT experience in ALL is with the use of HLA-matched sibling donors, these donors should generally be considered as first priority (20). The use of autologous marrow to support BMT is considered primarily for patients who lack suitable HLA-matched sibling donors. Because less than 30% of patients will have HLA-identical sibling donors, autologous BMT provides a feasible therapeutic option for the majority of patients who would not otherwise be considered eligible for BMT. The choice of alternative donors for BMT also depends somewhat on local studies and preferences. One approach, which is currently under evaluation at the University of Minnesota for patients who do not have an HLA-identical sibling donor, is to attempt to identify an HLA-matched unrelated donor within a 4-month period. If no donor is found through searches of donor banks, autologous BMT is utilized. Although allogeneic BMTs using partially HLA-mismatched related and unrelated donors have also been performed, these alternatives are most often reserved for patients not eligible for autologous BMT.

Marrow Purging to Remove Residual Leukemic Cells

In all patients undergoing autologous BMT, the attainment of a complete hematological remission is required prior to marrow harvest. Nevertheless, even though only morphologically normal marrow is used for autologous BMT, one theoretical limitation of autologous BMT is possible contamination of the harvested marrow with leukemia. As discussed previously, patients are eligible for autologous BMT only because they are at high risk for marrow relapse despite the fact that they have achieved a complete hematological remission. For this reason, virtually all BMT studies in ALL have utilized purging of autologous marrow with either monoclonal antibodies plus complement (3,25), immunotoxins (26,27), antibody-bead immunoconjugates (28), or pharmacological agents such as ASTA-Z or 4-hydroperoxycyclophosphamide (29,30). Use of these methods for purging residual leukemic cells is based on in vitro studies demonstrating the selective elimination of ALL tumor cells without depletion of normal marrow progenitor cells in model systems (29,31–33). Nevertheless, the need for purging autologous marrow from patients with ALL has not been proven definitively because there are no controlled trials to date specifically addressing this issue.

The purging of tumor cells from marrow using monoclonal antibodies was developed in 1980 and used for autologous BMT in ALL (2). Subsequently, many different methods for removing residual ALL cells have been developed and used extensively in autologous BMT for this disease. Although monoclonal antibodies selectively bind to target cells, cell-surface binding alone does not usually result in effective elimination of the tumor population. For this reason, monoclonal antibodies have been used to initiate complement-mediated cell lysis, as antibody/toxin conjugates (immunotoxins) or as antibody conjugated to physical particles such as plastic beads, magnetic beads, or iron particles. Because the desire is to eliminate clonogenic leukemic cells, monoclonal antibodies that recognize antigens selectively expressed on very early lymphoid cells have been utilized for in vitro treatment of autologous marrow in patients with ALL. B-cell precursor ALL antibodies directed against the CD9, CD10, CD19, and CD24 antigens have been demonstrated to bind leukemic cells but spare normal myeloid stem cells. Based on in vitro model systems, use of these antibodies in combination is more effective than when used individually (31,34,35). The CD19 antigen is one of the earliest cell-surface proteins to appear as lymphoid progenitor cells become committed to B-lineage differentiation, and this antigen is consequently expressed on leukemic cells from more than 95% of patients with B-lineage ALL (5). Several antibodies have been prepared against the CD19 determinant; one of these antibodies, when used as a pokeweed antiviral protein (PAP)/toxin immunoconjugate is very efficient in the removal of clonogenic leukemic cells in B-precursor ALL (36). Immunotoxin conjugates of anti-CD19 and blocked ricin have also been prepared and are now being used in clinical trials for purging autologous marrow in patients with ALL (37).

Most preclinical and clinical studies for purging T-precursor ALL have targeted antigenic determinants with broad (Pan T) reactivity. As with B-lineage ALL, monoclonal antibodies have been used individually and in combination to initiate complement-mediated lysis. Antibodies specific for CD5 have been studied extensively, and one CD5 antibody, T101, has proven very effective in the removal of clonogenic leukemic T cells when used as a ricin/immunotoxin conjugate (38). Monoclonal antibodies specific for CD7 have also been used; one CD7 antibody appears to be an effective immunotoxin for purging T leukemia (27,39). These antibodies have been utilized alone and also in combination with 4-hydroperoxycyclophosphamide (40).

Following autologous BMT for ALL, leukemic relapse is the most common cause of treatment failure. Recurrent leukemia following autologous BMT may be due to (1) inadequate removal of leukemic cells from the autologous marrow, (2) residual leukemia in the patient, and (3) absence of graft-versus-leukemia (GVL) effect in the autologous as compared with the allogeneic setting. Recently developed quantitative measures of minimal residual disease using polymerase chain reaction (PCR) may be helpful in evaluating the role of marrow purging as well as the effectiveness of different methods for in vitro depletion (41). In patients with non-Hodgkin's lymphomas, PCR detection of the tumor-specific *bcl-2* translocation has been used to evaluate the effectiveness of marrow purging with a combination of B-cell–specific monoclonal antibodies and complement (42). Patients whose marrows no longer contained PCR-detectable tumor cells after in vitro purging were found to have significantly better disease-free survival and lower relapse rate after autologous BMT. Although similar studies have not been carried out yet in patients with ALL, this finding clearly suggests that effective marrow purging may have a significant role in preventing relapse after autologous BMT. In addition, a leukemic progenitor cell colony assay was found to reflect accurately the clinically relevant residual leukemia burden and to have prognostic value for high-risk ALL patients undergoing autologous BMT (43).

BMT Preparative Regimens

Preparative regimens for patients undergoing autologous BMT have been similar to those regimens used for allogeneic BMT. In both, the majority of patients have received high-dose chemotherapy combined with total body irradiation (TBI) in an effort to eliminate residual leukemic cells. The combination of cyclophosphamide (CY) followed by either fractionated or single-dose TBI has been used in many patients with ALL. The use of fractionated rather than single-dose radiation may be associated with fewer long-term side effects in patients who are cured with this approach. As noted previously, the major obstacle to cure in patients with ALL undergoing autologous BMT has been relapse of leukemia after BMT. In an effort to decrease the post-BMT relapse rate, various modifications have been made in the standard CY/TBI preparative regimens. At the University of Minnesota, 3 sequential regimens have been utilized for patients undergoing autologous transplant over the past 10 years (40, 44–47). At the Dana Farber Cancer Institute (DFCI), several changes were also made in the BMT preparative regimen for pediatric patients over a similar period in attempts to provide more effective antileukemic therapy without concomitant increases in BMT-related toxicity (48). Regimens used at both centers are summarized in Table 55-2. Both centers have gradually escalated the dose of TBI by either varying the fractionation schedule or the total dose administered. Cytosine arabinoside (ara-C) has also been added in various schedules in an attempt to provide more effective high-dose chemotherapy. The regimen at the DFCI has also included teniposide or, more recently, etoposide (VP16). However, with the addition of high-dose VP16, high-dose ara-C was deleted from the BMT preparative regimen and used for intensive consolidation therapy 4 to 6 weeks prior to BMT conditioning. Although most of these changes have been made to reduce the rate of relapse in patients with ALL undergoing BMT, some changes were made to reduce regimen-related toxicity. In fact, it should be emphasized that the DFCI regimens summarized in Table 55-2 are used exclusively for pediatric patients. Adult patients (>18 yr) were not able to tolerate ara-C and teniposide in addition to CY

Table 55-2.
Acute Lymphoblastic Leukemia Bone Marrow Transplantation Preparative Regimens at the University of Minnesota and the Dana Farber Cancer Institute

Study Years	*Pretransplant Conditioning*
University of Minnesota	
1982–1984	CY (60 mg/kg × 2 d); 1,320 cGy fractionated TBI (165 cGy b.i.d. × 4 days)
1984–1986	850 cGy single-fraction TBI; ara-C (3 gm/m^2 b.i.d. × 6 days)
1987–1991	1,320 cGy hyperfractionated TBI (120 cGy × 11) with lung shielding; CY (60 mg/kg × 2 days)
Dana Farber Cancer Institute	
1980–1986	ara-C (500 mg/m^2/day × 5–7 days); teniposide (200 mg/m^2 × 2 days); CY (1,800 mg/m^2 × 2 days); TBI (850 cGy single fraction to 1,300 cGy in b.i.d fractions)
1986–1989	Teniposide (200 mg/m^2) days −8 and −6; ara-C (3 gm/m^2 b.i.d.) days −8, −7, and −6; CY (1,800 mg/m^2) days −5 and −4; 1,400 cGy fractionated TBI (175 cGy b.i.d. × 4 days)
1989–1992	1,400 cGy fractionated TBI (175 cGy BID × 4 days); etoposide (60 mg/kg × 1) day −4; CY (1,800 mg/m^2) days −3 and −2

CY = cyclophosphamide; TBI = total body irradiation; ara-C = cytosine arabinoside.

and TBI (49). As results of current regimens become known, it is likely that further changes in preparative regimens will be made.

Other conditioning regimens have been evaluated at other centers, including fractionated TBI, high-dose ara-C, and melphalan in a series of 26 autologous BMT recipients (50). These patients were either in complete remission (1st to 4th) or in relapse. The relapse probability in this group of patients was also high (62%). High-dose melphalan combined with TBI was evaluated in 24 children with ALL in second or third remission undergoing autologous BMT (51). In some patients, marrow was purged with the Campath-1 monoclonal antibody. All patients were in second or third remission; however, several of the patients had relapsed off therapy. The relapse rate was somewhat lower in this group of patients; only 8 of the 24 patients relapsed, and 12 patients remained alive in remission.

Despite the use of different conditioning regimens, the relapse rate has remained relatively high following autologous BMT. Regimens combining VP16 with TBI have been evaluated and are showing promise in patients undergoing allogeneic transplant for ALL (52,53). These regimens have not been tested extensively in the autologous setting but deserve further investigation based on recently reported studies.

Results of Autologous BMT

The use of autologous BMT at many centers has been reported extensively in the literature. Results from more than 15 centers reporting substantial numbers of patients are summarized in Table 55-3 (3,45,48, 49,54,55). Data from several European cooperative groups are also included (17,22,50,51,56–63); data in these reports may overlap with results reported from individual centers. As shown in this table, most centers utilize in vitro treatment of autologous marrow to deplete minimal residual disease, but a large number of different approaches to purging have been used. Similarly, most centers utilize TBI-based preparative regimens, but TBI is administered in many different ways and, as discussed previously, various chemotherapeutic agents have been added in attempts to provide more effective eradication of ALL in vivo. These differences in the way autologous BMT is carried out at different centers likely contribute to the wide variation in the clinical results achieved by this treatment approach. Clinical results also differ due to the wide variation in follow-up available for different studies.

Although many different purging methods have been utilized in the studies summarized in Table 55-3, engraftment of manipulated marrow is reported consistently. Delayed engraftment is noted in some individuals, which is more likely due to previous administration of prolonged and intensive chemotherapy than to marrow treatment and toxicity of this treatment to normal marrow progenitors. When compared with other types of BMT recipients, early myeloid engraftment appears more rapid than in patients with AML undergoing autologous BMT, but not as rapid as in patients receiving normal allogeneic marrow (64–66). Because GVHD does not develop in these patients and they do not require immunosuppressive medications, BMT-related morbidity is consistently less than that reported following allogeneic BMT. As a result, BMT-related mortality is generally low (<10%). Increased BMT-related mortality often reflects attempts to intensify the BMT ablative regimen and nonhematological toxicities associated with those agents. However, even in these instances, leukemic relapse is the predominant cause of failure following autologous BMT for ALL.

Perhaps the most important factors affecting outcome are patient selection criteria. Most centers have reported results for heterogeneous patient groups including adults as well as pediatric patients and patients with ALL in first remission as well as patients who have failed conventional-dose chemotherapy. As with other intensive combination chemotherapy regimens, the results of autologous BMT vary depending on stage of disease and age at time of BMT. When these various factors are taken into consideration, results of autologous BMT become somewhat more consistent.

As expected, patients undergoing autologous BMT in first remission generally do better than patients in second or subsequent remission, even though BMT is generally reserved for patients who continue to have chemotherapy-sensitive disease and are able to achieve complete hematological remission. Although criteria for high-risk first-remission ALL vary, 30 to 60% of such patients have been reported to have more than 2-year disease-free survival following autologous BMT (see

Table 55-3.
Clinical Results of Autologous Bone Marrow Transplantation

Center, Author, Ref	No. Patients	Age[a]	(Range)	*Status at BMT* CR1	CR2	CR≥3	*Marrow Purging* MAb	Drug
Minnesota, Ramsay (45)	155	9.5	(0.9–48)	14	78	63	CD9+CD10+CD24 or CD3+CD5+LFA-1	4HC
DFCI-Pediatric, Billet (48)	66	8	(3–18)	1	42	23	CD10+CD9	
DFCI-Adult, Soiffer (49)	22	22	(18–54)	1	11	10	CD10+CD9	
Jena, Zintl (58)	15	8	(2–11)	6	7	2	VIL-A1	
AIEOP, Coleselli (57)	56	11		0	36	20		VCR/4HC (32) Mafosfamide (16)
Royal Marsden, Schroeder (51)	24	. . .	(<16)	0	17	7	Campath-1 (6)	
ISG, Rizzoli (59)	82	21	(2–57)	37	45	0		Mafosfamide (56)
Uppsala,	21	27	(3–55)	21			CD10+CD19	
Simonsson (22)	32	9	(3–25)		29	3	or CD7	
Seattle, Doney (54)	89	18	(2–47)	10	27	52	anti-B (35) anti-T (10) none (39)	4HC (2)
Besancon, Cahn (50)	26	NA		6	16	4	(9)	Mafosfamide (13)
Goustave-Roussy, Pico (60)	24	10	(3–37)	0	14	10	CD10 (4)	Mafosfamide (17)
Genoa, Carella (61)	13	24	(NA)	7	4	2		Mafosfamide (7)
Marseille, Stoppa (62)	12	16	(4–47)	6	4	2	CD10+CD19	
Marseille, Blaise (68)	22	31	(7–47)	22			Multiple methods	Mafosfamide (4)
Charing Cross, Davis (63)	11	17	(9–25)	2	6	3	Campath-1	
Pittsburgh, Gonzales-Chambers (55)	10	33	(13–52)	1	6	3		4HC
Royal Free, Gilmore (56)	27	17	(13–45)	27			CD10+CD19 or CD7	
EORTC, Herve (23)	66	≤15	. . .	66			32%	Mafosfamide 36%
	17	≤15			177			
	242	>15		242				
	74	>15			74			

[a]Years median age.
MAb = Monoclonal antibody; NA = data not available; CR = complete remission; TBI = total body irradiation; ALL = acute lymphoblastic leukemia; CY = cyclophosphamide; 4HC = 4-hydroperoxycyclophosphamide; VCR = vincristine; ara-C = cytosine arabinoside; MEL = melphalan; BU = busulfan; BMT = bone marrow transplantation.

Table 55-3). Despite the fact that these patients are transplanted in first remission, leukemic relapse occurs in 30 to 70% of such patients and is the primary cause of failure.

The great majority of patients with ALL undergo autologous BMT in second or subsequent remission. Results for these patients also vary considerably; 15 to 40% have been reported to remain disease-free more than 2 years after BMT. Overall results for 155 patients treated at the University of Minnesota are shown in Figure 55-1. This study represents a very large series of patients treated over a 10-year period at a single institution. Disease-free survival at 5 years after BMT is 17%. The vast majority of failures occur in the first year after BMT and are predominantly due to leukemic relapse.

A large number of patients have also undergone autologous BMT in second or subsequent remission at DFCI. Analysis of the results in pediatric patients indicated that the duration of initial first remission is the most significant prognostic variable (48). In 20 patients whose first remission was less than 2 years, event-free survival at 4 years after BMT was only 10

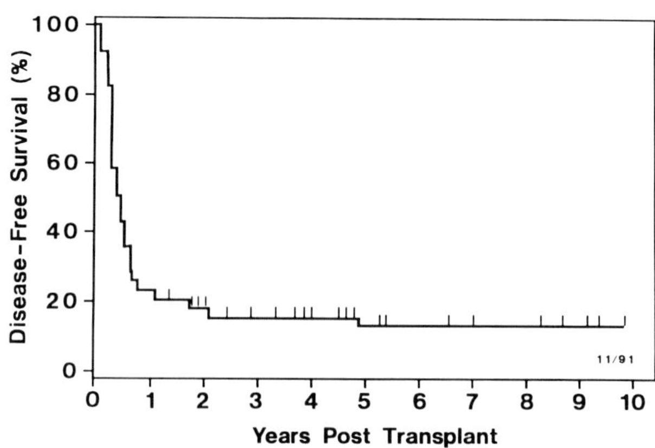

Figure 55-1. Disease-free survival following autologous bone marrow transplantation for acute lymphoblastic leukemia at the University of Minnesota (n=155).

Table 55-3. (continued)

BMT Regimen			% BMT Mortality	Relapse Rate (%)		DFS (%)		
TBI	*CY*	*Other*		*CR1*	*ALL*	*CR1*	*ALL*	*Positive Prognostic Factors*
Yes	Yes	+/− ara-C	9				17	
Yes	Yes	ara-C + VM-26	18		60		32	Duration 1st remission >24 months
Yes	Yes		18		75		20	Age <28
Yes	Yes	(2-BUCY)	7		27		67	
Yes	Yes	VCR (27) (14+TBI, 13-TBI)	8		45		21	Extramedullary relapse only
Yes	No	MEL	17		33		45	Duration 1st remission >18 months
Yes	Yes					38	33	>6 months from CR to BMT
Yes	Yes	+Ara-C (35) (4-MEL/TBI)	5	30	58	65	32	Off-therapy relapse; >6 months from CR to BMT
Yes	Yes		19	27	80	50	12	BMT in first remission
Yes		Ara-C + MEL			62		28	
	Yes	Ara-C + BCNU +MEL	21		63		16	
Yes	Yes	(2-BUCY)	15		77		8	
Yes	Yes	+/− MEL			50		50	
Yes	Yes	+/− MEL	9	52		40		
Yes		Ara-C + VM-26+prednisone	18		36		36	
Yes	Yes		20		60		30	
Yes	Yes	Ara-C (6)	8	67		32		
		Multiple regimens	6			46		
							33	
			8			45		
							24	

± 7%. In 51 patients whose first remission was 2 years or more, event-free survival at 3 years after BMT was 53 ± 7%. In all patients, autologous marrow was treated with anti-CD10 and anti-CD9 monoclonal antibodies and rabbit complement. Better results in patients with long first remissions were primarily due to the lower relapse rate in this group (35 vs 60%). This finding was further supported by the demonstration that even within the group of patients with initial remission of 2 years or longer, duration of longest remission prior to BMT continued to have further prognostic significance (Figure 55-2). In patients with prior remissions of 24 to 48 months, 3-year leukemia-free survival was 40 ± 11%. In patients with prior remissions 48 months or longer, 3-year leukemia-free survival was 81 ± 13%. Previous reports have suggested that some patients with very long remissions can be salvaged effectively with intensive conventional-dose chemotherapy regimens without the need for BMT (24); however, the excellent results of autologous BMT in second and third remission patients with very long prior remissions are comparable to that of current results in newly diagnosed children with ALL. Unfortunately, few relapsed patients have previously enjoyed very long prior remissions, and relapse after BMT continues to

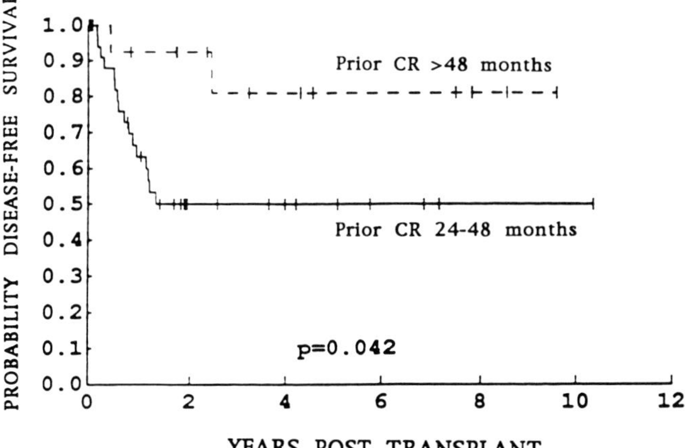

Figure 55–2. Disease-free survival following autologous bone marrow transplantation (BMT) for patients with acute lymphoblastic leukemia with long prior remissions. Fifty-one patients with prior remissions >2 years underwent autologous BMT at the Dana Faber Cancer Institute. All patients were transplanted in second or subsequent remission. Results in 38 patients with prior remissions of 24 to 48 months (*solid line*) are compared to results in 13 patients with prior remissions of >48 months (*broken line*).

be the predominant cause of failure following autologous BMT.

For pediatric patients with initial remission less than 2 years or who relapse while receiving chemotherapy, results of autologous BMT have generally been disappointing; only 10 to 20% of patients remain disease-free more than 2 years after BMT. Intensification of the transplant preparative regimen has been attempted in these individuals. Billet and colleagues (48) recently reported encouraging results. As discussed previously, the preparative regimens for pediatric patients at DFCI initially utilized VM26, ara-C, and CY, followed by TBI. In 1989, this was changed to TBI followed by VP16 and CY (see Table 55-2). High-dose ara-C was not included in the BMT preparative regimen but was used for pretransplant intensification. With this new preparative approach, 2-year disease-free survival for 11 patients is currently 61%, compared with only 10% for the previous regimen. Although accrual of additional patients and longer follow-up will be necessary to confirm these results, this study suggests that improved preparative programs may substantially improve clinical results for these patients.

Adult patients with ALL do not respond as well as pediatric patients to primary therapy, and results of autologous BMT parallel this distinction. At the DFCI, 3-year event-free survival was found to be 20% for 22 adult patients (age >18 yr) in second or third complete remission (49). However, within this group of adults, event-free survival was 45% for patients ages 18 to 28; there were no long-term survivors in patients older than 28 years. As in other studies of other age groups, leukemic relapse was the most frequent cause of failure following BMT.

Comparison of Autologous and Allogeneic BMT for ALL

There have been few controlled studies comparing results of autologous and allogeneic BMT in similar patients with ALL. One study from the University of Minnesota included 91 patients with high-risk or refractory ALL (44); 45 patients who did not have a matched donor received purged autologous marrow, whereas 46 patients who had matched donors received allogeneic marrow. All patients were given CY (60 mg/kg/day for 2 days) and fractionated TBI (1,320 cGy). Overall survival at 4 years did not differ between the two groups: 23% for autologous BMT and 31% for allogeneic BMT. However, the causes of failure were different. In the autologous BMT group, 31 patients (79%) failed due to leukemic relapse, and only 3 patients failed due to BMT-related toxicity. In contrast, failure following allogeneic BMT was evenly divided between leukemic relapse (15 patients) and toxicity (15 patients). However, the relapse rate in patients in whom GVHD did not develop following allogeneic BMT (75%) was similar to the relapse rate following autologous BMT (79%).

A second study from an Italian cooperative group (AIEOP) reported results in 65 high-risk pediatric patients with ALL who received either HLA-matched allogeneic marrow (30 patients) or autologous marrow (35 patients) (67). The conditioning regimen consisted of high-dose vincristine, fractionated TBI, and CY in all patients. Allogeneic BMT patients received cyclosporine for GVHD prophylaxis. Autologous marrow was purged with either vincristine and cortisone (17 patients), Asta-Z (7 patients), or monoclonal antibodies (one patient). As in the Minnesota study, fatal toxicities occurred more often following allogeneic BMT (17% mortality) than after autologous BMT (8% mortality). Similarly, the relapse rate was lower after allogeneic BMT (30%) than after autologous BMT (47%). As a result, overall disease-free survival following allogeneic and autologous BMT in children with relapsed ALL was similar (DFS 56% and 50%, respectively).

A third report from a French cooperative group summarized results in 47 patients with high-risk ALL who received either an allogeneic or an autologous BMT in first remission (68). Patients in both groups received similar induction therapy and were comparable in terms of age and characteristics at initial presentation. Autologous marrow was purged in all patients, but a variety of different in vitro treatment methods was used. Autologous BMT recipients received more consolidation chemotherapy before BMT. Nevertheless, the probability of relapse for patients receiving autologous BMT (52%) was substantially higher than in the group that underwent allogeneic BMT (9%). As a result, disease-free survival at 2 years after BMT was significantly better for the first remission patients who had allogeneic BMTs (71% DFS) than those who had autologous BMT (40% DFS). In comparison with other studies, this is one of the few reports to identify an overall advantage for allogeneic BMT. Although this study was restricted to patients in first remission, the factors responsible for these results are not known. Clearly, the very large difference in relapse rates was the primary factor and was not offset by differences in BMT-related toxicity. Many different marrow purging methods were used to treat autologous marrows, but the effectiveness of individual methods was not assessed. Inadequate marrow treatment may have contributed to the high relapse rate following autologous BMT in some patients. Alternatively, unknown factors may have contributed to enhanced eradication of residual leukemia in the patients who underwent allogeneic BMT.

New Approaches to Improve Results of Autologous BMT

As noted in other chapters, a variety of recent advances are likely to improve the effectiveness of BMT. In patients with ALL undergoing autologous BMT, the use of hematopoietic growth factors after marrow infusion can enhance hematopoietic engraftment and significantly reduce infectious complications and costs associated with this treatment (69). Although the mortality associated with autologous BMT in ALL is generally low (<10%), use of hematopoietic growth factors may result in further improvement.

Because relapse is the predominant cause of failure following autologous BMT in ALL, attempts to deal with this problem will likely have the greatest impact in improving the long-term results of treatment. Several studies have suggested that the rate of relapse can be reduced if autologous BMT is performed in first remission. However, identification of high-risk first remission patients remains difficult, and the vast majority of pediatric patients are therefore not candidates for autologous BMT until after relapse has occurred. Sensitive methods using PCR have been developed to identify patients with minimal residual disease (70–73), and these sensitive techniques may be useful in identifying additional high-risk individuals that may benefit from autologous BMT in first remission. As noted previously in this chapter, there have also been many attempts to improve BMT preparative regimens to provide more effective elimination of ALL cells in vivo. Most effective regimens have been based on the use of TBI, but the addition of ara-C, and more recently, VP16, may significantly improve the effectiveness of these regimens. Further clinical studies are now being carried out to assess the effectiveness of these regimens, and new regimens are continually being developed.

As noted previously, in vitro purging to remove residual leukemic cells from autologous marrow is used extensively in ALL (see Chapters 13 and 14). Despite the fact that different purging methods have been used for more than 12 years, there have been no clinical attempts to identify the most effective methods. Moreover, the role of purging itself remains controversial. Fortunately, the development of sensitive methods to assess the efficacy of marrow purging in individual patients (42,74) and the use of genetically marked marrow for autologous BMT (75) will allow investigators to address these issues. If genetically marked marrow is shown to contribute to leukemic relapse, this will provide strong evidence for the need to remove residual tumor cells prior to autologous BMT. Similarly, if more effective marrow depletion of tumor cells is shown to correlate with decreased relapse following BMT, the therapeutic role of marrow purging will be further substantiated.

Many studies are currently being carried out to develop new methods of eliminating residual leukemic cells after BMT. A GVL effect clearly contributes to the elimination of residual leukemic cells following allogeneic BMT (46,76). Although GVL has been associated with GVHD, the functional mechanism for GVL has not been defined clearly, and some animal models have suggested that GVL may, at least in part, be distinguished from GVHD (77–80). It has been widely assumed that GVL is restricted to allogeneic BMT, but evidence for this restriction is lacking. One of the effector mechanisms that may have a role in GVL is natural killer (NK) cells. The specificity of these cells is not restricted to allogeneic targets, and NK cells have been shown to be cytolytic to autologous leukemic cells in vitro. NK cells reconstitute early after both autologous and allogeneic BMT (81–83), and their function can be enhanced with interleukin-2 (IL-2) in vitro and in vivo (84). Clinical trials from several centers have demonstrated that IL-2 can be administered safely after autologous BMT and that IL-2 infusion enhances NK cell function in vivo. In Seattle, high-dose IL-2 has been administered with in vitro–generated lymphokine-activated killer (LAK) cells following autologous BMT (85). A prospective randomized trial of IL-2/LAK therapy following autologous BMT versus no further therapy is now being conducted. At the DFCI, IL-2 has been administered by outpatient continuous infusion at low doses for a 3-month period after full autologous reconstitution has been achieved (86). Low-dose infusions (2–4 $\times 10^5$ U/M^2/day) beginning 6 to 8 weeks after BMT are well tolerated and result in approximately 10-fold expansion of the total number of circulating NK cells. Further studies to assess the impact of this type of immunotherapy on leukemic relapse are now being conducted (see Chapter 19).

In addition to IL-2, other cytokines, such as interferon (87), or new immunomodulatory agents, such as linomide (88), may be able to induce or enhance GVL following autologous BMT. Attempts to induce GVL by initiating a GVHD-like syndrome after autologous BMT may also provide a novel method for eliminating minimal residual disease following BMT (89). The post-transplant setting may also provide a setting where immunotoxins directed at leukemia-associated antigens may be effective. Such studies are in progress in patients with B-cell non-Hodgkin's lymphomas following autologous BMT using an immunotoxin directed against the CD19 antigen conjugated to blocked ricin (B4-bR) (90). The CD19 antigen is widely expressed on all B-lineage leukemic cells and may also be particularly useful in patients with ALL following autologous BMT. A clinical trial using a CD19-specific antibody conjugated to pokeweed antiviral protein is being conducted in patients with ALL at the University of Minnesota. Given the intense interest in this approach and the variety of different methods that are being evaluated currently, it is very likely that effective methods for eliminating residual leukemic cells following autologous BMT will be developed in the near future. Because leukemic relapse remains the most frequent cause of failure following autologous BMT, effective elimination of residual leukemia should lead to significant improvement in disease-free survival following BMT.

References

1. McGovern J, Russell P, Atkins L, et al. Treatment of terminal leukemic relapse by total-body irradiation and intravenous infusion of stored autologous bone marrow obtained during remission. N Engl J Med 1959; 260:675–683.
2. Ritz J, Sallan SE, Bast RC, et al. Autologous bone

marrow transplantation in CALLA positive acute lymphoblastic leukemia following in vitro treatment with J5 monoclonal antibody and complement. Lancet 1982;2:60–63.

3. Ramsey NKC, LeBien T, Nesbit M, et al. Autologous bone marrow transplantation for patients with acute lymphoblastic leukemia in second or subsequent remission: results of bone marrow treated with monoclonal antibodies BA-1, BA-2, and BA-3 plus complement. Blood 1985;66:508–513.
4. Champlin R, Gale RP. Acute lymphoblastic leukemia: recent advances in biology and therapy. Blood 1989; 73:2051–2066.
5. Nadler LM, Korsmeyer SJ, Anderson KC, et al. The B cell origin of non-T cell acute lymphoblastic leukemia: a model for discrete stages of neoplastic and normal pre-B cell differentiation. J Clin Invest 1984;74:332–340.
6. Sallan SE, Ritz J, Pesando JM, et al. Cell surface antigens: prognostic implications in childhood acute lymphoblastic leukemia. Blood 1980;55:395–402.
7. Kurtzberg J, Waldman TA, Davey MD, et al. CD7+ CD4− CD8− acute leukemia: a syndrome of malignant pluripotent lymphohematopoietic cells. Blood 1989; 73:381–390.
8. Bloomfield CD, Goldman AI, Alimena G, et al. Chromosomal abnormalities identify high-risk and low-risk patients with acute lymphoblastic leukemia. Blood 1986;67:415–420.
9. Pui C, Crist WM, Look AT. Biology and clinical significance of cytogenetic abnormalities in childhood acute lymphoblastic leukemia. Blood 1989;76:1449–1463.
10. Chen Q, Cheng J-Y, Tsai L-H, et al. The *tal* gene undergoes chromosome translocation in a T cell leukemia and potentially encodes a helix-loop-helix protein. EMBO J 1990;9:414–424.
11. Macintyre EA, Smit L, Ritz J, Kirsch IR, Strominger JL. Disruption of the SCL locus in T-lymphoid malignancies correlates with commitment to the T-cell receptor $\alpha\beta$ lineage. Blood 1992;80:1511–1520.
12. Clavell LA, Gelber RD, Cohen HJ, et al. Four-agent induction and intensive asparaginase therapy for treatment of childhood acute lymphoblastic leukemia. N Engl J Med 1986;315:657–663.
13. Ramsay NKC, Kersey J. Indications for marrow transplantation in acute lymphoblastic leukemia. Blood 1990;75:815–818.
14. Hoelzer D, Thiel E, Loffler H, et al. Prognostic factors in a multicenter study for treatment of acute lymphoblastic leukemia in adults. Blood 1988;71:123–131.
15. Hussein KK, Dahlberg S, Head D, et al. Treatment of acute lymphoblastic leukemia in adults with intensive induction, consolidation, and maintenance chemotherapy. Blood 1989;73:57–63.
16. Linker CA, Levitt LW, O'Donnell M, Forman SJ, Ries CA. Treatment of adult acute lymphoblastic leukemia with intensive cyclical chemotherapy: a follow-up report. Blood 1991;78:2814–2822.
17. Henze G, Fengler R, Hartmann R, et al. Six year experience with a comprehensive approach to the treatment of recurrent childhood acute lymphoblastic leukemia (ALL-REZ BFM 85). A relapse study of the BFM Group. Blood 1991;78:1166–1172.
18. Thomas ED, Sanders JE, Flournoy N, et al. Marrow transplantation for patients with acute lymphoblastic leukemia: a long-term follow-up. Blood 1983;62:1139–1141.
19. Nesbit ME, Woods WG, Weisdorf D, et al. Bone marrow transplantation for acute lymphocytic leukemia. Semin Oncol 1985;12:149–159.
20. Barrett AJ, Horowitz MM, Gale RP, et al. Marrow transplantation for acute lymphoblastic leukemia: factors affecting relapse and survival. Blood 1989;74:862–871.
21. Kernan NA, Bartsch G, Ash RC. Analysis of 462 transplantations from unrelated donors facilitated by the National Marrow Donor Program. N Engl J Med 1993;328:593–602.
22. Simonsson B, Burnett AK, Prentice HG, et al. Autologous bone marrow transplantation with monoclonal antibody purged marrow for high risk acute lymphoblastic leukemia. Leukemia 1989;3:631–636.
23. Herve P, Labopin M, Plouvier E, Palut P, Tiberghien P, Gorin NC. Autologous bone marrow transplantation for childhood acute lymphoblastic leukemia—a European survey. Bone Marrow Transplant 1991;8(suppl): 72–75.
24. Rivera GK, Buchanan G, Boyett JM, et al. Intensive retreatment of childhood acute lymphoblastic leukemia in first bone marrow relapse: a pediatric oncology group study. N Engl J Med 1986;315:273–278.
25. Sallan SE, Niemeyer CM, Billett AL, et al. Autologous bone marrow transplantation for acute lymphoblastic leukemia. J Clin Oncol 1989;7:1–8.
26. Preijers FWMB, De Witte T, Wessels JMC, et al. Autologous transplantation of bone marrow purged in vitro with anti-CD7-(WT1-) ricin A immunotoxin in T-cell lymphoblastic leukemia and lymphoma. Blood 1989;74:1152–1158.
27. Uckun FM, Kersey JD, Vallera DA, et al. Autologous bone marrow transplantation in high-risk transmission T-lineage acute lymphoblastic leukemia using immunotoxins plus 4-hydroperoxycyclophosphamide for marrow purging. Blood 1990;76:1723–1733.
28. Kiesel S, Haas R, Moldenhauer G, Kvalheim G, Pezzutto A, Dorken B. Removal of cells from a malignant B-cell line from bone marrow with immunomagnetic beads and with complement and immunoglobulin switch variant mediated cytolysis. Leuk Res 1987;11:1119–1125.
29. Kaizer H, Stuart R, Brookmeyer R, et al. Autologous bone marrow transplantation in acute leukemia: a phase I study of in vitro treatment of marrow with 4 hydro-peroxycyclophosphamide to purge tumor cells. Blood 1985;65:1504–1510.
30. Gorin NC, Douay L, Laporte JP, et al. Autologous bone marrow transplantation using marrow incubated with Asta Z 7557 in adult acute leukemia. Blood 1986; 67:1367–1376.
31. Bast RC, DeFabritriis P, Lipton J, et al. Elimination of malignant clonogenic cells from human bone marrow using multiple monoclonal antibodies and complement. Cancer Res 1985;45:499–503.
32. Strong R, Uckun F, Youle R, Kersey J, Vallera D. Use of multiple T cell-directed intact ricin immunotoxins for autologous bone marrow transplantation. Blood 1985; 66:627–635.
33. Siena S, Castro-Malaspina H, Gulati S, et al. Effects of in vitro purging with 4-hydroperoxycyclophosphamide on the hematopoietic and microenvironmental elements of human bone marrow. Blood 1985;65:655–662.
34. LeBien T, Stepan D, Bartholomew R, Strong R, Anderson J. Utilization of a colony assay to assess the variables influencing elimination of leukemic cells from

human bone marrow with monoclonal antibodies and complement. Blood 1985;65:945–950.
35. Roy DC, Felix M, Cammady WG, Cannistra S, Ritz J. Comparative activities of rabbit complements of different ages using an in vitro marrow purging model. Leuk Res 1990;14:407–416.
36. Uckun FM, Jaxzcz W, Amburs JL, et al. Detailed studies on expression and function of CD19 surface determinant by using B43 monoclonal antibody and the clinical potential of anti-CD19 immunotoxins. Blood 1988; 71:13–29.
37. Roy D, Ish C, Blattler W, Lambert J, Ritz J. A new immunotoxin for purging of acute lymphoblastic leukemia cells prior to autologous bone marrow transplantation (abstract). Proc Am Assoc Cancer Res 1990;31:
38. Casellas P, Canat X, Fauser A, et al. Optimal elimination of leukemic T cells from human bone marrow with T101-ricin A-chain immunotoxin. Blood 1985;65:289–297.
39. Ramakrishnan S, Uckun F, Houston L. Anti-T cell immunotoxins containing pokeweed anti-viral protein: potential purging agents for human autologous bone marrow transplantation. J Immunol 1985;135:3616–3622.
40. Uckun FM, Kersey JH, Haake R, Weisdorf D, Ramsay NKC. Autologous bone marrow transplantation in high-risk remission B-lineage acute lymphoblastic leukemia using a cocktail of three monoclonal antibodies (BA-1/CD24, BA-2/CD9, and BA-3/CD10) plus complement and 4-hydroperoxycyclophosphamide for ex vivo bone marrow purging. Blood 1992;79:1094–1104.
41. Negrin RS, Kiem HP, Schmidt-Wolf IGH, Blume KG, Cleary ML. Use of polymerase chain reaction to monitor the effectiveness of ex vivo tumor cell purging. Blood 1991;77:654–660.
42. Gribben JG, Saporito L, Barber M, et al. Bone marrows of non-Hodgkin's lymphoma patients with a BCL-2 translocation can be purged of PCR detectable lymphoma cells using monoclonal antibodies and immunomagnetic bead depletion. Blood 1992;80: 1083–1089.
43. Miller C, Zehnbauer B, Piantadosi S, Rowley S, Jones R. Correlation of occult clonogenic leukemia drug sensitivity with relapse after autologous bone marrow transplantation. Blood 1991;78:1125–1131.
44. Kersey JH, Weisdorf D, Nesbit ME, et al. Comparison of autologous and allogeneic bone marrow transplantation for treatment of high risk refractory acute lymphoblastic leukemia. N Engl J Med 1987;317:461–467.
45. Ramsay N, LeBien T, Weisdorf D, et al. Autologous BMT for patients with acute lymphoblastic leukemia. In: Gale R, Champlin R, eds. Bone marrow transplantation: current controversies. New York: Alan R. Liss, 1989:57–66.
46. Weisdorf DJ, Nesbit ME, Ramsay NKC, et al. Allogeneic bone marrow transplantation for acute lymphoblastic leukemia in remission: prolonged survival associated with acute graft-versus-host-disease. J Clin Oncol 1987;5:1348–1355.
47. Woods WG, Ramsay NKC, Weisdorf DJ, et al. Bone marrow transplantation for acute lymphocytic leukemia utilizing total body irradiation followed by high doses of cytosine arabinoside. Bone Marrow Transplant 1990;6:9–16.
48. Billet AL, Kornmehl E, Tarbell NJ, et al. Autologous bone marrow transplantation after a long first remission for children with recurrent acute lymphoblastic leukemia. Blood 1993;81:1651–1657.
49. Soiffer RJ, Roy DC, Gonin R, et al. Monoclonal antibody-purged autologous bone marrow transplantation in adults with acute lymphoblastic leukemia at high risk for subsequent relapse. Bone Marrow Transplant 1993 (in press).
50. Cahn JY, Bordignoni P, Souillet G, et al. The TAM regimen prior to allogeneic and autologous bone marrow transplantation for high risk acute lymphoblastic leukemia: a cooperative study of 62 patients. Bone Marrow Transplant 1991;7:1–4.
51. Schroeder H, Pinkerton C, Powles R, et al. High dose melphalan and total body irradiation with autologous marrow rescue in childhood acute lymphoblastic leukemia after relapse. Bone Marrow Transplant 1991;7:11–15.
52. Chao NJ, Forman SJ, Schmidt GM, et al. Allogeneic bone marrow transplantation for high-risk acute lymphoblastic leukemia during first complete remission. Blood 1991;8:1923–1927.
53. Dopfer R, Henze G, Gotze-Bender C, et al. Allogeneic bone marrow transplantation for childhood acute lymphoblastic leukemia in second remission after intensive primary and relapse therapy according to the BFM- and CoALL-protocols: results of the German Cooperative Study. Blood 1991;78:2780–2784.
54. Doney K, Buckner C, Fisher L, et al. Autologous bone marrow transplantation for patients with acute lymphoblastic leukemia. Bone Marrow Transplant 1993 (in press).
55. Gonzales-Chambers R, Przepiorka D, Shadduck R, et al. Autologous bone marrow transplantation with 4-hydroperoxycyclophosphamide-purged marrow for acute lymphoblastic leukemia. Med Pediatr Oncol 1991;19: 160–164.
56. Gilmore MJML, Hamon MD, Prentice HG, et al. Failure of purged autologous bone marrow transplantation in high risk acute lymphoblastic leukemia in first complete remission. Bone Marrow Transplant 1991;8:19–26.
57. Colleselli P, Dini G, Andolina M, et al. Autologous bone marrow transplantation for acute lymphoblastic leukemia: the high dose vincristine study of AIEOP BMT group. Bone Marrow Transplant 1991;7(suppl 3):28–30.
58. Zintl F, Hermann J, Fuchs D, et al. Comparison of allogeneic and autologous bone marrow transplantation for treatment of acute lymphocytic leukemia in childhood. Haematol Blood Transfus 1990;33:692–698.
59. Rizzoli U, Mangoni L, Carella A, et al. Drug-mediated marrow purging: mafosfamide in adult acute leukemia in remission. The experience of the Italian Study Group. Bone Marrow Transplant 1989;4(suppl 1):190–194.
60. Pico J, Hartmann O, Maraninchi D, et al. Modified chemotherapy with carmustine, cytarabine, cyclophosphamide, and 6-thioguanine (BACT) and autologous bone marrow transplantation in 24 poor-risk patients with acute lymphoblastic leukemia. J Natl Cancer Inst 1986;76:1289–1293.
61. Carella A, Martinengo M, Santini G, et al. Autologous bone marrow transplantation for acute leukemia in remission: the Genoa experience. Haematologica 1988; 73:119–124.
62. Stoppa A, Hirn J, Blaise D, et al. Autologous bone marrow transplantation for B cell malignancies after in vitro purging with floating immunobeads. Bone Marrow Transplant 1990;6:301–307.

63. Davis H, Revell P, Ginangrande P, et al. Safe application of a 13-Gy split dose total body irradiation schedule prior to bone marrow transplantation. Bone Marrow Transplant 1988;3:349–356.
64. Hill RS, Mazza P, Amos D, et al. Engraftment in 86 patients with lymphoid malignancy after autologous marrow transplantation. Bone Marrow Transplant 1989;4:69–74.
65. Rowley S, Piantadosi S, Marcellus D, et al. Analysis of factors predicting speed of hematologic recovery after transplantation with 4-hydroperoxycyclophosphamide-purged autologus bone marrow grafts. Bone Marrow Transplant 1991;7:183–191.
66. Robertson MJ, Soiffer RJ, Griffin JD, et al. Human bone marrow depleted of CD33-positive cells mediates delayed but durable reconstitution of hematopoiesis: clinical trial of MY9 monoclonal antibody-purged autografts for the treatment of acute myeloid leukemia. Blood 1992;79:2229–2236.
67. Uderzo C, Coleselli P, Messina C, et al. Allogeneic BMT versus autologous BMT in childhood acute lymphoblastic leukemia (ALL): an Italian cooperative study of vincristine (VCR), F-TBI and cyclophosphamide. Bone Marrow Transplant 1991;7(suppl 2):132.
68. Blaise D, Gaspard MH, Stoppa AM, et al. Allogeneic or autologous bone marrow transplantation for acute lymphoblastic leukemia in first complete remission. Bone Marrow Transplant 1990;5:7–12.
69. Nemunaitis J, Rabinowe SN, Singer JW, et al. Recombinant granulocyte-macrophage colony-stimulating factor after autologous bone marrow transplantation for lymphoid cancer. N Engl J Med 1991;324:1773–1778.
70. Yokota S, Hansen-Hagge TE, Ludwig W-D, et al. Use of polymerase chain reactions to monitor minimal residual disease in acute lymphoblastic leukemia patients. Blood 1991;77:331–339.
71. Neale BAM, Menarguez J, Kitchingham GR, et al. Detection of minimal residual disease in T-cell acute lymphoblastic leukemia using polymerase chain reaction predicts impending relapse. Blood 1991;78:739–747.
72. Gehly G, Bryan E, Lee A, Kidd P, Thomas E. Chimeric BCR-abl messenger RNA as a marker for minimal residual disease in patients transplanted for Philadelphia chromosome-positive acute lymphoblastic leukemia. Blood 1991;78:458–465.
73. Yamada M, Wasserman R, Lange B, Riechard B, Womer R, Rovera G. Minimal residual disease in childhood B-lineage lymphoblastic leukemia. N Engl J Med 1990; 323:448–455.
74. Gribben JG, Freedman AS, Neuberg D, et al. Immunologic purging of marrow assessed by PCR before autologous bone marrow transplantation for B-cell lymphoma. N Engl J Med 1991;325:1525–1533.
75. Rill D, Moen R, Buschle M, et al. An approach for the analysis of relapse and marrow reconstitution after autologous marrow transplantation using retrovirus-mediated gene transfer. Blood 1992;79:2694–2700.
76. Weiden PL, Flournoy NS, Thomas ED, et al. Antileukemic effect of graft-versus-host-disease in human recipients of allogeneic-marrow grafts. N Engl J Med 1979;300:1068–1073.
77. Slavin S, Ackerstein A, Naparstek R, Weiss O, Weiss L. The graft-versus-leukemia (GVL) phenomenon: is GVL separable from GVHD? Bone Marrow Transplant 1990;6:155–161.
78. Sykes M, Romick M, Sachs D. Interleukin 2 prevents graft-versus-host disease while preserving the graft-versus-leukemia effect of allogeneic T cells. Proc Natl Acad Sci USA 1990;87:5633–5637.
79. Ackerstein A, Kedar E, Slavin S. Use of recombinant human interleukin-2 in conjunction with syngeneic bone marrow transplantation in mice as a model for control of minimal residual disease in malignant hematologic disorders. Blood 1991;78:1212–1215.
80. Horowitz MM, Gale RP, Sondel PM, et al. Graft-versus-leukemia reactions after bone marrow transplantation. Blood 1990;75:555–562.
81. Soiffer R, Bosserman L, Murray C, Cochran K, Daley J, Ritz J. Reconstitution of T cell function following CD6 depleted allogeneic bone marrow transplantation. Blood 1990;75:2076–2084.
82. Reittie JE, Gottlieb D, Heslop HE, et al. Endogenously generated activated killer cells circulate after autologous and allogeneic marrow transplantation but not after chemotherapy. Blood 1989;73:1351–1358.
83. Jacobs R, Stoll M, Stratmann G, Leo R, Link H, Schmidt RE. CD16− CD56+ natural killer cells after bone marrow transplantation. Blood 1992;79:3239–3244.
84. Higuchi CM, Thompson JA, Cox T, Lindgren CG, Buckner CD, Fefer A. Lymphokine-activated killer function following autologous bone marrow transplantation for refractory hematological malignancies. Cancer Res 1989;49:5509–5513.
85. Higuchi CM, Thompson JA, Peterson FB, Buckner CD, Fefer A. Toxicity and immunomodulatory effects of interleukin-2 after autologous bone marrow transplantation for hematologic malignancies. Blood 1991;77: 2561–2568.
86. Soiffer RJ, Murray C, Cochran K, et al. Clinical and immunologic effects of prolonged infusion of low-dose recombinant interleukin-2 after autologous and T-cell-depleted allogeneic bone marrow transplantation. Blood 1992;79:517–526.
87. Klingemann H-G, Grigg A, Wilkie-Boyd K, et al. Treatment with recombinant interferon α-2b early after bone marrow transplantation in patients at high risk for relapse. Blood 1991;78:3306–3311.
88. Bengtsson M, Simonsson B, Carlsson K, et al. Stimulation of NK cell, T cell, and monocyte functions by the novel immunomodulator linomide after autologous bone marrow transplantation. Transplantation 1992; 53:882–888.
89. Yeager A, Vogelsang G, Jones R, et al. Induction of cutaneous graft-versus-host disease by administration of cyclosporine to patients undergoing autologous bone marrow transplantation for acute myeloid leukemia. Blood 1992;79:3031–3035.
90. Grossbard ML, Gribben JG, Freedman AS, et al. Adjuvant immunotoxin therapy with anti-B4-blocked ricin after autologous bone marrow transplantation for patients with B-cell non-Hodgkin's lymphoma. Blood 1993;81:2263–2271.

Chapter 56
Autografting in Chronic Myeloid Leukemia

Michael J. Barnett, Connie J. Eaves, and Allen C. Eaves

This chapter focuses on the role of autografting procedures in the management of patients with chronic myeloid leukemia (CML). Autografting (i.e., intravenous infusion of autologous [the patient's own] hematopoietic stem cells after intensive therapy) allows administration of chemotherapy or chemoradiotherapy in doses that would otherwise result in prolonged or permanent myelosuppression. The rationale for such dose escalation is that it will result in a greater antitumor effect.

Conventional therapy of CML (with hydroxyurea or busulfan) can usually control the overall tumor burden (as assessed by the white cell count and size of the spleen) in patients in the chronic phase of disease. However, in the vast majority of patients managed with conventional therapy, there is no evidence of cytogenetic normalization of hematopoiesis (i.e., cells belonging to the Philadelphia chromosome [Ph]–positive neoplastic clone continue to predominate in both the blood and the marrow). More importantly, neither these two drugs nor combination chemotherapy significantly delays progression of the disease to blast phase. Because the blast phase is inevitably fatal, conventional therapy does little to improve survival, and the median life expectancy from diagnosis is approximately 4 years (1). In a proportion of patients with CML in chronic phase, induction of cytogenetic remission and the return of polyclonal hematopoiesis (2) can be achieved with combination chemotherapy in standard dosage (Table 56-1) (3–5). However, these remissions are invariably short-lived and do not confer substantial survival benefit. Prolonged administration of α-interferon can also induce the reappearance of normal hematopoiesis in some patients (see Table 56-1) (6). Whether this agent influences the natural history of CML is not yet known.

The only treatment protocol known to cure patients with CML involves the use of "myeloablative" doses of chemotherapy or chemoradiotherapy followed by transplantation of marrow from a histocompatible donor (7–9). Allogeneic bone marrow transplantation (BMT), however, has generally been restricted to patients who have a sibling with the same human leukocyte antigen (HLA) type to act as a marrow donor. In addition, these protocols are usually limited to patients under the age of 50 years because of the severity of graft-versus-host disease (GVHD) encountered in older individuals (10). Partially HLA-matched related marrow donors (11) and unrelated volunteer marrow donors (9) are now also being used, the latter increasingly so. Unfortunately, even with this expansion of the donor pool, most patients with CML are not considered eligible for allogeneic BMT due to either their age or the lack of an adequately matched donor. In addition, there is still a significant risk of fatality associated with the procedure, usually directly or indirectly associated with GVHD (7–9). Thus, although intensive therapy with marrow rescue offers the only current basis for cure, new strategies are being sought to make the procedure safer and to allow its extension to a larger proportion of patients.

Rationale for Autografting in CML

Use of an autologous rather than an allogeneic graft is, at least theoretically, attractive. In its simplest form, an autograft should provide the protective function of an allograft without any of the problems of donor availability or GVHD. For autografting to be a curative option, two conditions have to be met. First, the intensive therapy alone must eliminate every leukemic *stem* cell in the patient. Second, it must be possible to obtain an aliquot of autologous cells that is both free of leukemic stem cells and includes sufficient normal precursors to allow permanent resumption of normal blood cell formation in a time frame compatible with survival. Some information about each of these issues is currently available and is reviewed.

Efficacy of Intensive Therapy

A best estimate of the antileukemic effectiveness due exclusively to the intensive treatment regimens used in BMT protocols is obtained by comparing the results in recipients of allogeneic grafts and recipients of syngeneic grafts (from a normal identical twin donor) (12). For chronic-phase CML, such comparisons show the relapse rate after syngeneic BMT to be higher than after allogeneic BMT (approximately 50% versus

Table 56-1.
Cytogenetic Response to Treatment of CML Early in Chronic Phase

Treatment, Ref	No. Evaluable Patients	*Achievement of Cytogenetic Response (% of Patients)*[a]		*Median Survival After Diagnosis (mo)*		
		Complete	*Partial*	*All*	*Responders*[a]	*Failures*[a]
L-15(3,4)[b]	42	33	14	50	55	46
ROAP(5)[c]	34	29	24	52	NR	35
α-Interferon(6)[d]	96	19	7	62	NS	NS

[a]Defined by percent of Ph-negative marrow metaphases achieved: complete response = 100%; partial response = 66 to 99%; failure = <66%.
[b]Cytosine arabinoside, daunorubicin, 6-thioguanine, hydroxyurea, methotrexate, vincristine, cyclophosphamide, prednisone.
[c]Rubidazone or daunorubicin, cytosine arabinoside, vincristine, prednisone.
[d]Partially pure (n = 51); recombinant (n = 45).
CML = chronic myeloid leukemia; NR = not reached; NS = not stated.

approximately 20%). Nevertheless, cure of CML can be achieved with syngeneic BMT in approximately 40% of patients with chronic-phase disease (13,14). The reason for the significantly lower relapse rate in recipients of allogeneic BMT is that there is an additional antileukemic effect attributable to an as yet poorly defined immunological action of the allograft, which is referred to as the graft-versus-leukemia (GVL) effect (15–17). The phenomenon clearly has relevance to autografting, during which an antileukemic effect of the graft would not be expected. Thus, for autografting protocols to be as successful as those utilizing allogeneic BMT, it is likely that additional therapeutic approaches to replace the GVL effect will have to be incorporated.

Composition of the Autograft

Twenty years ago it was widely assumed that by the time of diagnosis, the original normal hematopoietic stem-cell population had become extinct in most patients. This perception was based on the general failure of any treatment at that time to elicit the reappearance of cytogenetically normal cells despite a marked reduction in the total size of the leukemic clone. Subsequently, with the testing of more aggressive treatment protocols, attainment of cytogenetic remissions in at least some patients suggested that normal hematopoietic stem cells were present, although functionally suppressed (18). However, it was difficult to develop these clinical observations further because quantitative assays for both normal hematopoietic stem cells and their leukemic counterparts were not available. An estimate of the number of these cells present in individual patients therefore could not be made, nor could potential differences in the sensitivities of normal and leukemic stem cells to particular agents be defined.

Initial attempts to address these questions involved the use of in vitro colony assays. These assays allowed the number of both normal and leukemic cells at an early stage of differentiation to be determined. In most patients with CML, virtually all of the progenitors detected by colony assays proved to be of leukemic origin (19,20). This finding reflects the significant amplification of leukemic cells that occurs at early stages of hematopoietic cell development during unregulated expansion of the CML clone. Moreover, this expansion affects early hematopoietic cells on all lineages equally, although at the level of mature blood cell production it is only the output of granulocytes and, to a lesser extent, platelets that is elevated (21). Thus, even a normal number of primitive normal hematopoietic cells are usually not detectable because of their dilution by leukemic cells. Quantitative measurements of the progenitor content of the peripheral blood of patients with CML have shown that the number of these cells increases *exponentially* with the white cell count (i.e., for every 10-fold increase in mature cells there is, on average, a 100 fold increase in leukemic progenitors). In the marrow, the concentration of progenitors is not correspondingly increased; in fact, the ratio of progenitors to nucleated cells remains approximately normal. However, because the overall cellularity of the marrow is usually increased (up to approximately 5-fold), the absolute number of leukemic progenitors in the marrow will also be increased by this factor. Conversely, in newly diagnosed patients with low white cell counts and in whom the leukemic progenitors have not yet expanded significantly, normal progenitors can be consistently detected and are found to be present at near-normal levels (22). However, even in such patients, the more mature hematopoietic cells appear to be exclusively of leukemic origin, reflecting the significant suppression of the latter stages of normal hematopoiesis in patients with CML. Evaluation of the ratio of the *total* number of normal and leukemic cells in patient blood or marrow samples must therefore be interpreted with caution, because such information is unlikely to reflect the relative numbers of the rare subpopulations of normal and leukemic cells at early stages of hematopoietic cell development.

Quantitation of Normal and Leukemic Stem Cells

Recently, a method was developed for measuring a very primitive type of hematopoietic cell (more primitive than the cells detected by conventional in vitro colony assays). These cells were given the operational name "long-term culture initiating cells" (LTC-IC) to reflect the procedure used for their detection. LTC-IC give rise to in vitro colony forming cells after a minimum of 5 weeks of culture on competent fibroblasts (23). The LTC-IC present in normal human marrow can also be physically separated from in vitro colony forming cells (24). Low numbers of LTC-IC are normally found in the peripheral blood as well.

The growth factors required to support production of in vitro colony forming cells from LTC-IC are not yet completely defined. Granulocyte colony stimulating factor (G-CSF), together with interleukin-3 (IL-3), appear able to support production of in vitro colony forming cells from LTC-IC, and this production is enhanced if Steel factor (also known as stem-cell factor [SCF], mast-cell growth factor [MGF], and *c-kit* ligand) is also present, although Steel factor alone is not effective. Cultured fibroblasts also have the ability to support production of in vitro colony forming cells from LTC-IC, but they appear to do this by virtue of their ability to produce other as yet unidentified growth factors (25,26).

The full functional potential of human LTC-IC is also not yet established. Several findings suggest that these cells at least overlap with transplantable hematopoietic stem cells. First, the same (or analogous) conditions used to detect (and maintain) LTC-IC in human marrow support extensive proliferation of some transplantable murine hematopoietic stem cells that can regenerate all lymphoid and myeloid lineages in lethally irradiated recipients (27). Second, LTC-IC are relatively resistant to 4-hydroperoxycyclophosphamide (24), a drug that is thought to spare stem cells. Third, intensively treated patients with CML who have been autografted with marrow previously maintained in culture for 10 days have shown rapid regeneration of normal hematopoiesis, indicating engraftment by normal cells from the cultured autograft (28,29). Analysis of the cell types present in these autografts has demonstrated that most of the in vitro colony forming cells were leukemic, whereas most of the LTC-IC were normal. This finding suggests that engraftment, at least in such circumstances, may be a function of the normal LTC-IC present, rather than being influenced by the number or type of in vitro colony forming cells also infused.

Studies of the genotype, properties, and behavior of LTC-IC in marrow and blood samples from patients with CML have shown that leukemic (Ph-positive) LTC-IC can also be quantitated and characterized using the LTC-IC assay (30). However, normal and leukemic LTC-IC have relatively low and high turnover rates, respectively (21); thus most leukemic LTC-IC are phenotypically different from normal LTC-IC with respect to properties associated with changes in cycling status (31,32).

Strategies to Optimize Selection of Normal Hematopoietic Stem Cells for Autografting

Quantitative assessment of normal and leukemic LTC-IC in the marrow of patients with CML has shown that, on average, both are markedly reduced; normal LTC-IC are usually more numerous. In blood, leukemic LTC-IC increase exponentially with the white cell count, as is the case for leukemic progenitors detected by in vitro colony assays (30). These findings suggest that the marrow would usually be a better choice than the blood as a source of cells for a CML autograft in any protocol seeking to restore normal hematopoiesis after delivery of intensive therapy. However, because of the absolute reduction in the number of normal stem cells in the marrow of most patients with CML, a conventional marrow harvest (approximately 2×10^{10} cells) may not contain sufficient normal hematopoietic stem cells to ensure rescue of the patient's hematopoietic system following myeloablative therapy. However, even single normal stem cells may have the capacity *eventually* to reconstitute the entire human hematopoietic system, although this capacity may not be myeloprotective and is rarely elicited clinically. In most BMTs, it is likely that many stem cells are transplanted and the hematopoietic cells reconstituted are then polyclonal in origin (33).

If leukemic stem cells are present in the autograft, even at very low numbers, they may have the potential to re-establish disease after infusion. Ultimately, questions of which and how many normal cells are required for successful engraftment and which and how many leukemic cells can re-establish disease can only be addressed in a definitive fashion by clinical studies involving genetic marking of the autograft. In approximately half the patients with chronic-phase CML, some Ph-positive LTC-IC can be detected in less than 10^8 marrow cells (i.e., $<1\%$ of a standard marrow harvest) (34). Methods for their further reduction (without simultaneous compromise of the normal hematopoietic stem-cell population) may therefore be important for many patients otherwise eligible for treatments requiring a marrow autograft. A number of centers are currently pursuing a variety of approaches that might allow normal and leukemic stem cells to be separated further. These approaches include the use of physical (32), pharmacological (35), biological (36), or cell culture-based (28) strategies. The latter is the most advanced, with achievement of a 30- to 50-fold purging effect of leukemic LTC-IC and full retention of normal LTC-IC (30,37). However, culture purging is a labor-intensive procedure, and its molecular basis remains a complete mystery. Both of these factors currently detract from its potential widespread use or improvement. Pharmacological purging of CML marrow cells with derivatives of cyclophosphamide achieves less of a selective effect (3-

to 5-fold reduction of leukemic LTC-IC under conditions that spare normal LTC-IC) (31,38), and a high degree of variability between patients is encountered. Some separation of normal and leukemic LTC-IC in CML marrow can also be obtained using physical methods (32); however, it is not yet clear whether this technique can be translated into a clinically useful protocol. Because of the reduced numbers of normal stem cells in CML marrow and the inevitable further losses associated with physical purification methods, applicability of this approach may be limited. Ultimately, it is hoped that all such limitations will be overcome when methods are devised to expand normal hematopoietic stem cells differentially in culture.

Summary

In patients with CML treated with conventional therapy, there is inexorable progression of the disease to a fatal outcome. Currently, the only curative treatment involves intensive therapy followed by allogeneic or syngeneic BMT, although only a minority of patients can be treated with this approach. The results of syngeneic BMT indicate that intensive therapy alone (i.e., without a GVL effect) has the capacity to eradicate the leukemic clone. This finding, together with the knowledge that functionally intact and probably quantitatively useful numbers of very primitive normal hematopoietic cells may be present in a substantial proportion of patients eligible for intensive therapy, provide strong impetus for the continued development and evaluation of autograft-based treatment modalities.

Clinical Results of Autografting in CML

Use of autografting to allow intensive treatment of CML was introduced two decades ago. As with the first allografts (39,40), the intention of these early studies was to improve on the dismal prognosis of patients with blast-phase disease; median survival with other therapies was approximately 4 months (41). Subsequent efforts, based in part on this early experience, included patients with chronic-phase CML. Currently, autografting in chronic phase is being undertaken with curative intent. Thus, over the last 20 years, the role of autografting in CML has changed.

Autografting after Transformation

In 1974, the Seattle group described the course of 2 patients with transformed CML treated with high-dose cyclophosphamide and total body irradiation (TBI) followed by infusion of autologous marrow cells that had been previously harvested and cryopreserved during chronic phase (42). A later report extended this experience to a total of 7 patients (43). The goal was to achieve a "second chronic phase" and therefore gain temporary respite from an otherwise imminently fatal situation. Although this study was unsuccessful due to transplant-related mortality, it introduced the feasibility of using marrow autografts in the treatment of CML. Subsequently, a study conducted at the Hammersmith Hospital in London demonstrated that cells collected from the peripheral blood by leukapheresis could also restore hematopoiesis following myeloablative therapy (44).

The strategy of harvesting autologous hematopoietic cells during chronic phase and then storing them frozen for later use to allow intensive therapy of transformed disease was then evaluated by a number of centers. The results of these studies, which utilized a variety of chemotherapy or chemoradiotherapy treatment regimens supported by an autograft of either marrow or blood cells, are summarized in Tables 56-2 and 56-3 (43,45–54). The intensity of treatment varied considerably, and some patients were autografted on more than one occasion either for recurrence of blast-phase disease or a consolidation of a second chronic phase. Despite the differences in these clinical studies, a number of general conclusions may be drawn. First, restoration of chronic-phase disease was achieved in most patients receiving autografts of blood cells and in approximately half the patients receiving autografts of marrow cells. Second, when a chronic phase was re-established, its duration prior to recurrence of blast-phase disease was usually relatively brief (i.e., months). Third, Ph-negative hematopoiesis was occasionally observed, but this was also transient. Finally, there was a meaningful prolongation of life in only a minority of patients, most likely because the transformed leukemic subclone responsible for the blast phase of CML is highly resistant to eradication by intensive therapy, as shown by the high recurrence rate seen in patients given a TBI-based regimen and an allogeneic BMT (7).

There have been several reports of patients with transformed CML who were autografted with marrow (48,49,55) or blood (54,56) cells that had been converted to Ph-negativity in vivo. Such cytogenetic remissions were induced by the use of chemotherapy in patients both before (48,56) and after (49,54,55) the onset of blast phase. These studies are important because they reinforce the concept that elimination of Ph-positive cells from the autograft allows at least initial regeneration of the marrow with normal cells.

Probably the most favorable result achieved to date in patients autografted for transformed CML is that reported by the Bordeaux group (53). In this study, a subset of patients underwent intensive therapy and autografting on 2 occasions: the first to re-establish chronic phase, followed by the second as consolidation. After recovery from the second procedure, α-interferon was given as maintenance therapy. The median duration of the second chronic phase was 18 months, which is an impressive result in such a patient group. However, the general inability of intensive therapy to eradicate the blast-phase subclone limits the current utility of autografting in patients with transformed disease.

Table 56-2.
Results of Autografting with Marrow Cells in Transformed CML

Authors, Year, Ref	No. Patients	Intensive Therapy	Achievement of Second Chronic Phase: % of Patients	Achievement of Second Chronic Phase: Median Duration, months (range)	% Ph-negative Marrow Metaphases (in Evaluable Patients)	Median Survival After Autografting, months (range)
Buckner et al. 1978 (43)	7[a]	CY + TBI (n = 4); BCNU + CY + TBI (n = 3)	43	2(1–3)	54 (in 1 of 4)	2(1–4.5)
Thomas et al. 1984 (45)	11[b]	TAD (n =4); MAdHAT (n = 7)	55	5.5(2.5–8.5)	NS	4(0.5–11)
Phillips and Herzig, 1984 (46)	4[c]	CY + TBI	50	6, 26	100 (in 1, otherwise NS)	7.5(2–32)
Lemonnier et al. 1986 (47)	13[d]	TACC (n = 10); TACC + TBI (n = 3)	46	4(1.5–26)	100 (in 1 of 5)	3(0.5–34)
Vellekoop et al. 1986 (48)	11[e]	PIP + TBI	56 (5 of 9, NA in 2)	5.5(4–12.5)	100 (in 3 of 6); 95 (in 1 of 6); 5 (in 1 of 6)	5.5(1–19)
Kantarjian et al. 1991 (49)	7[f]	CY + BCNU + ETOP	0 (0 of 2, NA in 5)	NA	100 (in 1 of 7); 80 (in 1 of 7); 45, 55 (in 2 of 7); 8 (in 1 of 7)	13(1–19)

[a]Five in blast phase (0 lymphoid); and 2 in accelerated phase (1 Ph-negative CML); all autografted once, 2 with additional blood cells.
[b]Eleven in blast phase (0 lymphoid); 10 autografted once and 1 twice (second for recurrent blast phase).
[c]Four in blast phase (1 lymphoid); all autografted once.
[d]Ten in blast phase and 3 in accelerated phase; 12 autografted once and 1 twice (second with CY + TBI and mafosfamide-treated cells as consolidation of third chronic phase).
[e]Eight in blast phase and 2 in second chronic phase (5 lymphoid), 1 in accelerated phase; all autografted once, 3 with Ph-negative cells (harvested after combination chemotherapy).
[f]One in blast phase and 5 in second chronic phase, 1 in accelerated phase; all autografted once, 2 with Ph-negative cells (harvested after combination chemotherapy).
CML = chronic myeloid leukemia; CY = cyclophosphamide in high dosage; TBI = total body irradiation; BCNU = carmustine in high dosage; TAD = 6-thioguanine, cytosine arabinoside, daunorubicin; MAdHAT = melphalan in high dosage, adriamycin, hydroxyurea, cytosine arabinoside, teniposide; TACC = 6-thioguanine, cytosine arabinoside, cyclophosphamide in high dosage, CCNU (lomustine) in high dosage; PIP = piperazinedione in high dosage; ETOP = etoposide in high dosage. NS = not stated; NA = not applicable.

Autografting in Chronic Phase

By the late 1970s, it was apparent that combination chemotherapy in standard dosage given early in chronic phase would not influence survival significantly (3,18). Thereafter, a few centers began to treat patients with chronic-phase CML with intensive therapy supported by an autograft of either marrow (49,57) or blood (58) cells that had been collected previously and cryopreserved. The rationale was that a reduction in the size of the leukemic stem-cell population would decrease the target population available for secondary mutational events. As a result, emergence of a blast-phase subclone might be delayed and survival prolonged.

The results of 3 studies of this type are summarized in Table 56-4 (49,57,58). They illustrate the following general points relevant to this approach. First, recovery of hematopoiesis has usually been satisfactory, although both early and late graft failures have been encountered occasionally. For example, in the Hammersmith study, where blood cell autografts were used, 3 incidents of graft failure occurred (58). Second, normal cells have been readily detectable during regeneration of the hematopoietic system in approximately half the patients, although their dominance had usually been short-lived. Third, in most patients it has not been possible to determine whether the natural history of the disease has been altered by the treatment. In the studies summarized in Table 56-4, one patient died of graft failure and blast-phase disease developed in 3 patients (one in each of the series) post-autograft and they died. In all but 2 of the 30 remaining patients, including those who initially showed some conversion to normal hematopoiesis, chronic-phase disease was re-established. The 2 exceptions continued in cytogenetic remission.

In one of these studies (57), the patients who were autografted were selected from a much larger initial group because they showed a hematological response and cytogenetic improvement on α-interferon. One of the other 2 reports (58) does not state how patients were selected but, given the small numbers involved, it seems unlikely that ineligibility for allogeneic BMT was the sole criterion used. Thus, probably a significant number of the patients in this combined experience could have belonged to a group with a good prognosis who would have survived for a longer period than average regardless of therapy received. Because of the broad range in survival times observed when large numbers of conventionally treated patients with CML are followed and the ability to identify clinical parameters that are associated with shorter or longer survival times (1), patient selection

Table 56-3.
Results of Autografting with Blood Cells in Transformed CML

Authors, Year, Ref	No. Patients	Intensive Therapy	Achievement of Second Chronic Phase: % of Patients	Achievement of Second Chronic Phase: Median Duration, months (range)	% Ph-negative Marrow Metaphases (in Evaluable Patients)	Median Survival After Autografting, months (range)
Haines et al. 1984 (50)	51[a]	DAT ± MEL (n = 9); DAT + TBI (n = 12); Super-RATE ± MEL (n = 30)	94	NS	14–36 (in 3 of 11)	6 (0.5–35)
Preisler et al. 1984 (51)	16[b]	ara-C + Dox + VC + Pred + ARA-C (n = 10); ARA-C (n = 4); ARA-C + BU (n = 2)	31	11 (1–12)	100 (in 1, otherwise NS)	7.5 (0.5–17)
Karp et al. 1985 (52)	7[c]	ara-C + BCNU (n = 4); BCNU (n = 3)	71	4 (2–7)	0 (in 7 of 7)	11(2–16)
Reiffers et al. 1991 (53)	47[d]	Group 1: Super-RATE (n = 4) *or* DAT + CY + TBI (n = 13)	91	3 (1–19)	100 (in 1 of 29); 66–99 (in 3 of 29)	~3.5 (NS–21)
		Group 2: ARA-C + CY + TBI (n = 13)		10 (1–48+)	36–65 (in 5 of 29)	~9.5 (1–49+)
		Group 3: BU + MEL (n = 17)		18 (1–39+)	10–35 (in 5 of 29)	~19 (NS–40+)
Carella et al. 1991 (54)	5[e]	ETOP + CY + TBI	NA	NA	100 (in 5 of 5)	NS (5+–15+)

[a]Forty five in blast phase (8 lymphoid) and 6 in accelerated phase; 30 autografted once, 13 twice, and 8 three times (16 for recurrent blast phase and 5 as consolidation of second chronic phase).
[b]Sixteen in blast phase (0 lymphoid); 15 autografted once and 1 twice (for resistant blast phase), and 3 given Ara-C + Dox± ARA-C as consolidation of second chronic phase.
[c]Seven in blast phase (1 lymphoid); 1 autografted once, 4 twice, and 2 three times (for recurrent blast phase).
[d]Twenty four in blast phase (2 lymphoid) and 23 in accelerated phase; 27 autografted once and 20 twice. Group 1 = single autograft; Group 2 = double autograft (second with MEL as consolidation of second chronic phase) in 8; Group 3 = double autograft (second with MEL as consolidation of second chronic phase) in 12, and given α-interferon after autografting.
[e]Five in complete (i.e., hematological and cytogenetic) remission after treatment of blast phase (3 lymphoid); all autografted once with Ph-negative cells (collected after combination chemotherapy) and given cyclosporine after autografting.
CML = chronic myeloid leukemia; DAT = daunorubicin, cytosine arabinoside, 6-thioguanine; MEL = melphalan in high dosage; TBI = total body irradiation; Super-RATE = DAT, vincristine, prednisolone; ara-C = cytosine arabinoside; Dox = doxorubicin; VC = vincristine; Pred = prednisone; ARA-C = cytosine arabinoside in high dosage; BU = busulfan in high dosage; BCNU = carmustine in high dosage; CY = cyclophosphamide in high dosage; ETOP = etoposide in high dosage; NS = not stated; NA = not applicable.

in any CML trial is an important confounding factor that may prevent independent assessment of the effectiveness of a given treatment modality.

Durable Ph-negative hematopoiesis (100 and 98% Ph-negative marrow metaphases) more than 3 years after autografting was achieved in 2 of the patients in the Hammersmith study (58). In both, however, hematopoiesis early after autografting was exclusively or predominantly Ph-positive, and only later did large numbers of normal hematopoietic cells emerge. Such a pattern is consistent with the presence in the autograft of leukemic cells with transient repopulating potential; origin of the late-appearing normal hematopoietic cells is attributed to the eventual expansion of small numbers of Ph-negative stem cells persisting in the patient after intensive therapy. This could be similar to the mechanisms believed to explain rare cases of cytogenetic conversion in patients recovering from marrow hypoplasia induced by busulfan (59).

Autografting with Cells Manipulated In Vitro

Direct evidence of transplantable Ph-positive stem cells comes from early experience with granulocyte transfusions. Ph-positive hematopoiesis developed in several individuals with acute leukemia or aplastic anemia as a complication of receiving transfusions of *unirradiated* granulocyte preparations obtained by leukapheresis from patients with CML (60,61). It can therefore be assumed that an unmanipulated blood or marrow autograft will likely contain some cells capable of re-establishing the disease after intensive therapy. Accordingly, if autografting is to be undertaken with curative intent, it will be necessary to establish methods that can reduce the content of leukemic stem cells ex vivo without compromising the numbers of normal hematopoietic cells needed to restore blood cell formation.

Several approaches to achieve this objective are currently being investigated clinically. McGlave and co-workers (36) are evaluating the use of a 36-hour in vitro exposure of marrow autografts to γ-interferon. This approach is based on their observation of a greater toxic effect of γ-interferon on leukemic as compared with normal progenitors detected by in vitro colony assays (62). The preliminary results of the clinical study (summarized in Table 56-5) suggest that this approach is unlikely to confer any advantage over an unmanipulated autograft. Brief (i.e., 30 min) in vitro exposures to cyclophosphamide derivatives have also been found to kill primitive Ph-positive progeni-

Table 56-4.
Results of Autografting in Chronic Phase CML

Authors, Year, Ref	No. Patients	Intensive Therapy	Graft Failure	% Ph-negative Marrow Metaphases (in Evaluable Patients)[a]	Continuation of Chronic Phase After Autografting: % of Patients	Continuation of Chronic Phase After Autografting: Median Duration, months (range)	Median Survival After Diagnosis, months (range)
Brito-Babapulle et al. 1989 (58)	14[b]	BU + MEL (n = 11); CY + TBI + Dauno (n = 2); CY + TBI (n =1)	3 (1 early, 2 late)	100 (in 1 of 13); 15–33 (in 5 of 13)	86[c]	40+ (25+–53+)	46+ (15–85+)
De Fabritiis et al. 1990 (57)	12[d]	BU + MEL	0	100 (in 2 of 12); 75–95 (in 4 of 12); 57 (in 1 of 12); 10, 14 (in 2 of 12)	92	18+ (16+–20+)	48+ (37+–57+)
Kantarjian et al. 1991 (49)	8[e]	CY + BCNU + ETOP	0	100 (in 1 of 8); 84, 96 (in 2 of 8); 8, 13 (in 2 of 8)	88	10+ (8+–19+)	NS

[a]One to 2 months after autografting.
[b]Fourteen in first chronic phase (duration = median 10, range 1–44 mo), 3 after T-cell–depleted allografts had failed to take; 8 autografted once; 4 twice, with second preceded by chemotherapy in high dosage (as treatment of chronic phase) and 1 of whom was subsequently allografted, 1 twice and 1 three times, with second and third not preceded by chemotherapy (for graft failure), all with blood cells.
[c]Includes 2 with durable Ph-negative hematopoiesis.
[d]Twelve in first chronic phase (duration = NS) of 14 selected from 44 patients by virtue of hematological response and cytogenetic improvement on α-interferon; all autografted once, 10 with marrow cells and 2 with blood cells, and all were given α-interferon after autografting.
[e]Eight in first chronic phase (duration = median 40, range 25–81 mo); all autografted once, all with marrow cells, 1 with Ph-negative cells (harvested after interferon therapy), and all were given α-interferon after autografting.
CML = chronic myeloid leukemia; BU = busulfan in high dosage; MEL = melphalan in high dosage; CY = cyclophosphamide in high dosage; TBI = total body irradiation; Dauno = daunorubicin; BCNU = carmustine in high dosage; ETOP = etoposide in high dosage; NS = not stated.

tors differentially (31,38). A clinical trial using autografts treated with one such derivative (mafosfamide) is underway (35).

Another approach is one that simply exploits the innately different behavior of normal and leukemic LTC-IC when incubated for extended periods (i.e., days) in vitro. Under standard LTC conditions, normal LTC-IC numbers remain unchanged for 10 days, whereas Ph-positive LTC-IC decline rapidly during this same initial period. This finding, together with the fact that the initial number of normal LTC-IC in CML marrow is usually already higher than the number of leukemic LTC-IC, explains the frequent appearance of normal progeny in CML marrow cultures within a few weeks, even though such cells may not be detectable in the starting (preculture) marrow specimen (22,28,37). The Vancouver group treated 20 patients with intensive therapy supported by a marrow autograft maintained in culture for 10 days. The results from this study (summarized in Table 56-5) indicate consistent restoration of Ph-negative hematopoiesis; some patients remained continuously disease-free for extensive periods. Culture of the autograft appears to have been important to achievement of these results because infusion of unmanipulated reserve cells as a backup treatment for graft failure was rapidly followed by regrowth of leukemic cells in 2 of 3 patients in whom this effect could be documented (34).

In the Vancouver study, eligibility for autografting required that the marrow of candidate patients be shown to have at least 2% of the average normal frequency of normal LTC-IC and that leukemic LTC-IC be undetectable at the end of 10 days of culture. These eligibility criteria resulted in the selection of approximately one-third of all patients considered from a heterogenous group (34). The purpose of imposing these entry criteria was to try to ensure that the therapy to be evaluated would be tested only in patients at least theoretically likely to benefit from it (i.e., those in whom the autograft would contain "sufficient" normal hematopoietic stem cells to achieve hematological rescue and negligible leukemic stem cells). However, this selection makes it difficult to interpret survival data, because there is no parallel or historical control group for comparison. Further studies will be needed to establish survival of the "eligible" subgroup (and the "excluded" subgroup) when managed with conventional therapy and whether it differs from that of the patients who underwent intensive therapy and autografting. Nevertheless, the fact that cultured autografts from at least a selected subgroup of patients with CML can result in sustained restoration of normal hematopoiesis is encouraging.

Future Directions

Currently, intensive therapy with autografting appears to offer little benefit to the majority of patients

Table 56-5.
Results of Autografting with Marrow Cells Manipulated In Vitro

Authors, Year, Ref	*No. Patients*	*Intensive Therapy*	*Manipulation of the Autograft*	*Graft Failure*	*% Ph-negative Marrow Metaphases (in Evaluable Patients)*[a]	*Achievement of Complete Remission*[b]	
						% of Patients	*Duration (mo)*
Barnett et al., 1989 (28); 1992 (34)	20[c]	ETOP + CY + TBI (n = 3); BU + CY + MEL (n = 16); BU + MEL (n = 1)	Long-term culture for 10 days	5	100 (in 12 of 14); 94 (in 1 of 4); 76 (in 1 of 14)	60	23+, 23+, 11+; <1+ (death in CR); 5–11 in 8
McGlave et al. 1990 (36)	10[d]	CY + TBI	Incubation with γ-interferon for 36 hours	1	100 (in 3 of 7); 35 (in 1 of 7); 5 (in 1 of 7)	30	<1+ (death in CR); 1, 2

[a]One to 2 months after autografting.
[b]Hematological and cytogenetic remission.
[c]Fourteen in first chronic phase, 1 in second chronic phase, 1 in third chronic phase, 4 in accelerated phase, of 33 selected from 88 patients on the basis of a preassessment of marrow in long-term culture; all autografted once.
[d]Six in first chronic phase, 4 in accelerated phase; all autografted once.
ETOP = etoposide in high dosage; CY = cyclophosphamide in high dosage; TBI = total body irradiation; BU = busulfan in high dosage; MEL = melphalan in high dosage; CR = complete remission.

with transformed CML. In contrast, there is reason to believe that this type of treatment could be developed into a curative approach for those with chronic-phase disease. The first step toward this goal—restoration of normal hematopoiesis—can now be achieved consistently. The challenge for the future will be to identify strategies that allow normal hematopoiesis to be sustained for the rest of the patient's life and to make this approach applicable to more patients.

As in other diseases treated with current intensive therapy regimens, the presence of malignant stem cells persisting in the patient rather than in the autograft is likely to be the major cause of recurrent disease. However, both problems must be overcome if cures are to be obtained. In this regard, manipulation of the immune system is one strategy that offers promise. Experience with allogeneic BMT in CML indicates that there are immunocompetent cells in the graft that can exert a potent antileukemic effect (i.e., GVL). Various strategies to evoke such an effect postautograft are now being evaluated (63). These strategies include use of cyclosporine to induce autologous GVHD (54,64), α-interferon to provide both direct and indirect antileukemic activity (49,53, 57,65), and IL-2 to generate lymphokine-activated killer cells (66,67). A second area of future clinical development lies in the exploitation of hematopoietic growth factors, which should help to reduce the problem of myelosuppression postautograft and may also be used to improve the antileukemic effect of current therapies.

In the future, it should become possible to manipulate the autograft for therapeutic advantage in more ambitious ways. High efficiency gene transfer to very primitive normal and Ph-positive hematopoietic cells (i.e., LTC-IC) is now feasible using recombinant retroviruses (68). Applied to autografting, this technique will allow the progeny of such genetically marked cells to be followed in the recipient and, in the event of disease recurrence, it may be possible to establish the origin of the reappearing leukemic cells. Eventually, these techniques may also be useful for eliminating residual leukemic stem cells (e.g., by inactivating BCR-ABL messenger RNA [69]) or for modifying normal hematopoietic stem cells to provide them with increased resistance to agents used for eradication of residual leukemic stem cells in the host.

There is reason to be optimistic that curative treatments for CML will be developed that may obviate the need for transplantation of allogeneic marrow. Indeed, one might envisage autograft-based protocols ultimately becoming a first-line treatment in patients with CML.

References

1. Sokal JE, Cox EB, Baccarani M, et al. Prognostic discrimination in "good-risk" chronic granulocytic leukemia. Blood 1984;63:789–799.
2. Singer JW, Arlin AZ, Najfeld V, et al. Restoration of nonclonal hematopoiesis in chronic myelogenous leukemia (CML) following a chemotherapy-induced loss of the Ph[1] chromosome. Blood 1980;56:356–360.
3. Goto T, Nishikori M, Arlin Z, et al. Growth characteristics of leukemic and normal hematopoietic cells in Ph'+ chronic myelogenous leukemia and effects of intensive treatment. Blood 1982;59:793–808.
4. Clarkson B. Chronic myelogenous leukemia: is aggressive treatment indicated? J Clin Oncol 1985;3:135–139.
5. Kantarjian HM, Vellekoop L, McCredie KB, et al. Intensive combination chemotherapy (ROAP 10) and splenectomy in the management of chronic myelogenous leukemia. J Clin Oncol 1985;3:192–200.
6. Talpaz M, Kantarjian H, Kurzrock R, Trujillo JM, Gutterman JU. Interferon-alpha produces sustained cytogenetic responses in chronic myelogenous leukemia. Ann Inter Med 1991;114:532–538.
7. Thomas ED, Clift RA, Fefer A, et al. Marrow transplantation for the treatment of chronic myelogenous leukemia. Ann Intern Med 1986;104:155–163.
8. Goldman JM, Apperley JF, Jones L, et al. Bone marrow transplantation for patients with chronic myeloid leukemia. N Engl J Med 1986;314:202–207.
9. McGlave PB, Beatty P, Ash R, Hows JM. Therapy for chronic myelogenous leukemia with unrelated donor bone marrow transplantation: results in 102 cases. Blood 1990;75:1728–1732.
10. Klingemann H-G, Storb R, Fefer A, et al. Bone marrow transplantation in patients aged 45 years and older. Blood 1986;67:770–776.
11. Beatty PG, Clift RA, Mickelson EM, et al. Marrow transplantation from related donors other than HLA-identical siblings. N Engl J Med 1985;313:765–771.
12. Fefer A, Cheever MA, Thomas ED, et al. Disappearance of Ph[1]-positive cells in four patients with chronic granulocytic leukemia after chemotherapy, irradiation and marrow transplantation from an identical twin. N Engl J Med 1979;300:333–337.
13. Fefer A, Thomas ED. Bone marrow transplantation for the treatment of chronic myelogenous leukemia. In: DeVita VT Jr, Hellman S, Rosenberg SA, eds. Important advances in oncology 1990. Philadelphia: J.B. Lippincott, 1990:143–158.
14. Gale RP, Goldman JM, Horowitz MM. Identical twin transplants in chronic myelogenous leukemia in chronic phase (abstract). Exp Hematol 1991;19:573.
15. Weiden PL, Flournoy N, Thomas ED, et al. Antileukemic effect of graft-versus-host disease in human recipients of allogeneic-marrow grafts. N Engl J Med 1979; 300:1068–1073.
16. Sullivan KM, Weiden PL, Storb R, et al. Influence of acute and chronic graft-versus-host disease on relapse and survival after bone marrow transplantation from HLA-identical siblings as treatment of acute and chronic leukemia. Blood 1989;73:1720–1728.
17. Horowitz MM, Gale RP, Sondel PM, et al. Graft-versus-leukemia reactions after bone marrow transplantation. Blood 1990;75:555–562.
18. Cunningham I, Gee T, Dowling M, et al. Results of treatment of Ph'+ chronic myelogenous leukemia with an intensive treatment regimen (L-5 protocol). Blood 1979;53:375–395.
19. Singer JW, Fialkow PJ, Steinmann L, Najfeld V, Stein SJ, Robinson WA. Chronic myelocytic leukemia (CML): failure to detect residual normal committed stem cells in vitro. Blood 1979;53:264–268.
20. Dube ID, Gupta CM, Kalousek DK, Eaves CJ, Eaves AC. Cytogenetic studies of early myeloid progenitor com-

partments in Ph[1]-chronic myeloid leukaemia (CML). I. Persistance of Ph[1]-negative committed progenitors that are suppressed from differentiating in vivo. Br J Haematol 1984;56:633–644.

21. Eaves CJ, Eaves AC. Cell culture studies in CML. In: Goldman JM, ed. Bailliere's clinical haematology, vol. 1,#4. Chronic myeloid leukaemia. London: Bailliere Tindall, 1987:931–961.
22. Kalousek DK, Eaves CJ, Eaves AC. In-vitro cytogenetic studies of haemopoietic malignancies. Cancer Surv 1984;3:439–463.
23. Sutherland HJ, Lansdorp PM, Henkelman DH, Eaves AC, Eaves CJ. Functional characterization of individual human hematopoietic stem cells cultured at limiting dilution on supportive marrow stromal layers. Proc Natl Acad Sci USA 1990;87:3584–3588.
24. Eaves CJ, Sutherland HJ, Udomsakdi C, et al. The human hematopoietic stem cell in vitro and in vivo. Blood Cells 1992;18:301–307.
25. Sutherland HJ, Eaves CJ, Lansdorp PM, Thacker JD, Hogge DE. Differential regulation of primitive human hematopoietic cells in long-term cultures maintained on genetically engineered murine stromal cells. Blood 1991;78:666–672.
26. Sutherland HJ, Reid D, Eaves CJ. Steel factor synergizes with IL-3 and G-CSF to replace marrow feeders in promoting differentiation of highly purified human hematopoietic cells (abstract). Exp Hematol 1992; 20:755.
27. Fraser CC, Szilvassy SJ, Eaves CJ, Humphries RK. Proliferation of totipotent hematopoietic stem cells in vitro with retention of long-term competitive in vivo reconstituting ability. Proc Natl Acad Sci USA 1992; 89:1968–1972.
28. Barnett, MJ, Eaves CJ, Phillips GL, et al. Successful autografting in chronic myeloid leukaemia after maintenance of marrow in culture. Bone Marrow Transplant 1989;4:345–351.
29. Turhan AG, Humphries RK, Eaves CJ, et al. Detection of breakpoint cluster region-negative and nonclonal hematopoiesis in vitro and in vivo after transplantation of cells selected in cultures of chronic myeloid leukemia marrow. Blood 1990;76:2404–2410.
30. Udomsakdi C, Eaves CJ, Swolin B, Reid DS, Barnett MJ, Eaves AC. Rapid decline of chronic myeloid leukemic cells in long-term culture due to a defect at the leukemic stem cell level. Proc Natl Acad Sci USA 1992;89:6192–6196.
31. Udomsakdi C, Eaves CJ, Lansdorp PM, Eaves AC. Unique characteristics of primitive neoplastic cells from patients with chronic myeloid leukemia (CML) assessed using the long-term culture-initiating cell (LTC-IC) assay (abstract). Blood 1991;78(suppl 1):29a.
32. Verfaillie CM, Miller WJ, Boylan K, McGlave PB. Selection of benign primitive hematopoietic progenitors in chronic myelogenous leukemia on the basis of HLA-DR antigen expression. Blood 1992;79:1003–1010.
33. Turhan AG, Humphries RK, Phillips GL, Eaves AC, Eaves CJ. Clonal hematopoiesis demonstrated by X-linked DNA polymorphisms after allogeneic bone marrow transplantation. N Engl J Med 1989;320:1655–1661.
34. Barnett MJ, Eaves CJ, Phillips GL, et al. Autografting in chronic myeloid leukemia with cultured marrow. Leukemia 1992;6(suppl 4):118–119.
35. Carlo-Stella C, Mangoni L, Piovani G, et al. In vitro marrow purging in chronic myelogenous leukemia: effect of mafosfamide and recombinant granulocyte-macrophage colony-stimulating factor. Bone Marrow Transplant 1991;8:265–273.
36. McGlave PB, Arthur D, Miller WJ, Lasky L, Kersey J. Autologous transplantation for CML using marrow treated ex vivo with recombinant human interferon gamma. Bone Marrow Transplant 1990;6:115–120.
37. Coulombel L, Kalousek DK, Eaves CJ, Gupta CM, Eaves AC. Long-term marrow culture reveals chromosomally normal hematopoietic progenitor cells in patients with Philadelphia chromosome-positive chronic myelogenous leukemia. N Engl J Med 1983; 308:1493–1498.
38. Degliantoni G, Mangoni L, Rizzoli V. In vitro restoration of polyclonal hematopoiesis in a chronic myelogenous leukemia after in vitro treament with 4-hydroperoxycyclophosphamide. Blood 1985;65:753–757.
39. Doney K, Buckner CD, Sale GE, Ramberg R, Boyd C, Thomas ED. Treatment of chronic granulocytic leukemia by chemotherapy, total body irradiation and allogeneic bone marrow transplantation. Exp Hematol 1978; 6:738–747.
40. Doney KC, Buckner CD, Thomas ED, et al. Allogeneic bone marrow transplantation for chronic granulocytic leukemia. Exp Hematol 1981;9:966–971.
41. Kantarjian HM, Keating MJ, Talpaz M, et al. Chronic myelogenous leukemia in blast crisis. Analysis of 242 patients. Am J Med 1987;83:445–454.
42. Buckner CD, Clift RA, Fefer A, Neiman PE, Storb R, Thomas ED. Treatment of blastic transformation of chronic granulocytic leukemia by high dose cyclophosphamide, total body irradiation and infusion of cryopreserved autologous marrow. Exp Hematol 1974; 2:138–146.
43. Buckner CD, Stewart P, Clift RA, et al. Treatment of blastic transformation of chronic granulocytic leukemia by chemotherapy, total body irradiation and infusion of cryopreserved autologous marrow. Exp Hematol 1978;6:96–109.
44. Goldman JM, Catovsky D, Hows J, Spiers ASD, Galton DAG. Cryopreserved peripheral blood cells functioning as autografts in patients with chronic granulocytic leukaemia in transformation. Br Med J 1979;1:1310–1313.
45. Thomas MR, Robinson WA, Dantas M, Koeppler H, Drebing C, Glode LM. Autologous marrow transplantation for patients with chronic myelogenous leukemia (CML) in blast crisis. Am J Hematol 1984;16:105–112.
46. Phillips GL, Herzig GP. Intensive chemotherapy, total body irradiation, and autologous marrow transplantation for chronic granulocytic leukemia—blast phase: Report of four additional cases. J Clin Oncol 1984; 2:379–384.
47. Lemonnier M-P, Gorin N-C, Laporte J-P, et al. Autologous marrow transplantation for patients with chronic myeloid leukemia in accelerated or blastic phase: report of 14 cases. Exp Hematol 1986;14:654–658.
48. Vellekoop L, Zander AR, Kantarjian HM, et al. Piperazinedione, total body irradiation, and autologous bone marrow transplantation in chronic myelogenous leukemia. J Clin Oncol 1986;4:906–911.
49. Kantarjian HM, Talpaz M, LeMaistre CF, et al. Intensive combination chemotherapy and autologous bone marrow transplantation leads to the reappearance of Philadelphia chromosome-negative cells in chronic myelogenous leukemia. Cancer 1991;67:2959–2965.
50. Haines ME, Goldman JM, Worsley AM, et al. Chemotherapy and autografting for chronic granulocytic leukaemia in transformation: probable prolongation of

survival for some patients. Br J Haematol 1984;58: 711–721.

51. Preisler HD, Raza A, Higby D, et al. Treatment of myeloid blastic crisis of chronic myelogenous leukemia. Cancer Treat Rep 1984;68:1351–1355.

52. Karp DD, Parker LM, Binder N, et al. Treatment of the blastic transformation of chronic granulocytic leukemia using high dose BCNU chemotherapy and cryopreserved autologous peripheral blood stem cells. Am J Hematol 1985;18:243–249.

53. Reiffers J, Trouette R, Marit G, et al. Autologous blood stem cell transplantation for chronic granulocytic leukaemia in transformation: a report of 47 cases. Br J Haematol 1991;77:339–345.

54. Carella AM, Gaozza E, Raffo MR, et al. Therapy of acute phase chronic myelogenous leukemia with intensive chemotherapy, blood cell autotransplant and cyclosporine A. Leukemia 1991;5:517–521.

55. Vogler WR, Winton EF, James S, O'Neill S, Granade S, Mallard G. Autologous marrow transplantation after karyotypic conversion to normal in blastic phase of chronic myelocytic leukemia. Am J Med 1983;75:1080–1084.

56. Korbling M, Burke P, Braine H, Elfenbein G, Santos G, Kaizer H. Successful engraftment of blood derived normal hemopoietic stem cells in chronic myelogenous leukemia. Exp Hematol 1981;9:684–690.

57. De Fabritiis P, Sandrelli A, Meloni G, et al. Prolonged suppression of myeloid progenitor cell numbers after stopping interferon treatment for CML may necessitate delay in harvesting marrow cells for autografting. Bone Marrow Transplant 1990;6:247–251.

58. Brito-Babapulle F, Bowcock SJ, Marcus RE, et al. Autografting for patients with chronic myeloid leukaemia in chronic phase: peripheral blood stem cells may have a finite capacity for maintaining haempoiesis. Br J Haematol 1989;73:76–81.

59. Finney R, McDonald GA, Baikie AG, Douglas AS. Chronic granulocytic leukemia with Ph[1] negative cells in bone marrow and a ten year remission after busulphan hypoplasia. Br J Haematol 1972;23:283–288.

60. Graw RG Jr, Buckner CD, Whang-Peng J, et al. Complication of bone-marrow transplantation: graft-versus-host disease resulting from chronic-myelogenous-leukaemia leukocyte transfusions. Lancet 1970;2:338–341.

61. Lowenthal RM, Grossman L, Goldman JM, et al. Granulocyte transfusions in treatment of infections in patients with acute leukaemia and aplastic anaemia. Lancet 1975;1:353–358.

62. McGlave P, Mamus S, Vilen B, Dewald G. Effect of recombinant gamma interferon on chronic myelogenous leukemia bone marrow progenitors. Exp Hematol 1987;15:331–335.

63. Klingemann H-G, Phillips GL. Immunotherapy after bone marrow transplantation. Bone Marrow Transplant 1991;8:73–81.

64. Jones RJ, Vogelsang GB, Hess AD, et al. Induction of graft-versus-host disease after autologous bone marrow transplantation. Lancet 1989;1:754–757.

65. Klingemann H-G, Grigg AP, Wilkie-Boyd K, et al. Treatment with recombinant interferon (α-2b) early after bone marrow transplantation in patients at high risk for relapse. Blood 1991;78:3306–3311.

66. Mackinnon S, Hows JM, Goldman JM. Induction of in vitro graft-versus-leukemia activity following bone marrow transplantation for chronic myeloid leukemia. Blood 1990;76:2037–2045.

67. Higuchi CM, Thompson JA, Petersen FB, Buckner CD, Fefer A. Toxicity and immunomodulatory effects of interleukin-2 after autologous bone marrow transplantation for hematologic malignancies. Blood 1991;77: 2561–2568.

68. Hughes PFD, Thacker JD, Hogge D, et al. Retroviral gene transfer to primitive normal and leukemic hematopoietic cells using clinically applicable procedures. J Clin Invest 1992;89:1817–1824.

69. Szczylik C, Skorski T, Nicolaides NC, et al. Selective inhibition of leukemia cell proliferation by BCR-ABL antisense oligodeoxynucleotides. Science 1991;253:562–565.

Chapter 57
Autologous Bone Marrow Transplantation for Multiple Myeloma

Bart Barlogie and Sundar Jagannath

Multiple myeloma accounts for approximately 10% of all hematological malignancies (1,2). Incidence of and mortality from this monoclonal B-cell tumor are increasing, especially among black Americans (3). The disease etiology is unknown, although associations with environmental and occupational exposure to certain chemicals and radiation have been reported (1,3). Recent research implicates *c-myc* (4–6), *ras* (6–8), and *bcl-2* oncogenes in myelomagenesis (9,10). Several cytokines exerting tumor growth stimulation are released by marrow stroma (11) and other normal accessory cells (12) (paracrine loop) or by tumor cells themselves (autocrine loop) (13). Some of these agents account for disease symptoms such as anemia (interleukin-6 [IL-6] [14], tumor necrosis factor-alpha [TNF-α]), lytic bone disease (IL-6 [15], IL-1-β [16], TNF-β [17]), and immune dysfunction (TGF-β [18]); renal failure is multifactorial but most often due to Bence Jones proteinuria and hypercalcemia (19). The hallmark of multiple myeloma is the plasma cell producing and secreting monoclonal immunoglobulin (20). Immunophenotype analysis indicates that myeloma cells express multiple lineage and differentiation markers, often in association with the mature plasma cell phenotype (21). This observation has led some authors to postulate that transformation occurs at an early hemopoietic stem-cell level, which would explain the association with myelodysplastic disease, acute leukemia, and myeloproliferative disorders, even without prior cytotoxic therapy.

A combination of melphalan and prednisone (MP) has been the mainstay of therapy for nearly 30 years, producing disease control in approximately one half of patients and yielding median survival expectations on the order of 3 years (22). True complete remissions, as defined by disappearance of monoclonal gammopathy on immunofixation analysis and of monoclonal marrow plasmacytosis, are attained infrequently with MP (<10%). Numerous trials evaluated the potential benefit from added alkylating agents and anthracyclins but failed to extend survival obtained with the MP regimen (23,24). Once refractoriness to alkylating agents in conventional doses had been established, tumor control could be achieved in only approximately 10% until the introduction of the VAD regimen (25): VAD combines continuous infusions of vincristine and adriamycin (doxorubicin) with added pulses of high-dose dexamethasone (26). Despite marked tumor regression by at least 75% in 40 to 50% of such patients, use of VAD in patients with previously untreated myelomas also failed to extend survival duration beyond results achieved with the MP regimen (27,28). Subsequent studies indicated that glucocorticoids were crucial to VAD's efficacy and possibly accounted for much of the standard alkylating agent regimens' activities as well (29). Recent data indicate that dexamethasone inhibits host cell production of cytokines, including IL-6 (30,31), and may thus induce tumor cell apoptosis (32).

The usually advanced age of patients with myelomas and their susceptibility to infections probably explain the lack of enthusiasm for investigation of intensive therapy (33). The erratic absorption of melphalan after oral administration (34) and the marked alkylating agent responsiveness of cultured human myeloma cells (35) finally prompted McElwain and Powles (36) to evaluate intravenous melphalan (MEL) at doses of 140 mg/m^2 in a small group of previously treated patients with myelomas and some newly diagnosed patients with high-risk features. Demonstration of frequent complete remissions motivated other investigators to pursue the high-dose therapy concept, eventually at myeloablative intensity requiring hematopoietic stem-cell support (37–49). Unlike the experience with standard-dose regimens, complete remissions could be obtained in up to 50% of patients, especially when such high-dose therapy was administered during stages of retained sensitivity to conventional dose regimens (49). The advanced age of patients with myelomas explains why trials with autologous transplants outpaced those using allotransplants, for which treatment-related mortality, mainly from graft-versus-host disease (GVHD), seems to increase with advancing age (50).

This chapter reviews currently available autotransplant results in patients with multiple myelomas and addresses the following issues: (1) evidence of clinical

Table 57-1.
Melphalan Dose Response in Refractory Myeloma

Regimen	Graft	GM-CSF	N	%ED	%R	%CR	*Median Months* RFS	*Median Months* Survival
MEL (100 mg/m²)	. . .	±	47	19	38	6	4	7
MEL (140 mg/m²) + TBI (850 cGy)	ABMT	–	18	28	72	11	12	14
MEL-1 (200 mg/m²)	ABMT PBSC	+	18	0	56	0	10	13
MEL-2 (200 mg/m²)	ABMT PBSC	+	19	0	74	16	23+	23+
p Values				0.02	0.02		0.0003	0.002
HD-CY	. . .	+	31	3	19	0	N/A[a]	N/A[a]
CBV	PBSC	–	15	13	60	0	4	8

[a]Most patients were transplanted subsequently.
MEL = melphalan; ABMT = autologous bone marrow transplantation; PBSC = peripheral blood stem cell; HD-CY = high-dose cyclophosphamide; GM-CSF = granulocyte-macrophage colony stimulating factor; ED = early death; R = remission; CR = complete remission; RFS = relapse-free survival.

benefit from increased dose intensity of cytotoxic agents; (2) choice of preparative regimens; (3) prognostic factors with intensive therapy; (4) source of autologous hemopoietic stem cells; and (5) removal of tumor cells from autografts (purging).

Dose Intensity

Increased antitumor activity should be recognized by an increase in the frequency of complete remission and an extension of event-free and overall survival durations. Due to their more homogeneous and limited clinical course, the issue of a dose response effect is best examined in patients with resistant myelomas. Marked increases were observed in overall and complete response rates, and remission and survival times were extended significantly as the MEL dose was increased from 100 to 200 to 400 mg/m² (administered in 2 cycles) or to 140 mg/m² with added total body irradiation (TBI; 850 cGy) (Table 57-1 and Figure 57-1) (51). Thus, MEL (140 mg/m²) with TBI and MEL (200 mg/m²) (especially with 2 cycles; MEL [400 mg/m²]) essentially doubled relapse-free and overall survival durations. Combined use of marrow (autologous BMT [ABMT]) and peripheral blood stem cells (PBSC) eliminated treatment-related mortality as a result of brisk hemapoietic engraftment (*vida infra*) (52). These data strongly indicate that resistance to standard doses of alkylating agents, usually including MEL, can be overcome by MEL dose escalation and addition of TBI (53). Because of its relative lack of extramedullary toxicity, MEL is an attractive transplant drug and lends itself to repeated application (54) or combination with TBI and other chemotherapeutic agents (55).

Choice of Preparative Regimen

Comparative trials of standard and intensive therapy regimens have not been reported, nor are there comparisons among different high-dose therapies. Because of a better end point definition, evaluation of preparative regimens should be more informative in refractory myelomas, emphasizing frequency of complete responses (see Table 57-1). The alkylator cyclophosphamide (CY), even at near-maximum tolerated doses of 6 gm/m² (high-dose CY [HD-CY]), effected responses (≥75% tumor regression) in only 19% and no CR among 31 subjects with alkylating agent-resistant myeloma that was frequently refractory also to VAD (56). Even the addition of nitrosourea and etoposide in the CBV regimen, conducted with PBSC support, yielded results comparable to those with MEL at a subtransplant dose of 100 mg/m² (57). There is only limited experience available with busulfan (BU), usually combined with HD-CY (BU-CY) (58), and multidrug combinations with MEL have been explored mainly in responsive myeloma (*vide infra*) (55).

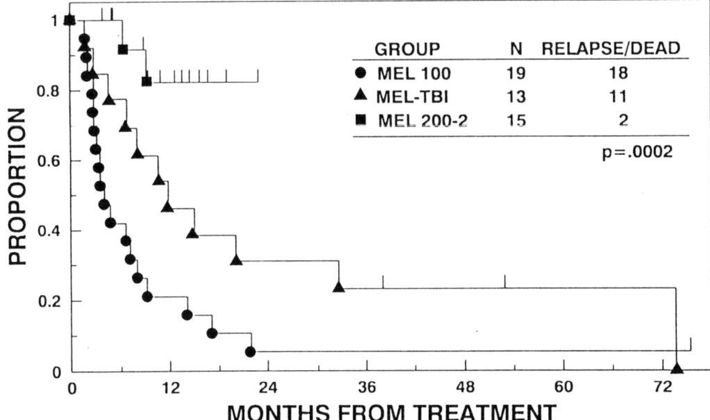

Figure 57-1. Relapse-free survival was extended progressively with increasing dose intensity of melphalan (MEL) from 100 mg/m² (MEL-100) to melphalan (140 mg/m²) plus total body irradiation (TBI) (850 cGy) (MEL-TBI) to MEL (400 mg/m²) applied with 2 transplants within one year (MEL-200–2).

Table 57-2.
TBI In Responsive Myeloma: Melphalan Versus Thiotepa

Regimen	N	Evaluable Patients	%ED	%R	%CR	Median Months RFS		Median Months Survival		Median Follow-up
MEL (140 mg/m²)	19	19	5	58	37	23	p = .003	38	p=.09	35
THIO (750 mg/m²)	15	15	0	47	13	7		23		44
MEL-1 (200 mg/m²)	31	29	0	86	7	20+		20+		8
MEL-2 (200 mg/m²)	22	18	0	89	28	19+		19+		11

ED = early death; R = remission; CR = complete remission; RFS = relapse-free survival; MEL = melphalan; THIO = thiotepa.

TBI was evaluated with MEL (140 mg/m²) or thiotepa (mainly at 750 mg/m²). Sufficient data, however, are available only in responsive myeloma (Table 57-2) (44). With minimum and median durations of follow-up of 28 and 40 months, respectively, the relapse-free survival duration of 23 months after MEL (140 mg/m²) with TBI significantly exceeded the 7-month survival after thiotepa and TBI. The much shorter follow-up of patients receiving one or two cycles of MEL (200 mg/m²) precludes formal comparisons with TBI-containing regimens (52,54). However, CR rates above 25% were observed only with either MEL (140 mg/m²) with TBI or 2 cycles of MEL (200 mg/m²), whereas thiotepa and TBI or a single course of MEL (200 mg/m²), effected CR rates of approximately 10%. Figure 57-2 depicts, for 36 evaluable patients, the additional tumor cytoreduction achieved from a second cycle of autograft-supported high-dose therapy administered within 6 months after the first transplant. Approximately two thirds had no change in their response category; 28% converted to partial or complete response; and one patient, relapsing prior to the second transplant, failed to respond to alternate therapy with MEL (140 mg/m²) with TBI or CY/VP16/TBI.

These data indicate that MEL is superior to both HD-CY and thiotepa (51,56). MEL (140 mg/m²) with TBI appears superior to a single course of MEL (200 mg/m²) in terms of CR rate; however, further follow-up is needed to estimate the contribution in responsive myeloma of a second treatment cycle, which had been beneficial in refractory disease (see Tables 57-1 and 57-2). The higher mortality with TBI may be due to a greater incidence of severe mucositis and attendant infectious complications, although speedier hematological recovery with added PBSC and GM-CSF may have accounted for the lack of mortality with MEL (200 mg/m²).

Most larger clinical trials have been conducted in recently diagnosed high-risk patients (Tables 57-3 and 57-4) (49,56,59). Median survival durations were approximately 3 to 3.5 years with MEL (200 mg/m²) (Royal Marsden, from diagnosis) (43,60), repeated cycles of MEL (140 mg/m²) (Harousseau, from diagnosis) (61), and with MEL (140 mg/m²) and added TBI (Reiffers and colleagues [47]; Jagannath and coworkers [52], from transplant). With a median follow-up of 35 months, two thirds of patients are alive in a trial of MEL (140 mg/m²) with TBI (1,200 cGy) and additional chemotherapeutic agents (55) (see Table 57-4). Although allogeneic transplant data in acute leukemia suggest a critical TBI dose of 1,200 cGy (at which mortalities from relapse and regimen toxicity appear minimized), the data in myeloma are currently inconclusive. Heterogeneity of disease, treatment, and source of autologous stem cells preclude conclusions as to the best preparative regimen.

Prognostic Factors Associated With Intensive Therapy

High-dose therapy regimens were initially developed for patients with advanced and refractory myelomas. Once efficacy and relative safety were established, untreated patients with high-risk features were offered autotransplant-supported consolidation therapy, and more recent trials employed such an approach for

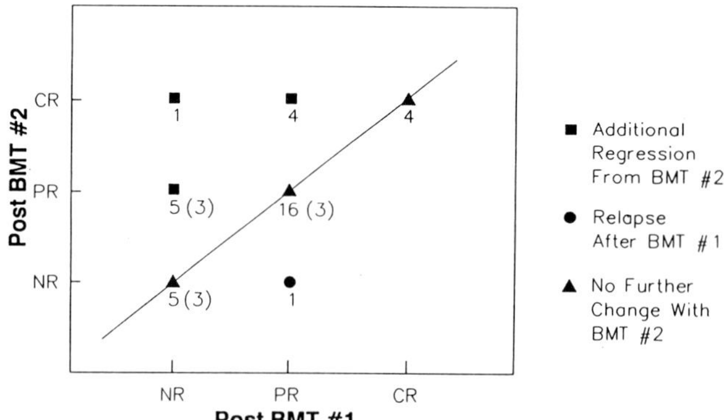

Figure 57-2. Additional responses can be obtained in the course of double transplants. Among 36 evaluable patients treated with 2 cycles of melphalan (MEL) (200 mg/m²) (or with total body irradiation [TBI] [850 cGy] plus MEL-140, or cyclophosphamide-etoposide [CY-VP16] with the second transplant, shown in parentheses), 6 of initially 10 unresponsive patients (<75% tumor regression) achieved remission including one complete remission; 4 of 21 patients in partial remission after one transplant achieved true complete remissions, whereas one patient with a relapse after the first transplant failed to respond after the second transplant.

Table 57-3.
ABMT for Multiple Myeloma

Institution	N	Regimen	Disease	%CR	%R	%ED	RFS: CR	RFS: PR	Survival
Royal Marsden (43)	50	MEL (200 mg/m^2)	Untreated; "VAMP" induction	50	74	0	24 mo	10 mo	3.5 years
	39	MEL (200 mg/m^2) ± IFN	Untreated; CY + VAMP ± verapamil induction	47	83	?	2/21 relapses with IFN; 7/18 relapses without IFN		
University of Nantes, France (61)	97	MEL (140 mg/m^2); no Tx	53 untreated; 44 advanced	25	71	8			Overall, 24 mo; 37 mo in untreated MM; 17 mo in advanced MM
	35	MEL (140 mg/m^2) (18 patients); MEL (140 mg/m^2) + TBI (850 cGy,) (17 patients)				6	28 mo		41 mo
University of Toulouse, France (45)	31	MEL (140 mg/m^2); TBI (800 cGy)	111, in remission	43	100	3	3 year projection		
							85%	24%	(81% alive)
University of Arkansas, Little Rock (44)	37	MEL (140 mg/m^2) + TBI (850 cGy)	Responsive, 19; resistant, 18	37 11	58 72	5 28	20 mo 12 mo	14 mo	60% projected at 4 yr; min F/U, 26 mo
	18	Thiotepa (750 mg/m^2) + TBI (850 cGy)	Responsive, 15; resistant, 3	13 0	47 100	0 0	8 mo 8 mo	23 mo 23 mo	
University of Arkansas, Little Rock (52)	27	MEL (200 mg/m^2) × 2[a]	Responsive, 18; resistant, 9	44 33	89 89	0 0	3 relapses 1 relapse	89% alive 100% alive	

[a]First transplant with MEL (200 mg/m^2), 27 patients; second transplant with MEL (200 mg/m^2), 25; MEL + TBI, 2.
ABMT = autologous bone marrow transplantation; CR = complete remission; R = remission; ED = extensive disease; RFS = relapse-free survival; PR = partial remission; MEL = melphalan; TBI = total body irradiation; VAMP = vincristine, methotrexate, 6-mercaptoprine, and prednisone; CY = cyclophosphamide; MM = multiple myeloma.

Table 57-4.
PBSC for Multiple Myeloma

Institution	Regimen for PBSC Mobilization	N	Disease Features	Transplantation N	Transplantation Regimen
Hopital Haut-Leveque, Bordeaux, France (47)	CY (7 gm/m^2)	26	III; 23 recent diagnosis	26	MEL (140 mg/m^2) TBI (1,350 cGy)
Hopital du Hasenrain, Mulhouse, France (46)	MEL (100–140 mg/m^2)	20	III; 20 recent diagnosis	10	MEL (280 mg/m^2) TBI (1,000 cGy)
Hopital Saint-Louis, Paris, France (48)	High-dose CHOP	73	46; ≤ 3 cycles of therapy	50	MEL (140 mg/m^2) TBI (1,200 cGy) CY 2,400 (43) VP16 (750 mg/m^2) CCNU (120 mg/m^2) Busulfan (16mg/kg) (7) + MEL (140 mg/m^2)
University of Arkansas, Little Rock (52)	CY (6 gm/m^2) ± GM-CSF	75	46; > 12 mo; 31, resistant to MP + VAD	60	MEL (200 mg/m^2) (57) MEL (140 mg/m^2) TBI (850 cGy) (3)

ABMT = autologous bone marrow transplantation; PR = partial remission; CR = complete remission; CY = cyclophosphamide; MEL = melphalan; CHOP = CY, hydroxydaunomycin, vincristine, prednisone; GM-CSF = granulocyte-macrophage colony stimulating factor; MP = methyl prednisone; VAD = vincristine, adriamycin, decadron; TBI = total body irradiation; CY = cyclophosphamide; VP16 = etoposide; CCNU = lomustine.

all individuals with symptomatic disease (see Tables 57-3 and 57-4). A critical question concerns any survival advantage from such consolidation therapy in first remission over salvage therapy for sensitive or resistant relapse. Such trials have not been conducted formally. Obviously, lack of a prospective assignment to transplantation for the different clinical circumstances is fraught with considerable selection bias. Figure 57-3A portrays the shorter survival from transplant for the 14 patients receiving MEL140-TBI or thiotepa-TBI for resistant relapse compared with the remaining 41 patients treated in remission (first, 14; second or later remission, 20) or during a phase of primary drug resistance (7 patients). Despite a survival advantage (time interval from diagnosis to transplant) of at least 2 years for all patients with resistant relapse as opposed to only 14 among the 41 other patients, the latter group had a similar survival from diagnosis (Figure 57-3B).

Because details of past therapy and response are not always readily available, other prognostic features were also surveyed (Table 57-5). Age 50 years or less, 24 months or less from initial treatment to transplant, beta$_2$-microglobulin (B2M) 2.5 mg/L or less prior to transplant, immunoglobulin G (IgG) isotype and kappa light chain, as well as TBI with MEL rather

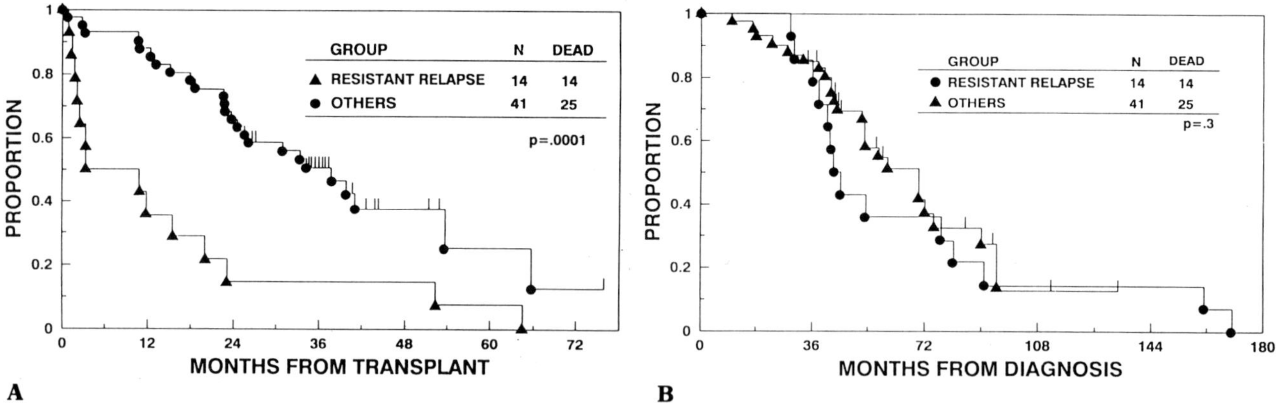

Figure 57-3. Inferior survival after total body irradiation (850 cGy) with melphalan (140 mg/m^2) (37 patients) or thiotepa (750 mg/m^2) (18 patients) was associated with resistant relapse (i.e., failure to respond to vincristine, adriamycin, decadron (VAD) salvage therapy [A]). All 14 patients with resistant relapse were transplanted more than 24 months since initial therapy. However, their survival from diagnosis (B) was not superior to results obtained in the remaining patients ("others"), although this guarantee time of 2 years applied to only 14 of these 41 patients.

Table 57-4. cont.

Added ABMT	Deaths: Pre-transplant	Deaths: During Transplant	Response: ≥ PR	Response: CR	Median Days to: Granulocyte >500/μL	Median Days to: Platelets >50,000/μL	Months of Follow-up	Outcome
7	0	0	23	13	13	28	18	Median survival, 36 mo; 65% alive
1	3	1	10	9	11	22	?	30% alive
0	5	3	39/39	20	15	29	35	Median survival 60 mo; 66% alive
57	3	0	45	12	15	19	12	84% alive

Table 57-5.
Prognostic Factors with Total Body Irradiation

Parameter	N	%ED	(p Value)	%R	(p Value)	(%CR)	(p Value)	Median Months: RFS	(p Value)	Median Months: Survival	(p Value)
Age (yr)											
≤ 50	24	8		71		(21)		21	(0.01)	52	(0.008)
> 50	31	13		55		(19)		9		19	
Performance status											
≤ 1	46	7		61		(24)		16	(0.1)	31	(0.02)
> 1	9	33		67		(0)		7		3	
Months from diagnosis											
≤ 24	27	4		74	(0.05)	(33)	(0.04)	21	(0.01)	54	(0.01)
> 24	28	18		50		(7)		9		19	
$Beta_2$- microglobulin											
≤ 2.5 mg/L	28	7		64		(25)		20	(0.0001)	40	(0.0003)
> 2.5 mg/L	27	15		59		(15)		7		15	
Ig Isotype											
G	30	10		63		(17)		18	(0.02)	40	(0.02)
Others	25	12		60		(24)		8		18	
Ig Isotype											
G	30	10		63		(17)		18	(0.007)	40	(0.007)
A	13	8		54		(23)		7		15	
Light chain											
Kappa	41	10		66		(22)		16	(0.04)	25	(0.5)
Lambda	14	14		50		(0)		8		24	
Status at treatment											
Resistant Relapse	14	36	(0.003)	64		(0)		8	(0.004)	7	(0.0001)
Others	41	2		61		(27)		18		38	
Type of therapy											
Melphalan + TBI	37	16		65		(24)		19	(0.009)	34	(0.7)
Thiotepa + TBI	18	0		56		(0)		8		23	

ED = early death; R = remission; CR = complete remission; RFS = relapse-free survival; TBI = total body irradiation.

Table 57-6.
Prognosis after TBI for Myeloma: Multivariate Regression Analysis

End Point	*Variable*	*p Value*
Early death	Resistant relapse;	0.03
	Performance status > 1	0.05
Complete Response	≤ 24 mo from diagnosis	0.02
Relapse-free survival	B2M ≤ 2.5 mg/L;	< 0.001
	age ≤ 50 yr;	0.004
	kappa light chain	0.02
Survival	Not resistant relapse;	0.003
	IgG isotype;	0.01
	age ≤ 50 yr	0.03

TBI = total body irradiation; B2M = beta$_2$-microglobulin.

Table 57-7.
Prognosis after TBI for Myeloma According to Number of Favorable Variables[a]

No. Favorable Variables	*N*	*%ED*	*%CR*	*Median Months RFS*	*Median Months Survival*
4–5	10	0	60	53+	54
3	15	13	20	18	34
0–2	30	13	7	8	17
p Values			0.001	0.0001	0.0007

[a]B2M ≤ 2.5; ≤ 24 mo from diagnosis; age ≤ 50 years; MEL; CR.
TBI = total body irradiation; ED = early death; B2M = beta$_2$-microglobulin; CR = complete remission; RFS = relapse-free survival; MEL = melphalan.

than thiotepa, were all favorable parameters. In multivariate analysis, early mortality was highest with resistant relapse and poor performance; less than 2 years of prior therapy favored higher CR rates; low pretransplant B2M, younger age, and kappa light chain were all associated independently with extended relapse-free survival; overall survival was prolonged in the absence of resistant relapse, with IgG myeloma and younger age (up to 50 years) (Table 57-6). Table 57-7 illustrates that the combined use of 5 prognostic variables (B2M ≤ 2.5 mg/L; ≤ 24 months from diagnosis; age ≤ 50 years; MEL rather than thiotepa with TBI; and achieving CR post-transplant) permitted segregation of patients into 3 risk groups, significantly affecting incidence of complete remission, relapse-free, and overall survival duration. The CR rate was 60% among patients exhibiting at least 4 favorable prognostic features, but only 7% when fewer than 3 of these variables were present. As expected, frequency of CR was linked to relapse-free and overall survival. Durable responses were observed only in the most favorable group of patients, whose CR rate was 60% (see Table 57-7; Figure 57-4). Thus, for cure to be a realistic goal, high CR rates in excess of 50% seem to be required.

When considering autotransplants as a treatment option for patients with myeloma, use of alkylating agents potentially damaging normal hemopoietic stem cells (especially MEL and nitrosoureas) should be restricted, and autografts procured at the time of maximum tumor cytoreduction. Initial therapy is best performed with the VAD regimen that affects rapid tumor cytoreduction and spares normal hemopoietic stem cells.

Source of Hemopoietic Stem Cells

The source of hemopoietic stem cells is not only pertinent to the management of patients with myeloma undergoing autologous transplants, but also to the entire spectrum of hematological malignancies, such as acute and chronic leukemias and lymphomas. Blood stem cells are the obvious choice in conditions in which normal marrow procurement is compromised by extensive radiation to the usual sites of marrow collection (i.e., posterior iliac crest). Similarly, patients with persistent marrow plasmacytosis will have a lower risk of tumor cell reseeding with blood stem cell grafts in the absence of marrow purging, although an adverse effect of up to 30%

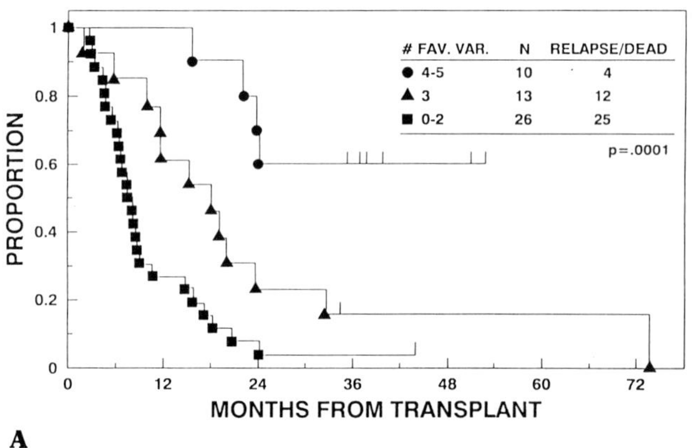

A

B

Figure 57-4. Relapse-free survival (A) and overall survival (B) from transplant were shortened progressively as the number of favorable variables declined. Favorable variables included beta$_2$-microglobulin (B2M) ≤ 2.5 mg/L; ≤24 months from initial diagnosis; age ≤ 50; melphalan rather than thiotepa with total body irradiation; and complete remission after transplant.

Table 57-8.
Hematological Recovery after High-dose CY

		Median Days to			
Parameter	*N*	*Granulocyte* > *500/μL*	(*p Value*)	*Platelets* > *50,000/μL*	(*p Value*)
Total	75	16		16	
Prior therapy					
≤ 12 mo	29	15		15	
> 12 mo	46	17	0.09	18	0.003
GM-CSF					
+	39	15	0.0003	15	
−	36	18		18	0.03
≤ 12 mo *and* GM-CSF	17	15		15	
> 12 mo *or* GM-CSF	33	16	0.003	15	0.004
> 12 mo *and no* GM-CSF	25	19		20	

CY = cyclophosphamide; GM-CSF = granulocyte-macrophage colony stimulating factor.

tumor cells in marrow autografts has not been documented (*vida infra*).

In the setting of remission consolidation therapy, in which marrow plasmacytosis is typically reduced to less than 5%, the relative roles of marrow and blood stem-cell grafts have not been evaluated. PBSCs seem to afford speedier hemopoietic engraftment in patients with lymphomas, perhaps due to a greater frequency of more mature progenitor cells (62). Other studies in myeloma with PBSC collected under steady-state conditions suggest comparable engraftment kinetics (57). However, faster engraftment was observed when PBSCs had been collected after chemotherapy priming (with high-dose [HD-CY] (52) or CHOP-like [cyclophosphamide, hydroxydaunomycin, vincristine, prednisone] regimens) (48,55), especially with added hemopoietic growth factor support (59).

In an extensive investigation of nearly 100 patients treated with HD-CY at 6 gm/m^2 with or without GM-CSF, the following principles were established (52). Recovery proceeded faster with less prior therapy (<12 mo) and with GM-CSF (Table 57-8). Similarly, PBSC procurement, as defined by CFU-GM or CD-34 antigen expression, was likewise more effective with less prior therapy and added GM-CSF (Table 57-9). Platelet recovery proved to be a reliable in vivo indicator of blood stem-cell function because it related both to quantity of stem cells collected and to post-transplant engraftment using MEL200 with both marrow and PBSC grafts. As expected, long duration of prior therapy (>12 mo) and lack of GM-CSF post-HD-CY, already shown to determine post-HD-CY recovery and PBSC procurement, were also crucial variables for post-transplant recovery of both neutrophils and platelets (Table 57-10). Post-transplant administration of GM-CSF shortened the duration of neutrophil recovery. Thus, under the ideal circumstance of limited prior therapy and GM-CSF both for PBSC procurement and post-transplantation, recovery to granulocyte levels greater than 500/μL and platelets greater than 50,000/μL occurred within 14 days from transplantation, so that the actual durations of neutropenia and thrombocytopenia were reduced to a median of only 4 days.

A further issue with ABMT versus PBSC concerns the extent of tumor cell reseeding. Several lines of investigation indicate clearly the presence of circulating tumor cells in myeloma even at diagnosis (63). Phenotypic and in vitro culture studies suggest the presence of myeloma progenitor cells in the peripheral blood, although quantitative comparisons with marrow have not been conducted (64–69). Comparison of clinical outcome following marrow or PBSC grafts are not feasible due to heterogeneity of preparative regimens and disease features (see Tables 57-3 and 57-4).

Finally, because of frequent post-transplant relapses, hematological tolerance of subsequent chemotherapy salvage regimens deserves consideration (44,70). Although precise data are currently not available, complete hematological reconstitution with combined marrow and blood stem-cell support (with

Table 57-9.
Peripheral Blood Stem-cell Mobilization[a]

Parameter	*N*	*% Patients with Good PBSC*	p *Value*
Total	72	56	
Prior therapy			
≤ 12 mo	28	85	
> 12 mo	44	40	0.0005
GM-CSF			
+	36	69	
−	36	44	0.03
Post-HD-CY platelet recovery (> 50,000/μL)			
Fast ≤ 14 days	39	85	
Slow > 14 days	33	24	< 0.0001
≤ 12 mo *and* GM-CSF	16	94	
≤ 12 mo *or* GM-CSF	31	58	< 0.001
> 12 mo *and no* GM-CSF	25	36	

[a]Good > 50 CFU-GM/10^5 cells.
PBSC = peripheral blood stem cell; GM-CSF = granulocyte-macrophage colony stimulating factor; HD-CY = high-dose cyclophosphamide.

Table 57-10.
Factors Influencing Engraftment after First Autotransplant

Parameter	N	Median Days to Granulocyte > 500/μl	(p Value)	Median Days to Platelets > 50,000/μl	(p Value)
Total	60	15		19	
PBSC Mobilization					
Good	37	14		15	
Poor	23	17	(0.04)	60	(0.0001)
Post-HD-CY platelet recovery (> 50,000/μL)					
Fast ≤ 14 days	35	14		15	
Slow > 14 days	25	15	(0.4)	62	(0.0001)
≤ 12 mo *and* GM-CSF post-HD-CY	15	14		15	
≤ 12 mo *or* GM-CSF post-HD-CY	27	15	(0.02)	20	(0.01)
> 12 mo *and no* GM-CSF post-HD-CY	18	20		32	
GM-CSF post-transplant					
+	38	14		17	
−	22	21	(0.003)	20	(0.8)

PBSC = peripheral blood stem cell; HD-CY = high-dose cyclophosphamide; GM-CSF = granulocyte-macrophage colony stimulating factor.

platelet levels exceeding 150,000/μL and normal bone marrow cellularity) (71) is consistent with the clinical experience that such patients tolerate further myelosuppressive regimens such as EDAP (etoposide, dexamethasone, ara-C, cisplatin) (72).

Bone Marrow Purging

Few studies have been performed with bone marrow purging using monoclonal antibodies (73), immunotoxins (74), or cytotoxic drugs (75). In vitro tumor cell removal has been documented with all of these methods, and hemopoietic engraftment does not appear impaired. Most investigators agree that a potential benefit from marrow purging can be ascertained only under ideal clinical conditions, when tumor cytoreduction is profound so that tumor cell reseeding might become an important variable. Relapses within 6 months have been noted even when such purging protocols were applied to patients in early remission. The advent of gene transfer technology hopefully will permit the assessment of the relative contributions to relapse of tumor cell reseeding and expansion of remaining disease (76). Available data from ABMT studies without purging indicate that the degree of myeloma cell contamination in autografts does not influence remission or survival times (Figure 57-5) (52).

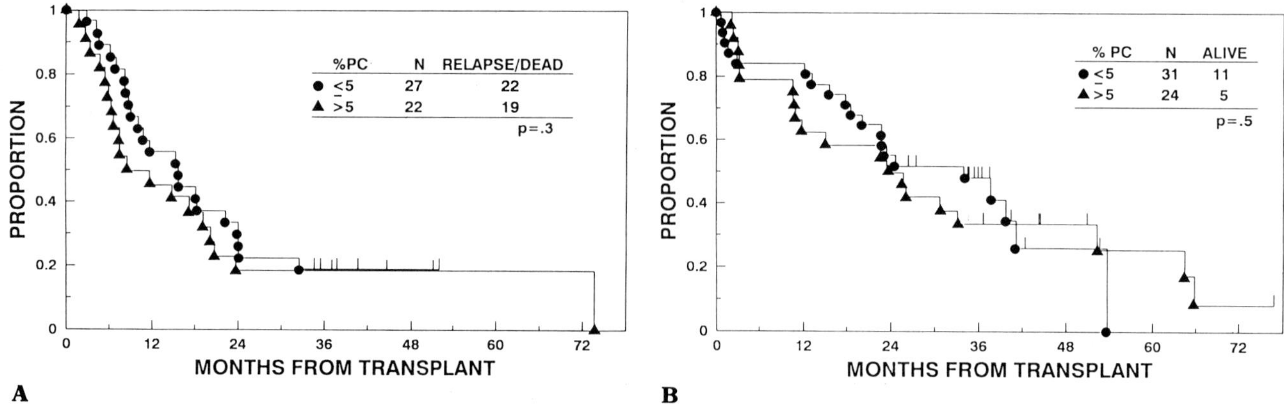

Figure 57-5. Relapse-free (A) and overall survival (B) were not influenced by the percentage of plasma cells (percent PC) present in bone marrow autografts.

The Next Steps

Several important trials are currently under way that deserve comment. Some are testing whether more intensive remission induction prior to transplantation with mutually noncross-resistant regimens (i.e., VAD; HD-CY; EDAP) followed by tandem transplants 3 to 6 months apart with subsequent interferon (IFN) maintenance will augment incidence and duration of complete remissions (71). This "total therapy" approach has enrolled 105 patients, of whom 69 received one and 42 patients two transplants to date (Table 57-11). Consistent with the study objective, there was a progressive increase in the incidence of tumor regression by at least 75% during the successive phases of induction therapy. Appreciable rates of complete remission (CR) were not observed until transplant doses of MEL alone or combined with TBI were administered. Thus, the CR rate reached 23% after the first and 50% after the second transplant with a treatment-related mortality of 1% and 5%, respectively.

The current Royal Marsden study addresses the role of post-transplant IFN therapy in a randomized fashion (60). Early results favor IFN maintenance (see Table 57-3). The European Bone Marrow Transplant (EBMT) group, together with the European Organization for Research and Treatment of Cancer (EORTC), launched a trial of MEL140 and TBI (800 cGy) for remission consolidation after VMCP-VBAP to be compared with standard dose chemotherapy (Durie BGM. Personal communication).

Summary and Perspective

Autotransplant experience in approximately 500 patients reported to date demonstrates the general feasibility of this approach in an attempt to deliver even myeloablative cytotoxic therapy at a high level of safety to elderly patients with myelomatosis, especially when recent advances in supportive care with blood stem cells and hemopoietic growth factors are utilized. From a safety point of view, low mortality in the 1 to 2% range can be anticipated when hemopoietic stem-cell function is preserved (52). This is the case when prior exposure to alkylating agents is limited to less than one year. Hemopoietic growth factor administration in conjunction with PBSC mobilization and after transplantation further accelerates engraftment (52,62).

Table 57-11.
Response to Total Therapy

Regimen	*Evaluable Patients*	*% Cumulative Response* ≥ 75%	≥ 90%	CR[a]
VAD-1	105	26	15	0
VAD-2/3	95	39	28	1
HD-CY	87	57	45	2
EDAP	80	68	59	10
MEL-200-1	69	83	78	23
MEL-200-2[a]	42	93	90	50

[a]By immunofixation.
VAD = vincristine, adriamycin, decadron; HD-CY = high-dose cyclophosphamide; EDAP = eptoside, dexamethasone, Ara-C, platinum; MEL-200-1 = melphalan 200 mg/m^2 first cycle; MEL-200-2 = melphalan 200 mg/m^2 second cycle.

Among the available preparative regimens, MEL alone at maximum tolerated doses (200 mg/m^2) can be administered twice with relatively limited extramedullary toxicity. However, the long-term effects of a strategy of employing such a well tolerated regimen repeatedly vis-a-vis more toxic therapy with TBI are not known. With a single application, MEL140 and TBI (1,020 cGy) seem to produce consistently high complete remission rates in the 40 to 50% range when applied for response consolidation.

If attainment of CR is considered a prerequisite for long-term disease control and eventually cure, autotransplants should not be used as a last resort for refractory myelomas because of limited antitumor effect and hemopoietic stem-cell damage sustained by prolonged exposure to agents like MEL and nitrosoureas (52). However, available data are insufficient to make specific recommendations as to which patients might benefit most. As with other malignancies, the greatest benefit is likely to be seen among patients at lowest risk, who, in the case of multiple myeloma, still have no prospect for cure. Hence, results of currently on-going clinical trials evaluating early response consolidation with myeloablative therapy and autotransplants are anxiously being awaited.

As additional autotransplant trials get underway, their overall benefit in relationship to standard dose therapies has to be addressed in comparative trials that are already in the planning or early accrual stage. Large myeloma referral centers should consider the issue of marrow- versus PBSC-supported high-dose therapy, incorporating gene transfer technologies to learn more about the nature of relapse after autologous transplantation as well as the relative contributions of marrow and blood to hemopoietic reconstitution and to relapse. As complete remissions by immunofixation and marrow immunocytochemical methods are attained more frequently, recent molecular techniques with polymerase chain reaction should be employed for semiquantitative assessment of minimal residual disease (77).

Post-transplant immunomodulating therapy has a sound biological rationale, and preliminary in vitro data with IL-2 in chronic myelogenous leukemia appear promising (78). There is an expansion in the marrow of natural killer (NK) cells in myeloma, the antitumor activity of which might be further enhanced by IL-2 administration (79). Reduction of marrow IL-6 levels, which have been demonstrated to render myeloma target cells more resistant to NK cell lysis (80), can be attempted with high doses of glucocorticoids (30,31). Thus, a number of different post-transplant options are available to achieve further tumor cytoreduction by appropriate manipulation of host cell immune responses. IFN-α displays antitumor activity in approximately one third of newly diagnosed patients (mainly those with low tumor stage) (81,82), extends remissions after induction therapy with standard doses of alkylating agents (83), and, when combined with such treatment for induction, has been shown to increase the incidence of marked tumor cytoreduction (84). These encouraging results of pilot trials, however, have not been confirmed (85). Yet, several on-going transplant trials employ IFN-α as post-transplant maintenance therapy.

Autologous bone marrow purging remains controversial in several diseases, especially in acute leukemia, for which few comparative trials without tumor cell removal have been conducted (86). Considering the aforementioned major issues, autograft purging probably assumes a relatively less urgent role.

In relationship to allogeneic transplants, autografts offer several advantages, including their applicability to patients up to the age of 70 (75% of patients accrued into large cooperative trials), low mortality under 5%, and relatively short hospitalization, even to the point of out-patient treatment, resulting in further cost reduction (52). By comparison, allogeneic transplants can be offered to approximately 1 of every 10 autotransplant candidates. The experience in the EBMT group demonstrates prolonged unmaintained remissions, although the issue of persistent monoclonal gammopathy in some of these relapse-free survivors is currently unknown (50). As with other hematological tumors, the question of a graft-versus-myeloma effect may be important, especially when considering myeloma as a malignancy involving an early hemopoietic stem cell. The potential of cyclosporine to induce self-limited autologous GVHD and possibly a graft-versus-tumor effect deserves clinical investigation in multiple myeloma (87).

A peculiar observation is the development of oligoclonal gammopathies after intensive therapy both with autologous and allogeneic transplants and the occasional switch in immunoglobulin heavy and light chain classes (88). Given the propensity of myeloma for evolution to myeloproliferative disorders, including acute myelogenous leukemia, even without cytotoxic therapy (21), the long-term effects of marrow-ablative chemotherapy and chemoradiotherapy have to be evaluated carefully. Thus, patients in whom secondary cytopenia develops should be scrutinized for the presence of myelodysplastic disease, especially by demonstration of cytogenetic abnormalities such as monosomy 5 or 7, which can also be recognized conveniently by fluorescence in situ hybridization technology in interphase cells (89).

Anticipating further progress in growth factor research, autografts may be replaced eventually by sequential use of several hemopoietic growth factors, including stem-cell factor, IL-1, IL-3, and IL-6. Some of these cytokines may exert growth stimulation of tumor cells (recruitment) and therefore render the kinetically relatively dormant myeloma cells more sensitive to cytotoxic agents. Stem-cell factor, IL-1, and G-CSF may also exert sufficient radioprotection and possibly chemoprotection; therefore, otherwise supralethal doses of treatment can be survived (90).

It is hoped that the recent advances in biological and therapeutic research will improve markedly the natural history of myelomas, which has not changed in more than 2 decades.

References

1. Barlogie B, Epstein J, Selvanayagam P, Alexanian R. Plasma cell myeloma—new biologic insights and advances in therapy. Blood 1988;73:865–879.
2. Barlogie B, Alexanian R, Jagannath S. Plasma cell dyscrasias. JAMA 1992;268:2946–2951.
3. Riedel DA, Pottern LM. The epidemiology of multiple myeloma In: Barlogie B, ed. Hematology/oncology clinics of North America: multiple myeloma. Philadelphia: W. B. Saunders, 1992:225.
4. Selvanayagam P, Blick M, Narni F, et al. Alteration and abnormal expression of the c-myc oncogene in human multiple myeloma. Blood 1988;71:30–35.
5. Greil R, Fasching B, Loidl P, Huber H. Expression of the c-myc proto-oncogene in multiple myeloma and chronic lymphocytic leukemia: *in situ* analysis. Blood 1991;78:180–191.
6. Ernst TJ, Gazdar A, Ritz J, Shipp MA. Identification of a second transforming gene, rasN, in a human multiple myeloma line with a rearranged c-myc allele. Blood 1988;72:1163–1167.
7. Neri A, Murphy JP, Cro L, et al. Ras oncogene mutation in multiple myeloma. J Exp Med 1989;170:1715–1725.
8. Tsuchiya H, Epstein J, Selvanayagam P, et al. Correlated flow cytometric analysis of H-ras p21 and nuclear DNA in multiple myeloma. Blood 1988;72:796–800.
9. Hamilton MS, Barker HF, Ball J, Drew M, Abbot SD, Franklin IM. Normal and neoplastic human plasma cells express bcl-2 antigen. Leukemia 1991;5:768–771.
10. Durie BGM, Mason DY, Giles F, et al. Expression of the bcl-2 oncogene protein in multiple myeloma. Blood 1990;76:1378a.
11. Caligaris-Cappio F, Bergui L, Gregoretti MG, et al. Role of bone marrow stromal cells in the growth of human multiple myeloma. Blood 1991;77:2688–2693.
12. Klein B, Zhang X-G, Jourdan M, et al. Paracrine but not autocrine regulation of myeloma-cell growth and differentiation by interleukin-6. Blood 1989;73:517–526.
13. Kawano M, Hirano T, Matsuda T, et al. Autocrine generation and requirement of BSF-2/IL-6 for human multiple myeloma. Nature 1988;332:83–85.
14. Bataille R, Jourdan M, Zhang XG, Klein B. Serum levels of interleukin-6, a potent myeloma cell growth factor, as a reflection of disease severity in plasma cell dyscrasias. J Clin Invest 1989;84:2008–2011.
15. Bataille R, Chappard D, Klein B. Mechanisms of bone lesions in multiple myeloma. In: Barlogie B, ed. Hematology/oncology clinics of North America. Philadelphia: W. B. Saunders, 1992:285.
16. Cozzolino F, Torcia M, Aldinucci D, et al. Production of interleukin-1 by bone marrow myeloma cells: its role in the pathogenesis of lytic bone lesions. Blood 1989;74:380–387.
17. Garrett LR, Durie BGM, Nedwin GE, et al. Production of the bone resorbing cytokine lymphotoxin by cultured human myeloma cells. N Engl J Med 1987;317:526–532.
18. Lynch RG. A role for TGF beta in the immunodeficiency of malignant plasmacell tumors. Second EURAGE symposium on monoclonal gammopathies: clinical

significance and basic mechanisms. Brussels, Belgium, Sept 18–20, 1991.

19. Alexanian R, Barlogie B, Dixon D. Renal failure in multiple myeloma: pathogenesis and prognostic implications. Arch Intern Med 1990;150:1693–1695.
20. Barlogie B, Alexanian R, Pershouse M, Smallwood L, Smith L. Cytoplasmic immunoglobulin content in multiple myeloma. J Clin Invest 1985;76:765–769.
21. Epstein J, Xiao H, He X-Y. Markers of multiple hematopoietic-cell lineages in multiple myeloma. N Engl J Med 1990;322:664.
22. Bergsagel DE, Sprague CC, Austin C, Griffith KM. Evaluation of new chemotherapeutic agents in the treatment of multiple myeloma IV: L-phenylalanine mustard. Cancer Chemother Rep 1962;21:87–99.
23. Boccadoro M, Marmont F, Tribalto M, et al. Multiple myeloma: VMCP/VBAP alternating combination chemotherapy is not superior to melphalan and prednisone even in high-risk patients. J Clin Oncol 1991;9:444–448.
24. Gregory WM, Richards MA, Malpas JS. Combination chemotherapy versus melphalan and prednisone in the treatment of multiple myeloma: an overview of published trials. J Clin Oncol 1992;10:334–342.
25. Barlogie B, Smith L, Alexanian R. Effective treatment of advanced multiple myeloma refractory to alkylating agents. N Engl J Med 1984;310:1353–1356.
26. Alexanian R, Barlogie B, Dixon D. High dose glucocorticoid treatment for resistant multiple myeloma. Ann Intern Med 1986;105:8–11.
27. Alexanian R, Barlogie B, Tucker S. VAD-based regimens as primary treatment for multiple myeloma. Am J Hematol 1990;33:86–89.
28. Samson D, Gaminara E, Newland A, et al. Infusion of vincristine and doxorubicin with oral dexamethasone as first-line therapy for multiple myeloma. Lancet 1989;2:882–885.
29. Alexanian R, Dimopoulos M, Barlogie B. Intermittent dexamethasone as initial chemotherapy for multiple myeloma. Blood 1991;78:688a.
30. Kishimoto T. The biology of interleukin-6. Blood 1990;74:1–10.
31. Ray A, LaForge S, Sehgal PB. On the mechanism for efficient repression of the interleukin-6 promoter by glucocorticoids: enhancer, TATA Box and RNA start site occlusion. Mol Cell Biol 1990;10:5736–5746.
32. Hardin JW, MacLeod SL, Hsu SM, Epstein J, Barlogie B. IL-6 prevents dexamethasone-induced apoptosis in a human myeloma cell line (ARP-1). Proc Am Assoc Cancer Res 1992;33:1674.
33. Barlogie B. Toward a cure for multiple myeloma? N Engl J Med 1991;325:1304–1306.
34. Alberts DS, Chang FY, Chen HSG, et al. Oral melphalan kinetics. Clin Pharmacol Ther 1979;6:737–745.
35. Dalton WS, Salmon SE. Drug resistance in myeloma: mechanisms and approaches to circumvention. In: Barlogie B, ed. Hematology/oncology clinics of North America. Philadelphia: W.B. Saunders, 1992:383–393.
36. McElwain TJ, Powles RL. High-dose intravenous melphalan for plasma cell leukemia and myeloma. Lancet 1983;1:822–823.
37. Barlogie B, Hall R, Zander A, Dicke K, Alexanian R. High dose melphalan with autologous bone marrow transplantation for multiple myeloma. Blood, 1986; 67:1298–1301.
38. Barlogie B, Alexanian R, Dicke K, Zagars G, Spitzer G, Jagannath S, Horowitz L. High dose chemoradiotherapy and autologous bone marrow transplantation for resistant multiple myeloma. Blood, 1987;70:869–872.
39. Harousseau JL, Milpied N, Garand R, Bourhis JH. High dose melphalan and autologous bone marrow transplantation in high risk myeloma. Br J Haematol 1987;67:493.
40. Selby P, McElwain TJ, Nandi AC, et al. Multiple myeloma treated with high dose intravenous melphalan. Br J Haematol 1987;66:55–62.
41. Barlogie B, Alexanian R, Smallwood L, et al. Prognostic factors with high dose melphalan for refractory multiple myeloma. Blood 1988;72:2015–2019.
42. Barlogie B, Jagannath S, Dixon D, et al. High-dose melphalan and GM-CSF for refractory multiple myeloma. Blood 76:677–680.
43. Gore ME, Selby PJ, Viner C, et al. Intensive treatment of multiple myeloma and criteria for complete remission. Lancet 1989;2:879–885.
44. Jagannath S, Barlogie B, Dicke KA, et al. Autologous bone marrow transplantation in multiple myeloma: identification of prognostic factors. Blood 1990;76: 1860–1866.
45. Attal M, Huguet M, Schlaifer D, et al. Intensive combined therapy for previously untreated aggressive myeloma. Blood 1992;79:1130–1136.
46. Henon PH, Beck G, Debecker A, Eisenmann JC, Lepers M, Kandel G. Autograft using peripheral blood stem cells collected after high dose melphalan in high risk myeloma. Br J Haematol 1988;71:253–254.
47. Reiffers J, Marit G, Boiron JM. Autologous blood stem cell transplantation in high-risk multiple myeloma. Br J Haematol 1989;72:296–297.
48. Fermand JP, Levy Y, Gerota J, et al. Treatment of aggressive multiple myeloma by high-dose chemotherapy and total body irradiation followed by blood stem cell autologous graft. Blood 1989;73:20–23.
49. Barlogie B, Gahrton G. Bone marrow transplantation in multiple myeloma—a review. Bone Marrow Transplant 1991;7:71–79.
50. Gahrton G, Tura S, Ljungman P, et al. Allogeneic bone marrow transplantation in multiple myeloma. N Engl J Med 1991;325:1267.
51. Jagannath S, Vesole D, Barlogie B. High dose therapy, autologous stem cells and hemopoietic growth factors for the management of multiple myeloma. In: Armitage J, Antmant K, eds. High-dose cancer therapy. Baltimore, MD: Williams & Wilkins, 1992.
52. Jagannath S, Vesole DH, Glenn L, Crowley J, Barlogie B. Low risk intensive therapy for multiple myeloma with combined autologous bone marrow and blood stem cell support. Blood 1992;80:1666–1672.
53. Jagannath S, Barlogie B. Autologous bone marrow transplantation for multiple myeloma. In: Barlogie B, ed. Hematology/oncology clinics of North America: multiple myeloma. Philadelphia: W. B. Saunders, 1992: 437–449.
54. Vesole D, Jagannath S, Glenn L, Barlogie B. Double autotransplantation (DAT) with melphalan (MEL) for multiple myeloma (MM). Blood 1991;78:238a.
55. Fermand JP, Chevret S, Levy Y, et al. The role of autologous blood stem cells in support of high dose therapy for multiple myeloma. In: Barlogie B, ed. Hematology/oncology clinics of North America. Philadelphia: W. B. Saunders, 1992:451–462.
56. Barlogie B, Jagannath S. Autotransplants in Myeloma. Bone Marrow Transplant 1992;10:27–44.
57. Ventura GJ, Barlogie B, Hester JP, et al. High dose cyclophosphamide, BCNU and VP-16 with autologous blood stem cell support for refractory multiple myeloma. Bone Marrow Transplant 1990;5:265–268.
58. Bensinger WI, Buckner CD, Clift R, et al. Allogeneic

marrow transplantation for patients with multiple myeloma. In: Pileri A, Boccadoro M, eds. III International workshop on multiple myeloma from biology to therapy. Torino, Italy, 1992.

59. Barlogie B, Fermand J-P, Henon P, Jagannath S. Peripheral blood stem cell transplants in multiple myeloma. In: Gale RP, ed. Blood stem cell transplants. Oxford: Cambridge University Press, 1993 (in press).
60. Cunningham D, Milan S, Millar B, et al. Strategies for the management of myeloma with conventional chemotherapy and high-dose melphalan (HDM) and ABMT-possible roles for verapamil and maintenance interferon. In: Pileri A, Boccadoro M, eds. III International workshop on multiple myeloma biology and therapy, Torino, Italy, 1991:133.
61. Harousseau JL, Milpied N, Laporte JP, et al. Double intensive therapy in high risk multiple myeloma. Blood 1992;79:2827–2833.
62. Gianni AM, Siena S, Bregni M, et al. Granulocyte-macrophage colony-stimulating factor to harvest circulating haemopoietic stem cells for autotransplantation. Lancet 1989;8663:580–584.
63. Barlogie B, Alexanian R. Cellular aspects of myeloma: Biologic and clinical implications. In: Delamore IW, ed. Multiple myeloma and other paraproteinemias. Edinburgh: Churchill Livingstone, 1986:154–168.
64. Pilarski LM, Mant MJ, Ruether BA. Pre-B cells in peripheral blood of multiple myeloma patients. Blood 1985;66:416–422.
65. Berenson J, Wong R, Kim K, Brown N, Lichtenstein A. Evidence for peripheral blood B lymphocyte but not T lymphocyte involvement in multiple myeloma. Blood 1987;70:1550–1553.
66. Berenson JR, Lichtenstein AK. Clonal rearrangement of immunoglobulin genes in peripheral blood of multiple myeloma patients. Br J Haematol 1989;73:425–427.
67. Mellstedt H, Hammarstrom S, Holm G. Monoclonal lymphocyte population in human plasma cell myeloma. Clin Exp Immunol 1974;17:371–384.
68. Bast E, van Camp B, Reynaert P, Wirniga G, Ballinx R. Idiotypic peripheral blood lymphocytes in monoclonal gammopathy. Clin Exp Immunol 1982;47:682.
69. Caligaris-Cappio F, Bergui L, et al. Identification of malignant plasma cell precursors in the bone marrow of multiple myeloma. J Clin Invest 1985;76:1243.
70. Jagannath S, Barlogie B. Repeated high dose therapy in refractory myelomatosis. In: Dicke K, Armitage J, Dicke-Evinger MJ, eds. Autologous bone marrow transplantation. Proceedings of the Fifth International Symposium, Omaha, Nebraska, August 25, 1990.
71. Barlogie B, Jagannath S, Vesole D, Glenn L. Total therapy (TT) for newly diagnosed or minimally treated multiple myeloma (MM). Blood 1991;78:489a.
72. Barlogie B, Alexanian R, Cabanillas F. Etoposide, dexamethasone, cytarabine, and cisplatin in vincristine, doxorubicin, and dexamethasone-refractory myeloma. J Clin Oncol 1989;7:1514–1517.
73. Anderson K, Barut B, Takvorian T, et al. Monoclonal antibody (MoAb) purged autologous bone marrow transplantation for multiple myeloma (MM). Blood 1991;77:712–720.
74. Gobbi M, Cavo M, Tazzari PL, et al. Autologous bone marrow transplantation with immunotoxin-purged marrow for advanced multiple myeloma. Eur J Haematol 1989;43:176–181.
75. Reece DE, Barnett MJ, Connors JM, et al. Intensive therapy with busulfan, cyclophosphamide and melphalan (bucy+mel) and 4-hydroperoxycyclophosphamide (4HC) purged autologous bone marrow transplantation (AUTOBMT) for multiple myeloma (MM). Blood 1989; 74:754a.
76. Buschle M, Campana D, Hoffbrand AV, Brenner MK. Transfection of human bone marrow B cell progenitors. Blood 1991;78:1235a.
77. Billadeau B, Blackstadt M, Greipp P, et al. Analysis of B-lymphoid malignancy using allele-specific polymerase chain reaction: a technique for sequential quantitation of residual disease. Blood 1991;78:3021–3029.
78. Mackinnon S, Hows JM, Goldman JM. Induction of in vitro graft-versus-leukemia activity following bone marrow transplantation for chronic myeloid leukemia, Blood 1990;76:2037–2045.
79. Hoover RG, Kornbluth J. Immunoregulation of murine and human myeloma. In: Barlogie B, ed. Hematology/oncology clinics of North America. Philadelphia: W. B. Saunders, 1992:407–424.
80. Bianchi A, Dodd L, Kornbluth J. Selective deficiency in the ability of LAK cells from patients with multiple myeloma to lyse myeloma tumor cells. Blood 1990; 76:796a.
81. Mellstedt H, Ahre A, Bjorkholm M, Holm G, Johansson B, Strander H. Interferon therapy in myelomatosis. Lancet 1979;1:245–248.
82. Alexanian R, Barlogie B, Gutterman J. α-Interferon combination therapy of resistant myeloma. Am J Clin Oncol 1991;14:188–192.
83. Mandelli F, Avvisati G, Amadori S, et al. Maintenance treatment with recombinant interferon alfa-2b in patients with multiple myeloma responding to conventional induction chemotherapy. N Engl J Med 1990; 322:1430–1434.
84. Oken MM, Kyle RA, Greipp PR, Kay NE, Tsiatis A, O'Connell MJ. Alternating cycles of VBMCP with interferon (gamma IFN-alpha2) in the treatment of multiple myeloma. Proc Am Soc Clin Oncol 1988;7:868a.
85. Salmon SE, Crowley J. Impact of glucocorticoids (GC) and interferon (FIN) on outcome in multiple myeloma. Proc Am Soc Clin Oncol 1992;11:1069a.
86. Gorin NC, Aegerter P, Auvert B, et al. Autologous bone marrow transplantation for acute myelocytic leukemia in first remission: a European survey of the role of marrow purging. Blood 1990;75:1660.
87. Geller RB, Esa AH, Beschorner WE, Frondoza CG, Santos GW, Hess AD. Successful in vitro graft-vs-tumor effect against an Ia-bearing tumor using cyclosporine-induced syngeneic graft-vs-host disease in the rat. Blood 1989;74:1165.
88. Barlogie B, Dicke K, Alexanian R. High dose melphalan for refractory myeloma—the M.D. Anderson experience. Hematol Oncol 1988;6:167–172.
89. Dao D, Epstein J, Barlogie B, Sawyer JR. Interphase cytogenetics in multiple myeloma. Proc Am Assoc Cancer Res 1992;33:1594a.
90. Waddick KG, Song CW, Souza L, Uckun FM. Comparative analysis of the in vivo radioprotective effects of recombinant granulocyte-colony-stimulating factor (G-CSF), recombinant granulocyte-macrophage CSF, and their combination. Blood 1991;77:2364–2671.

Chapter 58

Dose-intensive Therapy with Autologous Bone Marrow Transplantation in Solid Tumors

Karen H. Antman, Anthony Elias, and Howard A. Fine

Rationale for Dose-Intensive Therapy in Solid Tumors

Delivery of the highest possible doses of chemotherapy is essential to achieve cure in laboratory models of many solid tumors. However, the dose-response curve for most non-hormonal antitumor agents is steep for both toxic and therapeutic effects (1). In high growth rate experimental animal tumors there is a linear-log correlation between dose and tumor cytotoxicity (2). Doubling the dose increases tumor cell kill by a log or more (i.e., 10-fold) (3). Experiments indicate that the destruction of tumor stem cells may be much greater than the degree of tumor regression (4). Theory, experimental, and clinical data suggest that solid tumors recur despite an initial response to chemotherapy because of resistance to the chemotherapy drugs (5). In the laboratory, resistance to alkylating agents can often be overcome by using a 5- to 10-fold higher dose, doses feasible with autologous bone marrow transplantation (BMT).

Clinically, some correlation between chemotherapy dose and response has long been recognized (1). Systematic analysis of dose-response relationships in the clinic has proven problematic. Until recently, few attempts had been made to quantify dose-response relationships in patients treated with chemotherapy (6–13). In 1984, Hryniuk and Bush (14) introduced the concept of dose intensity for the purpose of quantifying dose-response effects. Dose was quantitated per unit time (i.e., dose intensity) expressed in drug dose administered per m^2 per week (14). These analyses assume that all drugs used are therapeutically equivalent and that cross-resistance or synergy between drugs, peak drug concentrations, or duration of drug exposure have no role. Their analyses in metastatic and adjuvant breast cancer and in ovarian cancer suggested that dose intensity correlated with response or survival. They concluded that chemotherapy regimens should be designed to maximize dose intensity. A corollary of this conclusion is that regimens should be designed to intensify dose per unit time, a strategy different from attempts to deliver a single cycle of high-dose chemotherapy with autologous BMT designed to avoid drug resistance.

The dose-intensity hypothesis and methodology have been debated extensively both practically and theoretically (15,16). Randomized clinical trials in which dose intensity is the sole or most important variable are difficult to interpret because the increased doses planned varied from 10% to 2- to 3-fold over the low dose arms. Because serum levels for a given dose of drug commonly vary 5-fold, drug serum levels achieved in these trials must overlap considerably. In addition, the actual doses delivered in the two arms of a study (often not included in the publication) may not be significantly different. Although some of these trials have shown an increased response rate for regimens with greater dose intensity, few trials demonstrate a significantly increased overall survival. The lack of improvement in survival for the higher dose-intensity regimens may reflect the relatively minor differences in dose administered or the lack of any major effect of conventional dose chemotherapy regimens on median survival. Randomized trials in a variety of solid tumors suggest that modest increments in dose intensity produce, at best, only modest effects on survival.

Because the limiting toxicity of higher chemotherapy doses is myelosuppression, many authors have used marrow, and more recently blood-derived hematopoietic stem cells, to ensure prompt marrow recovery after considerably higher doses of chemotherapy. Curative BMT requires a malignancy responsive to cytoreductive therapy, effective treatment whose limiting toxicity is marrow failure, performance of the procedure early in the course of disease when there is minimal tumor burden and resistance to drugs, and, finally, a source of hematopoietic stem cells free of clonogenic tumor cells (17).

Combination Chemotherapy

The laboratory observations of dose response and the need for combination chemotherapy were basic to the design of the initial treatment regimens for malignancies that are now curable with chemotherapy (i.e., leukemia, lymphoma, testis carcinoma, and breast cancer in the adjuvant setting) (18–21). Considerable variability in sensitivity to cytotoxic drugs has been demonstrated in vitro for a variety of animal and human tumors. Pleiotropic drug resistance has been described for selected groups of cytotoxic agents (e.g., antibiotics and vinca alkaloids) but has not been described for alkylating agents. Skipper and colleagues (2,4,22,23) estimated the spontaneous rate of mutation to resistance to a single drug as $1/10^6$ to 10^7 cancer cells. The likelihood of spontaneous mutations conferring resistance is high in patients with visually apparent tumor. Thus, combinations of active noncross-resistant agents are essential to decrease the emergence of drug resistance. When designing curative treatment regimens, maximally tolerated doses can be employed in combination only by selecting agents with different dose-limiting toxicities.

Characteristics of Alkylating Agents

Combinations of alkylating agents are particularly appropriate for high-dose therapy. First, alkylating agents at conventional doses are active against a variety of human malignancies. Even resistant diseases (e.g., malignant melanoma) consistently have demonstrated some low level of response to conventional doses of alkylating agents. Response rates at transplant doses indicate enhanced activity with the appearance of complete responses.

The alkylating agents have heterogeneous mechanisms of transport, biotransformation, and processes of DNA repair, although the site and structure of the DNA adduct formation and the formation of DNA-DNA crosslinks appear similar throughout this class. Alkylating agents have been shown to be noncross-resistant with each other and with antitumor agents of other classes (24,25). Substantial therapeutic synergy has been observed in a variety of murine tumor systems for alkylators combined with other alkylating agents, antimetabolites, or DNA-binding drugs (26).

At conventional doses, most alkylating agents share a common toxicity, myelosuppression. Marrow autografting ameliorates myelosuppression and permits further dose escalation to the development of dose limiting nonmyelosuppressive toxicity. The non-myelosuppressive dose-limiting toxicity of the various alkylating agents differs substantially when used at high dose with autologous BMT: stomatitis and enterocolitis for melphalan; cardiotoxicity for cyclophosphamide (CY); pulmonary fibrosis and hepatic toxicity for carmustine (BCNU); renal, hepatic, and ototoxicity for cisplatin; and renal and central nervous system (CNS) toxicity for ifosfamide. Hence, non-overlapping toxicity would be anticipated if these agents were combined at full or nearly full transplant doses.

Overview of Reported High-dose Experience in Solid Tumors

Solid tumors are common causes of morbidity and mortality in the United States (Table 58-1). The medical and fiscal impact of an effective (i.e., curative) new treatment for subsets of patients with even a few of these diseases would be substantial (see discussion of cost effectiveness). The number of transplants for solid tumors could very quickly exceed the number currently performed for treatment of leukemias and lymphomas. Patients with breast and ovarian cancer, sarcomas, melanoma, and testis cancer are frequently young and otherwise healthy, ideal candidates for intensive therapy.

A critical assessment of the transplant literature in many other solid tumors is hampered by small series with various primary malignancies treated with multiple regimens. However, a brief review of the available studies is worthwhile.

Table 58-1.
Incidence and Deaths per Year for Various Malignancies, Listed in Order of Mortality

	Incidence	*Deaths*
Lung	168,000	146,000
Colorectal	156,000	58,300
Breast	181,000	46,300
Non-Hodgkin's lymphoma	41,000	19,400
Leukemia	28,200	18,200
Ovarian	21,000	13,000
Brain and central nervous system	16,900	11,800
Melanoma	32,000	6,700
Sarcoma	7,900	4,350
Hodgkin's disease	7,400	1,600
Testis	6,300	350

Data from (27).

Testis, Other Genitourinary, and Germ-cell Primary Cancer

Most patients with newly diagnosed metastatic testis cancer respond readily to curative standard-dose regimens. The few patients who fail multiple regimens, and are therefore eligible for autologous BMT studies, represent an extensively treated group with refractory tumors. Early investigators of high-dose therapy in patients with refractory testis cancer reported high mortalities, particularly from renal or multi-organ failure in patients with extensive prior cisplatin exposure and borderline renal function (28–31). Indiana University investigators, however, designed a better tolerated carboplatin and etoposide regimen (32). Currently in cisplatin-refractory testis cancer (incurable with conventional dose therapy), high-dose therapy with platinum and etoposide–based regimens results in 10 to 30% disease-free survival at 2 years. Because testis cancer tends to relapse early, these patients are presumably cured (33–35). Data on high-dose therapy in germ-cell malignancy are summarized in Chapter 60.

Breast Cancer

Far more data exist for high-dose therapy in various stages of breast cancer (36). Reported data suggest a strong relationship between dose intensity of adjuvant chemotherapy and disease-free survival at conventional chemotherapy doses (6). High-dose regimens differ, but the major determinant of outcome appears to be disease status at the time of high-dose therapy. Although longer follow-up will be required before drawing any conclusions as to whether patients with high risk, stage II, locally advanced, or metastatic disease can be cured with high-dose therapy, disease-free survivals of up to 8 years have been observed in a few patients transplanted in early trials with metastatic breast cancer (36). Studies of autologous marrow transplantation in breast cancer are summarized in Chapter 59.

Ovarian Cancer and Other Gynecological Primary Cancers

With an incidence of 21,000 and a mortality of 13,000, ovarian cancer is a common malignancy in older women. Although front-line cisplatin-based chemotherapy can achieve a complete response in 30 to 50% of patients with residual tumor after surgical debulking of less than 2 cm, at least half of even this "good prognosis" group with complete response eventually relapse. Patients with larger than 2-cm lesions after first laparotomy, residual tumor after conventional cisplatin-based chemotherapy on second look laparotomy, or relapse after complete response have invariably fatal disease.

At conventional doses, response of ovarian cancer appears to correlate with cisplatin dose in retrospective analyses (37), Phase II studies (38,39), and in several randomized studies (12,40). Dose escalation of doxorubicin with hematopoietic growth factors has also been attempted (41), as well as modulation of agents such as melphalan with attempts at glutathione depletion (42–44). Autologous marrow transplantation is particularly attractive as a strategy to ameliorate myelosuppression in ovarian cancer because of infrequent marrow involvement (Table 58-2) (45–78).

These trials in ovarian cancer allow several conclusions. Responses after single agents such as high-dose melphalan or carboplatin in relapsed patients are generally short. However, occasional complete responses have been durable (30 or more mo). In Phase I trials of combinations in patients with relapsed or refractory ovarian cancer, many patients did not undergo disease evaluation for response, particularly if an invasive procedure was required. Nevertheless, for those with evaluable disease, the complete response rate was 38%, with an overall response rate of 69%.

Promising results were achieved in patients with persistent disease at second-look laparotomy (after conventional-dose chemotherapy). In this group with invariably fatal cancer with conventional-dose therapy, high-dose single-agent CY or melphalan resulted in 30 to 48% progression-free survival (63–66).

Third-look laparotomy in several series using high-dose combination chemotherapy with CY-, melphalan–or platinum–based regimens documented approximately 50% conversion from partial to complete response. Many of these responses have proven durable after 3 and 4 year follow-up (67,73,74,79). Thus, on the basis of Phase II studies with 2- to 4-year follow-up, a substantial percentage of patients who would be incurable with conventional-dose chemotherapy remains progression-free. Further follow-up is required to document whether any significant proportion of these patients can be cured with dose-intensive chemotherapy. Trials of high-dose therapy after several cycles of conventional therapy are underway for women with a poor prognosis, including women who have a pathologically documented complete response at second-look laparotomy.

Other Gynecological Malignancies

Only anecdotes exist for high-dose treatment of cervical and uterine carcinomas. Shea and associates (50) treated 2 patients with cervical and one with uterine cancer in their Phase I study of escalating carboplatin. None of the 3 responded (50). One patient with carcinoma of the fallopian tube treated with high-dose ifosfamide and carboplatin responded (78). Kessenger and co-workers (77) reported 6 patients treated for cervical cancer but provided no response data.

Respiratory Tract Primary Cancer

Lung cancer is a major public health problem in the United States and is currently the most common cause of death from cancer. Practical problems in dose-intensive therapy of patients with lung cancer include an older population with underlying smoking-related cardiovascular disease, metachronous cancers, and early metastatic spread of disease.

Small-cell Lung Cancer

Approximately 20% of lung cancers have small-cell histology. Although initially sensitive to chemotherapy, the disease almost always recurs. Five-year survival for disease limited (LD) to the ipsilateral chest is 5 to 10%; for more extensive disease (ED), there are only anecdotal survivors. Phase I and II studies differ in the status of the patients at the time of transplantation and the number of courses of intensification given (Table 58-3) (69,80–91). These studies document a high response rate and even complete responses; however, response duration was 2 to 5 months, with none lasting more than one year.

Souhami and colleagues (91,92), at the University College Hospital in London, treated 25 newly diagnosed, previously untreated patients given high-dose CY and radiotherapy to the primary site. Fifty-six percent of patients attained CR, with a median duration of 43 weeks and a median survival of 69 weeks. These results are comparable to standard

Table 58-2.
High-dose Chemotherapy with Autologous Bone Marrow Transplantation in Gynecological Cancers

Author	No. Patients	Status at Time of HDC	Conditioning Regimen	Response			Duration (mo) of Response	References
				CR	TR	Eval		
Ovarian								
Failed or refractory								
Single agents								
Marseilles	8	Refractory	M	1	5	8	1 toxic death; 2 PF 21+, 31+	(45)
NATG	7	Refractory	M	1	4	7	5(3–10+)	
Cleveland	2		M	0	0	0	5, 6.5	(46)
Royal Free, London	2		M	1	1	2	8,35	(47)
Total	19		M	3	10	17		
NATG	3	Refractory	T	1	2	3	8+, 9+	(48)
Seattle	3		C	3	3	3	4–12+ months' response	(49)
DFCI, Harvard	11	Refractory	Cb	1	6	11	Median, 3	(50)
Combinations (carboplatin then cyclophosphamide-based)								
San Diego	8	7 refractory	ipCb TE	4	6	7	6(3–7)	(51)
Tampa, Florida	6	Refractory	EICb	1	4	6		(52)
Paris	15	10 refractory	(E or VM26)ICb	1				(53)
DFCI, Harvard	6		DC	0	4	6		(54)
Dallas	1		TC					(55)
Duke	1	Failed	TPC	0	1	1		(56)
DFCI, Harvard	2	Relapsed	BPC	0	2	2	4	(57)
Vancouver	1	Relapsed	MEC	0	0	0		(58)
Duke	12	Refractory	ipP TC	0	6	8	6 (3–11+)	(59)
Chicago	3	Refractory	Mitox TC	1	1	1		(60)
Loyola, Tucson	6	5 refractory	Mitox CbC	4	5	6		(61)
Groningen, Neth	6		Mitox (M or C)	2	4	5	3, 5, 5+, 9+, 14+, 36+	(62)
Total				17	31	45		
Persistent disease at second look laparectomy (stages 3 and 4)								
Single agents								
Paris	16		C[a]			NA	30% PFS at 3 years	(63)
Clermont-Ferrand	14	9 macroscopic	M			NA	5 (36%) PFS 30, 30, 37, 52, 60 mo	(64)
Marseilles	27	9 in CR 10 PR <2 cm 8 PR > 2 cm	M				13 without progression 6 PFS 9–32 mo 3 PFS 13–54 mo; 1 death of AML 4 PFS 8–35 mo; 1 toxic death	(65, 66)

Combinations (cyclophosphamide based then platinum-based)								
Groningen, Neth	11	8 macroscopic	EC	6	6	11	Median CR: 15 (8–75+ mo); no response in 3 with > 2 cm disease	(67–69)
Dallas	13	+	CT±Cb	3	1	7	PFS 8 (2–19 mo)	(55)
Marseilles	12		MC				PFS: 50% at 3 yr	(45,70,71)
Vancouver	4		EMC			NA	3+, 9+, 10+, 29+	(58)
Paris	5		(P or M)C[a]					(63)
Tokai, Japan	34	19 macroscopic	2x APC			NA	44% PFS at 4 yr	(72)
Rome	13	13 macroscopic	EPCb	6	3	11	1 toxic death	(73)
Tampa, Florida	3	2 macroscopic	EICb	2	1	3		(74)
Transplanted (after several cycles of conventional dose therapy) as part of an initial therapy program								
Clermont-Ferrand	31	9 pathological CRs	Cb(M or C)				18 patients PF at median of 52 mo	(75)
Paris	37	8 pathological CRs	C(M or Cb)[a]				15 patients PF 32–47 mo	(76)
Other gynecological cancers								
Cervix								
DFCI, Harvard	2		Cb		0	2		(50)
Loyola, Tucson	1		CCbMitox	0	1	1		(61)
Nebraska	6		CPE				4–30	(77)
Uterine								
DFCI, Harvard	1		Cb		0	1		(50)
Fallopian tube								
DFCI, Harvard	1		ICb		1	1		(78)

[a]Abdominal irradiation

HDC = high-dose chemotherapy; A = doxorubicin; C = cyclophosphamide; Cb = carboplatin; E = etoposide; I = ifosfamide; M = melphalan; Mitox = mitoxantrone; P = cisplatin; T = thiotepa; NA = not available; PFS = progression-free survival after bone marrow transplantation; ip = intraperitoneal; CR = complete response; TR = total response; Eval = evaluable patients; NATG = North American Transplant Group; DFCI = Dana Farber Cancer Institute; AML = acute myeloid leukemia.

Table 58-3.
High-dose Chemotherapy with Autologous Bone Marrow Transplantation for Failed Small-cell Lung Cancer or as Initial Treatment

Author	*No. Patients*	*No. in Complete Response*	*No. Disease-free*	*Median Duration (mo)*	*No. Toxic Deaths*	*References*
Relapsed						
UCLA	1	1	0	2	0	(80)
Kanawaza, Japan	2	1	0	2	NA	(81)
Cleveland	3	1	0	5	0	(82)
NATG	4	0	0	0	0	(83)
Institut Gustave-Roussy, Villejuif	6	3	0	4	1	(84)
Groningen, Netherlands	5	0	0	5	2	(69)
Marshfield, Wisconsin	8	1	0	2	NA	(85)
DFCI, Harvard	1	0	0	2	0	(86)
M.D. Anderson, Houston	3	0	0	0	0	(87)
Vanderbilt, Nashville	3	0	0	. . .	0	(88)
M.D. Anderson, Houston	9	1	0	3	1	(89)
As initial treatment						
M.D. Anderson, Houston	14	7	1	10 (4–30)	0	(90)
University College Hospital	25	14	11	11	0	(91)
Total	39	21	12	. . .	0	

NATG = North American Transplant Group; DFCI = Dana Farber Cancer Institute; NA = not available.

repetitive dose regimens for small-cell lung cancer but were obtained with a single treatment. Thirty percent of the patients were disease-free at 20 or more months.

In the study by Farha and co-workers (90), at M.D. Anderson Hospital in Texas, untreated patients initially received high-dose therapy with marrow support. Patients then received prophylactic cranial irradiation and 4 courses of the same drugs at standard doses, followed by radiotherapy to the primary site. All patients responded (54% completely), with a median time to treatment failure and survival of 41 and 56 weeks, respectively. However, the authors stress that these results are also obtainable with conventional-dose regimens.

Studies of autologous BMT in responding small-cell lung cancer are reviewed in Table 58-4 (84,86,91–110). Sculier and colleagues (93), in the European Organization for Research on the Treatment of Cancer (EORTC), reported Phase I trials in small-cell lung cancer after a standard two-cycle induction regimen. At the time of transplant, 3 were complete responders and 10 were partial responders. Patients who received the "lower" etoposide doses did not receive an autologous marrow infusion. However, prolonged aplasia was observed when 2 gm/m^2 or more etoposide were administered without autologous marrow support. Five complete responses were obtained in 11 evaluable patients without CR before intensification. As in the other studies, these responses were of short duration. The authors concluded that "following the hypothesis of Norton and Simon, late intensification should be restricted to patients with a very small amount of residual tumor" (93).

In a follow-up study, Spitzer and colleagues (94), at M.D. Anderson Hospital, studied 32 patients with untreated, limited, small-cell lung cancer who received 3 cycles of induction therapy, followed by 2 courses of intensification with marrow support. Of the 13 patients who were in CR at the time of transplant, 5 (38%) remain disease-free at 4 or more years. One of 9 partial responders before transplant remains disease-free.

In a small study from Ravenna, Italy, patients were transplanted after a standard induction at the time of clinical or pathologically proven complete response (95,96). Two courses of high-dose etoposide were given, along with prophylactic cranial irradiation. Two patients remain disease-free more than 9 months (see Table 58-4).

In the only randomized study, by Humblet and colleagues (97) from the Ludwig Institute in Brussels, patients responding to standard induction treatment received either a further course of standard induction treatment or intensification with autologous marrow support. The median time to relapse was 8 weeks in the control group versus 42 weeks for the intensification arm. Four of 13 patients with LD in the intensification arm were disease-free at 30 to 164 weeks. The median survival for the control and ABMT patients with LD was 58 and 104 weeks, respectively ($p = 0.08$). Because of the only modest improvement in survival and the toxicity of the intensification therapy, the authors concluded that dose-intensive therapy should not be considered a standard therapy in small-cell lung cancer.

These small-cell lung cancer studies suggest several conclusions. In general, high-dose therapy in relapsed patients yields short responses at considerable costs in toxicity. The use of high-dose therapy as initial treatment results in a 54% complete response rate, with some patients surviving disease-free, results

Table 58-4.
High-dose Chemotherapy with Autologous Bone Marrow Transplantation as Intensification for Responding Small-cell Lung Cancer

	At Presentation			*Intensification*				*Response*				*Median Months*		*DFS*		
Author	*No. Patients*	*CTI (Gy)*	*PCI (Gy)*	*No. Patients*	*LD*	*ED*	*Regimen*	*CR*	*PR−>CR*	*PR*	*D*	*CR*	*S*	*2 yr*	*>2 yr*	*References*
Single agent studies																
Ravenna, Italy	34	45	30	15	10	5	E × 2	8	3	4	0	12	18	4	3	(95, 96)
University College Hospital	15	54	20	15	14	1	CY	2	4	4	2	8	8	2	0	(91, 92)
EORTC	36	0	20	36	21	7	CY	21	5	7	1	8	11	0	0	(98)
Glasgow Royal Infirmary	77	0	0	20	9	11	CY	7	2	11	1	...	...	...	...	(99–101)
Royal Marsden, London	25	45	30	4	4	0	(CY)L	4	0	0	0	17+	17+	0	0	(102)
Single alkylating agent studies																
National Cancer Institute	9	20	+	8	0	8	CE	3	1	2	2	10	11	0	0	(103, 104)
Glasgow Royal Infirmary	22	40	0	22	16	6	CE	11	2	3	0	...	...	1	...	(105)
EORTC	5	50	30	15	11	4	CE	3	5	5	1	9	10	0	0	(93)
M.D. Anderson, Houston	32	50	30	32	32	0	CAEVM × 2	13	9	10	0	...	12	7	6	(94)
EORTC	41	0	0	13	4	9	PAE	4	2	4	?	6	9	0	0	(106)
Combination alkylating agent studies																
DFCI, Harvard		0	0	3	3	0	CBE	0	2	0	2	...	...	0	0	(86)
Catholic University, Belgium	23	0	30	23	16	7	CBE	6	9	4	4	...	...	7	2	(97)
Seattle	10	0	30	10	3	7	CB/TBI	3	2	1	3	...	9	1	1	(107)
Combination alkylating agents, with chest RT																
Institut Gustave-Roussy, Villejuif	6	55	+	6	6	0	BEL	6	0	0	0	13	16+	2	2	(84, 108)
Institut Gustave-Roussy, Villejuif	7	45	+	7	0	7	BEL	4	2	1	0	6	9	0	0	(84, 108)
DFCI, Harvard	19	54	30	19	19	0	CBP	6	9	3	1	15+	18+	5	4	(109, 110)
DFCI, Harvard	9	54	30	9	0	9	CBP	2	3	3	1	11	16	1	1	(109, 110)

LD = limited disease; ED = extensive disease; CR = complete response; PR−>CR = conversion from partial to complete response; PR = partial response; D = toxic deaths; MS = median survival; DFS = disease-free survival; CY = cyclophosphamide; E = etoposide; A = doxorubicin (adriamycin); V = vincristine; M = methotrexate; P = cisplatin; L = melphalan (L-Pam); B = carmustine (BCNU); TBI = total body irradiation; CTI = chest/thoracic irradiation; PCI = prophylactic cranial irradiation; DFCI = Dana Farber Cancer Institute; EORTC = European Group for Research and Treatment of Cancer.

Table 58-5.
Consolidation of Responding Small-cell Lung Cancer with High-dose Chemotherapy with Autologous BMT

	No. Trials	*Subset with Chest RT*	*No. Patients*	*% Disease-free*	*% Mortality*
Single agents	5	3	84	14	5
Single alkylator and etoposide	5	2	90	12	7
Combination alkylators	3	0	36	22	25
with chest RT		2	41	46	5
Limited disease			25	52	4
Extensive disease			16	38	6

BMT = bone marrow transplantation; RT = radiotherapy.

similar to treatment with conventional therapy (90,91).

The best results have been achieved in patients with limited disease with complete responses to their initial chemotherapy regimen (Table 58-5). High-dose treatment for patients with LD already in CR after induction results in 40 to 70% disease-free survival at more than 2 years, whereas the same intensification in patients in partial response will usually achieve only short complete responses.

An important component of therapy for small-cell lung cancer is obtaining local control. Complete responders tend to recur in sites of prior bulk disease after conventional or high-dose therapy, and the addition of chest radiotherapy appears to enhance disease-free survival significantly in both settings (111,112).

Two trials combine both combination alkylator therapy with chest radiotherapy (84,108,110). The disease-free survival for 25 patients with LD transplanted in CR or near CR was 52% at a median follow-up of 3 years (110).

Non-small-cell Lung Cancer

Although occasional patients with other respiratory tract primary cancer have participated in Phase I development of high-dose regimens (113), only 2 trials with Phase II data have been published (Table 58-6). Williams and colleagues (114), from University of Chicago, treated 15 patients with and without prior chemotherapy for non-small-cell lung cancer with CY and thiotepa–based high-dose regimens. There were no complete responses, although 7 (47%) responded partially for a median duration of 12 weeks. There were 2 toxic deaths (114). Lazarus and associates (82) treated 26 patients with non-small-cell lung cancer with high-dose cisplatin (200 mg/m^2) and escalating high-dose etoposide. Responses were observed in 15 patients, including 2 complete responses. The median duration of response was 3 months (range, 1–22 + mo) (82). Better regimens are needed.

Brain Tumors

Primary brain tumors currently result in 11,800 deaths per year and are the third leading cause of cancer-related deaths in young adults age 15 to 34 years old (27). The median survival of patients treated with surgical resection alone is 4 months (115); with surgery and adjuvant radiotherapy it is approximately 9 months (116). Response rates for the most widely used chemotherapeutic agents at conventional doses, BCNU, range between 20 and 30% (117,118). Other agents with at least modest activity include other alkylating agents, some vinca alkaloids, and the semisynthetic epidophyllotoxins. Unfortunately, none of these agents has significantly prolonged survival.

Several aspects in the design of high-dose regimens for CNS primary cancer are unique. High-dose therapy of brain tumors is complicated by the theoretical risk of thrombocytopenia-associated CNS bleeding. Most of the published studies have attempted to maintain the platelet count at greater than 50,000/μL, rather than the usual 20,000/μL required to prevent spontaneous bleeding in other patients. A second consideration, the blood-brain barrier, diminishes the number of candidate drugs for use in combinations in those with significant CNS levels. Fortunately, nitrosoureas, the most active agents against gliomas, are

Table 58-6.
High-dose Chemotherapy with Autologous BMT in Non-small-cell Lung Cancer

Author	*No. Patients*	*Status at Time of HDC*	*Conditioning Regimen*	*Response* CR	TR	Evaluable	*Duration of Response (mo)*	*References*
Cleveland	26	Mixed	P+E	2	15	26	3	(82)
Chicago	15	Mixed	CY+T	0	7	15	3	(114)
San Antonio	5	Mixed	M	0	1	4	NA	(113)

BMT = bone marrow transplantation; CR = complete response; TR = total response; HDC = high-dose chemotherapy; CY = cyclophosphamide; T = thiotepa; P = cisplatin; E = etoposide; M = melphalan; NA = not available.

already fully permeable across the blood-brain barrier. Blood and spinal fluid levels of thiotepa are also approximately equivalent. Furthermore, in areas of tumor, the blood-tumor barrier is variably nonfunctional. One rational approach to increasing CNS tumor levels is dose intensification of agents that can penetrate the CNS.

Single-agent Studies in Recurrent Disease

On the basis of significant activity of BCNU at conventional dose, early trials studied high-dose BCNU (800 mg/m^2) in the treatment of patients with recurrent glioblastoma multiforme (119) (Table 58-7) (120–130).

In a study reported by Phillips and others (120), which used 1,050 to 1,350 mg/m^2 BCNU, the objective response rate was 44%. Two of 27 previously failed patients were disease-free 60 and 84 months after treatment, but 6 of 12 patients treated adjuvantly were disease-free between 7 and 59 months (120). Interstitial pneumonitis occurred in 5 patients, 3 of whom died. Of 4 patients in whom drug-induced severe hepatitis developed, 2 died. One patient died of complications of subacute encephalomyelopathy, whereas late, unexplained neurological deterioration developed in 2 patients despite continued CR. In all there were 6 treatment-related deaths (17%).

In the trial by Takvorian and colleagues (121), BCNU was used at doses varying between 600 to 1,400 mg/m^2. Toxicity was substantial; BCNU-associated pulmonary fibrosis developed in 8 patients, 4 of whom died of progressive pulmonary dysfunction. Severe hepatitis developed in 4 patients, 2 of whom died. Clinical bleeding secondary to thrombocytopenia occurred in 3. Renal function was reduced by more than 50% in 4 of 28 patients, but tended to improve with time. A total of 9 of 28 patients (32%) died of treatment-related causes (3 infectious, 4 pulmonary, 2 hepatic). One toxicity of particular concern was acute obtundation in 9 patients (usually transient) or late dementia. Although late CNS events were attributed to tumor recurrence, a late effect from the BCNU cannot be discounted.

Hildebrand and colleagues (122) in Brussels reported a small series of 7 patients treated with 390 mg/m^2 oral lomustine (CCNU) but observed no responses by computed tomography of the brain. Only 5 of the 7 patients received bone marrow support, suggesting that the total dose of chemotherapy was not as high as that achieved in other transplant trials. Four of the 7 patients had low-grade gliomas (one had a brainstem glioma, usually low grade) generally considered less responsive to chemotherapy. Furthermore, the bioavailability of oral agents, particularly in the setting of severe nausea and vomiting, may be variable.

Giannone and associates (123) studied etoposide at doses of 1,000 to 2,400 mg/m^2. Nine of the 16 patients (56%) had received previous chemotherapy. Hematological toxicity was especially severe, and 2 patients died of infection. Extramedullary toxicity consisted of mild gastrointestinal symptoms, including nausea, vomiting, and mucositis. The response rate was 19%.

Combination Studies in Recurrent Disease

Mortimer and associates (124) reported the use of high-dose BCNU alone or with 5-fluorouracil in recurrent high-grade astrocytomas. Toxicity included one case each of reversible hepatic veno-occlusive disease and interstitial pneumonia; there were 2 transplant-related deaths from sepsis. Of 10 evaluable patients, there were 2 complete responses and 6 partial responses (PR), for a total response rate of 80%. Although median survival was not reported, the median time to tumor progression was 7.3 months, compared with an expected survival after recurrence of 3 to 4 months.

The report by Nomura and co-workers (125) is difficult to interpret. Eight study patients with recurrent gliomas were treated with 2 different chemotherapy regimens, one of which may not have required bone marrow support (28). Nevertheless, 3 responses (one complete) were seen in patients with substantial prior treatment, suggesting that dose escalation can overcome drug resistance in vivo (125).

Adjuvant Trials

Investigators soon questioned whether the natural history of brain tumors might be altered by high-dose therapy used as part of the initial treatment regimen. Wolff and colleagues (127) reported 18 patients with high-grade astrocytomas treated initially with surgery followed by radiation (50–60 Gy). Within one to 2 months of completing radiation, patients received BCNU (900–1,005 mg/m^2) with an autologous marrow transplant. Four of 6 patients in whom interstitial infiltrates developed died. The median survival of the group was 18 months; the 2-year survival was 22%. Of the 4 long-term survivors (+25, +42, +60, +77 mo), 2 had progressive tumor, one had a severe encephalomyelopathy, and one was alive and well. The authors concluded that although long-term survival was observed in this trial, the 22% incidence of fatal pulmonary toxicity was unacceptable.

Of 25 patients treated in San Antonio with 1,050 mg/m^2 BCNU and 60 Gy whole-brain radiotherapy 3 weeks following craniotomy, 66% of the patients followed for more than one year achieved CR. The median survival was 26 months; 2- and 3-year survival was approximately 60 and 44%, respectively. Pulmonary toxicity developed in 3 patients (12%). There were 4 transplant-related deaths (16%), 2 of infections, one with pulmonary toxicity, and one of aspiration (128).

Ascensao and co-workers (126), at New York Medical College, studied high-dose thiotepa (600–900 mg/m^2) for grade III and IV astrocytomas followed by radiation (60 Gy) to the site of the tumor one to 4 weeks after transplantation. Of 5 evaluable patients, 3 responded

Table 58-7.
High-dose Studies with Autologous BMT for Brain Tumors

Author	No. Patients	No. Prior: Radio-therapy	No. Prior: Chemo-therapy	No. Grade III/IV	Drug	Dose (mg/m^2)	% Mortality	% Response: CR	% Response: TR	Months Survival: Median	Months Survival: 2 yr	References
Recurrent Disease												
Single agents												
Genova	4	+	0	0/4	BCNU	800	0	. . .	NR	NR	NR	(119)
DFCI, Harvard	28	+	6	NA	BCNU	600–1,400	32	NR	33	4.3	NR	(121)
NATG	36	+	5	7/28	BCNU	1,050–1,350	17	NR	44	4.0	. . .	(120)
Brussels	7	+	0	1/1	CCNU	390	0	0	0	3.5	NR	(122)
Vanderbilt	16	+	5	3/8	Etoposide	1,800–2,400	13	0	19	4.0	NR	(123)
Combinations												
Seattle	11	+	0	2/9	BCNU±5-FU	1,000–1,200	18	2	80	NR	NR	(124)
Japan	8	+	8	3/5	ACNU	50	1	38	NR	NR	. . .	(125)
					AVPE	17						
Totals								7	37	4.1		
Adjuvant Trials												
NY Medical College	7	–	0	NA	Thiotepa	600–900	0		57	NR	NR	(126)
Vanderbilt	18	+	0	3/15	BCNU	900–1,050	22		NR	17.5	22	(127)
San Antonio	25	–	0	12/13	BCNU	1,050	16		64	26.0	59	(128)
Royal Marsden	22	–	0	0/22	BCNU	800–1,000	27		NR	17.0	25	(129)
Lyon	98	–	0	20/75	BCNU	800	6		NR	12.0	NR	(130)
Totals									63	15.4	37	

BMT = bone marrow transplantation; NA = not available; BCNU = carmustine; CCNU = lomustine; NR = not reported. AVPE = doxorubicin, vincristine, cisplatin, cyclophosphamide (endoxan); CR = complete response; TR = total response; DFCI = Dana Farber Cancer Group.

completely and one partially. Acute toxicity included mild mucositis and a case of transient confusion. Thus, high-dose thiotepa appears to be a promising agent for further trials of malignant gliomas.

Mbidde and co-workers (129), from the Royal Marsden Hospital, described an adjuvant trial of high-dose BCNU (800–1,000 mg/m^2) given a median of 27 days postcraniotomy. Radiation therapy (55 Gy) was administered 15 to 43 days following autologous BMT. One of 3 patients with interstitial pneumonitis died, as did one of 2 patients with severe hepatitis. There were 6 early deaths (27%). Despite this rather high early mortality, median survival was 17 months. The 2- and 3-year survival was 25 and 13%, respectively.

The largest series of patients with malignant gliomas treated with high-dose chemotherapy comprised 98 patients who underwent cytoreductive surgery (800 mg/m^2 BCNU) (130). Whole-brain radiotherapy (24 Gy) was followed by a 21-Gy boost to the tumor bed 4 weeks after autologous marrow transplant. Toxicity was relatively low. Pulmonary infiltrates developed in 4 patients and was reversible in 2. Total transplant-related mortality was 6%. Median survival for the entire patient population was 12 months (14 and 11 for patients with grade III and IV astrocytomas, respectively).

Thus, although toxicity of high-dose therapy in patients with gliomas is substantial, it is not appreciably different from toxicities in patients with other types of tumors treated with similar regimens. The risk of intracranial hemorrhage was acceptable given the total of 3 episodes reported in these trials (perhaps because investigators attempted to keep platelet counts high).

The effect of previous radiation in sensitizing neural tissue to the neurotoxic effects of chemotherapy could increase effectiveness or toxicity of these regimens. Cisplatin-induced ototoxicity significantly increased in patients with prior radiation compared with those receiving radiation following cisplatin administration (131). Thus, increased CNS toxicity found in patients with malignant astrocytomas treated with high-dose BCNU may be related to previous cranial radiation rather than to the presence of a brain tumor.

The cumulative data from these trials suggest that the response rates of high-dose BCNU in patients with recurrent gliomas is generally higher than that for repeated conventional-dose BCNU, although the median survival of these patients does not appear to differ significantly. However, the appearance of a few long-term survivors is significant in a virtually invariably fatal tumor.

Thus, the strategy of dose-intensification using combination chemotherapy may prove useful in a patient population with less prior treatment, and the few published trials investigating the role of high-dose single-agent chemotherapy as part of the initial treatment are encouraging. Dose-intensive therapy in the postoperative setting is clearly feasible. Treatment-related mortality ranged between 0 and 27% in the 5 adjuvant trials reported; 16 of 190 patients (9.4%) died of treatment-related complications.

Because the median survivals in these 5 adjuvant trials (12,17,17, and 26 mo) compare favorably with median survivals of patients treated with radiation alone (8 mo) or with conventional-dose chemotherapy (11 mo) (132), such comparisons are hazardous because patients included in high-dose trials may be highly selected. Age, performance status, and tumor grade profoundly influence prognosis. The transplant trial with the lowest reported median survival (130) can be criticized for use of suboptimal doses of radiation. That an additional 1,000 to 1,500 cGy radiation can increase median survival has been suggested in several early radiation trials (133). Thus, adjuvant high-dose single-agent chemotherapy may prolong survival significantly in patients with malignant astrocytomas compared with standard multimodality treatment. Although a randomized trial would be required to test this hypothesis, such a trial would be premature until an optimal combination regimen is constructed and tested. Additional trials are needed to evaluate toxicities and activities of other single agents and the judiciously constructed combinations. CY and cisplatin, 2 agents with demonstrated activity at conventional doses in malignant gliomas, have been studied extensively in dose-intensification regimens for other tumors. Combinations including BCNU, thiotepa, cisplatin (or carboplatin), and CY appear most promising.

Recent advances in the delivery of high-dose focused radiation have made a substantial impact on local tumor control, but patients treated with brachytherapy and radiosurgery tend to relapse at sites in the CNS distant from the original tumor (134–136). High-dose chemotherapy to treat the entire CNS may prove most useful for high-grade astrocytomas treated with surgery and standard external beam radiation, followed by focused radiotherapy. This intensive, multidisciplinary approach may ultimately make an impact on the prognosis of patients with this devastating disease.

Sarcomas

Ewing's Sarcomas

Ewing's sarcomas are exquisitely sensitive to conventional-dose chemotherapy and radiotherapy. A high percentage of patients achieve complete response. Nevertheless, less than 30% of children with metastatic disease can be cured, and few if any adults with metastatic disease survive with conventional-dose therapy. On the basis of its sensitivity to available therapy but poor prognosis, Ewing's sarcoma appears to be an auspicious candidate for treatment with escalated doses of chemotherapy and radiation.

Initial trials studied single agents in recurrent Ewing's sarcomas. Two of 3 failed patients with Ewing's sarcomas treated in London with up to 250 mg/m^2 melphalan have remained disease-free at 12 and 14 months (137).

Graham-Pole and colleagues (138) reported 6 partial responders among 8 previously extensively treated

Table 58-8.
High-dose Therapy with Autologous BMT for Ewing's Sarcoma

Author	*No. Patients*	*Status at Time of HDC*	*Conditioning Regimen*	*Response*			*Duration of Response (mo)*	*References*
				CR	*TR*	*Evaluable*		
Failed or refractory								
Single agents								
Royal Marsden	3	Refractory	M	2	1	3	12+, 13+	(137)
NATG	10	Refractory	M	2	8	10	3(3–7)	(143)
Dublin	1	Failed	M		1	1	4	(144)
Gainesville, Florida	8	Refractory	M		6	8	Median 3(2–6)	(138)
EBMT	9	5 refractory	M	2	4	8	7(2–14)	(145)
NATG	1	Refractory	T		1	1	3	(48)
Combinations								
EBMT	12	5 responding	various	4	9	10	2 disease-free 4, 65 mo	(145)
EBMT	11	6 refractory	TBI/VM	1	4	9	2 disease-free 10, 54 mo	(145)
M.D. Anderson	7		CYBV		4	6	1–2 mo; 1 toxic death	(139)
Inst. Gustave-Roussy	3	Refractory	CYBU	1	1	3		(146)
Responding								
Single agents after relapse								
Royal Marsden	5	Partial response	M	1			1 disease-free at 77 mo	(147)
EBMTG	42	23 responding	Various				20% survival at 40 mo	(148)
Single agents in first response								
Royal Marsden	3	Partial response	M	2	2	2	1 toxic death; 2 relapsed	(147)
Royal Marsden	8	Complete response	M	8	8	8	2 disease-free at 54, 67 mo	(147)
							Median 18 mo	(147)
Gainesville, Florida	6	>8 cm primary/mets	M				1 DF at 40+ mo	(149)
Combinations in first response								
Inst. Gustave-Roussy	18	Stage 4; all in CR	Various				7 DF at 29 mo(3–63)	(146)
National Cancer Inst.	32	13 metastatic	TBI, CYAV				17 DF median 30 mo;	(142)
							13/18 primary only; 4/13 stage 4	(140,142,150)
Gainesville, Florida	20	>8 cm primary/mets	TBI, CYAV				63% disease-free at 3 yr	(149)
Gainesville, Florida	5	> 8 cm primary/mets	TBI, CYE					(149)
EBMTG	55	27 in CR	Various				30% survival at 40 months	(148)

BMT = bone marrow transplantation; HDC = high-dose chemotherapy; B = carmustine (BCNU); CY = cyclophosphamide; A = amsacrine doxorubicin; D = dacarbazine (DTIC); V = vincristine; TBI = total body irradiation; M = melphalan; Pc = procarbazine; BU = busulfan; CR = complete response; TR = total response; NATG = North American Transplant Group; EBMTG = European Bone Marrow Transplant Group.

patients with Ewing's sarcomas given up to 210 mg/m^2 melphalan and autologous BMT. The median time to treatment failure was short (3 mo). This experience was similar to that at the M.D. Anderson Hospital (139). Of 8 patients given 6 gm/m^2 CY, 300 mg/m^2 dacarbazine, and 720 mg/m^2 etoposide, 4 partially responded.

Of 32 high-risk patients with Ewing's sarcomas in first complete response given high-dose vincristine, CY, doxorubicin, and TBI at the National Cancer Institute (NCI), 17 were reported disease-free with a median follow-up of 30 months (140–142). (Table 58-8) (143–150).

Although short responses are generally achieved with high-dose therapy in relapsed patients, an occasional patient treated in second or subsequent response will have durable remission. More promising results are achieved in patients transplanted in first complete response with a combination chemotherapy regimen; 30 to 63% of patients are disease-free at 3 or 4 years.

Other Sarcomas

There are few reports of autologous transplantation in patients with osteogenic sarcomas. One failed patient, transplanted in Australia after 200 mg/m^2 melphalan, had stable pulmonary metastases but complete resolution of scalp lesions (151).

Forty-three children with soft-tissue sarcomas were treated with induction chemotherapy comprising 6 courses of vincristine, doxorubicin, and CY, given in most cases within 8 weeks (rapid VAC). Thirty-six patients then received high-dose melphalan with autologous marrow transplant; 26 also received irradiation to the site of the primary tumor. There was one toxic death 2 months after high-dose melphalan due to infection and possible anthracycline cardiomyopathy. Actuarial survival at 5 years for all stages was 57%, and event-free survival was 44%; for patients with nonmetastatic diseases, these values were 62 and 53%, respectively (152).

For adult soft-tissue sarcomas, the number of patients (generally with refractory disease) is still small. Ifosfamide combinations have been reported by Elias and colleagues (78) and Fields and associates (52) (Table 58-9) (153–159).

Melanomas

The relatively promising results in chemotherapy-sensitive cancers contrast with those of the chemotherapy-resistant tumor melanoma. The rationale for high-dose melphalan treatment of melanomas is based on a linear-log dose-response curve for human melanoma xenografts in nude mice. The response rate of human melanomas to a standard dose of melphalan is approximately 9%. Response rates in melanomas

Table 58-9.
High-dose Therapy for Other Sarcomas

Author	No. Patients	Status at Time of HDC	Conditioning Regimen	Response CR	TR	Evaluable	Duration of Response (mo)	References
Osteosarcoma								
Tampa, Florida	1	PR	ICbE	0	1	1		(153)
Oklahoma	1	Failed	CYB	0	1	1	2	(154)
New Zealand	1	Refractory	M		0	1	13+	(151)
Rhabdomyosarcoma, PNET								
Memorial, NYC	10	Relapsed, 5 CRs	ME				5 DF 2–17 mo (median 7)	(155)
Memorial, NYC	8	All in 1st CR	ME				7 DF 2–11 mo (median 4)	(155)
National Cancer Inst.	38		TBI, CYAV					(150)
Melbourne	4	Responding	CYAD	2	4	4	4(1–14)	(156)
EBMTG	46	Various	Various				20% DFS at 5 yrs	(147)
Other soft-tissue sarcomas								
NATG	4	Refractory	B	0	3	4	"Short"	(143)
Seattle	3	Refractory	CY					(157)
NATG	6	Refractory	T	0	1	6		(158)
NATG	7	Refractory	M	1	1	7	4+	(143)
EBMTG	43	Responding	M				44% DFS at 5 yr	(152)
Oklahoma	3	2 failed	CYB	0	1	1	4	(154)
DFCI, Harvard	8	Metastatic	CYBP	1	6	6	2–7	(57)
Duke	1		CYPM	0	1	1		(159)
DFCI, Harvard	10	Refractory	ICb	1	3	8	1 toxic death	(78)
Tampa, Florida	9	Refractory	EICb	0	2	2		(52)
EBMTG	49	Various	Various				20% DFS at 5 yrs	(152)

A = doxorubicin (adriamycin); B = carmustine (BCNU); CY = cyclophosphamide; D = dacarbazine (DTIC); M = melphalan; I = ifosfamide; Cb = carboplatin; TBI = total body irradiation; HDC = high-dose chemotherapy; CR = complete response; TR = total response; EBMT = European Bone Marrow Transplant Group; NATG = North American Transplant Group; DFCI = Dana Farber Cancer Institute; DFS = disease-free survival.

Table 58-10.
High-dose Therapy with Autologous BMT for Melanoma

Author	No. Patients	Status at Time of HDC	Conditioning Regimen	Response CR	Response TR	%RR	References
Single agents							
Marseilles	2		M	0	2	100	(70)
Royal Free, London	3		M	0	0	0	(47)
San Antonio	3		M	0	2	67	(113)
Cleveland	20		M	5	14	70	(160)
Royal Marsden	28	10 failed	M	2	11	43	(161, 162, 167)
NATG	26	16 failed; 10 untreated	M	6	18	69	(164, 168, 169)
						63	
						80	
NY Medical College	31		M	0	11	35	(170)
Total	113			13	62	55	
NATG	31	15 failed; 16 untreated	BCNU	4	14	45	(164, 168, 169)
						13	
						75	
M.D. Anderson	5		BCNU	0	1	20	(87)
RPMI	6		BCNU	0	1	17	(171)
Royal Marsden	9		BCNU	1	4	44	(172)
Total	51			5	20	39	
NATG	55	31 failed; 24 untreated	T	4	29	53	(164, 168, 169)
						52	
						54	
M.D. Anderson	4		AMSA	0	0	0	(173)
Colorado	4		Mustard	1	2	50	(174)
Seattle	2		CY	0	0	0	(49, 157)
Combinations							
Vanderbilt	7		TM	0	4	57	(169)
Colorado	17		BM	2	7	41	(174)
NATG	58		BM	8	36	59	(168)
Duke	6		CYPM	0	4	6	(159)
DFCI, Harvard	19		CYBP±M	1	11	65	(175)
Chicago	3		CYT±M	2	0	67	(176)
NATG	6		CYT	3	2	83	(168)
Oklahoma	5		CYB	0	2	40	(154)
Tampa, Florida	10		ICbE	1	0	10	(52)
Total	131			17	66	50	

BMT = bone marrow transplantation; HDC = high-dose chemotherapy; CR = complete response; TR = total response; CY = cyclophosphamide; B = carmustine (BCNU); P = cisplatin; M = melphalan; T = thiotepa; I = ifosfamide; Cb = carboplatin; E = etoposide; NATG = North American Transplant Group; RPMI = Roswell Park Memorial Institute; DFCI = Dana Farber Cancer Institute.

for high-dose melphalan are shown in Table 58-10 (160–176). Although there appears to be a dose-response in Lazarus and co-worker's (160) study of 180 and 225 mg/m^2, in a larger study by Cornbleet and others (161), patients treated with 260 mg/m^2 melphalan achieved only an 8% CR rate, with a 43% response rate overall. Melphalan or BCNU at standard doses produce responses in 10 to 20% of patients. When given at high doses with melphalan, response rates of 40 to 65% occur, and a significant percentage of complete responses is observed. Diarrhea and mucositis are dose-limiting for melphalan (160–162), whereas BCNU is limited by lung and liver toxicity (163,164).

Investigators at Duke University randomized 39 patients with more than 4 positive lymph nodes (estimated survival with conventional therapy at 5 years is 5%) to immediate dose-intensive therapy with CY, BCNU, and cisplatin or to observation with high-dose therapy in the event of relapse. Of 20 patients randomized to observation, 18 have relapsed versus 15 of 19 randomized to high-dose therapy. More than half the patients on both arms relapsed locally (165).

Melanoma cells circulating in peripheral blood have been detected with reverse transcriptase and polymerase chain reaction (166). Whether contamination of marrow could also be detected with these techniques is currently unknown.

Colon and Gastrointestinal Malignancies

Evidence of a dose-response curve has been reported for metastatic colon cancer treated with 180 mg/m^2 melphalan by Leff and colleagues (177) in San Antonio. Of 20 patients, 3 (15%) responded completely and 6 partially (30%). The median unmaintained time to treatment failure was 3 months.

Investigators in Cleveland studied melphalan and misonidazole in 14 patients with metastatic colorectal cancer. One patient died of toxicity; 6 patients achieved a partial remission of 3 to 10 months (median, 4 mo) (178).

Few optimal patients with untreated or responding metastatic colorectal cancer treated with a combination chemotherapy regimen have been studied. Of the 10 patients who received combinations, many had failed a prior regimen. Nevertheless, 6 of 8 evaluable patients responded with one complete response. The few patients treated, generally in phase I trials, for other gastrointestinal primary cancers are shown in Table 58-11 (179–182).

Cost Effectiveness

Major advances in supportive care in the last 2 years have decreased the time to engraftment, morbidity, and cost associated with transplant. In multiple randomized trials hematopoietic growth factors have been found to decrease the time to engraftment, days on antibiotics, and total hospital days (183). Even more effective in achieving these aims has been addition of peripheral blood stem cells (184–188). Indeed, for the first time, the strategies of increased dose can be tested efficiently and relatively safely. The use of regimens with 5- to 10-fold increments in dose can be compared with conventional-dose chemotherapy regimens, whereas in the past, even a 1.5- to 2-fold escalation in dose resulted in substantial myelosuppression.

Table 58-11.
High-dose Therapy with Autologous BMT for Gastrointestinal Malignancy

Author	*No. Patients*	*Status at Time of HDC*	*Conditioning Regimen*	*Response*			*Duration of Response (mo)*	*References*
				CR	*TR*	*Evaluable*		
Colorectal cancer								
Single agents								
San Antonio	20	Metastatic	M	3	6	20	Median 3 mo	(113, 177)
Royal Free	2	Failed	M	0	1	2	2	(47)
NATG	7	Metastatic	M	1	4	7	2.5(2–3)	(143)
Cleveland	14	Metastatic	Misonidazole + M		6	14	4 (3–10)	(178)
NATG	22	16 failed	T	1	13	22	5(2–9+)	(48, 179)
Cleveland	3	Metastatic	T	0	0			(180)
NATG	4	Metastatic	B	1	2	4	5, 24	(143)
DFCI, Harvard	1		Cb	0	0	1		(50)
Wayne State, Detroit	3		Mito C	0	1	3		(181)
Combinations								
DFCI, Harvard	2	Metastatic	CYBP	0	0	2		(57)
Duke	1	Failed	CYTP	0	1	1		(56)
Oklahoma	5	3 failed	CYB	1	4	4	2–11	(154)
Chicago	2	1 as initial therapy	TCY	0	1	1		(176)
Total	10			1	6	8		
Gastric cancer								
Single agents								
NATG	2	NA	B	0	0	2		(143)
NATG	1	NA	T	0	0	1		(48)
Wayne State, Detroit	1		Mito C	0	0	1		(181)
Combinations								
Groningen, Netherlands	1		CYMitox	0	1	1	3	(62)
Duke	1		CYPM	0	0	1		(159)
Pancreatic cancer								
NATG	1	NA	B	0	0	1	...	(143)
Chicago	1		CYTMitox	0	0	1	...	(60, 182)
Wayne State, Detroit	1		Mito C	0	0	1		(181)
Esophageal cancer								
NATG	1	NA	B	0	0	1		(143)
Hepatic/cholangiocarcinoma								
NATG	1	NA	B	0	0	1		(143)
DFCI, Harvard	1	failed	ICb	0	0	1		(78)

HDC = high-dose chemotherapy; CR = complete response; TR = total response; B = carmustine (BCNU); Cb = carboplatin; CY = cyclophosphamide; I = ifosfamide; M = melphalan; Mitox =mitoxantrone; Mito C = mitomycin C; NA = not available; P = cisplatin; T = thiotepa; NATG = North American Transplant Group; DFCI = Dana Farber Cancer Institute.

A preliminary analysis of costs was based on assumptions modeled on published series of patients with metastatic breast cancer with 2 to 3 year follow-up compared with conventional-dose therapy. The cost of conventional dose therapy was estimated at $36,100 and for marrow transplant $89,700. On the basis of a median survival of 27 months for high-dose therapy compared with 21 months for conventional-dose therapy, the estimated benefit is 6 months. Thus the $115,800 current cost per year of life saved was greater than most but not all acceptable therapies. However, if CRs prove to be durable and growth factors and peripheral blood progenitor cell support significantly lower the costs, dose-intensive therapy was estimated to be quite cost effective at $17,000 per year of life saved (compared with $45,000 per year of life saved for renal dialysis) (189,190).

Quality-of-life Issues

Most patients who do not relapse resume a normal lifestyle within 3 to 6 months after high-dose therapy and autologous BMT (191). A 10% incidence of herpes zoster in the year following treatment in the Dana-Farber Cancer Institute series was considerably below the 50% incidence after dose-intensive therapy for lymphomas. The only prospective evaluation published to date is a preliminary analysis from the Duke University marrow transplant team of 52 patients transplanted for metastatic breast cancer compared with similar patients receiving conventional therapy. Scores were significantly correlated with outcome of treatment (192).

Summary

High-dose therapy for solid tumors with autologous hematopoietic stem-cell support represents an active area of continued study in cancer therapy firmly based on laboratory and clinical observations. High-dose therapy has been facilitated by substantial progress in supportive care, such as hematopoietic growth factors and peripheral blood progenitor cells.

References

1. Frei III E, Canellos GP. Dose, a critical factor in cancer chemotherapy. Am J Med 1980;69:585–594.
2. Skipper HE, Schabel FM, Jary R, Wilcox WS. Experimental evaluation of potential anticancer agents. Cancer Chemother Rep 1964;35:1–111.
3. Hill RP, Stanley JA. The response of hypoxic B16 melanoma cells to in vivo treatment with chemotherapeutic agents. Cancer Res 1975;35:1147–1153.
4. Skipper HE. Criteria associated with destruction of leukemia and solid tumor cells in animals. Cancer Res 1967;27:2636–2645.
5. Frei III E, Antman K, Teicher B, Eder P, Schnipper L. Bone marrow autotransplantation for solid tumors—prospects. J Clin Oncol 1989;7:515–526.
6. Budman DR, Wood W, Henderson IC, et al. Initial findings of CALGB 8541: a dose and dose intensity trial of cyclophosphamide, doxorubicin, and 5-fluorouracil as adjuvant treatment of Stage II, node +, female breast cancer (abstract 29). Proc Am Soc Clin Oncol 1992;11:51.
7. Becher R, Wandl U, Kloke O, et al. Randomized study of different doses of epirubicin and identical doses of cyclophosphamide in advanced breast cancer. Proc Am Soc Clin Oncol 1990;9:47.
8. Bennett JM, Muss HB, Doroshow JH et al. A randomized multicenter trial comparing mitoxantrone, cyclophosphamide, and fluoruracil with doxorubicin, cyclophosphamide, and fluorouracil in the therapy of metastatic breast cancer. J Clin Oncol 1988;6:1611–1620.
9. Focan C, Closon MT, Andrien JM, et al. Dose response relationship with epirubicin as first line chemotherapy for advanced breast cancer. A randomized trial. Ann Oncol 1990;1(suppl):S18.
10. Habeshaw T, Jones R, Stallard S, et al. Epirubicin at 2 dose levels with prednisolone as treatment for advanced breast cancer: results of a randomised trial. Proc Am Soc Clin Oncol 1990;9:43.
11. Hortobagyi GN, Bodey SP, Buzdar AU, et al. Evaluation of high-dose versus standard FAC chemotherapy for advanced breast cancer in protected environment units: a prospective randomized study. J Clin Oncol 1987;5:354–364.
12. Ngan HYS, Choo YC, Cheung M, et al. A randomized study of high-dose versus low-dose cisplatinum combined with cyclophosphamide in the treatment of advanced ovarian cancer. Chemotherapy 1989;35:221–227.
13. Tannock IF, Boyd NF, Deboer G, et al. A randomized trials of two dose levels of cyclophosphamide, methotrexate, and fluorouracil chemotherapy for patients with metastatic breast cancer. J Clin Oncol 1988;6: 1377–1387.
14. Hryniuk WM, Bush H. The importance of dose intensity in chemotherapy of metastatic breast cancer. J Clin Oncol 1984;2:1281–1287.
15. Cohen M, Rajendra R, Ahuja N, Nguyen D. Chemotherapy dose intensity and median survival in advanced breast cancer: no apparent relationship. Proc Am Soc Clin Oncol 1990;9:34.
16. Henderson IC, Hayes DF, Gelman R. Dose-response in the treatment of breast cancer: a critical review. J Clin Oncol 1988;6:1501–1515.
17. Santos GW. Overview of autologous bone marrow transplantation. Int J Cell Cloning 1985;3:215–216.
18. Pinkel D. Ninth annual David Karnofsky lecture: treatment of acute lymphocytic leukemia. Cancer 1979;43:1128–1137.
19. Frei E III, Freireich EJ. Progress and perspectives in the chemotherapy of acute leukemia. Adv Chemother 1965;2:269–289.
20. Frei E III, Karon M, Levin RH, et al. The effectiveness of combinations of antileukemic agents in inducing and maintaining remission in children with acute leukemia. Blood 1965;26:642–656.
21. Freireich EJ, Henderson ES, Karon M, Frei E III. The treatment of acute leukemia with respect to cell population kinetics. The proliferation and spread of neoplastic cells; 21st Annual Symposium on Fundamental Cancer Research. Houston: University of Texas Press, 1968:441–452.
22. Skipper HE. Combination therapy: some concepts and results. Cancer Chemother Rep 1974;4:137–145.
23. Skipper HE. Stepwise progress in the treatment of disseminated cancers. Cancer 1983;51:1773–1776.
24. Frei E III, Cucchi C, Rosowsky A, et al. Alkylating agent

resistance: in vitro studies of human cell lines. Proc Natl Acad Sci USA 1985;82:2158–2162.
25. Schabel F. Patterns of resistance and therapeutic synergism among alkylating agents. Fundam Cancer Chemother 1978;23:200–215.
26. Schabel FM, Griswold DP, Corbett TH. Recent studies with surgical adjuvant chemotherapy or immunotherapy of metastatic solid tumors of mice. In: Jones SE, Salmon SE, eds. Adjuvant therapy of cancer II. New York: Grune and Stratton, 1979:3–17.
27. Boring CC, Squires TS, Tong T. Cancer statistics, 1992. CA 1992;42:19–38.
28. Blijham G, Spitzer G, Litam J, et al. The treatment of advanced testicular carcinoma with high dose chemotherapy and autologous marrow support. J Cancer 1981;17:443–444.
29. Champlin R. Autologous bone marrow transplantation for testicular carcinoma. Int J Cell Cloning 1985; 3:260–261.
30. Greco F, Johnson D, Wolff S, et al. A phase II study of high-dose VP16 and autologous bone marrow transplantation for refractory germinal neoplasms (abstract). Proc Am Assoc Clin Oncol 1983;2:138.
31. Wolff S, Johnson D, Hainsworth J, et al. High dose VP16-213 monotherapy for refractory germinal malignancies: a phase II study. J Clin Oncol 1984;2:271–274.
32. Nichols CR, Tricot G, Williams SD, et al. Dose-intensive chemotherapy in refractory germ-cell cancer—a phase I/II trial of high dose carboplatin and etoposide with autologous bone marrow transplantation. J Clin Oncol 1989;7:932–939.
33. Birch R, Williams SD, Cone A, et al. Prognostic factors for favorable outcome in disseminated germ cell tumors. J Clin Oncol 1986;4:400–407.
34. Linkesch W, Kuhrer I, Wagner A. rhu-GM-CSF after ultrahigh dose carboplatin, VP-16, cyclophosphamide with ABMT in refractory germ cell cancer (abstract). Proc Am Soc Clin Oncol 1990;9:141.
35. Pico JL, Ostronoff JP, Droz D, et al. High-dose chemotherapy with cisplatin, etoposide and cyclophosphamide (PEC Protocol) followed by autologous bone marrow support in non-seminomatous germ cell tumors (abstract 41). Proc Am Soc Clin Oncol 1989;8:12.
36. Antman K, Corringham R, de Vries E, et al. Dose intensive therapy in breast cancer. Bone Marrow Transplant 1992;10:67–73.
37. Levin L, Hryniuk WM. Dose intensity analysis of chemotherapy regimens in ovarian cancer. J Clin Oncol 1987;5:756–760.
38. Ozols R, Corden B, Jacob J, et al. High-dose cisplatin in hypertonic saline. Ann Intern Med 1984;100:19–24.
39. Ozols R, Ostchega Y, Gregory C, Young R. High-dose carboplatin in refractory ovarian cancer patients. J Clin Oncol 1987;5:197–201.
40. Boni C, Cocconi G, Lottici R, et al. Conventional vs high dose-intensity cisplatin in advanced ovarian cancer: preliminary report of a randomized trial (abstract 651). Proc Am Soc Clin Oncol 1990;9:168.
41. Bronchud MH, Howell A, Crowther D, Hopwood P, Souza LM, Dexter TM. The use of granulocyte colony-stimulating factor to increase the intensity of treatment with doxorubicin in patients with advanced breast and ovarian cancer. Br J Cancer 1989;60:121–125.
42. Robson CN, Lewis AD, Wold CR, et al. Reduced levels of drug-induced DNA crosslinking in nitrogen mustard-resistant Chinese hamster ovary cells expressing elevated glutathione S-transferase activity. Cancer Res 1987;47:6022.
43. Hamilton TC, Winker MA, Lovie KG, et al. Augmentation of adriamycin, melphalan and cisplatin cytotoxicity in drug-resistant and sensitive human ovarian carcinoma cell lines by buthionine sulfoximine mediated glutathione depletion. Biochem Pharmacol 1985; 34:2583.
44. Green JA, Vistica DT, Young RC, et al. Melphalan resistance in human ovarian cancer. Potentiation of ME cytotoxicity by nutritional and pharmacologic depletion of intracellular glutathione (GSH) levels (abstract). Proc Am Assoc Cancer Res 1984;25:290.
45. Viens P, Maraninchi D. High dose chemotherapy and autologous marrow transplantation for common epithelial ovarian carcinomas. In: Armitage J, Antman K, eds. High dose chemotherapy. Baltimore: Williams & Wilkins, 1992;729–734.
46. Lazarus J, Herzig R, Graham-Pole J, et al. Intensive melphalan chemotherapy and cryopreserved autologous bone marrow transplantation for the treatment of refractory cancer. J Clin Oncol 1983;2:359–367.
47. Corringham R, Gilmore M, Prentice H, Boesen E. High-dose melphalan with autologous bone marrow transplant: treatment of poor prognosis tumors. Cancer 1983;52:1783–1787.
48. Herzig RH, Fay JW, Herzig GP, et al. Phase I-II studies with high-dose thiotepa and autologous marrow transplantation in patients with refractory malignancies. In: Herzig GP, ed. Advances in cancer chemotherapy: high dose thiotepa and autologous marrow transplantation. New York: Park Row Publishers, 1987:17–33.
49. Buckner CD, Rudolph RH, Fefer A, et al. High dose cyclophosphamide therapy for malignant disease. Cancer 1972;29:357–365.
50. Shea TC, Flaherty M, Elias A, et al. A phase I clinical and pharmacological study of high-dose carboplatin and autologous bone marrow support. J Clin Oncol 1989;7:651–661.
51. Shea TC, Storniolo AM, Mason JR, Newton B, Mullen M, Hunger K. High-dose intravenous and intraperitoneal combination chemotherapy with autologous stem cell rescue for patients with advanced ovarian cancer (abstract 756). Proc Am Soc Clin Oncol 1992;11:236.
52. Fields KK, Zorsky PE, Heimenz J, et al. Ifosfamide, carboplatin and etoposide in the treatment of refractory malignancy (abstract 188). Proc Am Soc Clin Oncol 1992;11:90.
53. Lotz JP, Machover D, Malassagne B, Donsimoni R, Gerota J, Izrael V. Phase I/II study of two consecutive courses of intensive chemotherapy combining VP16 or VM 26 with carboplatin and ifosfamide with ABMT for treatment of solid tumors (abstract 45). Proc Am Soc Clin Oncol 1990;9:13.
54. Tobias J, Weiner R, Griffiths C. Cryopreserved autologous marrow infusion following high-dose cancer chemotherapy. Eur J Cancer 1977;13:269–277.
55. Collins RH, Pineiro L, Fay JW. High dose chemotherapy and autologous bone marrow transplantation for advanced ovarian cancer. Proc Am Soc Clin Oncol 1992;11:233.
56. Shpall E, Jones E, Egorin M, et al. A phase I trial of high-dose combination cyclophosphamide, cisplatin and thiotepa with autologous bone marrow support in the treatment of resistant solid tumors (abstract 544). Proc Am Soc Clin Oncol 1987;6:139.

57. Antman K, Eder JP, Elias A, et al. High-dose combination alkylating agent preparative regimen with autologous bone marrow support: the Dana-Farber Cancer Institute/Beth Israel Hospital experience. Cancer Treat Rep 1987;71:119–125.
58. Barnett M, Swenerton K, Hoskins P, et al. Intensive therapy with carboplatin, etoposide and melphalan and autologous stem cell transplantation for epithelial ovarian carcinoma. Proc Am Soc Clin Oncol 1990;9:168.
59. Shpall E, Clarke-Pearson D, Soper J, et al. High dose alkylating agent chemotherapy with autologous bone marrow support in patients with stage III/IV epithelial ovarian cancer. Gynecol Oncol 1990;38:386–391.
60. Ellis ED, Williams SF, Moormeier JA, Kaminer LS, Bitran JD. A phase I-II study of high dose cyclophosphamide, thiotepa and escalating doses of mitoxantrone with autologous stem cell rescue in patients with refractory malignancies. Bone Marrow Transplant 1990;6:439–442.
61. McKenzie R, Alberts D, Bishop M, et al. Phase I trial of high dose cyclophosphamide, mitoxantrone, and carboplatin with autologous bone marrow transplantation in female malignancies: pharmacologic levels of mitoxantrone and high response rate in refractory ovarian cancer (abstract). Proc Am Soc Clin Oncol 1991;10:186.
62. Mulder POM, Sleijfer DT, Willemse PH, de Vries EG, Uges DRA, Mulder NH. High dose cyclophosphamide or melphalan with escalating doses of mitoxantrone and autologous bone marrow transplantation for refractory solid tumors. Cancer Res 1989;49:4654–4658.
63. Extra J, Dieras V, Espie M, et al. Intensification therapeutique avec autogreffe medullaire au cours des adenocarcinomes ovariens: etude de phase I-II de 21 sujets. Cahiers Cancer 1989;1:81–84.
64. Dauplat J, Legros M, Condat P, Ferriere J, Ahmed SB, Plagne R. High-dose melphalan and autologous bone marrow support for treatment of ovarian carcinoma with positive second-look operation. Gynecol Oncol 1989;34:294–298.
65. Viens P, Maraninchi D, Legros M, et al. High dose melphalan and autologous marrow rescue in advanced epithelial ovarian carcinomas: a retrospective analysis of 35 patients treated in France. Bone Marrow Transplant 1990;5:227–233.
66. Stoppa AM, Maraninchi D, Niens P, et al. High doses of melphalan and autologous marrow rescue in advanced common epithelial ovarian carcinomas: a retrospective analysis in 35 patients. In: Dicke K, Spitzer G, Jagannath S, Evinger-Hodges MJ, eds. Autologous bone marrow transplantation. Houston, TX: The University of Texas M.D. Anderson Cancer Center, 1989:509–518.
67. Mulder P, Willemse P, Aalders JG, et al. High-dose chemotherapy with autologous bone marrow transplantation in patients with refractory ovarian cancer. Eur J Cancer Clin Oncol 1989;25:645–649.
68. Vriesendorp R, Aalders J, Sleijfer D, et al. Effective high dose chemotherapy with autologous bone marrow infusion in resistant ovarian cancer. Gynecol Oncol 1984;17:271–276.
69. Postmus PE, De Vries EGE, De Vries-Hospers HG, et al. Cyclophosphamide and VP16-213 with autologous bone marrow transplantation. A dose escalation study. Eur J Cancer Clin Oncol 1984;20:777–782.
70. Maraninchi D, Gastuat JA, Herve P, et al. High-dose melphalan and autologous marrow transplantation in adult solid tumors: clinical responses and preliminary evaluation of different strategies. In: McVie JG, Dalesio O, Smith IE, ed. Autologous bone marrow transplantation and solid tumors, vol 14. New York: Raven, 1984:145–150.
71. Maraninchi D, Abecasis M, Gastaut J, et al. High-dose melphalan with autologous bone marrow rescue for the treatment of advanced adult solid tumors. Cancer Treat Rep 1984;68:471–474.
72. Shinozuka T, Murakami M, Miyamoto Y, et al. High dose chemotherapy with autologous bone marrow transplantation in ovarian cancer (abstract). Proc Am Soc Clin Oncol 1991;10:193.
73. Panici PB, Scambia G, Baiocchi G, et al. High dose chemotherapy and autologous peripheral stem cell support in advanced ovarian cancer (abstract). Proc Am Soc Clin Oncol 1991;10:195.
74. Fields KK, Zorsky PE, Saleh RA, et al. A phase I-II study of high-dose ifosfamide, carboplatin and etoposide with autologous bone marrow rescue: preliminary results (abstract). Proc Am Soc Clin Oncol 1991;10:70.
75. Legros M, Fleury J, Cure H, et al. High-dose chemotherapy and autologous bone marrow transplant in 31 advanced ovarian cancers: long-term results (abstract 700). Proc Am Soc Clin Oncol 1992;11:222.
76. Extra JM, Giacchetti S, Bourstyn E, Colin P, Maylin C, Marty M. High dose chemotherapy with autologous bone marrow reinfusion as consolidation therapy for patients with advanced ovarian adenocarcinoma (abstract). Proc Am Soc Clin Oncol 1992;11:234.
77. Kessinger A, McIntosh D, Smith M. High dose chemotherapy and autologous hematopoietic stem cell transplantation for patients with refractory metastatic carcinoma of the uterine cervix (abstract 763). Proc Am Soc Clin Oncol 1992;11:237.
78. Elias AD, Ayash L, Eder JP, et al. A phase I study of high-dose ifosfamide and escalating doses of carboplatin with autologous bone marrow support. J Clin Oncol 1991;9:320–327.
79. Pierelli L, Menichella G, Foddai M, et al. High dose chemotherapy with cisplatin, VP16 and carboplatin with stem cell support in patients with advanced ovarian cancer. J Haema tologica 1991;76:63–65.
80. Douer YD, Champlin R, Ho W, et al. High-dose combined-modality therapy and autologous bone marrow rescue for refractory solid tumors. Am J Med 1981;71:973–976.
81. Harada M, et al. Combined-modality therapy and autologous bone marrow transplantation in the treatment of advanced non-hodgkin's lymphoma and solid tumors: the Kanawaza experience. Transplant Proc 1982;4:733–737.
82. Lazarus HM, Spitzer TR, Creger RT. Phase I trial of high-dose etoposide, high-dose cisplatin, and reinfusion of autologous bone marrow for lung cancer. Am J Clin Oncol 1990;13:107–112.
83. Phillips GL, Fay JW, Herzig GP, et al. A phase I-II study: intensive BCNU and cryopreserved autologous marrow transplantation for refractory cancer. Cancer 1983;52:1792–1802.
84. Pico JL, Baume D, Ostronoff M, et al. Chimiotherapie A Hautes Doses Suivie D'Autogreffe de Moelle Osseuse dans le Traitement du Cancer Bronchique a Petites Cellules. Bull Cancer 1987;74:587–595.
85. Rushing DA, Baldauf MC, Gehlsen JA, et al. High-dose BCNU and autologous bone marrow reinfusion in the treatment of refractory or relapsed small cell carcinoma of the lung (abstract 846). Proc Am Soc Clin Oncol 1984;3:217.

86. Stahel RA, Takvorian RW, Skarin AT, Canellos GP. Autologous bone marrow transplantation following high-dose chemotherapy with cyclophosphamide, BCNU, and VP-16 in small cell carcinoma of the lung and a review of current literature. Eur J Cancer Clin Oncol 1984;20:1233–1238.
87. Spitzer G, Dicke KA, Verma DS, et al. High-dose BCNU therapy with autologous bone marrow infusion: preliminary observations. Cancer Treat Rep 1979;63:1257–1264.
88. Wolff S, Fer M, McKay C. High-dose VP-16-213 and autologous bone marrow transplantation for refractory malignancies: a phase I study. J Clin Oncol 1983; 1:701–705.
89. Spitzer G, Dicke KA, Latam J, et al. High-dose combination chemotherapy with autologous bone marrow transplantation in adult solid tumors. Cancer 1980;45:3075–3085.
90. Farha P, Spitzer G, Valdivieso M, et al. High-dose chemotherapy and autologous bone marrow transplantation for the treatment of small cell lung carcinoma. Cancer 1983;52:1351–1355.
91. Souhami R, Harper PG, Linch D, et al. High dose cyclophosphamide with autologous bone marrow transplantation as initial treatment of small cell carcinoma of the bronchus. Cancer Chemother Pharmacol 1982;8:31–34.
92. Souhami RL, Hajichristou HT, Miles DW, et al. Intensive chemotherapy with autologous bone marrow transplantation for small cell lung cancer. Cancer Chemother Pharmacol 1989;24:321–325.
93. Sculier JP, Klastersky J, Stryckmans P, the EORTC. Late intensification in small cell lung cancer: a phase I study of high doses of cyclophosphamide and etoposide with ABMT. J Clin Oncol 1985;3:184–191.
94. Spitzer G, Farha P, Valdiviesco M, et al. High dose intensification therapy with autologous bone marrow support for limited small cell bronchogenic carcinoma. J Clin Oncol 1986;4:4–13.
95. Marangolo M, Rosti G, Ravaioli A, et al. Small cell carcinoma of the lung: high-dose VP-16 and autologous bone marrow transplantation as intensification therapy: preliminary results. Int J Cell Cloning 1985;3:277.
96. Marangolo M, Rosti G, Amadori D, et al. High-dose etoposide and autologous bone marrow transplantation as intensification treatment in small cell lung cancer: a pilot study. Bone Marrow Transplant 1989; 4:405–408.
97. Humblet Y, Symann M, Bosly A. Late intensification chemotherapy with ABMT in selected small cell carcinomas of the lung: a randomized study. J Clin Oncol 1987;5:1864–1873.
98. Smith IE, Evans BD, Harland SJ, et al. High dose cyclophosphamide with autologous bone marrow rescue after conventional chemotherapy in the treatment of small cell lung carcinoma. Cancer Chemother Pharmacol 1985;14:120–124.
99. Banham S, Burnett A, Stevenson R, et al. Pilot study of combination chemotherapy with late dose intensification and autologous bone marrow rescue in small cell bronchogenic carcinoma. Br J Cancer 1982;42:486.
100. Banham S, Loukop M, Burnett A, et al. Treatment of small cell carcinoma of the lung with late dosage intensification programmes containing cyclophosphamide and mesna. Cancer Treat Rev 1983;10(suppl A):73–77.
101. Burnett AK, Tansey P, Hills C, et al. Haematologic reconstitution following high dose and supralethal chemoradiotherapy using stored non-cryopreserved autologous bone marrow. Br J Haematol 1983; 54:309–316.
102. Cornbleet M, Gregor A, Allen S, Leonard R, Smyth J. High dose melphalan as consolidation therapy for good prognosis patients with small cell carcinoma of the bronchus. Proc Am Soc Clin Oncol 1984;3:210.
103. Ihde DC. Current status of therapy for small cell carcinoma of the lung. Cancer 1984;54:2722–2728.
104. Ihde DC, Diesseroth AB, Lichter AS, et al. Late intensive combined modality therapy followed by autologous bone marrow infusion in extensive stage small-cell lung cancer. J Clin Oncol 1986;4:1443–1454.
105. Cunningham D, Banham SW, Hutcheon AH, et al. High-dose cyclophosphamide and VP-16 as late dosage intensification therapy for small cell carcinoma of lung. Cancer Chemother Pharmacol 1985;15:303–306.
106. Klastersky J, Nicaise C, Longeval E, et al. Cisplatin, adriamycin and etoposide for remission induction of small-cell bronchogenic carcinoma: evaluation of efficacy and toxicity and pilot study of a "late intensification" with autologous bone marrow rescue. Cancer 1982;50:652–658.
107. Stewart P, Buckner CD, Thomas ED, et al. Intensive chemoradiotherapy with autologous marrow transplantation for small cell carcinoma of the lung. Cancer Treat Rep 1983;67:1055–1059.
108. Pico JL, Beaujean F, Debre M, et al. High dose chemotherapy (HDC) with autologous bone marrow transplantation (ABMT) in small cell carcinoma of the lung (SCCL) in relapse. Proc Am Soc Clin Oncol 1983;2:206.
109. Elias AD, Skarin AT, Herman T, et al. High dose combined alkylating agents with autologous bone marrow support followed by consolidative radiotherapy for responding small cell lung cancer. Lung Cancer 1991;7(suppl):109.
110. Elias AD, Ayash L, Wheeler C, et al. High dose combination alkylating agents supported by autologous marrow with chest radiotherapy for responding limited stage small cell lung cancer. Proc Am Soc Clin Oncol 1992;11:296.
111. Perry MC, Eaton WL, Propert KJ, Ware JH, et al. Chemotherapy with or without radiation therapy in limited small-cell carcinoma of the lung. N Engl J Med 1987;316:912–918.
112. Turrisi AT, Glover DJ, Mason BA. A preliminary report: concurrent twice-daily radiotherapy plus platinum-etoposide chemotherapy for limited small cell lung cancer. Int J Radiat Oncol Biol Phys 1988;15:183–187.
113. Knight W, Page CP, Kuhn JGMC, Newcomb TF, Audie L. High does L-PAM and autologous marrow infusion for refractory solid tumors (abstract C585). Proc Am Soc Clin Oncol 1984;3:150.
114. Williams S, Bitran J, Mick R, et al. High dose multiple alkylator chemotherapy with autologous bone marrow reinfusion in patients with advanced non small cell lung cancer. Cancer 1989;63:238–242.
115. Frankel SA, German WJ. Glioblastoma multiforme (review of 219 cases with regard to natural history, pathology, diagnostic methods and treatment). J Neurosurg 1958;15:489–503.
116. Walker MD, Alexander E, Hunt WE, et al. Evaluation of BCNU and/or radiotherapy in the treatment of anaplastic gliomas. J Neurosurg 1978;49:333–343.

117. Walker MD, Hurwitz BS. BCNU in the treatment of malignant brain tumor—a preliminary report. Cancer Chemother Rep 1970;54:364–371.
118. Wilson CB, Bladrey EB, Know KJ. 1,2-B13 (2-chloroethyl)-1-nitrosourea in the treatment of brain tumors. Cancer Chemother Rep 1970;54:273–281.
119. Carella A, Giordano D, Santini G, et al. High dose BCNU followed by autologous bone marrow infusion in glioblastoma multiforme. Tumori 1981;67:473–475.
120. Phillips G, Fay J, Herzig G, et al. Autologous bone marrow transplantation in malignant glioma (abstract). Int J Cell Cloning 1985;3:257.
121. Takvorian T, Parker LM, Hockberg FH, et al. Autologous bone marrow transplantation: host effects of high dose BCNU. J Clin Oncol 1983;1:610–620.
122. Hildebrand J, Badjou R, Collard-Ronge E, et al. Treatment of brain gliomas with high dose of CCNU and autologous bone marrow transplantation. Biomedicine 1980;32:71–75.
123. Giannone L, Wolff S. Phase II treatment of central nervous system gliomas with high dose etoposide and autologous bone marrow transplantation. Cancer Treat Rep 1987;71:759–761.
124. Mortimer J, Hewlett J, Bay J, et al. High dose BCNU with autologous bone marrow rescue in the treatment of recurrent malignant gliomas. J Neuro-oncol 1983; 1:269–273.
125. Nomura K, Watanabe T, Nakamura O, et al. Intensive chemotherapy with autologous bone marrow rescue for recurrent malignant gliomas. Neurosurg Rev 1984;7:13–22.
126. Ascensao J, Ahmed T, Feldman E, et al. High dose thiotepa with autologous bone marrow transplantation and localized radiotherapy for patients with astrocytoma grade III-IV (glioma): a promising approach. Proc Am Soc Clin Oncol 1989;8:90.
127. Wolff S, Phillips G, Herzig G, et al. High dose carmustine with autologous bone marrow transplantation for adjuvant treatment of high grade gliomas of the central nervous system. Cancer Treat Rep 1987;71:183–185.
128. Johnson DB, Thompson JM, Corwin JA, et al. Prolongation of survival for high grade malignant gliomas with adjuvant high dose BCNU and ABMT. J Clin Oncol 1987;5:783–789.
129. Mbidde E, Selby P, Perren T, et al. High dose BCNU chemotherapy with autologous bone marrow transplantation and full dose radiotherapy for grade IV astrocytomas. Br J Cancer 1988;58:779–782.
130. Biron P, Vial C, Cauvin F, et al. Strategy including surgery, BCNU high dose followed by ABMT and radiotherapy in supratentorial high grade astrocytomas—a report of 98 patients. In: Dicke KA, Armitage J, eds. Autologous bone marrow transplantation, proceedings of the Fifth International Symposium. Omaha: University of Nebraska, 1991:637–646.
131. Kretschmar C, Warren M, Lavolly, et al. Ototoxicity of preradiation cisplatin for children with central nervous system tumors. J Clin Oncol 1990;8:1191–1198.
132. Fine H, Dear K, Loeffler J, et al. Meta-analysis of adjuvant chemotherapy for malignant gliomas in adults. Cancer 1993 (in press).
133. Walker M, Strike T, Sheline G. An analysis of dose-effect relationship in the radiotherapy of malignant gliomas. Int J Radiat Oncol Biol Phys 1979;5:1725.
134. Loeffler J, Alexander E III, Wen P, et al. Results of stereotactic brachytherapy in the initial management of patients with glioblastomas. J Natl Cancer Inst 1990; 82:1918–1921.
135. Loeffler JS, Alexander E III, Hochberg FH, et al. Clinical patterns of failure following interstitial radiation for malignant gliomas. Int J Radiat Oncol Biol Phys 1990;19:1455–1462.
136. Alexander E III, Loeffler JS, Wen P, et al. Radiosurgery as part of the initial management of patients with high-grade gliomas. J Clin Oncol 1993 (in press).
137. Cornbleet M, Corringham R, Prentice H, et al. Treatments of Ewing's sarcoma with high-dose melphalan and autologous bone marrow transplantation. Cancer Treat Rep 1981;65:241–244.
138. Graham-Pole J, Lazarus H, Herzig R, et al. High-dose melphalan therapy for the treatment of children with refractory neuroblastoma and Ewing's sarcoma. Am J Pediatr Hematol Oncol 1984;6:17.
139. Papadopoulos N, Armen T, Chawla S, et al. High dose intravenous cytoxan, carmustine, etopside, and autologous bone marrow transplant for advanced refractory small round cell sarcomas in adults (abstract 533). Proc Am Soc Clin Oncol 1986;5:137.
140. Abrams R, Simon R, Glaubiger D, et al. Hemopoietic recovery in Ewing's sarcoma after intensive combination therapy and autologous marrow infusion. Lancet 1980;1:385.
141. Miser J, Steis R, Longo D, et al. Treatment of newly diagnosed high risk sarcomas and primitive neuroectodermal tumors in children and young adults (abstract C-935). Proc Am Soc Clin Oncol 1985;4:240.
142. Miser J. Kinsella T, Triche T, et al. Preliminary results of treatment of Ewing's sarcoma of bone in children and young adults: six months of intensive combined modality therapy without maintenance. J Clin Oncol 1988;6:484–490.
143. Herzig R, Phillips G, Lazarus H, et al. Intensive chemotherapy and autologous bone marrow transplantation for the treatment of refractory malignancies. In: Dicke K, Spitzer G, Zander A, eds. Autologous bone marrow transplantation; proceedings of the First International Symposium. Houston, TX: University of Texas M.D. Anderson Cancer Center Press, 1985:197–202.
144. McCann SR, Reynolds M, Meldrum R, et al. High dose melphalan with autologous bone marrow transplantation in the treatment of metastatic Ewing's Sarcoma. Irish J Med Science 1993 (in press).
145. Dini G, Hartmann O, Pinkerton R, Dallorso S, Philip T. Autologous bone marrow transplantation in Ewing's sarcoma. In: Dicke K, Spitzer G, Jagannath S, eds. Autologous bone marrow transplantation: proceedings of the Third International Symposium. Houston, TX: University of Texas M.D. Anderson Hospital Press, 1987:593–599.
146. Hartmann O, Bouffet E, Valteau D, et al. High dose chemo/radiotherapy and autologous bone marrow transplantation as consolidation therapy in children's metastatic Ewing's sarcoma. In: Dicke K, Spitzer G, Jagannath S, eds. Autologous bone marrow transplantation: proceedings of the Third International Symposium. Houston, TX: University of Texas M.D. Anderson Hospital Press, 1987:609–615.
147. Pinkerton CR. Megatherapy for soft tissue sarcomas. EBMT experience. Bone Marrow Transplant 1991; 3:120–122.
148. Philip T. EBMT working party solid tumor registry. In:

Report of European Bone Marrow Transplant Group, Lyon, France 1991.
149. Marcus R Jr, Graham-Pole J, Springfield D, et al. High-risk Ewing's sarcoma: end-intensification using autologous bone marrow transplantation. Int J Radiat Oncol Biol Phys 1988;15:53–59.
150. Bader JL, Horowitz ME, Dewan R, et al. Intensive combined modality therapy of small round cell and undifferentiated sarcomas in children and young adults. Radiother Oncol 1989;16:189–201.
151. Mauger D. Complete regression of osteogenic sarcoma scalp metastases following one pulse of high dose melphalan combined with a bone marrow autograft: case report. N Z Med J 1982;95:455–456.
152. Pinkerton CR, Groot LJ, Barrett A, et al. Rapid VAC high dose melphalan regimen, a novel chemotherapy approach in childhood soft tissue sarcomas. Br J Cancer 1991;64:381–385.
153. Fields KK, Saleh RA, Zorsky PE, et al. Treatment of refractory metastatic breast cancer with ifosfamide, carboplatin, and etoposide (ICE). Proc Am Soc Clin Oncol 1991;10:70.
154. Slease RB, Benear JB, Selby GB, et al. High-dose combination alkylating agent therapy with autologous bone marrow rescue for refractory solid tumors. J Clin Oncol 1988;6:1314–1320.
155. Ghavimi F, Kernan NA, Lindsley K, et al. Autologous bone marrow transplant in recurrent or poor risk rhabdomyosarcoma or undifferentiated sarcoma (abstract 1195). Proc Am Assoc Cancer Res 1992;33:200.
156. Ekert H, Ellis WM, Waters KD, Tauro G. Autologous bone marrow rescue in the treatment of advanced tumors of childhood. Cancer 1982;49:603–609.
157. Mortimer J, Collins C. High dose cyclophosphamide in refractory malignancy (abstract 185). Proc Am Soc Clin Oncol 1986;5:47.
158. Brown R, Herzig R, Fay J, et al. A phase I-II study of high-dose N, N1, N2 triethylenethiophosphoramide (thiotepa) and autologous marrow transplantation for refractory malignancies (abstract 494). Proc Am Soc Clin Oncol 1986;5:127.
159. Peters WP, Stuart A, Kloman M. High-dose combination cyclophosphamide, cisplatin, and melphalan with autologous bone marrow support. Cancer Chemother Pharmacol 1989;23:377–383.
160. Lazarus H, Herzig R, Wolff S, et al. Treatment of metastatic malignant melanoma with intensive melphalan and autologous bone marrow transplantation. Cancer Treat Rep 1985;69:473–477.
161. Cornbleet MA, McElwain TJ, Kumar PJ, et al. Treatment of advanced malignant melanoma with high-dose melphalan and autologous bone marrow transplantation. Br J Cancer 1983;48:329–334.
162. McElwain TJ, Hedley DW, Burton G, et al. Marrow autotransplantation accelerates hematologic recovery in patients with malignant melanoma treated with high dose melphalan. Br J Cancer 1979;40:72–80.
163. Herzig GP, Phillips GL, Herzig RH, et al. High dose nitrosourea and autologous bone marrow transplantation: a phase I trial. In: Prestaykoaw C, Baker LH, eds. Nitrosoureas, current status and new developments. New York: Academic Press, 1981:337–341.
164. Fay J, Levine M, Phillips GL, et al. Treatment of metastatic melanoma with intensive BCNU and autologous marrow transplantation (abstract 783). Proc Am Soc Clin Oncol 1981;22:532.
165. Meisenberg B, Ross M, Jones R, Vredenburgh J, Seigler H, Peters WP. Adjuvant high-dose combination alkylating agent chemotherapy with autologous bone marrow support in multi-node positive melanoma (abstract 1187). Proc Am Soc Clin Oncol 1992;11:345.
166. Smith B, Selby P, Southgate J, Pittman K, Bradsey C, Blair GE. Detection of melanoma cells in peripheral blood by means of reverse transcriptase and polymerase chain reaction. Lancet 1991;338:1227–1229.
167. McElwain TJ, Hadley DW, Jarman M, et al. High dose melphalan and noncryopreserved autologous bone marrow in treatment of malignant melanoma and neuroblastoma. Exp Hematol 1979;7:360–371.
168. Herzig RH, Brown RA, Wolf SN, et al. Dose intensive therapy for advanced melanoma. In: Dicke KA, Armitage JO, Dicke-Evinger MJ, eds. Autologous bone marrow transplantation: proceedings of the Fifth International Symposium. Omaha: University of Nebraska, 1991:661–668.
169. Wolff S, Herzig RH, Fay JW, et al. High dose thiotepa with ABMT for metastatic malignant melanoma: results of phase I and II studies of the North American BMT group. J Clin Oncol 1989;7:245–249.
170. Ariel I. Treatment of disseminated cancer by intravenous hydroxyurea and autogenous bone-marrow transplants: experiences with 35 patients. J Surg Oncol 1975;7:331–335.
171. Barbasch A, Higby D, Brass C, et al. High-dose cytoreductive therapy with autologous bone marrow transplantation in advanced malignancies. Cancer Treat Rep 1983;67:143–148.
172. Lakhani S, Selby P, Bliss JM, et al. Chemotherapy for malignant melanoma: combinations and high doses produce more responses without survival benefit. Br J Cancer 1990;61:330–334.
173. Zander A, Spitzer G, Legha S, et al. High-dose AMSA and bone marrow rescue in patients with solid tumors. Cancer Treat Rep 1982;66:385–386.
174. Thomas MR, Robinson WA, Glode M. Treatment of advanced malignant melanoma with high dose chemotherapy and ABMT. Am J Clin Oncol 1982;5:611–622.
175. Shea TC, Antman KH, Eder JP, et al. Malignant melanoma: treatment with high-dose combination alkylating agent chemotherapy and autologous bone marrow support. Arch Dermatol 1988;124:878–884.
176. Williams SF, Bitran JD, Kaminer L, et al. A I-II study of bialkylator chemotherapy, high-dose thiotepa, and cyclophosphamide with autologous bone marrow reinfusion in patients with advanced cancer. J Clin Oncol 1987;5:260–265.
177. Leff RS, Thompson JM, Johnson DB, et al. Phase II trial of high dose melphalan and autologous bone marrow transplantation for metastatic colon carcinoma. J Clin Oncol 1986;4:1586–1591.
178. Spitzer TR, Lazarus HM, Creager R, Berger N. High dose melphalan, misonidazole and autologous bone marrow transplantation for the treatment of metastatic colorectal carcinoma. Am J Clin Oncol 1989;12:145–151.
179. Fay JW, Herzig RH, Herzig GP, Wolf SN. Treatment of metastatic colon carcinoma with intensive thiotepa and autologous bone marrow transplantation. In: Herzig GP, ed. Advances in cancer chemotherapy. New York: Wiley and Sons, 1987:31–34.
180. Lazarus HM, Reed MD, Spitzer TR, Rabaa MS, Blumer JL. High-dose IV thiotepa and cryopreserved autolo-

gous bone marrow transplantation for therapy of refractory cancer. Cancer Treat Rep 1987;71:689–695.

181. Karanes C, Ratanatharathorn V. Schilcher RB, et al. High-dose mitomycin C with autologous bone marrow transplantation in patients with refractory malignancies. Am J Clin Oncol 1986;9:444–448.

182. Ellis E, Moormeier J, Kaminer L, Mick R, Williams S, Bitran J. Phase I-II study of high dose cyclophosphamide, thiotepa and mitoxantrone (CTM) with autologous bone marrow reinfusion (ABMR) in patients with refractory malignancies (abstract 61). Proc Am Soc Clin Oncol 1990;9:17.

183. Nemunaitis J, Rabinowe SN, Singer JW, et al. Recombinant granulocyte-macrophage colony-stimulating factor after autologous bone marrow transplantation for lymphoid malignancy: pooled results from three randomized double-blind, placebo controlled trials. N Engl J Med 1991;324:1773–1778.

184. Juttner CA, Haylock DN, Branford A, et al. Haemopoietic reconstitution using circulating autologous stem cells collected in very early remission from acute non-lymphoblastic leukemia (abstract 312). Exp Hematol 1986;14:465.

185. Gianni AM, Siena S, Bregni M, et al. Granulocyte-macrophage colony stimulating factor to harvest circulating hematopoetic stem cells for autotransplant. Lancet 1989;2:580–585.

186. Gianni AM, Bregni M, Siena S, et al. Recombinant human granulocyte-macrophage colony-stimulating factor reduces hematologic toxicity and widens clinical applicability of high-dose cyclophosphamide treatment in breast cancer and non-Hodgkin's lymphoma. J Clin Oncol 1990;8:768–778.

187. Elias A, Mazanet R, Wheeler C, et al. Peripheral blood progenitor cells: two protocols using GM-CSF potentiated progenitor cell collection. In: Dicke KA, Armitage J, eds. Autologous bone marrow transplantation, proceedings of the Fifth International Symposium. Omaha: University of Nebraska, 1991:875–880.

188. Elias A, Ayash L, Anderson K, et al. GM-CSF mobilized peripheral blood progenitor cell support after high dose chemotherapy for breast cancer: effect of GM-CSF post reinfusion. Blood 1993 (in press).

189. Hillner BE, Smith TJ, Desch CE. Estimating the cost-effectiveness of autologous bone marrow transplantation for metastatic breast cancer (abstract 60). Proc Am Soc Clin Oncol 1991;10:46.

190. Hillner BE, Smith TJ, Desch CE. Efficacy and cost-effectiveness of autologous bone marrow transplantation in metastatic breast cancer—estimates using decision analysis while awaiting clinical trial results. JAMA 1992;267:2055–2061.

191. Ferro N, Kusminsky G, Dictar M, et al. Assessment of psychosocial aspects influencing quality of life following autologous bone marrow transplantation (abstract 1422). Proc Am Soc Clin Oncol 1992;11:406.

192. Winer E, Gold D, Lees J, et al. Evaluation of quality of life (QL) in patients with metastatic breast cancer (MBC) undergoing high dose chemotherapy with autologous bone marrow support (HDC) (abstract). Proc Am Soc Clin Oncol 1991;10:62.

Chapter 59

Autologous Bone Marrow Transplantation for Breast Cancer

William P. Peters

Breast cancer is the second leading cause of cancer death among women, with 183,000 new cases annually, and 48,000 deaths. Early detection, surgery, radiation therapy, and chemotherapy have resulted in improvement in survival in patients with early-stage breast cancer. During the past decade, the paradigm for the standard-dose treatment of primary breast cancer has undergone considerable evolution. In the early 1980s, adjuvant chemotherapy for *node-positive* breast cancer was controversial and little evidence supported its use in postmenopausal women. Even in the late-1980s, some oncologists believed that little survival benefit would be derived from adjuvant chemotherapy for breast cancer (1). Currently, adjuvant chemotherapy and hormonal therapy for breast cancer is accepted as a standard of care for most patients with breast cancer, and a large statistical overview has demonstrated that polychemotherapy offers both a disease-free and overall survival advantage for women with node-positive or node-negative primary breast cancer (2).

However, little progress has occurred in metastatic disease, despite multiple clinical trials; in fact, during the past decade, therapeutic results in stage IV breast cancer appear to have worsened. The median time to treatment failure in randomized comparative trials conducted during the 1980s was between 4 and 8 months, compared with 12 to 16 months in the prior decade. The overall survival was between 12 and 16 months in these trials, compared with a median survival of 22 months in the prior decade. These outcomes probably reflect the widespread use of adjuvant chemotherapy in primary disease, which is a negative prognostic factor for treatment of metastatic disease. In premenopausal women with metastatic cancer, the inability of conventional dose chemotherapy to offer even a year of palliative response suggested that more aggressive approaches were reasonable to consider. In this regard, the evolution of high-dose therapy for breast cancer has been even more rapid. A decade ago, there was little support for the use of more intensive dose therapy in metastatic breast cancer. Treatment of the disease was for palliation, and high-dose therapy was associated with considerable morbidity and mortality. The available information came from Phase I trials in patients with advanced resistant breast cancer, and although responses were frequent, response durations were short. Approximately 40% of patients required critical care support, mortality was often in excess of 20%, and therapy was expensive. Currently, multicenter Phase III trials are underway; morbidity and mortality have been reduced markedly through the use of hematopoietic colony stimulating factors, peripheral blood progenitor cells, and better supportive care; and maturing results from large Phase II studies provide evidence that high-dose therapy produces a high frequency of complete remissions. Several centers report that some women with poor-prognosis breast cancer can remain continuously disease-free for extended periods after brief treatments that involve autologous bone marrow transplantation (BMT).

Rationale for High-dose Chemotherapy and Autologous Bone Marrow Support in Breast Cancer

Dose intensification with conventional chemotherapy and combined modality therapy have enabled the development of curative strategies for patients with acute leukemia (3–5), lymphoma (6–10), testicular cancer (11–16), head and neck cancer (17), and ovarian cancer (18–20). A major milestone in these efforts was the attainment of a *documented complete response* that marked the end point of systemic therapy. Results from trials of adjuvant chemotherapy for breast cancer have demonstrated that the eradication of microscopic tumor deposits is possible, even with regimens that are noncurative in metastatic disease (21–25). The absolute value of adjuvant therapy has been modest; on average, only between approximately 4 and 20% absolute improvement in overall 5-year disease-free survival has been achieved in most node number subsets. The absolute benefit appears larger in patients with higher numbers of involved lymph nodes compared with patients with small numbers of involved nodes. The odds reduction of recurrence and survival appears similar across each of the nodal subsets examined. The impact of conventional-dose adjuvant chemotherapy has been modest and has required a large meta-analysis of randomized clinical data to define clearly the therapeutic benefit (2). In metastatic disease, conventional-dose chemotherapy produces frequent disease shrinkage but seldom produces clinical complete remission. The use of dose intensification as a means to improve the frequency and quality of complete remissions is consistent with the results obtained in other diseases and could reasonably be expected to be associated with an improvement in outcome.

The approach to breast cancer treatment using high-dose chemotherapy and autologous BMT has been based on 4 principles: (1) that dose is a critical factor in treatment and that even minor compromises in administered dose may result in reduced treatment efficacy; (2) that combination chemotherapy is essential to overcome drug resistance in epithelial tumors; (3) that the alkylating agents are, for a variety of biological and biochemical reasons, ideal agents to form the core of high-dose therapeutic regimens; and (4) that tumor volume may be limiting for high-dose treatment to be effective.

Dose

Quantitative studies in both animal and human malignancies have demonstrated that drug resistance to the alkylating agents appear relative to the dose employed and that absolute resistance to the alkylating agents is unusual. In experimental systems, the dose-response relationship can be shown to be log-linear, even in the most resistant animal tumors. These effects continue over several logs of drug dose. Furthermore, the slope of the killing curves among various tumors remains essentially constant and does not appear to plateau within the clinically relevant dose range after a threshold dose for therapeutic efficacy has been reached. This relationship does not apply, however, to all classes of anticancer agents. Furthermore, although the major dose-limiting toxicity for most of the alkylating agents is myelosuppression, other drugs are toxic for other organs at or near the myelotoxic dose. The use of high-dose chemotherapy in breast cancer relies on an ability to escalate the drug dose substantially before toxicity in nonhematopoietic organs occurs.

During the past decade, there has been considerable controversy about the role of dose intensification in the treatment of breast cancer. Reviews of the literature by Hryniuk and Bush (26) and Henderson and colleagues (27) have come to different conclusions based on an analysis of similar data sets. These investigators reviewed the therapeutic responses of various treatment programs and recognized that, although the treatment programs contain similar agents, they are administered in varying dose intensities. Hryniuk and Bush noted a clear impact of dose intensity, both on disease-free survival and on overall survival, particularly when the dose actually administered was analyzed; the reviews by Henderson express caution about these therapeutic approaches and analytic methods.

Numerous investigators have demonstrated that steep dose-response curves can be seen in the treatment of malignancy. This concept was reviewed by Frei and Canellos (28), and the results of early therapeutic efforts in the treatment of breast cancer have been reviewed by Peters (29). The implication of these considerations is that dose escalation by one- or 2-fold may have a major effect on therapeutic outcome.

Fortunately, the evolving results of randomized comparative trials are beginning to settle these divergent opinions. In both primary and metastatic disease, where formal analysis of dose as a treatment variable has been undertaken, the use of more dose-intensive regimens not requiring BMT has led to an improvement in both disease-free and overall survival, as well as in the quality of life of patients who have been treated in these programs. Recent studies of standard-dose adjuvant chemotherapy in the treatment of primary breast cancer, reported by Budman and associates (30), suggested that doubling of the dose can lead to improved disease-free and overall survival in adjuvant chemotherapy of primary breast cancer. Similar results have been reported by Tannock and his colleagues (31) in metastatic disease. Unfortunately, these data are limited in applicability; the trials were conducted with doses of chemotherapy that are low by contemporary standards and may represent threshold dose effects. Randomized, clinical trials are underway evaluating the contribution of high-dose therapy with and without autologous BMT to outcome in both metastatic and high-risk primary breast cancer.

Combination Chemotherapy

The biological and biochemical heterogeneity of neoplastic cells suggest that combinations of agents will prove more efficient than single agents. This concept has become an established principle of curative regimens. In settings where the treatment program is designed for palliation, such as the general approach to metastatic breast cancer, the survival benefit of combinations over single agents is more difficult to demonstrate (32,33).

The frequent occurrence of some drug-resistant cells to any single agent at the time of clinical presentation generally mandates the use of multiple drugs in the treatment of breast cancer. Agents selected for use should have activity against breast cancer at the dose used. Many, indeed most, myelosuppressive agents have not, however, been tested adequately at high doses against most cancers, because myelosuppression has limited their usefulness in the absence of marrow support. Although total body irradiation (TBI) has a major role in conditioning programs used during allogeneic and autologous transplantation for acute leukemias and lymphomas, it appears to be of limited value in breast cancer because doses required for elimination of macroscopic and even microscopic disease often exceed the tolerable limits that can be administered.

Biological and Biochemical Properties of the Alkylating Agents

Alkylating agents have been generally included in high-dose regimens for breast cancer. The rationale for their use derives from both in vitro and preclinical in vivo studies that demonstrated a steep and direct dose-response effect in vitro for the alkylating agents. In various animal models, noncross-resistance can be demonstrated among selected agents. Observations by Schabel and colleagues (34,35) provided preclinical data demonstrating the utility of combined alkylating agent regimens. These investigators also demonstrated therapeutic synergy with the use of combined alkylating agents at standard doses. However, the importance of synergy is less clear in the high-dose setting. More important to the overall outcome appears to be the development of intrinsic resistance to many alkylating agents or, more specifically, to the cross-resistance pattern seen among the selected agents.

Selected alkylating agents have been demonstrated in single-agent, high-dose Phase I trials to differ in their nonmyelosuppressive toxicities. For example, the dose-limiting toxicity of cyclophosphamide (CY) is hemorrhagic myocarditis; for platinum, nephrotoxicity and neurotoxicity; for carmustine, hepatic and pulmonary toxicity. Thiotepa is limited by mucosal and organic nervous system toxicity; busulfan by enterocolitis and anorexia; melphalan by mucositis. Hence, it is possible to select agents that possess some apparent nonoverlapping toxicities for use in combination in high doses as long as the marrow is protected. In some patients, secondary major organ toxicity has been encountered at much lower doses with certain combinations of drugs. For example, attempts to combine carboplatin with CY and carmustine have reported dose-limiting hepatic toxicity at doses 40% of the single agent maximum tolerated dose of carboplatin (36). These toxicities may result in part from the perturbation of alkylating agent pharmacology in combination (37).

Some drugs are not amenable to dose escalation or do not have a linear dose-response effect. For example, antimetabolites such as 5-fluorouracil and methotrexate plateau in their dose response after only a limited dose escalation. Other agents that appear to possess a dose-response effect, such as doxorubicin, although limited predominantly by myelosuppression, have nonhematopoietic toxicities that quickly limit further dose escalation (38). Cardiotoxicity, mucosal and epithelial toxicity do not permit substantial dose escalation. Thus, it is unlikely that such compounds will have a major role in high-dose therapeutic regimens, unless synergy with other active agents is present, providing a role for these agents in high-dose programs. However, they are likely to be useful for induction or consolidation chemotherapy programs coupled with high-dose programs.

Volume of Disease as an Important Treatment Variable in Breast Cancer

The development of therapeutic strategies using high-dose therapy in breast cancer has paralleled the use of BMT in the leukemias and lymphomas. In these diseases, use of dose intensification has been successful in both acute and chronic leukemia, particularly when treated with allogeneic BMT. The initial efforts by Thomas and colleagues (39) to utilize high-dose CY and TBI in the treatment of relapsed leukemia resulted in cure in approximately 12% of treated patients, although as many as 50% of patients in certain series died from therapy-related complications and 35 to 40% of patients relapsed. A major conceptual break-through occurred with the application of the same therapy in an earlier stage of disease—the first complete remission—in an effort to decrease the risk of leukemic recurrence and perhaps also to decrease the incidence of therapy-related complications. This intervention resulted in a significant decrease in post-transplant leukemic recurrence to 20%; thus, approximately 50 to 75% of patients under the age of 20, and 25 to 50% of those ages 30 to 50 can be cured (40).

The situation in solid tumors may be similar. Conventional and even high-dose therapy of metastatic disease are less effective when large tumor volumes are present. However, therapeutic regimens capable of producing frequent, rapid, and complete responses in metastatic disease may be capable of producing cure in a minimal disease state. Surgery and radiation therapy may augment local control.

Metastatic and Primary Breast Cancer

Zambetti and co-workers (41) and Fisher and associates (23) demonstrated the importance of tumor volume in adjuvant chemotherapy in primary breast cancer. In primary disease, use of chemotherapy programs that are noncurative in the metastatic disease setting (e.g. cyclophosphamide, methotrexate, and 5-fluorouracil [CMF]; melphalan and 5-fluorouracil [PF]; or cyclophosphamide and doxorubicin [CA]) resulted in modest but consistent improvements in disease-free and overall survival.

The success of adjuvant chemotherapy can be attributed to several factors, including (1) treatment of early disease before the development of drug resistance, and (2) treatment at the time of minimal tumor burden. The importance of the latter is emphasized by the fact that adjuvant chemotherapy programs have proven successful in reducing the odds reduction for both recurrence and survival.

Conceptually, it should be possible to produce a condition of low tumor burden in patients with both metastatic and primary disease. In patients with metastatic disease, use of intensive induction therapy, coupled with other strategies, may enable reduction of the tumor burden to the point where a clinical complete remission could be obtained. In the primary disease setting, following surgical resection, patients have achieved an optimal complete remission, and the use of high-dose intensification, coupled with other strategies, may theoretically enable sufficient reduction of the tumor burden to allow complete cytoreduction.

Newer studies in both the metastatic disease setting and in primary breast cancer have supported the importance of dose intensification in treatment strategy. Studies by Tannock and colleagues (31) in metastatic disease demonstrated improvement in response rate, disease-free survival, and overall survival for patients with metastatic disease, as well as improvement in the quality of life for the more dose-intensive regimen. The Cancer and Leukemia Group B, in a large, multicenter, randomized comparative trial (protocol 8541) in primary breast cancer demonstrated the value of more dose-intensive therapy in all patient subsets, including both premenopausal and postmenopausal patients, high and low node–positive patients, and in hormone receptor–positive and –negative subsets (30).

High-dose Chemotherapy and ABMT in Advanced Breast Cancer

Phase I Trials of Toxicity

During the early 1980s, Phase I trials of high-dose single-agent and combination chemotherapy targeted at identifying active drug for breast cancer and identifying maximal tolerated doses were undertaken. These trials included primarily patients who had failed prior chemotherapy for metastases and were not expected to have either a significant response rate or durability of remission. In a compiled series (42) of 1,367 patients who had failed one or 2 prior chemotherapy programs, the use of *active second-line combinations* of drugs as standard doses (including doxorubicin in those not previously exposed) resulted in an overall objective response rate of 33 ± 14%. The average median duration of response in responders (only 23 of 35 reports [66%] provided duration of response) was 6.7 months, and average median survival was 8.5 months (17 of 35 reports [49%] provided information on survival). Patients included in the early Phase I/II high-dose therapy trials often had failed these second line approaches as well. In interpreting these data, it is important to note that the high-dose regimens were used once so that duration of response reflects duration of *unmaintained* response. Comparable data are not available from trials of standard-dose chemotherapy (particularly in advanced disease), because patients are generally repetitively treated until progression. Table 59-1 lists a summary compilation of the response data from these studies. Patients who received a standard high-dose regimen of CY, cisplatin, and carmustine (CY/cDDP/BCNU) are presented separately because data on this treatment program are available in multiple treatment settings.

These data indicate that the frequency of objective

Table 59-1.
Advanced Resistant Breast Cancer: Response Frequency to High Dose and Conventional Dose Chemotherapy Selected Programs

Drugs and/or RT	No. Trials	No. Patients	Complete Remission		Objective Response		Median Response Duration
			No.	%	No.	%	
Single high-dose treatment + ABMT							
Combination drugs (91)	27	214	36	17	147	69	4.2
CPB (92,93)	2	23	6	26	15	65	5
Combination drug + RT[a]	6	19	7	37	12	63	5
Single-agent drug[a]	17	140	6	4	36	26	6.8
Repetitive conventional-dose therapy							
Second line combined drugs (94)	35	1367	NR	NR		32	6.7
Single-agent drugs (94)	95	2224	NR	NR		6.6	Too few responses to determine
Single agent Phase II trials from DCT/CTEP[b]	61	1373	17	1	107	8	Too few responses to determine

[a]Adapted from Antman K, Bearman SI, Davidson et al. Dose intensive therapy in breast cancer: current status. In: Gale RP, Champlin RE, eds. New strategies in bone marrow transplantation. New York: Alan R Liss, 1990.
[b]Chesson B. Response rates in breast cancer on single-agent investigational phase II trials conducted by the DCT/CTEP from 1982–1989. Personal communication.
RT = radiotherapy; ABMT = autologous bone marrow transplantation; CPB = cyclophosphamide, cisplatin, carmustine (BCNU); DCT/CTEP = Division of Cancer Treatment/Cancer Therapy Evaluation Program; NR = not reported.
(Reproduced by permission from Antman K, Bearman SI, Davidson et al. Dose intensive therapy in breast cancer: current status. In: Gale RP, Champlin RE, eds. New strategies in bone marrow transplantation. New York: Alan R Liss, 1990).

response is substantially higher than standard-dose regimens, although median response duration and survival is similar. The overall objective response rate for high-dose therapy is 2 to 10 times greater than the response rate for conventional dose therapy, even compared with patients with, in general, less prior therapy. The median duration of response is similar to the second-line conventional-dose treatments. However, as with standard-dose therapy in the advanced disease setting, sustained remissions are rare. No studies evaluating quality of life in this patient category have been performed; thus, the palliative value of either of these therapeutic approaches is unknown.

High-dose Chemotherapy as First Treatment for Metastatic Breast Cancer

Because of the high frequency of objective response in patients with advanced resistant breast cancer, several groups treated a series of patients with a single high-dose therapy at the time of first relapse from primary disease. Patients in these series were young, premenopausal women, and most were estrogen receptor–negative, with measurable visceral disease. Patients were not excluded from high-dose trials if they received prior adjuvant chemotherapy, as occurred in many trials previously reported with standard-dose chemotherapy. These trial results, as well as a series of contemporary standard-dose trials reporting response duration and survival, are summarized in Table 59-2.

The data suggest that a single course of high-dose therapy produces a higher frequency of complete and partial remissions in patients with metastatic breast cancer than occurs with multiple courses of standard-dose chemotherapy. Furthermore, even though high-dose therapies are given only once, and therefore the appropriate analysis end point is progression from unmaintained remission (not available for standard-dose therapies), the median duration of response for high-dose and conventional-dose therapy is similar for both disease-free and overall survival.

Table 59-2.
Metastatic Breast Cancer: Treatment Results with Selected High-dose Therapy or Standard-dose Therapy Programs

			Complete Remission		*Objective Response*			
Drugs and/or RT	*No. Trials*	*No. Patients*	*No.*	*%*	*No.*	*%*	*Median Response Duration*	*Survival Duration*
Single high-dose treatment and ABMT								
Combination Drugs (91)	3	31	13	42	25	81	range: 13–82 mo	NA
CPB (95)	1	22	12	54	17	77	4	10
Coventional dose repetitive therapy								
CMF (94)	14	842	86	10	274	32	6	10
CMFp (96)	1	153	8	5	61	40	5	10
CMF (97)	1	106	3	6	22	21	NA	12
CMF (98)	1	40			25	62	8	17
CMFVb (99)	1	50			31	62	3	6
AF/AFC/AFCM (100)	1	313			141	45	7	14
CA (98)	1	152	6	4	63	41	5	11
CAF (101)	1	164			61	37	4	12
CAFVp (102)	1	52				52	16	25
FAC (103)	1	1424	221	16	924	65	14	22
CFP,CFPV A,CA,MA,AEA,MV,I (69)	9	438	49	11	NA	NA	NA	NA
Single high-dose treatment and ABMT after standard-dose induction chemotherapy								
Various[a]	17	229	132	58	204	89	2–42+	NA
AFM–> CPB[b]	1	45	27	60 (68% of patients receiving ABMT)[c]	43	96	18	20
CEP × 2 (104)	1	66	39	59	54	82	12	21
MFAVP –> CVp (105)	1	41	23	56	39	95	21	> 21

[a]Adapted from Antman K, Bearman SI, Davidson N, et al. Dose Intensive Therapy in Breast Cancer: Current Status. In: Gale RP, Champlin RE, ed. New strategies in bone marrow transplantation. New York: Alan R Liss, 1990.
[b]Adapted from Jones RB, Shpall EJ, Ross M, et al. AFM induction chemotherapy followed by intensive alkylating agent consolidation with autologous bone marrow support (ABMS) for advanced breast cancer. Current results. Proc Am Soc Clin Oncol 1990;7:121.
[c]40 of 45 patients enrolled actually were transplanted. Five patients did not proceed to ABMT because of progression of CNS or liver disease (3), hepatitis (1), or refusal (1). Thus, 60% of all enrolled patients or 68% of patients actually transplanted achieved complete remission.
Adapted from (44).
RT = radiotherapy; ABMT = autologous bone marrow transplantation; C = cyclophosphamide; M = methotrexate; F = 5-fluorouracil; p = prednisone; P = cisplatin; Vb = vinblastine; A = doxorubicin; V = vincristine; E = etoposide.

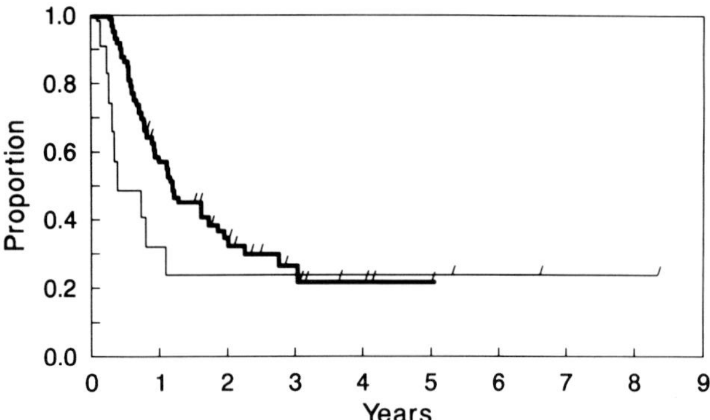

Figure 59-1. Event-free survival for women with metastatic breast cancer achieving a complete remission after a single treatment with high-dose CPA/cDDP/BCNU, and ABMS (*thin line*) or after induction therapy with doxorubicin, 5-fluorouracil, and methotrexate (AFM) followed by high-dose CPA/cDDP/BCNU and ABMS (*thick line*). *Ticks* represent censored observations.

Furthermore, the trials with upfront high-dose therapy indicate that a fraction of patients can remain disease-free for prolonged periods after a single high-dose treatment with autologous BMT. In data from Peters and colleagues, updated with follow-up now to 8 years (43) (Figure 59-1), 3 of 22 (14%) poor-prognosis patients who were premenopausal, estrogen receptor–negative, and had visceral disease remain continuously disease-free. The high complete response rate allowed patients to be followed without subsequent therapy until relapse. Because of the low frequency of complete response produced by standard-dose therapy, there are no previous reports available for comparison of patients with unresectable visceral metastatic disease in which a single treatment has been administered and followed until relapse without subsequent therapy. Other groups have reported similar findings (44).

High-dose Consolidation Therapy with Autologous BMT after Induction Chemotherapy in Metastatic Breast Cancer

Recognition of the limitations of high-dose therapy in patients with bulk tumor led to 2 strategies for extending the therapeutic results. In the first, induction chemotherapy was used to reduce tumor burden in metastatic disease prior to autologous BMT; in the second, high-dose chemotherapy and autologous BMT is used after surgery and standard-dose induction chemotherapy for high-risk primary breast cancer. A summary of the data for metastatic disease is presented in Table 59-2. The comparison control groups presented in general represent young, premenopausal, hormone receptor–negative patients similar to those enrolled in trials of high-dose chemotherapy.

The use of high-dose chemotherapy as consolidation in patients with metastatic breast cancer has produced consistent results. The overall response rate at the end of treatment approaches 90%. Complete responses will occur in 60% of all patients entering the study and 68% of patients actually completing transplantation. Furthermore, 30% of patients remain alive in continuous complete remission off therapy at a follow-up of 3 years (compared with 6% alive and none progression-free in the Tannock standard-dose trial (31)). Each of these trials has more than 20% of the complete responders remaining progression-free at 3 years; nearly twice the frequency obtained in the best standard-dose trials.

The major benefit from high-dose therapy occurs in patients who achieve a complete remission. Figure 59-1 shows the Kaplan-Meier estimate of event-free survival for patients achieving a complete remission with a program utilizing high-dose CY/cDDP/BCNU and autologous BMT, either as initial chemotherapy for metastatic breast cancer or as consolidation after intensive induction chemotherapy. Both series demonstrate a 23 to 25% durable remission rate in these patients at 5 years and beyond. Patients who do not achieve a complete remission generally have disease progression within 18 months. Randomized, comparative trials attempting to confirm these observations are ongoing.

High-dose Consolidation Therapy with Autologous BMT in High-risk Primary Disease

Combination chemotherapy has been demonstrated to provide long-term, disease-free survival for some patients with primary breast cancer in whom the disease has spread to the axillary lymph nodes. However, despite adjuvant chemotherapy, the prognosis for patients who have extensive involvement of the axillary lymph nodes at the time of primary therapy remains poor. Data from the Natural History Data Base and other studies indicate that, despite contemporary adjuvant chemotherapy, 55 to 87% of women with primary breast cancer involving 10 or more axillary lymph nodes will relapse within 5 years of diagnosis. For these reasons, efforts to utilize high-dose chemotherapy with autologous BMT in these patients have been undertaken, despite the recognized risks of high-dose therapy. Two studies (45,46) with sufficient patients and follow-up have been described. In these 2 studies, involving 133 patients with median follow-up of more than 2 years each (in the first, follow-up to beyond 5 years), 72 and 92% of patients remain event-free. These results are substantially better than historical or contemporary results obtained in similar prognosis patients treated without high-dose therapy. These data and comparison control groups are summarized in Table 59-3. Prospective randomized trials attempting to confirm these results have been initiated in the CALGB and SWOG cooperative group and in the ECOG cooperative cancer groups (Figure 59-2).

Table 59-3.
Autologous Bone Marrow Transplantation in Primary Breast Cancer Involving ≥ 10 Axillary Lymph Nodes

		Relapse-free Survival		
Series	*n*	*1 Year (%)*	*3 Years (%)*	*5 Years (%)*
Duke high-dose therapy with ABMT (45)	85	96	72	72
Milan HDSC	48	92	92	NA
Standard-dose regimens				
Duke standard dose	30	58	23	13
National Historical Data Base (106)	119	77	33	27
Milan CMF		75	52	37
Johns Hopkins Hospital-Abeloff, 16-week regimen (107)	52	88	54	
M.D. Anderson FAC (108)	149	92	56	45
SWOG 7436 Melphalan (109)	48	72	36	22
SWOG 7436 CMFVp ([a])	33	92	46	32
ECOG 5181 (CMFpTH) 4181 (CMFPT), 6177 (CMFp (T)), 5177 (CMF) ([b])	319	86	48	28
Selected CALGB 7581 CMFVP (45)[c]	48	78	37	28
Selected CALGB 8082 CMFVP/VATH (45)[c]	47	82	42	29

[a]Osborne CK. Personal communication.
[b]Robert N. Personal communication.
[c]Patients selected were less than or equal to 56 years old, with 10 or more nodes at surgery and did not relapse during the first 4 months of therapy, thus similar to those in Duke 10+ LN trial.
Modified from (29).
ABMT = autologous bone marrow transplantation; C = cyclophosphamide; M = methotrexate; F = 5-fluorouracil; A = doxorubicin; T = thiotepa; H = halotestin; CALBG = Cancer and Leukemia Group B; SWOG = Southwest Oncology Group; ECOG = Eastern Cooperative Oncology Group.

Bone Marrow Contamination

Breast cancer frequently involves the bone and bone marrow. Bone marrow metastases develop in more than 60% of patients with metastatic disease at some point in the course of their disease. The response of breast cancer involving the bone is difficult to evaluate because methods of following bone involvement in breast cancer are inadequate and insensitive. The development of new lytic lesions is an insensitive monitor of disease, and the development of increased intensity of uptake on bone scans is seen with both disease progression and response. Furthermore, bone disease correlates closely with detection of malignant cells in bone marrow biopsies. In addition to the difficulty in monitoring treatment results, studies using autologous BMT for breast cancer involving bone are complicated by the potential for bone marrow involvement with malignancy. Because autologous BMT is premised on the availability of a source of hematopoietic stem cells free of malignant contamination, the use of marrow or peripheral blood from patients with known bone involvement carries with it the risk of infusion of viable malignant cells in the cellular product obtained.

Studies concerning this problem have focused on efforts to detect malignant cells and on efforts to "purge" bone marrow (or peripheral blood) of malignant cells. The precise value of purging is difficult to assess in most disease settings, and, particularly in breast cancer, this area is extremely complicated. In general, techniques that have focused on the use of monoclonal antibodies recognizing either epithelial antigens or putative breast cancer–specific antigens have minimal or no detectable cross-reaction with normal bone marrow. Patients with early advanced breast cancer have been studied using immunohistochemical techniques (47,48), flow cytometry, immunofluorescence (49,50), and culture of cells from bone marrow harvest screens (51). Mansi and colleagues (52) reported that 26.4% of patients with primary breast cancer have immunohistochemically positive cells when studied with a monoclonal antibody to an epithelial antigen. With early follow-up, 26 of 75 patients (35%; 26 of 60 [43%] patients with distant metastases) had immunohistochemically positive cells at presentation. These results appeared to correlate with disease-free interval and survival, although others suggest that the differences are accountable by other more traditional prognostic factors (53). The technical aspects of detecting true malignant cells in the marrow is formidable. Although several groups have reported the presence of cells bearing epithelial or other antigens (54–56), there is no demonstration that

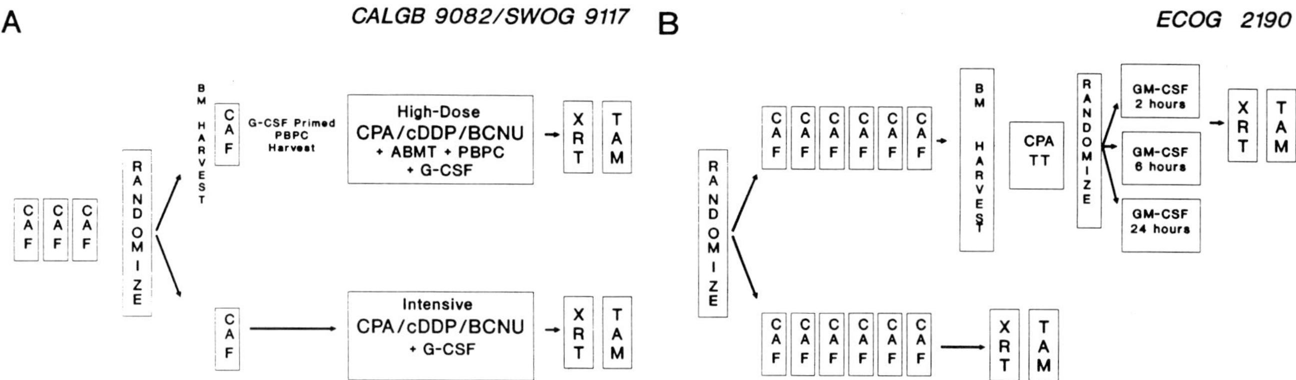

Figure 59-2. Trial designs for cooperative group studies in high-risk primary breast cancer conducted by the: (A) CALGB (9082)/SWOG (9017), and (B) ECOG cancer groups. In (A), C = cyclophosphamide, 600 mg/m^2 IV day 1; A = doxorubicin, 60 mg/m^2 day 1; F = 5-fluorouracil, 600 mg/m^2 day 1, day 8, with cycles repeated at 28-day intervals; PBPC = peripheral blood progenitor cells collected after G-CSF priming; high-dose CPA/cDDP/BCNU = cyclophosphamide, 5,625 mg/m^2; cDDP = cisplatin, 165 mg/m^2 by continuous infusion over 72 hours; BCNU = carmustine, 600 mg/m^2 IV over 2 hours; intensive CPA/cDDP/BCNU = cyclophosphamide, 900 mg/m^2; cDDP = cisplatin, 90 mg/m^2 by continuous intravenous infusion over 3 days; BCNU = carmustine, 90 mg/m^2 intravenously; XRT = radiation therapy to the chest wall and regional lymph nodes; and TAM = tamoxifen, 10 mg p.o. b.i.d. In (B), C = cyclophosphamide, 100 mg/m^2 p.o. q.d. × 14; A = doxorubicin, 30 mg/m^2 IV, day 1, day 8; F = 5-fluorouracil = 500 mg/^{2} IV day 1, day 8, with each cycle repeated every 28 days; CPA = cyclophosphamide, 6,000 mg/m^2 IV over 96 hours; TT = thiotepa, 800 mg/m^2 IV over 96 hours (patients are randomized to 3 schedules of GM-CSF administration, either as a 2-hour infusion, a 6-hour infusion, or a 24-hour infusion); XRT = radiation therapy to the regional lymph nodes; and TAM = tamoxifen, 10 mg p.o. b.i.d.

these are truly clonogenic cells. Recently, Diel and associates (57) reported identifying correlation between the presence of detection of antigen-positive cells using a tumor-associated glycoprotein, TAG-12, and subsequent recurrence. No study has been reported that confirms in vitro the biological capabilities of these cells, nor have samples been studied simultaneously with several techniques to establish the relative specificity of each method.

Several different purging methods have been reported, including the use of 4-hydroperoxycyclophosphamide (58,59), monoclonal antibodies (60–62), combination methodologies (63), and physical techniques. None have yet been tested in randomized trials, but therapeutic results so far do not appear meaningfully different from studies where no purging has been performed. Differences in the selected patient populations make comparisons difficult and relapses from involved marrow would not be expected for several years after transplantation because of the number of tumor doublings that would have to take place before tumor nodules become clinically detectable.

Toxicity Associated with High-dose Chemotherapy for Breast Cancer

The toxicities associated with high-dose chemotherapy for breast cancer display several unique features that differ from those generally encountered in other transplant settings. The chemotherapy programs often differ from those used with allogeneic BMT or with lymphoma and autologous BMT in that the treatment programs are almost always combination alkylating agents and generally do not employ TBI therapy. The doses and combinations of drugs in these programs have resulted in novel toxicities (64), although many toxicities are similar to those in other transplantation programs.

Myelosuppression

The average time to achieving a neutrophil count greater than 500/mm^3 after autologous BMT in most studies ranges between 15 and 25 days; thrombocytopenia lasts for a somewhat more extended period. In some patients, particularly those who have received extensive prior chemotherapy, hematopoietic recovery is slower, and persistent thrombocytopenia may become a major problem; some patients remain platelet-dependent for more than 100 days after transplantation.

Hematopoietic colony-stimulating factors (CSF), such as GM-CSF and G-CSF, have been utilized recently to accelerate hematopoietic recovery (65,66). The results using CSFs as adjuncts after BMT have been remarkably consistent. In each case, use of CSF accelerated the myeloid recovery after high-dose therapy with BMT. Platelet reconstitution was usually not improved. There consistently remained a period of absolute leukopenia and neutropenia that was not eliminated by the use of CSFs alone at any of the doses studied. This finding is likely to be related to a relative deficiency in cryopreserved marrow of the mature progenitors bearing CSF receptors responsive to late-acting CSFs. The addition of CSF-primed peripheral blood progenitor cells has resulted in a major reduction in both the duration of absolute leukopenia and in the toxicity associated with autologous BMT (67,68, 69). Hematopoietic recovery is accelerated and there is a reduction in the infectious complications seen. Some studies have noted a reduction in the need for platelet and red cell transfusions. These reductions in myelosuppression and toxicity offer the potential to reduce hospitalization after BMT, particularly when coupled with the use of prophylactic antibiotics.

Organ Toxicity

Organ system toxicity occurs following high-dose chemotherapy in the BMT setting as a direct effect of the chemotherapy and radiation therapy. It is likely that infectious complications, as well as medical treatment such as antibacterials and antifungals, contribute to these injuries.

Veno-occlusive disease (VOD) of the liver, reflecting endothelial damage from alkylating agents or radiation therapy with subsequent clot formation or fibrosis in the small hepatic venules occurs in as many as 20 to 40% of patients undergoing autologous BMT (70,71). The mechanism of injury presumably reflects the deposition of activated drug metabolites into the hepatic venules after metabolism in the liver, with subsequent injury to endothelial cells. The syndrome presents as right-quadrant pain, hepatomegaly, ascites, jaundice. No specific therapy has been shown to be effective after establishment of the syndrome. Efforts to utilize prostaglandin synthetase inhibitors or heparin to prevent the clot formation during the period of chemotherapy, diagnosis of VOD by ultrasonography (72,73), or treatment by tissue plasminogen activator (74) have been studied, with success reported in uncontrolled trials.

Nephrotoxicity occurring in the setting of autologous BMT can result from many causes, including the use of specific chemotherapeutic agents known to influence kidney function (cisplatin, nitrosoureas, phenylalanine mustard), coupled with nephrotoxic effects of antibiotics generally used during supportive care settings. Late renal dysfunction (75) probably related to radiation therapy can occur.

Pulmonary drug toxicity has been reported in the post-transplant setting (76,77). CY produces a characteristic pulmonary alveolitis in animal systems (78) and probably occurs in humans as a combined injury resulting from radiation therapy and CY as part of the preparative regimen. Pulmonary drug toxicity is commonly associated with carmustine when the acute or chronic dose exceeds 1,200 mg/m^2. The clinical syndrome is generally manifested by fever, interstitial infiltrates, and dyspnea. It is characterized pathologically by type II pneumocyte proliferation, fibrosis, and alveolar inflammation (79). Pulmonary insufficiency can be rapidly progressive, and diagnostic efforts should be instituted promptly. The clinical syndrome is often confused with an infectious etiology because of the complicating fever, and delay in making a specific diagnosis can lead to rapid progression of the toxicity. Although no controlled trials have been undertaken, empirical observations suggest that chemoradiation injury is worsened by exposure to high concentrations of oxygen. The use of corticosteroids in high doses is often useful in ameliorating this toxicity (72).

The most frequent serious cardiac complication associated with autologous BMT is hemorrhagic myocarditis, generally due to CY administration alone or in combination with other drugs. The pathology suggests that the lesion is due to endothelial injury and subsequent bleeding into the myocardium. Prior radiation therapy or extensive doxorubicin therapy may predispose children to this injury. Other reported cardiac complications include nonbacterial thrombotic endocarditis, catheter-associated right-sided endocarditis (81), and hypertension both during marrow infusion (82) and after chemotherapy, perhaps mediated through atrial natriure factor (83).

The use of high-dose agents has resulted in a variety of central nervous system complications during treatment for breast cancer, including organic brain syndrome from thiotepa (84), etoposide (85) and infectious complications (86).

Cutaneous toxicity is frequently noted during treatment ranging from drug allergies to a macular erythematous eruption called host-versus-host syndrome or autologous graft-versus-host disease (87), believed to be related to a type of graft-versus-host disease, although the mechanism is unclear.

Quality of Life

Systematic evaluation of quality of life has been undertaken in preliminary studies in patients undergoing autologous BMT for breast cancer. Winer and colleagues (88) found, using the Functional Living Index-Cancer (FLIC) and Symptom Distress Scale (SDS), that quality of life appears acceptable compared with previously reported nontransplant regimens, and few patients reported significant limitation a year or more after treatment (89).

Economics of ABMT for Breast Cancer

Recent studies of the cost-effectiveness of autologous BMT have indicated that the real cost of the procedure is dependent on how effective the treatments are and what time horizon is used for the analysis (90). It can be expected that, as the costs of the procedure decrease and the application to earlier disease settings is analyzed, cost-effectiveness will be more evident.

References

1. Henderson IC. Basic principles in the use of adjuvant therapy. Semin Oncol 1990;17:40–44.
2. Early Breast Cancer Trialist's Collaborative Group. Systemic therapy of early breast cancer by hormonal, cytotoxic, or immune therapy. Lancet 1992;1:71–85.

3. Gale RP. Progress in acute myeloid leukemia. Ann Intern Med 1984;101:702–705.
4. Buchner T, Hiddemann W, Loffler G, et al. Improved cure rate by very early intensification combined with prolonged maintenance chemotherapy in patients with acute myeloid leukemia: data from the AML Cooperative Group. Semin Oncol 1991;28:76–79.
5. Culbert SJ, Shuster JJ, Land VJ, et al. Remission induction and continuation therapy in children with their first relapse of acute lymphoid leukemia. A Pediatric Oncology Group Study. Cancer 1991;67:37–42.
6. Kilmo MP, Connors JM. MACOP-B chemotherapy for diffuse large-cell lymphoma. Ann Intern Med 1985; 102:596–602.
7. Armitage JO, Chesson BD. Interpretation of clinical trials in diffuse large-cell lymphoma. J Clin Oncol 1988;6:1335–1347.
8. Armitage JO. The place of third-generation regimens in the treatment of adult aggressive non-Hodgkin's lymphoma. Ann Oncol 1991;2:37–41.
9. DeVita VT Jr, Hubbard SM, Young RC, Longo DL. The role of chemotherapy in diffuse aggressive lymphomas. Semin Hematol 1988;25:2–10.
10. Diaz P, Cabanillas F. Treatment of non-Hodgkin's lymphoma. Curr Opin Oncol 1991;3:830–837.
11. Einhorn LH. Testicular cancer: a model for curable neoplasm. The Richard and Hilda Rosenthal Foundation Award Lecture. Cancer Res 1981;41:3275–3280.
12. Broun ER, Nichols CR, Kneebone P, et al. Long-term outcome of patients with relapsed and refractory germ cell tumors treated with high-dose chemotherapy and autologous bone marrow rescue. Ann Intern Med 1992;117:124–128.
13. Einhorn LH, Williams SD, Loehrer PJ, et al. Evaluation of optimal duration of chemotherapy in favorable-prognosis disseminated germ cell tumors: a Southeastern Cancer Study Group protocol. J Clin Oncol 1989;7:387–391.
14. Einhorn LH. Treatment of testicular cancer: a new and improved model. J Clin Oncol 1990;8:1777–1781.
15. Nichols CR, Tricot G, Williams SD. Dose-intensive chemotherapy in refractory germ cell cancer—a phase I/II trial of high-dose carboplatin and etoposide with autologous bone marrow transplantation. J Clin Oncol 1989;7:932–939.
16. Ianotti NI, Bosl GJ. A review of the management of germ cell tumors: evolution of a curative treatment program. Cancer Invest 1990;8:173–179.
17. Adelstein DJ, Sharan VM, Earle AS, et al. Long-term results after chemoradiotherapy for locally confined squamous-cell head and neck cancer. Am J Clin Oncol 1990;13:440–447.
18. Piver MS. Ovarian carcinoma. A decade of progress. Cancer 1984;54:2706–2715.
19. Young RC. Mechanisms to improve chemotherapy effectiveness. Cancer 1990;65:815–822.
20. DePree N, Wils J. Long-term survival of patients with advanced ovarian carcinoma treated with cisplatin-based chemotherapy regimens. Anticancer Res 1989; 9:1869–1871.
21. Henderson IC, Canellos GP. Cancer of the breast over the past decade. N Engl J Med 1980;302:78–90.
22. Early Breast Cancer Collaborative Group. Systemic treatment of early breast cancer by hormonal, cytotoxic, or immune therapy. Lancet 1992;1:1–15, 71–85.
23. Fisher B, Brown AM, Dimitrov NV, et al. Two months of doxorubicin-cyclophosphamide with and without interval reinduction therapy compared with 6 months of cyclophosphamide, methotrexate, and fluorouracil in positive-node breast cancer patients with tamoxifen-nonresponsive tumors: results from the National Surgical Adjuvant Breast and Bowel Project B-15. J Clin Oncol 1990;8:1482–1496.
24. Fisher B, Redmond C, Legault-Poisson S. Postoperative chemotherapy and tamoxifen compared with tamoxifen alone in the treatment of positive-node breast cancer patients aged 50 years and older with tumors responsive to tamoxifen: results from the National Surgical Adjuvant Breast and Bowel Project B-16. J Clin Oncol 1990;8:1005–1018.
25. Henderson IC. Adjuvant systemic therapy: state of the art, 1989. Breast Cancer Res Treat 1989;15:3–22.
26. Hryniuk W, Bush H. The importance of dose intensity in chemotherapy for metastatic breast cancer. J Clin Oncol 1984;2:1281–1288.
27. Henderson IC, Hayes DF, Gelman R. Dose response in the treatment of breast cancer. J Clin Oncol 1988; 6:1501–1515.
28. Frei E, Canellos GC. Dose—a critical factor in cancer therapy. Am J Med 1980;69:585–594.
29. Peters WP. High-dose chemotherapy and autologous bone marrow support for breast cancer. In: DeVita VT, Hellman S, Rosenberg SA, eds. Important advances in oncology, 1991. Philadelphia: J. B. Lippincott, 1991: 135–150.
30. Budman DR, Wood W, Henderson IC, et al. Initial findings of CALGB 8541: a dose and dose intensity trial of cyclophosphamide (C), doxorubicin (A), and 5-fluorouracil (F) as adjuvant treatment of stage II, node +, female breast cancer. Proc Am Soc Clin Oncol 1992;11:29a.
31. Tannock I, Boyd N, DeBoer G, et al. A randomized trial of two dose levels of cyclophosphamide, methotrexate, and fluorouracil chemotherapy for patients with metastatic breast cancer. J Clin Oncol 1988;6:1377–1387.
32. Powell TG, Sniff IE, Ford HT, Coombes RC, Jones JM, Gazet JC. Failure of chemotherapy to prolong survival in a group of patients with metastatic breast cancer. Lancet 1980;1:580–582.
33. Priestman T, Baum M, Jones V, Forbes J. Treatment and survival in advanced breast cancer. B Med J 1978;2:1673–1674.
34. Schabel FM, Trader MW, Laster WR, Wheeler GP, Witt MH. Patterns of resistance and therapeutic synergism among alkylating agents. Antibiot Chemother 1978; 23:200–215.
35. Schabel FM Jr, Skipper HE, Trader MW, et al. Establishment of cross resistant profiles for new agents. Cancer Treat Rep 1984;68:453–459.
36. Jones RB, Shpall EJ, Ross M, Coniglio D, Affronti ML, Peters WP: High-dose carboplatin, cyclophosphamide, and BCNU with autologous bone marrow support: excessive hepatic toxicity. Cancer Chemotherapy and Pharmacology 1990;26:155–156.
37. Egorin MJ, Cohen BE, Herzig RH, Ratain MJ, Peters WP. Human plasma pharmacokinetics and urinary excretion of thiotepa and its metabolites in patients receiving high-dose thiotepa therapy. In: Herzig GP, ed. Advances in cancer chemotherapy: high-dose thiotepa and autologous marrow transplantation. New York: Park Row Publishers, 1987.
38. Bronchchud M, Howell A, Crowther D, Hopwood P, Souza L, Dexter T. The use of granulocyte colony-stimulating factor to increase the intensity of treatment

with doxorubicin in patients with advanced breast and ovarian cancer. Br J Cancer 1989;60:121–125.
39. Thomas ED, Storve R, Clift RA, et al. Bone marrow transplantation. N Engl J Med 1975;292:832–895.
40. Thomas ED, Buckner CD, Clift RA, et al. Marrow transplantation for acute non-lymphoblastic leukemia in first remission. N Engl J Med 1979;301:597–599.
41. Zambetti M, Valugussa P, Bonadonna G. Eight-year results with adjuvant intravenous CMF in node-negative (N-) and estrogen receptor negative (ER-) breast cancer. Proc Am Soc Clin Oncol 1992;11:69a.
42. Henderson IC. Chemotherapy for advanced disease. In: Harris JR, et al. eds. Breast diseases. Philadelphia: J.B. Lippincott, 1987:428–279.
43. Peters WP, Shpall EJ, Jones RB, Ross M. High-dose combination cyclophosphamide, cisplatin, and carmustine with bone marrow support as initial treatment for metastatic breast cancer: three to six year follow-up. Proc Am Soc Clin Oncol 1990;9:10.
44. Antman K, Bearman SI, Davidson N, et al. Dose intensive therapy in breast cancer: current status. In: Gale RP, Champlin RE, eds. New strategies in bone marrow transplantation. New York: Alan R. Liss, 1990:423–436.
45. Peters WP, Ross M, Vredenburgh JJ, et al. High-dose chemotherapy and autologous bone marrow support as consolidation after standard-dose adjuvant therapy for high-risk primary breast cancer. J Clin Oncol 1993; 11:1132–1143.
46. Gianni AM, Siena S, Bregni M, et al. Growth factor-supported high-dose sequential (HDS) adjuvant chemotherapy in breast cancer with ≥ 10 positive nodes. Proc Am Soc Clin Oncol 1992;11:60.
47. Neville AM. Some immunobiochemical approaches for the detection of metastases. Invasion Metastasis 1981; 1:2–11.
48. Redding WH, Monoghan P, Imrie SF, et al. Detection of micrometastases in patients with primary breast cancer. Lancet 1983;2:1271–1274.
49. Ginsbourg M, Musset M, Misset JL, et al. Identification of mammary metastatic cells in the bone marrow as a marker of a minimal residual disease and of their proliferative index as a factor of prognosis—an immunocytologic study with monoclonal antibodies. Suppl J Med Oncol Tumor Pharmacother 1988;1:51–54.
50. Osborne MP, Asina S, Wong GY, et al. Immunofluorescent monoclonal antibody detection of breast cancer in bone marrow: sensitivity in a model system. Cancer Res 1989;49:2510–2513.
51. Sharp JG, Vaughan WP, Kessinger A, et al. Significance of detection of tumor cells in hematopoietic stem cell harvests of patients with breast cancer. In: Dicke K, Armitage JO, Dicke-Evinger MJ, eds. Autologous bone marrow transplantation, V. Omaha: University of Nebraska Medical Center, 1991:385–391.
52. Mansi JL, Berger U, Easton D, et al. Micrometastases in bone marrow in patients with primary breast cancer: evaluation as an early predictor of bone metastases. Br Med J 1987;295:1093–1096.
53. Blamey RW, Robertson JFR, Locker AP. Micrometastases in bone marrow in patients with breast cancer. Br Med J 1987;295:1487.
54. Cote RJ, Rosen PP, Lesser ML, et al. Detection of occult bone marrow micrometastases (BMM) in patients with operable breast cancer predicts early recurrence. Proc US Can Acad Pathol 1990;23A.
55. Schlimok G, Funke I, Holzmann B, et al. Micrometastatic cancer cells in bone marrow: in vitro detection with anti-cytokeratin and in vivo labeling with anti-17-1A monoclonal antibodies. Proc Natl Acad Sci USA 1987;84:8672–8676.
56. Untch M, Harbeck N, Eirmann W. Micrometastases in bone marrow in patients with breast cancer. Br Med J 1988;296:290.
57. Diel IJ, Kaufmann M, Goerner R, Costa SD, Kaul S, Bastert G. Detection of tumor cells in bone marrow of patients with primary breast cancer: A prognostic factor for distant metastasis. J Clin Oncol 1992;10:1534–1539.
58. Shpall EJ, Jones RB, Bast RC Jr. 4-Hydroperoxycyclophosphamide purging of breast cancer from the mononuclear cell fraction of bone marrow in patients receiving high-dose chemotherapy and autologous marrow support: a phase I trial. J Clin Oncol 1991;9:85–93.
59. Kennedy MJ, Beveridge R, Rowley S, et al. High dose consolidation chemotherapy and rescue with purged autologous bone marrow following dose-intense induction for metastatic breast cancer. Proc Am Soc Clin Oncol 1989;8:19.
60. Cooper KL, Shpall EJ, Peters WP, Bast RC. Elimination of clonogenic breast cancer cells from human bone marrow: comparison of immunotoxin treatment with chemoseparation and immunoseparation using 4-hydroperoxycyclophosphamide (4-HC) and immunomagnetic separation. Proc Am Assoc Cancer Res 1989;30:237.
61. Shpall EJ, Bast RC, Joines W, et al. Immunopharmacologic bone marrow purging in metastatic breast cancer patients receiving high-dose chemotherapy with autologous bone marrow support. Proc Am Soc Clin Oncol 1990;9:9.
62. Anderson I, Shpall EJ, Leslie D, et al. Elimination of malignant clonogenic breast cancer cells from human bone marrow. Cancer Res 1989;49:4659–4664.
63. Shpall EJ, Johnston C, Hami L. Bone marrow purging. In: Armitage JO, Antman KH, eds. High-dose cancer therapy. Pharmacology, hematopoietins, stem cells. Baltimore: Williams & Wilkins, 1992:249–275.
64. Peters WP, Eder JP, Henner WD, Bast RC, Schnipper L, Frei E. Novel toxicities associated with high-dose combination alkylating agents and autologous bone marrow support. In: Dicke KA, Spitzer G, Zander AR, eds. Autologous bone marrow transplantation: proceedings of the First International Symposium. Houston, TX: M.D. Anderson Hospital Press, 1985:231–235.
65. Brandt SJ, Peters WP, Atwater SK, et al. Effect of recombinant human granulocyte-macrophage colony-stimulating factor on hematopoietic reconstitution following high-dose chemotherapy and autologous bone marrow transplantation. N Engl J Med 1988; 318:869–876.
66. Sheridan WP, Morstyn G, Wolf M, et al. Granulocyte colony-stimulating factor and neutrophil recovery after high-dose chemotherapy and autologous bone marrow transplantation. Lancet 1989;2:891–895.
67. Gianni AM, Bregni M, Siena S, et al. Rapid and complete hemopoietic reconstitution following combined transplantation of autologous blood and bone marrow cells. A changing role for high dose chemo-radiotherapy? Hematol Oncol 1989;7:139–148.
68. Gianni AM, Siena S, Bregni M, et al. Granulocyte-macrophage colony-stimulating factor to harvest circulating haemopoietic stem cells for autotransplantation. Lancet 1989;2:580–585.
69. Decker DA, Ahmann DL, Bisel HF, et al. Complete

responders to chemotherapy in metastatic breast cancer. JAMA 1979;242:2075–2079.

70. Ayash LJ, Hunt M, Antman K, et al. Hepatic venoocclusive disease in autologous bone marrow transplantation of solid tumors and lymphomas. J Clin Oncol 1990;8:1699–1706.
71. McDonald GB, Sharma P, Matthews DE, et al. The clinical course of 53 patients with veno-occlusive disease of the liver after marrow transplantation. Transplantation 1985;39:603–608.
72. Matsuishi E, Anzal K, Dohmen K, et al. Sonographic diagnosis of venoocclusive disease of the liver and danazol therapy for autoimmune thrombocytopenia in an autologous marrow transplant patient. Japan J Clin Oncol 1990;20:188–192.
73. Herbetko J, Grigg AP, Buckley AR, Phillips GL. Venoocclusive liver disease after bone marrow transplantation: findings at duplex sonography. Am J Roentgenol 1922;158:1001–1005.
74. Baglin TP, Harper P, Marcus RE. Veno-occlusive disease of the liver complicating ABMT successfully treated with recombinant tissue plasminogen activator (rt-PA). Bone Marrow Transplant 1990;5:439–441.
75. Tarbell NJ, Guinan EC, Niemeyer B, Mauch P, Sallan SE, Weinstein HJ. Late onset of renal dysfunction in survivors of bone marrow transplantation. Int J Radiat Oncol Biol Phys 1988;15:99–104.
76. Jochelson M, Tarbell NJ, Freeman AS, et al. Acute and chronic pulmonary complications following autologous bone marrow transplantation in non-Hodgkin's lymphoma. Bone Marrow Transplant 1990;6:329–331.
77. Litam JP, Dail DH, Spitzer G, et al. Early pulmonary toxicity after administration of high-dose BCNU. Cancer Treat Rep 1981;65:39–44.
78. Blumenstock DA, Cannon FD, Hales CA, Vlahovic VL, Alpern H, Kazemi H. Pulmonary function of DLA-nonidentical lung allografts in dogs treated with lethal total-body irradiation, autologous bone marrow transplantation, and methotrexate. Transplantation 1979; 28:223–227.
79. Todd NW, Peters WP, Ost AH et al. Pulmonary drug toxicity in patients with primary breast cancer treated with high-dose combination chemotherapy and autologous bone marrow transplantation. Ann. Rev. Resp. Diseases 1993;147:1264–1270.
80. Ahmed T. Autologous marrow transplantation for Hodgkin's disease. Current techniques and prospects. Cancer Invest 1990;8:99–106.
81. Martino P, Micozzi A, Venditti M, et al. Catheter-associated right-sided endocarditis in bone marrow transplant recipients. Rev Infect Dis 1990;12:250–257.
82. Sugarman J, Bashore TM, Ohman EM, Jones R, Peters WP. Hypertension and reversible myocardial depression associated with autologous bone marrow transplantation. Am J Med 1990;88:52–55.
83. Graves SW, Eder JP, Schryber SM, et al. Endogenous digoxin-like immunoreactive factor and digitalis-like factor associated with the hypertension of patients receiving multiple alkylating agents as part of autologous bone marrow transplantation. Clin Sci 1989; 77:501–507.
84. Wolff SN, Herzig RH, Fay JW, et al. High-dose thiotepa with autologous bone marrow transplantation for metastatic malignant melanoma: results of phase I and II studies of the North American Bone Marrow Transplantation Group. J Clin Oncol 1989;7:245–249.
85. Leff RS, Thompson JM, Daly MB, et al. Acute neurologic dysfunction after high-dose etoposide therapy for malignant glioma. Cancer 1988;62:32–35.
86. Leff RS, Martino RL, Pollock WJ, Knight WA III. Pituitary abscess after autologous bone marrow transplantation. Am J Hematol 1989;31:62–64.
87. Jones RJ, Vogelsang GB, Hess AD, et al. Induction of graft-versus-host disease after autologous bone marrow transplantation. Lancet 1989;1:754–757.
88. Winer E, Lindley C, Hardee M, et al. Quality of life (QL) assessment in patients with breast cancer surviving 12 months or more following high dose chemotherapy with autologous bone marrow transplant (HDC-ABMT). Proc Am Soc Clin Oncol 1992;11:383.
89. Peters WP, Kurtzberg J, Romber G, et al. Comparative effects of G-CSF and GM-CSF on primary peripheral blood progenitor cells for use with autologous bone marrow after high-dose chemotherapy. Blood 1993;81: 1709–1719.
90. Hillner BE, Smith TJ, Desch CE. Efficacy and cost-effectiveness of autologous bone marrow transplantation in metastatic breast cancer—estimates using decision analysis while awaiting clinical trial results. JAMA 1992;267:2055–2016.
91. Antman K, Bearman SI, Davidson, et al. Dose intensive therapy in breast cancer: current status. In: Gale RP, Champlin RE, eds. New strategies in bone marrow transplantation. New York: Alan R. Liss, 1991:423–436.
92. Eder JP, Antman, Peters WP, et al. High dose combination alkylating agent chemotherapy with autologous bone marrow support for metastatic breast cancer. J Clin Oncol 1986;4:1592–1597.
93. Peters WP, Eder JP, Schryber S, et al. High-dose combination alkylating agents with autologous bone marrow support: a phase I trial. J Clin Oncol 1986;4:646–654.
94. Henderson IC. Chemotherapy for advanced disease. In: Harris JR, Hellman S, Henderson IC, Kinne DW, eds. Breast diseases. Philadelphia: J. P. Lippicott, 1988:442, 449.
95. Peters WP, Shpall EJ, Jones RB, et al. High-dose combination alkylating agents with bone marrow support as initial treatment for metastatic breast cancer. J Clin Oncol 1988;6:1368–1376.
96. Coates A, Gebski V, Bishop JF, et al. Improving the quality of life during chemotherapy for advanced breast cancer. N Engl J Med 1987;317:1490–1495.
97. Tannock I, Boyd N, DeBoer G, et al. A randomized trial of two dose levels of cyclophosphamide, methotrexate and fluorouracil chemotherapy for patients with metastatic breast cancer. J Clin Oncol 1988;6:1377–1387.
98. Bull JM, Tormey DC, Li SH, et al. A randomized comparative trial of adriamycin versus methotrexate in combination drug therapy. Cancer 1978;41:1649–1657.
99. Rubens RD, Knight RK, Hayward JL. Chemotherapy of advanced breast cancer: a controlled randomized trial of cyclophosphamide versus a four-drug combination. Br J Cancer 1975;32:730–736.
100. Tranum BL, McDonald B, Thigpen T, et al. Adriamycin combinations in advanced breast cancer. Cancer 1982; 49:835–839.
101. Bennett JM, HB Muss, Doroshow JH, et al. A randomized multicenter trial comparing mitoxantrone, cyclophosphamide, and fluorouracil with doxorubicin, cyclophosphamide, and fluorouracil in the therapy of metastatic breast carcinoma. J Clin Oncol 1988;6: 1611–1620.

102. Muss HB, Richards F, Cooper MR, et al. Chemotherapy versus chemoimmunotherapy with methanol extraction residue of bacillus Calmette-Guerin (MER) in advanced breast cancer: a randomized trial by the Piedmont Oncology Association. Cancer 1982;47: 2295–2301.
103. Hortobagyi GN, Frye D, Buzdar AU, et al. Complete remissions in metastatic breast cancer: a thirteen year follow-up report. Proc Am Soc Clin Oncol 1988;7:143a.
104. Dunphy FR, Spitzer G, Buzdar AU, et al. Treatment of estrogen receptor-negative or hormonally refractory breast cancer with double high-dose chemotherapy intensification and bone marrow support. J Clin Oncol 1990;8:1207–1216.
105. Mulder NH, DeVries EGE, Sleijfer DTH, Mulder POM, Willemse PHB. Intensive induction chemotherapy and intensification with autologous bone marrow reinfusion in patients with stage IIIB and IV breast cancer. Proc Am Soc Clin Oncol 1990;9:91a.
106. Jones SE, Moon TE, Bonadonna G, et al. Comparison of different trials of adjuvant chemotherapy in stage II breast cancer using a natural history data base. Am J Clin Oncol 1987;10:387–395.
107. Abeloff MD, Beveridge RA, Donehower RC, et al. Sixteen-week dose-intensive adjuvant chemotherapy for operable breast cancer with ten or more positive nodes. Proc Am Soc Clin Oncol 1990;9:86a.
108. Kau SW, Buzdar A, Fraschini G, Hug V, Holmes F, Hortobagyi G. Impact of adjuvant chemotherapy with FAC in patients with $\geq$ 10 positive nodes operable breast cancer. Proc Am Soc Clin Oncol 1989;8:114a.
109. Tormey DC, Weinberg VE, Holland JF, et al. A randomized trial of five and three drug chemotherapy and chemoimmunotherapy in women with operable node positive breast cancer. J Clin Oncol 1983;1:138–145.
110. Lichtman SM, Budman D, Bosworth S, et al. Adjuvant therapy of stage II breast cancer treated with CMFVP, radiation therapy and VATH following lumpectomy. Am J Clin Oncol 1991;14:317–321.

Chapter 60
Germ-cell Cancer

Craig R. Nichols and E. Randolph Broun

Overview

Germ-cell cancer is a relatively uncommon disease; it accounts for approximately 1% of all malignancies in men (1). However, it is an important disease in the field of oncology, because it represents a highly curable malignancy, and one in which the incidence is focused on young patients at their peak of productivity. Despite the infrequency of the diagnosis, the impact of cure in this population is enormous and has been the subject of a recent cost-benefit analysis; the annual economic value of cisplatin-based chemotherapy for this disease has been estimated at $150 million (2).

The development of effective therapy that can now cure the majority of patients is a product of several decades of rational drug development, well-planned clinical trials, and a small measure of serendipity. As a result, germ-cell cancer has truly become a "model" for the treatment of other malignancies (3). To understand the role of high-dose treatment in this unique malignancy, we review the important role of histopathology, serum tumor markers, and utility of surgical extirpation of residual cancer in management of these patients. An overview of the important clinical trials using conventional dose therapy forms a basis for understanding the value of high-dose treatments of this chemotherapy-sensitive tumor.

Histopathology

In the United States, classification of testicular malignancies is based on the system described initially by Dixon and Moore in 1952 (4). Approximately 95% of all testicular neoplasms are of germinal origin (Table 60-1).

Seminomas

Overall, the diagnosis of pure seminoma accounts for approximately 47% of all testicular malignancies, but its incidence is increased in cryptorchid testes, where it accounts for more than 60% of malignancies (5,6). Currently, seminoma is subclassified as either classic or spermatocytic. Formerly, a third category of "anaplastic seminoma" was distinguished histologically, based on a large number of mitoses per high-power field, an absence of trophoblastic elements, and a tumor appearing less well organized on low-power examination than its classic counterpart. Although patients with this anaplastic variant may present with more advanced disease, when stratified by stage of disease, survival rates are no different than those for patients with classic seminoma, and ultrastructural characteristics are identical (7–9).

Approximately 7% of classic seminomas contain true syncytial trophoblastic giant cells (as distinct from Langerhans' cells), which stain positively for human chorionic gonadotropin (HCG), and which may account for the low-level elevation of serum HCG in some patients with pure seminoma.

Clinically, classic seminomas present in the fourth or fifth decade, most commonly as an enlarging, painless testicular mass. Only one quarter of seminomas present with metastatic disease, and in a review of more than 2,300 cases, Smith (5) documented that 74.7% of patients presented with stage I disease, 19.5% with stage II, and only 5.8% with stages III and IV.

Lymphatic spread is to the para-aortic lymph nodes, then to the mediastinal or supraclavicular lymph nodes, usually only after development of significant infradiaphragmatic disease. Hematogenous dissemination to lung, liver, bone, or adrenal is a late occurrence in the natural history of this disease. Low-level HCG elevation can be seen in 5 to 10% of

Table 60-1.
Pathological Classification of Testicular Germ-cell Tumors

Primary Malignancies
- Germinal neoplasms (containing one or more of the following types)
  1. Seminoma
     a. Classic
     b. Anaplastic
     c. Spermatocytic
  2. Embryonal carcinoma
  3. Teratoma
     a. Mature
     b. Immature
  4. Choriocarcinoma
  5. Yolk sac tumor (formerly endodermal-sinus tumor)

pure seminomas, and is likely a result of the presence of syncytial trophoblastic elements within the tumor (10). The presence of such HCG elevation, however, does not appear to negatively influence prognosis (10–12). Seminomas do not secrete alpha-fetoprotein (AFP), however, and elevation of this serum marker denotes the presence of nonseminomatous elements.

Embryonal-cell Carcinomas

Embryonal carcinomas account for 20% of all testicular tumors. Macroscopically, pure embryonal carcinomas tend to be small (even in the presence of widespread metastases), although larger tumors can efface the normal testicular tissue. The cut surface is less homogenous than seminomas, with frequent areas of necrosis and hemorrhage. Direct invasion of the spermatic cord, the epididymis, and the tunica albuginea is common.

Clinically, these are aggressive tumors with a high metastatic potential. Embryonal carcinomas may contain differentiated components of extraembryonic structures, such as trophoblastic or yolk sac elements, with corresponding elevations of serum HCG or AFP levels, respectively.

Yolk-sac Carcinomas

Although yolk sac elements are frequently found in embryonal carcinomas, this pattern can also appear in a pure form. Formerly referred to as endodermal sinus tumors, they are the most common testicular malignancy in infants and young children (13–15). In children, they are occasionally designated as infantile embryonal carcinomas or orchidoblastomas, and they carry an excellent prognosis (16). In adults, pure yolk sac tumors are virulent neoplasms with early hematogenous dissemination and a particular affinity for development of hepatic metastases. Primary mediastinal germ-cell tumors are especially prone to exhibit this type of extraembryonic differentiation; the incidence in one series approached 50% (17). Serologically, patients with pure yolk sac tumors have elevated serum AFP levels, usually with normal serum HCG levels.

Choriocarcinomas

Although trophoblastic components are common components of mixed germ-cell tumors, pure choriocarcinomas of the adult testis are rare. Choriocarcinomas of the testis represent the most aggressive pathological variant of germ-cell tumors in adults, characteristically with early hematogenous and lymphatic spread. Large volume visceral metastases may be observed at presentation with an occult primary lesion. A poorer prognosis in these patients may result from the average volume of disease at presentation, as opposed to an inherent resistance to therapy with this pathological pattern. Serologically, these patients characteristically have extreme elevations of serum HCG levels, with normal serum AFP levels.

Teratocarcinomas

Teratocarcinomas refer to germ-cell tumors containing elements of mature teratomas mixed with other germ-cell elements. Macroscopically, there is a variegated appearance, with cystic areas of the mature teratoma admixed with areas of solid tumor, representing the malignant elements. Microscopically, separate areas of obviously malignant germinal elements (i.e., embryonal carcinomas) are in proximity to mature, adult-like structures. Clinically, the aggressiveness of this tumor lies somewhere between that of mature teratomas and pure embryonal carcinomas.

Teratomas

Teratomas refer to germ-cell tumors that contain elements of all 3 germ layers (endoderm, mesoderm, and ectoderm), and they present with varying degrees of differentiation. Although technically no malignant tissue exists in these terminally differentiated tumors, metastases can occur and death can result from slowly progressive, unresectable disease. Therefore, the label "benign" is misleading and should be avoided when referring to these tumors. Teratomas do not secrete either B-HCG or AFP and are not responsive to chemotherapy. In fact, the presence of an enlarging mass radiographically during chemotherapy in a serologically responding patient may connote the presence of teratomatous elements. Surgical extirpation represents the only known therapeutic option. Subcategories include mature teratomas, immature teratomas, or teratomas with malignant transformation.

Microscopically, mature (adult) teratomas are easily distinguished, with obvious epithelial-lined structures, as well as mature cartilage and striated or smooth muscle. Although each component is histologically mature, distribution of these elements appears haphazard. Overall, testicular teratomas are much less well organized at an organ level than their ovarian counterparts.

Several histological features may result in teratomas being labeled as "immature." The presence of a highly cellular stroma exhibiting mitotic figures is sufficient to make this diagnosis. More commonly, immature teratomas have areas of primitive mesoderm, endoderm, or ectoderm mixed with the more mature elements.

A relatively recent observation has been of a variant of teratoma that contains malignant non-germ-cell elements, presumably derived from somatic tissues within the teratoma (18–20). It is unclear whether these elements represent partial differentiation along somatic lines of the malignant totipotent germ cell, or malignant degeneration of a mature somatic element of the teratoma. This histopathological entity may include areas of adenosquamous carcinoma, multiple varieties of soft-tissue sarcomas, neuroblastomas, or nephroblastomas. The presence of these malignant somatic tissues either at the time of diagnosis or following induction chemotherapy is a poor prognostic sign in terms of relapse and overall survival.

Serum Tumor Markers

Management of testicular cancer has come to depend on accurate determination of levels of serum tumor markers and interpretation of these values in the clinical context. The most sensitive and specific markers are AFP and the beta subunit of HCG. AFP is a glycoprotein normally produced by the fetal yolk sac and is derived from yolk sac or embryonal carcinoma elements of germ-cell cancers. Levels of AFP are not detectable in normal adults; the half-life of this protein in the serum is approximately 5 days. HCG is a smaller glycoprotein that is normally produced by trophoblastic tissues. In germ-cell cancers, syncytiotrophoblastic components elaborate HCG. The protein is comprised of an alpha and a beta subunit, each of which are antigenically distinct. The serum half-life of the entire protein is 18 to 24 hours.

Clinical decisions in patients with germ-cell cancer are frequently dependent on precise measurement of serum tumor markers: beta subunit HCG, AFP, and lactate dehydrogenase (LDH). Overall, HCG will be elevated in 75% of patients with disseminated testicular and primary retroperitoneal nonseminomatous germ-cell tumors, and AFP is elevated in 40% of patients. Elevated LDH is a less specific marker and is probably a correlate of disease bulk. Pure seminomas are most frequently associated with normal AFP and HCG levels, but approximately 10% of all patients and up to 50% of patients with advanced disease may have low-level elevations of HCG (usually less than 100 ngU/mL). Any elevation of AFP in patients with seminomas must be viewed as evidence of nonseminomatous disease, and management should proceed accordingly.

The rate of disappearance of elevated tumor markers is very useful in determining response to treatment. HCG is the most useful marker in this regard; the most clinically helpful guideline is that a 10-fold decrease in HCG levels over a 3-week period is consistent with disease eradication. Less steep declines of HCG levels correlate with the emergence of drug-resistant disease, in the case of chemotherapy, or residual disease, in the case of surgery. Likewise, reappearance of marker elevation often predates the radiographic appearance of recurrent disease and as such is an invaluable method of detecting early relapse.

Although the presence of tumor markers and the accurate determination of these markers serve as a luxury in the management of patients with germ-cell cancer, the presence of these markers can lead to errors in clinical management if not interpreted with caution. First, HCG determination can be nonspecific, and there is some cross-reactivity in the radioimmunoassay with luteinizing hormone. Also, HCG can be falsely elevated in patients who use marijuana. Low levels of HCG elevation are consequently difficult to interpret. A conservative approach to this dilemma is to repeat the HCG determination to insure that the elevation is not a laboratory error. If the level is still high, the patient should be queried regarding drug usage. Testosterone should be given to insure that a hypogonadal state with resultant high levels of luteinizing hormone is not interfering with the determination of HCG levels. If the level remains increased, restaging procedures and investigation of sanctuary sites are in order.

False-positive elevations of AFP are quite rare. Differential considerations would include laboratory error; other tumor types, such as hepatomas; or liver inflammation from cirrhosis or hepatitis.

Clinical Staging

The most widely used staging system for seminomatous germ-cell tumors divides patients into clinical categories of local disease only (stage I); abdominal nodal metastasis of minimal extent (stage IIA) or bulky extent (stage IIB, C); nodal disease above the diaphragm (stage III); or extranodal metastasis (stage IV). In a similar manner, staging of nonseminomatous disease is divided into stage I (or A), referring to tumors confined to the testis; stage II (or B), indicating metastatic disease to the nodes of the periaortic or vena caval zone without pulmonary or visceral involvement; and stage III (or C), which denotes metastasis above the diaphragm or involving other viscera.

Standard procedures to establish clinical stage include abdominal and chest computed tomography (CT) scans with other studies (e.g., bone scan, brain CT) performed only as warranted by clinical symptoms. Bipedal lymphangiography has been recommended in earlier studies but is limited by the low sensitivity (75–80%) and specificity (up to 10% false-positive rate) and the invasive nature of the procedure. With CT-based staging, 25% of patients will be understaged and 10 to 20% will be overstaged. These limitations in clinical staging have led to a policy of surgical staging that provides accurate pathological parameters of disease extent and simplified follow-up.

Management of Disseminated Germ-cell Cancer

Early Studies

In 1974, investigators at Indiana University began studies using cisplatin, vinblastine, and bleomycin (PVB) in patients with disseminated testicular cancer. The initial study of 50 patients remains a landmark study in modern oncology (21). This study incorporated principles of combination chemotherapy as well as the concept of surgically resecting residual disease after the completion of chemotherapy. Induction chemotherapy was brief (3–4 courses), and maintenance chemotherapy was given for 2 years after induction therapy. Of this group of 47 patients, 33 (70%) obtained a complete remission with chemotherapy. Of the remaining 14 patients, 5 obtained a complete remission, with resection of residual disease after the completion of chemotherapy. Six of the patients obtaining remission have relapsed, but now with follow-up exceeding 10 years, it is gratifying to note that there seems to be little evidence of long-term toxicity from chemotherapy (22).

The initial study of PVB was very effective; yet there was substantial toxicity. In the next important series of studies, investigators at Indiana University, in conjunction with the Southeastern Cancer Study Group, designed a randomized trial comparing cisplatin plus bleomycin and either vinblastine (PVB) or etoposide (BEP) (23). Patients were randomly allocated to receive BEP or PVB, and 83 and 74%, respectively, achieved a disease-free status. In the combined subgroups of patients with minimal or moderate disease by the Indiana classification system, 90% achieved a disease-free status, with no difference between the 2 treatment arms. Although PVB and BEP gave equally good therapeutic results, there was a marked difference in neuromuscular toxicity; the PVB patients experienced significantly more paresthesias, myalgias, and abdominal cramping. Because BEP had substantially less neuromuscular toxicity with equal or superior therapeutic results, 4 courses of cisplatin, etoposide, and bleomycin became the new standard.

Prognostic Factors in Disseminated Disease

In recent years, primary therapeutic strategies have diverged for the treatment of patients with germ-cell tumors with a low versus high risk of relapse, with corresponding emphasis on less versus more intensive treatment, respectively. As increasingly aggressive (and toxic) regimens are developed for patients with a low likelihood of achieving a complete remission or who have a high risk of relapse, elucidation of prognostic factors to correctly identify such patients becomes increasingly important. Different prognostic factors (and the relative importance of each) have been reported by separate groups and have evolved into a number of staging systems for advanced disease. Such assignment of patients into "good-risk" and "poor-risk" categories have been undertaken by the National Cancer Institute (NCI) (24), the European Organization for the Research and Treatment of Cancer (EORTC) (25), Memorial Sloan-Kettering Cancer Center (26), the Southeastern Cancer Study Group (27), the Medical Research Council (28,29), and the Danish Testicular Carcinoma Study Group (30). A number of characteristics are uniformly identified in "poor-risk" patients and include a high volume of metastatic disease, significant elevations of serum tumor markers, extragonadal primary lesions, and visceral organ involvement. New prognostic factors are being identified and include measurements of the kinetics of tumor growth, with a higher proliferative index predictive of poor outcome of therapy (31).

Treatment of "Good Risk" Disseminated Disease

Although there is debate regarding the relative importance of a number of potential prognostic factors, in general those patients with serum marker elevation only, small volume infradiaphragmatic or supradiaphragmatic involvement, or both, without visceral involvement are highly curable and are categorized as good risk. This group of patients constitutes approximately 70% of patients presenting with disseminated disease.

Stratification by selected prognostic factors in a series of randomized clinical trials has confirmed their predictive value. In the mid-1980s, several clinical trials were designed specifically for this group of patients. Because virtually all these patients achieve complete remission with standard chemotherapy, these trials addressed the possibility of reducing the amount of chemotherapy administered (thus decreasing acute and chronic toxicity) while maintaining the excellent cure rate. Several approaches to this reduction in therapy have been employed, including a shortening of the duration of therapy, use of chemotherapeutic agents with less single-agent toxicity, or a reduction in the number of agents used. A number of trials have addressed the issue of less intensive therapy for patients with good-risk germ-cell tumors (32–35). Review of these trials suggests that good-risk germ-cell cancer can be reliably cured with either 3 courses of cisplatin, etoposide, and bleomycin, or 4 courses of the two-drug combination, cisplatin and etoposide. The current standard of therapy in this patient population has minimal acute and probably even less long-term toxicity. Further reductions in the amount of therapy are therefore unlikely to significantly reduce toxicity but certainly have the potential to reduce the cure rate in this stage of disease.

Treatment of "Poor Risk" Disseminated Disease

The one third of patients with disseminated testicular cancer who present with poor prognostic features remain a therapeutic challenge. Serial clinical trials have helped to define therapy for this less favorable clinical setting (36–38). Most investigators use 4 courses of cisplatin, etoposide, and bleomycin (BEP) or 3 to 4 courses of vinblastine, cyclophosphamide, actinomycin-D, cisplatin, and bleomycin (VAB-6) in patients with poor-risk germ-cell cancer. Such "standard treatment" cures approximately 60% of patients in this risk category. The current emphasis in the initial treatment of these poor-risk patients is exploration of dose-intense regimens and use of etoposide and other newer agents as initial therapy.

Postchemotherapy Surgery

Depending on the stage at diagnosis, 20 to 50% of patients who undergo induction chemotherapy for disseminated germ-cell tumor have significant residual radiographic abnormalities. In this subset of patients, post-chemotherapy resection of residual disease is often performed to remove residual teratomas or viable cancer. Several points bear emphasis in this setting. First, consideration of postchemotherapy surgery should be made only if serum AFP and HCG levels have normalized. Patients with persistently elevated serum markers should be considered for salvage chemotherapy rather than surgical "debulking." Second, postchemotherapy resection of residual abnormalities is rarely urgent, and sufficient time should be taken to allow the patient to recover from the effects of induction chemotherapy. Typically, patients are taken to surgery 6 weeks after the last round of treatment. Third, repeat imaging of the areas of abnormality should be performed prior to surgery. In many patients, continued involution of residual masses occurs after completion of therapy and surgical resection is not necessary.

The histopathological findings in postchemotherapy surgical specimens help define the need for further treatment. In earlier reports, approximately 40% of patients had teratomas, 40% had fibrous necrotic debris, and 20% had residual viable germ-cell cancer. Analysis of recent series suggests that the incidence of persistent cancer is decreasing (32,36).

Those patients with persistent cancer identified and totally removed at postchemotherapy surgery require special management. If the surgical margins are free of tumor, all sites of known disease are removed, and the serum tumor markers remain normal, patients should receive 2 postoperative cycles of cisplatin-based therapy similar to induction therapy. Those patients with unresectable disease, positive surgical margins, or elevated tumor marker levels should be considered for full salvage therapy using new agents and more prolonged courses of therapy. Approximately two thirds of patients receiving additional postoperative cisplatin-based chemotherapy after total resection of residual viable cancer will remain free of disease (39).

Salvage Chemotherapy

Despite the dramatic successes of chemotherapy in disseminated disease, 20 to 30% of all such patients will fail to achieve complete remission with first-line therapy. These individuals, as well as those who relapse from complete remission, are candidates for salvage chemotherapy. Because of the decreased efficacy and increased toxicity of second-line chemotherapy, this represents an important decision point in the treatment of such patients and requires the expertise of individuals well versed in the intricacies of therapeutic options for this stage of testicular cancer.

There are several clinical situations that may mimic progressive or recurrent disease, but salvage chemotherapy is not indicated in those patients. One such situation involves the appearance of nodular lesions on chest radiographs or chest CT scans at the end of chemotherapy or soon after completion of such therapy. These nodules may merely represent bleomycin-induced pulmonary injury and are characteristically located in a subpleural region. This possibility should be considered in patients who are otherwise responding serologically or radiographically.

Another clinical situation frequently mistaken for progressive disease is the syndrome of "growing teratoma." In patients with elements of teratomas in their primary lesion, radiographically enlarging metastatic lesions during chemotherapy concurrently with appropriately declining serological markers (as described), are likely to represent the presence of teratomatous elements in these growing lesions. Appropriate management of such patients includes completion of induction chemotherapy with subsequent surgical resection of residual radiographic abnormalities, not administration of salvage chemotherapy.

The therapeutic results with salvage chemotherapy have not been as dramatic as those for initial therapy, due primarily to the paucity of active single agents in patients refractory to cisplatin. During the 2 decades since the introduction of cisplatin, only 2 agents, etoposide (VP16) and ifosfamide, have demonstrated a 25% or greater response in this setting. European studies in the early 1980s established the activity of ifosfamide in testicular cancer, both in minimally and heavily pretreated patients (40–42). Subsequent trials from Indiana University evaluated the role of this agent in refractory disease. Ifosfamide as a single agent in third-line therapy had an objective response rate of 23%, although the median duration of remission was only 3.5 months (43). A trial evaluated combination chemotherapy with ifosfamide + cisplatin + either VP16 (VIP) or vinblastine (VeIP) as third- or fourth-line therapy; 30% of patients achieved a disease-free status (44). These remissions appeared durable, with a median duration of remission of 34 months, and 75% of complete responders remained alive and disease-free at the time of the report. On the basis of these results, ifosfamide combination chemotherapy is being evaluated as first-line therapy in patients with poor-risk disease in an intergroup trial.

High-dose Chemotherapy: Background and Rationale

Preliminary studies using high-dose chemotherapy in patients with refractory germ-cell cancer had mixed results. In early studies using high-dose cyclophosphamide, etoposide, or thiotepa, high rates of response were obtained, but these responses were uniformly brief (45). Subsequent studies in Europe and the United States using principles and chemotherapy combinations more specific to germ-cell cancer had more favorable results. We review recent and current studies using high-dose chemotherapy in germ-cell cancer using supportive autologous bone marrow transplantation, hematopoietic growth factors, and high-dose therapy without specific efforts to modulate myelosuppression. We also discuss implications of current clinical trials and future directions.

Phase II Clinical Trials of Intensive Chemotherapy

A variety of Phase II clinical trials have been performed with the goal of intensifying the dose of available agents in patients with poor-risk germ-cell cancer. Most of these protocols have used very high-dose cisplatin with etoposide, bleomycin, and, frequently, with the addition of agents of unknown efficacy in germ-cell cancer, such as vincristine and methotrexate. These trials have invariably reported superior outcome, and such trials have been held as validation of the concept of dose intensity in germ-cell cancer. These high-dose Phase II trials are summarized in Table 60-2. The dose intensity of the regimen is given relative to standard therapy with bleomycin (30 units weekly × 12), etoposide (100 mg/m^2 every day × 5 for 21 days), and cisplatin (20 mg/m^2 every day × 5 every 21 days) (BEP).

These trials illustrate some of the difficulties in drawing conclusions regarding dose intensity. The investigators used a myriad of classification systems to assign poor risk. Many trials include patients that by other classification systems would be good risk (particularly patients with bulky abdominal disease only). Inclusion of such patients into these poor-risk trials will apparently validate the newer regimen because such patients would have excellent outcome with standard therapy. When reclassified by other more stringent classification systems, response rates diminish and often are comparable to standard therapy. These trials are performed over a long period, thus allowing for other nontreatment-related factors to influence the comparison with historical control subjects (46).

Some of the randomized clinical trials in poor-risk germ-cell cancer require further discussion because they test some basic principles of dose intensity. One important randomized clinical trial of dose intensity in germ-cell cancer is the trial of the Southeastern Cancer Study Group and the Southwest Oncology Study Group (36). Over 4 years, 154 eligible patients with advanced germ-cell cancer were enrolled in this trial. This trial compared treatment with etoposide, bleomycin, and either standard-dose cisplatin (20 mg/m^2 daily × 5) (BEP) or high-dose cisplatin (40 mg/m^2 daily × 5) (BEP-2) every 3 weeks for 4 cycles of treatment.

Of 78 patients entered on the standard-dose cisplatin arm, 77 were eligible and evaluable for survival toxicity and response. Thirty-six patients (47%) had complete responses to chemotherapy, and an additional 20 patients (26%) became free of disease by total resection of teratoma (15 patients) or resection of residual cancer (5 patients). Of the 81 patients entered on the high-dose arm, 76 were eligible and evaluable for survival, toxicity, and response. Thirty-five high-dose patients (45%) obtained complete remission with chemotherapy alone, whereas 16 patients (21%) required surgery to obtain disease-free status (15 teratoma and one cancer). Overall, 73% of patients receiving standard-dose therapy became disease-free, whereas 67% of patients receiving high-dose therapy became disease-free.

Dose-intensity analysis as described by Levin and Hryniuk (47) was performed for each drug in the treatment regimen. Overall dose intensity was calculated for each arm, and comparisons were made for the most important single agent, cisplatin; the 2 most important agents, cisplatin and etoposide; and the overall dose intensity of all 3 agents. In all these analyses, the agents were given equal weight in consideration of dose intensity. The 3 univariate logistical regression analyses investigating the relationship between dose intensity and treatment were unable to conclude that dose intensity had an effect on response (cisplatin, $p = 0.42$; cisplatin and etoposide, $p = 0.33$; cisplatin, etoposide, and bleomycin, $p = 0.15$).

This trial provides one of the best examples of a prospective analysis of dose intensity. The straightforward comparison of one variable (cisplatin dose intensity) simplifies the analysis. The randomized format assured that poor prognostic features (and inherent inability to tolerate aggressive treatment) were distributed equally between the 2 treatment arms. There was a full accounting of dose actually delivered. The young age of the patients and the experience of the investigators allowed for maintenance of dose intensity in both treatment groups. Indeed, the median dose intensity for the entire chemotherapy combination in the standard arm was 0.97. The difference in dose intensity between the 2 arms (0.97 to 1.21) was substantially greater than the usual comparisons of dose intensity, which cluster in the range of 0.6 to 0.8 relative dose intensity. This difference is even more striking when the most important component in the BEP combination, cisplatin, is considered, for which the relative dose

Table 60-2.
Cisplatin/Etoposide-based Therapy in Poor-risk Germ-cell Cancer

Regimen	*Dose Intensity (Relative to BEP)*	*%NED*	*Reference*
Bop/BEP	0.82 + vincristine	66	(65)
BEP	1.00	88	(66)
BEP	1.00	63	(23)
BEP	1.00	73	(36)
BEP-2	1.33	68	(36)
PVeBV × 2 + PEC	1.13 + cytoxan	41	(38)
PVeBV	1.33 + vinblastine	88	(62)
PVeBV	1.33 + vinblastine	61	(38)
BEP	1.61	86	(67)

BEP = bleomycin, etoposide, and cisplatin; BoP = bleomycin vincristine, cisplatin; BEP-2 = bleomycin, etoposide, and double-dose cisplatin; PVeBV = cisplatin, vinblastine, bleomycin, and etoposide; PEC = cisplatin, etoposide, and cyclophosphamide; % NED = no evidence of disease.

intensity was 1.82 to 1.00 in the high dose and standard arm, respectively, or even when the comparison is made with the 2 most important drugs, cisplatin and etoposide, for which the difference in relative dose intensity was 1.35 to 1.00.

The impact of achieving high cisplatin dose intensity in this study was clear. There was a marked increase in ototoxicity, neurotoxicity, gastrointestinal complications, and severe myelosuppression. Therapy-related deaths, although rare, occurred more commonly in the high-dose arm. This increase in therapy-induced toxicity was not compensated by an increase in complete remission rate or survival. With identical therapeutic results achieved with much less toxicity, cisplatin (100–120 mg/m^2/course), etoposide, and bleomycin remains the standard combination for poor-risk germ-cell cancer. Higher doses of cisplatin should not be used outside the context of a controlled clinical trial.

The trials in patients with poor-risk germ-cell cancer highlight two important points in reference to very high-dose chemotherapy in this disease. First, with modern standard-dose chemotherapy, 75% of patients obtain disease-free status. The group at Indiana University has been unable to define any subgroup that had less than a 50% likelihood of successful outcome. Thus, it is extremely unlikely that very high-dose chemotherapy with the attendant risk and expense will impact on the primary care of patients with germ-cell cancer. Second, analysis of dose intensity in therapy of testis cancer suggests that the dose-response relationship is relatively shallow and that minor modifications of doses of existing therapy (20–50% increase in delivered dose intensity) are unlikely to improve therapeutic outcome. More likely, improved results will come with new drug combinations.

Autologous Bone Marrow Transplantation and High-dose Chemotherapy in Germ-cell Neoplasms

Indiana University Studies

Investigations into the use of high-dose carboplatin (CBDCA) and VP16 with autologous bone marrow support began at Indiana University in 1986. Initial investigations were in patients who were heavily pretreated and for whom no other curative therapeutic options existed. Subsequent studies have explored modification of the initial regimen in refractory patients and the efficacy of this regimen in patients in first relapse after conventional therapy. Important insights into the need for patient selection, the particular problem of primary nonseminomatous mediastinal germ-cell tumors, and the value of intervention early in the course of the disease for these toxic, expensive, yet potentially curative modes of therapy have been gained.

The initial Phase I/II dose escalation study examined the use of 2 courses of high-dose CBDCA and VP16 in patients with germ-cell tumors refractory to cisplatin (defined as progression on or within 4 weeks of the last cisplatin dose) or recurrent after a minimum of 2 prior regimens containing cisplatin (48). Thirty-three patients were entered in this trial. The initial 13 patients were treated with escalating doses of CBDCA to establish the maximum tolerated dose in combination with VP16 at a fixed dose of 1,200 mg/m^2. The subsequent 20 patients were treated with VP16 (1,200 mg/m^2) and the Phase II dose of CBDCA (1,500 mg/m^2, given in 3 divided doses on days -7, -5 and -3). Toxicities seen in the protocol were the expected severe myelosuppression, moderate enterocolitis, and stomatitis. Grade 3 hepatic toxicity (more than 5-fold increase in liver enzymes), usually in association with massive infections, was observed in 8 of 33 (24%) patients. Significant ototoxicity, neurotoxicity, or nephrotoxicity were not seen despite extensive prior exposure to cisplatin in this patient population.

Overall, 7 of 33 (21%) patients died as a consequence of treatment, 2 on the Phase II portion of the study. Deaths were primarily due to infection, although one patient died of veno-occlusive disease of the liver. This was a very heavily pretreated patient population; more than half the patients received 3 or more prior chemotherapy regimens, and 67% of patients were cisplatin-refractory. Eight patients obtained a complete remission (CR), and 6 obtained a partial remission (PR), for an overall response rate of 44% (95% confidence intervals, 27–63%). Of the 8 patients obtaining CR, 3 are long-term disease-free survivors, and a fourth patient died at 22 months (free of germ-cell cancer) from a therapy-related acute nonlymphocytic leukemia. Review of responding patients reveals that CR was achieved despite advanced stage or disease refractory to cisplatin.

More recently, an overview of the experience at Indiana University with the first 40 patients with multiple relapsed and refractory germ-cell cancer treated with double autologous transplant demonstrated a 15% long-term disease-free survival (49).

Following the Phase I/II study, a larger multi-institutional Phase II trial was carried out through the Eastern Cooperative Oncology Group (ECOG) utilizing the same dose and schedule of agents as in the Phase II portion of the initial study (50). Patients again had to have failed at least 2 prior cisplatin-based regimens, at least one of which contained ifosfamide, or be cisplatin-refractory. Forty patients were entered in this multi-institution cooperative group effort between July 1988 and September 1989. Two patients were ineligible due to insufficient prior therapy (1) and incorrect histological diagnosis (1). Twenty-two of 38 (58%) evaluable patients proceeded to a second course of high-dose therapy. Toxicity was similar to that seen in the Phase I trial; 5 of 38 (13%) patients died of treatment-related causes (infection, 1; hemorrhage, 2; hepatic toxicity, 2). All treatment-related deaths occurred during the first course of therapy. Other extramyeloid toxicities were comparable to those seen in the initial study. Nine patients (24%) achieved a CR, including 2 patients disease-free with post-BMT surgical resection; 8 achieved a PR, for an overall response rate of 45%. Three of the CRs occurred after the first BMT, and 4 patients converted to CR after the second BMT. Five of 9 are alive and free of disease with a minimum follow-up of 18 months. Of note, all PRs recurred, with a median duration of remission of 2.5 months. Achievement of a CR was associated with testicular rather than extragonadal primary disease, absence of liver metastases, and embryonal cell type.

A striking finding in this study was the poor outcome in patients with nonseminomatous mediastinal germ-cell tumors. Eleven patients with this diagnosis were enrolled in this study and none obtained durable remission. This finding parallels the institutional experience at Indiana University with patients with nonseminomatous mediastinal germ-cell tumors treated in second or greater relapse with high-dose chemotherapy and autologous BMT (51). Since 1987, 12 such patients were treated on serial protocols of high-dose CBDCA/VP16 ± ifosfamide. Seven of the 12 failed to receive the planned second course of therapy due to tumor progression or therapy-related toxicity. No patient achieved a CR, and the median survival after high-dose chemotherapy was 3.5 months. This subgroup has been identified as having poor outcome with other conventional salvage therapies, and such patients should be the focus of investigation of new approaches in treatment (52). At Indiana University, patients with primary mediastinal germ-cell tumors who fail primary therapy are treated with 2 rounds of high-dose CBDCA/VP16 with high-dose ifosfamide, as initial salvage therapy.

Results with high-dose CBDCA/VP16/autologous BMT in patients with recurrent and refractory germ-cell cancer indicate that a fraction of patients could be rendered permanently disease-free. In view of the known activity of ifosfamide in recurrent and refractory germ-cell tumors and its favorable side-effect profile for dose escalation in the setting of BMT, investigators at Indiana University added high-dose ifosfamide to the CBDCA/VP16 treatment template. Ifosfamide, as a single agent, has been shown to produce responses in patients with recurrent and cisplatin-resistant germ-cell cancer (43). Seven patients were entered in a Phase II trial of CBDCA/VP16 in the previously described doses and schedule with the addition of ifosfamide beginning at 10 gm/m^2 daily × 5 with mesna (53). The patients were treated with one or 2 courses of high-dose therapy. Due to excessive renal toxicity at the first dose level, escalation of the ifosfamide dose was impossible. Of the 7 patients treated, 4 had a marked decline in their renal function; 3 of the 4 required hemofiltration or hemodialysis. Six of the 7 patients had decline of serum biomarkers, indicating a response to treatment, but all responses have been brief, perhaps due to the truncated treatment course necessitated by the toxicity encountered.

Recent trials include further attempts to escalate doses of CBDCA and VP16 in patients with refractory germ-cell tumors. Escalation has been possible because patients currently undergoing this therapy are much less heavily pretreated than those in the initial Phase I trial. Thirty-two patients were on a careful dose escalation of each of these agents. The maximum tolerated dose level was 700 mg/m^2 carboplatin and 750 mg/m^2 VP16 given daily on days -6, -5, and -4. Dose-limiting toxicity for this regimen was mucositis. There were 5 treatment-related deaths; 4 due to sepsis and multiorgan failure and one due to central nervous system hemorrhage. Future directions in these patients will focus on attempts to improve the therapeutic index by exploring new agents, both alkylating agents and new platinum analogues, development of a second "noncross-resistant" regimen for use in the double autologous transplant setting, and use of newer cytokines to improve supportive care.

In the treatment of acute leukemia, bone marrow transplantation was used initially in end-stage, heavily treated patients with refractory disease. In this setting, a small response rate was observed with few long-term survivors (54). When this treatment was used in more favorable, less heavily treated patients, toxicity diminished, response rates improved, and more cures were seen. Similarly, use of high-dose therapy with autologous bone marrow transplantation in the treatment of multiply relapsed and refractory testicular cancer has resulted in an overall response rate of approximately 50% and approximately 15 to 20% cures. A logical extension of this concept is to employ high-dose therapy earlier in the sequence of treatment of recurrent germ-cell cancer.

Because the overall cure rate for recurrent testis cancer with ifosfamide-cisplatin–based therapy is 20 to 25%, the proper next investigation seems to be incorporation of high-dose chemotherapy as a component of initial salvage therapy. A recent pilot survey at Indiana University enrolled 25 patients with cisplatin-sensitive disease; they were treated with conventional salvage therapy (usually vinblastine, ifosfamide, and cisplatin [VeLP]) for 2 courses, followed by a single course of high-dose carboplatin and VP16. Several preliminary results of this trial merit emphasis.

First, only one patient suffered a therapy-related death, and this patient died due to acute renal failure associated with sepsis after the first course of VeLP. Thus, there were no transplant-related deaths in this series. Only 7 of the 25 patients enrolled did not enter the transplantation portion of the protocol (one VeLP death; 2 refusal, 2 progressive disease; 2 patients in whom insurance coverage was denied). Of the 18 patients completing the protocol, 10 (56%) obtained a CR, one obtained disease-free status by resection of residual cancer, and 5 (28%) obtained a PR, for an overall response rate of 88%. Two of the 18 patients proceeding to transplantation actually required 2 transplantations for sluggish decline in serum biomarkers. Of the 7 patients not proceeding to transplantation, onc obtained a CR and one patient a PR, for an overall response rate of 28%. The response rate for all patients entering the protocol was 16 of 25 (72%). Twelve of the 25 patients remain without disease at a median follow-up of 19 months. It is unclear that these results are superior to conventional salvage approaches because these patients were highly selected, but the excellent tolerance of therapy and the high response rate are encouraging.

A number of conclusions can be drawn from the series of studies performed at Indiana University. First, a small percentage of patients with multiply relapsed or cisplatin-resistant germ-cell cancer can be cured with high-dose chemotherapy. Second, the initial attempt to increase the therapeutic ratio of the regimen with the addition of ifosfamide was unsuccessful in this patient population. Furthermore, analysis of prognostic factors from these and other studies suggest that patients with primary mediastinal nonseminomatous germ-cell cancer have a particularly poor prognosis and such patients should be entered into clinical trials of more intense therapy or combinations with newer agents.

Institut Gustave-Roussy Studies

Similar studies from other institutions provide further substantiation of the curative potential of high-dose chemotherapy in refractory germ-cell cancer. Serial studies at the Institut Gustave-Roussy (IGR) demonstrated activity in recurrent germ-cell cancer. These investigators developed a regimen using cisplatin (40 mg/m^2, day 1–5), etoposide (350 mg/m^2, day 1–5), and cyclophosphamide (CY) (1,600 mg/m^2, day 2–5) (PEC). Sixteen patients with recurrent germ-cell cancer were enrolled (55). All had received prior therapy with cisplatin-based treatments. Five of the 15 evaluable for response were long-term survivors. The succeeding study enrolled untreated patients believed to be at high risk of treatment failure with conventional therapy (56). Brief conventional induction therapy was followed by a single round of high-dose chemotherapy with PEC. Of 32 poor-risk patients entered, 15 remain free of disease at a median follow-up of 18 months.

Other European Studies

Nichols and colleagues (57) expanded the CBDCA/VP16 skeleton with the addition of ifosfamide. In this study, 21 patients were entered after failing primary, and often, secondary chemotherapy. In addition to the CBDCA and VP16 as given at Indiana University, ifosfamide was added at a dose of 12 gm/m^2 over 3 days. No significant renal toxicity was encountered in this study. Thirteen of the 21 patients received one course, 7 received 2 courses, and one received 3 courses. There was one therapy-related death due to veno-occlusive disease. There were 8 CRs ranging from one to 33 months. Five of the CRs are ongoing.

A preliminary report from Linkesch and colleagues (58) in Austria combines features of the PEC protocol and the protocols from Indiana University along with recombinant granulocyte-macrophage colony stimulating factor (GM-CSF). In this study, high-dose chemotherapy with carboplatin (2,000 gm/m^2), VP16 (1,500 mg/m^2), and CY(60 mg/kg × 2) was given to patients with recurrent and refractory germ-cell cancer. All patients were deemed incurable with standard therapy and 62% had advanced disease by the Indiana University classification system. Twelve patients received the high-dose chemotherapy with autologous bone marrow rescue, and an additional 30 patients received the same treatment with hematopoietic growth factors along with autologous BMT. The hematological toxicity appeared to be successfully modulated by the use of recombinant GM-CSF or G-CSF. Of the 12 patients receiving therapy without the hematopoietic growth factor, the median time to an absolute granulocyte count greater than 500 was 20 days, compared with 13 days for the 30 patients receiving identical therapy plus GM-CSF. The median time of isolation was longer in the control group of patients (25 days), compared with 18 days in the group receiving hematopoietic growth factors. Nonhematological toxicity included grade 3 and 4 diarrhea in 9 patients, renal toxicity in 3 and liver toxicity in 2. There was no significant neurotoxicity or cardiac toxicity and there were 3 therapy-related deaths. Response was assessed in 38 patients and reported by state of disease at time of transplant. In patients with recurrent disease, 11 of 17 patients (64%) obtained remission, including 5 PRs and 6 CRs. In patients with refractory disease, 10 of 15 (67%) obtained a response, including 7 CRs. Of the 6 patients with progressive disease on chemotherapy, only one obtained a brief PR. Of the patients obtaining CR, 10 of 13 remain in CR, of whom 7 have been disease-free for more than one year.

High-dose Chemotherapy as Initial Salvage Treatment

There is now ample evidence that high-dose chemotherapy (PEC; high-dose CBDCA/VP16) can cure patients who are incurable with conventional salvage regimens. However, in this heavily pretreated population, the impact of such therapy has been small (15–20% long-term disease-free survivors) and toxicity has been substantial. The next logical step in the development of better therapy for patients with germ-cell cancer is to consider use of such high-dose treatments earlier in the course of recurrent disease, prior to the development of bulky drug-resistant disease and at a time when performance status and organ function are maintained.

One of the first reports of such an approach is from Barnett and colleagues (59) at the Cancer Control Agency of British Columbia. These investigators reported the results of using high-dose chemotherapy as part of initial salvage chemotherapy. In this trial, 18 patients with recurrent or persistent germ-cell cancer after cisplatin-based primary therapy were given conventional induction chemotherapy with cisplatin,

VP16, vincristine, and bleomycin, given on a weekly schedule, or vinblastine, ifosfamide, cisplatin combinations. At the completion of conventional salvage chemotherapy, consolidation with high-dose chemotherapy was given with autologous bone marrow support. Patients received high-dose carboplatin, VP16, and either high-dose CY or ifosfamide. There were 2 toxic deaths, 2 patients were too early to evaluate, and 8 of 14 remained free of germ-cell cancer progression.

Siegert and colleagues (60), in Germany, reported the results of high-dose carboplatin, VP16, and ifosfamide in the treatment of recurrent testicular cancer. Patients had received a median of 6 cycles of cisplatin-based chemotherapy. Patients were given 2 induction courses of conventional-dose cisplatin, VP16, and ifosfamide prior to receiving escalated therapy. Fifty-five patients received treatment with conventional therapy followed by carboplatin (1,500–2,000 mg/m^2), VP16 (1,200–2,400 mg/m^2), ifosfamide (0–10 gm/m^2). Two patients died related to treatment. Responses included 12 patients (21%) with CR and 16 patients (28%) with marker-negative PR. Twenty-one of these patients (38%) have maintained their response from 3+ to 26+ months. Although the precise degree of chemotherapy resistance in this patient population was not given, it is encouraging that a high percentage of recurrent patients remain progression-free.

The Eastern Cooperative Oncology Group has begun a similar trial in which patients with recurrent germ-cell cancer (noncisplatin-resistant) receive 2 courses of conventional salvage chemotherapy (VIP or PVB). Responding patients will then receive a single round of high-dose VP16 and carboplatin as described earlier. Relative to the preceding ECOG trial, this trial will enter a group of patients who have much less prior therapy, have better performance status, and have responding smaller volume disease.

High-dose Chemotherapy as Primary Treatment of Germ-cell Cancer

Memorial Sloan-Kettering Cancer Center has begun to use high-dose chemotherapy as a portion of initial treatment in selected patients (61). Patients are given conventional chemotherapy (VAB-6), and those patients in whom there is a suboptimal decline in serum HCG or AFP levels after 2 to 3 cycles of treatment are given CBDCA/VP16 with autologous marrow support. To date, the majority of patients entered in the protocol have required transplantation and there is early evidence of improved outcome relative to a comparable group of patients from earlier trials. To date, 16 patients have been treated with CBDCA/VP16 after suboptimal response to VAB-6. Nine patients (56%) have obtained a CR and 8 remain free of disease ranging from 8+ to 27+ months. These reports compare favorably to a similar prognostic group treated with VAB-6 alone, in whom only 14% had durable response to treatment.

Investigators at Institut Gustave-Roussy IGR recently completed a Phase III trial testing the addition of high-dose chemotherapy to conventional-dose induction therapy for patients with untreated poor-risk germ-cell cancer. Patients with poor-risk features as assigned by the IGR prognostic system were randomly allocated to receive PVeBV, as described by Ozols and colleagues (62), or a modified PVeBV × 2 cycles followed by high-dose intensification with PEC (62). Preliminary results suggest no benefit for patients receiving high-dose intensification. Of 49 patients randomized to receive PVeBV × 4, there were 2 early deaths and one refusal. Complete response was obtained in 30 of 49 (61%) patients, and 82% of patients were 2-year survivors. Of 53 patients randomized to 2 cycles of modified PVeBV plus consolidation, there were 8 early deaths and 2 refusals. Complete response was obtained in 21 of 53 (41%) patients, and 61% of patients were 2-year survivors. A statistically significant improvement in CRs ($p = 0.01$) and a trend toward improved survival ($p = 0.1$) were seen in the standard arm relative to the "dose-intense" arm.

Whether high-dose chemotherapy will become a component of standard initial therapy in poor-risk patients with germ-cell cancer remains to be seen. The difficulty in reliably identifying a subgroup of patients with very poor outcome and the relative rarity of these malignancies will complicate these clinical investigations. The growing concerns regarding the role of high-dose VP16 in the development of unique therapy-related leukemias may further diminish the enthusiasm for moving high-dose therapy into primary treatment for a group of patients who generally do well with conventional treatment (63,64). However, the poor results of currently available salvage treatments certainly justifies incorporation of newer higher risk approaches for this patient population.

References

1. Drain L. Testicular cancer in California from 1942–1969: the California Tumor Registry experience. Oncology 1973;27:45–51.
2. Shibley L, Brown M, Schuttinga J, Rothenberg M, Whalen J. Cisplatin-based combination chemotherapy in the treatment of advanced-stage testicular cancer: cost-benefit analysis. J Natl Cancer Inst 1990;82:186–192.
3. Einhorn L. Treatment of testicular cancer: a new and improved model. J Clin Oncol 1990;8:1777–1781.
4. Dixon F, Moore R. In: Dixon F, Moore R, eds. Atlas of tumor pathology. Washington, DC: Armed Forces Institute of Pathology, 1952:31B:section 8.
5. Smith R. Management of testicular seminoma. In: Skinner D, deKernion J, eds. Genitourinary cancer. Philadelphia: W.B. Saunders, 1978:460–468.
6. Sulak M. Testicular tumors. Classification of different pathologic types. JAMA 1970;213:91–93.
7. Johnson D, Gomez J, Ayala A. Anaplastic seminoma. J Urol 1975;114:80–82.
8. Janssen M, Johnston W. Anaplastic seminoma of the testis: ultrastructural analysis of 3 cases. Cancer 1978;41:538–544.
9. Jacobsen G, Nrgaard-Pederson B. Placental alkaline

phosphatase in testicular germ cell tumors and in carcinoma in-situ of the testis. An immunohistochemical study. Acta Pathol Microbiol Immunol Scand 1984;92:323–329.
10. Javadpour N, Mclntire K, Waldmann T, Bergman S. The role of alpha-fetoprotein and human chorionic gonadotropin in seminoma. J Urol 1978;120:687–690.
11. Kuber W, Kratzik C, Schwarz H, Susani, Spona J. Experience with beta-HCG-positive seminoma. Br J Urol 1983;55:555–559.
12. Swartz D, Johnson D, Hussey D. Should an elevated human chorionic gonadotropin titer alter therapy for seminoma? J Urol 1984;131:63–65.
13. Mostofi F. Testicular tumors: epidemiologic, etiologic and pathologic features. Cancer 1973;32:1186–1201.
14. Teilum G. Special tumors of ovary and testis. In: Comparative pathology and histological identification. Philadelphia: J.B. Lippincott, 1977:31.
15. Drago J, Nelson RP, Palmer J. Childhood embryonal carcinoma of the testis. Urology 1978;12:499–503.
16. Hessl J. Orchidoblastoma or infantile embryonal carcinoma. Urology 1975;5:265–269.
17. Nichols C, Saxman S, Wiliams S, et al. Primary mediastinal nonseminomatous germ cell tumors: a modern single institution experience. Cancer 1990; 65:1641–1646.
18. Ahlgren A, Simrell R, Triche T, Ozols R, Barsky S. Sarcoma arising in a residual testicular teratoma after cytoreductive chemotherapy. Cancer 1984;54:2015–2018.
19. Ahmed T, Bosl G, Hajdu S. Teratoma with malignant transformation in germ cell tumors in men. Cancer 1985;56:860–863.
20. Ulbright T, Loehrer P, Roth L, Einhorn L, Williams S, Clark S. The development of non-germ cell malignancies within germ cell tumor. A clinicopathologic study in 11 cases. Cancer 1984;54:1824–1833.
21. Einhorn L, Donohue J. Cis-diamminedichloroplatinum, vinblastine, and bleomycin combination chemotherapy in disseminated testicular cancer. Ann Intern Med 1977;87:293–298.
22. Roth BJ, Greist A, Kubilis PS, Williams SD, Einhorn LH. Cisplatin-based combination chemotherapy for disseminated germ cell tumors: long-term follow-up. J Clin Oncol 1988;6:1239–1247.
23. Williams S, Birch R, Einhorn L, Irwin L, Greco F, Loehrer P. Treatment of disseminated germ cell tumors with cisplatin, bleomycin, and either vinblastine or etoposide. N Engl J Med 1987;316:1435–1440.
24. Ozols R, Diesseroth A, Javadpour N, Barlock A, Messerschmidt G, Young R. Treatment of poor prognosis non-seminomatous testicular cancer with a "high-dose" platinum combination chemotherapy regimen. Cancer 1983;51:1803–1807.
25. Stoter G, Kaye S, Sleyfer D, et al. Preliminary results of BEP (bleomycin, etoposide, cisplatin) versus an alternating regimen of BEP and PVB (cisplatin, vinblastine, bleomycin) in high volume metastatic testicular nonseminomas. An EORTC study. Proc Am Soc Clin Oncol 1986;5:106.
26. Bosl G, Geller N, Cirrincione C, et al. Multivariate analysis of prognostic variables in patients with metastatic testicular cancer. Cancer Res 1983;43:3403.
27. Birch R, Wiliams S, Cone A, et al. Prognostic factors for favorable outcome in disseminated germ cell tumors. J Clin Oncol 1986;4:400–407.
28. Horwich A, Stenning S, Mead B, et al. Prognostic factors for survival in advanced non-seminomatous germ cell tumours. Proc Am Soc Clin Oncol 1990;9:132.
29. Medical Research Council Working Party on Testicular Tumours. Prognostic factors in advanced non-seminomatous germ-cell testicular tumours: results of a multicentre study. Lancet 1985;1:8–11.
30. Vaeth M, Schultz H, von der Maase H, Engelholm S, Krag Jacobsen G, Norgaard-Pedersen B. Prognostic factors in testicular germ cell tumours: experiences from 1058 consecutive cases. Acta Radiol Oncol 1984;23:271–285.
31. Sledge G, Eble J, Roth B, Wuhrman B, Fineberg N, Einhorn L. Relation of proliferative activity to survival in patients with advanced germ cell cancer. Cancer Res 1988;48:3864–3868.
32. Einhorn LH, Williams SD, Loehrer PJ, et al. Evaluation of optimal duration of chemotherapy in favorable-prognosis disseminated germ cell tumors: a Southeastern Cancer Study Group protocol. J Clin Oncol 1989;7:387–391.
33. Bosl G, Geller N, Bajorin D, et al. A randomized trial of etoposide + cisplatin versus vinblastine + bleomycin + cisplatin + cyclophosphamide + dactinomycin in patients with good-prognosis germ cell tumors. J Clin Oncol 1988;6:1231–1238.
34. Bajorin DF, Sarosdy MF, Bosl GJ, Weisen S, Heller G. A randomized trial of etoposide + carboplatin (EC) vs. etoposide + cisplatin (EP) in patients with metastatic germ cell tumors. Proc Am Soc Clin Oncol 1991;10:168.
35. Loehrer PJ, Elson P, Johnson DH, Williams SD, Trump DL, Einhorn LH. A randomized trial of cisplatin plus etoposide with or without bleomycin in favorable prognosis disseminated germ cell tumors. Proc Am Soc Clin Oncol 1991;10:169.
36. Nichols C, Williams S, Loehrer P, et al. Randomized study of cisplatin dose intensity in advanced germ cell tumors: a Southeastern Cancer Study Group and Southwest Oncology Group protocol. J Clin Oncol 1991;9:1163–1172.
37. Sampson MK, Rivkin SE, Jones SE, et al. Dose-response and dose-survival advantage for high versus low-dose cisplatin combined with vinblastine and bleomycin in disseminated testicular cancer. A Southwest Oncology Group study. Cancer 1984;53:1029–1035.
38. Droz J, Pico J, Biron P, et al. No evidence of a benefit of early intensified chemotherapy (HDCT) with autologous bone marrow transplantation (ABMT) in first line treatment of poor risk non seminomatous germ cell tumors. Proc Am Soc Clin Oncol 1992;11:197.
39. Fox E, Einhorn L, Weathers T, Williams S, Donohue J. Outcome analysis for patients with persistent germ cell carcinoma in post chemotherapy (PC) retroperitoneal lymph node dissections (RPLND). Proc Am Soc Clin Oncol 1992;11:198.
40. Schmoll H. The role of ifosfamide in testicular cancer. In: Brade WP, Nagel GA, Seevers S, eds. Ifosfamide in tumor therapy. Basel: Karger, 1987:234–255.
41. Scheulen M, Niederle N, Hoffken K, Schutte J, Seeber S, Schmidt C. Ifosfamide/Mesna alone or in combination with etoposide: salvage therapy for patients with metastasized nonseminomatous testicular cancer. Proc Am Soc Clin Oncol 1985;4:97.
42. Aiginger P, Schwartz H, Kuzmits R. Ifosfamide and cisplatin in testicular tumor patients resistant to vinblastine, bleomycin, cisplatinum. 13th International Cancer Congress 1982;13:180.
43. Wheeler B, Loehrer P, Williams S, Einhorn L. Ifos-

famide in refractory male germ cell tumors. J Clin Oncol 1986;4:28–34.

44. Loehrer PJ, Lauer R, Roth BJ, Williams SD, Kalasinski LA, Einhorn LH. Salvage therapy in recurrent germ cell cancer: ifosfamide and cisplatin plus either vinblastine or etoposide. Ann Intern Med 1988;109:540–546.
45. Cheson B, Lacerna L, Leyland-Jones B, Sarosy G, Wittes R. Autologous bone marrow transplantation: current status and future directions. Ann Intern Med 1989;110:51–65.
46. Bosl GJ, Geller NL, Chan EYW. Stage migration and the increasing proportion of complete responders in patients with advanced germ cell tumors. Cancer Res 1988;48:3524–3527.
47. Levin L, Hryniuk WM. Dose-intensity analysis of chemotherapy regimens in ovarian carcinoma. J Clin Oncol 1987;5:756–767.
48. Nichols CR, Tricot G, Williams SD, et al. Dose-intensive chemotherapy in refractory germ cell cancer—a phase I/II trial of high dose carboplatin and etoposide with autologous bone marrow transplantation. J Clin Oncol 1989;7:932–939.
49. Broun E, Nichols C, Kneebone P, et al. Long term outcome of patients with relapsed and refractory germ cell tumors treated with high dose chemotherapy and autologous bone marrow rescue. Ann Intern Med 1993; 117:124–128.
50. Nichols C, Andersen J, Lazarus H, et al. High-dose carboplatin and etoposide with autologous bone marrow transplantation in refractory germ cell cancer: an Eastern Cooperative Oncology Group protocol. J Clin Oncol 1992;10:558–563.
51. Broun E, Nichols G, Einhorn L, Tricot G. Salvage therapy with high dose chemotherapy and autologous bone marrow support in the treatment of primary nonseminomatous mediastinal germ cell tumors (EGG CT). Cancer 1991;68:1513–1515.
52. Munshi N, Loehrer P, Williams S, et al. Ifosfamide combination salvage chemotherapy in extragonadal germ cell tumors (EGGCT). Proc Am Soc Clin Oncol 1991;10:182.
53. Broun E, Nichols C, Tricot G, Loehrer P, Williams S, Einhorn L. High dose carboplatin/VP-16 plus ifosfamide with autologous bone marrow support in the treatment of refractory germ cell tumors. Bone Marrow Transplant 1991;7:53–56.
54. Thomas ED, Buckner CD, Banaji M, et al. One hundred patients with acute leukemia treated by chemotherapy, total body irradiation, and allogeneic marrow transplantation. Blood 1977;49:511–533.
55. Pico J, Droz J, Gouyette A, et al. 25 high dose chemotherapy regimens (HDCT) followed by autologous bone marrow transplantation for treatment of relapsed or refractory germ cell tumors. Proc Am Soc Clin Oncol 1986;5:111.
56. Droz J, Pico J, Ghosn M, et al. High complete remission (CR) and survival rates in poor prognosis (PP) non seminomatous germ cell tumors (NSGCT) with high dose chemotherapy (HDCT) and autologous bone marrow transplantation (ABMT). Proc Am Soc Clin Oncol 1989;8:130.
57. Nichols C, Rosti G. Dose-intensive therapy for germ cell neoplasms. Semin Oncol 1992;19:145–149.
58. Linkesch W, Krainer M, Wagner A. Phase I/II trial of ultrahigh carboplatin, etoposide, cyclophosphamide with ABMT in refractory or relapsed non-seminomatous germ cell tumors (NSGCT). Proc Am Soc Clin Oncol 1992;11:196.
59. Barnett M, Coppin C, Murray N, et al. Intensive therapy and autologous bone marrow transplantation (BMT) for patients with poor prognosis nonseminomatous germ cell tumors. Proc Am Soc Clin Oncol 1991;10:165.
60. Siegert W, Beyer J, Weisbach V, et al. High dose carboplatin (C), etoposide (E) and ifosfamide (I) with autologous stem cell rescue (ASCR) for relapsed and refractory non-seminomatous germ cell tumors (NSG CT). Proc Am Soc Clin Oncol 1991;10:163.
61. Motzer R, Gulati S, Crown J, et al. High-dose chemotherapy and autologous bone marrow rescue for patients with refractory germ cell tumors: early intervention is better tolerated. Cancer 1992;69:550–556.
62. Ozols RF, Ihde DC, Linehan M, Jacob J, Ostchega Y, Young RC. A randomized trial of standard chemotherapy vs a high-dose chemotherapy regimen in the treatment of poor prognosis nonseminomatous germ-cell tumors. J Clin Oncol 1988;6:1031–1040.
63. Nichols C, Breeden E, Loehrer P, Williams S, Einhorn L. Secondary leukemia associated with standard dose etoposide: review of serial germ cell tumor protocols. N Engl J Med 1993.
64. Pedersen-Bjergaard J, Hansen S, Larsen S, Daugaard G, Philip P, Rorth M. Increased risk of myelodysplasia and leukaemia after etoposide, cisplatin and bleomycin for germ cell-tumours. Lancet 1991;338:359–363.

Chapter 61
Neuroblastomas

Robert C. Seeger and C. Patrick Reynolds

Neuroblastoma, a tumor of the peripheral nervous system, is the most common extracranial solid tumor of childhood, with an incidence of 1 per 7,000 children under the age of 15 years (1). Forty percent of patients have low- or intermediate-risk tumors, and they nearly all become long-term, disease-free survivors with only observation or with conventional therapy, which includes surgery alone or surgery with local irradiation and chemotherapy. Sixty percent have high-risk tumors, and conventional treatment of these patients infrequently results in long-term survival (2). Recent studies utilizing autologous bone marrow transplantation (BMT) show that some high-risk patients can become long-term survivors after induction with chemotherapy and consolidation with myeloablative chemotherapy or chemoradiotherapy (3). However, recurrent tumor develops in many patients after myeloablative therapy even though they achieve a complete clinical remission. Further improvement in survival may result from intensifying induction and consolidation therapy and from developing complementary therapy that can be given with or after induction and consolidation therapy.

This chapter reviews the diagnosis of neuroblastomas and the definition of risk groups. It then discusses myeloablative consolidation therapy and autologous BMT in the context of combined modality treatment, which also includes induction chemotherapy, surgery, and local irradiation. Future strategies that may further improve survival, including postautologous BMT therapy, are also considered.

Diagnosis and Identification of Risk Groups

Neuroblastomas usually occur in early childhood; 85% of patients are diagnosed in the first 6 years and 50% in the first 2 years of life (4). The primary tumor arises within the sympathetic nervous system and can present as a neck, mediastinal, abdominal, or pelvic mass (4–7). Fifty percent of patients have metastases at diagnosis, most commonly in bone marrow, bone, liver, and lymph nodes (5–7). The histology of primary or metastatic tumor tissue is usually diagnostic, although the appearance can vary (8–10). If light microscopy reveals ganglion cells or pseudorosettes, the tumor is a neuroblastoma. In the absence of such features, electron microscopic demonstration of dense-core neurosecretory granules excludes Ewing's sarcoma, rhabdomyosarcoma, and lymphoma (10) but does not exclude peripheral primitive neuroectodermal tumors (PNETs), which can also have these ultrastructural features (11–13). However, increased catecholamine metabolites in the urine of a patient with histological evidence of a small, round-cell tumor (from tumor tissue or bone marrow metastases) establishes a diagnosis of neuroblastoma (7,8). Nearly 85% of patients with neuroblastomas have elevated levels of homovanillic acid (HVA), which is formed from dopamine, or vanylmandellic acid (VMA), which is formed from norepinephrine, in their urine; approximately 95% have elevations of one or the other (7). Peripheral PNETs (e.g., Askin's tumor, peripheral neuroepithelioma, esthesioneuroblastoma) do not produce catecholamines (13). Cell surface antigens, oncogene activation, karyotype, and morphology in vitro can aid in establishing a diagnosis for those few patients whose tumors are not readily identified (7).

Analysis of risk factors at the time of diagnosis is essential for selecting appropriate therapy (4,14–16). A major determinant of risk is the clinical stage of disease at diagnosis (4). Assessment of the extent of disease utilizes chest radiography; computed tomography or magnetic resonance imaging of the chest, abdomen, and pelvis; skeletal survey or ^{99m}Tc-diphosphonate bone scan; ^{131}I-metaiodobenzylguanidine (MIBG) scan; and bilateral iliac crest bone marrow aspiration and trephine biopsy (8). Although several clinical staging systems have been employed, the two most commonly used are defined in Table 61-1 (8,17,18). The International Neuroblastoma Staging System (INSS) was recently developed to provide common criteria for worldwide use (8).

Subsets of patients within the same clinical stage but with different risks can be defined according to age (4), tumor N-*myc* gene amplification (14), histopathology (9), tumor DNA ploidy (19,20), and serum markers (21,22). Recently, other prognostic markers also have been reported but have not been tested extensively. These markers include expression of *mdr-1* P-glycoprotein (23), c-*Ha ras* p21 (24), pp60$^{c\text{-}src}$ (25),

Table 61-1.
Clinical Staging Systems for Defining Extent of Disease at Diagnosis

Evans/CCSG Staging System[17,18]	
Stage I	Tumor confined to the organ or structure of origin.
Stage II	Tumor extending in continuity beyond the organ or structure of origin but not crossing the midline. Regional lymph nodes on the homolateral side may be involved.
Stage III	Tumors extending in continuity beyond the midline. Regional lymph nodes bilaterally may be involved.
Stave IV	Remote disease involving bone, parenchymatous organs, soft tissues, distant lymph node groups, or marrow.
Stage IV-S	Patients who would otherwise be stage I or II but who have remote disease confined to one or more of the following sites: liver, skin, or marrow (without evidence of bone metastases).
International Neuroblastoma Staging Systems (INSS)[8]	
Stage I	Localized tumor confined to the area of origin; complete gross excision, with or without microscopic residual disease; identifiable ipsilateral and contralateral lymph nodes negative microscopically.
Stage 2A	Unilateral tumor with incomplete gross excision; identifiable ipsilateral and contralateral lymph nodes negative microscopically.
Stage 2B	Unilateral tumor with complete or incomplete gross excision; with positive ipsilateral regional lymph nodes; identifiable contralateral lymph nodes negative microscopically.
Stage 3	Tumor infiltrating across the midline with or without regional lymph node involvement; or unilateral tumor with contralateral regional lymph node involvement; or midline tumor with bilateral regional lymph node involvement.
Stage 4	Dissemination of tumor to distant lymph nodes, bone, marrow; liver, or other organs (except as defined in stage 4-S).
Stage 4-S	Localized primary tumor as defined for stage 1 or 2, with dissemination limited to liver, skin, or marrow.

gp140[trk] (high-affinity nerve growth factor receptor (26–28), *nm23*/nucleoside diphosphate kinase (29); loss of heterozygosity for chromosome 1p (30); chromosome telomeric length (31); and occult marrow metastases (32).

Using clinical and laboratory analyses, low-, intermediate-, and high-risk groups can be identified among newly diagnosed patients (Table 61-2) (2,7). Approximately 60% of children with neuroblastomas are at high risk for development of fatal progressive disease. This group includes those older than 1 year at diagnosis with stage IV disease (INSS stage 4) and those with tumors that have amplification of the N-*myc* proto-oncogene. Fewer than 10% of patients with high-risk disease achieve long-term survival with conventional chemotherapy even though many initially respond (5,6,14,15). Thus, maximally intensive induction and consolidation therapy is currently appropriate for these patients.

Treatment of High-risk Neuroblastomas

Once it is determined that a newly diagnosed patient has a high-risk neuroblastoma, a comprehensive plan for intensive, multimodal therapy must be developed and initiated. Cure of high-risk neuroblastomas requires destruction or removal of 10^{11} to 10^{12} tumor cells by combined modality therapy (3). The usual plan includes an induction phase, during which chemotherapy, surgery, and local irradiation are used for reduction of mass disease, and a consolidation phase, during which high-dose therapy is given in an effort to eliminate remaining tumor cells. During the past 10 years, autologous or allogeneic BMT has been used for hematopoietic reconstitution after consolidation with high-dose, myeloablative chemotherapy or chemoradiotherapy (3). A plan for treating high-risk neuroblastomas, which utilizes autologous BMT, is shown in Table 61-3.

A number of studies performed in the 1980s that used myeloablative therapy and autologous BMT suggest that long-term disease-free survival (>5 years) may be achieved in 20 to 40% of patients (3). Although this rate of survival is better than that achieved in the 1970s with conventional chemotherapy (33), contem-

Table 61-2.
Definition of Risk Groups.

Low risk (survival > 80–100% with surgery alone)
- All stage I[a]
- Stage II
  - *without* amplification of N-*myc*
- Stage IV-S
  - *without* amplification of N-*myc*

Intermediate risk (survival > 80% with surgery, conventional chemotherapy, ± local irradiation)
- Stage III
  - *without* amplification of N-*myc*
  - *without* elevated serum ferritin or neuron-specific enolase
  - *with* no or few occult tumor cells in marrow by immunocytology
  - *with* favorable histopathology (Shimada)
- Stage IV (diagnosed < 1 year of age)
  - *without* amplification of N-*myc*
  - *without* elevated serum ferritin or neuron-specific enolase
  - *with* no or few of occult tumor cells in marrow by immunocytology
  - *with* hyperdiploid DNA content
  - *with* favorable histopathology

High risk (survival < 10–15% with conventional chemotherapy, surgery, ± local irradiation)
- Stage IV (diagnosed at 1 year of age or older)
- Any clinical stage or age
  - *with* N-*myc* amplification

[a]Evans/CCSG staging system[17,18].

Table 61-3.
General Plan for Treatment of High-risk Neuroblastomas

Induction phase
Chemotherapy
Bone marrow harvest, purging, and cryopreservation
Surgery and local irradiation
Consolidation phase
Myeloablative therapy + autologous bone marrow transplantation
Postconsolidation phase
No therapy or biological therapy

porary nonmyeloablative regimens utilizing hematopoietic growth factors for hematological support may give improved results (34–40). A randomized comparison of myeloablative versus nonmyeloablative consolidation therapy after uniform induction chemotherapy is being performed by the Childrens Cancer Group, but results will not be available until 1994 (Matthay K. Personal communication). Without question, however, patients with high-risk disease should receive aggressive induction and consolidation therapy, preferably in the context of a multi-institution clinical trial. Because there is a relatively large experience with myeloablative consolidation therapy and autologous BMT and because therapy-related mortality with this procedure is not substantially higher than aggressive nonmyeloablative consolidation therapy, it is reasonable to consider autologous BMT as one of the standard treatments for high-risk neuroblastomas.

Induction Phase: Induction Chemotherapy, Autologous Marrow Cryopreservation, Surgery, Local Irradiation

Induction-phase therapy aims for maximum tumor reduction without marrow ablation. This phase is usually limited to 4 to 6 months so that consolidation with high-dose therapy can be performed before large numbers of resistent tumor cells emerge and before normal organs are physiologically compromised (2,3,7). An intensive induction chemotherapy regimen is likely to achieve the greatest response in primary and metastatic tumors (34–40). The former facilitates surgical resection and the latter is important for preparing autologous marrow for autologous BMT (3). In addition, patients who have achieved a complete or very good partial remission at the conclusion of induction therapy have the best long-term survival after myeloablative consolidation and autologous BMT (41).

Chemotherapy

A number of drugs have been identified that are active against neuroblastomas as single agents and in combination, including cyclophosphamide, L-phenylalanine mustard, thiotepa, ifosfamide, cisplatin, carboplatin, doxorubicin, teniposide, etoposide, vincristine, and dacarbazine (5–7,40). Multiagent chemotherapy regimens have been based on tumor cell cycle, drug resistance, and toxicity considerations (34,35,37–39,42–47). A recent review of nonmarrow ablative regimens demonstrated that greater dose intensity of cyclophosphamide, doxorubicin, teniposide, and cisplatin (but not vincristine) was associated with improved response, progression-free survival, and survival (40). The more intensive chemotherapy regimens appear to be most effective, with more than 90% responses (complete plus partial remission) and 40 to 50% 2-year survival. These regimens include (1) high-dose cisplatin or carboplatin and etoposide (35,37,39); (2) high-dose cyclophosphamide (40); and (3) cyclophosphamide or ifosfamide, cisplatin, etoposide, and doxorubicin (38,48). Even greater chemotherapy dose intensity, which may result in improved antitumor efficacy, may now be possible with the availability of hematopoietic growth factors (49); however, drug doses and the interval between courses of chemotherapy may still be limited by acute or long-term toxicity to marrow stem cells. Administration of peripheral blood stem cells after chemotherapy could overcome this problem; however, neuroblastoma cells can circulate in blood and these would be reinfused with stem cells (50) (see Future Directions).

Harvest, Purging, Cryopreservation, and Evaluation of Autologous Marrow

Autologous marrow that is free of detectible tumor cells and that has sufficient normal cells for engraftment must be cryopreserved before myeloablative therapy is given. At diagnosis, marrow metastases are detectible in 85% of stage IV patients with immunocytology, which is sensitive enough to detect one tumor cell/10^5 normal cells (32). After 3 or 4 courses of intensive chemotherapy (e.g., cyclophosphamide, cisplatin, doxorubicin, and etoposide) (38), metastases are detectible in only 33% of patients, and the tumor contamination in these patients is generally less than 0.1% (51). Such in vivo purging of tumor cells by induction chemotherapy is essential before marrow is harvested for cryopreservation because currently available purging methods cannot reliably remove more than 2% of tumor cells (Reynolds CP, Seeger RC. Unpublished observations). If 3 or 4 courses of a given chemotherapy regimen do not reduce marrow metastases to this level, consideration should be given to alternative induction chemotherapy. In this situation, marrow should be re-evaluated after each subsequent course of chemotherapy to determine if the marrow is suitable for harvest.

To maximize the probability of prompt marrow engraftment, it is important to infuse at least 10^8 cells/kg after myeloablative therapy (52,53). Because of the cell losses associated with marrow processing, purging, cyropreservation, and thawing, we harvest 0.5 to 1×10^9 nucleated cells/kg. One week before marrow harvest, marrow cellularity and tumor content are assessed. We require at least 15×10^6 nucleated cells/mL and less than 2% tumor cells by immunocytology before proceeding with harvest. Overt pelvic bone metastases, if present at diagnosis, are re-evaluated, because their presence can contribute to contamination of harvested marrow (3). If a bone scan remains positive, we recommend avoiding the area during marrow harvest.

Neuroblastoma cells that are infused with autologous marrow could re-establish disease depending on their number and clonogenicity in vivo. If the assay for detecting tumor cells has low sensitivity, the number of malignant cells infused with apparently tumor-free marrow may be considerable. For example, if the marrow contained 0.1% tumor cells, a 15-kg child infused with 3×10^9 marrow cells (2×10^8 cells/kg) would receive 3×10^6 tumor cells. Thus, it is prudent to minimize this risk by using marrow for autologous BMT that has no detectible tumor cells at a test sensitivity of at least one tumor cell/10^5 normal cells (32). Clearing marrow to below this level can be accomplished for more than 90% of patients by a combination of in vivo and ex vivo tumor cell purging (51).

A number of different methods for ex vivo purging have undergone preclinical and clinical testing (Table 61-4) (54–57). Methods that use monoclonal antibodies that react with cell surface antigens of tumor but not normal cells are most selective and consequently the least likely to damage pluripotent stem cells. Most laboratories use a "cocktail" of antitumor antibodies in an effort to overcome intratumor and intertumor heterogeneity in expression of cell surface antigens (57–59). An alternative to removing tumor cells with antitumor antibodies is to select pluripotent stem cells positively with anti-stem-cell antibodies (60–63). Although this approach has the advantage that a single set of antibodies can be used for a variety of tumors, isolated stem cells need to be evaluated carefully for tumor contamination because malignant cells may be nonspecifically or specifically (if they express stem-cell antigens) included with normal cells.

The most common method for ex vivo purging of marrow from patients with neuroblastomas utilizes magnetic immunobeads. We use a multistep purging system and assess efficacy at each step by immunocytological examination (32,58,59,64). The first and second steps deplete tumor cell clumps by sedimentation in hetastarch (tumor clumps sediment at unit gravity with erythrocytes) and by passage of nonsedimented cells through 40- and 20-μm filters (64). The filtered marrow is then mixed with magnetic immunobeads that are coated with a cocktail of 5 monoclonal antibodies that bind to neuroblastomas but not to normal pluripotent stem cells. Bead-tumor cell conjugates form and are removed with high-energy magnets (58,59,65). This 3-step procedure can remove more than 3 logs of tumor cells (51,59). After purging, the marrow is cryopreserved in bags in tissue culture medium containing hetastarch, human serum albumin, and dimethyl sulfoxide (52,66) (see Chapter 23).

Surgery

Some stage III or IV neuroblastomas can be resected grossly at diagnosis. However, many are large and involve vital structures, and 4 to 6 courses of induction chemotherapy are often given before definitive resection is attempted (67–71). The presence of viable tumor cells in many neuroblastomas that are excised during the induction phase and frequent relapse at the primary site after autologous BMT both indicate the importance of local control through resection (72). Complete surgical removal is the local therapy of choice because local irradiation may be only partially effective and because it can cause late complications. However, if complete gross resection is not possible, local irradiation should be given in an attempt to prevent recurrence (73,74). Patients with stage III or IV disease who have residual gross tumor after delayed surgery appear to have a higher incidence of relapse than those who do not have tumor remaining (68).

Local Irradiation

Neuroblastomas are radio-sensitive (75), and a dose-response relationship appears to exist; doses of 2,500

Table 61-4.
Methods for Ex Vivo Removal (Purging) of Neuroblastoma Cells from Autologous Marrow

Method	*Principle*	*Estimated Efficacy (log_{10} Decrease in Tumor Cells)*	*Ref*
Physical			
Density sedimentation	Tumor cells more dense than normal cells	0.5–1	(64)
Velocity sedimentation	Tumor cells clumped	0.5–0.9	(152)
Filtration	Tumor cells clumped	0.1–0.6	(64)
Pharmacological			
Mafosfamide (Asta-Z-7557)	Tumor cells relatively more sensitive than normal cells	3	(153,154)
6-Hydroxydopamine	Specific uptake by adrenergic cells	1–2	(155,156)
Dye-mediated photolysis	Dye uptake by tumor causes photosensitivity	2–5	(157)
Immunological			
Monoclonal antibodies with complement	Specific lysis	2–4	(158)
Magnetic immunobeads	Specific removal	2–4	(57–59,159)

cGy or more yield superior results (76). Although a randomized clinical trial has not been performed to determine the contribution of irradiation to local control of high-risk tumors, one investigation suggests that 2,100 cGy local irradiation decreases recurrences for patients with stage IV disease (74). Local irradiation is usually given to patients with primary and metastatic tumor masses and with bone lesions that persist after induction chemotherapy and surgery (77,78). The dose given to patients with residual abdominal, chest, or cranial disease ranges from 1,000 to 2,100 cGy, depending on field size, location, and whether total body irradiation (TBI) will be given subsequently; the dose to residual bone lesions in the extremities usually is at least 2,000 cGy. These doses are given in 150- to 200-cGy fractions. For example, if a child is to receive TBI as part of myeloablative consolidation therapy, local irradiation to a residual abdominal tumor is usually limited to 1,000 cGy because higher doses, when combined with myeloablative chemoradiotherapy, can cause excessive intestinal mucosal damage (78,79). If TBI is not used, higher doses (e.g., 2,100 cGy) of abdominal and thoracic irradiation may be possible (74). Tumors adjacent to or invading the spine are treated with fields that include the entire width of the spine and adjacent soft tissues to minimize the risk of kyphosis/scoliosis (73). If marrow is to be harvested for autologous BMT, the pelvis should not be irradiated until after marrow has been harvested and cryopreserved because irradiation destroys marrow cells.

Consolidation Phase: Myeloablative Therapy and Autologous BMT

Rationale

The experimentally observed linear-log relationship between drug dose and tumor cell cytotoxicity for many chemotherapeutic agents, particularly alkylating agents, suggests that a 3- to 10-fold increase in drug dose will result in a multiple log increase in tumor cell killing (80,81). With autologous BMT to restore hematopoiesis, many drugs can be escalated well beyond their usual, nonmarrow ablative dose before nonhematopoietic toxicity becomes dose-limiting, and combining 3 or more noncross-resistant drugs at full or nearly full doses has curative potential (82,83). Even if 10^3 to 10^6 tumor cells remain after autologous BMT, treatment of this number of cells may be more successful than treatment of 10^7 to 10^9 cells. (see Future Directions).

Drug Selection and Dose

Drugs that are appropriate for high-dose therapy with autologous BMT should have activity for the tumor type, should be tolerable at 3 to 10 times the nonmarrow ablative dose, and should generate a steep and straight-line dose-response curve over many logs of tumor cell kill (83,84). Agents that have a shallow or curvilinear dose-response curve or that have unacceptable nonhematopoietic toxicity after modest escalation will probably not add efficacy to intensive regimens unless they augment effects of other drugs when given in conventional or nontoxic doses (83). Preclinical studies in vitro and in tumor bearing mice can guide selection of drugs and provide dose-response curves (80,85,86), but maximum tolerated dose and antitumor activity must be systematically determined in clinical trials (83,87).

Drug Combinations

The most effective myeloablative therapy is likely to result from using a combination of 3 or more agents that are individually effective (80,87). In choosing a combination of agents, noncross-resistance and nonoverlapping toxicities are important considerations. Tumor cells generally do not develop high-level resistance to alkylating agents even after prolonged in vitro selection, and when it does develop, resistance to one often does not impart resistance to another (80,83,88). Attention should also be given to pharmacology and drug interactions that could have antitumor or toxic effects. For example, a nephrotoxic drug given before L-phenylalanine mustard (L-PAM; melphalan) could significantly increase its toxicity because excretion is influenced by renal function (87). Ideally, each drug in a combination should be given at its full or nearly full individual dose. However, because there is no clear way to predict the toxicity of a combination from individual toxicities, dose escalation studies are necessary to determine the maximum tolerated dose of each agent in combination (80,87). In developing regimens for children, dose and toxicity data from studies in adults should be taken into account. A mathematical model has been described that may be useful for selecting cytotoxic drugs and doses for a combination regimen based on antitumor activities of drugs given as single agents and their organ-specific maximum tolerated dose (89,90).

Complications

Morbidity and mortality after intensive therapy and autologous BMT are regimen-related and can vary significantly (84,91). Careful assessment is necessary when new protocols are being tested, and a toxicity rating scale has been developed for this purpose (91). Acute complications that may occur during the first few months after autologous BMT are discussed in Chapter 8. Fatal toxicity, which can occur in 5 to 20% of patients depending on the therapeutic regimen, can result from marrow aplasia (failure of engraftment), encephalopathy and cerebral hemorrhage, cardiomyopathy, pulmonary hemorrhage, pneumonitis, renal failure, gastrointestinal hemorrhage, hepatic veno-occlusive disease (92,93), or infection (94–96). During the first year after marrow engraftment, complications are usually secondary to immunological deficiency (e.g., pneumocystis pneumonia can occur if trimethoprim-sulfamethoxazole is not given during the first year after autologous BMT) (see Chapter 27).

Long-term complications have not been studied extensively in children who have undergone autologous BMT for neuroblastoma (97,98). Some problems that are anticipated or that have been recognized include infertility; endocrine deficiencies causing impaired linear growth and delayed or absent secondary sex characteristics; high tone hearing loss (in patients receiving cisplatin before or during intensive therapy); abnormal dental development; and a second malignancy (see Chapters 38 and 39) (99–102). Two patients have been reported in whom a second malignancy developed among 509 children undergoing autologous BMT for neuroblastoma (103,104).

Myeloablative Therapy and Autologous BMT Before Disease Progression

Myeloablative therapy has been tested using one or more drugs with or without TBI (Table 61-5) (51,74,79, 103,105–118). Autologous bone marrow has been used to reconstitute hematopoiesis in nearly all studies because fewer than 25% of patients have a histocompatible sibling to donate allogeneic marrow. Initial investigations demonstrated the activity of L-PAM against neuroblastoma (115), and nearly all subsequent regimens have utilized L-PAM with additional drugs and usually with TBI. Most patients who undergo BMT in first complete response, very good partial response, or partial response maintain or achieve a complete remission; however, 45 to 60% have recurrence of tumor months to years afterward (51,105,112). Most relapses are in the first 2 years after BMT, but they can occur 3 to 5 years later (51,105,112). Even though multiple logs of kill must have been attained, recurrence of neuroblastoma after autologous BMT most likely is due to incomplete eradication of tumor cells in the body by intensive therapy. This hypothesis is supported by the high frequency of relapses in sites of known previous disease (119) and by the observation that patients undergoing allogeneic BMT, in which the infused marrow is tumor-free, have the same recurrence rate as those undergoing autologous BMT with purged marrow (Ramsay NKA, et al. Unpublished observations). Nonetheless, patients receiving autologous marrow are at risk for recurrence due to tumor contamination of the infused marrow, and use of marrow that has fewer than one tumor cell/10^5 normal cells minimizes the possibility of infusing tumorigenic cells with the autologous BMT. Overall, data obtained during the past 10 years suggest that long-term disease-free survival (>5 years) can be achieved in 20 to 40% of patients (see Table 61-5).

Table 61-5.
Intensive Therapy and Autologous BMT for High-risk Neuroblastomas

Regimen	*No. Patients*	*Estimated Survival (%)[a]* 2 yr	3 yr	*Follow-up, Median months (range)*	*Ref*
Autologous BMT before progressive disease					
L-PAM	12	25	NA	33 (18–35)	(115)
L-PAM	15	33	33	39 (29–54)	(108)
L-PAM	22	45	40	34 (21–49)	(114)
L-PAM/carm/tenip (x1 or 2)	33	51	38	28 (8–50)	(109)
L-PAM/TBI	54	37	37	14 (6–47)	(105, 121)
L-PAM/vinc/TBI	37	44	NA	6 (3–48)	(110)
L-PAM/vinc/TBI	62	40	25	55 (NA)	(160)
L-PAM/tenip/dox/cisplat/TBI	31	56	56	7 (1–44)	(79)
L-PAM/tenip/dox/cisplat/TBI	45	45	45	29 (17–44)	(51)
carm/tenip/carbo + L-PAM/vinc/TBI	32	34	34	7 (4–36)	(111)
Autologous BMT after progressive disease					
Bu/Cy	10	0	0	7 (1–15)	(107)
L-PAM/TBI	27	24	24	14 (6–47)	(105, 121)
L-PAM/vinc/TBI	7	14	NA	18 (18)	(113)
L-PAM/tenip/dox/TBI	23	32	32	30 (9–90)	(103, 120)
L-PAM/tenip/dox/cisplat/TBI	7	0	0	4 (1–10)	(79)

[a]Estimates are for progression-free survival 2 and 3 years after autologous BMT and are from Kaplan-Meier analyses; data cited from reference (160) are 2- and 5-year estimated survival. The survival data cited for references (109) and (110) are after diagnosis rather than after BMT; data for references (115) and (108) are actual percent surviving progression-free.
BMT = bone marrow transplantation; BU = busulfan; carbo = carboplatin; carm = carmustine (BCNU); cisplat = cisplatin; CY = cyclophosphamide; dox = doxorubicin (Adriamycin); L-PAM = L-phenylalanine mustard (melphalan); tenip = teniposide (VM-26); vinc = vincristine; TBI = total body irradiation; NA = not available.

Myeloablative Therapy and Autologous BMT after Disease Progression

Patients whose tumors do not respond to therapy or in whom progressive disease develops during or after therapy have the highest risk of succumbing to their disease. The best strategy is to prevent progressive disease with effective induction and consolidation regimens. However, when this approach fails, innovative therapies, including those that utilize autologous BMT, are warranted. Myeloablative therapy is appropriate for some of these patients, but others should be excluded if they are unlikely to benefit. Selection of patients who are most likely to benefit is justified because of the morbidity, potential mortality, and expense of autologous BMT. In addition, suitable autologous marrow must be cryopreserved and adequate function of vital organs must be documented. Activity of myeloablative therapy can be evaluated even with selection of patients because this group overall has less than 5% chance of survival with current nonmyeloablative therapy, even if an initial response occurs (119). Myeloablative therapy and autologous BMT can be successful for some patients in this group (103,120). However, long-term survival is not achieved as often as for those treated before disease progression (see Table 61-5) (79,105). Therapies that have activity in this patient population may lead to advances in therapy of neuroblastomas because they are likely to be even more effective in newly diagnosed patients whose tumors may be more responsive.

Identification of Risk Subsets Within the High-Risk Group

It is becoming apparent that there are subsets of patients who have different outcomes after autologous BMT within the high-risk group. Although, it is not yet possible to accurately identify these subsets, those who undergo autologous BMT after an initial complete or very good partial response and before disease progression have the greatest likelihood of success (41,79). Within this group, those without bone metastases at diagnosis are most likely to become long-term disease-free survivors (41). Survival of patients whose tumors do or do not have genomic amplification of N-*myc* is the same as that for patients given myeloablative consolidation therapy (41). For patients who undergo myeloablative therapy after disease progression, outcome is related to response to reinduction therapy and to disease status at the time of autologous BMT (103,105,121).

Conclusions

Investigations of myeloablative therapy and autologous BMT for neuroblastoma lead to a number of conclusions. First, the outcome for patients given myeloablative therapy before disease progression is better than for those treated afterward. Although the results for the latter group may be improved by more effective reinduction and myeloablative therapy, autologous BMT is recommended relatively soon after diagnosis, prior to development of progressive disease. Second, the role of TBI is not clear. Because of its potential for causing morbidity and mortality, it is important to test myeloablative regimens that do not utilize TBI (74); if activity is demonstrated, a randomized study comparing a given combination of drugs with and without TBI could be performed. Third, although results of these limited and uncontrolled studies do not prove an advantage of multiple agents compared to a single agent (i.e., L-PAM), considerable preclinical and clinical data for other malignancies support the use of multidrug therapy to overcome tumor heterogeneity and drug resistance (83,90). Fourth, recurrence of neuroblastoma after autologous BMT most likely is due to incomplete eradication of tumor cells in the body by intensive therapy rather than to infusion of tumor cells with autologous marrow. This hypothesis is supported by the high frequency of relapses in sites of known previous disease (119) and by the observation that patients undergoing allogeneic BMT, in whom the infused marrow is tumor-free, have the same recurrence rate as those undergoing autologous BMT with purged marrow. Finally, careful characterization of study populations with respect to prognostic factors at diagnosis and during therapy is necessary to compare myeloablative and nonmyeloablative therapy and to define new subgroups among high-risk patients. The latter would facilitate the design of future studies.

Future Directions

Chemotherapy and Targeted Radiotherapy

Further improvement in disease-free survival may be achieved by increasing the dose intensity of induction chemotherapy, particularly in combination with hematopoietic growth factors. Subsequent consolidation may also be more effective if dose intensity is increased maximally by utilizing hematopoietic growth factors or autologous BMT (40,89,90,122). For example, a second cycle of myeloablative therapy and autologous BMT (double autologous BMT) is being tested (109,111). This approach is based on the hypothesis that the second cycle will be as effective as the first and thus will eradicate the few remaining logs of tumor cells. Sufficient autologous marrow can be cryopreserved from a single harvest for 2 transplants for many patients; therefore this is not a limiting factor. Although morbidity and expense are currently considerable, hematopoietic growth factors and peripheral stem-cell supplementation of marrow stem cells may decrease cytopenia so that double autologous BMT becomes more feasible.

In the long term, more effective induction and myeloablative chemotherapy will depend on understanding the molecular and cellular basis for tumor resistance through studies of recurrent tumors and tumor-derived cell lines. Other than the possible contribution of P-glycoprotein–mediated multidrug resistance (123), little data exist to explain failure of intensive combination therapy and thus to provide a rational basis for developing more effective strategies. Neuroblastoma cell lines, which are established at diagnosis and again at disease progression, can be used for basic investigations as well as for preclinical testing of new therapeutic strategies (86,124).

New methods for targeting radiotherapy are being tested that take advantage of unique properties of neuroblastomas. For example, radiolabeled metaiodobenzylguanidine, which is a catecholamine analogue that is taken up by neuroblastoma cells, can induce responses (125–128). Monoclonal antibodies can also deliver radioisotopes to neuroblastomas (129,130). Hematopoietic suppression can be a limiting toxicity, which can be enhanced by localization of radiolabeled ligand to tumor cells in bone marrow (127,128). Thus, delivery of high doses of radiation to tumor sites will probably require radioprotective cytokines, peripheral stem-cell support, or marrow rescue. Both radiolabeled antibodies and metaiodobenzylguanidine could be used with myeloablative chemotherapy.

Postconsolidation Therapy

Regardless of how effective induction and consolidation therapies become, many patients will still have minimal residual disease after consolidation therapy. Cytokines can activate effector cells that alone or in combination with antitumor cell antibodies may have antitumor effects. Interleukin-2 (IL-2) can stimulate lymphokine-activated killer cell activity against neuroblastoma in vitro or in vivo (131–133). Granulocyte-macrophage colony stimulating factor (GM-CSF), G-CSF, M-CSF, and IL-2 can enhance antibody-dependent cellular cytotoxicity (ADCC)(134–136) by activating lymphoid and myeloid effector cells. They have been shown to augment anti-G_{D2} monoclonal antibody mediated ADCC against neuroblastoma cells in vitro (135). Because the G_{D2} ganglioside is strongly expressed on the surface of neuroblastoma cells and anti-G_{D2} antibody has antitumor activity in patients by itself (137,138), a combination of monoclonal anti-G_{D2} antibody and cytokines might have antitumor efficacy, especially if used in a setting of minimal residual disease. Although studies to date have utilized single monoclonal antibodies and single cytokines, future trials will likely employ combinations of antibodies and cytokines to maximize antitumor activity. Another strategy is to immunize patients using their own tumor cells. This approach is promising because the immunogenicity of tumor cells can be significantly increased by transducing them with cytokine genes (139–143).

Differentiation inducers can arrest cell proliferation and induce terminal differentiation. They are probably best suited for postautologous BMT therapy, during which tumor load is small and their effects on tumor cell proliferation will not negatively interfere with radiation or chemotherapy. One example of a potentially useful differentiation inducer is 13-cis-retinoic acid (144). Preclinical studies have shown that retinoic acid can induce differentiation, arrest cell proliferation, and decrease expression of the N-*myc* proto-oncogene by human neuroblastoma cell lines (124,144, 145); and clinical responses in neuroblastoma patients have been documented (124). The lack of hematopoietic toxicity of 13-cis-retinoic acid when given at maximum tolerable dose after autologous BMT allows it to be tested after consolidation therapy (3,124). The Childrens Cancer Group is performing a randomized study to determine the efficacy of 13-cis-retinoic acid in preventing tumor recurrence when given after myeloablative or nonmyeloablative consolidation therapy.

Autologous Bone Marrow and Peripheral Blood Stem Cells

Stem cells that restore hematopoiesis after intensive therapy can be obtained from bone marrow or from apheresed peripheral blood (146,147). Currently, bone marrow is utilized for most autologous BMTs because sufficient cells can be obtained in one harvest and can be more readily purged of detectible tumor cells. Collection of peripheral blood stem cells is facilitated by administration of G-CSF or GM-CSF after chemotherapy so that 2 aphereses usually provide sufficient cells for engraftment. However, apheresed peripheral blood stem cells may be contaminated by circulating tumor cells (146,148). Studies aimed at increasing the sensitivity of detection and the ease and efficacy of purging are warranted to improve removal of tumor cells from marrow and peripheral blood stem cells. Another strategy being developed to provide stem cells utilizes ex vivo expansion with hematopoietic growth factors (149–151). If peripheral blood–derived or ex vivo–expanded stem cells can be used to support patients through very intensive induction chemotherapy and myeloablative therapy, morbidity and hospitalization may be decreased even while dose intensity is increased.

Summary

Autologous BMT allows delivery of intensive, myeloablative chemotherapy or chemoradiotherapy to children with high-risk neuroblastomas. Results from several studies indicate that long-term survival can result for some patients, although relapses can occur months to years after complete clinical remission. The efficacy of nonmyeloablative versus myeloablative consolidation therapy is being addressed in one randomized study. Future investigations will aim to increase disease-free survival by intensifying induction and consolidation regimens and by developing therapies to be given after consolidation that are directed at minimal residual disease.

References

1. Young JL Jr, Miller RW. Incidence of malignant tumors in U. S. children. J Pediatr 1975;86:254–258.
2. Seeger RC, Reynolds CP. Neuroblastoma. In: Holland JF, Frei E III, Bast RC Jr, Kufe DW, Morton DL, Weichsenbaum RR, eds. Cancer medicine. Philadelphia: Lea and Febiger, 1993:2172–2184.
3. Seeger RC, Reynolds CP. Treatment of high-risk solid tumors of childhood with intensive therapy and autologous bone marrow transplantation. Pediatr Clin North Am 1991;38:393–424.
4. Breslow N, McCann B. Statistical estimation of prognosis for children with neuroblastoma. Cancer Res 1971;31:2098–2103.
5. Hayes FA, Smith EI. Neuroblastoma. Principals Practices Pediatr Oncol 1989;607–622.
6. Kushner BH, Cheung NK. Neuroblastoma. Pediatr Ann 1988;17:269–276, 278.
7. Reynolds CP, Selch MT, Seeger RC. Neuroblastoma. Cancer treatment, ed 3. Philadelphia: W.B. Saunders, 1990:489.
8. Brodeur GM, Seeger RC, Barrett A, et al. International criteria for diagnosis, staging, and response to treatment in patients with neuroblastoma. J Clin Oncol 1988;6:1874–1881.

9. Shimada H, Chatten J, Newton W Jr, et al. Histopathologic prognostic factors in neuroblastic tumors: definition of subtypes of ganglioneuroblastoma and an age-linked classification of neuroblastomas. J Natl Cancer Inst 1984;73:405–416.
10. Triche TJ, Askin FB. Neuroblastoma and the differential diagnosis of small-, round-, blue-cell tumors. Hum Pathol 1983;14:569–595.
11. Israel MA, Miser JS, Triche TJ, Kinsella T. Neuroepithelial tumors. In: Pizzo PA, Poplack DG, eds. Principals and practices of pediatric oncology. Philadelphia: J.P. Lippincott, 1989:623–634.
12. Jurgens H, Bier V, Harms D, et al. Malignant peripheral neuroectodermal tumors. A retrospective analysis of 42 patients. Cancer 1988;61:349–357.
13. Thiele CJ, McKeon C, Triche TJ, Ross RA, Reynolds CP, Israel MA. Differential protooncogene expression characterizes histopathologically indistinguishable tumors of the peripheral nervous system. J Clin Invest 1987;80:804–811.
14. Seeger RC, Brodeur GM, Sather H, et al. Association of multiple copies of the N-myc oncogene with rapid progression of neuroblastomas. N Engl J Med 1985;313: 1111–1116.
15. Evans AE, D'Angio GJ, Propert K, Anderson J, Hann HW. Prognostic factor in neuroblastoma. Cancer 1987; 59:1853–1859.
16. Sather HN. The use of prognostic factors in clinical trials. Cancer 1986;58:461–467.
17. Evans AE, D'Angio GJ, Randolph J. A proposed staging for children with neuroblastoma: Childrens Cancer Study group A. Cancer 1971;27:374–378.
18. D'Angio GJ, Evans AE, Koop CE. Special pattern of widespread neuroblastoma with a favorable prognosis. Lancet 1971;1046–1048.
19. Look AT, Hayes FA, Nitschke R, McWilliams NB, Green AA. Cellular DNA content as a predictor of response to chemotherapy in infants with unresectable neuroblastoma. N Engl J Med 1984;311:231–235.
20. Look AT, Hayes FA, Shuster JJ, et al. Clinical relevance of tumor cell ploidy and N-myc gene amplification in childhood neuroblastoma: a Pediatric Oncology Group study. J Clin Oncol 1991;9:581–591.
21. Hann HW, Evans AE, Siegel SE, et al. Prognostic importance of serum ferritin in patients with stages III and IV neuroblastoma: the Childrens Cancer Study Group experience. Cancer Res 1985;45:2843–2848.
22. Zeltzer PM, Marangos PJ, Parma AM, et al. Raised neuron-specific enolase in serum of children with metastatic neuroblastoma. A report from the Children's Cancer Study Group. Lancet 1983;2:361–363.
23. Chan HS, Haddad G, Thorner PS, et al. P-glycoprotein expression as a predictor of the outcome of therapy for neuroblastoma. N Engl J Med 1991;325:1608–1614.
24. Tanaka T, Slamon DJ, Shimada H, et al. A significant association of Ha-ras p21 in neuroblastoma cells with patient prognosis. A retrospective study of 103 cases. Cancer 1991;68:1296–1302.
25. Bjelfman C, Hedborg F, Johansson I, Nordenskjoeld M, Pahlman S. Expression of the neuronal form of pp60c-src in neuroblastoma in relation to clinical stage and prognosis. Cancer Res 1990;50:6908–6914.
26. Suzuki T, Bogenmann E, Shimada H, Stram D, Seeger RC. Aggresive neuroblastomas lack high affinity nerve growth factor receptors. J Natl Cancer Inst 1993;85: 377–384.
27. Suzuki T, Bogenmann E, Stram D, Seeger RC. Neuroblastomas lacking high affinity nerve growth factor (NGF) receptors (gp140proto-trk) rapidly progress (abstract). Proc Am Assoc Cancer Res 1992;32:210.
28. Suzuki T, Shimada H, Stram D, Seeger RC. Correlations between high affinity nerve growth factor receptor expression (gp140trk), N-myc proto-oncogene amplification, histopathologic classification, and survival in neuroblastoma. Lab Invest 1993;68:9.
29. Leone A, Seeger RC, Arboleda MJ, Slamon DJ, Stram D, Steeg PS. Evidence for nm23 overexpression, DNA amplification and mutation in aggressive childhood neuroblastomas. Oncogene 1993;8:855–865.
30. Fong CT, White PS, Peterson K, et al. Loss of heterozygosity for chromosomes 1 or 14 defines subsets of advanced neuroblastomas. Cancer Res 1992;52: 1780–1785.
31. Hiyama E, Hiyama K, Yokoyama T, Ichikawa T, Matsuura Y. Length of telomeric repeats in neuroblastoma: correlation with prognosis and other biological characteristics. Jpn J Cancer Res 1992;83:159–164.
32. Moss TJ, Reynolds CP, Sather HN, Romansky SG, Hammond GD, Seeger RC. Prognostic value of immunocytologic detection of bone marrow metastases in neuroblastoma. N Engl J Med 1991;324:219–226.
33. Finklestein JZ, Klemperer MR, Evans AE. Multiagent chemotherapy for children with metastastic neuroblastoma; a report from Childrens Cancer Study Group. Med Pediatr Oncol 1979;6:179.
34. Campbell LA, Seeger RC, Harris R, Villablanca JG, Matthay KK. Continuous infusion chemotherapy for refractory neuroblastoma. Proc Soc Clin Oncol 1991;32:197.
35. Castello MA, Clerico A, Jenkner A, Dominici C. A pilot study of high-dose carboplatin and pulsed etoposide in the treatment of childhood solid tumors. Pediatr Hematol Oncol 1990;7:129–135.
36. Cheung NK, Heller G, Kushner BH, Burch L, O'Reilly RJ. Stage IV neuroblastoma more than 1 year of age at diagnosis: major response to chemotherapy and survival durations correlated strongly with dose intensity. Prog Clin Biol Res 1991;366:567–573.
37. Hartmann O, Pinkerton CR, Philip T, Zucker JM, Breatnach F. Very-high-dose cisplatin and etoposide in children with untreated advanced neuroblastoma. J Clin Oncol 1988;6:44–50.
38. O'Leary M, Sather H, Ramsay N, et al. Intensive chemotherapy for poor prognosis neuroblastoma. Proc Am Assoc Cancer Res 1990;31:201.
39. Philip T, Ghalie R, Pinkerton R, et al. A phase II study of high-dose cisplatin and VP-16 in neuroblastoma: a report from the Societe Francaise d'Oncologie Pediatrique. J Clin Oncol 1987;5:941–950.
40. Cheung NV, Heller G. Chemotherapy dose intensity correlates strongly with response, median survival, and median progression-free survival in metastatic neuroblastoma. J Clin Oncol 1991;9:1050–1058.
41. Seeger RC, Matthay KK, Villablanca JG, et al. Intensive chemoradiotherapy and autologous bone marrow transplantation (ABMT) for high risk neuroblastoma (abstract). Proc Am Assoc Cancer Res 1991;10:310.
42. Bernard JL, Philip T, Zucker JM, et al. Sequential cisplatin/VM-26 and vincristine/cyclophosphamide/doxorubicin in metastatic neuroblastoma: an effective alternating non-cross-resistant regimen? J Clin Oncol 1987;5:1952–1959.
43. Hayes FA, Green AA, Mauer AM. Correlation of cell kinetic and clinical response to chemotherapy in disseminated neuroblastoma. Cancer Res 1977;37:3766–3770.

44. Ikeda K, Nakagawara A, Yano H, et al. Improved survival rates in children over 1 year of age with stage III or IV neuroblastoma following an intensive chemotherapeutic regimen. J Pediatr Surg 1989;24:189–193.
45. Kushner BH, Helson L. Coordinated use of sequentially escalated cyclophosphamide and cell-cycle-specific chemotherapy (N4SE protocol) for advanced neuroblastoma: experience with 100 patients. J Clin Oncol 1987;5:1746–1751.
46. Ninane J, Pritchard J, Malpas JS. Chemotherapy of advanced neuroblastoma: does adriamycin contribute? Arch Dis Child 1981;56:544–548.
47. Shafford EA, Rogers DW, Pritchard J. Advanced neuroblastoma: improved response rate using a multiagent regimen (OPEC) including sequential cisplatin and VM-26. J Clin Oncol 1984;2:742–747.
48. Campbell LA, Seeger RC, Harris R, Villablanca JG, Matthay KK. Continuous infusion chemotherapy for refractory neuroblastoma. J Clin Oncol 1993;11:-623–629.
49. Antman KS, Griffin JD, Elias A, et al. Effect of recombinant human granulocyte-macrophage colony-stimulating factor on chemotherapy-induced myelosuppression. N Engl J Med 1988;319:593–598.
50. Moss TJ, Sanders DG, Lasky LC, Bostrom B. Contamination of peripheral blood stem cell harvests by circulating neuroblastoma cells. Blood 1990;76:1879–1883.
51. Seeger RC, Villablanca JG, Matthay KK, et al. Intensive chemoradiotherapy and autologous bone marrow transplantation for poor prognosis neuroblastoma. Prog Clin Biol Res 1991;366:527–534.
52. Herzig GP. Autologous marrow transplantation for cancer therapy. Prog Clin Biol Res 1984;149:319–335.
53. Stewart FM, Kaiser DL, Ishitani KP. Progenitor cell numbers (CFU-GM, CFU-D, and CFU-Mix) and hemopoietic recovery following autologous bone marrow transplantation. Exp Hematol 1989;17:974–980.
54. Anderson KC, Nadler LM, Takvorian T. Monoclonal antibodies: their use in bone marrow transplantation. Prog Hematol 1987;15:137–181.
55. Janossy G. Bone marrow purging. Immunol Today 1989;8:253–258.
56. Santos GW, Colvin OM. Pharmacological purging of bone marrow with reference to autografting. Clin Hematol 1986;15:67–83.
57. Treleaven JG, Gibson FM, Ugelstad J, et al. Removal of neuroblastoma cells from bone marrow with monoclonal antibodies conjugated to magnetic microspheres. Lancet 1984;1:70–73.
58. Seeger RC, Reynolds CP, Vo DD, Ugelstad J, Wells J. Depletion of neuroblastoma cells from bone marrow with monoclonal antibodies and magnetic immunobeads. Prog Clin Biol Res 1985;175:443–458.
59. Reynolds CP, Seeger RC, Vo DD, Black AT, Wells J, Ugelstad J. Model system for removing neuroblastoma cells from bone marrow using monoclonal antibodies and magnetic immunobeads. Cancer Res 1986;46: 5882–5886.
60. Andrews RG, Singer JW, Bernstein ID. Percursors of colony-forming cells in humans can be distinguished from colony-forming cells by expression of the CD33 and CD34 antigens and light scatter properties. J Exp Med 1989;169:1721–1731.
61. Andrews RG, Singer JW, Bernstein ID. Human hematopoietic precursors in long-term culture: single CD34+ cells that lack detectable T cell, B cell, and myeloid cell antigens produce multiple colony-forming cells when cultured with marrow stomal cells. J Exp Med 1990;172:355–358.
62. Bensinger WI, Berenson RJ, Andrews RG, et al. Positive selection of hematopoietic progenitors from marrow and peripheral blood for transplantation. J Clin Apheresis 1990;5:74–76.
63. Berenson RJ, Andrews RG, Bensinger WI, et al. Antigen CD34+ marrow cells engraft lethally irradiated baboons. J Clin Invest 1988;81:951–955.
64. Reynolds CP, Billups CB, Moss TJ. Depletion of tumor cell clumps with with sedimentation and filtration of bone marrow prior to other purging modalities. Proc Am Soc Clin Oncol 1989;8:309.
65. Saur JW, Reynolds CP, Black AT. Magnetic depletion devices for rapid separation of cells in blood, bone marrow, or other tissues using immunomagnetic beads. US Patent No. 4710472, December 1, 1987.
66. Gorin NC. Collection, manipulation and freezing of haemopoietic stem cells. Clin Haematol 1986;15: 19–48.
67. Grosfeld JL, Ballantine TV, Baehner RL. Experience with "second-look" operations in pediatric solid tumors. J Pediatr Surg 1978;13:275–280.
68. Haase GM, Wong KY, deLorimier AA, Sather HN, Hammond GD. Improvement in survival after excision of primary tumor in stage III neuroblastoma. J Pediatr Surg 1989;24:194–200.
69. Moss TJ, Fonkalsrud EW, Feig SA, et al. Delayed surgery and bone marrow transplantation for widespread neuroblastoma. Ann Surg 1987;206:514–520.
70. Sitarz A, Finklestein J, Grosfeld J, et al. An evaluation of the role of surgery in disseminated neuroblastoma: a report from the Children's Cancer Study Group. J Pediatr Surg 1983;18:147–151.
71. Smith EI, Krous HF, Tunell WP, Hitch DC. The impact of chemotherapy and radiation therapy on secondary operation for neuroblastoma. Ann Surg 1980;191:561–569.
72. Nesbit M Jr. Advances and management of solid tumors in children. Cancer 1990;65:696–702.
73. Halperin EC, Cox EB. Radiation therapy in the management of neuroblastoma: the Duke University Medical Center experience 1967–1984. Int J Radiat Oncol Biol Phys 1986;12:1829–1837.
74. Kushner BH, O Reilly RJ, Mandell LR, Gulati SC, LaQuaglia M, Cheung NK. Myeloablative combination chemotherapy without total body irradiation for neuroblastoma. J Clin Oncol 1991;9:274–279.
75. Deacon JM, Wilson PA, Peckham MJ. The radiobiology of human neuroblastoma. Radiother Oncol 1985;3: 201–209.
76. Fontanesi J, Bowman L, Hancock M, et al. Impact of irradiation on local control in advanced neuroblastoma. Proc Am Assoc Cancer Res 1992;33:257.
77. D'Angio GJ, Matthay KK, Evans AE. Role of radiotherapy in neuroblastoma (letter). J Clin Oncol 1991;9: 2076–2077.
78. D'Angio GJ, August C, Elkins W, et al. Metastatic neuroblastoma managed by supralethal therapy and bone marrow reconstitution (BMRc). Results of a four-institution Children's Cancer Study Group pilot study. Prog Clin Biol Res 1985;175:557–563.
79. Seeger RC, Moss TJ, Feig SA, et al. Bone marrow transplantation for poor prognosis neuroblastoma. Prog Clin Biol Res 1988;271:203–213.
80. Teicher BA, Holden SA, Eder JP, Herman TS, Antman KH, Frei E. Preclinical studies relating to the use of

thiotepa in the high-dose setting alone and in combination. Semin Oncol 1990;17:18–32.
81. Frei E, Teicher BA, Holden SA, Cathcart KN, Wang YY. Preclinical studies and clinical correlation of the effect of alkylating dose. Cancer Res 1988;48:6417–6423.
82. Eder JP, Elias A, Shea TC. A phase I-II study of cyclophosphamide, thiotepa and carboplatin with autologous bone marrow transplantation in solid tumor patients. J Clin Oncol 1990;8:1239–1245.
83. Frei E, Antman K, Teicher B, Eder P, Schnipper L. Bone marrow autotransplantation for solid tumors—prospects. J Clin Oncol 1989;7:515–526.
84. Cheson BD, Lacerna L, Leyland Jones B, Sarosy G, Wittes RE. Autologous bone marrow transplantation. Current status and future directions. Ann Intern Med 1989;110:51–65.
85. Gulati SC, Kwon JH, Atzpodien J. In vitro chemosensitivity of two Ewing's sarcoma cell lines; implication for autologous bone marrow transplantation. Cancer Invest 1989;7:411–416.
86. Hill BT, Whelan RDH, Hosking LK. Use of human neuroblastoma continuous cell lines for in vitro drug sensitive screening. Invest New Drugs 1988;6:11–18.
87. Peters WP, Eder JP, Henner WD, et al. High-dose combination alkylating agents with autologous bone marrow support: a Phase 1 trial. J Clin Oncol 1986;4:646–654.
88. Teicher BA, Cucchi CA, Lee JB, Flatow JL, Rosowsky A, Frei E. Alkylating agents: in vitro studies of cross-resistance patterns in human cell lines. Cancer Res 1986;46:4379–4383.
89. Gelman RS. Keeping an open mind about the doses of chemotherapy (editorial; comment). J Natl Cancer Inst 1990;82:1446–1447.
90. Simon R, Korn EL. Selecting drug combinations based on total equivalent dose (dose intensity). J Natl Cancer Inst 1990;82:1469–1476.
91. Bearman SI, Appelbaum FR, Buckner CD, et al. Regimen-related toxicity in patients undergoing bone marrow transplantation. J Clin Oncol 1988;6:1562–1568.
92. Brugieres L, Hartmann O, Benhamou E, et al. Veno-occlusive disease of the liver following high-dose chemotherapy and autologous bone marrow transplantation in children with solid tumors: incidence, clinical course and outcome. Bone Marrow Transplant 1988;3:53–58.
93. Dulley FL, Kanfer EJ, Appelbaum FR, et al. Venocclusive disease of the liver after chemoradiotherapy and autologous bone marrow transplantation. Transplantation 1987;43:870–873.
94. Kirk JL, Greenfield RA, Slease RB. Analysis of early infectious complications after autologous bone marrow transplantation. Cancer 1982;62:2445–2450.
95. Schuchter LM, Wingard JR, Piantadosi S. Herpes zoster infection after autologous bone marrow transplantation. Blood 1989;74:1424–1427.
96. Wacker P, Hartmann O, Benhamou E. Varicella-zoster virus infections after autologous bone marrow transplantation in children. Bone Marrow Transplant 1989; 4:191–194.
97. Willi SM, Cooke K, Goldwein J, August CS, Olshan JS, Moshang TJ. Growth in children after bone marrow transplantation for advanced neuroblastoma compared with growth after transplantation for leukemia or aplastic anemia. J Pediatr 1992;120:726–732.
98. Hovi L, Saarinen UM, Siimes MA. Growth failure in children after total body irradiation preparative for bone marrow transplantation. Bone Marrow Transplant 1991;8(suppl 1):10–13.
99. Sanders J, Sullivan K, Witherspoon R, et al. Long term effects and quality of life in children and adults after marrow transplantation. Bone Marrow Transplant 1989;4(suppl 4):27–29.
100. Sanders JE, Buckner CD, Sullivan KM, et al. Growth and development in children after bone marrow transplantation. Horm Res 1988;30:92–97.
101. Sanders JE, Buckner CD, Sullivan K. Growth and development after bone marrow transplantation. Prog Clin Biol Res 1989;309:375–382.
102. Sanders JE, Buckner CD, Amos D. Ovarian function following marrow transplantation for aplastic anemia or leukemia. J Clin Oncol 1988; 6:813–818.
103. August CS, Auble B. Autologous bone marrow transplantation for advanced neuroblastoma at the Children's Hospital of Philadelphia. In: Dicke KA, Spitzer G, Jagannath S, Evinger-Hodges MJ, eds. Autologous bone marrow transplantation. Houston, TX: The University of Texas, M.D. Anderson Cancer Center, 1989:567.
104. Dini G, Philip T, Hartmann O, et al. Bone marrow transplantation for neuroblastoma: a review of 509 cases. EBMT Group. Bone Marrow Transplant 1989;4 (suppl 4):42–46.
105. Pole JG, Casper J, Elfenbein G, et al. High-dose chemoradiotherapy supported by marrow infusions for advanced neuroblastoma: a Pediatric Oncology Group study. J Clin Oncol 1991; 9:152–158. (Published erratum appears in J Clin Oncol 1991;9:1094).
106. Shuster JJ, Cantor AB, McWilliams N, et al. The prognostic significance of autologous bone marrow transplant in advanced neuroblastoma. J Clin Oncol 1991;9:1045–1049.
107. Hartmann O, Benhamou E, Beaujean F, et al. High-dose busulfan and cyclophosphamide with autologous bone marrow transplantation support in advanced malignancies in children: a phase II study. J Clin Oncol 1986;4:1804–1810.
108. Hartmann O, Kalifa C, Benhamou E, et al. Treatment of advanced neuroblastoma with high-dose melphalan and autologous bone marrow transplantation. Cancer Chemother Pharmacol 1986;16:165–169.
109. Hartmann O, Benhamou E, Beaujean F, et al. Repeated high-dose chemotherapy followed by purged autologous bone marrow transplantation as consolidation therapy in metastatic neuroblastoma. J Clin Oncol 1987;5:1205–1211.
110. Philip T, Bernard JL, Zucker JM, et al. High-dose chemoradiotherapy with bone marrow transplantation as consolidation treatment in neuroblastoma: an unselected group of stage IV patients over 1 year of age. J Clin Oncol 1987;5:266–271.
111. Philip T, Chauvin F, Michon J, et al. A pilot study of double ABMT in advanced neuroblastoma (32 patients). In: Dicke KA, Spitzer G, Jagannath S, Evinger-Hodges MJ, eds. Autologous bone marrow transplantation. Houston, TX: University of Texas, M.D. Anderson Cancer Center, 1989:799.
112. Philip T, Zucker JM, Bernard JL, et al. The LMCE1 unselected group of stage IV neuroblastoma revisited with a median follow up of 59 months after ABMT. Prog Clin Biol Res 1991;366:517–526.
113. Pinkerton CR, Philip T, Biron P, et al. High-dose melphalan, vincristine, and total-body irradiation

with autologous bone marrow transplantation in children with relapsed neuroblastoma: a phase II study. Med Pediatr Oncol 1987;15:236–240.
114. Pinkerton CR. ENSG 1-randomised study of high-dose melphalan in neuroblastoma. Bone Marrow Transplant 1991;7(suppl 3):112–113.
115. Pritchard J, McElwain TJ, Graham-Pole J. High-dose melphalan with autologous marrow for treatment of advanced neuroblastoma. Br J Cancer 1982;45:86–94.
116. Seeger RC, Moss TJ, Feig SA, et al. Autologous bone marrow transplantation for poor prognosis neuroblastoma. UCLA Symp Mol Cell Biol, New Series 1989;91:279–288.
117. Vossen JM. Autologous bone marrow rescue as part of a curative approach for pediatric solid tumors: the case of neuroblastoma. Pediatr Hematol Oncol 1990;7: iii–vii.
118. Yaniv I, Bouffet E, Irle C, et al. Autologous bone marrow transplantation in pediatric solid tumors. Pediatr Hematol Oncol 1990;7:35–46.
119. Matthay KK, Atkinson J, Reynolds CP, Selch M, Seeger RC. Patterns of relapse after autologous bone marrow transplantation (BMT) for neuroblastoma (abstract). Proc Am Soc Clin Oncol 1991;10:312.
120. August CS, Serota FT, Koch PA, et al. Treatment of advanced neuroblastoma with supralethal chemotherapy, radiation, and allogeneic or autologous marrow reconstitution. J Clin Oncol 1984;2:609–616.
121. Graham-Pole J, Pick T, Casper J, et al. Myeloablative treatment for children with metastatic neuroblastoma supported by bone marrow infusions: progress and problems. Autologous Bone Marrow Transplant, Proc 4th Int Symp 1989;559–566.
122. Kushner BH, O'Reilly RJ, LaQuaglia M, Cheung NK. Dose-intensive use of cyclophosphamide in ablation of neuroblastoma. Cancer 1990;66:1095–1100.
123. Chan HS, Haddad G, Thorner PS, et al. P-glycoprotein expression as a predictor of the outcome of therapy for neuroblastoma. N Engl J Med 1991;325:1608–1614.
124. Reynolds CP, Kane DJ, Einhorn PA, et al. Response of neuroblastoma to retinoic acid in vitro and in vivo. Prog Clin Biol Res 1991;366:203–211.
125. Claudiani F, Garaventa A, Scopinaro G, et al. Diagnostic and therapeutic use of 131I-metaiodobenzylguanidine in children with neuroblastoma. J Nucl Med Allied Sci 1988;32:1–6.
126. Feine U, Mueller Schauenburg W, Treuner J, Klingebiel T. Metaiodobenzylguanidine (MIBG) labeled with 123I/131I in neuroblastoma diagnosis and follow-up treatment with a review of the diagnostic results of the International Workshop of Pediatric Oncology held in Rome, September 1986. Med Pediatr Oncol 1987;15: 181–187.
127. Sisson JC, Hutchinson RJ, Carey JE, et al. Toxicity from treatment of neuroblastoma with 131I-metaiodobenzylguanidine. Eur J Nucl Med 1988;14:337–340.
128. Treuner J, Klingebiel T, Bruchelt G, Feine U, Niethammer D. Treatment of neuroblastoma with metaiodobenzylguanidine: results and side effects. Med Pediatr Oncol 1987;15:199–202.
129. Cheung NK, Yeh SD, Gulati S, et al. 131I-3F8: clinical validation of imaging studies and therapeutic applications. Prog Clin Biol Res 1991;366:409–415.
130. Cheung NK, Neely JE, Landmeier B, Nelson D, Miraldi F. Targeting of ganglioside GD2 monoclonal antibody to neuroblastoma. J Nucl Med 1987;28:1577–1583.
131. Atzpodien J, Gulati SC, Kwon JH, et al. Anti-tumor efficacy of interleukin-2-activated killer cells in human neuroblastoma ex vivo. Exp Cell Biol 1988;56: 236–244.
132. Favrot MC, Floret D, Negrier S, et al. Systemic interleukin-2 therapy in children with progressive neuroblastoma after high dose chemotherapy and bone marrow transplantation. Bone Marrow Transplant 1989;4:499–503.
133. Sosman JA, Hank JA, Sondel PM. In vivo activation of lymphokine-activated killer activity with interleukin-2: prospects for combination therapies. Semin Oncol 1990;17:22–30.
134. Hank JA, Robinson RR, Surfus J, et al. Augmentation of antibody dependent cell mediated cytotoxicity following in vivo therapy with recombinant interleukin 2. Cancer Res 1990;50:5234–5239.
135. Kushner BH, Cheung NK. GM-CSF enhances 3F8 monoclonal antibody-dependent cellular cytotoxicity against human melanoma and neuroblastoma. Blood 1989;73:1936–1941.
136. Munn DH, Cheung NK. Phagocytosis of tumor cells by human monocytes cultured in recombinant macrophage colony-stimulating factor. J Exp Med 1990;172: 231–237.
137. Cheung NK, Lazarus H, Miraldi FD, et al. Ganglioside GD2 specific monoclonal antibody 3F8: a phase I study in patients with neuroblastoma and malignant melanoma. J Clin Oncol 1987;5:1430–1440.
138. Handgretinger R, Baader P, Dopfer R, et al. A phase I study of neuroblastoma with the anti-ganglioside GD2 antibody 14.G2a. Cancer Immunol Immunother 1992; 35:199–204.
139. Pardoll DM, Golumbek P, Levitsky H, Jaffee L. Molecular engineering of the antitumor immune response. Bone Marrow Transplant 1992;9(suppl 1):182–186.
140. Golumbek PT, Lazenby AJ, Levitsky HI, et al. Treatment of established renal cancer by tumor cells engineered to secrete interleukin-4. Science 1991;254: 713–716.
141. Fearon ER, Pardoll DM, Itaya T, et al. Interleukin-2 production by tumor cells bypasses T helper function in the generation of an antitumor response. Cell 1990;60:397–403.
142. Gansbacher B, Bannerji R, Daniels B, Zier K, Cronin K, Gilboa E. Retroviral vector-mediated gamma-interferon gene transfer into tumor cells generates potent and long lasting antitumor immunity. Cancer Res 1990;50:7820–7825.
143. Gansbacher B, Zier K, Daniels B, Cronin K, Bannerji R, Gilboa E. Interleukin 2 gene transfer into tumor cells abrogates tumorigenicity and induces protective immunity. J Exp Med 1990;172:1217–1224.
144. Sidell N, Altman A, Haussler MR, Seeger RC. Effects of retinoic acid (RA) on the growth and phenotypic expression of several human neuroblastoma cell lines. Exp Cell Res 1983;148:21–30.
145. Thiele CJ, Reynolds CP, Israel MA. Decreased expression of N-myc precedes retinoic acid-induced morphological differentiation of human neuroblastoma. Nature 1985;313:404–406.
146. Lasky LC, Bostrom B, Smith J, Moss TJ, Ramsay NK. Clinical collection and use of peripheral blood stem cells in pediatric patients. Transplantation 1989;47: 613–616.
147. Stiff PJ, Koester AR, Eagleton LE, Hindman T, Braud E, Weidner MK. Autologous stem cell transplantation

using peripheral blood stem cells. Transplantation 1987;44:585–588.
148. Moss TJ, Sanders DG. Detection of neuroblastoma cells in blood. J Clin Oncol 1990;8:736–740.
149. McAlister IB, Teepe M, Gillis S, Williams DE. Ex vivo expansion of peripheral blood progenitor cells with recombinant cytokines. Exp Hematol 1992;20:626–628.
150. Muench MO, Moore MA. Accelerated recovery of peripheral blood cell counts in mice transplanted with in vitro cytokine-expanded hematopoietic progenitors. Exp Hematol 1992;20:611–618.
151. Schwartz RM, Emerson SG, Clarke MF, Palsson BO. In vitro myelopoiesis stimulated by rapid medium exchange and supplementation with hematopoietic growth factors. Blood 1991;78:3155–3161.
152. Figdor CG, Voute PA, de Kraker J, Vernie LN, Bont WS. Physical cell separation of neuroblastoma cells from bone marrow. Prog Clin Biol Res 1985;175:459–470.
153. Sindermann H, Peukert M, Hilgard P. Bone marrow purging with mafosfamide—a critical survey. Blut 1989;59:432–441.
154. Beaujean F, Hartmann O, Benhamou E, Lemerle J, Duedari N. Hemopoietic reconstitution after repeated autologous transplantation with mafosfamide-purged marrow. Bone Marrow Transplant 1989;4:537–541.
155. Reynolds CP, Reynolds DA, Frenkel EP, Smith RG. Selective toxicity of 6-hydroxydopamine and ascorbate for human neuroblastoma in vitro: a model for clearing marrow prior to autologous transplant. Cancer Res 1982;42:1331–1336.
156. Kushner BH, Gulati SC, Kwon JH, O'Reilly RJ, Exelby PR, Cheung NK. High-dose melphalan with 6-hydroxydopamine-purged autologous bone marrow transplantation for poor-risk neuroblastoma. Cancer 1991;68:242–247.
157. Sieber F, Rao S, Rowley SD, Sieber Blum M. Dye-mediated photolysis of human neuroblastoma cells: implications for autologous bone marrow transplantation. Blood 1986;68:32–36.
158. Juhl H, Petrella EC, Cheung NK, Bredehorst R, Vogel CW. Complement killing of human neuroblastoma cells: a cytotoxic monoclonal antibody and its F(ab')2-cobra venom factor conjugate are equally cytotoxic. Mol Immunol 1990;27:957–964.
159. Kemshead JT, Heath L, Gibson FM, et al. Magnetic microspheres and monoclonal antibodies for the depletion of neuroblastoma cells from bone marrow: experiences, improvements and observations. Br J Cancer 1986;54:771–778.
160. Philip T, Zucker JM, Bernard JL, et al. Improved survival at 2 and 5 years in the LMCE1 unselected group of 72 children with stage IV neuroblastoma older than 1 year of age at diagnosis: is cure possible in a small subgroup? J Clin Oncol 1991;9:1037–1044.

Part VI
Allogeneic Marrow Transplantation for Genetic Diseases

Chapter 62
Bone Marrow Transplantation in Thalassemia

Guido Lucarelli and Reginald A. Clift

Thalassemia syndromes are widely distributed throughout the Mediterranean, Middle Eastern and Asian countries, and occur with a significant incidence worldwide in populations that originated in these regions. Weatherall and Clegg (1) stated that the thalassemias probably represent the most common single gene disorder to cause a major public health problem in the world. In the Mediterranean area alone there are more than 200,000 patients with β-homozygous thalassemia. In certain areas, such as Greece, the Mediterranean littoral of Italy, in Iran, Southern Russia, India and Southeast Asia, where 10 to 15% of the population carry the β-thalassemia gene, the homozygous birthrate is between 1:150 and 1:200. According to the World Health Organization, approximately 180 million people are heterozygous for one of several forms of genetic disorders of hemoglobin synthesis (2). Thalassemia major is one of the major scourges of humankind.

Defective synthesis of the β-chains of adult hemoglobin A leads to an imbalance of chain production and the accumulation of free α-chains in red cell precursors and red blood cells. This accumulation in turn causes intramedullary destruction of red cell precursors and markedly ineffective erythropoiesis, which result in severe hemolytic anemia. Many patients with homozygous β-thalassemia die in childhood from chronic anemia and its complications if insufficiently transfused or from iron overload if adequate iron chelation therapy is not administered. Currently recommended nontransplant therapy is available in most countries and consists of hypertransfusion to maintain hemoglobin levels between 10 and 12 gm/dL, together with chelation therapy aimed at preventing iron accumulation as a consequence of the transfusion therapy. To be effective, it is recommended that chelation therapy should consist of continuous subcutaneous infusion for at least 12 hours daily. Successful implementation of such treatment has improved life expectancy over the second decade of life and dramatically improved the quality of life for children with thalassemia. However, the impact of this treatment on long-term survival is unclear, and consistent delivery of chelation is difficult to achieve and expensive. Patient compliance with the chelation regimen is frequently poor, and transfusion therapy is limited by the availability of "clean" blood.

Thalassemia major is most common in third-world countries, where the cost of instituting and maintaining hypertransfusion and chelation programs on a national scale is prohibitive. An alternative approach in dealing with this major public health problem is to invest heavily in preventive measures, such as genetic counseling and prenatal diagnosis with induced termination of affected pregnancies. Religious and social constraints conspire to restrict the wider application of such measures, which may ameliorate but cannot eliminate this public health problem.

Future treatment of patients with thalassemia may be easier and improved if and when highly efficient orally administered iron chelators are available. Eventually thalassemia, like all the single-gene disorders, will be treated by revising the underlying genetic malformation, which may be achieved by genetic manipulation of the hemopoietic stem cell. Although thalassemia is a disease with a well-defined genetic target, there are many daunting obstacles to success in this endeavor. Genetic engineering studies have had some limited success in animals and in the treatment of adenosine deaminase deficiency in humans, and autologous marrow transplantation will probably be the vehicle for the genetic treatment of thalassemia. Moreover, regimens derived from experience in eliminating leukemic marrow will probably be used to overcome the competitive advantage of rapidly proliferating, genetically abnormal cells (3). Much additional research will be necessary before clinical trials are warranted in this area.

It is against this background that allogeneic bone marrow transplantation has been used in attempts at curing thalassemia. The first successful marrow transplant for thalassemia was reported in 1982 by Thomas and colleagues (4), and the first reports of series of transplants were by Lucarelli and associates (5,6).

Conventional Therapy

Infants with thalassemia major who receive no treatment will die in early infancy from congestive heart failure or other complications of severe anemia. Red cell transfusion therapy designed to avert this outcome will reduce mortality derived directly from anemia, but complications resulting from severe and accelerating hemolytic anemia driven by almost completely ineffective erythropoiesis will develop. These complications include cardiomegaly, massive hypersplenism, and severe bone malformations resulting from marrow extension. In 1964, Wolman (7) reported that patients maintained at a higher baseline hemoglobin level had less severe complications and were in better health than those maintained at lower hemoglobin levels. Stimulated by this observation, Piomelli and colleagues (8) studied a tranfusion regimen designed to prevent the baseline hemoglobin from falling below 10 gm/DL. When this hypertransfusion regimen was instituted in infancy and rigorously implemented, cardiomegaly and bone malformation were greatly reduced, although normalization of growth was not achieved and the development of hypersplenism was not prevented (8). The target level of 10 gm/DL hemoglobin was designed to depress endogenous erythropoiesis and thereby avoid marrow hypertrophy with accompanying marrow space extension. This objective was partially achieved, but complete suppression of endogenous red cell production requires that hemoglobin levels be maintained at levels greater than 13 gm/DL (9). There are major obstacles in the way of achieving these levels. It was demonstrated that raising the baseline hemoglobin level from 10 to 11 gm/DL produced a 20% increase in the red cell transfusion requirement (10), and there are many reasons for minimizing transfusion in patients with thalassemia.

Hypertransfusion regimens have a major impact on iron traffic and distribution in patients with severe hemolytic anemia, and the complications of iron overload, such as endocrine deficiency, liver and pancreatic damage, and heart disease, are the principal causes of death in patients with thalassemia receiving this form of therapy. As a result, attempts have been made to enhance iron mobilization and excretion with the use of chelating agents. The agent currently used is deferoxamine, which is not currently available in a form suitable for oral administration (11). Because maintenance of steady plasma levels of this agent is essential to effective management of iron traffic, the drug is continuously administered either intravenously or subcutaneously, and the most common regimen is 8 to 10 hours daily of continuous subcutaneous administration with the aid of a portable infusion pump (12). This therapy, when rigorously adhered to, substantially reduces but does not eliminate the iron overload for patients on hypertransfusion therapy.

The diagnosis of β-thalassemia is usually made within the first year of life, and red cell transfusions are usually initiated soon afterwards. To maintain a hemoglobin level between 10 and 12 gm/dL, transfusions are usually required every 15 to 21 days. There are 2 common causes for failure of conventional therapy in the treatment of thalassemia. The first is the inadequate supply of safe blood even in well-developed countries; the second is irregular and discontinuous administration of deferoxamine, which is usually due to the high cost of chelation therapy and poor patient compliance.

The development of a regimen of hypertransfusion combined with regular iron chelation has transformed the prognosis for thalassemic children (13). If good compliance is obtained, patients rarely die from anemia, and children with thalassemia are sick mainly because of complications arising from treatment with blood transfusions. Their clinical state depends primarily on the degree of transfusional iron overload but is compounded by exposure to hepatitis viruses and other blood-borne infectious agents. There is a dearth of good follow-up data, and the cohort of patients that has received this treatment since early infancy is only now approaching young adulthood. The first patient treated with the regimen is now in his mid-twenties, and statistics are not available that assess the outcome of treatment on the basis of intent to treat. It is abundantly clear that compliance rates for chelation therapy vary enormously, and, even with strong parental support, many children find this cumbersome and unpleasant therapy completely unacceptable, particularly as they grow older.

In conclusion, patients with homozygous β-thalassemia, if properly transfused and chelated, have a reduced but not abolished organ iron overload. In children with poor compliance with the medical prescription, iron overload is more severe, creating endocrine, cardiac, and hepatic lesions. Several authors have reported a high incidence of growth retardation due to impairment of the pituitary-gonadal axis and of diabetes mellitus due to iron deposits in the pancreas, as well as liver disease due to iron overload and viral hepatitis (14–17). In the majority of centers treating thalassemia, adequate chelation with deferoxamine was initiated in 1976 to 1977, and all observations reported by clinicians treating thalassemia refer to groups of patients heterogeneous for age and duration of chelation therapy. The situation for patients who have not received optimal chelation therapy was described by Gabutti and associates (14) in 1988 in a report of complications in a group of 183 patients who were 20 years old. Of these, 20% had cardiac disease, 43% had diabetes, 26% had liver disease, 28% had hypothyroidism, and 22% had hypoparathyroidism. Sixty percent of these patients had more than one complication, which is indicative of a very poor prognosis, with a 50% probability of death within 10 years of the appearance of the first complication. It is certain that patients who have received regular chelation therapy will have less iron overload than those reported by Gabutti and colleagues (14), together with significantly improved survival. Unfortunately, there is no way of determining from the literature what the complication rate will be in a population of patients entered into a study of modern chelation therapy. Therefore, it is impossible to draw conclusions on the contemporary frequency of complications due to iron overload.

The difficulties in achieving compliance with hypertransfusion/chelation regimens are greater in patients of low economic and educational status. Moreover, thalassemia is most common in developing and third-world countries, where delivery of such therapy (or of marrow transplantation) to a significant proportion of the affected population is problematic.

Bone Marrow Transplantation

Slavin and colleagues (18) noted that in the absence of specific gene therapy, allogeneic marrow transplantation represents the only rational therapeutic modality for the eradication of β-thalassemia major. However, the early mortality and morbidity associated with marrow transplantation discouraged its use in a situation where hypertransfusion and chelation provided palliation without substantial early mortality. The results of marrow transplantation have improved steadily, with major progress in the management of transplant-related complications, and by 1981 it appeared that "good-risk" candidates could be treated by marrow transplantation from suitable donors with a high probability of survival from the procedure (19). The decision was then made to undertake studies of marrow transplantation as an alternative to hypertransfusion and chelation for the treatment of β-thalassemia.

Because any risks associated with marrow transplantation might be enhanced by the iron overload and sensitization to human leukocyte antigens (HLA) induced by hypertransfusion, it was considered desirable to conduct early clinical studies in very young patients. In December 1981, a 14-month-old child with β-thalassemia major who had been transfused with a total of 250 mL packed red blood cells received a bone marrow transplant from his HLA-identical sister in Seattle (4). This procedure was successful and the child is now 12 years old and in excellent health, without the hematological manifestations of thalassemia. Two weeks later, the Pesaro team performed the first of an extensive series of transplants for thalassemia.

Preparatory Regimens

Preparatory regimens for marrow transplantation of patients with diseases other than aplastic anemia must achieve 2 objectives. One is elimination of the (disordered) marrow, and the other is establishment of a tolerant environment that will permit transplanted marrow to survive and thrive. Although total body irradiation (TBI) can accomplish both these objectives, there are many reasons to avoid the use of this marrow-ablative modality. These reasons include the known growth-retarding effects of TBI in young children and the increased risk of secondary malignancies, which has been reported in patients treated for leukemia (20), lymphoma, and aplastic anemia (21, 22), and which are particularly objectionable in very young patients with a hopefully long anticipated lifespan. The risk of these toxicities has not yet been determined for cytotoxic regimens that do not involve TBI.

There is a considerable body of experience with the use of busulfan (BU) and its derivatives in ablating marrow in patients undergoing marrow transplantation for the treatment of nonmalignant conditions, such as the Wiskott-Aldrich syndrome (23,24) and inborn errors of metabolism (25). Cyclophosphamide (CY) is an agent that is well established as providing adequate immunosuppression to permit allogeneic engraftment of patients with aplastic anemia (26,27). Experience in the use of chemotherapy-only transplant regimens for the treatment of malignancy (28–33) has been pivotal in developing regimens appropriate for the treatment of thalassemia.

BU is an alkylating agent with exquisite specificity for the most primitive precursors of the myeloid-erythroid axis. It has been used in low doses for more than 30 years for the treatment of patients with chronic myeloid leukemia, and its toxicity and effectiveness have been well documented in that setting. Studies in rodents demonstrated that marrow-lethal doses of BU have minor toxicity to the lymphoid system and cause little immunosuppression (34). Canine studies of transplants between DLA-identical littermates demonstrated 50% engraftment after BU alone and 95% engraftment when antithymocyte serum was added to the conditioning regimen (35). Clinical experience with the use of BU in very high doses was delayed due to the lack of an acceptable preparation suitable for intravenous use. The first clinical trials of very high-dose BU in the context of marrow transplantation were reported by Santos and associates (30). In these studies, patients with acute myeloid leukemia (AML) received allogeneic marrow transplants after immunosuppression with CY (200 mg/kg over 4 days), and oral BU (16 mg/kg over 4 days) was administered as additional antitumor therapy. Early results with this therapy were encouraging, and, in successful attempts to reduce early transplant-related toxicity, Tutschka and colleagues (36) reduced the CY dose to 120 mg/kg over 2 days. Although there are no clinical studies of the issue, it is widely believed that 120 mg/kg CY does not provide adequate immunosuppression to permit consistent allogeneic engraftment in recipients with normal immune competence. Successful allogeneic engraftment after the Tutschka regimen suggests that BU can enhance the immunosuppressive properties of CY.

CY has been a component of most conditioning regimens for transplanting patients with hematological malignancies. Santos and associates (28) reported on its use in high doses (200 mg/kg over 4 days) as the sole antitumor agent in patients receiving allogeneic transplants for leukemia and demonstrated that it was sufficiently immunosuppressive to permit sustained allogeneic engraftment. CY is most commonly employed for the treatment of lymphoid malignancies and solid tumors and it has been used as a component of combination chemotherapy for the treatment of acute leukemia. It is not regarded as a highly effective agent against myeloid malignancies, but single-drug studies are not available in this context. The dose-limiting toxicity of CY is to the heart and not to the marrow. Mice, monkeys, and humans recover hematopoiesis promptly after the highest doses of CY because CY does not eliminate hematopoietic stem cells. Therefore, CY alone is not an appropriate conditioning modality for marrow transplantation for the treatment of thalassemia because the thalassemic marrow would regrow rapidly. In contrast, BU is an agent that has a good possibility of eradicating a diseased erythron but when used alone is not likely to be sufficiently immunosuppressive to permit sustained allogeneic engraftment. In summary, a combination of BU and CY is likely to eradicate the thalassemia and to facilitate sustained allogeneic engraftment.

Disease Eradication

Many of the hematopoietic manifestations of thalassemia resemble those of hematopoietic malignancy. The extreme myeloid hyperplasia with aggressive extension of a rapidly proliferating erythron into intramedullary and extramedullary areas not usually occupied by marrow results in major bone remodeling, together with extreme hepatomegaly and splenomegaly. By analogy with the behavior of malignant tissue, it might be supposed that this large mass of rapidly proliferating hematopoietic tissue would be more difficult to eradicate than normal hematopoietic tissue, and more likely to recur after transplantation. Although post-transplant thalassemic recurrence is a problem, it occurs in circumstances that differ from those usually observed with leukemic relapse. The most common presentation of leukemic relapse is return of the leukemia in the presence of a persisting immune system of donor origin. In contrast, the recurrence of thalassemia usually occurs in the context of a return of host-type immune reconstitution. Thus, this event has aspects of both relapse and rejection. However, it is customary to speak of this phenomenon as rejection.

Engraftment

Most patients undergoing transplantation for the treatment of thalassemia have been transfused repeatedly. Experience with marrow transplantation for the treatment of aplastic anemia in heavily transfused patients demonstrated that a history of many pretransplant transfusions increased the probability of graft rejection (37,38). There is a substantial incidence of graft rejection in patients with thalassemia after most preparatory regimens for marrow grafting, and this incidence seems to be related to the stage of disease at the time of transplant. As discussed, in most cases of graft rejection, the thalassemic marrow will regrow and subsequent survival will be long (albeit with thalassemia). Occasional patients reject their grafts without recurrence of thalassemia. Unless rescued by a second transplant, these patients will die from the consequences of marrow aplasia. These diverse scenarios suggest the possibility that proliferation and persistence of a donor-type immune system reduces the probability of recurrence of thalassemia. It is not known whether this is a consequence of early graft-versus-host disease (GVHD) eradicating residual host hemopoietic precursors.

Transplant-related Morbidity and Mortality

Marrow transplantation is a dangerous undertaking. The regimen necessary to eradicate a diseased marrow and to facilitate persistent engraftment is necessarily toxic, and the consequences of successful allogeneic marrow engraftment are acute and chronic GVHD, syndromes associated with severe immune incompetence. Both prophylaxis against GVHD and methods for its treatment are immunosuppressive. There is interaction between the toxic effects of the preparative regimen and of GVHD or measures aimed at its prevention, but transplant-related toxicity can be conveniently categorized as either regimen-related toxicity (RRT) or GVHD.

The regimens used to prepare patients with thalassemia for transplantation are similar to those used in the treatment of aplastic anemia or leukemia. RRT from these or similar regimens has been well described in studies of marrow transplantation for the treatment of hematological malignancies (39,40). The lungs and the liver are the organs most at risk for toxicity generated by TBI and BU, whereas the heart is the main site for CY-induced damage. These toxicities are enhanced by patient age, previous exposure to cytotoxic agents, and the presence of latent viruses such as hepatitis C and cytomegalovirus. Patients transplanted for the treatment of thalassemia should derive some benefit from the fact that they are usually young and have no previous exposure to cytotoxic agents, but because of previous intensive transfusion therapy they will have a high probability of carrying harmful viruses and will have organ damage induced by extreme iron overload.

Clinical Transplant Experience

The Seattle Experience

The Seattle team transplanted 5 patients using a regimen of a single dose of 5 mg/kg dimethylbusulfan (DMB), a relatively soluble derivative of BU that can be administered parenterally, followed by CY (200 mg/kg over 4 days) with methotrexate (MTX) administered over 102 days as prophylaxis against acute GVHD (41–43). Two of these patients died within the first 100 days of transplant from veno-occlusive disease (VOD) of the liver and from adenovirus interstitial pneumonia (IP), and 3 survive more than 5.5, 9.3 and 10 years after transplantation with normal hematopoiesis and Karnofsky performance

Table 62-1.
HLA-identical Transplants Through January 1992: Pretransplant Characteristics

Patients	
Males	280
Females	211
Age (yr)	
Range	1–32
25th percentile	5
Median	9
75th percentile	13
No β-globin synthesis	276
Trace β-globin synthesis	215
Splenectomy	101
Donors	
Normal	159
Thalassemia heterozygotes	332
HLA-identical siblings	475
HLA-identical parents	16
Red Cell ABO groups	
Compatible	281
Minor incompatibility	76
Major incompatibility	134

HLA = human leukocyte antigen.

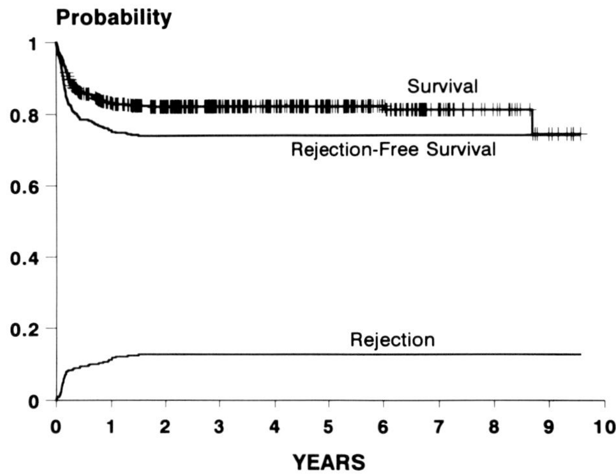

Figure 62-1. The probabilities of survival, rejection, and rejection-free survival for 491 patients with β-homozygous thalassemia who received transplants from human leukocyte antigen–identical family members between December 1981 and February 1992.

scores (KPS) of 100. After the Pesaro group demonstrated the feasibility of using oral BU in very young children, the Seattle group prepared 3 additional patients for transplantation with BU (14 mg/kg), CY (200 mg/kg), and GVHD prophylaxis consisting of a short course of MTX and cyclosporine (CSP). All 3 patients are alive more than 2.4, 5.2, and 5.3 years later. One of these patients has had recurrence of thalassemia (KPS = 90), and the other 2 are well (KPS = 100).

The Pesaro Experience

By far the largest body of experience in the treatment of thalassemia with marrow transplantation has been accumulated in Pesaro. From December 1981 through January 1992, 491 patients with homozygous β-thalassemia received marrow transplants from HLA-identical related donors (475 siblings, 16 parents). Some of the characteristics of these patients and their donors are described in Table 62-1. Figure 62-1 presents the statistics for survival, rejection-free survival, and rejection for these patients. The latest rejection occurred on day 548, and the latest death occurred nearly 9 years after transplantation. Twelve different conditioning regimens were used to prepare these patients for transplantation, but most patients were treated with one of two regimens: (1) protocol 6 (295 patients) and (2) protocol 12 (35 patients). These protocols are described in Table 62-2.

In the early experience, the best results were obtained in younger patients (5,44,45). Of the first 6 patients over the age of 16 years, 4 died of GVHD-related causes within the first 100 days, one died of infection on day 235, and one had recurrence of thalassemia on day 48 and died of consequent cardiac damage more than 6 years after transplantation. In view of this experience, the early studies concentrated on patients under the age of 17 years.

Children and Adolescents

Results in young patients were very encouraging, and in 1990, Lucarelli and colleagues (6) reported experience through August 1988 in treating 222 consecutive patients under the age of 16 years. All these patients received HLA-identical marrow (10 from parents, the rest from siblings). All patients were prepared for transplantation with a regimen that consisted of BU (3.5 mg/kg on each of 4 consecutive days; total dose, 14

Table 62-2.
Treatment Regimens

Protocol 6
Busulfan, 14 mg/kg over 4 days
Cyclophosphamide, 50 mg/kg/day × 4
Protocol 12
Busulfan, 14 mg/kg over 4 days
Cyclophosphamide, 60 mg/kg/day × 2
Antilymphocyte globulin, 10 mg/kg/day days −5 to +5
Cyclophosphamide, 7.5 mg/kg day + 1
Methotrexate, 10 mg/m² days + 3, 6, and 11
In both protocols
Cyclosporine, 5 mg/kg/day intravenously day −5 to day +5
Cyclosporine, 3 mg/kg/day intravenously day +6 to day +21
Cyclosporine, 12.5 mg/kg/day orally from day +22
Prednisolone, 0.5 mg/kg intravenously from day −1
Acyclovir, 15 mg/kg/day intravenously from day −1
Amikacin, 15 mg/kg/day intravenously from day −1
Immunoglobulin, 500 mg/kg intranvenously on day −1
Immunoglobulin, 250 mg/kg intravenously on days +8 and +22
Amphotericin B, 0.3 mg/kg/day intravenously from day +8

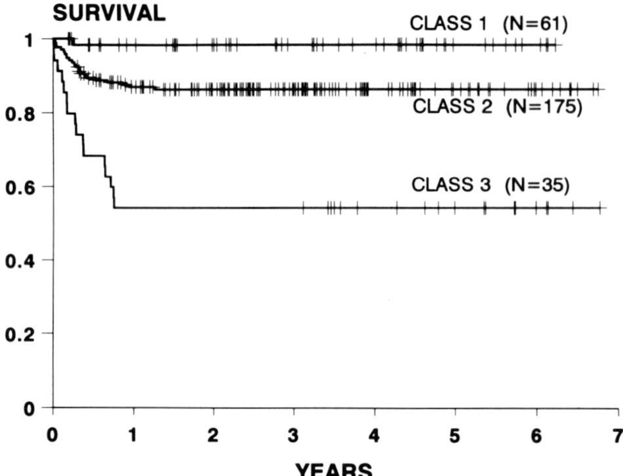

Figure 62-2. The probabilities of survival for 271 patients younger than 17 years with thalassemia who received marrow transplants from human leukocyte antigen–identical family members after conditioning with protocol 6. The categorization into risk classes is described in the text.

mg/kg), followed by CY (50 mg/kg on each of 4 consecutive days). One hundred forty-one donors were heterozygous for β-thalassemia, and 81 were normal homozygotes. Five different regimens were used to prevent acute GVHD. Protocol 6 was employed for 116 patients.

Analysis of the influence of pretransplant characteristics on the outcome of transplantation was conducted in the 116 patients who received treatment according to protocol 6. It was demonstrated that hepatomegaly and portal fibrosis were associated with a significantly reduced probability of survival. In multivariate analysis, a history of poor compliance with the chelation regimen could not be distinguished from hepatomegaly as a predictor of survival and rejection-free survival. The degree of hepatomegaly and the presence of portal fibrosis were used to assign patients to 3 classes according to the absence of both factors (class 1), the presence of one factor (class 2), or the presence of both factors (class 3). Patients in class 1 had significantly higher probabilities of survival and rejection-free survival than the patients in classes 2 or 3. Patients in class 3 had lower probabilities of survival and rejection-free survival than those in class 2, but the differences were not statistically significant (6).

The influence of pretransplant characteristics on the outcome of transplantation was re-examined in late 1989, by which time 161 patients under the age of 17 had been treated with protocol 6. The quality of chelation was characterized as regular when deferoxamine therapy was initiated not later than 18 months after the first transfusion and administered subcutaneously for 8 to 10 hours continuously for at least 5 days each week. The chelation variable was defined as irregular for any deviation from this requirement. The degree of hepatomegaly (≥ 2 cm), the presence or absence of portal fibrosis in the pretransplant liver biopsy, and the quality of chelation (regular or irregular) given through the years before transplant were identified as variables to be used in categorizing patients into 3 risk classes. Class 1 patients had none of these adverse risk factors, class 3 patients had all 3, and class 2 patients had one or 2 adverse risk factors. This analysis confirmed previous findings on the prognostic significance of risk class, but the influence of the quality of chelation therapy was greater than in the first analysis.

As of February 1992, 288 patients younger than 17 years received HLA-identical transplants using protocol 6. For 17 patients, it was not possible to assign a risk class because one or more risk variables were not known. There were 61 class 1 patients, 175 class 2 patients, and 35 class 3 patients. The probabilities of survival, rejection, and rejection-free survival are displayed in Figures 62-2, 62-3, and 62-4, respectively. Figure 62-5 depicts the probabilities of dying for patients in the three classes who had not rejected their grafts and shows that the survival differences between the classes were not exclusively associated with different rejection rates. Figure 62-6 presents the probabilities for development of acute GVHD graded by established criteria (46,47), and Table 62-3 presents the causes of death for patients in each class. There were no significant differences between the classes in the incidence of moderate (Figure 62-6A) or severe (Figure 62-6B) acute GVHD, suggesting that the differences in mortality between the classes may be a consequence of a reduced tissue tolerance for the cytotoxic agents in the conditioning regimen rather than a consequence of a reduced compliance with the GVHD prophylaxis regimen.

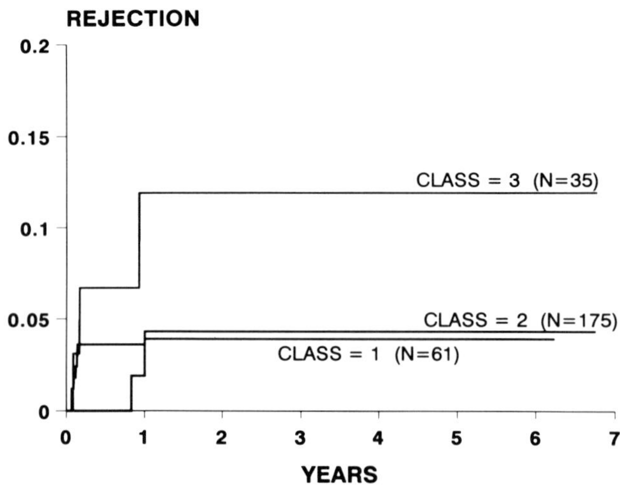

Figure 62-3. The probabilities of graft rejection for 271 patients younger than 17 years with thalassemia who received marrow transplants from human leukocyte antigen–identical family members after conditioning with protocol 6. The categorization into risk classes is described in the text.

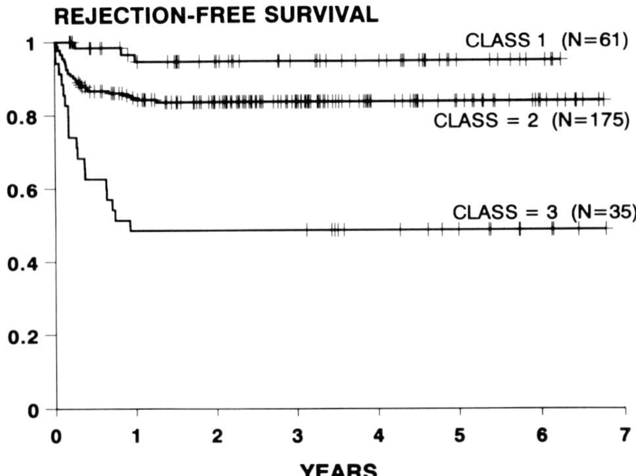

Figure 62-4. The probabilities of rejection-free survival for 271 patients younger than 17 years with thalassemia who received marrow transplants from human leukocyte antigen–identical family members after conditioning with protocol 6. The categorization into risk classes is described in the text.

Table 62-3.
Mortality by Risk Category[a]

	Class 1	*Class 2*	*Class 3*
Number of transplants	61	175	35
Number of deaths	1	23	16
Rejection			
With Aplasia	0	2	0
With Thalassemia	0	0	1
With acute GVHD			
Bacterial or fungal infection	1	9	5
Interstitial pneumonia	0	3	1
Interstitial pneumonia (idiopathic)	0	1	0
Without acute GVHD			
Bacterial or fungal infection	0	5	3
Cardiac tamponade	0	1	5
Varicella zoster	0	1	0
Chronic GVHD and infection	0	1	0
Lymphoma	0	0	1

[a]Includes 271 patients under 17 years on protocol 6.
GVHD = graft-versus-host disease.

It was concluded that class 1 patients have a very high probability of cure following marrow transplantation with a very low risk of complications. In contrast, it is also clear that, for the most part, these are patients who respond well to conventional therapy. The risks associated with transplantation are greater for patients who have liver damage (usually as a result of transfusions with inadequate chelation therapy or hepatitis). The one-year survival for young class 3 patients treated with protocol 6 was 54%. In an attempt to improve results in class 3 patients, a new treatment regimen was devised that used a lower dose of CY (see Table 62-2, protocol 12). Early experience with this regimen in patients less than 17 years of age is illustrated in Figure 62-7. With a minimum follow-up of one year, there have been no deaths in 19 patients treated with this regimen, although there is no difference in the rejection rate.

Adult Patients

As described, early experience with transplantation for patients older than 16 years was disastrous. Most adult patients presenting for transplantation have disease characteristics that place them in class 3, and because of the improved results in treating young class 3 patients using protocol 12, transplantation studies were resumed for patients older than 16 years. From October 1988 through November 1991, 29 consecutive patients, aged 17 through 32, were transplanted using preparative regimens assigned on the basis of disease class. Twenty-two patients were assigned to class 3 and received the regimen of protocol 12 (14 patients) or another modification of the Tutschka regimen (BU, 16 mg/kg + CY, 120 mg/kg). Seven patients were categorized as class 2 and were treated according to protocol 6. All patients had damage associated with thalassemia and its treatment with transfusion and iron chelation to organs other than the marrow. In the class 3 patients, these complications were very severe and indicated a poor prognosis with continued conventional therapy. All 29 patients achieved engraftment. One class 2 patient died of the complications of severe VOD, and the other patients survive disease-free. One (class 3) patient rejected the graft on day 42 and survives with thalassemia 16 months after transplantation. Four class 3 patients died from infection and GVHD within the first 100 days after transplantation, and one class 3

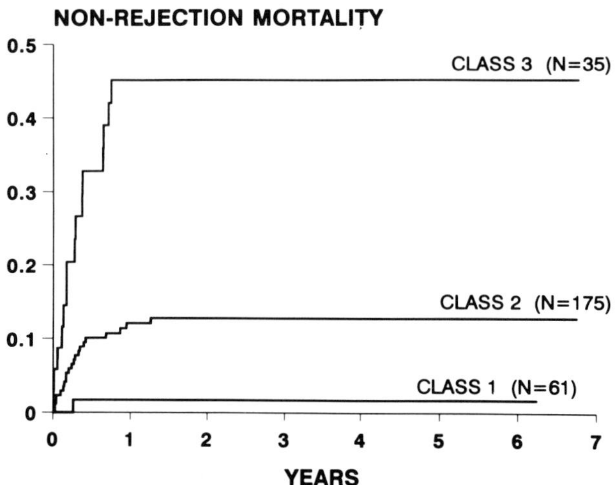

Figure 62-5. The probabilities of rejection-free mortality for 271 patients younger than 17 years with thalassemia who received marrow transplants from human leukocyte antigen–identical family members after conditioning with protocol 6. The categorization into risk classes is described in the text. Patients who rejected their grafts were censored at the time of rejection.

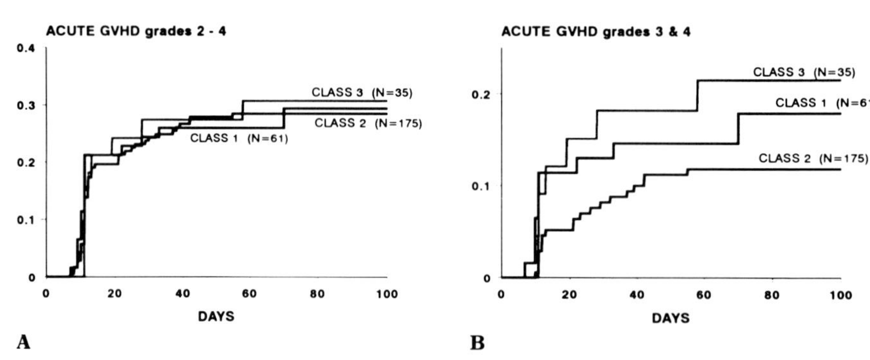

Figure 62-6. (A) The probabilities for development of acute graft-versus-host disease (GVHD) more severe than grade 1 for 271 patients younger than 17 years with thalassemia who received marrow transplants from human leukocyte antigen (HLA)–identical family members after conditioning with protocol 6. The categorization into risk classes is described in the text. (B) The probabilities of developing acute GVHD more severe than grade 2 for 271 patients younger than 17 years with thalassemia who received marrow transplants from HLA-identical family members after conditioning with protocol 6. The categorization into risk classes is described in the text.

patient died as a result of ingesting poisonous mushrooms 18 months after transplantation. Figure 62-8 shows the probabilities of survival, rejection-free survival, and rejection for all 29 patients (the mushroom poisoning patient was censored on the day of death). Transplantation provided what is probably a permanent cure for the marrow defect in nearly all these patients, but prolonged follow-up is necessary to determine the long-term outcome. It is reasonable to hope that removal of the continuing cause for the extramedullary organ damage will modify disease progression and permit healing of the damaged organs.

Mismatched Related Transplants

Experience with the use of mismatched related donors in marrow transplantation for the treatment of malignancy primarily has involved transplants between donors and recipients identical for one haplotype. When donor and recipient differed for one antigen determined by the unshared haplotype, the outcomes of transplantation were not greatly different from those obtained with genotypically identical sibling transplants. With this in mind, 11 patients were transplanted from family members with whom they were one antigen mismatched. Of two class 1 recipients, one died from complications of acute GVHD and one survives without thalassemia more than 9.5 years after transplantation. In 6 class 2 recipients, there were 2 early deaths (one each from interstitial pneumonia and infection) and of the 4 survivors, 2 have rejected their grafts and survive with recurrent thalassemia. Among two class 3 recipients, there was one early death from infection, and the survivor rejected the graft and survives with recurrent thalassemia.

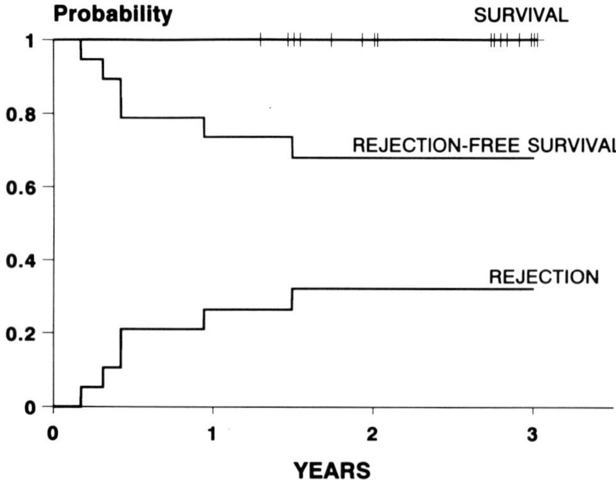

Figure 62-7. The probabilities of survival, rejection, and rejection-free survival for 19 patients with thalassemia in risk class 3, less than 17 years of age at the time of transplant, who were prepared for transplantation with protocol 12.

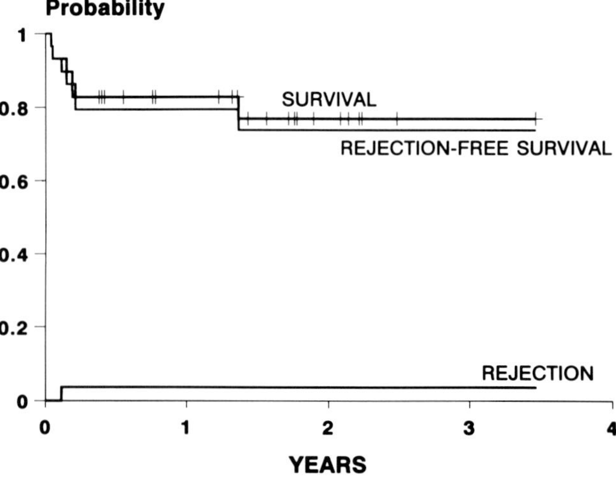

Figure 62-8. The probabilities of survival, rejection, and rejection-free survival for 19 patients with thalassemia older than 16 years of age who were transplanted between October 1988 and December 1991.

Seven patients received transplants from donors with whom they were 2 or 3 antigens mismatched. Although 5 of these patients survive between 2 and 5 years after transplantation, only one is thalassemia-free (at 5 years), and the others survive with recurrent thalassemia. There were 2 early deaths, one from infection and the other from the complications of acute GVHD.

Experience at Other Transplant Centers

Several reports describe the experience of other groups in transplanting patients for the treatment of thalassemia (18,48–53). In Italy, the Pescara group has been particularly active, reporting 52 patients transplanted through November 1990 (53). Seven of these patients were older than 16 years and 6 survived from 3+ months to 35+ months after transplantation. The group in Israel reported 10 patients who received total lymphoid irradiation (TLI) as well as BU and CY (18). The marrow was T-cell–depleted with the CAMPATH-1 monoclonal antibody. With a follow-up of 3 to 46 months, 7 patients were alive and well. The 3 deaths were due to intracranial hemorrhage, interstitial pneumonia, and chronic GVHD after a second transplant (the first having been rejected). At Stanford University, 3 children with thalassemia/hemoglobin E disease (double heterozygotes) were transplanted from HLA-identical siblings after preparation with a regimen identical to the Pesaro protocol 6. One patient survives without thalassemia and 2 had rejection with recurrent thalassemia. One was successfully transplanted after TBI and CY, and the other survives with thalassemia and awaits retransplantation. All three patients have KPS of 100% (Amylon MD. Personal communication).

Use of Unrelated Donors

We know of only 2 instances of the use of unrelated donors for the treatment of patients with thalassemia. One child was transplanted in Paris (Gluckman E. Personal communication) after a regimen of BU (16 mg/kg over 4 days) followed by CY (200 mg/kg over 4 days). The other patient was transplanted in Seattle after BU (24 mg/kg over 4 days) followed by CY (120 mg/kg over 4 days) (Thomas ED. Unpublished data). In each case, the unrelated donor was HLA-identical with the recipient. Both patients promptly rejected the grafts, and recurrent thalassemia developed.

Long-term Follow-up of Transplanted Patients

Currently, only myeloablative regimens followed by marrow transplantation can eradicate hematological thalassemia. However, thalassemic patients who have acquired normal bone marrow as a result of transplantation are not accurately described as cured. Such patients have homozygosity for the mutant gene in every cell in the body except the hematopoietic system. We do not yet know whether disease syndromes will be uncovered as a result of prolonged survival with this abnormality. Moreover, there is uncertainty about the reversibility of the various lesions suffered by different organs as a result of the thalassemia and its treatment. In particular, we do not yet know how effectively excess iron deposits can be mobilized and excreted from the body once the patient's marrow is functioning normally and transfusions are no longer needed. We do not know whether this sessile iron will continue to engender disease. Some of the pre-existing lesions, such as persistent and aggressive chronic hepatitis initiated by the hepatitis C virus, may progress or may not be readily reversed.

After successful transplantation, the body is left with a severe iron overload. Even under the best of circumstances, normal homeostatic mechanisms would take a long time to return the iron load and distribution to normal. The use of chelating agents to hasten clearance is likely to be inefficient, and periodic bleeding may help resolve this problem. The latter option is currently being studied in Pesaro. There is some evidence that class 1 patients will achieve relatively normal iron distribution within one or 2 years, but early indications are that this distribution will be more difficult to achieve in patients with advanced disease. The need to retain the option for reversing thalassemia-induced lesions to organs other than marrow is one of the factors that favors early rather than late transplantation.

There are long-term complications that arise from the allogeneic transplant itself. Thus, chronic GVHD develops in small proportion of patients, which may occasionally be severely disabling. There are indications that gonadal function of some patients who have undergone marrow transplantation for thalassemia is impaired, but it is not clear how much of this effect is a result of previous iron overload (16,17) or a consequence of the preparatory regimen.

Role of Transplantation

The results of transplantation from HLA-identical family members are clear. Class 1 patients have a very high probability of cure, with very low early and late morbidity and mortality. There is no reason for denying these patients the advantages of a life free from daily tedious, expensive, and uncomfortable therapy. We do not know the probability that a patient receiving conventional therapy will deteriorate into a worse risk category, but the fact is that every day transplant centers are confronted with patients in risk classes 2 and 3 who represent failures of conventional treatment. Delay of transplantation until the patient is in a risk category beyond class 1 substantially reduces the probability of transplant success and jeopardizes the reversibility of liver and cardiac damage. We therefore believe that patients with β-thalassemia who have HLA-identical donors should be transplanted as soon as possible.

Approximately 60% of thalassemic children do not

have HLA-identical family members. The use of family member donors genotypically identical for one HLA haplotype with minimal mismatching on the other haplotype has not been very rewarding, with only 3 successes in 11 patients mismatched for one antigen and only one success of 7 patients mismatched for more than one antigen. Clearly more studies are needed of partially matched transplants, but they are currently not an attractive option in the early management of patients who can obtain and tolerate conventional therapy. There is no extensive experience with the use of unrelated donors, but results in the first 2 such transplants, and results of transplants from partially matched related donors, indicate that unrelated donor transplants should not be performed except in the context of a well-defined research environment.

References

1. Weatherall DJ, Clegg JB. The thalassaemia syndromes. Oxford: Blackwell Scientific, 1981:744.
2. Anonymous. Community control of hereditary anemias. Bulletin of the World Health Organization 1981;61:63.
3. Thomas ED. Marrow transplantation and gene transfer as therapy for hematopoietic diseases. In: Molecular biology of homo sapiens; Cold Spring Harbor Symposia on Quantitative Biology, vol. 51, no. 2. 1986:1009–1012.
4. Thomas ED, Buckner CD, Sanders JE, et al. Marrow transplantation for thalassaemia. Lancet 1982;2:227–229.
5. Lucarelli G, Galimberti M, Polchi P, et al. Marrow transplantation in patients with advanced thalassemia. N Engl J Med 1987;316:1050–1055.
6. Lucarelli G, Galimberti M, Polchi P, et al. Bone marrow transplantation in patients with thalassemia. N Engl J Med 1990;322:417–421.
7. Wolman IJ. Transfusion therapy in Cooley's anemia: growth and health as related to long-range hemoglobin levels, a progress report. Ann NY Acad Sci 1964; 119:736–747.
8. Piomelli S, Danoff SJ, Becker MH, Lipera MJ, Travis SF. Prevention of bone malformations and cardiomegaly in Cooley's anemia by early hypertransfusion regimen. Ann NY Acad Sci 1969;165:427–436.
9. Piomelli S, Hart D, Graziano J, Grant G, Karpatkin M, McCarthy K. Current strategies in the management of Cooley's anemia. Ann NY Acad Sci 1985;445:256–267.
10. Piomelli S, Graziano J, Karpatkin M, et al. Chelation therapy, transfusion requirement, and iron balance in young thalassemic patients. Ann NY Acad Sci 1980; 344:409–417.
11. Hershko C, Weatherall DJ. Iron chelating therapy. Clin Lab Sci 1988;26:303–345.
12. U.S. Department of Health, Education and Welfare Public Health Service, National Institutes of Health. Assessment of Cooley's anemia research and treatment. DHEW Publ. No. (NIH) 79-1653, 1979.
13. Piomelli S. Cooley's anemia management: 25 years of progress. In: Buckner CD, Gale RP, Lucarelli G, eds. Advances and controversies in thalassemia therapy: bone marrow-transplantation and other approaches. New York: Alan R. Liss, 1989:23–26.
14. Gabutti V, Piga A, Sacchetti L, et al. Quality of life and life expectancy in thalassemic patients with complications. In: Buckner CD, Gale RP, Lucarelli G, eds. Advances and controversies in thalassemia therapy: bone marrow transplantation and other approaches. New York: Alan R. Liss, 1989:35–41.
15. Politis C. Complications of blood transfusions in thalassemia. In: Buckner CD, Gale RP, Lucarelli G, eds. Advances and controversies in thalassemia therapy: bone marrow transplantation and other approaches. New York: Alan R. Liss, 1989:67–76.
16. Manenti F, Galimberti M, Lucarelli G, et al. Growth and endocrine function after bone marrow transplantation for thalassemia. In: Buckner CD, Gale RP, Lucarelli G, eds. Advances and controversies in thalassemia therapy: bone marrow transplantation and other approaches. New York: Alan R. Liss, 1989:273–280.
17. De Sanctis V, Galimberti M, Lucarelli G, Polchi P, Ruggiero L, Vullo C. Gonadal function after allogeneic bone marrow transplantation for thalassaemia. Arch Dis Child 1991;66:517–520.
18. Slavin S, Or R, Cividalli G, et al. Bone marrow transplantation in β-thalassemia with prevention of graft-vs-host disease. In: Fucharoen S, Rowley PT, Paul NW, eds. Birth defects: original article series. Thalassemia: pathophysiology and management. Part B. New York: Alan R. Liss, 1987:313–316.
19. Thomas ED. Allogeneic bone marrow transplantation for blood cell disorders. In: Cao A, Carcassi U, Rowley PT, eds. Thalassemia: recent advances in detection and treatment, birth defects: original article series, vol. 18. New York: Alan R. Liss, 1982:361–369.
20. Witherspoon RP, Fisher LD, Schoch G, et al. Secondary cancers after bone marrow transplantation for leukemia or aplastic anemia. N Engl J Med 1989;321:784–789.
21. Socie G, Henry-Amar M, Cosset JM, Devergie A, Girinsky T, Gluckman E. Increased incidence of solid malignant tumors after bone marrow transplantation for severe aplastic anemia. Blood 1991;78:277–279.
22. Witherspoon RP, Storb R, Pepe M, Longton G, Sullivan KM. Cumulative incidence of secondary solid malignant tumors in aplastic anemia patients given marrow grafts after conditioning with chemotherapy alone (letter). Blood 1992;79:289–290.
23. Parkman R, Rappeport J, Geha R, et al. Complete correction of the Wiskott-Aldrich syndrome by allogeneic bone-marrow transplantation. N Engl J Med 1978;298:921–927.
24. Kapoor N, Kirkpatrick D, Blaese RM, et al. Reconstitution of normal megakaryocytopoiesis and immunologic functions in Wiskott-Aldrich syndrome by marrow transplantation following myeloablation and immunosuppression with busulfan and cyclophosphamide. Blood 1981;57:692–696.
25. Hobbs JR, Hugh-Jones K, Shaw PJ, Downie CJC, Williamson S. Engraftment rates related to busulphan and cyclophosphamide dosages for displacement bone marrow transplants in fifty children. Bone Marrow Transplant 1986;1:201–208.
26. Thomas ED, Buckner CD, Storb R, et al. Aplastic anaemia treated by marrow transplantation. Lancet 1972;1:284–289.
27. Storb R, Champlin RE. Bone marrow transplantation for severe aplastic anemia. Bone Marrow Transplant 1991;8:69–72.
28. Santos GW, Sensenbrenner LL, Burke PJ, et al. Marrow transplantation in man following cyclophosphamide. Transplant Proc 1971;3:400–404.

29. Tutschka PJ, Elfenbein GJ, Sensenbrenner LL, et al. Preparative regimens for marrow transplantation in acute leukemia and aplastic anemia. Baltimore experience. Am J Peiatr Hematol Oncol 1980;2:363–370.
30. Santos GW, Tutschka PJ, Brookmeyer R, et al. Marrow transplantation for acute nonlymphocytic leukemia after treatment wth busulfan and cyclophosphamide. N Engl J Med 1983;309:1347–1353.
31. Appelbaum FR, Storb R, Ramberg RE, et al. Allogeneic marrow transplantation in the treatment of preleukemia. Ann Intern Med 1984;100:689–693.
32. Tutschka PJ, Copelan EA, Kapoor N. Replacing total body irradiation with busulfan as conditioning of patients with leukemia for allogeneic marrow transplantation. Transplant Proc 1989;21:2952–2954.
33. Tutschka PJ, Copelan EA, Kapoor N, Avalos BR, Klein JP. Allogeneic bone marrow transplantation for leukemia using chemotherapy as conditioning: 6-year results of a single institution trial. Transplant Proc 1991;23: 1709–1710.
34. Floersheim GL, Elson LA. Restoration of hematopoiesis following a lethal dose of dimethyl myleran by isologic bone marrow transplantation in mice. Experiments on modifications of intolerance to homologous bone marrow by 6-mercaptopurine, amino-chlorambucil and cortisone. Acta Haematol 1961;26:233–245.
35. Storb R, Weiden PL, Graham TC, Lerner KG, Nelson N, Thomas ED. Hemopoietic grafts between DLA-identical canine littermates following dimethyl myleran. Evidence for resistance to grafts not associated with DLA and abrogated by antithymocyte serum. Transplantation 1977;24:349–357.
36. Tutschka PJ, Copelan EA, Klein JP. Bone marrow transplantation for leukemia following a new busulfan and cyclophosphamide regimen. Blood 1987;70:1382–1388.
37. Storb R, Thomas ED, Buckner CD, et al. Marrow transplantation in thirty "untransfused" patients with severe aplastic anemia. Ann Intern Med 1980;92:30–36.
38. Storb R, Prentice RL, Thomas ED, et al. Factors associated with graft rejection after HLA-identical marrow transplantation for aplastic anaemia. Br J Haematol 1983;55:573–585.
39. Bearman SI, Appelbaum FR, Buckner CD, et al. Regimen-related toxicity in patients undergoing bone marrow transplantation. J Clin Oncol 1988;6:1562–1568.
40. Bearman SI, Appelbaum FR, Back A, et al. Regimen-related toxicity and early posttransplant survival in patients undergoing marrow transplantation for lymphoma. J Clin Oncol 1989;7:1288–1294.
41. Thomas ED, Sanders JE, Buckner CD, et al. Marrow transplantation for thalassemia. Ann NY Acad Sci 1985;445:417–427.
42. Thomas ED, Lucarelli G. Marrow transplantation for thalassemia major. In: Fucharoen S, Rowley PT, Paul NW, eds. Thalassemia: pathophysiology and management. Birth defects: original article series, vol. 23, 5B. New York: Alan R. Liss, 1988:303–306.
43. Storb R, Anasetti C, Appelbaum F, et al. Marrow transplantation for severe aplastic anemia and thalassemia major. Semin Hematol 1991;28:235–239.
44. Lucarelli G, Polchi P, Izzi T, et al. Allogeneic marrow transplantation for thalassemia. Exp Hematol 1984; 12:676–681.
45. Lucarelli G, Polchi P, Galimberti M, et al. Marrow transplantation for thalassemia following busulphan and cyclophosphamide. Lancet 1985;1:1355–1357.
46. Thomas ED, Storb R, Clift RA, et al. Bone-marrow transplantation. N Engl J Med. 1975;292:832–843,895–902.
47. Shulman HM, Sullivan KM, Weiden PL, et al. Chronic graft-versus-host syndrome in man. A long-term clinicopathologic study of 20 Seattle patients. Am J Med 1980;69:204–217.
48. Brochstein JA, Kirkpatrick D, Giardina PJ, et al. Bone marrow transplantation in two multiply transfused patients with thalassemia major. Br J Haematol 1986;63:445–456.
49. Borgna-Pignatti C. Marrow transplantation for thalassemia. Annu Rev Med 1985;36:329–336.
50. Lin KH, Lin KS. Allogeneic bone marrow transplantation for thalassemia in Taiwan: factors associated with graft failure. Am J Pediatr Hematol Oncol 1989;11: 417–423.
51. Frappaz D, Gluckman E, Souillet G, et al. Allogeneic bone marrow graft in thalassemia major. The French experience. Arch Fr Pediatr 1990;47:97–102.
52. Di Bartolomeo P, Di Girolamo G, Angrilli F, et al. Bone marrow transplantation for adult patients with thalassemia major. Bone Marrow Transplant 1991;7 (suppl 2):73.
53. Di Bartolomeo P, Di Girolamo G, Angrilli F, et al. Bone marrow transplantation for thalassemia in Pescara. In: Buckner CD, Gale RP, Lucarelli G, eds. Advances and controversies in thalassemia therapy: bone marrow transplantation and other approaches. New York: Alan R. Liss, 1989:193–199.

Chapter 63
Bone Marrow Transplantation for Sickle Cell Disease

Ernest Beutler and Keith M. Sullivan

It is one of the ironies of modern medicine that more effort has been invested in the study of sickle cell disease than any other genetic disorder, and that despite the hard work and resources expended, management of the disorder is still very unsatisfactory.

This is not to suggest that much has not been achieved. Sickle cell disease was the first anemia of humans in which the mutation was understood at the amino acid level (1); after the triplet code was deciphered, the nucleotide substitution was deduced, even before confirmation by actual sequencing was possible. The biophysical properties of sickle hemoglobin have been characterized extensively (2). Some of the factors that may be responsible for the marked variability in phenotype expression of the same mutation have been identified (3–7). This increased understanding has led to a host of therapeutic suggestions, including pH modification (8), the use of methemoglobin-forming agents (6), carbon monoxide (9–11), pyridoxine (12), urea (13–15), cyanate (16,17), zinc (18), dimethyl adipimidate (19,20), 5-azacytidine (21,22), ticlopidine (23), hydroxyurea (24–26), cetiedil (27), bepridil (28), pentoxifylline (29), desmopressin (30), butyrate (31), and erythropoietin (32). Nonetheless, the mainstay of therapy has remained blood transfusions (33–37), antibiotic prophylaxis (38–40), and analgesic drugs (41–43).

Although the search for new agents to control the sickling process continues, there is increasing interest in modalities that might eliminate the underlying disorder by correcting the defect at the hematopoietic stem-cell level. Such a strategy consists of destroying the patient's own abnormal stem cells and replacing them with stem cells from a normal person or with the patient's own, genetically corrected stem cells. The latter approach is still beyond our technical capabilities; thus, allogeneic bone marrow transplantation (BMT) remains the only modality that can be expected to cure sickle disease today.

However, the risk intrinsic to BMT must be balanced against the risks of the expected morbidity and mortality of the disease that one is attempting to cure. Weighing these risks has been difficult because the clinical course of sickle cell disease is quite variable. Unlike patients with severe aplastic anemia or acute leukemia, patients with sickle disease have a high likelihood of surviving for many years, and, in rare cases, with very little morbidity. Thus, it is essential to have an understanding of the pathogenesis and natural history of sickle cell disease if rational decisions are to be made regarding BMT.

Pathogenesis of Sickling

The sickle mutation is a substitution of a thymine for an adenine in codon 6 of the β-globin coding sequence, changing a GAG to GTG. This process results in the substitution of valine for glutamic acid at amino acid 6. Sickle cell anemia is the homozygous (SS genotype) state for this mutation. Other sickle diseases result from the compound heterozygous state of the sickle mutation and another abnormal β-globin gene. Examples are SC disease, the heterozygous state for the sickle mutation and the hemoglobin C mutation, and sickle-thalassemia, the heterozygous state for sickle hemoglobin and β-thalassemia. Hemoglobin tetrameres containing the mutant chain behave quite normally in the oxyconformation, but in the deoxy state, they tend to aggregate into rigid rods that deform the red cell into a characteristic sickle shape.

Blood with sickled red cells has markedly abnormal rheological properties, which leads to obstruction of small blood vessels throughout the body, with consequent organ dysfunction and pain. Sickling apparently leads to a considerable number of secondary abnormalities of the erythrocytes, such as decreased levels of nicotinamide adenine dinucleotide (44), development of vesicles (45), and increased adhesiveness (46,47). The sickled red cells have a shortened intravascular life span, leading to anemia and reticulocytosis. Increased susceptibility to infection is another common manifestation of the sickle diseases (48,49). It may result from the functional asplenia that commonly occurs because of repeated splenic thromboses and from ill-defined abnormalities of leukocyte function (50).

Clinical Course

The clinical manifestations of sickle cell disease vary enormously from patient to patient. A very few go through life with only occasional problems that can be attributed to their disease. This condition seems to be particularly common in some Arab populations (51,52). In contrast, most patients with sickle disease suffer a range of adverse effects, ranging from mild anemia and occasional bouts of pain in some, to catastrophic strokes, fatal infections, splenic sequestration, acute chest syndrome, and organ failure in the less fortunate.

Manifestations of the disease are to a large extent age-related. In the neonatal period, there are usually no stimata of disease. The β-globin chain bears the mutation, but it is the γ-globin chain of fetal hemoglobin that is produced in the late antenatal period. Thus, sickling does not begin to occur until β-chain production results in a sufficient concentration of adult sickle hemoglobin to deform the red cells.

Neurological Damage

As the sickle hemoglobin concentration begins to increase, some of the characteristic stigmata of early childhood sickle disease become apparent. Findings include anemia, dactylitis, painful crises, recurrent infections, acute sequestration of red cells in an enlarged spleen, and cerebrovascular accidents (53). The latter complication is greatly feared, because the residua of a stroke are often serious and permanent. Approximately 8% of children with sickle disease will experience a stroke (54), and more subtle brain damage may exist in a larger number of patients examined by magnetic resonance scanning (55). The 5- to 10-year age group has the highest prevalence of this complication, but the first stroke can occur as early as the second year of life or as late as the eighteenth year (54). It is not possible to predict with any accuracy in which children this complication will develop, but if one stroke has occurred, development of subsequent strokes is observed in 67% of patients (56).

Chronic transfusion therapy has been shown to reduce the rate of recurrent stroke (37,57,58). However, red-cell alloimmunization, infection, and iron overload may develop in frequently transfused patients (54,59,60). Moreover, even after 5 to 12 years of treatment, strokes may recur after discontinuation of transfusion therapy (54). Of further concern, investigations over the last several years reveal subclinical brain damage in many patients with sickle cell anemia (55). Even in the absence of overt stroke and motor deficit, a substantial number of children with sickle cell disease demonstrate significant impairment in neuropsychological testing (61).

Organ Failure

Sequestration crises, in which a large proportion of the red-cell mass is sequestered in an enlarged spleen, is another devastating and unpredictable event in sickle cell disease (62). Treatment consists of transfusion and, in selected patients, splenectomy (39). Older patients with sickle cell disease tend to have a clinical course in which painful vaso-occlusive crises have a predominant role, and vasculopathy leads to failure of the brain, kidneys, or lungs (Figure 63-1). Painful crises generally involve the skeleton and are characterized by pain that may be very severe and accompanied by fever. Precipitating factors are not always evident, although there is a tendency for attacks to occur after infections and sometimes after exposure to cold. Painful episodes usually persist for several days and then gradually abate. Hip pain may be a symptom of osteonecrosis of the femoral head, although nearly half the patients with osteonecrosis have no pain at initial diagnosis (63). Among 2,590 patients older than 5 years of age who entered the Cooperative Study of Sickle Cell Disease (CSSCD) between 1979 and 1981, osteonecrosis of the hip was estimated to develop in 40% with SS genotype by age 30. The results of hip athroplasty were poor; two thirds of patients continued to experience pain and three quarters continued to have limited range of movement after surgery (63).

Changes in the central nervous system in older patients may range from subtle cognitive disabilities to massive, fatal hemorrhagic or thrombotic infarctions. As shown in Table 63-1, the onset of neurological events tends to be earlier than that of other forms of organ failure, but may occur well into adult life (64). Chronic renal failure with glomerulosclerosis is also observed in older patients with sickle disease. Accompanying features include hypertension, proteinuria, and nephrotic syndrome. Despite dialysis, median survival after the diagnosis of sickle renal failure is 4

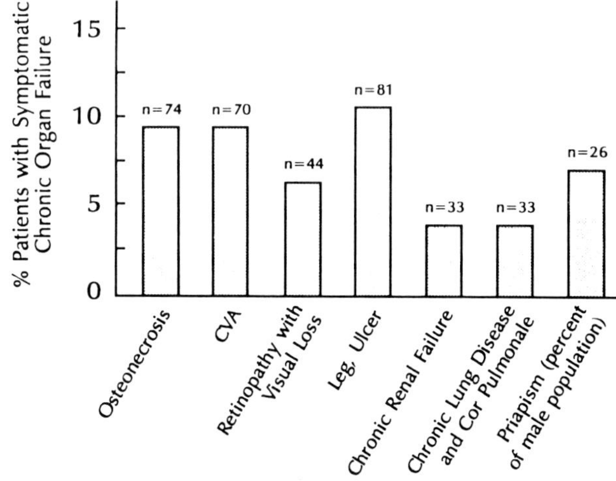

Figure 63-1. Irreversible organ failure in 785 patients with sickle cell anemia (SS genotype) followed in the Los Angeles area. CVA = cerebrovascular accident. Adapated from Powers D, Chan LS, Schroeder WA. The variable expression of sickle cell disease is genetically determined. Semin Hematol 1990; 27:360–376.)

Table 63-1.
Age at Onset of Irreversible Organ Failure in Sickle Cell Anemia

	Age at Diagnosis (yr)	
Clinical Failure	*Median*	*Range*
Cerebral infarction of hemorrhage	13.1	0.6–47.1
Chronic renal failure	25.1	12.8–62.9
Chronic lung disease	24.2	6.0–43.3
Leg ulcer	24.5	4.0–52.5
Osteonecrosis	23.1	1.3–60.9
Retinopathy	25.8	8.9–65.3
Priapism	22.3	6.2–47.9

Adapted from Powars D, Chan LS, Schroeder WA. The variable expression of sickle cell disease is genetically determined. Semin Hematol 1990;27:360–376.

years (65). Chronic restrictive lung disease, pulmonary hypertension, and cor pulmonale are observed in some patients with sickle cell disease (66). An acute chest syndrome characterized by pulmonary infiltrate, hypoxia, chest pain, fever, and leukocytosis has also been described (67). This syndrome may result from rib infarction and pain, leading to hypoventilation and atelectasis (68).

Pain

A report from the CSSCD detailed the natural history of pain in sickle cell disease (69). The average pain rate was 0.8 episodes per patient-year. One third of all pain episodes occurred in 5.2% of patients, with 3 to 10 episodes per year. Among patients more than 20 years of age, the probability of survival to age 40 was 38% in patients with 3 or more episodes of pain per year, compared with an 80% probability in patients with fewer episodes of pain.

Prognosis

Historical Perspective

Half a century ago, sickle cell trait was known to be common in Africa, but the disease was so rare that the relationship between the trait and the disease seemed to be obscure. The lack of homozygotes was no doubt a consequence of poor health care conditions in Africa. Under these circumstances, few sickle patients survived early childhood. This situation has changed markedly, particularly in areas of the developed world, where the standards of health care are high. Indeed, if survival of patients with sickle cell disease was as uncommon now as it once was, decisions regarding BMT would be easier to make.

Mortality Rates

In one 1979 to 1981 cohort of patients, the mortality of sickle disease was 7% by 36 months of age and 15% by 20 years of age (70). A high proportion of deaths were due to infection (71). Figure 63-2 presents data collected from a cohort of patients in the Los Angeles area (5). In a recent update of the CSSCD experience, the median age at death for patients with sickle cell disease (SS genotype) was 40 years for men and 49 years for women (72). Compared with the entire African-American population, this represents a 30-year reduction in life expectancy for patients with sickle cell disease.

Modifying Factors

A number of factors have been found to be correlated with prognosis in sickle cell disease. Analysis of children entering the CSSCD before 12 years of age found that a low hematocrit or a low fetal hemoglobin value in the first 2 years of life predicted an increased risk of subsequent morbidity (73). Among 519 patients in the newborn cohort who entered the study before 0.6 years of age, 43 (8%) had factors developing by the second year of life that predicted an increased risk of subsequent severe medical complications. Predictive factors included a low age-adjusted fetal hemoglobin or hematocrit level and the onset of dactylitis, painful crisis, or acute chest syndrome before the second year of life (73).

It was suggested more than 30 years ago that the presence of fetal hemoglobin should ameliorate the sickling process (6,74), and a number of studies of the natural course of the disease have shown that such a correlation exists (7), although it seems to be fairly weak at lower levels of fetal hemoglobin (75).

The presence of α-thalassemia, a common genetic trait in African populations, ameliorates the course of sickle cell disease (3,75–79). Patients with a single or double α-locus deletion have a distinctly lower mean corpuscular hemoglobin concentration, which may be responsible for the decreased severity of their disease; on the average, hematocrit values are higher and

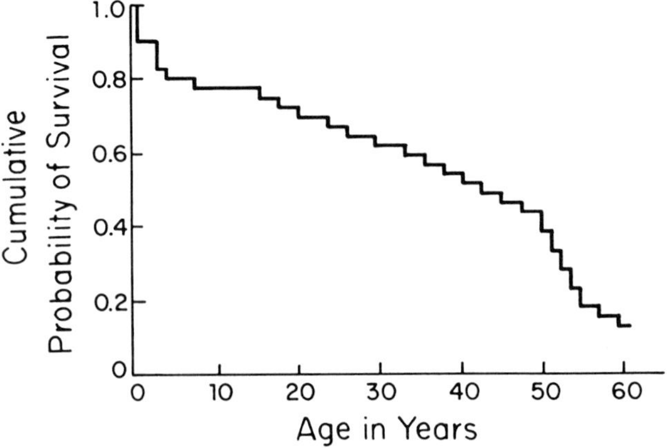

Figure 63-2. Mortality in patients presented in Figure 63-1. (Adapted from D, Chan LS, Schroeder WA. The variable expression of sickle cell disease is genetically determined. Semin Hematol 1990;27:360–376.)

reticulocyte counts are lower. However, there is considerable individual variation and marked overlap between groups.

The sickle gene has apparently arisen independently several times and is found in the context of different β-globin gene haplotypes as defined by restriction polymorphisms. The 4 major haplotypes are designated Senegal, Benin, Bantu (or Central African Republic), and Arab-India. The first 2 originate in Western Africa, the Bantu type in central Africa, and the Arab-India from the Arabian Peninsula and the Indian subcontinent. Some of these haplotypes may influence the clinical severity of the disease, either by affecting the production of the γ-globin chains of fetal hemoglobin or in some other manner. The haplotypes are strongly correlated with the production of one of the 2 types of γ-chains, $^{G}\gamma$ (80). The total amount of fetal hemoglobin is also correlated with the β-globin haplotype; SS patients homozygous for the Senegal or the Arab-Indian haplotype manifest higher concentrations of hemoglobin F (81,82). Some differences seem to exist between the severity of clinical disease and the haplotype (64). Table 63-2 summarizes data on the incidence of complications in patients with and without a sickle gene found in the context of the Bantu haplotype, which is associated, on average, with lower fetal hemoglobin levels. Although differences exist in frequency, it is clear that all of the complications occur, albeit at different frequencies in those with and without the Bantu haplotype.

Indications for BMT

In view of the relatively good initial survival that attends sickle cell disease in many patients and the relative weakness of predictors of the clinical course for individual patients, the decision whether to transplant a patient can be very difficult. There are currently no generally agreed on criteria that physicians can consult when making this recommendation.

Table 63-2.
Effect of the Bantu (CAR) Haplotype on Symptomatic Organ Damage in Sickle Cell Anemia

	Age-adjusted Incidence/100 Person Years	
Complication	*"Bantu" Present (n = 82)*	*"Bantu" Absent (n = 139)*
Stroke	1.59	0.79
Glomerulosclerosis	0.65	0.13
Chronic restrictive lung disease	0.23	0.18
Composite soft-tissue damage (CNS/lung/kidney/retina/leg ulcers)	5.05	2.24
Death	0.81	0.30

CAR = Central African Republic; CNS = central nervous system.
Adapted from Powars DR. Sickle cell anemia. β-gene-cluster haplotypes as prognostic indicators of vital organ failure. Semin Hematol 1991;28:202–208.

Factors that must be taken into account are age, complications that have already occurred, the prognostic factors mentioned, and the availability of a human leukocyte antigen (HLA)–identical donor. A review of patients in the Northern California Comprehensive Sickle Cell Center revealed that only 18% of patients had an HLA-identical sibling free of sickle cell anemia (83). Recruitment of minority volunteers for the United States National Marrow Donor Program (NMDP) has received widespread support, but as of early 1992, only 18,456 (3.7%) of the 491,215 NMDP donors were of African-American origin (84).

Patients and physicians must also consider the availability of alternative therapies for sickle cell disease. To date, no comparative trials have been conducted to test the risks and benefits of standard supportive care, hydroxyurea, chronic transfusion therapy, and BMT. However, most investigators agree that based on cost alone, BMT would be more cost-effective than chronic transfusion and iron chelation therapy for sickle cell patients with stroke (85,86).

The ideal patient for transplantation, therefore, is a small child who has had a stroke, but not a very severe one, and who has an HLA-identical sibling without sickle cell disease. Adults with sickle disease would ordinarily not be candidates for BMT. Existing organ damage and the higher incidence of graft-versus-host disease (GVHD) would put them at higher risk (87). Patients who do not have an HLA-matched family donor should not be transplanted until there is further experience with family donors for sickle disease and matched unrelated BMTs for patients with leukemia. Currently, selection criteria and timing of BMT remain controversial, and several symposia have been held to explore these issues (88–93). It remains unrealistic to expect no risk associated with BMT (93); however, given the considerable morbidity associated with sickle cell anemia, some sickle cell experts have argued for early transplantation of asymptomatic children (94). Others have proposed selection of children with severe symptomatic sickle disease before onset of organ failure (95). Parental choice is a key factor in these discussions. To gain cure for their children, a survey found that 54% of parents were willing to accept a 5% risk of mortality with BMT and 37% were willing to risk a 15% mortality (96).

Results of BMT in Sickle cell Disease

Although it has long been clear that transplantation would cure sickle cell disease (97), there has until recently been reluctance to offer this treatment modality to patients because of the risk inherent in the BMT procedure. Indeed, the first patients to be treated were transplanted, not for the sickle cell disease itself, but rather for acute leukemia (98,99) or a second genetic disorder (100).

Results of HLA-identical BMT for sickle cell anemia alone have been reported by investigators in Belgium

(101,102). Initial patients were children of parents from Zaire or Cameroon studying in Brussels. Due to concern for transfusion support and medical care in Africa, 12 patients were transplanted from HLA-matched donors. Ages ranged from 11 months to 23 years. None had evidence of chronic organ failure; however, the median number of vaso-occlusive crises was 4 (range, 1–6) episodes per year. All were prepared with 16 mg/kg busulfan (BU) and 200 mg/kg cyclophosphamide (CY) and received cyclosporine (CSP) as GVHD prophylaxis. Those patients older than 12 years of age received additional thoracoabdominal irradiation (750 cGy with lung shielding) conditioning and methotrexate (MTX) combined with CSP for GVHD prophylaxis. One patient had a small amount of Hb S present 36 months after transplantation, which is consistent with mixed chimerism, and the other 11 had full donor engraftment confirmed by hemoglobin electrophoresis. Grade I to II acute GVHD in 4 patients developed and one had chronic GVHD, which resolved with treatment. All 12 patients survive a median of 27 months after transplantation, and 7 have returned home to Africa. A second series of 5 patients transplanted in another center in Belgium provided similar results (103).

The combined Belgian and French experience has now increased to 42 patients transplanted for sickle cell anemia (104). Patients ranged in age from 1 to 23 (median, 8) years. Prior clinical features included acute chest syndrome (6 patients), chronic transfusion therapy (7 patients), and stroke (6 patients). Preparative conditioning included BU (14–16 mg/kg or 500–600 mg/m^2) and CY (200–260 mg/kg). Nine patients received additional irradiation (750 cGy). GVHD prophylaxis included MTX and CSP (25 patients) or CSP alone (17 patients). One patient died on day 92 of GVHD and a combined cytomegalovirus and *aspergillus* infection. The other 41 survive from 1 to 75 months after transplantation. Graft rejection was noted in 5 (12%) patients 2, 2, 14, 15, and 23 months after BMT. Two were successfully retransplanted, and 38 of the 42 (90%) patients currently survive with donor engraftment (Table 63-3).

The experience in the United States is still very limited (105). Three patients have been transplanted for complications of sickle cell disease (2 with prior strokes and one with recurrent severe pain crises and acute chest syndrome) and 2 for other disorders (acute myeloid leukemia and Morquio's disease). The 5 patients ranged in age from 3 to 10 (median, 4) years. Preparative regimens included BU and CY with or without antithymocyte globulin (ATG) in 4 patients and total body irradiation in the patient with leukemia. Various combinations of MTX, CSP, and prednisone were used for GVHD prophylaxis. The patient with Morquio's disease failed to engraft but was successfully retransplanted. All patients have hemoglobin of the donor pattern. Grade II–IV acute GVHD developed in 2 patients, and transient chronic GVHD developed in one. The median duration of hospitalization was 6 (range, 4–10) weeks. Subsequent transient neurological events developed in both patients transplanted for stroke: one suffered transient ischemic episodes between 6 and 9 months after BMT, and seizures, aphasia, and hemiparesis developed in one 5 and 7 weeks after BMT. Symptoms have resolved in both patients, and all 5 survive in good to excellent clinical condition a median of 16 (range, 8–112) months following BMT.

Future Directions

As described in Chapters 43 and 62, considerable progress has been observed in BMT for children with nonmalignant diseases such as severe aplastic anemia and thalassemia. More than 90% survival has been observed in good-risk patients given marrow grafts from HLA-identical donors (106,107). Whether these results will be obtained in patients with sickle cell anemia is unknown, but the initial experience in Europe and the United States appears encouraging

Table 63-3.
BMT for Sickle Cell Anemia

Factor	*European Experience*		*United States Experience*		
Author, reference	Vermylen (104)	Milpied (99)	Johnson (98)	Mentzer (100)	Johnson (105)
No. patients	42	1	1	1	3
Disease	SCA	SCA/ALL	SCA/AML	SCA/MD	SCA
Median age (range, yr)	8 (1–23)	22	8	4	4 (3–10)
Preparatory regimen (mg/kg)	BU (14–16 + CY (200–260) ± TAI	CY (120) + TBI	CY (120) + TBI	BU/CY/ATG CY/ATG/TBI	BU (14–16) + CY ± ATG
Graft rejection	5	1	0	1	0
Acute GVHD	13	0	1	0	1
Chronic GVHD	6	0	1	0	0
Number surviving	41	0	1	1	3
Follow-up (mo)	1–75	. . .	112	37	8–16

ALL = acute lymphoid leukemia; AML = acute myeloid leukemia; ATG = antithymocyte globulin; BMT = bone marrow transplantation; BU = busulfan; CY = cyclophosphamide; GVHD = graft-versus-host disease; MD = Morquio's disease; SCA = sickle cell anemia; TAI = thoracoabdominal irradiation; TBI = total body irradiation.

Table 63-4.
Selection of Patients with Sickle Cell Disease for BMT

Inclusion
Homozygous patients with sickle cell disease < 16 years old
One or more of the following complications
- Stroke or CNS hemorrhage
- Impaired neurological function and abnormal MRI scan
- Recurrent acute chest syndrome
- Stage I to II sickle lung disease
- Sickle nephropathy (GFR 30–50% predicted)
- Bilateral proliferative retinopathy and visual impairment
- Osteonecrosis of multiple joints
- Chronic priapism or recurrent debilitating pain
- Alloimmunization (≥ 2 antibodies) on chronic transfusion therapy

Exclusion
Patients ≥ 16 years old
HLA-nonidentical donor
One or more of the following conditions
- Karnofsky performance < 70%
- Hepatitis or moderate/severe portal fibrosis
- Renal impairment (GFR < 30% predicted)
- Stage III to IV sickle lung disease

BMT = bone marrow transplantation; CNS = central nervous system; GFR = glomerular filtration rate; MRI = magnetic resonance imaging.

(104,105). It is also unknown whether sickle cell vasculopathy will reverse with BMT and what effect the vascular abnormalities will have on the outcome of transplantation. Future prospective trials comparing BMT with alternative therapies and conventional supportive treatment of sickle cell anemia will be required to answer these important questions.

Criteria for patient selection remain problematic given the uncertainty in predicting the clinical course of individual patients. An approach decided at recent conferences was to offer BMT to children who have already demonstrated significant morbidity from sickle cell disease (88,92). To assure safety in the initial pilot study, marrow donors would be restricted to HLA-identical siblings, and patients with advanced organ failure would be excluded (Table 63-4). A national United States collaborative trial has been established to test a standard preparatory regimen in these patients with symptomatic sickle cell anemia (95). Conditioning with BU, CY, and ATG will be employed to test the efficacy of this regimen in safely ablating sickle marrow. This experience, in turn, will be important in designing future trials of autologous BMT of genetically corrected hematopoietic stem cells, as outlined in Chapter 7.

References

1. Ingram VM. Gene mutations in human haemoglobin: the chemical difference between normal and sickle cell haemoglobin. Nature 1957;180:326–328.
2. Noguchi CT, Schechter AN. The intracellular polymerization of sickle hemoglobin and its relevance to sickle cell disease. Blood 1981;58:1057–1068.
3. Embury SH, Dozy AM, Miller J, et al. Concurrent sickle-cell anemia and alpha-thalassemia. Effect on severity of anemia. N Engl J Med 1982;306:270–274.
4. Nagel RL. Severity, pathobiology, epistatic effects, and genetic markers in sickle cell anemia. Semin Hematol 1991;28:180–201.
5. Powars D, Chan LS, Schroeder WA. The variable expression of sickle cell disease is genetically determined. Semin Hematol 1990;27:360–376.
6. Beutler E. The effect of methemoglobin formation in sickle cell disease. J Clin Invest 1961;40:1856–1871.
7. Powars DR, Weiss JN, Schroeder WA. Is there a threshold level of fetal hemoglobin that ameliorates morbidity in sickle cell anemia? Blood 1984;63:921–926.
8. Greenberg MS, Kass EH. Studies on the destruction of red blood cells. XIII. Observations on the role of pH in the pathogenesis and treatment of painful crisis in sickle-cell disease. Arch Intern Med 1958;101:355–363.
9. Beutler E. The effect of carbon monoxide on red cell life span in sickle cell disease. Blood 1975;46:253–259.
10. Sirs JA. The use of carbon monoxide to prevent sickle-cell formation. Lancet 1963;1:971–972.
11. Purugganan HB, McElfresh AE. Failure of carbonmonoxy sickle-cell haemoglobin to alter the sickle state. Lancet 1964;1:79–80.
12. Beutler E, Paniker NV, West CJ. Pyridoxine administration in sickle cell disease: an unsuccessful attempt to influence the properties of sickle hemoglobin. Biochem Med 1972;6:139–143.
13. Treatment of sickle-cell crises. Lancet 1974;2:762–765.
14. Cooperative Urea Trials Group. Therapy for sickle cell vaso-occlusive crises. JAMA 1974;228:1129–1131.
15. Nalbandian RM, Shulta G, Lusher JM, Anderson JW, Henry RL. Sickle cell crisis terminated by intravenous urea in sugar solutions, a preliminary report. Am J Med Sci 1971;261:309–324.
16. De Furia FG, Miller DR, Cerami A, Manning JM. The effects of cyanate in vitro on red blood cell metabolism and function in sickle cell anemia. J Clin Invest 1972;51:566–574.
17. Peterson CM, Tsairis P, Ohnishi A, et al. Sodium cyanate induced polyneuropathy in patients with sickle-cell disease. Ann Intern Med 1974;81:152–158.
18. Brewer GJ, Oelshlegel FJ Jr, Prasad AS. Zinc in sickle cell anemia. Prog Clin Bio Res 1975;1:417–432.
19. Lubin BH, Pena V, Mentzer WC, Byman E, Bradley TB, Packer L. Dimethyl adipimidate: a new antisickling agent. Proc Natl Acad Sci USA 1975;72:43–46.
20. Guis MS, Lande WM, Mohandas N, et al. Prolongation of sickle cell survival by dimethyl adipimidate is compromised by immune sensitization. Blood 1984;64:161–165.
21. Charache S, Dover G, Smith K, Talbot CC Jr, Moyer M, Boyer S. Treatment of sickle cell anemia with 5-azacytidine results in increased fetal hemoglobin production and is associated with nonrandom hypomethylation of DNA around the gamma-delta-beta globin gene complex. Proc Natl Acad Sci USA 1983;80:4842–4846.
22. Ley TJ, DeSimone J, Noguchi C, et al. 5-Azacytidine increase gamma-globin synthesis and reduces the proportion of dense cells in sickle cell anemia. Blood 1983;62:370–380.
23. Semple MJ, Alhasani SF, Kioy P, Savidge GF. A double-blind trial of ticlopidine in sickle-cell disease. Thromb Haemost 1984;51:303–306.

24. Platt OS, Orkin SH, Dover G, Beardsley GP, Miller B, Nathan DG. Hydroxyurea enhances fetal hemoglobin production in sickle cell anemia. J Clin Invest 1984; 74:652–656.
25. Veith R, Galanello R, Papayannopoulou T, Stamatoyannopoulos G. Stimulation of F-cell production in Hb S patients treated with ara-C or hydroxyurea. N Engl J Med 1985;313:1571–1575.
26. Dover GJ, Humphries RK, Moore JG, et al. Hydroxyurea induction of hemoglobin F production in sickle cell disease: relationship between cytotoxicity and F-cell production. Blood 1986;67:735–738.
27. Benjamin LJ, Berkowitz LR, Orringer E, et al. A collaborative, double-blind randomized study of cetiedil citrate in sickle cell crisis. Blood 1986;67:1442–1447.
28. Reilly MP, Asakura T. Antisickling effect of bepridil. Lancet 1986;1:848.
29. Teuscher T, Weil von der Ahe C, Baillod P, Holzer B. Double-blind randomized clinical trial of pentoxiphyllin in vaso-occlusive sickle cell crisis. Trop Geogr Med 1989;41:320–325.
30. Baldree LA, Ault BH, Chesney CM, Stapleton FB. Intravenous desmopressin acetate in children with sickle trait and persistent macroscopic hematuria. Pediatrics 1990;86:238–243.
31. Perrine SP, Swerdlow P, Faller DV, et al. Butyric acid modulates developmental globin gene switching in man and sheep. Adv Exp Med Biol 1989;271:177–183.
32. Goldberg MA, Brugnara C, Dover GJ, Schapira L, Charache S, Bunn HF. Treatment of sickle cell anemia with hydroxyrea and erythropoietin. N Engl J Med 1990;323:366–372.
33. Green M, Hall RJC, Huntsman RG, Lawson A, Pearson TC, Wheeler PCG. Sickle cell infarctive crises treated by exchange transfusion. JAMA 1975;231:948–950.
34. Davey RJ, Esposito DJ, Jacobson RJ, Corn M. Partial exchange transfusion as treatment for hemoglobin SC disease in pregnancy. Arch Intern Med 1978;138:937–939.
35. Rifkind S, Waisman J, Thompson R, Goldfinger D. RBC exchange pheresis for priapism in sickle cell disease. JAMA 1979;242:2317–2318.
36. Bischoff RJ, Williamson A III, Dalali MJ, Rice JC, Kerstein MD. Assessment of the use of transfusion therapy perioperatively in patients with sickle cell hemoglobinopathies. Ann Surg 1988;207:434–438.
37. Piomelli S. Chronic transfusions in patients with sickle cell disease. Indications and problems. Am J Pediatr Hematol Oncol 1985;7:51–55.
38. Gaston M, Verter J, Woods G, et al. Prophylaxis with oral penicillin in children with sickle cell anemia. A randomized trial. N Engl J Med 1986;314:1593–1599.
39. Vichinsky E, Lubin BH. Suggested guidelines for the treatment of children with sickle cell anemia. Pediatr Hematol 1987;1:483–501.
40. Evans JPM. Practical management of sickle cell disease. Arch Dis Child 1989;64:1748–1751.
41. Shapiro BS. The management of pain in sickle cell disease. Pediatr Clin North Am 1989;36:1029–1046.
42. McPherson E, Perlin E, Finke H, Castro O, Pittman J. Patient-controlled analgesia in patients with sickle cell vaso-occlusive crisis. Am J Med Sci 1990;299:10–12.
43. Beutler E. The sickle cell diseases and related disorders. In: Williams WJ, Beutler E, Erslev AJ, Lichtman MA, eds. Hematology. New York: McGraw-Hill, 1990:613–644.
44. Zerez CR, Lachant NA, Lee SJ, Tanaka KR. Decreased erythrocyte nicotinamide adenine dinucleotide redox potential and abnormal pyridine nucleotide content in sickle cell disease. Blood 1988;71:512–515.
45. Lew VL, Hockaday A, Sepulveda MI, et al. Compartmentalization of sickle-cell calcium in endocytic inside-out vesicles. Nature 1985;315:586–589.
46. Hebbel RP, Ney PA, Foker W. Autoxidation, dehydration, and adhesivity may be related abnormalities of sickle erythrocytes. Am J Physiol 1989;256:C579–C583.
47. Hebbel RP, Schwartz RS, Mohandas N. The adhesive sickle erythrocyte; cause and consequence of abnormal interactions with endothelium, monocytes/macrophages and model membranes. Clin Haematol 1985;14:141–161.
48. Barrett-Conner E. Bacterial infection and sickle cell anemia. Medicine (Baltimore) 1971;50:97.
49. Boghossian SH, Wright G, Webster AD, Segal AW. Investigations of host defense in patients with sickle cell disease. Br J Haematol 1985;59:523–531.
50. Boghossian SH, Nash G, Dormandy J, Bevan DH. Abnormal neutrophil adhesion in sickle cell anaemia and crisis: relationship to blood rheology. Br J Haematol 1991;78:437–441.
51. Padmos MA, Roberts GT, Sackey K, et al. Two different forms of homozygous sickle cell disease occur in Saudi Arabia. Br J Haematol 1991;79:93–98.
52. Perrine RP, Pembrey ME, John P, Perrine S, Shoup F. Natural history of sickle cell anemia in Saudi Arabs. Ann Intern Med 1978;88:1–6.
53. Smith JA. The natural history of sickle cell disease. Ann NY Acad Sci 1989;565:105–108.
54. Ohene-Frempong K. Stroke in sickle cell disease: demographic, clinical, and therapeutic considerations. Semin Hematol 1991;28:213–219.
55. Pavlakis SG, Bello J, Prohovnik I, et al. Brain infarction in sickle cell anemia: magnetic resonance imaging correlates. Ann Nuerol 1988;23:125–130.
56. Powars D, Wilson B, Imbus C, Pegelow C, Allen J. The natural history of stroke in sickle cell disease. Am J Med 1978;65:461–471.
57. Russell MO, Goldberg HI, Reis L. Transfusion therapy for cerebral vascular abnormalities in sickle cell disease. J Pediatr 1976;88:382–387.
58. Russell MO, Goldberg HI, Hodson A, et al. Effect of transfusion therapy on arteriographic abnormalities and on recurrence of stroke in sickle cell disease. Blood 1984;63:162–169.
59. Vichinsky EP, Earles A, Johnson RA, Hoag S, Williams A, Lubin B. Alloimmunization in sickle cell anemia and transfusion of racially unmatched blood. N Engl J Med 1990;322:1617–1621.
60. Rosse WF, Gallagher D, Kinney TR, et al. Transfusion and alloimmunization in sickle cell disease. Blood 1990;76:1431–1437.
61. Swift A, Cohen M, Hynd G, et al. Neuropsychologic impairment in children with sickle cell anemia. Pediatrics 1989;84:1077–1085.
62. Kinney TR, Ware RE, Schultz WH, Filston HC. Long-term management of splenic sequestration in children with sickle cell disease. J Pediatr 1990;117:194–199.
63. Milner PF, Kraus AP, Sebes JI, et al. Sickle cell disease as a cause of osteonecrosis of the femoral head. N Engl J Med 1991;325:1476–1481.
64. Powars DR. Sickle cell anemia: β^s-gene-cluster haplotypes as prognostic indicators of vital organ failure. Semin Hematol 1991;28:202–208.

65. Powars DR, Elliot-Mills DD, Chan L, et al. Chronic renal failure in sickle cell disease: risk factors, clinical course, and mortality. Ann Intern Med 1991;115:614–620.
66. Powars D, Weidman JA, Odom-Maryon T, Niland JC, Johnson C. Sickle cell chronic lung disease: prior morbidity and the risk of pulmonary failure. Medicine (Baltimore) 1988;67:66–76.
67. Charache S, Scott JC, Charache P. "Acute chest syndrome" in adults with sickle cell anemia. Microbiology, treatment, and prevention. Arch Intern Med 1979; 139:67–69.
68. Rucknagel DL, Kalinyak KA, Gelfand MJ. Rib infarcts and acute chest syndrome in sickle cell diseases. Lancet 1991;337:831–833.
69. Platt OS, Thorington BD, Brambilla DJ, et al. Pain in sickle cell disease. Rates and risk factors. N Engl J Med 1991;325:11–16.
70. Leikin SL, Gallagher D, Kinney TR, et al. Mortality in children and adolescents with sickle cell disease. Pediatrics 1989;84:500–508.
71. Gill FM, Brown A, Gallagher D, et al. Newborn experience in the cooperative study of sickle cell disease. Pediatrics 1989;83:827–829.
72. Platt O, for the Cooperative Study of Sickle Cell Disease. The natural history of sickle cell disease: life expectancy. Am J Pediatr Hematol Oncol. 1993 (in press).
73. Muenz LR, Bray GL, Makris NG, Lessin LS, for the Cooperative Study of Sickle Cell Disease. Prediction of severity in sickle cell disease. Am J Pediatr Hematol Oncol 1993 (in press).
74. Jackson JF, Odom JL, Bell WN. Amelioration of sickle cell disease by persistent fetal hemoglobin. JAMA 1961;177:867–869.
75. Powars DR, Schroeder WA, Weiss JN, Chan LS, Azen SP. Lack of influence of fetal hemoglobin levels or erythrocyte indices on the severity of sickle cell anemia. J Clin Invest 1980;65:732–740.
76. Serjeant BE, Mason KP, Kenny MW, et al. Effect of alpha-thalassemia on the rheology of homozygous sickle cell disease. Br J Haematol 1983;55:479–486.
77. Noguchi CT, Dover GJ, Rodgers GP, et al. Alpha thalassemia changes erythrocyte heterogeneity in sickle cell disease. J Clin Invest 1985;75:1632–1637.
78. Steinberg MH, Embury SH. Alpha-thalassemia in blacks: genetic and clinical aspects and interactions with the sickle hemoglobin gene. Blood 1986;68:985–990.
79. Stevens MCG, Maude GH, Beckford M, et al. Alpha thalassemia and the hematology of homozygous sickle cell disease in childhood. Blood 1986;67:411–414.
80. Labie D, Pagnier J, Lapoumeroulie C, et al. Common haplotype dependency of high gamma-globin gene expression and high Hb F levels in β-thalassemia and sickle cell anemia patients. Proc Natl Acad Sci USA 1985;82:2111–2114.
81. Nagel RL, Ranney HM. Genetic epidemiology of structural mutations of the β-globin gene. Semin Hematol 1990;27:342–359.
82. Miller BA, Oliveri N, Salameh M, et al. Molecular analysis of the high-hemoglobin-F phenotype in Saudi Arabian sickle cell anemia. N Engl J Med 1987;316:244–250.
83. Mentzer WC, Heller S, Pearle P, Whitmer S, Hackney E, Vichinsky E. Availability of related donors for bone marrow transplantation in sickle cell anemia. Am J Pediatr Hematol Oncol 1993 (in press).
84. Perkins H, Hansen JA. The U.S. National Marrow Donor Program. Am J Pediatr Hematol Oncol 1993 (in press).
85. Kirkpatrick DV, Barrios NJ, Humbert JH. Bone marrow transplantation for sickle cell anemia. Semin Hematol 1991;28:240–243.
86. Cohen AR. Transfusion therapy and iron chelation in patients with sickle cell disease and stroke. Am J Pediatr Hematol Oncol 1993 (in press).
87. Sullivan KM, Agura E, Anasetti C, et al. Chronic graft-versus-host disease and other late complications of bone marrow transplantation. Semin Hematol 1991; 28:250–259.
88. Sullivan KM, Reid CD. Introduction to a symposium on sickle cell anemia: current results of comprehensive care and the evolving role of bone marrow transplantation. Semin Hematol 1991;28:177–179.
89. Kodish E, Lantos J, Siegler M, Kohrman A, Johnson FL. Bone marrow transplantation in sickle cell disease: the trade-off between early mortality and quality of life. Clin Res 1990;38:694–700.
90. Weatherall DJ. Bone marrow transplantation for sickle cell anemia. Lancet 1988;2:328–329.
91. Nagel RL. The dilemma of marrow transplantation in sickle cell anemia. Semin Hematol 1991;28:233–234.
92. Kirkpatrick D. The selection and timing of bone marrow transplantation in sickle cell disease. Am J Pediatr Hematol Oncol 1993 (in press).
93. Thomas ED. The pros and cons of bone marrow transplantation for sickle cell anemia. Semin Hematol 1991;28:260–262.
94. Piomelli S. Bone marrow transplantation in sickle cell diseases: a plea for a rational approach. Bone Marrow Transplant 1992;10(suppl 1):58–61.
95. Sullivan KM. National collaborative study of marrow transplantation for symptomatic sickle cell anemia. Am J Pediatr Hematol Oncol 1993 (in press).
96. Kodish E, Lantos J, Stocking C, et al. Bone marrow transplantation for sickle cell disease: a study of parent's decisions. N Engl J Med 1991;325:1349–1353.
97. Thomas ED. Marrow transplantation for nonmalignant disorders (editorial). N Engl J Med 1978;298: 963–964.
98. Johnson FL, Look AT, Gockerman J, Ruggiero MR, Dalla-Pozza L, Billings FT III. Bone-marrow transplantation in a patient with sickle-cell anemia. N Engl J Med 1984;311:780–783.
99. Milpied N, Harrouseau JL, Garand R, David A. Bone-marrow transplantation for sickle-cell anaemia. Lancet 1988;2:328–329.
100. Mentzer W, Packman S, Wara W, Cowan M. Successful bone marrow transplantation in a child with sickle cell anemia (SCA) and Morquio's disease (abstract). Blood 1990; 76(suppl 1):69a.
101. Vermylen C, Fernandez-Robles E, Ninone J, Cornu G. Bone marrow transplantation in five children with sickle cell anaemia. Lancet 1988;1:1427–1428.
102. Vermylen C, Cornu G, Phillips M, et al. Bone marrow transplantation in sickle cell anemia. Arch Dis Child 1991;66:1195–1198.
103. Ferster A, De Valck C, Azzi N, Fondu P, Toppet M, Sariban E. Bone marrow transplantation for severe sickle cell anaemia. Br J Haematol 1992;80:102–105.
104. Vermylen C, Cornu G. Bone marrow transplantation in sickle cell anemia: the European experience. Am J Pediatr Hematol Oncol 1993 (in press).

105. Johnson FL, Mentzer WC, Kalinyak KA, Sullivan KM, Abboud MR. Marrow transplantation for sickle cell disease: U.S. experience. Am J Pediatr Hemotol Oncol 1993 (in press).

106. Lucarelli G, Galimberti M, Polchi P, et al. Bone marrow transplantation in patients with thalassemia. N Engl J Med 1990;322:417–421.

107. Storb R, Sanders JE, Pepe M, et al. Graft-versus-host disease prophylaxis with methotrexate/cyclosporine in children with severe aplastic anemia treated with cyclophosphamide and HLA-identical marrow grafts. Blood 1991;78:1144–1149.

Chapter 64

Transplantation Approaches for Severe Combined Immunodeficiency Disease, Wiskott-Aldrich Syndrome, and Other Lethal Genetic, Combined Immunodeficiency Disorders

Richard J. O'Reilly, Wilhelm Friedrich, and Trudy N. Small

In 1968, Gatti and colleagues (1) and Bach and associates (2) reported the first successful applications of an allogeneic bone marrow transplantation (BMT) for the curative correction of lethal diseases in humans. These successes were attributable to the use of sibling donors compatible on the basis of human leukocyte antigen (HLA) serology and mutual nonresponsiveness in mixed lymphocyte culture (MLC). The disorders targeted in these transplants were severe combined immunodeficiency disease (SCID) and Wiskott-Aldrich syndrome (WAS), 2 lethal genetic disorders of immunity. Since that time, several important advances in clinical BMT have been achieved through experimental transplants applied to these disorders, such as the initial successful applications of unmodified marrow transplants from HLA-partially matched (1,3) and HLA-compatible unrelated donors (4) and T-cell–depleted HLA haplotype–disparate marrow grafts for patients lacking a compatible donor (5). The requirement for myeloablation as well as immunosuppression to ensure full hematopoetic chimerism and correction of genetic disorders involving nonlymphoid lineages was also initially demonstrated in a series of transplants for WAS (6,7).

In this chapter, we review the current results of BMT in the treatment of the different variants of SCID, the other lethal combined immunodeficiencies, and WAS. The focus is on the improvements made in providing curative allogeneic BMT to affected children lacking an HLA-matched sibling. Current knowledge regarding the mechanisms of graft-resistance, graft-host tolerance, and donor-host co-operation, which limit or potentiate durable chimerism and reconstitution of immunity in these uniquely informative hosts, is summarized.

Severe Combined Immunodeficiency Disease

SCID is a heterogeneous, lethal, congenital disorder of lymphoid progenitors that results in the failure of T cells to respond to mitogens, specific antigens, and allogeneic cells, and the inability of B cells to produce specific antibody (8,9). Clinically, 3 major isolated forms of SCID have been identified (9): classic SCID, characterized by T and B lymphopenia and agammaglobulinemia; the more common SCID with B lymphocytes, in which normal to increased numbers of circulating serum immunoglobulin (Ig)–positive cells and variable levels of nonspecific serum immunoglobulins are observed; and SCID secondary to adenosine deaminase deficiency (ADA), which may present with either of the preceeding lymphoid phenotypes (10). This latter form of SCID is considered to result from the loss of lymphoid progenitors and their differentiated progeny secondary to accumulation of deoxyadenosine and its phosphorylated metabolites dATP and S-adenosylhomocysteine, substances toxic to lymphocytes that cannot be metabolized in the absence of ADA activity (11).

In addition to these types, SCID may also be associated with reticular dysgenesis (12), a rare and poorly understood disorder of hematopoeisis, in which affected infants demonstrate severe neutropenia and lymphoid hypoplasia, with preservation of red cell and platelet production; and Omenn's syndrome (13), a disorder presenting with scaling erythroderma, leukocytosis, eosinophilia, hepatosplenomegaly, and lymphadenopathy, with lymphoid replacement by Langerhans and reticulum cells (14). Cases of SCID also have been described in association with short-limbed dwarfism and ectodermal dysplasia (15). Rarer forms of SCID, in which patients have nonfunctional T lymphocytes that demonstrate capping defects (16), lack of CD7 expression (17), or abnormal CD3 subunit expression, have been described (18).

SCID associated with ADA deficiency (10,19), short-limbed dwarfism (15), Omenn's syndrome (13), or a capping defect (16) are inherited as autosomal recessive disorders; the classic form of SCID, SCID with B cells, and probably reticular dysgenesis can be inherited as either a sex-linked or an autosomal recessive disorder (9,12,20). Despite the heterogeneity of SCID, of 238 evaluated children from Europe (n = 183) or at Memorial Sloan-Kettering Cancer Center (MSKCC) (n = 55), the distribution of SCID phenotypes was surprisingly similar, with reticular dysgenesis representing 3 and 2%, ADA deficiency 16 and 15%, classical SCID 27 and 25%, SCID with B cells 44 and 49%, and SCID with nonfunctional T cells 9 and 9% of the 2 patient populations, respectively (21).

Patients presenting with specific variants of SCID may exhibit significant differences in the functional or phenotypic characteristics of their lymphoid cells, even when the patients are derived from the same pedigree. The basis for these variations in the expression of presumed single gene disorders is unclear but may, in part, reflect postzygotic events altering the environment in which these cells grow. In the ADA-deficient form of SCID, the disorder has usually been ascribable to a point mutation in the ADA gene resulting in the generation of an inactive or unstable enzyme (22,23), although a large deletion within the ADA gene has also been reported (24). Overall, approximately 30% of affected children have T lymphocytes that can be induced to respond to mitogens and to allogeneic cells when supplied with a source of ADA activity, such as infusion of ADA+ normal red cells (25,26) or polyethylene glycol polymerized ADA (27). Surprisingly, this variation in response to ADA can also be found in single families (28). Among both ADA+ and ADA− variants of SCID, considerable heterogeneity has also been observed in such parameters as the number and function of natural killer (NK) cells (29–32), the capacity of monocytes to produce interleukin-1 (IL-1) (33) and to provide accessory signals for T-cell responses to mitogens and superantigens (34), the ability of their thymus to secrete thymic peptide hormones such as thymulin (35,36) and thymosin alpha-1 (37), and the capacity of their lymphocytes to acquire phenotypic or functional characteristics of T lymphocytes when cocultured with thymic epithelium (38,39).

One other feature of many patients with SCID that may contribute significantly to this phenotypic variation, misguided definition of the host's HLA haplotype (thereby potentially confusing selection of a transplant donor) and otherwise impact transplant results is engraftment with transplacentally derived maternal T cells. Early studies by Kadowaki and colleagues (40) and O'Reilly and associates (41) implicated these maternal T lymphocytes in the pathogenesis of a lethal disorder distinguishable but pathologically similar to Omenn's syndrome, which was consistent with graft-versus-host disease (GVHD) but was observed in untransfused patients with SCID. It is now recognized that a high proportion of patients with SCID are engrafted with maternal T cells. In most instances, these cells do not initiate GVHD (42). In our own series, maternal T lymphocytes have been detected in 50% of the patients with ADA^+ forms of SCID, either by HLA serotyping or karyotyping primarily isolated or IL-2-expanded T lymphocytes (42,43). A skin rash and transient hepatitis suggestive of GVHD developed in only one patient. The maternal T cells fail to respond to host antigens in MLC and cell-mediated lympholysis assays (42,44), even in patients with features consistent with GVHD (41). Indeed, in most reported patients, these cells also fail to respond to third-party alloantigens (41,44,45). In certain patients, maternal cells have been shown to suppress B-cell immunoglobulin synthesis in vitro (2). Whether these cells also modulate B-cell development in these patients is unknown.

HLA-matched Transplants for SCID

The first successful allogeneic BMT in humans was reported in 1968 by Gatti and colleagues (1), who grafted marrow from an HLA-compatible normal sister to treat a patient with SCID. This patient remains a full hematopoetic and lymphoid chimera, with normal immunological function 24 years after transplantation. Since then, BMT has emerged as a treatment of choice for children with SCID. Over the intervening years, the results of such transplants have improved significantly. In a review by Kenny and Hitzig (46) of 31 reported patients transplanted from HLA-identical siblings through 1977, 48% achieved long-term survival. In our own compilation of results through 1983, 34 of 59 (58%) patients transplanted from HLA-identical relatives survive with reconstitution (47). A survey of the European experience through 1986 indicated that the probability of a successful outcome had improved to 68% (48). In an update of 32 patients transplanted between 1983 and 1989, this success rate had increased to more than 90% (21).

The continuing improvements observed in the results of HLA-matched BMTs cannot be ascribed to more effective conditioning regimens, because these regimens are rarely used to prepare patients with SCID for unmodified HLA-matched grafts. In fact, these patients regularly achieve durable donor T-lymphocyte chimerism without conditioning. Although only 50% of these patients are chimeric for donor B lymphocytes, these patients usually also achieve full reconstitution of both T- and B-cell function (48–51).

Advances in the drug prophylaxis of GVHD cannot be cited as a basis for current successes either, because it is also rarely used. Although acute GVHD has been observed in up to 70% of patients, it has been severe in less than 10% and has been associated with less than 10% mortality (21). Chronic GVHD following HLA-matched sibling grafts has been rare.

The basis for this low incidence likely reflects, in part, the young age of the patients as well as the absence of tissue injury that would be induced if a conditioning regimen was used.

Because of these considerations, improvements in the results of HLA-matched grafts for SCID have been ascribed principally to advances in the treatment and prevention of infections in the post-transplant period. In the review by Kenny and Hitzig (46), interstitial pneumonias caused by viruses or *Pneumocystis carinii* that developed early after BMT accounted for more than half the fatalities. Introduction of effective prophylaxis for *Pneumocystis carinii* (52) and the recent development of useful antiviral agents for respiratory syncytial virus (53) and for cytomegalovirus (CMV) (54) have reduced the incidence and mortality associated with these infections. Similarly, introduction of techniques permitting long-term systemic treatment with antifungal agents and total parenteral nutrition has reduced mortality in patients who present with severe inanition due to chronic mucocutaneous candidiasis.

Diagnostic approaches for SCID have also radically improved. For example, the T-lymphocytopenia characteristic of SCID can now be established by examination of fetal blood cells at 16 to 18 weeks' gestation (55,56). ADA-deficient SCID can also be detected by enzymatic analysis of cells cultured from chorionic villous biopsies as early as 8 weeks (57,58). Such cells have also been used to diagnose the X-linked form of SCID by virtue of distinctive restriction-length polymorphisms of the X chromosome bearing the defective gene (59). Such approaches permit elective abortion of affected progeny. Alternatively, HLA phenotyping can be performed on these cells, permitting identification of suitable donors from within or outside the family, and decisions regarding delivery, infection prophylaxis, and postnatal transplant approach can be made months before the child is born. As a result of these diagnostic advances, second affected infants have been referred for BMT before they acquired serious infections. Indeed, in some instances, BMT has been undertaken within the first 1 to 2 weeks of life. The probability of a successful BMT in such patients has been in excess of 90%.

Unfortunately, large scale application of sensitive genetic, enzymatic, or immunological techniques for diagnosis of these rare diseases has not been found to be sufficiently cost-effective for screening all newborns. First affected children continue to be diagnosed only after the development of viral (53) or *Pneumocystis carinii* pneumonias, CMV or adenovirus hepatitis (60), or refractory mucocutaneous candidiasis (61). Furthermore, although disseminated *Vaccinia* infections have been eliminated since smallpox vaccinations were discontinued, patients with SCID continue to present with disseminated infection secondary to prior immunization with bacillus Calmette-Guerin (BCG) (62) and polio vaccine–related viral infections of the central nervous system (63). Such infections often stimulate a marked inflammatory response during the early stages of immune reconstitution. As a result, these patients continue to have a high (30%) risk of death in the first 6 months after transplantation.

Summarizing this experience with HLA-matched transplants, it is clear that for most variants of SCID, transplants of unmodified, HLA-matched marrow can be administered without cytoreductive preparation and will result in engraftment of donor T lymphocytes and, to a variable degree, B lymphocytes, permitting full reconstitution of immunological function. Exceptions do exist, however. For example, some patients with ADA- SCID have required multiple HLA-matched transplants to achieve engraftment (64); for such patients, administration of immunosuppressive drugs may be indicated to facilitate engraftment of lymphoid progenitors in a secondary transplant. For those variants involving more than the lymphoid lineage, such as Omenn's syndrome (65) or reticular dysgenesis (66), preparative regimens incorporating both myeloablative and immunosuppressive agents have also been required to insure rapid and full hematopoietic and lymphoid chimerism and correction of the lymphoid and myeloid abnormalities observed.

Unmodified Marrow Transplants from HLA-nonidentical Related Donors

Following the demonstration that BMT from HLA-matched siblings could induce durable chimerism and restore both T- and B-cell function to patients with SCID, several groups began to explore the use of alternative HLA-nonidentical related donors for the 60 to 80% of patients lacking an HLA-matched sibling (67). Initial studies focused on the use of HLA-haploidentical but MLC-compatible related donors, because studies in murine models of BMT suggested that recipients with class II major histocompatibility complex (MHC) disparities at H-2 were at particular risk for lethal GVHD (68). Early clinical experiences also supported this approach because disparities for HLA-A or B on one haplotype were tolerated without lethal GVHD. Of 9 children with SCID engrafted with HLA-A or B disparate MLC-compatible marrow, reviewed by Kenny and Hitzig (46), 2 achieved immunoreconstitution and long-term disease-free survival. GVHD developed in 6, but it was severe in only 2. However, 5 patients succumbed to infection within 3.5 months of transplantation, precluding assessments of the ultimate incidence and severity of chronic GVHD. In these early studies, 3 additional patients received grafts mismatched only for HLA-D. Unfortunately, none of these patients survived long enough to assess GVHD fully (46). Of 21 patients with SCID who received marrow grafts from HLA-nonidentical donors who were at least MLC-compatible reported by 1983, 7 were long-term survivors with reconstitution (47).

Although most unmodified HLA-nonidentical related donor marrow grafts administered to children with SCID have been MLC-compatible with the recipient, it is no longer clear that a single disparity for a class II allele constitutes a greater risk than a disparity for a class I allele. Indeed, in a large series of leukemic patients who received BMTs from related partially mismatched donors for HLA-D, reported by Beatty and co-workers (69), the incidence and severity of GVHD and the probability of survival for patients possessing unique HLA-D determinants did not differ from those recorded for patients transplanted from donors mismatched for 1 HLA-A or HLA-B allele.

When incompatible donors whose cells are able to recognize both class I and II determinants unique to the host have been used, unmodified BMTs for SCID have invariably failed, either because the transplants failed to engraft or because they were complicated by severe GVHD or infection in the early post-transplant period. Thus, of 31 patients reviewed by Kenny and Hitzig (46), 3 of 19 evaluable patients failed to engraft; of the 16 who did engraft, severe GVHD developed in 10. None survived. Similarly, survival among leukemic patients transplanted with unmodified marrow derived from donors disparate for two HLA alleles or a full haplotype has been poor. The incidence of graft failure has been high despite preparation with total body irradiation (TBI) and cyclophosphamide (CY). Furthermore, severe GVHD and associated infections have developed in 90% of these patients despite the use of cyclosporine (CSP) and methotrexate (MTX) prophylaxis, a regimen clearly effective in reducing the risk of severe GVHD and associated mortality in HLA-matched leukemic recipients (70).

Unmodified Marrow Transplants from Histocompatible Unrelated Donors

In the mid 1970s, it was recognized that within specific ethnogeographic groups, certain HLA-A and HLA-B determinants were coassociated at frequencies far in excess of those predicted by the frequencies of the individual HLA-A and HLA-B alleles (71). Identification of such HLA haplotypes in genetic disequilibrium suggested the feasibility of finding an unrelated donor for patients inheriting 2 such common haplotypes from a relatively limited donor pool (72). Acting on this principle, our group identified an HLA phenotypically compatible MLC nonreactive unrelated donor for a child with SCID. A series of transplants from this donor, which were initiated in 1973, ultimately led to durable lymphoid engraftment and full immunological reconstitution (4). Unfortunately, severe chronic GVHD developed, and the patient ultimately succumbed to metastases from an associated squamous-cell carcinoma of the skin 10 years later. Nevertheless, subsequent successful applications of BMTs from unrelated donors to patients with aplastic anemia or leukemia inheriting common haplotypes confirmed the feasibility of this approach (73,74). With the recent development of a large marrow donor program, it has been possible to secure HLA phenotypically matched donors for 10 to 20% of patients lacking a sibling donor (75,76). The incidence of grade II to IV GVHD following BMT for HLA-matched serologically MLC-compatible unrelated donors is equal to that observed in recipients of marrow grafts from related donors differing for 2 HLA alleles on one haplotype (77). However, cumulative results of such BMTs applied to children with leukemia have been encouraging, with a disease-free survival (DFS) rate of more than 50% at 1.5 years for patients transplanted in first or second remission of acute leukemia or chronic-phase CML (78).

Filipovich and associates (79) recently reported a series of 8 patients (SCID, (n=4); combined immunodeficiency disease [CID], n=4) transplanted with unmodified marrow from unrelated donors identified in these volunteer donor programs. Again, most of the patients inherited haplotypes in linkage disequilibrium. To achieve consistent engraftment, these patients were pretreated with busulfan (BU), cyclophosphamide (CY), and antithymocyte globulin (ATG). All received drug prophylaxis against GVHD. Strikingly, grade III acute GVHD developed in only one of the 7. Of the 8 patients, 6 are alive with immunological reconstitution 1 to 3.8 years after BMT. These encouraging early results indicate the potential of this approach for those children with SCID inheriting common haplotypes for whom a donor can be readily identified. They are particularly appealing for patients with CID syndromes who have too frequently failed to engraft with parental HLA haplotype–disparate T-cell–depleted BMTs despite preparation with regimens containing BU and CY. However, it is still unclear whether such grafts offer any significant advantage over parental T-cell–depleted HLA-nonidentical marrow grafts in the treatment of SCID when comparable preparative regimens are used. Indeed, given the protracted time (4–6 mo) still required to identify and recruit most donors, the attendant duration of infectious risks to a child with SCID may be justified only for patients inheriting very common haplotypes and when use of parental donors would itself impose an undue risk of infection (e.g., active CMV infection).

Fetal Tissue Transplants for SCID

In the mouse, the liver is the major hematopoietic organ from day 11 to 19 of gestation (80,81), whereas in many strains, the thymus does not become lymphoid until after birth (82). In 1958, Uphoff (83) demonstrated that hematopoietic cells derived from the fetal liver of parental strain mice could be used to reconstitute hematopoietic function in lethally irradiated F1 hybrid mice without lethal GVHD. This finding contrasted with the consistent development of lethal GVHD in such hybrids after transplants of spleen cells from adult parental strain donors. Yunis and colleagues (84) subsequently demonstrated that neonatal thymectomy also abrogated the potential of spleen cells derived from adult animals to induce GVHD. These studies indicate that lymphocytes developing in the thymus were essential to the pathogenesis of this disorder.

In humans, the liver constitutes the main source of blood-forming cells from the 8th to 19th week of gestation (85). However, by 11 to 12 weeks' gestation, lymphocytes responsive to mitogens are already detected in the thymus (86,87). By 12 to 14 weeks, the normal lymphoid architecture of the thymus is established (86). Thereafter, thymic lymphocytes are capable of responding to allogeneic cells in MLC (88,89) and can initiate local GVH reaction in xenogeneic hosts (90). On the basis of these observations in humans, together with studies in murine models, investigators have used 8 to 14 week gestational aged fetal liver for transplantation to eliminate the possibility of concurrently transplanting post-thymic T cells capable of inducing lethal GVHD. In fact, no instances of lethal GVHD have been recorded in recipients of fetal liver of 14 weeks' gestation or less (91), although moderately severe skin rashes pathologically indistinguishable from GVHD have been recorded in recipients of transplants of liver from fetuses as early as 7 weeks' gestation (92).

In 1973, Keightly and associates (93) performed the first successful fetal liver transplant and thereby restored immune function to a patient with SCID with ADA deficiency. Thereafter, fetal liver and thymus grafts were evaluated extensively at several centers experienced in the diagnosis and treatment of SCID. In 1983, we reviewed 64 patients who had received a total of 105 fetal liver transplants at these centers (94). Of these transplants, only 22 produced durable engraftment of fetal lymphoid cells confirmed by karyotype or HLA phenotype. Of these 22 engrafted patients, 18 achieved a full or partial reconstitution of T-cell function; however, only 10 were ultimately able to generate antibody responses to immunization. Thirteen (20%) of these patients were surviving one year after transplantation. GVHD was severe in only 2 patients, both of whom received liver and thymus grafts from fetuses of 16 weeks' gestation.

In our own series, eight patients with SCID received a total of 23 separate transplants of liver with or without thymus derived from electively aborted cadaveric fetuses of 9 to 12 weeks' gestation (94). Sustained engraftment of lymphoid precursors was documented in only 6. As has been observed in murine models of fetal tissue transplants (95,96), concurrent administration of liver cells and thymus from the same fetus appeared to increase the incidence of engraftment. Immunological reconstitution was inconsistent. Of the 6 patients durably engrafted, normal proliferative responses to mitogens, antigens, and allogeneic cells developed in only 2. Only one of the 8 patients transplanted with fetal liver and thymus survives with engraftment of fetal cells. However, this patient remains fully reconstituted more than 16 years after transplantation. In a larger and continuing single center series, Touraine and colleagues (97) treated 19 patients with SCID with a combined transplant of liver and thymus from 8 to 12 week gestationally aged fetuses. As in our series, engraftment has been achieved following less than one third of the transplants. Of 19 patients with SCID who have been summarized, 8 are durably engrafted and surviving, with evidence of at least partial reconstitution of T and B cells.

Because the fetal donors for these transplants are fully allogeneic to their hosts, concerns have been raised as to whether effective antigen-specific immune responses could ever develop in such patients because of the lack of any HLA sharing between the donor and host (98). Although such disparities likely contribute to the low incidence of engraftment and persisting immunodeficiencies in some engrafted patients, the level of immunocompetence achieved by several long-term allogeneic fetal liver chimeras is impressive. For example, the T cells in our patient that are derived from the fetal donor are able to recognize and lyse *Influenza* virus–infected cells bearing host-specific haplotypes but are unable to recognize virus in the context of the fetal donor. This patient also produces antibody, although his B cells are of host origin. Roncarolo and associates (99) reported a similar experience in a patient with SCID transplanted by Touraine and colleagues (100) who has sustained engraftment of fully allogeneic fetal liver–derived T cells for more than 10 years. These fetal T cells proliferate in response to tetanus antigen presented by host-type antigen-presenting cells (99) and provide help to the patient's own B cells for the production of virus-specific antibody (101). These cases indicate that fully allogeneic lymphoid cells can be re-educated within the host environment to recognize antigen in the context of host HLA determinants. Such interactions between engrafted T cells and fully allogeneic host cells are similar to those documented in a proportion of lethally irradiated normal mice (98,102) or mice with SCID (103) reconstituted with allogeneic, T-cell–depleted marrow.

Although the few patients with SCID who have achieved durable engraftment and long-term immunological reconstitution following fetal liver transplants have demonstrated that fully allogeneic hematopoietic cells lacking T lymphocytes can be used to achieve functional immune reconstitution without lethal GVHD, the cumulative results with this approach have been inferior to those achieved with either T-cell–depleted haplotype-disparate parental marrow grafts or unmodified transplants from histocompatible unrelated donors (79,104). Engraftment of allogeneic fetal hematopoietic cells has been difficult to achieve in patients with SCID, even though these patients lack T cells and are unable to reject skin allografts. Furthermore, the results suggest that in humans, as in murine models (98), only a small proportion of durably engrafted recipients of fully allogeneic fetal liver or T cell–depleted marrow achieve full reconstitution of antigen-specific cell-mediated immune functions.

HLA-nonidentical T-cell–depleted Transplants for SCID

In 1975, von Boehmer and colleagues (105) demonstrated that pretreatment of parental murine spleen cells with an antithymocyte antibody and complement (C') abrogated their capacity to induce lethal

GVHD after transplantation into H2-incompatible hybrids. These studies were rapidly confirmed in other mouse and rat models of allogeneic transplantation (106,107). In an alternative approach, Reisner and associates (108) used the plant lectins soybean agglutinin and peanut agglutinin to separate hematopoietic progenitors from mature T cells in murine spleen and marrow. The progenitor-rich marrow fraction could then be transplanted into fully allogeneic or hemiallogeneic irradiated hosts to produce stable hematopoietic and lymphoid chimerism without GVHD.

In 1981, Reisner and co-workers (5) reported a patient with leukemia who received an HLA-A, B nonidentical parental graft that had been depleted of T cells by differential agglutination with soybean lectin and by E-rosette depletion (SBA⁻ E⁻). The patient achieved full lymphoid and hematopoietic chimerism, and no GVHD was observed. Subsequently, our group reported 3 patients with SCID who were successfully transplanted with HLA-A,B,D haplotype–disparate marrow from a parental donor after depletion of T cells by a further modification of this approach (109,110). Each of these patients achieved durable lymphoid engraftment without pretransplant cytoreduction or post-transplant drug prophylaxis against GVHD. Neither acute nor chronic GVHD was observed. These patients remain stable lymphoid chimeras, with normal T-cell immunity 11.5 years after transplantation. In 1982, Reinherz and co-workers (111) described a patient with SCID who also achieved reconstitution of cell-mediated immunity following a series of 3 HLA-A,B,D haplotype–disparate parental marrow grafts depleted of T cells by treatment with the T-cell–specific murine monoclonal antibody, OKT12, and complement. Engraftment was achieved after the third graft, for which the patient was cytoreduced with BU and CY. GVHD was observed but was transient and of only moderate severity. This patient is also well 11 years after BMT.

These initial studies fostered widespread application of HLA-A,B,D haplotype–disparate T-cell–depleted marrow grafts to the treatment of patients with SCID and other lethal immune deficiencies. The techniques for T-cell depletion that have been used include soybean lectin agglutination and E-rosette depletion (109,110,112–120), multiple E-rosette depletions alone (121), treatment with cytotoxic T-cell–specific murine monoclonal antibodies and rabbit complement (122–126), and treatment with the rat monoclonal antibody CAMPATH-1 and human complement (127). The differences between these techniques in terms of the specific types of cells eliminated from the graft by the treatment used and the degree of T-cell depletion have been reported (128). The most commonly employed techniques for T-cell depletion of HLA haplotype–disparate marrow grafts applied to the treatment of SCID have been either those of Reisner and colleagues (109), in which marrow is depleted of T cells by soybean agglutination followed by E-rosetting, or use of the rat pan-T-cell monoclonal antibody CAMPATH-1 and donor serum as a source of complement (127). These techniques reproducibly achieve 2.8 to 3.0 and 2.3 to 2.5 log depletions of clonable T cells, respectively (128,129). Both techniques also deplete the graft of B cells and most NK cells, although their progenitors are preserved. This finding may in part explain the significantly lower incidence of donor-type Epstein-Barr virus (EBV) lymphomas that have complicated these transplants (130,131). Over the past 11 years, HLA haplotype–disparate parental marrow grafts depleted of T cells by SBA⁻ E⁻ have been used to treat nearly 200 children with SCID, CAMPATH-1 + C′ an additional 50+ patients, and E-rosette alone, 26+ patients.

In a recent review of the European experience with HLA-nonidentical marrow grafts depleted by one or another of these techniques (21), of 100 children with SCID, 56 are surviving with full immunological reconstitution of at least T-cell function up to 10 years after transplantation. Of these 56, grade II or greater GVHD developed in 27%. In the combined experience with SBA⁻ E⁻ T-cell–depleted mismatched marrow from MSKCC and the University of Ulm, of 91 patients transplanted, 64 survive engrafted with reconstitution of T-cell, and in a smaller fraction, B-cell immunity at a median of 5 years after BMT (Kaplan-Meier probability estimate = 69%; Figure 64-1). In this combined series, grade II or greater GVHD ascribable to the E-rosette–depleted HLA haplotype–disparate T-cell–depleted transplant developed in only 4 patients. In our own series (n = 46), the probability of survival with immunological reconstitution at 5 years (76%) cannot be distinguished from that recorded for HLA-matched marrow grafts (78%). Furthermore, for pa-

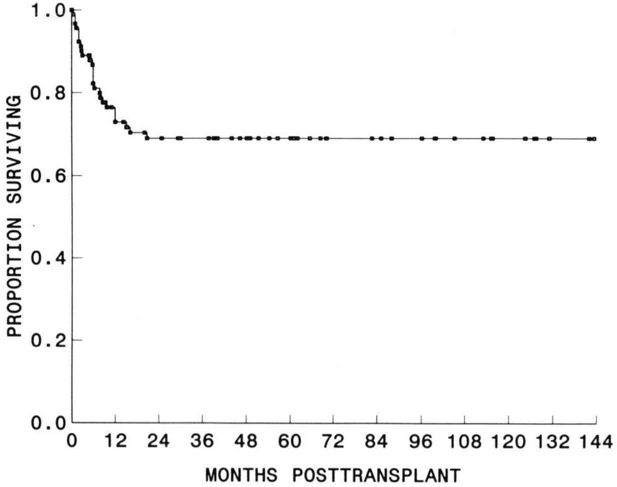

Figure 64-1. Kaplan-Meier plot of the probability of survival with immune reconstitution in the combined Memorial Sloan-Kettering Cancer Center and Ulm University series of 91 children with severe combined immunodeficiency disease transplanted with SBA⁻E⁻ T-cell–depleted marrow grafts from human leukocyte antigen–haploidentical parental donors.

tients without antecedent CMV or adenovirus infection at the time of transplant, the DFS rate is more than 90%.

The Distinctive Immunobiology of BMT in SCID

The increasing recent success of HLA haplotype–disparate T-cell–depleted marrow grafts applied to patients with SCID reflects significant advances in our understanding of SCID and the biological systems in such patients that may obstruct or limit engraftment. The unique states of chimerism and the immunological function of these long-term chimeras have also provided insights into the nature of graft/host tolerance and the capacity of normal donor lymphoid progenitors to develop and function in an allogeneic host environment. The accumulated information regarding these aspects of HLA-disparate T-cell–depleted marrow grafts when applied to patients with SCID is reviewed.

Engraftment

When parental HLA haplotype–disparate T-cell–depleted marrow grafts were initially applied to the treatment of children with SCID, the patients were grafted without preparatory cytoreduction. It was reasoned that patients with SCID lack functional T cells and had consistently failed to reject an organ or skin allograft. Furthermore, preparatory cytoreduction had not been required to secure engraftment of at least donor lymphoid cells when unmodified, HLA-matched grafts had been used. However, it was soon recognized that a proportion of patients with SCID could resist engraftment of HLA-disparate T-cell–depleted marrow grafts. The frequency of this complication has been markedly lower than that observed following allogeneic fetal liver transplants (132). However, in our compilation of the first 75 patients with SCID transplanted with T-cell–depleted grafts without cytoreduction, 23 (30%) failed to achieve sustained engraftment (104). In the recent compilation of the European experience reported by Fischer and colleagues (21), graft failures were reported in 50% of the patients transplanted without prior cytoreduction.

In most instances, failure to achieve engraftment may ultimately be ascribed to an active cell-mediated process, because patients who have failed initial BMT without preparatory cytoreduction have, in 86% of patients (21), achieved durable engraftment and reconstitution after secondary BMT administered following intensive treatment with immunosuppressive drug combinations, such as CY coupled with ATG, cytosine arabinoside, or BU. Attempts to identify specific mechanisms whereby patients with SCID can resist engraftment of allogeneic hematopoietic cells have not always yielded consistent results, most likely because of the limited numbers and heterogeneity of the patients evaluated. However, cumulative evidence supports at least 4 possible mechanisms of graft resistance.

Patients with SCID associated with ADA deficiency who have received transplants of T-cell–depleted marrow without cytoreduction have experienced a particularly high incidence of graft failure. In our recent compilation, 60% of patients failed to engraft, compared with a 24% incidence of graft failure in ADA+ forms of SCID (104). This high incidence of graft failure has been hypothesized to be due to the presence of alloreactive ADA− host T lymphocytes, which can be induced in the presence of donor ADA+ cells in sufficient numbers to initiate immunological rejection (48). It is well recognized that up to one third of patients with ADA− SCID can generate T cells capable of some response to mitogens or allogeneic cells if they are supplied with ADA, either by transfusion of ADA+ red cells (26) or by infusions of polyethylene glycol-linked ADA enzyme (27). On the basis of this observation, it has been suggested that a T-cell–depleted marrow graft may also supply sufficient ADA activity to permit the generation of host T cells capable of rejecting the transplant. A similar mechanism can be proposed to explain graft failures occasionally reported in patients with ADA− SCID following unmodified HLA-matched marrow transplants (64). To date, donor-reactive host T cells have not been demonstrated in ADA− patients who have failed such transplants. However, the consistent durable engraftment that has recently been achieved in patients with ADA− SCID prepared for T-cell–depleted BMT with BU and CY is in accord with this hypothesis (114).

For patients with ADA+ forms of SCID, the basis for graft resistance is less clear. One possibility that has been proposed is that T lymphocytes of maternal origin, which presumably gain access to the patient by transplacental infusion, might restrict engraftment of marrow from a nonmaternal donor. As noted earlier, maternal T cells have been detected in 20 to 50% of patients with SCID by karyotypic or HLA serotypic analyses of T cells separated from peripheral blood (42), sorted with fluorescent antibodies by cytofluorography (133), or expanded in the presence of IL-2 (134). In our own series, 50% of patients with ADA+ forms of SCID have been found to be engrafted with maternal T cells. Parenthetically, maternal cells have not been detected in any of the 7 patients with ADA− SCID, again suggesting that some capacity to reject allogeneic lymphoid cells may develop in these patients during embryonal life when toxic metabolites can be removed by diffusion into the maternal circulation. Following an HLA-matched, unmanipulated marrow graft from a sibling, maternal cells are eliminated early after engraftment and initiation of functional immune reconstitution (135,136). Although it is reasonable to suggest that transplacentally derived maternal T cells might prevent engraftment of a T-cell–depleted BMT transplant from a paternal or sibling donor, evidence for this hypothesis is still meager and indirect. Fischer and associates (48), reviewing the European transplant experience, reported that the presence of maternal T cells before transplantation is associated with a reduced incidence of engraftment and should be considered an indication for pretransplant cytoreduction. Unfortunately, this report does not specify the incidence of graft failure observed or the parental donor used. In the combined MSKCC–Ulm series, 2 of 5 patients with maternal cell chimerism failed to achieve durable engraftment following an initial BMT from a paternal donor and were reconstituted only after secondary transplants from the mother. In contrast, when the mother has been used as the donor for a T-cell–depleted BMT for such chimeric patients, functional reconstitution has been consistently achieved following BMT administered without preparatory cytoreduction. Indeed, Barrett and colleagues (137) reported data indicating that transplacentally derived maternal T cells may hasten establishment and functional development of a maternal T-cell–depleted graft. Strikingly, such grafts have also not been associated with any increase in the incidence or severity of GVHD.

In murine models, NK cells have been identified as effectors of the resistance of certain hybrid mice to parental strain marrow grafts (138–140). This form of marrow graft resistance is genetically determined (138,141). The target specificity of this form of resistance has been ascribed to alloantigens selectively expressed on hematopoietic cells, termed *H-h antigens*, which are encoded by genes linked to but distinct from the H-2 complex (142). It is hypothesized that resistance is directed only against hematopoietic cells homozygously expressing an H-h determinant. Although the specificity of graft resistance has been confirmed repeatedly, it has been demonstrated only recently that the putative NK cell effectors can exhibit allospecificity reacting against hematopoetic cells (143). That T and B cells do not contribute to this allospecific resistance has been demonstrated by Murphy and associates (140), who showed that NK cells derived from mice with SCID that are unable to generate antibodies or alloreactive T cells can mediate this specific form of marrow graft resistance.

NK cells have also been implicated in the pathogenesis of graft failure or delayed and incomplete immune reconstitution complicating HLA-nonidentical T-cell–depleted BMTs for SCID. Approximately 30 to 50% of patients with ADA+ forms of SCID have normal to elevated numbers of functional NK cells (29–32). Our group (112,144) and Peter and coworkers (145), who each reported large series of patients with ADA+ SCID transplanted with SBA^-E^- T-cell–depleted grafts, found that patients who have normal to high NK cell activity have a higher incidence of either graft failure or delayed immunological reconstitution. In a prospective analysis of our series, this association between host NK activity and graft resistance is highly significant. Similarly, Buckley and associates (115) noted delayed reconstitution in the 2 patients of their series of 10 ADA+ SCIDs who had normal to high levels of NK cells. In the review of European cases by Fischer and colleagues (48), this relationship has not been observed. However, in this series, several patients received posttransplant prophylaxis with agents such as CSP, which may inhibit NK cell functions.

Abnormalities of accessory cells or their functions have also been implicated in the pathogenesis of graft failures. Sahdev and colleagues (33), examined the function of circulating monocytes in patients with SCID. Of 21 patients examined, 5 had monocytes that were unable to generate IL-1 in response to endotoxin stimulation. In 3 of these patients, this deficiency could be ascribed to an NK-mediated prostaglandin-induced inhibition. However, an irreversible deficiency was documented in the other 2 patients. When these latter 2 patients received T-cell–depleted marrow grafts without preparatory cytoreduction, one failed to engraft; the other remained immunodeficient despite engraftment of donor T cells. Immune functions were restored only when donor monocyte/macrophage populations were established after cytoreductive therapy and a secondary transplant.

In summary, at least 4 mechanisms may contribute to explain the graft resistance observed in certain patients with SCID: (1) alloreactive host T cells, which can be induced in some ADA-deficient patients; (2) host NK cells; (3) transplacentally derived maternal cells; and (4) accessory cell dysfunctions.

For patients with ADA− SCID, preparative cytoreduction with a combination of CY and BU prior to primary grafts has already been recommended to ensure engraftment (113). In the combined MSKCC–Ulm experience, this approach has resulted in consistent engraftment; 8 of 10 patients so treated are surviving with full immune reconstitution. The relative significance of the other mechanisms of graft resistance discussed is still being assessed in prospective analyses. In our own series, the presence of NK cell function in a patient with SCID has been highly correlated with graft failure. For this reason, such patients are now receiving cytoreduction prior to their first BMT as a standard approach. Other centers are cytoreducing all patients with SCID, arguing that this approach also ensures engraftment of donor B cells. It can be questioned however, whether this is the correct approach in a severely ill patient with SCID who does not possess characteristics associated with graft resistance. A secondary BMT administered to a healthy older child who has functioning donor T cells following a primary BMT without cytoreduction might carry a markedly lower cumulative risk.

T-cell Reconstitution After BMT

Following an unmanipulated HLA-matched related BMT for SCID without preparatory chemotherapy, T cells of donor origin can be detected 1 to 2 weeks after transplantation. Immune reconstitution has been observed as early as 2 to 4 weeks after BMT; normalization of both T- and B-cell function developed at a mean of 6 and 9 weeks, respectively, in 18 reported patients (146). Normal T-cell mitogen responses have been documented 6 to 24 months after BMT in 6 patients with SCID prepared with BU and CY who received unmodified, unrelated, matched, or partially mismatched marrow transplants (79). Patients receiving TBI, BU, cytosine arabinoside, or thiotepa coupled with CY prior to a T-cell–depleted HLA-nonidentical marrow graft enjoy rapid engraftment of donor hematopoietic cells; neutrophil and platelet recovery generally occurs 3 to 5 weeks after BMT. However, engraftment of donor T cells is usually not detectable until 9 to 12 weeks following a T-cell–depleted BMT, usually after the development of donor B cells and NK cells in cytoreduced patients (Figure 64-2). In our series, no major differences in quality and tempo of T-cell reconstitution were demonstrated between patients receiving T-cell–depleted haplotype-disparate grafts who did or did not receive cytoreduction prior to the graft. This finding contrasts to results of Wijnaedts and associates (146), who report faster reconstitution in cytoreduced patients. In both our cytoreduced and noncytoreduced patients, recovery of normal numbers of circulating T cells is usually achieved by the third to fourth post-BMT month (Figure 64-3), followed rapidly by T-cell proliferation to mitogens and common antigens (Figure 64-4). These results are similar to those reported for noncytoreduced patients (115). The earliest CD3+

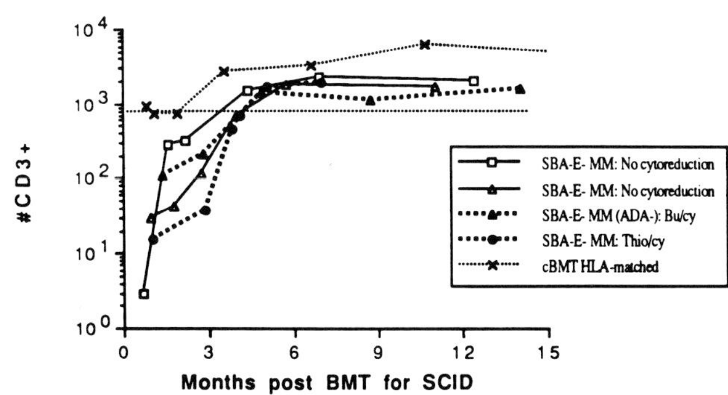

Figure 64-3. Comparison of the return of absolute numbers of circulating CD3+ T cells following bone marrow transplantation for severe combined immunodeficiency disease (SCID). The figure demonstrates the rapid return of T cells (1 mo) following an unmodified, human leukocyte antigen (HLA)–matched sibling transplant (cBMT). Patients receiving SBA$^-$E$^-$ HLA-mismatched (MM) transplants with or without cytoreduction (cyclophosphamide with busulfan or thiotepa) generally experience development of normal numbers of CD3+ T cells 3 to 4 months after transplantation. Lower limit of normal CD3+ cells is indicated by the *horizontal dashed line.*

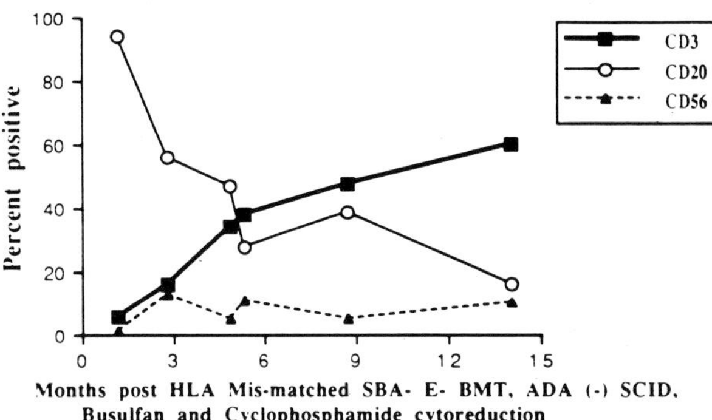

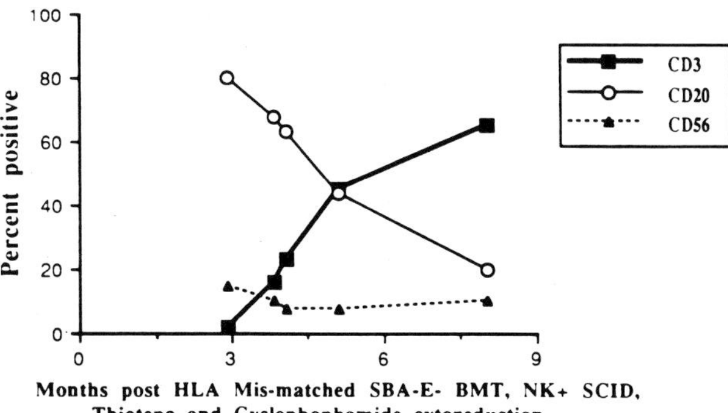

Figure 64-2. Percent of circulating donor T (CD3), natural killer (NK) (CD56), and B (CD20) cells following SBA$^-$ E$^-$ haploidentical marrow transplants in a patient with ADA-severe combined immunodeficiency disease (SCID) (top) and NK + SCID (bottom).

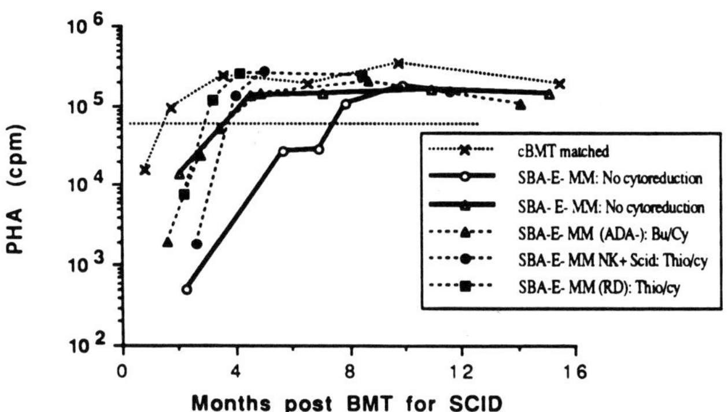

Figure 64-4. Proliferative response to phytohemagglutamin A (PHA) following transplantation for severe combined immunodeficiency disease (SCID). The figure demonstrates the rapid normalization of the PHA response in a recipient of an unmodified, human leukocyte antigen (HLA)–matched sibling transplant (cBMT), compared with the development of the PHA response in patients receiving SBA$^-$ E$^-$ HLA-mismatched (MM) transplants with or without cytoreduction (3–7 mo). The recipients of an SBA$^-$E$^-$ HLA-mismatched related transplant without cytoreduction (n=2) and the patient who received an unmodified HLA-matched transplant had B-cell-positive SCID. Cytoreduction with busulfan and cyclophosphamide (CY) was given before transplantation to a patient with adenosine deaminase deficiency (ADA$^-$). Thiotepa and CY cytoreduction was given to 2 patients, one with natural killer cell–positive SCID and one with reticular dysgenesis (RD). Lower limit of normal PHA (tritiated thymidine: cpm ^{3}H) is indicated by the *horizontal dashed line.*

cells often show a marked predominance of CD4+ T cells, particularly in patients who receive cytoreduction. In addition, a significant population of CD3+, CD4− and CD8− T cells bearing the gamma/delta receptor have been detected early after transplantation and may persist for months after grafting (147).

The basis for the time necessary to achieve functional reconstitution of T cells following an unmodified transplant administered after cytoreduction or a T-cell–depleted marrow graft is only partially understood. The functional T cells detected early after transplantation after an unmanipulated, HLA-matched BMT administered after cytoreduction are likely expanded from the mature T cells transferred in the marrow inoculum because transplants of peripheral blood leukocytes have restored function with similar rapidity (148,149). In addition, passive transfer of antigen-specific cell-mediated immune functions expressed by the donor has been documented early after transplantation, likely reflecting the function of transferred mature lymphocytes (150). Cells other than these mature T cells must also be involved, however, because reconstitution of immune function in cytoreduced children with leukemia or WAS receiving matched marrow grafts is usually not recorded until 4 to 6 months after BMT.

In untreated or cytoreduced patients transplanted with T-cell–depleted marrow, it is possible that the delay in the reconstitution of T cells reflects the time necessary to expand the small number of mature T cells transferred in such a graft. However, it is more likely that this delay is a manifestation of the time required for marrow-derived lymphoid precursors to differentiate and expand within the host's microenvironment. Several lines of evidence support this latter hypothesis, including changes in the host thymus that predate development of T-cell functions; the characteristics of the state of tolerance achieved; and the restriction patterns of the antigen-reactive T cells that emerge after BMT. The thymic epithelium of most patients with SCID is embryonal in anatomical structure (151), and regardless of the variant under study, deficient in production of thymosin alpha and thymulin (36,37). Iwata and co-workers (152) and Incefy and associates (153) observed increments in circulatory thymulin activity occurring shortly after initial documentation of lymphoid chimerism following both unmanipulated HLA-matched and T-cell–depleted mismatched transplants for SCID. Although recipients of unfractionated marrow grafts may have significant responses to mitogens by this time (152), such responses develop in recipients of T-cell–depleted grafts only after recovery of near-normal levels of serum thymulin (153). These results, coupled with histological studies of the thymus following immune reconstitution after T-cell–depleted BMT (154), suggest that recovery of immune function follows the migration of donor lymphoid precursors to the thymus, maturation of that organ's architecture and supportive function, and subsequent differentiation of donor lymphocytes within this host environment. Consistent with this concept is the fact that, in contrast to recipients of unmanipulated marrow grafts, even short-term acquisition of donor cell–mediated immunity following T-cell–depleted grafts has been minimal (155). Furthermore, the restriction patterns of antigen-reactive T cells and their responses to host alloantigens are quite different from those of the donor's own mature T lymphocytes.

The quality and degree of T-cell immunity ultimately achieved following haplotype-disparate T-cell–depleted marrow grafts have been reported to be comparable to that achieved following matched unmanipulated grafts. Normal T-cell numbers and subsets develop, which respond appropriately to mitogens, antigens, and allogeneic cells (104,109,114,115, 146,156). Furthermore, patients regularly generate strong delayed-type hypersensitivity reactions following antigenic challenge (115). Consistent development of intact cell-mediated immune functions following HLA haplotye–disparate T-cell–depleted marrow grafts contrasts with the relatively low frequency of such responses in recipients of fully allogeneic fetal liver transplants (91). This difference in the incidence of immune reconstitution in human transplant recipients is similar to that recorded in murine models comparing the incidence and integrity of T-cell immune reconstitution in lethally irradiated hosts transplanted with H-2 haplotype–disparate or fully allogeneic T-cell–depleted marrow (98). The immune competence in recipients of haplotype disparate marrow grafts likely reflects the homology for one HLA haplotype that facilitates the generation of antigen-reactive T cells restricted to that shared haplotype (157).

Although sharing of one haplotype may be adequate to insure the capacity of the transplanted host to respond to a variety of antigenic stimuli, estimates regarding the capacity of these human hosts to generate antigen-reactive donor T cells restricted to the haplotype unique to the host are extremely limited. In murine models, the T cell's recognition of "self" antigens and its "self" restriction have been shown to be based not on its own H-2 genotype, but rather on the genetic background of other cells within the thymus in which the T cell develops (158). The nature of the cells imprinting "self" recognition on the developing T cells remains controversial. Studies by Ron and associates (159) and Zinkernagel and colleagues (160) suggested that the thymic epithelial cell is critical to this imprinting, whereas studies by Longo and Schwartz (161) implicated antigen-presenting cells within the thymus. The unique states of chimerism that develop in patients transplanted for SCID facilitate clarification of this issue. Patients who have received no preparative cytoreduction are usually selectively engrafted with donor T cells and their progenitors. Monocyte/macrophages, B cells, and other hematopoietic cells are of host origin. In contrast, in patients prepared with myeloablative doses of BU and CY, all hematopoietic cells, including T and B lymphocytes and macrophages, may be of donor origin. Recently, 3 studies examined the restriction patterns of antigen-reactive donor-type T cells cloned from circulating lymphocytes of patients transplanted for SCID. In the patients described by Roberts and co-workers (162) and Roncarolo and associates (99), who achieved reconstitution of cell mediated immune function following selective engraftment of T-cell precursors derived from an $SBA^- E^-$ haplotype-disparate marrow and a fully allogeneic fetal liver, respectively, donor T cells proliferated in response to tetanus antigen only when presented by EBV-transformed B cells bearing either the shared HLA haplotype or the haplotype unique to the host. Cells restricted to the donor's unique haplotype were not identified. These studies thus demonstrated that donor T-cell progenitors developing within a fully allogeneic or haploidentical host can recognize antigens in the context of MHC determinants unique to the host. However, the cells defining this restriction (i.e., thymic epithelial cells or antigen-presenting cells in the macrophage lineage) cannot be distinguished.

Reports by Chu and associates (163) and Geha and colleagues (164), however, provide important new evidence addressing this issue. These investigators examined a patient with SCID who had received an HLA haplotype–disparate transplant depleted of T cells with the T12 monoclonal antibody and complement after cytoreduction with BU and CY. In this patient, tetanus antigen–reactive T-cell clones generated in response to immunizations 6 weeks and one year after transplantation were restricted to both unique donor and unique host HLA determinants as well as to the shared haplotype. At these periods after transplantation, the patient's T cells were found to be exclusively of donor type; monocytes were of a mixed donor and host origin. This patient was subsequently studied 4 years later, at which time the monocytes were exclusively of donor origin (164). Tetanus antigen–specific T-cell responses restricted to the host-specific haplotype were still detectable, although at much lower magnitude than those restricted to the unique haplotype of the donor. However, when this patient was then immunized with a different antigen, Keyhole limpet hemocyanin (KLH), to which neither the donor nor the recipient had been previously exposed, the antigen-specific T-cell responses were exclusively observed when the antigen was presented by cells bearing either the shared or the donor haplotype. This study thus suggests that the restriction patterns developed by the donor T cells emerging after BMT are defined according to the origin of accessory cell populations in the thymus of the host rather than that of the thymic epithelium.

Further studies of patients with SCID who are either lymphoid or full hematopoietic chimeras are needed to confirm these findings. In future studies, it will also be important to determine to what degree antigen-reactive T cells restricted to the unique donor or host HLA haplotypes contribute to the overall response to a given antigen. Recent studies suggest that the capacity of T cells to respond to a given antigen may depend in part on similarities between the antigen and MHC determinants on the antigen presenting cell (165,166). If, in cytoreduced full chimeras, donor T cells capable of recognizing antigen in association with the unique HLA haplotype of the host constitute only a small fraction of responding clones, some limitation to the intensity and diversity of responses to viruses infecting host tissues might be incurred.

GVHD and Tolerance

The incidence of grade II to IV acute GVHD following T-cell–depleted haplotype–disparate marrow grafts has been low. Of 24 patients transplanted with marrow depleted of T cells with monoclonal antibodies and complement or by E-rosette depletion alone, grade II to IV acute GVHD developed in 11 (45%), although this process was reversed in all but one (124). In the combined MSKCC–Ulm series, grade II to IV GVHD developed in 4% of the patients with SCID engrafted with $SBA^- E^-$ transplants. One patient died of this complication. Because the incidence of GVHD has been shown to be correlated with the dose of T cells in the marrow graft (167), the lower incidence of clinically significant GVHD may reflect the greater degree of T cell depletion achieved with the latter technique.

The tolerance that develops in patients with SCID reconstituted with haplotype–disparate T-cell–depleted marrow has been well described (109,168–170). In mixed leukocyte cultures and in cell-mediated lympholysis assays, engrafted and functional T cells consistently fail to react against host alloantigens, yet they are fully reactive to third-party cells (109,168–170). In cell-mediated lympholysis assays in which the engrafted donor T cells have been admixed with the donor's own T lymphocytes before or after sensitization with host cells or cells from the nondonor parent, the engrafted donor T cells failed to suppress the alloreactivity of the donor's own T cells against the host, suggesting that the tolerance observed is not based on the dominance of a suppressor cell system (168–170). In limiting dilution analyses, suppressors of donor antihost cytotoxic activity have been detected, but at frequencies comparable to those of the suppressor T cells that regulate autocytotoxic T-cells detected in normal individuals (171,172). Thus, the tolerance observed appears to be largely based on a deletion of host-reactive clones, and suppressor mechanisms have a less prominent role.

This state of tolerance may also extend to alloantigens not expressed by the donor or host if the patient with SCID is already engrafted with other cells at the time of transplantation. Functional T cells derived from only one parent developed in 2 patients in our series who had received sequential transplants from both parents, but they were chimeric with B cells derived from the host and from both parental donors. In these 2 patients, the functional donor T cells failed to respond to either host cells or cells derived from the other parent (168).

Among patients in whom a state of split lymphoid chimerism develops or is maintained, in which T cells are of donor type but B cells and macrophages are of host type, it has been found repeatedly that the donor T cells exhibit a significant proliferative (but not cytotoxic) response to Ia+ cells of donor origin that greatly exceeds the low or absent level of reactivity against Ia+ cells of the host (168–170). The studies by von Boehmer and Hafen (173) and by Lo and Sprent (174) documented an essential role for antigen-presenting cells in the thymus in defining those alloantigens to which developing T cells will be tolerant. Because these cells, like the circulating monocytes in patients with SCID, are likely of host origin, it has been hypothesized that the donor antidonor proliferative responses represent the response of donor T cells made tolerant to the host against the "allogeneic" Ia specificities of the donor. The significance of these responses to the functional development of a haplotype-disparate marrow graft is still unclear. However, the possibility that these responses might contribute to restrict or to prevent the development of donor type Ia+ B lymphocyte populations cannot be discarded. Indeed, in at least one patient, such donor-reactive populations were found to be suppressive to B cell Ig production in vitro (169).

B-Cell Engraftment and Function

Although full reconstitution of cell mediated function has been observed regularly in the majority of patients with SCID transplanted with T-cell–depleted, HLA-disparate marrow grafts, humoral immunity develops in roughly half the patients (21,109–118,121, 126,127). In part, this deficiency reflects the failure to engraft donor B cell precursors (21,104,146). Whereas preparative regimens with CY alone or in combination with cytosine arabinoside markedly improve the incidence of engraftment of donor T-cell precursors in patients with evidence of graft resistance, consistent engraftment of donor B cells has been observed only in patients prepared with myeloablative therapy, such as BU coupled with CY (21,104,146). Humoral immunity has been restored in a minority of patients whose B cells remain exclusively of host origin. Indeed, of 32 long-term, durably engrafted patients receiving T-cell–depleted haplotype-disparate grafts for SCID at MSKCC, specific IgG antibody production developed in only 2 of 18 evaluated patients with exclusively host B cells, compared with each of the 14 engrafted with donor B cells. Similar results have recently been reported by Fischer and colleagues (21), who reported that of 23 patients with host B cells, full B-cell immunity developed in only one patient and partial B-cell immunity developed in 6, compared with 33 of 34 patients with donor B cells (19 full, 14 partial).

It has been hypothesized that failure to engraft donor B cells is due to inadequacies of "space" resulting from the prior expansion of nonfunctional B cells detected in the majority of patients with SCID. However, several patients in our series with classic SCID who lack serum Ig+ cells by definition failed to engraft donor B cells in the absence of cytoreduction (175). In our series, failure to engraft or expand donor B-cell progenitors has not correlated with patient characteristics associated with resistance to T-cell engraftment, such as NK cell activity or IL-1 deficiencies, nor is it more frequently observed in any specific variant of SCID. Furthermore, although our initial studies suggested a correlation between pretransplant engraftment of maternal T cells and a failure to engraft donor B cells (175), subsequent analysis of our larger series has failed to support this relationship. It is likely that failure to engraft or expand donor B-cell progenitors reflects other as yet undefined resistance mechanisms that are sensitive to myeloablative therapy. For example, failure to develop donor B cells might be due to deficiencies in the capacity of host accessory cell systems to provide factors necessary to expand or differentiate donor B-cell progenitors within the host environment. If such is the case, preparation with BU and CY might ensure engraftment of both B-cell progenitors and these essential accessory cells.

The basis for the deficiencies of host B cells observed both prior to and following HLA-disparate marrow grafts is still poorly understood. Pretransplant, the circulating host serum Ig+ lymphocytes, when present, express HLA-DR, CD19, CD20, serum Ig, CD21, Leu-8, and lack expression of CD10. In addition, these cells often express CD1c, CD38, CD5, and CD23 (176). This phenotype is similar to that of normal cord blood B cells, which also express CD1c, CD38, CD5, and CD23. In normal individuals, however, this B-cell population decreases with age, representing a minor population in older children (>2 yr) and adults (176,177). Donor B cells of this phenotype can also be isolated from patients during the first year following T-cell–depleted, or conventional BMT for leukemia (177). However, in patients receiving transplants for either SCID or leukemia, after pretransplant cytoreduction, expression of these antigens on the circulating donor B cells decreases during the second and third post-transplant year, coincident with the normalization of serum Ig levels and generation of specific antibody responses (177; Small TN. Unpublished observations). In contrast, the host B cells of patients with SCID in whom humoral immunity fails to develop after transplantation continue to express the CD1c, CD5, CD38, and CD23 antigens, suggesting an inability to differentiate in response to signals provided by functional donor-derived T cells (Small TN. Unpublished observations). In addition, recent studies have demonstrated that unlike donor-engrafted CD23+ B cells, the residual host CD23+ SCID B cells do not up-regulate CD23 in response to IL-4 (156). Despite these abnormalities, pretransplant SCID B cells proliferate following stimulation with *Staphylococcus aureus* Cowan strain I (SAC), anti-μ, and B-cell growth factor (BCGF), as do normal cord blood B cells (156,176).

Assays of in vitro Ig production, utilizing a synergistic combination of pokeweed mitogen and SAC, demonstrate that whereas circulating B cells derived from normal adults produce both IgG and IgM, SCID B cells cocultured with donor or third party T cells produce only IgM (176). Following transplantation, host B cells produce IgM in vitro (Keever CA. Unpublished observations) and may generate specific IgM antibody. However, no patient with exclusively host B cells has produced IgG in vitro until a minimum of 5 years after transplantation, whereas the majority of patients with donor B cells have produced IgM during the first transplant year and subsequently produce IgG (Keever CA. Unpublished observations). These in vitro findings are consistent with the serum levels of IgG and IgM detected in our patients. Although the provision of normal helper T-cell function in vitro does not induce antibody production in the majority of patients, the B cells of certain patients do generate plaque-forming cells under these conditions (178).

These in vitro findings suggest that SCID B cells are intrinsically defective. Paradoxically, however, despite the lack of donor B cells in 50 to 70% of patients with SCID transplanted with unmodified HLA-identical or partially matched marrow (48,179,180), only rare patients are antibody-deficient (181). Indeed, in the review by Kenny and Hitzig (46), only 4 of 25 patients reconstituted with HLA-matched marrow grafts remained antibody-deficient. That host B cells can indeed form antibodies in these split lymphoid chimeras was first demonstrated by Griscelli and colleagues (49), who documented that the antibodies generated had the distinctive Gm allotype of the host. Similarly, isohemagglutinin production against the donor red-cell antigens has been documented in patients with host B cells, suggesting that they are functional B cells (182). Given these observations, the fact that patients with SCID who lack donor B cells following BMT of HLA haplotype–mismatched T-cell–depleted marrow remain hypogammaglobulinemic and unable to generate specific antibodies suggests persistent defects in those interactions between host B cells and donor T cells necessary for the development of the host B cells' capacity to generate specific antibody.

Until recently, studies in animal models of BMT provided no precedents for such selective deficits of B-cell function following an H-2 haplotype–disparate T-cell–depleted marrow graft. Indeed, H-2 haplotype–disparate, T-cell–depleted marrow grafts administered to lethally irradiated mice have regularly produced full restorations of both humoral and cell-mediated immune function. However, in these radiation chimeras, B cells are of donor origin. Thus, the humoral immune reconstitution observed does not reflect the development of host B cells in the presence of haplotype-disparate donor T cells. Recently, however, Zinkernagel and colleagues (103) used T-cell–deficient marrow cells derived from allogeneic nude mice to reconstitute immune function in unirradiated C.B-17 mice with SCID. In the resultant mixed lymphoid chimeras, cell-mediated immune responses were fully restored. The donor T cells that develop exhibit virus-specific cytolytic activity that is restricted to infected targets of host type. However, like the patients with SCID transplanted with HLA haplotype–disparate T-cell–depleted marrow, these chimeras are not able to generate T-cell–dependent IgG antibody.

Several hypotheses raised to explain the residual humoral immune deficits observed in these patients have been examined in our series. It has been demonstrated that engrafted donor CD4+ helper cells can provide effective help to freshly isolated donor B cells in the production of IgM, IgG, and in the generation of SRBC plaques (Keever CA. Unpublished observations). Evidence previously reviewed indicates that the engrafted T cells are also able to interact with antigen-presenting accessory cells bearing the unique host haplotype. In contrast, host B cells isolated after reconstitution of donor T-cell function are unable to produce IgG in the presence of either the donor's own freshly isolated helper T cells or engrafted donor-type helper T cells. Thus, unless the donor-derived helper T cells developing within the host are uniquely deficient in their interaction with host B cells, the host B cells are more likely responsible for the lack of effective cooperation observed. Whether the abnormalities of SCID B cells make them more stringent in their requirements for HLA homologies is currently unknown.

It is also possible that the residual deficiencies of humoral immunity are due to an active process that suppresses the development of antibody-forming cells. Such suppressor functions might be a manifestation of a subclinical GVHD, analogous to that described by Hurtenbach and Shearer (183) in the parent to newborn F1 model of GVHD. Subclinical GVHD could be initiated either by residual T cells in the T-cell–depleted graft or by transplacentally derived maternal T cells already established in the host prior to transplantation. Indeed, as previously noted, suppressors of Ig secretion have been detected among the maternally derived T cells detected in at least one patient with SCID (136).

Two other pathological states reflecting disturbed B-cell regulation have been observed at increased frequency in recipients of HLA haplotype–disparate T-cell–depleted marrow grafts: antibody-mediated autoimmune cytopenias and EBV-associated lymphoproliferative disorders, including lymphomas.

The incidence of autoimmune cytopenias among patients with SCID receiving HLA-nonidentical T-cell–depleted BMT can be significant. In a series of 10 patients reported by Morgab and colleagues (184), autoimmune thrombocytopenia developed in 2 patients and an autoimmune hemolytic anemia developed in one. Autoantibodies developed in 6 of 15 patients reported by Wijnaedts and associates (146), leading to overt disease in 4. By comparison, autoantibodies developed in 4 of 15 patients receiving unmodified HLA-matched related transplants, clinical disease developed in none (146). In our own series, autoimmune hemolytic anemias developed in 2 of 37 engrafted patients early in the course of immunological reconstitution. Thus, the incidence of such complications may range from 5 to 40%. These disorders have, in our experience, necessitated intensive treatment with corticosteroids to achieve initial control but have ultimately resolved. Maintenance immunosuppressive therapy has not been required, nor have these disorders recurred.

EBV-associated B-cell lymphoproliferative disorders, particularly polyclonal lymphomas, have been reported at a significant frequency both in leukemic patients treated for GVHD with certain T-cell–specific monoclonal antibodies (185) and among leukemic recipients of marrow T-cell–depleted with monoclonal antibodies (186). Strikingly, the lymphomas that developed in the leukemic patients have usually been found to be of donor rather than host origin (185). This complication is rare among leukemic patients transplanted with marrow depleted by techniques that remove both T and B lymphocytes from the graft, such as lectin agglutination or treatment with CAMPATH-1 (130,131). Thus, removal of cells that might serve as targets for transformation by EBV may reduce the risk for this complication.

Lymphomas among patients with SCID who have received T-cell–depleted haplotype-disparate marrow grafts have also been reported. Similar to the lymphomas observed in leukemic BMT recipients, these processes developed early after transplantation (3–9 mo), in patients either who had failed to engraft or whose graft had achieved only rudimentary evidence of T-cell function (123,187). All but one of these lymphomas were EBV antigen–positive. However, in contrast to the findings in leukemic patients, of the 6 lymphomas described, 4 have been documented to be of host origin (104). Such lymphomas have not been observed among SCID recipients of unfractionated, HLA-matched marrow grafts.

Several factors may predispose SCID recipients of HLA haplotype–disparate grafts to these aberrations of B-cell growth and function. First, patients with SCID who have not received transplants are at increased risk for lymphoreticular malignancies (188). Second, it has been observed repeatedly that the B cells in the circulation of patients with SCID may be stimulated to undergo benign oligoclonal expansions early in the course of T-cell engraftment and functional reconstitution, which may render them more susceptible to EBV-induced transformation (189–191). Such oligoclonal expansions normally resolve as donor-type T-cell populations, including T suppressor cells, gain normal function in the host (191). In our experience, the rare autoimmune hemolytic anemias or thrombocytopenia that develop occur early in the course of immune reconstitution, and resolve once reconstitution of T-cell function is achieved. Similarly, polyclonal lymphoproliferations and lymphomas have developed consistently at a time when the donor T-cells have achieved only rudimentary function or have declined both in number and activity. This finding suggests that if functional reconstitution of regulatory T cells is impeded or aborted, uncontrolled expansion of activated EBV-susceptible B cells or autoreactive clones may continue, thereby placing such patients at particular risk for severe autoimmune disorders or EBV-associated lymphomatous transformations.

The EBV lymphomas reported to date among patients with SCID have been fulminant, refractory to chemotherapy and radiation and ultimately fatal. Recently, however, new approaches have been developed that may prevent these processes or reverse them early in their course. Although in vitro studies have shown that EBV DNA polymerase is sensitive to acyclovir (192) and other nucleoside analogues (193), it has little effect on latent infection, will not inhibit the growth of EBV-transformed cells (194), and has little effect on the course of established EBV-associated lymphomas (195). However, the incidence of EBV-associated lymphomas has been reported to be dramatically reduced or eliminated among recipients of HLA-nonidentical T-cell–depleted grafts who have received prolonged acyclovir prophylaxis (196). Fischer and colleagues (197) reported effective therapy of polyclonal EBV-induced lymphoproliferative disorders with in vivo administration of anti-CD21 and CD24 monoclonal antibodies. Of 6 patients with WAS who received T-cell–depleted HLA-disparate grafts and in whom this complication developed, resolution of the lymphoproliferative disorder was observed in all 5 patients with polyclonal disease (198). Therapy with alpha-interferon and gammaglobulin has also been reported to induce durable remissions (199).

Combined Immunodeficiency

The diagnostic category of "combined immunodeficiency with T-cell predominance" (9), or Nezelof syndrome (200), refers to a heterogenous group of patients who present with a history of severe recurrent, acute, and chronic infections and who have profound but not absolute deficiencies of T- and B-cell function. In this group of disorders, T lymphocytes may be deficient or normal in number. Lymphocyte transformation responses to mitogens and allogeneic cells are markedly abnormal in vitro but are not absolutely deficient as they are in patients with SCID. In several of these CID syndromes, B cells are prominent and immunoglobulins may be normal or increased. However, except in nucleoside phosphorylase deficiency, antibody responses to antigenic stimulation are usually absent.

In recent years, the pathogenetic basis for several CID syndromes have been described. These include a congenital deficiency of the IL-1 receptor (201); congenital disorders of T-cell activation, which result in the inability to generate T-cell–derived cytokines (202) or specifically IL-2 (203,204); defects in the expression of the T cell CD3 receptor (18) and the IL-2 receptor (205); severe forms of nucleoside phosphorylase deficiency (206); and the bare lymphocyte syndromes (207,208), a series of genetic disorders resulting in defective transcription and ultimate expression of HLA class I or II, or both, determinants on the surface of lymphoid and hematopoetic cells. Recently, a distinct syndrome characterized by selective deficiencies of CD8+ T cells with functionally abnormal CD4+ T cells has also been recognized (209).

Experience with the application of BMT to the treatment of these disorders is extremely limited. It is clear, however, that the function of the alloreactive T lymphocytes detected in these disorders is usually sufficient to prevent engraftment of either an unmodified HLA-identical or partially matched marrow transplant and consistently prevents engraftment of T-cell–depleted HLA-nonidentical grafts. Experience with HLA-matched BMT applied to these disorders is largely limited to single case reports recording disappointing results. Three patients with Nezelof syndrome received transplants of HLA-matched marrow with (n = 1) or without (n = 2) cytoreduction. Each achieved durable engraftment and reconstitution (48,210). In contrast, none of 3 patients receiving HLA-matched grafts for nucleoside phosphorylase deficiency (48,206) and only 1 of 6 patients grafted for bare lymphocyte syndrome achieved reconstitution despite preparative cytoreduction.

There has been considerably more experience with HLA haplotype–disparate T-cell–depleted BMT in these disorders. Among patients transplanted for unspecified CID syndromes in Europe prepared with BU and CY with or without ATG, engraftment rates have been poor, ranging from 14 to 36%, depending on the post-transplant GVHD prophylaxis used. Long-term survival rates of less than 10% have been recorded (48). Preparation with BU or TBI and CY permitted engraftment and reconstitution in at least one patient transplanted for nucleoside phosphorylase deficiency (206) and in one of 2 patients with bare lymphocyte syndrome (211; Friedrich W. Unpublished observations). Two patients with IL-2 deficiency failed to engraft despite cytoreduction with CY with BU or cytosine arabinoside (204; Small TN. Unpublished observations). Recently, encouraging results have been achieved with HLA-nonidentical T-cell–depleted marrow transplants administered after cytoreduction with BU and CY when the patients also received anti-LFA-1 in the post-transplant period (198). Of 11 transplanted patients reported by Fischer and colleagues (198), 7 (3/4 with bare lymphocyte syndrome, 4/7 with CID) achieved engraftment, immunological reconstitution, and long-term DFS (198).

These results indicate a pressing need for new and more effective preparative regimens and post-transplant treatment strategies to ensure full and durable chimerism and reconstitution of immunological function in patients afflicted with these rare combined immunodeficiency disorders.

Wiskott-Aldrich Syndrome

Wiskott-Aldrich Syndrome, an X-linked recessive disorder, is characterized by progressive T-cell immunodeficiency, impaired antipolysaccharide antibody production, eczema, and thrombocytopenia (212). Laboratory studies demonstrate variable but generally reduced responses to T-cell mitogens and allogeneic cells, markedly decreased serum IgM and isohemagglutinins (212–216), normal serum IgG2 levels (217), and small platelet volume associated with impaired platelet aggregation (9). Patients with WAS exhibit aberrant expression of CD43, a sialoglycoprotein (218,219) found on all circulating lymphoid and hematopoetic cells except red cells (220). Because CD43 is encoded on chromosome 16 (221,222), a structural abnormality within this gene cannot be the primary defect in X-linked WAS, which maps to the proximal short arm of the X chromosome between the TIMP and DXS146 loci (223). Nevertheless, the specific absence of proliferation of WAS T cells in response to anti-CD43 and periodate, which activates normal T cells by interaction with the CD43 molecule, can be particularly helpful in making the diagnosis of WAS, especially in individuals with mild or unusual clinical presentations (224).

The CD43 ligand is ICAM-1 (225), whose other ligands include the integrins LFA-1 and LFA-3, molecules important in lymphocyte and myeloid cell adhesion, respectively (226,227). Experiments demonstrating both mitogenicity of anti-CD43 antibodies (228) and enhancement of antigen-specific activation following transfection of complementary DNA encoding CD43 into murine T-cell hybridomas (229) have led to the hypothesis that the immunodeficiency associated with WAS is related to impaired activation or cell adhesion mediated through these surface molecules.

It has been demonstrated that CD43 is abnormally glycosylated on WAS lymphocytes (220,230). This finding, as well as reports of aberrant expression of platelet GP 1b (218) (also an O-glycosylated molecule) in 2 patients with WAS, led to experiments that revealed abnormal patterns of activity of certain developmentally regulated glycosyltransferases in platelets, resting and activated T cells, and EBV-transformed B-cell lines derived from WAS patients (230–232). These studies suggest that the hematopoetic and immunological abnormalities of WAS may ultimately be ascribed to a gene broadly affecting the regulation of O-glycosylation (230–232) of proteins expressed on the surface of hematopoetic cells.

BMT for WAS

In 1968, Bach and associates (2) reported correction of the immunological abnormalities associated with WAS following a marrow graft from an HLA-matched sibling. However, despite preparation with high-dose CY, this patient did not achieve engraftment of hematopoetic elements and remained thrombocytopenic. In 1978, Parkman and colleagues (6) induced a full correction of both lymphoid and platelet abnormalities associated with WAS by administering an HLA-matched marrow graft after treating the patient with a myelosuppressive and immunosuppressive regimen consisting of TBI, procarbazine, and ATG. On the basis of the success of this BMT, these authors suggested that myeloablation as well as immunosuppression might be required to correct disorders involving other nonlymphoid lineages to provide "space" or a niche in which their progenitors could proliferate and develop. Subsequently, Kapoor and co-workers (7) demonstrated that BU, when combined with CY, provided a myeloablative and immunosuppressive chemotherapeutic regimen adequate to insure full hematopoetic chimerism, thereby providing full correction of both lymphoid and thrombocyte defects for a series of children with WAS. Currently, results from large centers in the United States and Europe indicate that such regimens, when used to prepare patients for HLA-matched marrow grafts, have led to full correction and long-term DFS for 36 of 41 (88%) patients transplanted (48,144,233–235; Friedrich W. Unpublished observations). Strikingly, long-term chimeras have not only experienced full reconstitution of immune function and production of normal platelets, but have also enjoyed sustained freedom from autoimmune hemolytic anemias and EBV-associated lymphoproliferative disorders, to which patients with WAS are so susceptible. Thus, HLA-matched marrow grafts administered after appropriate myeloablation and immunosuppression clearly constitute the treatment of choice for this disorder.

More problematic are children with WAS who lack an HLA-identical sibling. A review of mismatched transplants for WAS prior to 1987 reported 3 of 13 (23%) survivors (236). Since then, the outcome of 28 additional patients with WAS who lack an HLA-identical sibling (79,198,235,237) has been reported (Table 64-1). Of 25 patients who receivied a T-cell–depleted mismatched transplant, 9 (36%) are alive and well with full (n = 7) or partial (n = 2) immunoreconstitution. Obstacles to successful outcome in these patients include graft rejection despite intensive cytoreduction, EBV-associated lymphoproliferative disorders, and GVHD. Of these 25 patients, 5 patients (20%) experienced graft failure, and EBV lymphomas developed in 9 (36%). In addition, grade II or greater GVHD developed in 45% of engrafted patients. The increased incidence of GVHD in these patients despite even rigorous T-cell depletion is unusual. At MSKCC, moderate to severe GVHD developed in 3 of 6 patients receiving HLA-mismatched marrow T-cell–depleted with soybean agglutination followed by rosetting with sheep red blood cells, in contrast to 1 of 19 patients with SCID durably engrafted with SBA$^-$ E$^-$ haploidentical transplants after cytoreduction. This finding suggests that target cell populations that trigger GVHD may be different in these 2 patient groups. Despite these problems, efforts to improve engraftment (e.g., in vivo anti-LFA-1 antibody treatment, different cytoreductive regimens, method of T-cell

Table 64-1.
Bone Marrow Transplantation for Patients With Wiskott-Aldrich Syndrome who Lack an HLA-matched Related Marrow Donor

Institution	*T-cell Depletion*	*Donor (Related vs. Unrelated)*	*Cytoreduction*	*Durable Engraftment*
University of Wisconsin (125,236) (n = 5)	CT-2 (anti-CD2) + C	Related donors: n = 1, HLA-B MM (G[b]); n = 3, HLA-A, B MM (DR typing not included); n = 1, HLA-DR MM	n = 1; BU 4 mg/kg × 4; CY 50 mg/kg × 4 n = 3; ara-C 2 gm/m² × 6; CY 45 mg/kg × 2; TBI 1,320 cGy in 8 fractions n = 1; ara-C 2 gm/m² × 6; CY 45 mg/kg × 2; BU 4 mg/kg	
Hopital des Enfants-Malades (198) (n = 14)	9: E-rosetting 5: CAMPATH-1 + C	Related donors: n = 8, HLA- A,B DR MM; n = 4, HLA-B, DR MM; n = 1, HLA-A, B MM; n = 1, DR MM	BU 4 mg/kg × 4; Cy 50 mg/kg × 4 Post-transplant anti-CD11a infusion for graft rejection prophylaxis (n = 14)	7/9 E-rosette 3/5: Campath; 3/3 are mixed chimeras
MSKCC (233) (n = 6)[a]	SBA-E−	Related donors; n = 3, HLA-A, B, DR MM; n = 2, HLA-B, DR MM; (R)[c]; haplotype MM (G); n = 1, HLA-B MM (R); A,B,DR MM (G)	TBI 1375 cGy in 11 fractions; ara-C 3 gm/m² × 8 Secondary graft; thiotepa, CY, ATG 2/6 received ATG post-BMT for rejection prophylaxis	5/6 1 patient rejected primary graft and required secondary BMT
University of Minnesota (79) (n = 3)[a]	None	Unrelated donors: n = 1, HLA-A MM; n = 1, HLA-B MM; n = 1, HLA-matched	BU 4 mg/kg × 4; CY 50 mg/kg × 4; ATG for graft rejection prophylaxis, pre- and post-BMT	3/3

[a]One patient in each group received treatment prior to BMT for an EBV lymphoproliferative disorder.
[b]HLA-mismatched donor toward host.
[c]HLA-mismatched host toward donor.

depletion) and the ability to treat polyclonal EBV-induced lymphoproliferative disorders successfully (e.g., CD21 and CD24 antibody administration [198] or alpha-interferon with intravenous gammaglobulin [199]) are likely to improve the results of subsequent BMTs. In addition, preliminary results with unmodified transplants, utilizing HLA-matched or one antigen–mismatched unrelated donors appear promising (79). Nevertheless, the decision when to transplant patients with WAS who lack an HLA-matched related donor is likely to remain an area of controversy until results are markedly improved, particularly for splenectomized patients with WAS who are no longer thrombocytopenic and may be maintained infection-free for extended periods with aggressive antibiotic and gammaglobulin prophylaxis.

Future Directions

Exploration of the use of HLA-partially matched related and compatible unrelated donors and the subsequent development of highly efficient techniques for depleting T cells from marrow cells have extended the applications of curative BMT to all children afflicted with SCID, regardless of the variant under treatment. At our own center, long-term results of HLA haplotype–disparate T-cell–depleted parental marrow grafts have shown durable engraftment with correction of the deficiencies of T-cell function associated with SCID at rates comparable to those achieved with unmodified grafts from HLA-matched siblings. Future improvements in the application of these approaches to patients with the different CID syndromes and WAS await the development of more consistently effective preparatory regimens, which will insure durable and complete engraftment with low early and long-term toxicity. Such regimens may employ more targeted agents, such as monoclonal antibodies specific to effectors of resistance, as well as the use of cytokines such as IL-1, IL-2, and certain of the B-cell–promoting cytokines to facilitate earlier recovery of immunological function, thereby reducing the period of risk from infection during the post-transplant period. The quality, intensity, and diversity of both T- and B-cell immune responses generated in patients with SCID reconstituted with marrow derived from unrelated HLA-compatible or HLA haplotype–disparate donors need to be explored further and compared with those achieved by recipients of HLA-matched grafts. In murine models, the use of biparental T-cell–depleted marrow grafts has been shown to be effective in reconstituting both hematopoeisis and immune function in lethally irradiated hosts (105). In the future, this approach might be considered if antigen-reactive HLA haplotype–disparate lymphocytes from one parental donor developing within children transplanted for SCID are found to exhibit limited diversity due to preferential selec-

Table 64-1. cont.

GVHD Prophylaxis	*Acute GVHD O/I/II/II I/IV*	*Chronic GVHD O/llm/ext*[a]	*Outcome*	*EBV Lymphoma*	*Immune Function*
2/5: none 1/5: ALG +steroids 2/5: CSP	0/1/2/1/0	2/1/1	n = 4: alive, well n = 1: died day +37 with staphylococcal sepsis	None	T&B cell reconstitution (n = 3)
CSP (recipients of E-rosetted BM) None (recipients of Campath-treated BM)	7/0/2/1/0	9/1/0	n = 7, alive (10+ to 56+ months); 2 with autologous recovery	n = 6; All treated with anti-CD21 and CD24 MoAb, 5/6 CR	T &B cell reconstitution (n = 3)
None	2/0/1/2/0	2/0/3	n = 1: alive, well 66+ months 5 deaths (pulmonary hemorrhage, disseminated candidiasis, sepsis, EBV lymphoma [2])	n = 3: 3 deaths. One died of pulmonary hemorrhage; no evidence of lymphoma	T &B cell reconstitution (n = 1)
1: MTX, steroids, CSP 1:MTX, ATG, steroids 1: not reported	2/0/1/1/0	0	n = 2: alive, well 20+, 33+ months; 1 death from VOD and *Aspergillosis*	None	T& B cell reconstitution (n = 2)

[a]O = overall; llm = limited; Ext = extensive.

tion of clones restricted to the haplotype shared by the donor and the host.

The lethal congenital immune deficiency disorders will likely continue to be important models for future developments in BMT. The first applications of gene therapy in humans have been introduced to correct the ADA-deficient form of SCID (238). The development of approaches utilizing retroviral vectors to insert the normal ADA gene into both lymphoid and hematopoetic cells first in animals and then in humans dramatically accelerated research in this important area. Within the next 5 years, it is expected that the genes responsible for certain X-linked variants of SCID and WAS will be cloned. Correction of these disorders by insertion of their normal gene counterparts into early hematopoetic cells could lead to consistent reversals of these lethal disorders with genetically manipulated autologous hematopoetic cells.

Advances in the molecular genetics of several of these lethal immune deficiencies, such as ADA deficiency, X-linked forms of SCID, and WAS, now permit prenatal diagnosis from analysis of fetal cells isolated from chorionic villous biopsies as early as 8 weeks' gestation (58). Autosomal forms of SCID can also be diagnosed as early as 18 weeks' gestation (55,56). Currently, cells from an affected fetus are used to establish diagnosis and to identify the HLA genotype to permit selection of a donor and a transplant approach long before a child is born. However, several investigators are now exploring the possibility of correcting these lethal genetic disorders of immunity before birth by infusions of fetal liver or adult bone–marrow derived T-cell–depleted primitive hematopoetic progenitor cells into the peritoneal sac of an affected fetus as early as 11 weeks' gestation. Preliminary results in at least 2 patients documented engraftment and immunological reconstitution mediated by these prenatal hematopoetic grafts, indicating the feasibility of this approach (239). Prenatal correction probably will also be used for certain of the other CID syndromes. Whether the "physiological space" necessary for development of lymphoid and nonlymphoid cells in individuals, such as patients with WAS, is adequate in early embryonal life to permit engraftment and correction of the deficits in these lineages remains to be determined.

The authors gratefully acknowledge the helpful advice and critical review of Dr Katherine A. Siminovitch for the section on Wiskott-Aldrich syndrome.

References

1. Gatti RA, Meeuwissen HJ, Allen HD, Hong R, Good RA. Immunological reconstitution of sex-linked lymphopenic immunological deficiency. Lancet 1968;2:1366–1369.
2. Bach FH, Albertini RJ, Anderson JL, et al. Bone marrow transplantation in a patient with the Wiskott-Aldrich syndrome. Lancet 1968;2:1364–1366.
3. Copenhagen Study Group of Immunodeficiencies. Bone-marrow transplantation from an HL-A nondentical but mixed-lymphocyte-culture identical donor. Lancet 1973;2:1146–1150.
4. O'Reilly RJ, Dupont B, Pahwa S, et al. Reconstitution in severe combined immunodeficiency by transplantation of marrow from an unrelated donor. N Engl J Med 1977;297:1311–1318.
5. Reisner Y, Kapoor N, Kirkpatrick D, et al. Transplantation for acute leukemia with HLA-A and B non-identical parental marrow cells fractionated with soybean agglutinin and sheep red cells. Lancet 1981;2:327–331.
6. Parkman R, Rapperport J, Geha R, et al. Complete correction of the Wiskott-Aldrich syndrome by allogeneic bone marrow transplantation. N Engl J Med 1978;298:921–927.
7. Kapoor N, Kirkpatrick D, Blaese RM, et al. Reconstitution of normal megakaryocytopoiesis and immunological functions in Wiskott-Aldrich syndrome by marrow transplantation following myeloablation and immunosuppression with busulfan and cyclophosphamide. Blood 1981;57:692–696.
8. Rosen FS, Cooper MD, Wedgewood RJP. The primary immunodeficiencies. N Engl J Med 1984;311:235–242.
9. Rosen FS, Aiuti F, Hitzig W, et al. Meeting report: primary immunodeficiency disease. Clin Immunol Immunopathol 1983;28:450–475.
10. Giblett ER, Anderson JE, Cohen F, Pollara B, Meeuwissen HJ. Adenosine-deaminase deficiency in two patients with severely impaired cellular immunity. Lancet 1972;2:1067–1069.
11. Carson DA, Kaye J, Seegmiller JE. Lymphospecific toxicity in adenosine deaminase deficiency and urine nucleoside phosphorylase deficiency: Possible role of nucleoside kinase(s). PNAS 1977;74:5677–5682.
12. DeVaal OM, Seynhaeve V. Reticular dysgenesis. Lancet 1959;2:1123–1125.
13. Omenn G. Familial reticuloendotheliosis. N Engl J Med 1965;273:427–432.
14. Ruco LP, Stoppacciaro A, Pezzella F, et al. The Omenn's syndrome: histological, immunohistochemical and ultrastructural evidence for a partial T cell deficiency evolving in an abnormal proliferation of T lymphocytes and S-100+/T_6+ Langerhans-like cells. Virchow's Arch 1985;407:69–82.
15. Gatti RA, Platt N, Pomerance HH, et al. Hereditary lymphopenic agammaglobulinemia associated with a distinctive form of short-limbed dwarfism and ectodermal dysplasia. J Pediatr 1969;75:675–684.
16. Gelfand EW, Oliver JM, Schuurman RK, Matheson DS, Dosch HM. Abnormal lymphocyte capping in a patient with severe combined immunodeficiency disease. N Engl J Med 1979;301:1245–1249.
17. Jung LKL, Fu SM, Hara T, Kapoor N, Good RA. Defective expression of T cell associated glycoprotein in severe combined immunodeficiency. J Clin Invest 1986;77:940–946.
18. Alarcon B, Regueiro JR, Arnaiz-Villena A, Terhorst C. Familial defect in the surface expression of the T-cell receptor-CD3 complex. N Engl J Med 1988;319:1203–1208.
19. Parkman R, Gelfand EW, Rosen FS, Sanderson A, Hirschhorn R. Severe combined immunodeficiency and adenosine deaminase deficiency. N Engl J Med 1975; 14:714–719.
20. Ownby DR, Pizzo S, Blackmon L, Gall SA, Buckley RH. Severe combined immunodeficiency with leukopenia

(reticular dysgenesis) in siblings: immunologic and histopathologic findings. J Pediatr 1976;89:382–387.
21. Fischer A, Landais P, Friedrich W, et al. European experience of bone-marrow transplantation for severe combined immunodeficiency. Lancet 1990;336:850–854.
22. Valerio D, Dekker BMM, Duyvesteyn MGC, et al. One adenosine deaminase allele in a patient with severe combined immunodeficiency contains a point mutation abolishing enzyme activity. EMBO J 1986;5:113–119.
23. Bonithron DT, Markham AF, Ginsburg D, Orkin SH. Identification of a point mutation in the adenosine deaminase gene responsible for immunodeficiency. J Clin Invest 1985;76:894–897.
24. Markert ML, Hershfield MS, Wiginton DA, et al. Identification of a deletion in the adenosine deaminase gene in a child with severe combined immunodeficiency. J Immunol 1987;138:3203–3206.
25. Polmar SH, Stern RC, Schwartz AL, et al. Enzyme replacement therapy for adenosine deaminase deficiency and severe combined immunodeficiency. N Engl J Med 1976;295:1337–1343.
26. Polmar SH. Enzyme replacement and other biochemical approaches to the therapy of adenosine deaminase deficiency. In: Ciba Foundation Symposium. Enzyme defects and immune dysfunction, vol. 68. Amsterdam: Excerpta Medica, 1979:213.
27. Hershfield MS, Buckley RH, Greenberg ML, et al. Treatment of adenosine deaminase deficiency with polyethyene glycol-modified adenosine deaminase. N Engl J Med 1987;316:589–596.
28. Hitzig WH, Landolt R, Muller G, Bodner P. Heterogeneity of phenotypic expression in a family with Swiss-type agammaglobulinemia: Observations in the acquisition of agammaglobulinemia. J Pediatr 1971;78:968–980.
29. Messina C, Kirkpatrick D, Fitzgerald PA, et al. Natural killer function and interferon generation in patients with primary immunodeficiencies. Clin Immunol Immunopathol 1986;39:394–404.
30. Peter HH, Friedrich W, Dopfer R, et al. NK cell function in severe combined immunodeficiency (SCID): evidence of a common T and NK cell defect in some but not all SCID patients. J Immunol 1983;131:2332–2339.
31. Ten Berge RJM, Schellekens PTA, Budding-Koppenol A, Dooren LJ, Vossen JM. Natural killer (NK)-cell activity in sorted subsets of peripheral blood monoclonal cells from patients with severe combined immunodeficiency. J Clin Immunol 1987;7:198–202.
32. Sindel LJ, Buckley RH, Schiff SE, et al. Severe combined immunodeficiency with natural killer-cell predominance: abrogation of graft-versus-host disease and immunologic reconstitution with HLA-identical bone marrow cells. J Allergy Clin Immunol 1984;73:829–836.
33. Sahdev I, O'Reilly J, Hoffman MK. Correlation between interleukin-1 production and engraftment of transplanted bone marrow stem cells in patients with lethal immunodeficiencies. Blood 1989;73:1712–1719.
34. Denning D, O'Reilly RJ. Effect of IL-7 on the function of B lineage cells. Proc Am Assoc Cancer Res 1992;33:302.
35. Incefy GS, Darofnne M, Pahwa S, et al. Thymic activity in severe combined immunodeficiency disease. PNAS 1977;74:1250–1253.
36. Incefy G, Flomenberg N, Small T, et al. Evidence that appearance of thymulin in plasma follows lymphoid chimerism and precedes development of immunity in patients with lethal combined immunodoeficiency transplanted with T cell depleted haploidentical marrow. Transplantation 1990;50:55–61.
37. Lewis V, Twomey J, Goldstein G, et al. Circulating thymic hormone activity in congenital immunodeficiency. Lancet 1977;2:471–475.
38. Pyke KW, Dosch HM, Ipp MM, Gelfand EW. Demonstration of an intrathymic defect in a case of severe combined immunodeficiency disease. N Engl J Med 1975;293:424–428.
39. Pahwa RN, Pahwa SG, Good RA. T-lymphocyte differentiation in vitro in severe combined immunodeficiency. J Clin Invest 1979;64:1632–1641.
40. Kadowaki J, Thompson RI, Zuelzer WW, et al. XX/XY lymphoid chimaerism in congenital immunological deficiency syndrome with thymic alymphoplasia. Lancet 1965;2:1152–1156.
41. O'Reilly RJ, Patterson JH, Bach FH, et al. Chimerism detected by HLA typing. Transplantation 1973;15:505–507.
42. Pollack MS, Kirkpatrick D, Kapoor N, O'Reilly RJ. Identification by HLA typing of intrauterine-derived maternal T-cells in four patients with severe combined immunodeficiency. N Engl J Med 1982;307:662–666.
43. Flomenberg N, Dupont B, O'Reilly RJ, Hayward A, Pollack MS. The use of T cell culture techniques to establish the presence of an intrauterine-derived maternal T cell graft in a patient with severe combined immunodeficiency (SCID). Transplantation 1983;36: 733–735.
44. Pollack MS, Kapoor N, Sorell M, Morishima Y, Dupont B, O'Reilly RJ. Absence of demonstrable suppressor cell activity in a severe combined immunodeficiency patient with a sustained engraftment of DR-positive maternal T cells. Transplant Proc 1981;13:270–273.
45. Barret M, Buckley RH, Schiff SE, Kidd PC, Ward FE. Accelerated development of immunity following transplantation of maternal marrow stem cells into infants with severe combined immunodeficiency and transplacentally acquired lymphoid chimerism. Clin Exp Immunol 1988;72:118–123.
46. Kenny AB, Hitzig WH. Bone marrow transplantation for severe combined immunodeficiency. Eur J Pediatr 1979;131:155–177.
47. O'Reilly RJ, Kapoor N, Kirkpatrick D, et al. Transplantation of hematopoietic cells for lethal congenital immunodeficiencies. Birth Defects 1983;19:129–137.
48. Fischer A, Friedrich W, Levinsky R, et al. Bone marrow transplantation for immunodeficiencies and osteopetrosis: European survey, 1968–1985. Lancet 1986; 2:1080–1083.
49. Griscelli C, Durandy A, Virellizier JL, Baues JJ, Daguillard F. Selective defect of precursor T cells associated with apparently normal B lymphocytes in severe combined immunodeficiency disease. J Pediatr 1978;93:404–411.
50. Bortin MM, Rimm AA. Severe combined immunodeficiency disease: characterization of the disease and results of transplantation. JAMA 1977;238:591–600.
51. Korver K, Delange GG, Van Der Bergh ER, et al. Lymphoid chimerism after allogeneic bone marrow transplantation. Transplantation 1987;44:643–650.
52. Leggiadro RJ, Winkelstein JA, Hughes WT. Prevalence of *Pneumocystis carinii* pneumonitis in severe combined immunodeficiency. J Pediatr 1981;99:96–98.
53. Hall CB, McBride JT, Walsh EE, et al. Aerosolized ribavirin treatment of infants with respiratory syncitial viral infection: a randomized double-blind study. N Engl J Med 1983;308:1443–1447.
54. Emanuel D, Cunningham I, Jules-Elysea K, et al.

Cytomegalovirus pneumonia after bone marrow transplantation successfully treated with the combination of ganciclovir and high dose intravenous immune globulin. Ann Intern Med 1988;109:777–782.
55. Durandy A, Dumez Y, Guy-Grand D, Oury C, Henrion R, Griscelli C. Prenatal diagnosis of severe combined immunodeficiency. J Pediatr 1982;101:995–997.
56. Linch DC, Rodeck CH, Simmonds HA, Levinsky RJ. Prenatal diagnosis for severe combined immunodeficiency. Birth Defects 1983;19:121–123.
57. Hirschhorn R, Beratis N, Rosen FS, Parkman R, Stern R, Polmar S. Adenosine deaminase deficiency in a child diagnosed prenatally. Lancet 1975;1:73–75.
58. Dooley R, Fairbanks LD, Simmonds HA, et al. First trimester diagnosis of adenosine deaminase deficiency. Prenat Diagn 1987;7:561–565.
59. Goodship J. Lau YL, Malcolm S, Pembrey ME, Levinsky RJ. Use of X chromosome inactivation to establish carrier status for X-linked severe combined immunodeficiency. Lancet 1988;1:729–732.
60. South MA, Dolen J, Beach DK, et al. Fatal adenovirus hepatic necrosis in severe combined immunodeficiency. Pediatr Infect Dis 1982;23:416–419.
61. Edwards JE, Lehrer RI, Stiehm ER, et al. Severe candidial infections: clinical perspective, immune defense mechanisms, and current concepts of therapy. Ann Intern Med 1978;89:91–106.
62. Carlgren LE, Hansson CG, Henricsson L, et al. BCG infection in an infant with congenital, lymphocytopenic aggamaglobulinemia. ACTA Pediatr Scand 1966;55:636.
63. Feigin RD, Guggenheim MA, Johnson SD. Vaccine-related paralytic poliomyelitis in an immunodeficient child. J Pediatr 1971;79:642–647.
64. Biggar WD, Park BY, Good RA. Compatible bone marrow transplant and immunologic reconstitution of combined immunodeficiency disease. Birth Defects 1975;11:385–390.
65. Junker AK, Chan KJ, Massing BG. Clinical and immune recovery from Omenn's syndrome after bone marrow transplantation. J Pediatr 1989;114:596–600.
66. Levinsky RJ, Tiedman K. Successful bone-marrow transplantation for reticular dysgenesis. Lancet 1983; 1:671–673.
67. Dupont B, O'Reilly RJ, Pollack MS, Good RA. Use of genotypically different donors in bone marrow transplantation. Transplant Proc 1979;11:219–224.
68. Klein J, Park JM. Graft-versus-host reaction across different regions of the H-2 complex of the mouse. J Exp Med 1973;137:1213–1225.
69. Beatty PG, Clift RA, Michelson EM, et al. Marrow transplantation from related donors other than HLA-identical siblings. N Engl J Med 1985;313:765–771.
70. Storb R, Deeg HJ, Whitehead J, et al. Methotrexate and cyclosporine compared with cyclosporine alone for prophylaxis of acute graft versus host disease after marrow transplantation for leukemia. N Engl J Med 1986;314:729–735.
71. Cavalli N, Sforza LL, Bodmer WF. The genetics of human populations. San Francisco: Freeman and Company, 1971.
72. L'Esperance P, Hansen JA, O'Reilly RJ, et al. Bone marrow donor selection among unrelated four-locus identical individuals. Transplant Proc 1975;7:823–833.
73. Duqesnoy RJ, Zevvi A, Marrari M, et al. Bone marrow transplantation for severe aplastic anemia using a phenotypically HLA identical SB-compatible unrelated donor. Transplantation 1983;35:566–569.
74. Hansen JA, Clift RA, Thomas ED, et al. Transplantation of marrow from an unrelated donor to a patient with acute leukemia. N Engl J Med 1980;303:565–570.
75. McCullough J, Hansen JA, Sororcek D, Bertsch G. The national marrow donor program: how it works, accomplishments to date. Oncology 1989;3:63–72.
76. Sonnenberg FA, Eckman MH, Pauker SG. Bone marrow donor registries: the relation between registry size and the probability of finding complete and partial matches. Blood 1989;74:2569–2573.
77. Kernan NA, Bartsch G, Ash RC, et al. Analysis of 462 transplantations from unrelated donors facilitated by the National Marrow Donor Program. N Engl J Med 1993;328:593–602.
78. Beatty PG, Hansen JA, Longton GM, et al. Marrow transplantation from HLA matched unrelated donors from treatment of hematologic malignancies. Transplantation 1991;51:443–448.
79. Filipovich AH, Shapiro RS, Ramsay NKC, et al. Unrelated donor bone marrow transplantation for correction of lethal congenital immunodeficiencies. Blood 1992; 80:270–276.
80. Niewisch H, Hajdik I, Sultanian I, Vogel H, Matioli G. Hemopoietic stem distribution in tissues of fetal and new born mice. J Cell Physiol 1970;76:107–116.
81. Moore MAS, McNeill TA, Haskill JS. Density distribution analysis of in vivo and in vitro colony forming cells in developing fetal liver. J Cell Physiol 1970;75:181–192.
82. Jenkinson EJ, Owen JJT, Aspinall R. Lymphocyte differentiation and major histocompatibility complex antigen expression in the embryonic thymus. Nature 1980;284:177–179.
83. Uphoff D. Preclusion of secondary phase of irradiation syndrome by inoculation of fetal hematopoietic tissue following lethal total body X-irradiation. J Natl Cancer Inst 1958;20:625–632.
84. Yunis EJ, Good RA, Smith J, Stutman O. Protection of lethally irradiated mice by spleen cells from neonatally thymectomized mice. PNAS 1974;71:2544–2548.
85. Thomas DB, Yaffey JM. Human fetal hematopoiesis II: hepatic hematopoiesis. Br J Haematol 1964;10:193–197.
86. August CS, Berkel AI, Driscoll S, Merier E. Onset of lymphocyte function in the developing human fetus. Pediatr Res 1971;5:539–547.
87. Kay HEM, Doe J, Hockley A. Response of human foetal thymocytes to phytohaemagglutinin (PHA). Immunology 1970;18:393–396.
88. Carr MC, Stites DP, Fudenberg HH. Dissociation or responses to phytohaemagglutinin and adult allogeneic lymphocytes in human foetal lymphoid tissues. Nature 1973;241:279–281.
89. Pirofsky B, Davies GH, Ramirez-Mateos JC, Newton BW. Cellular immune competence in the human fetus. Cell Immunol 1973;6:324–323.
90. Asantila T, Sorvari T, Hirvonen T, Toivanen P. Xenogeneic reactivity of human fetal lymphocytes. J Immunol 1973;111:984–987.
91. O'Reilly RJ, Kapoor N, Kirkpatrick D. Fetal tissue transplants for severe combined immunodeficiency: their limitations and functional potential. In: Seligman M, Hitzig WH, eds. Primary immunodeficiencies. Amsterdam: Elsevier/North Holland Biomedical Press, 1980:419.
92. Buckley RH, Whisnant JK, Schiff RI, Gilbertson RB, Huang AT, Platt MS. Correction of severe combined

immunodeficiency by fetal liver cells. N Engl J Med 1976;294:1076–1081.
93. Keightly RG, Lawton AA, Cooper M. Successful fetal liver transplantation in a child with severe combined immunodeficiency. Lancet 1975;2:850–853.
94. O'Reilly RJ, Pollack MS, Kapoor N, et al. Fetal liver transplantation in man and animals. In: Gale RP, ed. Recent advances in bone marrow transplantation. New York: Alan R. Liss, 1983:799–830.
95. Saltzstein EC, Bortin MM, Rimm AA. Long lived canine allogeneic radiation chimera produced with combined fetal liver and thymus cells. Proc Soc Exp Biol Med 1974;18:461–463.
96. Lowenberg B. Fetal liver transplantation. Holland: Radiobiologic Institute/Rijswyk, 1976:56–88.
97. Touraine JL, Laplace S, Rezzoug F, et al. The place of fetal liver transplantation in the treatment of inborn errors of metabolism. J Inherited Metab Dis 1991; 14:619–626.
98. Zinkernagel RM, Althage A, Callahan G, Welsh RM. On the immunocompetence of H-2 incompatible irradiation bone marrow chimeras. J Immunol 1980;124: 2356–2365.
99. Roncarolo MG, Yssel H, Touraine JL, et al. Antigen recognition by MHC-incompatible cells of a human mismatched chimera. J Exp Med 1988;168:2139–2152.
100. Touraine JL. Bone marrow and fetal liver transplantation in immunodeficiencies and inborn errors of metabolism: lack of significant restriction of T cell function in long term chimeras despite HLA match. Immunol Rev 198;71:103–120.
101. Roncarolo MG, Touraine JL, Banchereau J. Cooperation between major histocompatibility complex mismatched mononuclear cells from a human chimera in the production of antigen-specific antibody. J Clin Invest 1986;77:673–680.
102. Singer A, Hathcock KS, Hodes RJ. Self recognition in allogeneic radiation bone marrow chimeras: a radiation-resistant host element dictates the self specificity and immune response phenotype of T-helper cells. J Exp Med 1981;153:1286–1301.
103. Zinkernagel RM, Ruedi E, Althage A, Hengartner H, Reimann G. Thymic selection of H-2-incompatible bone marrow cells in SCID mice. J Exp Med 1988;168:1187–1192.
104. O'Reilly RJ, Keever CA, Small TN, Brochstein J. The use of HLA-non-identical T-cell-depleted marrow transplants for correction of severe combined immunodeficiency disease. Immunodef Rev 1989;1:273–309.
105. von Boehmer H, Sprent J, Nabholz M. Tolerance to histocompatibility determinants in tetraparental bone marrow chimeras. J Exp Med 1975;141:322–334.
106. Onoe K, Fernandez G, Good RA. Humoral and cell-mediated immune responses in fully allogeneic bone marrow chimera in mice. J Exp Med 1980;151:115–132.
107. Muller-Rochholtz W, Wottge HU, Muller-Hermerlink HK. Bone marrow transplantation in rats across strong histocompatibility barriers by selective elimination of lymphoid cells in donor marrow. Transplant Proc 1976;8:537–541.
108. Reisner Y, Itsicovitch L, Meshorer A, Sharon N. Hematopoietic stem cell transplantation using mouse bone marrow and spleen cells fractionated by lectins. PNAS 1978;75:2933–2936.
109. Reisner Y, Kapoor N, Kirkpatrick D, et al. Transplantation for severe combined immunodeficiency with HLA-A.B.D. Dr incompatible parental marrow fractionated by soybean agglutinin and sheep red blood cells. Blood 1983;61:341–348.
110. O'Reilly RJ, Kapoor N, Kirkpatrick D, et al. Transplantation for severe combined immunodeficiency using histoincompatible parental marrow fractionated by soybean agglutinin and sheep red blood cells: experience in six consecutive cases. Transplant Proc 1983; 17:455–459.
111. Reinherz E, Geha R, Rappeport JM, et al. Reconstitution after transplantation with T-lymphocyte-depleted HLA haplotype-mismatched bone marrow for severe combined immunodeficiency. PNAS 1982;79:6047–6051.
112. O'Reilly RJ, Brochstein J, Collins N, et al. Evaluation of HLA-haplotype disparate parental marrow grafts depleted of T lymphocytes by differential agglutination with a soybean lectin and E-rosette depletion for the treatment of severe combined immunodeficiency. Vox Sang 1986;51:81–86.
113. Friedrich W, Goldmann SF, Ebell W, Blutters-Sawatzki R. Severe combined immunodeficiency: treatment by bone marrow transplantation in 15 infants using HLA-haploidentical donors. Eur J Pediatr 1985;144:125–130.
114. Blütters-Sawatzki R, Friedrich W, Ebell W, et al. HLA-haploidentical bone marrow transplantation in three infants with adenosine deaminase deficiency: stable immunological reconstitution and reversal of skeletal abnormalities. Eur J Pediatr 1989;149:104–109.
115. Buckley RH, Schiff SE, Sampson HA, et al. Development of immunity in human severe primary T-cell deficiency following haploidentical bone marrow stem cell transplantation. J Immunol 1986;136:2398–2407.
116. Cowan MJ, Wara DW, Weintrub PS, Pabst H, Ammann A. Haploidentical bone marrow transplantation for severe combined immunodeficiency disease using soybean agglutinin-negative, T-depleted marrow grafts. J Clin Immunol 1985;5:370–376.
117. Levinsky RJ, Morgan G, Davies C, et al. Mismatched bone marrow transplantation for severe combined immunodeficiency: the Great Ormond Street experience. In: Griscelli C, Vossen J, eds. Progress in immunodeficiency research and therapy. Amsterdam: Elsevier Science Publishers, 1984:393–399.
118. Filipovitch AH, Ramsay NKC, McGlave P, et al. Mismatched bone marrow transplantation at the University of Minnesota: use of related donors other than HLA MLC identical siblings and T-cell depletion. In: Gale RP, ed. Recent advances in bone marrow transplantation. New York: Alan R. Liss, 1983:769–783.
119. Gotoh YI, Yamaguciti Y, Minegishi M, et al. Deficiency of NK activity and HNK-1^+ cells after transplantation of fetal thymus and liver or haploidentical soybean agglutinin treated marrow cells in two severe combined immunodeficiency patients. Clin Exp Immunol 1985;61:608–613.
120. Kapoor N, Jung LKL, Engelhard D, et al. Lymphoma in a patient with severe combined immunodeficiency with adenosine deaminase deficiency, following unsustained engraftment of histoincompatible T-cell depleted bone marrow. J Pediatr 1986;100:435–438.
121. Fischer A, Durandy A, De Villartay JP, et al. HLA-haploidentical bone marrow transplantation for severe combined immunodeficiency using E-rosette fractionation and cyclosporine. Blood 1986;67:444–449.

122. Ritz, J. Use of monoclonal antibodies in autologous and allogeneic bone marrow transplantation. Clin Hematol 1983;12:813–832.
123. Shearer WT, Ritz J, Finegold MJ, et al. Epstein-Barr virus-associated B-cell proliferations of diverse clonal origins after bone marrow transplantation in a 12-year-old patient with severe combined immunodeficiency. N Engl J Med 1985;312:1151–1159.
124. Hayward AR, Murphy S, Githens J, Troup G, Ambruso D. Failure of a pan-reactive anti-T cell antibody, OKT3, to prevent graft versus host disease in severe combined immunodeficiency. J Pediatr 1982;100:665–668.
125. Trigg ME, Billing R, Sondel PM, et al. Clinical trial depleting T lymphocytes from donor marrow for matched and mismatched allogeneic bone marrow transplants. Cancer Treat Rep 1985;69:377–386.
126. Moen RC, Horowitz SD, Sondel PM, et al. Immunologic reconstitution after haploidentical bone marrow transplantation for immune deficiency disorders: treatment of bone marrow cells with monoclonal antibody CT-2 and complement. Blood 1987;70:664–669.
127. Morgan G, Linen DC, Knott LT, et al. Successful haploidentical mismatched bone marrow transplantation in severe combined immunodeficiency: T-cell removal using CAMPATH-1 monoclonal antibody and E-rosetting. Br J Haematol 1986;62:421–430.
128. Frame J, Collins NH, Cartagena T, et al. T-cell depletion of human bone marrow: comparison of CAMPATH-1[a] plus complement, anti-T cell ricin A chain immunotoxin and soybean agglutinin alone or in combination with sheep erythrocytes or immunomagnetic beads. Bone Marrow Transplant 1993 (in press).
129. Kernan NA, Flomenberg N, Collins NH, O'Reilly RJ, DuPont B. Quantitation of T-lymphocytes in human bone marrow by a limiting dilution assay. Transplantation 1985;40:317–322.
130. O'Reilly RJ, Kernan NA, Cunningham I, et al. Allogeneic transplants depleted of T-cells by soybean lectin agglutination and E rosette depletion. Bone Marrow Transplant 1988;3:3–6.
131. Hale G, Cobbold S, Waldmann H. T cell depletion with CAMPATH-1 in allogeneic bone marrow transplantation. Transplantation 1988;45:753–759.
132. O'Reilly RJ, Kirkpatrick D, Kapoor N, et al. A comparative review of the results of transplants of fully allogeneic fetal liver and HLA-haplotype mismatched, T-cell depleted marrow in the treatment of severe combined immunodeficiency. In: Gale RP, Touraine JL, Lucarelli G, eds. Fetal liver transplantation. New York: Alan R. Liss, 1985:327–342.
133. Geha RS, Reinherz E. Identification of circulating maternal T and B lymphocytes in uncomplicated severe immunodeficiency by HLA typing of subpopulations of T-cells separated by the fluorescence-activated cell sorter and of Epstein-Barr virus-derived B cell lines. J Immunol 1983;130:2493–2495.
134. Flomenberg N, DuPont B, O'Reilly RJ, Hayward A, Pollack MS. The use of T-cell culture techniques to establish the presence of an intrauterine-derived maternal T cell graft in a patient with severe combined immunodeficiency (SCID). Transplantation 1983;36: 733–735.
135. Burzy MS, Magenis E, Tomar D. Bone marrow transplantation for severe combined immune deficiency in an infant with chimerism due to intrauterine-derived maternal lymphocytes: donor engraftment documented by chromosomal marker studies. Am J Med Genet 1984;18:527–539.
136. Le Deist F, Raffoux C, Griscelli C, Fischer A. Graft vs. graft reaction resulting in the elimination of maternal cells in a SCID patient with maternofetal GvHD after an HLA identical bone marrow transplantation. J Immunol 1987;138:423–427.
137. Barrett M, Buckley RH, Schiff SE, Kidd PC, Ward FE. Accelerated development of immunity following transplantation of maternal marrow stem cells into infants with severe combined immunodeficiency and transplacentally required lymphoid chimerism. Clin Exp Immunol 1988;72:118–123.
138. Cudkowicz G, Bennett M. Peculiar immunobiology of bone marrow allografts. II: rejection of parental grafts by resistant F_1 hybrid mice. J Exp Med 1971;134:1513–1528.
139. Keissling R, Hochman PS, Haller O, Shearer GM, Wigzell H, Cudkowicz G. Evidence for a similar or common mechanism for natural killer cell activity and resistance to hemopoietic grafts. Eur J Immunol 1977;7:655–663.
140. Murphy WJ, Kumar V, Bennett M. Rejection of bone marrow allografts by mice with severe combined immune deficiency (SCID). J Exp Med 1987;165:1212–1217.
141. Petranyi GG, Kiessling R, Klein G. Genetic control of "natural killer" lymphocytes in the mouse. Immunogenetics 1975;2:53–61.
142. Daley JP, Nakamura I. Natural resistance of lethally irradiated F_1 hybrid mice to parental marrow grafts is a function of H-2, H-h restricted effectors. J Exp Med 1984;159:1132–1148.
143. Ciccone E, Pende D, Viale O, et al. Evidence of a natural killer (NK) cell repertoire for (allo) antigen recognition: Definition of five distinct NK-determined allospecificities in humans. J Exp Med 1992;175:709–718.
144. O'Reilly RJ, Brochstein J, Kernan NA, et al. HLAA, B, D disparate, SBA-E marrow grafts for severe combined immunodeficiency disease (SCID). Blood 1988; 72:399a.
145. Peter HH, Kliche A, Drager R, et al. NK-cell function in severe combined immunodeficiency (SCID): possible relevance for classification and prognosis. In: Vossen J, Griscelli C, eds. Progress in immunodeficiency research and therapy II. Amsterdam: Elsevier Science Publishers, 1986:287–295.
146. Wijnaendts L, Le Deist C, Griscelli C, Fischer A. Development of immunologic functions after bone marrow transplantation in 33 patients with severe combined immunodeficiency. Blood 1989;74:2211–2219.
147. Small TN, Keever CA, O'Reilly RJ, Flomenberg N. Presence of circulating CD3+ T-cells expressing the gamma-delta T-cell receptor following HLA-mismatched T-cell depleted BMT for severe combined immunodeficiency. Blood 1988;72:408A.
148. Polmar SH, Schacter BZ, Sorensen RV. Long-term immunological reconstitution by peripheral blood leukocytes in severe combined immune deficiency disease: implications for the role of mature lymphocytes in histocompatible bone marrow transplantation. Clin Exp Immunol 1986;64:518–525.
149. Rich KC, Richman CM, Mejias E, Daddona P. Immunoreconstitution by peripheral blood leukocytes in adenosine deaminase deficient severe combined immunodeficiency. J Clin Invest 1980;66:389–395.

150. Lum LG, Seigneuret MC, Storb R. The transfer of antigen specific immunity from marrow donors to marrow recipients. J Clin Immunol 1986;6:389–396.
151. Burzy MS, Schulte-Wisserman H, Gilbert E, Horowitz SD, Pellet J, Hong R. Thymic morphology in immunodeficiency diseases: results of thymic biopsies. Clin Immunol Immunopathol 1979;12:31–51.
152. Iwata T, Incefy GS, Good RA, et al. Circulating thymic hormone levels in severe combined immunodeficiency. Clin Exp Immunol 1983;53:1–9.
153. Incefy GS, Flomenberg N, Small T, et al. Evidence of thymulin in plasma follows lymphoid chimerism and precedes development of immunity in patients with lethal combined immunodeficiency transplanted with T-cell depleted haploidentical marrow. Transplantation 1990;50:55–61.
154. Hong R, Horowitz S, Moen R, et al. Thymus and B cell reconstitution in severe combined immunodeficiency after transplantation of monoclonal antibody depleted parental mismatched bone marrow. Bone Marrow Transplant 1987;1:405–409.
155. Wimperis JZ, Berry NJ, Prentice HG, Lever A, Griffiths PD, Brenner MK. Regeneration of humoral immunity to Herpes simplex virus following T cell depleted allogeneic bone marrow transplantation. J Med Virol 1987;23:93–99.
156. Small TN, Gardner S, Weiner-Fedus S, O'Reilly RJ, Flomenberg NF. In vitro cytokine production and responsiveness following T-cell depleted haplo-identical bone marrow transplantation for severe combined immunodeficiency disease (SCID). Blood 1991; 78:248a.
157. Katz DH, Skidmore BJ, Katz LR, Bogowitz CA. Adaptive differentiation of murine lymphocytes. I: both T and B lymphocytes differentiating in F_1 parental chimeras manifest preferential cooperative activity for parmer lymphocytes derived from the same parental type corresponding to the chimeric host. J Exp Med 1978;148:727–745.
158. Bevan M, Fink P. The influence of thymus H-2 antigens on the specificity of maturing killer and helper cells. Immunol Rev 2978;42:3–19.
159. Ron Y, Lo D, Sprent J. T cell specificity in twice irradiated F_1 parent bone marrow chimeras: failure to detect a role for immigrant marrow-derived cells in imprinting intrathymic H-2 restriction. J Immunol 1986;137:1764–1771.
160. Zinkernagel RM. Selection of restriction specificities of virus-specific cytotoxic T cells in the thymus: no evidence for a crucial role of antigen-presenting cells. J Exp Med 1982;156:1842–1847.
161. Longo DL, Schwartz RH. T-cell specificity for H-2 and Ir gene phenotype correlates with the phenotype of thymic antigen-presenting cells. Nature 1980;287: 44–46.
162. Roberts JL, Volkman DJ, Buckley RH. Modified MHC restriction of donor-origin T cells in human severe combined immunodeficiency transplanted with haploidentical bone marrow stem cells. J Immunol 1989;143:1575–1579.
163. Chu E, Umetsu D, Rosen F, Geha RS. Major histocompatibility restriction of antigen recognition by T-cells in a recipient of haplotype mismatched human bone marrow transplantation. J Clin Invest 1983;72:1124–1129.
164. Geha RS, Rosen FS. The evolution of major histocompatibility complex (MHC) restrictions in antigen recognition by T-cells in a haploidentical bone marrow transplant recipient. J Immunol 1989;143:84–89.
165. Guillet JG, Lai MZ, Briner TJ, et al. Immunological self, non-self discrimination. Science 1987;235:865–870.
166. Buus S, Sutte A, Colon SM, Miles C, Grey HM. The relation between major histocompatibility complex (MHC) restriction and the capacity of Ia to bind immunogenic peptides. Science 1987;235:1353–1358.
167. Kernan NA, Collins NH, Juliano L, Cartagena T, DuPont B, O'Reilly RJ. Cloneable T lymphocytes in T-cell depleted bone marrow transplants correlate with development of graft- versus-host disease. Blood 1986;68:770–773.
168. Keever CA, Flomenberg N, Brochstein J, et al. Tolerance of engrafted donor T-cells following bone marrow transplantation for severe combined immunodeficiency. Clin Immunol Immunopathol 1988;48:261–276.
169. De Villartay JP, Griscelli C, Fischer A. Self tolerance to host and donor following HLA-mismatched bone marrow transplantation. Eur J Immunol 1986;16:117–122.
170. Schiff SE, Buckley RH. Modified responses to recipient and donor B-cells by genetically donor T cells from human haploidentical bone marrow chimeras. J Immunol 1987;138:2088–2094.
171. Rosenkrantz K, Keever C, Kirsch J, et al. In vitro correlates of graft-host tolerance after HLA-matched and mismatched marrow transplants: suggestions from limiting dilution analysis. Transplant Proc 1987;19:98–103.
172. Rosenkrantz K, Keever C, Bhimani K, et al. Both ongoing suppression and clonal elimination contribute to graft-host tolerance following transplantation of HLA mismatched T-cell depleted marrow for severe combined immunodeficiency. J Immunol 1990;144: 1721–1728.
173. von Boehmer H, Hafen K. Minor but not major histocompatibility antigens of thymic epithelium tolerize precursors of cytolytic T cells. Nature 1986; 320:626–628.
174. Lo D, Sprent J. Identity of cells that imprint H-2 restricted T cell specificity in the thymus. Nature 1986;319:672–675.
175. O'Reilly RJ, Keever C, Kernan NA, et al. Investigation of humoral immune deficiencies following T cell-depleted, HLA-haplotype mismatched parental marrow transplants for the treatment of severe combined immunodeficiency. In: Eibl MM, Rosen FS, eds. Primary immunodeficiency diseases. Amsterdam: Elsevier Science Publishers, 1986:301–307.
176. Small TN, Keever CA, Dupont T, Collins NH, O'Reilly RJ, Flomenberg N. Phenotypic and functional characterization of B cells from patients with severe combined immunodefiency disease. Hum Immunol 1989; 25:181–193.
177. Small TN, Keever CA, Weiner-Fedus S, Heller G, O'Reilly RJ, Flomenberg N. B cell differentiation following autologous, conventional, or T-cell depleted bone marrow transplantation: a recapitulation of normal B cell ontogeny. Blood 1990;76:1647–1656.
178. Pahwa S, Pahwa RN, Good RA. Heterogeneity of B lymphocyte differentiation in severe combined immunodeficiency disease. J Clin Invest 1980;66:543–550.
179. Korver K, DeLange GG, van Den Bergh RL, et al. Lymphoid chimerism after allogeneic bone marrow transplantation. Transplantation 1987;44:643–650.

180. Vossen JM, Asma GEM, van Den Bergh RL, et al. HLA-identical and haploidentical bone marrow transplantation for severe combined immunodeficiency: chimerism and immunological reconstitution in vitro and in vivo. In: Griscelli G, Vossens J, eds. Progress in immunodeficiency research and therapy I. Amsterdam: Elsevier Science Publishers, 1984:417–424.
181. Geha RS. Is the B-cell abnormality secondary to T-cell abnormality in severe combined immunodeficiency? Clin Immunol Immunopathol 1976;6:102–106.
182. Vossen JM, De Koning J, van Bekkum DW, et al. Successful treatment of an infant with severe combined immunodeficiency by transplantation of bone marrow cells from an uncle. Clin Exp Immunol 1973;13:9–20.
183. Hurtenbach V, Shearer GM. Analysis of murine T lymphocyte markers during the early phases of GvH-associated suppression of cytotoxic T-lymphocyte responses. J Immunol 1983;130:1561–1566.
184. Morgab G, Strobel S, Levinsky RJ. Immune dysregulation following bone marrow transplantation for severe combined immunodeficiency. In: Vossen J, Griscelli C, eds. Progress in immunodeficiency research and therapy II. Amsterdam: Excerpta Medica, 1986:359–364.
185. Martin PJ, Shulman HM, Schubach WH, et al. Fatal Epstein-Barr virus-association proliferation of donor B cells after treatment of acute graft-versus-host disease with a murine anti-T cell antibody. Ann Intern Med 1984;101:310–315.
186. Trigg ME, Billing R, Sondel PM, et al. Clinical trial depleting T lymphocytes from donor marrow for matched and mismatched allogeneic bone marrow transplants. Cancer Treat Rep 1985;69:377–386.
187. Lymphoma in a patient with severe combined immunodeficiency with adenosine deaminase deficiency, following unsustained engraftment of histoincompatible T-cell-depleted bone marrow. J Pediatr 1986;108:435–438.
188. Spector BD, Perry GS, Kersey JH. Genetically determined immunodeficiency diseases (GDID) and malignancy: report from the immunodeficiency cancer registry. Clin Immunol Immunopathol 1978;11:12–29.
189. De Fazio SR, Criswell BS, Kimzey SL, South MA, Montgomery JR. A paraprotein in severe combined immunodeficiency disease detected by immunoelectrophoretic analysis of plasma. Clin Exp Immunol 1975;19:563–570.
190. De Koning J, Van Bekkum DW, Dicke KA, Dooren LJ, Van Rood JJ, Raol J. Transplantation of bone marrow cells and fetal thymus in an infant with lymphopenic immunological deficiency. Lancet 1969;1:1223–1227.
191. Ghory P, Schiff S, Buckley R. Appearance of multiple benign paraproteins during early engraftment of soy lectin T-cell depleted haploidentical bone marrow cells in severe combined immunodeficiency. J Clin Immunol 1986;6:161–169.
192. Datta AK, Colby BM, Shaw JE, Pagano JS. Acyclovir inhibition of Epstein-Barr virus replication. PNAS 1980;77:5163–5166.
193. Lin JC, Smith MC, Pagano JS. Comparative efficacy and selectivity of some nucleoside analogs against Epstein-Barr virus. Antimicrob Agents Chemother 1985;27:971–973.
194. Hanto DW, Frizszera G, Gajl-Peczalska KJ, et al. Acyclovir therapy of Epstein-Barr virus (EBV)-induced post-transplant lymphoproliferative diseases. Transplant Proc 1985;17:89–92.
195. Sullivan JL, Medveczky P, Forman SJ, Baker SM, Monroe C. Epstein-Barr virus induced lymphoproliferation. N Engl J Med 1984;311:1163–1167.
196. Moen RC, Horowitz SD, Sondel PM, et al. Immunologic reconstitution after haploidentical bone marrow transplantation for immune deficiency disorders: treatment of bone marrow cells with monoclonal antibody CT-2 and complement. Blood 1987;70:664–669.
197. Fischer A, Blanche S, Le Bidois J, et al. Anti-B-cell monoclonal antibodies in the treatment of severe B-cell lymphoproliferative syndrome following bone marrow and organ transplantation. N Engl J Med 1991;324:1451–1456.
198. Fischer A, Friedrich W, Fasth A, et al. Reduction of graft failure by a monoclonal antibody (anti-LFA-1 CD11a) after HLA nonidentical bone marrow transplantation in children with immunodeficiencies, osteopetrosis, and Fanconi's anemia: a European Group for Immunodeficiency/European Group for Bone Marrow Transplantation report. Blood 1991;77:249–256.
199. Shapiro RS, Chauvenet A, McGuire W, et al. Treatment of B-cell lymphoproliferative disorders with interferon alfa and intravenous gamma globulin (letter). N Engl J Med 1988;318:1334.
200. Lawlor GJ, Ammann AJ, Wright WC, La Franchi SH, Bilstrom D, Stiehm ER. The syndrome of cellular immunodeficiency with immunoglobulins (type Nezelof 1964). J Pediatr 1974;84:183–192.
201. Chu E, Rosenwasser LH, Dinareud CA, Rosen FS, Gena RS. Immunodeficiency with defective T-cell response to interleukin-1. PNAS 1984;81:4945–4949.
202. Chatila T, Castigli E, Pahwa R, et al. Primary combined immunodeficiency resulting from defective transcription of multiple T-cell lymphokine genes. PNAS 1990;87:10033–10037.
203. Disanto JP, Keever CA, Small TN, Nichols GL, O'Reilly RJ, Flomenberg N. Absence of interleukin-2 production if a severe combined immunodeficiency disease syndrome with T-cells. J Exp Med 1990;171:1697–1704.
204. Weinberg K, Parkman R. Severe combined immunodeficiency due to a specific defect in the production of IL-2. N Engl J Med 1990;322:1718–1723.
205. Weinberg KI, Parr T, Annett GM, et al. Severe combined immunodeficiency (SCID) due to defective interleukin-2 receptor alpha (IL-2R alpha). Pediatr Res 1989;170a.
206. Markert ML. Purine nucleoside phosphorylase deficiency. Immunodeficiency Rev 1991;3:45–81.
207. Touraine JL, Betuel H, Souillet G, Jeune M. Combined immunodeficiency disease associated with absence of cell surface HLA-A and B antigens. J Pediatr 1978; 93:47–51.
208. Hadam MR, Dupfer R, Peter HH, Niethammer D. Congenital agammaglublinemia associated with lack of expression of HLA-D-region antigens. In: Griscelli C, Vossen J, eds. Progress in immunodeficiency research and therapy. Amsterdam: Excerpta Medica, 1984:43–50.
209. Roifman CM, Hummel D, Martinez-Valdez H, et al. Depletion of CD8+ cells in human thymic medulla results in selective immune deficiency. J Exp Med 1989;170:2177–2182.
210. Businco L, Rossi P, Paganelli R, et al. Immunologic reconstitution with bone marrow transplantation and thymic hormones in two patients with severe pure T-cell defects. Birth Defects 1983;19:281–285.

211. Ash RC, Casper JT, Chitambar CR, et al. Successful allogeneic transplantation of T-cell depleted bone marrow from closely HLA-matched unrelated donors. N Engl J Med 1990;322:486–494.
212. Aldrich RA, Steinberg AGI, Campbell DC. Pedigree demonstrating a sex-linked recessive condition characterized by draining ears, eczematous dermatitis and bloody diarrhea. Pediatrics 1954;13:133–138.
213. Wolff JA. Wiskott-Aldrich syndrome: clinical, immunologic and pathologic observations. J Pediatr 1967; 70:221–232.
214. Cooper MD, Chase HP, Lowman JT, Krivit W, Good RA. The Wiskott-Aldrich syndrome: an immunologic deficiency disease involving the afferent limb of immunity. Am J Med 1968;44:499–513.
215. Blaese RM, Strober W, Brown RS, Waldmann TA. The Wiskott-Aldrich syndrome: a disorder with possible defect in antigen processing or recognition. Lancet 1968;1:1056–1061.
216. Ochs HD, Slicher SJ, Harker LA, Von Behrens WE, Clark RA, Wedgewood RJ. The Wiskott-Aldrich syndrome: studies of lymphocytes, granulocytes and platelets. Blood 1980;55:243–252.
217. Nahm MH, Blaese RM, Crain MJ, Briles DE. Patients with Wiskott-Aldrich syndrome have normal IIgG2 levels. J Immunol 1991;137:3484–3487.
218. Parkman R, Remold-O'Donnell E, Kenney DM, Perrine S, Rosen FS. Surface protein abnormalities in lymphocytes and platelets from patients with Wiskott-Aldrich syndrome. Lancet 1981;2:1387–1388.
219. Remold-O'Donnell E, Kenney DM, Parkman R, Cairns L, Savage B, Rosen FS. Characterization of a human lymphocyte surface sialoglycoprotein that is defective in Wiskott-Aldrich syndrome. J Exp Med 1984;159: 1705–1710.
220. Remold-O'Donnell E, Zimmerman C, Kenney D, Rosen FS. Expression on blood cells of sialophorin, the surface glycoprotein that is defective in Wiskott-Aldrich syndrome. Blood 1987;70:104–109.
221. Pallant AA, Eskenazi MG, Mattei REK, et al. Characterization of cDNAs encoding human leukosialin and localization of the leukosialin gene to chromosome 16. PNAS 1989;86:328–331.
222. Shelley CS, Remold-O'Donnel E, Davis III AE, et al. Molecular characterizations of sialophorin (CD43), the lymphocyte surface sialoglycoprotein defective in Wiskott-Aldrich syndrome. PNAS 1989;86:819–822.
223. Greer WL, Peacocke M, Siminovitch KA. The Wiskott-Aldrich syndrome: refinement of the localization on Xp and identification of another closely linked marker locus, OATL1. Hum Genet 1992;88:453–456.
224. Puck JM, Siminovitch KA, Poncz M, Greenberg CR, Rottem M, Conley ME. Atypical presentation of Wiskott-Aldrich syndrome: diagnosis in two unrelated males based on studies of maternal T cell X chromosome inactivation. Blood 1990;75:2369–2374.
225. Rosenstein Y, Park JK, Hahn WC, Rosen FS, Bierer BE, Burakoff SJ. CD43, a molecule defective in Wiskott-Aldrich syndrome, binds ICAM-1 (letter to the editor). Nature 1991;354:233–235.
226. Springer TA, Dustin ML, Kishimoto TK, Martin SD. The lymphocyte function associated with LFA-1, CD2, and LFA-3 molecules: cell adhesion receptors of the immune system. Ann Rev Immunol 1987;5:223–252.
227. Diamond MS, Staunton DE, de Fougerolles AR, et al. ICAM-1 (CD54): a counter-receptor for Mac1 (CD11b/CD18). J Cell Biol 1990;111:3129–3139.
228. Axelsson B, Youseffi-Etemad R, Hammarstrom S, Perlmann P. Induction of aggregation and enhancement of proliferation and IL-2 secretion in human T cells by antibodies to CD43. J Immunol 1988; 141:2912–2917.
229. Park JK, Rosenstein YJ, Remold-O'Donnell E, Bierer BE, Rosen FS, Burakoff SJ. Enhancement of T-cell activation by the CD43 molecule whose expression is defective in Wiskott-Aldrich syndrome. Nature 1991; 350:706–709.
230. Greer WL, Higgins E, Sutherland DR, et al. Altered expression of leucocyte sialoglycoprotein in Wiskott-Aldrich syndrome is associated with a specific defect in *O*-glycosylation. Cell Biol Biochem 1989;67:503–509.
231. Higgins EA, Siminovitch KA, Zhuang D, Brockhausen I, Dennist JW. Abberant *O*-linked oligosaccharide biosynthesis in lymphocytes and platelets from patients with the Wiskott-Aldrich syndrome. J Biol Chem 1991;266:6280–6290.
232. Piller F, LeDeist F, Weinberg KI, Parkman R, Fukuda M. Altered *O*-glycan synthesis in lymphoctyes from patients with Wiskott-Aldrich syndrome. J Exp Med 1991;173:1501–1510.
233. O'Reilly RJ, Brochstein J, Dinsmore R, Kirkpatrick D. Marrow transplantation for congenital disorders. Semin Hematol 1984;21:188–221.
234. Rimm IJ, Rappeport JM. Bone marrow transplantation for the Wiskott-Aldrich syndrome: long-term follow-up. Transplantation 1990;50:617–620.
235. Brochstein JA, Gillio AP, Ruggiero M, et al. Marrow transplantation from human leukocyte antigen-identical or haploidentical donors for correction of Wiskott-Aldrich syndrome. J Pediatr 1991;119–907.
236. Buckley RH. Advances in the correction of immunodeficiency by bone marrow transplantation. Pediatr Ann 1987:16:412–421.
237. Rumelhart SL, Trigg ME, Horowitz SD, Hong R. Monoclonal antibody T-cell-depleted HLA-haploidentical bone marrow transplantation for Wiskott-Aldrich syndrome. Blood 1990;75:1031–1035.
238. Blaese RM. Progress toward gene therapy. Clin Immunol Immunopathol 1991;61:547–555.
239. Touraine JL. *In utero* transplantation of fetal liver stem cells in humans. Blood Cells 1991;17:379–387.

Chapter 65
Bone Marrow Transplantation for Osteopetrosis

Peter F. Coccia

Osteopetrosis is a rare inherited disorder characterized by generalized skeletal sclerosis that occurs in various mammals including humans (1,2). Osteopetrosis is a result of the dysfunction of osteoclasts, the multinucleated giant cells that resorb bone and mineralized cartilage (3,4). The osteoclast is a specialized macrophage derived from the bone marrow stem cell (4,5). Some variants of osteopetrosis in laboratory animals and humans can be corrected by bone marrow transplantation (BMT) (1,6).

Osteopetrosis in Humans

Historically, two major forms of osteopetrosis have been described. The benign or "adult" form is usually inherited in an autosomal dominant pattern and is associated with minimal disability and a normal life expectancy. The malignant or "infantile" form is inherited in an autosomal recessive pattern and has widespread systemic manifestations. However, both forms have been found to be heterogeneous, and other specific variants have been described.

The adult-benign autosomal dominant form was first described by the German radiologist Albers-Schönberg in 1904 (7) by radiographic demonstration of the characteristic dense, radiopaque bones (Albers-Schönberg syndrome or marble bone disease). Diagnosis is usually made by radiographic demonstration of diffuse skeletal sclerosis. Most patients are asymptomatic and have a normal life expectancy. Minimal disability has been reported, secondary to an increased susceptibility to fractures, and occasionally bone pain, osteomyelitis of the mandible, and cranial-nerve palsies (8). This autosomal dominant form has been reviewed recently, and 2 distinct types have been described based on clinical, radiological, and biochemical criteria (9,10).

A number of variants with autosomal recessive inheritance have also been described. A syndrome of mild osteopetrosis with renal tubular acidosis and cerebral calcification characterized by a profound deficiency of carbonic anhydrase isoenzyme II has been reported in 12 families (11). Another variant of interest is a rare syndrome of severe osteopetrosis with parathyroid hormone resistance and induction of bone resorption after administration of bovine parathyroid hormone (12). Other variants continue to be described (13), but further discussions in this chapter will be confined to the infantile malignant variant.

Infantile Malignant Osteopetrosis

The classic form of infantile malignant osteopetrosis is characterized by autosomal recessive inheritance and is almost always diagnosed in early infancy (14,15). The inability to resorb and remodel bone due to osteoclast dysfunction, in the presence of normal bone formation by osteoblasts, results in deposition of excessive mineralized osteoid and cartilage (16). All bones are uniformly dense, sclerotic, and radiopaque. Medullary cavities are absent on long bone radiographs (17). Bone biopsy reveals encroachment of medullary cavities by bone and mineralized cartilage, thick trabeculae, and decreased medullary spaces. The residual medullary cavities are occupied with large numbers of nonfunctional osteoclasts and there is usually increased marrow fibrosis (15,18–20). Osteoclasts are reported to be normal in size in some patients (18,19) and increased in size in others; the large osteoclasts have increased numbers of nuclei (18,20). Electron microscopy of osteoclasts has been reported to demonstrate normal ruffled borders at the bone junction in some patients examined (18,20,21) and complete absence of ruffled borders in others (18–21).

Encroachment of marrow spaces leads to extramedullary hematopoiesis, progressive hepatosplenomegaly, and hypersplenism. The result is anemia with reticulocytosis, leukoerythroblastosis, and thrombocytopenia.

Encroachment of cranial-nerve foramina leads to retinal atrophy, which progresses to blindness (22), auditory nerve damage, and oculomotor and facial nerve palsies (23). Defective bone resorption also leads to progressive macrocephaly, frontal bossing, hypertelorism, exophthalmos, and other craniofacial abnormalities. Hydrocephalus, ventricular enlargement, increased intracranial pressure, cerebral vascular occlusive complications, and seizures are also reported (8,23,24). Nasal stuffiness is a common presenting symptom that is secondary to progressive narrowing and obstruction of nasal airways (14). Excessive tearing may occur secondary to nasolacrimal duct stenosis

(25). Other reported complications are osteomyelitis of the mandible and the maxilla, retarded tooth eruption, and rampant caries.

Sclerotic bones are brittle, and pathological fractures occur frequently. Linear growth is retarded and dwarfism has been reported in survivors to the second decade.

Infections are common in children with infantile malignant osteopetrosis. A variety of subtle defects in neutrophil and monocyte function as well as a decrease in natural killer cell function have been reported (6,15,26–28). Included are defects in phagocytosis (6), decreased intracellular killing (6,26), abnormal nitroblue tetrazolium reduction by both neutrophils and monocytes (27,28), and decreased response to stimuli of neutrophil activation (28).

Children become progressively severely debilitated, and, until recently, survival beyond the first decade was not reported. Infection, bleeding, and severe anemia are the usual reported causes of death. Improvements in supportive care, antibiotics, and ready availability of blood components have prolonged survival in recent years.

The Osteoclast and Bone Resorption

There is an extensive amount of literature concerning the origin, structure, and function of the osteoclast and its role in bone resorption (1,3,4,29,30). A brief overview is provided to clarify issues important to an understanding of the pathophysiology of osteopetrosis and the role of BMT in its correction.

The cell of origin of the osteoclast is the pluripotent hematopoietic stem cell. The monoblast is likely the committed progenitor cell of origin of the osteoclast, as well as the circulating monocyte, the tissue macrophage, and the foreign body giant cell. Osteoclasts are thought to form from repeated fusions of these mononuclear precursors, which migrate to skeletal sites via vascular pathways. Bone-resorbing osteoclasts have from one to more than 20 nuclei.

Degradation (2,29) of collagenous bone matrix and bone mineral complexes requires activation of the osteoclast. Activation involves elaboration of cytoplasmic infoldings of the plasma membrane next to the bone surface, which is known as the ruffled border. Once the ruffled border is formed, plasma and lysosomal membranes fuse and lysosomal contents, including carbonic anhydrase isoenzyme II and acid hydrolases, are released to the extracellular space. Matrix and mineral are digested and the products of resorption are then endocytosed for additional intracellular processing. Bone resorption is confined to a small area of osteoclast-bone interface by a circumferential seal of the plasma membrane, which is defined as the clear zone.

Differentiation, maturation, fusion, activation, and function are controlled by various lymphokines, monokines, and hormones, including macrophage colony stimulating factor (M-CSF), interleukins, osteoclast-activating factor, parathyroid hormone, 1,25-dihydroxyvitamin D, calcitonin, prostaglandins, and glucocorticoids.

Osteopetrotic Mutations in Animal Models

Congenital osteopetrosis is a well-known mutation in a variety of mammalian species, including mouse, rat, and rabbit (1,2,31). There are 8 well-studied animal mutations (Table 65-1). In all variants, the mode of inheritance is autosomal recessive. All variants demonstrate osteoclast hypofunction, generalized skeletal sclerosis, absent or poorly developed marrow cavities,

Table 65-1.
Mammalian Osteopetrosis

Mutation	*Symbol*	*Osteoclasts*[a] *Number*	*Size*	*Ruffled Borders*	*Survival*	*Effective Treatment*
Mouse						
Grey-lethal	gl/gl	↓	↓	+	Lethal	BMT
Microphthalmia	mi/mi	N	↓↓	−	Normal	BMT
Osteosclerosis	oc/oc	↑	↓	−	Lethal	None
Osteopetrosis	op/op	↓↓	↓	+	Normal	M-CSF
Rat						
Incisorsabsent	ia/ia	↑↑	N	−	Normal	BMT
Osteopetrosis	op/op	↓	↑	+	Lethal	BMT
Toothless	tl/tl	↓↓↓	↓	−	Reduced	M-CSF
Rabbit						
Osteopetrosis	os/os	↓	↓	−	Lethal	None
Humans						
Infantile malignant		↑↑	N, ↑	±	Lethal	BMT

[a]Increases or decreases with respect to normal littermates/control subjects are indicated by *arrows*.
N = same as normal littermate/control. Presence or absence of ruffled borders is indicated by + or −, respectively.
Modified, expanded and updated from the reports of Marks SC Jr (1,2). Bibliography available upon request.
BMT = bone marrow transplantation; M-CSF = macrophage colony stimulating factor.

reduced size of osseous foramina, defective bone modeling and remodeling, and weak bone susceptible to pathological fracture. All mutants are resistant to the hypercalcemic effects of parathyroid hormone and 1,25-dihydroxyvitamin D; all have increased blood levels of 1,25-dihydroxyvitamin D. All of these characteristics are associated with the infantile malignant form seen in young children.

The major differences among the variants described in the current literature have been compiled (1,2). Included are remarkable differences in osteoclast numbers, from virtually absent in the tl/tl rat to significant hyperplasia in the ia/ia rat and humans; differences in osteoclast size from primarily mononuclear forms in the mi/mi mouse to very large (many nuclei) in the op/op rat; and differences in the appearance of the ruffled border at the osteoclast-bone interface from absent to normal in the various mutants. Disease severity as measured by survival past infancy and known effective treatment are detailed in Table 65-1.

Bone Marrow Transplantation

In a series of elegant experiments, Walker (32,33) demonstrated that osteopetrosis can be cured in the gl/gl and mi/mi mouse strains by either temporary parabiosis or stem-cell transplantation. Infusions of marrow or spleen cells from normal littermates into lethally irradiated osteopetrotic mice resulted in complete correction of osteopetrosis and normal survival. Conversely, infusion of spleen cells from osteopetrotic mice to lethally irradiated normal littermates led to the development of osteopetrosis. Similar experiments have demonstrated complete correction after BMT in the ia/ia (34) and op/op (35) rat mutations.

Correction or induction of osteopetrosis in these 4 strains by transplantation of stem cells suggest defects intrinsic to the osteoclast progenitor or the osteoclast itself. Studies in the mi/mi mouse, which demonstrate that the bone-resorbing osteoclasts are of donor origin after transplantation, support this viewpoint (36,37). Beige mice, which have giant lysosomes in their hematopoietic cells, were used as stem-cell donors for transplants into irradiated mi/mi mice. After transplantation, giant lysosomes were present in the functional osteoclasts of the recipients. In most reported studies, the preparative regimen utilized has been a single fraction of total body irradiation (TBI) of 600 cGy delivered by a Cobalt-60 source for recipient osteopetrotic mutants and 900 cGy for recipient normal littermates, considered to be the marrow lethal dose for each group. Marrow or spleen cells at 10 to 50 $\times$ 10^6 nucleated cells/animal were given intravenously or intraperitoneally 2 hours later. Donors were highly inbred littermates, full engraftment was routine, and graft-versus-host disease (GVHD) was not reported.

In the other 4 mutants, BMT is unable to correct osteopetrosis, and spleen cells from normal littermates do not transmit osteopetrosis. These observations suggest that the defects in these mutants are not intrinsic to the osteoclast progenitor or the osteoclast. Recent reports described the cure of osteopetrosis in both the op/op mouse (38,39) and the tl/tl rat (40) with infusions of recombinant human M-CSF. Both mutants appear to be severely deficient in M-CSF and have markedly decreased numbers of monocytes, macrophages, and osteoclasts. In the op/op mouse, a mutation involving the insertion of a single base pair in the coding region of the M-CSF gene has been described (41). No effective therapy has been reported for the lethal mutations in the oc/oc mouse and the os/os rabbit (2).

An additional observation has been reported. Targeted disruption (deletion) of the *c-src* proto-oncogene in transgenic mice produces an autosomal recessively inherited osteopetrotic mutation (42,43). It has also been shown that *c-src* is a tyrosine kinase present in high levels in osteoclasts that is critical to osteoclast function but not osteoclast development (44,45). Mutant mice have abundant osteoclasts that lack ruffled borders and fail to remodel bone. Furthermore, the mice develop osteopetrotic skeletal changes (43,45).

Treatment of Infantile Malignant Osteopetrosis

Historically, treatment of infantile malignant osteopetrosis consisted of supportive care measures and attempts to control mineral intake. Anemia and thrombocytopenia were treated with transfusions and occasionally splenectomy (46). Dietary manipulations to reduce calcium intake, increase phosphate intake, or both, were employed in an attempt to mobilize bone calcium without success. Attempts to induce bone resorption with infusions of parathyroid hormone, vitamin D, and calcitonin were also unsuccessful. Treatment with corticosteroids results in decreased hepatosplenomegaly, decreased leukoerythroblastosis, increased hemoglobin and platelet counts, and decreased need for transfusion. However, there is no significant effect on the underlying process, and patients deteriorate when corticosteroids are discontinued (47). Treatment with corticosteroids and a low calcium, high phosphate diet has been reported to ameliorate symptoms and to improve bone density in 4 infants (48), but this observation has not been confirmed by other investigators.

Bone Marrow Transplantation

Reports of successful correction of osteopetrosis in mouse and rat mutants in the mid 1970s by BMT led to attempts to utilize allogeneic BMT to treat children with infantile malignant osteopetrosis. In the past 15 years, numerous reports have appeared in the literature concerning BMT for osteopetrosis. Certainly, the published material under-represents the number of transplants performed, because investigators tend not to publish their failures.

In 1977, Ballet and colleagues (49,50) reported the first BMT for osteopetrosis. A 3-month-old infant girl was transplanted without immunosuppression with marrow from a human leukocyte antigen (HLA)–identical 2-year-old sister. Although durable engraftment was not demonstrated, radiological and other evidence for significant bone resorption was present. O'Reilly and associates (51) speculated that extended short-term engraftment may have occurred because the patient and her donor were part of a highly inbred family. These investigators also reported 3 other children given transplants without immunosuppression from less well-matched donors. None of the recipients showed evidence of engraftment or clinical improvement (50).

In 1980, Coccia and co-workers (6) reported a 5-month-old girl transplanted from her HLA-identical, mixed leukocyte culture (MLC)–compatible brother after preparation with cyclophosphamide (CY) (200 mg/kg) and modified TBI (400 cGy with head and lung shielding). Engraftment was documented by chromosomal analysis. Anemia, thrombocytopenia, leukoerythroblastosis, and metabolic abnormalities were corrected within 12 weeks of BMT. Comparison of bone biopsies before BMT and 13 weeks after BMT showed complete correction (Figure 65-1). Serial radiographs revealed bony remodeling and new nonsclerotic bone formation (Figure 65-2). Fluorescent Y-body analysis after BMT demonstrated that the nuclei were of donor origin (male) in osteoclasts (Figure 65-3) but remained of recipient origin (female) in osteoblasts. Subsequent follow-up showed progressive loss of the graft (16). Dense new bone formation can be appreciated on the last 3 panels of Figure 65-2, but with preservation of marrow cavities. Since 18 months after BMT, no male karyotypes have been detected in peripheral blood or marrow cells. The patient is now more than 14 years after transplantation. Bones are extremely sclerotic and she is short, but no other evidence of osteopetrosis remains. She sees and hears, development and intelligence are normal, she is an excellent student, and she is pubertal. She has no hepatosplenomegaly, and blood counts and chemistries are normal. In this child, it appears that once marrow cavities and foramina were remodeled, the correction was permanent despite sclerotic new bone formation.

Our BMT group subsequently transplanted 3 additional infants. The first, utilizing an unrelated donor, died 10 days after BMT of overwhelming sepsis without evidence of engraftment. The other 2 patients, both girls, were transplanted after preparation with

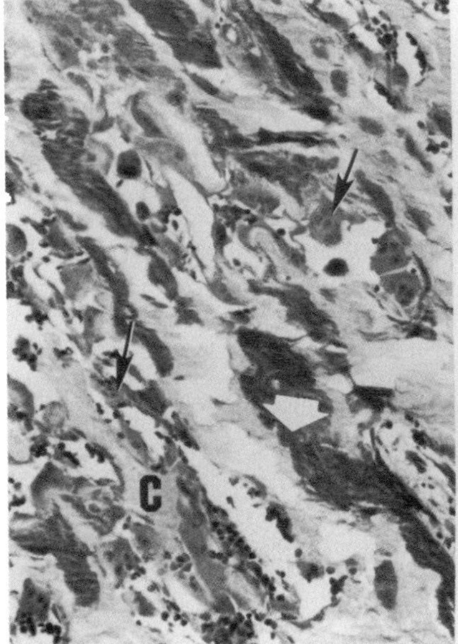

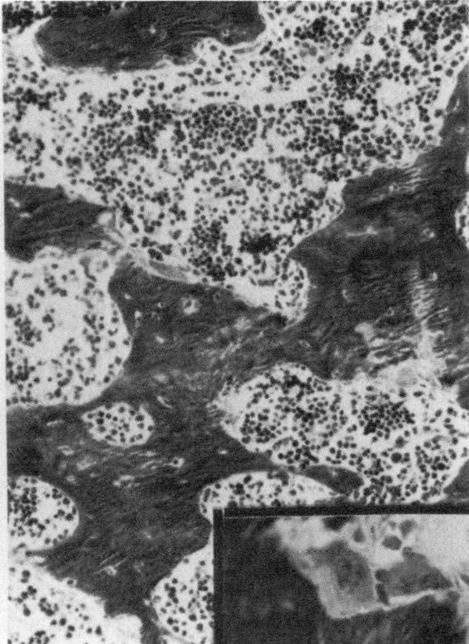

Figure 65-1. Bone histology before bone marrow transplantation (BMT) (left) and 13 weeks after BMT (right). The biopsy specimen studied before BMT had the characteristic features of osteopetrosis. The trabecular matrix mass was markedly increased and composed of mineralized cartilage (C) as well as bone (*white arrow*). Numerous nonresorbing osteoclasts (*black arrows*) were present in the residual marrow space and contained few hematopoietic precursors (undecalcified; modified Masson X100). The biopsy specimen obtained 13 weeks after BMT showed virtual normalization of the bone and marrow. The trabecular matrix mass was markedly reduced and there were few residual cartilaginous bars. The marrow space contained abundant, normal hematopoietic precursors, and the osteoclasts, the number of which was markedly reduced, were actively resorbing bone, as evidenced by their presence in resorption bays (*insert*). (Undecalcified, modified Masson, X100; insert, X450, before 30% reduction.) (Reprinted, by permission of The New England Journal of Medicine, from Coccia PF, Krivit W, Cervenka J, et al. Successful bone marrow transplantation for infantile malignant osteopetrosis. N Engl J Med 1980;302:701–708.)

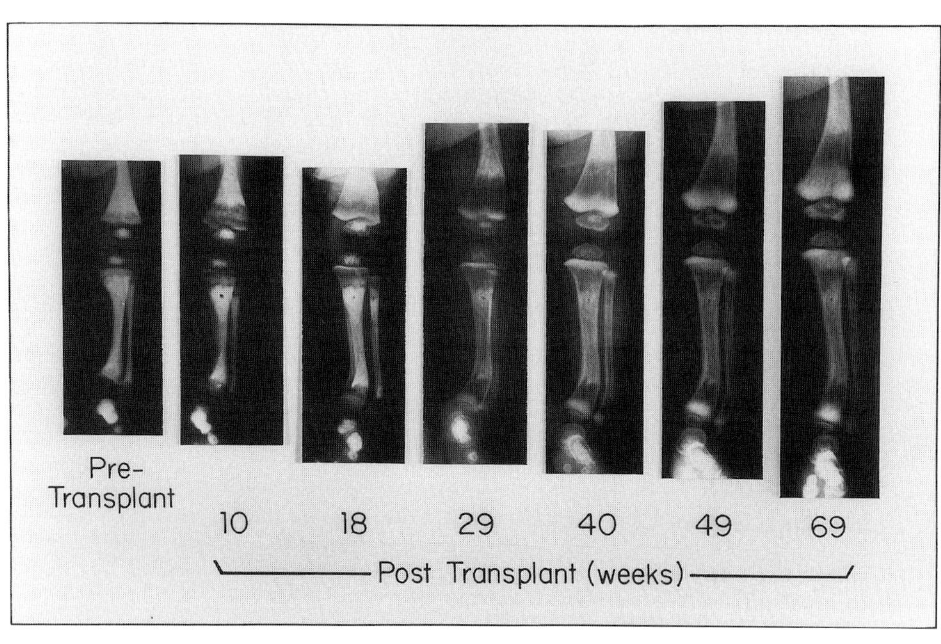

Figure 65-2. Representative radiographs of the left leg obtained before bone marrow transplantation (BMT) and 10 to 69 weeks after BMT. Before BMT, the bones were very dense. The fraying of the ends of the long bones is typical of rachitic change. Ten weeks after transplantation, metaphyseal and periosteal remodeling and new bone formation of nearly normal density were seen. The rachitic changes were resolving, and the provisional zone of calcification was reestablished. At 18 and 29 weeks, there was a marked increase in the thickness of normal-appearing new bone as a result of longitudinal and appositional growth. Metaphyses and epiphyses had a normal appearance, and no evidence of rickets was seen. Dense remnants of the original bone were seen within the normal-appearing new bone. At 40, 49, and 69 weeks, new bone formation is again of increased density, suggesting recurrence of the osteopetrotic process. Marrow cavities have not been replaced by dense bone. The small round hole seen in the proximal tibia within the dense remnant of original bone is at the site of a trephine needle biopsy performed 6 weeks after BMT.

busulfan (BU) (16 mg/kg), CY (200 mg/kg), and 1,000 cGy splenic irradiation given as daily 200-cGy fractions (52). Marrow from parental donors without T-cell depletion was used. In the second patient, a one HLA-B antigen–mismatched mother, and in the third patient, a phenotypically identical father, were donors. Both patients engrafted promptly and are fully chimeric, with complete correction of all manifestations of osteopetrosis. Both patients had severe optic atrophy before transplantation and remain blind. Severe acute and chronic GVHD developed in one child (Patient 2), which slowly responded to therapy. The other child has not had GVHD. They are now 5 and 9 years after transplantation, and both have normal development and intelligence.

Sorell and colleagues (26) and O'Reilly and associates (51) reported 3 children, one with transient engraftment, one with complete correction, and one with partial correction. Both engrafted children have durable mixed chimerism. Detailed case reports (53–56) describe an additional 5 patients successfully engrafted from HLA-matched siblings in 2, and mismatched relatives in 3. Three patients (53,55) have shown complete correction. The fourth patient (54) received a T-cell–depleted transplant, demonstrated sustained engraftment and correction of osteopetrosis, but died of an *Aspergillus* brain abscess 9 months after BMT. The fifth patient (56) was transplanted from a phenotypically identical maternal grandfather who was subsequently proven to be the child's father.

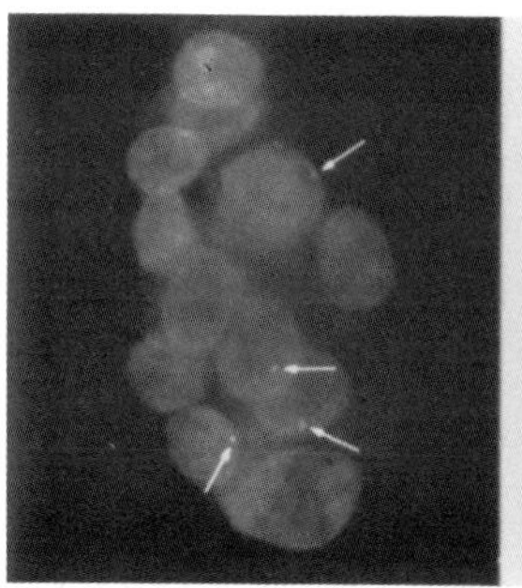
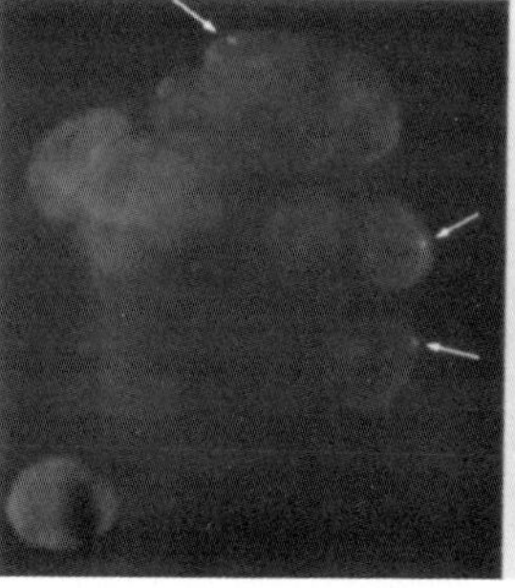
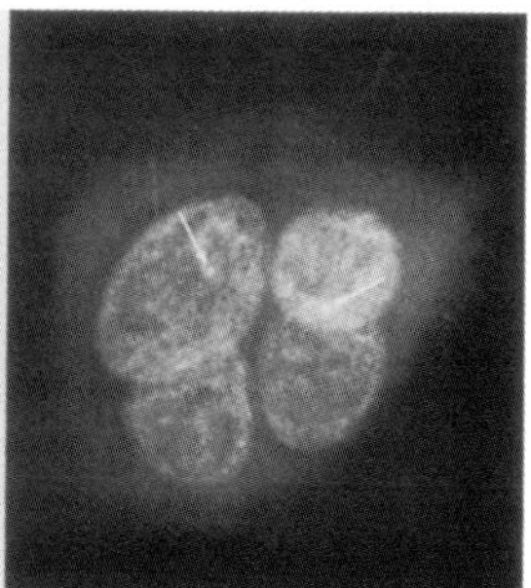

Figure 65-3. Osteoclasts with fluorescent Y bodies after bone marrow transplantation (BMT). The osteoclasts were stained with quinacrine dihydrochloride. *Arrows* indicate the Y bodies in nuclei that are seen in this focal plane (fluorescence microscopy, X 1,000, before 30% reduction; right panel enlarged for clarity). Reprinted, by permission of The New England Journal of Medicine, from Coccia PF, Krivit W, Cervenka J, et al. Successful bone marrow transplantation for infantile malignant osteopetrosis. N Engl J Med 1980;302:701–708.

Restriction fragment length polymorphism analysis demonstrated mixed chimerism and slow progressive loss of the graft and recurrence of osteopetrotic bone formation, but correction of other manifestations of osteopetrosis, similar to the previously described case (6,16).

Fischer and co-workers (57,58) summarized the European experience with BMT for osteopetrosis to 1990. Six of 9 patients (57) with HLA-identical donors have shown complete correction of bone lesions and hematopoietic abnormalities. Two of 6 have persistent neurosensory defects. Eight of 17 patients (58) with T-cell–depleted HLA-nonidentical donors are alive and engrafted 9 to 56 months after transplantation. Most have mixed chimerism and all are well. Five of 8 are reported to have full correction of their disease, whereas 3 of 8 are reported as having partial correction. Nine patients died: 5 with no engraftment, 2 with sepsis, and 2 with interstitial pneumonitis.

Twenty-seven patients have been registered with the International Bone Marrow Transplantation Registry who underwent BMT for osteopetrosis between 1978 and 1990. Some representative patients are cited above. The group includes 17 boys and 10 girls. Thirteen had matched sibling donors and 14 had mismatched related donors. Preliminary analysis reveals 15 of 27 are alive, with disease status reported as cured or improved in all.

Transplantation Issues

In general, BMT for osteopetrosis is similar to BMT for other nonmalignant inherited disorders detailed in this book. However, there are certain unique issues that must be understood for better analysis of the data and improvement of outcome.

Pretransplant Evaluation

The typical infant with osteopetrosis will present with anemia and thrombocytopenia. Transfusion may be necessary, and red cell and platelet survival may be short secondary to hypersplenism. A course of corticosteroid therapy may stabilize the patient hematologically and reduce transfusion requirements (47). Some patients will present with, or develop, severe bone pain, progressive debilitation, and poor oral intake, requiring narcotic analgesics and hyperalimentation. Evaluation for optic atrophy, including funduscopic examination, visual evoked-response electroencephalograms, and optic foramina imaging, should be completed quickly because early optic nerve decompression may preserve vision (22). Baseline evaluation of calcium/phosphorus homeostasis, alkaline and acid phosphatase levels, and parathyroid hormone studies (12) should be obtained. Imaging studies should include long bone radiographs (17), measurements of liver and spleen size, and cranial computed tomography scans (24). In addition, magnetic resonance imaging (59), radionucleotide marrow scans, and bone densitometry may be useful to assess sites of hematopoiesis and to quantitate bone resorption and development of marrow cavities.

An open wedge bone biopsy from the iliac crest should be obtained and processed for routine histology and transmission electron microscopy (18–21). Light microscopic analysis of osteoclast number, size, nucleation, and morphology should be performed. Marrow cellularity and the degree of myelofibrosis should be determined. Quantitative histomorphometry may be useful (19–21). Electron microscopic analysis for the presence, size, and frequency of ruffled borders, clear zones, and alkaline phosphatase activity at the membrane-matrix interface should be evaluated (18–21). Routine determination of these parameters is extremely important both to provide further clues to the etiology and heterogeneity of human osteopetrosis and as a baseline indicator of BMT outcome.

It has been reported and frequently cited that patients with either advanced marrow fibrosis (60) or markedly increased marrow osteoclasts (i.e., "hyperosteoclastic state" [20,21]) have more severe disease and poor response to BMT due to poor engraftment. Caution must be exercised in interpreting these data. The type (open wedge versus trephine needle), location, depth, and quality of the biopsy all influence interpretation. Also, biopsies in infants tend to have more osteoclasts and less fibrosis than in older children, in whom massive marrow accumulation of bone and cartilage tends to obliterate marrow spaces (20).

The experience of our BMT group does not support this pessimistic view. The first patient we transplanted (6,18) had markedly increased marrow osteoclasts (see Figure 65-1) and minimal fibrosis. She engrafted promptly, and all longitudinal and oppositional new bone formation was of normal density, but a sclerotic core of original bone persisted (see Figure 65-2). The next patient successfully transplanted (52) had small densely fibrotic marrow cavities with a minimal increase in osteoclasts. She also engrafted promptly, but new bone formation was of the same density as the original bone. Her long bones gradually decreased in density over 4 to 6 months, and no sclerotic core was seen. Normal marrow cavities were appreciated only when the overall bone density was normal. The third child had moderate fibrosis and increased numbers of large abnormal-appearing osteoclasts. She engrafted promptly. New bone formation was of normal density, and the dense core of original bone progressively decreased in density to normal over a few months.

Donor Selection

An HLA-matched nonaffected sibling is the preferred donor. If a matched sibling is unavailable, it is likely that a matched or minimally mismatched family donor can be identified due to the high incidence of parental consanguinity. Obligate heterozygote relatives are suitable donors. Because progression of the disease is relatively slow, unrelated donor search and transplantation are reasonable options.

Leukoerythroblastosis makes interpretation of mixed lymphocyte culture results difficult due to high autologous proliferation. Isolation of recipient mononuclear cells may allow for interpretation (52). However, new molecular techniques for determination of HLA-D-region identity can be performed with small numbers of nucleated cells and obviate the need for mixed lymphocyte culture studies (see Chapter 4).

Preparative Regimens and Engraftment

Most reported patients have been prepared with BU at either 2 mg/kg/day for 4 days (51,55) or 4 mg/kg/day for 4 days (53,56–58) followed by CY at 50 mg/kg/day for 4 days. Engraftment was prompt, with the development of hematopoietic mixed chimerism in most children. Failure of engraftment has been reported only with mismatched, T-cell–depleted grafts. Late graft failure has been reported in at least 3 well-studied patients (6,26,56). Hepatosplenomegaly dramatically regresses after high-dose therapy but redevelops with engraftment, probably as a temporary site of extramedullary hematopoieses. When marrow cavities develop, the spleen again regresses. In one patient, liver and spleen size were maximal 12 weeks after BMT but were normal in size 22 weeks after BMT, with concomitant appearance of medullary cavities in long bones on radiographs (6). The addition of splenic irradiation to BU/CY in these 2 patients with mismatched donors resulted in sustained full hematopoietic chimerism.

Post-transplant Evaluations and Complications

Serial re-evaluations to document engraftment and bone resorption are valuable to assess efficacy of therapy. An open bone biopsy 3 to 6 months after BMT is valuable to assess osteoclast function.

The only unusual complication after BMT referable to osteopetrosis is hypercalcemia. A 30-month-old boy (Gluckman AE. Personal communication) received a marrow graft in 1980 from his HLA-identical sister after preparation with CY and 400 cGy modified TBI. He engrafted rapidly, and mild acute GVHD developed. The child demonstrated both histological and radiological improvement and grew 5 cm in the first 2 months after BMT. Severe hypercalcemia developed on day +60 and was refractory to saline diuresis, furosemide, corticosteroids, calcitonin, and dialysis. Death from hypercalcemia occurred on day +165. O'Reilly and associates (51) reported 2 additional cases of severe hypercalcemia in patients 120 and 15 months old at the time of BMT who responded to prolonged (6–10 weeks), intensive saline diuresis. They speculated that hypercalcemia was a problem in older patients who had massive bony deposition of calcium, which was released with rapid resorption of bone after BMT (51). The current availability of agents that selectively inhibit calcium resorption from bone should provide effective options to control this serious complication. Diphosphonate derivatives selectively inhibit osteoclast-mediated bone resorption. Side effects of concern are myelosuppression and nausea. Gallium nitrate inhibits bone resorption by the incorporation of gallium into bone mineral, which interferes with the ability of the osteoclast to acidify and solubilize bone mineral. Gallium nitrate has few side effects other than hypophosphatemia and is not myelosuppressive. Titration of these agents should allow controlled resorption of sclerotic bone without severe life-threatening hypercalcemia.

Other Therapeutic Options

No other curative therapies have been reported for infantile malignant osteopetrosis. One patient was treated with high-dose calcitriol (1,25-dihydroxyvitamin D) for 3 months while being maintained on a low calcium diet (61). Increased bone matrix and mineral turnover were demonstrated, and osteoclasts developed ruffled borders. Markedly improved monocyte resorption of bone was demonstrated in vitro, but only slight clinical improvement was demonstrated.

Eight patients with osteopetrosis have been treated with recombinant human interferon-gamma (62). Interferon-gamma increases superoxide production, which is known to be deficient in osteopetrotic patients (28). Interferon-gamma was administered 3 times a week by subcutaneous injection for 6 months. Improved bone resorption was documented biochemically, trabecular bone volume decreased on bone biopsy, osteoclasts developed ruffled borders, and radionucleotide marrow scans improved. Patients demonstrated significant increases in hemoglobin concentration and platelet counts, and transfusion requirements decreased. No changes in bone density on radiographs were reported. Although some clinical improvement was demonstrated, it appears that the underlying disease process remained unchanged.

Clinical trials utilizing M-CSF have been proposed (Wang WC. Personal communication). A recent report (63) of measurements of M-CSF in 13 patients with infantile osteopetrosis demonstrated normal to increased levels in all patients. Furthermore, in 6 patients studied, the M-CSF present was biologically active. It is unlikely that infantile osteopetrosis will respond like the M-CSF–deficient op/op mouse (38,39) and tl/tl rat (40). However, pharmacological levels of M-CSF may stimulate osteoclast function and improve bone resorption.

In patients undergoing evaluation for BMT, treatment with high-dose calcitriol (61), recombinant interferon-gamma (62), or M-CSF may be beneficial, especially if there is a delay secondary to difficulties in finding a donor. These strategies may stabilize patients, decrease transfusion requirements, and produce less side effects than a trial of corticosteroids (47) or parathyroid hormone (12).

Future Directions

It appears that allogeneic BMT remains the only curative therapy available for children with malignant osteopetrosis. Rapid and complete correction is possible even when BMT results in durable mixed chimerism. Curiously, some patients with late graft failure remain corrected aside from redevelopment of sclerotic bone formation. However, full chimerism should still be the objective even if it requires more intensive preparative regimens. All reported patients with sustained grafts were cured. The addition of splenic irradiation to BU/CY may result in full chimerism, even with less than fully matched donors, without increasing morbidity. Certainly, the donor pool for these patients should be expanded to include unrelated donors.

The etiology of infantile malignant osteopetrosis remains obscure. The finding of increased numbers of multinucleated osteoclasts in essentially all patients studied suggests the disorder is not one of stem-cell differentiation, maturation, or cell fusion. Osteoclast hyperplasia suggests a disorder of function and explains the observed increases in humoral stimulators of bone resorption. Possible etiologies include defective activation by these humoral stimulators due to an abnormal receptor on the cell surface, defective recognition of effete bone, or digestive incompetence secondary to abnormalities in intracellular enzyme systems (16). The recent observation (43) that osteopetrosis can be induced in transgenic mice by disruption of the *c-src* proto-oncogene provides encouragement that the defective gene in infantile malignant osteopetrosis in humans will soon be identified and cloned. The knowledge gained may provide direction for future therapeutic approaches, such as gene therapy.

Many lessons have been learned from studies of stem-cell transplantation of osteopetrotic mutants in animals and humans. In addition to curing the rare infant with this disorder, the knowledge gained in the area of osteoclast function and bone resorption may benefit the many patients with disorders of excessive bone resorption, such as osteoporosis, hypercalcemia of malignancy, periodontal disease, and abnormal fracture healing.

References

1. Marks SC Jr. Congenital osteopetrotic mutations as probes of the origin, structure, and function of osteoclasts. Clin Orthop 1984;189:239–263.
2. Marks SC Jr. Osteoclast biology: lessons from mammalian mutations. Am J Med Genet 1989;34:43–54.
3. Hall BK, ed. Bone, vol 2, the osteoclast. Boca Raton, FL CRC Press, 1991.
4. Mundy GR, Roodman GD. Osteoclast ontogeny and function. In: Peck W, ed. Bone and mineral research/5. New York: Elsevier Science, 1987;209–279.
5. Teitelbaum SL, Kahn AJ. Mononuclear phagocytes, osteoclasts and bone resorption. Miner Electrolyte Metab 1980;3:2–9.
6. Coccia PF, Krivit W, Cervenka J, et al. Successful bone-marrow transplantation for infantile malignant osteopetrosis. N Engl J Med 1980;302:701–708.
7. Albers-Schönberg H. Roentgenbilder einer seltenen knochener-krankung. Munch Med Wochenschr 1904;51: 365–368.
8. Johnston CC Jr, Lavy N, Lord T, Vellios F, Merritt AD, Deiss WP. Osteopetrosis: a clinical, genetic, metabolic, and morphologic study of the dominantly inherited, benign form. Medicine (Baltimore) 1968;47:149–167.
9. Bollerslev J. Autosomal dominant osteopetrosis: bone metabolism and epidemiological, clinical, and hormonal aspects. Endocr Rev 1989;10:45–67.
10. Warpole IR, Nicoll A, Goldblatt J. Autosomal dominant osteopetrosis type II with "malignant" presentation: further support for heterogeneity? Clin Genet 1990;38: 257–263.
11. Sly WS, Whyte MP, Sundaram V, et al. Carbonic anhydrase II deficiency in 12 families with the autosomal recessive syndrome of osteopetrosis with renal tubular acidosis and cerebral calcification. N Eng J Med 1985;313:139–145.
12. Glorieux F, Pettifor J, Marie P, Delvin EE, Travers R, Shephard N. Induction of bone resorption by parathyroid hormone in congenital malignant osteopetrosis. Metab Bone Dis Rel Res 1981;3:143–150.
13. Monaghan BA, Kaplan FS, August CS, Fallon MD, Flannery DB. Transient infantile osteopetrosis. J Pediatr 1991;118:252–256.
14. Loriá-Cortés R, Quesada-Calvo E, Cordero-Chaverri C. Osteopetrosis in children: a report of 26 cases. J Pediatr 1977;91:43–47.
15. Reeves J, Arnaud S, Gordon S, et al. The pathogenesis of infantile malignant osteopetrosis. Bone mineral metabolism and complications in five infants. Metab Bone Dis Rel Res 1981;3:135–142.
16. Coccia, PF. Cells that resorb bone. N Engl J Med 1984;310:456–458.
17. Kolawole TM, Hawass ND, Patel PJ, et al. Osteopetrosis; some unusual radiological features with a short review. Eur J Radiol 1988;8:89–95.
18. Teitelbaum SL, Coccia PF, Brown DM, Kahn AJ. Malignant osteopetrosis: a disease of abnormal osteoclast proliferation. Metab Bone Dis Rel Res 1981;3:99–105.
19. Helfrich MH, Aronson, DC, Everts V, et al. Morphologic features of bone in human osteopetrosis. Bone 1991;12: 411–419.
20. Shapiro F, Key LL, Anast C. Variable osteoclast appearance in human infantile osteopetrosis. Calcif Tissue Int 1988;43:67–76.
21. Cournot G, Trubert-Thil CL, Petrovic M, et al. Mineral metabolism in infants with malignant osteopetrosis: heterogeneity in plasma 1,25-dihydroxyvitamin D levels and bone histology. J Bone Mineral Res 1992;7:1–10.
22. Haines SJ, Erickson DL, Wirtschafter JD. Optic nerve decompression for osteopetrosis in early childhood. Neurosurgery 1988;23:470–475.
23. Lehman RAW, Reeves JD, Wilson WB, Wesenberg RL. Neurological complications of infantile osteopetrosis. Ann Neurol 1977;2:378–384.
24. Bartynski WS, Barnes PD, Wallman JK. Cranial CT of autosomal recessive osteopetrosis. AJNR 1989;10:543–550.
25. Orengo SD, Patrinely JR. Dacryocystorhinostomy in osteopetrosis. Ophthalmic Surg 1991;22:396–398.
26. Sorell M, Kapoor N, Kirkpatrick D, et al. Marrow transplantation for juvenile osteopetrosis. Am J Med 1981;70:1280–1287.

27. Reeves JD, August CS, Humbert JR, Weston WL. Host defense in infantile osteopetrosis. Pediatrics 1979;64: 202–206.
28. Beard CJ, Key L, Newburger PE, et al. Neutrophil defect associated with malignant infantile osteopetrosis. J Lab Clin Med 1986;108:498–505.
29. Marks SC Jr, Popoff SN. Bone cell biology: the regulation of development, structure and function in the skeleton. Am J Anat 1988;183:1–44.
30. Chambers TJ. The origin of the osteoclast. Bone Mineral Res 1989;6:1–25.
31. Marks SC, Walker DG. Mammalian osteopetrosis—a mode for studying cellular and humoral factors in bone resorption. In: Bourne GH, ed. The biochemistry and physiology of bone. New York: Academic Press, 1976: 227–301.
32. Walker DG. Bone resorption restored in osteopetrotic mice by transplants of normal bone marrow and spleen cells. Science 1975;190:784–785.
33. Walker DG. Spleen cells transmit osteopetrosis in mice. Science 1975;190:785–787.
34. Marks SC Jr. Studies of the cellular cure for osteopetrosis by transplanted cells: specificity of the cell types in *ia* rats. Am J Anat 1978;151:131–137.
35. Milhaud G, Labat ML, Graf B, et al. Démonstration cinétique, radiographique et histologique du la guérison de l'osteopetrose congenitale du rat. CR Acad Sci Paris 1975;280:2485–2488.
36. Ash P, Loutit JF, Townsend KMS. Osteoclasts derived from haematopoietic stem cells. Nature 1980;283:669–670.
37. Marks SC Jr, Walker DG. The hematogenous origin of osteoclasts: experimiental evidence from osteopetrotic (microphthalmic) mice treated with spleen cells from beige mouse donors. Am J Anat 1981;16:1–10.
38. Felix R, Cecchini MG, Fleisch H. Macrophage colony stimulating factor restores in vitro bone resorption in the *op/op* osteopetrotic mouse. Endocrinology 1990; 127:2592–2594.
39. Kodama H, Yamasaki A, Nose M, et al. Congenital osteoclast deficiency in osteopetrotic (op/op) mice is cured by injections of macrophage colony stimulating factor. J Exp Med 1991;173:269–272.
40. Marks SC Jr, Wojtowicz A, Szperl M, et al. Administration of colony stimulating factor-1 corrects some macrophage, dental, and skeletal defects in an osteopetrotic mutation (toothless, tl) in the rat. Bone 1992; 13:89–93.
41. Yoshida H, Hayashi S, Kunisada T, et al. The murine mutation osteopetrosis is in the coding region of the macrophage colony stimulating factor gene. Nature 1990;345:442–443.
42. Marks SC Jr. Congenital Osteopetrosis in mammals—new windows on osteoclast biology. In: Sabkin H, Price P, eds. Chemistry and biology of mineralized tissues. Amsterdam: Elsevier Science, 1992:475–482.
43. Soriano P, Montgomery C, Geske R, Bradley A. Targeted disruption of the c-src proto-oncogene leads to osteopetrosis in mice. Cell 1991;64:693–702.
44. Baron R, Chatterlee D, Horne W, Levy J, Lomri A, Neff L. Osteoclasts express high-levels of the c-src proto-oncogene. J Bone Mineral Res 1991;6(suppl 1):S197.
45. Kato I, Yoneda T, Izbicka E, et al. Osteoclasts deficient in c-src tyrosine kinase fail to resorb bone in vitro and in vivo. J Bone Mineral Res 1991;6(suppl 1):S197.
46. Tesluk GC, Thomas CG Jr, Benjamin JT, McMillan CW. Fatal overwhelming postsplenectomy sepsis following autologous splenic transplantation in severe congenital osteopetrosis. J Pediatr Surg 1984;19:269–272.
47. Reeves, JD, Huffer WE, August CS, Hathaway WE, Koerper M, Walters CE. The hematopoietic effects of prednisone therapy in four infants with osteopetrosis. J Pediatr 1979;94:210–214.
48. Dorantes LM, Mejia AM, Dorantes S. Juvenile osteopetrosis: effects on blood and bone of prednisone and a low calcium, high phosphate diet. Arch Dis Child 1986;61:666–670.
49. Ballet JJ, Griscelli C, Coutris C, Milhaud G, Maroteaux P. Bone marrow transplantation in osteopetrosis. Lancet 1977;2:1137.
50. Ballet JJ, Griscelli C. Lymphoid cell transplantation in human osteopetrosis. In: Horton JE, Tarpley TM, Davis WF, eds. Mechanisms of localized bone loss. Arlington, VA: Information Retrieval, 1978:399–414.
51. O'Reilly RJ, Brochstein J, Dinsmore R, Kirkpatrick D. Marrow transplantation for congenital disorders. Semin Hematol 1984;21:188–221.
52. Warkentin PI, Strandjord SE, Schacter B, et al. Successful bone marrow transplantation (BMT) for infantile malignant osteopetrosis (OP) using a mismatched parental donor. Blood 1985;66:255a.
53. Seiff CA, Levinsky R, Rogers D, et al. Allogenenic bone-marrow transplantation in infantile malignant osteopetrosis. Lancet 1983;1:437–441.
54. Orchard PJ, Dickerman JD, Mathews CHE, et al. Haploidentical bone marrow transplantation for osteopetrosis. Am J Pediatr Hematol Oncol 1987;9:335–340.
55. Kaplan FS, August CS, Fallon MD, Dalinka M, Axel L, Haddad JG. Successful treatment of infantile malignant osteopetrosis by bone-marrow transplantation. J Bone Joint Surg [Am] 1988;70:617–623.
56. Schroeder RE, Johnson FL, Silberstein MJ, et al. Longitudinal follow up of malignant osteopetrosis by skeletal radiographs and restriction fragment length polymorphism analysis after bone marrow transplantation. Pediatrics 1992;90:986–989.
57. Fischer A, Friedrich W, Levinsky R, Vossen J, Griscelli C, Kubanek B. Bone-marrow transplantation for immunodeficiencies and osteopetrosis: European Survey. Lancet 1986;1:1080–1084.
58. Fischer A, Friedrich W, Fasth A, et al. Reduction of graft failure by a monoclonal antibody (Anti-LFA-1 CD11a) after HLA nonidentical bone marrow transplantation in children with immunodeficiencies, osteopetrosis, and Fanconi's anemia: a European Group for Immunodeficiency/European Group for Bone Marrow Transplantation report. Blood 1991;77:249–256.
59. Rao VM, Dalinka MK, Mitchell DG, et al. Osteopetrosis: MR characteristics at 1.5 T^1. Radiology 1986; 161:217–220.
60. Blazar BR, Teitelbaum SL, Fallon MD, et al. Malignant osteopetrosis (OP): observations on the disease spectrum. Pediatr Res 1984;18:291A.
61. Key L, Carnes D, Cole S, et al. Treatment of congenital osteopetrosis with high-dose calcitriol. N Engl J Med 1984;310:409–415.
62. Key LL Jr, Ries WL, Rodriguiz RM, Hatcher HC. Recombinant human interferon gamma therapy for osteopetrosis. J Pediatr 1992;121:119–124.
63. Orchard PJ, Dahl N, Aukerman SL, Blazar BR, Key LL Jr. Circulating macrophage colony-stimulating factor is not reduced in malignant osteopetrosis. Exp Hematol 1992;20:103–105.

Chapter 66
Bone Marrow Transplantation for Storage Diseases

William Krivit and Elsa G. Shapiro

Enzymatic deficiency is the common characteristic of the storage diseases discussed in this chapter. The resultant failure to hydrolyze specific substrate produces an organelle dysfunction that eventually causes destruction of the involved cell. Thereafter, changes occur in specific tissues, which lead to the clinical course produced by the pathological process. The phenotypes of these diseases, although quite variable in expression, can be identified by the presence of the abnormal cellular metabolites due to the original enzymatic deficiency. Bone marrow transplantation (BMT) has changed our thinking concerning the possibility of treatment of children with these storage diseases.

Heretofore, no methods were available for sustained correction of the deficient enzymatic activity. Currently, normalization of enzymatic deficiency can be obtained following successful engraftment of allogeneic BMT. However, quantification is needed to compare risk factors associated with BMT with the measured clinical benefits derived from enzymatic correction. A prospective study of the value of BMT has been planned to provide answers. A consortium has been formed that includes 25 institutions and 100 investigators. Standard methods of analysis have been developed and disseminated to these centers. The logo of the consortium (Figure 66-1) illustrates the complex and overlapping elements to be studied.

Physiology of BMT

Treatment of storage diseases, including BMT, has the conceptual goal of providing normal enzymatic activity (1). New and normal enzymatic activity has been found in all patients who were engrafted. The level of enzymatic activity in the leukocytes is the same as that in the donor. The monocyte-phagocytic system provides the cellular machinery for this enzymatic replacement (2). The monocyte-phagocytic system consists of marrow-derived cell systems in the liver (Kupffer's cells), bone (osteoclasts), lung (pulmonary macrophages), lymph nodes (fixed and wandering histiocytes), and skin (Langerhans cells) (Figure 66-2). Transfer of enzyme from donor monocyte-phagocytic cell to recipient cell has been demonstrated in several disease states. Substrate accumulation decreases as a result of enzymatic replenishment as shown both in vitro and in vivo. Permanence of new enzyme has been noted for more than 10 years, and engraftment continues without need of continued immunosuppressive medication.

Storage Diseases

Maroteaux-Lamy Syndrome

Maroteaux-Lamy syndrome (MLS), a mucopolysaccharidosis inherited in an autosomal recessive manner, is caused by an enzymatic deficiency of arylsulfatase B (*N*-acetylgalactosamine-4-sulfatase). Hepatosplenomegaly, dysostosis multiplex with later development of pulmonary and cardiac insufficiency, delayed onset of hydrocephalus, and demise in the second or third decade of life comprise the clinical aspects. Most, but not all, patients with MLS have normal intelligence. The initial patient with storage disease undergoing BMT at the University of Minnesota had MLS (3). The

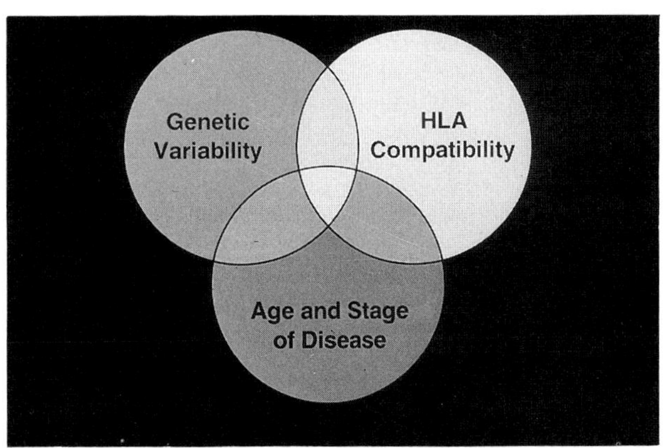

Figure 66-1. The focus of the consortium will be on those individual patients who have appropriate genetic disease qualifications as analyzed by molecular biology. The descriptive definition of stage of disease is denoted by degree of pathology present and patient accomplishments. An excellent histocompatible donor match is considered as a balance essential for providing the low mortality and morbidity risks compatible with known long-term difficulties and multisystem complications.

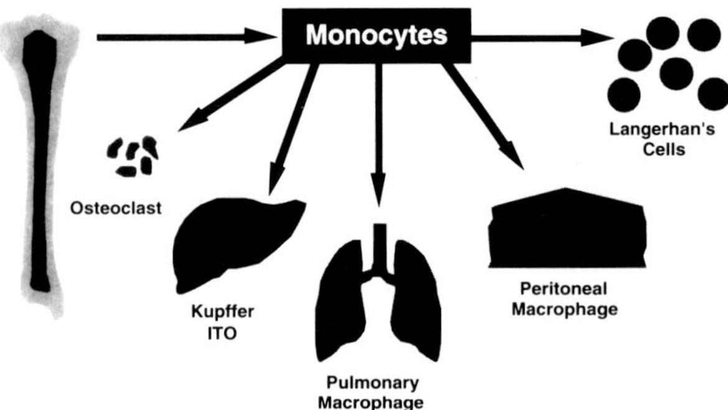

Figure 66-2. The monocyte-macrophage system from the newly derived marrow transplanted hematopoietic system involves many systems. Fibroblasts, hepatocytes, muscles, osteoblasts, and chondrocytes have different origins.

arylsulfatase B enzyme activity in the leukocytes has remained within normal levels for 10 years since BMT, and the patient recently graduated from college with Phi Beta Kappa honors. Heart failure, pulmonary hypertension, hepatosplenomegaly, and severe sleep apnea all disappeared after BMT. The facial dysmorphological aspects characteristic of mucopolysaccharidosis noted before BMT have improved. There has been no evidence of deterioration of the central nervous system (CNS), as has been reported in other patients with MLS.

Engraftment by allogeneic BMT has resulted in successful correction of the enzymatic defect in 5 other patients (4). Improvement in aspects of the visceral disease as characterized by cardiopulmonary dysfunction and hepatosplenomegaly has been noted in each patient. None of the BMT patients have had deterioration of CNS function. The normalcy of enzymatic activity and the example of our first patient would predict that the secondary problem of hydrocephalus will be prevented. Stiffness of several joints and difficulty in walking have all shown lessening of severity, although skeletal disease has not changed significantly.

The MLS gene has been cloned and inserted into deficient fibroblasts. The opportunity for gene insertion in the experimental arylsulfatase B deficient feline model is now under active investigation. Clinical application of gene insertion must be delayed until demonstration of continued gene expression in this animal model. Until then, BMT should be considered in most patients with MLS who have a histocompatible donor.

Metachromatic Leukodystrophy

Metachromatic leukodystrophy (MLD) is a demyelinating disorder of the white matter resulting from failure of degradation of sulfatide. Arylsulfatase A enzymatic activity is deficient in peripheral white cells, tissues, and fibroblasts. The clinical presentation and prognosis can be distinguished by the age of onset and are classified as late infantile, juvenile, adolescent, and adult forms (5). The late infantile form is characterized by rapid disease progressing to decerebration and death. The juvenile, adolescent, and adult forms of MLD present with a behavioral disturbance. Frequently, there is an attention deficit and problems with behavior, and then dementia becomes more prominent (6). The length of time from onset to diagnosis is frequently several years, followed by another period of years before the patient becomes decerebrate and dies.

Sulfatide loading studies on fibroblasts are capable of distinguishing between these several forms of MLD. Fibroblasts from late infantile, juvenile, adolescent, and adult forms cleave the sulfatide load in increasing amounts, respectively. Each patient should undergo fibroblast sulfatide loading studies.

Late Infantile MLD

A patient, engrafted 8 years ago at 4 years of age, has normal levels of arylsulfatase A (Figure 66-3). Neuropsychological results indicate gains in intelligence (6), and neuroelectrophysiological measurements have remained stable at the level of abnormality present at the time of transplant (7). Peripheral sensory nerve biopsies have not shown degeneration. The child now requires the use of a walker because she cannot use lower extremities for ambulation. There is cerebellar dysfunction as noted by continuous tremor, nystagmus, and truncal ataxia. Magnetic resonance imaging (MRI) studies have shown a remarkable decrease of intensity of T2-weighted signals, so that only a minimal degree of demyelination is now observed as compared with initial studies. Her sister with the same enzyme defect died at 8 years of age.

A review of 7 such patients, engrafted for at least one year, indicates disease progression despite normalization of enzymatic activity (8). BMT changed the

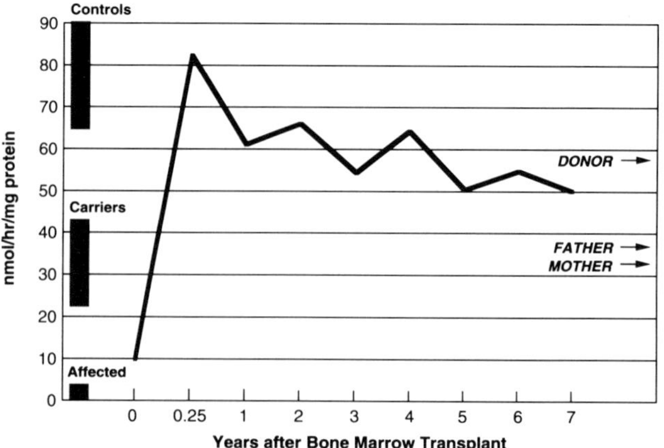

Figure 66-3. The arylsulfatase A enzyme as measured in the circulating leukocytes has continued to be in normal range for the 8 years since transplantation. The arysulfatase A enzyme was measured by Dr David Wenger.

disease pattern and prolonged the lifespan when compared with nontransplanted patients with MLD in these families and in the literature. This experience has provided a basis for considering the use of BMT for infants or younger children prior to onset of clinical MLD. Presymptomatic patients are detected on a biochemical basis after an older affected sibling has the diagnosis confirmed. This special group should be considered treatable so as to arrest the disease process, because the pattern of disease would be similar to that of their affected sibling.

Marshaling all needed data as quickly as possible represents a challenge. Urinary sulfatide should be measured immediately to detect abnormal amounts. Fibroblast culture should be completed as soon as possible. Separation of pseudodeficiency from true MLD must be determined expeditiously. In addition, differentiation between enzymatic deficiency as opposed to protein activator deficiency must be established (9).

Priority should be given to initiation of BMT when a histocompatible donor has been found. One patient has shown engraftment for 2 years without clinical progression of disease (10). A critical caveat concerning these presymptomatic patients lies in the high frequency of pseudodeficiency in families with a truly affected patient. Even though other family members may have similarly low arylsulfatase A levels in the leukocytes as the patient with MLD, these pseudodeficient individuals have normal life expectancy and are asymptomatic. The sulfatide loading studies are necessary for correct interpretation of the genetic defect.

Juvenile MLD

A 13-year-old girl with juvenile MLD was transplanted successfully at the University of Minnesota 3 years ago. She was initially referred for major behavioral problems with inappropriate social behavior and verbal belligerence. She was spatially disoriented, and her school work had deteriorated. Before BMT, a low-normal IQ with perceptual, attentional, and organizational difficulties was noted. Three years after BMT, she is alert and improved with regard to new learning and conceptual tasks. She is much less disinhibited and impulsive, and her social skills are improving. There is no progression of disease, in contrast to the same disease in her 21-year-old sister, who died, and her 12-year-old brother, who is now bed-ridden. Early detection of juvenile, adult disease or presymptomatic infants provides a window of opportunity for BMT. Because of the prolonged latency before significant progression, BMT should be effective. Conversely, the presence of overt symptomatology and neurological impairment in patients with the late infantile type are considered as contraindications for BMT. These important differences in rates of progression need to be emphasized in discussing benefits of BMT in MLD (11).

BMT continues to be the only treatment modality available despite extensive knowledge of the molecular basis of MLD (12). Earlier diagnosis and improved long-term outcome will be accomplished as knowledge concerning the differential diagnosis of disease and the results of treatment with BMT are reported.

Globoid Cell Leukodystrophy

Globoid cell leukodystrophy (GLD), inherited in an autosomal recessive manner, is caused by a deficiency of galactocerebrosidase. Pathognomonic observation of globoid cells in the CNS is the distinguishing characteristic of this disease. These large globoid cells contain the linear inclusion bodies secondary to accumulation of the unmetabolized lipids.

The term *Krabbe's disease* pertains to the original description of a clinical syndrome in infants. Rapid deterioration occurs within a few months after birth, and continued seizures and decerebration lead to an early death. The comparison of infantile GLD or Krabbe's disease to the "twitcher" mouse model is quite apt. BMT provides complete correction of enzymatic deficiency in both human and mouse models. The changes and amelioration that occur in the clinical, pathological, and neurological behavior pattern have been noted (13,14). There is morphological evidence of loss of globoid cells and attendant substrate accumulation. Ultimately, however, both in the human disease and in the mouse model, there is demise, with symptoms of CNS disorder still present.

Juvenile and adult forms of GLD are to be contrasted to the infantile form. Late-onset GLD is entirely different and is frequently mistaken for other neurological and psychological diseases (15). Positive response following BMT in one patient with the juvenile form of GLD gives credence to the potential for treatment. This 12-year-old girl has had full enzymatic recovery for the last 2.5 years. She has had major clinical changes: improvement in ataxia, tremor, memory, and ability to do school work. MRI lesions, which had been progressive until BMT, have subsequently shown less prominence. She demonstrates continued verbal growth and improvement in IQ, short-term memory, verbal fluency, and spatial orientation. Her visual agnosia, although improved, has not completely resolved. Progression of the disease appears to be arrested. This case report provides the basis for recommending BMT as a method for ameliorating and preventing further deterioration in the juvenile and adult forms of GLD.

Adrenoleukodystrophy

Adrenoleukodystrophy (ALD), a peroxisomal sex-linked storage disease in which very long chain fatty acids (VLCFA) accumulate in plasma and in the CNS, is caused by a deficiency of a specific ligase. The childhood cerebral form of ALD is malignant in its course; death occurs at the end of the first decade of life if untreated.

Dietary restriction and supplementation with GTE: GTO (Lorenzo's oil) will readily reduce the elevated

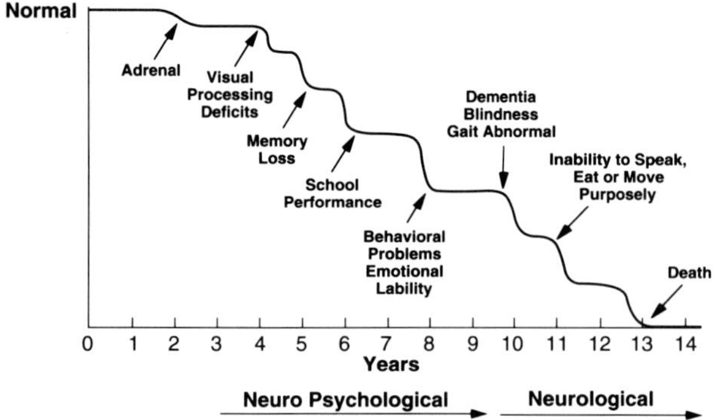

Figure 66-4. The theoretical construct of the changes that occur in the cerebral form of adrenoleukodystrophy. Early detection as a result of loss of cerebral function is measured by neuropsychological testing. The presence of overt neurological disease is a manifestation of a more severe process.

plasma VLCFA to normal. Dietary restriction and supplementation should be instituted in all patients diagnosed with ALD (16). Preliminary data suggest that if treatment with strict dietary restriction and oil supplementation is started early enough, the onset of neurological disease may be retarded (16). Unfortunately, despite normalization of VLCFA, there is evidence of ongoing neuropsychological deterioration. The sensitivity of the extensive neuropsychological testing in discerning changes in patients with ALD indicates ongoing cognitive compromise and early dementia which is rarely suspected in school work (Figure 66-4) (Shapiro, et al, personal communication).

In 9 patients in Minnesota and France, BMT provided a return to normalcy in the cognitive aberrations seen on neuropsychological tests (17). Improvement occurred within months after BMT and has continued. BMT is indicated for those boys who, despite normalcy of VLCFA in plasma, have progression of abnormalities on neuropsychological testing. For instance, one boy scored better than before BMT on a test of visual motor integration (Beery VMI), with an increase from 90 to 98. Another patient had a marked improvement in visual processing (Benton Judgment of Line Orientation Test); his score changed in 6 months after BMT from a 54 to 119. Visual learning and memory (Wide Range Assessment of Memory and Learning) standard score rose from a low of 75 to 95. Similar data have been obtained in the tests of components of attentional functioning.

In contrast, patients whose neuropsychological evaluation or clinical symptomatology showed moderately advanced abnormalities have not fared well. Continued neurological deterioration occurred in one of the 7 boys who had significant hearing impairment and major deficits in the neuropsychological tests prior to BMT at the University of Minnesota. Elsewhere, similar data indicate poor prognosis after BMT if seizures and severe neuropsychological impairment have already occurred. Because of late disease with progression, 2 deaths occurred immediately after BMT.

For patients with a suitable human leukocyte antigen (HLA)–compatible donor, earlier decision making for BMT is part of the prospective plans in the collaborative study. In contrast, adrenomyeloneuropathy, the adult male form of ALD, has a predilection for the spinal cord and a lifespan prognosis measured in decades; therefore, BMT has not been recommended.

Hurler's Syndrome

Hurler's syndrome (type I), inherited in an autosomal recessive manner, is caused by deficiency of α-L-iduronidase (α-L-iduronide iduronohydrolase) (IDUA), which is the characteristic laboratory diagnostic observation (18). Clinical, biochemical, and genetic molecular biology features of IDUA-deficient individuals vary widely between severe and milder forms (Hurler, Hurler-Scheie, and Scheie). The latter 2 forms have a better outcome than the more severe Hurler type (19).

In the Minnesota series, 13 patients were transplanted with an HLA-identical sibling donor, with 3 deaths (Figure 66-5). Thirteen additional patients with Hurler's syndrome were transplanted from donors other than HLA-identical siblings, with 7 deaths (Figure 66-6). Engraftment continues in all 16 survivors. The first patient in this series was engrafted 8 years ago. The initial BMT resulted in autogenous regeneration after several months. She was retransplanted successfully, is currently attending special school, and has an intelligence score of 80.

The relative rate of intellectual gain continues to fall below normal in each of the individuals studied. One third of the children have IQs in the severely retarded range (<50). The second third have mild mental deficiency, with IQs between 69 and 51. The remainder are between 70 and 85, which is within the lower second standard deviation. Despite continued increase in some capabilities, eventual intelligence

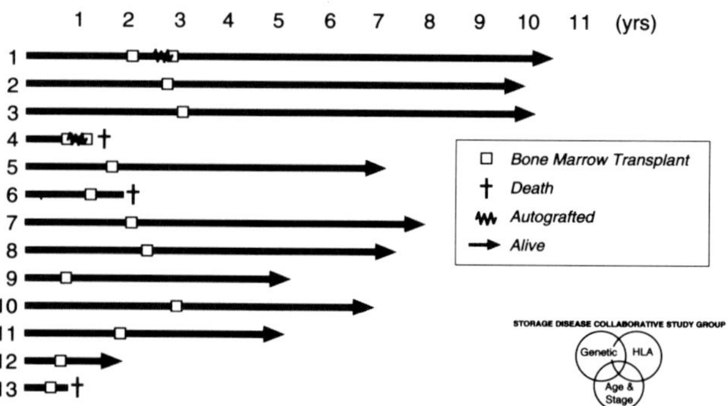

Figure 66-5. The course of disease of 13 patients with Hurler's syndrome transplanted with human leukocyte antigen–identical sibling donors. The specific details of death and long-term complications are described in the text.

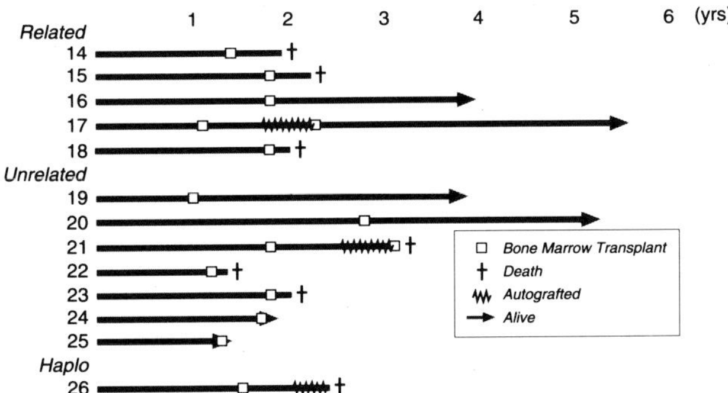

Figure 66-6. The disease course of 13 patients with Hurler's syndrome transplanted with other than human leukocyte antigen–identical sibling donors. The increased incidence of severe graft-versus-host disease and other long-term complications is described in the text.

scores of approximately 100 have been reported. What factors can help explain the differences in intellectual outcomes? Inclusion of Hurler-Scheie or Scheie genotypic patients is the most likely reason. The classic clinical description of infants with hepatosplenomegaly and dysostosis multiplex in the first years of life has been assumed to represent the more severe or Hurler phenotype. However, there is a strong possibility that the Hurler-Scheie and Scheie genotype, which have an inherent better prognosis, could be hidden within the clinical Hurler phenotype.

A study of the biochemical basis of distinguishing between Hurler and Hurler-Scheie by examination of IDUA has been published (20–23). Measurements of the differences in urinary excretion of heparan and dermatan sulfate, as well as degree of hydrolysis of desulfated natural heparin, have been available as a means of classification (Table 66-1) (24,25).

Unfortunately, these tests and other gene probes have not been used or were not available in any of the prior experiences with BMT. The current challenge will be to utilize all the expertise available for appropriate genotype classification. Bias due to possible inclusion of Hurler-Scheie type needs to be carefully evaluated. Utilization of gene analysis as well as the function tests will be required to distinguish between classes of clinical disease. These tests will be mandated for each new patient in the consortium study.

Whether the donor is a carrier with half levels of enzyme or normal with 100% levels does not appear to explain the wide range of intellectual outcomes. In animal BMT studies, results are not different when comparing use of carrier donors versus normal donors (13).

The degree of clinical severity before BMT as noted by hepatosplenomegaly or skeletal defects has failed to indicate prognosis. Severe heart failure and associated cardiac disease, an increase in intracranial pressure, and development of hydrocephalus with need for a shunt are poor prognostic signs. These complications in the natural course of the disease need to be accommodated in the prospective study.

Graft-versus-host disease (GVHD) has been quite prominent in the 13 patients with Hurler's syndrome transplanted with HLA-identical siblings; one death was due to grade IV GVHD.

The most common conditioning regimen for BMT was busulfan (BU) and cyclophosphamide (CY). The problems relating to BU pharmacokinetics are important. In young infants and children, BU levels in the plasma have an area under the curve less than that in older children and adults (26), suggesting the need to adjust BU dosage on an individual basis. A prospective study is planned to evaluate this concept.

Coronary artery stenosis is a major cause of morbidity and mortality in patients with severe forms of IDUA deficiency. The lack of cardiac symptoms and disease several years after BMT is in contradistinction to that anticipated in nontransplanted patients. In an attempt to demonstrate changes in coronary artery stenosis subsequent to BMT, coronary arteriography and echocardiological examination were completed (27). Coronary arteriography was found to be incapable of distinguishing normal from abnormal. It seems advisable to follow patients with noninvasive procedures (28).

Orthopedic problems still occur following long-term engraftment (29,30). Surgical interventions for femoral-acetabular dislocation, carpal tunnel syndrome, and medial tibial epiphyseal abnormal growth have been required. Although there is growth in the long bones, there is significant retardation in the vertebral column. Braces and surgery have been needed to prevent ongoing distortion of kyphoscoliosis in the lumbar region. Myelopathy from such distortion of the spinal column represents a significant threat to ambulation of these patients in later years. In addition, low self-esteem will occur when the abnormal growth and skeletal problems set patients apart from their peers as cognitive ability to discern differences improves.

BMT for IDUA deficiency has been accomplished in

Table 66-1
α-L-iduronidase–Deficient Individuals

	Hurler Syndrome (n = 9)	*Hurler-Scheie Syndrome (n = 4)*	*Scheie's Syndrome (n = 4)*	*Control Subjects (n = 6)*
Urinary qualitative AMPS analysis				
AMPS (mg/ 24 kr) (SD)	48.6 (12.8)	44.2 (5.3)	41 (4.2)	2.5 ± 07
Dermatan sulfate (%)	61–70	>90	>90	<2
Heparan sulfate (%)	30–39	<10	<10	<3
Fibroblast Hydrolysis of natural substrate[a]				
Dermatan sulfate	None	None	None	7.4
Heparin[b]	None	6.3	5.4	6.8

[a]Umole of iduronic acid produced in 24-hour period/mg protein.
[b]Desulfated.
AMPS = acidic mycopolysaccharides.

many institutions (31,32). Ophthalmological data on patients with Hurler's syndrome indicate improvement in conjunctival inclusion bodies, retinal responses, and glaucoma (33,34). Additional case reports have noted in situ morphological clearance of glycosaminoglycans from skin fibroblasts (35). A preliminary report on psychomotor development of patients with Hurler's syndrome was published (36). Clearance of glycosaminoglycans by morphological assay in hepatic biopsies from patients with Hurler's syndrome has been reported (37).

As discussed, careful pretransplant assessment of patients with IDUA deficiency is necessary to aid physicians and parents in assessing realistic prognostic outlooks.

Hunter's Syndrome

Hunter's Syndrome (type II), inherited as a sex-linked recessive disorder, is caused by the deficiency of iduronate sulfatase. Clinically, there are 2 distinct patterns of neurological disease, severe and mild. Mental retardation with low IQ levels in the range of 30 to 40 at 4 to 6 years of age is present in the severe form. The milder form is associated with a lesser mental deficit. Indeed, there are individuals who are quite capable of successfully completing education and earning a living (38). The molecular biological tools now available can detect the major gene deletion in the severe form (39,40). Detection of this deletion in leukocytes and fibroblasts of such individuals is available on a practical basis.

The results of BMT for Hunter's syndrome for 7 children has been detailed (2). Identification of severe or mild form in these transplanted patients had not been determined on a molecular basis. Some of the patients were transplanted at an older age. Therefore, a major impact on the ongoing process of mental retardation was not to be anticipated. Without an appropriately conducted study, the potential for providing amelioration or stabilization of mental retardation or severe skeletal dysplasia cannot be evaluated readily in these few patients.

Results of BMT for patients with Hunter's syndrome should be more favorable if only fully HLA-compatible donors are selected to reduce the incidence of severe GVHD (Krivit W, personal communication). Skeletal and cardiac late complications would be less common if BMT were carried out for patients under the age of 3 before late complications were established. For example, one patient died of coronary sclerosis at 8 years after being transplanted at 5 years.

Specific neuropsychological tests are now available to measure the particularly aggressive behavioral problems of these patients and should be undertaken in any prospective studies. Two transplanted patients are now so aggressive that special care is required.

Sanfilippo's Syndromes

Sanfilippo's syndromes (type III), inherited in an autosomal recessive manner, are comprised of 4 distinct enzymatic disorders. Differences in clinical manifestations are apparent in each of these entities and variation has been observed within families.

Twenty-eight patients have been transplanted worldwide. Four patients died, 3 failed to engraft, one suffered a CNS catastrophe, and one required a liver transplant because of hepatic failure. The data do not confirm the initial report of the United States experience (2). Of the successfully engrafted patients, none have had stabilization of intelligence. There has been major deterioration in all patients followed for more than 18 months after transplantation; many are profoundly mentally deficient and unstable. The most telling experience is that of twins who had an elder sibling with the disease. On the basis of biochemical data, they were transplanted in an asymptomatic state before their second birthday. At 10 years of age, one is untestable and the other has an IQ in the 30 range. This finding confirms previous reports that patients with Sanfilippo's syndrome experience continued loss of intelligence despite persistent engraftment and normalcy of enzyme activity (41,42). Two other patients transplanted after preparation with radiation and chemotherapy suffered immediate neurological decline that led to incapacitation in one and death in the other.

Clearance of glycosaminoglycan from hepatic tissue is much less complete and takes longer in patients with Sanfilippo's syndrome than in those with Hurler syndrome (37). This slower clearance may be explained by their different rates of enzymatic incorporation (20,43).

The need for earlier identification of children with Sanfilippo's syndrome is critical if BMT is to be tested in a rational manner. A questionnaire study was directed to parents of children with Sanfilippo's syndrome (44). Clearly, significant delay was apparent in accomplishing normal milestones in the first year of life. Large head circumference and skeletal dysplasia were also noted early in the first year of life. Encouragement and training of physicians to utilize the enzymatic leukocyte assay or measurement of urinary glycosaminoglycans, or both, will allow for earlier diagnosis.

Choice of whether to transplant patients with Sanfilippo's syndromes should be guided by the difficulties noted in these results.

Gaucher's Disease

Gaucher's disease types can be defined by gene analysis (45). The extraordinary success of the CEREDASE enzyme infusion program has revolutionized therapy for this disease (46). The discussion concerning dosages is important (47–49). Type II, which is the least common, is clinically diagnosed in infancy after a rapid onset of severe neurological deterioration. There are no data that indicate treatment is helpful. Type III is more difficult to distinguish from the severe form of type I. The neuropathological type characteristically found in Swedish families has been studied most extensively. The patient reported by Ringden and colleagues (50) has remained neuropsychologically stable and is now attending high school. Other investigators presented results indicative of continued improvement in patients with type III after BMT for periods of 2 to 3 years (51). Kyphoscoliosis has been noted and represents a severe problem in several of these patients.

Several patients with type III have been treated with CEREDASE who have not had CNS disease progression. Because of these findings, Gaucher's disease has been removed from the eligibility listing of diseases to be considered for BMT by the consortium study. The absoluteness of the blood-brain barrier needs to be reviewed carefully in view of data indicating that large molecular weight molecules do enter the CNS to a greater extent than previously thought (52–56).

Niemann-Pick Disease

Niemann-Pick disease (type IA) following BMT engraftment with normal leukocyte enzymatic assay has not improved in 2 patients (57). Postmortem biopsy tissue of liver and brain of one patient did not demonstrate enzymatic activity. There was also no decrease in spleen or liver size or a change in the extensive neurological disease.

Wolman Disease

Three patients with Wolman disease have been transplanted; 2 had enzymatic reconstitution of the deficient acid lipase (cholesterol esterase) activity. Unfortunately, both died within the first months following BMT due to sepsis and renal dysfunction; the third failed to engraft. A review of Wolman disease provides the rationale for considering BMT for future patients (58).

Glycogen Storage Disease (Type II)

Despite normalization of acid maltase enzymatic activity in the leukocytes of 2 patients transplanted for glycogen storage disease, there was no resolution of the abnormal lysosomal storage disease (59). Whether the outlook would be better if the more late infantile or juvenile form were transplanted is only conjectural.

I-cell Disease

Patients with I-cell disease (mucolipidosis type II) have inclusion bodies in the lysosomes of fibroblasts. An increase in lysosomal enzymes in plasma is the characteristic biochemical marker. Pathophysiology relates to the "leakiness" into the plasma from the lysosome due to specific transferase deficiency. The one patient transplanted in Japan demonstrated a remarkable decrease in serum lysosomal enzymatic activity (60). Unfortunately, the CNS symptoms included severe psychomotor retardation, which was not changed. Patients with I-cell disease should be considered as a potential BMT recipients if they have normal CNS function.

Farber Disease

Farber disease is defined by the accumulation of ceramide in large lumps over the extremities due to deficiency of ceramidase. After BMT in one patient, the ceramidase deficiency was corrected and the large masses of ceramide accumulation totally disappeared (61). Unfortunately, the patient had a severe CNS disorder and died.

Fucosidosis

Patients with fucosidosis should be considered for BMT based on the remarkable data accumulated in the canine model by Taylor and associates (62). These investigators clearly demonstrated clearance of fucoside and enzymatic reconstitution in brain as well as in other organs. Furthermore, neurological disabilities were totally controlled and prevented if the BMT was performed early in the life of the dog. This is clearly a disease that needs consideration for BMT.

Mannosidosis

Mannosidosis has been treated with BMT in one patient without success; however, recent data by Walkley and colleagues (63) prove that mannosidase enters the neurons after BMT in a feline model.

Morquio's Disease

Morquio's disease (type IV) has been treated with BMT (64). Current data are inconclusive as to the benefit derived because the enzyme may not be able to enter into abnormal chondrocytes.

Batten Disease

Batten disease, an autosomal recessive inherited condition, is characterized by lysosomal accumulation of "ceroid-lipofuscin." The abnormal lysosomes are best appreciated in the CNS in humans. In the ovine and canine models, lysosomes of the hepatic, pancreatic, and renal tissues are also commonly involved. The most appropriate theory as to etiology concerns subunit C of mitochondrial adenosine triphosphate synthase. Initial investigations by Palmer and associates (65) indicate that the ovine model is most likely due to an accumulation of the subunit C secondary to failure of its catabolism. Subunit C accumulates in the tissues of patients with juvenile ceroid lipofuscinosis in brain, liver, and skeletal muscle. BMT should be considered for this disease.

Choice of Marrow Donor

HLA-identical Sibling Donor

Eighteen patients with different storage diseases (excluding Hurler's syndrome) have been successfully engrafted from sibling donors without mortality due to transplantation (Krivit W. Unpublished data.). Each has had documentation of engraftment by blood genetic markers and by equivalency of enzymatic assay of the recipient leukocytes to that of the donor. Engraftment has been persistent. Acute GVHD, although frequently present, was readily treated by use of steroids and antithymocyte globulin (ATG). Chronic GVHD developed in one patient.

The preparative regimen consisted of BU and CY. The dosage of BU varied throughout the study. Our initial patient received 12 mg/kg; the next 7 patients received 16 mg/kg. Because of the data from our pharmacokinetic study (26), BU dosage was escalated to 24 mg/kg in 4 patients. This dosage was discontinued because of severe pneumonitis. BU used for the last 6 patients was 20 mg/kg given orally every 6 hours for 4 days. The CY total dosage was 240 mg/kg. The marrow inoculum varied from 2.0 to 4.0 $\times$ 10^8 nucleated marrow cells/kg of recipient weight. Initial GVHD prevention consisted of prednisone, methotrexate, and ATG. Cyclosporine (CSP) and methylprednisolone have been used for the past 6 years.

Of the 13 patients with Hurler's syndrome who underwent BMT from a matched sibling donor, 3 died following BMT (Figure 66-5). One died of overwhelming GVHD, one from pneumonia, and one from aplasia secondary to failure of engraftment. Two demonstrated autogenous regeneration after transient donor engraftment. Both were retransplanted with CY and total body irradiation (TBI). One died of pneumonia; the other is our longest living engrafted survivor, who has maintained a chimeric status of 50% engraftment. GVHD has been quite prominent and severe. The preparative regimen, prevention, and treatment protocols for GVHD for these 13 patients were the same as the non-Hurler group described.

Other Related Donors

Ten patients at the University of Minnesota received BMTs from family members who were not matched siblings. Three patients received marrow from siblings who were one antigen–mismatched. The mixed leukocyte culture (MLC) rejection reactivity was quite low (8, 0, and 3%). Severe acute GVHD developed in the patient with Hurler's syndrome, who died from chronic GVHD at 140 days. The patient with ALD had a prolonged course of moderate acute and chronic GVHD, including bronchiolitis obliterans. The patient with infantile Krabbe's disease engrafted. At the end of 2 years, engraftment was absent by enzymatic assay. This is our only incidence of such a late loss of engraftment after BMT, presumably due to use of a T-cell–depleted marrow. Krabbe's disease caused death.

Five patients were transplanted whose donors were parents with one antigen mismatched. The patient with Gaucher's disease received the father's marrow. There was no engraftment, and the patient died 75 days after BMT. The patient with Hurler's syndrome received marrow from the father, and engraftment and post-BMT course have been excellent, with no complications. The patient with Sanfilippo A received the mother's marrow and engraftment continues over 18 months with a moderate degree of GVHD. The other patient with Sanfilippo A received the mother's marrow but died of a massive CNS bleed within the first month of transplant due to thrombocytopenia. The latest patient with Hurler's syndrome had acute and chronic GVHD; pulmonary hemorrhage and death occurred on day 70.

Two patients with Hurler's syndrome were transplanted with marrow from grandparents. Major complications during transplant secondary to acute GVHD developed in one. Chronic GVHD developed and she died 130 days after transplantation. The other had autogenous marrow regeneration after a previous unrelated transplant. He therefore received CY and TBI as the preparative regimen and marrow from his grandfather, who was HLA phenotypically identical. There were no complications with GVHD, and engraftment has continued for 4 years.

Unrelated Donors

Fourteen patients received marrow from an unrelated donor (8, Hurler's syndrome; 2, adult GLD; 1, Sanfilippo C; 1, Wolman disease; 1, MLD; 1, ALD). Engraftment occurred in all 14 patients. Two patients with Hurler's syndrome lost the graft with subsequent autogenous regeneration. One died after retransplantation with the CY and TBI protocol. GVHD caused death in 7 patients (2, adult GLD; 3, Hurler's syndrome; 1, MLD; 1, Wolman disease). Severe chronic GVHD persists in 5 patients (4, Hurler's syndrome; 1, Sanfilippo C). Minimal chronic GVHD continues in 2 patients who are fully engrafted.

Haploidentical donors were used in 3 patients (1, Hurler's syndrome; 1, Gaucher's disease; 1, Wolman disease). These BMTs were unsuccessful and all three patients died.

In summary, the risk of transplant death was 3 of 31 (9.6%) when HLA-matched sibling donors were used. With other donors, the risk of transplant death was 10 of 27 (37%).

Ethics

The quality of life after BMT is of utmost importance (see Chapter 42). In aplastic anemia and malignancies, although decrements in IQ and growth are noted, there is the expectation of comparatively adequate status after BMT. Conversely, quality of life, as measured by growth, skeletal difficulties, and neuropsychological outcome for patients with storage diseases, is gradually being defined. Because of these long-term problems, criteria for eligibility for BMT should not be applied in a manner similar to that for malignancy or aplastic anemia.

Paramount in establishing eligibility has been the consideration of whether there is a matched donor available for the BMT (see Chapter 4). In addition to serological histocompatibility typing, we have restricted BMT to those with lower MLC reactivity (Krivit W, personal communication). In the National Marrow Donor Program, the MLC is now being replaced by molecular typing; however, the MLC should be considered as an adjunct to molecular typing.

The preparative regimen methodology needs special comment. Leukoencephalopathy or demyelination within currently utilized extensive preparative regimens for aplastic anemia and malignancies have been reported (66). There are other articles that indicate development of CNS complications when extensive preparative regimens are used (67–75). Patients with ongoing CNS disorders, as is the case in patients with storage diseases, merit specific and special considerations.

BMT for treatment of any disease is one of the most involved and complex decisions ever to face parents, patients and physicians responsible for providing guidance. Survival is only one aspect to be considered (70–74). Quality of life and future independence of the patient must be considered. The potential for burdening parents and the family with an individual not able to be independent needs to be kept constantly in mind. Even though parents and families willingly assume this responsibility out of desperation, years from time of transplantation they will become more knowledgeable and frequently may regret their decisions. Cost, ethics, and the future for BMT were discussed extensively in 1986 (75). Cautions noted then are still important and need to be reviewed by anyone participating in these studies.

Conclusions

Some doubt the value of BMT as an effective therapeutic modality and regard the opportunity provided by BMT with continued skepticism because of the considerable risks and costs. There is expectant anticipation that molecular biology will provide better and less expensive therapy. Use of enzyme in treatment for Gaucher's disease has provided an excellent example of this potential.

Conversely, enzymatic replenishment by BMT has support from those who note that, for the next several years, this will be the only readily available method of treatment. Without such treatment, continued morbidity and certain death due to disease will occur. Parents and physicians still wish to do everything possible for patients, even though long-term events are not known. Several have had clinical success in retrieving children from otherwise certain demise using donors other than HLA-identical siblings (see Chapter 51).

The role of BMT in the treatment of storage diseases must be defined by careful collection and analysis of data by physicians dedicated to pursuing the best treatment options. The risk of BMT mortality and morbidity is minimized by the use of donors who are excellent histocompatible matches. This criterion should provide an expectation of mortality and morbidity of approximately 10 to 15%. Operationally, this appears to be a level that the majority of physicians and parents find acceptable.

Limiting BMT to those patients with least risk is justified because the clinical results have shown many residual complications despite correction of enzyme deficiency. The added problems of BMT-engendered growth retardation (76) and secondary malignancies (77,78) need to be considered. Because long-term results cannot be predicted, there should be grave concern that the eventual caretakers will have to assume complex and serious problems in these children in the decades ahead.

Because of the many unknowns and variables present, a prospective study of the value of BMT is now underway in as many as 25 major centers in the United States and Canada. Active participation in these studies will result in data that could indicate the best methods for future care and the most appropriate recommendations for children with storage disorders.

References

1. Krivit W. Lysosomal storage diseases. In: Hoffman R, Benz EJ, Shattil SJ, Furie B, Cohen HJ, eds. Hematology. New York: Churchill-Livingstone, 1991:615–627.
2. Krivit W, Shapiro EG. BMT for storage diseases. In: Desnick RJ, ed. Treatment of genetic diseases. New York: Churchill-Livingstone, 1991:203–221.
3. Krivit W, Shapiro EG. Bone marrow transplantation in Maroteaux-Lamy syndrome (mucopolysaccharidosis type VI). Biochemical and clinical status 24 months after transplantation. N Engl J Med 1984;311:1601–1611.
4. Krivit W. Maroteaux-Lamy syndrome (mucopolysaccharidosis type VI) treatment by allogeneic BMT in 6 patients and potential for autotransplantation bone marrow gene insertion. Int Pediatr 1992;7:47–52.
5. Krivit W, Shapiro E, Kennedy E, et al. Treatment of late infantile metachromatic leukodystrophy by bone marrow transplantation. N Engl J Med 1990;322:28–32.
6. Shapiro EG, Lipton ME, Krivit W. White matter dysfunction and its neuropsychological correlates: longitudinal study of a case of metachromatic leukodystrophy treated with bone marrow transplant. Clin Exp Neuropsychol 1992;14:610–624.
7. Dhuna A, Toro C, Torres F, Kennedy WR, Krivit W. Longitudinal neurophysiologic studies in a patient with MLD following BMT. Arch Neurol 1992;49:1088–1092.
8. Krivit W, Shapiro EG, Lockman L, et al. Recommendations for treatment of MLD by BMT based on a review of seven patients who have been engrafted for at least a year. In: Hobbs JR, Riches PG, eds. COGENT II, correction of certain genetic diseases by transplantation. Westminster Medical School Press, 1992:57–73.
9. Wenger DA, Williams C, Considine E, Rafi MA. Research developments on lysosomal disorders. MLD and Gaucher disease. Int Pediatr 1992;7:34–39.

10. Goldberg KL, Barrios NJ, McNeil J, Kirkpatrick DV, Shapira E, O'Byrne C. Treatment of MLD with partially matched BMT. Pediatr Res 1992;31:140.
11. Shapiro EG, Lockman LA, Krivit W. Metachromatic leukodystrophy is treatable with BMT: the importance of early identification in patients with psychiatric symptoms. Neurology 1993 (in press).
12. Polten A, Fluharty AL, Fluharty CB, Kappler J, Von Figura K, Gieselmann V. Molecular basis of different forms of metachromatic leukodystrophy. N Engl J Med 1991;324:18–22.
13. Haskins M, Baker HJ, Birkenmeier E, et al. Transplantation in animal model systems. In: Desnick RJ, ed. Treatment of genetic diseases. New York: Churchill-Livingstone, 1991:183–201.
14. Shapiro E, Lockman L, Kennedy W, et al. BMT as treatment for globoid cell leukodystrophy. In: Desnick RJ, ed. Treatment of genetic disease. New York: Churchill-Livingstone, 1991:221–236.
15. Kolodny EH, Raghavan S, Krivit W. Late-onset Krabbe disease (globoid cell leukodystrophy) and clinical and biochemical features of 15 cases. Dev Neurosci 1991; 13:232–239.
16. Moser HW, Moser AB, Smith KD, et al. Adrenoleukodystrophy: phenotypic variability: implications for therapy. J Inherited Metab Dis 1992;15:645–664.
17. Krivit W, Shapiro EG, Lockman LA, et al. Recommendations for treatment of childhood cerebral form of adrenoleukodystrophy. In: Hobbs JR, Riches PG, eds. COGENT II, correction of GEN diseases by transplantation. Westminster Medical School, 1992:38–49.
18. Freeman C, Hopwood JJ. Human alpha-L-iduronidase. Catalytic properties and an integrated role in the lysosomal degradation of heparan sulphate. Biochem J 1992;282:899–908.
19. Hopwood JJ, Moraris CP. The mucopolysaccharidosis. Mol Biol Med 1990;7:381–404.
20. Bach G, Friedman R, Weismann B, Neufeld EF. The defect in the Hurler and Scheie syndromes: deficiency of α-L-iduronidase. Proc Natl Acad Sci USA 1972; 69:2048.
21. Ullrich K, Grobe H, Von Figuara K, Hopwood JJ, Muller V. Late onset form of mucopolysaccaridosis type I: clinical aspect and biochemical characterization of residual α-L-iduronidase activity. J Inherited Metab Dis 1981;4:171–172.
22. Taylor JA, Gibson GJ, Brooks DA, Hopwood JJ. α-L-iduronidase in normal and mucopolysaccharidosis-type I human skin fibroblasts. Biochem J 1991;274:263–268.
23. Fujibayashi S, Minami R, Ishikawa Y, Wagatsuma K, Nakao T, Tsugawa S. Properties of α-L-iduronidase in cultured skin fibroblasts from α-L-iduronidase-deficient patients. Hum Genet 1984;65:268–272.
24. Matalon R, Deanching M, Omura K. Hurler, Hurler-Scheie and Scheie compound: residual activity of α-L-iduronidase toward natural substrate suggesting allelic mutations. J Inherited Metab Dis 1983;6(suppl 2):133.
25. Matalon R. Characteristics of urinary glycosaminoglycan excretion in Hurler, Hurler-Scheie, and Scheie patients: congenital metabolic disease New York: Dekker, 1985:253–254.
26. Grochow LB, Krivit W, Whitley CB, Blazar B. Busulfan disposition in children. Blood 1990;75:1723–1727.
27. Braunlin EA, Hunter DW, Krivit W, et al. Evaluation of coronoary artery disease in the Hurler syndrome by angiography. Am J Cardiol 1992:69:1487–1489.
28. Taylor DB, Blaser S, Burrows PE, Stringer DA, Clarke JTR, Thorner P. Arteriopathy and coarctation of the abdominal aorta in children with mucopolysaccharidosis: imaging findings. Am J Roentgenol 1991;157: 819–824.
29. Hugh-Jones K, Hobbs JR, Vellodi A, Hancock M, Sheldon J, Jones S. Long-term follow-up of children with Hurler's disease treated with BMT. In: Hobbs JR, ed. COGENT I. London: Westminster Medical Trust, 1989;103–111.
30. Downie C, Hancock MR, Hobbs JR. Long term outcome after BMT in Hurler's disease. In: Hobbs JR, Riches PG, eds. COGENT II. London: Westminster Medical Trust, 1992;1–13.
31. Ciocci GH, Downey JH, Pettigrew AL, Miara C, Morrow J. Update on outcome following allogeneic bone marrow transplant for patients with Hurlers syndrome using alternative marrow donors. Keystone Symposium, UCLA Bone Marrow Transplantation, Jan 1992.
32. Saunders EF, Kirby MA, Solh HS, Clarke JTR. Enzyme replacement in Hurler's syndrome using BMT. Keystone Symposium, UCLA Bone Marrow Transplantation, Jan 1992.
33. Summers CG, Purple RL, Whitley CE, Krivit W. Ocular changes in mucopolysaccharidosis following BMT. Ophthalmology 1990;96:977.
34. Christiansen SP, Smith TJ, Henslee-Downey PJ. Normal intraocular pressure after a bone marrow transplant in glaucoma associated with mucopolysaccharidosis type I-H. Am J Ophthalmol 1990;109:230–231.
35. Navarro C, Dominguez C, Costa M, Ortega JJ. Bone marrow transplant in a case of mucopolysaccharidosis I Scheie phenotype: skin ultrastructure before and after transplantation. Acta Neuropathol 1991;82:33–38.
36. Hugh-Jones K. Psychomotor development of children with mucopolysaccharidosis type I-H following BMT. Birth defects 1986;22:1, 25–29.
37. Resnick JM, Krivit W, Snover DC, et al. Pathology of the liver in the mucopolysaccharidoses a light and electron microscopic assessment before and after BMT, 1992; 10:273–280.
38. Neufeld E, Muenzer J. The mucopolysaccharidosis. In: Scriver CR, Beaudet A, Sly WS, Valle D, eds. The metabolic basis of inherited disease. New York: McGraw-Hill, 1989;1565–1588.
39. Palmeri G, Hopwood JJ. The iduronate sulfatase gene: identification of heterogenous deletions in patients with Hunter syndrome. Genomics 1992;12:52–57.
40. Meunzer J, Tutera AM. Molecular analysis of iduronate sulfatase mutations in Hunter syndrome (MPSII). Pediatr Res 1992;31:134A.
41. Hugh-Jones K, Hobbs JR, Vellodi M, et al. Long term followup of twins with Sanfilippo B disease treated with BMT. In: Hobbs JR, ed. COGENT I. London: Westminster Medical School Trust, 1989;112–113.
42. Bordigoni P, Vidailhet M, Lena M, Maire I, Gelot S. BMT for Sanfilippo syndrome. In: Hobbs JR, ed. COGENT I. London: Westminster Medical School Trust, 1989:114–119.
43. O'Brien JS, Miller AL, Loverde AW, Veath ML. Sanfilippo disease type B: enzyme replacement and metabolic correction in cultured fibroblasts. Science 1973;181:753–755.
44. Nidiffer FD, Kellyu TE. Developmental and degenerative patterns associated with cognitive, behavioural and motor difficulties in the Sanfilippo syndrome: an epidemiological study. J Ment Def Res 1983;27:185–203.

45. Beutler E. Gaucher's disease. N Engl J Med 1991; 325:1354–1359.
46. Barton NW, Brady RO, Dambrosia JM, et al. Replacement therapy for inherited enzyme deficiency: macrophage-targeted glucocerebrosidase for Gaucher's disease. N Engl J Med 1991;324:1464–1470.
47. Barton NW, Brady RO, Dambrosia JM, et al. Dose-dependent responses to macrophage targeted glucocerebrosidase in a child with Gaucher disease. J Pediatr 1992;120:277–280.
48. Beutler E, Kaye A, Garver P, Thurston D, Dawson A, Rosenbloom B. Enzyme replacement for Gaucher's disease. Blood 1991;78:1183–1189.
49. Abrahamov A, Hadas-Halpern I, Levy-Lahad E, Zimran A. Enzyme replacement therapy for children with Gaucher disease: low dose, high frequency, lower cost, high efficacy. Pediatr Res 1992;31:137A.
50. Ringden O, Groth CG, Erikson A. Mansson E-E, Svennerholm L. BMT in the Norrbottnian type of Gaucher disease. Acta Pediatr Scand 1990;79:680–685.
51. Tsai P, Lipton JM, Sahdev I, et al. Allogenic bone marrow transplantation in severe Gaucher disease. Pediatr Res 1992;31:503–507.
52. Dermietzel R, Krause D. Molecular anatomy of the blood-brain barrier as defined by immunocytochemistry. Int Rev Cytol 1991;127:57–105.
53. Liu HM, Atack JR, Rapoport SI. Immunohistochemical localization of intracellular plasma proteins in the human CNS. Acta Neuropathol 1989;78:16–21.
54. Link H, Tibbling G. Principles of albumin and IgG analyses in neurological disorders. II. Relation of the concentration of the proteins in serum and cerebrospinal fluid. Scand J Clin Lab Invest 1977;37:391–396.
55. Tibbling G, Link H, Ohman S. Principles of albumin and IgG analysis in neurological disorders. I. Establishment of reference values. Scand J Clin Lab Invest 1977;37:385.
56. Kondo A, Nakano T, Suzuki K. Blood-brain barrier permeability to horseradish peroxidase in twitcher and cuprizone-intoxicated mice. Brain Res 1987;425:186–190.
57. Bayever E, August CS, Jamani N, Ferreira P, Wenger D, Krivit W. Allogeneic bone marrow transplantation for Niemann-Pick disease (type IA). Bone Marrow Transplant 1992;10(suppl 1):85–86.
58. Krivit W, Freese D, Chan KW, Kulkarni R. Wolman's disease: a review of treatment with bone marrow transplantation and considerations for the future. Bone Marrow Transplant 1992;10(suppl 1):97–101.
59. Harris RE, Hannon D, Vogler C, Hug G. BMT in type IIA glycogen storage disease. In: Krivit W, Paul W, eds. Bone Marrow Transplantation for treatment of lysosomal storage diseases. March of Dimes Original Article Series. New York: Alan R. Liss, 1986;22:119–134.
60. Kurobane I, Aikawa J-i, Narisawa K, Tada K. BMT in I-cell disease. In: Hobbs JR, ed. COGENT I. London: Westminster Medical School Trust, 1989:132–136.
61. Souillet G, Guibaud P, Fensom AH, Maire I, Zabot MT. Outcome of displacement BMT in Farber's disease. In: Hobbs JR, ed. COGENT I. London: Westminster Medical School Trust, 1989:137–141.
62. Taylor RM, Farrow BRH, Stewart GJ. Amelioration of clinical disease following BMT in fucosidase-deficient dogs. Am J Med Genet 1992;42:628–632.
63. Walkley SU, Thrall MA, Dobrenis K, et al. Evidence for correction of enzyme defect in CNS neurons in a lysosomal storage disease following bone marrow transplant. Presented at the Annual Meeting of the Society for Inherited Metabolic Disorders, Pine Mountain, GA, Mar 20–23, 1992.
64. Kato S, Kubota C, Yabe H, Yamamura M, Kurobane E, Orii T. BMT in Morquio's disease. In: Hobbs JR, ed. COGENT I. London: Westminster Medical Trust Fund, 1989:120–126.
65. Palmer DN, Fearnley IM, Walker JE, et al. Mitochoncrial ATP synthase subunit c storage in the ceroid-lipofuscinosis (Batten disease) Am J Med Genet 1992; 42:561–567.
66. Lockman LA. Sung JH, Krivit W. Acute parkinsonian syndrome with demyelinating leukoencephalopathy in bone marrow transplant recipients. Pediatr Neurol 1991;7:457–463.
67. Thompson CB, Sanders JE, Flournoy N, Buckner CD, Thomas ED. The risks of CNS relapse and leukoencephalopathy in patients receiving marrow transplants for acute leukemia. Blood 1986;67:195–199.
68. Wiznitzer M, Packer RJ, Augusut CS, Burkey ED. Neurologic complications of BMT in childhood. Ann Neurol 1984;16:569–576.
69. Atkinson K, Clink H, Lawler S, et al. Encephalopathy following BMT. Eur J Cancer 1977;13:623–625.
70. Lenarsky C, Kohn DB, Weinberg KI, Parkman R. Bone marrow transplant for genetic disease. Hematol Oncol Clin North Amer 1990;4:589–602.
71. Schaison G, Bordigoni P, Leverger G. BMT for genetic and metabolic disorders. Nouv Rev Fr Hematol 1989;31:119–123.
72. Cowan MJ. BMT for the treatment of genetic diseases. Clin Biochem 1991;24:375–381.
73. Ringden O, Groth CG, et al. BMT for metabolic disorders in Hudinge Hospital. Transplant Proc 1990; 22:198–202.
74. Hobbs JR. Displacement bone marrow transplantation and immunoprophylaxis for genetic diseases. Adv Intern Med 1988;33:81–118.
75. Krivit W. Ethics, cost and future of BMT for lysosomal storage diseases. Birth Defects 1986;22:1, 189–194.
76. Wingard JR, Plotnick LP, Fraeemer CS, et al. Growth in children after BMT: busulfan plus cyclophosphamide versus cyclophosphamide plus total body irradiation. Blood 1992;1068–1073.
77. Witherspoon RP, Fisher LD, Schoch G, et al. Secondary cancers after bone marrow transplantation for leukemia or aplastic anemia. N Engl J Med 1989;321:784–789.
78. Socie G, Henry-Amar M, Cosset JM, Devergie A, Girinsky T, Gluckman E. Increased incidence of solid malignant tumors after BMT for severe aplastic anemia. Blood 1991;78:277.

Chapter 67
White Blood Cell Disorders

Kenneth Weinberg

Inborn errors of granulocyte production or function are rare diseases that can be cured by bone marrow transplantation (BMT). Unlike the majority of patients with acquired neutrophil disorders, who are usually adults, patients with genetic disorders of the myeloid compartment typically present in childhood with serious bacterial or fungal infections (1,2). Cutaneous, oral, middle ear, and sinus infections are probably more common in the congenital white blood cell disorders than in patients who are neutropenic following chemotherapy and may be more difficult to treat because the neutropenia or dysfunction is sustained. Conventional treatment for myeloid disorders consists of aggressive management of established infections and use of prophylactic antibiotics to decrease the incidence of new infections (1–4). However, chronic or recurrent infections develop despite conventional therapy. The use of BMT or recombinant cytokine therapy to treat myeloid disorders now offers the opportunity to correct the underlying defects.

General Considerations

Role of BMT in the Therapy of White Blood Cell Disorders

Because BMT results in the engraftment of donor hematopoietic stem cells, it is a logical treatment of genetic defects of myeloid differentiation or function (5). If the defect in granulocyte number or function is intrinsic to the neutrophils, replacement of the patient's hematopoietic stem cells with those from a healthy donor will result in the production of normal myeloid progenitors and, ultimately, normal numbers of functional neutrophils (Table 67-1).

Timing of BMT

The timing of BMT is not clearly established for myeloid disorders. For some diseases, laboratory testing or previous experience can be used to predict the clinical course. For example, patients with the severe phenotype of CD11/CD18 deficiency have an extremely poor prognosis with conventional supportive care alone. BMT for these patients should be undertaken as soon as possible. Unfortunately, prognostication for other myeloid disorders is less clear-cut. Because the risks of BMT (nonengraftment, infection, graft-versus-host disease [GVHD]) are serious, there is a tendency to observe patients with myeloid disorders to determine the severity of the disease before making a decision regarding BMT. The potential risks of delays must also be weighed. First, it is possible that the patient will die from infection before definitive therapy is instituted. Second, the risks of BMT for myeloid disorders are increased in older compared with younger patients. In a survey of 14 European BMT centers treating immune deficiencies, age was a significant factor in predicting the outcome of BMT (6). Phagocytic defects were present in 14 of the 41 patients who did not have severe combined immunodeficiency disorders (SCID). Among the patients with defects other than SCID, disease-free survival was 60% for patients less than 2 years of age at the time of BMT, 66.7% for patients between 2 and 4 years of age, and 18.2% for patients older than 4 years of age. The potential risks and benefits of both BMT and conventional therapy should be discussed with families early in the course of leukocyte disorders. If conventional therapy is initially chosen as the preferred treatment, then BMT should be reconsidered promptly if serious or persistent complications develop.

Preparative Regimens

As for other genetic diseases, successful treatment of myeloid disorders with BMT requires administration of chemotherapy or radiation therapy, or both, to ablate the recipient hematopoietic stem cells and to suppress the immune system to allow engraftment of

Table 67-1.
White Blood Cell Disorders Treated with Bone Marrow Transplantation

Congenital neutropenias
Infantile agranulocytosis (Kostmann's syndrome)
Neutrophil actin defects
Neutrophil actin dysfunction
Deficient actin polymerization
Chronic granulomatous disease
CD11/18 deficiency
Chediak-Higashi syndrome

donor marrow (5,7). Initial attempts to treat myeloid disorders were not successful because marrow ablation was inadequate, allowing recovery of the patients' abnormal stem cells (8–10).

The first successful transplants for myeloid disorders used total body irradiation (TBI) as part of the conditioning regimen (7,11). Selection of a pretransplant conditioning regimen should take into account the potential developmental sequelae of the treatment. Because of the deleterious effects of TBI on central nervous system (CNS), skeletal, and endocrine development, regimens that contain only chemotherapy are preferable. The combination of busulfan (BU) and cyclophosphamide (CY) is the preferred conditioning regimen for transplantation of histocompatible marrow to patients with myeloid disorders. Additional immunosuppression may be required for patients who have become alloimmunized by transfusion or for those receiving marrow from haploidentical or matched unrelated donors (12,13).

The optimal dose of BU for pretransplant conditioning of children with white cell diseases remains unclear. Oral BU is absorbed and metabolized differently in young children than in adults (14,15). Early BMTs for genetic diseases used low doses of BU (e.g., 8 mg/kg) (16,17). However, recovery of autologous hematopoietic cells was observed with these low doses, suggesting that the failure to engraft was due to inadequate ablation of recipient hematopoiesis, not insufficient immunosuppression. Even when the BU dose was increased to 16 mg/kg, nonengraftment and autologous recovery were observed. In addition to the age-related differences in BU disposition, patients with myeloid disorders may have abnormalities of gastrointestinal function that could affect BU pharmacokinetics. For example, patients with chronic granulomatous disease frequently have granuloma formation in the stomach, which could interfere with motility or absorption (1–3). Therefore, patients with myeloid disorders receiving BU for pretransplant conditioning should have plasma BU levels measured to verify that the dose is adequate to achieve hematopoietic ablation.

Risks, Complications, and Alternate Treatments

The risks and complications of BMT may be modified by the nature of the primary myeloid defect and previous treatment. For example, patients with leukocyte adhesion deficiency may also have lymphoid defects (12,18). The resulting immune deficits may result in worsened pretransplant clinical status but may also decrease the risk of immunological rejection of the marrow graft. The type of primary defect may be important in determining the types of infections likely to complicate BMT. For example, chronic granulomatous disease results almost exclusively in infection with catalase-positive micro-organisms. Treatment received prior to BMT may have a negative effect on the outcome of BMT. Some patients have received white blood cell (WBC) transfusions to treat severe infections (3,19). WBC transfusions increase the risks of cytomegalovirus (CMV) infection and alloimmunization (20).

Therapy with recombinant cytokines is an alternate to BMT for some WBC disorders. Congenital neutropenias respond to recombinant human granulocyte colony stimulating factor (G-CSF) treatment, and chronic granulomatous disease can be ameliorated by recombinant interferon-gamma (INF-γ) therapy (21–24). Cytokine therapy is less risky than BMT but is noncurative and requires repeated administration of the cytokines. The long-term efficacy and complications of cytokine therapy are currently unknown.

Gene therapy approaches to WBC disorders have been proposed but have not been tested clinically. For congenital neutropenias, neutrophil actin defects, and Chediak-Higashi syndrome, gene therapy is not possible because the defective genes are unknown. Chronic granulomatous disease and CD11/18 deficiency are candidate diseases for gene therapy because the defective gene is known. In these diseases, transduction of normal copies of the genes into hematopoietic stem cells and appropriate expression in myeloid cells has not been demonstrated in vivo.

Congenital Neutropenias

Patients with mild (1,000–1,500 neutrophils/mm^3), moderate (500–1,000 neutrophils/mm^3), and severe (<500 neutrophils/mm^3)) neutropenia have been described (1). Attempts to classify congenital neutropenias have been limited by an inadequate understanding of the mechanisms for neutropenia. Some patients have severe neutropenia, with profound marrow and peripheral blood depletion of mature neutrophils (1). Patients with infantile (Kostmann's) agranulocytosis have severe neutropenia, with an apparent block in myeloid differentiation. Marrow examination of patients with Kostmann's agranulocytosis shows promyelocytes, myelocytes, eosinophils, and monocytes, but not mature neutrophils. Other neutropenic patients have periodic oscillations of the neutrophil count between normal and neutropenic levels (cyclic neutropenia). A group of ill-defined patients with mild to severe neutropenia and no characteristic marrow abnormality has been classified as having chronic benign neutropenia.

The frequency and severity of infection is directly related to the degree of neutropenia. Patients with mild to moderate neutropenia may be asymptomatic, or occasional skin or oral infections may develop. More significant infections develop in patients with severe neutropenia, including cellulitis, skin abscesses and furuncles, stomatitis and gingivitis, pneumonia, and sepsis (1). The course of even severe neutropenia can vary, probably because most patients with chronic neutropenia derive some degree of protection from circulating monocytes and lymphocytes. Pyogenic organisms cause most of the infections that develop in patients with inborn errors of neutrophil production.

Kostmann's agranulocytosis was the first myeloid disorder to be treated successfully by BMT (11). The first patient had severe neutropenia and infections with *Klebsiella pneumoniae, Staphylococcus aureus,* and *Pseudomonas aeruginosa.* BMT was performed at 20 months of age after conditioning with TBI and rabbit antithymocyte serum (ATS). Mild GVHD developed but the patient ultimately survived with completely normal neutrophil counts. The addition of TBI to the conditioning regimen illustrates the importance of adequate ablation of the recipient's hematopoietic system. A patient with Kostmann's agranulocytosis has also been treated successfully by BMT of human leukocyte antigen (HLA)–mismatched T-cell–depleted marrow (6).

Although BMT is an effective therapy for Kostmann's agranulocytosis, therapy with recombinant human G-CSF has supplanted BMT as the primary treatment. G-CSF therapy has been shown to increase neutrophil counts and to decrease the infectious complications in most patients (21). Patients with cyclic neutropenia have also shown improvement in WBC counts and clinical condition with G-CSF therapy (22), which is generally well tolerated with few serious side effects. Because of its efficacy and safety, G-CSF treatment should be front-line therapy in the treatment of patients with Kostmann's agranulocytosis. BMT should be considered in patients who fail to respond to G-CSF, have serious side effects, or who are unwilling or unable to comply with chronic G-CSF administration.

Neutrophil Actin Defects

In addition to defects in neutrophil production, patients have been described with inborn errors of neutrophil function. These patients are also susceptible to infection. Because the defects are intrinsic to the neutrophil, BMT from normal donors can correct the disorders.

In 1974, Boxer and colleagues (25) described a male infant with a defect in neutrophil actin, with diminished actin polymerization. Actin polymerization is required as the "motor" of the neutrophil and is essential for such activities as migration and degranulation. The patient had abnormal migration and particle ingestion. Analysis of the neutrophils from the mother and the father of the patient demonstrated that they both have abnormally low levels of actin filaments in their neutrophils (26). The data from the parents' leukocytes suggest that the primary defect is one of actin assembly, and the mode of inheritance is autosomal recessive. As a consequence of the defect, the patient had severe staphylococcal infections of skin and eyes, massive hepatosplenomegaly, and intestinal fistula formation.

The first patient described with actin dysfunction received a BMT after conditioning with CY, ATS, and procarbazine (9). There was no evidence of donor engraftment, and autologous recovery of his abnormal neutrophils developed. A second BMT was performed after conditioning with TBI, CY, ATS, and procarbazine. After the second BMT, engraftment was demonstrated cytogenetically and by correction of neutrophil function. However, the patient died 53 days after BMT from pneumonia and respiratory failure. Although unsuccessful, this transplant indicates the importance of pretransplant conditioning to ablate the abnormal stem cell in myeloid disorders.

A second type of defect of actin polymerization has been described and successfully treated by BMT. The child was a Tongan infant who presented at 2 months of age to Childrens Hospital in Los Angeles with severe ulcerative infection of the palate and tongue with *Candida tropicalis,* pulmonary infiltrates, and thrombocytopenia (27). His infections responded to treatment with amphotericin B and broad-spectrum antibiotics, but the thrombocytopenia persisted. Three of his 7 siblings had died of infection in infancy.

Analysis of the patient's neutrophils demonstrated multiple defects in neutrophil function (27), including failure to migrate randomly or to respond to chemotactic stimuli. Spreading, phagocytosis, and killing, which all depend on neutrophil motility, were also abnormal. Induction of actin polymerization by chemotactic factor was abnormal. Polyacrylamide gel analysis of neutrophil proteins showed increased amounts of a 47-kd protein and decreased amounts of an 89-kd protein. Both of his parents had increased amounts of the 47-kd protein and decreased amounts of the 89-kd protein in their neutrophils but normal chemotaxis, suggesting that the disease is autosomal recessively inherited. The disease is probably distinct from the original case of neutrophil actin dysfunction because gel electrophoresis was reportedly normal in the first patient. The patient was successfully engrafted with marrow from an HLA-identical sibling with normal neutrophil function. He was conditioned for BMT with BU (16 mg/kg), CY (200 mg/kg), and antithymocyte globulin (ATG). The patient's posttransplant course was complicated by CMV pneumonia and respiratory failure, which resolved with ganciclovir, intravenous immunoglobulin, and ventilatory support. Engraftment was confirmed by cytogenetic analysis and by normalization of the patient's neutrophil motility. The patient is now 4 years post-BMT and is thriving without further serious infections.

Currently, the therapeutic options for children with neutrophil actin defects are supportive care or BMT. On the basis of the severity of the infections, supportive care alone is unlikely to result in long-term survival. Therefore, BMT is the preferred treatment for these patients. Matched unrelated donor or haploidentical T-cell–depleted BMT should be considered for patients who lack a histocompatible sibling donor, although the transplant-associated mortality and potential for chronic GVHD will be higher. Future gene therapy will require identification of the primary defect and an understanding of the regulation and expression of the primary gene.

Chronic Granulomatous Disease

Chronic granulomatous disease is caused by a defect in the oxidase of phagocytic cells, including both neutrophils and monocytes (1–3,28). A variety of primary genetic defects leads to the phenotype of chronic granulomatous disease, resulting in abnormal function of NADPH oxidase, which is needed to generate superoxide, the reduced oxygen species used by phagocytic cells for killing of microbes. NADPH oxidase contains a membrane-bound heterodimeric complex, cytochrome b_{558}. After neutrophil activation, 2 cytosolic proteins translocate to the cell membrane and become associated with the cytochrome b_{558}. NADPH oxidase catalyzes the reduction of oxygen to superoxide. Patients with the X-linked form of chronic granulomatous disease have a variety of mutations of the 91-kd component of the cytochrome b_{558}. Other patients have autosomal dominant or recessive chronic granulomatous disease due to mutations of either the 22-kd component of the cytochrome b_{558} or of the 67 or 47 kd cytosolic components (28). The standard diagnostic test for chronic granulomatous disease detects oxidation of the dye, nitroblue tetrazolium (NBT).

Patients with chronic granulomatous disease have increased susceptibility to infection because of defective oxidase function. Infections with catalase-positive micro-organisms are most common because such organisms destroy any hydrogen peroxide they generate (1–3). In contrast, catalase-negative micro-organisms, such as *Streptococci*, are unable to destroy their own hydrogen peroxide. Phagocytic cells that have ingested catalase-negative micro-organisms utilize the hydrogen peroxide to kill the ingested micro-organism. Infection with *Staphylococcus aureus*, *Aspergillus* species, *Chromobacterium violaceum*, *Pseudomonas cepacia*, *Nocardia* species, and *Serratia marcescens* are common in these patients (3). The tendency toward infection with catalase-positive organisms must be considered in the supportive care of patients with chronic granulomatous disease undergoing BMT. Many of the species causing infection are rare and may be treated inadequately by routine broad-spectrum antibiotic regimens employed for other BMT recipients.

In addition to the infectious complications of chronic granulomatous disease, patients may have significant problems caused by widespread granuloma formation (1–3). Monocytes and macrophages in chronic granulomatous disease are also defective in oxidative killing. Micro-organisms that are ingested but not killed by macrophages may be sequestered within granulomas. The granulomas can cause severe obstructive lesions in the lungs, esophagus, stomach, and ureters. Chronic inflammation of the gums and mouth, lymphadenopathy, and liver abscesses are common.

The first attempts at BMT for chronic granulomatous disease were performed without TBI or BU to ablate recipient hematopoietic stem cells (8,10) and did not result in sustained hematopoietic engraftment. A patient who received BU (8 mg/kg) and CY (200 mg/kg) as pretransplant conditioning showed initial clinical improvement but did not achieve long-term engraftment, probably because of the low dose of BU employed (16). A 15-year-old patient with chronic granulomatous disease was completely engrafted after conditioning with TBI and ATS but died of chronic GVHD and interstitial pneumonitis (29). In a series from European transplant centers, none of the 3 patients transplanted for chronic granulomatous disease were successfully engrafted (6). One of the patients died and the other 2 had autologous recovery.

Therapy with recombinant human IFN-γ is a beneficial treatment for chronic granulomatous disease. A large randomized trial of IFN-γ in patients with a variety of subtypes of chronic granulomatous disease demonstrated decreased incidence and severity of infection (23). The beneficial effect of IFN-γ is not due to an improvement of neutrophil NADPH oxidase function but may be a result of monocyte stimulation (24). Side effects of IFN-γ have been minimal in the reported studies.

A trial of IFN-γ is indicated in all patients with chronic granulomatous disease. Lack of clinical response, occurrence of serious side effects, or inability to comply with chronic IFN-γ therapy are possible indications for BMT. Some patients may be unwilling to accept the risks of BMT, whereas others may choose to have a BMT because they find chronic, noncurative therapy with IFN-γ unacceptable. BMT is most likely to be successful in chronic granulomatous disease if undertaken before significant organ damage has developed. No data are currently available on whether IFN-γ treatment prior to transplantation will increase the risks of BMT complications (e.g., graft rejection).

CD11/18 Deficiency

After neutrophils have migrated to an area of inflammation, adherence to target cells is required before killing can occur. A heterodimeric surface glycoprotein molecule, CD11/CD18, mediates neutrophil adherence (18,30). The CD11 molecule is a 150 to 180-kd glycoprotein expressed by neutrophils, monocytes, lymphocytes and natural killer cells. There are 3 known forms of the CD11 molecule (CD11a, CD11b, CD11c), which are differentially expressed by hematopoietic cells. The CD11 molecule is associated on the cell surface of leukocytes with the 94-kd CD18 molecule. CD11/CD18 complexes form the leukocyte integrin family of surface proteins. The complex of CD11a/CD18 is also called LFA-1, whereas the CD11b/CD18 complex is also known as Mo1. A third type of CD11 molecule, CD11c, has been described on neutrophils and monocytes, but its function in adhesion is less well characterized than that of CD11a/CD18 and CD11b/CD18. The CD11/CD18 complex is necessary for leukocyte adherence to target tissues via interactions with the ICAM-1 adhesion molecules. The CD11b/CD18 complex is also the complement receptor type 3 (CR3), which binds to C3bi, a stable opsonin. C3bi binding by neutrophil CD11b/CD18 is an important stimulus of degranulation and the oxidative burst.

Since 1979, patients have been described whose leukocytes lack expression of CD11/CD18 (18). The primary defect in these patients is an abnormal gene for the CD18 molecule. Patients with deficiency of CD18 have defective assembly and surface expression of the Mo1 and LFA-1 complexes. The term *leukocyte adhesion deficiency* (LAD) has been proposed for patients lacking CD18, because the defect of CD18 results in defects of adhesion in all leukocytes (18). Patients with LAD have been divided into 2 groups, based on the severity of the defect in CD11/CD18 expression (18,31). Some patients have complete absence of the CD11/CD18 complex (severe LAD). Others have low baseline levels of CD11/18, which are not properly up-regulated by normal stimuli, such as C5b or chemotactic peptides (moderate LAD). The severity of the defect tends to be similar within families (18).

Complications of LAD include infections and poor wound healing (1–3,18,31). Many patients have a history of delayed separation of the umbilical cord. Leukocytosis is frequently present, but infected sites lack neutrophils. Skin infections commonly develop, which are characteristically ulcerative and slow to heal (pyoderma gangrenosum). Oral and dental infections are also common. The infections can become invasive, resulting in peritonitis from perirectal infections, head and neck abscesses from oral infections, and sepsis. Unlike chronic granulomatous disease, formation of granulomas has not been observed. Healing of surgical wounds has been poor in several patients. Because the CD11/CD18 complex is also needed for lymphocyte function, patients with LAD would be expected to be immunodeficient. Consistent with this hypothesis, one patient has been reported to have died of disseminated picornavirus infection, and aseptic meningitis has been observed in 3 others (18).

The risk of infection in LAD is related to the severity of the CD11/CD18 defect (18,31). Patients with severe deficiency of CD11/CD18 have a higher risk of dying in infancy than patients with moderate deficiency. The beneficial effects of moderate deficiency are not absolute—2 affected siblings of a moderately deficient patient died at ages 19 and 32 years (18).

BMT is a potentially curative treatment for LAD. The first patient to be transplanted with histocompatible marrow was a 15-month-old girl who received conditioning with BU (8 mg/kg) and CY (200 mg/kg) (17). The patient did not have successful engraftment, probably because of the inadequate dose of BU employed. The patient was successfully engrafted at age 27 months following administration of CY and TBI. The patient's neutrophil, monocyte, and natural killer cell function normalized. A second patient received a BMT at age 3 months following conditioning with BU (16 mg/kg) and CY (200 mg/kg) (17). Although the patient engrafted, she died from severe chronic GVHD, obstructive bronchitis, and respiratory failure. One of 2 other patients with LAD was engrafted successfully with histocompatible marrow (6). Three subsequent patients, who received HLA-haploidentical or two-locus-mismatched marrow after T-cell depletion, have been reported (12). The patients were conditioned with either BU (16 mg/kg), CY (200 mg/kg), and ATG (one patient), or BU (16 mg/kg), CY (200 mg/kg), and etoposide (900 mg/m^2) (2 patients). The first patient had autologous recovery but engrafted after a second BMT with CY and TBI conditioning. Engraftment of donor marrow in all 3 patients resulted in normalization of neutrophil adhesion. Because LFA-1 is probably involved in graft rejection, the authors of the report on mismatched BMT hypothesize that patients with LAD may not have a high risk of graft rejection with T-cell–depleted mismatched marrow (12).

The alternative to BMT is supportive care. Treatment with IFN-γ in one patient did not result in improvement in leukocyte adhesion or clinical status (32). Because of the severity of the disease, BMT with either histoincompatible parental or histocompatible unrelated donor marrow should be considered. The occurrence of death in the second and third decades of life in patients with moderate deficiency suggests that such patients should be considered for histocompatible BMT.

The cloning of the CD18 gene has permitted research on gene therapy approaches to LAD. Gene therapy will require efficient transduction of a normal CD18 gene into human hematopoietic stem cells and appropriate levels of lineage-specific expression. Successful transfer of the CD18 gene into lymphocytes from patients with LAD and murine marrow cells has been demonstrated (33–35). Clinical application will depend on future studies of CD18 gene transfer into the hematopoietic stem cells of these patients.

Chediak-Higashi Syndrome

Chediak-Higashi syndrome is a generalized membrane disorder in which the most serious pathology is hematological (1,36). Patients with Chediak-Higashi syndrome have abnormal neutrophils, monocytes, lymphocytes, and platelets (37). Neutrophils and myeloid precursors have abnormal giant azurophilic and specific granules (36). The abnormal myeloid precursors have poor survival in the marrow, resulting in moderate neutropenia (38). The neutrophils that enter the circulation have defective chemotaxis, adherence, degranulation, and killing. Giant granules are also found in the monocytes, lymphocytes, natural killer cells, and platelets and are probably associated with the defects in monocyte-mediated killing, cell-mediated immune functions, natural killer cell cytotoxicity and clotting (39–42).

In addition to the hematological abnormalities, these patients have abnormalities of the CNS and other neural crest–derived tissues. Cells in the CNS, like the abnormal blood cells, contain giant granules. Muscle weakness and abnormal motor neuron conduction, ataxia, and seizures develop in older patients with Chediak-Higashi syndrome (43). Melanocytes contain giant melanosomes, resulting in the characteristic partial albinism of affected patients (44). An autosomal recessive disease resembling Chediak-Higashi syndrome has been described in several species of animals, such as the beige mouse (45).

Clinically, the course of Chediak-Higashi syndrome can be divided into a chronic stable phase and a rapidly progressive accelerated phase, which is fatal (1,24). During the stable phase, patients are susceptible to gram-positive and gram-negative bacterial infections, especially *Staphylococcus aureus* infections. Management of the stable phase is based on aggressive diagnosis and treatment of infection. In some patients, administration of high doses of ascorbic acid can improve neutrophil function and decrease the severity or frequency of infection (46). The accelerated phase is marked by a lymphohistiocytic proliferation, which resembles the viral-associated hemophagocytic syndrome (47). Lymphohistiocytic infiltration of the marrow and reticuloendothelial system in the accelerated phase results in pancytopenia. In addition, patients have fevers, wasting, organomegaly, and severe infections. Although the accelerated phase is fatal, there is no evidence that the lymphohistiocytic proliferation is comprised of malignant cells. Treatment with glucocorticoids or vincristine has not been effective in controlling the accelerated phase.

In 1976, BMT from normal histocompatible congenic donors was shown to cure the hematological abnormalities of beige mice (48). The first BMT for Chediak-Higashi syndrome in a human was described in 1983 (49,50). The patient first received a BMT during accelerated phase after pretransplant conditioning with CY alone. Sustained hematopoietic engraftment was not achieved. A second BMT after conditioning with CY and TBI resulted in normalization of the patient's hematological function, immune and natural killer cell function, and clinical status. Successful BMT of 4 other patients with histocompatible donors has been reported; one other patient died after transplantation (6). Two attempts at haploidentical BMT for Chediak-Higashi syndrome were unsuccessful (6). Two patients in accelerated phase were transplanted successfully with marrow from matched unrelated donors (13). One patient was conditioned with CY and TBI, whereas the other patient received CY, TBI, etoposide, and ATG.

BMT is the recommended therapy for patients in accelerated phase of Chediak-Higashi syndrome. Because of the poor outcome of conventional therapy of the accelerated phase, both histocompatible and haploidentical BMT are justified. Matched unrelated donor transplants should be considered, but some patients in accelerated phase may not survive long enough to find a donor and to arrange for BMT. Histocompatible BMT can also be recommended for patients in stable phase. The question of whether haploidentical or unrelated donor BMT should be performed for patients in stable phase is problematic. Currently, there is no prognostic test for prediction of the length of stable phase in individual patients. Therefore, it is difficult to assess whether the higher risks of nonhistocompatible BMT are justified in patients who otherwise may survive for years in stable phase. There is insufficient experience to determine the long-term neurological outcome of patients with Chediak-Higashi syndrome following successful BMT.

Conclusions

Disorders of neutrophil production and function are debilitating, potentially life-threatening genetic diseases that can be cured by BMT. Factors contributing to the outcome of BMT include the type of primary WBC defect, the age and condition of the patient at the time of BMT, the conditioning regimen, and the degree of histocompatibility between donor and recipient. BMT is successful when pretransplant conditioning is adequate to provide ablation of abnormal hematopoietic stem cells and adequate immunosuppression. BU dose must be based on the patient's age and on absorption. BMT from histoincompatible donors requires more intensive pretransplant immunosuppressive therapy. BMT carries the risks of nonengraftment and severe GVHD, especially when nonhistocompatible donor bone marrow is used. The development of alternative therapies (e.g., G-CSF for Kostmann's agranulocytosis or INF-γ for chronic granulomatous disease) has dramatically changed the treatment for some patients with myeloid disorders. The conundrum in the treatment of myeloid disorders, as for other genetic diseases, is that delaying BMT may decrease the immediate risks to the patient but ultimately increase the risks of BMT.

References

1. Curnutte JT, Boxer L. Disorders of granulopoiesis and granulocyte function. In: Nathan DG, Oski FA, eds. Hematology of infancy and childhood. Philadelphia: W.B. Sanders, 1987;797–847.
2. Yang KD, Hill HR. Neutrophil function disorders: Pathophysiology, prevention and therapy. J Pediatr 1991;119:343–354.
3. Gallin JI, Buescher ES, Seligmann BE, Nath J, Gaither T, Katz P. Recent advances in chronic granulomatous disease. Ann Intern Med, 1983;99:657–674.
4. Jacobs RF, Wilson CD. Activity of antibiotics in chronic granulomatous disease leukocytes. Pediatr Res 1983; 17:916–919.
5. Parkman R. The application of bone marrow transplantation to the treatment of genetic disease. Science 1986;232:1373–1378.
6. Fischer A, Friedrick W, Levinsky R, et al. Bone-marrow transplantation for immunodeficiencies and osteopetrosis: European survey, 1968–1985. Lancet 1986;2:1080–1084.
7. Parkman R, Rapport JM, Hellman S, et al. Busulfan and total body irradiation as antihematopoietic stem cell agents in the preparation of patients with congenital bone marrow disorders for allogeneic bone marrow transplantation. Blood 1984;64:852–857.
8. Goudemand J, Aussens R, Delams-Marsalet Y, Farriaux JP, Fontaine G. Attempt to treat a case of chronic

familial granulomatous disease by allogeneic bone marrow transplantation. Arch Fr Pediatr 1976;33:121–129.

9. Camitta BM, Quesenberry PJ, Parkman R, et al. Bone marrow transplantation for an infant with neutrophil dysfunction. Exp Hematol 1977;5:109–116.
10. Foroozonfar N, Hobbs JR, Hugh-Jones D, et al. Bone-marrow transplant from an unrelated donor for chronic granulomatous disease. Lancet 1977;1:210–213.
11. Rappeport JM, Parkman R, Newburger, Camitta BM, Chusid MJ. Correction of infantile agranulocytosis (Kostmann's Syndrome) by allogeneic bone marrow transplantation. Am J Med 1980;68:605–609.
12. Le Deist F, Blanche S, Keable H, et al. Successful HLA nonidentical bone marrow transplantation in three patients with the leukocyte adhesion deficiency. Blood 1989;74:512–516.
13. Filipovich AH, Shapiro RS, Ramsay NKC, et al. Unrelated donor bone marrow transplantation for correction of lethal congenital immunodeficiencies. Blood 1992;80:270–276.
14. Grochow LB, Krivit W, Whitley CB, Blazar B. Busulfan disposition in children. Blood 1990;75:1723–1727.
15. Vassal G, Deroussent A, Challine D, et al. Is 600 mg/m^2 the appropriate dosage of busulfan in children undergoing bone marrow transplantation? Blood 1992;79:2475.
16. Kamani N, August CS, Douglas SD, Burkey E, Etzioni A, Lischner HW. Bone marrow transplantation in chronic granulomatous disease. J Pediatr 1984;105:42–46.
17. Fischer A, Descamps-Latscha B, Gerota I, et al. Bone-marrow transplantation for inborn error of phagocytic cells associated with defective adherence, chemotaxis, and oxidative response during opsonised particle phagocytosis. Lancet 1983;2:473–476.
18. Anderson DC, Springer TA. Leukocyte adhesion deficiency: An inherited defect in the Mac-1, LFA-1, and pl50,95 glycoproteins. Ann Rev Med 1987;38:175–194.
19. Yomtovian R, Abramson J, Quie P, McCullough J. Granulocyte transfusion therapy in chronic granulomatous disease: report of a patient and review of the literature. Transfusion 1981;21:739–743.
20. Hersman J, Meyers JD, Thomas ED, Buckner CD, Clift R. The effect of granulocyte transfusions on the incidence of cytomegalovirus infection after allogeneic marrow transplantation. Ann Intern Med 1982;96:149–152.
21. Boxer LA, Hutchinson R, Emerson S. Recombinant human granulocyte—colony stimulating factor in the treatment of patients with neutropenia. Clin Immunol Immunopathol 1992;62:539–546.
22. Hammond WP, Price TH, Souza LM, Dale DC. Treatment of cyclic neutropenia with granulocyte colony-stimulating factor. N Engl J Med 1989;320:1306–1311.
23. The International Chronic Granulomatous Disease Cooperative Study Group. A controlled trial of interferon gamma to prevent infection in chronic granulomatous disease. N Engl J Med 1991;324:509–516.
24. Woodman RC, Erikson RW, Rae T, Jaffe HS, Curnutte JT. Prolonged recombinant interferon-γ therapy in chronic granulomatous disease. Evidence against enhanced neutrophil oxidase activity. Blood 1992;79: 1558–1562.
25. Boxer LA, Hedley-White T, Stossel TP. Neutrophil actin dysfunction and abnormal neutrophil behavior. N Engl J Med 1974;291:1093–1099.
26. Southwick FS, Dabiri GA, Stossel TP. Neutrophil actin dysfunction is a genetic disorder associated with partial impairment of neutrophil actin assembly in three family members. J Clin Invest 1988;82:1525–1531.
27. Coates TD, Torkildson JC, Torres M, Church JA, Howard TH. An inherited defect of neutrophil motility and microfilamentous cytoskeleton associated with abnormalities in 47-Kd and 89-Kd proteins. Blood 1991;78:1338–1346.
28. Curnutte JT. Classification of chronic granulomatous disease. Hematol/Oncol Clin North Am 1988;2:241–252.
29. Rappeport JM, Newburger PE, Goldblum RM, Goldman AS, Nathan DG, Parkman R. Allogeneic bone marrow transplantation for chronic granulomatous disease. J Pediatr 1982;101:951–956.
30. Arnaout MA. Structure and function of the leukocyte adhesion molecules CD11/CD18. Blood 1990;75:1037–1050.
31. Anderson DC, Schmalsteig FC, Finegold MJ, et al. The severe and moderate phenotypes of heritable Mac-1, LFA-1 deficiency: their quantitative definition and relation to leukocyte dysfunction and clinical features. J Infect Dis 1985;152:668–669.
32. Weening RS, Bredius RGM, Vomberg PP, et al. Recombinant human interferon-γ treatment in severe leucocyte adhesion deficiency. Eur J Pediatr 1992;151:103–107.
33. Wilson J, Ping AJ, Krauss JC, et al. Correction of CD18-deficient lymphocytes by retrovirus-mediate gene transfer. Science 1990;248:1413–1416.
34. Hibbs ML, Wardlaw AJ, Stacker SA, et al. Transfection of cells from patients with leukocyte adhension deficiency with an integrin beta subunit (CD18) restores lymphocyte function-associated antigen-1 expression and function. J Clin Invest 1990;85:674–681.
35. Krauss JC, Mayo-Bond LA, Rogers CE, et al. An in vivo model of gene therapy for leukocyte adhesion deficiency. J Clin Invest 1991;88:1412–1417.
36. White JG, Clawson CC. The Chediak-Higashi syndrome: the nature of the giant neutrophil granules and their interactions with cytoplasm and foreign particulates. I. Progressive enlargement of the massive inclusions in mature neutrophils. Am J Pathol 1980;98:151–196.
37. Blume RS, Wolff S. The Chediak-Higashi syndrome: studies in four patients and a review of the literature. Medicine 1972;51:247–280.
38. Blume RS, Bennett JM, Yankee RA, et al. Defective granulocyte regulation in Chediak-Higashi syndrome. N Engl J Med 1968;279:1009–1015.
39. Gallin JI, Klimerman JA, Padgett GA, et al. Defective mononuclear leukocyte chemotaxis in the Chediak-Higashi syndrome of humans, mink and cattle. Blood 1975;45:863–870.
40. Klein M, Roder J, Haliotis T, et al. Chediak-Higashi gene in humans. II. The selectivity of the defect in natural-killer and antibody dependent cell-mediated cytotoxicity function. J Exp Med 1980;151:1049–1058.
41. Nair MPN, Gray RH, Boxer LA, et al. Deficiency of inducible suppressor cell activity in the Chediak-Higashi syndrome. Am J Hematol 1987;26:55–66.
42. Buchanan GB, Handin RI. Platelet function in the Chediak-Higashi syndrome. Blood 1976;47:941–948.
43. Pettit RE, Berdal KG, Chediak-Higashi syndrome. Neurologic appearance. Arch Neurol 1984;41:1001–1007.
44. Witop CJ Jr, Quevedo WC Jr. Albinism and other disorders of pigment metabolism. In: Stanbury JB, Wyngaarden JB, Fredrickson DS, et al, eds. The meta-

bolic basis of inherited disease, ed 5. New York: McGraw-Hill, 1983:301.
45. Padget EA. The Chediak-Higashi syndrome. Adv Vet Sci 1968;12:239–284.
46. Boxer LA, Watanabe AM, Rister M. Correction of leukocyte function in Chediak-Higashi syndrome by ascorbate. N Engl J Med 1976;295:1041–1045.
47. Rubin CM, Burke BA, McKenna RW, et al. The accelerated phase of Chediak-Higashi syndrome. An expression of the virus-associated hemophagocytic syndrome. Cancer 1985;56:524–530.
48. Kazmierowski JA, Elin RJ, Reynolds HY, et al. Chediak-Higashi syndrome; reversal of increased susceptibility to infection by bone marrow transplantation. Blood 1976;47:555–559.
49. Griscelli C, Virelizier JL. Bone marrow transplantation in a patient with Chediak-Higashi syndrome. In: Wedgewood RJ, Rosen FS, Paul NW, eds. Primary immunodeficiency diseases. New York: Alan R. Liss, 1983:333.
50. Virelizier JL, Lagrue A, Durandy A. Reversal of natural killer defect in a patient with Chediak-Higashi syndrome after bone marrow transplantation. N Engl J Med 1982;306:1055–1056.

Chapter 68
Bone Marrow Transplantation in Fanconi's Anemia

Eliane Gluckman and Jill Hows

Fanconi's anemia (FA) was originally described as an autosomal recessive disorder characterized by progressive pancytopenia, diverse congenital abnormalities, and increased predisposition to malignancy. The gene frequency is approximately 1:200 to 300 in the European and North American populations (1–3).

The FA phenotype is so variable that diagnosis based on clinical manifestation alone is difficult and often unreliable (4,5). Hypersensitivity of FA cells to random chromatid breakage when stressed by DNA cross-linking agents provides a unique marker for the FA phenotype (6–9). Study of stressed chromatid breakage can be used both prenatally and postnatally for diagnosis of FA (10–16), and different rates of removal of DNA cross-links can be shown by electron microscopy (17). These tests are not sufficiently reliable for determining the complementation groups of a given patient, nor is there any apparent correlation between clinical phenotype and genetic class.

It has been shown that affected cells are highly sensitive to oxidative stress (18). Cultured FA cells also exhibit a highly specific endogenous cell cycle defect with a G2 phase of approximately twice the normal length (19). This defect is oxygen-sensitive in FA fibroblasts and can be exacerbated by exposure of these cells to low oxygen concentrations (20).

Two genetic complementation groups were originally described, which differed in their phenotype (21,22). FA cell lines can currently be classified into 4 different complementation groups, which correspond to phenotypic differences resulting in variable rates of recovery of DNA synthesis after treatment with DNA cross-linking agents in culture (22–24). These differences provided evidence for at least 4 FA genes. One of these genes, designated FACC, has been cloned and resides on chromosome 9 (24,25). Also, a genetic linkage study supports the provisional assignment of an FA gene to chromosome 20q (26).

Progressive pancytopenia and marrow hypoplasia are the main hematological features of FA. Bone marrow studies including clonogenic assays for burst-forming units erythroid (BFU-E), colony forming units of granulocyte and macrophage lineages (CFU-GM), and long-term marrow cultures, show a decrease of progenitor cell numbers, with no evidence of a gross microenvironmental defect (27). These findings suggest the main mechanism of aplasia is related to a stem-cell defect.

Although the molecular expression of the *c-kit* proto-oncogene and *kit* ligand in long-term marrow culture is normal in patients with FA, there is evidence for a subtle microenvironmental defect consisting of dysregulation of cytokines, such as interleukin-6 (IL-6), tumor necrosis factor (TNF), and GM-CSF, which may contribute to marrow failure (28,29). It is not yet known if in vivo administration of these cytokines will correct the aplasia.

Another characteristic of the disease is the development of myelodysplastic syndrome and leukemia (30). Bone marrow clonal cytogenetic abnormalities have been reported in some cases of leukemic transformation, as well as in patients lacking morphological evidence of leukemia at the time of the study. Several patients have been reported in whom acute myeloid leukemia (AML) or myelodysplastic syndrome were presenting hematological features, with a high frequency of monosomy 7 and duplications involving 11q. There have been no reports of acute lymphoblastic leukemia (ALL) in FA. An analysis of the International Fanconi Anemia Registry has shown a 9% incidence of myelodysplasia and leukemia. The mean age at leukemic transformation was 15 years. These patients had very poor prognosis; none were reported to achieve long-term complete remission. It is not known whether FA heterozygotes are at increased risk for development of leukemia because there is no reliable test for identifying heterozygotes in the population. The genetic defect in FA that predisposes to leukemia is unknown but is probably related to the chromosomal instability and to increased sensitivity to DNA cross-linking agents.

Nonhematological malignant tumors have been reported in FA, which are mainly hepatic and not always induced by androgen therapy, and adenocarcinoma of the oral cavity has also been described (4,5,29,31).

Diagnosis

Clinical Features

FA is usually diagnosed around the age of 5 to 10 years when the first hematological symptoms arise. It is characterized by progressive cytopenias with macrocytosis. Marrow aspiration and trephine biopsy at the time of diagnosis often show mild hypoplasia, with dyserythropoiesis. These findings are usually associated with a significant increase of hemoglobin F levels detected by electrophoretic studies. Initially, aplasia is usually responsive to low-dose androgenic steroids (e.g., oxymetholone, 0.5–1.0 mg/kg/day). Many patients can be maintained transfusion-free on oxymetholone for several years, with minimal side effects. Despite this maintenance, progressive pancytopenia occurs in most patients who, without bone marrow transplantation (BMT), die before adulthood of hemorrhage, infection, liver tumors, or leukemia.

The diagnosis of FA is straightforward when there is a family history of aplasia or when the typical malformations are present. The most frequent malformations are thumb and radial abnormalities, growth retardation, abnormal skin pigmentation with café au lait spots and melanoderma, kidney or urinary tract abnormalities, microphthalmia, small face, and cardiac malformations (32). The phenotype is variable from patient to patient and within the same family.

Approximately one third of patients with FA do not present with these classic features. In a study of the International Fanconi Anemia Registry, it was reported that 7% of patients were at least 16 years of age at the time of diagnosis. We have recently seen a man aged 31 years presenting for the first time with FA (Hows J. Unpublished data). This finding indicates that the diagnosis should be considered in younger adults as well as children presenting with aplastic anemia. Approximately 16% of patients with FA have normal stature, with minimal or absent associated malformations.

Other constitutional aplastic anemias may mimic FA (e.g., dyskeratosis congenita [33], Schwachman-Diamond syndrome, and xeroderma pigmentosa) (Table 68-1).

Table 68-1.
Clinical and Genetic Features of Fanconi's Anemia Contrasted with Other Inherited Bone Marrow Failure Syndromes

Disorder	*Inheritance*	*Associated Abnormalities*
Fanconi's anemia	Autosomal recessive	Described in text
Dyskeratosis congenita	Sex-linked recessive (sometimes autosomal recessive)	Nail and skin atrophy; skin cancer
Schwachman syndrome	Autosomal recessive	Exocrine pancreatic abnormalities; short stature
Xeroderma Pigmentosa	Autosomal recessive	Skin sensitivity to ultraviolet light; skeletal abnormalities
Late onset aplasia with proximal radioulnar fusion	Autosomal dominant	Aplasia in adult life; restricted pronation and supination of forearms

Diagnostic Tests

FA can be confirmed by in vitro testing. Diagnosis can be made by demonstration of spontaneous chromatid breaks in preparations of phytohemagglutinin-stimulated peripheral blood lymphocytes. In some patients with FA, spontaneous breaks do not occur. Therefore, in all patients, blood lymphocytes must be incubated with a DNA cross-linking agent, such as diepoxybutane (9), in parallel with a normal control sample to look for stress-induced chromatid breaks. Cytogenetic preparations may show chromatid breaks, gaps, fragmentation, and triradial and quadriradial figures (Figure 68-1). Other agents used in vitro to increase chromatid breakage include mitomycin C and nitrogen mustard (10). Because cytogenetics are not always easy to interpret, it is essential to perform the test in an experienced laboratory on patient and donor blood lymphocytes before BMT. Identification of FA in a patient with severe aplasia influences the method of pretransplant conditioning and graft-versus-host disease (GVHD) prophylaxis, as well as the advice given to the family. A simpler method of diagnosis has been described (34) based on the observation that addition of nitrogen mustard modifies the cell cycle due to an accumulation of cells in the G2/M phase. The method consists of treating FA cells with nitrogen mustard and comparing the DNA content of these cells with untreated FA cells, cells from normal subjects, and patients with other forms of aplastic anemia. In this simple test, cells are stained with the DNA dye, propidium iodide, followed by flow cytometric analysis of the cell cycle. Preliminary analysis has shown good correlation with classic cytogenetic results. Because this method can be standardized for use in routine laboratories, diagnosis of FA will be simplified, thus leading to more accurate data on the frequency of the condition.

Initial Management

In contrast to patients with acquired aplastic anemia, patients with FA usually show an excellent initial response to low-dose androgens. Treatment with oxymetholone (0.5–1.0 mg/kg/day) is sufficient, and patients can be maintained for months to years on doses as small as 0.25 mg/kg on alternate days. It is important to check marrow cytology and cytogenetics regularly to detect leukemic transformation. Liver function tests should be monitored to anticipate hepatic toxicity of androgen therapy. Although the exact incidence of liver adenoma or adenocarcinoma is not well documented, regular liver scans and measurement of blood alphafetoprotein levels are good early indicators of hepatic malignancy. It is likely that the hepatic toxicity of androgens is rare except when high doses are used for

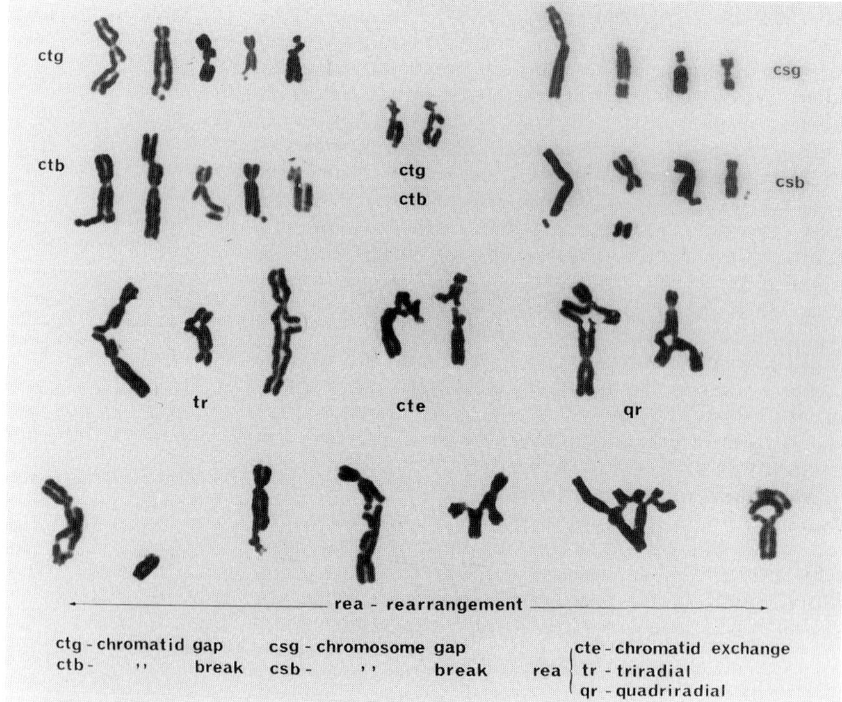

Figure 68-1. A typical karyotype from a patient with Fanconi's anemia. Examples of chromatid and chromosome gaps and breaks are shown, as well as chromatid exchange and triradial and quadroradial rearrangements.

prolonged periods. The existence of liver adenoma is not a contraindication to BMT, as tumor regression has been observed after androgens are discontinued (35).

Because FA is ultimately a fatal disease, it is reasonable to advise early BMT if there is a cytogenetically normal human leukocyte antigen (HLA)–identical sibling. In patients with mild hypoplasia, easily controlled with low-dose androgens, BMT can be planned electively, provided the patient is monitored routinely. There is a subset of very mildly affected patients with stable disease who do not require androgen therapy in whom BMT may safely be delayed for months or even years.

BMT for Fanconi's Anemia

Conditioning

In contrast to patients with acquired aplastic anemia, patients with FA are abnormally sensitive to high-dose cyclophosphamide (CY) (50 mg/kg/day for 4 days) used in BMT protocols for acquired aplastic anemia. Five patients with FA treated with high-dose CY have been reported, with only one long-term survivor. The other 4 patients died early after BMT of severe skin toxicity, gastrointestinal hemorrhage, hemorrhagic cystitis, and infection. It was postulated that the abnormal sensitivity to alkylating agents was the in vivo equivalent of the increased sensitivity of FA cells in vitro to DNA cross-linking agents (36).

The effect of CY metabolites was studied on chromosomes of patients with FA, their parents, and healthy controls subjects. A high susceptibility of FA cells was observed when low concentrations of serum from a CY-treated patient were added to phytohemagglutamin A (PHA)–stimulated lymphocyte cultures. No effect was observed with comparable concentrations on cells from FA heterozygotes or control subjects (8). It was concluded from this study that caution must be exercised in the use of alkylating agents in patients with FA. Sensitivity was particularly marked in tissues with a high rate of cell turnover, such as bladder and gut epithelia. Because the reduction of CY to 100 mg/kg in the conditioning protocol did not reduce toxicity, studies were conducted to explore the use of doses of CY ranging from a total dose of 20 to 40 mg/kg (5–10 mg/kg/day for 4 successive days).

Other components of the conditioning régimen have also been studied in vitro. Procarbazine and its azo derivative were found to be much weaker inducers of sister chromatid exchanges and weaker inducers of DNA cross-linkage than CY (37). It was concluded from this study that procarbazine could be used safely for BMT in patients with FA, but there are no clinical data to support this hypothesis (37). The toxicity of other drugs commonly used in conditioning regimes for leukemia, such as cytosine arabinoside, busulfan (BU), and etoposide, have not been studied on FA cells.

Irradiation is known to increase the number of chromosome breaks in FA cells, but to a lesser extent than alkylating agents (38,39). Lymphocytes from patients with FA exposed to 1 Gy irradiation show a higher rate of chromosome breaks per cells than normal control lymphocytes ($P<0.01$). An in vivo test of radiosensitivity and cell repair as a predictor of a patient's response to irradiation for BMT conditioning was described more than a decade ago (40,41). Cell repair was evaluated by comparing the reaction of the skin to a single dose of irradiation with the reaction after irradiation given in 2 equal fractions separated by an interval of 3 to 4 hours. Cell repair was considered normal if the skin reaction to a single 10-Gy dose of irradiation was similar to that of a 2 × 6 Gy fractionated dose. The most consistent abnormality was a delay in the peak skin reaction, ranging from 40 to 55 days in comparison with 30 days in normal control subjects. The second abnormality was an increased sensitivity to a single dose of 10 Gy irradiation. As a result of these studies, it was suggested that all patients with FA should receive a reduced dose of thoracoabdominal irradiation (5 Gy) and that there was no need for fractionation. To decrease further the toxicity of the conditioning regimen, cyclosporine (CSP) alone was given for prophylaxis of GVHD. Methotrexate (MTX) was not given because of its toxicity to mucosa, lung, and liver.

Results of BMT with Matched Sibling Donors

Paris Experience

The largest single center experience of BMT in patients with FA has been accumulated in Paris. Since the first studies of the toxic effect of high-dose CY, 34 patients have been transplanted using an HLA-identical sibling donor and a conditioning regimen with 20 mg/kg CY and 5 Gy thoracoabdominal irradiation. Thirty-one patients received a BMT and 3 cryopreserved cord blood cells (42,43). Currently, 25 patients (81%) are alive and well, with a follow-up ranging from 3 months to 11 years (median follow-up, 4 yr) (Figure 68-2).

Clinical Characteristics of Recipients and Donors of Matched Sibling BMT for FA

The median age of the BMT recipients was 9 years (range, 4–19 yr); most had typical malformations and had been previously transfused. All patients had received androgens or corticosteroids. Typical cytogenetic abnormalities enhanced by incubation of lymphocytes with DNA cross-linking agents were present in all patients. Two patients had additional clonal abnormalities as possible markers of leukemic transformation. These 2 patients received 40 mg/kg CY instead of 20 mg/kg. All donors were studied for the absence of malformations, the normality of blood counts, and the absence of chromosome breaks on cytogenetic analysis.

Results of Identical Sibling BMT

The patients received a mean cell dose of 4.9×10^8 nucleated cells/kg (range, $2.3–9.8 \times 10^8$/kg). The

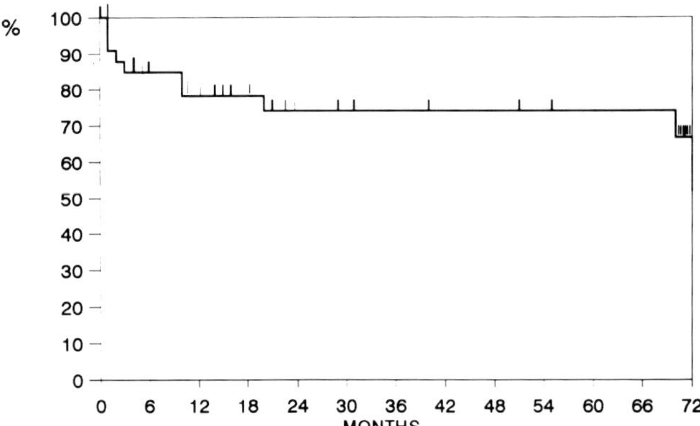

Figure 68-2. Actuarial survival curve for human leukocyte antigen–identical sibling bone marrow transplantation for Fanconi's anemia at Paris using a low-dose cyclophosphamide and thoracoabdominal irradiation protocol.

conditioning regimen was well tolerated except for esophagitis, which was severe in the first patients but which was prevented subsequently by the use of H_2-antagonists.

Despite the low dose conditioning regimen, only one patient rejected his graft and died on day +40 of *Candida* sepsis. This patient had severe infection at the time of BMT. Three patients had transient mixed hemopoietic chimerism soon after BMT. On long-term follow-up, all patients tested had a complete hematological reconstitution with donor cells and absence of chromosome breaks on cytogenetic analysis.

Acute GVHD, grade II to IV, was observed in 14 patients (47%). Chronic GVHD was observed in 12 of 26 patients surviving more than 120 days. Chronic GVHD was limited to skin in 10 patients and was more extensive, involving other organs, in 2. On long-term follow-up, none of the patients had sequelae of chronic GVHD. Among surviving patients, one has asymptomatic human immunodeficiency virus infection transmitted by an infected blood transfusion at or before BMT. Nine years after BMT, she has had no opportunistic infections. Eleven patients died, 6 during the first 6 months of rejection or severe GVHD associated with infection. Three patients died between 1 and 2 years after BMT of interstitial pneumonia or infection associated with chronic GVHD. Two late deaths were observed. Chronic hepatitis developed in one patient, who died of cirrhosis 9 years after BMT. Squamous cell carcinoma of the tongue developed in the other 6 years after BMT, which was resistant to treatment. A pharyngeal adenocarcinoma developed in one additional patient 8 years after BMT.

Cincinnati Experience

At the Cincinnati Children's Hospital, 12 patients with FA received BMTs from HLA-identical siblings (Harris R. Personal communication). The preparative regimen consisted of CY (5 mg/kg × 4) and thoracoabdominal irradiation (400 cGy). GVHD prophylaxis consisted of CSP, ATG, and prednisone. All patients were successfully engrafted, toxicity consisted of mild to moderate mucositis, and mild GVHD developed in only one. With a median follow-up of 1.5 years, all 12 patients are living and well. The addition of ATG to the regimen seemed to reduce the risk of GVHD. The low dose preparative regimen provided adequate immunosuppression and myeloablation with minimal toxicity.

The results in Paris and Cincinnati show that reduction of the dose of alkylating agents in the preparative regimen for BMT in FA is associated with decreased toxicity. Survival is excellent when the donor is an HLA-matched sibling.

Seattle Experience

The first patient with FA was transplanted in 1973 from an HLA-identical donor after preparation with CY (50 mg/kg × 4) (44). The patient is alive 19 years later. She is of small stature but otherwise normal, with a Karnofsky score of 100%.

A total of 17 patients have been reported by the Seattle group (45,46). Twelve patients with FA and aplastic anemia were conditioned with CY (140–200 mg/kg over 4 days) followed by marrow grafts from HLA-identical siblings (n = 11) or a phenotypically matched parent (n = 1). All patients engrafted except one whose donor was found retrospectively to have cytogenetic abnormalities consistent with the diagnosis of FA. Toxicities associated with BMT included oral mucositis (n=11), ranging from mild to severe; hemorrhagic cystitis (n = 8); and transient cardiac abnormalities (n = 3). Acute GVHD grade III developed in 4 and contributed to mortality in 3. Eight patients had either no (n = 4) or grade I acute GVHD (n = 4). Four had chronic GVHD, including the one with poor graft function, who received 3 consecutive transplants. In 2 of the 4 patients, chronic GVHD has resolved. One of the 4 died at 10.4 years of a squamous-cell carcinoma, and one died from poor graft function. Currently, 7 of the 12 are living from 2 to 19 years after BMT. All have Karnofsky scores of 100%. Actuarial survival at 5 years is 65% (Figure 68-3).

Five patients had FA with evidence of leukemic transformation, and they were conditioned for BMT either with CY (60 mg/kg × 2), and total body irradiation (TBI) (1,200 cGy) (n = 4) or with BU (14 mg/kg) and CY (50 mg/kg × 2). Grafts were from HLA-identical siblings (n = 3) or from fathers (n = 2), one of whom was HLA phenotypically identical. Two died of fungal infection, one of interstitial pneumonia, and one of renal failure. One patient is alive more than 10 years after BMT.

These results differ somewhat from the experience in Paris in showing that CY can be used as a conditioning regimen for patients with FA who do not have evidence of leukemia. It is possible that doses of CY lower than 140 mg/kg could still provide sufficient immunosuppression for successful grafts from HLA-identical donors. These data confirm the poor outcome of patients transplanted with evidence of leukemia, indicating the need for consideration of BMT before leukemic transformation occurs.

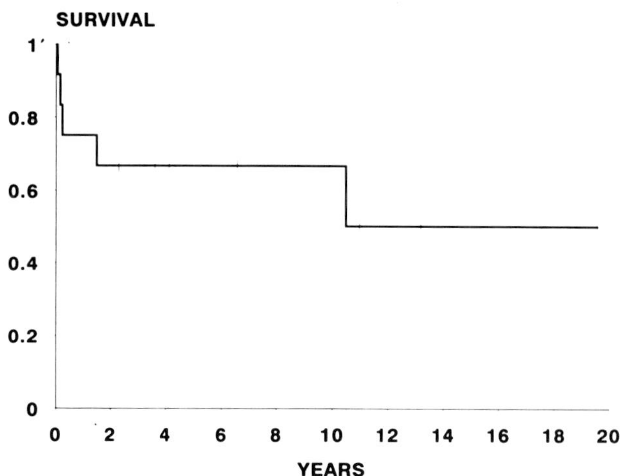

Figure 68-3. Actuarial survival curve for 12 patients with Fanconi's anemia without evidence of leukemia given a human leukocyte antigen–identical sibling bone marrow transplantation at Seattle after preparation with a cyclophosphamide regimen.

Conclusions from Experience with HLA-matched Sibling BMT for FA

It can be concluded from these reports that the toxicity of the conditioning regimen can be decreased by the use of low-dose CY. However, questions still remain about the necessity of using radiotherapy to achieve myeloablation. BU has not been systematically tested in clinical BMT for FA, and there is some concern about the risk of rejection if a single agent is used. The risk of secondary malignancy observed after BMT for acquired severe aplastic anemia was higher with than without irradiation (47,48). In the two FA series reported herein, 3 cases of late development of carcinoma were seen. In 2 cases, the patient was irradiated and the other received CY alone. Clearly, more patients and longer follow-up are needed to evaluate the incidence of secondary malignancy after BMT for FA. Surprisingly, autologous reconstitution followed by leukemia has not yet been reported despite the use of low-intensity conditioning protocols and the fact that FA is a preleukemic syndrome. With long-term follow-up, patients with FA do not differ markedly from patients with acquired severe aplastic anemia except for growth and developmental retardation, which is in part due to the genetic defect.

Given the good results of BMT, the adverse effect of previous blood transfusions, the possible toxicity of long-term high-dose androgen therapy, and the risk of leukemic transformation, it is reasonable to transplant all patients with an HLA-identical sibling as soon as pancytopenia requiring androgen therapy develops.

Results of BMT in patients with leukemic transformation are poor. Most patients do not tolerate the standard induction regimen and die early of regimen-related toxicity. Agents such as cytosine arabinoside, etoposide, and BU have not been tested adequately in preparatory protocols for BMT of FA in leukemic transformation.

Alternative Donor Transplants

Phenotypically Matched Parental Donors

BMTs with marrow from phenotypically HLA-identical parents are usually successful (46,49). In patients with family consanguinity, additional HLA and non-HLA-histocompatible antigens may be matched fortuitously.

Mismatched Related Donors

Mismatched related donors have been used in a very limited number of patients. In Paris, 6 partially matched related donor BMTs have been performed, but there are no survivors. In the Hammersmith group, one of 5 patients with related mismatched donors survived (49). Such results are similar to mismatched family donor transplants for acquired severe aplastic anemia (50).

Matched Unrelated Donor BMT for FA

The experience with unrelated donor transplants for FA, as for aplastic anemia (50,51), is extremely limited. In Paris, 2 of 6 patients survived after unrelated donor BMTs, one for 4 years, whereas in the other patient, follow-up is too short for evaluation. At the Hammersmith Hospital, 5 unrelated donor BMTs for FA have been performed. In all patients, a low-dose CY regimen was used, with 200 cGy TBI for 3 days, oropharyngeal shielding, and CSP administered for GVHD prophylaxis after BMT. Three patients, 2 heavily sensitized to blood products, died in the early post-BMT period. Two deaths were from graft failure and one was from bacterial sepsis and acute GVHD. The two survivors are well, with normal blood counts and without chronic GVHD 3 and 8 years after BMT. Of note, both had pretransplant Karnofsky scores of 100% and were transfusion-independent at the time of BMT. They received pretransplant courses of the monoclonal antibody Campath 1-G , with either in vivo or ex vivo T-lymphocyte depletion using Campath monoclonal antibodies. In both patients, the donor-recipient pairs were fully HLA-A, B, and DR "matched" by serology. Mild steroid-responsive acute GVHD developed in both patients.

The probability of clinically significant GVHD and graft failure may be increased for patients with FA transplanted with unrelated donor marrow compared with sibling donor BMTs (49). Despite this probability, "matched" unrelated donor BMT should be considered in well-selected patients without suitable related donors. In newly diagnosed patients without leukemic transformation, transfusion independence can usually be maintained with low-dose androgen therapy while an unrelated donor search is being performed. In minimally sensitized patients, T-lymphocyte depletion should be considered to reduce the risk of clinically significant GVHD. Monoclonal antibodies such as Campath 1-G and antilymphocyte globulin appear to be well tolerated by patients with FA.

Cord Blood Transplants for FA

The first HLA-matched sibling cord blood transplant was performed in a patient with FA (43) after it was demonstrated that cord blood collected and cryopreserved at birth contained an adequate number of stem cells for engraftment (52). FA was the first model used in humans because of the availability of prenatal diagnosis for FA and HLA typing of the fetus. Four families were selected because the fetus was HLA-identical (16). Patients received the same conditioning regimen described by the Paris group. Three of 4 patients who engrafted had minimal grade I GVHD, no chronic GVHD, and complete hematological reconstitution, with a follow-up ranging from 2 to 3 years. This new method of stem-cell transplantation prevents the need for subsequent marrow harvest under generalized anesthesia of infant donors.

Conclusions

The exact genetic defect of FA is not fully understood. However, the finding by cytogenetic analysis that DNA cross-linking agents increased cell damage in culture led to the modification of the preparative regimens and improved the results of BMT for FA. Further progress should be achieved by location of the gene or genes involved, leading to the potential for gene transfer therapy. More knowledge of the mechanisms responsible for development of aplasia and leukemia will be important for selection of patients and development of protocols for BMT for FA.

References

1. Fanconi G. Familial constitutional panmyelocytopathy Fanconi anemia. Clinical aspects. Semin Hematol 1967;4:233–240.
2. Swift MR, Hirschorn K. Fanconi anemia inherited susceptibility to chromosome breakage in various tissues. Ann Intern Med 1966;65:496–503.
3. Schroeder TM, Tilgen D, Kruger J, Vogel F. Formal genetics of Fanconi anemia. Hum Genet 1976;32:257–288.
4. Glanz A, Fraser FC. Spectrum of anomalies in Fanconi anemia. J Med Genet 1982;19:412–416.
5. Alter BP. The bone marrow failure syndromes. In: Nathan DG, Oski FA, eds. Hematology of infancy and childhood. Philadelphia: W.B. Saunders, 1987:159–241.
6. Sasaki MS, Tonomura A. A high susceptibility of Fanconi anemia to chromosome breakage by DNA cross-linking agents. Cancer Res 1973;33:1829–1836.

7. Auerbach AD, Wolman SR. Susceptibility of Fanconi anaemia fibroblasts to chromosome damage by carcinogens. Nature 1976;261:494–496.
8. Berger R, Bernheim A, Gluckman E. In vitro effect of Cyclophosphamide metabolites on chromosomes of Fanconi anaemia patients. Br J Haematol 1980;45:565–568.
9. Auerbach AD, Adler B, Chaganti RSK. Prenatal and postnatal diagnosis and carrier detection of Fanconi anemia by a cytogenetic method. Pediatrics 1981; 67:128–135.
10. Berger R, Bernheim A, Le Coniat M, Vecchione D Schaison G. Nitrogen-induced chromosome breakage. A tool to Fanconi anemia diagnosis. Cancer Genet Cytogenet 1980;2:269–274.
11. Cervenka J, Hirsch BA. Cytogenetic differentiation of Fanconi anemia, idiopathic aplastic anemia and Fanconi anemia heterozygotes. Am J Med Genet 1983; 15:221–224.
12. Duckworth-Rysieki G, Hulten M, Mann J, Taylor AM. Clinical and cytogenetic diversity in Fanconi's anemia. J Med Genet 1984;21:197–203.
13. Joenje H, Oostra AB. Clastogenicity of cyclophosphamide in Fanconi's anemia lymphocytes without exogenous metabolic activation. Cancer Genet Cytogenet 1986;22:339–345.
14. Auerbach AD, Sagi M, Adler B. Fanconi anemia: prenatal diagnosis in 30 fetuses at risk. Pediatrics 1985;76:794–800.
15. Auerbach AD, Zhang M, Ghosh R, et al. Clastogen-induced chromosomal breakage as a marker for first trimester prenatal diagnosis of Fanconi anemia. Hum Genet 1986;73:86–88.
16. Auerbach AD, Liu Q, Ghosh R, Pollack MS, Douglas GW, Broxmeyer HE. Prenatal identification of potential donors for umbilical cord blood transplantation for Fanconi anemia. Transfusion 1990;30:682–687.
17. Rousset S, Nocentini S, Revet B, Moustacchi E. Molecular analysis by electron microscopy of the removal of Psoralen-photoinduced DNA cross-links in normal and Fanconi anemia. Cancer Res 1990;50:2443–2448.
18. Joenje H, Gille JJP. Oxygen metabolism and chromosomal breakage in Fanconi anaemia. In: Schroeder T, Obe G, Auerbach AD, eds. Clinical, cytogenetic and experimental aspects of Fanconi anemia. Berlin: Springer-Verlag, 1989:174–178.
19. Dutrillaux B, Aurias A, Fosse AM, Buriot D, Prieur M. The cell cycle of lymphocytes in Fanconi anemia. Hum Genet 1982;62:327–332.
20. Hoehn H, Kubbies M, Schindler D, Poot M, Rabinovitch PS. BrdU-Hoechst flow cytometry links the cell kinetic defect of Fanconi anemia to oxygen hypersensitivity. In: Schroeder-Kurth TM, Auerbach AD, Obe G, eds. Fanconi anemia: clinical, cytogenetic and experimental aspects. Berlin: Springer-Verlag, 1989:161–173.
21. Duckworth-Rysiecki G, Cornish G, Clarke CA, Buckwald M. Identification of two complementation groups in Fanconi anemia. Som Cell Mol Genet 1985;11:35–41.
22. Moustacchi E, Papadopoulo D, Diatloff-Zito C, Buckwald M. Two complementation groups of Fanconi anemia differ in their phenotypic response to a DNA-cross-linking agent. Hum Genet 1987;75:45–47.
23. Papadopoulo D, Porfirio B, Moustacchi E. Mutagenic response of Fanconi's anemia cells from a defined complementation group after treatment with photoactivated bifunctional psoralens. Cancer Res 1990;50:3289–3294.
24. Strathdee CA, Duncan AMV, Buchwald M. Evidence for at least four Fanconi anaemia genes including FACC on chromosome nine. Nature Genet 1992;1:196–198.
25. Strathdee CA, Gavish H, Shannon WR, Buchwald M. Cloning of cDNAs for Fanconi's anaemia by functional complementation. Nature 1992;356:763–767.
26. Mann WR, Venkatraj VS, Allen RG, et al. Fanconi anemia: evidence for linkage heterogeneity on Chromosome 20q. Genomics 1991;9:329–337.
27. Alter BP, Knobloch ME, Weiberg RS. Erythropoiesis in Fanconi anemia. Blood 1991;78:602.
28. Stark R, Andre C, Thierry D, et al. Expression of C-kit and Kit ligand in LTBMC's in congenital and acquired aplastic anemia. Blood 1991;78(suppl 1):370.
29. Rosselli F, Sanceau J, Wietzerbin J, Moustacchi E. Abnormal lymphokine production: a novel feature of the genetic disease Fanconi anemia: I. Involvement of interleukin-6. Hum Genet 1992;89:42–48.
30. Auerbach AD, Allen RG. Leukemia and preleukemia in Fanconi anemia patients. A review of the literature and report of the International Fanconi Anemia Registry. Cancer Genet Cytogenet 1991;51:1–12.
31. German J. Patterns of neoplasia associated with the chromosome-breakage syndromes. In: German J, ed. Chromosome mutation and neoplasia. New-York: Alan R. Liss, 1983:1983–1997.
32. Auerbach AD, Rogatko A, Schroeder-Kurth TM. International Fanconi anemia Registry: relation of clinical symptoms to diepoxybutane sensitivity. Blood 1989; 73:391–396.
33. Hanada T, Abe T, Nakazawa M, Aoki Y, Uyeno K. Bone marrow failure in dyskeratosis congenita. Blood 1984; 64:496–500.
34. Miglierina R, Le Coniat M, Gendron M, Berger R. Diagnosis of Fanconi anemia by flow cytometry. Nouv Rev Fr Hematol 1990;32:391–393.
35. Johnson FL, Feagler JR, Lerner KG, et al. Association of androgenic-anabolic steroid therapy with development of hepatocellular carcinoma. Lancet 1972;2:1273–1276.
36. Gluckman E, Devergie A, Schaison G, et al. Bone marrow transplantation in Fanconi anaemia. Br J Haematol 1980;45:557–564.
37. Auerbach AD, Adler B, O'Reilly RJ, Kirkpatrick D, Chaganti RSK. Effect of procarbazine and cyclophosphamide on chromosome breakage in Fanconi anemia cells: relevance to bone marrow transplantation. Cancer Genet Cytogenet 1983;9:25–36.
38. Higurashi M, Conen P. In vitro chromosomal radiosensitivity in Fanconi anemia. Blood 1971;38:336–342.
39. Knox SJ, Wilson FD, Greenberg BR, et al. Increased radiosensitivity of a subpopulation of T lymphocyte progenitors from patients with Fanconi anemia. Blood 1981;57:1043–1048.
40. Dutreix J, Gluckman E. Skin test of radiosensitivity. Application to Fanconi anemia. J Eur Radiother 1983;4:3–8.
41. Gluckman E, Devergie A, Dutreix J. Radio sensitivity in Fanconi anemia: application to the conditioning for bone marrow transplantation. Br J Haematol 1983; 54:431–440.
42. Gluckman E. Bone marrow transplantation for Fanconi anemia Baillière's Clin Haemato 1989;2:153–162.
43. Gluckman E, Broxmeyer HE, Auerbach AD, et al. Hematopoietic reconstitution in a patient with Fanconi anemia by means of umbilical cord blood from an HLA identical sibling. N Engl J Med 1989;321:1174–1178.

44. Storb R, Thomas ED, Buckner CD, et al. Allogeneic marrow grafting for treatment of aplastic anemia. Blood 1974;43:157–180.
45. Deeg HJ, Storb R, Thoms ED, et al. Fanconi's anemia treated by allogeneic marrow transplantation. Blood 1983;61:954–959.
46. Flowers MED, Doney KC, Storb R, et al. Marrow transplantation for Fanconi anemia with or without leukemic transformation: an update of the Seattle experience. Bone Marrow Transplant 1992;9:167–173.
47. Socie G, Henry-Amar M, Cosset JM, Devergie A, Girinsky T, Gluckman E. Increased incidence of solid malignant tumors after bone marrow transplantation for severe aplastic anemia. Blood 1991;78:277–279.
48. Witherspoon RP, Storb R, Pepe M, Longton G, Sullivan KM. Cumulative incidence of secondary solid malignant tumors in aplastic anemia patients given marrow grafts after conditioning with chemotherapy alone. Blood 1992;79:289–290.
49. Hows JM, Chapple M, Marsh JCW, Durrant S, Yin JL, Swirsky D. Bone marrow transplantation for Fanconi anaemia: the Hammersmith experience 1977–89. Bone Marrow Transplant 1989;4:629–634.
50. Storb R, Longton G, Anasetti C, et al. Changing trends in marrow transplantation for aplastic anemia. Bone Marrow Transplant 1992;10(suppl 1):45–52.
51. Hows J, Szydlo R, Anasetti C, Camitta B, Gajewski J, Gluckman E. Unrelated donor marrow transplants for severe acquired aplastic anemia. Bone Marrow Transplant 1992;10(suppl 1):102–107.
52. Broxmeyer HE, Douglas GW, Hangoc G, et al. Human umbilical cord blood as a potential source of transplantable stem/progenitor cells. Proc Natl Acad Sci USA 1989;86:3828–3832.

Part VII
Recent Advances and Future Directions

Chapter 69

Mobilization and Collection of Peripheral Blood Progenitor Cells for Support of High-dose Cancer Therapy

Elizabeth J. Shpall and Roy B. Jones

Peripheral blood progenitor cells (PBPCs) may soon replace bone marrow as the major source of autologous hematopoietic progenitor cell support for patients receiving high-dose chemotherapy. This trend is due, in part, to the perception that multiple leukapheresis procedures are less morbid than a marrow harvest. Additionally, several non-randomized studies have demonstrated improvements in the rate of platelet recovery for patients who received PBPCs alone (1, 2), or in combination with bone marrow (3-5), when compared to patients who received bone marrow alone or with post-transplant growth factor support. Finally, several studies with multi-year follow-up have confirmed the durability of hematopoietic reconstitution produced using only PBPCs (1, 6–8).

Collection of Peripheral Blood Progenitor Cells

PBPCs are collected during out-patient leukapheresis procedures using a continuous-flow blood cell separator such as the COBE-Spectra or the Fenwall CS-3000 equipment. Approximately 9–14 liters of blood are processed over two to four hours. The vast majority of the processed blood elements are returned to the patient. A final PBPC volume of approximately 200 ml is collected and cryopreserved.

When the leukapheresis procedures are completed, patients receive high-dose chemotherapy and/or radiotherapy followed by infusion of the thawed PBPCs alone or with marrow that was previously harvested and cryopreserved. The time to hematopoietic reconstitution, commonly defined as a granulocyte count of 500/μl and a platelet count of 20,000/μl, reflects the quality of the infused progenitors.

What constitutes an adequate leukapheresis product has not been universally accepted. Time to hematopoietic reconstitution has been shown to correlate with the number of colony-forming units granulocyte-macrophage (CFU-GM) (9, 10), and CD34-positive (+) cells (11) contained in the pheresis product. Given the lack of standardization of the latter two assays among laboratories, however, the total mononuclear cell (MNC) count is probably the most consistent (although not necessarily the most predictive) parameter to discuss. Generally transplant centers attempt to collect a total of $4.0–6.0 \times 10^8$ MNCs per kilogram of patient body weight. As summarized in Table 69-1, the number of leukapheresis procedures performed depends upon whether the cells are collected from patients in a "steady state" or following chemotherapy and/or growth factor treatment which mobilizes the hematopoietic progenitors into the peripheral blood. Whether tumor cells are also mobilized with chemotherapy and/or growth factors is still unknown and requires investigation.

Collection of PBPCs in the Steady State

In the steady state, six or more leukaphereses may be required to reach the target MNC number described above. This approach was employed initially, before the development of PBPC mobilization techniques. Kessinger et al. showed that patients who received non-mobilized PBPCs had a median recovery of granulocytes in 8 days and platelets in 23 days (1), a result comparable to that of patients who received autologous marrow support (12). Williams et al. reported median granulocyte and platelet recoveries of 15 and 42 days, respectively, with non-mobilized PBPCs (13). In the latter study delayed platelet recovery was noted in 22% of patients, which stimulated interest in developing mobilization techniques that would improve platelet recovery. Steady state collections are now generally reserved for patients who fail to mobilize PBPCs due to extensive prior therapy or because of substantial tumor contamination of the marrow (14).

Mobilization with Chemotherapy

Chemotherapy-induced mobilization occurs after administration of non-myeloablative high-dose chemo-

Table 69-1.
Hematopoietic recovery following transplantation of autologous peripheral blood progenitor cells

PBPC Mobilization	*Number of Chereses*	*Median days to ANC ≥ 500/μL*	*Median days to Platelet Independence or ≥ 20–50K/μL*	*Reference*
None	8	8	23	Kessinger (1)
None	NR	15	42	Williams (13)
Chemotherapy	3–6	11	14	To (15)
Chemotherapy	NR	12	17	Reiffers (7)
*G-CSF	3	9	15	Sheridan (3)
*G-CSF	3	9	14	Shpall (17)
G-CSF	3	9	9	Shpall (42)
GM-CSF	4	14	12	Elias (18)
*Chemo+GM-CSF	NR	NR	10	Spitzer (27)

PBPC = peripheral blood progenitor cells, ANC = absolute neutrophil count, NR = data not reported.
*Patients received autologous marrow in addition to the PBPCs.

therapy, most commonly 4–7 grams/m^2 of cyclophosphamide (CY) (7, 15, 16). Leukapheresis procedures are carried out as the peripheral leukocyte count is recovering. Generally 3–4 pheresis procedures are performed, beginning on the first day that the leukocyte count reaches 1,000/μl. Chemotherapy-mobilized PBPCs have been shown to contain a significantly higher content of CFU-GM than those collected in the steady state (6). Juttner et al. reported that patients who received chemotherapy-mobilized PBPCs had a significantly faster recovery of both granulocytes and platelets (11 and 13.5 days, respectively) than patients who received either autologous marrow support (22 and 32 days, respectively) or allogeneic marrow grafts (24.5 and 33 days, respectively) (6). Other studies reported similar data with hematopoietic recovery occurring approximately one week earlier when chemotherapy-mobilized PBPCs are compared to marrow (10, 16). The drawback to this technique is the lack of standardization with respect to the chemotherapy mobilization regimens employed and the optimal timing of collections. With patient to patient variability in the time to marrow recovery, it can be difficult to predict when to schedule the leukapheresis procedures. Finally, high doses of CY without growth factor support have been associated with neutropenic fevers which have rarely resulted in toxic death (6).

Mobilization with Recombinant Growth Factors

The recombinant growth factors granulocyte colony stimulating factor (G-CSF) (3, 4, 17), granulocyte-macrophage colony stimulating factor (GM-CSF) (4, 18–20) and more recently interleukin-3 (IL-3) (21) have been administered for PBPC mobilization. Typically, the growth factor is administered for 6-14 days, with 3–6 leukaphereses performed during the final days of therapy (i.e. days 5, 6, and 7 of a 6-day growth factor course). As with chemotherapy-induced mobilization, the number of CFU-GM in the peripheral blood is substantially higher following treatment with G-CSF (22) and GM-CSF (23) when compared to those collected in the steady state. The reproducibility of growth factor-induced mobilization makes this approach logistically easier to arrange than mobilization with chemotherapy.

As summarized in Table 69-1, a consistent finding among studies which employed G-CSF or GM-CSF mobilized PBPCs is shortening of the time to platelet recovery compared to studies of patients who did not receive PBPCs. Examples are the studies by Sheridan et al. in which time to reach a platelet count of 50,000/μl was shortened significantly from 39 days in patients who received marrow support to 15 days with G-CSF mobilized PBPCs in addition to marrow (3). Of interest in that study were the bone marrow biopsy results at engraftment, which showed normal or increased numbers of megakaryocytes in 7 of 11 patients (64%) who received G-CSF-mobilized PBPCs, compared to 18 control patients whose biopsies showed no evidence of megakaryocyte production (3).

The reason platelet recovery is superior when PBPCs are used has not been fully explained. It is likely that megakaryocyte precursors in the peripheral blood are elicited by the growth factor and/or chemotherapy mobilization regimens. Further study of this issue is warranted.

Strategies to improve PBPC mobilization are in progress utilizing combinations of growth factors (24–26), as well as chemotherapy plus growth factor regimens (27). Additionally, the development of newer growth factors such as stem cell factor (SCF) may open new avenues of PBPC support (28). In animal studies SCF has been shown to stimulate more primitive hematopoietic cells than the other recombinant growth factors in current clinical use (29). The most impressive effects, however, have been demonstrated when SCF and G-CSF are combined. With a low dose schedule of SCF plus G-CSF, synergistic increases in the number of PBPCs, CFU-GM, and the more primitive high proliferative potential colony forming cells have been demonstrated (30). Andrews et al. reported similar data in primate studies (31). These pre-clinical data suggest that SCF plus G-CSF may produce a PBPC product which requires fewer leukaphereses and contains higher numbers of both myeloid and megakaryocytic precursors than PBPCs mobilized with the individual growth factors described above. Thus, mobilization studies with low doses of SCF plus G-CSF have been initiated to evaluate the clinical efficacy of this combination. Phase I trials reported mast cell-related adverse effects with high doses of SCF (32, 33).

Tumor Cell Contamination of Peripheral Blood Progenitors

Over the past few years PBPCs have been employed as a substitute for bone marrow in patients with known marrow metastases because of the belief that peripheral blood contained fewer tumor cells than the corresponding marrow (34). Although this may still be the case, the recent development of sensitive detection techniques have revealed that contamination of peripheral blood with malignant cells is common, and much more prevalent than routine histology would suggest (17, 35–38).

Infusion of bone marrow containing residual tumor detected by polymerase chain reaction (PCR) was associated with a significantly higher relapse rate in non-Hodgkin's lymphoma (NHL) patients than infusion of autologous marrow which was normal by PCR analysis (39). Whether infusion of tumor in PBPCs will have an impact on clinical outcome remains to be determined. Because of potential toxicity to the progenitors, chemical or immunologic purging of PBPCs has not been extensively studied. We therefore investigated a method for the positive selection of hematopoietic precursors, where the depletion of breast cancer cells was anticipated without toxicity to normal progenitors.

Positive Selection of CD34+ Hematopoietic Progenitor Cells

The CD34 antigen is expressed on the pluripotent hematopoietic progenitors, but not on the neoplastic cells of patients with NHL, myeloma and most solid tumors. CD34+ hematopoietic progenitors have been isolated from marrow fractions using an immunoadsorption method developed by Berenson et al. (40). This positive selection method was employed for patients receiving high-dose chemotherapy at the University of Colorado Bone Marrow Transplantation Unit. As shown in Figure 69-1, patients with high-risk breast cancer received three cycles of adriamycin, 5-fluorouracil and methotrexate (AFM) as reported by Jones et al. (41). Following recovery from the final cycle of AFM, marrow was harvested and incubated with the biotinylated anti-CD34 antibody 12.8. The coated cells were then applied to a column of avidin-coated beads (Cell-Pro Inc., Bothell, WA), and the CD34+ cells were isolated and cryopreserved (42). The first three cohorts of patients received CD34+ marrow alone. Following the harvest, cohorts 4 and 5 received a seven day course of G-CSF. Leukapheresis was performed on days 5, 6 and 7. The CD34+ PBPCs were isolated from each leukapheresis product and cryopreserved. Patients in cohorts 4 and 5 received PBPCs alone (n=11) or in combination with CD34+ marrow (n=12) (42). As shown in Table 69-1, granulocyte recovery, defined as the number of days to reach a granulocyte count of 500/μl, was achieved in an average of 9 days (range 8–10) for both groups. Platelet transfusion independence, defined as a sustained platelet count >10,000/μl, was achieved in 14 (range 8–18) and 9 (range 8–10) days, respectively, for patients who received CD34+ PBPCs alone or in combination with CD34+ marrow. This result is compared to the engraftment rates for cohorts 1–3, summarized in Table 69-2, who received a CD34+ marrow fraction alone, or in combination with systemic growth factors (42). Patients who received CD34+ marrow alone had an average time to both granulocyte recovery and platelet transfusion independence of 23 days. Patients who received CD34+ plus G-CSF achieved granulocyte and platelet recovery in 13 and 16 days, respectively. Patients who received CD34+ marrow plus GM-CSF achieved both granulocyte and platelet independence in 18 days. One

Table 69-2.
Hematopoietic recovery following transplantation of autologous CD34+ hematopoietic progenitor cells

Patient Cohort (n)	*CD34+ Marrow*	*CD34+ PBPC*	*Growth Factor*	*Days to ANC>500/μL*	*Days to Platelet Independence*
1 (7)	+	−	None	23	23
2 (10)	+	−	G-CSF	13	16
3 (8)	+	−	GM-CSF	18	18
4 (12)	+	+	G-CSF	9	9
5 (11)	−	+	G-CSF	9	14

Five sequentially treated cohorts were included in this study. Cohorts 1–3 received CD34+ marrow on day +1. Cohorts 4 and 5 received CD34+ peripheral blood progenitor cells (PBPCs), on days −1, 0, and +1. Granulocyte colony stimulating factor (G-CSF) was instituted on day +1 for cohort 2, and day −1 for cohorts 4 and 5. Granulocyte-macrophage colony stimulating factor (GM-CSF) was instituted on day +1 for cohort 3. The median time to an ANC of >500 cells/μL and platelet transfusion independence is described for each cohort.
PBPC = peripheral blood progenitor cells. ANC = absolute neutrophil count. NR = data not reported. + = patients received CD34 = selected bone marrow or G-CSF-mobilized PBPCs which were CD34-selected following leukapheresis.

patient who received CD34+ marrow plus GM-CSF still requires bi-monthly platelet transfusions, 5 months following transplant. The patient has a normal granulocyte count and bone marrow biopsies showed decreased numbers of megakaryocytes, with no evidence of breast cancer. This patient received her "backup" marrow 2 months post-transplant with no improvement in her platelet transfusion requirement. To date there have been no granulocyte engraftment failures observed with a median follow-up of 9 months (range 1–23 months).

Using a sensitive immunohistochemical technique (43), breast cancer was detected in the unpurified PBPCs of five of the 23 patients (22%) in Table 69-1 who underwent leukapheresis (17, 42). Using the same technique, breast cancer was detected in the unpurified marrow of 13 of the 37 patients (35%) summarized in Table 69-2. Following CD34+ purification of the marrow and PBPCs, 1.3 to >4.0 logs of breast cancer cell depletion was documented.

The preliminary data suggest that CD34+ PBPCs alone or in combination with CD34+ marrow, produce faster granulocyte and platelet recovery than CD34+ marrow. CD34+ PBPCs alone are capable of restoring hematopoiesis following high-dose chemotherapy. Contamination of PBPCs with breast cancer cells is common. CD34+ selection is an effective method for removing tumor from both the PBPCs and the marrow. Longer follow-up will be required to assess the durability of engraftment produced with the CD34+ PBPCs, as well as the ultimate therapeutic effect of this approach.

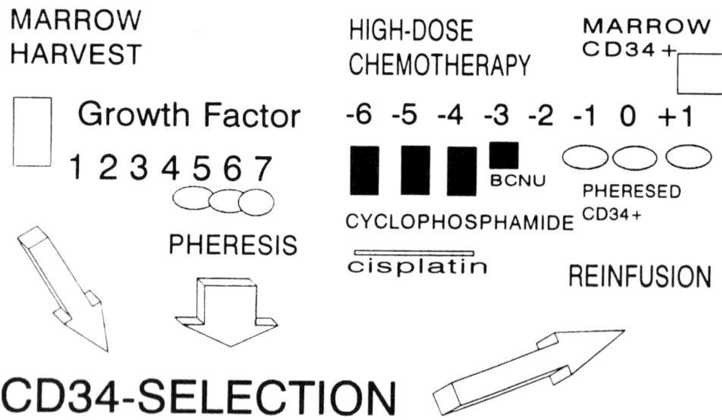

Figure 69–1. Breast cancer patients at the University of Colorado received high dose cyclophosphamide, cisplatin, and BCNU on days -6 through -3 (4). Five sequentially treated cohorts were included in this study. Cohorts 1–3 received CD34+ marrow on day +1. Cohorts 4 and 5 received CD34+ peripheral blood progenitor cells (PBPCs), on days -1, 0, and +1. Granulocyte colony stimulating factor (G-CSF) was instituted on day +1 for cohort 2, and day -1 for cohorts 4 and 5. Granulocyte-macrophage colony stimulating factor (GM-CSF) was instituted on day +1 for cohort 3.

Ex Vivo Expansion of CD34+ Progenitor Cells

Recently several potential applications of ex vivo PBPC expansion have been considered. Haylock et al. described the use of "expanded" hematopoietic progenitors to supplement a standard autograft (44). This technique would provide mature functional neutrophils within days of the infusion, potentially decreasing the period of neutropenia further. In their preclinical studies with a combination of SCF, IL-1, IL-3, IL-6, GM-CSF, and G-CSF the investigators demonstrated a 29–30 fold expansion of CFU-GM by day 7 of culture (44). They postulated that with their approach sufficient CFU-GM to accomplish the goal of hastening marrow recovery could be achieved. Using a variety of SCF-based growth factor combinations, other investigators have reported similar results, demonstrating a 20–200 fold expansion of CFU-GM (45).

Large scale ex vivo studies at the University of Colorado SCF, IL-3, IL-6, and G-CSF produced an average of 8.65 x 10^5 CFU-GM when 1×10^6 G-CSF mobilized CD34+ PBPCs were cultured for seven days. The degree of expansion of PBPC and marrow CFU-GM was comparable when either fresh or thawed CD34+ progenitors were used. CD34-purification appears to be essential for this procedure, as insufficient expansion was achieved when unpurified hematopoietic progenitors were used. In CD34-selection trial described above, patients in cohort 5, who received CD34+ PBPCs alone received a mean total of 11 x 10^6 CFU-GM (range $5–20\times10^6$). All patients engrafted successfully, suggesting that the CFU-GM content of the infused product was sufficient. Based on the pre-clinical results with ex vivo expansion procedure, $>5\times10^6$ total CFU-GM should consistently produce by culturing less than one CD34-selected leukapheresis product.

Although CFU-GM is only a surrogate marker of hematopoietic reconstitutive ability, it is currently the most commonly employed measurement of graft function. Preliminary data suggest that the long-term culture initiating cell colony (46) may be more predictive of graft function than CFU-GM, but this assay is also only a surrogate end-point and may not be clinically relevant. The reconstitutive capability of an autograft can only be evaluated in a clinical trial where it is infused into a patient following high-dose therapy. Thus, a clinical study will be performed using CD34+ PBPCs from a single leukapheresis product which are expanded ex vivo, to answer the question of whether these cells can support high-dose chemotherapy.

With expansion of small number of PBPCs it may be possible to produce quantities sufficient to support multiple cycles of high-dose therapy. Long-term cultures of marrow from patients with chronic myeloid leukemia have been shown to support the growth and expansion of normal progenitors differentially, while leukemic cells did not survive (47). Thus, there may be a beneficial purging effect of ex vivo PBPC expansion for a variety of hematologic malignancies and solid tumors. This ex vivo approach will give investigators more freedom to manipulate the PBPC fractions. For example, growth factor regimens could be designed to favor the development of megakaryocyte-rich PBPCs, or fractions containing predominately myeloid progenitors (or both), as clinically indicated. Finally, there is substantial interest in developing ex vivo PBPC expansion techniques for use in conjunction with gene insertion experiments (48–50). Studies to optimize ex vivo expansion procedures are in progress in a number of centers, and clinical studies to assess this technology are being designed.

References

1. Kessinger A, Armitage JO, Landmark JD, Smith DM, Weisenburger D. Autologous peripheral hematopoietic stem cell transplantation restores hematopoietic function following marrow ablative therapy. Blood 1988; 71:723–727.
2. Juttner CA, To LB, Ho JQ, et al. Early lymphohematopoietic recovery after autografting using peripheral blood stem cells in acute nonlymphoblastic leukemia. Transplant Proc 1988;20:40–42.
3. Sheridan W, Begley CG, Juttner CA, et al. Effect of peripheral blood progenitor cells mobilized by filgrastim (G-CSF) on platelet recovery after high-dose chemotherapy. Lancet 1992;1:640–644.
4. Peters WP, Ross M, Vredenburgh J, et al. High-dose chemotherapy and autologous bone marrow support as consolidation after standard-dose adjuvant therapy for high-risk primary breast cancer. J Clin Oncol 1993; 11:1132–1143.
5. Gianni AM, Bregni M, Siena S, et al. Rapid and complete hematopoietic reconstitution following combined transplantation of autologous blood and bone marrow cells. A changing role for high-dose chemoradiotherapy? Hematol Oncol 1989;7:139–143.
6. Juttner CA, To LB, Roberts MM, et al. Comparison of hematologic recovery, toxicity, and supportive care of autologous PBSC, autologous BM, and allogeneic BM transplants. Int J Cell Cloning 1992;10:160.
7. Reiffers J, Castaigne S, Tilly H, et al. Hematopoietic reconstitution after autologous blood stem cell transplantation. A report of 46 cases. Plasma Ther Transfus Technol 1987;8:360-364.
8. Stiff PJ, Murgo AJ, Wittes RE, et al. Quantification of peripheral blood colony forming unit-culture rise following chemotherapy: could leukocytaphereses replace bone marrow for autologous transplantation? Transfusion 1983;23:500–503.
9. Juttner C, To LB. Peripheral blood stem cells: mobilization by myelosuppressive chemotherapy. In: Dicke K, Armitage J, Dicke-Evinger M, eds. Proceedings of the 5th International Symposium on Autologous Bone Marrow Transplantation. University of Nebraska Press, 1991:783–788.
10. Reiffers J, Faberes C, Commenges D, et al. The CD34 assay is not of predictive value for engraftment after PBSC transplantation. In: Proceedings of the 2nd International Symposium on Peripheral Blood Stem Cell Autografts. Mulhouse, France, 1991.
11. Sienna S, Bregni M, Brando B, et al. Flow cytometry for clinical estimation of circulating hematopoietic progenitors for autologous transplantation in cancer patients. Blood 1991;77:400–406.
12. Kessinger A, Armitage JO. The evolving role of autologous peripheral stem cell transplantation following high-dose therapy for malignancies. Blood 1991; 77:211–213.
13. Williams SF, Bitran JD, Richards JM, et al. Peripheral blood-derived stem cell collections for use in autologous transplantation after high-dose chemotherapy: an alternative approach. Bone Marrow Transplant 1990; 5:129–133.
14. Cantin G, Marchand-Laroche D, Bouchard MM, Leblond PF. Blood-derived stem cell collection in acute nonlymphoblastic leukemia: predictive factors for a good yield. Exp Hematol 1989;17:991–996.
15. To LB, Shepperd KM, Haylock DN, et al. Single high doses of cyclophosphamide enable the collection of high numbers of stem cells from the peripheral blood. Exp Hematol 1990; 18: 442–447.
16. Kessinger A, Armitage JO, Smith DM, Landmark JD, Bierman PJ, Weisenburger D. High-dose therapy and autologous marrow peripheral blood stem cell transplantation for patients with lymphoma. Blood 1989;74: 1260–1265.
17. Shpall EJ, Jones RB, Franklin W, et al. CD34+ marrow and/or peripheral blood progenitor cells provide effective hematopoietic reconstitution of breast cancer patients following high-dose chemotherapy with autologous hematopoietic progenitor cell support. Blood 1992;80(Suppl 1):24a.
18. Elias A, Mazanet R, Anderson K, et al. GM-CSF mobilized stem cell autografts. In: Proceedings of the 2nd International Symposium on Peripheral Blood Stem Cell Autografts. Mulhouse, France, 1991.
19. Gianni AM, Siena S, Bregni M, et al. Granulocyte-macrophage colony stimulating factor to harvest circulating hematopoietic stem cells for autotransplantation. Lancet 1989;2:580–586.
20. Haas R, Ho AD, Bredthauer U, et al. Successful autologous transplantation of blood stem cells mobilized with recombinant human granulocyte-macrophage colony stimulating factor. Exp Hematol 1990;18: 94–98.
21. Vose JM, Kessinger A, Bierman P, Sharp G, Garrison L, Armitage JO. The use of rh-IL-3 for mobilization of peripheral blood stem cells in previously treated patients with lymphoid malignancies. In: Proceedings of the 2nd International Symposium on Peripheral Blood Stem Cell Autografts. Mulhouse, France, 1991.
22. Duhrsen U, Villeval JL, Boyd J, Kannourakis G, Morstyn G, Metcalf D. Effects of recombinant granulocyte colony stimulating factor on hematopoietic progenitor cells in cancer patients. Blood 1988;72:2074–2081.
23. Socinski MA, Cannistra SA, Elias A, Antman KH, Schnipper L, Griffin JD. Granulocyte-macrophage colony stimulating factor expands the circulating hematopoietic progenitor cell compartment in man. Lancet 1988;1:1194–1198.
24. McNiece I, Langley KE, Zsebo KM. Recombinant SCF synergizes with GM-CSF, G-CSF, IL-3 and epo to stimulate human progenitor cells of the myeloid and erythroid lineages. Exp Hematol 1992;19:226–231.
25. Hara H, Namiki M. Mechanism of synergy between GM-CSF and G-CSF in colony formation from human marrow cells in vitro. Exp Hematol 1989;17:816–821.
26. Brucher J, Martin H, Hess U, et al. Interleukin-3

combined with rGM-CSF efficiently mobilizes circulating hematopoietic progenitor cells without prior chemotherapy. In: Proceedings of the 2nd International Symposium on Peripheral Blood Stem Cell Autografts. Mulhouse, France, 1991.

27. Spitzer G, Huan SD, Hester J, et al. Influence of mobilized peripheral blood cells on the hematopoietic recovery from autologous marrow and recombinant granulocyte-macrophage colony stimulating factor (rhGM-CSF) following high-dose cyclophosphamide, etoposide, and cisplatin. In: Proceedings of the 2nd International Symposium on Peripheral Blood Stem Cell Autografts. Mulhouse, France, 1991.
28. Zsebo K, Williams D, Geissler EN, et al. Stem cell factor is encoded at the S1 locus of the mouse and is the ligand for the c-kit tyrosine kinase receptor. Cell 1990;63:213–219.
29. Andrews RG, Bartelmez SH, Knitter GH, et al. A c-kit ligand, recombinant human stem cell factor mediates reversible expansion of CD34+ colony-forming cell types in blood and marrow of baboons. Blood 1992; 80:920–927.
30. Briddell RA, Hartley CA, Smith KA McNiece IK. Recombinant rat SCF synergizes with recombinant human G-CSF in vivo to mobilize PBPCs which have enhanced repopulating potential. Blood, 1993 (in press).
31. Andrews RG, Appelbaum FR, Bensinger WI, McNiece IK, Bernstein ID, Zsebo K. Stem cell factor stimulates the in vivo expansion of hematopoietic progenitor cells and stimulates circulation of cells that engraft and rescue lethally irradiated recipients. In: Dicke K, ed. Proceedings of the 6th International Symposium on Autologous Bone Marrow Transplantation. Houston, 1992.
32. Crawford J, Lau D, Erwin R, Rich B, McGuire B, Meyers F. A phase I trial of recombinant methionyl human stem cell factor (SCF) in patients with advanced non-small cell lung carcinoma. Proc Am Soc Clin Oncol 1993;12: 135.
33. Demetri G, Costa J, Hayes D, et al. A phase I trial of recombinant methionyl human stem cell factor in patients with advanced breast cancer pre and post chemotherapy with cyclophosphamide and doxorubicin. Proc Amer Soc Clin Oncol 1993;12:142.
34. Sharp JG, Armitage J, Grouse D, et al. Are occult tumor cells present in peripheral stem cell harvests of candidates for autologous transplantation? In: Dicke K, Spitzer G, Jagannath S, Evinger-Hodges M, eds. Proceedings of the 4th International Symposium on Autologous Bone Marrow Transplantation. Houston: M.D. Anderson Press, 1989:693–696.
35. Horning SJ, Galili N, Cleary M, et al. Detection of Non-Hodgkin's Lymphoma in the peripheral blood by analysis of antigen receptor gene rearrangements: results of a prospective study. Blood 1990;75:1139–1145.
36. Sharp J, Kessinger A, Mann S, et al. Detection and clinical significance of minimal tumor cell contamination of peripheral blood stem cell harvests. Int J Cell Cloning 1992;10:92–94.
37. Osborne MP, Wong GY, Gonzalez A, Potter C, Vlamis V, Cote RJ. Bone marrow micrometastases (BMM) in breast cancer: the effect of tumor cell (TC) burden on early relapse. Proc Am Soc Clin Oncol 1993;12:75.
38. Ross AA, Cooper BW, Lazarus H, et al. Incidence of tumor cell contamination in peripheral blood stem cell (PBSC) collections from breast cancer patients. Proc Am Soc Clin Oncol 1993;12:68.
39 Gribben JG, Freedman AS, Neuberg D, et al. Immunologic purging of marrow assessed by PCR before autologous bone marrow transplantation for B-cell lymphoma. N Engl J Med 1991;325:1525-1533.
40. Berenson R, Bensinger W, Kalamasz D. Positive selection of viable cell populations using avidin-biotin immunoadsorption. J Immunol Methods 1986;91:11–19.
41. Jones RB, Shpall EJ, Shogan J, et al. The Duke AFM Program: intensive induction chemotherapy for metastatic breast cancer. Cancer 1990;66:431–436.
42. Shpall E, Jones R, Franklin W, et al. Transplantation of autologous CD34 positive hematopoietic progenitor cells into breast cancer patients following high-dose chemotherapy. Proc Am Soc Clin Oncol 1993;12: 105.
43. Johnston CS, Shpall EJ, Williams S, et al. Detection of minimal residual breast cancer in bone marrow. Prog Clin Biol Res 1992;377:637–642.
44. Haylock DN, To LB, Dowse CA, Juttner CA, Simmons PJ. Ex vivo expansion and maturation of peripheral blood CD34+ cells into the myeloid lineage. Blood 1992; 80:1405–1412.
45. Muench M, Schneider J, Moore MA. Interactions among colony-stimulating factors, IL-1 beta, IL-6, and Kit-ligand in the regulation of primitive murine hematopoietic cells. Exp Hematol 1992;20:339–349.
46. Coulombel L, Eaves AC, Eaves CJ. Enzymatic treatment of long-term human marrow cultures reveals the preferential location of primitive hematopoietic progenitors in the adherent layer. Blood 1983;62:291–297.
47. Barnett M, Eaves CJ, Phillips GL, et al. Successful autografting in chronic myeloid leukemia after maintenance of marrow in culture. Bone Marrow Transplant 1989;4:345–351.
48. Smith C. Retroviral vector-mediated gene transfer into hematopoietic cells: prospects and issues. J Hematotherapy 1992;1:155–166.
49. Bregni M, Magni M, Siena S, Nicola MD, Bonadonna G, Gianni AM. Human peripheral blood hematopoietic progenitors are optimal targets of retroviral-mediated gene transfer. Blood 1992;80:1418–1422.
50. Nolta JA, Crooks GM, Overell RW, Williams DE, Kohn DB. Retroviral vector-mediated gene transfer into primitive human hematopoietic progenitor cells: effect of mast cell growth factor (MGF) combined with other cytokines. Exp Hemat 1992;20:1065-1071.

Chapter 70
Bone Marrow Transplantation in the Twenty-first Century

Martin J. Cline

It is my intention to discuss some of the current problems of bone marrow transplantation (BMT) and to suggest potential solutions that may evolve in the twenty-first century. Some of the solutions will be obvious extrapolations of research that is already well advanced. Development of new antiviral agents and isolation of useful new hematopoietic hormones are examples of already "mature" research fields. In contrast, some of the proposed solutions will involve fields that are still embryonic in evolution. Construction of tailor-made molecules to block lymphoid cell surface receptors, isolation of human pluripotent hematopoietic stem cells, and introduction of cancer suppressor genes by retroviral vectors are examples of these new fields. As I complete my analysis of each of the current problems and foreseeable solutions, I present several hypothetical case studies of BMT in the twenty-first century that will reflect and summarize my vision of what lies ahead.

What are the major problems that now confront patients who have a disease potentially treatable by BMT? My summary encapsulated in Table 70-1 includes the following problem list: infection in the immunocompromised host; graft-versus-host disease; a limited ability to destroy malignant cells in the bone marrow and in the patient; the toxicity of conditioning regimens used to eradicate malignant disease or obliterate the transplant recipient's immune system; and the high technology and cost of current procedures, which limit application of BMT to a relatively few economically and geographically favored patients. I use this problem list as a point of departure for considering the technology we are apt to develop in the years ahead to enhance the success rate and to decrease the complexity of BMT. Almost identical problems in BMT were identified in the antecedent volume published nearly one decade ago (1), and a very similar problem list could have been published 2 decades ago if anyone had chosen to encapsulate the field at that time. This is not to say that we have not made substantial progress in these 20 years, but that progress has been slow and achieved at the cost of enormous effort and sacrifice for those involved.

Will we solve these major problems of BMT and will we progress more quickly toward solutions in the future? It seems reasonable to be optimistic that the major problems of BMT will be solved in the century that lies ahead. Almost certainly, the reagents and the technologies that will be used in the future will originate from the remarkable recent advances in

Table 70-1.
Bone Marrow Transplantation: Current Problems and Potential Solutions in the Twenty-first Century

Problem	*Potential Solutions (in order of development)*
Infection in the immunocompromised host	1. Better antimicrobial antibiotics 2. Hematopoietins to accelerate production of phagocytes 3. Lymphokines to accelerate immunological reconstitution
Graft-versus-host disease	1. More effective immunological suppression 2. Fine tuning of immunological ablation 3. Fine-tuning of cross-matching by DNA typing of donor and recipient 4. The construction of receptor blocking agents 5. Isolation of hematopoietic stem cells 6. Universal storage of autologous stem cells
Eradication of malignant disease	1. The "right" combination of conventional therapy 2. More effective purging of autologous marrow a. Detection of minimal residual disease b. Isolation of hematopoietic stem cells c. Universal storage of autologous stem cells d. Gene therapy with antioncogenes, blocking genes, or drug-activating genes
Nonhematopoietic toxicity of conditioning regimens	1. More selective agents 2. Detection of minimal residual disease with reduced drug dosage 3. Gene therapy

knowledge and techniques of modern biology. There is every reason to assume that these advances will continue at an undiminished rate; however, the pace of acquisition of fundamental insights into biological mechanisms has recently been measured in years or fractions of years, whereas fundamental changes in our therapeutic armamentarium often require decades. Consequently, we should be optimistic about progress and eventual success, but it is unlikely that we will get the "quick fix" for the problems of BMT.

Infection

Infection in the immunocompromised host is still an important complication of BMT, although the magnitude of this problem is diminishing as a consequence of improved antimicrobial antibiotics and introduction of hematopoietic hormones. Infections in transplant recipients result from disease- and therapy-induced abnormalities of blood phagocytes, of immunoglobulin-producing B lymphocytes, and of cytotoxic T lymphocytes. The immunodeficiency of BMT (see Chapter 36) results in a diversity of opportunistic disease syndromes, some of which are well characterized, and others of which may have multiple ill-defined etiologies. The disease syndrome of interstitial pneumonitis is an example of the latter.

New Antimicrobial Agents

Currently, viruses present the most challenging infectious problems in BMT recipients even though considerable progress has been made in the past decade as a result of introduction of effective antiviral agents. Moreover, we are using these new antibiotics earlier and more effectively in the course of viral illness. One need only cite the prophylactic use of ganciclovir in BMT recipients who are either cytomegalovirus (CMV)-positive or who have CMV-positive donors (2). In the future, we can anticipate continued introduction of new antiviral agents from the pharmaceutical companies based on the success of acyclovir, ganciclovir, and azidothymidine.

I have plotted a rough curve of development of new antiviral agents over the last 30 years by using 2 relatively crude sources of data. I counted the number of abstracted important articles on antiviral drugs summarized on a yearly basis in the *YearBook of Medicine,* and I measured with a ruler the space devoted to references on antiviral agents in the Index Medicus. Both follow a roughly similar pattern. In 1960, there were no articles on antiviral agents that were thought to be sufficiently important to merit abstracting in the *YearBook of Medicine.* In 1968, there was a single article on the treatment of herpes simplex encephalitis with iodo-2′-deoxyuridine. In 1991, there were 6 articles on 4 different antiviral agents, excluding vaccines. On the basis of this limited data, I would surmise that the search for new antiviral agents is following a sigmoidal curve and that we are now on the exponential part of that curve.

Similarly, BMT recipients have benefited from the introduction of new antibacterial antibiotics that are generally effective in neutropenic patients. As an example, ciprofloxacin has been shown to be highly effective in preventing bacterial infections in BMT recipients (3). Ciprofloxacin represents a departure from many of the traditional classes of antibacterial antibiotics. It is reasonable to assume, therefore, that antibacterial agents of novel classes as well as new antiviral drugs will be developed in the future, and that these will continue to decrease infection as a problem in BMT.

Hematopoietic Hormones

In 1966, Bradley and Metcalf (4), in Australia, and Pluznick and Sacks (5), in Israel, first reported observing colonies of hematopoietic cells growing in soft agar. At that time, few people would have predicted that these observations would lead to clinically useful biological reagents. By the early 1970s, however, it was already clear that the presence of hematopoietic hormones was driving the proliferation of stem cells in the soft agar cultures and that there were probably several classes of "hemopoietins," each directed at a target cell of a specific lineage (6). By the early 1980s, the research observations of the academic centers were taken up by several of the newly emerging biotechnology companies and a few of the established pharmaceutical companies and were soon translated into cloned DNA sequences and then into reagents for testing in clinical trials (7,8). By the end of the 1980s, granulocyte colony stimulating factor (G-CSF) and granulocyte-macrophage CSF (GM-CSF), had a clearly established role in alleviating the bone marrow suppression induced by cytotoxic drugs and irradiation and their use in BMT is likely to be routine in the foreseeable future.

It is not difficult to project the continuing trajectory of the hemopoietins from the first observation of colonies grown in soft agar in 1966 to their ultimate clinical application. Eighteen different hematopoietic growth factors have been cloned and characterized to date, and new receptors continue to be identified (9). One can predict that more hematopoietic hormones will be identified, cloned, and tried on patients, singly and in combinations, in the future (10–14). There must be hormones that will stimulate very primitive hematopoietic stem cells, because, after all, we must all develop a hematopoietic system from the single cell of a fertilized egg. The *c-kit* ligand may be a candidate for such a "multipoietin" (13). Other hormones will surely stimulate megakaryopoiesis (14), and still others will stimulate specific classes or specific stages in differentiation of B and T cells and perhaps natural killer cells. By using such hormones, it is possible that we can accelerate development of primitive hematopoietic stem cells and accelerate the rate of immunological reconstitution in BMT recipients. Twenty years would appear to be a reasonable time to identify, clone, and test all of the major human hematopoietic hormones, and not many years later we should see routine use of stimulants of primitive stem cells in marrow transplant clinics.

I now consider the first of the clinical scenarios in which the scientific advances of the twenty-first century will be applied to the problems of BMT. Although the case histories are entirely imaginary constructs, the general picture will be familiar to contemporary transplanters. The therapeutic strategies described in these cases represent my own speculations about the future of our field of endeavor. The choice of cases 10 to 70 years in the future reflects my own estimates of the pace of introduction of new developments into clinical practice.

Case 1—The Year 2002

A 28-year-old mother of 2 was referred to UCLA Medical Center for allogeneic BMT for acute myelocytic leukemia (AML). The disease was diagnosed 4 months earlier and a remission was induced with a 12-day/4-drug regimen that included a new anthracycline antibiotic, high-dose cytarabine, etoposide, and a newly introduced myelosuppressive platinum compound. However, on the basis of blast-cell phenotype and oncogene analysis, the patient was considered to have poor prognosis AML and allogeneic BMT was recommended. Among her 4 siblings, 2 were human leukocyte antigen (HLA)–identical potential donors. By DNA genotyping, one was considered a "best match."

The pretransplantation conditioning regimen included fractionated total body irradiation, high-dose cytarabine, etoposide, and busulfan. After BMT, the patient received *c-kit* ligand, interleukin-11 (IL-11), and GM-CSF intravenously. There had been 3 episodes of herpes virus infection on the transplant unit within the previous 6 months; consequently, beginning pretransplantation, the patient received not only ganciclovir but also a second-generation acyclovir.

Engraftment was documented by day 6; neutrophils reached 600/μL by day 8, and platelets reached 50,000/μL by day 9. On day 7, the patient had a brief febrile episode, which was treated with a third-generation ciprofloxacin analogue. She was discharged from the hospital on day 19.

Comment:

This clinical history, set 10 years in the future, is based on the concept that total body irradiation and myelosuppressive agents will continue to be the foundation of antileukemic therapy for BMT. However, better donor selection methods based on DNA genotyping will be in use, and new antimicrobials and hormones to accelerate functional engraftment will be available. In this case, BMT was recommended rather than intensive consolidation therapy because her leukemia was considered to have a poor prognosis on the basis of genetic analysis of the leukemic cells. By the year 2002, genetic markers should largely have replaced chromosomal analysis in predicting clinical responses.

Graft-versus-Host Disease

Graft-versus-host disease (GVHD) has been a nagging problem for patients and transplanters since the first attempts at allogeneic BMT several decades ago (15,16). The importance of this problem is attested to by the number of chapters in this text that address different aspects of GVHD (see Chapters 17–19, 26, 51), and is emphasized more cogently by statistics which indicate that 20% or more of some categories of recipients of allogeneic grafts from family members may die of GVHD or its complications. The problem is even more severe in recipients of matched bone marrow from unrelated donors and recipients of imperfectly matched bone marrow (17,18). Statistics relative to the control of GVHD have improved somewhat over the past decade as a consequence of more effective immunological agents, such as cyclosporine. Nevertheless, the impact of GVHD is such that allogeneic BMT is still limited in the last decade of the twentieth century to a relatively small group of patients with well-matched donors and with catastrophic diseases, such as malignancy, bone marrow aplasia, or severely disabling genetic diseases (19).

I believe we are still hampered in precisely defining the clinical and histological features of GVHD and in separating these features with certainty from derangements induced by the toxicity of drugs and high levels of irradiation or by infectious agents that are difficult to identify. We are still ignorant of the precise subset of lymphoid cells that are the initial instigators of GVHD, and we are ignorant of the interactions of these instigating cells with other cells that amplify the pathogenic process. We are only beginning to identify the noncellular biological mediators of GVHD. We do have some clues as to the characteristics of the cells involved from animal model systems and from analyses of cell surface antigens of lymphoid subpopulations (see Chapters 17, 18). These presumed culprits in GVHD are the targets of current trials aimed at suppressing GVHD by manipulating the donor bone marrow to expunge the offending cells (20,21). The manipulations are, however, relatively crude and utilize physical or immunological means that cannot possibly be highly cell-type specific. The thought that a particular plant lectin or a monoclonal antibody that reacts with all CD5-containing lymphoid cells will have a high specificity for the subset of cells mediating GVHD must surely be founded either on extreme naivety or an overwhelmingly optimistic view of biology. After all, 10 to 12 years ago investigators were already using physical separation of cell subsets and monoclonal antibodies to remove specific lymphoid populations from donor marrow and to remove lymphoid tumor cells (22–26). The fact that these procedures are still not used in a uniform and widely accepted manner suggests that this approach has inherent limitations. There is little doubt that with sufficiently vigorous application of monoclonal antibodies directed against multiple subsets of T cells, one can effectively ablate the immune system of the donated marrow; however, the complications are those one would anticipate: prolonged immunological deficiency, frequent lack of engraftment because of the failure of production of hematopoietic lymphokines, and an increased rate of recurrence of leukemia because of loss of the antileukemic activity of the graft. Similarly, the intense application of immunosuppression with both cyclosporine and methotrexate after transplantation diminishes the frequency of acute GVHD, but leukemic relapse is more frequent than with less intensive immunosuppression, and survival is not improved.

What then are the answers to this nagging problem of GVHD, and the compounding problems associated with total lymphoid annihilation? The answers to these questions cannot be provided with certainty, but one can certainly suggest lines of inquiry that may bear fruit in the future. My own choice for preventing GVHD is never to have to use foreign marrow in a BMT recipient. If each had a portion of their pluripotent hematopoietic stem cells stored frozen at birth, the need for allogeneic bone marrow need never arise, except perhaps in those few individuals unfortunate enough to have a serious genetic defect affecting hematopoietic cells. Cord blood might be a source of such stem cells. In making this suggestion, I am presuming either that enough stem cells normally exist in the fetal/newborn circulation to repopulate an adult hematopoietic system, or that enough stem cells can be induced to circulate by the appropriate hematopoietic hormonal manipulation (27,28). This hypothesis is easily testable, and, if correct, one could readily envision banks of frozen cord blood stem cells waiting ready for use in the mid-twenty-first century. Of course, there would be significant economic and social implications for such an undertaking, and we would have ignored the allogeneic graft-versus-leukemia effect, but these considerations are best left unexamined until we test the hypothesis.

Are there other avenues open for the control of GVHD for those of us unfortunate enough not to have frozen autologous stem cells? Several possibilities come to mind: (1) enrichment of hematopoietic stem cells for infusion; (2) "fine tuning" of immunological ablation of the donor marrow; (3) tailoring molecules to block selected lymphoid receptors; and (4) pharmacological agents that block the mediators of GVHD. In addition, better matching of donor and patient by DNA cross-matching would seem to be a natural application of the rapidly evolving field of genotyping.

The physical and immunological techniques for hematopoietic stem-cell isolation are sufficiently advanced in mouse studies that between 10 and 100 highly purified marrow cells can reconstitute the hematopoietic system of an irradiated animal (29). What we can do in the mouse we should ultimately be able to do in humans. Suppose we could infuse 20 cells that only contained multipotent hematopoietic stem cells and no partially differentiated pre-T cells. When such primitive stem cells from a donor matched by the methods of the twenty-first century (30) are infused into a recipient, they might reconstitute hematopoiesis without recognizing the environment as foreign. Of course, several questions arise with regard to the experiment. Would the T-lymphocyte system evolve from the primitive stem cells in the absence of a fully functional thymus gland, and, if not, would appropriate T-lymphocyte differentiation occur if recombinant thymic hormones were supplied? As the cells differentiate, would they recognize the host tissues as foreign? Could one selectively ablate undesirable subsets of evolving cytotoxic T cells by cell-specific cytotoxic molecules? The answers to these questions are not known, but they suggest important avenues to explore as the technology for isolating human hematopoietic stem cells improves.

What about the alternative approach of fine-tuning the ablation of cells that mediate GVHD? For this approach we need to know more about the cells that mediate this process. Once they are identified, there are several strategies available for elimination of reactive subsets of cells, such as monoclonal antibodies with a linked toxic molecule or amplification of the subset by in vitro exposure to both antigens of the recipient and hematopoietic hormones, followed by exposure to cell-cycle–specific toxins. Other possibilities come to mind, and I suspect that the future will reveal to us many sophisticated techniques for eliminating undesirable cells once they have been identified.

As I scanned the pages of *Science* and *Nature* during the past year, I was increasingly impressed by the current ability of science to define the three-dimensional structure of receptor molecules and other proteins from their primary amino acid sequence. It seems certain that we shall be able sometime in the future to routinely tailor-make ligand agonists and antagonists to fit into the external pockets of these receptors. Ultimately, therefore, we should be able to manipulate the behavior of specific lymphoid populations without the necessity of searching them out and destroying them.

As still another approach to controlling GVHD, it is conceivable that therapy aimed at the secondary mediators of GVHD may be sufficiently effective as to reduce mortality of allogeneic transplantation and to allow its application to a wider range of individuals. For example, it has been suggested that tumor necrosis factor-alpha (TNF-α) and IL-1 may be mediators of GVHD, and there is a recent report that an IL-1 receptor antagonist may prevent GVHD in mice receiving BMTs (31). We will consider the use of such agents in reducing toxicity of conditioning regimens.

Case 2—The Year 2012

A 19-year-old woman was referred to Tokyo University Medical Center for BMT for malignant myelofibrosis. Multiple marrow samplings suggested a primary clonal population of cells with an abnormality of the platelet-derived growth factor-3 receptor gene and a secondary clonal population with loss of the chromosome 11p anti-oncogene. The patient had no siblings, and a search for a "best match" was conducted in the Japanese DNA-genotyping registry containing 59×10^6 DNA samples.

Pretransplantation, the patient's own long-lived T lymphocytes were stored frozen for subsequent reinfusion. She was prepared for transplantation with fractionated total body irradiation. Peripheral blood stem cells were collected from a genotype-matched unrelated individual. After transplantation, the patient received human "multipoietin" and GM-

CSF, as well as a new compound that blocks CD8 lymphocyte effector function.

During the course of engraftment, the ratio of suppressor and helper subpopulations of lymphocytes was carefully monitored and was manipulated by in vivo administration of cloned lymphokines and the specific lymphocyte receptor blocker. As anticipated, clinical recovery was uneventful and there was no evidence of GVHD. She was discharged from the hospital on day 16 and continued to receive anti-TNF-α and anti-TNF-β agents for 2 months. Marrow samples were obtained periodically to monitor for the recurrence of malignant fibrosis. None was observed at 18 months after transplantation.

Comment

Better cross-matching of unrelated donors and post-transplant use of more specific immunosuppressives and blockers of pharmacological mediators of inflammation will largely have eliminated GVHD early in the twenty-first century.

Case 3—The Year 2032

A 4-year-old boy was admitted to Middlesex-University College Hospital, London, for treatment of severe aplastic anemia. The disease was thought to have arisen from an accidental exposure to a new tricyclic antidepressent, which the child found in his mother's medicine chest. Flow cytometric analysis of his peripheral blood large mononuclear cells revealed none with the phenotype of multipotent hematopoietic stem cells, and his prognosis for spontaneous recovery from aplasia was therefore judged to be poor. Consequently, he was given an intravenous infusion of 103 hematpoietic stem cells isolated from the bone marrow of his 8-year-old sister. No conditioning program was used prior to infusion. The patient's thymus gland was considered to be still functional and he was not given thymic hormones after transplantation; however, human multipoietin, IL-11, and GM-CSF were given after transplantation and engraftment was uneventful. The child was discharged home on day 16.

Comment

Purification of hematpoietic stem cells for transplantation is likely to be mature technology in the first half of the twenty-first century.

Eradication of Malignant Diseases

Our current strategies for eliminating malignant disease from the bone marrow and from patients are not very effective. Even under optimal circumstances of allogeneic BMT, recurrences are not uncommon in acute and chronic myeloid leukemias and are frequent in acute lymphoblastic leukemia, suggesting there is often disease outside the bone marrow that is not eradicated. Although some would suggest otherwise, the results are worse with autologous than with allogeneic BMT, either because of a lack of an allogeneic antileukemic effect or because of residual leukemic cells in the autologous marrow. The results of autologous BMT for refractory or high-risk leukemias do not encourage me to believe that this will be the therapy of the future, except perhaps in a few categories of diseases (see Chapters 52–57). The results of autologous or allogeneic BMT in solid tumors are very poor when viewed from any perspective.

The main problem with current therapy of malignancy by BMT can be summarized as a failure to eliminate malignant disease by means that do not cause irreversible damage to the host. How will this problem be addressed by bone marrow transplanters in the twenty-first century?

One approach is already obvious: to determine whether autologous marrow is free of tumor cells before it is reinfused. Several techniques are already being applied to this problem of detecting "minimal residual disease." The polymerase chain reaction (PCR) is already being used to detect immunoglobulin gene rearrangements in B-cell tumors, T-cell receptor gene rearrangement in T-cell tumors, and oncogene rearrangements such as *bcr-abl* in other specific types of malignancy (32,33). Flow cytometry and labeled monoclonal antibodies can detect a few neoplastic cells among many normal cells in certain leukemias. Similarly, antibodies to epithelial markers can detect a few malignant epithelial cells among many hematopoietic cells. The current limit of sensitivity of antibody and nucleic acid approaches to detecting minimal residual disease is approximately one malignant cell among 10^4 or 10^5 normal cells (33,34). Probably the sensitivity of analysis will increase before we enter the next century, and we should be able to tell with confidence whether we are infusing a single malignant cell along with each 10^6 or 10^7 normal marrow cells. This degree of sensitivity may not be necessary, however, as we improve our abilities to enrich hematopoietic stem cells from mixed populations of cells. As discussed earlier, we may be able to reconstitute hematopoiesis with less than 100 cells, and certainly with less than 10^4 cells, in the future. When this improvement is accomplished, current levels for detection of minimal residual disease will suffice to assure that no cancer cells are being infused along with the hematopoietic stem cells.

Undoubtedly, it will take several years to develop the technology for isolating multipotent human hematopoietic stem cells from a mixed population of blood or marrow cells. Until we can isolate them, how do we get rid of malignant cells that contaminate the marrows we infuse in autologous BMTs? And, more importantly, how do we get rid of tumor cells in the patient's body outside of the bone marrow? One approach might involve the development of new chemotherapeutic agents or the use of the "right" combination of existing agents. Clinically useful new chemotherapeutic agents have been introduced into our therapeutic arsenal at the rate of approximately one per year since the mid 1960s. Etoposide, carboplatin, taxol, and retinoic acid are examples of recent useful additions to our armamentarium. New and old anticancer drugs have enhanced our abilities to control and, in a few patients, to eradicate malignant disease. In recent years, they have been used in aggressive combinations in experimental programs of autologous BMT aimed at eradicating neoplasia.

These programs, however, have thus far been generally disappointing in achieving their goals. We do not yet understand why certain drugs in the "right" combination frequently eradicate certain malignancies, such as Hodgkin's disease, germ-cell tumors of the testis, and acute lymphoblastic leukemia (ALL) of childhood. Consequently, we are left to search for the right combination of drugs using very crude guidelines of drug effectiveness or guided only by the limits of a patient's tolerance. The story of the development of retinoic acid analogues for treatment of progranulocytic leukemia (35,36) may, however, be a paradigm for the rational development of drugs based on specific molecular defects in cancer. It is hoped that this principle can be applied more frequently in the future, and there may be grounds for limited optimism in this area.

Let us consider another approach. The problem of eliminating malignant cells from bone marrow would be greatly simplified if one could be absolutely certain that there were no such cells present at the time of bone marrow harvest. This brings us back to the ideas, discussed previously, of isolating a few pluripotent stem cells for the purposes of reconstituting hematopoiesis or of freezing everyone's stem cells at or near the time of birth. The cord blood would be expected to be free of tumor cells except for some rare ALLs and a few other childhood neoplasms. Not only would the hematopoietic stem cells be tumor-free but, as previously noted, they probably would not generate GVHD. Of course, the problem of eradication of malignant cells from the rest of the body would remain even if one infused tumor-free marrow. Therefore, one must ask if there are strategies by which a disseminated malignancy can be eradicated from somatic tissues. Many investigators are currently pessimistic about the chances that conventional cytotoxic chemotherapy can ever achieve this objective for common tumors, such as colon cancer and nonsmall-cell lung cancers. No matter what new cytotoxic agents come along, most cancers seem to be capable of evolving drug-resistant subpopulations. Furthermore, the anticancer drugs, whether they be DNA-intercalating agents, antimetabolites, or cell-spindle poisons, seem to lack sufficient specificity for tumor cells. Similarly, there is no great expectation that current strategies of immunotherapy will prevail, whether these strategies involve toxins linked to idiotype-specific monoclonal antibodies or lymphokine-activated killer cells. Tumors appear to be too heterogeneous and too prone to undergo antigenic modulation to be so easily conquered. More than 2 decades of failure of clinical immunotherapy does not engender much optimism. It would seem that we need innovative new approaches to anticancer therapy. Fortunately, these new approaches may be emerging from the recent extraordinary advances in understanding the molecular mechanisms of neoplasia. The discovery and characterization of oncogenes and antioncogenes are very likely to contribute to novel therapeutic approaches in the twenty-first century. We can already see the beginnings of a new therapeutic strategy based on gene therapy in the current literature. One such strategy is to inhibit the expression of an activated oncogene; another is to introduce into tumor cells the product of a missing anti-oncogene.

Gene Therapy of Cancer

Oncogenes are generated when normal proto-oncogenes are altered by mutations, structural rearrangements, or viral activation (37). They act dominantly so that only a single proto-oncogene needs to be altered for its products to induce a tumor phenotype. One can conceive of blocking the expression of such an altered gene by introducing into cells an "anti-sense" nucleic acid sequence that ties up either its DNA or its messenger RNA (mRNA) by sequence-specific hybridization. This approach has already been tried in vitro with chronic myelocytic leukemia (CML) blast cells and the leukemogenic *bcr-abl* fusion gene. In one study, leukemic cells were exposed to an 18 base pair "anti-sense" oligodeoxynucleotide complementary to the junctions of the fused BCR and ABL genes. Leukemic colony formation was suppressed, whereas granulocyte-macrophage colony formation from normal progenitors was unaffected (38). This approach is said to demonstrate "the feasibility of gene-targeted selected killing of neoplastic cells."

Another novel approach involves anti-oncogenes. Antioncogenes are tumor suppressor genes; when their products are lost or inactivated, tumors progress (39). Inactivation may occur by mutations or structural rearrangements of the anti-oncogenes themselves or when their products are bound to some proteins of DNA tumor viruses. In general, the mutations or structural rearrangements must inactivate the 2 antioncogenes on both chromosomes before the tumor progresses in vivo. This phenomenon offers the possibility of gene therapy based on the introduction of one or more copies of the missing antioncogene into tumor cells. There are numerous descriptions of this strategy in tumor model systems. In successful models, expression of the introduced normal antioncogene results in suppression of the tumor phenotype (40). The usual vector used for introduction of the antioncogene is a modified retrovirus that can infect the tumor cell but does not replicate to spread and harm the host.

In still another approach to gene therapy of tumors, a recombinant retrovirus containing a gene specifically transcribed only by the tumor cells is used to activate a drug, which will then kill the tumor. This approach has been called "virus-directed enzyme/prodrug therapy." In one example, replication-defective retroviruses were constructed containing a viral thymidine kinase gene that was transcriptionally regulated by a regulatory sequence for the alpha-fetoprotein gene. Alpha-fetoprotein is produced in hepatoma cells but not in normal liver cells. Consequently, when the virus was introduced into hepatoma cells, thymidine kinase was produced.

It in turn metabolically activated the nontoxic "prodrug" 6-methoxypurine arabinonucleoside (araM) to a cytotoxic derivative, ara-adenosine triphosphate (41).

What are the likely hurdles to be overcome in the development of these strategies for gene therapy of cancer? Almost certainly, there will be difficulty getting the retroviral vectors with anticancer genes into every single malignant cell. Some tumor cells will lack the appropriate viral receptors; others will be remote from a blood supply at the time of viral infusion. A second potential problem is that most advanced tumors have cellular populations with several different abnormal oncogenes and antioncogenes. For example, as blast crisis evolves in CML, alterations in the *p53* gene, the *Rb* gene, or the *N-ras* gene may be engrafted on the underlying abnormality in the ABL gene (42). In breast cancer, several genes may be involved: RAS, MYC, *Neu*, *Int-2*, and a gene on chromosome 17q12-q23. Therefore, introduction of one molecular agent may not suffice to revert the malignant cell to normal. This will almost certainly be the case for most tumors, because carcinogenesis is in molecular terms a multistep process. These observations suggest that gene therapy of cancer will probably be most effective when the tumor is small and the numbers of clonal cell populations are few. If this thesis is correct, gene therapy will be used either when the tumor is in its preclinical stages or when it has been reduced in size by other therapeutic maneuvers. At least in the early part of the twenty-first century, gene therapy will probably be part of a multimodality approach to cancer.

Case 4—The Year 2052

A 20-year-old man from a wealthy New York family was diagnosed as having CML. He was referred to North Shore Cornell Medical Center for bone marrow ablation and replacement. The patient's disease had been diagnosed one week earlier on a routine blood count using automated analysis of ABL gene mRNA. CML cells constituted less than 5% of the nucleated cell population in the bone marrow at diagnosis. At the medical center, multiagent myelosuppressive drugs were administered, which reduced the CML content of the marrow to less than 0.01%. At that time, a BCR-ABL antisense 18 base pair nucleic acid fragment was infused intravenously. Because of the anticipation of severe myelosuppression from drugs, the patient was given an infusion of his own cord blood hematopoietic stem cells, which had been frozen at the time of his birth at the New York Medical Center in Manhattan.

Engraftment of the autologous marrow was prompt. There was no evidence of leukemic recurrence detected by enhanced sensitivity PCR- ligation chain reaction by the year 2059, when the patient was lost to follow-up.

Comment

Early detection of leukemia will almost certainly be possible using automated nucleic acid analytic techniques. Nucleic acid blocking agents may nulify acquired defects 60 years in the future, and stem-cell storage may well be a reality for the affluent.

Toxicity of Conditioning Regimens

The toxicity of conditioning regimens is currently an important problem in BMT and is apt to be an increasing problem as we seek to rid patients and their bone marrows of carcinomas and sarcomas in protocols of autologous BMT. Target organs may include heart, lung, liver, kidney, gastrointestinal tract, central nervous system, skin, gonads, endocrine organs, as well as the hematopoietic and vascular systems. To this list must be added the general problem of retardation of growth in young patients and the occurrence of second malignancies. These complications of BMT will become less acceptable as we improve survival statistics in the devastating malignancies.

One approach to this problem is to develop more tumor-selective chemotherapeutic agents. However, the experience of the past 30 years is not encouraging in this regard. Each new agent, whether it be a classic drug or a "biological response modifier," has had its associated toxicity. Although there is currently no basis for optimism with regard to the future development of highly tumor-specific agents, unforeseen developments may of course occur in the century ahead.

Another strategy for reducing tissue toxicity of conditioning programs is to use agents that interfere with the mediators of GVHD, which is akin to using anti–inflammatory agents in rheumatoid arthritis: They do not subvert the basic disease process, but they block the amplification events that may increase tissue injury. Recently, a trial with an agent that down-regulates TNF-α production has been described (43). TNF-α is presumed to be one of the mediators of certain complications of BMT, including GVHD, veno-occlusive disease, and diffuse noninflammatory idiopathic pneumonia. This trial is clearly a step in the direction of using pharmacological agents to modify the mediators of tissue injury in BMT.

Another approach to reducing tissue toxicity is to reduce the dosage of drugs used in conditioning, which can only be done if one is certain of eradicating the malignancy at lesser doses. This approach may be achievable as our skills in detecting minimal residual disease improve in the future. Moreover, aggressive post-transplant immunosuppression may not be required if purified allogeneic stem cells or autologous cord blood stem cells are infused to re-establish hematopoiesis. Finally, aggressive pretransplant and post-transplant immunosuppression may not be necessary if BMT is avoided altogether and the simpler technique of gene therapy becomes a reality. In a sense, BMT may be an intermediary technology that will be used until more specific approaches are developed for eliminating malignant diseases and for treating inborn errors of metabolism.

Gene Therapy for Inherited Disease

Gene therapy is likely to become the standard technique for treating certain hereditary diseases in the next century. One can readily envision removing some long-lived T lymphocytes from the blood of a patient with a genetic defect and infecting these cells in vitro with a retrovirus containing a normal version of the defective gene. The T cells could then be reinfused without the necessity of conditioning regimens. If all goes well, the T cells would make the key enzyme in sufficient quantity to have clinical utility for the patient. This idealized procedure is obviously far simpler than BMT and avoids the toxicity of conditioning regimens and the possibility of GVHD.

Target cells in gene therapy need not be limited to the hematopoietic system, because viruses could be targeted to other organs. The procedure need not be delayed until the patient develops clinical manifestations of the gene defect. Recombinant retrovirus-carrying genes of interest could be inserted in utero, into the liver of the fetus (44), and the resultant baby would be born with a normal genetic makeup.

Case 5—The Year 2032

An 8-year-old Hispanic boy from a poor family was referred to the outpatient clinic of Children's Hospital of Los Angeles for gene therapy of Gaucher's disease. According to the mother, the child's only complaint was of mild knee pain. He was in the 5th percentile for height and weight. A liver tip was palpable and a spleen tip was felt 3 cm below the left costal margin.

After blood and urine were obtained for routine laboratory analysis, a 35-mL sample of peripheral blood was drawn into heparin. The child was observed in the clinic for one hour after phlebotomy and was then sent home.

The patient's blood was sedimented with dextran and the nucleated cells were concentrated by centrifugation. Multipotent and GM stem cells were collected by flow cytometry using appropriate monoclonal antibodies. The cells were suspended in tissue culture medium and were exposed overnight to a replication-defective retrovirus containing a novel "minigene." This gene consisted of the transcriptional control domains and a complementary DNA fragment corresponding to the coding sequences of the human glucocerebrosidase gene.

The next morning, the child and his mother returned to the clinic, where he received an intravenous infusion of his own cells that had been exposed to retrovirus. During the next 6 weeks, he was given biweekly injections of *c-kit* ligand, IL-11, and human multipoietin. Blood glucocerebrosidase reached 60% of median normal levels by week 5 and remained at levels of 30 to 70% over the next 6 months. Neither liver nor spleen were palpable at 6 months; however, the gene-treated GM stem cells were thought to be exhausted and it was decided to repeat the process. Follow-up appointments were given for 3-month intervals.

Comment

Forty years from now, gene therapy should be a simple procedure because of the availability of techniques for enriching hematopoietic cell populations and a series of tailor-made genes on the shelf. The regimen should have little or no toxicity. Some transplantation technology will be sufficiently simple and inexpensive that wide application may be possible.

Case 6—The Year 2062

A 32-year-old school teacher from Chongqing, China, was found to have a spherical nodule of 0.4 cm diameter in the left breast on routine enhanced nuclear magnetic resonance screening. The lesion was suctioned through a medium-bore hollow tube and found to be a ductal carcinoma with molecular abnormalities of Int-2/FGF complex, mutations in the p53 gene, and loss of both alleles of the 17q12 breast cancer anti-oncogene. The mutation in the p53 gene was characteristic of that due to aflotoxin exposure. The patient was given a high titer trivalent "antitumor vaccine" containing several engineered retroviruses with an Int-2/FGF antisense DNA, normal gene sequences for the p53 gene, and the 17q12 breast cancer anti-oncogene. Each of the viruses also contained a "self-destruct" signal that could be activated by injection of a protein sequence derived from a rare marine organism. A public health officer was dispatched to locate the source of aflotoxin and traced it to rice grown on her grandparent's farm 90 km south of Chongqing.

Comment

Seventy years in the future, BMT may not be necessary at all.

References

1. Cline MJ. Future considerations in bone marrow transplantation. In: Blume K, Petz L, eds. Clinical bone marrow transplantation. New York: Churchill-Livingstone, 1983:359–372.
2. Schmidt GH, Horak DA, Niland JC, et al. A randomized control trial of prophylactic ganciclovir for cytomegalovirus pulmonary infections in recipients of allogeneic bone marrow transplants. N Engl J Med 1991;324:1005–1011.
3. Lew MA, Kehoe K, Ritz J, et al. Prophylaxis of bacterial infections with ciprofloxacin in patients undergoing bone marrow transplantation. Transplantation 1991;51:630–635.
4. Bradley TR, Metcalf D. The growth of mouse bone marrow cells in vitro. Aust J Exp Biol Med Sci 1966;44:287–300.
5. Pluznik DH, Sachs L. The cloning of normal "mast" cells in tissue culture. J Cell Physiol 1965;66:319–324.
6. Golde DW, Cline MJ. Regulation of granulopoiesis. N Engl J Med 1974;291:1388–1395.
7. Moore MS. Clinical implications of positive and negative hematopoietic stem cell regulators. Blood 1991;78:1–19.
8. Metcalf D. The molecular control of blood cells. Cambridge, MA: Harvard University Press, 1988.
9. Matthews W, Jordan CT, Wiegand GW, Pardoll D, Lemischka IR. A receptor tyrosine kinase specific to hematopoietic stem and progenitor cell-enriched populations. Cell 1991;65:1143–1152.
10. Migliaccio G, Migliaccio AR, Valinsky J, et al. Stem cell factor induces proliferation and differentiation of highly enriched murine hematopoietic cells. Proc Natl Acad Sci USA 1991;88:7420–7424.
11. Keller JR, Jacobsen SEW, Sill KT, Ellingsworth LR, Ruscetti FW. Stimulation of granulopoiesis by transforming growth factor beta: Synergy with granulocyte/macrophage-colony stimulating factor. Proc Natl Acad Sci USA 1991;88:7190–7194.
12. Demetri GD, Griffin JD. Granulocyte colony-stimulating factor and its receptor. Blood 1991;78:2791–2808.
13. Andrews RG, Knitter GH, Bartelmez SH, et al. Recombinant human stem cell factor, a c-kit ligand, stimulates hematopoiesis in primates. Blood 1991;78:1975–1980.
14. Teramura M, Kobayashi S, Hoshino S, Oshimi K, Mizoguchi H. Interleukin-11 enhances human megakaryocytopoiesis in vitro. Blood 1992;79:327–331.

15. Thomas ED, Lochte HL, Lu WC, Ferrebee JW. Intravenous infusion of bone marrow in patients receiving radiation and chemotherapy. N Engl J Med 1957; 257:491–496.
16. Santos GW. History of bone marrow transplantation. Clin Hematol 1983;12:611–639.
17. Beatty PG. The use of unrelated donors for bone marrow transplantation. Marrow Transplant Rev 1991;1:1–6.
18. Van Rood JJ, Zwaan FE, Willenze R. The unrelated bone marrow donor. Bone Marrow Transplant 1988;3: 371–377.
19. Parkman R. The application of bone marrow transplantation to the treatment of genetic diseases. Science 1986;232:1373–1378.
20. Marmont AM, Horowitz MN, Gale RP, et al. T-cell depletion of HLA identical transplants in leukemia. Blood 1991;78:2120–2130.
21. Antin JH, Bierer BE, Smith BR. Selective depletion of bone marrow T-lymphocytes with anti-CD5 monoclonal antibodies: effective prophylaxis for graft versus host disease in patients with hematologic malignancies. Blood 1991;78:2139–2149.
22. Prentice HG, Janossy G, Skeggs D, et al. Use of anti-T-cell monoclonal antibody OKT3 to prevent acute graft versus host disease in allogeneic bone marrow transplantation for acute leukemia. Lancet 1982;1:700–703.
23. Ritz J, Schlossman SF. Utilization of monoclonal antibodies in the treatment of leukemia and lymphoma. Blood 1982;59:1–11.
24. Nadler LM, Stashenko P, Hardy R, et al. Serotherapy of a patient with a monoclonal antibody directed against a human lymphoma-associated antigen. Cancer Res 1980;40:3147–3154.
25. Blythman HE, Casellas P, Gros O, et al. Immunotoxins: hybrid molecules of monoclonal antibodies and a toxin subunit specifically kill tumor cells. Nature 1981; 290:145–146.
26. Krolick KA, Uhr JW, Vitetta ES. Selective killing of leukemia cells by antibody-toxin conjugates: implications for autologous bone marrow transplantation. Nature 1982;295:604–605.
27. Haas R, Ho AD, Bredthauer U, et al. Successful autologous transplantation of blood stem cells mobilized with recombinant human granulocyte-macrophage colony stimulating factor. Exp Hematol 1990; 18:94–98.
28. Gianni AM, Sienna S, Bregni M, et al. Granulocyte-macrophage colony stimulating factor to harvest circulating hematopoietic stem cells for autotransplantation. Lancet 1989;2:580–585.
29. Spangrude GJ, Smith L, Uchida N, et al. Mouse hematopoietic stem cells. Blood 1991;78:1395–1402.
30. Piercy JM, Morel C, Freidel AC, et al. Selection of unrelated donors for bone marrow transplantation is improved by HLA class II genotyping with oligonucleotide hybridization. Proc Natl Acad Sci USA 1991;88:7121–7125.
31. McCarthy PL, Abhyankar S, Neden S, et al. Inhibition of interleukin-1 by an interleukin-1 receptor antagonist prevents graft versus host disease. Blood 1991;78: 1915–1918.
32. Billadeau D, Blackstadt M, Greipp P, et al. Analysis of B-lymphoid malignancies using allele-specific polymerase chain reaction: a technique for sequential quantitation of residual disease. Blood 1991;78:3021–3029.
33. Gribbon JG, Freedman AS, Nuberg D, et al. Immunologic purging of marrow assessed by PCR before autologous bone marrow transplantation for B-cell lymphoma. N Engl J Med 1991;325:1525–1533.
34. Cline MJ. Molecular diagnosis of human cancer. Lab Invest 1989;61:368–380.
35. Huang ME, Ye YC, Chen SR, et al. Use of all-trans retinoic acid in the treatment of acute promyelocytic leukemia. Blood 1988;72:567–572.
36. de The H, Chomienne C, Lanotte M, Degos L, Dejean A. The t(15;17) translocation of acute promyelocytic leukaemia fuses the retinoic acid receptor alpha gene to a novel transcribed locus. Nature 1990;347:558–561.
37. Bishop JM. The molecular genetics of cancer. Science 1987;235:305–311.
38. Szczylik C, Skorski T, Nicolaides NC, et al. Selective inhibition of leukemia cell proliferation by BCR-ABL antisense oligodeoxynucleotides. Science 1991;253: 562–565.
39. Findley CA, Hinds PW, Levine AJ. The p53 proto-oncogene can act as a suppressor of transformation. Cell 1989;57:1083–1093.
40. Huang HJ, Yee JK, Shew JY, et al. Suppression of the neoplastic phenotype by replacement of the Rb gene in human cancer cells. Science 1988;242:1563–1566.
41. Huber BE, Richards CA, Krenitsky TA. Retrovial-mediated gene therapy for the treatment of hepatocellular carcinoma: an innovative approach for cancer therapy. Proc Natl Acad Sci USA 1991;88:8039–8043.
42. Cline MJ, Jat PS, Foti A. Molecular mechanisms in the evolution of chronic myelocytic leukemia. Leuk Lymph 1992;7:283–287.
43. Bianco JA, Appelbaum FR, Neumonitis J, et al. Phase I-II trial of pentoxifylline for the prevention of transplant-related toxicities following bone marrow transplantation. Blood 1991;8:1205–1211.
44. Clapp DW, Deumenco LL, Hatzoglou M, Gearson SL. Fetal liver hematopoietic stem cells as a target for in utero retroviral gene transfer. Blood 1991;78:1132–1139.

INDEX